MOSBY's Paramedic Textbook

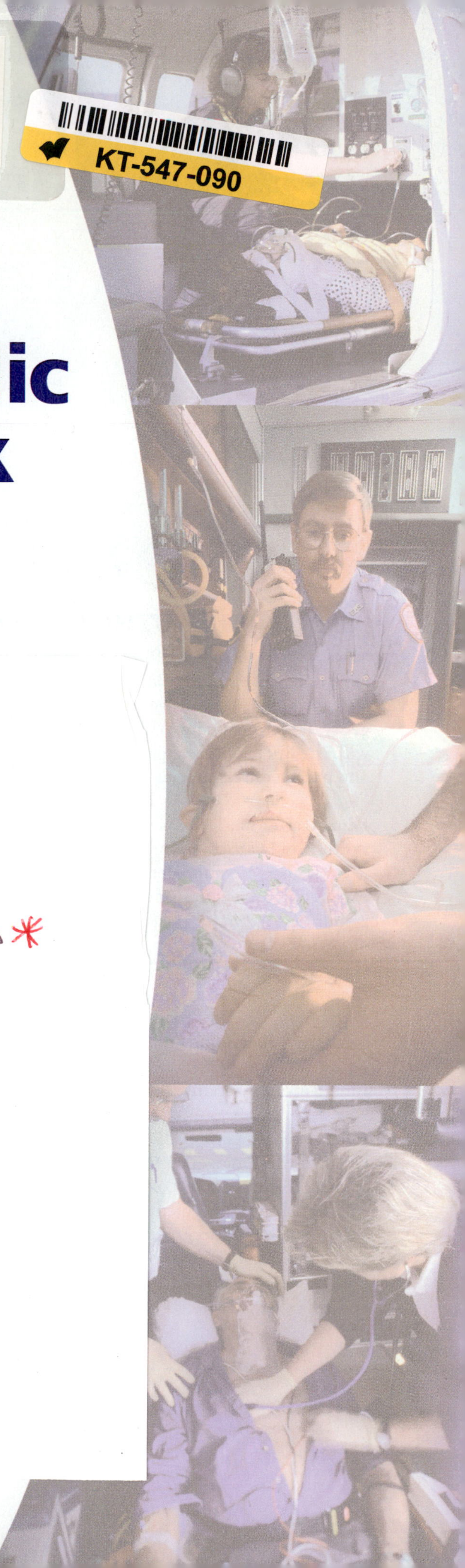

ABOUT THE AUTHOR AND CONTRIBUTORS

Mick J. Sanders, EMT-P, MSA, received his paramedic training in 1978 from St. Louis University Hospitals. He earned a Bachelor of Science degree and a Master of Science degree from Lindenwood College in St. Charles, Missouri. He has worked in various health care systems as a field paramedic, emergency department paramedic, and EMS instructor. For 12 years, Mr. Sanders served as Training Specialist with the Bureau of Emergency Medical Services, Missouri Department of Health, where he oversaw EMT and paramedic training and licensure in St. Louis city and the surrounding metropolitan areas.

Kim McKenna, RN, BSN, CEN, EMT-P, is the Chief Medical Officer for the Florissant Valley Fire Protection District in Florissant, Missouri, and an Adjunct Instructor for St. Louis Community College in St. Louis, Missouri. Her past experiences include intensive care and emergency nursing. She has been involved in prehospital education since 1985, including 4 years as the primary instructor of a paramedic training program.

Gary Quick, MD, FACEP is a previous Associate Professor and prior Chair of the Department of Emergency Medicine at the University of Oklahoma Health Sciences Center in Oklahoma City, Oklahoma. Dr. Quick is a career emergency physician with over 30 years in clinical practice, as well as extensive educational and research experience. He is widely published and serves the specialty of emergency medicine in several capacities at the national and state level for the American College of Emergency Physicians.

Lawrence M. Lewis, MD, FACEP, is Associate Professor of Emergency Medicine and Medicine and Chief of the Emergency Medicine Division at Washington University School of Medicine and Barnes-Jewish Hospital in St. Louis, Missouri. He completed his medical school training at the University of Miami School of Medicine before attending a residency at Washington University. He is an active researcher in emergency medicine with over 40 publications and serves on several national and state emergency medicine committees.

labelled overleaf →

PART EIGHT

30 Pulmonary Emergencies, *816*

31 Neurology, *836*

32 Endocrinology, *864*

33 Allergies and Anaphylaxis, *882*

34 Gastroenterology, *892*

35 Urology, *908*

36 Toxicology, *920*

37 Hematology, *970*

38 Environmental Conditions, *984*

39 Infectious and Communicable Diseases, *1004*

40 Behavioral and Psychiatric Disorders, *1042*

41 Gynecology, *1062*

42 Obstetrics, *1072*

PART NINE

43 Neonatology, *1100*

44 Pediatrics, *1116*

45 Geriatrics, *1160*

46 Abuse and Neglect, *1184*

47 Patients with Special Challenges, *1196*

48 Acute Interventions for the Home Health Care Patient, *1210*

PART TEN

49 Ambulance Operations, *1230*

50 Medical Incident Command, *1240*

51 Rescue Awareness and Operations, *1256*

52 Crime Scene Awareness, *1276*

53 Hazardous Materials Incidents, *1286*

54 Bioterrorism and Weapons of Mass Destruction, *1306*

EMERGENCY DRUG INDEX (EDI), 1321

GLOSSARY, 1366

CCT APPENDIX: ADVANCED PRACTICE PROCEDURES FOR THE CRITICAL CARE PARAMEDIC, 1418

ILLUSTRATION CREDITS, 1424

ELSEVIER

evolve

To access your Student Resources, visit the Web address below:

http://evolve.elsevier.com/Sanders/paramedic/

- **Chapter Challenges**
  540 graded multiple-choice questions are included to test student knowledge.

- **Body Spectrum**
  80 anatomy illustrations are available to color online or print out for coloring and studying offline. Students can use this interactive format to test their knowledge by completing quizzes after each part is colored.

- **Anatomy Challenges**
  Approximately 200 interactive director engines enhance the anatomy and physiology provided in the textbook.

- **Lecture Notes from the PowerPoint Slides**
  Students can view and print these for additional study.

- **Chapter Objectives and Summaries**
  Taken from each chapter in the book, these are excellent quick-reference tools when reviewing textbook concepts.

MOSBY'S Paramedic Textbook

THIRD EDITION

Mick J. Sanders, EMT-P, MSA

PHYSICIAN ADVISERS

Lawrence M. Lewis, MD, FACEP
Associate Professor of Emergency Medicine
Chief, Emergency Medicine Division
Washington University School of Medicine/
Barnes-Jewish Hospital
St. Louis, Missouri

Gary Quick, MD, FACEP
Attending Emergency Physician
Oklahoma Heart Hospital
Prior Associate Professor and Chief
of Emergency Medicine
University of Oklahoma
Oklahoma City, Oklahoma

CONTRIBUTING EDITOR

Kim McKenna, RN, BSN, CEN, EMT-P
Chief Medical Officer
Florissant Valley Fire Protection District
Florissant, Missouri

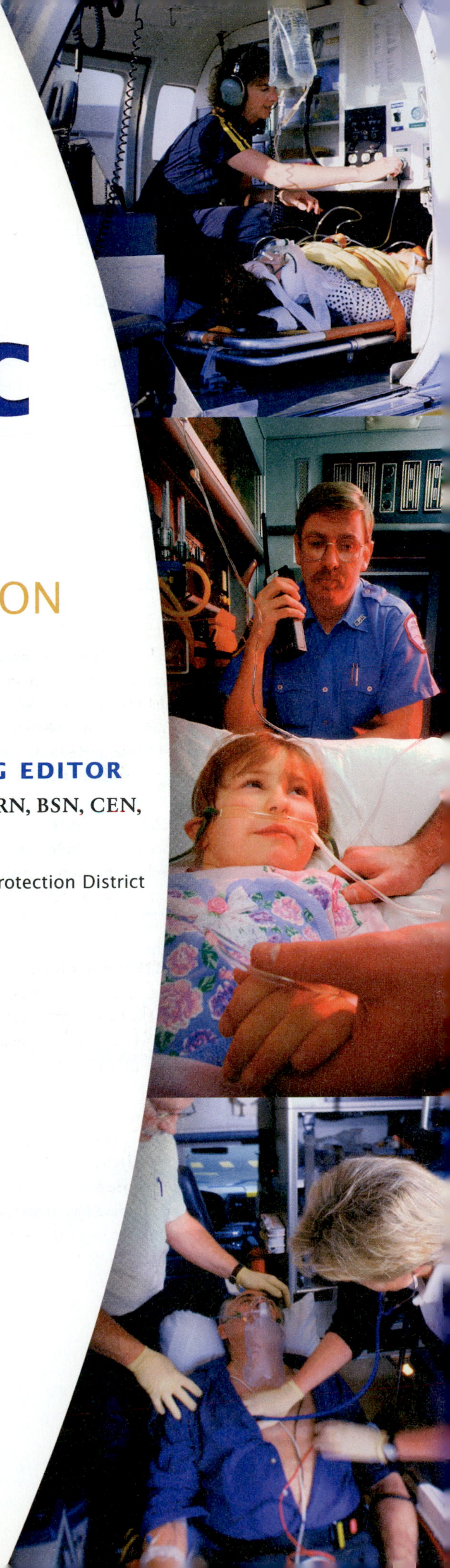

With more than 1000 illustrations

ELSEVIER
MOSBY

MosbyJems

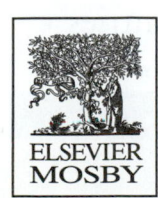

ELSEVIER
MOSBY

11830 Westline Industrial Drive
St. Louis, Missouri 63146

MOSBY'S PARAMEDIC TEXTBOOK, EDITION 3 0-323-02786-5

NOTICE

Knowledge and best practice in this field are constantly changing. As new research and experience broaden our knowledge, changes in practice, treatment, and drug therapy may become necessary or appropriate. Readers are advised to check the most current information provided (i) on procedures featured or (ii) by the manufacturer of each product to be administered, to verify the recommended dose or formula, the method and duration of administration, and contraindications. It is the responsibility of the practitioner, relying on their own experience and knowledge of the patient, to make diagnoses, to determine dosages and the best treatment for each individual patient, and to take all appropriate safety precautions. To the fullest extent of the law, neither the publisher nor the authors assumes any liability for any injury and/or damage to persons or property arising out or related to any use of the material contained in this book.

Previous editions copyrighted 1994, 2001

International Standard Book Number 0-323-02786-5

Acquisitions Editor: Linda Honeycutt
Developmental Editor: Laura Bayless
Publishing Services Manager: Melissa Lastarria
Project Manager: Rich Barber
Designer: Teresa McBryan

Printed in China

Last digit is the print number: 9 8 7 6 5 4 3 2 1

To my family,
and
in loving memory of my father,
James H. Sanders.

FOREWORD

When we reviewed our foreword to the second edition of *Mosby's Paramedic Textbook,* we noted that in certain areas, our vision for the future of EMS was on the mark. Very few individuals anticipated the cataclysmic watershed events of September 11, 2001. Like airline security changes and daily broadcasts of the color-coded terror threat levels, paramedic and medical textbooks will likely be divided into two categories for some time to come: pre-9/11 and post-9/11. To be fair, our foreword mentioned the "increasing threats of chemical and biological terrorism," but this has moved from an important footnote to a "front-and-center" issue. After "anthrax by mail" and the World Trade Center attack, there will be a strong emphasis on disaster and mass casualty incidents for the foreseeable future. Paramedics, firefighters, and police must be taught and continuously trained in disease pattern recognition, scene safety, crowd control, medical triage, communications, and early management (including isolation precautions and decontamination). Additionally, the Institute of Medicine report has elevated patient safety to a rightful position of importance in the design and operation of medical systems and medical personnel.

We also discussed the changing role of the paramedic, including the potential to "greet and treat" patients. In the past 5 years, however, the increasing problems with emergency department (ED) overload (long delays to evaluation and treatment) and ED diversion have made front-page news regularly. The ability to care for an aging population with complicated acute and chronic conditions, as well as the uninsured and underinsured, have stretched the limits of the system nearly to the breaking point, even without epidemics or mass casualty incidents.

Thus the challenges for health care in this first decade of the new millennium must go beyond learning new science, developing new clinical skills, and improving bedside technologies. Surely these issues will be of critical importance, but we must take a broader look at health care in this country and improve the way it is delivered to the entire population, not just those patients we happen to transport or evaluate when they arrive in the ED. Optimum management of health care will require a paradigm shift in how we view the spectrum of health care providers and rethink resource utilization. There are already serious workforce shortages, rationing of various drugs (e.g., antibiotics, antiemetics, and steroids), and almost daily physical limitations in inpatient, ICU, and specialty (e.g., psychiatry) beds.

How might this affect those who have chosen a career in prehospital emergency care? No one can be certain, but it is already true that emergency medical technicians and paramedics are being charged with increasing responsibility to recognize serious conditions (such as stroke, MI, hypoglycemia, congestive heart failure, and asthma) and to initiate specific and appropriate treatment. If demand for ED and inpatient services continues to outstrip supply, the impact on prehospital providers is likely to be profound. The future paramedic must be prepared for the increasing responsibility and the rising complexity of diseases he or she will confront, in order to provide more care in the home, at the scene, and to triage accurately across the spectrum of health care facilities from Level I specialty EDs to non-emergency referrals.

Finally, the greatest future challenge will perhaps come from newly emerging diseases. West Nile fever is an epidemic in many states and is expanding its endemic territory. More dangerous viruses such as Ebola virus or Marburg virus may emerge at any time in epidemic proportions naturally or at the hands of terrorists. Sudden acute respiratory syndrome (SARS) is a recent example of an emerging disease springing from an unanticipated source. Paramedics occupy a focal point for first contact with patients with these diseases. Most importantly, the first responder personnel contact will presumably be the key point for controlling the epidemic promptly or the linchpin for unchecked spread of the contagion.

This is a challenging time for all health care providers, as the rules change in so many areas simultaneously. But it is a particularly challenging time for those on the "front line" who must recognize and treat those traditional emergencies that we will continue to see day by day, but who also must be prepared to provide an expanded scope of prehospital practice, once considered primarily the domain of hospital and emergency department medicine.

Simultaneously, our future paramedics must always remain vigilant for the unexpected attacks of weapons of mass destruction and the appearance of emerging highly contagious and potentially lethal diseases.

We hope that this third edition of *Mosby's Paramedic Textbook* provides much of the information, instruction, and guidance to aid you in your professional practice. Your goal should be to provide the highest quality of prehospital care while maintaining optimal personal and patient safety.

Lawrence M. Lewis, MD, FACEP
Gary Quick, MD, FACEP

FOREWORD

Emergency medical services is the modern way of obtaining help for the victim of a sudden illness or traumatic injury. Since the inception of EMS in the 1970s, the complexity and sophistication of these vital services have expanded rapidly. The 1980s were a time of growth and maturation for EMS providers. New skills, such as cardiac pacing, intraosseous infusion, and advanced airway techniques, were added to the repertoire and toolboxes of the early EMS providers. The 1990s was the decade of technological explosion, implementation of sophisticated patient monitoring systems, and advanced communications and transportation systems. Advanced treatments delivered in the prehospital setting for debilitating diseases, such as stroke and heart attack, changed the outcome of these devastating events for thousands of people.

Today, paramedics face the call for help armed with highly technical equipment, advanced pharmacological agents, and vast communications and transportation systems that could only be viewed as science fiction in the 1970s. Virtual hospitals, telehome care, Internet health care sites, and access to telemedicine exist in limited areas today but will probably be the norm in the next decade. Demands for timely and effective out-of-hospital care by a population better educated in every aspect of health care will force changes in all areas of our current EMS systems, including the providers, the types of services available, and the distribution of every type of resource needed to run an EMS system.

In the journey ahead, EMS will undergo a revolution. To date, this revolution in technology and knowledge has led to an expansion in the scope and complexity of the U.S. Department of Transportation's EMT-Paramedic national standard curriculum. The educational preparation needed to meet the roles and responsibilities of today's paramedic is becoming increasingly sophisticated, compared to what was required of our predecessors of the 1970s. The demand for an increase in our knowledge and competencies has in turn linked the professional paramedic to the health care education setting—the days of "on-the-job" training have passed. The EMS educational experience must facilitate the integration of the reality of "street practice" with the expanded educational preparation required of the paramedic.

The second edition of *Mosby's Paramedic Textbook* is the ideal source to facilitate the integration of "book knowledge" and "street practice." It is based on the 1998 national standard paramedic curriculum and is an excellent source of information. The textbook is appropriate and suitable for use in the primary classroom setting and also to bring the experienced EMS provider "up to the minute" with the latest information regarding prehospital emergency care. Areas of anatomy, physiology, and pathophysiology required to understand complex illness and injury have been expanded and cover both customary and fresh topics. Woven into the text is the author's well-thought-out rationale for how the new information included in the revised curriculum will assist paramedics as they become part of the EMS team.

As a professional educator, I know that each student learns in a different manner. However, it is a well-accepted tenet that the more senses involved in the learning process—the more likely it is that learning will take place. The innovative design of the third edition of *Mosby's Paramedic Textbook* is coupled with the latest in computer and interactive learning technologies to form a complete learning experience. Accompanying ancillaries include CD-ROM presentations, color slides, and Internet support to assist the students as they advance through the well-organized text. Practice examinations and case scenarios are provided to help both the instructor and student in bridging the gap between classroom experience and the world of work experience. Mick J. Sanders has taken his years of experience as a paramedic, educator, and author and brought together a text that will serve as a benchmark for excellence in paramedic education.

The promise of the future in EMS is exciting—fundamental changes, driven by new technology and medical advances, will occur. With these changes comes the opportunity for fulfillment in one of the most rewarding health care professions: EMS. For those of you willing to commit your talent, compassion, and experience to the tasks associated with completing the paramedic education program, an exciting and rewarding career awaits you.

Judith A. Ruple, PhD, RN, NREMT-P
Associate Professor
College of Health and Human Services
The University of Toledo
Toledo, Ohio

FOREWORD

A student walked into my office the other day and asked me a question I have answered many times before. "Which paramedic book is the best choice for me to use as I study for my refresher course?" In an automatic motion, I went to my bookshelf and pulled down the first edition of *Mosby's Paramedic Textbook.* I answered with my usual response, citing the strengths of the book compared to the others available. After copying the title and author, the student thanked me and left my office to go to class.

After she left, I pondered my response. Why is it that I automatically recommend Mick Sanders' book to anyone who asks? Is it because I have many friends who were involved in the process, and I have known the author since I started in this field many years ago? Is it because I have such great respect for Mick and his incredible knowledge of the EMS field? Is it because I was a reviewer for the workbook before publication? Is it because the book has been our primary text for the paramedic program since it was published?

Well, yes. But that alone isn't enough to get my recommendation. There has to be more than association. There has to be quality, accuracy, and something deep down that goes beyond just being a good book.

In today's changing world of EMS, being "good" just isn't enough. Do you know anybody who works hard to be "average," who strives to be called "adequate," who yearns to be told "Your medical performance during that clinical save was 'sufficient'?" If you needed advanced medical care, would you look around for someone who did the minimum required, or would you search for the most qualified, experienced, and excellent provider available? You wouldn't settle for anything less. When you go to work as an EMT, a nurse, a paramedic, do you not strive to provide excellent care to those whose lives you touch?

As I reviewed the chapters for this edition of the textbook, one theme came across as I pored over each page. Excellence. As chapters were rewritten and revised, that theme remained. Excellence. It needs to be a word in our daily vocabulary in EMS. As our profession grows, so too must our body of knowledge. As reflected in the new D.O.T. guidelines, the EMS Education Agenda for the Future, and the National EMS Education and Practice Blueprint, more is being required from us as EMS professionals, both in knowledge base and in functional problem-solving ability. We must be able to *think,* and we must equally be able to *do.*

In order to be able to do our jobs both today and in the future, we need the tools to help us achieve excellence. But functioning equipment and state-of-the-art technology only meet half of our needs. A house built on a foundation of sand soon crumbles, while the house built on rock will withstand a thousand storms. In your hands, you hold the rock. The foundation of your education as a paramedic. The tool to fill in the gaps and to enhance an already strong foundation. This book is solid. It is complete. It is accurate. But more importantly, it is excellent.

In these pages, you, the student, will find a thorough discussion of every aspect of prehospital care presented in a logical, readable format. The objectives and chapter summaries will help you study, and the verbal and pictorial illustrations will help you understand. You, the instructor, will find not only a superb tool for your students, you will notice that this book follows and often, enhances, the latest D.O.T. curriculum and is very easy to work with as you teach. My initial anxieties about teaching the new curriculum vanished into thin air as I read through the pages of this text. This book has been the standard for paramedic education, and this second edition continues in that tradition of excellence.

I was excited when I read through the new T-method in Chapter 18. Mick's thoughtful consideration of students' math challenges has led to his creation of a new method for dosage calculations. To me, this is one more example of his dedication to quality in prehospital education, a commitment which he makes very seriously. In your hands rests the most excellent source of paramedic core material that is available today, a work I am proud to have been affiliated with.

This book took over 25 years in the making, as Mick Sanders brings his extensive background in EMS to the pages of this text. It is the culmination of his years as provider, educator, administrator, and writer. It is his personal commitment to excellence in prehospital care. I challenge you, the reader, to commit yourself likewise to excellence in whatever you choose to do, whether EMS is your career or avocation. You would want only the best EMS providers caring for you. Go and do likewise. Be the best. Be excellent!

Janet Fitts, RN, BSN, CEN, EMT-P
EMS Coordinator
East Central College
Union, Missouri

PREFACE

As a paramedic student, you have chosen to work in an exciting and rewarding area of health care—prehospital emergency care. Few professions can provide the same type of opportunities that lie before you. Through your training, you will meet the educational demands of a profession that requires knowledge in anatomy and physiology, mathematics, pharmacology, advanced education in the health sciences, and physical skills in using highly technical and sophisticated equipment. You will have an opportunity to play an important role in injury prevention, to participate in research, and to be a role model in your community. And most importantly, you will be entrusted with the lives of the people you serve. This describes today's paramedic—a member of a unique profession composed of highly-trained men and women dedicated to making a difference in people's lives.

CONTENT AND ORGANIZATION

The third edition of *Mosby's Paramedic Textbook* has been extensively reviewed by physicians, nurses, paramedics, educators, and national and international experts in the field of emergency care—people who know and value the important role of the paramedic in health care delivery. The text was developed from the 1978 Department of Transportation's National Standard Curriculum for EMT-Paramedic and meets *every* cognitive objective as defined in that document. The third edition has also been enhanced to address recent advances and important issues in emergency medical services (EMS), including new equipment and procedures; critical care transport (CCT); and special considerations for dealing with bioterrorism and weapons of mass destruction (WMD).

Part One explains the paramedic's role and the unique aspects of the profession, such as an overview of EMS systems and the importance of personal well-being. It also introduces the paramedic student to methods of injury prevention, medical/legal issues, and ethics. Personal safety is emphasized in Part One and throughout the text.

Part Two provides a review of human systems and is an easily located reference for anatomical structures and their functions. The general principles of pathophysiology lay the foundation for the textbook and are presented here. In addition, there is a new chapter that maps life span development and special considerations for specific age groups.

Part Three focuses on patient assessment and the importance of caring for both the physical and emotional needs of the patient. Separate chapters have been included for therapeutic communications, history taking, techniques of physical examination, and an overview of patient assessment. Clinical decision making, assessment-based management, communications, and documentation are also presented here.

Part Four introduces the paramedic student to pharmacology and venous access and medication administration. The pharmacology chapter has been enhanced to include an appendix on herbal products, their common uses, indications, and possible interactions with medications.

Part Five is devoted to airway management and ventilation. The physiology of the respiratory system is presented in depth, and basic and advanced methods of managing a patient's airway are illustrated in this chapter.

Part Six is a thorough presentation of trauma. It begins with a discussion of trauma systems and mechanism of injury. This is followed by separate chapters on hemorrhage and shock; soft tissue trauma; burns; head and facial trauma; and injury to the spine, thorax, abdomen, and musculoskeletal system.

Part Seven covers cardiology in detail. Electrophysiology of the heart and electrocardiogram (ECG) interpretation is presented first and is followed by cardiovascular emergencies such as cardiac rhythm disturbances, myocardial infarction, and stroke. Techniques in managing cardiac emergencies, including basic and advanced cardiac life support, follow the current guidelines established by the American Red Cross (ARC) and the American Heart Association (AHA).

Part Eight addresses the many types of medical conditions that can lead to a medical emergency. Separate chapters are included for pulmonary, neurology, endocrinology, allergies and anaphylaxis, gastroenterology, urology, toxicology, and hematology. In addition, environmental conditions, infectious and communicable diseases, behavioral and psychiatric disorders, gynecology, and obstetrics are covered in detail.

Part Nine describes special considerations for select patient groups such as neonates, pediatrics, and geriatrics. It also addresses the needs of patients who have been victims of abuse and neglect, those with special challenges, and home care patients who may require acute interventions.

Part 10 deals with the various aspects of advanced EMS systems, such as ambulance operations, medical incident command, rescue operations, crime scene awareness, and hazardous materials incidents. A new chapter that provides an overview of bioterrorism and weapons of mass destruction has been included here, reflecting new hazards and responsibilities important to today's emergency provider.

Each chapter of *Mosby's Paramedic Textbook* begins with an introduction and a list of objectives that provide an overview of the material to be presented. This allows the student to review the content and progression of each chapter in an easy-to-follow format. Key terms are included to highlight terminology and concepts critical to providing emergency care, and boldfaced items identify terms that are included in the glossary. Each chapter concludes with references that can be used as a resource for supplemental reading and a bulleted summary that reviews the most important material presented in the chapter. The textbook also is accompanied by a student workbook to help measure understanding of the core material. The third edition of *Mosby's Paramedic Textbook* also includes the following features that help make this textbook a leader in EMS education:

- Emergency Drug Index. The Emergency Drug Index (EDI) details specific information on more than 70 emergency drugs. It provides a quick source of reference for a drug's description, onset and duration, indications, contraindications, adverse reactions, drug interactions, packaging, dosage and administration for adult and pediatric patients, and special considerations. Drugs in the textbook that are found in the EDI are denoted with a bold italic font as a reminder to the reader of their importance and easy location of reference.
- Critical Thinking Questions. Critical thinking questions are found in each chapter to aid in understanding concepts and how information presented in the text can impact day-to-day activities and "real life" patient care.
- Advanced ECG Rhythm Interpretation. All cardiac rhythms and dysrhythmias are presented in lead I, II, III, and MCL1 to enhance assessment of the cardiac patient. In addition, the text includes advanced electrophysiology, multi-lead ECG monitoring (including 12-lead monitoring), fibrinolytic therapy, and current treatment modalities as recommended by the American Heart Association.
- Full-Color Illustrations. More than 1500 tables, charts, line drawings, and photographs are included in the text to illustrate anatomy, physiology, and patient management guidelines. State-of-the-art equipment and step-by-step demonstrations of practical skills also are presented in full color to demonstrate emergency care procedures.
- Text Boxes. Boxes in each chapter expand on interesting and relevant information, such as unusual facts and figures, "nice-to-know" data, and "need-to-know" material, such as the rights of terminally ill patients and the possible effects of biological terrorism.
- Box Notes. Box notes are presented in each chapter to highlight vital information and words of warning.
- Expanded Glossary. The glossary has been expanded to include definitions on hundreds of medical terms presented in the textbook chapters.
- Index. The thorough and detailed index makes it easy to find information that was presented in the text.

I hope reading this preface reinforces the decision you made to choose this textbook. Whether you're a paramedic student, practicing paramedic, nurse, administrator, or educator, I think you will find this textbook to be a valuable EMS resource.

Mick J. Sanders

AUTHOR ACKNOWLEDGMENTS

The third edition of *Mosby's Paramedic Textbook* resulted from the combined efforts of many talented and dedicated individuals. In addition to my physician advisers, Larry Lewis and Gary Quick, and the many experts who reviewed the manuscript, I would like to acknowledge a few others who helped make this textbook possible: Kim McKenna, my friend, colleague, contributor, and the author of the workbook. She's been my "can't-do-without" partner since the first edition of the text. Her devotion to this project has been invaluable. (Kim, I owe you.) Laura Bayless, my developmental editor. Her support and her daily emails helped remind me that there was light at the end of the tunnel. Kim and I are grateful for her involvement. Rich Barber, my project manager, who made the book "come to life." Linda Honeycutt, my executive editor. Taz Meyer, who worked with Kim on the revision to the Instructor Resource Kit and ancillaries. Their contributions and attention to detail were wonderful and greatly improved the product. Don McKenna and Rick Brady for their excellent photography. Jeanne Robertson, who provided beautiful illustrations. Ray Kemp who provided many of the scene photos for this edition.

I also want to thank those people who were instrumental in the success of the first and second editions, and for their contributions that are still an important part of this edition, especially Julie Long, Claire Merrick, Nancy Peterson, and Mark Weiber. Others include Barb Aehlert, Rich Barber, Catherine Parvenski Barwell, Amy Buxton, Lin Dempsey, Jen Etling, Janet Fitts, William Greenblatt, Larry Hatfield, Jon King, Dana Knighten, Tina Kult, Christa Lenk, Yavilah McCoy, Linda McKinley, Gayle Morris, Ronald Olshwanger, Darrell Paranich, Janice Ratchie Saia, James Silvernail, Karen Snyder, Nadine Sokol, Rob Thriault, Derril and Kelly Trakalo, Elaine Steinborn, Lana VanLaningham, and Kellie White. Models Chris Arter, Larry Ashby, Tim Dorsey, Mark Flauter, Rosalyn Golden, Jason Herin, Julie Hull, Diane Kaatman, Sue Lakebrink, Frank Lipski, Mindy McCoy, the McKenna family (Don, Becky, Ginny, Grant, Kim, Maggie, and Bill), Dan Peters, Steve Sanneman, John Taylor, Lance Varga, Joel Vanderploeg, and Monroe Yancie. Creve Coeur Fire Protection District, Eureka Fire Protection District, Tom Fitts (Alliance Medical), Chris Shanks (Armstrong Medical), Rob Kuchick (Medtronic-PhysioControl), St. Charles County Ambulance, St. John's Mercy Medical Center, St. Louis City EMS and other physicians, hospitals, and equipment manufacturers who supplied illustrations and scene photos to accompany the text.

Finally, I want to mention a few special people whose interest in me and whose support of this project was something I could always count on: Dixie Allen (my mother), Ruby Hagood (my grandmother), Randy Sanders (my brother), and Will Denney (a great friend).

Mick J. Sanders

PUBLISHER ACKNOWLEDGMENTS

The editors wish to acknowledge and thank the many reviewers of this book, who devoted countless hours to intensive review. Their comments were invaluable in helping to develop and fine tune the revision of this textbook.

Organizations and individuals who took part in this extensive project were:

Beth Lothrop Adams, MA, RN, NREMT-P
Quality Manager
Fairfax County Fire & Rescue Department
Fairfax, Virginia

Patrick Black, BS, NREMT-P
Director of EMT-Paramedic Technology
East Central Community College
Decatur, Mississippi

Chip Boehm, RN, EMT-P/FF, EMS I/C
Paramedic/Firefighter
Portland Fire Department
Portland, Maine

Kristen Borchelt, NREMT-P
Paramedic, PALS Instructor
Cinicinnati Children's Hospital
Cincinnati, Ohio

Angel Clark Burba, MS, NREMT-P
Associate Professor and EMS Program Director
Howard Community College
Columbia, Maryland

Heather Micholene Davis, MS, NREMT-P
County of Los Angeles Fire Department
Los Angeles, California

Bill Doss, EMT-P
Miami Township Fire & EMS
Clermont County, Ohio

Steven Dralle, BA, EMT-P
American Medical Response-South Texas
San Antonio, Texas

James W. Drake, MS, NREMT-P
EMS Coordinator
Jameson Memorial Hospital
New Castle, Pennsylvania

Peter Glaeser, MD
University of Alabama at Birmingham
Birmingham, Alabama

Thomas James Gottschalk, NREMT-P, I/C, CCEMT-P
Platinum Educational Group LLC
Grand Rapids, Michigan

Shawn Harthorn, EMT, MACS
Doña Ana Branch Community College
Las Cruces, New Mexico

Robert Hawkes, BA, BS, NREMT-P, CCEMTP
Southern Maine Community College
South Portland, Maine

Seth Collings Hawkins, MD
EMS Coordinator
Blue Ridge HealthCare/Mountain Emergency Physicians
Morganton, North Carolina

Attila Hertelendy, MHSM, CCEMT-P, NREMT-P, ACP
University of Mississippi Medical Center
Jackson, Mississippi

John C. Hopkins, EMT-P
Voridian Inc
Lexington County EMS
Lexington, South Carolina

Arthur Hsieh, MA, NREMT-P
Program Director
Hospital Consortium Education Network
San Mateo, California

I. Kevin Johnson, AS, BS, NREMT-P
Emergency Health Services Faculty
Inver Hills Community College
Inver Grove Heights, Minnesota

Mark Lockhart, NREMT-P
Deputy Chief-EMS
Maryland Heights Fire Protection District
Maryland Heights, Missouri

Joanne McCall, RN, MA, CEN
Educator Emergency Services
Providence Hospital and Medical Centers
Novi, Michigan

Kirk E. Mittleman, AAS, BS, NREMT-P/Utah EMT-P
Mt. Nebo Training Association
Provo, Utah

Taz Meyer, BS, EMT-P
Operations Coordinator
St. Charles County Ambulance District
St. Peters, Missouri

Susan M. Caley Opsal, MS
Illinois Valley Community College
Oglesby, Illinois

David S. Pecora, MS, PA-C, NREMT-P
Chief, Physician Assistant
Clinical Instructor
West Virginia University
Department of Emergency Medicine
Morgantown, West Virginia

Eric Powell, EMT-P
Emerald Isle, North Carolina

Virginia K. Riedy, RN, NREMT-P
EMS Education Manager
Columbus Division of Fire
Columbus, Ohio

Becky Ridenhour, PharmD
Troy, Missouri

Blaine Riggleman, EMT-P
Program Director
Holmes Community College
Ridgeland, Mississippi

Judith A. Ruple, PhD, RN, NREMT-P
Professor
College of Health and Human Services
The University of Toledo
Toledo, Ohio

Gordon M. Sachs, EFO, MPA
Fire/EMS Chief (retired)
Fairfield, Pennsylvania

Gail Saxowsky, RNC, MPH
Clinical Coordinator
EMT Program
Chemeketa Community College
Salem, Oregon

Roberta J. Secrest, PhD, PharmD, RPh
Global Medical Communications
Eli Lilly and Company
Indianapolis, Indiana

Wayne Snyder, MPA, EMT-P
EMS and Emergency Preparedness Coordinator
Mercy Memorial Hospital
Monroe, Michigan

Robert Swor, DO, FACEP
Director, EMS Programs
Department of Emergency Medicine
William Beaumont Hospital
Royal Oak, Michigan

Rob Theriault, EMCA, RCT(Adv), CCP(F)
Manager, Education and Professional Development
Sunnybrook-Osler Centre for Prehospital Care
Ontario, Canada

Mike Turner
General Manager
Central County Fire Alarm
St. Louis, Missouri

Anne Walters
Front Range Community College
Westminster, Colorado

Robert B. Wylie, BS, EFO, CFI
Assistant Chief
Central County Fire & Rescue
St. Peters, Missouri

And we offer a special thanks to those who helped on the previous editions of this text:

First edition: National Association of EMTs Society of Paramedics Instructor/Coordinators Society; National Council of State EMS Training Coordinators; National Association of EMS Physicians; Thomas F. Anderson, PhD, RRT; Doug Austin, Jr.; Vatche H. Ayvazian, MD; John Barrett, MD; David S. Becker; John E. Blue, II, EMT-P, BS; Chip Boehm, RN, EMT-P; Kevin Brown, MD, MPH; Jeffrey A. Crill, RN, EMT-P; David DaBell, MD; Alice "Twink" Dalton; Theodore R. Delbridge, MD; Linda D. Dodge; Robert Elling, MPA, NREMT-P; Franklin E.Foster, JD; Bill Garcia, MICP; Mike Gray; Janet A. Head, RN, MS; Kenneth

Hines; Steven Kidd; Mark A. Kirk, MD; Kevin Kraus, BS, EMT-P; Richard A. Lazar; Mark Lockhart, NREMT-P; Julie Long; Glenn H. Luedtke, NREMT-P; Mary Beth Michos, RN; Gary P. Morris; Keith Neely, EMT-P, MPA; Gregory Noll; Michael P. Peppers, PharmD; Dwight Polk, BA, NREMT-P; William Raynovich; Lou E. Romig, MD, FAAP; José V. Aalazar, BA, NREMT; Randy L. Sanders; Carol J. Shanaberger; JoAnn Shew, RN, CS, MSN; John Sinclair; Todd M. Stanford, BS, PA-C, MICP; Andrew W. Stern, NREMT-P, MPA; Mike Taigman; Vickie H. Taylor; Michael W. Turner; Patricia L. Westbrook, MS, CCC; Jason T. White; Sherrie C. Wilson, EMT-P, I/C; Monroe Yancie, NREMT-P; and Rodney C. Zerr.

Second edition: Joseph J. Acker, AHT, EMT-P; Richard Alcorta, MD, FACEP; Chandra Aubin, MD; Alan J. Azzara, Esq, BA, JD, EMT-P; Catherine A. Parvensky Barwell, RN/EMT-P, MEd; James P. Boedeker, MD; William Brandes; David H. Brisson, RN, EMCA; Lawrence R. Brown, MD, PhD; Roy Edward Cox, Jr., MEd, EMT-P; Kevin Cunningham, BS, EMT-P; John Czajkowski; Heather Micholene Davis, MS, NREMT-P; Jeff G. DeGraffenreid, MEd, Paramedic; William H. Dribben, MD; William J. Dunne, MS, NREMT-P; Lisa Susan Etzwiler, MD, FAAP; Daryl Eustace; Edward Ferguson, MD; Janet Fitts, RN, BSN, CEN, EMT-P; Ken Fowke, BSc, EMA-II; Timothy Gridley; Larry Hatfield; Shirley A. Jones, MS Ed, MHA, EMT-P; Antoinette Kanne, RN, MS; Lisa Keenly, MD; Anthony C. Kessels; J. Steven Kidd; Jeffrey Levine, MD, FACS; James Linardos, MS, EMT-I; Michael Mullins, MD; Scott Mullins; Robert E. O'Connor, MD, MPH; Nathan Piemann, MD; Denise S. Pope, RN, MSN, BSN, MSN; John Eric Powell, MS, NREMT-P; Chris Richter, MD; Becky Ridenhour, PharmD; Cleeve Robertson, MD; S. Rutherford Rose, PharmD, FAACT; Stanley Sakabu, MD, FACS; Robert J. Schappert III; Roberta J. Secrest, PhD, PharmD; Sharon Smith, MD; Karen Snyder; Andrew W. Stern, NREMT-P, MPA, MA; Gail Stewart, BS, EMT-P, CHES; Robert Thieriault, RCT (Adv), CCP (F); Eric Thompson, MD; Bryan Troop, MD, FACS, FCCM; Christina Wagner, MD; Bruce J. Walz, PhD; Roxanne Ward, RN; A. Keith Wesley, MD, FACEP; and Brian S. Zachariah, MD, MBA.

SPECIAL FEATURES

Chapter Openers set the stage for learning with **Objectives** and **Key Terms** with definitions.

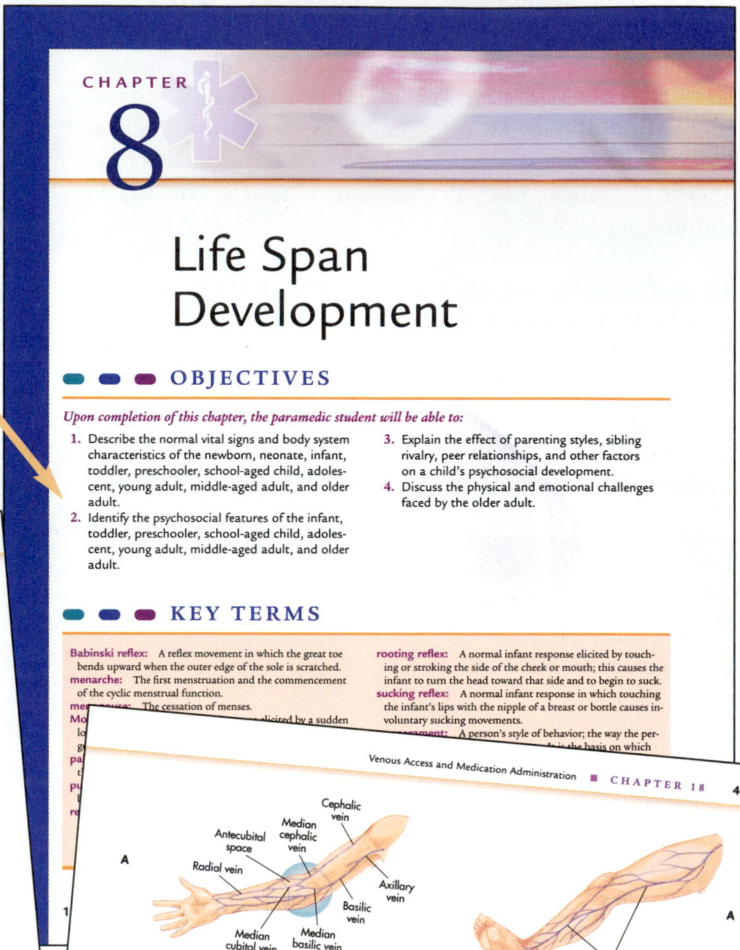
CHAPTER 8

Life Span Development

OBJECTIVES

Upon completion of this chapter, the paramedic student will be able to:

1. Describe the normal vital signs and body system characteristics of the newborn, neonate, infant, toddler, preschooler, school-aged child, adolescent, young adult, middle-aged adult, and older adult.
2. Identify the psychosocial features of the infant, toddler, preschooler, school-aged child, adolescent, young adult, middle-aged adult, and older adult.
3. Explain the effect of parenting styles, sibling rivalry, peer relationships, and other factors on a child's psychosocial development.
4. Discuss the physical and emotional challenges faced by the older adult.

KEY TERMS

Babinski reflex: A reflex movement in which the great toe bends upward when the outer edge of the sole is scratched.
menarche: The first menstruation and the commencement of the cyclic menstrual function.
rooting reflex: A normal infant response elicited by touching or stroking the side of the cheek or mouth; this causes the infant to turn the head toward that side and to begin to suck.
sucking reflex: A normal infant response in which touching the infant's lips with the nipple of a breast or bottle causes involuntary sucking movements.

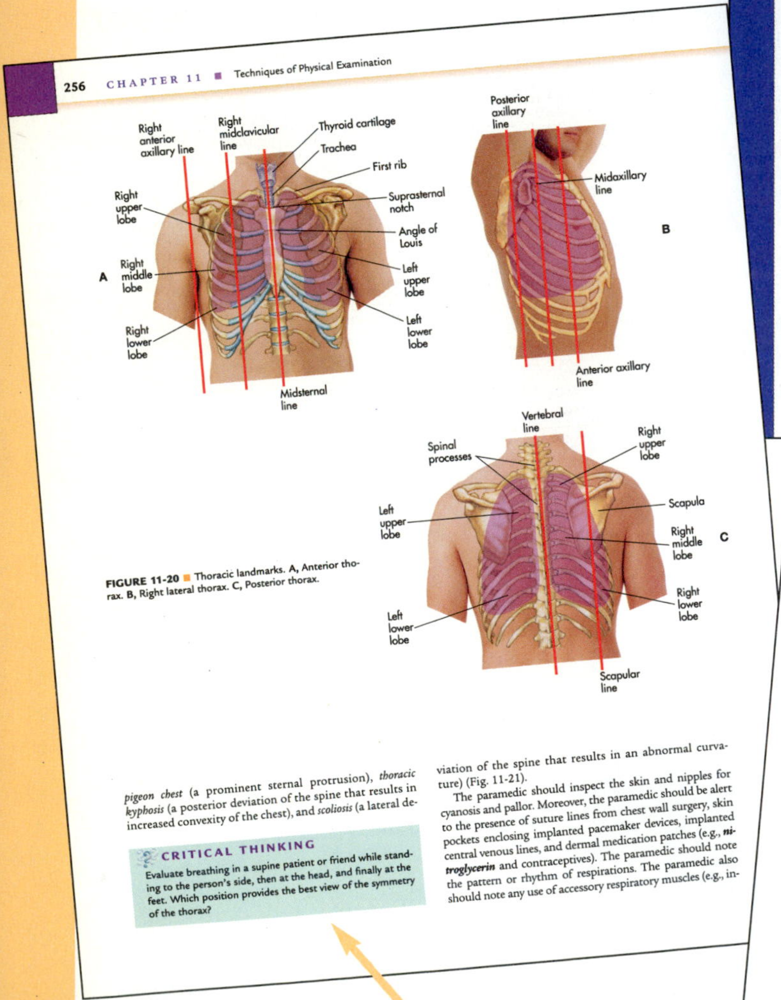

FIGURE 11-20 ■ Thoracic landmarks. A, Anterior thorax. B, Right lateral thorax. C, Posterior thorax.

pigeon chest (a prominent sternal protrusion), thoracic kyphosis (a posterior deviation of the spine that results in increased convexity of the chest), and scoliosis (a lateral deviation of the spine that results in an abnormal curvature) (Fig. 11-21).

The paramedic should inspect the skin and nipples for cyanosis and pallor. Moreover, the paramedic should be alert to the presence of suture lines from chest wall surgery, skin pockets enclosing implanted pacemaker devices, implanted central venous lines, and dermal medication patches (e.g., nitroglycerin and contraceptives). The paramedic should note the pattern or rhythm of respirations. The paramedic also should note any use of accessory respiratory muscles (e.g., in-

CRITICAL THINKING

Evaluate breathing in a supine patient or friend while standing to the person's side, then at the head, and finally at the feet. Which position provides the best view of the symmetry of the thorax?

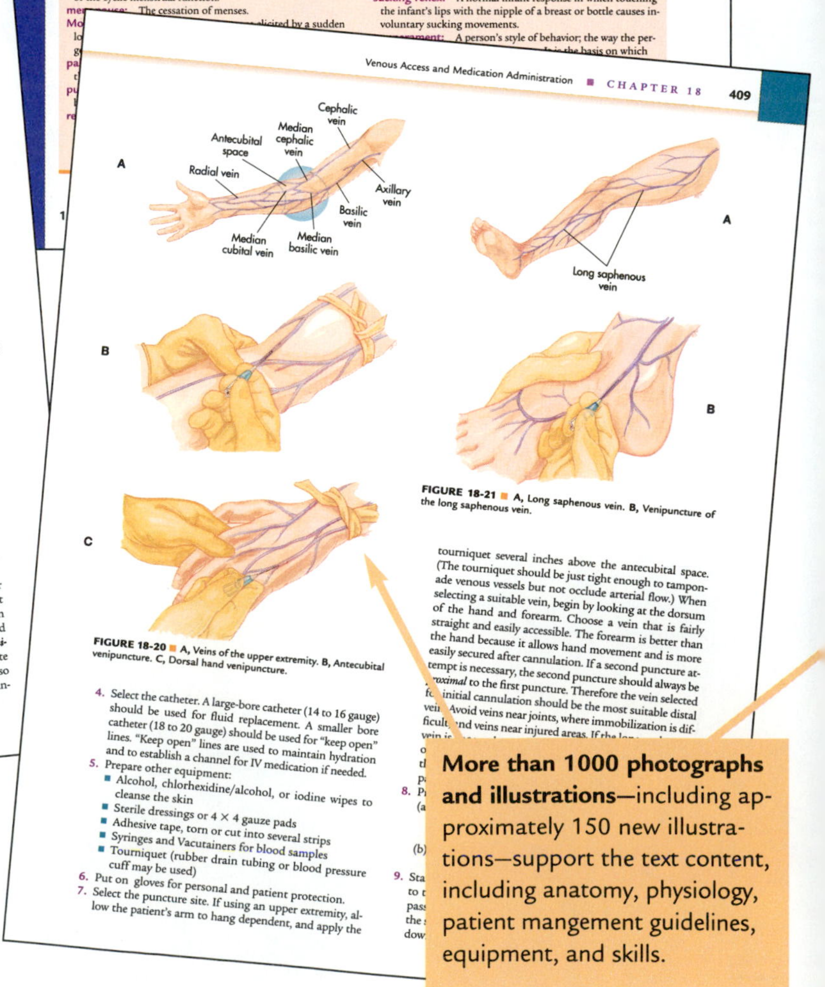

FIGURE 18-20 ■ A, Veins of the upper extremity. B, Antecubital venipuncture. C, Dorsal hand venipuncture.

FIGURE 18-21 ■ A, Long saphenous vein. B, Venipuncture of the long saphenous vein.

4. Select the catheter. A large-bore catheter (14 to 16 gauge) should be used for fluid replacement. A smaller bore catheter (18 to 20 gauge) should be used for "keep open" lines. "Keep open" lines are used to maintain hydration and to establish a channel for IV medication if needed.
5. Prepare other equipment:
   - Alcohol, chlorhexidine/alcohol, or iodine wipes to cleanse the skin
   - Sterile dressings or 4 × 4 gauze pads
   - Adhesive tape, torn or cut into several strips
   - Syringes and Vacutainers for blood samples
   - Tourniquet (rubber drain tubing or blood pressure cuff may be used)
6. Put on gloves for personal and patient protection.
7. Select the puncture site. If using an upper extremity, allow the patient's arm to hang dependent, and apply the

tourniquet several inches above the antecubital space. (The tourniquet should be just tight enough to tamponade venous vessels but not occlude arterial flow.) When selecting a suitable vein, begin by looking at the dorsum of the hand and forearm. Choose a vein that is fairly straight and easily accessible. The forearm is better than the hand because it allows hand movement and is more easily secured after cannulation. If a second puncture attempt is necessary, the second puncture should always be proximal to the first puncture. Therefore the vein selected for initial cannulation should be the most suitable distal vein. Avoid veins near joints, where immobilization is difficult, and veins near injured areas.

Boxed **Critical Thinking** questions aid in understanding concepts and how chapter content impacts patient care.

More than 1000 photographs and illustrations—including approximately 150 new illustrations—support the text content, including anatomy, physiology, patient mangement guidelines, equipment, and skills.

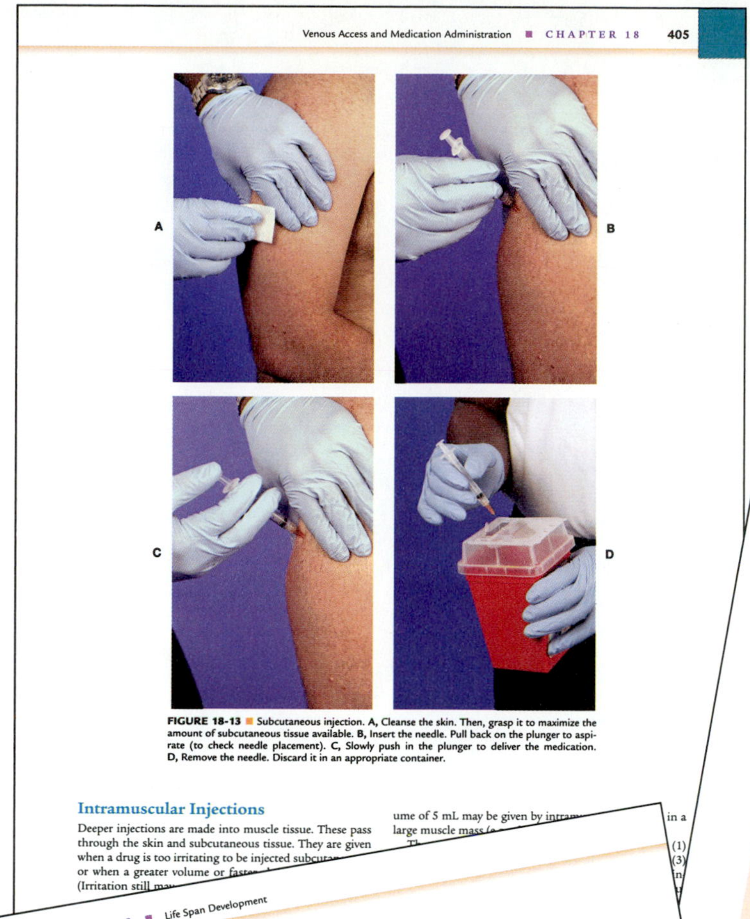

FIGURE 18-13 ■ Subcutaneous injection. **A,** Cleanse the skin. Then, grasp it to maximize the amount of subcutaneous tissue available. **B,** Insert the needle. Pull back on the plunger to aspirate (to check needle placement). **C,** Slowly push in the plunger to deliver the medication. **D,** Remove the needle. Discard it in an appropriate container.

Intramuscular Injections

Deeper injections are made into muscle tissue. These pass through the skin and subcutaneous tissue. They are given when a drug is too irritating to be injected subcutan... or when a greater volume or faster ... (Irritation still ma...

ume of 5 mL may be given by intram... in a large muscle mass ...

ALS skills are presented step-by-step in full-color to demonstrate emergency care procedures.

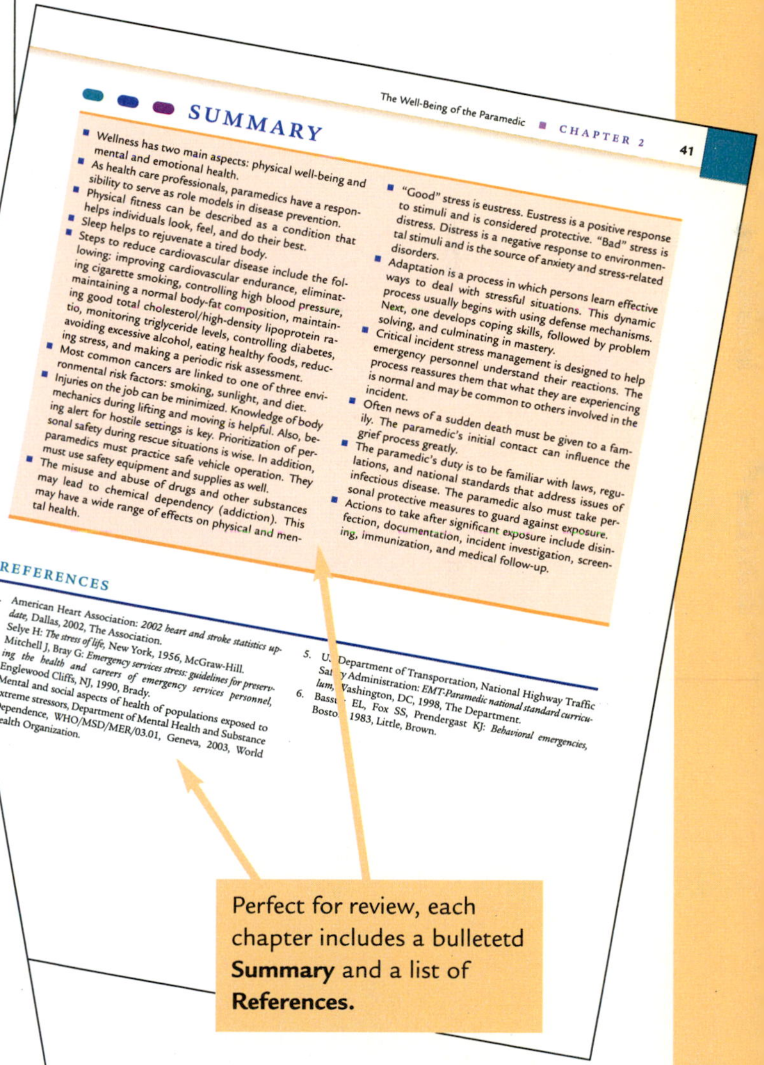

SUMMARY

- Wellness has two main aspects: physical well-being and mental and emotional health.
- As health care professionals, paramedics have a responsibility to serve as role models in disease prevention.
- Physical fitness can be described as a condition that helps individuals look, feel, and do their best.
- Sleep helps to rejuvenate a tired body.
- Steps to reduce cardiovascular disease include the following: improving cardiovascular endurance, eliminating cigarette smoking, controlling high blood pressure, maintaining a normal body-fat composition, maintaining good total cholesterol/high-density lipoprotein ratio, monitoring triglyceride levels, controlling diabetes, avoiding excessive alcohol, eating healthy foods, reducing stress, and making a periodic risk assessment.
- Most common cancers are linked to one of three environmental risk factors: smoking, sunlight, and diet.
- Injuries on the job can be minimized. Knowledge of body mechanics during lifting and moving is helpful. Also, being alert for hostile settings is key. Prioritization of personal safety during rescue situations is wise. In addition, paramedics must practice safe vehicle operation. They must use safety equipment and supplies as well.
- The misuse and abuse of drugs and other substances may lead to chemical dependency (addiction). This may have a wide range of effects on physical and mental health.
- "Good" stress is eustress. Eustress is a positive response to stimuli and is considered protective. "Bad" stress is distress. Distress is a negative response to environmental stimuli and is the source of anxiety and stress-related disorders.
- Adaptation is a process in which persons learn effective ways to deal with stressful situations. This dynamic process usually begins with using defense mechanisms. Next, one develops coping skills, followed by problem solving, and culminating in mastery.
- Critical incident stress management is designed to help emergency personnel understand their reactions. The process reassures them that what they are experiencing is normal and may be common to others involved in the incident.
- Often news of a sudden death must be given to a family. The paramedic's initial contact can influence the grief process greatly.
- The paramedic's duty is to be familiar with laws, regulations, and national standards that address issues of infectious disease. The paramedic also must take personal protective measures to guard against exposure.
- Actions to take after significant exposure include disinfection, documentation, incident investigation, screening, immunization, and medical follow-up.

REFERENCES

1. American Heart Association: *2002 heart and stroke statistics update*, Dallas, 2002, The Association.
2. Selye H: *The stress of life*, New York, 1956, McGraw-Hill.
3. Mitchell J, Bray G: *Emergency services stress: guidelines for preserving the health and careers of emergency services personnel*, Englewood Cliffs, NJ, 1990, Brady.
4. Mental and social aspects of health of populations exposed to extreme stressors, Department of Mental Health and Substance Dependence, WHO/MSD/MER/03.01, Geneva, 2003, World Health Organization.
5. U... Department of Transportation, National Highway Traffic Sa...y Administration: *EMT-Paramedic national standard curriculum*, Washington, DC, 1998, The Department.
6. Bass... EL, Fox SS, Prendergast KJ: *Behavioral emergencies*, Bosto... 1983, Little, Brown.

Perfect for review, each chapter includes a bulletetd **Summary** and a list of **References.**

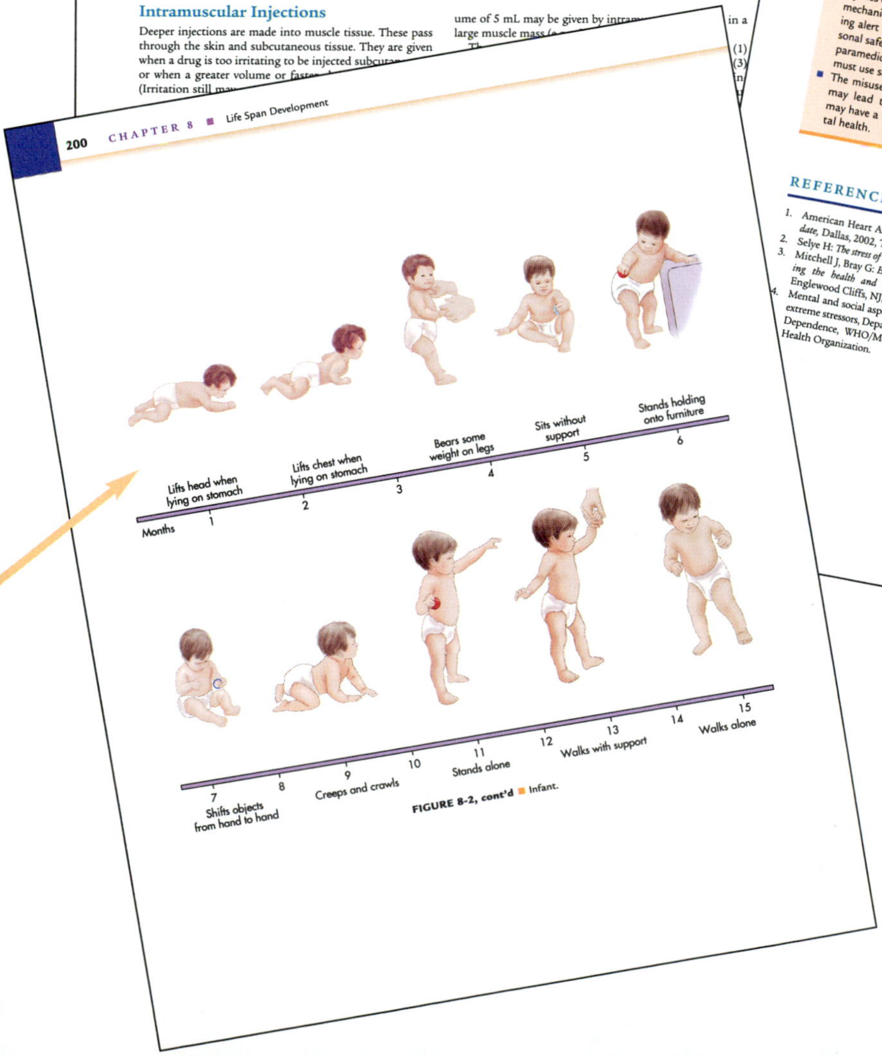

FIGURE 8-2, cont'd ■ Infant.

CONTENTS

PART ONE

1 Emergency Medical Services Systems: Roles and Responsibilities, *2*
Emergency Medical Services System Development, *3*
Current Emergency Medical Services Systems, *7*
National Emergency Medical Services Group Involvement, *10*
Paramedic Education, *11*
Licensure, Certification, and Registration, *11*
Professionalism, *11*
Roles and Responsibilities of the Paramedic, *13*
Medical Direction for Emergency Medical Services, *15*
Improving System Quality, *16*
Emergency Medical Services Research, *16*

2 The Well-Being of the Paramedic, *22*
Wellness Components, *23*
Stress, *32*
Dealing with Death, Dying, Grief, and Loss, *37*
Prevention of Disease Transmission, *39*

3 Injury Prevention, *42*
Injury Epidemiology, *43*
Overview of Injury Prevention, *43*
Feasibility of Emergency Medical Services Involvement, *46*
Participation in Prevention Programs, *50*

4 Medical/Legal Issues, *54*
Legal Duties and Ethical Responsibilities, *55*
The Legal System, *55*
Legal Accountability of the Paramedic, *58*
Paramedic-Patient Relationships, *61*
Resuscitation Issues, *65*
Crime Scene Responsibilities, *69*
Documentation, *69*

5 Ethics, 72
Ethics Overview, *73*
A Rapid Approach to Emergency Ethical Problems, *76*
Ethical Tests in Health Care, *76*
Resolving Ethical Dilemmas, *76*
Ethical Issues in Contemporary Paramedic Practice, *77*

PART TWO

6 Review of Human Systems, *82*
Terminology, *83*
Cell Structure, *84*
Tissues, *90*
Organ Systems, *92*
Special Senses, *144*

7 General Principles of Pathophysiology, *150*
SECTION ONE Cellular Physiology, *152*
Basic Cellular Review, *152*
Cellular Environment, *152*

SECTION TWO Cellular Injury and Disease, *172*
Alterations in Cells and Tissues, *172*
Hypoperfusion, *176*
Self-Defense Mechanisms, *181*
Variances in Immunity and Inflammation, *185*
Stress and Disease, *187*
Genetics and Familial Diseases, *189*

8 Life Span Development, *196*
Newborn, *197*
Toddler and Preschool Years, *201*
School-Age Years, *203*
Adolescence, *204*
Early Adulthood, *206*
Middle Adulthood, *206*
Late Adulthood, *207*

PART THREE

9 Therapeutic Communication, *214*
- Communication, *215*
- Internal Factors in Effective Communication, *216*
- External Factors in Effective Communication, *217*
- Patient Interview, *218*
- Strategies for Obtaining Information, *219*
- Methods of Assessing Mental Status During the Interview, *220*
- Special Interview Situations, *221*

10 History Taking, *226*
- Content of the Patient History, 227
- Techniques of History Taking, 228
- Special Challenges, 231

11 Techniques of Physical Examination, *234*
- Physical Examination: Approach and Overview, *235*
- Mental Status, *238*
- General Survey, *240*
- Anatomical Regions, *250*
- Physical Examination of Infants and Children, *274*
- Physical Examination of Older Adults, *277*

12 Patient Assessment, *280*
- Scene Size-Up and Assessment, *281*
- Patient Assessment Priorities, *282*
- Initial Assessment, *282*
- Focused History and Physical Examination: Medical Patients, *286*
- Focused History and Physical Examination: Trauma Patients, *286*
- Rapid Trauma Physical Examination, *287*
- Detailed Physical Examination, *287*
- Ongoing Assessment, *287*
- Care of Medical Versus Trauma Patients, *288*

13 Clinical Decision Making, *290*
- The Spectrum of Prehospital Care, *291*
- Critical Thinking Process for Paramedics, *291*
- Fundamental Elements of Critical Thinking for Paramedics, *293*
- Field Application of Assessment-Based Patient Management, *293*
- Putting it all Together: The Six R's, *294*

14 Assessment-Based Management, *298*
- Effective Assessment, *299*
- The Right Stuff, *302*
- Optional Take-in Equipment, *302*
- General Approach to the Patient, *303*
- Presenting the Patient, *303*

15 Communications, *306*
- Phases of Communications during a Typical Emergency Medical Services Event, *307*
- Role of Communications in Emergency Medical Services, *308*
- Communications Systems, *310*
- Components and Functions of Dispatch Communications Systems, *314*
- Regulation, *315*
- Procedures for Emergency Medical Services Communications, *315*

16 Documentation, *318*
- Importance of Documentation, *319*
- General Considerations, *320*
- The Narrative, *320*
- Elements of a Properly Written Emergency Medical Services Document, *326*
- Systems of Narrative Writing, *326*
- Special Considerations of Documentation, *327*
- Document Revision/Correction, *328*
- Consequences of Inappropriate Documentation, *328*

PART FOUR

17 Pharmacology, *332*
- SECTION ONE Drug Information, *334*
- Historical Trends in Pharmacology, *334*

- SECTION TWO Mechanisms of Drug Action, *337*
- General Properties of Drugs, *337*
- Drug Interactions, *347*
- Drug Forms, Preparations, and Storage, *348*
- Drug Profiles and Special Considerations in Drug Therapy, *348*

- SECTION THREE Drugs that Affect the Nervous System, *351*
- Review of Anatomy and Physiology, *351*

SECTION FOUR Drugs that Affect the Cardiovascular System, *364*
Review of Anatomy and Physiology, *364*

SECTION FIVE Drugs that Affect the Blood, *368*
Anticoagulants, Fibrinolytics, and Blood Components, *368*

SECTION SIX Drugs that Affect the Respiratory System, *370*
Review of Anatomy and Physiology, *370*

SECTION SEVEN Drugs that Affect the Gastrointestinal System, *372*
Review of Anatomy and Physiology, *372*

SECTION EIGHT Drugs that Affect the Eye and Ear, *374*
Treatment of Eye Disorders, *374*

SECTION NINE Drugs that Affect the Endocrine System, *375*
Review of Anatomy and Physiology, *375*

SECTION TEN Drugs that Affect the Reproductive System, *376*
Treatment of Disorders of the Reproductive System, *376*

SECTION ELEVEN Drugs Used in Neoplastic Diseases, *377*
Antineoplastic Agents, *377*

SECTION TWELVE Drugs Used in Infectious Disease and Inflammation, *378*
Treatment of Infectious Disease and Inflammation, *378*

SECTION THIRTEEN Drugs that Affect the Immunological System, *381*
Review of Anatomy and Physiology, *381*

APPENDIX Herbs, *385*
Herbal Products, *385*
Herbal Supplements, *385*

18 Venous Access and Medication Administration, *388*
Mathematical Equivalents Used in Pharmacology, *389*
Drug Calculations, *391*
Drug Administration, *396*
Medical Asepsis, *397*
Universal Precautions in Medication Administration, *397*
Enteral Administration of Medications, *397*
Parental Administration of Medications, *399*
Administration of Percutaneous Medications, *420*
Special Considerations for Pediatric Patients, *423*
Obtaining a Blood Sample, *423*
Disposal of Contaminated Items and Sharps, *425*

APPENDIX Universal Precautions: Measures to Prevent Transmission of the Human Immunodeficiency Virus (HIV), *427*

PART FIVE

19 Airway Management and Ventilation, *430*
SECTION ONE Respiratory Physiology, *431*
Mechanics of Respiration, *431*
Measurement of Gases, *437*
Pulmonary Circulation, *438*

SECTION TWO Respiratory Pathophysiology, *449*
Foreign Body Airway Obstruction, *449*
Aspiration by Inhalation, *452*

SECTION THREE Airway Evaluation, *453*
Essential Parameters of Airway Evaluation, *453*
Supplemental Oxygen Therapy, *455*
Ventilation, *459*
Airway Management, *464*
Suction, *466*
Mechanical Adjuncts in Airway Management, *469*
Advanced Airway Procedures, *472*
Pharmacological Adjuncts to Airway Management and Ventilation, *490*
Translaryngeal Cannula Ventilation, *492*
Cricothyrotomy, *494*

PART SIX

20 Trauma Systems and Mechanism of Injury, *501*

Epidemiology of Trauma, *501*

SECTION ONE Kinematics, *503*

Energy, *503*

SECTION TWO Blunt Trauma, *504*

Blunt Trauma, *504*

Restraints, *506*

Organ Collision Injuries, *508*

Other Motorized Vehicular Collisions, *510*

Pedestrian Injuries, *511*

Other Causes of Blunt Trauma, *511*

SECTION THREE Penetrating Trauma, *513*

Penetrating Trauma, *513*

21 Hemorrhage and Shock, *520*

Hemorrhage, *521*

Definition of Shock, *522*

Tissue Oxygenation, *522*

The Body as a Container, *523*

Capillary-Cellular Relationship in Shock, *524*

Classifications of Shock, *526*

Stages of Shock, *527*

Uncompensated Shock, *527*

Management and Treatment Plan for the Patient in Shock, *529*

Integration of Patient Assessment and the Treatment Plan, *536*

22 Soft Tissue Trauma, *538*

Anatomy and Physiology, *539*

Pathophysiology, *540*

Pathophysiology and Assessment of Soft Tissue Injuries, *542*

Management Principles for Soft Tissue Injuries, *547*

Hemorrhage and Control of Bleeding, *549*

Dressing Materials Used with Soft Tissue Trauma, *551*

Management of Specific Soft Tissue Injuries Not Requiring Closure, *552*

Special Considerations for Soft Tissue Injuries, *556*

23 Burns, *558*

Incidence and Patterns of Burn Injury, *559*

Classifications of Burn Injury, *561*

Pathophysiology of Burn Shock, *565*

Assessment of the Burn Patient, *566*

General Principles in Burn Management, *567*

Inhalation Burn Injury, *569*

Chemical Burn Injury, *570*

Electrical Burn Injuries, *573*

Radiation Exposure, *576*

24 Head and Facial Trauma, *580*

Maxillofacial Injury, *581*

Ear, Eye, and Dental Trauma, *585*

Anterior Neck Trauma, *590*

Head Trauma, *593*

Brain Trauma, *596*

Injury Rating Systems, *603*

25 Spinal Trauma, *606*

Spinal Trauma: Incidence, Morbidity, and Mortality, *607*

Traditional Spinal Assessment Criteria, *607*

Review of Spinal Anatomy and Physiology, *609*

General Assessment of Spinal Injury, *609*

Classifications of Spinal Injury, *611*

Evaluation and Assessment of Spinal Cord Injury, *614*

General Management of Spinal Injuries, *615*

Cord Injury Presentations, *626*

Nontraumatic Spinal Conditions, *627*

Assessment and Management of Nontraumatic Spinal Conditions, *628*

26 Thoracic Trauma, *630*

Skeletal Injury, *631*

Closed Pneumothorax, *633*

Heart and Great Vessel Injury, *638*

Other Thoracic Injuries, *640*

27 Abdominal Trauma, *644*

Mechanisms of Abdominal Injury, *645*

Specific Abdominal Injuries, *646*

Vascular Structure Injuries, *649*

Assessment of Abdominal Trauma, *649*

Management of Abdominal Trauma, *649*

28 **Musculoskeletal Trauma,** *652*
Classifications of Musculoskeletal Injuries, *653*
Inflammatory and Degenerative Conditions, *656*
Signs and Symptoms of Extremity Trauma, *658*
Assessment of Musculoskeletal Injuries, *658*
Upper Extremity Injuries, *660*
Lower Extremity Injuries, *664*
Open Fractures, *668*
Straightening Angular Fractures and Reducing Dislocations, *669*
Referral of Patients with Minor Musculoskeletal Injury, *670*

PART SEVEN

29 **Cardiology,** *674*
Risk Factors and Prevention Strategies, *676*

SECTION ONE Anatomy and Physiology of the Heart, *676*
Anatomy, *676*
Physiology, *677*

SECTION TWO Electrophysiology of the Heart, *681*
Electrical Activity of Cardiac Cells and Membrane Potentials, *681*
Cell Excitability, *682*
Electrical Conduction System of the Heart, *685*

SECTION THREE Assessment of the Patient with Cardiac Disease, *688*
Assessment, *688*

SECTION FOUR Electrocardiogram Monitoring, *691*
Basic Concepts of Electrocardiogram Monitoring, *691*
Relationship of the Electrocardiogram To Electrical Activity, *699*

SECTION FIVE Electrocardiogram Interpretation, *702*
Steps in Rhythm Analysis, *702*

SECTION SIX Introduction to Dysrhythmias, *713*
Classification of Dysrhythmias, *713*
Dysrhythmias Originating in the Sinoatrial Node, *714*
Dysrhythmias Originating in the Atria, *722*
Dysrhythmias Sustained or Originating in the Atrioventricular Junction, *735*
Dysrhythmias Originating in the Ventricles, *738*
Dysrhythmias that Are Disorders of Conduction, *763*

SECTION SEVEN Specific Cardiovascular Diseases, *778*
Pathophysiology and Management of Cardiovascular Disease, *778*

SECTION EIGHT Techniques of Managing Cardiac Emergencies, *799*
Basic Cardiac Life Support, *799*
Defibrillation, *802*
Implantable Cardioverter Defibrillators, *804*
Synchronized Cardioversion, *805*
Transcutaneous Cardiac Pacing, *806*
Cardiac Arrest and Sudden Death, *807*
Termination of Resuscitation, *808*

PART EIGHT

30 **Pulmonary Emergencies,** *816*
Pathophysiology, *817*
Scene Size-up and Rescuer Safety, *818*
Obstructive Airway Disease, *820*
Pneumonia, *825*
Adult Respiratory Distress Syndrome, *828*
Pulmonary Thromboembolism, *830*
Upper Respiratory Infection, *831*
Spontaneous Pneumothorax, *831*
Hyperventilation Syndrome, *832*
Lung Cancer, *832*

31 **Neurology,** *836*
Anatomy and Physiology of the Nervous System, *837*
Neurological Pathophysiology, *842*
Pathophysiology and Management of Specific Central Nervous System Disorders, *847*

32 **Endocrinology, 864**
Anatomy and Physiology of the Endocrine System, *865*
Specific Disorders of the Endocrine System, *866*
Disorders of the Pancreas: Diabetes Mellitus, *867*
Disorders of the Thyroid Gland, *877*
Disorders of the Adrenal Glands, *878*

33 Allergies and Anaphylaxis, *882*
Antigen-Antibody Reaction, *883*
Allergic Reaction, *883*
Localized Allergic Reaction, *884*
Anaphylaxis, *884*

34 Gastroenterology, *892*
Gastrointestinal Anatomy, *893*
Assessment of the Patient with Acute Abdominal Pain, *893*
Management of the Patient with an Abdominal Emergency, *897*
Specific Abdominal Emergencies, *897*

APPENDIX Nasogastric Tube Insertion, *906*
Necessary Equipment, *906*
Procedure, *906*
Possible Complications, *906*

35 Urology, *908*
Anatomy and Physiology Review, *909*
Physical Examination for Patients with Genitourinary Disorders, *912*
Management and Treatment Plan, *912*
Management, *917*

36 Toxicology, *920*
SECTION ONE Poisonings, *921*
Poison Control Centers, *921*
General Guidelines for Managing a Poisoned Patient, *922*
Poisoning by Ingestion, *922*
Poisoning by Inhalation, *932*
Poisoning by Injection, *935*
Poisoning by Absorption, *944*

SECTION TWO Drug Abuse, *945*
Toxic Effects of Drugs, *945*

SECTION THREE Alcoholism, *955*
Alcohol Dependence, *955*
Ethanol, *956*
Medical Consequences of Chronic Alcohol Ingestion, *956*
Alcohol Emergencies, *959*

SECTION FOUR Management of Toxic Syndromes, *961*
General Management Principles for Toxic Syndromes, *961*

APPENDIX Toxicology in Emergency Cardiac Care, *966*
Guidelines for Severe Poisoning, *966*

37 Hematology, *970*
Blood and Blood Components, *971*
Specific Hematological Disorders, *972*
General Assessment and Management of Patients with Hematological Disorders, *980*

38 Environmental Conditions, *984*
Thermoregulation, *985*
Hyperthermia, *988*
Hypothermia, *990*
Frostbite, *993*
Submersion, *995*
Diving Emergencies, *997*
High-Altitude Illness, *1000*

39 Infectious and Communicable Diseases, *1004*
Public Health Principles Related to Infectious Diseases, *1005*
Pathophysiology of Infectious Disease, *1009*
Physiology of the Human Response to Infection, *1011*
Stages of Infectious Disease, *1016*
Human Immunodeficiency Virus, *1016*
Hepatitis, *1021*
Tuberculosis, *1023*
Meningococcal Meningitis, *1025*
Pneumonia, *1026*
Tetanus, *1027*
Rabies, *1028*
Hantavirus, *1028*
Viral Diseases of Childhood, *1029*
Other Viral Diseases, *1031*
Sexually Transmitted Diseases, *1032*
Lice and Scabies, *1036*
Reporting an Exposure to an Infectious or a Communicable Disease, *1038*
Paramedic's Role in Preventing Disease Transmission, *1039*

40 Behavioral and Psychiatric Disorders, 1042
Understanding Behavioral Emergencies, 1043
Assessment and Management of Behavioral Emergencies, 1045
Specific Behavioral and Psychiatric Disorders, 1048
Special Considerations for Patients with Behavioral Problems, 1057

41 Gynecology, 1062
Organs of the Female Reproductive System, 1063
Menstruation and Ovulation, 1063
Specific Gynecological Emergencies, 1066

42 Obstetrics, 1072
Normal Events of Pregnancy, 1073
Specialized Structures of Pregnancy, 1073
Fetal Growth and Development, 1074
Obstetrical Terminology, 1077
Patient Assessment, 1077
Complications of Pregnancy, 1080
Delivery Complications, 1091

PART NINE

43 Neonatology, 1100
Risk Factors Associated with the Need for Resuscitation, 1101
Physiological Adaptations at Birth, 1102
Assessment and Management of the Neonate, 1103
Resuscitation of the Distressed Newborn, 1106
Postresuscitation Care, 1108
Neonatal Transport, 1108
Specific Situations, 1109
Psychological and Emotional Support, 1113

44 Pediatrics, 1116
The Paramedic's Role in Caring for Pediatric Patients, 1117
Emergency Medical Services for Children, 1117
Growth and Development Review, 1118
Anatomy and Physiology Review, 1120
General Principles of Pediatric Assessment, 1122
General Principles of Patient Management, 1125
Specific Pathophysiology, Assessment, and Management, 1125
Infants and Children with Special Needs, 1153

APPENDIX Recommended Childhood Immunization Schedule, 1159

45 Geriatrics, 1160
Demographics, Epidemiology, and Societal Issues, 1161
Living Environments and Referral Sources, 1161
Physiological Changes of Aging, 1162
General Principles in Assessment of the Geriatric Patient, 1166
System Pathophysiology, Assessment, and Management, 1166

46 Abuse and Neglect, 1184
Battering, 1185
Elder Abuse, 1188
Child Abuse, 1189
Sexual Assault, 1192

47 Patients with Special Challenges, 1196
Physical Challenges, 1197
Mental Challenges, 1200
Pathological Challenges, 1201
Culturally Diverse Patients, 1205
Terminally Ill Patients, 1207
Patients with Communicable Diseases, 1207
Financial Challenges, 1207

48 Acute Interventions for the Home Health Care Patient, 1210
Overview of Home Health Care, 1211
General Principles of and Management, 1213
Specific Acute Home Health Care Interventions, 1214

PART TEN

49 Ambulance Operations, 1230
Ambulance Standards, 1231
Checking Ambulances, 1231
Ambulance Stationing, 1231
Safe Ambulance Operation, 1232
Aeromedical Transportation, 1236

50 Medical Incident Command, *1240*
Incident Command System, *1241*
Mass Casualty Incidents, *1248*
Principles and Technology of Triage, *1250*
Critical Incident Stress Management, *1253*

51 Rescue Awareness and Operations, *1256*
Appropriate Training for Rescue Operations, *1257*
Phases of a Rescue Operation, *1258*
Rescuer Personal Protective Equipment, *1260*
Surface Water Rescue, *1260*
Hazardous Atmospheres, *1263*
Highway Operations, *1265*
Hazardous Terrain, *1270*
Assessment Procedures During Rescue, *1273*

52 Crime Scene Awareness, *1276*
Approaching the Scene, *1277*
Dangerous Residence, *1278*
Dangerous Highway Encounters, *1278*
Violent Street Incidents, *1279*
Violent Groups and Situations, *1279*
Safety Tactics, *1281*
Tactical Patient Care, *1283*
EMS at Crime Scenes, *1284*

53 Hazardous Materials Incidents, *1286*
Scope of Hazardous Materials, *1287*
Laws and Regulations, *1287*
Identification of Hazardous Materials, *1288*
Personal Protective Clothing and Equipment, *1291*
Health Hazards, *1293*
Response to Hazardous Materials Emergencies, *1295*
Medical Monitoring and Rehabilitation, *1298*
Emergency Management of Contaminated Patients, *1299*
Decontamination of Rescue Personnel and Equipment, *1301*
APPENDIX Overview of Training Requirements for EMS Personnel Responding to a Hazardous Materials Incident as Established by OSHA/EPA and the NFPA, *1304*
OSHA/EPA Training Requirements, *1304*
NPFA 473: Competencies for EMS Personnel Responding to Hazardous Materials Incidents, *1304*

54 Bioterrorism and Weapons of Mass Destruction, *1306*
History of Biological Weapons, *1307*
Critical Biological Agents, *1308*
Methods of Dissemination, *1308*
Specific Biological Threats, *1309*
Nuclear and Radiological Threats, *1312*
Incendiary Threats, *1313*
Specific Chemical Threats, *1313*
Explosive Threats, *1316*
Department of Homeland Security, *1316*
General Guidelines for Emergency Response, *1317*
APPENDIX Personal Protective Equipment for Chemical, Biological, Radiological, and Nuclear Agents, 1319

EMERGENCY DRUG INDEX (EDI), 1321

GLOSSARY, 1366

CCT APPENDIX: ADVANCED PRACTICE PROCEDURES FOR THE CRITICAL CARE PARAMEDIC, 1418

ILLUSTRATION CREDITS, 1424

PART ONE

IN THIS PART

CHAPTER 1 Emergency Medical Services Systems: Roles and Responsibilities

CHAPTER 2 The Well-Being of the Paramedic

CHAPTER 3 Injury Prevention

CHAPTER 4 Medical/Legal Issues

CHAPTER 5 Ethics

CHAPTER

1

Emergency Medical Services Systems: Roles and Responsibilities

OBJECTIVES

Upon completion of this chapter, the paramedic student will be able to:

1. Outline key historical events that influenced the development of emergency medical services (EMS) systems.
2. Identify the key elements necessary for effective EMS systems operations.
3. Differentiate among training and roles and responsibilities of the four nationally recognized levels of EMS licensure/certification: first responder, EMT-Basic, EMT-Intermediate, and EMT-Paramedic.
4. List the benefits of membership in professional EMS organizations.
5. Describe the benefits of continuing education.
6. Differentiate among professionalism and professional licensure, certification, and registration.
7. Describe the paramedic's role in patient care situations as defined by the U.S. Department of Transportation.
8. Describe the benefits of each component of off-line (indirect) and online (direct) medical direction.
9. Outline the role and components of an effective, continuous quality improvement program.
10. Identify the key components of prehospital research and its benefits to the EMS system.

KEY TERMS

advanced life support: The provision of care that paramedics or allied health professionals render, including advanced airway management, defibrillation, intravenous therapy, and medication administration.

basic life support: Care provided by persons trained in first aid, cardiopulmonary resuscitation, and other noninvasive care.

capitation: A method of payment to cover all health care expenses for each member of a managed care organization.

continuous quality improvement: A management approach to customer service and organizational performance that includes constant monitoring, evaluation, decisions, and actions.

emergency medical services: A national network of services coordinated to provide aid and medical assistance from primary response to definitive care; the network involves personnel trained in rescue, stabilization, transportation, and advanced management of traumatic and medical emergencies.

EMT-Paramedic: A person who has completed training based on the EMT-Paramedic National Standard Curriculum, including advanced training in patient assessment, cardiac rhythm interpretation, defibrillation, drug therapy, and airway management.

extended scope of practice: The expansion of health care services provided by emergency medical technicians and paramedics in the prehospital setting.

managed care organizations: Networks that provide patient care services to their members, including health maintenance organizations and preferred provider organizations.

off-line (indirect) medical direction: The establishment and monitoring of all medical components of an EMS system, including protocols, standing orders, educational programs, and the quality and delivery of online (direct) medical direction.

online (direct) medical direction: The medical direction physician or designee who directly supervises prehospital care activities via radio or phone. Online (direct) medical direction also may be responsible for the activities of the emergency department staff and others at the medical direction hospital.

reciprocity: The practice of granting an individual licensure or certification/registration based on licensure or certification/registration by another state, agency, or association.

standing orders: Specific treatment protocols used by prehospital emergency care providers in the absence of online (direct) medical direction when delay in treatment would harm the patient.

treatment protocols: Guidelines that define the scope of prehospital intervention practiced by emergency care providers.

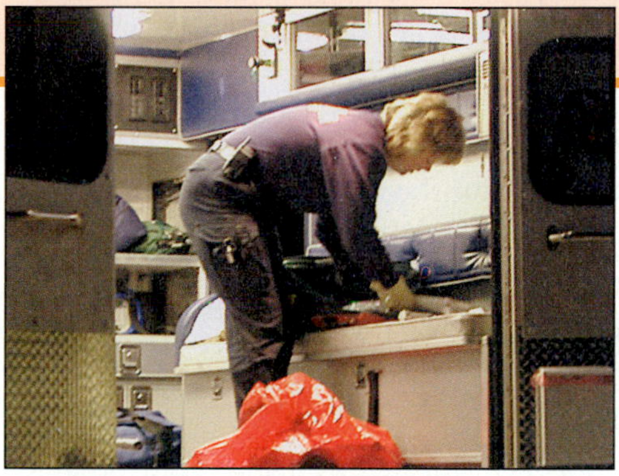

The role of the emergency medical technician–paramedic (EMT-Paramedic, or EMT-P) has evolved. The role differs from the ambulance driver of the past. The paramedics of today work in complex emergency medical services systems. Paramedics take part in an array of professional activities. These activities help paramedics provide quality service in the field. The activities also help paramedics to provide state-of-the-art patient care in less traditional health care settings.

EMERGENCY MEDICAL SERVICES SYSTEM DEVELOPMENT

Assigning a time and place to the birth of organized prehospital emergency care is difficult. To understand the emergency medical services (EMS) system development, one must first consider certain events from ancient times to the present.

Before the Twentieth Century

The ancient Egyptians used herbs and drugs as medicine. They also splinted fractured bones, and they performed some surgeries. The Edwin Smith papyrus (circa the seventeenth century BC) depicted medical practice in Egypt. This system referred to the beat of the heart, palpation, and abnormal motor functions associated with brain injury. Other ancient texts show that surgery was practiced by the Babylonians of Mesopotamia, an ancient area of Asia, as early as 1700 BC.[1] At this time Hammurabi, a King of Babylonia, created a set of laws known as the Code of Hammurabi. These laws set forth fees and penalties for surgeons who offered health care to some social classes (Box 1-1).

Organized prehospital emergency care has its roots in military history. Paintings of Roman battlefields suggest that some of the warriors cared for the injured. The first "ambulance" is thought to have been a covered cart. The ambulance was used by one of Napoleon's surgeons, Jean Larry. He moved injured soldiers to treatment areas during the Napoleonic wars in the 1800s.[1] In the American Civil

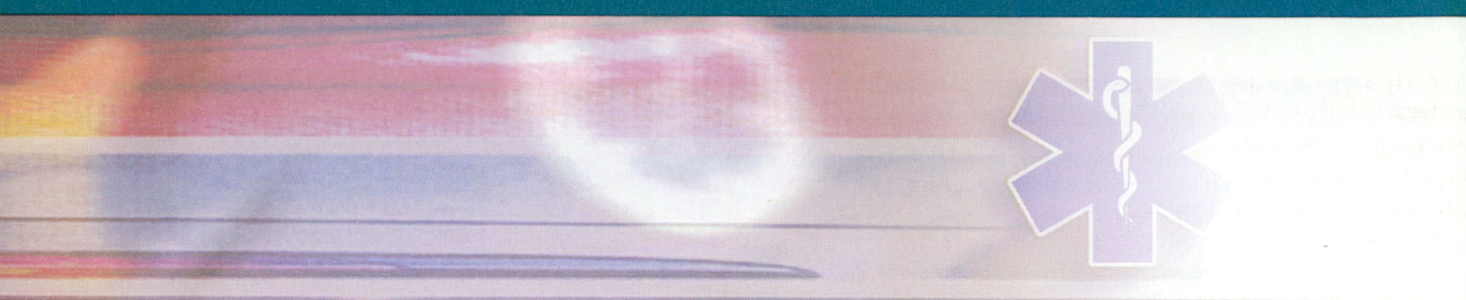

BOX 1-1 Code of Hammurabi (1700 BC)

- If a doctor has treated a freeman with a metal knife for a severe wound, and has cured the freeman, or has opened a freeman's tumor with a metal knife, and cured a freeman's eye, then he shall receive 10 shekels of silver.
- If the son of a plebeian, he shall receive 5 shekels of silver.
- If a man's slave, the owner of the slave shall give 2 shekels of silver to the doctor.
- If a doctor has treated a man with a metal knife for a severe wound, and has caused the man to die, or has opened a man's tumor with a metal knife and destroyed the man's eye, his hands shall be cut off.
- If the doctor has treated the slave of a plebeian with a metal knife for a severe wound and caused him to die, he shall render slave for slave.
- If he has opened his tumor with a metal knife and destroyed his eye, he shall pay half his price in silver.
- If a doctor has healed a freeman's broken bone or has restored diseased flesh, the patient shall give the doctor 5 shekels of silver.
- If he be the son of a plebeian, he shall give 3 shekels of silver.
- If a man's slave, the owner of the slave shall give 2 shekels of silver to the doctor.
- If a doctor of oxen or asses has treated either ox or ass for a severe wound, and cured it, the owner of the ox or ass shall give to the doctor one sixth of a shekel of silver as his fee.

War a nurse set up care for the wounded. This nurse, Clara Barton, also brought the American Red Cross (a Swiss organization) to the United States in 1905. The first civilian ambulance services were begun in Cincinnati and New York City in the 1860s.

Twentieth Century

During World War I, medical care made rapid progress. Wounded soldiers needed urgent care. Their injuries often were caused by machine guns and bombs. Thus the military developed battlefield ambulance corps. During World War II, the military moved wounded soldiers by air. Then during the Korean conflict, the military evacuated soldiers with helicopters. During the Vietnam conflict, the military improved urgent care and rapid evacuation with well-trained corpsmen. These efforts became the basis of the prehospital emergency care of today.

In the early twentieth century through the mid-1960s, prehospital care in the United States was provided in several ways. Care mostly was provided by urban, hospital-based systems. These systems later developed into municipal services. Care also was provided by funeral directors and volunteers who had little or no training in emergency care.

CRITICAL THINKING

How would you feel about moving to an area with this minimal level of emergency medical services?

BOX 1-2 Eleven Recommendations for Emergency Medical Services Identified in the White Paper

1. Extension of basic and advanced first aid training to greater numbers of the lay public
2. Preparation of nationally acceptable texts, training aids, and courses of instruction for rescue squad personnel, police officers, firefighters, and ambulance attendants
3. Implementation of recent traffic safety legislation to ensure completely adequate standards for ambulance design and construction, ambulance equipment and supplies, and the qualifications and supervision of ambulance personnel
4. Adoption at the state level of general policies and regulations pertaining to ambulance services
5. Adoption at district, county, and municipal levels of ways and means of providing ambulance services applicable to the conditions of the locality, control and surveillance of ambulance services, and coordination of ambulance services with health departments, hospitals, traffic authorities, and communication services
6. Initiation of pilot programs to determine the efficacy of providing physician-staffed ambulances for care at the site of injury and during transportation
7. Initiation of pilot programs to evaluate automotive and helicopter ambulance services in sparsely populated areas and in regions where many communities lack hospital facilities adequate to care for seriously injured persons
8. Delineation of radio frequency channels and equipment suitable to provide voice communication between ambulances, emergency departments, and other health-related agencies at the community, regional, and national levels
9. Initiation of pilot studies across the nation for evaluation of models of radio and telephone installations to ensure effectiveness of communication facilities
10. Day-to-day use of voice communication facilities by the agencies serving emergency medical needs
11. Active exploration of the feasibility of designating a single nationwide telephone number to summon an ambulance

From National Academy of Sciences, National Research Council: *Accidental death and disability: the neglected disease of modern society,* Washington, DC, 1996, National Academy Press.

Most patients received minimal stabilization at the scene. Then they were transported quickly to the nearest hospital.

Two landmarks in EMS development occurred in 1966:

1. The National Academy of Sciences-National Research Council Committee on Trauma and Shock published *Accidental Death and Disability: The Neglected Disease of Modern Society* (the "white paper"). This document lists recommendations to improve care for victims. Eleven of these recommendations are related directly to EMS (Box 1-2).
2. The U.S. Congress passed the Highway Safety Act of 1966. This act created the U.S. Department of Transportation. Congress also created the National Highway Traffic Safety Administration (NHTSA). The act provided legislative authority and funds to improve

BOX 1-3 Fifteen Required Components of the Emergency Medical Services System

1. Manpower
2. Training
3. Communications
4. Transportation
5. Facilities
6. Critical care units
7. Public safety agencies
8. Consumers
9. Access to care
10. Transfer of patients
11. Medical record keeping
12. Consumer information and education
13. Review and evaluation
14. Disaster linkage
15. Mutual aid

EMS. The act directed states to develop an effective EMS program as well. If the states did not develop effective EMS programs, they were subject to a loss of up to 10% of their federal highway construction funds. As a result of this act, states gave more than $142 million between 1968 and 1979 to develop EMS and early **advanced life support** (ALS) pilot programs.

Emergency medical services also emerged as a nationwide system because of death rate comparisons from World War I to Vietnam. Death rates for battlefield casualties were 8% in World War I. In World War II, they were 4.5%. In Korea, they decreased to 2.5%. Then in Vietnam, they were less than 2%. This decline was due to advances in field care for trauma patients.[2] These and other factors helped formulate the blueprint for improving prehospital emergency medical care in the United States. During 1972 and 1973, federal and private sources provided $31 million to fund EMS programs in 37 states and Puerto Rico.

In 1973 Congress passed the Emergency Medical Service Systems (EMSS) Act. This act paved the way for states to benefit from federal funds. The states could obtain the funds by forming regional EMS agencies. The act listed 15 vital parts of the EMS system (Box 1-3). Plus, the act required emergency care programs funded by the U.S. Department of Health and Human Services to plan and put into practice a regional approach for emergency response and immediate care for trauma patients. This act played a major role in creating regional EMS systems from 1974 to 1981.

CRITICAL THINKING

How does the "age" of the emergency medical services profession compare with the "age" of your parents' or grandparents' professions?

In 1981, funding for EMS development changed. This change was due to the Consolidated Omnibus Budget Reconciliation Act. This act consolidated EMS funding into state preventive health services block grants. As a result, funding under the EMSS Act was eliminated. These block grants were paid to state health departments instead of regional EMS organizations. Because these grants could be spent on projects other than EMS, the grants fell victim to politics. Thus direct funding for EMS declined. Through cuts in funding and staff, the ability of the NHTSA to support the U.S. Department of Health and Human Services effort diminished. As a result, each state had to develop and fund their EMS systems. Thus the great growth that EMS experienced in the 1960s and 1970s declined. The NHTSA continues to assist EMS development.[3] In fact, in 1988 the NHTSA established "10 System Elements" (the Statewide EMS Technical Assistance Program) as a recommended standard for EMS systems (Box 1-4).

BOX 1-4 The 10 System Elements of the National Highway Traffic Safety Administration

1. Comprehensive emergency medical services and trauma system legislation
2. Resource management and administration
3. Professional training
4. A communication system (911, communication centers, equipment, and the ability to communicate among ambulances, hospitals, fire departments, and police)
5. A transportation system (air, ground, and water)
6. Facilities (hospitals, trauma centers, specialty centers)
7. An inclusive trauma system fully integrated with emergency medical systems
8. Physician involvement (medical oversight)
9. Public information, education, and prevention
10. Data collection, quality improvement and evaluation, and research

From National Highway Traffic Safety Administration: *Emergency medical services: NHTSA leading the way,* Washington, DC, 1995, The Administration.

In 1996 the NHTSA and the Health Resources and Services Administration published a consensus paper that was held in high regard. This document, the *Emergency Medical Services Agenda for the Future,* was referred to as the *Agenda.* The Agenda was federally funded. Moreover, the Agenda was completed by the National Association of EMS Physicians and the National Association of State EMS Directors. These organizations created the Agenda to be used by government and private organizations at the national, state, and local levels. The Agenda was intended to build a common vision for the future of EMS. The Agenda also was meant to help guide planning, decision making, and policy for EMS (Fig. 1-1).

The Agenda made 14 suggestions for EMS. These aspects focused on principles of public health and safety systems. The principles included the EMS education system (described later in this chapter). The 14 attributes for EMS identified by the Agenda are the following:

1. Integration of health services
2. EMS research
3. Legislation and regulation
4. System finance
5. Human resources

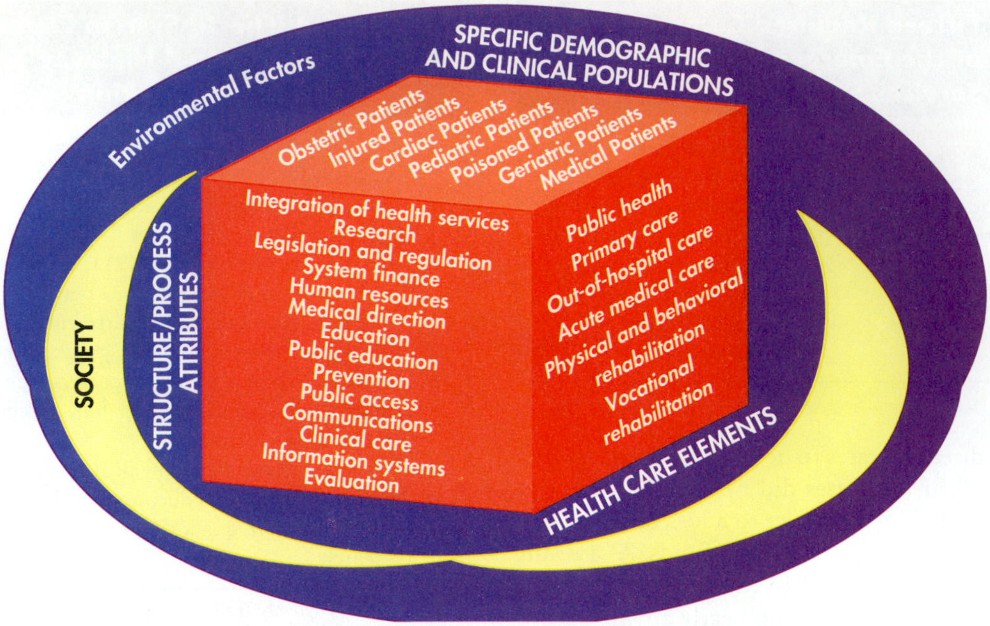

FIGURE 1-1 ■ Emergency medical services: part of the health care system.

6. Medical direction
7. Education systems
8. Public education
9. Prevention
10. Public access
11. Communication systems
12. Clinical care
13. Information systems
14. Evaluation

Box 1-5 outlines other landmarks in EMS development.

Recent changes in federal health care reform have begun to affect paramedics. These changes affect the way health care, including emergency care, is provided. The newer ideas of managed care and **extended scope of practice** are most relevant. *Managed care* refers to patient care services that are provided to members by **managed care organizations** (e.g., health maintenance organizations, preferred provider organizations, and other provider networks). These plans now cover about 40% of the U.S. population. The plans pay health care providers and some ambulance services a flat sum per member per month. This sum is paid up front to cover all health care expenses **(capitation).** If patient care expenses are less than the monthly payment received, then the provider keeps the difference. If expenses exceed the monthly payment received, then the provider absorbs the costs. (Other types of reimbursement plans also can be used.) This reform affects EMS systems in the way that they provide patient care choices for their clients (e.g., emergency versus nonemergency response, resources, and personnel; transportation modes; and health care facility options). Such reform also affects the type and amount of care given at the scene for those patients whose condition does not mandate transportation to a hospital for physician evaluation.

NOTE Medicare and Medicaid are the two insurance programs of the U.S. government. These plans have rules that affect how patients qualify for emergency medical services transportation. The rules also decide the conditions under which reimbursement for transportation will occur. This reimbursement became standardized throughout the country in 2002. Standardization occurred through a consensus process involving national emergency medical services agencies and the Center for Medicare Services. The new Medicare fee structure has caused major reductions in payment for some emergency medical services agencies. Yet, fees have increased for others.

Extended scope of practice came out of the cost-containment setting of managed care. As it relates to EMS, extended scope of practice refers to expanding services of emergency medical technicians (EMTs) and paramedics in the prehospital setting (EMS primary care). One example is providing health screenings and physical examinations. Another is triaging patients to a proper level of treatment. Giving follow-up examinations and immunizations are other examples. This expanded scope is driven not by what paramedics *can* do. Rather, it is driven by what they *should* do within a given system. This expanded scope also is driven by the availability of other factors. These factors may include health care resources and transportation times. Expanded scope for EMS providers most likely will continue to evolve. Emergency medical services agencies and managed care programs will develop other useful patient services to enhance revenues, to further injury-prevention programs, and to reflect changes in how medical care is delivered. Expanded scope also will ensure that EMS survives as a vital part of the health care system.

BOX 1-5 Other Landmarks in the Development of Emergency Medical Services

- 1958: Dr. Peter Safar demonstrates the efficacy of mouth-to-mouth ventilation.
- 1960: Cardiopulmonary resuscitation is shown to be effective.
- 1967: Dr. Eugene Nagel trains Miami firefighters as paramedics at the University of Miami School of Medicine.
- 1968: The American Telephone and Telegraph Company designates 911 as the universal emergency telephone number.
- 1969: The U.S. Department of Transportation and National Highway Traffic Safety Administration (NHTSA) develop the basic training course for emergency medical technicians (EMTs).
- 1969: The Committee on Ambulance Design develops Ambulance Design Criteria, a report to the U.S. Department of Transportation and the NHTSA to complement the National Academy of Sciences–National Research Council Medical Requirements for Ambulance Design and Equipment (1968). This document recommends ambulance design standards and emergency equipment. The NHTSA agrees to issue matching federal funds to states that purchase vehicles meeting these standards.
- 1970: The National Registry of Emergency Medical Technicians is organized to standardize education, examinations, and certification of EMTs on a national level.
- 1972: President Nixon directs the U.S. Department of Health, Education, and Welfare to develop new ways to organize emergency medical services (EMS), which results in $8.5 million in contracts being awarded to develop a model EMS system.
- 1972: The University of Cincinnati establishes the first residency program to train new physicians exclusively for the practice of emergency medicine.
- 1973: The star of life is adopted as the official symbol for EMS. The six blue bars of the star of life represent the six system functions of EMS: detection, reporting, response, on-scene care, care in transit, and transfer to definitive care.
- 1974: President Gerald Ford proclaims the first National EMS Week.
- 1975: The National Association of Emergency Medical Technicians is founded.
- 1975: The American Medical Association accepts and approves the EMT-Paramedic role as an emergency health occupation.
- 1977: More than 40 EMT training agencies throughout the United States develop and test the national training standards for the paramedic for 2 years.
- 1980: The U.S. Department of Health and Human Services releases the *Position Paper on Trauma Center Designation,* which describes trauma centers within EMS systems. The paper also categorizes facilities.
- 1984: The EMS for Children program, under the Public Health Act, provides funding for enhancing the EMS system to serve pediatric patients better.
- 1986: The 1979 Public Safety Officer's Act (SB 1479) is amended to expand the $50,000 compensation to include survivors of rescue squads, ambulance crew members, and public safety department volunteers killed in the line of duty (amended in 1990).
- 1990: President George Bush signs the Trauma Care Systems Planning and Development Act (HR 1602), which provides for annual grants to states based on geographical and population size to help establish and improve trauma systems. In 1995 Congress does not reauthorize funding for this act.
- 1991: Occupational Exposure to Blood-Borne Pathogens; Final Rule (CFR 29 1910.1030) establishes standards for workplace protection from blood-borne diseases.
- 1993: The Institute of Medicine publishes *Emergency Medical Services for Children,* which points out deficiencies in the ability of the health care system to address the emergency medical needs of pediatric patients.
- 1995: Congress does not reauthorize funding under the Trauma Care Systems and Development Act.
- 1997: The NHTSA publishes *A Leadership Guide to Quality Improvement for Emergency Medical Services Systems.*
- 1998: The U.S. Department of Transportation revises the national standard curriculum for paramedics.

CURRENT EMERGENCY MEDICAL SERVICES SYSTEMS

The EMS system of today is a network of coordinated services that provides aid and medical care to the community. The coordination is defined by the NHTSA Technical Assistance Program Standards. This coordination ensures that patients are treated quickly and properly. The coordination also ensures that resources are used efficiently, which reduces health care costs (Fig. 1-2). All of this improves patient outcome and reduces hospital stays.[4]

State EMS systems usually are made up of local and regional agencies that manage the delivery of prehospital care. The local agencies are responsible for providing day-to-day EMS to the community. Local agencies also work with regional and state agencies to create protocols and help set standards and guidelines. Local agencies provide data collection services and coordinate mutual aid and disaster planning. Most state EMS agencies have advisory councils to help organize EMS programs and activities. These councils are made up of medical professionals, paraprofessionals, consumers, and public and private agencies with an interest in EMS. The state agency is responsible for licensing and certification. In addition, the state enforces state EMS regulations and develops public education programs. Moreover, the state agency acts as a liaison with national agencies. Some of these national agencies include the NHTSA and the Federal Emergency Management Agency.

Emergency Medical Services System Operations

The operations of an effective EMS system include citizen activation, dispatch, prehospital care, hospital care, and rehabilitation.

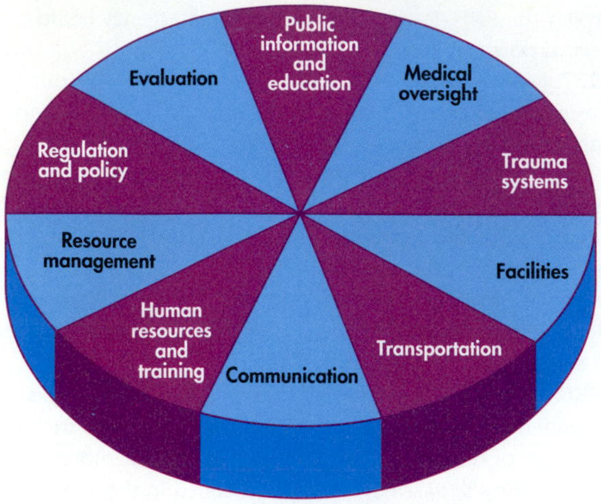

FIGURE 1-2 ■ Ten components of the emergency medical services system.

CITIZEN ACTIVATION

Emergency public safety services are highly visible in the community. However, the public is not always aware of the complex nature of these services. Citizens expect to have police and fire protection. They also expect to get a fast response with skilled personnel in an emergency. This is due to years of available public-safety service, public relations, press coverage, and national media. The public also expects such service because of public support in the form of taxes, donations, subscriptions for service, and user fees.

Public involvement in EMS goes beyond funding. Citizens often are at the scene of an injury or illness. They play an important role in recognizing the need for emergency services. Citizens sometimes administer first aid, help secure the scene and gain access to the patient, and can be instrumental in managing a crisis. Educating the public is fundamental to the development of an effective EMS system. Paramedics help prepare the public to respond to a medical emergency. They also build support for EMS by helping to develop and present public health care education and prevention programs (see Chapter 3).

> **CRITICAL THINKING**
> How is the emergency medical services system funded in your community?

Once citizens recognize that an emergency exists, the response is coordinated. Citizens contact communication centers and dispatching services by emergency phone numbers or radio. The number 911 offers access to public safety services in most of the country. These services include fire service, law enforcement, and EMS. The availability of emergency access through 911 continues to expand across the country as areas adopt the system. In areas that do not have 911, citizens should have easy access to other emergency phone numbers. These numbers can be promoted through public awareness programs, phone stickers, and phone book covers. Other ways of engaging an emergency response include firebox pull stations, citizen band radios, and cell phones. Chapter 15 covers 911 in more detail.

PREHOSPITAL CARE

Ill or injured patients may need prehospital intervention and stabilization. Interventions may involve **basic life support** and ALS skills. Depending on the situation (e.g., entrapment, distance to the hospital, and availability of ALS), initial prehospital care may be limited. The care may consist of giving only comfort and reassurance. Care also may require spinal immobilization, airway protection, endotracheal intubation, intravenous therapy, medication administration, defibrillation, and external cardiac pacing.

HOSPITAL CARE

When the patient is brought to the emergency department, patient care resources expand. This care may include physicians, physician assistants, nurse practitioners, nurses, technicians, ancillary support staff (allied health counselors, social workers, and others), secretaries, and medical record staff. The care also may include diagnostic services. These services may be provided by laboratory, radiology, and cardiopulmonary departments. Resources available beyond the emergency department include surgery, intensive care, physical therapy, pharmacy, nutrition services, and many others.

REHABILITATION

After hospital delivery and definitive care, many patients receive some type of rehabilitation services. Rehabilitation often occurs before and after hospital discharge. The services may be in the form of education and physical and occupational therapy that help the patient to recover. Rehabilitation also can help the patient to maintain maximal independence. One example of such therapy is helping patients and families adjust to required changes in lifestyle after a heart attack. Another example is retraining in activities of daily living. Job rehabilitation also allows one to adapt to limb impairment or loss.

Emergency Medical Services Provider Levels

Various levels of providers and medical direction come together to make an effective prehospital EMS system. The levels include dispatchers, first responders, EMT-Basics (EMT-Bs), EMT-Intermediates (EMT-Is), and **EMT-Paramedics** (EMT-Ps).

DISPATCHER

A dispatcher is a telecommunicator. This person serves as the primary contact with the public. The dispatcher directs the proper agencies to the scene. These agencies may include ground and air ambulances, fire departments, law en-

NOTE A move is underway by the National Highway Traffic Safety Administration, the Health Resources and Services Administration, and the National Association of State EMS Directors to create a new EMS National Scope of Practice Model. This project ultimately may define new emergency medical services provider levels and the skills each level of provider can perform.

More information can be found at *http://www.EMSScopeofPractice.org*

forcement, utility services, and others. The term *telecommunicator* applies to call takers, dispatchers, radio operators, data terminal operators, or any combination of such functions in a public service answering point located in a fire, police, or EMS communications center (see Chapter 15). An effective EMS dispatch communications system includes the following functions:

- *Receive and process calls for EMS assistance.* The dispatcher receives and records calls for EMS assistance and selects an appropriate course of action for each call. To do this, the dispatcher must obtain as much information as possible about the emergency event. This information includes name, call-back number, and address. The dispatch also may have to deal with distraught callers.
- *Dispatch and coordinate EMS resources.* The dispatcher directs the proper emergency vehicles to the correct address. This person also coordinates the emergency vehicles while en route to the scene, to the medical facility, and back to the operations base.
- *Relay medical information.* The dispatch center can provide a telecommunications channel among appropriate medical facilities and EMS personnel; fire, police, and rescue workers; and private citizens. The channel can consist of phone, radio, or biomedical telemetry.
- *Coordinate with public safety agencies.* The dispatcher aids communications between public safety (fire, law enforcement, rescue) and the EMS system. This aid coordinates services such as traffic control, escort, fire suppression, and extrication. The dispatcher must know the location and status of all EMS vehicles and whether support services are available. In larger systems, computer-aided dispatching is used. This provides for one or more of the following abilities:
  - Automatic entry of 911
  - Automatic interface to vehicle location with or without map display
  - Automatic interface to mobile data terminal
  - Computer messaging among multiple radio operators, call takers, or both
  - Dispatch note taking, reminder aid, or both
  - Ability to monitor response times, response delays, and on-scene times
  - Display of call information
  - Emergency medical dispatch review
  - Manual or automatic updates of unit status
  - Manual entry of call information
  - Radio control and display of channel status
  - Standard operating procedure review
  - Telephone control and display of circuit status

Many EMS and public service agencies require specialized training for their dispatch personnel. The personnel then can give directions to the caller while the caller waits for EMS arrival. The training may include the USDOT training program for the emergency medical dispatcher, which is described further in Chapter 15.

NOTE A curriculum is a specific blueprint for learning. A curriculum is derived from content and performance standards.

FIRST RESPONDER

First responders may be the first trained personnel in an EMS system to arrive on a scene. These responders may include personnel from fire departments and law enforcement agencies. They also may include designated commercial medical response teams, athletic trainers, and others. The first responder has satisfied training based on the *First Responder National Standard Curriculum* and is capable of the following:

1. Recognizing the seriousness of the patient's condition or extent of injuries
2. Assessing requirements for emergency medical care
3. Administering appropriate emergency medical care for life-threatening injuries relative to airway, breathing, and circulation
4. Performing safely and effectively the expectations of the job description as defined in the national curriculum

Because first responders often are the first to arrive at the scene of an injury or an illness, they are an integral part of an effective EMS response team.

CRITICAL THINKING

What type of dispatching is done in your community? Are dispatchers trained to the level of emergency medical directors?

EMT-BASIC

The EMT-B has finished training based on the *EMT-Basic National Standard Curriculum.* The EMT-B is trained in all phases of basic life support. This training includes the use of automated external defibrillators. The training also includes giving some emergency medications. Some EMT-Bs also are trained in advanced airway procedures that include orotracheal intubation. In addition to patient care training, EMT-Bs receive training in emergency vehicle operations. This training includes driving responses, tactics, and maintenance. They also play a role in educating the public and promoting health awareness.

EMT-INTERMEDIATE

The EMT-I is an EMT-B who has finished training based on the *EMT-Intermediate National Standard Curriculum*. This curriculum comes from the training curriculum for EMT-Ps. The degree of training and skills that the EMT-I practices varies between states and EMS systems. Training can include ALS procedures such as advanced airway adjuncts, intravenous therapy, defibrillation, cardiac rhythm interpretation, and administration of some emergency medications. Like the EMT-B, the EMT-I takes part in public education and health promotion programs.

EMT-PARAMEDIC

The EMT-P is an EMT-B or EMT-I who has finished training based on the *EMT-Paramedic National Standard Curriculum*. Paramedics are trained in all aspects of basic life support and ALS procedures that are relevant to prehospital emergency care. The paramedic has advanced training in patient assessment, cardiac rhythm interpretation, defibrillation, drug therapy, and airway management (Box 1-6). The paramedic's specific roles and duties are discussed later in this chapter.

BOX 1-6 Description of the Paramedic Profession

The description of the paramedic profession provides the philosophy and rationale for the depth and breadth of coverage:

- Paramedics have fulfilled requirements prescribed by an accrediting agency to practice the art and science of out-of-hospital medicine under medical direction. Through performing assessments and providing medical care, their goal is to prevent and reduce mortality and morbidity caused by illness and injury. Paramedics primarily provide care to emergency patients in an out-of-hospital setting.
- Paramedics possess knowledge, skills, and attitudes consistent with the expectations of the public and the profession. Paramedics recognize that they are an essential component of the continuum of care and serve as linkages among health resources.
- Paramedics strive to maintain high-quality, reasonable-cost health care by delivering patients directly to appropriate facilities. As an advocate for patients, paramedics seek to be proactive in affecting long-term health care by working with other provider agencies, networks, and organizations. The emerging roles and responsibilities of the paramedic include public education, health promotion, and participation in injury- and illness-prevention programs. As the scope of service continues to expand, the paramedic will function as a facilitator of access to care and as an initial treatment provider.
- Paramedics are responsible and accountable to medical direction, the public, and their peers. Paramedics recognize the importance of research and actively participate in the design, development, evaluation, and publication of research. Paramedics seek to take part in lifelong professional development, perform peer evaluation, and assume an active role in professional and community organizations.

From US Department of Transportation, National Highway Transportation Administration: *EMT-Paramedic national standard curriculum,* Washington, DC, 1998, The Department.

NATIONAL EMERGENCY MEDICAL SERVICES GROUP INVOLVEMENT

Many groups and organizations help to set the standards of EMS (Box 1-7). These groups exist at the national, state, regional, and local levels. They take part in development, education, and implementation. Being a member of such a group helps to promote the status of the paramedic by exposing the paramedic to trends in emergency care, continuing education, and to resource experts. The organizations also provide for national representation and a means for a unified voice in other health care organizations and issues of national matters.

One such organization is the National Registry of Emergency Medical Technicians. The National Registry helps develop professional standards in the EMS industry. This organization verifies competencies for EMTs and paramedics by preparing and conducting examinations. The organization also simplifies the process of state-to-state mobility and **reciprocity** for its members.

CRITICAL THINKING

What issue do you think your national emergency medical services association should work on to enhance patient care in your area?

The EMS standard-setting groups have many roles. Their primary role is to set standards with input from the profession and the community. By doing so, they help ensure that the public is protected from individuals and agencies that do not meet professional standards for licensure or certification.

BOX 1-7 Sampling of National Emergency Medical Services Organizations and Associations

American Ambulance Association
American College of Emergency Physicians
Association of Air Medical Services
Emergency Nurses' Association
National Association of EMS Educators
National Association of EMS Physicians
National Association of Emergency Medical Technicians
National Association of Search and Rescue
National Association of State EMS Directors
National Council of State EMS Training Coordinators
National Flight Nurses' Association
National Flight Paramedic Association
National Registry of Emergency Medical Technicians

PARAMEDIC EDUCATION

Initial Education

The national standard curriculum for paramedics was revised in 1998. That same year the NHTSA revised a portion of the *Agenda* (the *National Emergency Medical Services Education and Practice Blueprint* [the *Blueprint*]). This revision revealed the future of EMS education. The text was titled the *EMS Education Agenda for the Future: A Systems Approach* (the *Education Agenda*). The Education Agenda named core content for each provider level. The Education Agenda also stressed the integration of EMS within the overall health care system. Figure 1-3 is a diagram of a model that came from the revision.[5] Based on this model, the paramedic student must have competency in math, reading, and writing. This competency must occur before the student enrolls in a paramedic training program. Prerequisites (also called corequisites) are classes that must be taken before or at the same time as the paramedic program. These classes include EMT-B training and human anatomy and physiology. The model defines minimum content for a standard program of study. The program of study requires 1000 to 1200 hours of instruction.[6] The amount of instruction, however, can depend on state requirements and local needs. The amount of instruction also can depend on current practices, individual training sites, and clinical programs. New to this revision was the definition of cognitive (knowledge), psychomotor (skills), and affective (attitude) objectives.

When choosing a training site, the student should consider the resources of the program. These resources include accreditation, facilities, quality of instructors, equipment, clinical experiences, references from past students, text requirements, and other instructional materials.

Continuing Education

Continuing education provides a way for all health care providers to retain primary technical and professional skills. Continuing education also aids in learning new and advanced skills and knowledge. Some skills learned during the initial course of study are not used often. However, new data, procedures, and resources are being developed continuously.

Continuing education can take many forms, including the following:

- Conferences and seminars
- Lectures and workshops
- Quality-improvement reviews
- Skill laboratories
- Certification and recertification programs
- Refresher training programs
- Journal studies
- Multimedia presentations
- Internet-based learning
- Case presentations
- Independent study

LICENSURE, CERTIFICATION, AND REGISTRATION

Paramedics are granted permission to practice their skills by three processes. These processes are licensure, certification, and registration. The exact wording of granting this permission varies by state.

Licensure

Licensure is a process of regulating occupations. In this process a license is granted by a government authority. The license allows a person to engage in a profession or activity that otherwise would be unlawful. Some states and local authorities require that paramedics have a license.

Certification

Certification grants authority to a person so that the person can take part in an activity. This person has to meet certain qualifications. As a result, the person receives a document from a government or nongovernment entity. The document shows that the person has met basic requirements to practice in a field. Some states or local authorities require that paramedics be certified.

> **NOTE** Some persons believe that licensed professionals have greater status than those who are certified or registered. This belief is unfounded. A certification granted by a state and conferring a right to engage in a trade or profession is in fact a license.

Registration

Registration is the act of enrolling one's name in a register, or book of record. For example, paramedics can be licensed or certified in their state and can be registered with the National Registry of Emergency Medical Technicians.

PROFESSIONALISM

Training and performance standards have helped to define EMTs and paramedics as health care professionals. The term *profession* refers to a body of knowledge or expertise. The members of such a field are often self-regulated through a license or certification that confirms competence. In addition, most professions adhere to standards. These standards include initial and continuing education requirements. *Professionalism* refers to the way in which a person follows the standards of a profession. These standards may include conduct and performance standards. These standards also usually include adhering to a code of ethics approved by the profession (see Chapter 5).

Health Care Professional

Health care professionals conform to the standards of their profession. They instill pride in the profession. They earn the respect of others by providing quality patient care and striving for high standards. Emergency medical services pro-

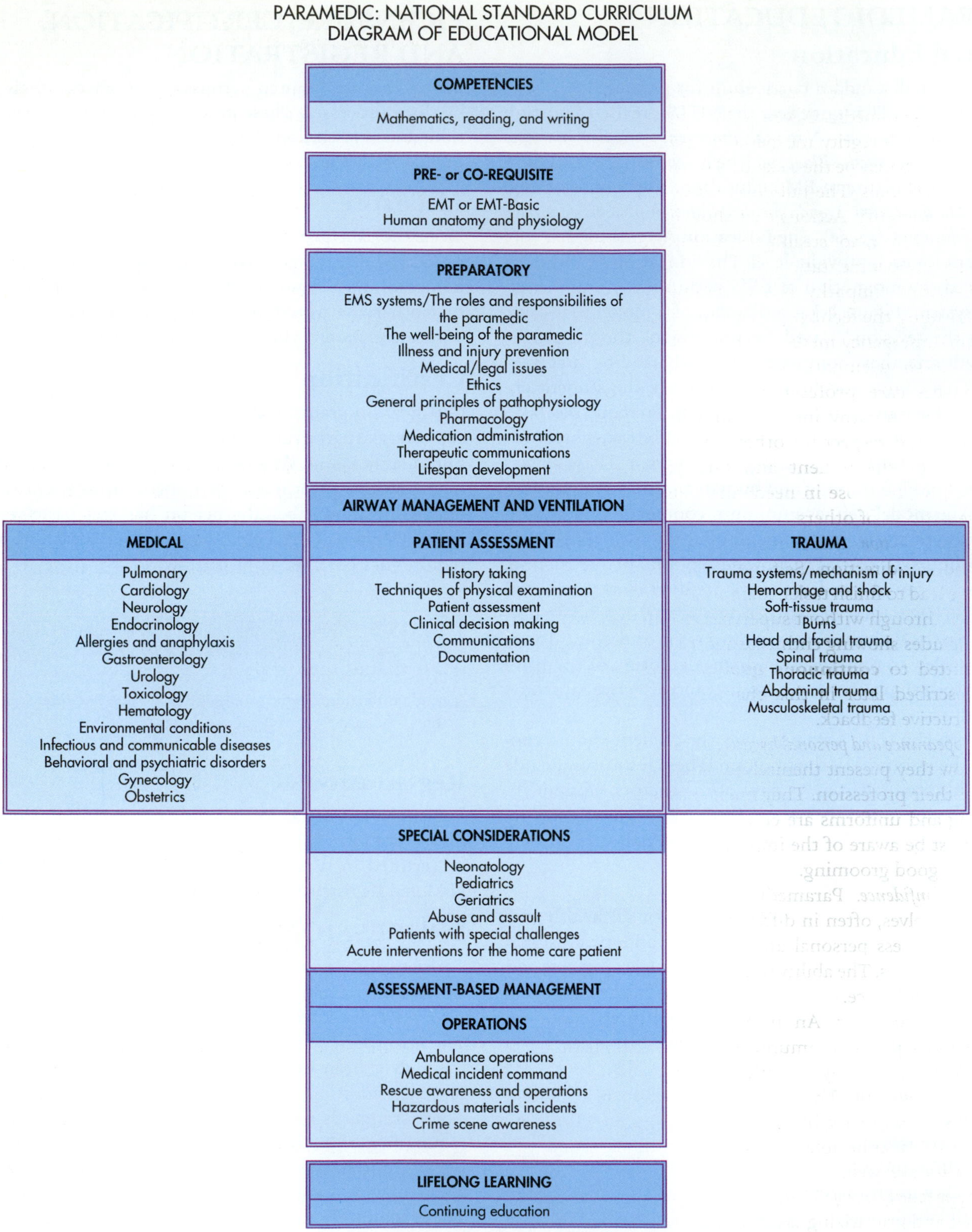
PARAMEDIC: NATIONAL STANDARD CURRICULUM
DIAGRAM OF EDUCATIONAL MODEL
COMPETENCIES
Mathematics, reading, and writing
PRE- or CO-REQUISITE
EMT or EMT-Basic
Human anatomy and physiology
PREPARATORY
EMS systems/The roles and responsibilities of the paramedic
The well-being of the paramedic
Illness and injury prevention
Medical/legal issues
Ethics
General principles of pathophysiology
Pharmacology
Medication administration
Therapeutic communications
Lifespan development
AIRWAY MANAGEMENT AND VENTILATION
MEDICAL
Pulmonary
Cardiology
Neurology
Endocrinology
Allergies and anaphylaxis
Gastroenterology
Urology
Toxicology
Hematology
Environmental conditions
Infectious and communicable diseases
Behavioral and psychiatric disorders
Gynecology
Obstetrics
PATIENT ASSESSMENT
History taking
Techniques of physical examination
Patient assessment
Clinical decision making
Communications
Documentation
TRAUMA
Trauma systems/mechanism of injury
Hemorrhage and shock
Soft-tissue trauma
Burns
Head and facial trauma
Spinal trauma
Thoracic trauma
Abdominal trauma
Musculoskeletal trauma
SPECIAL CONSIDERATIONS
Neonatology
Pediatrics
Geriatrics
Abuse and assault
Patients with special challenges
Acute interventions for the home care patient
ASSESSMENT-BASED MANAGEMENT
OPERATIONS
Ambulance operations
Medical incident command
Rescue awareness and operations
Hazardous materials incidents
Crime scene awareness
LIFELONG LEARNING
Continuing education

FIGURE 1-3 ■ Diagram of Department of Transportation education model.

fessionals occupy positions of public trust and are highly visible role models. Because EMS professionals are role models, the public has high expectations of EMTs and paramedics while they are on and off duty. Therefore professional conduct at all times and a commitment to excellence in daily activities complement the image of the EMS professional. Image and behavior are vital to establishing credibility and instilling confidence. The professional paramedic represents his or her employer; the EMS agency; the state, county, city, or district EMS office; and his or her peers.

Attributes of the Professional Paramedic

Many aspects of being professional can be applied to the role of the paramedic. Eleven of these attributes follow[6]:

1. *Integrity.* Integrity means being honest in all actions. Integrity may be the most important behavior for EMS professionals. The public assumes EMS professionals have integrity. Actions that show integrity include being truthful, not stealing, and providing complete and correct documentation.
2. *Empathy.* Empathy is identifying with and understanding the feelings, situations, and motives of others. Emergency medical services professionals always must show empathy to patients, families, and other health care professionals. Behavior that demonstrates empathy includes showing caring, compassion, and respect for others; understanding the feelings of the patient and family; being calm and helpful to those in need; and being supportive and reassuring of others.
3. *Self-motivation.* Self-motivation is the push for merit and self-direction. Self-motivation can mean taking the lead to finish tasks, to improve behavior, and to follow through without supervision. Self-motivation also includes showing enthusiasm for learning, being committed to **continuous quality improvement** (CQI; described later in this chapter), and accepting constructive feedback.
4. *Appearance and personal hygiene.* Paramedics are aware of how they present themselves. They are representatives of their profession. They must ensure that their clothing and uniforms are clean and in good repair. They must be aware of the importance of personal hygiene and good grooming.
5. *Self-confidence.* Paramedics must trust and rely on themselves, often in difficult situations. One key task is to assess personal and professional strengths and weaknesses. The ability to trust personal choices shows self-confidence.
6. *Communications.* An important part of the paramedic's job is communicating. The paramedic must be able to convey key information to others verbally and in writing. The paramedic must be able to speak clearly, write legibly, and listen actively. The paramedic must be able to adjust strategies to various situations as well.
7. *Time management.* Time management refers to organizing and prioritizing tasks to make the best use of time. Examples include being punctual and completing tasks and assignments on time.
8. *Teamwork and diplomacy.* The paramedic must be able to work with others well. In fact, the paramedic must be able to use tact and interpersonal skills to achieve a common goal. As a member of the EMS team, the paramedic must place the success of the team above personal success. A paramedic does this by supporting and respecting other team members, being flexible and open to change, and communicating with co-workers to resolve problems.
9. *Respect.* Respect means having regard for others and showing consideration and appreciation. Paramedics are polite to others and avoid the use of derogatory or demeaning terms. They know that showing respect brings credit to themselves, their association, and their profession.
10. *Patient advocacy.* The paramedic must always act as the patient's advocate. The paramedic must be an advocate even when the patient disagrees with the care. Paramedics should not attempt to impose their beliefs on patients. They also should not allow biases (religious, ethical, political, social, legal) to influence care. The paramedic must always place the needs of the patient above self-interests. The paramedic must protect the patient's confidentiality as well.
11. *Careful delivery of service.* Paramedics deliver the highest quality of patient care. With this care comes attention to detail and proper prioritization of care. Plus, paramedics review their actions and attitude on every call. As part of the careful delivery, paramedics master and refresh their skills; perform full equipment checks; and ensure safe ambulance operations. Paramedics also follow policies, procedures, and protocols and comply with the orders of their supervisors.

CRITICAL THINKING

Which of these professional attributes represent your strengths? Which ones do you think you need to work on?

ROLES AND RESPONSIBILITIES OF THE PARAMEDIC

The paramedic's roles and duties can be divided into two groups: primary responsibilities and additional responsibilities[6] (Box 1-8).

Primary Responsibilities

The paramedic must be prepared physically, mentally, and emotionally for the job. Preparation includes being committed daily to positive health practices (see Chapter 2). In addition, the paramedic must have the proper equipment and supplies. Moreover, the paramedic must maintain adequate knowledge and skills of the profession. The paramedic must respond to the scene in a safe and timely manner. During scene assessment, the paramedic must consider his or her own safety; safety of the crew, patients, and bystanders; and the mechanism of injury or probable cause of illness.

The paramedic must assess the patient at once to determine the injury or illness. At that point, the paramedic can set priorities of care and transportation. Managing an emergency often entails following protocols and also calls for working with medical direction as needed. After stabi-

BOX 1-8 Roles and Responsibilities of the Paramedic

Primary Responsibilities	Additional Responsibilities
Preparation	Community involvement
Response	Support of primary care efforts
Scene assessment	Advocation of citizen involvement in emergency medical services
Patient assessment	Participation in leadership activities
Recognition of injury or illness	Personal and professional development
Patient management	
Appropriate patient disposition	
Patient transfer	
Documentation	
Returning to service	

BOX 1-9 Sampling of Specialized Care Facilities

- Burn specialization center
- Cardiac treatment center
- Clinical laboratory service
- Emergency department
- Facility with acute hemodialysis capability
- Facility with acute spinal cord or head injury management capability
- Facility with reperfusion capability
- Facility with special radiological capabilities
- High-risk obstetrical facility
- Hyperbaric treatment center
- Intensive care unit for trauma patients
- Neurology center
- Operating suite
- Pediatric facility
- Postanesthesia recovery room or surgical intensive care unit
- Psychiatric facility
- Rehabilitation facility
- Stroke center
- Toxicology (including hazardous material or decontamination) service
- Trauma center

lizing the patient in the field, the paramedic should supply proper transport to the receiving facility. Transportation may include ground or air transport and may be based on the patient's condition. Choosing the facility calls for knowing which ones are available. The paramedic must know hospital designation and categorization as well (Box 1-9). Knowledge of transfer agreements and payers insurance systems also is helpful. Paramedics are also called upon for critical care transport (see the Appendix on p. 1418).

The paramedic is the patient's advocate as responsibility for care shifts to the staff at the facility. The paramedic needs to brief the staff about the patient's condition at the scene and during transportation. The paramedic also needs to provide thorough and accurate documentation in the patient care report. The paramedic should complete required documentation in a timely manner so that the EMS crew can return to service. The crew should prepare the ambulance for return to service. The crew does this by replacing equipment and supplies (per agency protocol). The crew also should review the call openly. Such review helps to identify ways to improve the patient care services that were provided at the scene and during transportation.

Additional Responsibilities

Other duties of the paramedic include community involvement, support of primary care efforts, advocating citizen involvement in the EMS system, participation in leadership activities, and personal and professional development.

A paramedic can be involved in the community and can be a role model for the profession in many ways. The paramedic can advocate injury prevention programs (see Chapter 3). The paramedic also can participate as a leader in community activities. A few ways to improve the health of the community include teaching cardiopulmonary resuscitation, first aid, and injury prevention. These activities also help to ensure proper use of EMS resources. The activities improve the integration of EMS with other health care and public safety agencies.

A few communities and their health care organizations use paramedics to aid in primary care efforts. These communities also use paramedics to aid in injury prevention and wellness programs. Paramedics can help to inform the public of the best use of prehospital and other non-EMS health care resources. Paramedics can offer options other than ambulance transportation. They can explain nonhospital emergency department clinical providers and freestanding emergency clinics as well. Programs on when, where, and how to use EMS and emergency departments promote the best use of the resources.

Getting citizens involved in EMS improves the system as a whole. Citizens can help to set the needs and parameters for EMS use in the community. They offer an objective view into quality improvement and problem solving. In addition, having involved citizens creates informed, independent advocates for the EMS system.

> **NOTE** Some emergency medical services agencies organize community emergency response teams. These teams help to prepare citizens to respond to emergencies. Members are trained to provide instant help to victims. The agencies also can organize volunteers in time of disaster. Plus, the agencies can collect disaster intelligence to support first responder efforts.

Paramedics can take part in leadership activities in their communities in many ways. They can conduct injury prevention initiatives (activities and risk surveys). They can help with media drives to promote EMS issues. They also can distribute materials about EMS and other health programs.

A paramedic must work to develop in personal and professional ways. Methods to accomplish this include continuing education, student mentoring, membership in professional organizations, becoming involved in work-related issues that affect career growth, exploring alternative career paths in the EMS profession, conducting and supporting research initiatives, and being actively involved in legislative issues related to EMS.

MEDICAL DIRECTION FOR EMERGENCY MEDICAL SERVICES

Many of the services that paramedics offer to patients come from practices in which paramedics act as "physician extenders." This means that paramedics extend the services of a physician to patients in the field, which is made possible through medical direction. The medical direction physician acts as the medical leader for the EMS system. The physician also serves as a resource and patient advocate for the EMS system. This relationship between the physician and paramedic is critical. The relationship allows for the delivery of advanced prehospital care. The ideal medical direction physician is properly educated as an EMS medical director. The physician also is motivated to provide the following[7]:

- EMS system design and operations
- Education and training of EMS personnel
- Participation in personnel selection
- Participation in equipment selection
- Development of clinical protocols in cooperation with expert EMS personnel
- Participation in CQI and problem resolution
- Direct input into patient care
- Interface between EMS systems and other health care agencies
- Advocacy within the medical community
- Guidance as the "medical conscience" of the EMS system (advocating for quality patient care)

Types of Medical Direction

The two types of medical direction are **online (direct) medical direction** and **off-line (indirect) medical direction.**[7] Both types ensure that the quality of medical care is in check in an EMS system. When the paramedic crew contacts online medical direction by radio or phone, the paramedics convey the patient's information. Then the paramedics receive orders through direct consultation with a physician or physician designee. This designee may be a registered nurse or physician assistant. The designee also may be a paramedic trained to give ALS orders in the medical direction system. Online medical direction allows for instant and specific care, telemetry, and CQI while paramedics are on the scene. As a rule, online medical direction supersedes off-line medical direction.[8]

An advisory group often is the voice behind the off-line direction. It also can be provided by a medical director. This director must have full medical direction authority. He or she also must have knowledge of the way in which the EMS system operates. This type of direction can be *prospective* or *retrospective.*[6] Prospective off-line direction covers the authority to set **treatment protocols** and **standing orders** (Box 1-10). Such knowledge includes training for care and triage in the prehospital arena (see Chapters 12 and 50). Such knowledge can involve the choice of the equipment, supplies, and personnel. Retrospective off-line direction includes any actions that are done after the EMS call. An example is reviewing a patient care report and providing CQI.

> **BOX 1-10 Protocols**
>
> *Treatment protocols* are written guidelines that define the scope of prehospital care for emergency medical services (EMS) providers. The medical director of the EMS service or members of a regional EMS advisory group create them. The paramedic must adhere to these protocols. The paramedic must follow the protocols unless advised otherwise by medical direction.
>
> *Standing orders* are more specific than protocols. Standing orders usually are included in a protocol when a delay in treatment would harm the patient. Most protocols and standing orders comply with national standards. They also comply with state EMS medical practice arts and regional guidelines. An example of a national standard is the American Heart Association guidelines for advanced cardiac life support. Another is the American College of Surgeons standards for advanced trauma life support. Protocols define the standard of care for paramedic crews and online physicians. The cases in which the paramedic acts strictly by standing orders usually are few. These situations may include intubation of a nonbreathing patient or first-line medication administration in cardiac arrest. Situations also may include events in which radio contact has failed and a delay could threaten the patient outcome.

On-Scene Physicians

Some of the first ambulance personnel were physicians. Yet, rarely is a medical direction physician on the scene providing direct field supervision of EMS personnel. At times, however, a physician (physician intervenor) may witness the injury or illness. Perhaps the patient's private physician is on the scene already. When this occurs, interaction between the on-scene physician and the EMS crew is essential.

> **NOTE** A physician intervenor may or may not be familiar with emergency medical services function. The physician also may not be familiar with the training in medical oversight responsibilities. The lines of authority for these physicians vary from state to state. The lines of responsibility vary as well.

If a nonmedical direction physician or the patient's physician is on the scene, EMS personnel must follow protocols. If no protocols are in place, the EMS personnel should contact online direction quickly. The policies of many EMS agencies require that the physician on the scene make contact with the online medical direction physician. Together the physicians can make choices about the legal responsibility for the patient's care. With permission of medical direction, a physician on the scene may take control of the patient's care. A physician on the scene may try to direct care that opposes the medical direction. Then EMS personnel on the scene must ask law officers to ensure that the scene is safe and the EMS care goes uninterrupted.

IMPROVING SYSTEM QUALITY

A major goal of any EMS system is to evaluate and improve care continually. One way to meet this goal is through a modified form of quality assurance. This form of quality assurance is known as *continuous quality improvement,* which is the ongoing study and improvement of a process, system, or organization (Box 1-11).

A CQI program identifies and attempts to improve problems in certain areas. These areas may include medical direction, financing, training, communication, prehospital management and transportation, interfacility transportation, receiving facilities, specialty care units, dispatch, public information and education, audit and quality assurance, disaster planning, and mutual aid. Continuous quality improvement is a process that involves all caregivers in the problem-solving aspect. Continuous quality improvement stresses the value of enabling frontline personnel to perform their jobs well. With this group approach, all parties can be involved in elaborating on the cause of the problem. They can work together to develop remedies and can design a course of action to correct the problem. Then they can enforce the plan and reexamine the issue to see whether the problem has been resolved to satisfaction.

BOX 1-11 Quality Assurance and Continuous Quality Improvement

Quality assurance (QA) is a system of quality management that by tradition was linked with spotting deviations from a standard (e.g., protocols). Quality assurance also altered these deviations through some type of punitive action. Continuous quality improvement (CQI) is a modified form of QA. Continuous quality improvement focuses on the system and not the individual. Thus this removes much of the punitive aspect associated with a QA program. Continuous quality improvement is less rigid than QA. In addition, CQI considers many factors that often apply to EMS. Continuous quality improvement includes the entire medical direction system and involves all health providers in the problem-solving process.

The EMS worker should use input taken from CQI activities to adapt treatment protocols and educational activities when needed. The goal of CQI is to find and fix problems in a positive manner. Continuous quality improvement also is aimed at improving the overall system. Example CQI activities include a review of the following:

- Outcome measures of prehospital care (e.g., scene times, procedure completion rates, and mortality reviews)
- Care while treatment is ongoing (concurrent reviews)
- Written EMS patient care paperwork (retrospective reviews)
- Random or selected radio communication tapes
- New procedures, equipment, or therapies

CRITICAL THINKING

The number of needle-stick injuries in your agency has increased. How might the continuous quality improvement process affect this situation?

Key actions or categories for EMS leaders to improve quality within their organization are as follows[8]:

1. *Leadership* has to do with the efforts of senior leadership and management. These persons lead by example to add CQI into the strategic planning process. They also integrate CQI into the entire organization. Such integration promotes quality values and CQI techniques in work practices.
2. *Information and analysis* deal with managing and using the data needed for effective CQI. Continuous quality improvement is based on management by fact. Thus information and analyses are critical to CQI success.
3. *Strategic quality planning* has three main parts. The first is developing long- and short-term goals for structural, performance, and outcome quality standards. The second is finding ways to achieve those. The third is measuring the effectiveness of the system in meeting quality standards.
4. *Human resource development and management* has to do with developing the full potential of the EMS workforce. This effort is guided by the principle that the entire EMS workforce is motivated to achieve new levels of service and value.
5. *Emergency medical services process management* has to do with the creation of high-quality services and with maintaining those services. Within the context of CQI, process management refers to the improvement of work activities. Process management also refers to improving work flow *across* functional or departmental boundaries.
6. *Emergency medical systems results* have to do with the assessment of the quality results achieved. These results also have to do with examining the success of the organization at achieving CQI.
7. *Satisfaction of patients and other stakeholders* involves ensuring ongoing satisfaction. Those internal and external to the EMS system must be satisfied with the services provided.

Benefits gained by applying these seven guidelines and recommendations include improvements in service and patient care delivery, economic efficiency and profitability, patient and community satisfaction and loyalty, and healthful outcomes.

EMERGENCY MEDICAL SERVICES RESEARCH

Emergency medical services research is a desirable activity for an EMS system. In fact, research is essential to the continued evolution of EMS. Quality EMS research helps shed light on the intended effects and cost-effectiveness of EMS interventions. This research is based on data and can lead to changes in professional standards, training, equipment, and procedures. In the health care climate of managed care and reduced spending by government agencies, future EMS funding may depend on proving the value of EMS services. Thus outcome studies are needed to ensure continued funding for EMS. The paramedic of today must have a basic knowledge of how to conduct research. This knowledge will help the paramedic to interpret published studies and to determine their value to EMS practice. The paramedic also must be willing to take part in collecting research data required for the continued development of EMS care. In addition, EMS research boosts respect for EMS professionals.

CRITICAL THINKING

How do you feel about research?

Basic Principles of Research

Emergency medical services research begins with stating a problem or question. The research then is carried out through standard research methods (Box 1-12). The research is reviewed by peers. The findings then are published in a professional journal for peer evaluation (Box 1-13). Emergency medical services research has many applications. One application includes gathering of research to draw conclusions about which procedures, techniques, and equipment are sound. Another includes gathering research to answer clinically valuable questions. And yet another includes gathering research to find results that lead to system improvements (Box 1-14).

After identifying a problem or question to be studied, a statement to be tested by the study must be defined. This statement is called the hypothesis. The problem might be the ability of a drug to lower a patient's blood pressure more effectively than another. A hypothesis for the drug study might be that drug A lowers blood pressure better and with fewer side effects than drug B.

The next step in the research process is to define the population for the study. The population can be any group

NOTE A hypothesis states the relationship between two or more variables. A variable is anything that varies in the amount or type.

of persons (e.g., all patients with a diastolic pressure greater than 100 mm Hg), places, or things. If the population group is large, the researcher can use a sample (e.g., all patients over 50 years of age who have a diastolic pressure greater than 100 mm Hg). The researcher should draw the sample *randomly*. That way, the patients in the study have an equal chance of being assigned to one group (Drug A Study) or the other (Drug B Study).

Drawing a random sample prevents selection bias (placing the best or worst patients in a study group). The researcher can make sure to get a random sample by using computer software programs. A statistical table of random digits may be helpful. The researcher can even flip a coin. Another way to limit bias is with systematic sampling. With

BOX 1-12 Types of Research

Descriptive (observational): A research design in which events are monitored and analyzed without an attempt to manipulate or alter the outcome

Experimental: A research design in which an intervention is introduced and the effects are monitored for an outcome

Prospective: A research design in which the specific question, hypothesis, and data collection are defined before the study begins

Retrospective: A research design in which the specific question, hypothesis, and data collection are defined after the data already exists

Cross-sectional: A research design in which a group of subjects is studied during a specified (usually short) period of time

BOX 1-13 Steps in Conducting Research

1. Prepare a question.
2. Write a hypothesis.
3. Decide what to measure and the best way to measure it.
4. Define the population.
5. Identify study limitations.
6. Seek study approval.
7. Obtain informed consent.
8. Gather data after conducting pilot trials.
9. Analyze the data with an awareness of the pitfalls in interpreting the data.
10. Determine what to do with the research product (publish, present, perform follow-up studies).

From Menegazzi J: *Research: the who, what, why, when and how,* Wilmington, Ohio, 1994, Ferno-Washington.

BOX 1-14 The Utstein Style: Reporting Outcomes of Out-of-Hospital Cardiac Arrests

In the past, emergency medical services (EMS) research on cardiac arrest (out of the hospital) has been hard to gather on a national level. This may be due to the variations in terms and definitions between EMS systems. For example, do the data that the EMS system reports make a distinction among arrests in which bystander cardiopulmonary resuscitation was begun before the arrival of EMS? The Utstein Style is a set of uniform templates to be used for reporting outcomes of prehospital cardiac arrest. These guidelines define many terms and activities used by EMS systems. These guidelines ensure that all members who are reporting data in a study are speaking the same language. With these templates, researchers now can make sound comparisons between the results published by EMS systems.

this method, patients are put into groups in the order in which they are encountered in the prehospital setting. For example, the first patient seen is put into group A, the second into group B, and the third into group A. The researcher also can use alternative time sampling to prevent bias by assigning a treatment group based on the day, week, or month in which patients are encountered in the study. Convenience sampling is the least preferred method. With this method, patients are assigned to groups when a particular person or crew is working. Even with carefully designed methods, sampling errors occur. Errors result from the fact that even the best sample will not work perfectly to represent the population because of the chance inclusion of one person in the study group rather than the chance inclusion of someone else.

▶NOTE A *parameter* is an aspect of a population that is hard or impossible to measure. For example, to find out the exact age (hour of birth) of all patients in a group would be nearly impossible. Nuisance variables are, for example, the use of audible and visual warning devices that can contribute to a rise in a patient's blood pressure. These variables also can make it hard to draw accurate conclusions from a study. Parameters and nuisance variables are hard to identify, control, avoid, or eliminate.

In addition to the bias of the researcher, bias can occur on the part of the participants in the study as well. Bias may be a result of the expectations of the participants. To lessen bias, the researcher can use blinding (either single, double, or triple). In a single blind method, one party (the patient, the health care provider, or the person gathering the data) is unaware (blinded) of the treatment at the time that it is given. That party is also unaware of the effect to be measured during the study. In a double blind study, two parties are blinded. A triple blind study occurs when all parties are blinded. *Unblinding* refers to all parties being made aware of the study, treatment, and outcome to be measured.

Statistics

The term *statistics* refers to numerical facts or data. These facts or data are classified and put into a chart to present key details about a subject. Statistics can be descriptive or inferential.

DESCRIPTIVE STATISTICS

Descriptive statistics does not try to infer anything about a subject that goes beyond the data. This type of statistics can be qualitative or quantitative. Qualitative analysis is nonnumerical; it is the organization and interpretation of observations. Qualitative analysis is used for finding key underlying dimensions and patterns. An example would be that it would show the age and gender of a sample. Qualitative analysis is not as precise as quantitative analysis.

Quantitative analysis in descriptive statistics uses *mean, median,* and *mode* to describe the most commonly occurring values within a sample. The mean is the arithmetic average of the group (e.g., the average age of the persons in the sample). The median is found first by arranging the measurement according to size from smallest to largest and then by choosing the one in the middle (or the mean of the two that are nearest to the middle). The median sometimes is referred to as the *fiftieth percentile.* The median frequently is used to divide a sample into two halves. The mode is the number that occurs more often than any other number in a set of data.

The following is an example of quantitative analysis:

Your sample has 13 participants. Their ages are 53, 53, 53, 54, 55, 55, 56, 57, 59, 60, 64, 71, and 79. The mean (average) age of the group is 59.15 years, the median (middle) age is 56, and the mode age is 53.

▶NOTE A *standard deviation* describes how much the scores in a set of numbers differ from the mean. The standard deviation also can be seen as how much the group varies from the average. A standard deviation is a single number that is derived through mathematical equations. The number tells how much deviation from the mean is typical of a given group. In a standard distribution, about 65% (two thirds) of all the numbers in the sample will be within 1 standard deviation of the mean. About 95% will be within 2 standard deviations of the mean. If the standard deviation is large, it points to an abnormal or skewed distribution of variability in the data or population under study.

INFERENTIAL STATISTICS

Inferential statistics offers a means to infer whether the relationships seen in a sample are likely to occur in the larger population. The researcher can use these statistics to decide whether the results of the study support or contradict the initial hypothesis. To do this, one must assume the opposite of what one may want to prove. One does this by stating a null hypothesis, or an exact statement that the results are a chance of variation. This is done in court where the accused is assumed to be innocent until proved guilty beyond a reasonable doubt. The assumption that the accused is not guilty is a null hypothesis. If the assumption cannot be rejected, the accused will go free. However, this does not always mean that the accused is really innocent. A research hypothesis is the opposite of the null hypothesis (e.g., the accused is guilty until proved innocent).

▶NOTE A *null hypothesis* states that no difference exists between two or more treatments. The sureness with which a null hypothesis can be rejected is called *confidence.*

When a statistical test reveals that the probability is rare that a set of results is attributable to chance alone, this result is called *statistically significant.* Statistically significant means that the observed phenomenon represents a significant departure from what might be expected by chance alone.

The *level of significance* is the probability of a Type I error that an investigator is willing to risk in rejecting a null hypothesis. Generally, the level of significance refers to the probability of the event occurring due to chance. The level of significance is the acceptable risk of sampling errors. The level of significance is established through mathematic equations. The level of significance is usually 0.05 (1 chance in 200) or 0.01 (1 chance in 100) that the difference between two groups is larger than expected as a result of chance alone (too large to be reasonably attributed to chance). If the level of significance is lowered from 0.05 to 0.01, the probability of rejecting a true hypothesis is decreased and the probability of accepting a false hypothesis is increased. A Type II error occurs when an investigator fails to accept the alternative hypothesis when in fact the alternative hypothesis was true. In other words, the null hypothesis was accepted when it was not true.

NOTE In statistics, rejecting the null hypothesis when it is true (a false alarm) is referred to as a *Type I error.* Accepting the null hypothesis when it is false (failing to detect a real phenomenon) is a Type II error. A Type II error occurs when the phenomenon is too small to see.

Research Ethics

When planning for research, researchers should think of using an institution review board (IRB). The wide use of IRBs came from a mandate in 1966 by the U.S. Public Health Services. This mandate required a review by a "committee of institutional associates" for any federally funded research that used human subjects. Today most IRBs involved in EMS research consist of many persons. These may include physicians, attorneys, psychologists, allied health professionals, and lay members of the community. In fact, many peer-reviewed EMS journals ask for a record that the research was approved by an IRB. The IRBs seek to reduce the risk of patients unknowingly entering into research that could harm them in any way. In 1981 (revised in 2001), the U.S. Department of Health and Human Services established regulations (CFR title 45, part 46) for research practice that are followed by most IRBs:

> In order to approve research covered by this policy the IRB shall determine that all of the following requirements are satisfied:
>
> (1) Risks to subjects are minimized: (i) by using procedures which are consistent with sound research design and which do not unnecessarily expose subjects to risk, and (ii) whenever appropriate, by using procedures already being performed on the subjects for diagnostic or treatment purposes.
>
> (2) Risks to subjects are reasonable in relation to anticipated benefits, if any, to subjects, and the importance of the knowledge that may reasonably be expected to result. In evaluating risks and benefits, the IRB should consider only those risks and benefits that may result from the research (as distinguished from risks and benefits of therapies subjects would receive even if not participating in the research). The IRB should not consider possible long-range effects of applying knowledge gained in the research (e.g., the possible effects of the research on public policy) as among those research risks that fall within the purview of its responsibility.
>
> (3) Selection of subjects is equitable. In making this assessment the IRB should take into account the purposes of the research and the setting in which the research will be conducted and should be particularly cognizant of the special problems of research involving vulnerable populations, such as children, prisoners, pregnant women, mentally disabled persons, or economically or educationally disadvantaged persons.
>
> (4) Informed consent will be sought from each prospective subject or the subject's legally authorized representative, in accordance with, and to the extent required by *46.116*.
>
> (5) Informed consent will be appropriately documented, in accordance with, and to the extent required by *46.117*.
>
> (6) When appropriate, the research plan makes adequate provision for monitoring the data collected to ensure the safety of subjects.
>
> (7) When appropriate, there are adequate provisions to protect the privacy of subjects and to maintain the confidentiality of data.
>
> (8) When some or all of the subjects are likely to be vulnerable to coercion or undue influence, such as children, prisoners, pregnant women, mentally disabled persons, or economically or educationally disadvantaged persons, additional safeguards have been included in the study to protect the rights and welfare of these subjects.[9]

CRITICAL THINKING
Why do you think the development of institution review boards was needed for research?

Consent

With informed consent, the subject voluntarily agrees to take part in the research project. The subject is also legally competent and understands what is being presented. With respect to EMS research and the problems associated with obtaining informed consent in emergency situations, alternatives to informed consent have been developed,[10] including the following:

- *Consent at a distance.* The base-station physician administers informed consent to the subject via radio or telephone.
- *Consent by proxy.* The paramedic administers informed consent to the subject.
- *Stepped consent.* The paramedic provides the subject with a brief overview of the experimental therapy. Full informed consent is obtained at the hospital.
- *Cohort consent.* Permission is obtained to enter into the study at some future time (e.g., during an asthma exacerbation or sickle cell crisis).
- *Deferred consent.* This consent is used during resuscitation, whereby the subject is stabilized and receives experimental therapy without permission, after which the family is approached for traditional informed consent.
- *Surrogate consent.* Lay persons are presented with the experimental protocol and are asked to rule if they feel that the treatment is appropriate.

- *Consent jury.* A lay panel determines certain aspects of the experimental protocol, particularly potential risks and complications that must be presented during a request for consent.

Research Format

The format for writing a manuscript for scientific literature has five basic sections:

1. The introduction provides a brief, historical background of the research. The introduction also relates any previously published research. The introduction provides a rationale for the study and the research hypothesis as well.
2. The methods section describes how the experiment was done. That way, the experiment can be replicated by others. This section also should define the inclusion or exclusion criteria for the study (how patients were chosen). This section also should contain the statistical methods used to analyze the data.
3. The results section provides answers to study questions and data (e.g., tables and figures). This information supports the research findings.
4. The discussion section lets the author interpret the research findings. Limitations of the project usually are given here as well. This section often has suggestions for improving the study through follow-up research.
5. The conclusion provides a brief and succinct summary of the four previous sections (Box 1-15).

BOX 1-15 Fifteen Steps in Evaluating and Interpreting Research

1. Was the research peer reviewed?
2. What was the research hypothesis?
3. Was the study approved by an institutional review board and conducted ethically?
4. What was the population being studied?
5. What were the inclusion and exclusion criteria for the study?
6. What method was used to draw a sample of patients?
7. How many patient groups participated?
8. How were patients assigned to groups?
9. What type of data was gathered?
10. Does it appear that the study had a sufficient number of patients enrolled?
11. Do there appear to be any potential confounding variables that are not accounted for?
12. Were the data properly analyzed?
13. Is the author's conclusion logical and based on the data?
14. Could the results apply in local EMS systems?
15. Are patients in the study similar to those in the local EMS system?

SUMMARY

- The roots of prehospital emergency care may date back to the military.
- In the early twentieth century through the mid-1960s, prehospital care in the United States was provided in a few ways. Care was provided mostly by urban hospital-based systems. These systems later developed into municipal services. Care also was provided by funeral directors and volunteers who were not trained in these services.
- The operations of an effective EMS system include citizen activation, dispatch, prehospital care, hospital care, and rehabilitation.
- The various levels of providers have their own distinct roles and duties. These roles include telecommunicators (dispatchers), first responders, EMT-Basics, EMT-Intermediates, and EMT-Paramedics. These levels combine to make an effective prehospital EMS system.
- Many professional groups and organizations help to set the standards of EMS. These groups exist at the national, state, regional, and local levels. The groups take part in development, education, and implementation. Being active in such a group helps to promote the status of the paramedic.
- Continuing education is crucial. It provides a way for all health care providers to maintain basic technical and professional skills.
- Professionalism refers to the way in which a person conducts himself or herself. Professionalism also refers to how one follows the standards of conduct and performance established by the profession.
- The roles and duties of the paramedic can be divided into two categories. These groups are *primary* and *additional* duties.
- The two types of medical direction are online (direct) and off-line (indirect) medical direction. Both are equally important. They help to ensure that the components of quality medical care are in place in an EMS system.
- A CQI program identifies and attempts to resolve problems in areas such as medical direction, financing, training, communication, prehospital management and transportation, interfacility transfer, receiving facilities, specialty care units, dispatch, public information and education, audit and quality assurance, disaster planning, and mutual aid.

- Quality EMS research helps shed light on the efficacy, effects, and cost-effectiveness of EMS interventions. The research is based on experimental data. Such research can lead to changes in professional standards and training. The research also can lead to changes in equipment and procedures.
- When planning research, the researcher should consider involving an institutional review board.

REFERENCES

1. Lyons A, Petrucelli J: *Medicine: an illustrated history,* New York, 1987, Harry N Abrams.
2. McNeil E: *Airborne care of the ill and injured,* New York, 1983, Springer-Verlag.
3. National Highway Traffic Safety Administration, US Department of Health and Human Services, Health Resources and Services Administration, Maternal and Child Health Bureau: *Emergency medical services agenda for the future,* Washington, DC, 1999, National Highway Traffic Safety Administration.
4. National Highway Traffic Safety Administration, US Department of Transportation: *Emergency medical services: NHTSA leading the way,* Washington, DC, 1995, The Administration.
5. National Registry of Emergency Medical Technicians: *National emergency medical services education and practice blueprint,* Columbus, Ohio, 1993, The Registry.
6. US Department of Transportation, National Highway Traffic Safety Administration: *EMT-Paramedic national standard curriculum,* Washington, DC, 1998, The Department.
7. National Association of EMS Physicians, National Highway Traffic Safety Administration, Maternal and Child Health Bureau: *National standard curriculum for medical direction,* Washington, DC, 1998, The Administration.
8. National Highway Traffic Safety Administration: *A leadership guide to quality improvement for emergency medical services (EMS) systems,* Washington, DC, 1997, The Administration.
9. Office for Human Research Protections. Code of Federal Regulations. http://ohrp.osophs.dhhs.gov/humansubjects/guidance/45cfr46.htm. Accessed March 4, 2003.
10. Menegazzi J: *Research: the who, what, why, when and how,* Wilmington, Ohio, 1994, Ferno-Washington.

CHAPTER 2

The Well-Being of the Paramedic

OBJECTIVES

Upon completion of this chapter, the paramedic student will be able to:

1. Describe the components of wellness and associated benefits.
2. Discuss the paramedic's role in promoting wellness.
3. Outline the benefits of specific lifestyle choices that promote wellness, including proper nutrition, weight control, exercise, sleep, and smoking cessation.
4. Identify risk factors and warning signs of cancer and cardiovascular disease.
5. Identify preventive measures to minimize the risk of work-related illness or injury associated with exposure, lifting and moving patients, hostile environments, vehicle operations, and rescue situations.
6. List signs and symptoms of addiction and addictive behavior.
7. Distinguish between normal and abnormal anxiety and stress reactions.
8. Give examples of stress-reduction techniques.
9. Outline the 10 components of critical incident stress management.
10. Given a scenario involving death or dying, identify therapeutic actions you may take based on your knowledge of the dynamics of this process.
11. List measures to take to reduce the risk of infectious disease exposure.
12. Outline actions to be taken following a significant exposure to a patient's blood or other body fluids.

KEY TERMS

addiction: A compulsive, uncontrollable dependence on a substance, habit, or practice to such a degree that cessation causes severe emotional, mental, or physiological reactions.

adrenaline: An endogenous adrenal hormone that helps prepare the body for energetic action.

anxiety: A state or feeling of apprehension, uneasiness, agitation, uncertainty, or fear resulting from the anticipation of some threat or danger.

autonomic nervous system: The part of the nervous system that regulates involuntary vital functions, including the activity of cardiac muscle, smooth muscle, and glands.

circadian rhythm: A pattern based on a 24-hour cycle, especially repetition of certain physiological phenomena, such as sleeping and eating.

distress: Negative, debilitating, or harmful stress.

eustress: Positive, performance-enhancing stress.

stress: A nonspecific mental or physical strain caused by any emotional, physical, social, economic, or other factor that initiates a physiological response.

universal precautions: Infection control practices in health care that are observed with every patient and procedure and that prevent exposure to blood-borne pathogens.

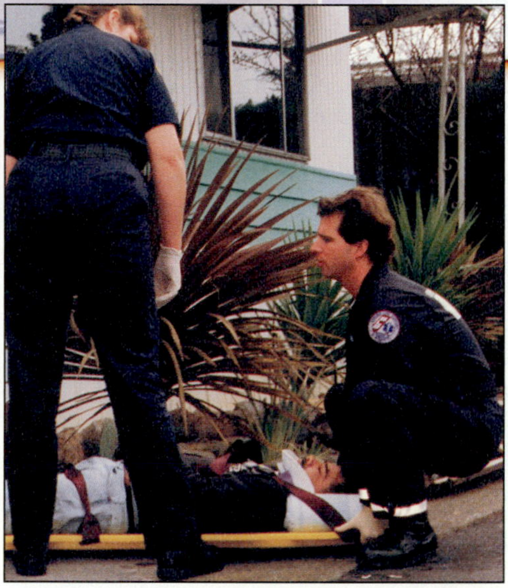

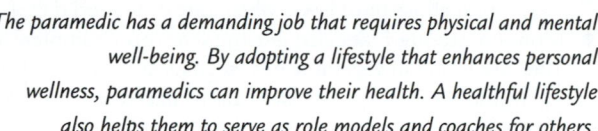

The paramedic has a demanding job that requires physical and mental well-being. By adopting a lifestyle that enhances personal wellness, paramedics can improve their health. A healthful lifestyle also helps them to serve as role models and coaches for others.

WELLNESS COMPONENTS

Wellness has two main aspects: physical well-being and mental and emotional health. Both aspects are key to the paramedic's health to deliver emergency care safely. Both aspects also help the paramedic to manage stressful events that are a natural part of the profession.

Physical Well-Being

Several factors play a major role in maintaining physical health. These factors include good nutrition, physical fitness, ample sleep, and the prevention of disease and injury.

NUTRITION

Nutrients are foods that hold the elements necessary for body function. The six categories of nutrients are carbohydrates, fats, proteins, vitamins, minerals, and water.

Carbohydrates are composed of carbon, hydrogen, and oxygen. Carbohydrates are obtained primarily from plant foods. The only important source of animal carbohydrates is lactose (milk sugar). Plants store carbohydrates as starch. Starch is made up of granules enclosed by cellulose walls that swell and burst when cooked. This feature makes cooked starchy foods easier to digest than raw, uncooked starchy foods.

All dietary fats contain a mixture of saturated and unsaturated fatty acids. Saturated fats are found mainly in meat and dairy products and in some vegetable fats. These fats raise the cholesterol levels in the blood by shutting down the process that normally removes excess cholesterol from the body. Unsaturated fats are subdivided further into polyunsaturated and monounsaturated fats. Polyunsaturated fats are found in safflower, sunflower, corn, soybean, and cottonseed oils and in some fish. These fats help rid the body of newly formed cholesterol. Omega-3 fatty acids are found mainly in cold-water fish such as tuna, salmon, and mackerel. These fats are a form of polyunsaturated fats. All polyunsaturated fats, including the omega-3 fats, are considered important to human health. Monounsaturated fats are liquid vegetable oils. Examples of these fats include canola and olive oil. Like polyunsaturated fats, these also may decrease blood cholesterol levels (Box 2-1). Trans fats are unsaturated fatty acids formed when vegetable oils are processed and made more solid or into a more stable liquid. Trans fats are present in a wide range of foods, including most foods made with partially hydrogenated oils, such as baked goods and fried foods, and some margarine products. Trans fats also occur

NOTE Cholesterol is present in all foods of animal origin and is concentrated heavily in fat and in poultry skin. Cholesterol is a white, waxy substance found in every cell and is needed by the body for normal functioning. Not all cholesterol is harmful; an adequate amount of cholesterol is needed for body functions. Cholesterol is manufactured in the liver and is carried through the bloodstream. Adding cholesterol to the diet can raise blood cholesterol levels and increase the risk of heart disease and stroke.

BOX 2-1 Fat and Cholesterol Control

Tips for a Healthful Eating Plan

- Select lean cuts of meat, such as loin and round cuts, and trim all visible fat.
- Buy lower-fat versions of your favorite dairy products, such as skim milk and skim milk–based cheeses.
- For added flavor, use herbs and spices in place of high-fat flavorings or sauces on vegetables, meats, poultry, and fish.
- Chill soups and stews and skim off the fat that collects on the surface.
- Choose low-fat or nonfat versions of your favorite salad dressings, mayonnaise, yogurt, and sour cream.
- Use low-fat or fat-free marinades to tenderize and add flavor to leaner cuts of meat.

Tips to Reduce Saturated Fats

- Use polyunsaturated or monounsaturated oil when a recipe calls for melted shortening or butter.
- Use vegetable oil margarine in place of butter or lard. Look for whipped, lower-fat tub margarine.

Tips to Be "Fat" Smart

- Saturated fats usually are solid at room temperature. They mainly come from animal foods such as meat, poultry, butter, and whole milk. Coconut, palm, and palm kernel oils are also high in saturated fat. Saturated fat is responsible for raising blood cholesterol levels.
- Polyunsaturated fats usually are liquid at room temperature. They are found in vegetable oils. Safflower, sunflower, corn, and soybean oils contain the highest amounts of these polyunsaturated fats. Polyunsaturated fats can help decrease high blood cholesterol levels when part of a good diet.
- Monounsaturated fats also are liquid at room temperature. They are found in vegetable oils, such as canola and olive oil. Monounsaturated fats can help to decrease high blood cholesterol levels if they are part of a lower-fat diet.
- Dietary cholesterol comes only from animal sources such as the fat in dairy products, egg yolks, meats, poultry, and seafood. Vegetables, fruits, and grains do not contain cholesterol.
- Hydrogenation is a process that makes an oil more solid at room temperature. Hydrogenated vegetable oils give some processed foods a longer shelf life. Examples of those foods include margarine and crackers.

From the American Dietetic Association, National Center for Nutrition and Dietetics: *The ABCs of fats, oils, and cholesterol,* Chicago, 1994, The Association.

naturally in low amounts in meats and dairy products. Although trans fats are unsaturated, they appear similar to saturated fats in terms of their effect on blood cholesterol levels.

Proteins are made of hydrogen, oxygen, carbon, and nitrogen (and most contain sulfur and phosphorus). Proteins are vital to building body tissue during growth, maintenance, and repair. When proteins are digested, they break down into amino acids (classified as *essential* or *nonessential*). Essential amino acids are needed for body growth and cellular life. They must be obtained in food because they are not made in the body. Nonessential amino acids are *not* needed for body health and growth and can be made in the body. Proteins that contain all the essential amino acids are complete proteins and are found in meats and dairy products. Proteins that are missing one or more essential amino acids are incomplete proteins (e.g., those in grains and vegetables). Proteins can be used as a source of energy but should be spared for their more important role in body health by the sufficient intake of carbohydrates.

Vitamins are organic substances that are present in minute amounts in foods. Because vitamins are crucial for metabolism and cannot be made in adequate amounts by the body, they must be gained through food or vitamin supplements. (An ample intake of vitamins through a balanced diet should make vitamin supplements unnecessary in healthy individuals.) Vitamins are water soluble or fat soluble. Vitamins C and B complex contain eight water-soluble vitamins. Water-soluble vitamins cannot be stored in the body. They must come from the daily diet. Fat-soluble vitamins (vitamins A, D, E, and K) can be stored in the body. Therefore a daily dietary intake of these vitamins is not required (Box 2-2).

BOX 2-2 Free Radicals and Antioxidants

Free radicals are natural by-products of chemical reactions in the body that can produce cellular injury. The buildup of these free radicals increases with age. The buildup is thought to be the cause of many diseases, including heart disease, diabetes, and some cancers. Substances that can generate free radicals can be found in fried foods, alcohol, tobacco smoke, pesticides, and air pollution. Other substances to which persons often are exposed also may create free radicals.

Antioxidants are known as free radical scavengers. They are compounds that reduce the formation of free radicals or react with and neutralize them, making them nontoxic to cells. Antioxidants occur naturally in the body. They also occur naturally in certain foods such as fruits, vegetables, and whole grains. Beta carotene (a form of vitamin A), and vitamins C and E are popular antioxidant supplements. These may benefit a person's health.

Minerals are elements that are inorganic; they occur naturally in the earth. Minerals play a key role in biochemical reactions in the body. Minerals include calcium, chromium, iron, magnesium, potassium, selenium, sodium, and zinc. Like vitamins, minerals come from the diet (Table 2-1).

Water is the most important nutrient because cellular function depends on a fluid environment. Water composes

TABLE 2-1 The ABCs of Nutrition

	FUNCTION	SOURCE
Vitamins		
A	Proper eye function; keeps skin, hair, and nails healthy; helps maintain healthy gums, glands, bones, teeth; helps ward off infection; may protect against lung cancer	Liver,* dairy products,* fish, carrots, yellow squash, dark-green leafy vegetables, corn, tomatoes, papaya
B_1 (thiamine)	Helps convert carbohydrates into biological energy; promotes proper nerve function	Pork,* unrefined and enriched cereals, organ meats,* legumes, nuts*
B_2 (riboflavin)	Crucial in the production of body energy	Milk,* cheese,* yogurt,* green leafy vegetables, fruits, bread, cereals, meats*
B_3 (niacin)	Lowers cholesterol levels in blood only in very high doses; may protect against cardiovascular disease	Yeast, meats* including liver,* cereals, legumes, seeds*
B_6	Essential for protein breakdown and absorption	Beef,* poultry,* fish, pork,* bananas, nuts,* whole grains, vegetables
B_{12}	Essential for the healthy function of nerve tissue	Meats,* meat products,* shellfish, fish, poultry,* eggs*
Biotin	Needed for breakdown of glucose (a type of sugar) and formation of certain fatty acids necessary for several important body functions	Meats,* poultry,* fish, eggs,* nuts,* seeds,* legumes, vegetables
C (ascorbic acid)	Strengthens blood vessel walls; keeps gums healthy; promotes healing of cuts and wounds	Strawberries, citrus fruits, tomatoes, cabbage, cauliflower, broccoli, greens
D	Helps build and maintain teeth and bones; needed for body to absorb calcium	Egg yolks,* fish and cod liver oil,* fortified milk and butter*
E	Helps form red blood cells, muscle tissue, and other tissues; may protect against heart disease	Poultry,* seafood, seeds,* nuts,* cooked greens, wheat germ, fortified cereals, eggs*
K†	Needed for normal clotting of blood	Spinach, broccoli, brussels sprouts, kale, turnip greens
Minerals		
Calcium	Helps build strong bones and teeth; promotes proper muscle and nerve function; helps blood to clot; helps activate enzymes needed to convert food to energy; may protect against the development of fragile, porous bones	Milk,* cheese,* yogurt,* buttermilk, other dairy products,* green leafy vegetables
Chromium	Works with insulin to maintain normal blood sugar	Whole-grain cereals, condiments (black pepper, thyme), meat products,* cheeses*
Iron	Essential to make hemoglobin, the oxygen-carrying component of red blood cells	Red meat* and liver,* shellfish and fish, legumes, dried apricots, fortified breads and cereals
Magnesium	Activates enzymes needed to release energy in body; promotes bone growth; needed to make cells and genetic material	Green leafy vegetables, beans, nuts,* fortified whole-grain cereals and breads, oysters, scallops
Potassium	With sodium, helps to regulate body's fluid balance; plays a major role in muscle contraction, nerve conduction, beating of the heart	Bananas, citrus fruits, dried fruits, deep yellow vegetables, potatoes, legumes, milk,* bran cereal
Selenium	Interacts with vitamin E to prevent breakdown of cells in body	Organ meats,* seafood, meats,* cereals and grains, egg yolks,* mushrooms, onions, garlic
Sodium	Helps maintain body fluid balance	Salt, processed foods, foods in brine, salted crackers and chips, cured meats, soy sauce (Note: sodium is so prevalent that low intake is very rare. The problem is avoiding excessive intake of sodium.)
Zinc	Boosts the immune system and helps fight disease; element in more than 100 enzymes—proteins that are essential to digestion and other functions	Red meats,* some seafoods, grains

U.S. Department of Agriculture's Center for Nutrition Policy and Promotion, Washington, D.C. www.usda.gov.
*These foods are high in fat and/or cholesterol. Use sparingly or substitute low-fat versions, where possible.
†Green leafy vegetables and other foods rich in vitamin K can contribute to blood clotting. If you take a drug that prevents blood clotting, talk to your physician before changing your diet.

NOTE Diseases caused by vitamin deficiency (e.g., scurvy, rickets, or beriberi) are rare in the United States. Making proper food choices can help to prevent them.

CRITICAL THINKING
Does your average diet meet these guidelines? If not, in what areas do you need to make changes?

50% to 60% of the total body weight. (Infants have the greatest percentage of body water; older adults have the least.) Water is obtained through consumption of liquids and fresh fruits and vegetables. Water also is produced when food is oxidized during digestion.

Dietary Recommendations. Various health care groups make recommendations for a healthful diet. These groups include the U.S. Department of Agriculture, the U.S. Department of Health and Human Services, and the Food and Drug Administration. Box 2-3 lists the dietary recommendations of the American Heart Association.

BOX 2-3 Dietary Guidelines

Achieve an Overall Healthful Eating Pattern
- Choose an overall balanced diet with foods from all major food groups, emphasizing fruits, vegetables, and grains.
- Consume a variety of fruits, vegetables, and grain products.
- Consume at least five daily servings of fruits and vegetables.
- Consume at least six daily servings of grain products, including whole grains.
- Include fat-free and low-fat dairy products, fish, legumes, poultry, and lean meats.
- Eat at least two servings of fish per week.

Achieve a Healthful Body Weight
- Maintain a level of physical activity that achieves fitness and balances energy expenditure with caloric intake; for weight reduction, expenditure should exceed intake.
- Limit foods that are high in calories and low in nutritional quality, including those with a high amount of added sugar.

Achieve a Desirable Cholesterol Level
- Limit foods with a high content of saturated fat and cholesterol. Substitute with grains and unsaturated fat from vegetables, fish, legumes, and nuts.
- Limit cholesterol to 300 mg a day for the general population and 200 mg a day for those with heart disease or its risk factors.
- Limit trans-fatty acids. Trans-fatty acids are found in foods containing partially hydrogenated vegetable oils, such as packaged cookies, crackers, and other baked goods and commercially prepared fried foods and some margarines.

Achieve a Desirable Blood Pressure Level
- Limit salt intake to less than 6 g (2400 mg sodium) per day, slightly more than 1 tsp a day.
- If you drink, limit alcohol consumption to no more than one drink per day for women and two drinks per day for men.

From American Heart Association. Dietary Guidelines: At-a-Glance. http://www.americanheart.org/presenter.jhtml?identifier=810. Accessed July 10, 2003.

Principles of Weight Control. Persons who are overweight tend to be at higher risk for developing certain illnesses. These illnesses include high blood pressure, diabetes mellitus, heart disease, and some cancers. The tenets of weight control are to eat the right balance of foods in moderation, limit fat consumption, and exercise regularly (Box 2-4).

Anyone committed to weight control for a healthier life should set realistic goals. For example, the general recommendation is a steady weight loss goal of ½ to 1 lb per week. A healthful lifestyle is balanced with proper nutrition and exercise. A healthful diet includes a variety of foods that are low in fat, saturated fat, and cholesterol. A healthful diet also includes plenty of grain products, vegetables, and fruit (Box 2-5). A diet also should be moderate in simple sugars, salt, and sodium. Alcoholic beverages should be avoided or consumed only in moderation. Finally, a system for checking weight control progress is essential. Adjustments and

BOX 2-4 Getting a Handle on Fat

Eat foods that are less than 30% fat. Try to aim for no more than 3 g of fat per 100 calories, which provides about 27% of the total calories from fat. This is important for the following reasons:
- Each gram of fat has more than double the calories of a gram of protein or carbohydrates.
- The body uses fewer calories to store the fat as excess weight.
- In complex carbohydrates, 23% of the calories are burned to make them into a usable form in the body; only 3% of fat calories are burned before they are "worn" on the hips or abdomen.
- Decreasing fat intake to less than 30% of daily calories helps reduce cholesterol, decreases risk of heart disease, helps with weight loss, and reduces risk of diabetes.

Fat content of various foods

More than 90% fat: whipped cream, pork sausage, cooking oils, margarine, butter, gravy, mayonnaise

More than 80% fat: spare ribs, bologna, cream cheese, salad dressing, high-fat steaks (T-bone, porterhouse, tenderloin, filet mignon)

More than 70% fat: half and half, peanuts, hot dogs, pork chops, most cheeses and nuts, sirloin steak, bacon, lamb chops

More than 60% fat: potato and corn chips, regular ground beef, ham, eggs

More than 50% fat: round steak, pot roast, creamed soup, ice cream, sweet rolls

More than 40% fat: whole milk, cake, doughnuts, french fries

More than 30% fat: muffins, cookies, fruit pies, low-fat milk, cottage cheese, tuna, chicken, turkey

More than 20% fat: lean fish, beef liver, ice milk

More than 10% fat: bread, pretzels, whole grains, legumes

Less than 10% fat: sherbet, nonfat milk, most fruits and vegetables, baked potato professional advice sometimes may be needed to achieve weight-control goals.

PHYSICAL FITNESS

Physical fitness can be described as a condition that helps persons look, feel, and do their best. Physical fitness is individual and varies from person to person. Physical fitness also is influenced by age, sex, heredity, personal habits, exercise, and eating habits. Being physically fit offers many benefits, which include the following:

- Decreased resting heart rate and blood pressure
- Increased oxygen-carrying capacity
- Enhanced quality of life
- Increased muscle mass and metabolism
- Increased resistance to injury
- Improved personal appearance and self-image
- Maintenance of motor skills throughout life

Cardiovascular Endurance. A physical examination is the first step before starting a fitness program. A physician should perform this exam. Another step is to have a fitness assessment performed by a certified physical trainer. The purpose of these assessments is to evaluate a person's present physical condition. These exams also create baseline assessments for weight, including body mass index (Box 2-6); high blood pressure; heart trouble (including family history); arthritis or other bone problems; muscular, ligament, or tendon problems; and other known or suspected diseases. These assessments help to establish a heart rate target zone as well. This is a measure used to improve cardiovascular endurance through exercise. Ideally, the heart rate target zone should be maintained during exercise for 20 minutes to increase cardiovascular endurance.

Muscle Strength. Another part of the fitness assessment tests muscular strength and endurance. Muscular strength is the ability of a muscle to exert force for a brief period. Muscle endurance is the ability of a muscle or a group of muscles to sustain repeated contractions or to continue applying force against a fixed object. Many exercises improve muscle strength and endurance.

The tenets of training for muscle strength and endurance should consider isometric and isotonic exercises, resistance, repetitions, sets, and frequency. *Isometric* exercises are those that do not result in any movement of a joint. An example of this is a contraction performed against an immovable object such as a wall or door frame. These exercises do not increase muscle bulk very much. However, they do strengthen the muscle at the joint angle at which the contraction is performed. *Isotonic* exercises move a joint through a range of motion against resistance of a fixed weight. An example of this is lifting a barbell. These exercises add muscle bulk by creating tension within the muscle. *Resistance* refers to the amount of weight moved or lifted during isotonic exercises. A *repetition* ("rep") refers to the full execution of an exercise from start to finish. A *set* is the number of times an exercise (rep) is done start to finish, one after another, without any rest time. *Frequency* refers to the least number of workouts that will have a positive effect on muscle strength and endurance.

Muscular Flexibility. Flexibility refers to the ability to move joints and use muscles through their full range of motion. The fitness assessment tests flexibility in several ways. A lack of normal flexibility may lead to muscle strains and other injuries.

Muscular flexibility can be improved by stretching exercises. These exercises must be done slowly, without a

CRITICAL THINKING

Calculate your body mass index. Does it fall within the recommendations?

NOTE There is a simple way to determine the heart rate target zone. First, multiply the established maximum heart rate of 220 minus a person's age in years. Then multiply this number by 70%.

Example for a 25-year-old:
Maximum heart rate (220 − 25) = 195
195 × 70% = 136 beats/min

BOX 2-5 Fiber

The human body requires fiber to maintain good health and to fight disease. Fiber (found only in plant foods) may be soluble or insoluble. Examples of soluble fiber include fiber obtained from peas, beans, oats, barley, and some fruits and vegetables. This type of fiber helps control the level of blood sugar. Soluble fiber also may lower the level of blood cholesterol. Insoluble fiber (found in whole grains and many vegetables) helps hold water in the colon and can reduce or prevent constipation. This type of fiber also may help prevent intestinal disease (e.g., diverticulosis, hemorrhoids, and certain cancers). Many authorities recommend a dietary intake of 20 to 35 g of fiber each day.

BOX 2-6 The Body Mass Index

The body mass index (BMI) is a widely used measurement of body fat that corrects for height. The BMI is the only body fat index that conveys the risk of disease or death. A healthful BMI is 19 to 25. A BMI of 25 to 29 indicates "moderately overweight." A BMI of 30 or more indicates "severely overweight." To calculate your body mass index, use the following formula:

Step 1: Multiply your weight in pounds by 0.45.
Example: 150 pounds × 0.45 = 67.5
Step 2: Multiply your height in inches by 0.025.
Example: 5 ft 9 in, or 69 inches × 0.025 = 1.725
Step 3: Square the answer from step 2.
Example: 1.725 × 1.725 − 2.976
Step 4: Divide the answer in step 1 by the answer in step 3.
Example: $\frac{67.5}{2.976}$ = BMI of 22.7

bouncing motion. The intensity of these exercises should be mild. A person should not strain or hold the breath and should feel no pain or discomfort. How often these exercises are done should match an individual's specific level of activity. For example, if daily work on an ambulance requires lifting patients, then regular stretching exercises specific to the paramedic's arms, back, thighs, calves, and hips would help.

> **CRITICAL THINKING**
>
> How many minutes per week do you perform physical activities that raise your heart rate? What benefits does a paramedic gain by maintaining a high level of personal fitness?

THE IMPORTANCE OF SLEEP

Sleep plays an important role in being physically fit because it helps to rejuvenate a tired body. The average adult needs 7 to 8 hours of sleep each day. In emergency medical services (EMS), where rotating shifts and 24-hour work shifts are common, sleep deprivation may occur and interrupt the normal **circadian rhythm.**

Circadian is Latin for "about a day." The circadian rhythm is the physiological ebb and flow of the body as it relates to the rotation of the earth. This timing system is based roughly on the solar day as the earth rotates in its course around the sun. For example, a person gets hungry or tired, energetic or moody, at fairly set times each day as the body systems change. The level of melatonin and cortisol affects the periods of sleepiness and wakefulness. The pineal gland secretes melatonin. The adrenal glands secrete cortisol. Release of these hormones is stimulated by the dark and is suppressed by light. Thus when the line between night and day is disrupted on an ongoing basis (e.g., working rotating work shifts or responding to emergency calls in the early morning hours during a 24-hour shift), irritability, depression, and illness can result (Box 2-7). Research is under way to help shift workers and their employers modify work schedules. Then changes in normal biorhythms will have the least adverse effects on employee health and productivity.

> **BOX 2-7 Getting Your Z's**
>
> Working nights, 24-hour shifts, and rotating shifts can inhibit getting enough rest. The following are some helpful tips:
>
> - Allow some time to unwind and relax before trying to go to sleep.
> - Consider exercise before sleeping as a way to reduce stress.
> - Avoid stimulants (e.g., caffeine in coffee, soda, tea, and chocolate) during the last few hours of your work shift.
> - Eat simple carbohydrates (e.g., cookies or candy bar) to release serotonin (a hormone that may help induce sleep).
> - Keep your sleeping area cool and dark so that your body will think it is nighttime.
> - Make sure your family and friends know about your work shifts and your sleeping schedule to minimize interruptions.
> - Try to maintain a "normal" period of dedicated sleep time each day.
> - Consult a physician about your sleep difficulties when needed.

> **CRITICAL THINKING**
>
> Do you get enough sleep? If not, which of these strategies should you try in an attempt to increase your hours of sleep?

> **NOTE** The circadian rhythm causes the jet lag that occurs during air travel to a distant time zone. Studies suggest that the symptoms of jet lag may be relieved by the administration of melatonin.

DISEASE PREVENTION

A paramedic can do a lot to help prevent serious personal illness. As health care professionals, paramedics must serve as role models in helping to prevent disease.

Cardiovascular disease. This disease accounts for more than 950,000 deaths each year in the United States.[1] For most persons, cardiovascular disease can be altered through living a healthful life. Boosting cardiovascular endurance can help to prevent this disease. However, other steps also are needed in the fight. These steps include the following:

- Eliminating cigarette smoking
- Controlling high blood pressure
- Maintaining a favorable body fat composition through regular exercise
- Maintaining a good total cholesterol/high-density lipoprotein ratio (Box 2-8)
- Monitoring triglyceride levels
- Controlling diabetes
- Avoiding excessive alcohol intake
- Eating healthful foods
- Reducing stress
- Obtaining risk assessments periodically

Cancer. The term *cancer* includes more than 100 diseases affecting nearly every part of the body. All these diseases are potentially life threatening. The main cause of all cancer is a change or mutation in the nucleus of a cell. Most common cancers are linked to one of three environmental risk factors: smoking, sunlight, or diet. Dietary factors are associated with some cancers of the gastrointestinal tract and may be linked to others, such as cancer of the breast, prostate, or uterus. A lack of dietary fiber is believed to be a risk factor for these cancers. Steps in preventing cancer include the following:

- Elimination of smoking
- Dietary changes
- Limitation of sun exposure; use of sunscreen

- Regular physical examinations
- Attention to the warning signs (Box 2-9)
- Periodic risk assessment

Infectious disease. Most infectious diseases can be avoided by doing two things. The first is practicing good personal hygiene, including hand washing. The second is following **universal precautions** and other guidelines in the workplace. These guidelines are established by the Centers for Disease Control and Prevention, the Occupational Safety and Health Administration, the National Fire Protection Association, the Federal Emergency Management Agency, the United States Fire Administration, and others (Table 2-2).

At a minimum, personal protective equipment to guard against the spread of infectious diseases should include the following:

- Disposable gloves when contact with blood or other body fluids is likely
- Masks and protective eye wear when blood splashing is likely to occur
- Gowns to protect clothing from spurting blood (e.g., during emergency childbirth)
- HEPA (high-efficiency particulate air filter) and N-95 respirators when tuberculosis is confirmed or suspected

BOX 2-8 Understanding the Cholesterol Numbers

Cholesterol moves through the body attached to various sizes of fat-carrying proteins. These proteins are called lipoproteins. Low-density lipoproteins (LDLs) are more common. They are thought to carry cholesterol to the cells where they can promote blood vessel disease. Smaller high-density lipoproteins (HDLs) are thought to carry cholesterol to the liver. They may help prevent or slow down blood vessel disease. Very low-density lipoproteins are made mostly of triglycerides (the main fatty substance in the fluid portion of blood) that are absorbed by the intestines and therefore are affected by fasting. (Fasting is abstaining from all or certain foods.)

Cholesterol
High blood cholesterol: 240 mg/dL or higher
Borderline high blood cholesterol: 220 to 239 mg/dL
Desirable blood cholesterol: less than 200 mg/dL

LDL Cholesterol: The "Bad" Cholesterol
Very high LDL cholesterol: 189 mg/dL or higher
High LDL cholesterol: 160 to 189 mg/dL or higher
Borderline high LDL cholesterol: 130 to 159 mg/dL
Desirable LDL cholesterol in healthy persons: less than 100 mg/dL
Desirable LDL cholesterol in persons at risk for heart disease: less than 90 mg/dL

HDL Cholesterol: Higher Is Better
Low HDL cholesterol: less than 40 mg/dL
Desirable HDL cholesterol: greater than 60 mg/dL

Very Low-Density Lipoproteins/Triglyceride: Lower Is Better
Should not exceed 200 to 300 mg/dL

A potential exposure to an infectious disease may occur. When exposure occurs, the paramedic should report it as soon as possible. Exposure needs to be reported to the receiving hospital. Exposure also should be reported to the proper designated officer in the local agency. That way, an exchange between the hospital and the emergency response organization can be set up (see Chapter 39). To defend against such diseases, the Occupational Safety and Health Administration has some provisions that require that a periodic risk assessment be offered to staff. The risk assessment includes regular testing for diseases such as tuberculosis and also testing for vaccinations for diseases. One such vaccination is for hepatitis B.

INJURY PREVENTION

The number of injuries that occur on the job can be reduced. Knowledge of proper body mechanics during lifting and moving is helpful. Staying alert for hostile settings also is essential. A paramedic must prioritize personal safety during rescue situations. Finally, one must practice safe vehicle operations and use safety equipment and supplies.

Body Mechanics During Lifting and Moving. Proper body mechanics during lifting and moving are crucial. They help to avoid personal injury and to avoid injury to a partner or patient (Box 2-10). The paramedic should consider the following guidelines when lifting and moving patients or equipment:

- Only move a victim you can handle safely; get additional help if needed.
- Look where you are walking or crawling.
- Move forward rather than backward when possible.
- Take short steps, if walking.
- Bend at the hips and knees.
- Lift with the legs, not the back.
- Keep the load close to the body.
- Keep patient's body in line when moving.

Hostile Environments. Paramedics may not be able to avoid being placed in hostile situations. Such situations may include responding to violent crimes of murder, rape, robbery, acts of terrorism, and aggravated assault. These crimes often are linked with the use of illegal drugs. This environment may threaten one's personal safety. When these situations occur, paramedics should do the following:

BOX 2-9 The Seven Warning Signs of Cancer (CAUTION) as Designated by the American Cancer Society

*C*hange in bowel or bladder habits
A sore throat that does not heal
*U*nusual bleeding or discharge
*T*hickening or lump in the breast or elsewhere
*I*ndigestion or difficulty swallowing
*O*bvious change in a wart or mole
*N*agging cough or hoarseness

TABLE 2-2 Personal Equipment for Protection Against Transmission of HIV and Hepatitis B Virus

ACTIVITY	DISPOSABLE GLOVES	GOWN	MASK	PROTECTIVE EYEWEAR
Bleeding control (spurting blood)	Yes	Yes	Yes	Yes
Bleeding control (minimal blood)	Yes	No	No	No
Emergency childbirth	Yes	Yes	Yes*	Yes*
Intravenous therapy	Yes	No	No	No
Endotracheal intubation	Yes	No	Yes*	Yes*
Oral or nasal suctioning	Yes	No	No	No
Administration of an injection	No	No	No	No

*If splashing is likely.

BOX 2-10 Prevention and Rehabilitation of Low Back Pain

The back is a complex system of ligaments, muscles, bones, nerves, and intervertebral disks. All of these parts can be injured by improper lifting techniques. Emergency medical services workers are highly vulnerable to low back pain and injury. An area of the back that often is a source of low back pain and injury is lordosis (an inward curvature in the lumbar spine that is normally present to some degree). Abnormal curvature in this area can result from poor posture and from being overweight with associated weak abdominal muscles. Back injury can be prevented or lessened to a significant degree by being physically fit, performing regular stretching exercises, and following some general rules of lifting:

1. Know the weight (ask the patient's weight if you can, and add the weight of the equipment). Two persons should work together to lift objects that weigh more than 60 lb.
2. Know your physical ability and limitations.
3. Keep your back positioned with a normal curvature.
4. Use your legs and abdominal muscles to support the weight; use your back muscles to maintain balance.
5. Keep the weight close to your body.
6. Communicate clearly and frequently with your partner.

If back pain or injury occurs when lifting, pushing, pulling, or stretching, tell a supervisor as soon as possible. Treatment for back pain usually begins with rest and ice or cold packs to lessen swelling. Treatment also can include pain medicine and muscle relaxants. A rehabilitatioin program usually will follow the injury. Rehabilitation often includes exercises to improve abdominal muscle strength. The exercises also help to improve the control of the pelvis and flexibility of the lower back.

From *EMT: injury free,* Wilmington, Ohio, 1991, Ferno-Washington.

- Carefully check the scene for safety concerns and do not enter the scene until it is safe.
- Coordinate all actions with law enforcement personnel.
- Follow protocols for establishing a medical incident command (see Chapter 50).
- Plan entrance and escape routes.
- Above all, stay alert and be prepared for the unexpected.

Safely managing a violent scene requires special training. The situation also calls for unity among many emergency response agencies. As members of the response team, paramedics should take part in planning, training, and practice sessions. These sessions help to ensure provider safety in hostile settings (see Chapter 52).

Rescue Situations. Many personal safety issues arise in the case of rescue. Examples include exposure to hazardous materials, bad weather, extremes in temperature, fire, toxic gases, unstable structures, heavy equipment, road hazards, and sharp edges and fragments. For every rescue response the key is to assess the scene for hazards first. One also must take personal protective measures. In addition, the scene should be monitored constantly during the operation. A safe rescue requires proper use of protective gear, special training, and safe rescue practices (see Chapter 51).

Safe Vehicle Operation. Safe operation of all vehicles is essential. Emergency vehicles must be operated properly as well to ensure personal safety and the safety of the crew and patient (see Chapter 49). Many factors affect safe vehicle operations, including the following:

- Safe driving of the vehicle
- Safe and appropriate use of escorts to and from emergency scenes
- Adverse environmental conditions (e.g., inclement weather)
- Appropriate use of audible and visual warning devices
- Proceeding through intersections safely
- Parking at the emergency scene
- Maintaining due regard for the safety of all others

CRITICAL THINKING

Is there any patient situation that would call for using unsafe vehicle operations? Keep in mind that this could risk the safety of those in the ambulance or in other vehicles.

Some EMS agencies require their employees to take a specialized driver's training class. One such program is the U.S. Department of Transportation Emergency Vehicle Operation Course. A program such as this allows EMS providers to practice driving in a safe and controlled setting.

Safety Equipment and Supplies. Proper use of safety equipment and supplies is key to injury prevention for EMS providers. Standards for protective clothing and equipment are required by Occupational Safety and Health Administration. These and other standards (such as those set by National Fire Protection Association) are used by many states, cities, and fire and EMS agencies. These standards help to ensure employee safety (see Chapter 51). Safety equipment and supplies include the following:

- Body substance isolation equipment
- Head protection
- Eye protection
- Hearing protection
- Respiratory protection
- Gloves
- Boots
- Coveralls
- Turnout coat and pants
- Specialty equipment
- Reflective clothing

Mental and Emotional Health

Many factors play a role in mental and emotional health. An important factor is to be aware of warning signs that could signal a potential problem (e.g., signs of substance misuse and health disorders caused by **anxiety** and **stress**). Also key to maintaining good emotional health is realizing the value of having personal time; being connected with family, peers, and the community; and accepting the personal differences that make individuals unique.

SUBSTANCE MISUSE AND ABUSE CONTROL

The misuse and abuse of drugs and other substances may lead to chemical dependency **(addiction)**. Such dependency may have a wide range of effects on physical and mental health (Box 2-11). Warning signs of addiction and addictive behavior include the following:

- Using a substance to relieve tension
- Using an increasing amount of the substance
- Lying about using the substance
- Experiencing guilt about using the substance
- Avoiding discussion about using the substance
- Experiencing interference with daily activities as a result of substance abuse

BOX 2-11 Common Drugs and Substances That Are Misused or Abused

- Alcohol
- Central nervous system stimulants (e.g., cocaine and amphetamines)
- Cigarettes and other tobacco products
- Hallucinogens
- Inhalants
- Marijuana
- Narcotics and related drugs
- Sedative-hypnotics
- Tranquilizers
- Nonprescription substances
- Sedatives
- Appetite suppressants
- Laxatives
- Cough and cold preparations
- Nasal sprays
- Analgesics

CRITICAL THINKING

Do you know anyone with these behaviors?

Methods used to manage substance abuse depend on the type of substance being misused. Substance misuse or abuse control may call for professional counseling. Physician-controlled drug therapy and support programs also may be necessary.

SMOKING CESSATION

Cigarette smoking is a major health hazard. Smoking is responsible for more than 400,000 deaths each year in the United States.[1] The health ramifications of cigarette smoking are numerous, including an increased risk of the following:

- Coronary heart disease
- Myocardial infarction
- Chronic obstructive pulmonary disease
- Sudden death
- Dying from a variety of diseases
- Miscarriage, premature birth, and birth defects

Smokers often name many reasons for continuing to smoke. These reasons may include peer pressure, relief of stress, weight control, and others. Regardless, most persons continue to smoke because of the addictive nature of nicotine. Nicotine is the stimulant in tobacco, but there are other harmful chemicals. These chemicals include hydrocarbons (tar) and carbon monoxide. Exposure to these chemicals is considered a health hazard for nonsmokers also. Nonsmokers have an increased risk of developing smoking-related illnesses through "passive smoking," or secondhand smoke.

Many resources and smoking cessation programs are available to those who want to quit smoking. Support groups and quit smoking campaigns are sponsored by the American Heart Association, the American Cancer Society, the American Red Cross, government health agencies, and local health care organizations. Other methods one may use alone or with these programs include the use of prescription and nonprescription drugs. Some examples include bupropion, dermal patches, and nicotine chewing gum. These products decrease the physical effects of smoking cessation. In a sense, they help to wean the smoker off of nicotine (Box 2-12).

ANXIETY AND STRESS

Anxiety can be defined as the worry or dread about future uncertainties. *Stress* can result from the interaction of events that cause anxiety and the coping abilities of the person. Stress can be positive (described later in this chapter). However, stress usually is thought of as having a negative effect (e.g., fear, depression, and guilt). Recognizing and coping with anxiety and stress is important for a lasting career in the EMS profession.

PERSONAL TIME FOR MEDITATION AND CONTEMPLATION

Setting aside some personal time can boost mental and perhaps even physical health. This time can be spent meditating or contemplating. *Meditation* is a form of relaxation. To med-

BOX 2-12 Body Changes When You Stop Smoking

Within 20 Minutes of Your Last Cigarette
Pulse and blood pressure drop to normal.
Body temperature of hands and feet increases to normal.

Within 8 Hours of Your Last Cigarette
Carbon monoxide level in blood drops to normal.
Oxygen level in blood increases to normal.

Within 24 Hours of Your Last Cigarette
Chance of heart attack decreases.

Within 48 Hours of Your Last Cigarette
Nerve endings begin to regenerate.
Ability to smell and taste is enhanced.

Within 72 Hours of Your Last Cigarette
Bronchial tubes relax, making breathing easier.
Lung capacity increases.

Within 2 Weeks to 3 Months after Your Last Cigarette
Circulation improves.
Walking becomes easier.
Lung function increases up to 30%.

Within 1 to 9 Months after Your Last Cigarette
Coughing, sinus congestion, fatigue, and shortness of breath decrease.
Cilia regrow in lungs, increasing the ability to handle mucus, clean the lungs, and reduce infection.

Within 5 Years of Your Last Cigarette
Lung cancer death rate for the average smoker (one pack per day) decreases.

Within 10 Years of Your Last Cigarette
Lung cancer death rate drops to 12 deaths per 100,000—almost the rate of nonsmokers.
Precancerous cells are replaced.
Risk for other cancers—such as those of the mouth, larynx, esophagus, bladder, kidney, and pancreas—decreases (20 chemicals in tobacco smoke cause cancer).

When smokers quit—the health benefits over time. http://www.cancer.org/docroot/SPC_1 when smokers_quit.asp

itate, a person limits his or her awareness to a repeated or constant focus. The person may focus on something that holds some attraction (e.g., controlled breathing, a pleasant site, fragrance, or a mantra). This quiet time provides an uninterrupted period for thoughtful introspection (contemplation) of important things in a person's life. Most who practice meditation do so once or twice a day for 10 to 20 minutes.

NOTE Spirituality is a unique quality of human existence. Spirituality should not be overlooked as a means for some to achieve mental and physical well-being.

FAMILY, PEER, AND COMMUNITY CONNECTIONS

Belonging to a group can affect a person's motivation and performance in a positive way. Persons tend to associate with others most like themselves. These may be family members, co-workers, and members of community and religious organizations. These groups provide a connection with others who share similar values and interests. As a rule, these bonds are healthful and raise self-esteem. They provide a way for one to contribute to group activities and goals. They also allow persons to interact in decision making, communication, and cooperative work.

FREEDOM FROM PREJUDICE

Accepting cultural differences gives persons the chance to learn about other cultures. Such acceptance also helps them to see cultural variations in a positive light. Moreover, one affirms the values of these differences. The four major ethnic minority groups in the United States are Hispanic/Latinos (Mexican-American, Puerto Rican, Cuban, Central and South American), Asians (Chinese, Korean, Japanese), Southwest Asians (Vietnamese, Laotians, Cambodians), and African Americans. Providing health care to patients of some cultures may call for special communication skills. Provision of care also may require some further education to understand the customs and beliefs of that culture. Getting this education can be fulfilling and worthwhile, and it allows the paramedic to see life from another viewpoint.

STRESS

As previously stated, stress can be positive and negative. The responses to stress may be physical, emotional, or both. "Good" stress **(eustress)** is a positive response to stimuli. Eustress is considered protective. "Bad" stress **(distress)** is a negative response to environmental stimuli. Distress is the source of anxiety and stress-related disorders.

Phases of the Stress Response

Hans Selye was an Austrian-born professor at the University of Montreal. He coined the term *stress* in its medical usage in 1950. The three stages of the stress response he found are the alarm reaction, resistance, and exhaustion (Fig. 2-1).[2] Selye called these phases the general adaption syndrome. He gave them this name to describe the attempt of body and mind to deal with stressful events.

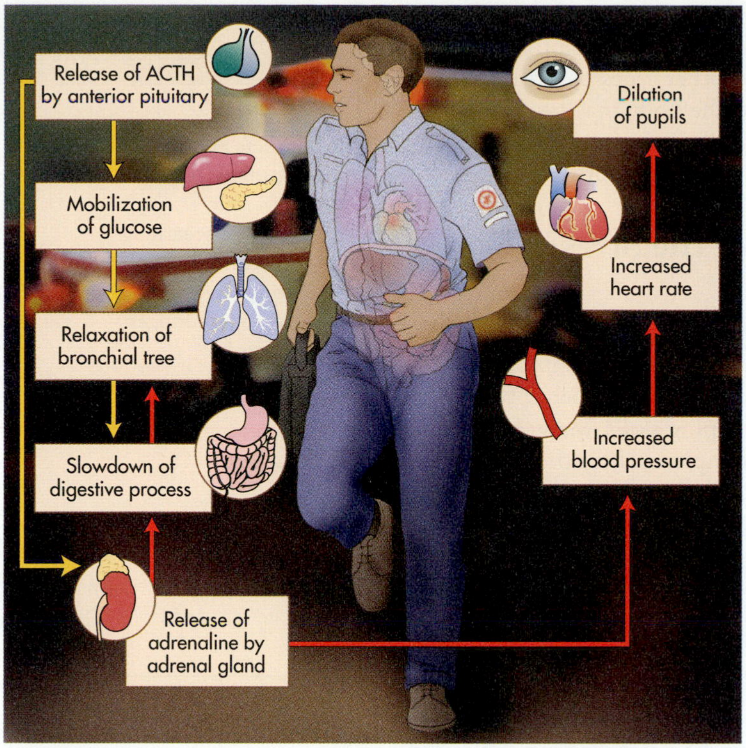

FIGURE 2-1 ■ Physiological response to stress. During the alarm reaction, the release of adrenocorticotropic hormone *(yellow)* results in a sympathetic discharge of adrenaline *(red)*. These stress hormones stimulate glucose production and cause the heart rate to increase, blood pressure to rise, and pupils to dilate. The bronchial tree relaxes for deep breathing, the digestive process slows, and the blood supply shifts to accommodate clotting mechanisms in case the body is wounded.

ALARM REACTION

The human body can prepare itself quickly to do battle or run from danger. This fight-or-flight reaction occurs when a situation threatens one's safety or comfort. This reaction is considered positive (eustress). The stress prepares individuals to be alert and to defend themselves. At first, the response of the body to stress is unaffected by the type of situation. The body reacts equally to events that are pleasant or unpleasant, dangerous or exciting, happy or sad. The purpose of the response is to achieve top physical preparedness rapidly to cope with the event. Examples would be an argument with a co-worker, performing an unfamiliar patient care procedure, and taking part in the delivery of a healthy infant.

The alarm reaction is set off by the **autonomic nervous system.** This reaction is coordinated by the hypothalamus. The hypothalamus triggers the pituitary gland to release adrenocorticotropic hormone into the bloodstream. This stress hormone stimulates the production of glucose. The hormone also increases the concentration of nutrients in the blood that provide energy. These nutrients are needed for the response to stress. Adrenocorticotropic hormone also activates the adrenal glands for an intense sympathetic discharge of **adrenaline** and noradrenaline. These hormones cause the heart rate to increase, blood pressure to rise, and the pupils of the eyes to dilate, which improves vision. Together these hormones relax the bronchial tree for deeper breathing, increase blood sugar for total energy, slow the digestive process, and shift blood supply to accommodate the clotting mechanism in case the body is wounded. After these physiological events, the body is ready for an emergency (fight or flight). The body can perform feats of strength and endurance far beyond its normal capacity. The alarm reaction takes only seconds. The reaction occurs to some extent at the first exposure of the body to a stressor. When the body realizes that an event is not dangerous or does not require the alarm reaction, the response stops. The individual begins to adapt to the situation. Then bodily functions return to normal.

RESISTANCE

The stress response raises the level of resistance to the agent that provoked it and others like it. That is, if a particular stress persists long enough, a person's reactions change. For example, a paramedic becomes accustomed to responding to emergency scenes in an ambulance using audible and visual warning devices. Thus the alarm reaction that once occurred is no longer elicited. Therefore reactions to stressors may change over time.

EXHAUSTION

As stress continues, coping mechanisms weaken. Then resistance fails. For example, paramedics may appear to be unaffected by the stress of life-threatening emergencies. However, all of their adaptive resources have been used to reach this stage of resistance. When any reservoir of adaptive resources no longer exists, resistance to other types of stress tends to decline as well. At that point, the body may become at risk for physical and psychological ills. Rest and recovery usually are needed before a person is ready for another emergency.

Factors That Trigger the Stress Response

Each person has unique means to deal with stressful situations. Individual reactions to stress are customized based on previous exposure to a specific type of stress, perception of the stressful event, and personal coping skills. Many factors can trigger the stress response. Examples include the following:

- Loss of something that is of value
- Injury or threat of injury
- Poor health or nutrition
- Frustration
- Ineffective coping skills

PHYSIOLOGICAL AND PSYCHOLOGICAL EFFECTS OF STRESS

Anxiety is a common symptom of stress. Feeling anxious in certain situations or unusual circumstances is normal and healthy. This response provides a warning system that protects persons from being overwhelmed by a sudden stimulation. Anxiety also prepares persons for action in critical situations. This adaptive response to stress prepares the paramedic to make quick, correct decisions regarding the emergency. Anxiety also allows the paramedic to perform at maximal efficiency.

Sometimes stress is not reduced by a solution to the conflict or emergency. This may lead to an ongoing state of vigilance and alertness beyond the initial event. The paramedic then may begin to feel chronic anxiety. This kind of anxiety fails to stimulate effective coping. In addition, a person may respond to conflict or stress by anxious behavior alone. Anxiety interferes with thought processes and with relationships and work performance. A person may develop problems concentrating, lose the ability to trust others, or become isolated or withdrawn.

Individuals who often are exposed to stressful situations or who are unable to cope with stressful events may experience a chronic state of anxiety. This state may lead to physical, emotional, cognitive, and behavioral effects (Box 2-13). Some warning signs may call for immediate evaluation and medical care. These signs include chest pain and difficulty breathing. Others call for less immediate action. The presence of one or more warning signs is an indicator of distress. However, absence of warning signs does not preclude the chance of a stress reaction.

BOX 2-13 Warning Signs and Symptoms of Stress

Physical
- Cardiac rhythm disturbances
- Chest pain
- Difficulty breathing
- Nausea
- Profuse sweating
- Sleep disturbances
- Vomiting

Cognitive
- Confusion
- Decreased level of awareness
- Difficulty making decisions
- Disorientation
- Distressing dreams
- Memory problems
- Poor concentration

Emotional
- Anger
- Denial
- Fear
- Feeling of being overwhelmed
- Inappropriate emotions
- Panic reactions

Behavioral
- Changes in eating habits
- Crying spells
- Excessive silence
- Hyperactivity
- Increased alcohol consumption
- Increased smoking
- Withdrawal

CAUSES OF STRESS IN EMERGENCY MEDICAL SERVICES

A variety of sources can produce stress in EMS work. Environmental stress includes noise, bad weather, confined spaces, poor lighting, spectators, rapid response to the scene, and life-and-death decision making. Psychosocial stress may arise from family relationships and can come from conflicts with co-workers, abusive patients, and similar sources. Personality stress relates to the way a person thinks and feels. For example, this kind of stress can include the need to be liked. Personality stress can include one's expectations and feelings of guilt and anxiety as well. Choosing a career in EMS requires developing an understanding of job-related stress and effective stress management.

REACTIONS TO STRESS

Certain types of persons may be attracted to certain types of careers. For example, some believe that EMS providers, firefighters, police officers, and others in public safety are inclined to stressful and demanding jobs.[3] However, no one is free from all conflict in managing stress.

ADAPTATION

Adaptation is a process that involves learning ways to deal with stressful situations. This process usually begins with using defense mechanisms. Next, adaptation focuses on developing coping skills, followed by problem solving. Finally, adaptation concludes with mastery.

Defense mechanisms are adaptive functions of the personality (Box 2-14). They assist a person in adjusting to stressful situations. They also help a person to avoid dealing with problems. *Denial,* for example, is a defense mechanism. Denial might be used to separate a person from the event long enough to deal with a problem that normally would be overwhelming.

Coping is an active process of confronting. Coping involves gathering information and using the information to change or adjust to a new situation. Taking part in regular physical

BOX 2-14 Common Defense Mechanisms

Repression
Repression is thought to be the mechanism underlying all other defense mechanisms. Repression is the involuntary attempt to keep certain feelings or memories from reaching conscious awareness. Traumatic events, intolerable and dangerous impulses, and other unacceptable ideas are forced out of consciousness. This defense mechanism may be seen as a result of an approach-avoidance conflict. This is a conflict between trying to recall or think about something and trying to avoid the topic because it creates fear. Once repressions form, they usually are difficult to abolish. The individual must be reassured that no danger exists in recalling the event. For example, an emergency medical services (EMS) co-worker is killed while on duty. The partner has no recall of the event from the time they arrived at the scene until after the event.

Regression
Regression is a return to earlier levels of emotional adjustment. Of all the reactions to anxiety and danger, regression may be the most dramatic and debilitating. A person returns to an earlier developmental phase of life. This phase may have been a time when tension and conflict could be avoided. For example, an EMS worker throws a temper tantrum because he was assigned driver status on a work shift when he thought he would have direct patient care duties.

Projection
Projection involves attributing one's own undesirable qualities, feelings, motives, or desires to someone else. Projection may appear as aggression toward others. However, the problem is actually self-anger. Often individuals are wrong in labeling their own motives and the motives of others. For example, a paramedic crashes an emergency vehicle en route to a call. Because of guilt, she feels that others blame her for the crash. In fact, she is blaming herself.

Rationalization
Rationalizations occur when persons feel the need to explain their behavior. This need may be a result of social training. They feel the need to explain because the true explanation would cause anxiety or guilt. A person is trying to prove that the behavior is "rational" and therefore worthy of the approval of self and others. Rationalization is a commonly used defense mechanism. For example, a paramedic performs a poor physical examination on a trauma patient. She fails to discover a femur fracture. When questioned by medical direction, she justifies her actions by saying that the police were hurrying her to clear the scene.

Compensation
Compensation is trying to cover up for a real or imagined weakness. One compensates by stressing a more positive trait or skill. This conceals frustration and anxiety by focusing attention on other behavior. For example, an EMS crew member has weak clinical skills and feels inadequate at emergency scenes. He compensates by becoming an instructor in water rescue.

Reaction Formation
Reaction formation is a defensive behavior that prevents desires that are undesirable from being expressed. The person exaggerates opposing attitudes and behavior, thereby expressing the opposite of the true motive. The original impulse is still present. However, the impulse is masked by actions or attitudes that do not cause anxiety or stress. For example, a paramedic is outwardly friendly to a co-worker whom she dislikes.

Sublimation
Sublimation is a form of substitution. Sublimation entails changing undesirable urges so that they are socially acceptable. Sublimation is a defense mechanism. However, the functions of sublimation are thought to extend beyond that of protection. Sublimation requires changing one's focus or energy. In this change, instinctual drives are substituted for ones that may result in a higher cultural achievement. For example, a paramedic may become angry from seeing people die in drunk-driving crashes. Thus he starts a public awareness program on the hazards of drinking and driving.

Denial
Denial is another defense mechanism. In denial the person rejects elements of reality that knowingly would be intolerable. The person gains protection from unpleasant reality by refusing to see it. The person may deny the event itself or the memory of it. For example, a person who has just lost a loved one may be unable to accept the reality of death. (Denial differs from repression. Persons who use repression as a defense mechanism seem deliberately to keep their feelings or memories at a distance from the conscious mind.)

Substitution
This defense mechanism switches another activity or goal for one that is desired but unreachable. Substitution may involve the redirection of an emotion from the first object to a more acceptable one. Substitution often results from frustration. For example, a co-worker is having marital problems. He feels that it is unacceptable to argue with his spouse. He substitutes and displaces his anger at work by being irritable, grouchy, and hostile toward other crew members.

Isolation
Isolation involves the separation of unacceptable impulses, acts, or ideas from their origin in memory. This defense mechanism removes the emotional charge from the event. Isolation prevents feelings from being linked to the memory. Isolation may be helpful to the EMS providers who must turn off feelings until after a call. For example, an EMS provider also may be a parent. This provider may have to give care to a dying child without being overcome by emotions.

activity is a great way to cope. Getting involved in activities at work that result in financial rewards and increased productivity is another. Finding humor in personal crises can be helpful. Moreover, talking though stressful events with family, friends, and co-workers is a good way to cope.

Persons also may use harmful or negative coping mechanisms. An individual may become withdrawn or use alcohol or other drugs. Some may have angry outbursts toward family members and co-workers. Others may become silent. These negative coping mechanisms threaten interpersonal relationships with co-workers and loved ones. They should be seen as signs that an individual is having trouble dealing with stress.

NOTE Burnout can be the result of cumulative stress. Burnout is defined by physical and emotional exhaustion and negative attitudes. Burnout can develop when one is exposed to chronic stress that cannot be managed with usual coping mechanisms.

Problem solving involves analyzing a problem and finding options to deal with the issue now and in the future. Problem solving allows a person to identify the problem clearly and come up with a course of action. This is a healthful approach to everyday concerns.

Mastery refers to the ability to see many options and solutions for problem situations. Mastery results from extensive experience and the use of effective coping mechanisms with situations that are similar. Mastery may be difficult to achieve.

STRESS MANAGEMENT TECHNIQUES

To manage stress well, a person must recognize the early warning signs of anxiety. Some of the physical effects of anxiety an individual may notice include the following:

- Heart palpitations
- Difficult or rapid breathing
- Dry mouth
- Chest tightness or pain
- Anorexia (lack of appetite), nausea, vomiting, diarrhea, abdominal cramps, flatulence, "butterflies"
- Flushing, diaphoresis (profuse sweating), body temperature fluctuation
- Urgency and frequency in urination
- Dysmenorrhea (painful menstruation), decreased sexual drive or performance
- Aching muscles, joints

Physical effects that may not be as noticeable include the following:

- Increased blood pressure and heart rate
- Blood shunting (diversion of the flow) to muscles
- Increased blood glucose levels
- Increased adrenaline production by adrenal glands
- Reduced gastrointestinal peristalsis
- Pupillary dilation

CRITICAL THINKING

Compare your reactions while on a highly stressful call in the field to those you experience when stressed about school. How are those feelings similar or different from each other?

Many warning signs appear during the emergency response or within 24 hours after the event. Some responses, however, may be delayed for some time. The responses may not appear for months or years after the event. If signs and symptoms of stress-related illness appear, the person should seek appropriate medical or psychological help.

Intervening to relieve stress is as key as recognizing the warning signals. Methods one may use initially to manage stress include reframing, controlled breathing, progressive relaxation, and guided imagery. All of these methods require practice to perform them properly. Reframing involves first looking at the situation from a different emotional viewpoint and then placing it in a different "frame" that fits the facts of another situation equally well. This acts to change the meaning of the situation. Controlled breathing is a natural stress control technique. A person concentrates on depth and rate of breathing to achieve a calming effect. Controlled breathing may begin with deep breathing, followed by less deep breathing, and finally normal breathing. Progressive relaxation is a stress reduction strategy in which the person systematically tightens and relaxes particular muscle groups (from head to toe or toe to head). This fools the brain into initiating muscle relaxation throughout the body. Guided imagery is used with meditation. Another person familiar with the technique acts as a guide during a stress response. The person experiencing stress then can focus on an image that helps relieve stress. (Once guided imagery is learned, a person can use the technique without prompting.)

Other ways to fight stress include being aware of personal limitations, peer counseling, and group discussions. Proper diet, sleep, and rest also help to relieve stress. In addition, pursuing positive activities outside of EMS can balance work and recreation. Ultimately, the individual must maintain personal health and well-being. However, intervention programs may be available through EMS agencies, hospitals, and other groups.

CRITICAL INCIDENT STRESS MANAGEMENT

Critical incident stress management (CISM) evolved from the early 1970s concept of critical incident stress debriefing. This program aimed to help emergency workers exposed to a major incident. Created by Jeff Mitchell, CISM is based on a partnership between mental health professionals and peer group support. Although the benefits of CISM as a form of psychological first aid are debated,[4] CISM is designed to give emergency workers a chance to vent their feelings about a call or event that had a major impact (Box 2-15).

BOX 2-15 Potential Situations for Critical Incident Stress Management

- Line-of-duty injury or death
- Disaster
- Emergency worker suicide
- Infant/child death
- Extreme threat to emergency worker
- Prolonged incident that ends in loss or success
- Victims known to operations personnel
- Death/injury of civilian caused by operations
- Other significant event

NOTE Defusing usually takes place within 8 hours after an event to allow an initial release of feelings. This also provides an opportunity for persons to share their experiences. Defusing is an informal gathering of the persons involved in the event and two-person teams trained in critical incident stress management who are also peers. A defusing usually lasts less than 1 hour.

Debriefing is more formal than defusing. Debriefing is conducted in a private setting and usually takes place 24 to 72 hours after the event. The debriefing is conducted by a specially trained critical incident stress management team of other emergency services personnel and mental health workers. Only those present at the incident are allowed to attend a debriefing.

Critical incident stress management aims to help emergency workers understand their reactions. It reassures them that what they are experiencing is normal. It also reassures them that what they are feeling may be common to others involved in the incident. The process may be for one person or may include various members of the emergency team (e.g., police, EMS crew members, firefighters, and emergency department staff). The 10 attributes of CISM are the following[5]:

1. Preincident stress training for all personnel
2. On-scene support for obviously distressed personnel
3. Individual consultations when only one or two personnel are affected by an incident
4. Defusing services immediately after a large-scale incident
5. Mobilization services after a large-scale incident
6. Critical incident stress debriefing 24 to 72 hours after an event for any emergency personnel involved in a stressful incident
7. Follow-up services to ensure that personnel are recovering
8. Specialty debriefings to nonemergency groups when no other timely resources are available within the community
9. Support during routine discussions of an incident by emergency personnel
10. Advice to command staff during large-scale events

In addition to CISM, other efforts can help manage stress. These efforts include employee assistance programs, counseling, spouse support programs, family life programs, pastoral services, and periodic stress evaluations. These efforts and others can be good resources to the paramedic in dealing with stress on the job (Box 2-16).

BOX 2-16 Techniques for Reducing Crisis-Induced Stress

- Allow adequate rest for emergency workers
- Provide food and fluid replacement
- Limit exposure to the incident
- Change assignments
- Provide postevent defusing/debriefing

CRITICAL THINKING

Imagine which type of call would be a critical incident for you personally.

DEALING WITH DEATH, DYING, GRIEF, AND LOSS

Death and dying always will be part of health care delivery. Medical science has given society the ability to postpone death in some instances and perhaps lessen its physical pain. However, the fight for self-preservation is still inevitably lost.

Patient and Family Needs

In the delivery of EMS, paramedics at times will give care to a dying person surrounded by loved ones. In such cases, the emotional needs of the dying patient, family, and loved ones should be of utmost importance. The patient and significant others will need to be comforted, given privacy, and treated with respect and dignity. Loved ones may need to express feelings of rage, anger, despair, and guilt. They may need the paramedic to provide control and direction for this solemn event. The paramedic's role in these cases is important and may be a determining factor in the way survivors adjust to their loss (Box 2-17).

Stages of the Grieving Process

In 1968 Elizabeth Kübler-Ross began her work on the psychological aspects of death and dying. Her studies identified five predictable stages of dying: denial, anger, bargaining, depression, and acceptance. Kübler-Ross found that patients and loved ones dealing with the death process generally experience the following five stages[6]:

1. *Denial* is characterized by the feeling "No, not me." Denial is an expected response to news of a life-threatening illness or situation. The news is so overwhelming that it must be absorbed slowly. The patient seeks other opinions, verifies the accuracy of medical reports, or

BOX 2-17 Hospice Programs

Hospice programs began in England in 1967. They since have become a standard service of many health care institutions in the United States. Their goal is to help the terminally ill patient, family, and loved ones cope when death is expected. The hospice philosophy supports home care for the patient. Home care provides for a more natural environment. In addition, volunteers and health care professionals provide counseling and other psychological support to the patient and family during the death process. Hospice programs are well respected in the medical community. The programs play an important role in helping patients and their families accept death as a natural event in life.

simply seems to ignore what he or she has been told. Denial is a valuable defense mechanism. Denial is troubling only when no indication exists that the patient understands the seriousness of the situation. Most patients, families, and friends deny death to some degree to continue with the daily business of living.

2. *Anger* can be viewed as the "Why me?" phase. Anger is probably the most difficult for persons who care about or are trying to help the dying person. In this phase, the person rejects all efforts to help or console. This anger is really the anger of the dying person toward all the persons who continue to live. More accurately, anger may be anger directed toward God because He does not appear to have acted fairly or justly with the dying person.
3. *Bargaining* is reflected in a "Yes, me, but . . ." frame of mind. The person admits the reality of being sick and of probably dying, but the person tries to bargain for extension or quality of life. These bargains usually are secret, frequently are made with God, and rarely are kept. For example, a father promises to be a "perfect patient" if only he can live to see his son's wedding.
4. *Depression* is the "Yes, me" reaction to anticipated death. Depression involves preparing to say and saying goodbye to everything and everyone a person has known and loved. The inherent sadness of this phase is appropriate and should be respected.
5. *Acceptance,* the simple and quiet "Yes," grows out of individuals' convictions that they have done what they could to be ready to die. Personal energy and interpersonal interests decrease significantly. During this phase, relatives and friends usually need more help than the dying person. The dying person's most important wish at this point is not to die alone.

NOTE Dying patients and their loved ones may fluctuate between these stages and may or may not experience all five stages.

Paramedics rarely are involved in a patient's process of coming to terms with death. However, they often see the reactions of patients and families going through the death process. For example, denial may be obvious in some family members. These people may not appear to see or acknowledge the seriousness of a situation in which decisions about resuscitation must be made. Anger may be directed at the paramedic crew or other health care workers. Bargaining may occur in the form of a mother who says, "Please save my child, and I promise that I'll always make her wear her seat belt!" The paramedic must realize the psychological aspects of the stages of grief (Box 2-18).

BOX 2-18 Recommended Communication Strategies

A situation involving death and dying is uncomfortable. Communication with the patient and loved ones may be difficult. The following recommendations for communications and activities may help a paramedic deal with dying patients and their families:

- Answer questions honestly for the patient and family and explain all activities.
- Do not initiate the subject of dying; let it come from the patient or family.
- If the patient or family asks you whether the patient is going to die, advise that you are doing everything you possibly can but that the situation is critical. This allows a brief time for the patient and family to prepare themselves.
- Do not falsely reassure the patient or family (e.g., "everything's going to be okay").
- Use compassionate, nonverbal communication (facial expression, touching).
- Offer to contact someone if the patient is alone.
- If family is not present, assure the patient that emergency department personnel will notify them. If they are nearby, encourage the family to come to the patient immediately or to meet the patient at the emergency department.
- Allow the family to stay with the patient when appropriate.

When it is necessary to give news of a sudden death to a family, the paramedic's initial contact can influence the grief response greatly. The paramedic should gather the family in a private area and advise them of the patient's death, with a brief account of the situation causing the death. The paramedic should use the words *death* or *dead* and should avoid euphemisms such as "he's passed on" or "she's no longer with us." The paramedic should be compassionate and allow time for the news to be absorbed and for questions to be asked. The family members should be allowed to see the relative if they choose. They should be told in advance if resuscitation equipment is still connected to the patient. These efforts, along with empathic interaction with the family, help relatives deal with the loss of a loved one.

Common Needs of the Paramedic When Dealing with Death and Dying

Dealing with death is difficult for everyone. Thus the paramedic's feelings and emotions also must be considered. The paramedic may experience some of the same stages of grief described earlier. These reactions are normal. In fact, the paramedic may expend a great deal of effort to disguise or suppress these emotions at the scene or while rendering care. However, the paramedic should discuss these feelings as soon as possible with friends, coworkers, and family. The paramedic should discuss these emotions in a constructive way that will lessen the emotional burden. Like others, the paramedic will need a chance to process the incident and obtain closure. Available resources, such as employee assistance programs and counseling and pastoral services, help avoid the effects of cumulative stress.

CRITICAL THINKING

What personal experiences have you had with death? How did you or others who were close to the deceased react to the initial news of the death?

BOX 2-19 Disease Transmission Terminology

Airborne and blood-borne pathogens are organisms carried through air or blood (and other body fluids). These organisms create disease in the human body or host. Some pathogens (e.g., certain bacteria) can survive outside a host. Others (such as viruses) can survive only in the human cell (see Chapter 39). Exposure occurs in cases of contact with a likely infectious body fluid or other infectious agent. Certain steps are used to destroy infectious organisms that may have come in contact with equipment and instruments. These steps include cleaning, disinfection, and sterilization. Body substance isolation is also known as universal precautions. These precautions are practices to prevent or reduce contact with body substances and other infectious agents.

Developmental Considerations When Dealing with Death and Dying

The way persons cope with their own death or the death of a loved one depends on their age, maturity, and understanding of death. The paramedic should be sensitive to the emotional needs of all age groups during this crisis. The following guidelines may be helpful when offering advice to family members who will be helping the young or elderly cope with the death of a loved one.[5]

Children up to age 3 probably will sense that something has happened in the family. They will realize that others are sad and crying. They also may be aware of increased activity in the household. The family should be urged to watch for changes in eating or sleeping patterns and for an increase in irritability. In addition, the family should be sensitive to the child's needs and try to maintain consistency in the child's routines and with significant persons in the child's life.

Children 3 to 6 years of age do not have a concept of the finality of death. They may believe that the person will return and may ask "when" continually. This age group believes in magical thinking and may feel that they are responsible for the death. They also may believe that everyone else they love will die too. The family should watch for changes in the child's behavior patterns with friends and at school, for difficulty sleeping, and for changes in eating habits. The family should emphasize that the child is not responsible for the death. The family should reinforce the fact that crying is normal when persons are sad and should encourage children to talk about their feelings.

Children 6 to 9 years of age are beginning to understand the finality of death. They want detailed explanations for the death and can differentiate fatal illness from just "being sick." Like the 3- to 6-year-olds, these children may be afraid that other loved ones will die too. This age group may be uncomfortable with expressing their feelings and may act silly or embarrassed when talking about death. The paramedic should suggest to the family that they talk about the normal feelings of anger, sadness, and guilt and that they share their own feelings about death with the child. The family members should not hesitate to cry because crying will let the child know that expression of feelings is acceptable.

Children 9 to 12 years of age are aware of the finality of death. They may want to know the details surrounding the event. They will be concerned with practical matters involving their lifestyle and may try to "act like an adult." (Most of these children, however, will show regression to an earlier stage of emotional response.) The paramedic should suggest to the family that they set aside time to talk to the child about feelings and encourage the sharing of memories to aid in the grief response.

Older adults usually show concern for other family members. In addition, they may be worried about their further loss of independence and about financial matters at hand. Family members should be sensitive and understanding about these issues because they are real for this age group.

PREVENTION OF DISEASE TRANSMISSION

Emergency workers often manage ill and injured patients. Thus prevention of disease transmission must be a priority in daily practice. Specific concerns arise for personal health and safety. One concern includes being aware of common sources of exposure. Another includes using personal protection. Finally, one must know what to do if an exposure has occurred (Box 2-19).

Common Sources of Exposure

Common sources of exposure to infectious agents in the prehospital setting include needlesticks and broken or scraped skin. Mucous membranes such as those that line the eyes, nose, and mouth also are a source for entry of infectious agents or microorganisms. As a result, the paramedic must practice universal precautions during all patient care encounters.

Protection from Airborne and Blood-Borne Pathogens

The following list contains some general guidelines to help prevent exposure to infectious diseases (a more complete discussion of infectious disease is presented in Chapter 39):

1. Follow engineering and work practices. Maintain good personal health and hygiene habits. (Wash hands frequently and pay attention to general cleanliness.)
2. Maintain immunizations for tetanus, diphtheria, polio, hepatitis B, MMR (measles, mumps, and rubella), and influenza.
3. Conduct a periodic screening for tuberculosis.
4. Practice body substance isolation (universal precautions) in all encounters with patients.
5. Properly clean, disinfect, and dispose of used materials and equipment immediately.
6. Use puncture-resistant containers to dispose of needles and other sharp objects.
7. Separate and label all soiled laundry (clothes, bed linens). Also separate and label all equipment. Do this until the items can be cleaned and disinfected properly.
8. Conduct a periodic risk assessment of health.

Documentation and Management of an Exposure

The paramedic must learn how to document and manage an exposure. The paramedic must be familiar with laws, regulations, and national standards that address issues of infectious disease. The paramedic also must take personal protective measures. In the event of a potential exposure to an infectious disease or a significant exposure to a patient's blood or body fluids, the paramedic should do the following:

1. Wash the area of contact with soap and water thoroughly and immediately.
2. Immediately document the situation in which the exposure occurred.
3. Describe actions taken to reduce chances of infection.
4. Comply with all required reporting responsibilities and time frames.
5. Cooperate with incident investigation.
6. Be screened for antibody titers and potential infectious diseases.
7. Obtain proper immunization boosters.
8. Obtain a full medical follow-up.

SUMMARY

- Wellness has two main aspects: physical well-being and mental and emotional health.
- As health care professionals, paramedics have a responsibility to serve as role models in disease prevention.
- Physical fitness can be described as a condition that helps individuals look, feel, and do their best.
- Sleep helps to rejuvenate a tired body.
- Steps to reduce cardiovascular disease include the following: improving cardiovascular endurance, eliminating cigarette smoking, controlling high blood pressure, maintaining a normal body-fat composition, maintaining good total cholesterol/high-density lipoprotein ratio, monitoring triglyceride levels, controlling diabetes, avoiding excessive alcohol, eating healthy foods, reducing stress, and making a periodic risk assessment.
- Most common cancers are linked to one of three environmental risk factors: smoking, sunlight, and diet.
- Injuries on the job can be minimized. Knowledge of body mechanics during lifting and moving is helpful. Also, being alert for hostile settings is key. Prioritization of personal safety during rescue situations is wise. In addition, paramedics must practice safe vehicle operation. They must use safety equipment and supplies as well.
- The misuse and abuse of drugs and other substances may lead to chemical dependency (addiction). This may have a wide range of effects on physical and mental health.
- "Good" stress is eustress. Eustress is a positive response to stimuli and is considered protective. "Bad" stress is distress. Distress is a negative response to environmental stimuli and is the source of anxiety and stress-related disorders.
- Adaptation is a process in which persons learn effective ways to deal with stressful situations. This dynamic process usually begins with using defense mechanisms. Next, one develops coping skills, followed by problem solving, and culminating in mastery.
- Critical incident stress management is designed to help emergency personnel understand their reactions. The process reassures them that what they are experiencing is normal and may be common to others involved in the incident.
- Often news of a sudden death must be given to a family. The paramedic's initial contact can influence the grief process greatly.
- The paramedic's duty is to be familiar with laws, regulations, and national standards that address issues of infectious disease. The paramedic also must take personal protective measures to guard against exposure.
- Actions to take after significant exposure include disinfection, documentation, incident investigation, screening, immunization, and medical follow-up.

REFERENCES

1. American Heart Association: *2002 heart and stroke statistics update,* Dallas, 2002, The Association.
2. Selye H: *The stress of life,* New York, 1956, McGraw-Hill.
3. Mitchell J, Bray G: *Emergency services stress: guidelines for preserving the health and careers of emergency services personnel,* Englewood Cliffs, NJ, 1990, Brady.
4. Mental and social aspects of health of populations exposed to extreme stressors, Department of Mental Health and Substance Dependence, WHO/MSD/MER/03.01, Geneva, 2003, World Health Organization.
5. US Department of Transportation, National Highway Traffic Safety Administration: *EMT-Paramedic national standard curriculum,* Washington, DC, 1998, The Department.
6. Bassuk EL, Fox SS, Prendergast KJ: *Behavioral emergencies,* Boston, 1983, Little, Brown.

CHAPTER 3

Injury Prevention

OBJECTIVES

Upon completion of this chapter, the paramedic student will be able to:

1. Identify roles of the emergency medical services community in injury prevention.
2. Describe the epidemiology of trauma in the United States.
3. Outline the aspects of the emergency medical services system that make it a desirable resource for involvement in community health activities.
4. Describe community leadership activities that are essential to enable the active participation of emergency medical services in community wellness activities.
5. List areas with which paramedics should be familiar to participate in injury prevention.
6. Evaluate a situation to determine opportunities for injury prevention.
7. Identify resources necessary to conduct a community health assessment.
8. Relate how alterations in the epidemiological triangle can influence injury and disease patterns.
9. Differentiate among primary, secondary, and tertiary health prevention activities.
10. Describe strategies to implement a successful injury prevention program.

KEY TERMS

community health assessment: An assessment of a target community to identify needs and resources required to provide prevention and wellness promotion activities.

injury risk: Real or potentially hazardous situations that put individuals at increased risk for sustaining an injury.

injury surveillance: The ongoing systematic collection, analysis, and interpretation of injury data essential to the planning, implementation, and evaluation of public health practice.

primary injury prevention: The practice of preventing an injury from occurring.

teachable moment: The time after an injury has occurred when the patient and observers remain acutely aware of what has happened and may be more receptive to being taught ways that the event or illness could have been prevented.

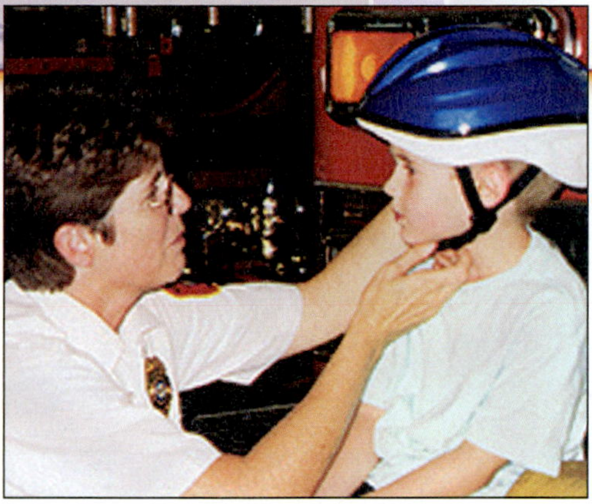

A community has a duty to provide injury prevention to its citizens. This prevention can occur in the form of leadership and educational activities. One goal of injury prevention is to decrease the incidence of preventable illness and injury. Another is to preserve life and function. A final goal is to prevent persons from needing costly medical care. As a member of the health care system the EMS provider can be a key resource in injury prevention programs (Box 3-1).

INJURY EPIDEMIOLOGY

Injuries that are unintentional are the leading cause of death among all persons 1 to 33 years of age. Unintentional injuries are the fifth leading cause of death overall. This cause is exceeded only by heart disease, cancer, stroke, and chronic obstructive pulmonary disease.[1] In 2001, 98,000 injury-related deaths occurred in the United States.

Injuries that are unintentional result in more years of life lost before 65 years of age than any other cause of death. From a financial view the effect of fatal and nonfatal unintentional injuries was $516.9 billion in 2001. This equaled about $5,000 per household (Fig. 3-1). The quality of life lost from these injuries is valued at another $1,172.3 billion. This makes the total cost $1,689.2 billion in 2001[1] (Table 3-1). About 37% of all emergency department visits in the United States are related to injury. This percentage accounts for more than 40 million visits to emergency departments in 2000 (Box 3-1).

▶ **NOTE** While you are reading this chapter, at least 4 persons will be killed by unintentional injury. Another 390 will be disabled. A death caused by unintentional injury occurs in the United States every 6 minutes.

OVERVIEW OF INJURY PREVENTION

For the most part, emergency medical services (EMS) has been a reactionary medical discipline. This means that EMS is not used until after patients are injured or ill. Reactionary medical care is termed *the acute care phase of injury control.* Reactionary medical care also is called *tertiary injury prevention.* Although EMS excels in acute care, a full system of injury control is made up of several facets of which acute care is one. The injury control strategy of preventing rather than simply treating an injury is known as **primary injury prevention.**

Preventive strategies yield better outcomes than treatment strategies in terms of lives saved and money spent. The success of these strategies weighs heavily on data collection. Success also depends on giving injury prevention information to patients. Paramedics are respected in the community and generally are welcomed into homes and businesses. Thus paramedics have a unique chance to find injury patterns and intervene on behalf of persons at risk.

Injury Concepts

DEFINITION OF INJURY

A puzzling factor that hindered the study of injury and therefore injury prevention was the seeming unrelatedness of injuries. On the surface, no relationship seemed to exist between a vehicle crash and a poisoning or a gunshot wound and a drowning. However, it now is known that all injuries are the result of either of two things. One is tissue damage caused by the transfer of energy to the human body. This energy may be mechanical, thermal, electrical, chemical, or radiation. The second is tissue damage caused by the absence of needed energy elements. These elements include things such as heat or oxygen. (See Chapter 20.)

THE INJURY TRIANGLE AND HADDON'S MATRIX

Injury is also a disease process. Three factors are necessary to cause a disease: host, agent, and environment. Together these three factors are known as *the injury triangle.* In the in-

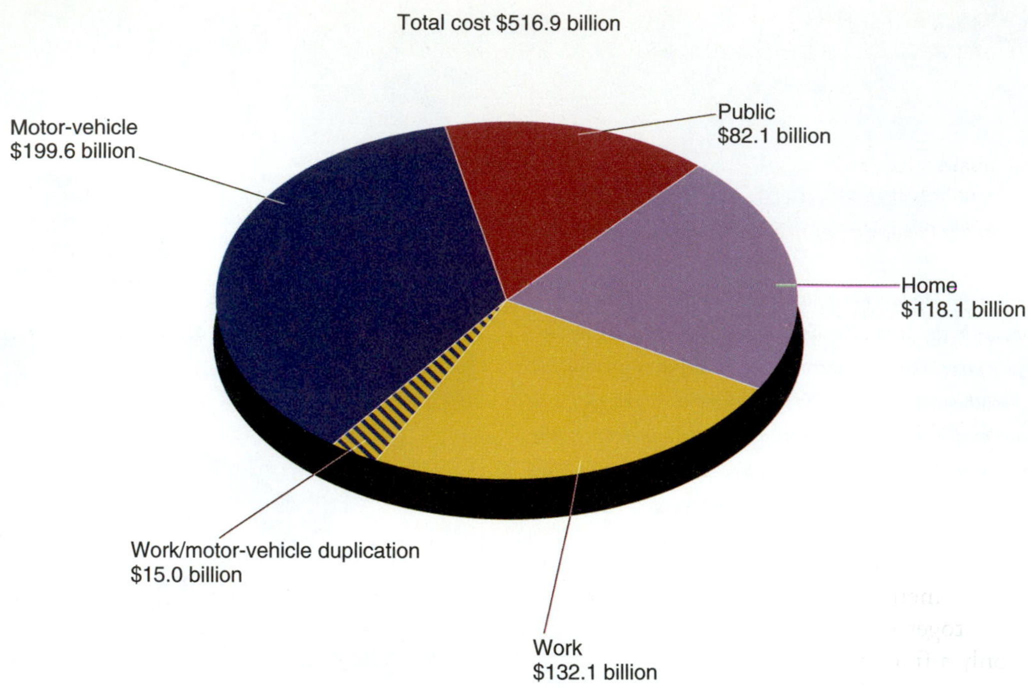

FIGURE 3-1 ■ Cost of unintentional injuries by class in 2001.

TABLE 3-1 Cost Equivalents, 2001

THE COST OF	IS EQUIVALENT TO
All injuries ($516.9 billion)	52 cents of every dollar paid in federal personal income taxes, **or** 52 cents of every dollar spent on food in the United States.
Motor vehicle crashes ($199.6 billion)	Purchasing 590 gallons of gasoline for each registered vehicle in the United States, **or** More than $1,000 per licensed driver, **or** Nearly 11 times greater than the combined profits reported by ExxonMobil and Chevron Texaco.
Work injuries ($132.1 billion)	32 cents of every dollar of corporate dividend to stockholders, **or** 19 cents of every dollar of pre-tax corporate profits, **or** Exceeds the combined profits reported by the top 15 Fortune 500 companies.
Home injuries ($118.1 billion)	A $94,000 rebate on each new single-family home built, **or** 46 cents of every dollar of property taxes paid.
Public injuries ($82.1 billion)	A $91 million grant to each public library in the United States, **or** A $99,600 bonus for each police officer and firefighter.

Courtesy National Safety Council estimates.

BOX 3-1 Injury and Illness Prevention Terminology

Injury: Intentional or unintentional damage to the person resulting from acute exposure to thermal, mechanical, electrical, or chemical energy or the absence of essentials such as heat and oxygen

Injury risk: Real or potentially hazardous situations that put individuals at increased risk for sustaining an injury

Injury surveillance: The ongoing collection, analysis, and interpretation of injury data essential to the planning, implementation, and evaluation of public health practice, closely integrated with the timely dissemination of these data to those who need to know, with the final link in the chain being the application of these data to prevention and control

Primary injury prevention: The practice of preventing an injury from occurring

Secondary and tertiary prevention: The care and rehabilitation activities, respectively, that are intended to prevent further problems from an event that has occurred already

Teachable moment: The time after an injury has occurred when the patient and observers remain acutely aware of what has happened and may be more receptive to being taught ways that the event or illness could be prevented

Years of productive life: The calculation obtained by subtracting the age of the victim's death from 65 (the average age of retirement)

TABLE 3-2 Haddon's Matrix for Automobile Crashes

	FACTOR		
PHASE	**HOST**	**AGENT**	**ENVIRONMENT**
Pre-event	Impaired capabilities, age, fatigue, alcohol/drug use, driving experience, adherence to driving laws	Defective equipment, dirty windows, improper maintenance, equipment design	Road shoulder too narrow, poor lighting, weather conditions, highway not divided, inadequate notification signs, road design, and construction
Event	Injury threshold due to aging, chronic disease, alcohol, use of restraints, ejection	Failure of doors, impact with sharp objects in the vehicle, vehicle size	Lack of guardrails, large trees near roadside, oncoming traffic
Post-event	Type or extent of injury, knowledge of first aid, alcohol	Bursting gas tanks, entrapment	Quality of rescue, EMS, hospitals, rehabilitation

jury triangle the host is the victim, the agent of injury is energy, and the environment provides a place for the agent and host to come together over time. The actual injury event may take only a fraction of a second, but the events that lead up to an injury and the events that occur as a result of an injury may take place over seconds, months, or even years.

In the mid-1960s, William Haddon (the "father" of injury prevention) came up with a tool to aid in understanding the entire injury sequence. This analytical tool is now known as *Haddon's matrix.* The three factors of the injury triangle are placed in a table on a timeline that is divided into three phases. These phases are pre-event, event, and postevent. For example, the Haddon's matrix in Table 3-2 charts the events that may occur before, during, and after a car crash. The table helps one to see that injuries often result from a predictable and therefore preventable chain of events. The matrix also affirms that most injuries are linked with many causes.

The *pre-event phase* is the period before the release of injury-causing energy. During this time the person's performance is greater than the task demands and energy is under control. Events in this phase tend to influence the *likelihood* that an injury will occur. Because the injury has yet to occur, primary injury prevention can take place in this phase. The time frame can be seconds to years, depending on what events come into play to cause the injury.

The *event phase* is the period during which the person's performance falls below the demands of the task. The result is the release of uncontrolled energy. The time frame usually is a fraction of a second to a few minutes. Events in this phase affect the transmission of energy. *Secondary injury prevention* recognizes that injuries are going to occur and is centered on reducing the severity of the injury as it is occurring.

The *postevent phase* is the period after the injury has occurred. This phase can last from a few seconds to years. In this time frame, tertiary injury prevention takes place and traditional EMS exists. The focus of tertiary injury prevention is to lessen the long-term adverse effects of the injury.

The Three E's of Injury Prevention

Three broad practices typically have been used to establish injury prevention programs. The first *E* of injury prevention is education. The second *E* is enforcement. The third *E* is engineering. A proactive, prevention-oriented EMS professional can play a key role in all three strategies.

EDUCATION

The purpose of education is to persuade high-risk persons or groups to change risky behavior. Education also is meant to teach these persons to adopt safety precautions. These precautions may include using personal restraints or wearing crash helmets. Education is considered an active countermeasure. Education requires the person to do something to take advantage of knowledge learned. Education often requires the person to make a behavioral change. Education is the most often used approach in injury prevention. Education is most effective when used with enforcement and engineering.

ENFORCEMENT

Enforcement requires that persons adopt certain behaviors that reduce risk. Enforcement occurs through force of law. Mandatory personal restraint (e.g., lap and shoulder restraints) and motorcycle helmet use laws are examples of this approach. Like education, enforcement is seen as an active countermeasure. Enforcement requires the person to adhere to the law to benefit from it. The success of this approach depends on compliance of individuals. Success also depends on the ability to enforce these laws. Even so, enforcement is more effective than education alone.

ENGINEERING

Engineering refers to product or environmental design. This design automatically provides protection or decreases the likelihood that an injury-producing incident will occur. This approach builds safety into a product. Thus a person does not have to do anything to benefit from engineering. Engineering is a passive countermeasure. Examples include air bags in cars and sprinkler systems in buildings. Engineering has proved to be the most effective of the three

E's. However, engineering also is the most expensive approach to undertake.

FEASIBILITY OF EMERGENCY MEDICAL SERVICES INVOLVEMENT

The United States has more than 600,000 EMS providers. As noted in *Emergency Medical Services: Agenda for the Future,* "People attracted to the EMS service are among society's best, and desire to contribute to their community's health. The composition of the EMS workforce reflects the diversity of the population it serves."[2] Thus it seems fitting that EMS plays a role in educating the public as a part of promoting health. The EMS workforce is a valuable human resource. The following points support the feasibility of EMS involvement in community health and injury prevention:

- Emergency medical services providers are often the most medically educated persons in rural settings.
- Emergency medical services providers are role models with high profiles.
- Emergency medical services providers often are seen as the champions of the customer.
- Emergency medical services providers are welcome in homes, schools, and other settings.
- Emergency medical services providers are seen as authorities on injury and prevention.
- Emergency medical services providers are often the first to spot situations that pose a risk for illness or injury (e.g., unsanitary conditions and unsafe home environments).

CRITICAL THINKING

Can you remember any program that a firefighter or paramedic taught you when you were a child? How did you feel about the firefighters and paramedics?

NOTE As managed care evolves, a demand on emergency medical services for supportive care and intervention will increase. Paramedics and emergency medical services agencies must adapt to their new role in the health care delivery system (Box 3-2).

BOX 3-2 Effects of Health Care Reform on Emergency Medical Services

To control costs, managed care reduces the number and length of hospitalizations. Because sicker patients are released from hospitals earlier, the chance for repeat emergency medical services calls to the same homes or sites is increased. These calls are for emergencies and nonemergency transportations to convalescent care. They also are for readmission to or follow-up services at hospitals. The need to provide some supportive medical care and intervention in the patient's home is also growing (see Chapter 48). Examples of services that paramedics and other health care workers provide to patients in their homes include the following:

- Caring for patients on monitors, ventilators, infusion pumps, and other complex medical equipment
- Drawing blood samples
- Providing wound care
- Measuring blood pressure
- Performing 12-lead electrocardiograms
- Performing other duties traditionally done before patients were released from the hospital

Many patients now take their own intravenous antibiotics and other intravenous medications at home. Premature infants ("premie graduates") often go home with advanced monitoring and life support equipment. Paramedics must be ready to help these patients with their special needs.

BOX 3-3 Essential Community Leadership Activities

Communities have the responsibility to assist and support emergency medical services (EMS) providers in the following activities:

- Protect the EMS provider from injury.
- Provide primary injury prevention education to EMS providers.
- Support and promote collection and use of injury data.
- Obtain support and resources for primary injury prevention activities.
- Empower individual EMS providers to conduct primary injury prevention activities.

Note: Emergency medical services, through expanded scope of practice, will be performing these leadership activities for injury prevention and wellness.

Essential Community Leadership Activities

Emergency medical services providers need to play an active role in community health and injury prevention programs. Other personnel in public service need to have active roles as well. The community must take the following steps to make sure of successful participation among these groups (Box 3-3).

PROTECT THE EMERGENCY MEDICAL SERVICES PROVIDER FROM INJURY

A basic first step for preventing injury and promoting wellness in a community is to protect the well-being of EMS personnel. Policies should help to ensure EMS safety during an emergency response, while the provider is at the scene, and during patient transportation. Protection can be accomplished with traffic safety laws and public education. Protection also can be enhanced with the help of law enforcement, fire service personnel, and other public service agencies.

All EMS workers must have access to personal protective equipment. This equipment helps to lessen eye, back, and skin injury. Other valuable safety tactics also are available. One is to reduce exposure to communicable diseases. Protection from hazardous chemicals also is crucial.

Communities can reduce injuries related to work through personal safety programs. Communities also can reduce injuries by creating a wellness program for EMS workers. (See Chapter 2.)

PROVIDE EDUCATION TO EMERGENCY MEDICAL SERVICES PROVIDERS

Primary and continuing education programs for emergency medical services personnel should include the basics of primary injury prevention. Community leaders should help to create a liaison between EMS programs and public and private specialty groups. These groups may include hospitals, other public health and safety agencies, safety councils, social services, religious organizations, colleges, and universities. This link will help to aid in specific education and training. Cooperation among these groups can help to find targets for prevention activities. Cooperation also encourages sharing the tasks of establishing programs.

SUPPORT AND PROMOTE COLLECTION AND USE OF INJURY DATA

Communities should create policies that encourage EMS providers to record all injuries. Communities should review and at times modify the tools for data collection. Such modification will make prompt recording of data feasible and realistic. The data collected should contribute to local, state, and national surveillance programs. For instance, these programs may include head and spinal cord injury registries.

OBTAIN SUPPORT AND RESOURCES FOR PRIMARY INJURY PREVENTION ACTIVITIES

The community needs to set up budgetary support for injury prevention programs. In addition, the community may need to seek other financial resources for fees and equipment, publicity, networking with other injury prevention organizations, and initiating or attending meetings of local organizations that are involved or that are requesting involvement in injury prevention. The community can get grants from state and national groups to help fund these initiatives. Examples of such organizations include the Centers for Disease Control and Prevention and Emergency Medical Services for Children. Communities also can get grants from private donors, community block grants, and institutions. The funding may not always be easy to obtain. Regardless of how funding is obtained, EMS workers have a duty to provide prevention initiatives on any call where a preventable event has occurred.

EMPOWER INDIVIDUAL EMERGENCY MEDICAL SERVICES PROVIDERS TO CONDUCT PRIMARY INJURY PREVENTION ACTIVITIES

The community must support injury prevention programs financially to support and promote interest and involvement in injury prevention activities from EMS providers. This support can influence individual EMS provider participation in the following ways:

- Providing rotating assignments to prevention programs
- Providing salary for off-duty injury prevention activities
- Rewarding and/or remunerating participation for on- and off-duty prevention activities

Essential Provider Activities

Activities that are essential for EMS workers are based on education. These activities include knowing and practicing the personal injury prevention strategies. Box 3-4 lists these strategies. The EMS provider also needs to know about illnesses and injuries common to various age groups, recreational activities, workplaces, and other facilities in the community (Box 3-5).

BOX 3-4 Personal Injury Prevention Strategies

Appropriate use of audible and visual warning devices
Availability and use of law enforcement
Exercise and conditioning
Practice of on-scene survival techniques
Proper driving techniques
Recognition of health hazards and high-profile crime areas
Restraint use (self, patient, passengers)
Safe approach to, parking at, and exiting the scene
Safe driving
Scene safety precautions
Stress management (personal, family, work)
Traffic control (vehicles, bystanders)
Use of on-scene survival resources
Use of personal protective equipment (reflective clothing, helmets)
Use of proper lifting and moving techniques
Wellness

BOX 3-5 Other Essential Provider Activities

Other essential provider activites include review of illness and injuries common to the following:
Infancy (low birth weight; mortality and morbidity)
Childhood (intentional, unintentional, or alleged intentional events)
Childhood violence to self and others
Adults
Geriatric patients
Recreation activities
Work hazards
Day care centers (licensed and nonlicensed)
Early release from hospital
Discharge from urgent care or other outpatient facilities
Signs of emotional stress that can lead to intentional, unintentional, or alleged events
Self-medication
Dangers of noncompliance (borrowing, not taking medicines on time or finishing the regimen)
Storage
Overmedication and polypharmacy

Implementation and Prevention Strategies

In addition to the primary personal injury prevention strategies described in Box 3-4, there are other key strategies. The EMS provider needs to use these prevention strategies for patient care considerations. The EMS provider needs to recognize the signs and symptoms of exposure to danger and the need for outside assistance. The EMS provider must document primary care and injury data as well. Finally, on-scene education is essential.

PATIENT CARE CONSIDERATIONS

The EMS provider needs to identify signs and symptoms of suspected abuse. The EMS provider also must recognize potentially abusive situations. Such recognition helps to ensure the safety of the EMS crew and the patient (see Chapter 46). Preplanning for these events helps to identify outside resources. These sources may include support programs. Such programs may be sponsored by municipal, community, and religious organizations (Box 3-6).

RECOGNITION OF DANGEROUS SITUATIONS

A priority for the paramedic is personal safety. Thus the EMS worker must stay alert for signs of dangerous situations. This includes recognizing general and specific environmental parameters. These parameters will help the paramedic to assess a patient's need for preventive information. These parameters also will help the paramedic to assess a patient's need for direction. Examples include the following:

- Safety hazards in the home
- Inadequate housing conditions
- Inadequate food and clothing
- Absence of protective devices (e.g., smoke detectors)
- Hazardous materials (e.g., lead-based paint and dangerous chemicals)
- Communicable disease (and potential for transmission)
- Signs of abuse or neglect

BOX 3-6 Sampling of Outside Resources and Services

Municipal
Animal control services
Child protective services
Fire service personnel
Law enforcement personnel
Social services

Community
Abuse support groups for spouses, children, and older adults
Alternative health care services (e.g., free clinics)
Alternative means of transportation
Alternative modes of education
Assistance for food, shelter, and clothing
Day care services
Disaster services (e.g., American Red Cross)
Immunization programs
Managed care organizations
Mental health resources and counseling
Rape or crisis intervention
Rehabilitation programs
Services for the disabled
Work-study programs

Religious
Family counseling
Grief support
Pastoral services
Support groups

CRITICAL THINKING

Do you know an emergency medical services provider who was injured on the job? How did the injury occur? Can you identify any measures that could have prevented it?

RECOGNITION OF THE NEED FOR OUTSIDE RESOURCES

Most communities have outside resources that can be helpful. The providers of these resources and services usually are eager to work with the community to develop injury prevention strategies.

DOCUMENTATION

Taking precise notes of patient care and primary injury data is crucial. This documentation offers a record of the events of the encounter. The notes are also helpful to others who will be taking part in the patient's care (see Chapter 16). Gathering primary injury data can be useful in designing injury prevention strategies. For example, one might study a large number of patients who received head injuries while riding a horse. This study may help one to observe that helmet use was notably absent in all seriously injured patients. Primary injury data include the following:

- Scene conditions
- Mechanism of injury
- Use of protective devices
- Absence of protective devices
- Risks at the scene
- Other factors as noted by the EMS agency

On-Scene Education

The EMS response to an injury or near-injury may provide for a **teachable moment.** This is a moment in which the patient and the family may be open to injury prevention tips and strategies. The paramedic can use this opportunity to assess hazards in an environment. The paramedic also can provide on-scene, one-on-one injury prevention education. The teachable moment involves a three-step process[3]:

1. *Observe the scene:* The first step is to look for contributing factors or hazards at the scene that may have caused or could cause an injury event. Examples include floor rugs without a nonslip backing and smoke detectors that are not working.
2. *Gather information:* The next step is to gather information from individuals and observers. What did they see? Why do they think the injury occurred? Has this been a common occurrence? Patients, family members or bystanders, and first responders may have valuable insight about a situation that caused an injury event.

3. *Make assessments:* The final step is to make decisions from the information that has been gathered. The first assessment is to decide whether the situation is critical or noncritical. If the situation is critical, the focus must be on patient care. If the situation is noncritical, a teachable moment exists. This is the opportunity to conduct one-on-one injury prevention counseling that may help to prevent another injury. Another assessment uses the information gathered through observation and history taking. The paramedic uses this step to decide whether high-risk persons, high-risk behaviors, or a high-risk setting exists. Based on the assessment of risks, the paramedic can create a remedy.

Three common on-scene remedies are *discussion*, *demonstration*, and *documentation.* Discussion involves talking about proper behavior or action with the person at risk. Injury prevention discussions are a 30- to 60-second process. The message must be offered in a patient-appropriate manner. This manner depends on age, education, and socioeconomic status. The message should be conveyed in a nonjudgmental, "here are the facts" tone of voice. Although discussion may not always work, the paramedic should attempt it.

It may be possible to demonstrate proper behavior as an injury prevention strategy. For example, a paramedic could replace a safety cap on a pill bottle and explain the importance of doing so. The paramedic could put a fresh battery in a smoke detector. Or the paramedic could move a throw rug on a slippery floor to a safer location. These demonstrations on the scene draw attention to likely hazards and can work to prevent future injury.

The paramedic should document what was seen, heard, and done at the scene. Written histories allow for follow-up by the receiving personnel. Other injury prevention groups also can use these histories in their data-gathering efforts. Lastly, histories make it easier for review in the EMS organization to improve injury prevention.

Other Injury Prevention Roles in Emergency Medical Services

In addition to the injury prevention strategies just listed, EMS personnel can play a major role in improving public health and safety. They can do this through supporting legislative change. Involvement in primary prevention programs also can help. Box 3-7 lists a sampling of these other injury prevention roles.

CRITICAL THINKING

At some point, you probably will visit an older adult family member or friend. See whether you can identify any potential hazards that exist in that person's home.

BOX 3-7 A Sampling of Injury Prevention Strategies*

Bicycle Safety
Bicycle helmet programs

Brain Injury
Brain injury prevention programs

Burns
Fire prevention programs
Smoke detector programs

Children
Babysitter training classes
Child abuse prevention programs
Child safety seat programs
Child safety programs
Drowning prevention programs
Emergency medical services (EMS) for children programs
Parenting classes
Playground safety programs
Safe kids programs
Safe school programs
Swimming classes
Youth advocacy groups

Community Safety
Safe communities programs

Elderly
Programs to reduce elderly falls

Firearm Safety
Gun safety programs

Home Safety
Home assessment programs

Legal/Political
Being involved as an expert or advisor in the political process during the debate over laws dealing with the following:
- Child and adolescent safety laws
- Drunk driving laws
- Engineering regulations (building safety into a product)
- Gun legislation
- Helmet laws

*This box should encourage the paramedic student to search for prevention programs that are of personal interest because the work likely will be voluntary and without pay.
This list is compiled from programs already in place. Some of these are national and some are local. The student should seek those programs that already exist in his or her area. If a program does not exist locally, chances are it exists somewhere in the United States. If interested, the student should search the Internet or other sources and find a comparable guide for starting a local program.

Continued

BOX 3-7 A Sampling of Injury Prevention Strategies*—cont'd

Many Internet sites have information on ways to prevent medical illness. Some of this material can be passed on to the EMS provider's patients. The information can be provided informally or through a program with handouts or public service activities. Sites include the following:

- Acquired immunodeficiency syndrome
- Cancer
- Cardiovascular health
- Childhood illnesses
- Flu
- Healthful lifestyle
- Heat disorders
- Medical conditions A to Z (Centers for Disease Control and Prevention site)
- Parenting
- Premenstrual syndrome
- Senior citizen illnesses
- Stroke

Most local physician offices have brochures that EMS personnel can hand out in cooperation with the local doctor.

Neurological Injury
Head injury prevention programs

Nutrition
Proper nutrition programs

Occupational Safety
Occupational illness and injury prevention programs

Pedestrian Safety
Pedestrian safety programs

Poisoning
National Poisoning Prevention Week

Posttraumatic Stress Syndrome
Programs for the community
Programs for EMS and other public safety personnel

Public Driving
Programs to prevent driving while intoxicated
Programs to prevent running of red lights
Programs to promote seat belt use

Rehabilitation
Rehabilitation support groups

Research
Universities throughout the United States research many illness and injury prevention strategies. These schools often welcome input from EMS personnel. This input may be in the form of volunteer work in data collection. Input also may be ride-alongs by the researchers. Input can even help in the actual writing of the research documents. Emergency medical services personnel should search for injury prevention centers, illness prevention centers, EMS research centers, and schools of public health within colleges and universities in their local area.

Smoking
Smoking cessation programs

Substance Abuse
Addiction programs
Substance abuse prevention programs
Substance abuse prevention programs for youth

Suicide
Suicide prevention programs

Trauma
National Trauma Awareness Week

Violence
Violence prevention programs
Violence survivor programs

*This box should encourage the paramedic student to search for prevention programs that are of personal interest because the work likely will be voluntary and without pay.
This list is compiled from programs already in place. Some of these are national and some are local. The student should seek those programs that already exist in his or her area. If a program does not exist locally, chances are it exists somewhere in the United States. If interested, the student should search the Internet or other sources and find a comparable guide for starting a local program.

PARTICIPATION IN PREVENTION PROGRAMS

Prevention programs that are effective first call for a **community health assessment.** This assessment is needed before the intervention can take place. The assessment also is required before the education can get under way.

Community Health Assessment

Paramedics most likely have limited time. They also have limited resources to allot to prevention and wellness promotion. Thus the EMS worker must maximize time and resources. Paramedics can perform a community health assessment to identify the target for community health education (Fig. 3-2). This assessment often is a large undertaking and may be conducted more effectively through a group effort with other health agencies (see Box 3-8) to evaluate the following:

- Population demographics
- Morbidity statistics
- Mortality statistics
- Crime and fire information
- Community resource allocation

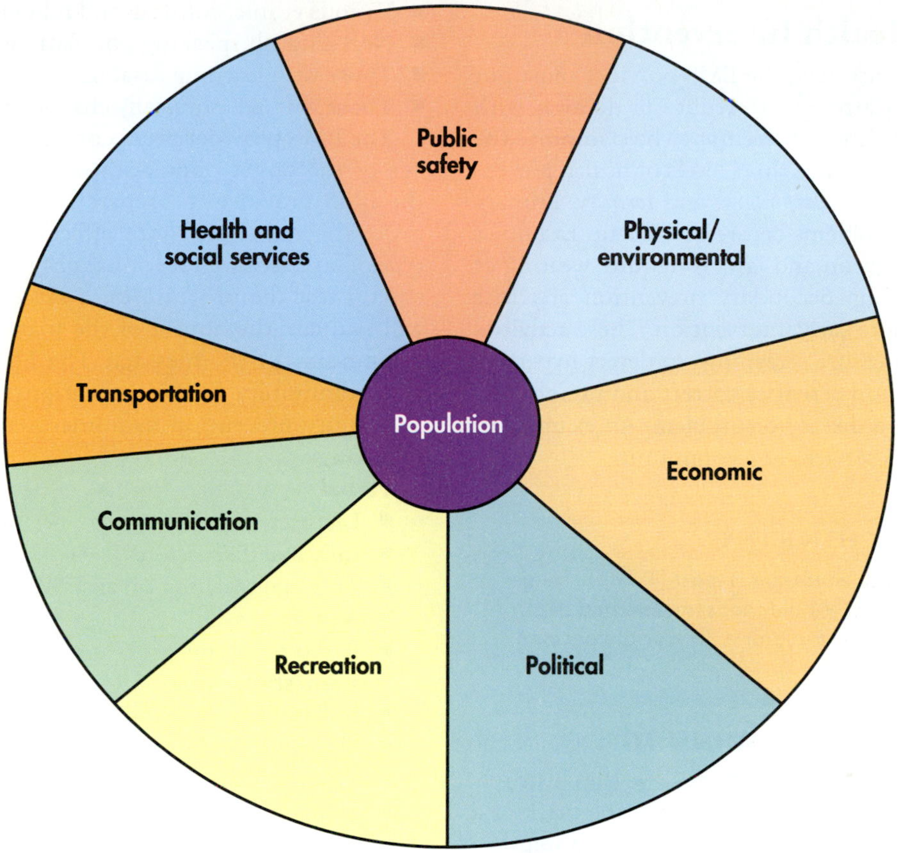

FIGURE 3-2 ■ Community health assessment.

BOX 3-8 Sampling of Community Health Information Sources

- American Red Cross
- Births and deaths (including cause)
- Call types and response times
- Census data (public library, Internet)
- Centers for Disease Control and Prevention
- Chamber of commerce
- Clustering of illnesses and injuries
- Communication
- Crime rate statistics
- Disaster planning
- Distribution of age, sex, race, ethnicity
- Distribution of grant monies
- Education and literacy rates
- Emergency coordinating council
- Emergency medical services
- Employment statistics
- Environmental hazards (sanitation, air quality)
- Federal Emergency Management Agency
- Federal government
- Fire service
- Fire-related injuries and fatalities
- Form of government
- Geographic distribution
- Health departments (city, county, state, Internet)
- Health services and school lunch programs
- Hospitals
- Housing and tax information
- Industry and economic figures
- Infectious disease statistics
- Law enforcement
- Local government
- Location and frequency of fires
- National Safety Council
- Newspapers, radio, and television stations
- Parks and recreation
- Population demographics
- Religious organizations
- Response times
- School board
- Socioeconomic status
- State trauma registry statistics

- Hospital data (e.g., emergency department visits and length of stay)
- Senior citizen needs
- Education standards
- Recreational facilities
- Environmental conditions
- Other factors

This "landscape" view of the health of a community can yield data that are valuable, and sometimes unexpected, about the target population. The assessment also can identify factors that relate or contribute to certain health risks. After the assessment the EMS provider should choose the target for health education carefully. The provider then should use a fitting intervention. Ideally, the EMS provider should compare the data from the assessment with those of another population (Box 3-8). This population should have similar demographics. For example, a city of similar size within the state would be a good choice.

Community Health Intervention

After identifying a health risk, the EMS provider must put into place a plan that attempts to reduce or do away with the risk. This plan also should attempt to help improve the health of the community. The three levels of health prevention activities are *primary, secondary,* and *tertiary*. Primary prevention prevents problems before they occur. Examples include seat belt education and laws to require wearing of helmets while bicycling. Secondary prevention activities find issues and promote early intervention. These activities may include blood pressure screenings to detect hypertension. Tertiary prevention activities correct and prevent further deterioration of a disease or problem. An example of this is providing EMS services in a community.

> **CRITICAL THINKING**
>
> What method of health education is most likely to change your personal behaviors? Would that same method be equally effective for a 5-year-old or a 70-year-old person?

Community Health Education

A good injury prevention program must serve the entire target population in a community. This also is the mark of a successful program. The community must try to improve the education and training for EMS and other public service agencies. In that way special groups can be included in the prevention program. Examples include training emergency personnel to communicate effectively with the following:

- Various ethnic, cultural, and religious groups
- Non-English-speaking populations
- Those with learning disabilities
- Those who are physically challenged

The EMS provider must consider the reading level and age of the target population. These considerations help the EMS provider to prepare educational materials and make the materials more effective. Before starting any type of large-scale educational program, the EMS provider should test the program on a target audience. This test will evaluate the appeal of the materials and ensure understanding of the message. The EMS provider can provide community health education to promote wellness and injury prevention in numerous ways, including the following:

Verbal
- Lectures
- Informal discussions
- Informal teaching on an EMS call
- Audiotapes
- Radio programs

Written/static visual
- Bulletin boards, exhibits
- Flyers, pamphlets, posters
- Models
- Slides, photographs

Dynamic visual
- Videotapes
- Television
- Internet resources

SUMMARY

- Emergency medical services providers are members of the community health care system. They can be an important resource in injury prevention.
- Unintentional injuries are the fifth leading cause of death. This cause is exceeded only by heart disease, cancer, stroke, and chronic obstructive pulmonary disease.
- The United States has more than 600,000 EMS providers. This valuable human resource plays a major role in public education. This component of health promotion seems only fitting.
- For EMS workers to play an active role in the health of a community is crucial. Thus the community must protect the EMS worker from injury. The community also needs to provide education to EMS workers. The community should supply support and promote the collection and use of injury data as well. In addition, the community must obtain resources for primary injury prevention activities. Lastly, the community needs to empower EMS providers to conduct primary injury prevention.

- All EMS workers must have a basic knowledge of personal injury prevention. They also should know about maladies and injuries common to various age groups, recreation activities, workplaces, and other facilities in the community.
- The paramedic needs to spot the signs and symptoms of abuse and abusive situations. In addition, the paramedic should notice exposure to danger.
- Paramedics should identify and use outside community resources. Plus they should document primary injury data properly. Moreover, they should identify and properly use the teachable moment.
- The EMS provider must maximize time and resources. Thus the EMS provider should identify targets for community health education. The EMS provider can do this by performing a community health assessment.
- To identify community education goals, the paramedic must understand several factors: (1) illness or injury is related to the extent or exposure to an agent; (2) illness or injury also is related to the strength of the agent; (3) illness or injury is linked to the susceptibility of the individual (host); and (4) illness or injury is related to the biological, social, and physical environment.
- Primary injury prevention involves preventing an injury from occurring. Secondary and tertiary prevention help to prevent further problems from an event that has already occurred.
- A good injury prevention program must serve the whole target population in a community. An effective program also takes into account reading level and age. These aspects are the mark of a successful program. The EMS provider can provide community health education in diverse ways, such as verbal, written/static material, and dynamic visual.

REFERENCES

1. National Safety Council: *Injury facts,* Itasca, Ill, 2002, The Council.
2. National Highway Traffic Safety Administration: *Emergency medical services: agenda for the future,* Washington, DC, 1996, The Administration.
3. Martinez R, Harter P: *Accidents aren't,* Stanford, Calif, 1993, Stanford University.

SUGGESTED READINGS

American Academy of Pediatrics, Committee on Injury and Poison Prevention: *Injury prevention and control for children and youth,* ed 3, Elk Grove Village, Ill, 1997, The Academy.

Christoffel T, Gallagher SS: *Injury prevention and public health: practical knowledge, skills, and strategies,* Gaithersburg, Md, 1999, Aspen.

Garrison HG, Foltin GL, Becker LR, et al: The role of emergency medical services in primary injury prevention, *Ann Emerg Med* 30:80-91, July 1997.

Institute of Medicine, Division of Health Promotion and Disease Prevention, Committee on Injury Prevention and Control: *Reducing the burden of injury,* Washington, DC, 1999, National Academy Press.

Kellerman AL, Todd KH: Injury control. In Tintinalli JE, Kelen GD, Stapczynski JS, eds: *Emergency medicine: a comprehensive study guide,* New York, 1999, McGraw-Hill.

Kinnane JM, Garrison HG, Coben JH, et al: Injury prevention: is there a role for out-of-hospital emergency medical services? *Acad Emerg Med* 4:306-312, 1997.

National Safety Council: *Injury fact book*, Chicago. 1999, The Council. US Department of Transportation, National Highway Traffic Safety Administration: *Emergency medical services agenda for the future implementation guide,* Pub No DOT HS 808 711, Washington, DC, 1998, Government Printing Office.

CHAPTER 4

Medical/Legal Issues

OBJECTIVES

Upon completion of this chapter, the paramedic student will be able to:

1. Describe the basic structure of the legal system in the United States.
2. Relate how laws affect the paramedic's practice.
3. List situations that the paramedic is legally required to report in most states.
4. Describe the four elements involved in a claim of negligence.
5. Describe measures paramedics may take to protect themselves from claims of negligence.
6. Describe the paramedic's responsibilities regarding patient confidentiality.
7. Outline the process for obtaining expressed, informed, and implied consent.
8. Describe legal complications relating to consent.
9. Describe actions to be taken in a refusal-of-care situation.
10. Describe legal considerations related to patient transportation.
11. Outline legal issues related to specific resuscitation situations.
12. List measures the paramedic should take to preserve evidence when at a crime or accident scene.
13. Detail the components of the narrative report necessary for effective legal documentation.
14. Define common medical-legal terms that apply to prehospital situations involving patient care.

KEY TERMS

abandonment: Terminating medical care without legal excuse or turning care over to personnel who do not have training and expertise appropriate for the medical needs of the patient.

assault: Creating apprehension, or unauthorized handling and treatment of a patient.

battery: Physical contact with a person without consent and without legal justification.

expressed consent: Verbal or written consent to the treatment.

false imprisonment: Intentional and unjustifiable detention of a person.

implied consent: The presumption that an unconscious or incompetent person would consent to lifesaving care.

informed consent: Consent obtained from a patient after explaining all facts necessary for the patient to make a reasonable decision.

involuntary consent: Treatment that is granted by authority of law.

negligence: Failure to use such care as a reasonably prudent emergency medical services provider would use in similar circumstances.

In the past, only hospitals and physicians were affected by medical malpractice. This is because EMS workers were not expected to meet professional standards of patient care. However, with state and national certification, licensure, and the paramedic's role as a health care professional, medical liability for EMS personnel is now a real concern.

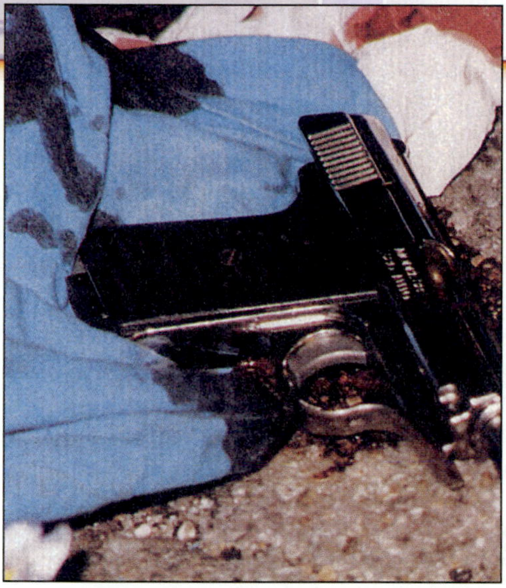

LEGAL DUTIES AND ETHICAL RESPONSIBILITIES

The paramedic's legal duties are to the patient, the employer, the medical director, and the public. These duties are defined by statutes and regulations. These duties are based on commonly accepted standards of medical care. Like other health care professionals, in addition to legal duties, paramedics have ethical responsibilities that include the following:

- Responding with respect to the physical and emotional needs of every patient
- Maintaining mastery of skills
- Participating in continuing education/refresher training
- Critically reviewing performance and seeking improvement
- Reporting honestly
- Respecting confidentiality
- Working cooperatively and with respect for other emergency workers and health care professionals
- Staying current with new concepts and modalities

Failing to perform emergency medical services (EMS) duties in a proper way can result in civil or criminal liability. As described in this chapter, the best legal protection is providing proper assessment and care to the patient. This care should be coupled with correct and full written documentation.

> **NOTE** Laws pertaining to patient care delivery vary by state. Every paramedic should be aware of the medical practice act in his or her state. The paramedic also should be aware of other regulatory statutes that pertain to emergency medical services (EMS). If necessary, the paramedic should consult with a private attorney experienced in EMS law or the state attorney general's office (or its equivalent) to clarify state laws and their application to EMS activities. The information contained in this chapter is general information and is not intended to be a complete guide to the legislative system, EMS laws, or regulations of any state.

THE LEGAL SYSTEM

The structure of the legal system in the United States is composed of five types of law. These types are legislative law, administrative law, common law, criminal law, and civil law.

Legislative law is made by legislative branches of government. Examples of these branches are city councils, district boards, general assemblies, and Congress. The power of these bodies to make law is defined by statutes, state constitutions, and in the case of Congress, the U.S. Constitution.

Administrative law refers to regulations that are developed by a governmental agency to provide details about the function and process of the law. (A good example is the criteria for paramedic licensure.) These regulations may address areas such as examinations, licenses, and maintenance of records. Regulatory agencies may hold disciplinary hearings on the revocation or suspension of licenses. An example of a regulatory agency is a state EMS bureau.

Common law is also known as case or judge-made law. This law comes from societal acceptance of customs or norms of behavior over time. This kind of law is based on the decisions of judges within the state and federal judicial systems. Regarding patient care activities, these court decisions may offer guidance in defining acceptable conduct and **negligence.** The decisions also may help one to interpret state statutes and regulations applicable to EMS.

Criminal law is a type of law in which the federal, state, or local government prosecutes persons for violating a law. Criminal laws are enacted to protect society (a "public" complaint). Violation of criminal law may be punishable by fine, imprisonment, or both.

Civil law (tort law) is an area of law that deals with "private" complaints brought by one person (plaintiff) against another person (defendant). These complaints are for an illegal act or wrongdoing (tort) for which the plaintiff requests the court to award damages. Most EMS activities that result in litigation are civil suits.

How Laws Affect the Paramedic

As stated before, the U.S. legal system has been active on issues relating to medical malpractice. To avoid litigation, the paramedic must know about these issues. The paramedic also must know how these issues can affect patient care activities.

SCOPE OF PRACTICE

Scope of practice refers to the range of duties and skills that a paramedic is allowed and expected to perform when needed. These duties are set by state law or regulation and by local medical direction. For example, the scope of practice for most paramedics in most states would include endotracheal intubation, defibrillation, the administration of medications, and other basic life support and advanced life support procedures.

CRITICAL THINKING

Why is it necessary to define the scope of practice for a profession?

MEDICAL DIRECTION

As explained in Chapter 1, medical direction is a key part of paramedic practice. Medical direction may be provided online (direct) or off-line (indirect). This depends on state and local requirements. Emergency medical services systems also should have a policy to guide paramedics in dealing with physicians on the scene. These persons may be known as *bystander physicians.* Some states, for example, have cards for paramedics to issue to these physicians. The cards officially prohibit interference with paramedics performing their job. (Use of these cards often requires legislative or regulatory support.)

MEDICAL PRACTICE ACT

A *medical practice act* refers to a law that governs the practice of medicine. This legislation varies by state. A medical practice act prescribes how and to what extent a physician may delegate authority to paramedics to perform medical acts.

LICENSURE AND CERTIFICATION

As explained in Chapter 1, paramedic licensure and certification may be required by state or local authorities. Licensure is a way to regulate an occupation. In this process an agency of the government gives consent to a person to engage in a profession. The agency may be, for example, a state medical board. The person must meet set criteria. Certification may be granted by a governmental body (e.g., city, county, or state) or a nongovernmental certifying agency. Certification also may be granted by a professional association. An example of such a group is the National Registry of Emergency Medical Technicians. Certification is granted to a person who has met certain criteria to take part in an activity. The terms *certification* and *license* often are used to refer to the same process. A certification, granted by a state, conferring a right to engage in a trade or profession is in fact a license.

CRITICAL THINKING

How does licensure/certification help to ensure the safety of your community?

MOTOR VEHICLE LAWS

For the most part, motor vehicle laws define the standards for operating emergency vehicles. These laws also define the standards for equipping the vehicles[1] (see Chapter 49). Like most laws, these codes vary by state.

▶NOTE Criminal statutes do not always require intent for an action to be seen as criminal. For example, an emergency vehicle crash may occur from reckless driving. The crash may result in civil and criminal lawsuits. High speeds, failure to judge road and weather conditions, and improper use or nonuse of audible and visual warning devices are key areas of liability. The paramedic should be well aware of state motor vehicle codes. The paramedic also should be aware of laws that apply to emergency vehicle operations.

MANDATORY REPORTING REQUIREMENTS

Paramedics and health care workers may be required by law to report certain cases. These include cases of abuse or neglect of children and older adults and spouse abuse. They also include cases that involve rape, sexual assault, gunshot wounds, stab wounds, animal bites, and some communicable diseases (Box 4-1). The content of the report and to whom it must be made is set by law, regulation, or policy. Local protocols set by medical direction and the EMS agency give guidance in these areas. Some states have penal-

BOX 4-1 Cases Reportable under Law in Most States

- Neglect or abuse of children
- Neglect or abuse of older adults
- Spouse abuse
- Rape, sexual assault
- Gunshot wounds
- Stab wounds
- Animal bites
- Certain communicable diseases

ties if mandatory reporting is not satisfied. Many reporting statutes provide immunity for the person reporting the situation. Immunity helps lessen the fear of legal consequences from such reporting should the report be false or unfounded. These statutes prohibit lawsuits against persons who file reports or offer a defense in court in the event of a lawsuit.

CRITICAL THINKING

Imagine that your state requires the reporting of gunshot wounds. Your patient has a small-caliber flesh wound. This patient also refuses care and begs you not to tell anyone so that her privacy will be protected. What will you do?

PROTECTION FOR THE PARAMEDIC

Some state and federal regulations provide legal protection for the paramedic. Examples include how paramedics are notified of exposure to infectious disease, protection provided by immunity statutes, and laws that describe special crimes against EMS personnel. These regulations vary by state and local jurisdictions.

Notification of Infectious Disease Exposure

The *Ryan White Comprehensive AIDS Resources Emergency Act of 1990* (PL 101-381) requires that emergency responders be advised if they have been exposed to infectious diseases. These diseases include hepatitis, tuberculosis, bacterial (meningococcal) meningitis, rubella (German measles), and human immunodeficiency virus. The act also requires that employers name a designated officer to coordinate communications between the hospital and the emergency response organization in case of an exposure. The responder must be notified within 48 hours of the exposure being determined. That way, postexposure management steps can be taken (see Chapter 39).

CRITICAL THINKING

Reflect on the time before the Ryan White law of 1990. At that time, why would some health care facilities not report significant infectious disease exposures to EMS personnel?

Immunity Statutes. Protecting state and other governmental entities from lawsuits came from an ancient English common law. This immunity was based on the idea that "the king can do no wrong." In modern law, this means that governmental agencies cannot be held liable for the negligent acts of their employees. Since the 1950s the trend in many states has been to discard this doctrine or limit its application. In some states, for example, immunity, if exercised, may apply only to the governmental agency. Immunity does not apply to the employee or operator of an emergency vehicle. Governmental immunity statutes vary throughout the country. Thus EMS providers may or may not be protected by this statute.

Good Samaritan laws exist in some form in all 50 states. The intent of these laws is to encourage persons to help others in an emergency without fear of a lawsuit. As a rule a person who gives emergency first aid in good faith, without expecting to be paid, and in a manner that another person with similar training would, is covered by these laws. For the most part, though, these laws do not protect health care workers from acts of gross negligence, reckless disregard, or willful or wanton misconduct. These laws also generally do not apply to paid, on-duty EMS workers.

CRITICAL THINKING

Imagine that there are no Good Samaritan laws in your state. Would this affect your decision about whether to stop and give aid to an ill or injured person while off duty?

Special Crimes Against a Paramedic. Paramedics may become victims of **assault** or **battery** while doing their job. To deter crimes against paramedics, some localities have enacted ordinances that provide the same level of protection for EMS providers as for law enforcement personnel. These ordinances make it illegal to harm or threaten to harm EMS crews or to obstruct patient care. The paramedic should use good judgment and work closely with the dispatch center and police so as to avoid risky situations. *One must remember that if the scene is not safe and it cannot be made safe, the EMS crew should retreat from the scene. In fact, the EMS crew should not enter the area until it has been secured properly.*

The Legal Process

An injury lawsuit against a paramedic consists of a series of steps[1] (Fig. 4-1). The lawsuit begins with an incident in which a person feels that he or she has been injured as a result of negligent patient care. This person is the plaintiff. The plaintiff then hires a lawyer. The lawyer conducts a case investigation to decide the merit of the complaint. The investigation may include examining patient care reports, textbooks, journal articles, and local protocols. If the lawyer thinks the plaintiff's case has merit, the lawyer prepares and files a complaint in court. The complaint outlines the negligent conduct that resulted in the alleged injury. After the complaint is filed in court, the complaint and a summons are served on the defendant, and the litigation process is initiated. The summons usually is served by a sheriff or other authorized person. The summons requires that the defendant answer the complaint or risk automatically losing the

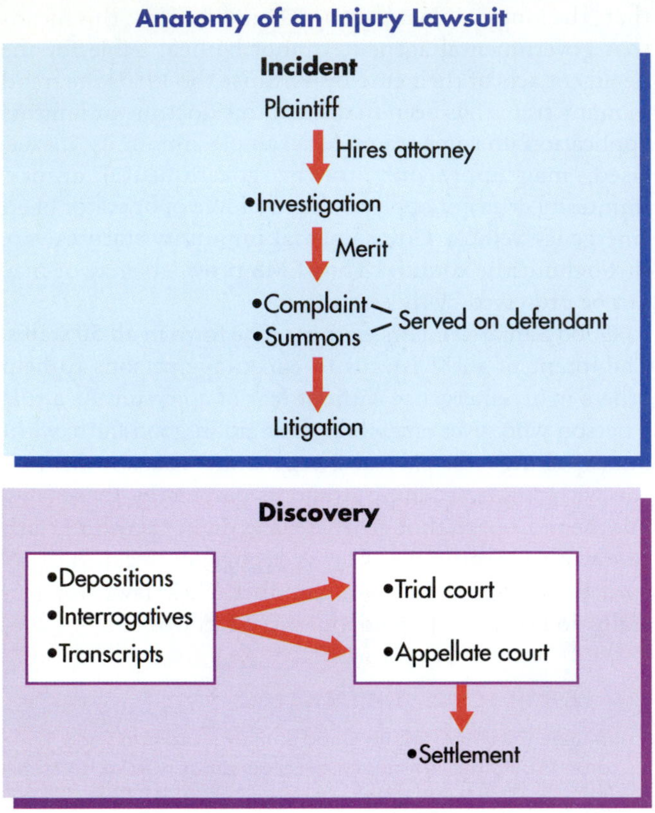

FIGURE 4-1 ■ Anatomy of a lawsuit.

case. At this point the defendant and all parties involved (e.g., the paramedic, ambulance service, and hospital) usually retain an attorney to defend against the lawsuit.

The next step in the legal process is known as *discovery*. This step usually involves the exchange of documents and the taking of depositions and interrogatives. Depositions are testimonies that are taken under oath outside of a courtroom. The person giving the deposition answers a list of questions from the lawyer for the other side. A court reporter types the questions and answers. This transcript may be used during the trial. When giving a deposition, the lawyer should always be present. An interrogative is a set of questions about the lawsuit that is answered in consultation with the party's lawyer. The interrogative then is given to the lawyer for the other side. During discovery, each side is entitled to receive all key information having to do with the lawsuit. Other documents that may be gathered during discovery are patient care reports, computer dispatch records, and tape recordings of radio messages related to the incident. After discovery, the case will be settled out of court or will go to trial. Quality improvement materials are discoverable in some states.

CRITICAL THINKING

Consider a case that occurred 5 years ago. How important will your written documentation be regarding that case?

During the trial, each party presents its side of the case. Based on the evidence, a judge or jury determines liability and any damages to be awarded to the plaintiff. Either side may appeal the decision of the trial court, but the appeal usually can be based only on errors in law made by the trial court.

Settlement may occur at any stage during the litigation. In settlement the plaintiff agrees to accept an amount of money in exchange for a promise not to pursue the claim. After the case is settled, it is dismissed.

NOTE The legal process may involve trial and appellate courts. A trial court determines the outcome of individual cases. The outcome may be determined by a judge or by a jury. The appellate court hears appeals of decisions by trial courts or other appeals courts. Decisions reached in the appellate court may set precedent for later cases of a similar nature.

LEGAL ACCOUNTABILITY OF THE PARAMEDIC

Paramedics should act in a way that is reasonable and prudent. They should provide a level of care and transportation that matches their education, training, and local protocol. If paramedics fail to meet these standards, the result may be legal liability.

NOTE Nearly anyone can be sued, regardless of the validity of the complaint. A lawsuit itself is not an indication of guilt or wrongdoing unless the allegations are proved.

Components of Negligence

Lawsuits involving patient care usually result from civil claims of negligence: the failure to act as a reasonable, prudent paramedic would act in similar circumstances. In most states, four elements must be proved for negligence to exist: (1) a duty to act existed; (2) actions performed were at a level below the standard of care (a breach of duty); (3) damage to the patient or other individual (plaintiff) occurred; and (4) the breach was the proximate cause of the damage.

CRITICAL THINKING

Certain advanced life support interventions have an increased risk of causing harm to the patient compared with basic life support skills. As a paramedic, what advanced life support interventions do you think that you will perform that have this increased risk?

DUTY TO ACT

Paramedics assume a duty to provide emergency care when requested while working for an EMS service. This duty may be formal, or contractual. The duty also may be informal, or volunteer. Once a paramedic takes on the duty to act, the paramedic must *continue to act* until patient care has been transferred to another health care worker who has training and experience meeting the needs of the patient, until it is abundantly clear that the patient no longer needs assistance, or until the patient/caregiver relationship is terminated by the patient. Duties include the following:

- To respond and render care
- To obey laws and regulations
- To operate emergency vehicles reasonably and prudently
- To provide care and transportation to the expected standard
- To provide care and transportation consistent with the scope of practice and local medical protocols
- To continue care and transportation through to its appropriate conclusion

> **NOTE** The delegation of scope of practice between a physician and a paramedic usually is only effective when the paramedic is on duty. Therefore an off-duty paramedic who provides emergency care usually must act in a basic life support capacity unless the paramedic has specific authorization from medical direction to perform advanced life support procedures.

BREACH OF DUTY

For negligence to exist, plaintiffs must prove that the paramedic had a duty to act and that the duty was breached. The paramedic must use the care, skill, and judgment that any other similarly trained paramedic would use in such a position. This standard of care is established by court testimony. This standard of care also is established by referring to codes, standards, criteria, and guidelines related to the case. Many states take into account national standards when defining acceptable care. If the paramedic did not meet written national or state standards, it may be easier for the plaintiff to prove breach of duty.

> **NOTE** *Standard of care* is a measure of competence of a professional. Standard of care differs from *scope of practice.* Scope of practice identifies specific medical practices that are permitted by licensure and certification.

Breach of duty may occur by *malfeasance* (performing a wrongful or unlawful act), *misfeasance* (performing a legal act in a manner that is harmful or injurious), or *nonfeasance* (failure to perform a required act or duty). In some cases, negligence may be so obvious that it does not require extensive proof. *Res ipsa loquitur* is a Latin phrase that means "the thing speaks for itself" and implies that the facts are so clear, that without a doubt the injury could have been caused only by negligence. *Negligence per se* means that negligence is shown by the fact that a statute or ordinance was violated and injury resulted.

DAMAGE TO THE PATIENT OR OTHER INDIVIDUAL (PLAINTIFF)

The third element of negligence is proof of damage; in other words, proof that the plaintiff suffered compensable damages. These damages include medical expenses, lost earnings, conscious pain and suffering, and wrongful death. Punitive damages also may be awarded in excess of compensable damages. These damages are meant to punish the person at fault and to deter others from causing such harm in the future. Punitive damages usually are not covered by malpractice insurance (described later in this chapter).

PROXIMATE CAUSE

Finally, the plaintiff must prove that the negligent act or lack of action caused the injury or made an existing injury worse. The plaintiff also must prove that the injury or further harm was foreseeable by the paramedic. The element of proximate cause is hard to establish at times. Proof of proximate cause often calls for expert witnesses. These witnesses address issues of duty, standard of care, and conflicting views of causation. For example, was a cervical spine injury caused by the car crash or was it the result of rescue efforts by the EMS crew? Other than direct patient care, there are three areas for negligent conduct. The first is patient transportation to a medical facility contrary to medical direction advice, trauma center designation, or other known special patient care needs and facility capabilities. The second is failure to maintain equipment, supplies, or vehicles. The third area is driving negligently or recklessly.

> **CRITICAL THINKING**
> Do you think that an effective quality management program can decrease the risk for negligent lawsuits? How?

Defenses to Negligence Claims

Most experts stress three items to protect health care workers against claims of negligence. These include training, competent patient care skills, and full documentation of all patient care activities. The following list gives other defenses to negligence and their pros and cons:

1. Good Samaritan laws
   - Generally do not protect providers from acts of gross negligence, reckless disregard, or willful or wanton misconduct
   - Generally do not prohibit the filing of a lawsuit
   - May provide coverage for paid or volunteer providers
   - Vary from state to state
2. Governmental immunity
   - Trend is toward limiting protection
   - May protect only governmental agency, not provider
   - Varies from state to state
3. Statute of limitations
   - Limit the number of years after an incident during which a lawsuit can be filed

- Set by law and may differ for cases involving adults and children
- Varies from state to state

4. Contributory negligence
   - Plaintiff may be found to have contributed to his or her own injury
   - Damages awarded may be reduced or eliminated based on the plaintiff's contribution to the injury

LIABILITY INSURANCE

All active health care workers need to have adequate liability insurance. This is also known as malpractice insurance. These policies offer coverage for legal defense and judgments against the person who holds the policy. Malpractice insurance falls into two groups: *primary* and *umbrella* policies. Primary policies are personal policies. They offer certain limits of coverage for the types of risks insured against. For example, a policy with a $100,000 limit pays up to that amount for covered damages caused by the insured.

> **CRITICAL THINKING**
>
> What kind of liability insurance protects you now as an Emergency Medical Technician-Basic provider? What type of liability insurance protects you as a student paramedic in a clinical experience?

Umbrella policies are liability policies for groups of workers. Employers of paramedics carry umbrella policies. For example, an ambulance service or a hospital may carry such a policy. These policies often have extra limits of coverage for workers who are on duty. These workers must act within the scope of practice. This scope is set by the employer with policy or protocol. A $1 million umbrella policy, for example, covers damages caused by the insured in excess of those limits in the underlying primary policy. The amount of coverage of such umbrella policies may vary by hospital and EMS agency. The umbrella policy may not cover the employee's liability. In such a case, a separate individual policy may be desirable. A variety of companies offer the individual coverage. Group plans often are cheaper, though, and may offer better coverage than the more costly individual ones.

SPECIAL LIABILITY CONCERNS

Regarding liability, a few issues are unique to prehospital care. One issue is the liability of the medical director. Another issue is the liability for "borrowed servants." Finally, issues arise relating to civil rights.

LIABILITY OF THE PARAMEDIC MEDICAL DIRECTOR

The medical direction physician delegates authority for care of patients to a paramedic. As a result, the physician has to assume legal responsibility for the patient. This also is known as *vicarious liability*. The physician assumes this responsibility for the care that is given out of the hospital. This liability may hold for actions that are performed through online (direct) medical direction. Liability also may hold for off-line (indirect) medical direction. In the latter, care is guided by the use of physician-developed protocols and standing orders. Therefore negligence on the part of a paramedic may become the responsibility of the medical direction physician (and the paramedic's employer), even in the absence of direct supervision.

Vicarious liability comes into play by virtue of the relationship between the employer and employee. It also arises because of one's being an agent who is approved to perform for the benefit of another. The paramedic is not an employee of the physician per se. Still, the paramedic acts as an agent in place of the physician. For this reason, the law may regard the actions of the paramedic as a legal responsibility of the physician.

LIABILITY FOR BORROWED SERVANTS

Borrowed servants is another key legal doctrine. The doctrine refers to a servant who serves two masters. An example of this is an EMT-Basic who is employed by a city. Yet the EMT also is supervised by a paramedic. This doctrine can create liability for the supervising paramedic. The doctrine also can create liability for the employer and the medical direction physician. (This is vicarious liability.) The amount of liability for the supervising paramedic depends on the degree of supervision. Liability also depends on the control given to the paramedic by the employer.

The borrowed servant doctrine is based on a theory that when a person has control over someone else's employee, that person should be liable for that person's acts. This is the case even though no employer-employee bond exists. Paramedics who have full supervisory control over EMT-Basics must protect the patient by making sure the EMT-Basics perform patient care properly.

CIVIL RIGHTS

The first civil rights law was enacted in 1866. This law prohibited discrimination based on race. Since then, civil rights laws have been changed many times. They have been changed to make it illegal to discriminate by reason of race, color, sex, religion, national origin, and in the case of health care, the ability to pay (Box 4-2). In the case of a municipal ambulance service, a patient could bring claim under the civil rights act for a number of violations in addition to those of discrimination. These violation could include treatment and transport without proper consent.

Another key civil rights law was passed in 1973. This law is the *Rehabilitation Act of 1973*. This act prohibits discrimination against handicapped persons solely based on the handicap. This act applies to any program or activity that receives federal financial help. These programs may include EMS agencies that receive Medicare or Medicaid reimbursement. Title II of the *Americans with Disabilities Act* also allows for equal accessibility for public services by persons with disabilities. This includes receiving good patient care regardless of disease condition. For example, these conditions may include acquired immunodeficiency syndrome,

BOX 4-2 COBRA/OBRA

The Consolidated Omnibus Budget Reconciliation Act (COBRA) became effective in 1986. The act is now known as the Emergency Medical Treatment and Active Labor Act. The act addressed the medical screening, stabilization, and transfer of patients with emergency medical conditions or who are in active labor for Medicare-participating hospitals. The act also addressed the issue of "patient dumping." (This dumping referred to the transfer, diversion, or premature discharge of patients from a hospital because of their inability to pay.) The act set penalties of up to $20,000 for each violation. The act was amended as the Omnibus Budget Reconciliation Act (OBRA 1989, 1990, and 1993). This amendment gave clarity and greater enforcement to the COBRA rules. The amendment also raised the possible fine to $50,000 per infraction. The major provisions of OBRA include the following:

- Medical screening as it relates to the capabilities of the sending and receiving hospitals
- Stabilization of the patient at a referring hospital (legal and financial responsibility)
- Provision of appropriate transfer methods, ensuring that the patient is stable and has consented to the transfer
- Definition of "appropriate transfer" as the provision of the needed level of care and resources available during the transfer
- Whistle-blower protection for physician and hospital staff

human immunodeficiency virus infection, tuberculosis, and other communicable diseases.

Protection Against Negligence Claims

Paramedics must be aware of how caring for a patient can pose a threat of litigation for negligence. The best protections against such claims are the following:

- Education/training/continuing education and skills retention
- Appropriate quality improvement
- Appropriate medical direction, online and off-line
- Accurate, thorough documentation (see Chapter 16)
- Professional attitude and demeanor

CRITICAL THINKING

Think back to a call you took as an emergency medical technician that did not go well and the patient did not do well. Did that call meet any of the elements of negligence? What measures could you take to prevent the recurrence of that type of situation?

PARAMEDIC-PATIENT RELATIONSHIPS

The relationship formed between the paramedic and the patient during a patient care encounter is a legal one. Thus legal issues may arise from providing patient care. These issues include confidentiality (Box 4-3), consent,

BOX 4-3 Health Insurance Portability and Accountability Act

The privacy provisions of the Health Insurance Portability and Accountability Act of 1996 (HIPAA) were published in 2003 by the Department of Health and Human Services. Compliance to the privacy rule is mandatory. The act requires all health care providers to do the following:

- Protect the privacy of patients' protected health information, disclosing the minimum amount needed for treatment, billing, and operations.
- Safeguard that information physically and administratively.
- Grant certain rights to patients regarding that information.

Compliance with HIPAA is required for health plans (payers of health care), health care clearinghouses (facilitators of electronic data exchange between standard and nonstandard formats for payers and providers), and health care providers who conduct certain financial and administrative transactions electronically. These groups are known as *covered entities*. They have to comply with certain standards regarding the protection of personal health information. They also have to comply with the coding of electronic transactions. In addition, they must keep proper security measures for electronic information. Emergency medical services provider agencies are direct providers of health care to patients. They generate protected health records that have information that identifies a person. (This may be a name, Social Security number, and address.) These records also contain medical information about that person. (This may include injury or illness and treatments provided.) If emergency medical services agencies transmit or have ever transmitted this protected health information electronically in connection with any of the transactions designated under HIPAA—such as billing or fund transfers—they are a covered entity and are subject to HIPAA.

From National EMS Data Analysis Resource Center: The Application of HIPAA Privacy to Emergency Medical Service Providers. http://www.nedarc.org/HIPAA/hipaa_and_ems.htm. Accessed June 8, 2003.

transportation, and the occasional use of force for restraining patients.

Confidentiality

Paramedics have a legal duty to protect a patient's privacy. This also is an ethical duty. Information from a patient usually can be shared with other health care workers involved in the patient's care. These details can be shared without the patient's permission. For example, such information may include a history of communicable disease. Likewise, details from a patient about an injury or crime may be reported to law enforcement. One may testify to these details in court as well. A potential liability exists, however, for invasion of privacy and defamation (libel or slander; see p. 62) in some cases. For example, potential liability exists in cases in which information is released with malicious intent or reckless disregard. Potential liability also exists in cases in which information is released to persons not legally entitled to the information.

DEFINITION OF CONFIDENTIALITY

What is confidential information? In general, it is defined as any details about a patient related to his or her history. Any assessment findings also are included. Any treatment given is included as well. This information can be in an electronic, written, or verbal format. As a rule, the release of this information for purposes other than treatment, payment (such as filing insurance claims), or ambulance service operations requires written permission from the patient or legal guardian. Exceptions to this general rule include the following:

- Federal, state, or local law that requires release of information
- Health care fraud and abuse detection
- Certain public health activities such as reporting a birth, death, or disease as required by law, as part of a public health investigation; to report child or adult abuse or neglect or domestic violence; to report adverse events such as product defects; or to notify a person about exposure to a possible communicable disease as required by law
- Health oversight activities including audits or government investigations, inspection, disciplinary proceedings, and other administrative or judicial actions undertaken by the government by law to oversee the health care system
- Judicial and administrative proceedings as required by a court or administrative order or in some cases in response to a subpoena or other legal process
- Law enforcement activities in limited situations, such as when there is a warrant for the request, or when the information is needed to locate a suspect or stop a crime
- Military, national defense and security, and other special government functions
- To avert a serious threat to the health and safety of a person or the public at large
- Workers' compensation purposes and in compliance with workers' compensation laws
- Coroners, medical examiners, and funeral directors who need information to identify a deceased person, determine the cause of death, or to carry out their duties as authorized by law
- If the patient is an organ donor: to organizations that handle organ procurement or organ, eye, or tissue transplantation; or to an organ donation bank, as necessary to facilitate organ donation and transplantation
- Research purposes (subject to strict oversight)
- Patients who are inmates or in custody of a law enforcement official, as needed (1) for the correctional institution to render health care; (2) to protect the patient's health or the health and safety of others; or (3) for the safety and security of the correctional institution or law enforcement

In some cases it may be necessary to release a patient's information. These confidential details may need to be released without the patient's written permission. The paramedic must adhere to all reporting requirements and procedures. These rules are set by state/local laws, the EMS agency, and medical direction. The paramedic should release only the minimum necessary details.

IMPROPER RELEASE OF INFORMATION

Improper release of confidential information can result in liability. Liability also can result if the information is wrong. Liability may come into play in two areas: invasion of privacy and defamation. Defamation is libel and/or slander.

Invasion of Privacy. Invasion of privacy is the release, without legal cause, of details about a patient's private life that might expose the person to ridicule, notoriety, or embarrassment. For example, a paramedic is caring for a public official who was in a car crash. After the call the paramedic tells everyone at the ambulance base that the official had a Nazi tattoo on his left shoulder. A custodian at the base hears the discussion and tells his wife. The wife works in the official's office. The next day, a flyer is passed around with a drawing of the official in the back of an ambulance with this tattoo. Within a few days, the EMS agency is contacted by the official's attorney, who claims an invasion of privacy. (The fact that the information released is true is not a defense for invasion of privacy.)

> **CRITICAL THINKING**
>
> Have you ever been in a situation where you or a colleague said something about a patient that you think may have violated confidentiality? What did you do about it?

Defamation. *Defamation* refers to saying something untrue about someone's character or reputation. The remark is said without legal privilege or consent of the person. *Libel* refers to false statements about a person. These statements may be made in writing or through the mass media. In addition, these statements are made with malicious intent or reckless disregard for the falsity of the statements. *Slander* refers to false verbal statements about a person. These statements are made with malicious intent or reckless disregard for the falsity of the statements. If the paramedic in the previous example had lied about the official's tattoo, he and the office worker who made and handed out the flyer could be sued for libel and slander.

Consent

Patient rights have been defined and clarified by legislation and by the judicial system through malpractice litigation. A basic concept of law and medical practice is a patient's rights. These include a competent patient's right to choose what medical care and transport to receive.

> **CRITICAL THINKING**
>
> Imagine being called to care for a patient who clearly is having signs and symptoms of a heart attack but is alert and refusing care. How will you feel? What strategies will you use to try to persuade the patient to allow your care and transport?

For consent to be given, the patient must be of legal age and must be able to make a reasoned decision regarding the following:

- Nature of the illness or injury
- Treatment recommended
- Risks and dangers of treatment
- Alternative treatments and associated risks
- Dangers of refusing treatment (including transport)

TYPES OF CONSENT

Informed consent is patient consent signifying that the patient knows, understands, and agrees to the care rendered. This consent is given based on full disclosure of the information. Verbal or written consent to the treatment is called **expressed consent.** (Consent also can be expressed nonverbally by actions or simply by the patient allowing care to be rendered.)

> **NOTE** For the most part, the paramedic must obtain consent before initiating treatment. However, paramedics do not have to obtain the same degree of informed consent as other health care providers. For example, in-hospital staff have to obtain a higher degree of consent. Because the paramedic is working in an emergency situation, the patient must only agree or at least must not object to the general nature of the care.

Implied consent involves unconscious or mentally impaired persons. Such consent presumes that these persons who need emergency care would consent to lifesaving care if they were able to do so. Unconscious patients and victims of shock, head injury, and alcohol or other drug intoxication are examples of patients to whom emergency care should be delivered in the absence of informed consent. One should note, however, that a competent adult who regains consciousness can revoke consent at any time during the care and transport. This often occurs in cases of diabetic patients and those with seizure disorders; they may choose to refuse insulin or anticonvulsant medicines.

Involuntary consent refers to care that is granted by the authority of law. An example is caring for patients who are held involuntarily for mental health evaluation. Another example is patients who may be held under arrest or who are in protective custody. The paramedic must follow all policies when giving care to these patients. One should note that officers of the law may not order an EMS provider to treat a patient who is competent and who objects to the care.

SPECIAL CONSENT SITUATIONS

Situations may arise in which obtaining consent for treatment is difficult. Such cases may involve minors, mentally incompetent adults, patients in an institution, or prisoners. In such cases, the EMS worker may need to obtain consent for medical care elsewhere. This may include a parent, legal guardian, representative of a state agency, or other legal authority. If a delay would threaten life, however, the EMS worker should treat the patient. Emergency medical services workers should be familiar with state laws governing such situations. In addition, EMS systems should have protocols for such situations. When a situation arises with consent issues, the paramedic should always contact medical direction. The paramedic should involve medical direction in the decision-making process. Finally, the paramedic should record all events carefully.

Minors. In most states a person is a minor until age 18. This is the case unless the person is emancipated. Emancipation means being legally released from parental control and supervision. Emancipation may include minors who are married, who are parents, who are in the armed forces, and who are living independently and are self-supporting. An example of the latter is college students not living at home or not receiving financial aid.

Unemancipated minors are those who are under parental control and supervision. These minors are not legally able to give *or* to withhold consent. Still, the paramedic must seek consent before giving treatment. The consent of a parent, legal guardian, or court-appointed custodian is needed. If a delay in getting consent would threaten life, then the emergency doctrine of treating and transporting the patient without consent applies. Although the courts will assume that the parents would have consented, the paramedic should document the nature of the emergency fully. The paramedic also should note the reason the minor needed urgent care.

Mentally Incompetent Adults. Providing emergency care for mentally incompetent adults is similar to caring for minors. This is the case at least regarding obtaining consent. These patients may not be able legally to give or refuse consent. Competence may be impaired by a number of factors, such as disease, injury, anxiety, mental illness, mental retardation, and alcohol or other drug use. The patient may not be mentally or emotionally able to make sound decisions about the care. Thus the emergency doctrine of treating and transporting without consent should be applied. Giving emergency care without consent should occur only when a life-threatening illness or injury exists. Emergency care also should be given only when a legal guardian is not present to grant or refuse consent. The paramedic should always involve medical direction in these cases.

Prisoners or Arrestees. As a rule, being incarcerated or in detention does not deny a person certain rights. The person still is allowed the right to make choices about medical care. However, a prisoner or arrestee may have a limb- or life-threatening injury or illness and may refuse to give consent. The court or police who have the patient in custody may (in some cases) authorize treatment. The authority of law provides consent through the emergency doctrine. Paramedics who often provide care in prison settings should be aware of local and state laws regarding consent for this population.

Refusal of Care or Transport. A mentally competent adult has the right to refuse medical care. This is the case even if the choice could result in death or permanent disability. Refusal of care may be due to religious beliefs, inability to pay, fear, or lack of understanding of medical procedures. The paramedic should be sensitive to these concerns. The paramedic should explain a procedure carefully and answer any questions the patient has. Documentation of this effort on the patient care report is prudent.

Involvement of medical direction, law officers, family members, and friends at the scene may help persuade the patient to accept care and transportation. Despite these efforts, however, some patients still refuse care. If this occurs, the paramedic should make sure the patient knows that he or she can call again for help, despite the first refusal. In addition, family members or friends should be encouraged to stay with the patient, if possible. Cases involving refusal of care are a major cause of lawsuits against EMS agencies. The paramedic should always consult with medical direction regarding these cases.

When dealing with any patient who refuses care, the paramedic should document the event completely. The paramedic should obtain the names and addresses of others who witnessed the event. The paramedic should record all attempts to obtain consent. In addition, the paramedic should advise the patient of the medical risks of refusing care. The paramedic should record this advice on the patient care report. The paramedic should ask law enforcement officers and other allied health professionals at the scene to make similar records of the event. Many EMS systems require the paramedic to obtain a release of liability. The patient and a disinterested witness sign the release, thus recording the refusal of care, transportation, or both.

Some EMS systems require EMS crews to contact medical direction while at the scene. At that time, the paramedics review the case with the physician or physician designee. Medical direction personnel may discuss the situation with the patient while the call is recorded. This policy may be useful in suppressing legal action. However, the most critical legal document of refusal is the written patient care report prepared by the paramedic.

LEGAL COMPLICATIONS RELATED TO CONSENT

Four other key legal issues are related to consent. These may result in a civil or criminal violation. Definitions and examples of these areas of liability follow:

Abandonment: Improper termination of care or turning care over to personnel who do not have training and expertise appropriate for the medical needs of the patient. Abandonment may occur at the scene. Abandonment also may occur when the patient is delivered to the emergency department. Examples include allowing a first responder to provide care for a patient who requires advanced life support care and placing a critical patient in the care of an unlicensed emergency department "tech" at the receiving hospital.

False imprisonment: Intentional and unjustifiable detention of a person. Examples include charges brought by a patient who was transported without consent or who was restrained without proper cause or authority.

Assault: Creating apprehension, or unauthorized handling and treatment of patients. An example is threatening to restrain a patient unless the patient quiets down.

Battery: Physical contact with persons without their consent and without legal cause. An example is drawing a patient's blood without permission.

The paramedic can avoid these other areas of liability by using good judgment. In addition, the paramedic must be sensitive to any special needs of the patient in crisis. The paramedic should always record any unusual situations or actions on the patient care report. The paramedic also should involve medical direction and law officers when needed.

Use of Force

One may have to use reasonable force or restraints when dealing with unruly or violent patients. These patients may be unable to make sound decisions about their care. An example is patients with behavioral emergencies. Another example is those with altered levels of consciousness caused by injury, substance abuse, or illness.

Most law enforcement agencies have the authority to place a patient in protective custody. This permits EMS workers to treat the patient. Emergency medical services personnel should become involved in restraining patients only when it can be done safely. Paramedics should apply restraints only when they have reason to suspect that patients are a threat to themselves or others. Most EMS agencies have protocols that must be followed when restraint of patients is necessary. Some protocols require that violent patients be put in protective custody by law enforcement personnel before paramedics get involved in patient care. Using reasonable force to restrain a patient must always be humane. Force should never be punitive. Physical restraint and the use of sedative drugs (chemical restraint) to help subdue a patient are described in Chapter 40.

Transportation

As stated before, once the paramedic has assumed the duty to act and has begun patient care, the paramedic must continue care until (1) the patient is transferred to another health care worker with training and expertise appropriate for the medical needs of the patient, (2) the patient clearly no longer needs care, or (3) the patient ends the patient-caregiver relationship. A key aspect of this continuum of care is related to patient transport.

USE OF EMERGENCY VEHICLE OPERATING PRIVILEGES

The driver of the emergency vehicle must operate the vehicle safely. The driver must conform to laws, regulations, and policies. The driver also must operate the vehicle in a manner that safeguards the patient, crew, and public. Right-of-way privileges usually given to operators of emergency vehicles include the following:

- The driver may travel slightly faster than the posted speed limit.
- The driver may move safely from one lane into the opposite lane of traffic.
- The driver may safely enter and pass through intersections on a red light.
- The driver may use audible and visual warning devices appropriately.
- The driver may park in unauthorized areas.

CRITICAL THINKING

Your supervisor decides that exceeding the posted speed limit (even with audible and visual warning devices) is too dangerous to the community. The supervisor disallows it on all but cardiac arrest calls. What will you do?

Paramedics should be aware of the laws in their state regarding right-of-way. Vehicle operating privileges can be abused. One example includes use of excessive speed. Another is the improper use or nonuse of audible and visual warning devices. As a rule, emergency vehicles should not exceed 10 miles per hour faster than the posted limits during response or patient transport (see Chapter 49).

CHOICE OF PATIENT DESTINATION

The choice of hospital should be based on patient needs and hospital capability. As a rule, the paramedic should honor the patient's choice. This is the case unless situations or the patient's condition dictates otherwise. Examples of hospital selection include hospitals that are on diversion status because of patient load and the need for specialty care that can be provided only at designated facilities (Box 4-4). Protocols for hospital selection must be established. Medical direction should be involved in cases in which a patient's choice of hospital cannot be honored. For example, some EMS services use a nearest hospital rule. This may be the case even if the nearest hospital is not the patient's choice of facility.

PAYER PROTOCOLS

At times, restrictions of health care plans may affect when and where a patient can be taken for medical care. For example, Medicare is the largest single payer of ambulance services in the United States. Medicare has complex rules as to what types of services and patient transports are eligible for reimbursement (Box 4-4). Paramedics need a basic understanding of these programs so that the EMS agency can be paid for their services. In addition, such knowledge assists paramedics to help patients decide what services are likely to be covered by their insurance policies. The majority of patients transported by ambulance are covered by Medicare, Medicaid, Blue Shield, or a combination of the three.[2]

In emergencies with threats to life or limb, payer protocols should not be a factor. Payer protocols should not play a role in providing patient care or transportation to the closest appropriate facility. However, the paramedic must provide a full description of patient care activities on the patient care report. This is crucial; some claims are rejected for reimbursement because of poor documentation.

BOX 4-4 Categorization of Hospital Resource Capabilities

Categorization of hospital emergency services was recommended by the American Medical Association in the early 1970s. In 1990, *Resources for Optimal Care of the Injured Patient* was published by the Task Force of the American College of Surgeons Committee on Trauma (revised in 1999 and amended in 2000). The publication described three levels of trauma centers based on resources, admissions, staff, research, and education involvement.

A level I institution can provide total care for every aspect of injury. The trauma center is qualified to care for the most severely injured patient, especially in the surgical critical care setting. Level II institutions provide care that supplements treatment in level I facilities or serve as the primary care institutions in less populated areas. Level III institutions provide services such as assessment, resuscitation, emergency surgery, and stabilization. Patients may be transferred to higher-level institutions as needed. Categorization of hospital resources identifies hospitals capable of handling trauma patients. Categorization also enables EMS providers to transport patients rapidly to the right medical facilities. Based on American College of Surgeons guidelines, some state governmental agencies have designated certain institutions as trauma centers. Other specialized care facilities—such as pediatric trauma centers, burn centers, hyperbaric centers, and poison treatment centers—provide care for critically ill or injured patients with special needs. (Note: A level IV facility [primarily a referral center] also has been designated by American College of Surgeons. Level IV is recognized by some states.)

In 1991 the Department of Health and Human Services and EMS division provided financial grants for states to develop comprehensive statewide trauma systems as part of the 1990 Trauma Systems Planning and Development Act (PL 101-590). These grants were last awarded in 1994.

RESUSCITATION ISSUES

Issues that deal with resuscitation are complex. They often involve certain legal and ethical considerations for the patient, family, EMS crew, and medical direction. Resuscitation issues that relate directly to EMS include withholding or stopping resuscitation, advance directives, potential organ donation, and death in the field.

Withholding or Stopping Resuscitation

As stated before, competent and informed adult patients have the right to refuse medical care. They can even refuse cardiopulmonary resuscitation (CPR). This right does not depend on the presence or absence of terminal illness, the agreement of family members, or approval of physicians. As a rule, patients who are pulseless should be resuscitated (unless directed otherwise by a physician), unless one or more of the following apply[3]:

- When a person lies dead, with obvious clinical signs of irreversible death
- When attempting to perform CPR would place the rescuer at risk of physical injury
- When the patient or surrogate has indicated that resuscitation is not desired

According to the American Heart Association, unwitnessed deaths in the presence of known serious, chronic, debilitating disease or in the terminal state of fatal illness may be a reliable criterion in some settings to believe that CPR is not indicated. Cardiopulmonary resuscitation also is not indicated for traumatic arrests with extended response or transport times after a patient's airway is ensured.[3] At times, it may be difficult for the paramedic to determine whether resuscitation should be initiated. An example would be a family member who requests CPR for a patient despite the presence of a no CPR order (Box 4-5). In this situation (or if the paramedic suspects that the no CPR order is invalid), the paramedic should initiate resuscitation and contact medical direction.

CRITICAL THINKING

You are called to care for a debilitated older adult patient in full cardiac arrest. The family members tell you that they want nothing done and are sobbing and begging you not to resuscitate the patient. They do not have the written documentation needed by your agency to permit the do not resuscitate order. What will you do? How will you feel about your decision?

In general, paramedics should err on the side of providing resuscitation and life support. They should do this in most cases in which any issue is unclear. If evidence later indicates that resuscitation should be withheld, life-support measures can be stopped.

Steps for determining when to stop resuscitation should be set by local protocols. The role of medical direction also should be defined clearly in these cases. As a model, the American Heart Association has recommended that resuscitation be discontinued in the prehospital setting when the patient cannot be resuscitated after an adequate trial of basic life support along with advanced cardiac life support. This determination should be made by EMS authorities and medical directors, who generally should ensure the following:

- The patient's airway has been successfully secured.
- Intravenous access has been achieved, and rhythm-appropriate medications and countershocks for ventricular fibrillation or pulseless ventricular tachycardia have been administered according to advanced cardiac life support protocols.
- Persistent asystole or agonal electrocardiographic patterns are present, and no reversible causes are identified (Box 4-6).

BOX 4-5 Definitions

Orders for no CPR, do not resuscitate, and do not attempt resuscitation represent a decision made between the patient and the physician. The decision is that cardiopulmonary resuscitation should be withheld in the event of cardiac arrest. These orders carry no limitation for other forms of treatment such as oxygen, fluid replacement, and drug administration. Some nursing home orders will specify levels of care/support to be provided. For example, the orders may specify no intubation.

Advance Directives

In 1991 a federal law was passed known as the Patient Self-Determination Act of 1990. The law required all facilities that accept Medicare or Medicaid to recognize any kind of advance directive. Examples of such directives are a durable power of attorney for health care or a do not resuscitate order[4] (Fig. 4-2). These legal documents are executed to let health care workers know of a person's wishes in the event the person becomes incapacitated. In such a case, the person would be unable to convey these wishes directly. The person's wishes may include treatment or the withholding of treatment. Many states also have passed legislation regarding living wills and the right to die with dignity. These laws are for patients with a terminal illness. The EMS service must work closely with medical direction to develop procedures and protocols that help EMS providers contend with these laws and policies.

No CPR orders should not be confused with advance directives. A physician must interpret an advance directive. An advance directive needs to be formulated into a treatment plan (which may include no CPR orders) that is consistent with the patient's wishes. Medical direction must establish and implement policies for dealing with advance directives.

The EMS crew may be dispatched to a dying patient who has asked not to be resuscitated. In such a case, the crew should contact medical direction immediately. That way, medical direction can decide about any patient care activities. If medical direction determines that the patient is not to receive medical intervention to prolong life, paramedics should give reasonable measures of comfort. Paramedics

BOX 4-6 Definitions*

Agonal: A cardiac rhythm frequently seen as the last rhythm in an unsuccessful resuscitation and otherwise known as "dying heart" rhythm

Asystole: The absence of mechanical and electrical activity in the heart

Countershock: A high-intensity, short-duration electrical shock applied to the area of the heart

Ventricular fibrillation/pulseless ventricular tachycardia: Pulseless rhythms of the heart

*See Chapter 29 for more discussion.

DO NOT RESUSCITATE (DNR) REQUEST

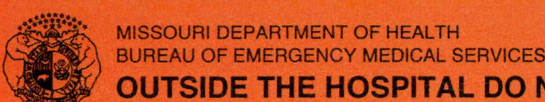

MISSOURI DEPARTMENT OF HEALTH
BUREAU OF EMERGENCY MEDICAL SERVICES

OUTSIDE THE HOSPITAL DO NOT RESUSCITATE (DNR) REQUEST

DNR # 13132

I, ________________________________, request limited emergency care as herein described.
(name)

I understand DNR means that if my heart stops beating or if I stop breathing, no medical procedure to restart breathing or heart functioning will be instituted.

I understand this decision will <u>not</u> prevent me from obtaining other emergency medical care by outside the hospital care providers and/or medical care directed by a physician prior to my death.

I understand I may revoke this directive at any time.

I give permission for this information to be given to the outside the hospital care providers, doctors, nurses, or other health personnel as necessary to implement this directive.

I hereby agree to the "Do Not Resuscitate" (DNR) order.

▶ Patient/Appropriate Surrogate Signature **(Mandatory)**	Date
▶ Witness **(Mandatory)**	Date

REVOCATION PROVISION

I hereby revoke the above declaration.

Signature	Date

I AFFIRM THIS DIRECTIVE IS THE EXPRESSED WISH OF THE PATIENT/PATIENT'S APPROPRIATE SURROGATE, IS MEDICALLY APPROPRIATE, AND IS DOCUMENTED IN THE PATIENT'S PERMANENT MEDICAL RECORD.

In the event of a cardiac or respiratory arrest, no cardiopulmonary resuscitation will be initiated.

▶ Physician's Signature **(Mandatory)**	Date
Physician - Printed Name	Physician's Telephone Number
Address	Facility or Agency Name

MO 580-1936 (8-94) EMS-21

THIS DNR REQUEST FORM SHOULD BE KEPT WITH THE PATIENT IN A VISIBLE LOCATION AT ALL TIMES.
THIS FORM WILL NOT BE ACCEPTED IF IT HAS BEEN AMENDED OR ALTERED IN ANY WAY.

DO NOT RESUSCITATE (DNR) REQUEST

FIGURE 4-2 ■ Advance directive.

also should give emotional support to family members and loved ones.

> **NOTE** Emergency medical services (EMS) and medical direction should work closely with the families and physicians of terminally ill patients in private homes and hospice programs. That way, these persons will make the best use of the EMS system. For instance, they will know when to call 911. Even though resuscitation may not be indicated, EMS personnel may be needed to manage pain. Emergency medical services personnel may be needed to treat acute medical illness or traumatic injury as well. In addition, EMS personnel may be needed to transport to a hospital. Policies must be set and adopted by local or state EMS authorities to allow persons to decline resuscitation attempts but still have access to other emergency medical care and ambulance transport.

Potential Organ Donation

Each day about 70 persons receive organ transplants. Another 16 persons on the waiting list die because not enough organs are available[5] (Box 4-7). The donation of organs and tissues and the transplantation process are complex. Donation and transplantation require the effort of many health care professionals. Paramedics can play a key role in the evaluation of potential donors. They can do this by identifying a patient as a potential donor. They also can establish communication with medical direction. Finally, they can provide emergency care that will help maintain viable organs.

Identifying likely donors who are dead or near dead is a key role for EMS in organ procurement. One can identify a donor by looking for a donor card. Paramedics also can look for a notation on a driver's license that indicates the person's intent to be a donor or not to be a donor. Other actions include talking with next of kin about the patient's intent to donate tissue or organs at death. Even if the patient has no donor card or other document, the family still has the right to make the decision to donate (Box 4-8). Special training is available to EMS workers from tissue procurement organizations. This training teaches them how to approach the family about organ donation.

Once the patient has been identified as a potential donor, paramedics should contact medical direction. Then the proper organ procurement agencies should be notified. These agencies are staffed 24 hours a day to assist in all aspects of the donation. These agencies help in gathering the proper documentation. The paramedic should record carefully and fully all patient care activities, vital sign assessments, and scene events (e.g., presence of drug paraphernalia) that may affect the evaluation of the potential donor by the agency.

Donations usually are separated into two groups. The groups are vital, or heartbeating, donors and the more common donor who has no heartbeat (nonvital tissue donor). Vital donors may donate the heart, liver, kidneys, lungs, and pancreas. These donors must meet the criteria for brain death (Box 4-9). In addition, the donor's heartbeat and circulation must be maintained until the vital organs are harvested. The nonvital (no heartbeat) tissue donor can donate corneas, skin, bones, tendons, heart valves, and saphenous veins up to 24 hours after cardiac death.

The paramedic plays a key role in helping to maintain viable organs in the prehospital setting. The paramedic's role is to preserve organ function. This is best done by airway management and by proper fluid resuscitation. The paramedic needs to maintain blood pressure and organ perfusion (see Chapter 7). The paramedic should give eye care to

BOX 4-7 United Network for Organ Sharing Transplant Statistics

Every 16 minutes a new name is added to the national transplant waiting list.

On December 16, 2002, the United Network for Organ Sharing national patient waiting list for organ transplant included the following:

Type of Transplant	Patients Waiting for Transplant
Heart	3,918
Heart-lung	198
Intestine	198
Kidney	53,532
Kidney-pancreas	2,492
Liver	17,294
Lung	3,859
Pancreas	1,330
TOTAL	80,838*

NOTE: United Network for Organ Sharing policies allow patients to be listed with more than one transplant center (multiple listing); therefore the number of registrations is greater than the actual number of patients.

*Some patients are waiting for more than one organ; therefore the total number of patients is less than the sum of patients waiting for each organ.

BOX 4-8 Legal Next of Kin

When a patient dies in the prehospital setting, organ and tissue donation should be offered as the final option for the surviving family. This option should be offered regardless of the decision to transport the patient to the hospital. Obtaining consent for organ or tissue donation is a delicate subject. The paramedic should approach the issue with compassion and in a positive manner. When approaching a family for organ donation, the paramedic must obtain consent from the next of kin. This relationship is defined by law. The accepted legal order is as follows:

1. Spouse (even if separated but not divorced)
2. Adult son or daughter (over age 18)
3. Parents (for any unmarried child)
4. Siblings (in the event both parents are deceased and the donor is unmarried or divorced with no adult children)
5. Legal guardian

BOX 4-9 Brain Death Criteria

Brain death is defined as the loss of all brain function, including that of the brainstem.[6] Brain dead patients are dependent on a ventilator. They make no spontaneous respiratory effort. In addition, they have lost all spontaneous movement. The clinical findings are usually confirmed in the hospital by electroencephalogram or a brain-flow scan. In most states, brain death must be declared by two separate physicians. Neither of these physicians can be involved in the removal or transplantation of the organs.

all nontransported persons who die at the scene using lubrication/saline solution or a commercial product (e.g., Lacri-Lube). The paramedic should tape the eyes closed so that donation of the cornea can continue to be an option for the family.

Death in the Field

In the field, determination of death usually is confirmed by the following signs:

- No spontaneous electrical activity in the heart as confirmed by electrocardiogram in several leads
- No spontaneous respirations
- Absent cough and gag reflex
- No spontaneous movement
- No response to painful stimuli
- Fixed and midpoint pupils

Other signs are used in determining death. These signs include the presence of dependent lividity and rigor mortis (Box 4-10). When an apparent death is encountered in the field, the paramedic should do the following:

- Contact medical direction for guidance and follow established state and local protocols.
- Document any observations or unusual findings at the scene.
- Notify appropriate authorities per protocol (e.g., police and coroner).
- Disturb the scene as little as possible.
- Provide emotional support to surviving family and friends at the scene.

CRIME SCENE RESPONSIBILITIES

Paramedics play two key roles when managing crime and other incident scenes. The first is providing patient care (the primary focus). The second is helping to preserve evidence at the scene when possible. Personal safety is always the first priority in any emergency response. If the scene is not safe and cannot be made safe, the EMS crew should not enter the area until it has been secured by appropriate personnel.

CRITICAL THINKING

Consider this scenario. At the scene of a shooting, you see a patient with slow, gasping respirations, but the police will not let you enter the crime scene. How do you think you will feel?

When responding to a crime scene, paramedics should be in direct radio communication with law enforcement at the scene. Communication will provide the paramedic with information on scene safety, the number of patients, and the need for more resources. These resources may include more EMS vehicles or personnel, aeromedical transport, fire service or specialized rescue units, and hazardous materials teams. If police are not on the scene or if the EMS crew is the first to respond, paramedics should maintain contact with the dispatch center. Thus proper information can be relayed to law enforcement. One should remember that law enforcement is in charge of the crime scene. Emergency medical services is in charge of patient care. Emergency medical services crews should work closely with police who will be protecting them. In addition to providing patient care, the paramedic should observe and document the overall scene and make an effort to protect potential evidence (Box 4-11). Scene safety considerations include the following:

- Approaching the scene only after it has been secured
- Approaching the scene from a direction that appears safe and allows for easy exit
- Maintaining constant radio contact with police or dispatch
- Surveying and assessing the scene before approaching the patient
- Keeping all unnecessary persons away from the patient
- Initiating conversations with bystanders only when necessary

DOCUMENTATION

The patient care report serves several functions. Of particular importance is that it provides a legal record of the patient care delivered in the field. The report also becomes a permanent part of the patient's hospital record.

BOX 4-10 Physiological Changes That Occur after Death

Within minutes after death, postmortem changes begin to occur in the body. The surface of the skin becomes pale and yellowish; body temperature falls and reaches that of the environment within 24 hours; blood pressure and muscle tension decrease; and the pupils become dilated. Blood and fluids begin to drain away from the face, nose, and chin as gravity causes blood to settle in the most dependent, lowest tissues. This drainage results in a bluish-purple discoloration in the tissues known as postmortem lividity.

Within 6 hours after death, muscle stiffening occurs from chemical changes in the body. This is known as rigor mortis. Smaller muscles in the face usually are affected first. This is followed by a stiffening of the entire body within 12 to 14 hours. Signs of tissue decay are usually obvious within 24 to 48 hours after death, depending on environmental temperatures. The rigor mortis diminishes and the body becomes flaccid within 12 to 14 hours. As the body decays, the skin loosens from the underlying tissues, and swelling and bloating become evident.

BOX 4-11 Crime Scene Preservation

Lifesaving procedures always take precedence over forensic considerations. However, the paramedic should disturb the scene as little as possible to help preserve evidence. Some forensic considerations include the following:

- Park the ambulance away from skid marks, tire prints, or other evidence.
- Follow the same path to and from the ambulance and patient.
- Avoid stepping on blood stains.
- Do not touch or move weapons or other environmental clues unless absolutely necessary for patient care.
- Document the exact condition of the patient and wound appearance on arrival at the scene, including environment of the patient and body position in relation to objects and doorways.
- If possible, cut or tear clothing along a seam to avoid altering tears made by a penetrating object. Avoid cutting through a hole made in the clothing by a wounding object.
- Do not shake clothing; keep all clothing in a paper bag rather than a plastic bag that may alter evidence; do not give clothing to the victim's family members.
- Save any avulsed tissue for forensic pathological examination.
- If a bullet is retrieved, place it in a padded container to prevent marring and secure the evidence until it is delivered to the authorities; obtain a receipt.
- Document any dying declarations made by patients.
- Report all actions and alterations made to the crime scene to the police.

In the legal field the general belief is that "if it was not written down, it was not done." The paramedic's record of an emergency call will be one of the first items reviewed in the case of a lawsuit for negligence or malpractice. Memory is faulty. Moreover, claims may not be filed until years after an event. As a result, EMS personnel may be expected to testify to events years after they occurred. The paramedic will be allowed to refer to written reports to refresh his or her memory about details while testifying. Therefore accuracy and attention to detail are crucial in documentation (see Chapter 16). Characteristics of an effective patient care report include the following:

- Completed promptly. The patient care report is a record made "in the course of business" not long after the event. Timely completion is essential to the patient care report becoming part of the hospital record.
- Completed thoroughly. The patient care report should cover assessment, treatment, and other relevant facts. The report should paint a complete, clear picture of the patient's condition and the care provided.
- Completed objectively. The paramedic should make observations and not assumptions or conclusions. The paramedic should avoid the use of emotional and value words or phrases.
- Completed accurately. Descriptions should be as precise as possible; the paramedic should avoid using abbreviations or jargon that is not common.
- Written with confidentiality maintained. The paramedic should follow policy for the release of patient information. When possible, the paramedic should get patient consent before the release. Records should be stored in a secure location with access limited by departmental policy. This applies to paper or electronic records.

All patient care records need to be maintained at least for the extent of the statute of limitations. This statute varies by state from 2 to 6 years for personal injury lawsuits. Patient records involving minors may need to be kept for a longer time because the statute of limitations may not begin until the minor is 18 years of age. (This also varies from state to state.)

CRITICAL THINKING

Think back to the first call you were on when a patient refused medical care. Can you remember exact details about his level of consciousness, what you told him about the risks of refusing care, and what you told him to do if the problem got worse? Do you think all of those facts are in the written documentation of that call in the event of litigation?

SUMMARY

- The structure of the legal system in the United States is composed of five types of law: legislative law, administrative law, common law, criminal law, and civil law.
- To safeguard against litigation, the paramedic must be knowledgeable of legal issues. The paramedic also must know about the effects of these issues.
- Paramedics and health care workers may be required by law to report some cases. These include cases of abuse or neglect of children and older adults and spouse abuse. They also include cases that involve rape, sexual assault, gunshot wounds, stab wounds, animal bites, and some communicable diseases.
- Lawsuits that have to do with patient care usually result from civil claims of negligence. This refers to the failure to act as a reasonable, prudent paramedic would act in such circumstances.
- Most legal authorities stress that protection against claims of negligence has three elements. The first is training. The second is competent patient care skills. The third is full documentation of all patient care activities.
- Some state and federal regulations provide protection for the paramedic with respect to notification of infectious disease exposure, immunity statutes, and special crimes against EMS personnel.

- Confidential information is threefold. For the most part, confidential information includes any details about a patient that are related to the patient's history. Any assessment findings also are included. Any treatment given is included as well. As a rule, the release of these details requires written permission from the patient or legal guardian. (There are some exceptions.)
- A mentally competent adult has the right to refuse medical care. This is the case even if the decision could result in death or permanent disability.
- Four other legal complications related to consent are abandonment, false imprisonment, assault, and battery.
- A competent patient has certain rights. The patient has the right to decide what medical care (and transportation) to receive. This is a basic concept of law and medical practice.
- Legal responsibilities for the patient continue until patient care is transferred to another member of the health care system (or it is clear that the patient no longer requires care). Legal issues related to patient transport include level of care during transportation, use of the emergency vehicle operating privileges, choice of patient destination, and payer protocols.
- Resuscitation issues that relate directly to EMS include withholding or stopping resuscitation, advance directives, potential organ donation, and death in the field.
- Emergency medical services play two important roles when responding to crime scenes: (1) focusing on patient care and (2) preserving evidence at the scene when possible.
- In the legal field the general belief is that "if it was not written down, it was not done." Thus thoroughness and attention to detail are vital in documentation.

REFERENCES

1. US Department of Transportation, National Highway Traffic Safety Administration: *EMT-Paramedic national standard curriculum,* Washington, DC, 1998, The Department.
2. Fitch J, Keller R, Raynor D et al: *EMS management beyond the street,* ed 2, Carlsbad, Calif, 1993, JEMS.
3. American Heart Association: Guidelines 2000 for cardiopulmonary resuscitation and emergency cardiovascular care, International Consensus on Science, *Circulation* 102(8):16, 2000.
4. Hall S: New act compels EMS to define new roles, *J Emerg Med Serv JEMS* 17(1):19, 1992.
5. US Department of Health and Human Services: Organ Donation. http://www.organdonor.gov. Accessed November 19, 2004.
6. Winmill D, Clawson J: Seize the moment: the EMS role in organ donation, *J Emerg Med Serv JEMS* 15(11):48, 1990.

CHAPTER

5

Ethics

OBJECTIVES

Upon completion of this chapter, the paramedic student will be able to:

1. Define ethics and bioethics.
2. Distinguish between professional, legal, and moral accountability.
3. Outline strategies to use to resolve ethical conflicts.
4. Describe the role of ethical tests in resolving ethical dilemmas in health care.
5. Discuss specific prehospital ethical issues including allocation of resources, decisions surrounding resuscitation, confidentiality, and consent.
6. Identify ethical dilemmas that may occur related to care in futile situations, obligation to provide care, patient advocacy, and the paramedic's role as physician extender.

KEY TERMS

bioethics: The systematic study of moral dimensions including moral vision, decisions, conduct, and policies of the life sciences and health care.

ethics: The discipline relating to right and wrong, moral duty and obligation, moral principles and values, and moral character; a standard for honorable behavior designed by a group with expected conformity.

morals: Social standards or customs; dealing with what is right or wrong in a practical sense.

unethical: Conduct that fails to conform to moral principles, values, or standards.

Ethical dilemmas will always be a part of prehospital care. At times paramedics will have to perform duties that may involve conflicts in moral judgment. An example includes issues of patient confidentiality or patient rights. Another is field testing of experimental drugs or procedures. Another example is honoring a do not resuscitate order. Such ethical issues are dynamic. The ethical dilemmas of today may be decided by law tomorrow.

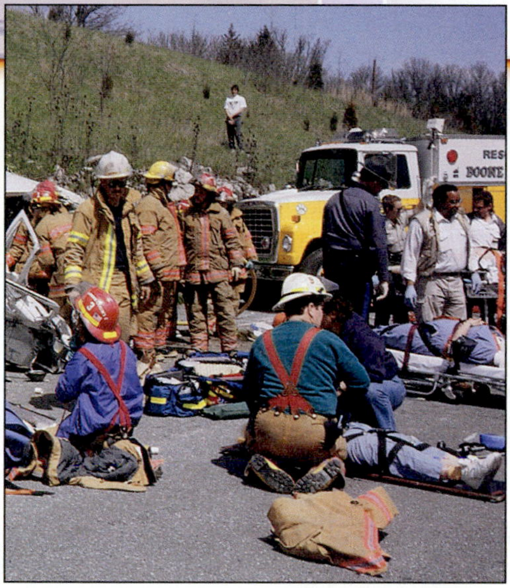

ETHICS OVERVIEW

Ethics is the field relating to right and wrong, duty and obligation, principles and values, and character.[1] Ethics is a basis for honorable actions designed by a group with expected conformity. **Morals** refers to social standards or customs, or dealing with what is right or wrong in a practical sense. The term **unethical** refers to conduct that fails to conform. Unethical conduct does not meet moral principles, values, or standards.[2] Ethical decisions are based on an appraisal of moral judgments. This idea places the responsibility on individuals.

The idea of ethics dates back to the ancient Greek philosophers. These include persons such as Hippocrates, Socrates, Plato, and Aristotle. These philosophers turned the Greek focus toward questions of ethics and virtue (how should one live?) for moral accountability and away from choice and fate that traditionally had been guided by astrology (Box 5-1). These philosophers laid the basis for a science of medical ethics **(bioethics)**, the analysis of choice in medicine.[3]

Bioethics is the systematic study of moral dimensions. Bioethics includes moral vision, decisions, conduct, and policies of the life sciences and health care. Bioethics uses a variety of ethical methodologies in an interdisciplinary setting.

One can make many ethical and other value choices instinctively. One makes these choices by drawing on longstanding personal beliefs, commitments, and habits. For example, most persons believe it is wrong to steal, to be deceitful, or to commit murder. In health care, however, paramedics are faced with life issues that involve a patient. The patient may have beliefs, commitments, and habits that may be different from the paramedic's personal experience. Throughout history, guidance in these situations has been provided through a variety of professional codes. These codes represent the collective wisdom of a group. The EMT Code of Ethics and the Principles of Medical Ethics of the American Medical Association are examples of professional codes (Boxes 5-2 and 5-3).

As with professional codes, a person's personal code of ethics is made up of principles of proper conduct. These values can assist one in making moral choices. A personal code is a critical reflection on one's life. For the paramedic, this code must take into account professional, legal, and moral responsibility (Box 5-4).

CRITICAL THINKING

Which of these quotes of ethical living best speaks for your personal philosophy?

Professional Accountability

As professionals, paramedics conform to a standard set by their level of training and regional practice. Paramedics are accountable to the patient, the medical director, and the emergency medical services system for meeting the

BOX 5-1 The Hippocratic Oath (Fourth Century BC)

The Oath of Hippocrates is a brief statement of principles. The oath is thought to have been conceived during the fourth century BC. The oath protected the rights of the patient. The oath also addressed the moral character of the physician as a healer. The Hippocratic oath was modified in the tenth or eleventh century to eliminate reference to pagan gods. The oath remains an expression of ideal conduct for the physician. *I swear by Apollo Physician and Asclepius and Hygieia and Panaceia and all the gods and goddesses, making them my witnesses, that I will fulfill according to my ability and judgment this oath and this covenant:*

To hold him who has taught me this art as equal to my parents and to live my life in partnership with him, and if he is in need of money to give him a share of mine, and to regard his offspring as equal to my brothers in male lineage and to teach them this art—if they desire to learn it—without fee and covenant; to give a share of precepts and oral instruction and all the other learning to my sons and to the sons of him who has instructed me and to pupils who have signed the covenant and have taken an oath according to the medical law, but to no one else.

I will apply dietetic measures for the benefit of the sick according to my ability and judgment; I will keep them from harm and injustice.

I will neither give a deadly drug to anybody if asked for it, nor will I make a suggestion to this effect. Similarly I will not give to a woman an abortive remedy. In purity and holiness I will guard my life and my art.

I will not use the knife, not even on sufferers from stone, but will withdraw in favor of such men as are engaged in this work.

Whatever houses I may visit, I will come for the benefit of the sick, remaining free of all intentional injustice, of all mischief and in particular of sexual relations with both female and male persons, be they free or slaves.

What I may see or hear in the course of treatment or even outside of the treatment in regard to the life of men, which on no account one must spread abroad, I will keep to myself, holding such things shameful to be spoken about.

If I fulfill this oath and do not violate it, may it be granted to me to enjoy life and art, being honored with fame among all men for all time to come; if I transgress it and swear falsely, may the opposite of all this be my lot.

BOX 5-2 The EMT Code of Ethics

Professional status as an Emergency Medical Technician and Emergency Medical Technician-Paramedic is maintained and enriched by the willingness of the individual practitioner to accept and fulfill obligations to society, other medical professionals, and the profession of Emergency Medical Technician. As an Emergency Medical Technician at the basic level or an Emergency Medical Technician—Paramedic, I solemnly pledge myself to the following code of professional ethics:

A fundamental responsibility of the Emergency Medical Technician is to conserve life, to alleviate suffering, to promote health, to do no harm, and to encourage the quality and equal availability of emergency medical care.

The Emergency Medical Technician provides services based on human need, with respect for human dignity, unrestricted by consideration of nationality, race, creed, color, or status.

The Emergency Medical Technician does not use professional knowledge and skills in any enterprise detrimental to the public well-being.

The Emergency Medical Technician respects and holds in confidence all information of a confidential nature obtained in the course of professional work unless required by law to divulge such information.

The Emergency Medical Technician, as a citizen, understands and upholds the law and performs the duties of citizenship; as a professional, the Emergency Medical Technician has the never-ending responsibility to work with concerned citizens and other health care professionals in promoting a high standard of emergency medical care to all people.

The Emergency Medical Technician shall maintain professional competence and demonstrate concern for the competence of other members of the Emergency Medical Services health care team.

An Emergency Medical Technician assumes responsibility in defining and upholding standards of professional practice and education.

The Emergency Medical Technician assumes responsibility for individual professional actions and judgment, both in dependent and independent emergency functions, and knows and upholds the laws which affect the practice of the Emergency Medical Technician.

An Emergency Medical Technician has the responsibility to be aware of and participate in matters of legislation affecting the Emergency Medical Technician and the Emergency Medical Services System.

The Emergency Medical Technician adheres to standards of personal ethics which reflect credit upon the profession.

Emergency Medical Technicians, or groups of Emergency Medical Technicians, who advertise professional services, do so in conformity with the dignity of the profession.

The Emergency Medical Technician has an obligation to protect the public by not delegating to a person less qualified any service which requires the professional competence of an Emergency Medical Technician.

The Emergency Medical Technician will work harmoniously with, and sustain confidence in, Emergency Medical Technician associates, the nurse, the physician, and other members of the emergency medical services health care team.

The Emergency Medical Technician refuses to participate in unethical procedures and assumes the responsibility to expose incompetence or unethical conduct of others to the appropriate authority in a proper and professional manner.

BOX 5-3 American Medical Association Principles of Medical Ethics*

Principles of Medical Ethics

- A physician shall be dedicated to providing competent medical care, with compassion and respect for human dignity and rights.
- A physician shall uphold the standards of professionalism, be honest in all professional interactions, and strive to report physicians deficient in character or competence, or engaging in fraud or deception, to appropriate entities.
- A physician shall respect the law and also recognize a responsibility to seek changes in those requirements which are contrary to the best interests of the patient.
- A physician shall respect the rights of patients, colleagues, and other health professionals, and shall safeguard patient confidences and privacy within the constraints of the law.
- A physician shall continue to study, apply, and advance scientific knowledge, maintain a commitment to medical education, make relevant information available to patients, colleagues, and the public, obtain consultation, and use the talents of other health professionals when indicated.
- A physician shall, in the provision of appropriate patient care, except in emergencies, be free to choose whom to serve, with whom to associate, and the environment in which to provide medical care.
- A physician shall recognize a responsibility to participate in activities contributing to the improvement of the community and the betterment of public health.
- A physician shall, while caring for a patient, regard responsibility to the patient as paramount.
- A physician shall support access to medical care for all people.

Adopted by the American Medical Association House of Delegates June 17, 2001.

* The Principles of Medical Ethics also have been adopted by the American College of Emergency Physicians.

BOX 5-4 Statements for Ethical Living

Socrates: The unexamined life is not worth living. Know thyself. Morality is the necessity of the heart. The soul is that which is.

Plato: Justice is the harmony of all virtues. Truth belongs to the mind.

Aristotle: Sense reveals only individual existence. The universal is immanent in the individual. Man finds his ethic only in his natural self-realization.

Zoroastrianism and Parsis: Good thoughts, good words, good deeds. The Reality is one, the wise by many men call it.

Buddhism: Let a man lift himself up by his own self; let him not depress himself; for he himself is his friend and he himself is his enemy.

Confucianism: Seek to be in harmony with all your neighbors.

Taoism: Being in one's inmost heart in kindly sympathy with all things.

Christianity: Love thy neighbor as thyself.

Judaism: Perform righteousness on earth that ye may find treasures in heaven.

Islam: Do what God likes, and avoid what He dislikes.

standard of care. Duties include commitment to high-quality patient care; continuing education; skill proficiency; and licensure, certification, or both. The paramedic is accountable by law to that level of training and that standard of care. A paramedic who is accountable to the profession is more likely to provide good patient care and make decisions that are ethically sound.

Legal Accountability

Through patient care the paramedic also assumes a role in the health care legal system (see Chapter 4). Legal issues often are entwined with ethical issues. However, ethics is not synonymous with law. (Ethics deals with moral actions; law deals with legal actions.) Many ethical decisions occur outside the boundaries of the law, and many legal decisions may not be ethical. (An example is a patient who has a living will in a state in which the legality of advance directives has not been resolved.) The paramedic should consider the importance of legal accountability as it relates to medical ethics and abide by the law when ethical conflicts occur.

Moral Accountability

Moral accountability refers to *personal* ethics, that is, personal values and beliefs. Combining moral, legal, and professional accountability may be difficult in an emergency. At times, the paramedic will have to draw on personal ethics to resolve conflicts among these roles and duties. Moreover, the paramedic will have to decide on a course of action. When dealing with ethical questions, the paramedic should remember the following key points[4,5]:

1. Emotion may not be a reliable determinant for ethical decision making. One should monitor the conscience. The conscience can be a good guide if one's conscience is well-informed concerning right or wrong. Rational decision making is making decisions that rely on research and prudence regarding what is right. However, some knowledge deficit may permit the paramedic to come to a flawed decision.
2. Decisions must not be based solely on the opinions of others. The decisions also must not be based on global protocols that were meant to guide, not dictate (e.g., codes of the profession). If paramedics come across a situation that they have never dealt with before, they are likely to make a poor, or even unethical, decision. In these cases, paramedics should consult with medical direction, a supervisor, or a set of guidelines or other resources. Consultation is better than limiting oneself to one's own knowledge base or principles. At times, input from patients and their loved ones can be a key source of information and can lead to a better decision.
3. Once the ethical question has been answered, the answer becomes a "rule" to guide behavior, at least in the particular setting. Once the rule has been identified, it should become a barrier to acting in opposition to the

rule. Paramedics are expected not to break the rule without a strong reason for their actions.

> **NOTE** In reference to answering ethical questions, no one knows all the answers. In addition, none of the tools or techniques will work in every case to arrive at the "right" decision. Nonetheless, health care providers are accountable for personal and professional actions and decisions. Seeking counsel and guidance with such decisions is always wise.

A RAPID APPROACH TO EMERGENCY ETHICAL PROBLEMS

A method of ethical case analysis has been designed. This method works as a way to deal with emergency ethical problems rapidly.[6] The rules of thumb process involves the following steps:

1. Ask yourself if you have experienced a similar ethical problem in the past. If so, use that experience as a precedent for this problem and follow the rule. (Periodically the paramedic must evaluate these rules.)
2. If you have not experienced a similar ethical problem in the past, buy time for deliberation and for consulting with co-workers and medical direction.
3. If there is no option to buy time for deliberation, use a set of three tests to help you make a decision[7] (Fig. 5-1):
   - Test 1: Impartiality Test—Would you accept the action if you were in the patient's place?
   - Test 2: Universalizability Test—Would you feel comfortable having this action performed in all relevantly similar circumstances?
   - Test 3: Interpersonal Justifiability Test—Are you able to provide good reasons to justify and defend your actions to others?

The first test is a good way to correct one's personal bias. The second test helps to do away with moral decision difficulty. The final test makes sure that the paramedic has reasons for proceeding. The final test also requires that others would approve of the reasons. If the paramedic can answer all three tests in the affirmative, then the paramedic has a fair probability that the action falls within the scope of being ethically acceptable. Even though there may be disagreement about a specific set of values, there often is general agreement over what may comprise wrong actions.

ETHICAL TESTS IN HEALTH CARE

The most basic question of ethical tests in health care is, "What is in the patient's best interest?" However, doing what is best, or what one thinks is best, is not enough to justify actions. One must determine what the patient wants. The paramedic can do this using statements by the patient (if the patient is mentally competent) and written statements. Family input is also helpful (if the patient shows altered mental status or incompetence). The role of "good faith" in making ethical decisions ("Am I doing my best to help and not harm my patient?") should be balanced with the wishes of the patient and the family. The

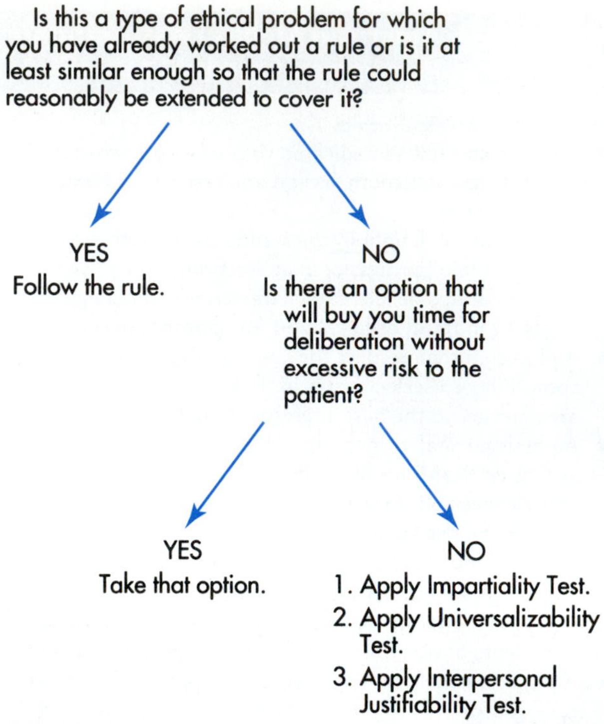

FIGURE 5-1 ■ A rapid approach to emergency ethical problems.

> **BOX 5-5 Global Concepts of Ethical Health Care**
>
> Therapeutic activity of the Greek doctor was subject to the following rules:
> - To help the patient, or at least to do no harm
> - To refrain from interfering if the illness were incurable and inevitably mortal
> - Insofar as possible, to attack the cause of the disease therapeutically
>
> Today, these global concepts of ethical health care can be stated as follows:
> - Provide patient benefit.
> - Do no harm.

global concept of health care (providing patient benefit and avoiding harm) recognizes and respects the patient's autonomy. The concept also recognizes the various legal issues that affect the delivery of health care (Box 5-5).

RESOLVING ETHICAL DILEMMAS

At times, resolving ethical dilemmas can be difficult. This may be the case when global concepts of health care are in conflict. Thus the resolution can be guided by the health care community and by the public. The role of the health care community in resolving these conflicts is to set standards of care. The health care community also must provide research and treatment protocols. Finally, the health care community must make prospective and retrospective reviews of decisions and policies. Reviews are done with the intent of educating the paramedic and improving the quality of patient care. The role of the public in managing ethical conflicts in medicine includes creating laws and setting public policy. This role also includes allocating resources to protect patient rights. Lastly, the role of the public includes participating in the use of advance directives and other self-determination documents to make patient wishes known.

ETHICAL ISSUES IN CONTEMPORARY PARAMEDIC PRACTICE

Paramedics will face some ethical issues during the span of their careers. Most issues deal with the patient's right to self-determination and the paramedic's duty to provide patient care (Box 5-6). The first concept is known as autonomy and the latter as beneficence. Some of the more common issues (and sample case studies) are described in this section. For each case study, the paramedic should apply the rapid approach to emergency medical problems (described previously in this chapter) and should answer the following ethical questions:

1. What is in the patient's best interest?
2. What are the patient's rights?
3. Does the patient understand the issues at hand?
4. What is the paramedic's professional, legal, and moral accountability?

BOX 5-6 Commonly Accepted Bioethical Values

Allocation of resources: The consistent access to quality medical services; distributing health-related services among various persons and uses.

Autonomy: Self-determination; a person's ability to make moral decisions, including those affecting personal medical care. The three components of autonomy are agency (awareness of oneself as having desires and intentions and acting on them); independence (absence of influences that so control what a person does that it cannot be said the person wants to do it); and rationality (rational decision making).

Beneficence: A duty to confer benefits; the practice of good deeds; obligation to benefit others or seek their good.

Confidentiality: The presumption that confidential information will not be revealed to others without the patient's permission. Confidentiality, like privacy, is valued because it protects individual preferences and rights.

Nonmaleficence: The prevention of harm, from Hippocratic tradition that established *primum non nocere* ("Above all, do no harm"); a prohibition on actions with foreseeable harmful effects.

Personal integrity: Adhering to a personal set of values and moral standards.

Allocation of Resources

Fairness in the allocation of resources and obligations is a commonly accepted bioethical value. Fairness is integrated into society-wide health care policies. This perceived right to universal access to an adequate level of health care is a complex economic issue. The issue is affected by the need to contain health care costs. Two factors affect true parity in the allocation of resources. The first is a person's access to health insurance. This may define what medical services are covered or excluded. The second is treatment decisions made when resources are inadequate to meet patient care needs. This may occur, for example, during a multiple-casualty disaster. When rationing of care is required, it should be based on ethically oriented criteria.[8]

The allocation of resources is more of a policy than a clinical concept. However, allocation can pose ethical dilemmas in prehospital care, as illustrated in the following case study:

CASE STUDY 1

A paramedic crew has been dispatched to the home of a 74-year-old man. The man is complaining of chest pain and shortness of breath. The patient is in obvious distress and provides a significant cardiac history. He asks to be taken to the Veterans Hospital (30 miles away). This is where he had heart surgery several years ago. Based on the patient's history, physical exam, and electrocardiogram findings, the paramedic crew (in consultation with medical direction) elects to take the patient to a closer hospital to be stabilized. The patient becomes anxious and complains of increasing chest pain. He tells the paramedic crew that he has no medical insurance and demands to be taken to the Veterans Administration hospital.

Decisions Surrounding Resuscitation

Advance directives, living wills, and other self-determination documents can help the paramedic. The paramedic can use these documents to make decisions about the appropriateness of resuscitation in the prehospital setting. The presence of the proper document often makes resuscitation decisions much easier. Having knowledgeable family members also makes such decisions easier. In other cases, however, the decision to initiate or withhold resuscitation measures is not so clear, as illustrated in the following case study:

CASE STUDY 2

The paramedic crew has been dispatched to a restaurant where an elderly woman has collapsed. She has suffered cardiac arrest, and a waiter is performing cardiopulmonary resuscitation. The electrocardiogram monitor reveals ventricular fibrillation. Defibrillatory shocks are delivered, but the rhythm remains unchanged. As resuscitation measures are continued, the woman's husband says to the paramedics, "She said she didn't want this. Her living will is at home. Please stop what you're doing and let her go."

Confidentiality

Most persons are seen as having a basic right to privacy. The notion of confidentiality refers to one's private and personal information. This information should not be disclosed by a health care worker to other persons without the patient's consent.

In some cases, the release of such information is required by law. An example of such a case is the disclosure of positive human immunodeficiency virus infection status to others involved in the patient's care. Conflict between ethics and confidentiality may arise, however, particularly if the public health would benefit from the disclosure of confidential information, as described in the following case study:

CASE STUDY 3

The paramedic crew has been dispatched to a motor vehicle crash. A young man has struck another car head-on, killing the driver of the other car. The patient is shaken but has only minor injuries. While preparing the patient for transport, the patient confides to the paramedic that he had used cocaine shortly before the crash occurred. The patient asks the paramedic, however, to keep the information confidential and not to tell the law enforcement officers at the scene.

> **CRITICAL THINKING**
>
> Your partner contacts a former patient to ask for a date using the phone number from the patient care report. Do you think that action violates any ethical principles? If so, which ones?

Consent

As explained in Chapter 4, competent patients have a legal right to decide on the medical care they will receive. This right is a basic element of the relationship between the patient and physician. This right is described in the Principles of Medical Ethics of the American Medical Association. The right also can be inferred from the EMT Code of Ethics. Cases in which patients refuse lifesaving care can produce legal and ethical conflicts, as illustrated in the following case study:

CASE STUDY 4

The paramedic crew has been dispatched to an office building. A 55-year-old woman collapsed at a business meeting. She is alert and oriented, complains of chest pain, and is pale and diaphoretic. The paramedics advise the patient of the possibility of a heart attack and the need for immediate care and transport for physician evaluation. The patient insists on waiting until after the meeting has concluded to seek medical care on her own, and she asks the EMS crew to leave.

Other Ethical Principles for Patient Care Situations

Other ethical principles for patient care situations relate to care in futile situations, legal obligations to provide care, patient advocacy and paramedic accountability, and the paramedic's role as a physician extender.

CARE IN FUTILE SITUATIONS

An action is seen as *futile* if it serves no purpose or is totally ineffective. When a paramedic is providing care in a case that may be futile, the paramedic should consult with medical direction. Consultation can help the paramedic to decide on a course of action. An example of a futile situation in health care is continuing resuscitation initiated by bystanders when the patient clearly has expired. Another example is providing life support measures for a patient who has fatal injuries. The definition of *futility* may pose an ethical dilemma. This may be especially true when a dispute or lack of agreement exists about the goals of treatment. Not all futility judgments are controversial. For example, cardiopulmonary resuscitation is futile and should not be provided to patients with obvious signs of death. Some obvious signs are decapitation, rigor mortis, tissue decompensation, or extreme dependent lividity.[8]

> **CRITICAL THINKING**
>
> You arrive at a home where you find a 3-month-old baby who obviously has been dead for several hours. The mother is screaming, "Help her, help her." Your partner decides to proceed with advanced life support care even though it is clearly futile. Is this decision ethical?

OBLIGATION TO PROVIDE CARE

In the prehospital arena the paramedic's duty to provide care seldom is an issue. (The patient's request for emergency service presents a legal duty to act.) In other areas of health care, though, an obligation to provide care may be affected by a few factors. The obligation may be affected by a patient's ability to pay. The obligation also may be shaped by the patient's insurance or other economic factors. Laws protect well-meaning caregivers from liability (e.g., Good Samaritan legislation). These laws also protect patients from unethical health care practices. Examples of such practices are "economic triage" and "patient dumping" (see Chapter 4).

PATIENT ADVOCACY AND PARAMEDIC ACCOUNTABILITY

While providing care, the paramedic serves as the patient's advocate. This advocacy may conflict at times with the paramedic's accountability to the patient, the physician medical director, and the health care system (e.g., health maintenance organization protocols). In such a case, the paramedic should discuss all options with medical direction. *As a rule, it is prudent and ethical to err on the side of providing the needs of the patient when conflict arises.* Examples of ways in which a paramedic can serve as the patient's advocate include the following:

- Educating patients on the delivery of health care and the role that they can play to affect change in the nation's health care system
- Ensuring that health care decisions are made by patients and their doctors and are based on the medical needs of patients, not financial considerations
- Informing patients of federal, state, and private sector health care reform initiatives

- Promoting patient access to reliable information about state-of-the-art medical technologies and treatments
- Promoting fairness and equality in America's health care system

ROLE AS PHYSICIAN EXTENDER

As a physician extender the paramedic has a role to fulfill. For the most part, the paramedic is to follow the orders of the medical director or the director's designee. Yet there may be times when these orders may not seem appropriate. For example, the paramedic may believe that a medication order is contraindicated for the patient. Also, a medication may be medically acceptable but not in the patient's best interest. A third example of such a case is a medication that is medically acceptable but morally wrong.

The converse can also occur. For example, a paramedic might request treatment for a case in which the field impression is unsure. Or the physician may lack information to approve the request. When a conflict occurs between medical direction and the paramedic, communication is the key. Communication can resolve short-term and long-term concerns.

CRITICAL THINKING

Your patient is in critical condition, and you cannot secure the airway. Medical direction tells you to divert because the hospital has no open beds in the intensive care unit. You repeat the urgency of your patient's condition and are still told to divert. You elect to override the physician's order and transport the patient to that hospital. Can you justify disobeying the physician's order?

SUMMARY

- Ethics is the discipline relating to right and wrong, moral duty and obligation, moral principles and values, and moral character. Bioethics is the science of medical ethics. Morals refers to social standard or customs.
- Paramedics must meet a standard established by their level of training and regional practice. Paramedics must abide by the law when ethical conflicts occur.
- A paramedic must act in a way that is seen as morally acceptable.
- The rapid approach to ethical issues is a process. The process involves reviewing past experiences; deliberation (if possible); and performing the impartiality test, universalizability test, and interpersonal justifiability test to reach an acceptable decision.
- Two concepts of ethical health care are to provide patient benefit and to do no harm.
- All resources must be allocated fairly. This is an accepted bioethical value.
- Advance directives, living wills, and other self-determination documents can help the paramedic to make decisions about the appropriateness of resuscitation in the prehospital setting.
- A health care professional is not allowed to reveal details supplied by the patient to others without the patient's consent. This is the principle of confidentiality.
- In some cases, patients refuse lifesaving care. These cases can produce legal and ethical conflicts.
- Other areas that are likely to raise ethical questions in the prehospital setting include providing care in futile situations, the paramedic's obligation to provide care, patient advocacy, and the paramedic's role as physician extender.

REFERENCES

1. Sanderson B: *History of ethics to 30 BC: ancient wisdom and folly.* Santa Barbara, Calif., 2002, World Peace Communications.
2. American Medical Association, Council on Ethical and Judicial Affairs: *Code of medical ethics: current opinions with annotations,* Chicago, 1997, The Association.
3. Veatch R: *Medical ethics,* ed 2, Sudbury, Mass, 1997, Jones and Bartlett.
4. US Department of Transportation, National Highway Traffic Safety Administration: *EMT-Paramedic national standard curriculum,* Washington, DC, 1998, The Department.
5. Bourn S: Through traffic keep right, *J Emerg Med Serv JEMS* 21(5):26, 1996.
6. Rosen P, Barkin R: *Emergency medicine: concepts and clinical practice,* ed 4, St Louis, 1998, Mosby.
7. Iserson K et al: *Ethics in emergency medicine,* ed 2, Tucson, Ariz, 1995, Galen Press.
8. American Heart Association: Guidelines 2000 for cardiopulmonary resuscitation and emergency cardiovascular care, International Consensus on Science, *Circulation* 102(8):14, 2000.

PART TWO

IN THIS PART

CHAPTER 6 Review of Human Systems

CHAPTER 7 General Principles of Pathophysiology

CHAPTER 8 Life Span Development

CHAPTER

6

Review of Human Systems

OBJECTIVES

Upon completion of this chapter, the paramedic student will be able to:

1. Discuss the importance of human anatomy as it relates to the paramedic profession.
2. Describe the anatomical position.
3. Properly interpret anatomical directional terms and body planes.
4. List the structures that compose the axial and appendicular regions of the body.
5. Define the divisions of the abdominal region.
6. List the three major body cavities.
7. Describe the contents of the three major body cavities.
8. Discuss the functions of the following cellular structures: the cytoplasmic membrane, the cytoplasm (and organelles), and the nucleus.
9. Describe the process by which human cells reproduce.
10. Differentiate and describe the following tissue types: epithelial tissue, connective tissue, muscle tissue, and nervous tissue.
11. For each of the 11 major organ systems in the human body, label a diagram of anatomical structures, list the functions of the major anatomical structures, and explain how the organs of the system interrelate to perform the specified functions of the system.
12. For the special senses, label a diagram of the anatomical structures of the special senses, list the functions of the anatomical structures of each sense, and explain how the structures of the senses interrelate to perform their specialized functions.

KEY TERMS

afferent division: Nerve fibers that send impulses from the periphery to the central nervous system.

anatomical position: A position standing erect with the feet and palms facing the examiner.

anterior: The front, or ventral, surface.

capillaries: Tiny vessels that connect arterioles to venules.

central nervous system: The brain and spinal cord.

efferent division: Nerve fibers that send impulses from the central nervous system to the periphery.

homeostasis: A state of equilibrium in the body with respect to functions and composition of fluids and tissues.

inferior: Toward the feet; below a point of reference in the anatomical position.

integumentary system: The largest organ system in the body, consisting of the skin and accessory structures.

limbic system: The part of the brain involved with emotions and olfaction.

lymphatic system: The network of vessels, ducts, nodes, valves, and organs involved in protecting and maintaining the internal fluid environment of the body.

organ: A structure made up of two or more kinds of tissues organized to perform a more complex function than any one tissue alone.

parasympathetic nervous system: The subdivision of the autonomic nervous system usually involved in activating vegetative functions such as digestion, defecation, and urination.

peripheral nervous system: A subdivision of the nervous system consisting of nerves and ganglia.

plasma membrane: The outer covering of a cell that contains the cellular cytoplasm; also known as the cell membrane.

posterior: The back, or dorsal, surface.

prone: The position in which the patient is lying on the stomach (face down).

reticular activating system: A functional system in the brain essential for wakefulness, attention, concentration, and introspection.

somatic nervous system: The part of the nervous system composed of nerve fibers that send impulses from the central nervous system to skeletal muscle.

superior: Situated above or higher than a point of reference in the anatomical position.

supine: The position in which the patient is lying on the back (face up).

system: Interconnected functions or organs in which a stimulus or an action in one area affects all other areas.

Human anatomy is the study of how the human body is organized. The paramedic must know anatomy to assess a patient by body region. This knowlege also will help the paramedic to communicate well with medical direction and other members of the health care team.

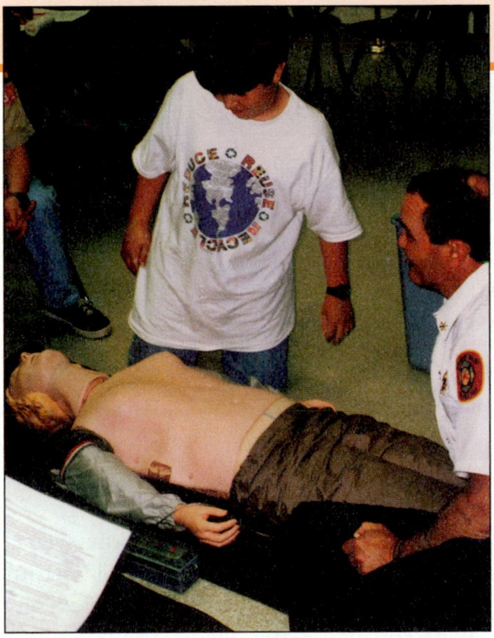

TERMINOLOGY

Directional terms used by the medical field refer to the human body in the **anatomical position.** This position describes a person standing erect with the feet and palms facing the examiner. A patient in the **supine** position is lying on the back (face up). A patient in the **prone** position is lying on the stomach (face down). A patient in the lateral recumbent position is on the right or left side. Regardless of the patient's position, the paramedic should always convey patient information with reference to the anatomical position (Fig. 6-1).

Directional terms, such as *up* or *down, front* or *back,* and *right* or *left,* also are expressed in anatomical terminology. The terms always refer to the patient, not the examiner (e.g., the patient's left arm). (Table 6-1 lists important directional terms.)

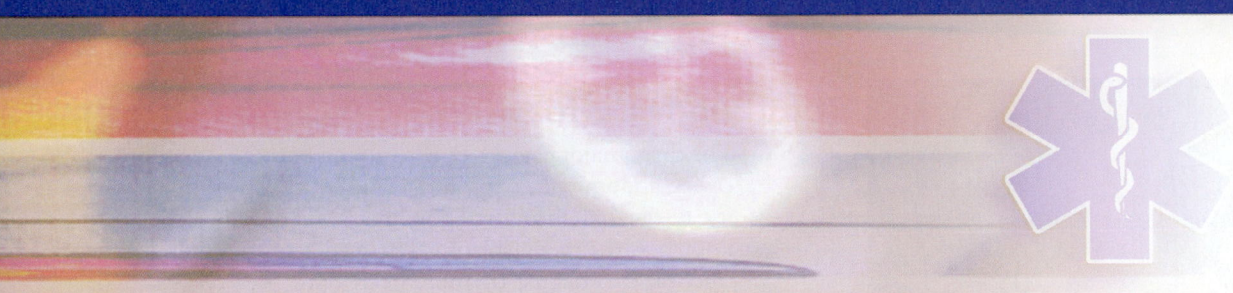

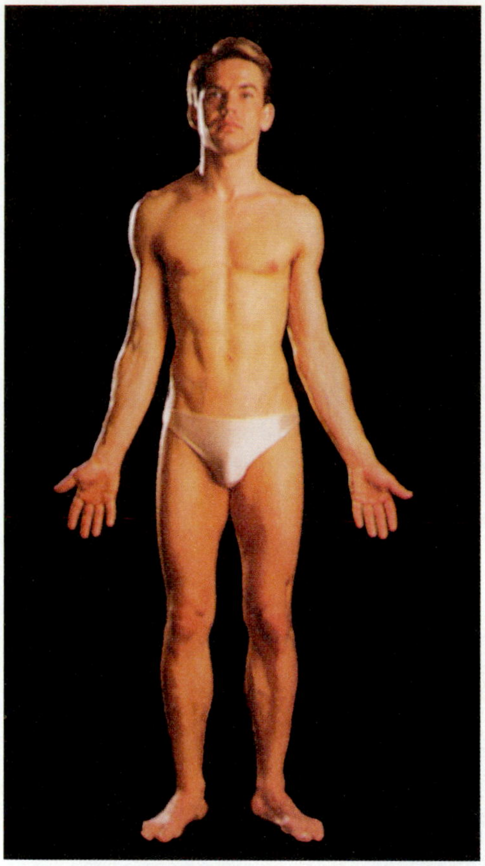

FIGURE 6-1 ■ Anatomical position. A human being in the anatomical position is standing with the feet and palms of the hands facing forward with the thumbs to the outside.

Anatomical Planes

Internal body structure relationships are classified into anatomical planes. These planes may be viewed as imaginary straight-line divisions of the human body (Fig. 6-2). The sagittal plane runs vertically through the middle of the body, creating right and left sections. A plane that is to one side of the midline is said to be parasagittal. The transverse, or horizontal, plane divides the body into top and bottom sections. These are known as **superior** and **inferior** sections. The frontal, or coronal, plane divides the body into front and back. These are known as **anterior** and **posterior** sections.

Body Regions

The human body is divided into a number of regions. This division helps to organize anatomical structures. The appendicular region is made up of the limbs, or extremities. The axial region is made up of the head, neck, thorax, and abdomen. The abdomen usually is divided into four quadrants. These are the upper right, lower right, upper left, and lower left. The dividing lines consist of two imaginary divisions. These divisions run horizontally through the umbilicus and vertically from the xiphoid process through the symphysis pubis (Fig. 6-3).

Body Cavities

The three major cavities of the human body are the thoracic cavity, abdominal cavity, and pelvic cavity. The thoracic cavity is divided into two portions by a midline structure known as the mediastinum. The mediastinum includes the trachea, esophagus, thymus, heart, and great vessels. The lungs are located on either side of this midline structure. The thoracic cavity is surrounded by the rib cage. This cavity is separated from the abdominal cavity by the diaphragm. The thorax contains two pleural cavities (which contain the lungs) and a pericardial cavity (which contains the heart). These cavities are lined with a serous membrane. The serous membrane that comes in contact with the **organ** is visceral. The serous membrane that comes in contact with the cavity wall is parietal. A thin, lubricating film of fluid is produced by these membranes. This fluid reduces the friction that occurs during movement of organs against other organs or body cavities.

An imaginary plane divides the abdominal cavity from the pelvic cavity. The division is drawn between the symphysis pubis and the sacral promontory. The latter is the projecting portion of the pelvis at the base of the sacrum. The abdominal and pelvic cavities are lined with a thin sheet of membranous tissue. This thin sheet of tissue secretes serous fluid. The serous membrane that covers the abdominal organs is known as visceral peritoneum. The serous membrane that covers the body cavity wall is known as the parietal peritoneum. Peritoneal organs are held in place by connective tissue. This tissue is called mesentery. The mesentery holds some of the abdominal organs to the body wall. The mesentery also offers a pathway for nerves and vessels to reach the organs. Abdominopelvic organs that do not have mesentery or peritoneum are said to be retroperitoneal. This means that they are behind the peritoneum. These organs include the kidneys, adrenal glands, pancreas, portions of the colon, and the urinary bladder. The pelvic cavity is enclosed by the bones of the pelvis. The abdominal and pelvic cavities often are referred to collectively as the peritoneal or abdominopelvic cavity (Fig. 6-4).

CELL STRUCTURE

Cells are the basic unit of life. They are highly organized units composed of protoplasm, or living matter. The three main parts of all human cells are the cytoplasmic membrane **(plasma membrane)**, cytoplasm, and nucleus.

Cytoplasmic Membrane

The cytoplasmic membrane encloses the cytoplasm. The membrane forms the outer boundary of the cell. The cytoplasmic membrane is believed to have two layers of phosphate-containing fat molecules. These molecules are known as phospholipids. The layers form a fluid framework for the cytoplasmic membrane (Fig. 6-5). Substances outside this membrane are considered extracellular (outside of cells) or intercellular (between cells). Substances

TABLE 6-1 Directional Terms

TERM	DEFINITION	TERM	DEFINITION
Left	Toward the left side	Distal	Farther than another structure from the point of attachment to the trunk
Right	Toward the right side	Medial	Toward the midline of the body
Superior	Situated above another structure (usually synonymous with "cephalic")	Lateral	Away from the midline of the body
Inferior	Situated below another structure (usually synonymous with "caudal")	Anterior	The front of the body (synonymous with "ventral")
Cephalic	Toward the head of the body	Posterior	The back of the body (synonymous with "dorsal")
Caudal	Toward the distal end of the spine	Ventral	Pertaining to the front
Proximal	Closer than another structure to the point of attachment to the trunk	Dorsal	Pertaining to the back

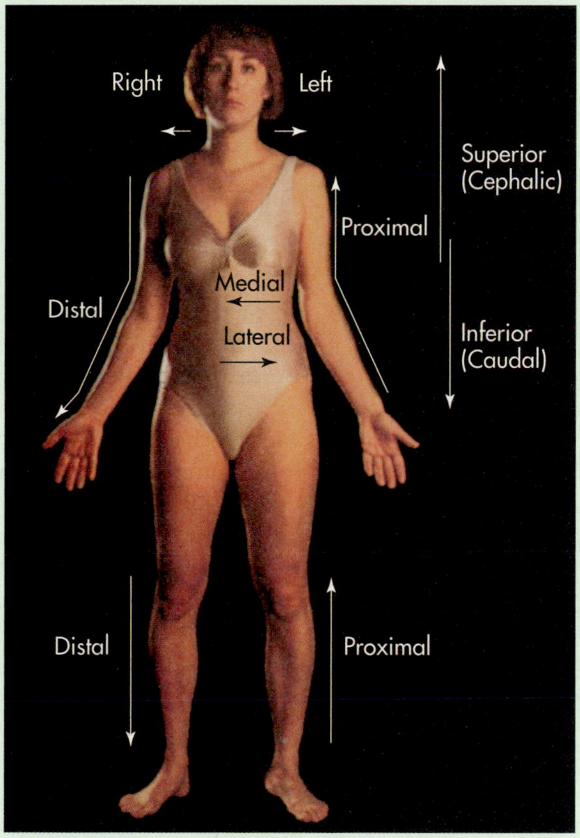

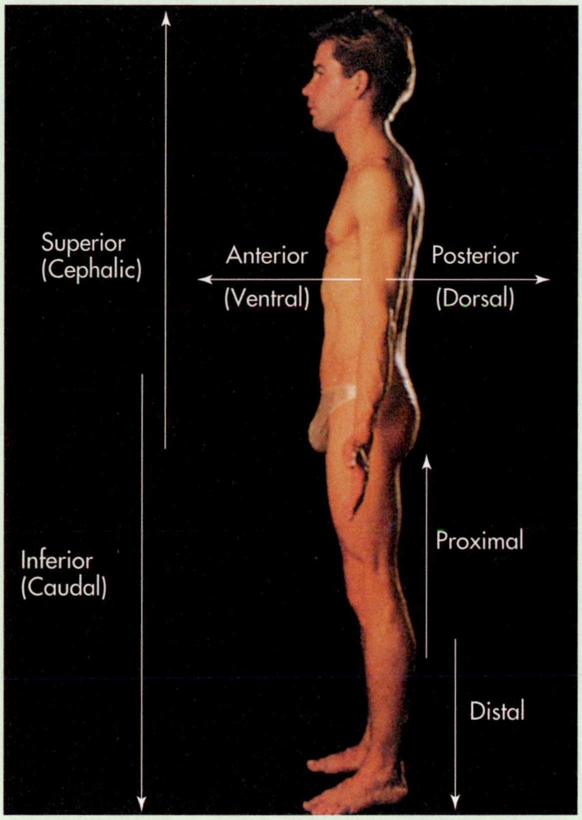

inside this membrane are intracellular. The functions of the cytoplasmic membrane are to enclose and support the cell contents and regulate what moves into and out of the cell.

The central layer of the cytoplasmic membrane is a lipid bilayer. This layer is composed of a double layer of lipid molecules. The lipid bilayer has a liquid quality. In fact, protein molecules "float" on the inner and the outer surfaces. Some of these proteins have carbohydrate molecules bound to them. The protein molecules are thought to function as membrane channels, carrier molecules, receptor molecules, enzymes, or structural supports in the membrane (see Chapter 8).

Cytoplasm

The cytoplasm lies between the cytoplasmic membrane and the nucleus. The nucleus can be viewed as a round or spherical structure in the center of the cell. Specialized structures in the cell, known as organelles, are located in the cytoplasm. These structures perform functions important to the survival of the cell (Table 6-2 and Fig. 6-6).

The endoplasmic reticulum is a chain of connecting sacs or canals. It winds through the cytoplasm of the cell. In essence, the endoplasmic reticulum serves as a tiny circulatory system for the cell. The tubular passages or canals in the endoplasmic reticulum carry proteins and other substances through the cytoplasm of the cell from one area to

Text continued on p. 89

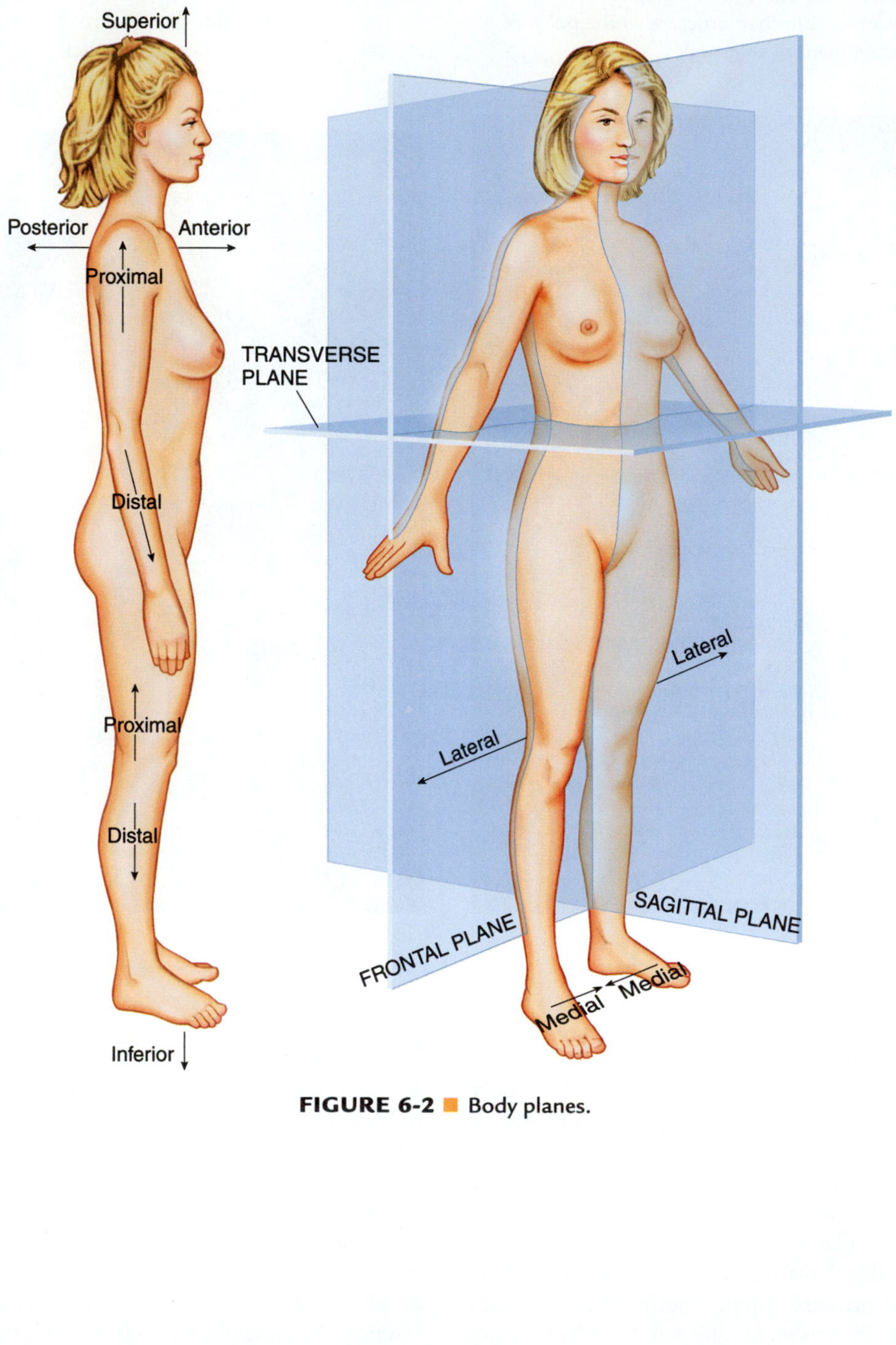

FIGURE 6-2 ■ Body planes.

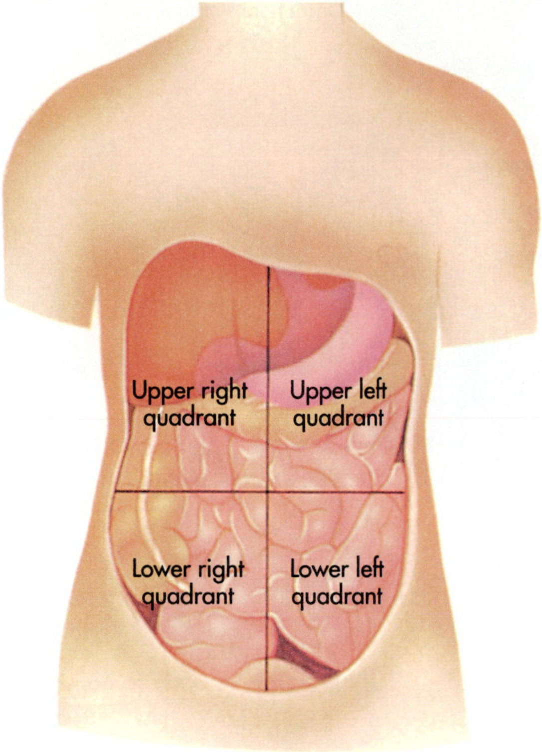

FIGURE 6-3 ■ Abdominal quadrants.

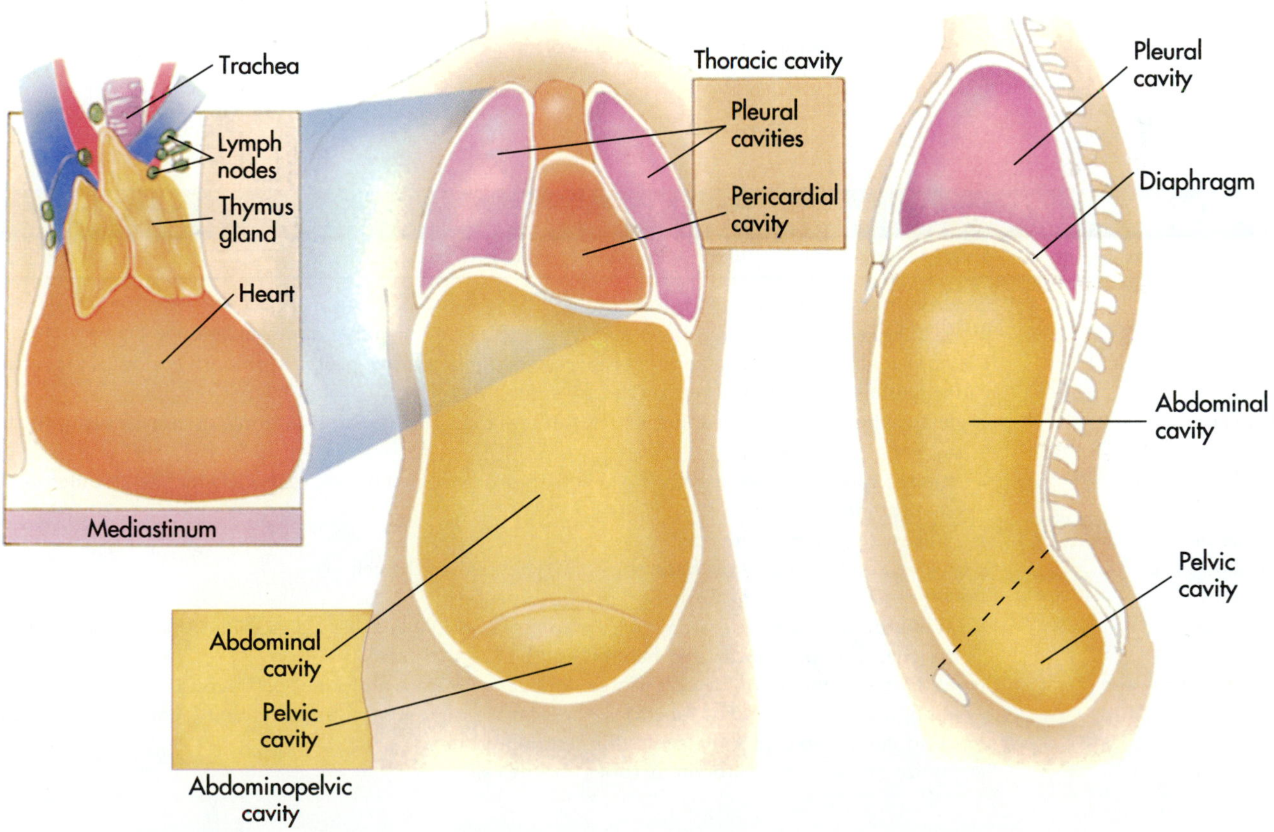

FIGURE 6-4 ■ Body cavities. The thoracic cavity includes the two pleural cavities and the pericardial cavity. Some of the contents of the mediastinum are shown on the left. The abdominopelvic cavity contains the abdominal cavity and the pelvic cavity.

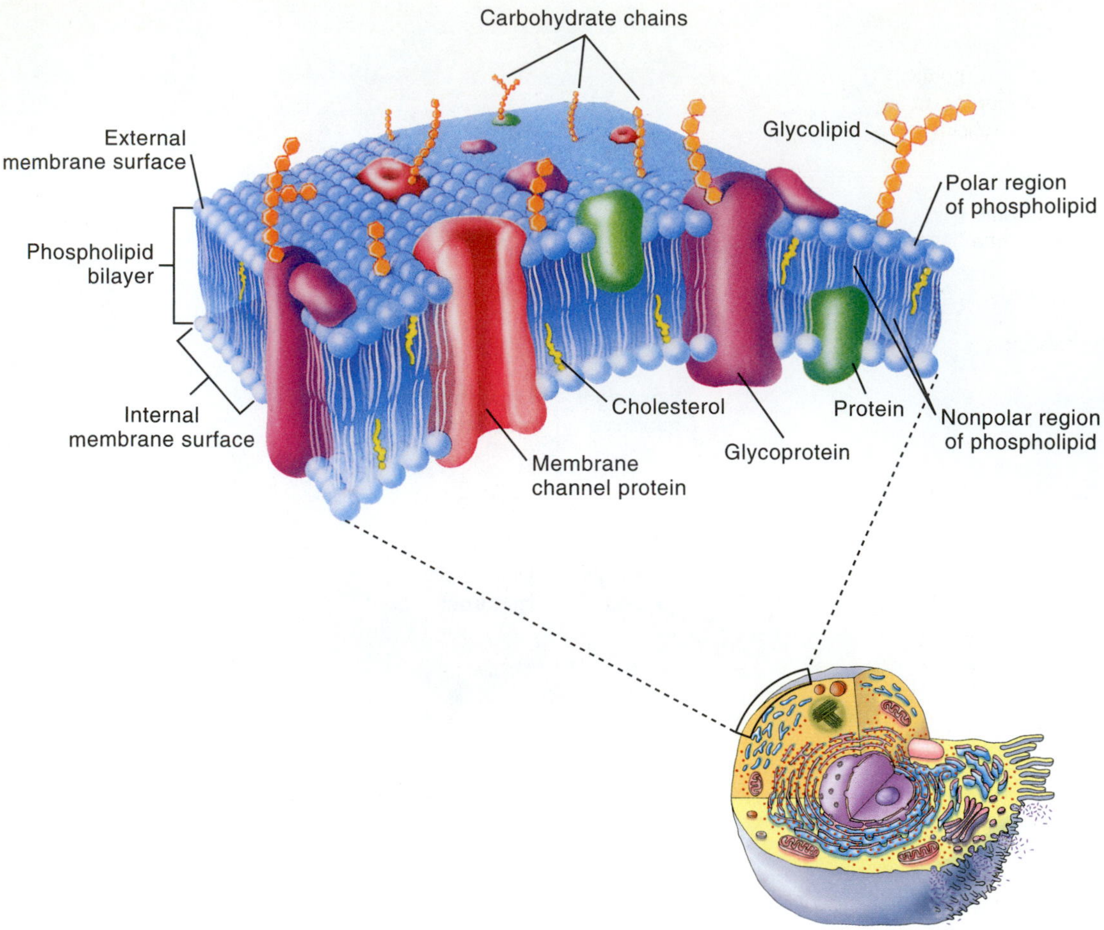

FIGURE 6-5 ■ Fluid mosaic model of the plasma membrane.

TABLE 6-2 Some Major Cell Structures and Their Functions

CELL STRUCTURE	FUNCTION
Centrioles	Function in cell reproduction
Cilia	Short, hairlike extensions on the free surfaces of some cells capable of movement
Endoplasmic reticulum	Ribosomes attached to rough endoplasmic reticulum synthesize proteins; smooth endoplasmic reticulum synthesizes lipids and certain carbohydrates
Flagella	Single and much larger projections of cell surfaces than cilia; the only example in human beings is the "tail" of a sperm cell
Golgi apparatus	Synthesizes carbohydrates, combines them with proteins, and packages the product as globules of glycoproteins
Lysosomes	The "digestive system" of the cell
Mitochondria	Synthesize adenosine triphosphate; the "powerhouses" of the cell
Nucleoli	Play an essential role in the formation of ribosomes
Nucleus	Dictates protein synthesis, thereby playing an essential role in other cell activities, namely active transport, metabolism, growth, and heredity
Plasma membrane	Serves as the boundary of the cell; protein and carbohydrate molecules on the outer surface of plasma membrane perform various functions; for example, they serve as markers that identify cells of each individual or as receptor molecules for certain hormones
Ribosomes	Synthesize proteins; the "protein factories" of the cell

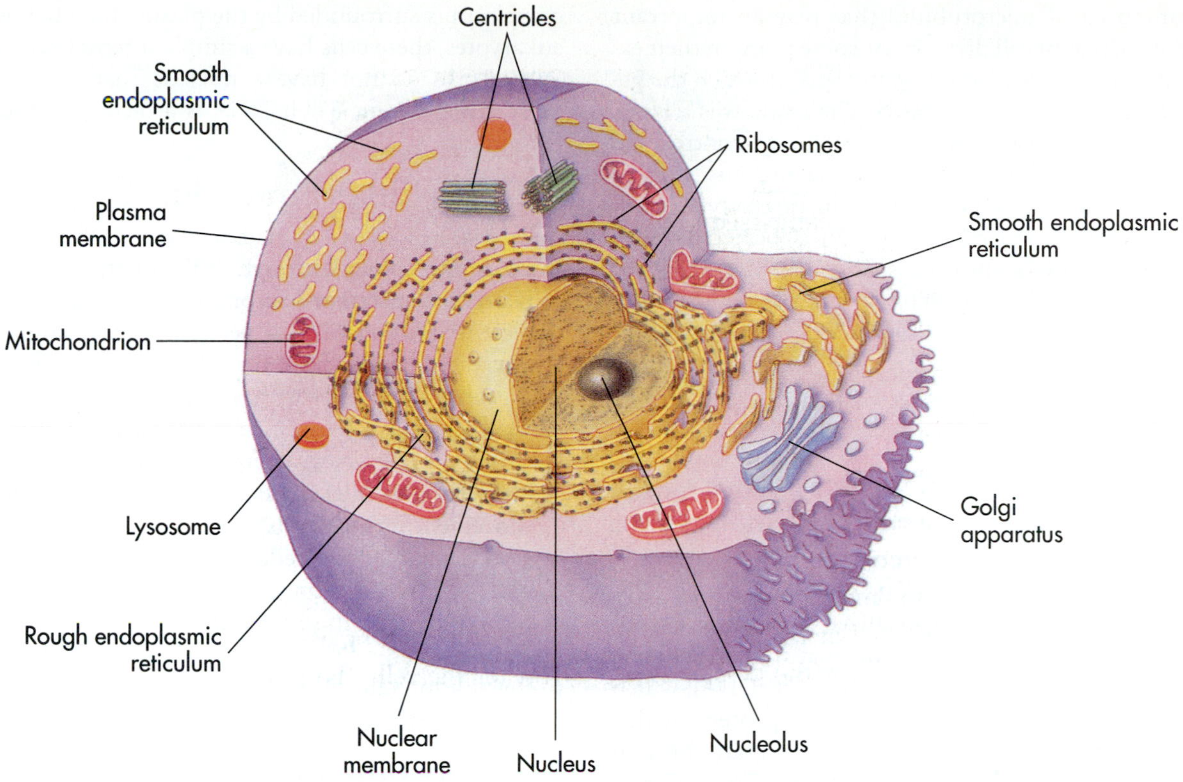

FIGURE 6-6 ■ Artist's interpretation of cell structure.

another. The two types of endoplasmic reticulum are smooth and rough. Smooth endoplasmic reticulum is found in cells that handle or produce fatty substances. This organelle also plays a part in detoxification processes through the chemical action of enzymes. Rough endoplasmic reticulum is found in cells that produce proteins to be secreted for use outside the cell.

Ribosomes are the "factories" in the cells where protein is synthesized. Ribosomes are macromolecules of protein and ribonucleic acid (RNA) composed of thousands of atoms. Ribosomes usually are bound to the endoplasmic reticulum but also are found free in cytoplasm. Ribosomes form complexes with strands of RNA, which through the genetic code provide the blueprint for the new protein. Individual amino acids are attached in long chains with peptide bonds to form the new proteins.

The Golgi apparatus concentrates and packages materials for secretion from the cell. This organelle consists of tiny sacs composed of smooth endoplasmic reticulum. These sacs are stacked one on the other near the nucleus. The Golgi apparatus concentrates and in some cases chemically modifies the proteins. It does this by synthesizing and attaching carbohydrate molecules to the proteins to form glycoproteins or attaching lipids to the proteins to form lipoproteins. These concentrated globules move slowly outward to and through the cell membrane. At this point, the globules break open and spill their contents. An example of a Golgi apparatus product is mucus.

Lysosomes are membranous-walled organelles that contain enzymes enabling them to function as intracellular digestive systems. These enzymes include those that digest nucleic acids, proteins, polysaccharides, and lipids. Certain white blood cells (leukocytes) have large numbers of lysosomes that contain enzymes to digest engulfed bacteria. If tissues are damaged, these powerful enzymes may escape from ruptured lysosome sacs into the cytoplasm, digesting damaged and healthy cells. Lysosomes also digest organelles of the cell that are no longer functional (autophagia).

The mitochondria are the power plants of the cell. These organelles are found throughout the cell. They are the site of aerobic oxidation. In the mitochondria, energy derived from the efficient metabolism of nutrients and oxygen via the Krebs cycle (further described in Chapter 8) is used to synthesize high-energy triphosphate bonds (e.g., adenosine triphosphate, or ATP). These triphosphate bonds are the energy source for the muscles, nerves, and overall function of the body.

> **CRITICAL THINKING**
> Your patient has bad lung disease and poor oxygenation. What effect will this have on cellular energy production?

Centrioles are paired, rod-shaped organelles that lie at right angles to each other in a specialized zone of cytoplasm. This zone is known as the centrosome. Each centriole is composed of microtubules that play an important role in the process of cell division. At some point in their existence, all human cells contain a nucleus in which the genetic material of the cell is located. The nucleus is a large, membrane-bound organelle that ultimately controls all other organelles in the cytoplasm. The nucleus may be spherical, elongated, or lobed, depending on the type of cell in which it is found. The nucleus usually is located near the center of the cell, but some cells, such as red blood cells (or erythrocytes), lose their nucleus as they develop. Other cells, such as certain bone cells, have more than one nucleus. The most significant categorizing feature of cells is the presence or absence of a nucleus.

Nucleus

The nucleus is a relatively large structure that is not always near the center of the cell. The cell nucleus is surrounded by a nuclear membrane. This membrane encloses a special type of protoplasm known as nucleoplasm. The nucleoplasm contains a number of specialized structures. Two of these are the nucleolus and the chromatin granules. The nucleolus consists of deoxyribonucleic acid (DNA), which "programs" the formation of RNA, and protein, which makes ribosomes. These ribosomes then migrate through the nuclear membrane into the cytoplasm of the cell and produce proteins. Chromatin granules are threadlike structures made up of proteins and DNA. During cell division, the chromatin condenses to form the 23 pairs of chromosomes characteristic of human cells. The information within nuclear DNA determines most of the chemical events that occur within the cell. The basic functions of the nucleus are cell division and control of genetic information. Not all cells are capable of continuous division, and some cells (e.g., nerve cells) cannot reproduce.

Major Classes of Cells

Free-living cells of multicellular "social" organisms are divided into two major classes. They are divided by the way genetic material is organized inside them. The two main types are eukaryotes ("true nucleus") and prokaryotes ("before nucleus").

Eukaryotes are larger than prokaryotes. In addition, they have more extensive intracellular anatomy. They have a separate membrane-bound nucleus. The nucleus holds the genetic material (chromosomes, DNA). The fluid filling of the eukaryotes is divided into the nucleoplasm and the cytoplasm. The nucleoplasm is inside the nuclear membrane. The cytoplasm is outside the nuclear membrane. Nearly all human body cells are eukaryotes, as are those of all living organisms. Exceptions to this are bacteria, cyanobacteria (blue-green algae), and mycoplasms. These are prokaryotes. Bacteria and mycoplasms cause many diseases in human beings and other animals. Viruses have a close association with cells but are not classified as cells.

In the simpler prokaryote cells the genetic material and enzymes required for energy production, cell growth, and cell division are contained in the jellylike cytoplasm. The cytoplasm is surrounded by the plasma membrane. Unlike eukaryotes, these cells have a simple internal organization. Prokaryotes do not have a nucleus that is bound by a plasma membrane. Their DNA is attached to the plasma membrane.

Chief Cellular Functions

Cells have evolved in a myriad of ways to fulfill specific tasks in the human body. Through differentiation (maturation), cells become specialized in one type of function or act in concert with other cells to perform a more complex task. For example, red blood cells only carry out one function. They transport respiratory gases around the body. The cells in the pancreas, for instance, synthesize and secrete large quantities of the digestive enzymes required to break down foods. The seven chief cellular functions are as follows[1]:

1. Movement (muscle cells)
2. Conductivity (nerve cells)
3. Metabolic absorption (kidney and intestinal cells)
4. Secretion (mucous gland cells)
5. Excretion (all cells)
6. Respiration (all cells)
7. Reproduction (most cells)

Cell Reproduction

All human cells, with the exception of reproductive (sex) cells, reproduce by a process known as mitosis. In this process, cells divide to multiply: one cell divides to form two cells. Many cell types in the body (e.g., epithelial, liver, and bone marrow cells) undergo cell division throughout an individual's life. Other cell types (e.g., nerve and skeletal muscle cells) divide until near the time of birth.

TISSUES

Characteristics of cell structure and composition are used to classify tissue types. Four main types of tissue make up the many organs of the body. They are epithelial, connective, muscle, and nervous tissue.

Epithelial Tissue

Epithelial tissue covers surfaces or forms structures (e.g., glands) derived from body surfaces. This tissue consists almost entirely of cells that have little or no intercellular material between them. The tissue forms continuous sheets that contain no blood vessels. Epithelium covers the outside of the body. Epithelium also lines the digestive tract, the vessels, and many body cavities.

Epithelial tissues can be subdivided by the shape and arrangement of the cells found in each type. If classified ac-

CRITICAL THINKING

Think about the role of each of the tissue types. Compare these roles with the types of materials used to construct a building. Imagine each tissue type as a component of building a body.

cording to shape, epithelial cells can be squamous (flat and scalelike). They can be cuboidal (cube shaped). They also can be columnar (more tall than wide). If classified according to arrangement, epithelial cells are simple (a single layer of cells of the same shape). They are stratified (multiple layers of cells of the same shape). They also are transitional (several layers of cells of differing shapes).

Connective Tissue

Connective tissue is the most abundant type of tissue in the body. Connective tissue is also the most widely distributed type. It consists of cells separated from each other by intercellular material. This material is known as the extracellular matrix. This nonliving matrix gives most connective tissue its fundamental characteristics and is the basis for separating connective tissue into the following seven subgroups:

1. Areolar connective tissue is a loose tissue. It consists of delicate webs of fibers and a variety of cells embedded in a matrix of soft, sticky gel. Areolar connective tissue is the "loose packing" material of most organs and other tissues. It attaches the skin to the underlying tissues. The areolar connective tissue contains three major types of protein fibers: *collagen, reticulum*, and *elastin*.
2. Adipose, or fat, tissue is a specialized connective tissue that stores lipids. Lipids take up less space per calorie than carbohydrates or proteins. Thus this tissue not only acts as an insulator and protector but also as a site of energy storage.
3. Fibrous connective tissue is made up mainly of bundles of strong, white collagenous fibers in parallel rows. Tendons are composed of this type of connective tissue. Fibrous connective tissue is characterized by strength and inelasticity.
4. Cartilage is made up of cartilage cells (chondrocytes). These cells are located in tiny spaces and are distributed throughout a somewhat rigid matrix. The makeup of cartilage varies by its location and ultimate role. For example, hyaline cartilage is found at articulating surfaces and is firm and smooth. Yet fibrocartilage is more flexible and supple. Cartilage makes up part of the human skeleton and covers the articulating surfaces of bones. In addition, cartilage forms the major skeletal tissue of the embryo before it is replaced by bony tissue. The type of cartilage depends on the relative amounts of collagen, elastin, and ground substance. Ground substance is composed of nonfibrous protein and other organic molecules and fluid. Increased amounts of collagen or elastin allow cartilage to spring back after being compressed. Blood vessels do not penetrate the substance of cartilage. Thus cartilage heals slowly after injury.
5. Bone is a highly specialized form of hard, connective tissue. Bone consists of living cells and mineralized matrix. The strength and rigidity of this matrix allow bone to support and protect other tissues and organs.

Bones are classified according to their shape (Fig. 6-7). Long bones are longer than they are wide. Examples of

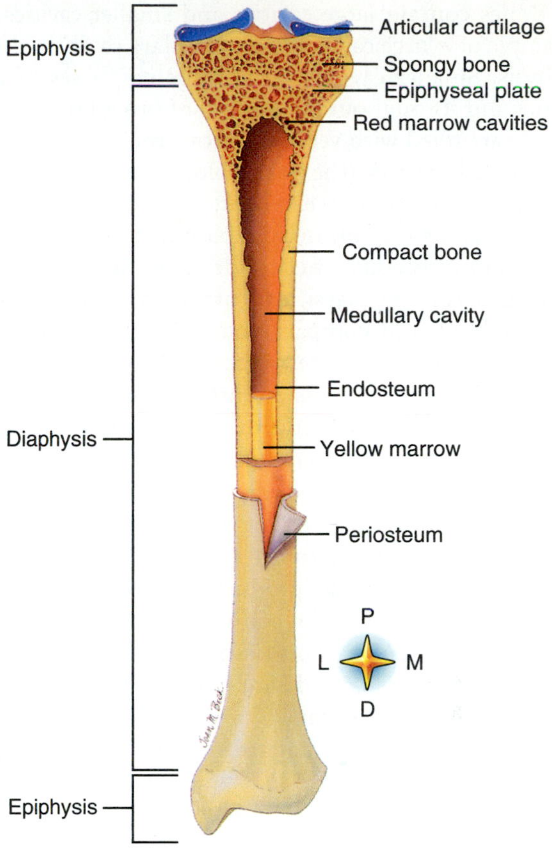

FIGURE 6-7 ■ Long bone.

long bones are the humerus, ulna, radius, femur, tibia, fibula, and phalanges. Short bones are about as broad as they are long. Examples of short bones are the carpal bones of the wrist and the tarsal bones of the ankle. Flat bones have a thin, flattened shape. Examples of flat bones are certain skull bones, ribs, sternum, and scapulae. Irregular bones are those that do not fit the other three categories. Examples of irregular bones include vertebrae and facial bones.

Each growing long bone consists of a diaphysis (shaft), an epiphysis at the end of each bone, and an epiphyseal or growth plate. The epiphyseal plate is the site of bone elongation. When bone growth stops, the epiphyseal plate becomes ossified. Then the plate is called the *epiphyseal line*. Injury to this area can impair bone growth if not recognized and treated properly (see Chapter 28).

CRITICAL THINKING

Intraosseous infusion is a critical intervention that can save a life. Intraosseous infusion is used to administer fluids and drugs. In children, such infusion requires the insertion of a needle into the bone of the leg. Why could the failure to identify anatomical landmarks or place the needle correctly in the epiphysis be harmful?

Bones contain large cavities and smaller cavities. An example of a large cavity is the medullary cavity in the diaphysis. Smaller cavities include the epiphyses of long bones and throughout the interior of other bones. These spaces are filled with yellow marrow (mainly adipose tissue) or red marrow (the site of blood formation). Blood supply to most bones is excellent. So some bones, such as the tibia and sternum, are suitable choices for venous access via intraosseous infusion (described in Chapter 18).

Bones can be classified further as cancellous or spongy bone and compact bone. Cancellous bone has spaces between the plates of the bone and resembles a sponge. Compact bone is essentially solid. Unlike cartilage, bone has a rich blood supply and can repair itself much more readily than cartilage.

6. Blood is a unique connective tissue because the matrix between the cells is liquid. The liquid matrix of blood allows it to flow rapidly through the body. Blood carries nutrients, oxygen, waste products, and other materials.
7. Hemopoietic tissue is the connective tissue in the marrow cavities of bones. This tissue also is in organs such as the spleen, tonsils, and lymph nodes. This tissue is responsible for the formation of blood cells and cells of the **lymphatic system** that are important in the defense against disease.

Muscle Tissue

Muscle tissue is a contractile tissue and is the force behind all movement. Muscle tissue is highly specialized to contract or shorten forcefully. It is behind all processes that provide motion for the body. Muscle tissue is grouped by anatomical location and function. Muscle tissue is skeletal, cardiac, and smooth or visceral muscle. When classified by appearance, muscle is striated or nonstriated. When classified by function, muscle is voluntary (consciously controlled) or involuntary (not normally consciously controlled). The three types of muscles are striated voluntary (skeletal) muscle, striated involuntary (cardiac) muscle, and nonstriated involuntary (smooth) muscle.

Skeletal muscle attaches to bones. It represents a large portion of the total weight of the human body. Contraction of these muscles is responsible for body movement. Cardiac muscle is the muscle of the heart. Contraction of the cardiac muscle pumps blood throughout the body. Smooth muscle is widespread throughout the body and is responsible for a variety of functions. Examples include movement in the digestive, urinary, and reproductive systems.

Nervous Tissue

The nervous tissue is characterized by the ability to conduct electrical signals, which are known as action potentials. The nervous tissue consists of two basic kinds of cells: neurons and neuroglia.

Neurons, or nerve cells, are the actual conducting cells of nervous tissue. They are composed of three major parts: cell body, dendrite, and axon. The cell body contains the nucleus and is the site of general cell functions. Dendrites and axons are nerve cell processes (projections of cytoplasm surrounded by membrane). Dendrites receive electrical impulses and conduct them toward the cell body. Axons usually conduct impulses away from the cell body. Neurons have many different sizes and shapes, especially in the brain and spinal cord.

Neuroglia are the support cells of the brain, spinal cord, and peripheral nerves. These cells are divided into several subgroups that nourish, protect, and insulate neurons.

ORGAN SYSTEMS

An **organ** is a structure made up of two or more kinds of tissues organized to perform a more complex job than any one tissue can perform. A **system** is a group of organs arranged to perform a more complex job than any one organ can perform (Fig. 6-8). The human body contains 11 major organ systems:

1. Integumentary
2. Skeletal
3. Muscular
4. Nervous
5. Endocrine
6. Circulatory
7. Lymphatic
8. Respiratory
9. Digestive
10. Urinary
11. Reproductive

Integumentary System

The **integumentary system** is the largest organ system of the body. It consists of the skin and accessory structures such as hair, nails, and a variety of glands. The functions of this system include protecting the body against injury and dehydration. The integumentary system also defends against invading microorganisms and regulates temperature.

> **CRITICAL THINKING**
>
> Consider your knowledge of the functions of the skin. What signs, symptoms, or complications would you expect in a patient with burns covering half the body?

SKIN

The skin is a sheetlike organ composed of two distinct layers of tissue: the epidermis and the dermis (Fig. 6-9). The epidermis is the outermost layer of skin. It consists of tightly packed epithelial cells. Cells of the innermost layer of the epidermis can undergo mitosis and can repair themselves if injured. Because of this characteristic, the body can maintain an effective barrier against infection, even when subjected to injury and normal wear and tear.

The dermis is the deeper of the two layers of skin. The dermis is made up largely of connective tissue. The dermis is much thicker than the epidermis. It contains collagenous and elastic fibers. The dermis also contains a specialized network

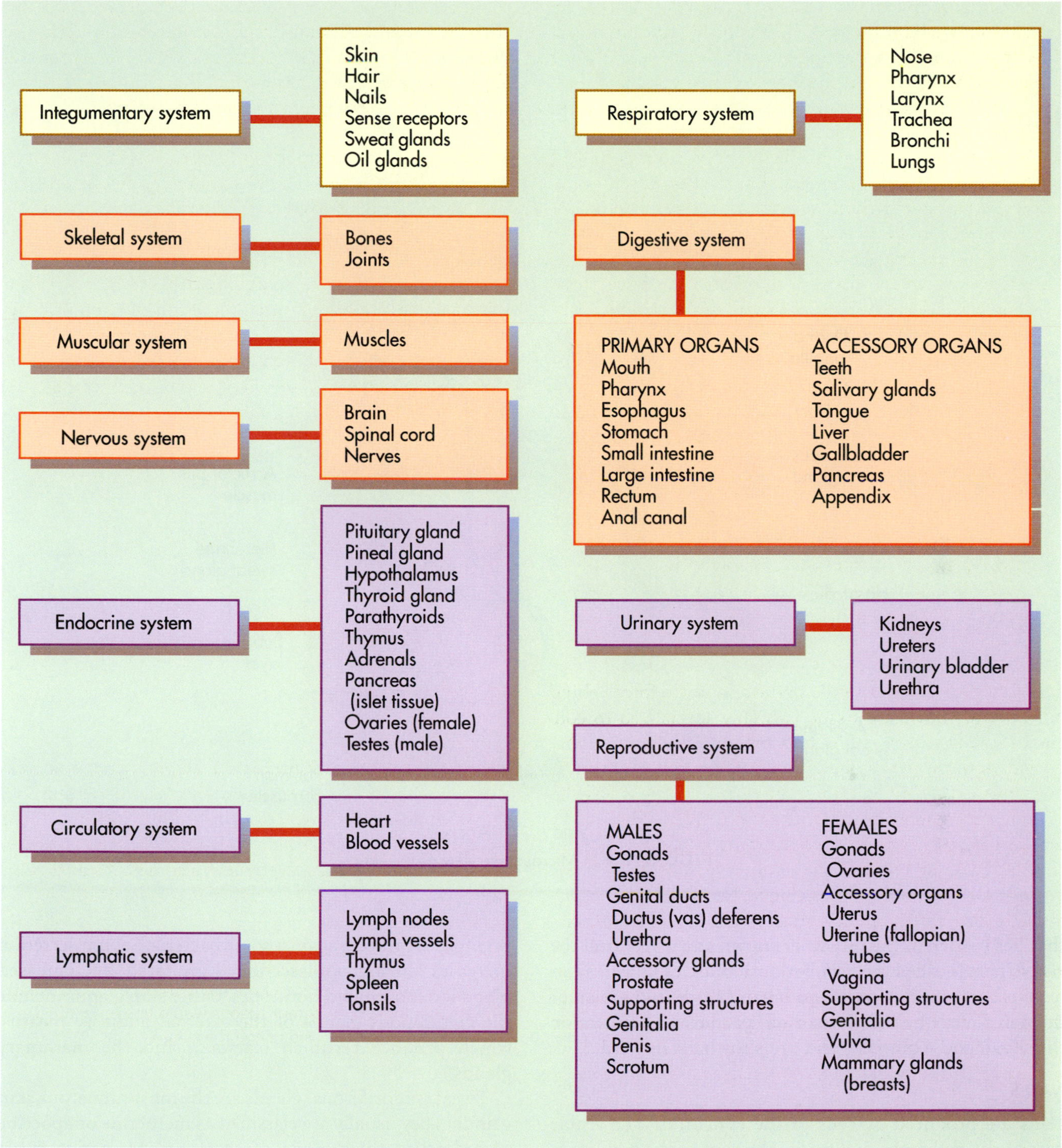

FIGURE 6-8 ■ Body systems and their organs.

of nerves and nerve endings. These nerves provide sensory information about pain, pressure, touch, and temperature. At various levels of the dermis are muscle fibers, hair follicles, sweat and sebaceous glands, and many blood vessels.

The layers of skin are supported by a thick layer of loose connective tissue and fat. This is known as subcutaneous tissue. Subcutaneous tissue insulates the body from temperature extremes. It serves as a source of stored energy as well. In addition, subcutaneous tissue acts as a shock absorber to protect underlying tissue from injury.

HAIR

Hair growth begins when cells of the epidermal layer of the skin grow into the dermis, forming a small tube called the *hair follicle.* Hair growth begins from a small, cap-shaped cluster of cells called the *hair papilla.* The part of the hair

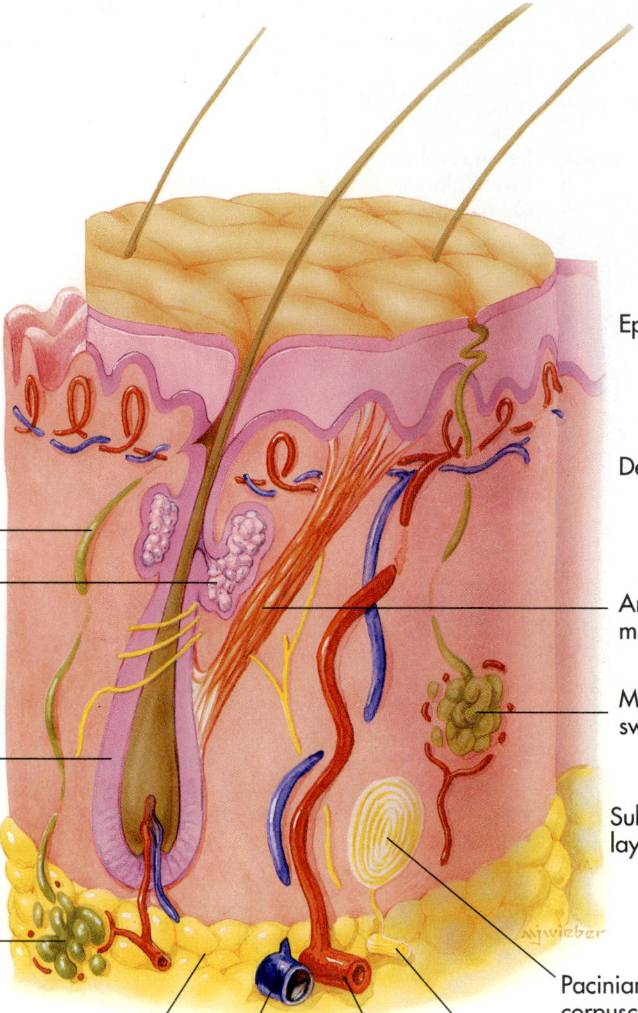

FIGURE 6-9 ■ Microscopic view of the skin.

that lies hidden in the follicle is known as the *root,* and the visible part is called the *shaft.* Smooth muscles known as *arrector pili* are associated with each hair follicle. Movement of the hair follicle by the arrector pili produces a pressure on the skin ("goose bumps") and pulls the hairs upward.

NAILS

Nails are produced by cells in the epidermis. The visible part of the nail is the nail body. The root of the nail lies in a groove and is hidden by a fold of skin known as the *cuticle.* The crescent-shaped white area of the nail is called the *lunula* and is most visible on the thumbnail. The nail bed that lies under the nail contains many blood vessels. In healthy individuals, this layer of epithelium appears pink through the translucent nail body.

GLANDS

The major glands of the skin are the sebaceous and sweat glands. Most sebaceous glands are found in the dermis and secrete oil (sebum) for the hair and skin. This oil prevents drying and protects against some bacteria. Sebum secretion increases during adolescence, stimulated by increased blood levels of the sex hormones. Other skin glands include the ceruminous glands of the external auditory meatus, which produce cerumen (earwax), and the mammary glands.

Sweat (sudoriferous) glands are the most numerous skin glands. They usually are classified as merocrine or apocrine according to their mode of secretion. Merocrine sweat glands are the most common. They open directly onto the surface of the skin through sweat pores. The coiled portion of the gland produces a fluid that is mostly water but also contains some salts (mainly sodium chloride) and small amounts of ammonia, urea, uric acid, and lactic acid. As the body temperature rises, the sweat glands produce sweat. The sweat evaporates and cools the body. Apocrine glands usually open into hair follicles. These glands are found in the axillae and genitalia and around the anus. These glands become active at puberty through the influence of sex hormones. Apocrine glands secrete an organic substance that is odorless when released but is quickly metabolized by bacteria to cause body odor.

CRITICAL THINKING

The ability to sweat is impaired in the elderly. What implications does this have?

Skeletal System

The skeletal system consists of bones and associated connective tissues. These tissues include cartilage, tendons, and ligaments. The skeletal system offers a rigid framework for support and protection. It also provides a system of levers on which muscles act to produce body movements. The skeletal system contains 206 bones. Bones are divided into two groups: the axial skeleton and the appendicular skeleton (Fig. 6-10).

AXIAL SKELETON

The axial skeleton is made up of the skull, hyoid bone, vertebral column, and thoracic cage. The skull is composed of 28 bones. These bones are divided into the following groups: the auditory ossicles, cranial vault, and facial bones (Fig. 6-11). The 6 auditory ossicles (3 on each side of the head) are located inside the cavity of the temporal bone. The auditory ossicles function in hearing.

The cranial vault consists of six bones that surround and protect the brain. They are the parietal, temporal, frontal, occipital, sphenoid, and ethmoid bones.

The 14 facial bones form the structure of the face in the anterior skull. These bones do not contribute to the cranial vault, however. The bones include the maxilla, mandible, and zygomatic, palatine, nasal, lacrimal, vomer, and inferior nasal concha bones. The frontal and ethmoid bones contribute to the cranial vault and the face.

The hyoid bone is attached to the skull by muscles and ligaments and "floats" in the superior aspect of the neck, just below the mandible. The hyoid bone serves as the attachment point for several important neck and tongue muscles.

The vertebral column consists of 33 bones. These bones can be divided into five regions: 7 cervical vertebrae, 12 thoracic vertebrae, 5 lumbar vertebrae, 5 sacral vertebrae (fused), and 4 coccygeal vertebrae (fused) (Fig. 6-12).

The weight-bearing portion of the vertebra is a bony disk called the *body*. Intervertebral disks are located between the bodies of adjacent vertebrae. The disks serve as shock absorbers for the vertebral column. They provide additional support for the body as well. In addition, the disks prevent the vertebral bodies from rubbing against each other. The spinal cord is protected by the vertebral arch and the dorsal portion of the body. A transverse process extends laterally from each side of the arch, and a single spinous process is present at the point of junction. Much vertebral movement is accomplished by the contraction of skeletal muscles attached to the transverse and spinous processes.

The thoracic cage protects vital organs within the thorax. It also prevents the collapse of the thorax during respiration. The thoracic cage consists of the thoracic vertebrae, ribs with their associated costal cartilages, and sternum (Fig. 6-13).

The 12 pairs of ribs can be divided into *true* or *false* ribs. The superior 7 (the true ribs) articulate with the thoracic vertebrae and attach directly through their costal cartilages to the sternum. The inferior 5 (the false ribs) articulate with the thoracic vertebrae but do not attach directly to the sternum. The eighth, ninth, and tenth ribs are joined to a common cartilage, which is attached to the sternum. The eleventh and twelfth ribs are "floating" ribs that have no attachment to the sternum.

The sternum is divided into three parts: the manubrium, body, and xiphoid process. At the superior margin of the manubrium is the jugular notch. One can palpate this notch easily at the anterior base of the neck. The point at which the manubrium joins the body of the sternum is the sternal angle (also known as the angle of Louis). The second rib is found lateral to the sternal angle and is used clinically as a starting point for counting the other ribs.

APPENDICULAR SKELETON

The appendicular skeleton consists of the bones of the upper and lower extremities. It also consists of their girdles, by which they are attached to the body.

The scapula and clavicle form the pectoral girdle. This girdle attaches the upper limbs to the axial skeleton. The direct point of attachment between the bones of the appendicular and axial skeleton occurs at the sternoclavicular joint between the clavicle and the sternum.

The humerus is the second longest bone in the body. The head of the humerus articulates with the scapula. The greater and lesser tubercles are on the lateral and anterior surfaces of the proximal end of the humerus. There the tubercles act as sites of muscle attachments. The humerus articulates with the radius and ulna at its distal end. The capitulum (lateral aspect of the humerus) articulates with the head of the radius. The trochlea (medial aspect of the humerus) articulates with the ulna. Proximal to the trochlea and capitulum are the medial and lateral epicondyles, respectively. These sites act as muscle attachments for the muscles of the forearm. (Figure 6-14 illustrates the bones of the upper extremity.)

The large bony process of the ulna (the *olecranon process*) can be felt at the point of the elbow. This process fits in a large depression on the posterior surface of the humerus known as the *olecranon fossa*. The structural relationship between these two processes makes movement of the joint possible. The distal end of the ulna has a small head that articulates with the radius and wrist bones. The posterior-medial side of the head has a small styloid process to which the ligaments of the wrist are attached. The proximal end of the radius articulates with the humerus. The medial surface of the head constitutes a smooth cylinder where the radius rotates against the radial notch of the ulna. Major anterior arm muscles (biceps brachii) are attached to the radial tuberosity.

Text continued on p. 99

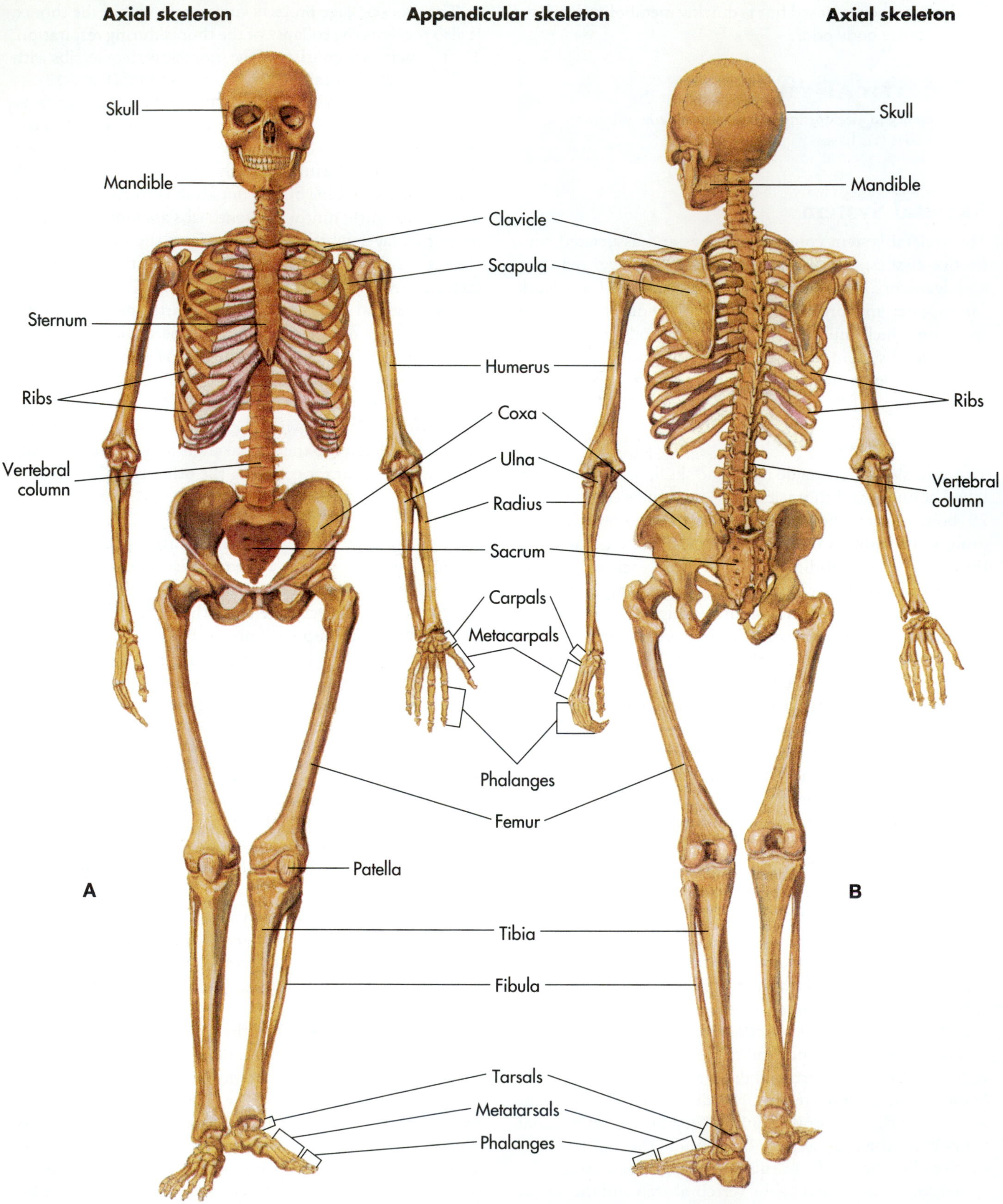

FIGURE 6-10 ■ Anterior (A) and posterior (B) views of the skeleton.

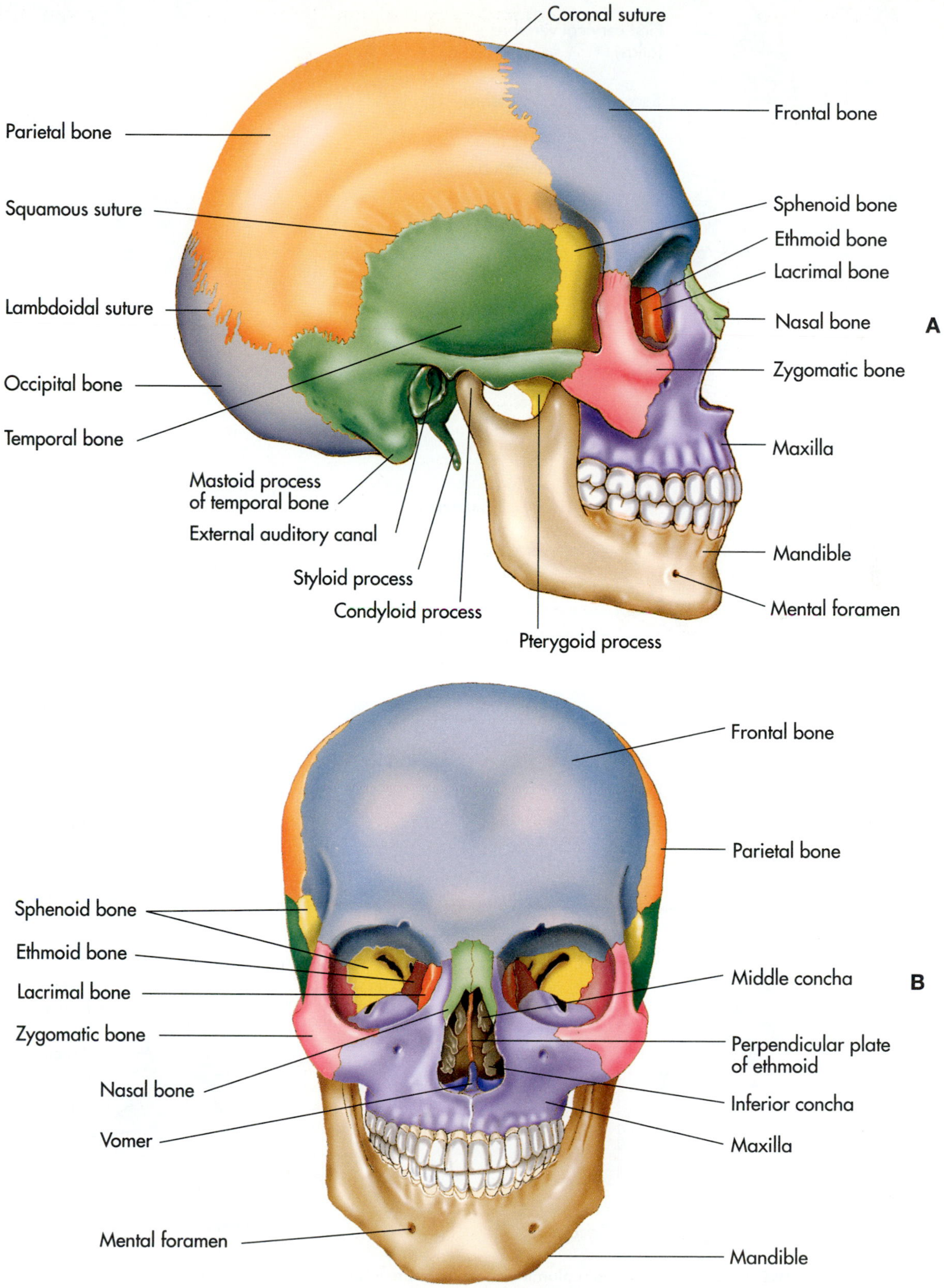

FIGURE 6-11 ■ Skull viewed from the right side **(A)** and the front **(B)**.

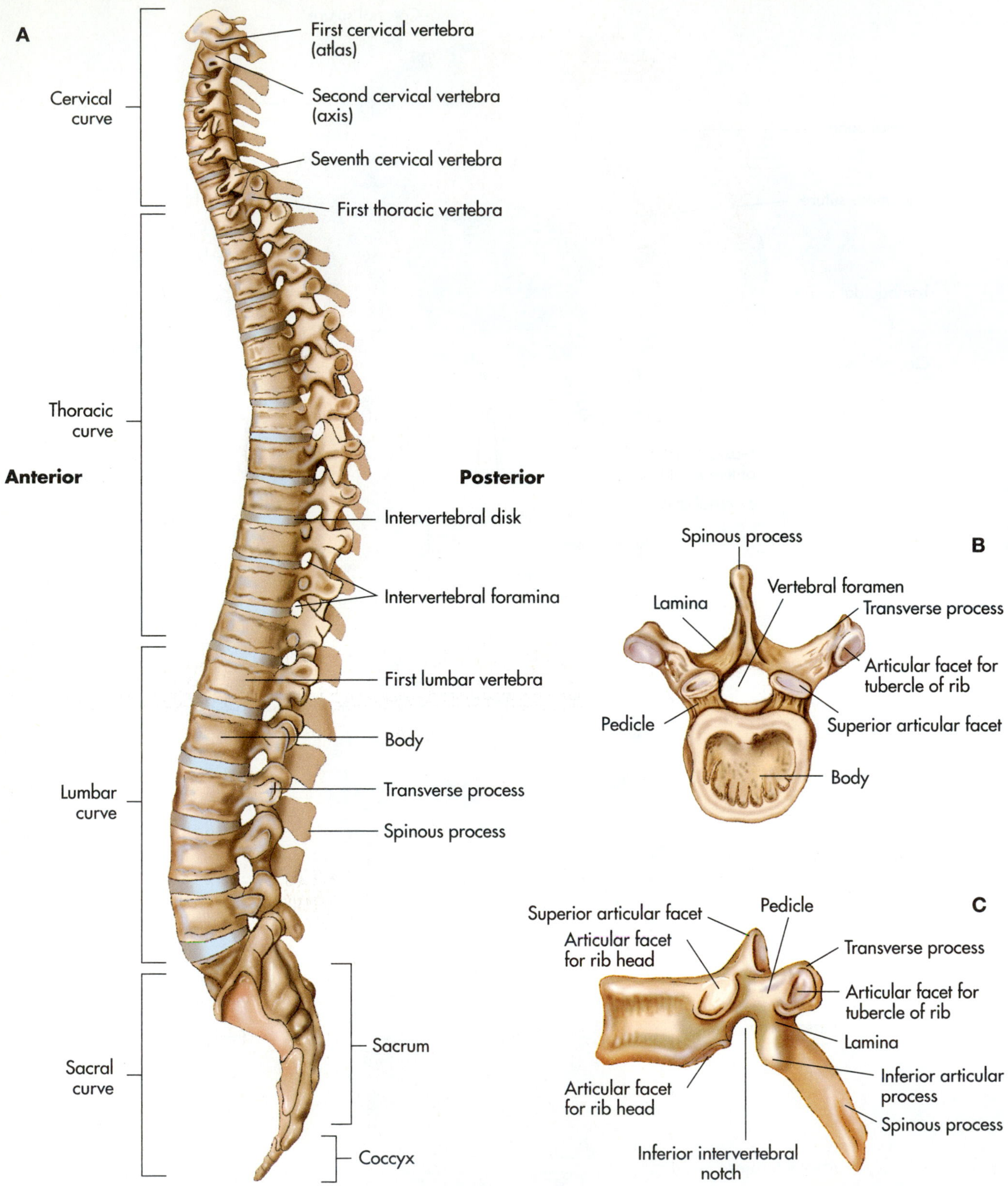

FIGURE 6-12 ■ **A,** Vertebral column viewed from the left side. **B,** Superior view of the vertebrae. **C,** Lateral view of the vertebrae.

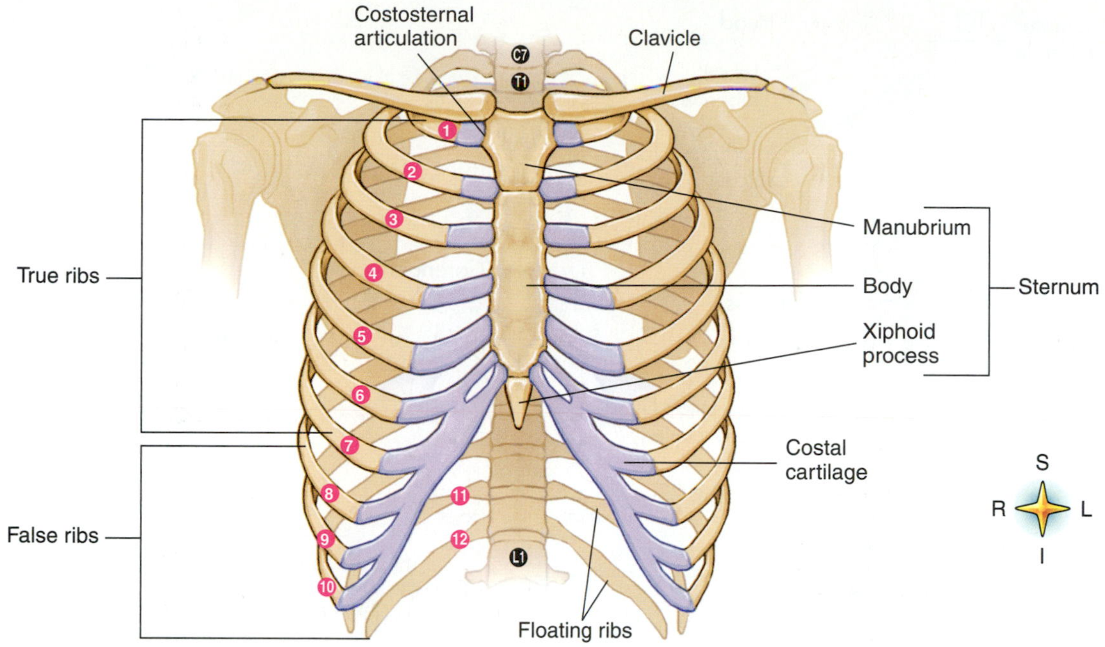

FIGURE 6-13 ■ Thoracic cage. Note the costal cartilages and their articulations with the body of the sternum.

The wrist is composed of 8 carpal bones, which are arranged in two rows of 4 each. Five metacarpals are attached to the carpal bones and constitute the bony framework of the hand. Twenty-eight phalanges make up the 10 digits of the hands. Each thumb has 2 phalanges, and each finger has 3 phalanges.

The pelvic girdle attaches the legs to the trunk (Fig. 6-15). The girdle consists of two coxae (hip bones). One is located on each side of the pelvis. Each coxa surrounds a large obturator foramen, through which muscles, nerves, and blood vessels pass to the leg. A fossa called the acetabulum is located on the lateral surface of each coxa. The acetabulum is the point of articulation of the lower limb with the girdle. During development, each coxa is formed by the fusion of three separate bones: the ilium, ischium, and pubis. The superior portion of the ilium is the iliac crest. The crest ends anteriorly as the anterior-superior iliac spine and posteriorly as the posterior-superior iliac spine.

The femur is the longest bone in the body. The femur has a neck that is well defined. It also has a prominent rounded head that articulates with the acetabulum. The proximal shaft has two tuberosities: a greater trochanter lateral to the neck and a smaller or lesser trochanter inferior and posterior to the neck. Both trochanters are attachment sites for muscles that attach the hip to the thigh. The distal end of the femur has medial and lateral condyles that articulate with the tibia. Located laterally and proximally to the condyles are the medial and lateral epicondyles. These are sites of muscle and ligament attachment. (Figure 6-16 illustrates the bones of the lower extremity.)

> **CRITICAL THINKING**
>
> Why should you anticipate blood loss when large bones are fractured?

Distally, the femur also articulates with the patella, which is located in a major tendon of the thigh muscle. The patella allows the tendon to turn the corner over the knee.

The two bones of the leg are the tibia and the fibula. The tibia is the larger of the two and supports most of the weight of the leg. A tibial tuberosity can be seen and palpated just inferior to the patella. The proximal end of the tibia has flat medial and lateral condyles that articulate with the condyles of the femur. The distal end of the tibia forms the medial malleolus, which helps to form the medial side of the ankle joint.

The fibula does not articulate with the femur. However, the fibula does have a small proximal head that articulates with the tibia. The distal end of the fibula forms the lateral malleolus to create the lateral aspect of the ankle joint.

The foot consists of seven tarsal bones (Fig. 6-17). The talus articulates with the tibia and the fibula to form the ankle joint. The calcaneus is located inferior and just lateral to the talus, supporting the bone. The calcaneus protrudes posteriorly where the calf muscles attach to it. The calcaneus is identified easily as the heel. The foot consists of tarsals, metatarsals, and phalanges. These bones are arranged in a manner similar to the metacarpals and phalanges of the hand, the great toe being analogous to the thumb. The ball of the foot is the junction between the metatarsals and the phalanges. Strong ligaments and leg muscle tendons normally hold the foot bones firmly in their arched position.

Text continued on p. 103

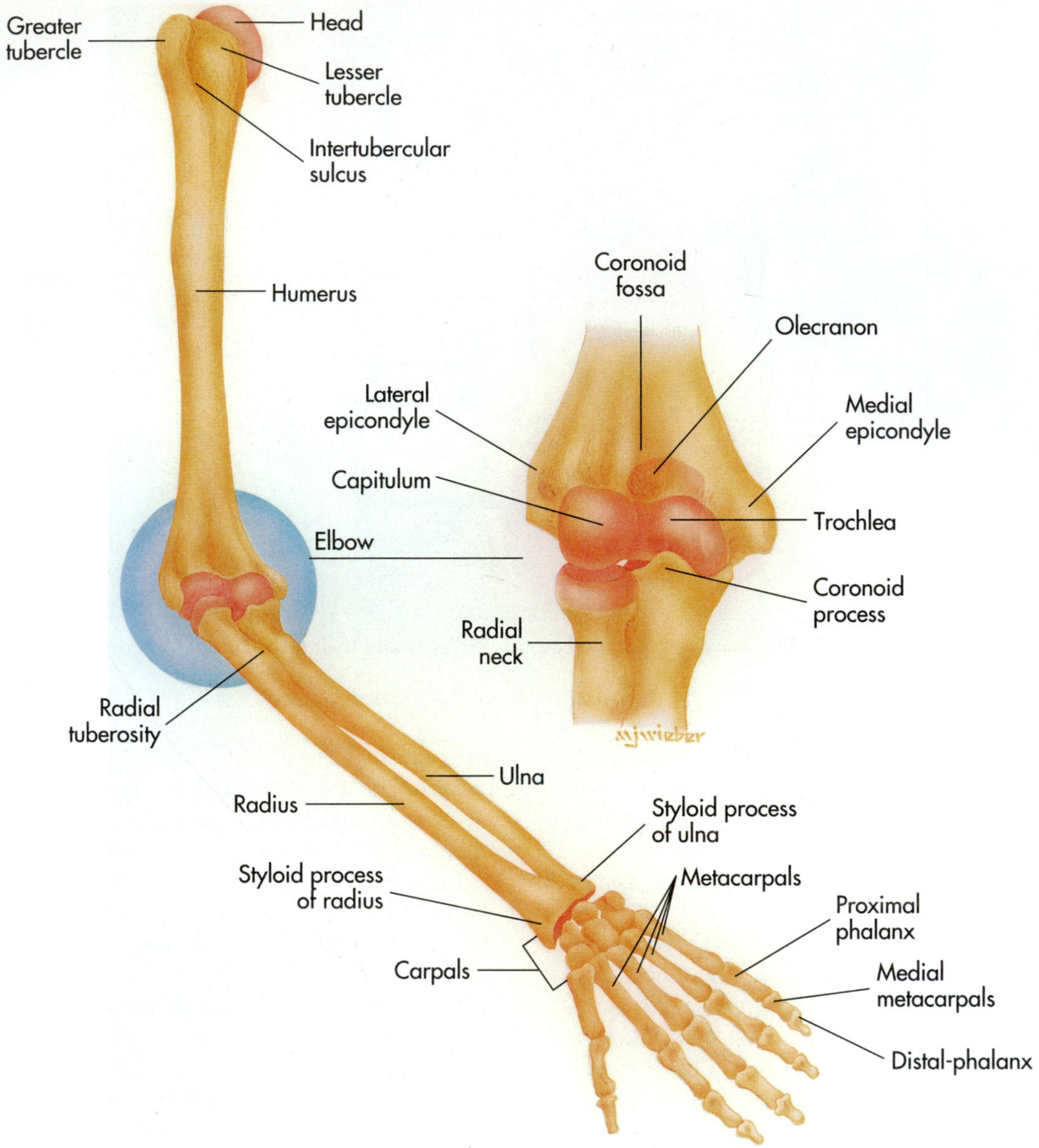

FIGURE 6-14 ■ Bones of the upper extremity.

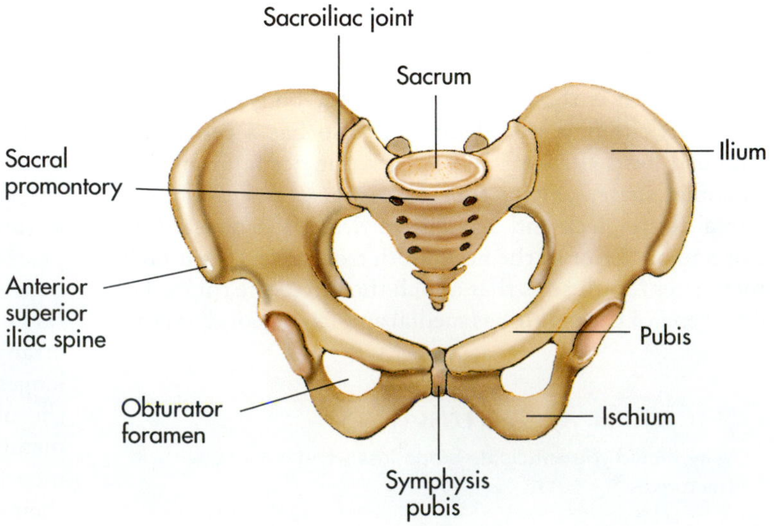

FIGURE 6-15 ■ Complete pelvic girdle, anterior view.

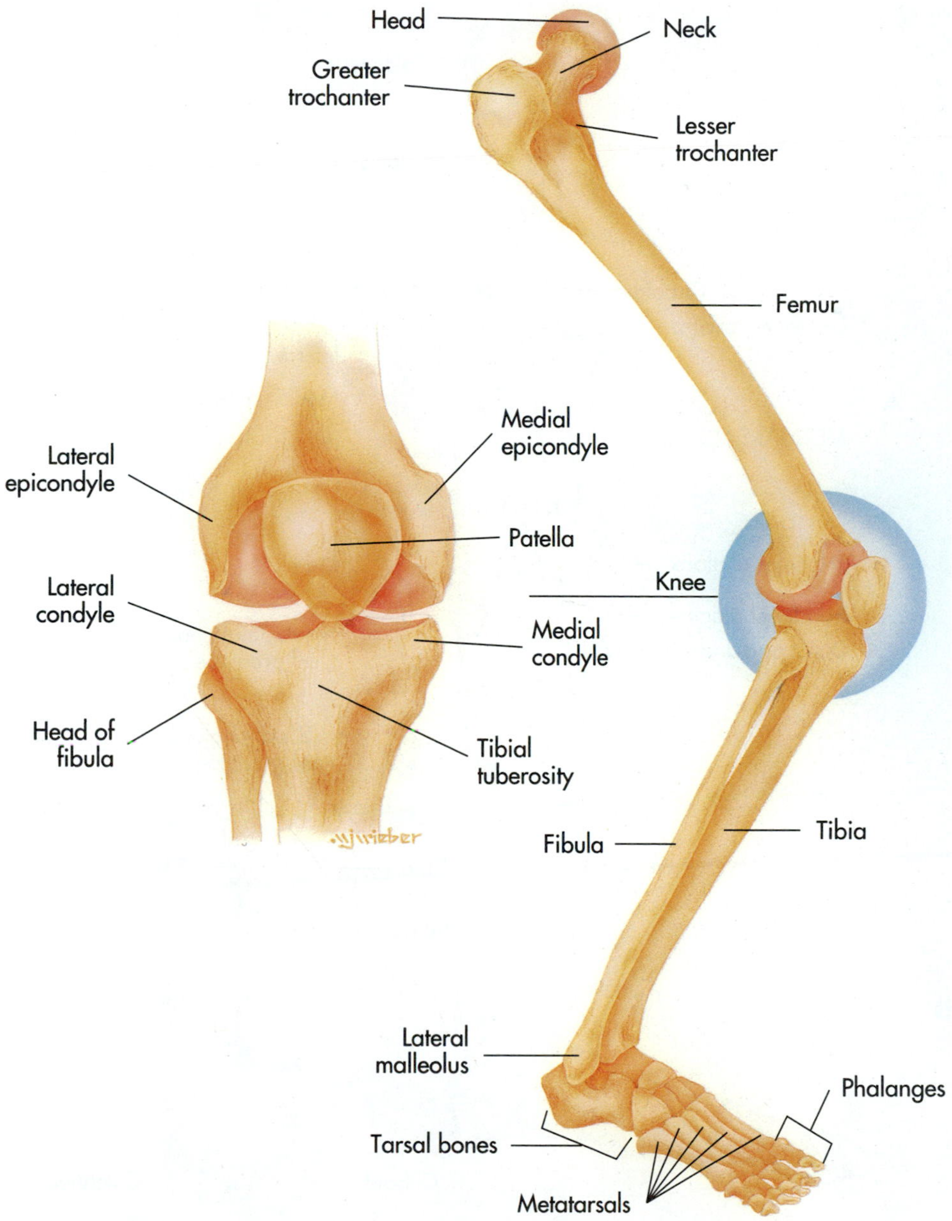

FIGURE 6-16 ■ Bones of the lower extremity.

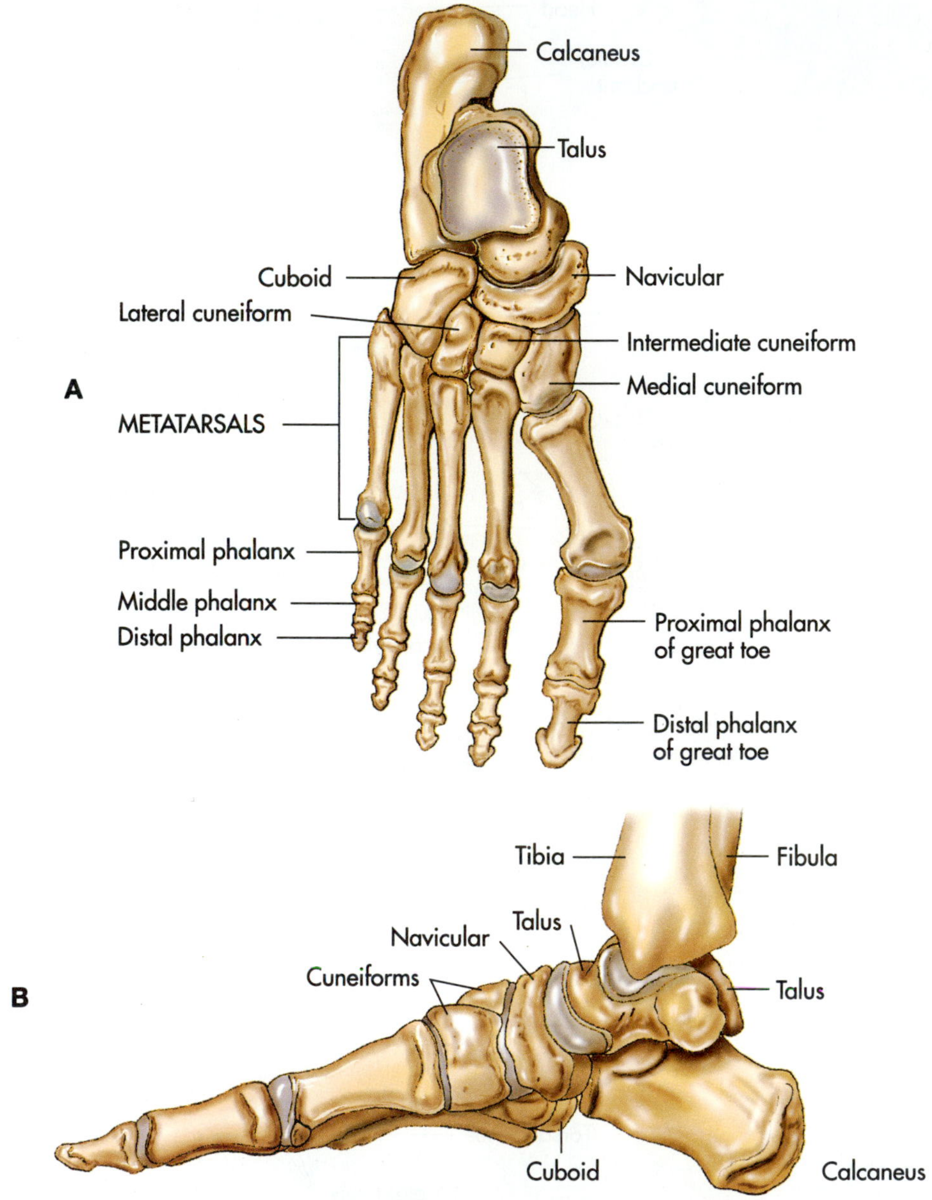

FIGURE 6-17 ■ Bones of the right ankle and foot. **A,** Dorsal view. **B,** Medial view.

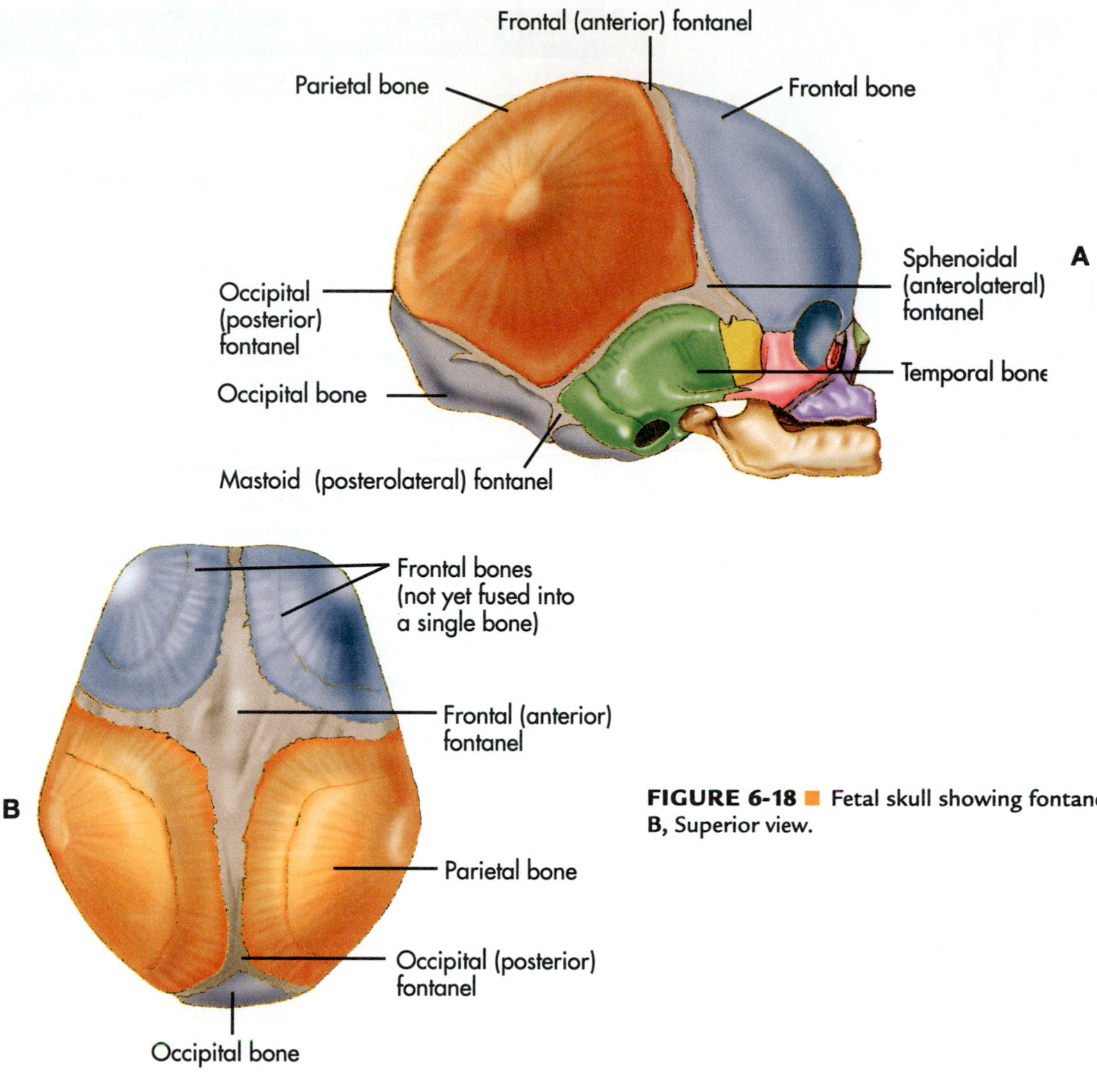

FIGURE 6-18 ■ Fetal skull showing fontanels. **A,** Lateral view. **B,** Superior view.

BIOMECHANICS OF BODY MOVEMENT

With the exception of the hyoid bone, every bone in the body connects to at least one other bone.

The connections or joints commonly are named according to the bones or portions of bones that are united at the joint. The three major classifications of joints are fibrous, cartilaginous, and synovial.

Fibrous joints. Fibrous joints consist of two bones united by fibrous tissue and have little or no movement. The joints are divided further based on structure into sutures, syndesmoses, or gomphoses. Sutures (seams between flat bones) are located in the skull bones and may be completely immobile in adults. In newborns, the sutures have gaps between them, called fontanels; these gaps are fairly wide to allow "give" to the skull during birth and to allow growth of the head during development (Fig. 6-18).

A syndesmosis is a fibrous joint in which the bones are separated by a greater distance than in a suture and are joined by ligaments. These ligaments may provide some movement of the joint. An example of this joint is the radioulnar syndesmosis that binds the radius and ulna together (Fig. 6-19).

A gomphosis consists of a peg that fits into a socket. The peg is held in place by fine bundles of collagenous connective tissue. The joints between the teeth and the sockets along the processes of the mandible and maxilla are examples of gomphoses.

Cartilaginous joints. Cartilaginous joints unite two bones by means of hyaline cartilage (synchondroses) or fibrocartilage (symphyses). A synchondrosis allows only slight movement at the joint. A common example of this type of joint is the epiphyseal plate of a growing bone. Another example is the cartilage rod between most of the ribs and the sternum. Symphysis joints are slightly movable

> **CRITICAL THINKING**
>
> **Why might the structure of the skull sutures be a disadvantage after trauma to the head of an adult?**

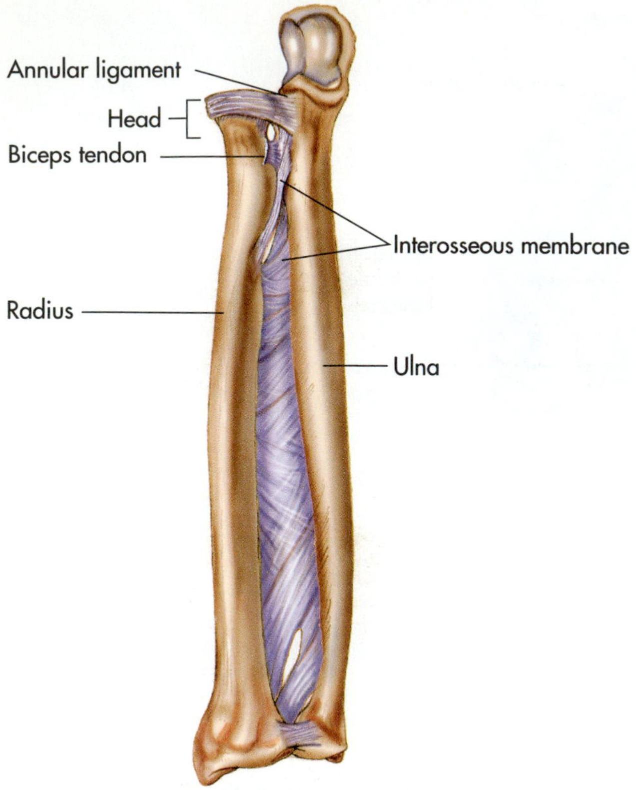

FIGURE 6-19 ■ Radioulnar syndesmosis of right forearm.

TABLE 6-3 Body Movement Terminology

TERM	DEFINITION
Flexion	Bending
Extension	Stretching out
Protraction	Movement in the anterior direction
Retraction	Movement in the posterior direction
Abduction	Movement away from the midline
Adduction	Movement toward the midline
Inversion	Turning inward
Eversion	Turning outward
Excursion	Movement from side to side
Rotation	Movement of a structure about its axis
Circumduction	Movement in a circular motion
Pronation	Rotation of the forearm so that the anterior surface is down
Supination	Rotation of the forearm so that the anterior surface is up
Elevation	Movement of a structure in a superior direction
Depression	Movement of a structure in an inferior direction
Opposition	Movement of the thumb and little finger toward each other
Reposition	Movement of a structure to its original position

because of the flexible nature of the fibrocartilage. Symphyses include the junction between the manubrium and the body of the sternum in adults, the symphysis pubis of the coxae, and the intervertebral disks.

Synovial joints. Synovial joints contain synovial fluid. This fluid is a thin lubricating film that allows considerable movement between articulating bones. Most joints that unite the bones of the appendicular skeleton are synovial. The articular surfaces of bones within synovial joints are covered with a thin layer of hyaline cartilage. This cartilage provides a smooth surface where the bones meet. The joint is enclosed by a joint capsule. This capsule consists of an outer fibrous capsule and an inner synovial membrane. The synovial membrane lines the joint and produces synovial fluid. Synovial joints are classified into six divisions according to the shape of the adjoining articular surfaces (Fig. 6-20):

1. Plane or gliding joints consist of two opposed flat surfaces that are about equal in size. Examples of these joints are the articular processes between vertebrae.
2. Saddle joints consist of two saddle-shaped articulating surfaces oriented at right angles to each other. Movement in these joints can occur in two planes. An example of a saddle joint is the carpometacarpal joint of the thumb.
3. Hinge joints consist of a convex cylinder in one bone applied to a corresponding concavity in another bone. These joints permit movement in one plane only. Examples of hinge joints are those of the elbow and knee.
4. Pivot joints consist of a relatively cylindrical bony process. This process rotates within a ring composed partly of bone and partly of ligament. An example of a pivot joint is the head of the radius articulating with the proximal end of the ulna.
5. Ball-and-socket joints consist of a ball (head) at the end of one bone and a socket into an adjacent bone into which a portion of the ball fits. These joints allow wide ranges of movement in almost any direction. Examples are the shoulder and hip joints.
6. Ellipsoid joints are modified ball-and-socket joints. The articular surfaces are ellipsoid rather than spherical. The shape of the joint limits movement, making it similar to a hinge motion, but the motion occurs in two planes. The atlantooccipital joint is an ellipsoid joint.

Types of movement. Movement may be described as it relates to the position of the body. In other words, movement can be described by motion away from the anatomical position or motion toward it. (Table 6-3 lists examples of each type of movement; also see Figures 6-21 to 6-25.)

CRITICAL THINKING

Why would it be an asset to use movement terms in your radio report or written patient care report?

Muscular System

The three primary functions of the muscular system are movement, postural maintenance, and heat production. As previously discussed, the major types of muscles are skeletal, cardiac, and smooth muscle. Skeletal muscle is far more

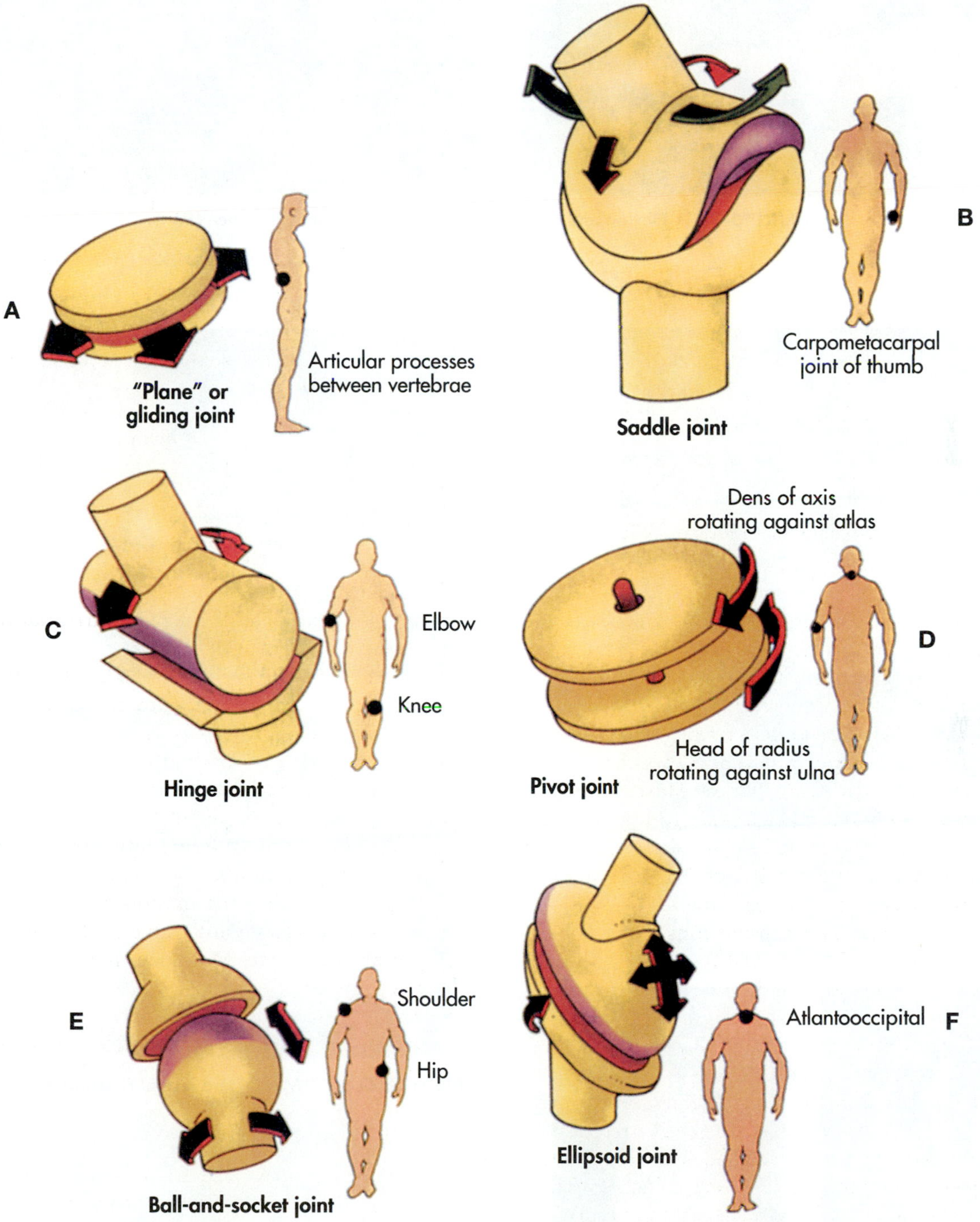

FIGURE 6-20 ■ Types of synovial joints and selected examples. **A**, Plane. **B**, Saddle. **C**, Hinge. **D**, Pivot. **E**, Ball-and-socket. **F**, Ellipsoid.

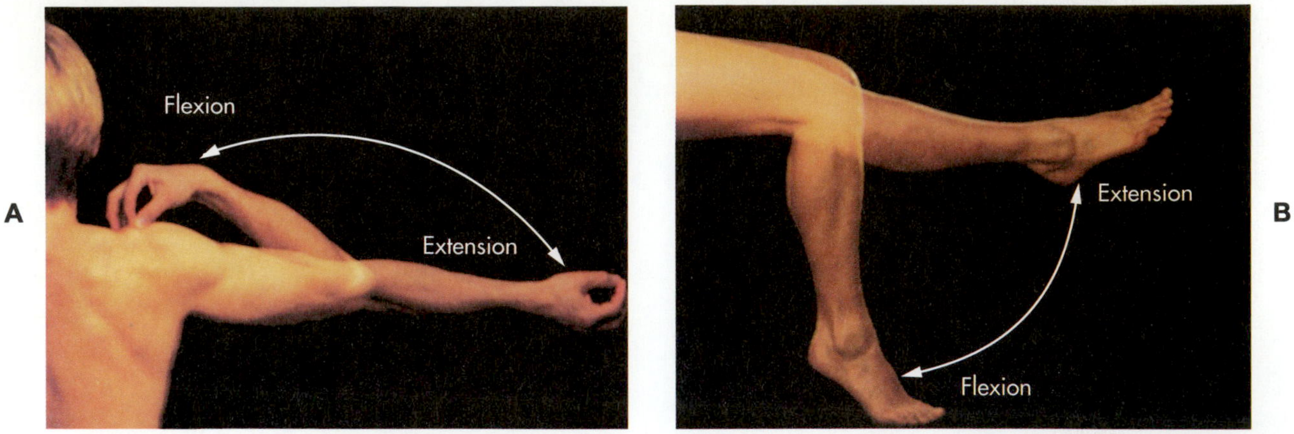

FIGURE 6-21 ■ Flexion and extension of the elbow (A) and the knee (B).

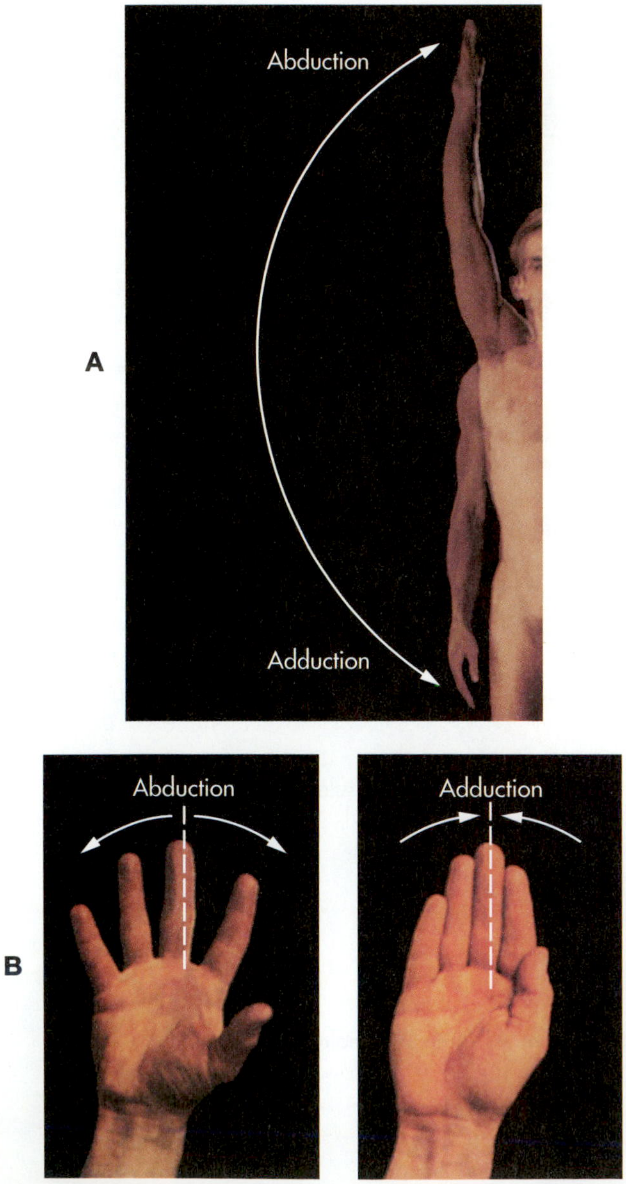

FIGURE 6-22 ■ Abduction and adduction of the upper extremity (A) and the fingers (B).

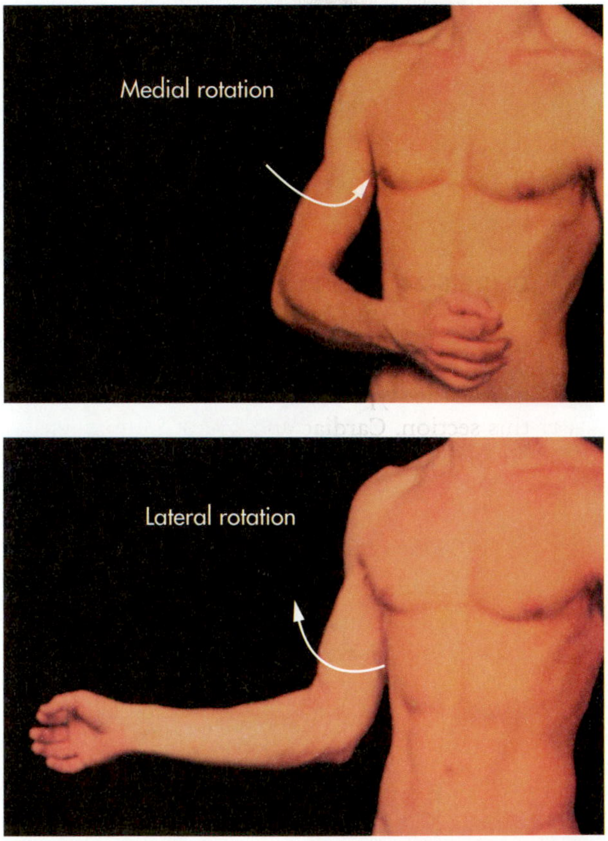

FIGURE 6-23 ■ Medial and lateral rotation of the humerus.

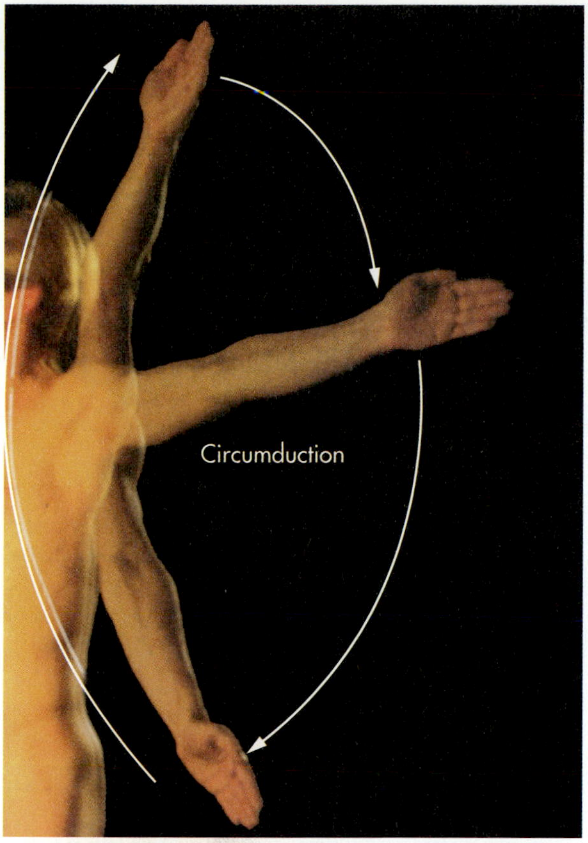

FIGURE 6-24 ■ Circumduction of the shoulder.

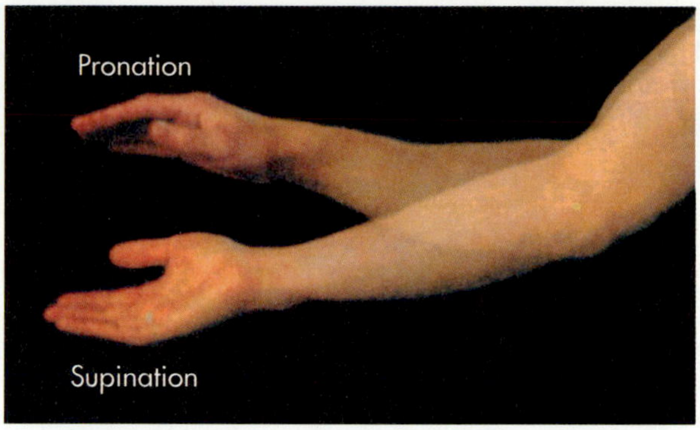

FIGURE 6-25 ■ Pronation and supination.

common than other types of muscle in the body and is the focus of this section. Cardiac and smooth muscle are presented later in this text. (Table 6-4 compares these muscle types.)

PHYSIOLOGY OF SKELETAL MUSCLE

Muscle tissue is made up of specialized contractile cells or muscle fibers. Skeletal muscle contracts in response to electrochemical stimuli. Nerve cells regulate the function of skeletal muscle fibers by controlling the series of events that results in muscle contraction.

Each skeletal muscle fiber is filled with thick and thin myofilaments. These are fine, threadlike structures. The thick myofilaments are formed from the protein myosin. The thin myofilaments are composed of the protein actin. The sarcomere is the contractile unit of skeletal muscle, containing thick and thin myofilaments. During the contraction process, energy obtained from ATP molecules enables the two types of myofilaments to slide toward each other and shorten the sarcomere and eventually the entire muscle.

A nervous impulse enters the muscle fiber through a specialized nerve known as a motor neuron. The point of contact between the nerve ending and the muscle fiber is the neuromuscular junction or synapse (Fig. 6-26). Each muscle fiber receives a branch of an axon. Each axon innervates more than a single muscle fiber. When a nerve impulse passes through this junction, specialized chemicals are released, causing the muscle to contract.

> **CRITICAL THINKING**
>
> Consider that exposure to a chemical nerve weapon caused too much chemical stimulation at the synapse for the muscles of the eye. What might you find in your examination of the eye?

SKELETAL MUSCLE MOVEMENT

Most muscles extend from one bone to another and cross at least one joint. Muscle contraction causes most body movements by pulling one of the bones toward the other across the movable joint. The points of attachment of each muscle are the origin and insertion. The origin is the end of the muscle attached to the more stationary of the two bones. The insertion is the end of the muscle attached to the bone undergoing the greatest movement. Some muscles of the face are not attached to bone at both ends but attach to the skin, which moves when muscles contract.

As some muscles contract and others relax at the same time, movement is created. Muscles that work together to cause movement are called *synergists.* A muscle that opposes another muscle (moves the structure in an opposite direction) is called an *antagonist.* The muscle that is the main cause of a movement is called the *prime mover.* For example, the biceps brachii, brachialis, and triceps brachii muscles are involved in flexion and extension of the forearm at the elbow joint. The biceps brachii is the prime mover during flexion. The brachialis is the synergistic muscle. When the biceps brachii and the brachialis muscles flex the forearm, the triceps brachii relaxes. The triceps is the antagonist. During extension of the forearm, the triceps brachii is the prime mover. The biceps and brachialis are the antagonistic muscles. The synergists and antagonists coordinate their activity, making movement smooth (Fig. 6-27).

Types of muscle contraction. Muscle contractions can be labeled as *isometric* or *isotonic.* This depends on the type of contraction that predominates. In isometric contractions the length of the muscle does not change. However,

TABLE 6-4 Comparison of Muscle Types

FEATURES	SKELETAL MUSCLE	CARDIAC MUSCLE	SMOOTH MUSCLE
Location	Attached to bones	Heart	Walls of hollow organs, blood vessels, eyes, glands, and skin
Cell shape	Long and cylindrical (1-40 mm in length and may extend the entire length of a muscle; 10-100 μm in diameter)	Cylindrical and branched (100-500 μm in length; 100-200 μm in diameter)	Spindle-shaped (15-200 μm in length, 5-10 μm in diameter)
Nucleus	Multiple, peripherally located	Single, centrally located	Single, centrally located
Special features		Intercalated disks join the cells to each other	
Striations	Yes	Yes	No
Control	Voluntary	Involuntary	Involuntary
Capable of spontaneous contraction	No	Yes	Yes
Function	Body movement	Pumps blood	Food movement through the digestive tract, emptying of the urinary bladder, regulation of blood vessel diameter, change in pupil size, contraction of many gland ducts, movement of hair, and many other functions

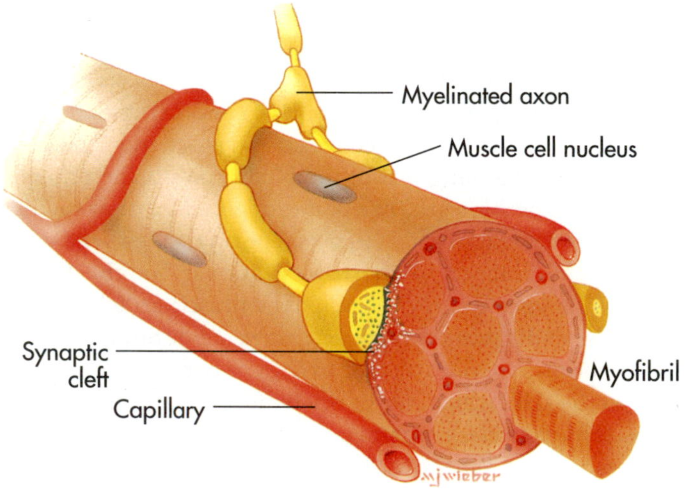

FIGURE 6-26 ■ Neuromuscular junction.

the amount of tension increases during the contraction. Isometric contractions are responsible for the constant length of the postural muscles of the body. During isotonic contractions, the amount of tension created by the muscle is constant during contraction, but the length of the muscle changes. An example of isotonic contraction is the movement of the arms or fingers. Most muscle contractions are a mix of both types of contractions.

Postural maintenance. Postural maintenance is a result of muscle tone, the constant tension produced by muscles of the body for long periods. This tone keeps the back and legs straight, the head in an upright position, and the abdomen from bulging. These positions balance the distribution of weight. Therefore they put less strain on muscles, tendons, ligaments, and bones.

Heat production. The energy needed to create muscle contraction is derived from ATP. Most of the energy released in the breakdown of ATP during a muscular contraction is used to shorten the muscle fibers. Some energy, though, is lost as heat during the chemical reaction. The normal body temperature comes in large part from this metabolism in skeletal muscle. If the body temperature drops below a certain level, the nervous system induces shivering. Shivering is rapid contractions of skeletal muscle that produce shaking rather than coordinated movements. The muscle movement increases heat production up to 18 times that of resting levels. The heat made during shivering can exceed that from moderate exercise. This helps to raise the body temperature to its normal range.

CRITICAL THINKING

Children under 3 months cannot shiver. How will you account for that in your prehospital care for patients in this age group?

Nervous System

The nervous system and the endocrine system are the main regulatory and coordinating systems of the body. The nervous system rapidly sends out information. This occurs by means of nerve impulses conducted from one area of the body to another. The endocrine system sends out information more slowly. This takes place by means of chemicals secreted by ductless glands into the bloodstream. These

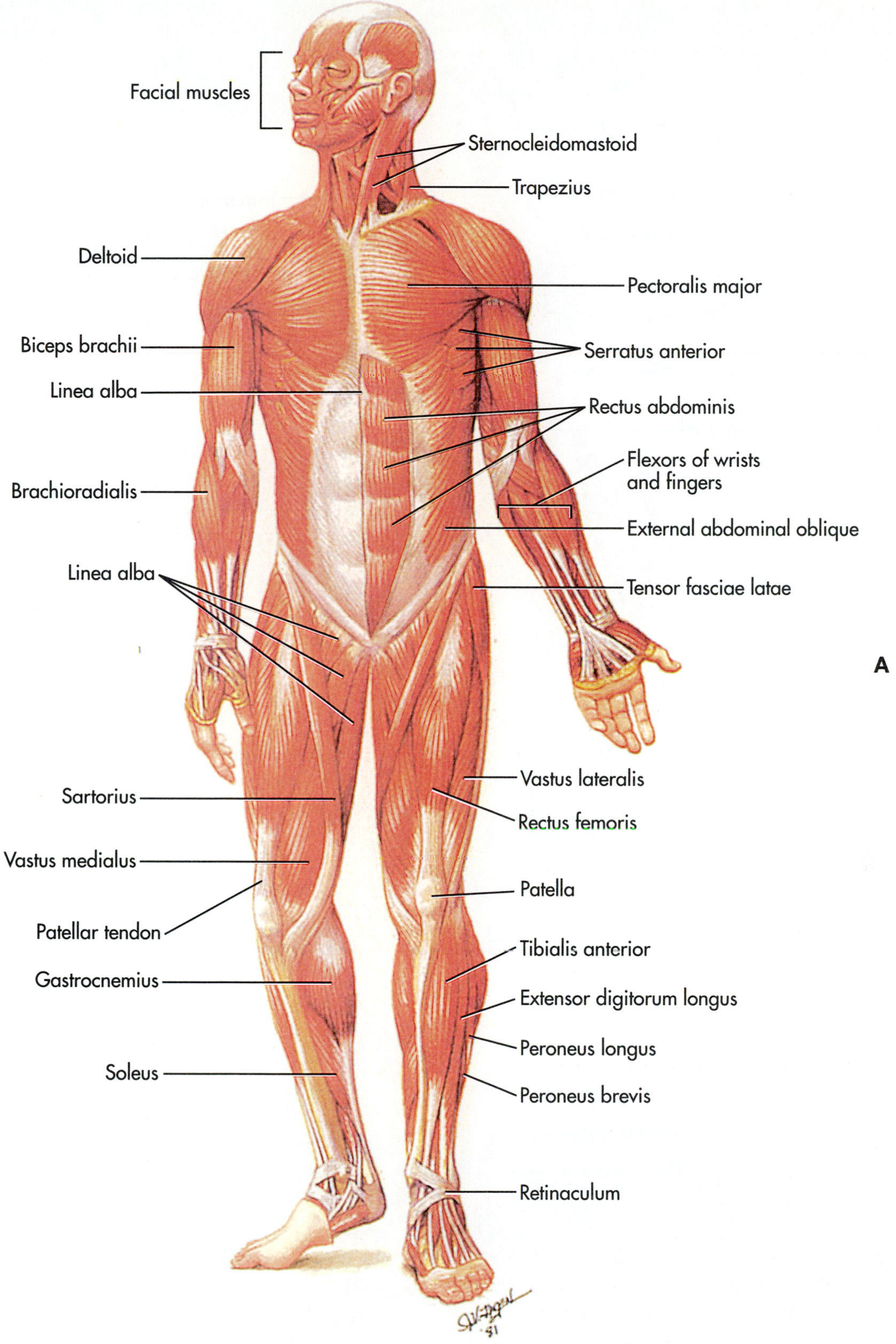

FIGURE 6-27 ■ **A,** Anterior view of body musculature.

Continued

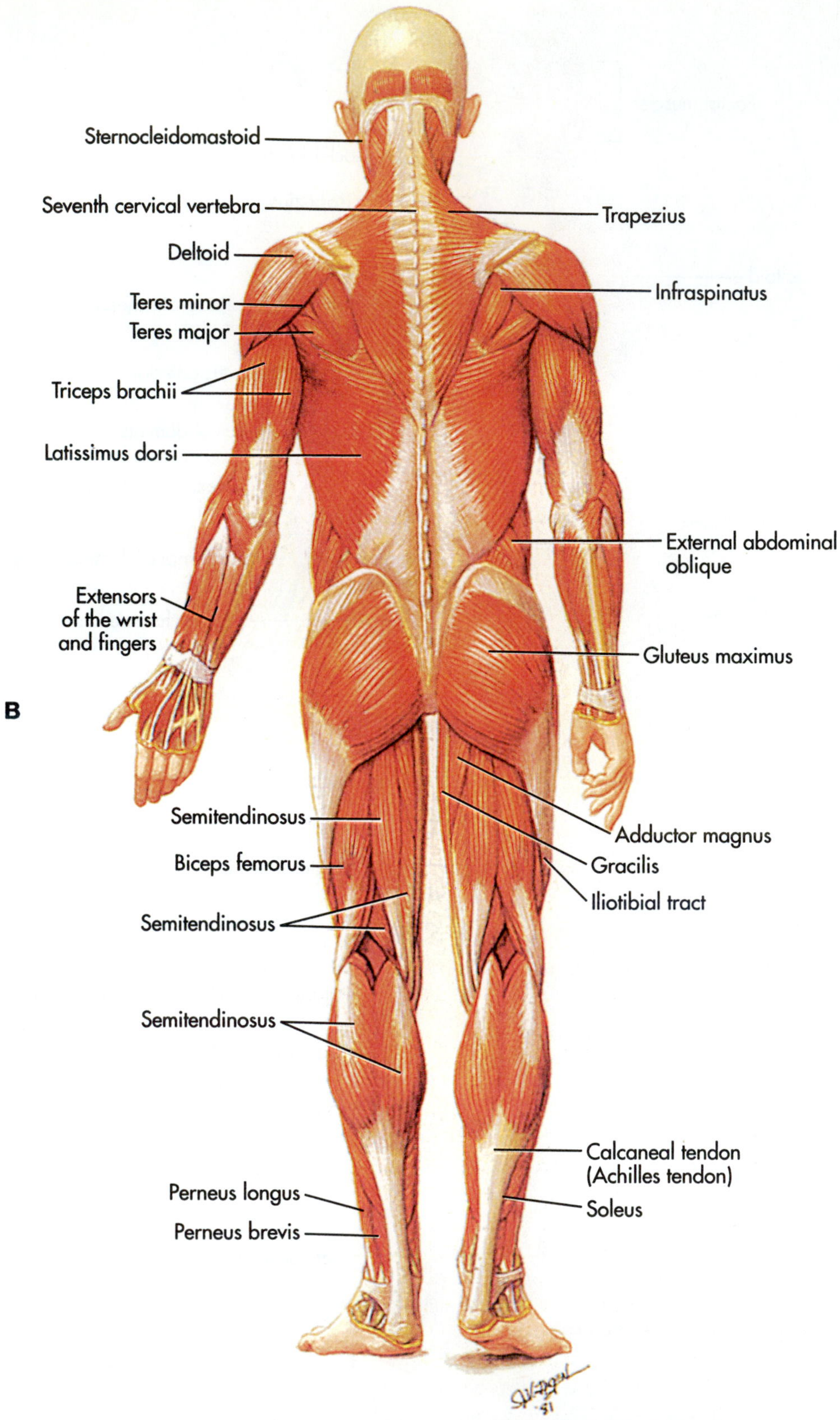

FIGURE 6-27, cont'd ■ **B,** Posterior view of body musculature.

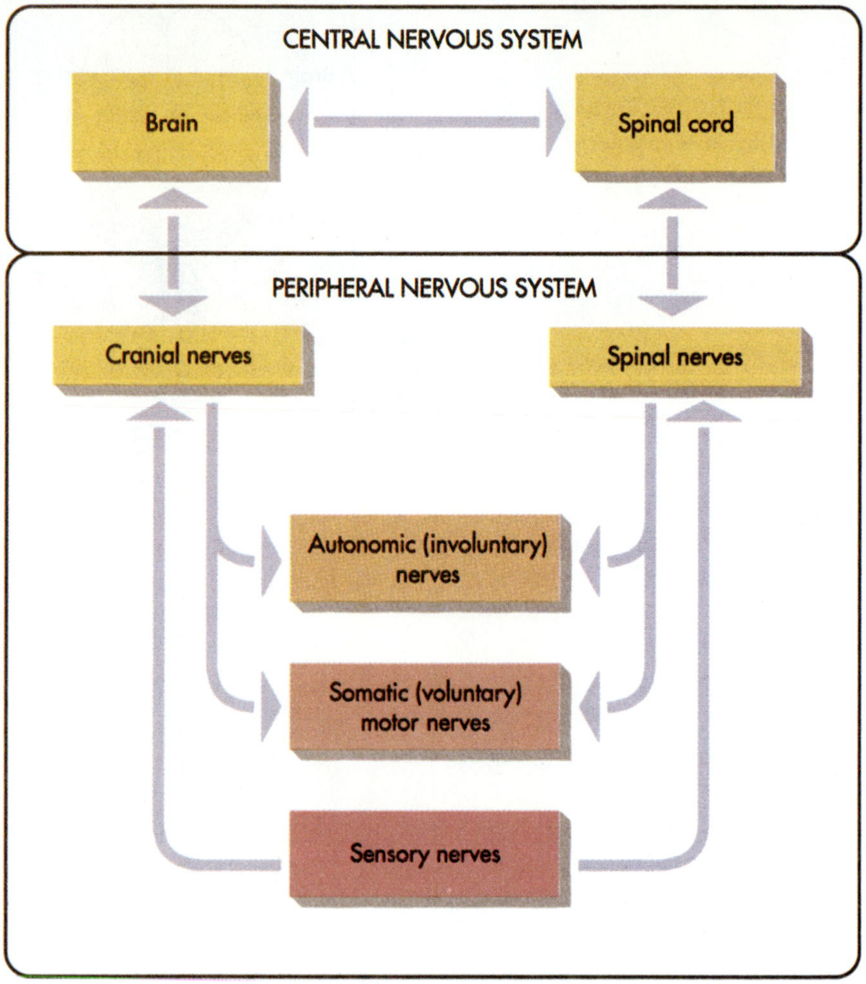

FIGURE 6-28 ■ Divisions of the nervous system.

chemicals and hormones then are circulated to other parts of the body. The constancy of the internal environment of the body is **homeostasis.** This constancy is sustained to a large degree by these regulatory and coordinating actions.

DIVISIONS

The human body has a single nervous system. This is the case even though some of its subdivisions are referred to as separate systems. Each subdivision has structural and functional aspects that separate it from the others (Fig. 6-28).

The **central nervous system** (CNS) is made up of the brain and spinal cord. These organs are encased in and protected by bone. The brain and spinal cord are continuous with each other. The **peripheral nervous system** (PNS) consists of the nerves and ganglia. The ganglia are collections of nerve cell bodies located outside the CNS. Forty-three pairs of nerves originate from the CNS to form the PNS; 12 pairs, the cranial nerves, originate from the brain, and the remaining 31 pairs, the spinal nerves, originate from the spinal cord. The **afferent division** transmits action potentials from the sensory organs to the CNS. The **efferent division** transmits action potentials from the CNS to effector organs such as muscles and glands (Fig. 6-29). The efferent division is divided further into the **somatic nervous system** and the autonomic nervous system. The somatic nervous system transmits impulses from the CNS to skeletal muscle. The autonomic nervous system transmits action potentials from the CNS to smooth muscle, cardiac muscle, and certain glands.

> **CRITICAL THINKING**
> How are the cranial nerves like the Supreme Court?

CENTRAL NERVOUS SYSTEM

As stated before, the CNS consists of the brain and spinal cord. There are four major regions of the adult brain. The first is the brainstem (consisting of the medulla, pons, and midbrain). Second is the diencephalon (which includes the thalamus and hypothalamus). Third and fourth are the cerebrum and the cerebellum, respectively (Fig. 6-30). (Table 6-5 describes the functions of these divisions.)

Brainstem. The medulla, pons, and midbrain constitute the brainstem. The brainstem connects the spinal cord to the remainder of the brain and is responsible for many es-

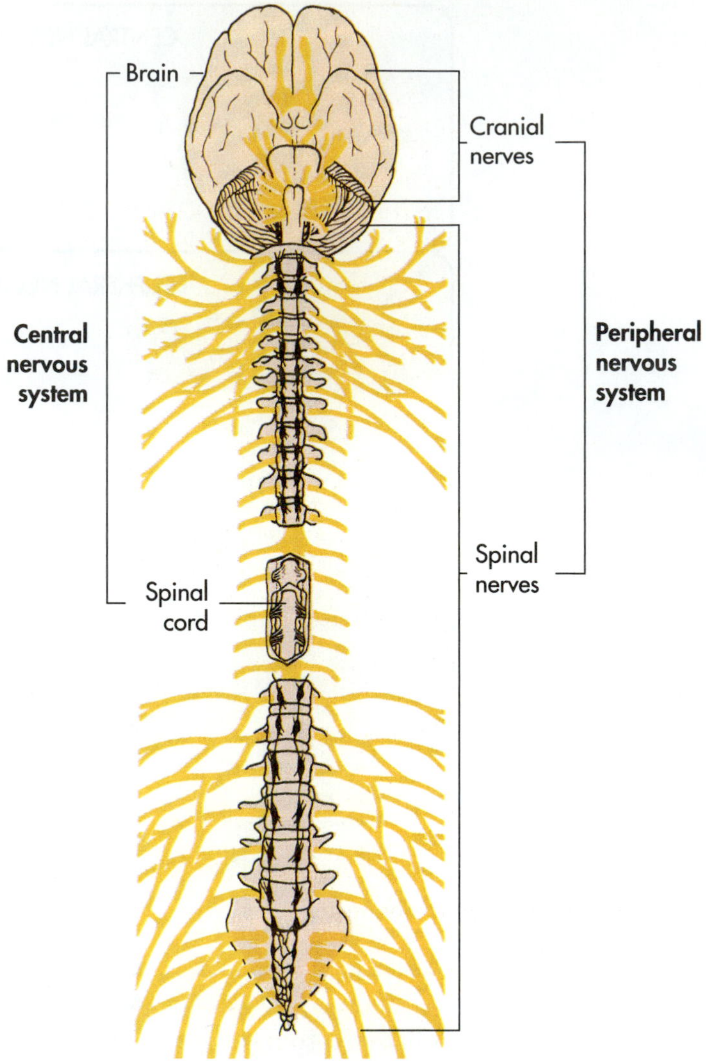

FIGURE 6-29 ■ The central nervous system consists of the brain and spinal cord. The peripheral nervous system consists of cranial nerves, which arise from the brain, and spinal nerves, which arise from the spinal cord.

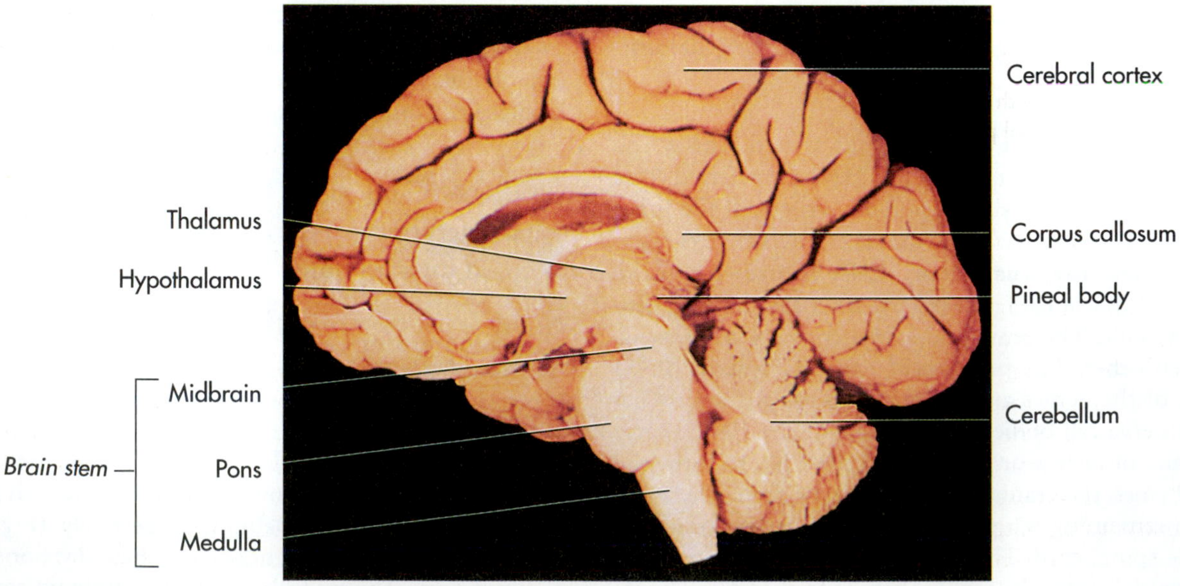

FIGURE 6-30 ■ Section of preserved brain.

TABLE 6-5 Functions of Major Divisions of the Brains

BRAIN AREA	FUNCTION
Brainstem	
Medulla	Two-way conduction pathway between the spinal cord and higher brain centers; cardiac, respiratory, and vasomotor control centers
Pons	Two-way conduction pathway between areas of the brain and other regions of the body; influences respiration
Midbrain	Two-way conduction pathway; relay point for visual and auditory impulses
Diencephalon	
Hypothalamus	Regulation of body temperature, water balance, sleep-cycle control, appetite, and sexual arousal
Thalamus	Sensory relay station from various body areas to cerebral cortex; emotions and alerting or arousal mechanisms
Cerebellum	Muscle coordination; maintenance of equilibrium and posture
Cerebrum	Sensory perception, emotions, willed movements, consciousness, and memory

sential functions. All but 2 of the 12 cranial nerves enter or exit the brain through the brainstem.

The medulla is also known as the *medulla oblongata.* The medulla is the most inferior portion of the brainstem. The medulla acts as a conduction pathway for ascending and descending nerve tracts. The medulla controls several body functions. Examples are regulation of heart rate, blood vessel diameter, breathing, swallowing, vomiting, coughing, and sneezing.

CRITICAL THINKING

You have a patient with an injury that affects the medulla. What will be the initial prehospital management priority? Why?

The pons contains ascending and descending nerve tracts. The pons relays information from the cerebrum to the cerebellum. In addition, the pons houses the sleep center and respiratory center that, along with the medulla, help control breathing.

The midbrain, or mesencephalon, is the smallest region of the brainstem. The midbrain is involved in hearing through audio pathways in the CNS. The midbrain also is involved in visual reflexes such as visual tracking of moving objects and turning of the eyes. Other parts of the midbrain help regulate the automatic functions that require no conscious thought. These functions include, for example, coordination of motor activities and muscle tone.

TABLE 6-6 Hypothalamic Functions

FUNCTION	DESCRIPTION
Autonomic	Helps control heart rate, urine release from the bladder, movement of food through the digestive tract, and blood vessel diameter
Endocrine	Helps regulate pituitary gland secretions and influences metabolism, ion balance, sexual development, and sexual functions
Muscle control	Controls muscles involved in swallowing and stimulates shivering in several muscles
Temperature regulation	Promotes heat loss when the hypothalamic temperature increases by increasing sweat production (anterior hypothalamus) and promotes heat production when the hypothalamic temperature decreases by promoting shivering (posterior hypothalamus)
Regulation of food and water intake	Hunger center promotes eating, and satiety center inhibits eating; thirst center promotes water intake
Emotions	Large range of emotional influences over body functions; directly involved in stress-related and psychosomatic illnesses and with feelings of fear and rage
Regulation of the sleep-wake cycle	Coordinates responses to the sleep-wake cycle with other areas of the brain (e.g., the reticular activating system)

The reticular formation is a group of nuclei scattered throughout the brainstem. It receives axons from a large number of sources, especially from the nerves that innervate the face. The reticular formation and its connections are known as the **reticular activating system.** This system is involved in the sleep-wake cycle. The reticular activating system also is important in arousing and maintaining consciousness. Coma after head injury results from damage to the this system.

Diencephalon. The diencephalon is the part of the brain between the brainstem and the cerebrum. Major components of this organ include the thalamus and hypothalamus. The thalamus is the largest portion of the diencephalon. The thalamus receives sensory input from various sense organs of the body. It relays these impulses to the cerebral cortex. The thalamus also has other functions, such as influencing mood and general body movements linked with strong emotions such as fear or rage.

The hypothalamus is a major controller in the brain. It acts as a gatekeeper to decide what information is passed along to the cerebrum. The hypothalamus is an active participant in emotions, hormonal cycles, and sexuality. (Table 6-6 gives a summary of the various hypothalamic functions.)

Cerebrum. The cerebrum is the largest portion of the brain. The cerebrum is divided into left and right hemispheres, and each hemisphere is divided into lobes named for the bones that lie over them (Fig. 6-31).

The frontal lobe is important in voluntary motor function, motivation, aggression, and mood. The parietal lobe is the major center for the reception and evaluation of most sensory information. This excludes smell, hearing, and vision. The occipital lobe functions in the reception and integration of visual input. The occipital lobe is not distinctly separate from other lobes. The temporal lobe receives and evaluates olfactory and auditory input. The temporal lobe plays a key role in memory. A thin layer of gray matter made up of neuron dendrites and cell bodies composes the surface of the cerebrum (cerebral cortex).

The **limbic system** is made up of portions of the cerebrum and diencephalon. This system influences emotions, visceral responses to those emotions, motivation, mood, and sensations of pain and pleasure.

Cerebellum. The cerebellum is the second largest part of the human brain. The cerebellum is involved in gross motor coordination and helps produce smooth movements. A major job of the cerebellum is to compare impulses from the motor cortex with those from moving structures (e.g., position of the body or body parts that innervate the joints and tendons of the structure being moved). The cerebellum compares the intended movement with the actual one. If a difference is detected, the cerebellum sends impulses to the motor cortex and the spinal cord to correct the discrepancy. Loss of cerebellum functioning results in an inability to make exact movements.

Spinal cord. The spinal cord lies within the spinal column and extends from the occipital bone to the level of the second lumbar vertebra. The spinal cord has a central gray portion and a peripheral white portion. The white matter consists of nerve tracts, and the gray matter consists of nerve cell bodies and dendrites. The dorsal root conveys afferent nerve processes to the cord, and the ventral root conveys efferent nerve processes away from the cord. Spinal ganglia, or dorsal root ganglia, contain the cell bodies of sensory neurons (Fig. 6-32).

CRITICAL THINKING

An older adult patient has a new onset of staggering gait. What area of the brain do you suspect has altered function?

The spinal cord is the main reflex center of the body. Many of these reflexes are autonomic or visceral. An example of this is increased heart rate in response to decreased blood pressure. Another example is the stretch reflex (knee-jerk reflex). Then there are also withdrawal reflexes (removing a limb or other body part from a painful stimulus). In addition to acting as a primary reflex center, the spinal cord tracts carry impulses to the brain in afferent, ascending tracts. These tracts also carry motor impulses from the

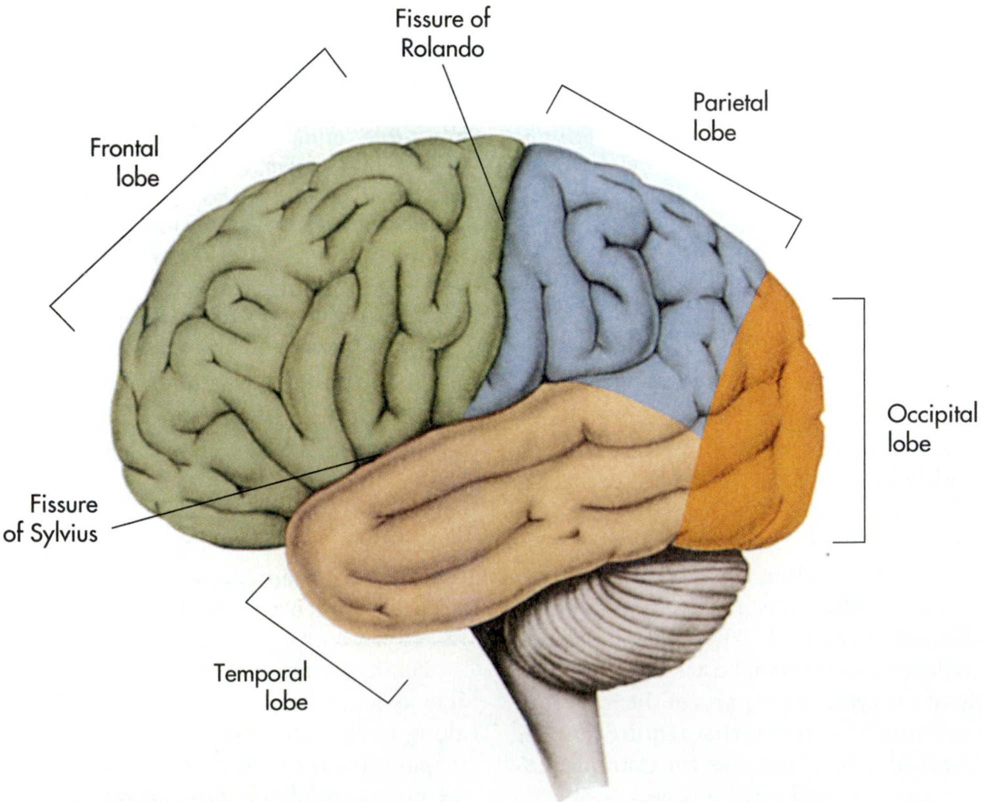

FIGURE 6-31 ■ Lobes of the cerebrum.

brain in efferent, descending tracts. (Ascending and descending pathways are addressed further in Chapter 31.)

The organs of the nervous system are surrounded by a tough, fluid-containing membrane. This membrane is known as the meninges. The meninges are surrounded by bone and have three connective tissue layers. The most superficial and thickest layer is the dura mater. It consists of two layers around the brain and one layer around the spinal cord. The two layers of the dura mater are fused around most of the brain but are separate in several places. The dura mater of the brain is attached tightly and is continuous with the periosteum of the cranial vault, whereas the dura mater of the spinal cord is separated from the periosteum of the vertebral canal by the epidural space.

The arachnoid layer is the second meningeal layer. The space between this layer and the dura mater is known as the subdural space, which contains a small amount of serous fluid. The third meningeal layer is the pia mater. The pia mater lies external to a basement membrane formed by special cells called the *glia limitans,* which completely envelops the CNS. The space between the pia mater and the arachnoid layer is the subarachnoid space. This space is filled with blood vessels and cerebrospinal fluid (Fig. 6-33).

The cerebrospinal fluid is similar to plasma and interstitial fluid (fluid that occupies the space outside the blood vessels). Cerebrospinal fluid bathes the brain and spinal cord and acts as a cushion around the CNS. Cerebrospinal fluid is formed continually from fluid filtering out of the blood in a network of brain capillaries and cells known as the choroid plexus. This special fluid fills the ventricles of

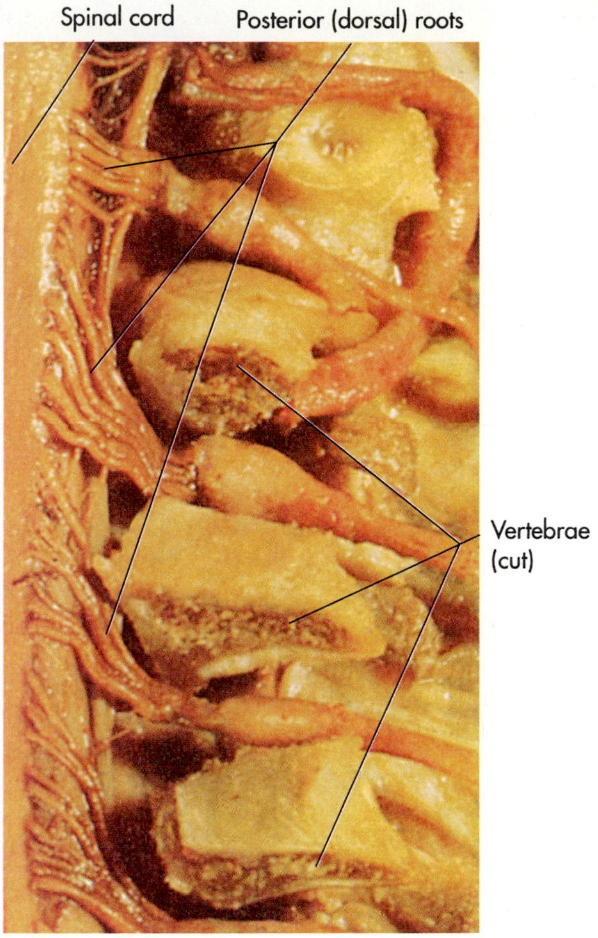

FIGURE 6-32 ■ Dissection of the cervical segment of the spinal cord.

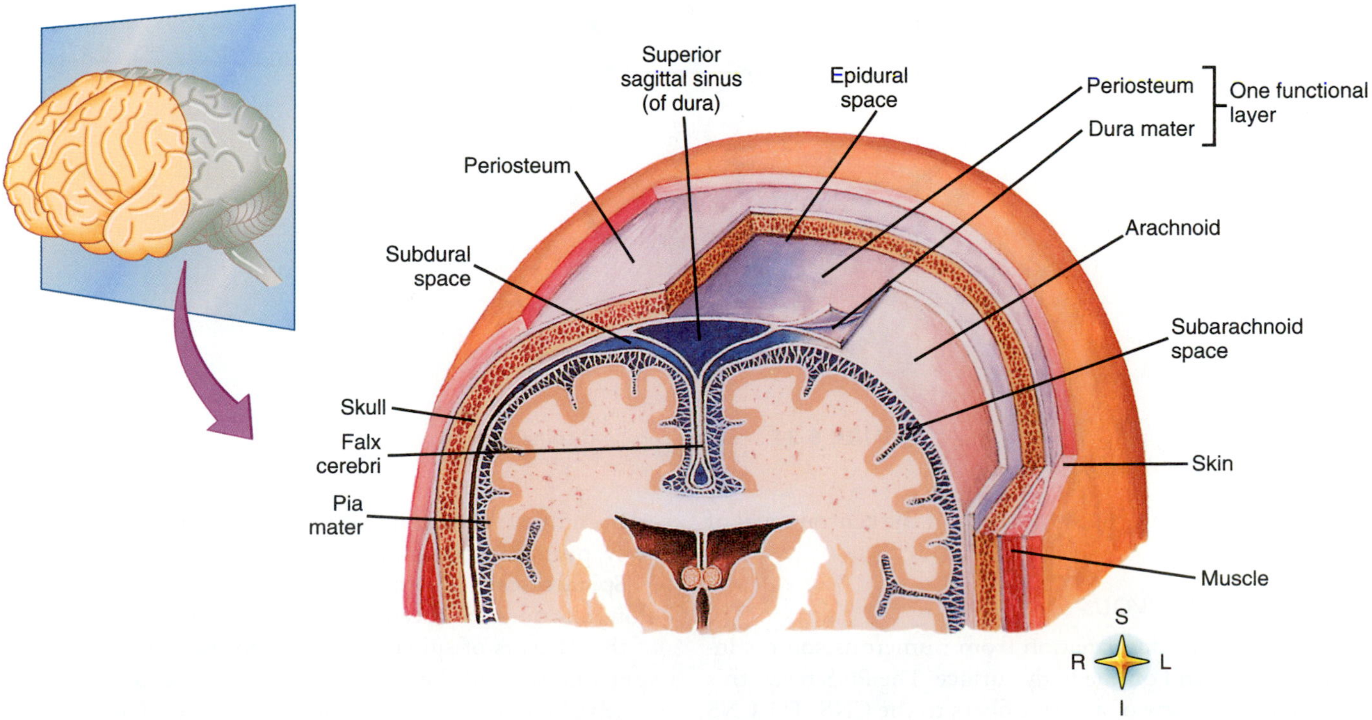

FIGURE 6-33 ■ Meningeal coverings of the brain and spinal cord.

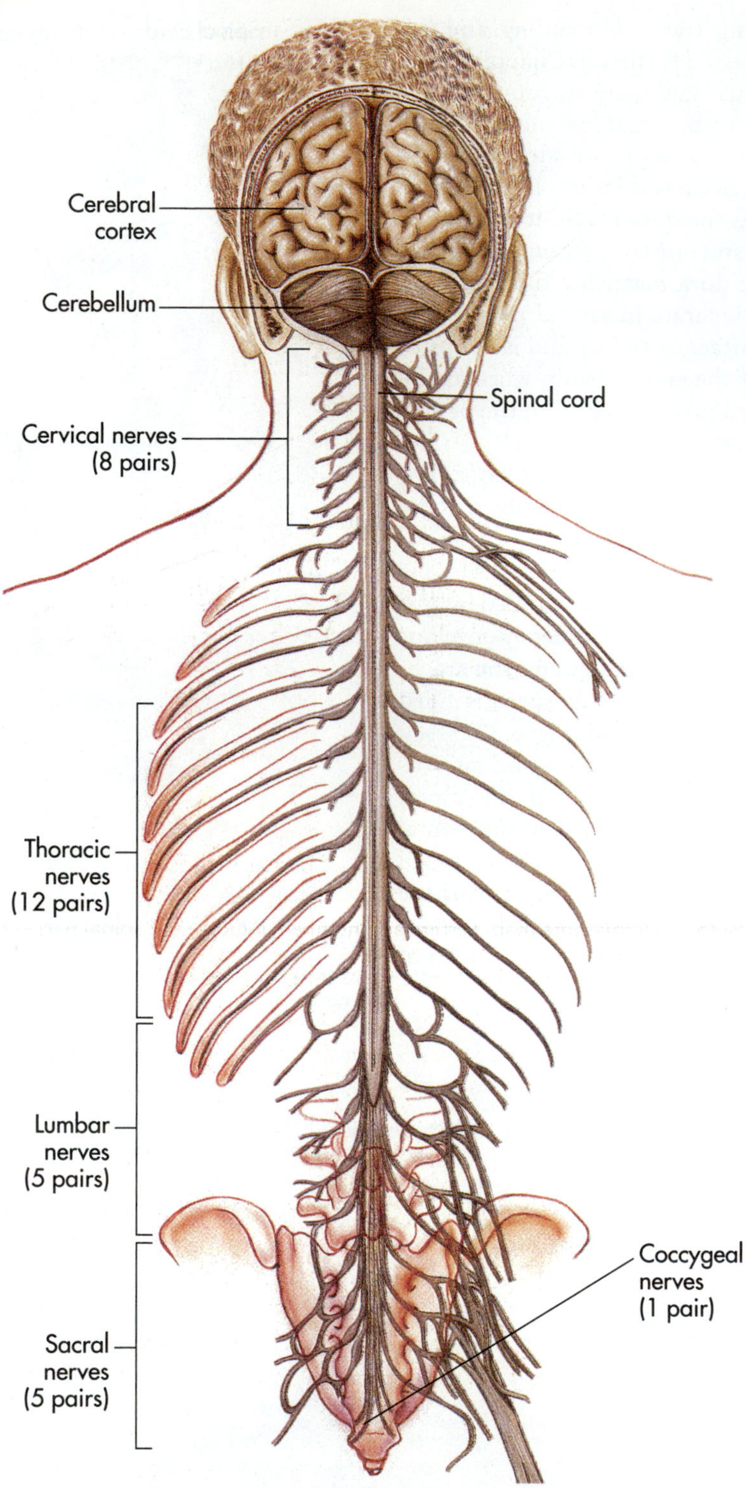

FIGURE 6-34 ■ Spinal cord and spinal nerves.

the brain, the subarachnoid space, and the central canal of the spinal cord.

PERIPHERAL NERVOUS SYSTEM

The PNS collects information from numerous sources inside the body and on the body surface. The PNS relays this information by way of afferent fibers to the CNS. The CNS then evaluates the information. Efferent fibers in the PNS relay information from the CNS to various parts of the body, primarily to muscles and glands.

Spinal nerves. The spinal nerves arise from many *rootlets* along the dorsal and ventral surfaces of the spinal cord. All of the 31 pairs of spinal nerves, except for the first pair of spinal nerves and the spinal nerves in the sacrum, exit the vertebral column though adjacent vertebrae. The first pair of spinal nerves exits between the skull and the first cervical

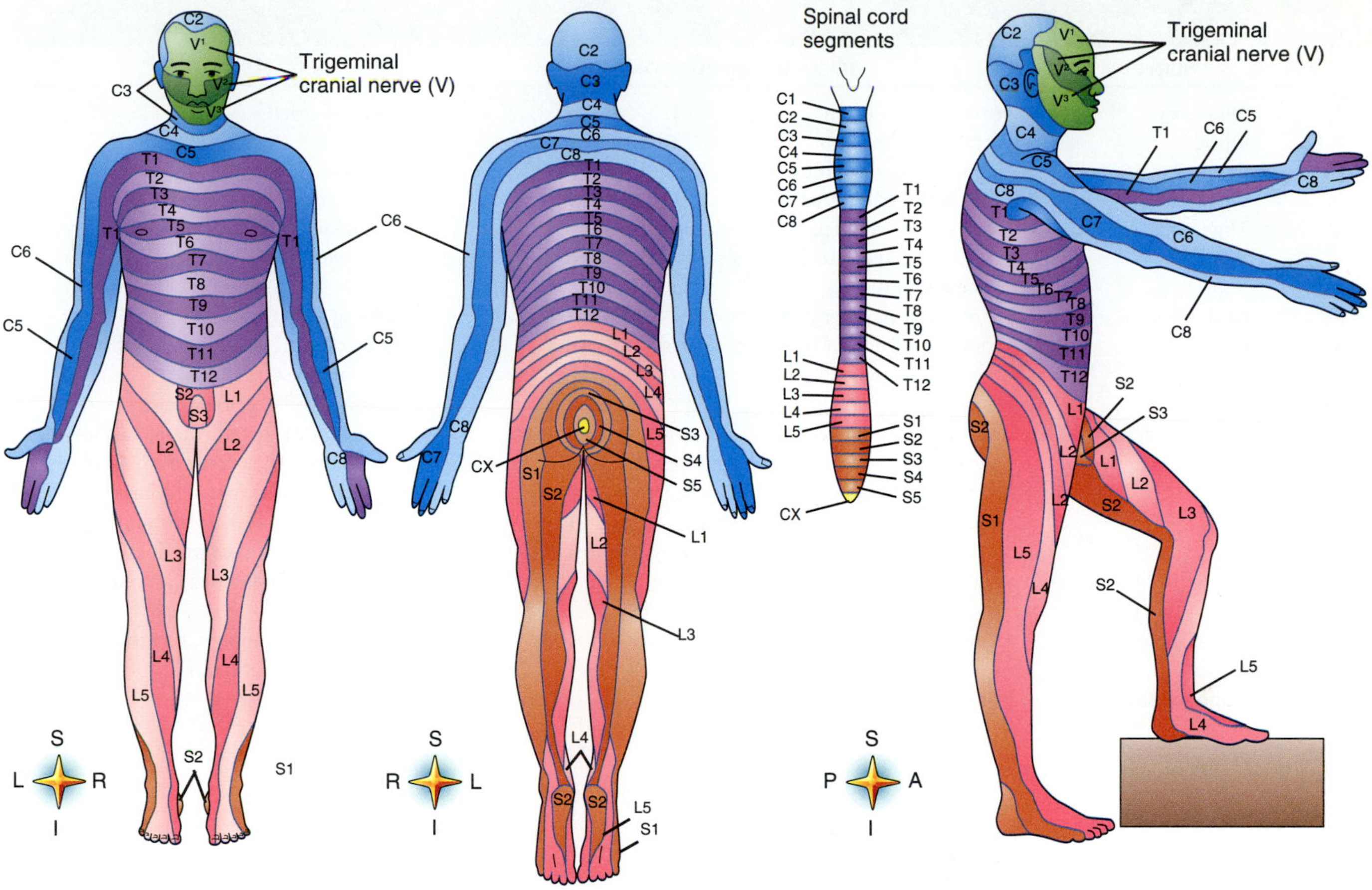

FIGURE 6-35 ■ Dermatome map. Letters and numbers indicate the spinal nerves innervating a given region of the skin.

vertebrae. The spinal nerves in the sacrum exit through the bone. Eight spinal nerve pairs exit the vertebral column in the cervical region, 12 in the thoracic region, 5 in the lumbar region, 5 in the sacral region, and 1 in the coccygeal region (Fig. 6-34).

Each spinal nerve except the first has a specific cutaneous sensory distribution. Detailed mapping of the skin surface reveals a close relationship between the source on the cord of each spinal nerve and the level of the body it innervates. (A grasp of this relationship is key when one examines a patient with a spinal cord injury.) The skin surface areas supplied by a single spinal nerve are known as dermatomes. (Figure 6-35 illustrates a dermatome map of the body.)

> **CRITICAL THINKING**
>
> Will the person with a spinal cord injury at the level of C5 have movement in the hands?

Cranial nerves. The 12 cranial nerves are divided into three general groups. These are sensory, somatomotor and proprioception, and parasympathetic. Sensory functions include the special senses, such as vision. They also include the more general senses, such as touch and pain. Somatomotor functions control the skeletal muscles through motor neurons. Proprioception provides the brain with information about the position of the body and its various parts, including joints and muscles. Parasympathetic function involves the regulation of glands, smooth muscle, and cardiac muscle (functions of the autonomic nervous system). Some cranial nerves have only one of the three functions. However, other cranial nerves have more than one function (Table 6-7). (Figure 6-36 illustrates the origin of cranial nerves.)

AUTONOMIC NERVOUS SYSTEM

As stated before, the PNS is made up of afferent and efferent neurons. Afferent neurons carry action potentials from the periphery to the CNS. Efferent neurons carry action potentials from the CNS to the periphery. Afferent neurons give information to the CNS. These data may stimulate somatomotor and autonomic reflexes. Thus afferent neurons cannot be put easily into groups by function. However, efferent neurons clearly differ structurally and functionally. They can be put into the somatomotor nervous system or the autonomic nervous system.

Somatomotor neurons innervate skeletal muscles. These neurons play a key role in locomotion, posture, and equilibrium. The movements controlled by the somatomotor nervous system usually are conscious movements. The effect of these neurons on skeletal muscle is always excitatory. Neurons of the autonomic nervous system innervate smooth muscle, cardiac muscle, and glands. These neurons

TABLE 6-7 Cranial Nerves

	NERVE	IMPULSE CONDUCTION	FUNCTIONS
I	Olfactory	From nose to brain	Sense of smell
II	Optic	From eye to brain	Vision
III	Oculomotor	From brain to eye muscles	Eye movements
IV	Trochlear	From brain to external eye muscles	Eye movements
V	Trigeminal	From skin and mucous membranes of head and from teeth to brain; also from brain to chewing muscles	Sensations of face, scalp, and teeth; chewing movements
VI	Abducens	From brain to external eye muscles	Turning eyes outward
VII	Facial	From taste buds of tongue to brain; from brain to face muscles	Sense of taste; contraction of muscles of facial expressions
VIII	Acoustic	From ear to brain	Hearing; sense of balance
IX	Glossopharyngeal	From throat and taste buds of tongue to brain; also from brain to throat muscles and salivary glands	Sensation of throat, taste, swallowing movements; secretion of saliva
X	Vagus	From throat, larynx, and organs in thoracic and abdominal cavities to brain; also from brain to muscles of throat and to organs in thoracic and abdominal cavities	Sensations of throat and larynx and of thoracic and abdominal organs; swallowing, voice production, slowing of heartbeat, acceleration of peristalsis
XI	Spinal accessory	From brain to certain shoulder and neck muscles	Shoulder movements, turning movements of head
XII	Hypoglossal	From brain to muscles of tongue	Tongue movements

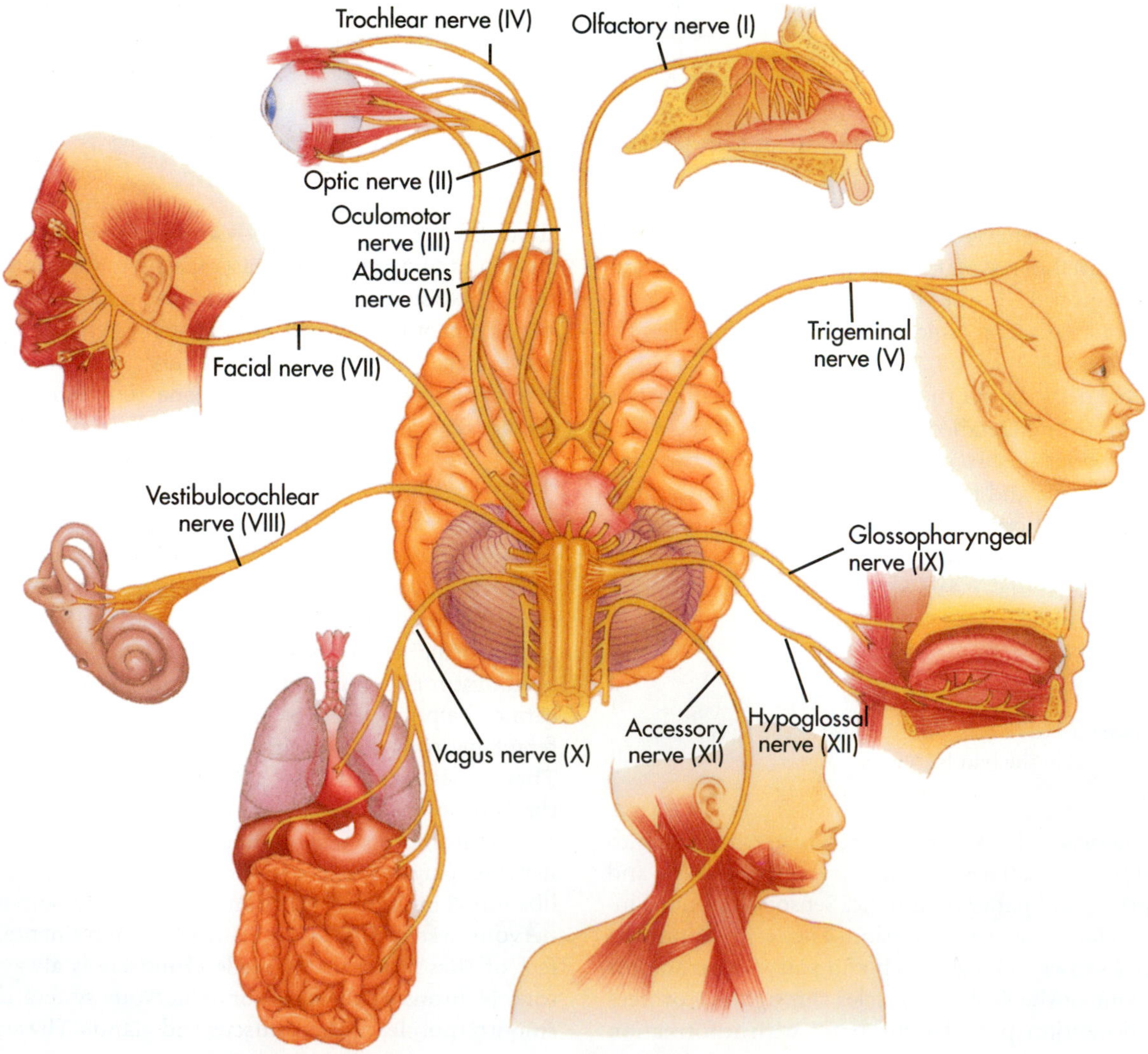

FIGURE 6-36 ■ Origin of cranial nerves.

TABLE 6-8 Functions of the Autonomic Nervous System

VISCERAL EFFECTORS	SYMPATHETIC CONTROL	PARASYMPATHETIC CONTROL
Heart Muscle	Accelerates heartbeat	Slows heartbeat
Smooth Muscle		
Of most blood vessels	Constricts blood vessels	None
Of blood vessels in skeletal muscles	Dilates blood vessels	None
Of the digestive tract	Decreases peristalsis; inhibits defecation	Increases peristalsis
Of the anal sphincter	Stimulates—closes sphincter	Inhibits—opens sphincter for defecation
Of the urinary bladder	Inhibits—relaxes bladder	Stimulates—contracts bladder
Of the urinary sphincters	Stimulates—closes sphincter	Inhibits—opens sphincter for urination
Of the eye:		
Iris	Stimulates radial fibers—dilation of pupil	Stimulates circular fibers—constriction of pupil
Ciliary	Inhibits—accommodation for far vision (flattening of lens)	Stimulates—accommodation for near vision (bulging of lens)
Of hairs (pilomotor muscles)	Stimulates—goose bumps	No parasympathetic fibers
Glands		
Adrenal medulla	Increases epinephrine secretion	None
Sweat glands	Increase sweat secretion	None
Digestive glands	Decrease secretion of digestive juices	Increase secretion of digestive juices

usually are controlled unconsciously. The effect of autonomic neurons on their target tissue is inhibitory or excitatory.

The autonomic nervous system is made up of two divisions: the sympathetic nervous system and **parasympathetic nervous system.** Both of these divisions in turn consist of autonomic ganglia and nerves. The action potentials in sympathetic neurons generally prepare a person for physical activity. Parasympathetic stimulation, however, activates vegetative functions such as digestion, defecation, and urination.

The functions of the autonomic nervous system help to maintain homeostasis. Or they quickly restore homeostasis (Table 6-8). Many internal organs receive fibers from parasympathetic and sympathetic divisions (Fig. 6-37). Thus sympathetic and parasympathetic impulses continually bombard them. These impulses influence the function of these organs in opposite or antagonistic ways. For example, the heart receives sympathetic impulses that increase the heart rate. The heart also receives parasympathetic impulses that decrease the heart rate. The ratio between these two forces determines the actual heart rate.

CRITICAL THINKING

You administer a drug that blocks the action of the parasympathetic nervous system. What would happen to the patient's heart rate?

Endocrine System

The endocrine system is made up of glands. These glands secrete hormones into the circulatory system (Fig. 6-38). The endocrine and nervous systems have a large amount of overlap. The overlap is functional and anatomical. Some neurons secrete regulatory chemicals (neurohormones) that function as hormones, such as antidiuretic hormone, into the circulatory system. Other neurons innervate endocrine glands and influence their secretory activity. However, some hormones secreted by the endocrine glands affect the nervous system.

Hormones, including neurohormones, are classified as proteins, polypeptides, derivatives of amino acids, or lipids. Lipid hormones are steroids or derivatives of fatty acids. Hormones are dissolved in blood plasma. Hormones are distributed quickly throughout the body. In general, the amount of hormone that reaches the target tissue directly correlates with the concentration of the hormone in the blood. (Table 6-9 lists endocrine glands, hormones, and their functions.)

Some hormones are present in fairly constant levels in the circulatory system. Amounts of other hormones change suddenly in response to certain stimuli. Still others change in fairly constant cycles. For example, thyroid hormones in the blood vary within a small range of concentrations. Their concentration is maintained continuously. Epinephrine is released in large amounts in response to stress or exercise. The concentration of epinephrine changes greatly. Reproductive hormones increase and decrease cyclically in women during their reproductive years.

Circulatory System

Blood vessels extend throughout the body. These vessels carry blood to and from all tissues. Blood transports nutrients and oxygen to tissues. Blood also carries carbon dioxide and waste products away from tissues. In addition, blood carries hormones produced in the endocrine

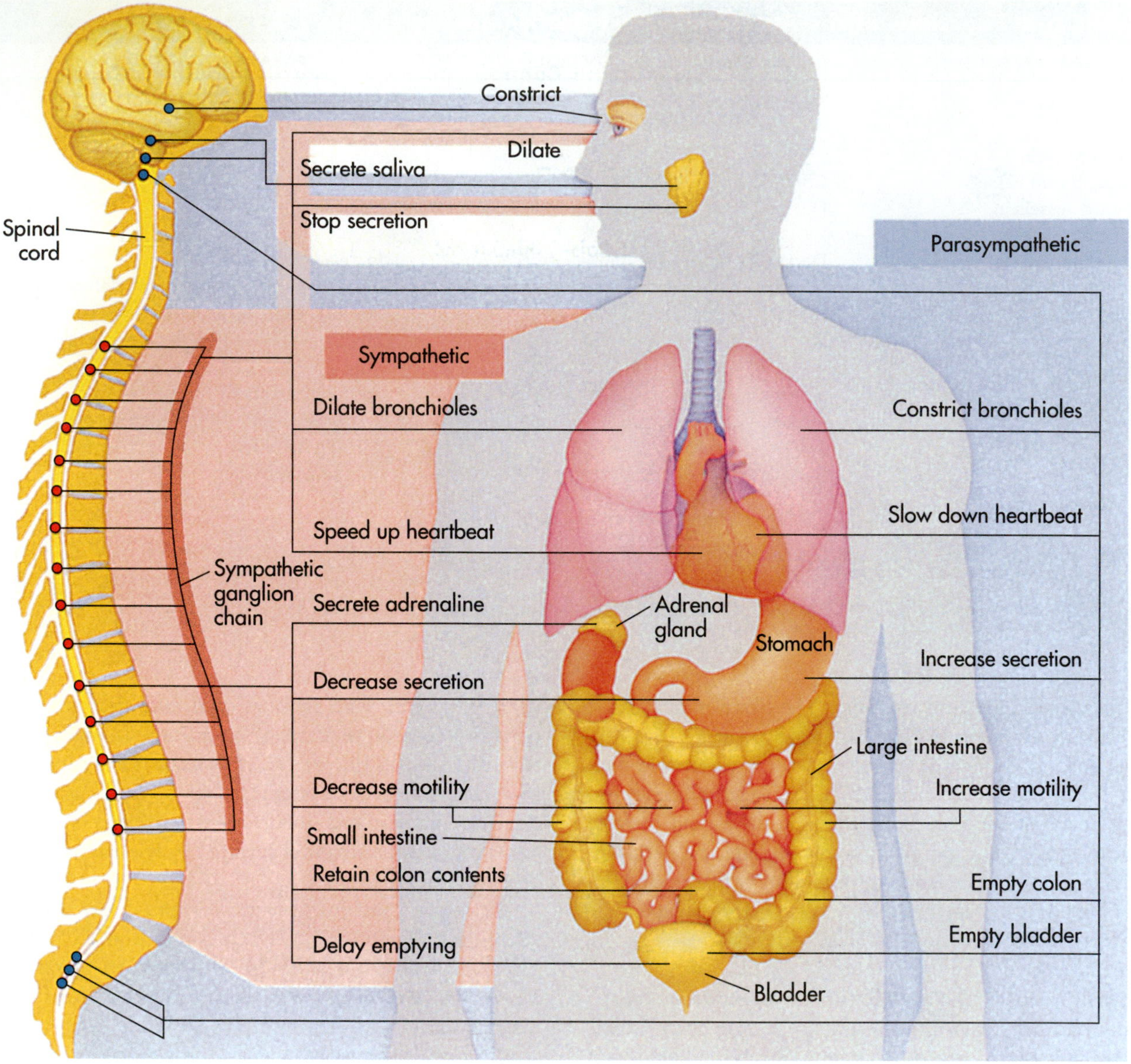

FIGURE 6-37 ■ Innervation of major target organs by the autonomic nervous system. The sympathetic fibers are highlighted with red, and the parasympathetic are highlighted with blue.

glands to their target tissues. Moreover, blood plays a key role in temperature regulation and fluid balance. Blood also protects the body from bacteria and foreign substances. These and other functions of blood help to maintain homeostasis.

BLOOD COMPONENTS

Blood is a special form of connective tissue. Blood consists of cells and cell fragments (formed elements) surrounded by a liquid intercellular matrix (plasma). About 95% of the volume of formed elements consists of red blood cells (erythrocytes). The remaining 5% consists of white blood cells (leukocytes) and cell fragments called platelets.

Plasma. Plasma is a pale yellow fluid composed of about 92% water and 8% dissolved or suspended molecules. Plasma contains proteins such as albumin, globulins, and fibrinogen. When the proteins that produce clots are removed from the plasma, the remaining fluid is called serum.

Formed elements. Three formed elements of blood are erythrocytes, leukocytes, and platelets or thrombocytes (cell fragments) (Table 6-10). Formed elements are produced in the embryo and fetus. They are also produced in tissues such as the liver, thymus, spleen, lymph nodes, and red bone marrow.

1. Erythrocytes are the most numerous of the formed elements. About 5.2 million erythrocytes are in one drop of male blood. About 4.5 million erythrocytes are in one drop of female blood. The major erythrocyte contents include lipids, ATP, and the enzyme carbonic anhydrase. The main component of erythrocytes is hemoglobin.

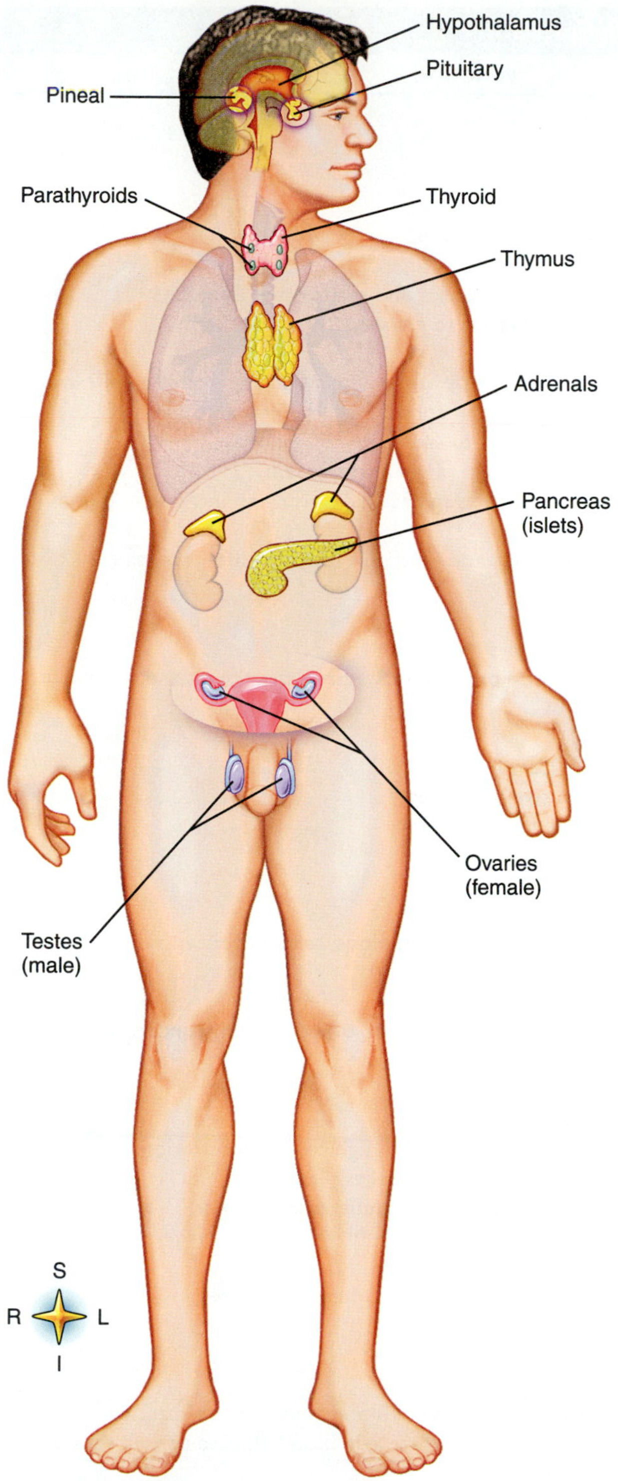

FIGURE 6-38 ■ Locations of major endocrine glands.

This is the protein that gives blood its red color. The primary functions of erythrocytes are to transport oxygen from the lungs to the various tissues of the body and to transport carbon dioxide from the tissues to the lungs. Under normal conditions, about 2.5 million erythrocytes are destroyed and replaced by the body each second. The average erythrocyte circulates for 120 days.

> **CRITICAL THINKING**
> If the number of erythrocytes drops, a person may become short of breath during mild exertion. Why will this happen?

2. Leukocytes are white blood cells that do not contain hemoglobin (thus they are clear). The several types of leukocytes are involved in guarding the body against invading microorganisms. They also remove dead cells and debris. Some leukocytes are grouped by their appearance. This is based on the presence or absence of cytoplasmic granules. The classifications include neutrophils, eosinophils, and basophils. Other types of leukocytes are nongranular. These leukocytes are named according to nuclear morphology and major site of proliferation. These include lymphocytes and monocytes.

   Neutrophils are the most common type of leukocyte in the blood. These cells normally remain in the circulation for 10 to 12 hours. Then they move into tissue to seek out and destroy bacteria and other foreign matter (phagocytosis). Neutrophils also secrete lysosomes that can destroy certain bacteria. Neutrophils usually survive for 1 to 2 days after leaving the circulation.

   Eosinophils leave the circulation to enter the tissues during an inflammatory reaction. Their numbers usually are elevated in the blood of persons who have allergies and certain parasitic infections. These cells have phagocytic properties. However, they are not thought to be as important in this function as neutrophils.

   Basophils are the least common of all leukocytes. They also are called mast cells when in tissues. Like eosinophils, basophils leave the circulation and migrate through tissues to play a role in allergic and inflammatory reactions. They also release heparin, which inhibits blood clotting. In addition, they release histamine, which is important to the inflammatory response.

   Lymphocytes are the smallest of all leukocytes. They are capable of migrating through the cytoplasm of other cells. The many different types of lymphocytes play a major role in immunity, including antibody production. Lymphocytes originate in bone marrow. They are most abundant in lymphoid tissues: the lymph nodes, spleen, tonsils, lymph nodules, and thymus.

   Monocytes are the largest of the leukocytes. They remain in the circulation for about 3 days before changing into macrophages. These large "eating" cells migrate through various tissues. An increase in the number of monocytes is common in patients with chronic infections.
3. Platelets are produced within bone marrow. They are 40 times as common in blood as leukocytes. Platelets play a key role in preventing blood loss by forming plugs that seal holes in small vessels and by forming clots that seal off larger wounds in the vessels.

TABLE 6-9 Endocrine Glands, Hormones, and Their Functions

GLAND/HORMONE	FUNCTION
Anterior Pituitary	
Thyroid-stimulating hormone	Tropic hormone Stimulates secretion of thyroid hormones
Adrenocorticotropic hormone	Tropic hormone Stimulates secretion of adrenal cortex hormones
Follicle-stimulating hormone	Tropic hormone Female: stimulates development of ovarian follicles and secretion of estrogens Male: stimulates seminiferous tubules of testes to grow and produce sperm
Luteinizing hormone	Tropic hormone Female: stimulates maturation of ovarian follicle and ovum; stimulates secretion of estrogen; triggers ovulation; stimulates development of corpus luteum (luteinization) Male: stimulates interstitial cells of the testes to secrete testosterone
Melanocyte-stimulating hormone	Stimulates synthesis and dispersion of melanin pigment in the skin
Growth hormone	Stimulates growth in all organs; mobilizes food molecules, causing an increase in blood glucose concentration
Prolactin (lactogenic hormone)	Stimulates breast development during pregnancy and milk secretion after pregnancy
Posterior Pituitary*	
Antidiuretic hormone	Stimulates retention of water by the kidneys
Oxytocin	Stimulates uterine contractions at the end of pregnancy; stimulates the release of milk into the breast ducts
Hypothalamus	
Releasing hormones (several)	Stimulate the anterior pituitary to release hormones
Inhibiting hormones (several)	Inhibit secretion of hormones by the anterior pituitary
Thyroid	
Thyroxine, triiodothyronine	Stimulate the energy metabolism of all cells
Calcitonin	Inhibits the breakdown of bone; causes a decrease in blood calcium concentration
Parathyroid	
Parathyroid hormone	Stimulates the breakdown of bone; causes an increase in blood calcium concentration
Adrenal Cortex	
Mineralocorticoids: aldosterone	Regulate electrolyte and fluid homeostasis
Glucocorticoids: cortisol (hydrocortisone)	Stimulate gluconeogenesis, causing an increase in blood glucose concentration; also have antiinflammatory, antiimmunity, and antiallergy effects
Sex hormones (androgens)	Stimulate sexual drive in the female but have negligible effects in the male
Adrenal Medulla	
Epinephrine (adrenaline), norepinephrine	Prolong and intensify the sympathetic nervous response during stress
Pancreatic Islets	
Glucagon	Stimulates liver glycogenolysis, causing an increase in blood glucose concentration
Insulin	Promotes glucose entry into all cells, causing a decrease in blood glucose concentration
Ovary	
Estrogens	Promotes development and maintenance of female sexual characteristics
Progesterone	Promotes conditions required for pregnancy
Testis	
Testosterone	Promotes development and maintenance of male sexual characteristics
Thymus	
Thymosin	Promotes development of immune-system cells

TABLE 6-9 Endocrine Glands, Hormones, and Their Functions—cont'd

GLAND/HORMONE	FUNCTION
Placenta	
Chorionic gonadotropin, estrogens, progesterone	Promote conditions required during early pregnancy
Pineal	
Melatonin	Inhibits tropic hormones that affect the ovaries; may be involved with the internal clock of the body
Heart (Atria)	
Atrial natriuretic hormone	Regulates fluid and electrolyte homeostasis

*Posterior pituitary hormones are synthesized in the hypothalamus but are released from axon terminals in the posterior pituitary.

TABLE 6-10 Classes of Blood Cells

BLOOD CELL	FUNCTION
Erythrocyte 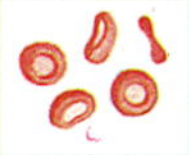	Oxygen and carbon dioxide transport
Neutrophil 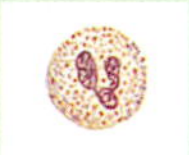	Immune defenses (phagocytosis)
Eosinophil 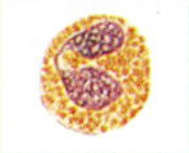	Defense against parasites
Basophil 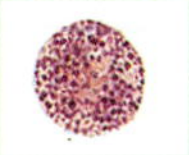	Inflammatory response
B lymphocyte 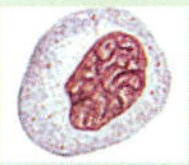	Antibody production (precursor of plasma cells)
T lymphocyte 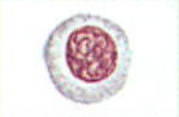	Cellular immune response
Monocyte 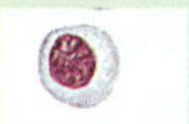	Immune defenses (phagocytosis)
Platelet 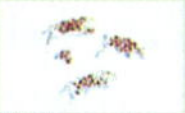	Blood clotting

CARDIOVASCULAR SYSTEM

The heart and cardiovascular system are responsible for circulating blood throughout the body. (The cardiovascular system is discussed more thoroughly in Chapters 21.)

Anatomy of the heart. The heart is a muscular pump consisting of four chambers: two atria and two ventricles. The adult heart is shaped like a blunt cone and is about the size of a closed fist. The heart is located in the mediastinum of the thoracic cavity in the pericardial cavity. The blunt, rounded point of the heart is the *apex,* and the larger, flat portion at the opposite end is the *base.*

The heart lies obliquely in the mediastinum. The base is directed posteriorly and slightly superiorly. The apex is directed anteriorly and slightly inferiorly. Two thirds of the mass of the heart lies to the left of the midline of the sternum (Figs. 6-39 and 6-40).

Pericardium. The pericardium is also known as the pericardial sac. The pericardium has a fibrous outer layer and a thin inner layer that surrounds the heart. These layers are the fibrous pericardium and the serous pericardium, respectively. The portion of the serous pericardium that lines the fibrous pericardium is the parietal pericardium. The portion that covers the heart surface is the visceral pericardium or the epicardium. The cavity between the parietal pericardium and the visceral pericardium normally contains a small amount of pericardial fluid. This fluid reduces friction as the heart moves within the pericardial sac.

> **CRITICAL THINKING**
>
> Why would a sudden increase in the amount of pericardial fluid be harmful?

Coronary vessels. Seven large veins normally carry blood to the heart: four pulmonary veins carry blood from the lungs to the left atrium, the superior and inferior venae cavae carry blood from the body to the right atrium, and the coronary sinus carries blood from the walls of the heart to the right atrium. Two arteries, the aorta and pulmonary

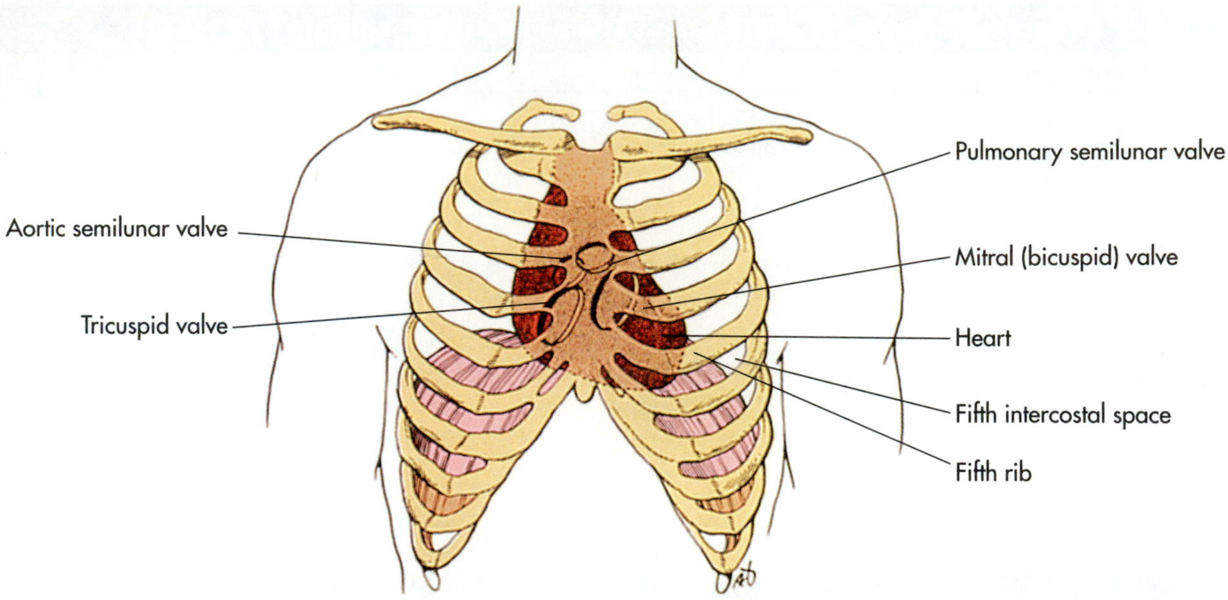

FIGURE 6-39 ■ Location of the heart in the thorax.

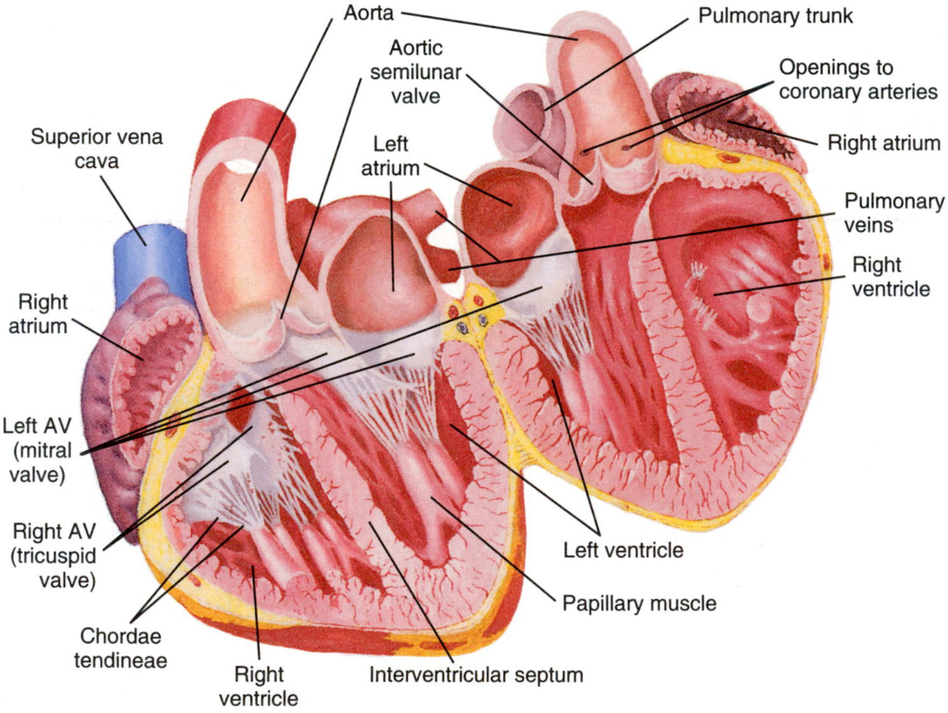

FIGURE 6-40 ■ Internal view of the heart.

trunk, exit the heart. The aorta carries blood from the left ventricle to the body. The pulmonary trunk carries blood from the right ventricle to the lungs. The right and left coronary arteries exit the aorta near the point where the aorta leaves the heart. They supply the heart muscle with oxygen and nutrients (Fig. 6-41).

Heart chambers and valves. The right and left chambers of the heart are separated by a septum. The *interatrial septum* separates the right and left atria. The *interventricular septum* separates the two ventricles. The atria open into the ventricles through the *atrioventricular canals.* An atrioventricular valve on each atrioventricular canal is composed of cusps or flaps. These valves allow blood to flow from the atria into the ventricles. Yet they prevent blood from flowing back into the atria. The atrioventricular valve between the right atrium and right ventricle has three cusps; it is called the tricuspid valve. The atrioventricular valve between the left atrium and left ventricle has two cusps and is called the bicuspid, or mitral, valve.

The aorta and pulmonary trunk possess aortic and pulmonary semilunar valves. These valves meet in the center of the artery to block blood flow. Blood flowing out of the

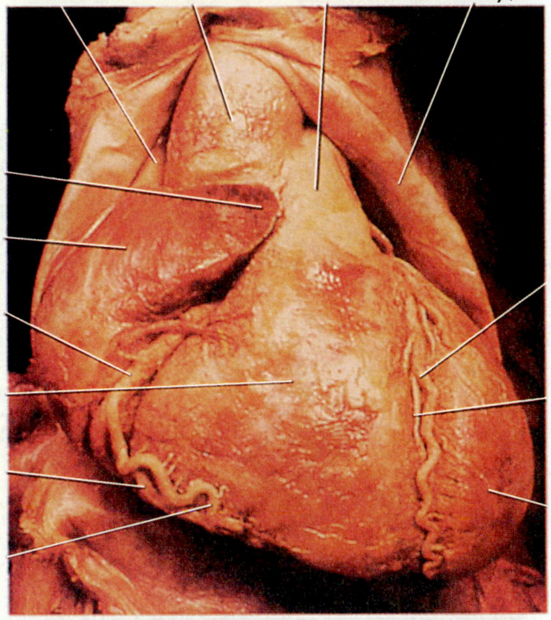

FIGURE 6-41 ■ Anterior surface of the heart.

ventricles pushes against each valve, forcing it open. However, when blood flows back from the aorta or pulmonary trunk toward the ventricles, the valves close.

Conduction system of the heart. The muscle tissue of the heart has the unique ability for spontaneous, rhythmic self-excitation. This excitation occurs by way of four structures embedded in the wall of the heart. These structures are the sinoatrial node, the atrioventricular node, the bundle of His, and the Purkinje fibers (Fig. 6-42).

An impulse conduction normally begins in the sinoatrial node. From there the impulse spreads in all directions through both of the atria, causing an atrial contraction. As the electrical impulses reach the atrioventricular node, they are relayed to the ventricles through the bundle of His and the Purkinje fibers. This impulse conduction causes both of the ventricles to contract shortly after the atrial contraction.

Route of blood flow through the heart. This text presents blood flow through the heart with a look at circulation of the right and left sides of the heart (Fig. 6-43). A key is to recall that both atria contract at the same time. This contraction is followed shortly thereafter by essentially simultaneous contraction of both ventricles. Knowing this is key to understanding clearly the electrical impulses of the heart, pressure changes, and heart sounds that are discussed in other chapters.

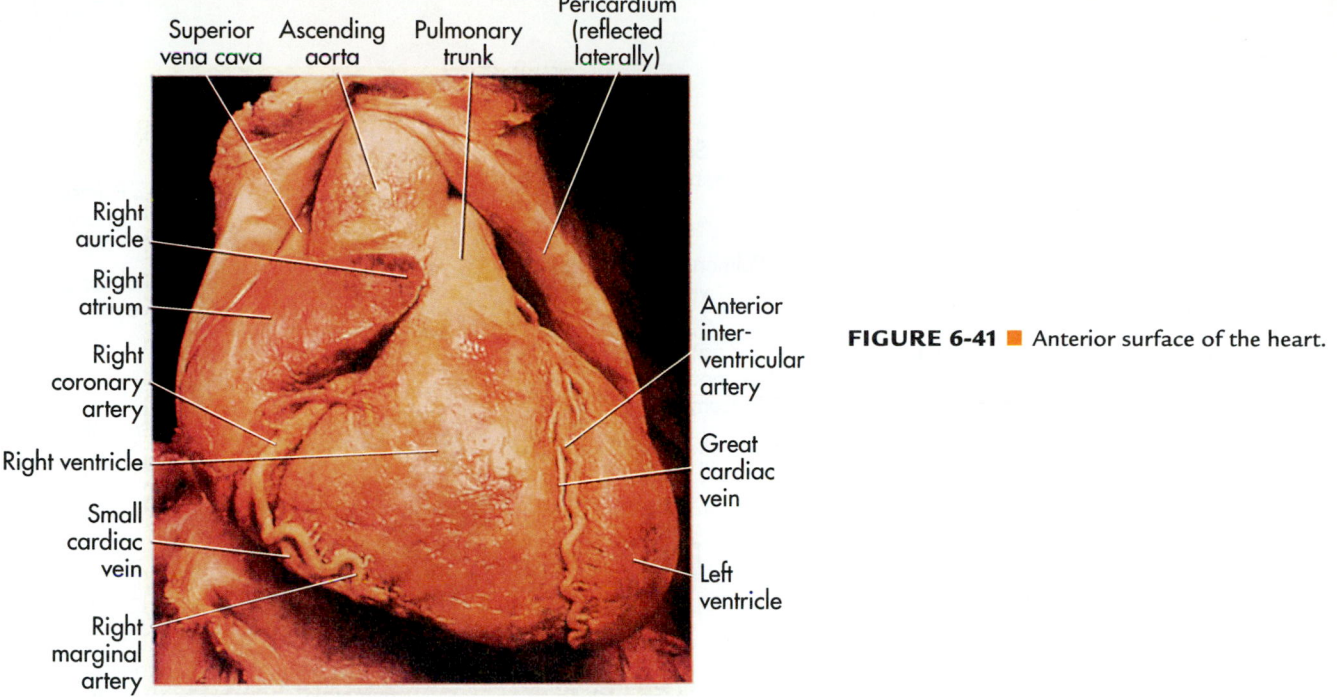

Blood enters the right atrium from the systemic circulation via the inferior and superior venae cavae. Blood enters from the heart via the coronary sinus. Most of this blood passes into the right ventricle as the ventricle relaxes after the previous contraction. When the right atrium contracts, the blood left in the atrium is pushed into the ventricle. The contraction of the right ventricle pushes blood against the tricuspid valve, forcing it closed. The contraction also pushes blood against the pulmonary semilunar valve, forcing the valve open. This flow allows blood to enter the pulmonary trunk. The pulmonary trunk divides into left and right pulmonary arteries that carry blood to the lungs. In the lungs the blood releases carbon dioxide and picks up oxygen.

CRITICAL THINKING

A clot forms in the right atria of the heart. Will it be circulated to the extremities? Why?

Blood returning from the lungs enters the left atrium through four pulmonary veins. The blood passing from the left atrium to the relaxed left ventricle opens the bicuspid valve. The contraction of the left atrium completes the filling of the left ventricle.

Contraction of the left ventricle pushes blood against the bicuspid valve, closing the valve. The pressure of the blood against the aortic semilunar valve causes it to open. This allows blood to enter the aorta. Blood flowing through the aorta is distributed to all parts of the body except for the pulmonary vessels in the lungs.

PERIPHERAL CIRCULATION

Blood is pumped from the ventricles of the heart into large elastic arteries. These arteries branch repeatedly to form many gradually smaller arteries. As these vessels become smaller, the amount of elastic tissue in the arterial wall decreases. At the same time, the amount of smooth muscle increases.

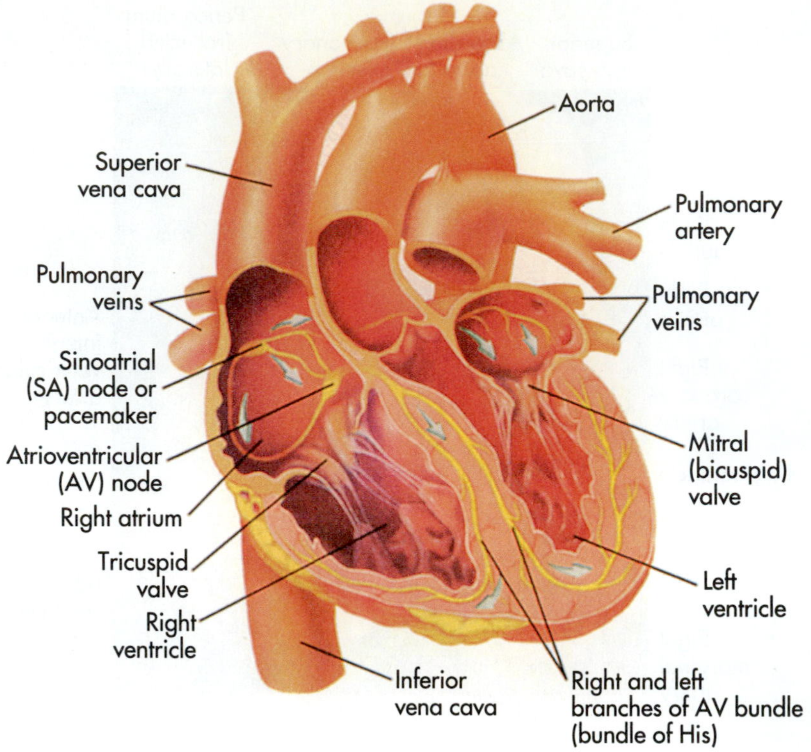

FIGURE 6-42 ■ Conduction system of the heart.

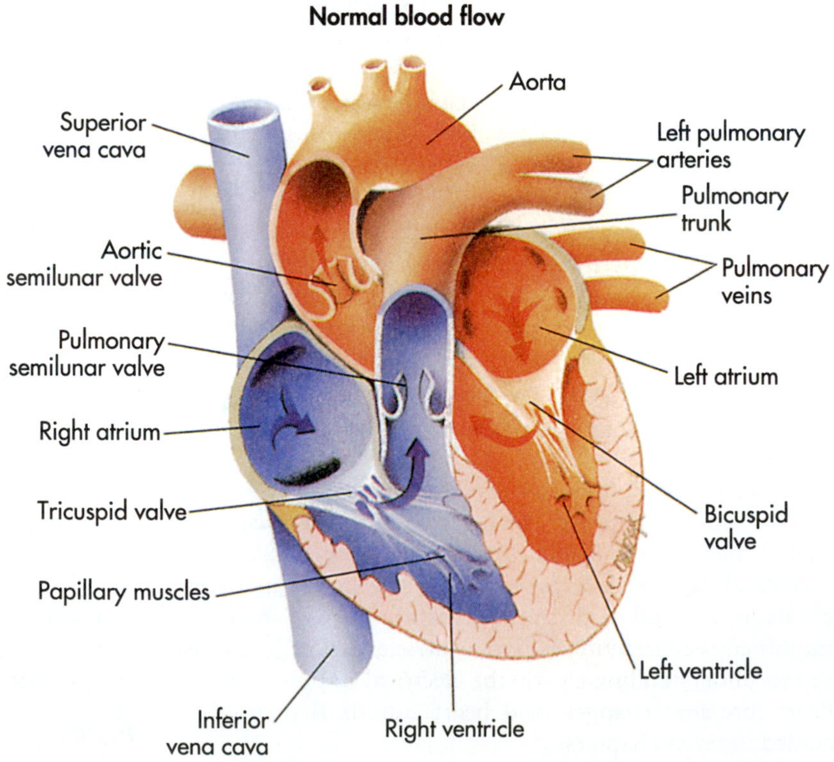

FIGURE 6-43 ■ Frontal section of the heart revealing the four chambers and direction of blood flow through the heart.

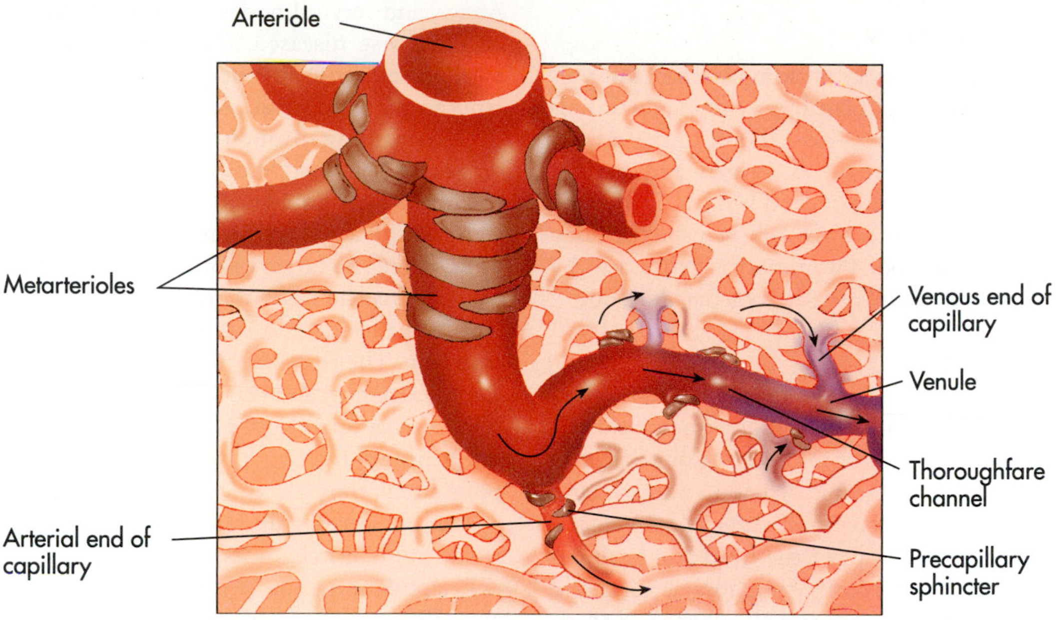

FIGURE 6-44 ■ Capillary network. The metarteriole, giving rise to the network, feeds directly from the arteriole into the thoroughfare channel, which feeds into the venule. The network forms numerous branches that transport blood from the thoroughfare channel and may return to the thoroughfare channel.

Blood flows from the arterioles into **capillaries** and from capillaries into the venous system. Compared with artery walls, vein walls are thinner and contain less elastic tissue and fewer smooth muscle cells. As veins approach the heart, the walls increase in diameter and thickness.

Capillary network. Arterioles supply blood to each capillary network (Fig. 6-44). Blood flows through this network and into the venules. The ends of the capillaries closest to arterioles are arterial capillaries. The ends closest to venules are venous capillaries.

Blood flow through arterioles may continue through metarterioles and into a thoroughfare channel to a venule in a relatively constant way. Or blood may enter the capillary circulation. Flow in the capillaries is regulated by smooth muscle cells. These cells are known as precapillary sphincters. Nutrient and product waste exchange is the major role of capillaries.

Arteries and veins. Blood vessel walls are made up of three layers of elastic tissue and smooth muscle. (Capillaries and venules are the exception.) These layers also are known as tunics. The layers are the tunica intima (inner layer), the tunica media (middle layer), and the tunica adventitia (outer layer). The thickness and composition of each layer vary with the type and diameter of the blood vessel.

Large elastic arteries often are called *conducting arteries* because they are the arteries that are largest in diameter. These vessels have more elastic tissue and less smooth muscle than any other arteries. Medium and small arteries have fairly thick muscular walls. These arteries also have elastic membranes that are well developed. These vessels are called *distributing arteries* because the smooth muscle allows these vessels partially to regulate blood supply to various body regions. The vessels do this by constriction or dilation. Arterioles are the smallest arteries in which the three tunics can be detected. Like small arteries, arterioles are capable of vasodilation and vasoconstriction.

Venules have only a few isolated smooth muscle cells and are similar in structure to the capillaries. Venules collect blood from the capillaries and transport it to small veins. These veins in turn transport the blood to the medium-sized veins. Nutrient exchange occurs across the walls of the venules, but as the small veins increase in thickness, the degree of nutrient exchange decreases.

As venules increase in diameter, the vessels become veins with walls that are a continuous layer of smooth muscle cells. Medium-sized and large veins collect blood from small veins and deliver it to the large venous trunks. Large veins transport blood from the medium-sized veins to the heart.

Veins with large diameters have valves that allow blood to flow to but not from the heart. Medium-sized veins have many valves, and more valves are present in the veins of the lower extremities than of the upper extremities. These valves help prevent the backflow of blood, especially in dependent tissues.

Arteriovenous anastomoses allow blood to flow from arteries to veins without passing through capillaries. Natural arteriovenous shunts occur in large numbers in the sole of the foot, palm, and nail bed, where they regulate body temperature. Pathological shunts can result from injury or tumors. These shunts can cause a direct flow of blood from arteries to veins. Severe shunts may lead to "high output" heart failure from increased venous return to the heart and its resultant demand on cardiac output.

PULMONARY CIRCULATION

Blood from the right ventricle is pumped into the pulmonary trunk. This trunk splits into the right and left pulmonary arteries. These arteries move blood to the respective lungs. After the exchange of oxygen and carbon dioxide, two pulmonary veins exit each lung and enter the left atrium. Pulmonary veins are the only veins in the body that carry oxygenated blood. Pulmonary arteries are the only arteries in the body that carry deoxygenated blood.

SYSTEMIC CIRCULATION

Oxygenated blood enters the heart from the pulmonary veins. The blood passes through the left atrium into the left ventricle. Then the blood passes from the left ventricle into the aorta. From the aorta, blood is distributed to all parts of the body. The arteries of systemic circulation include the aorta, coronary arteries, arteries of the head and neck, arteries of the upper and lower limbs, the thoracic aorta and its branches, the abdominal aorta and its branches, and arteries of the pelvis (Fig. 6-45).

The veins of systemic circulation include coronary veins, veins of the head and neck, veins of the upper and lower limbs, veins of the thorax, veins of the abdomen and pelvis, and the hepatic portal system, which transports blood from the digestive tract to the liver (Fig. 6-46).

Lymphatic System

The lymphatic system is considered part of the circulatory system because it consists of a moving fluid that comes from the body and returns to the blood. Unlike the circulatory system, the lymphatic system only carries fluid away from the tissues.

The lymphatic system includes lymph, lymphocytes, lymph nodes, tonsils, spleen, and the thymus gland. The lymphatic system has three basic functions. The first role is to help maintain fluid balance in tissues. The second role is to absorb fats and other substances from the digestive tract. The third role is as part of the immune defense system of the body.

The lymphatic system begins in the tissues as lymph capillaries. These capillaries differ in structure from blood capillaries. Lymph capillaries have a series of one-way valves. These valves allow fluid to enter the capillary. However, the valves prevent fluid from passing back into the interstitial spaces. Lymph capillaries are in almost all tissues of the body, except the CNS, bone marrow, and tissues without blood vessels (e.g., cartilage, epidermis, and cornea). Lymph capillaries join to form larger lymph capillaries that resemble small veins.

Lymph nodes are distributed along various lymph vessels. Most lymph passes through at least one node before entering the blood. The node filters the lymph as it passes through the node. Filtering removes microorganisms and foreign substances to prevent them from entering the general circulation. Three major collections of lymph nodes are located on each side of the body: inguinal nodes, axillary nodes, and cervical nodes. If a part of the body is inflamed or otherwise diseased, the nearby lymph nodes become swollen and tender as they limit the spread of microorganisms and foreign substances.

After passing through lymph nodes, lymph vessels converge toward the right or left subclavian vein. Vessels from the upper right limb and the right side of the head enter the right lymphatic duct. Lymph vessels from the rest of the body enter the larger thoracic duct. The right lymphatic duct drains the right thorax, right upper limb, and right side of the head and neck and opens into the right subclavian vein. The thoracic duct drains the left thorax, the left upper extremity, and the left side of the head and neck. The duct ends by entering the left subclavian vein. Thus all fluid drained from the tissue spaces eventually returns to the venous circulation.

Lymph serves a unique transport role. Lymph returns tissue fluid, proteins, fats, and other substances to the general circulation. The lymphatic system does not form a closed ring or circuit like the true circulatory system. Once lymph is formed, it flows only once through its system of lymphatic vessels before draining into the right and left subclavian veins.

CRITICAL THINKING

A woman has had a radical mastectomy (removal of breast and lymph tissue). Why might she have a chronically swollen arm?

Respiratory System

Oxygen is a basic element needed for normal cell metabolism. Carbon dioxide is a major waste product of this process. The organs of the respiratory system and the cardiovascular system transport oxygen to individual cells. These organs then transport carbon dioxide from the cells to the lungs. In the lungs the carbon dioxide is released into the air.

The respiratory system is a complex part of the human body. The aim of this section is to familiarize the reader with respiratory anatomy. (Further discussion of the respiratory system is presented in Chapter 19.)

AIRWAY ANATOMY

The structures of the respiratory system are divided into upper airway and lower airway. They are divided by their locations relative to the glottic opening. (This is the vocal cords and the space between them.) For the purpose of this text, all airway structures located above the glottis are considered to be upper airway. All structures located below the glottis are considered to be lower airway (Fig. 6-47).

UPPER AIRWAY STRUCTURES

The entrance to the respiratory tract begins with the nasal cavity. This cavity includes the nasopharynx, oropharynx, laryngopharynx, and larynx.

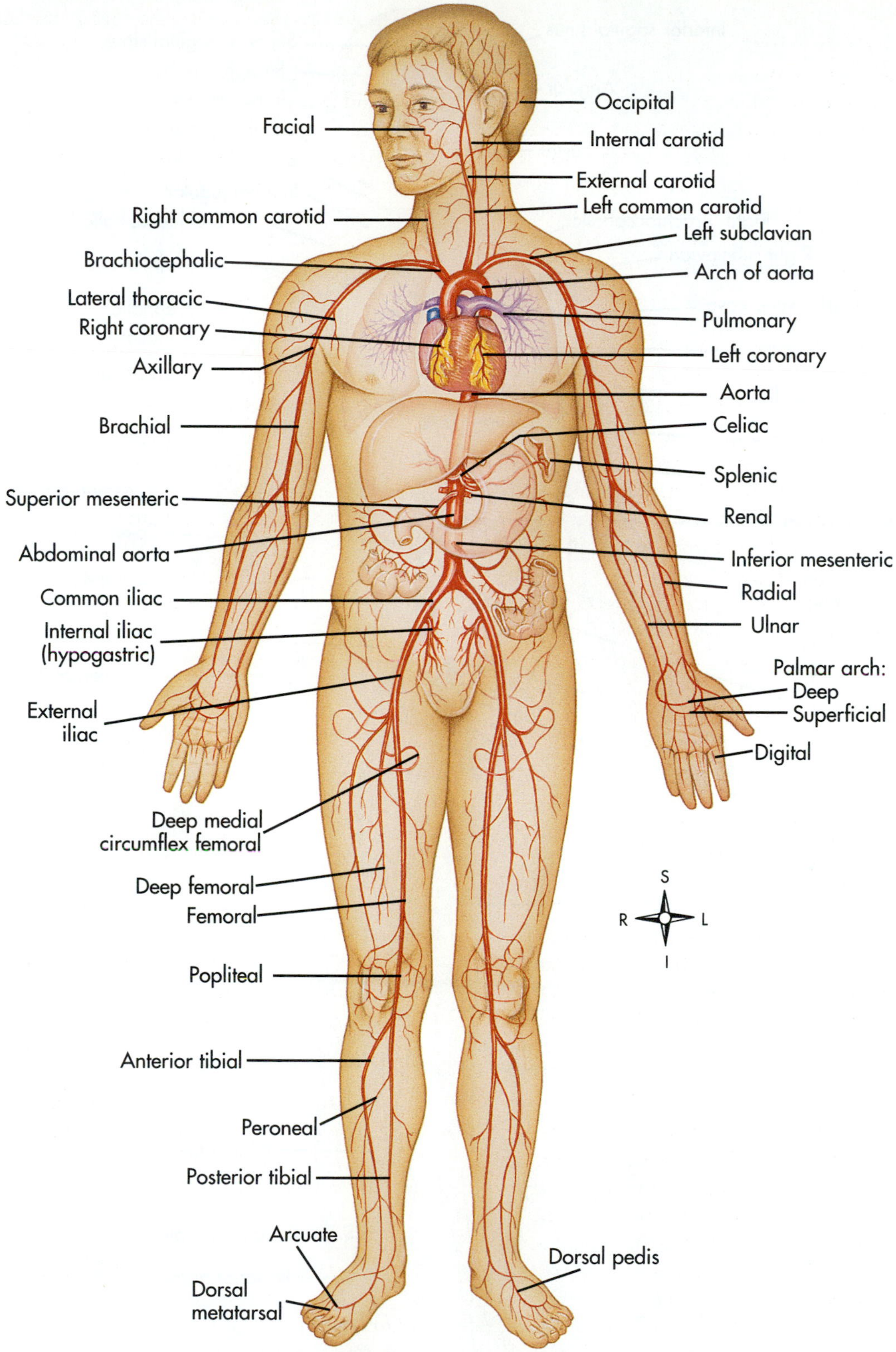
Occipital
Facial
Internal carotid
External carotid
Right common carotid
Left common carotid
Left subclavian
Brachiocephalic
Arch of aorta
Lateral thoracic
Right coronary
Pulmonary
Left coronary
Axillary
Aorta
Brachial
Celiac
Splenic
Superior mesenteric
Renal
Abdominal aorta
Inferior mesenteric
Radial
Common iliac
Ulnar
Internal iliac
(hypogastric)
Palmar arch:
Deep
Superficial
External
iliac
Digital
Deep medial
circumflex femoral
S
R
L
I
Deep femoral
Femoral
Popliteal
Anterior tibial
Peroneal
Posterior tibial
Arcuate
Dorsal pedis
Dorsal
metatarsal

FIGURE 6-45 ■ Principal arteries of the body.

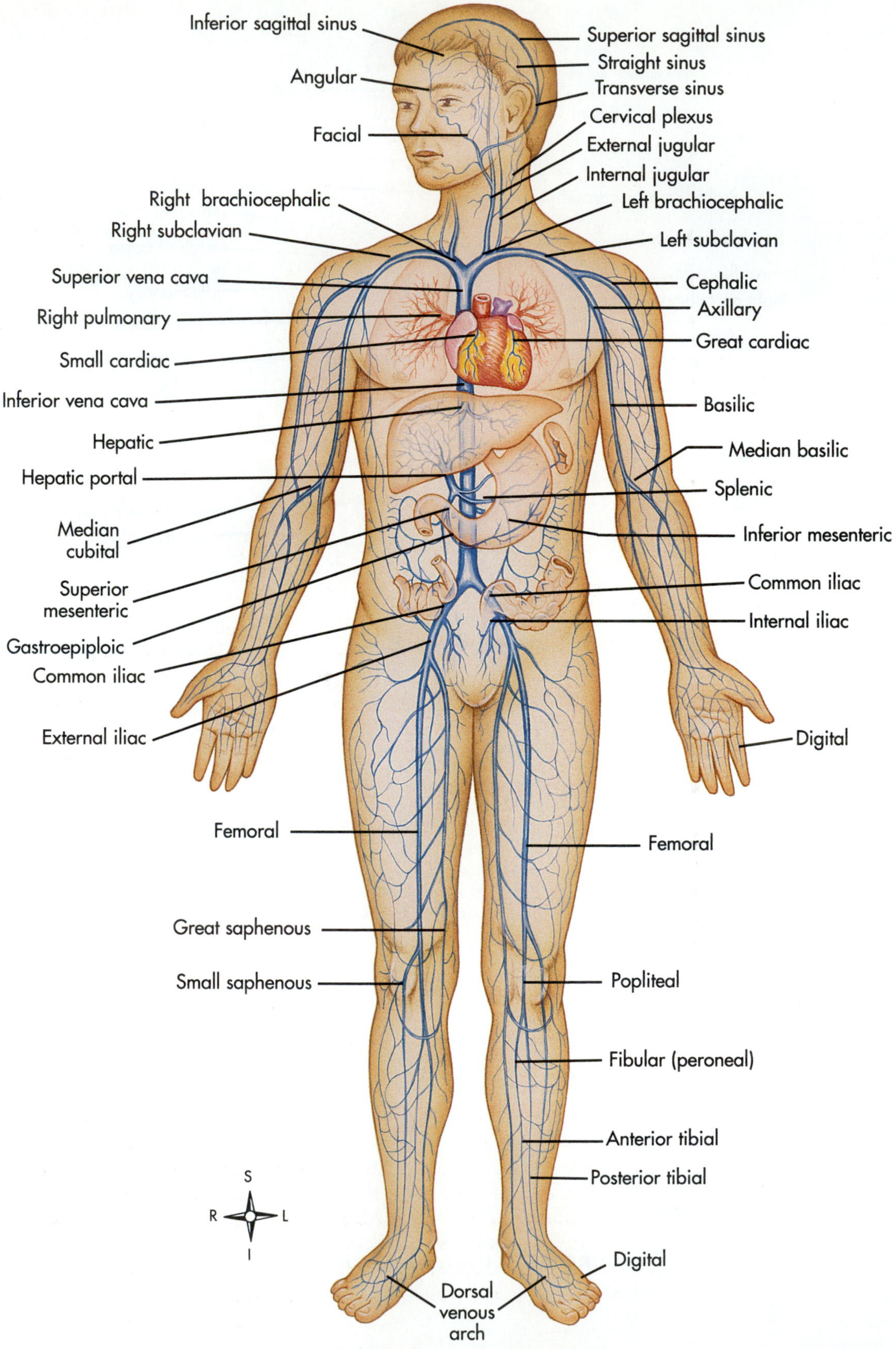
Inferior sagittal sinus
Angular
Facial
Right brachiocephalic
Right subclavian
Superior vena cava
Right pulmonary
Small cardiac
Inferior vena cava
Hepatic
Hepatic portal
Median cubital
Superior mesenteric
Gastroepiploic
Common iliac
External iliac
Femoral
Great saphenous
Small saphenous
Superior sagittal sinus
Straight sinus
Transverse sinus
Cervical plexus
External jugular
Internal jugular
Left brachiocephalic
Left subclavian
Cephalic
Axillary
Great cardiac
Basilic
Median basilic
Splenic
Inferior mesenteric
Common iliac
Internal iliac
Digital
Femoral
Popliteal
Fibular (peroneal)
Anterior tibial
Posterior tibial
Digital
Dorsal venous arch
S
R
L
I

FIGURE 6-46 ■ Principal veins of the body.

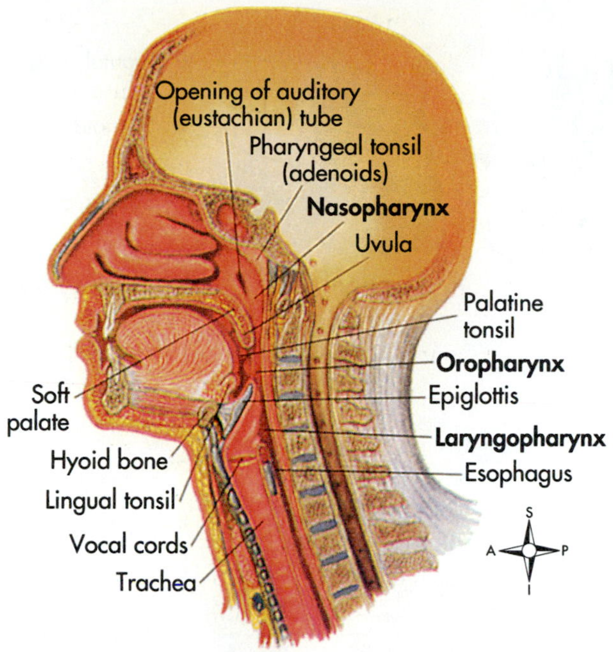

FIGURE 6-47 ■ Airway structures.

Nasopharynx. Air passes into the nasal cavity through the nostrils or *nares.* The right and left nasal cavities are separated by the nasal septum, a bony partition covered with a mucous membrane. This membrane has a rich blood supply that warms and humidifies the nasal lining and the inspired air as it passes through the nose. Inside each nostril a slight enlargement known as the *vestibule* is lined with coarse hairs that trap foreign substances carried into the nasal cavity by inspired air. The floor of the nasal cavity is composed of the hard palate; the lateral walls are formed by bony ridges coated with respiratory mucosa. These ridges are known as *conchae,* or *turbinates.*

Two patches of yellow-gray tissue lie just beneath the bridge of the nose. These patches compose the olfactory membranes. Located in the roof of the nasal cavity, these membranes contain the receptors for the sense of smell. The nasal cavities also connect to the middle ear cavities through the auditory (or eustachian) tubes.

> **CRITICAL THINKING**
>
> Why might a chronic cocaine abuser have a higher risk of sinus infection?

Sinuses are cavities in the bones of the skull that connect to the nasal cavities by small channels (Fig. 6-48). Four groups of sinuses, each named for the skull bone in which it lies, are the frontal sinuses, above the eyebrows; maxillary sinuses (the largest sinuses), in the cheekbones; ethmoid sinuses, just behind the bridge of the nose; and sphenoid sinuses, in a bone that cradles the brain, slightly anterior to the pituitary gland. These hollow chambers are lined with mucous membranes that secrete mucus into the nasal cavities. These chambers are thought to aid in adding resonance to the voice and decreasing the weight of the skull.

The back of each nasal cavity opens into the nasopharynx. This is the superior part of the pharynx. The nasopharynx extends from the internal nares to the level of the uvula. Like the nasal cavity, the nasopharynx is lined with mucous membrane.

Oropharynx. At the level of the uvula, the nasopharynx ends and the oropharynx begins. The oropharynx extends down to the level of the epiglottis. Anteriorly, the oropharynx opens into the oral cavity. The oral cavity is made up of the lips, cheeks, teeth, tongue (which is attached to the mandible), hard and soft palates, and palatine tonsils. The palatine tonsils and the pharyngeal tonsils (located in the roof and posterior wall of the nasopharynx) form a partial ring of lymphoid tissue. This tissue surrounds the respiratory tract. This ring is completed by the lingual tonsils. The tonsils lie on the floor of the oropharyngeal passageway at the base of the tongue.

Laryngopharynx. The laryngopharynx extends from the tip of the epiglottis to the glottis and the esophagus. The laryngopharynx is lined with mucous membrane. The mucous membrane protects the internal surfaces from abrasion.

Larynx. The laryngopharynx opens into the larynx, which lies in the anterior neck (Fig. 6-49). The larynx serves three main functions. The larynx is the air passageway between the pharynx and the lungs. The larynx is a protective sphincter to prevent solids and liquids from passing into the respiratory tree. Lastly, the larynx is involved in producing speech.

The larynx consists of an outer casing of nine cartilages connected to each other by muscles and ligaments. Six of the nine cartilages are paired; three are unpaired. The largest, most superior of the cartilages is the unpaired thyroid cartilage, or Adam's apple. This prominence is hardly visible in children or adult females but is visible in males after puberty.

The most inferior cartilage of the larynx is the unpaired cricoid cartilage. This is the only complete cartilaginous ring in the larynx. This cartilage forms the base of the larynx on which all other cartilages rest. The third unpaired cartilage is the epiglottis.

The six paired cartilages are stacked in two pillars between the cricoid cartilage and the thyroid cartilage. The largest inferior cartilages are ladle shaped and are known as the *arytenoid cartilages.* The middle pair are horn shaped and are known as *corniculate cartilages.* The smallest, most superior cartilages are wedge shaped and are known as *cuneiform cartilages.*

The U-shaped hyoid bone is tucked beneath the mandible. As previously mentioned, the hyoid is the only bone of the human body that does not articulate with another bone. The hyoid bone helps to suspend the airway by anchoring the muscles (particularly those of the tongue) to the jaw. The fibrous membrane that joins the hyoid and the thyroid cartilage is called the *thyroid membrane.* The

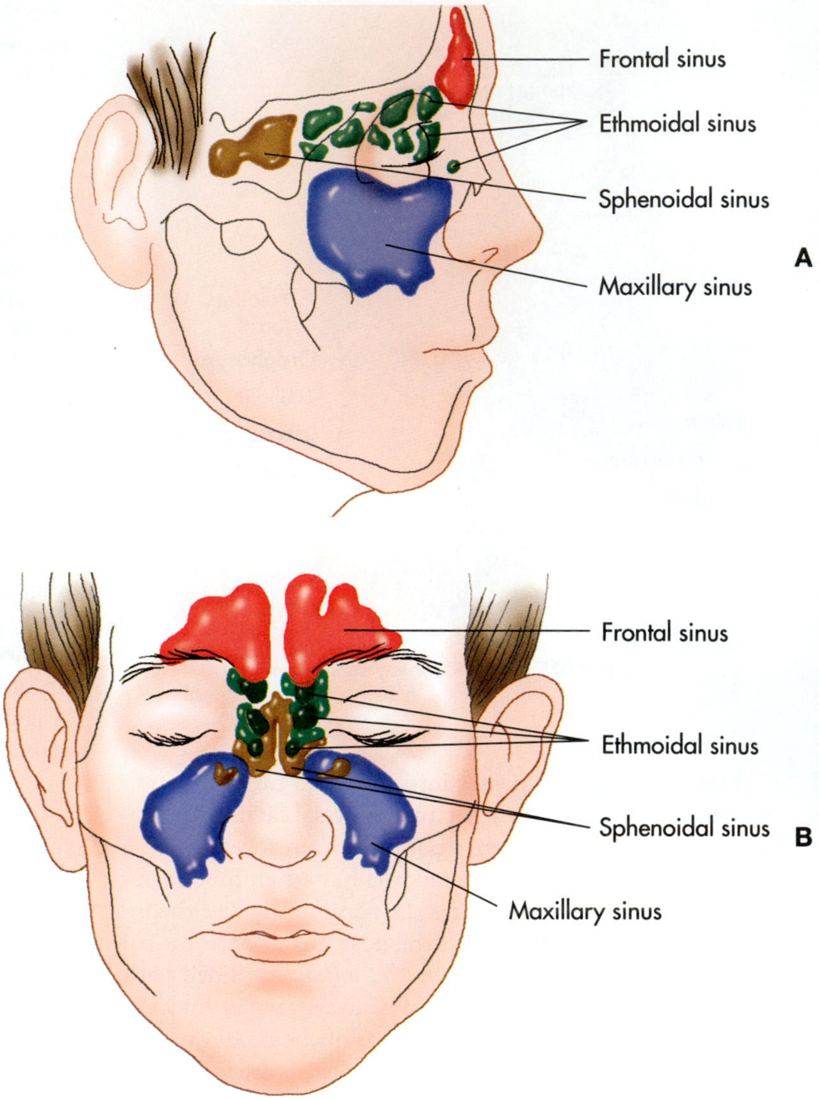

FIGURE 6-48 ■ Paranasal sinuses. Side **(A)** and front **(B)** views.

membrane joining the thyroid and cricoid cartilages is called the cricothyroid membrane.

Two pairs of ligaments extend from the anterior surface of the arytenoid to the posterior surface of the thyroid cartilage. The superior pair forms the vestibular folds, or false vocal cords, which are not involved directly in the production of voice sounds. The inferior pair of ligaments composes the vocal cords, or true vocal cords, which participate directly in producing voice sounds. In talking, air expelled from the lungs rushes up the throat to the larynx. In the larynx the air creates sound by vibrating the vocal cords. Muscles tighten the folds of the cords to produce the high-pitched tones and relax the cords to produce the deeper tones. The lip, tongue, and jaw further modify the sounds into intelligible words.

CRITICAL THINKING

Why can't a person talk when an endotracheal tube is correctly positioned in the trachea?

LOWER AIRWAY STRUCTURES

Below the glottis are the structures of the lower airway and lungs. These structures include the trachea, the bronchial tree (primary bronchi, secondary bronchi, and bronchioles), the alveoli, and the lungs (Fig. 6-50).

Trachea. The trachea is the air passage from the larynx to the lungs. The trachea is composed of dense connective tissue and smooth muscle reinforced with 15 to 20 C-shaped pieces of cartilage that form an incomplete ring. This ring protects the trachea and maintains an open passage for air. The adult trachea is about 1.5 cm in diameter and 9 to 15 cm in length. The trachea is located anterior to the esophagus and extends from the larynx to the fifth thoracic vertebra.

The trachea is lined with ciliated epithelium that contains many goblet cells. These cilia protect the lower airway.

NOTE A centimeter is equal to 0.4 inch. One inch is equal to 2.54 cm.

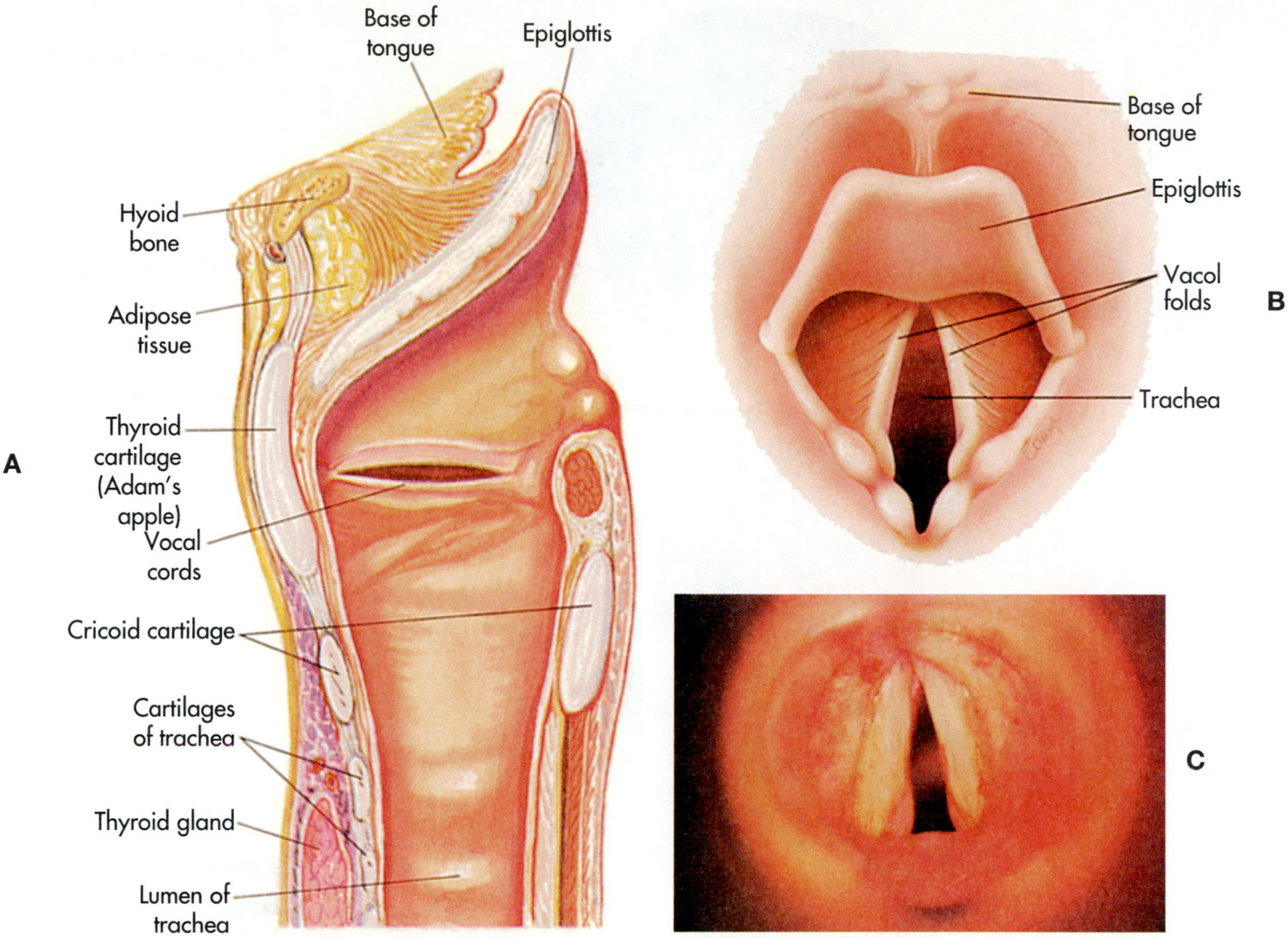

FIGURE 6-49 ■ Larynx. **A,** Sagittal section. **B,** Superior view. **C,** Photograph taken with an endoscope.

They sweep mucus, bacteria, and other small particles toward the larynx. At the larynx the mucus and its contents may be expelled through coughing. Or they may enter the esophagus, where they are swallowed and digested. Constant exposure to some irritants (e.g., cigarette smoke) may produce a tracheal epithelium that lacks cilia and goblet cells. When this protective mechanism is disrupted, the mucus and bacteria may contribute to disease.

Bronchial tree. The lower airway may be thought of as an inverted tree; the many subdivisions become narrower and shorter until they terminate at the alveoli. The large branches are primary bronchi; they divide into smaller secondary bronchi and bronchioles.

The trachea divides into the right and left primary bronchi at the level of the angle of Louis (the sternomanubrial joint). The point of bifurcation of the trachea into the right and left mainstem bronchi is called the *carina.* The right primary bronchus is shorter, wider, and more vertical. Like the trachea, the primary bronchi are lined with ciliated epithelium. They are supported by C-shaped cartilage rings. As the bronchi sequentially branch into smaller subdivisions, the amount of cartilage decreases. The bronchi also become more and more muscular until there is no cartilage. The primary bronchi extend from the mediastinum to the lungs.

The primary bronchi divide into the secondary bronchi as they enter the right and left lungs. Two secondary lobar bronchi in the left lung conduct air to its two lobes; three in the right lung conduct air to its three lobes. The secondary bronchi then divide into the tertiary segmental bronchi, of which there are 10 in the right lung and 9 in the left. The tertiary bronchi extend to the individual segments of each lobe of the lung (lobule). The bronchial tree continues to branch several times. As the cartilage continues to decrease and the diameter is reduced to about 1 mm, the bronchi become bronchioles.

CRITICAL THINKING

What is the benefit of having many bronchiole branches?

NOTE A millimeter is equal to 0.04 inch. One inch is equal to 25.40 mm.

The bronchiole walls are devoid of cartilage. Their muscles are sensitive to certain circulating hormones, such as epinephrine. Contraction and relaxation of these muscles alter

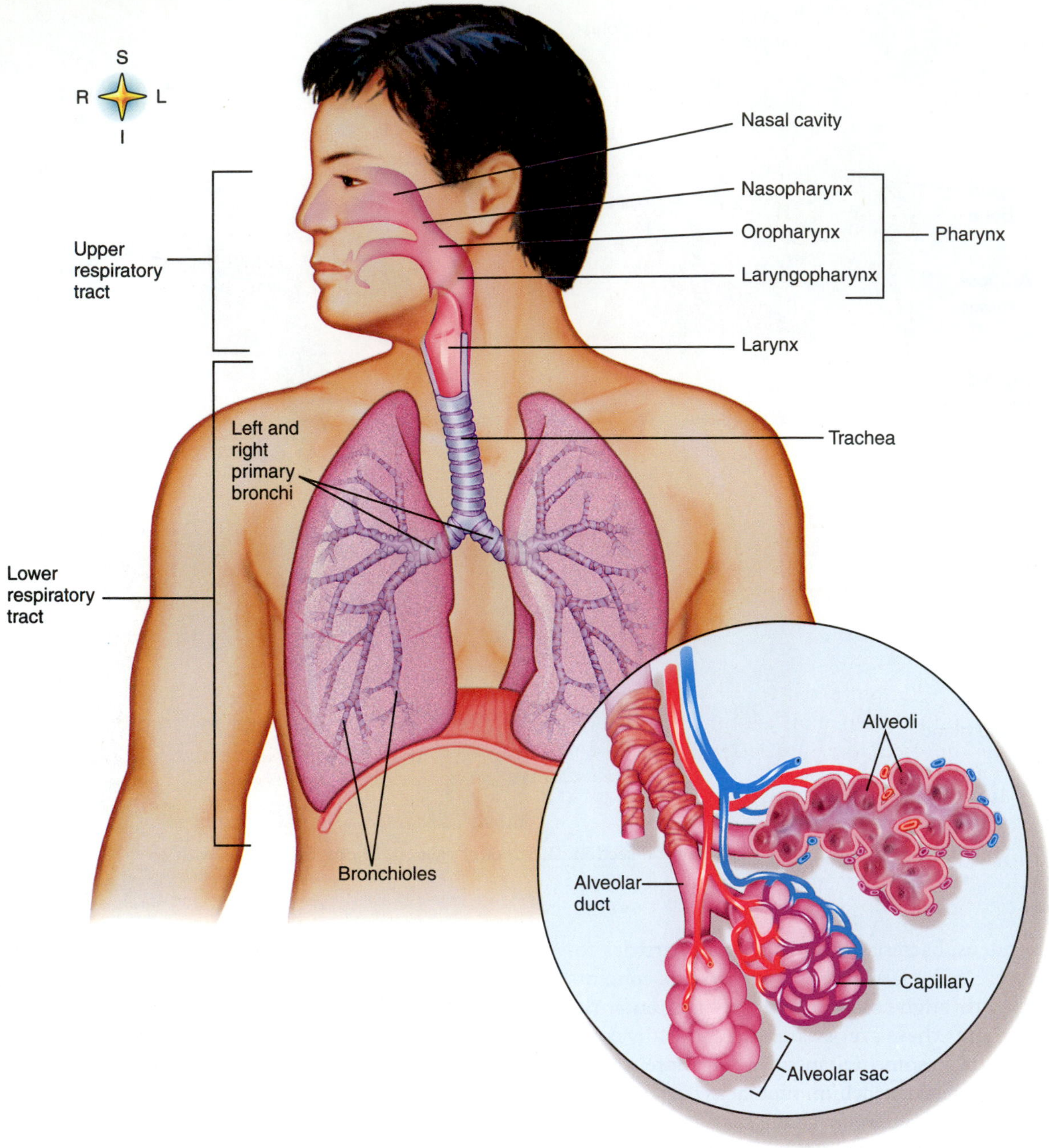

FIGURE 6-50 ■ Structural plan of the respiratory system. Inset shows alveolar sacs where the interchange of oxygen and carbon dioxide takes place through the walls of the grapelike alveoli.

resistance to air flow. The bronchioles can constrict if the smooth muscle contracts forcefully. (An example of this is an asthma exacerbation.) Bronchioles continue to divide. In time they become terminal bronchioles. Finally, they become respiratory bronchioles. Each respiratory bronchiole divides to form alveolar ducts. These ducts end as grapelike clusters of tiny, hollow air sacs. These sacs are called alveoli. The majority of respiratory gas exchange takes place in the alveoli.

Alveoli. The alveoli are the functional units of the respiratory system. They are the main constituent of lung tissue. Some 300 million alveoli exist in the two lungs. The wall of an alveolus consists of a single layer of epithelial cells and elastic fibers. These fibers permit the alveolus to stretch and contract during breathing. The exchange of oxygen and carbon dioxide in the lungs takes place in the alveoli (see Chapter 19).

Each alveolus is surrounded by a fine network of blood capillaries. These capillaries are arranged so that air within the alveolus is separated by a thin respiratory membrane from the blood contained within the alveolar capillaries. The large surface area of the respiratory membrane may be decreased by respiratory diseases. Examples of such diseases are emphysema and lung cancer. Such diseases restrict the exchange of oxygen and carbon dioxide.

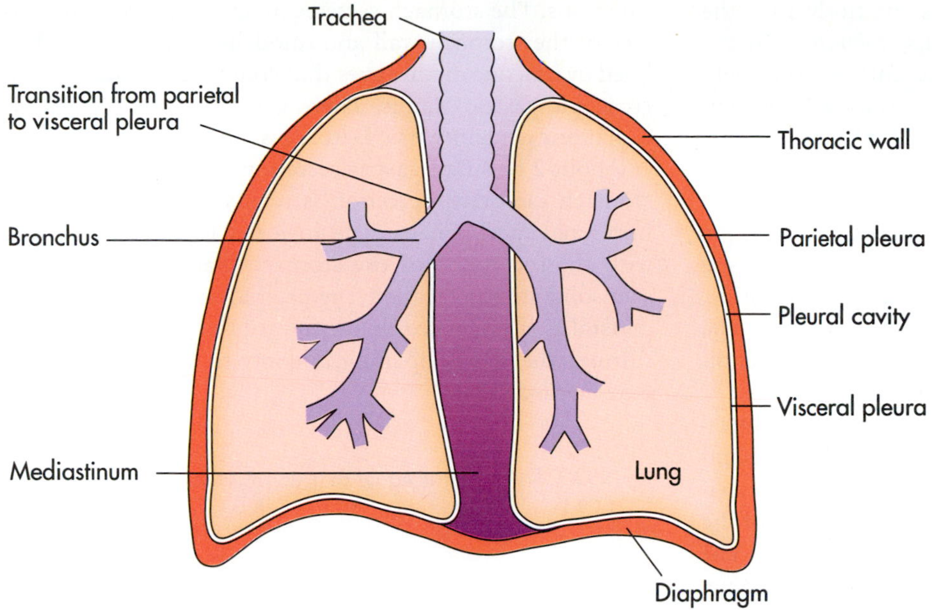

FIGURE 6-51 ■ Lungs surrounded by pleural cavities.

Alveoli are coated with pulmonary surfactant, which is a thin film made by alveolar cells. This fluid keeps the alveoli from collapsing. In addition, pores in the alveolar membrane allow for a limited flow of air between alveoli. This collateral ventilation offers some protection for the alveolus that is occluded by disease.

> **CRITICAL THINKING**
> One effect of toxic smoke inhalation is destruction of pulmonary surfactant. Why won't oxygen therapy alone always help? What do you think might help?

Lungs. The lungs are large, paired, spongy organs the main function of which is respiration. Although there is smooth muscle in the bronchioles of the lungs, the lungs expand and contract during the respiratory cycle as a result of the expansion of the thoracic cavity during inspiration and elastic recoil during expiration. The lungs are attached to the heart by the pulmonary artery and veins. The two lungs are separated by the mediastinum and its contents (the heart, blood vessels, trachea, esophagus, lymphatic tissues, and vessels). The point of entry for the bronchi, vessels, and nerves of each lung is known as the *hilum,* or root, of each lung. At birth the color of the lungs is rose pink. However, by adulthood, the color of the lungs changes to slate gray with dark patches as particulate matter is inhaled and deposited in the tissues. An adult lung weighs less than 2 lb.

Each lung is conical, with its base resting on the diaphragm and its apex extending to a point about 2.5 cm superior to each clavicle. The right lung is divided into three lobes. The left lung is slightly smaller than the right and is divided into two lobes. Each lobe is divided into lobules separated by connective tissue. Major blood vessels and bronchi do not cross this connective tissue, allowing for a diseased lobule to be removed surgically, leaving the remaining lung relatively intact. The left lung has 9 lobules, and the right lung has 10 lobules.

Both lungs are surrounded by a separate pleural cavity. The lungs are attached to each other only at the point of entry of the bronchi, vessels, and nerves of each lung (Fig. 6-51). The two layers of pleura (*visceral* and *parietal*) are so close that they are virtually in contact with each other. The pleurae are separated by a thin fluid that acts as a lubricant. This fluid allows the pleural membranes to slide past each other during respiration.

Between the two pleurae is a potential space known as the pleural space. When significant chest wall injury or pathologic pulmonary condition occurs, the pleural space may become filled with air (pneumothorax) or blood (hemothorax). Another fluid that may accumulate in the pleural space is transudates. Transudates most commonly accumulate because of congestive heart failure. Another fluid collection is exudates. Such fluid collection can result from infectious or malignant conditions.

Digestive System

The digestive system provides the body with water, electrolytes, and other nutrients used by cells. To accomplish this task, the digestive system is specialized to ingest food. Then the system propels the food through the gastrointestinal tract (digestive tract). Lastly, the digestive system absorbs nutrients across the wall of the lumen of the gastrointestinal tract.

The gastrointestinal tract is an irregularly shaped tube. Associated accessory organs (mainly glands) secrete fluid into the digestive tract. The first part of the digestive tract is the oral cavity. The salivary glands and tonsils are accessory organs of the oral cavity. The oral cavity opens posteriorly into the pharynx. The pharynx opens inferiorly into the esophagus. The esophagus opens inferiorly into the stomach (through the muscular *cardiac sphincter*). In the stomach small glands secrete acids and enzymes that help with digestion. The cardiac sphincter stops food from reentering the esophagus when the stomach contracts.

The stomach opens into the duodenum, the first section of the small intestine. Important accessory structures in this segment of the gastrointestinal tract are the liver, the gallbladder, and the pancreas. The jejunum, the major site of absorption, is the next segment of the small intestine. The last segment of the small intestine is the ileum. The ileum is similar in function to the jejunum but has fewer digestive enzymes and provides less absorption.

The last section of the digestive tract is the large intestine, the major functions of which are to absorb water and salts and to concentrate undigested food into feces. The major accessory glands secrete mucus. The first segment of the large intestine is the cecum with its attached appendix. The cecum is followed by the ascending, transverse, descending, and sigmoid portions of the colon and the rectum. The rectum joins the anal canal, which ends at the anus.

FUNCTIONS OF THE DIGESTIVE TRACT

As food moves through the digestive system, secretions are added to liquefy and digest the food. These secretions also provide lubrication. The processes of secretion, movement, and absorption are regulated by nervous and hormonal mechanisms.

ORAL CAVITY

Saliva contains a digestive enzyme referred to as salivary amylase. This enzyme begins the chemical digestion of carbohydrates. In addition, saliva prevents bacterial infection in the mouth. Saliva does this by washing the oral cavity with certain substances. These substances offer a weak antibacterial action. Salivary gland secretion is stimulated by the parasympathetic and sympathetic nervous systems. The parasympathetic controls salivation in the relaxed state.

The teeth chew food in the mouth to break up the food to aid swallowing and processing. Food then is swallowed by voluntary and involuntary actions. The pharynx elevates to receive the food from the mouth. As the pharyngeal muscles contract, the upper esophageal sphincter relaxes, the esophagus opens, and food is pushed into the esophagus. During this phase of swallowing, the vocal folds are moved medially. The epiglottis is tipped posteriorly to close the entrance of the airway and prevent aspiration.

Muscular contractions in the esophagus occur in peristaltic waves. These waves push the food through the esophagus toward the stomach. The contractions cause the cardiac sphincter (also known as the *lower esophageal sphincter*) to relax. The contractions push the food into the stomach.

STOMACH

The stomach acts primarily as a storage area and mixing chamber for ingested food. Although some digestion and absorption occur in the stomach, these are not its major functions. The stomach secretes mucus to protect the surface of the stomach wall and duodenum. The stomach is lined by mucous membranes that contain thousands of microscopic gastric glands. These gastric glands secrete hydrochloric acid, intrinsic factor, gastrin, and pepsinogen.

About 2 to 3 L of gastric secretions are produced by the stomach each day. Secretion is regulated by nervous and hormonal mechanisms. The ingested food is mixed well with the secretions of the stomach glands to produce a semisolid mixture called chyme. Movements resembling peristalsis slowly force chyme toward the pyloric sphincter, through the pyloric opening, and into the duodenum (Figs. 6-52 and 6-53).

▶NOTE A liter is equal to 1.06 qt. One gallon is equal to 3.79 L.

SMALL INTESTINE

The mucosa of the small intestine produces secretions that contain mucus, electrolytes, and water. These substances lubricate the intestinal wall. They also protect the intestine from the acidic chyme and digestive enzymes. In addition, secretions of the liver and pancreas enter the small intestine to aid in the digestive process.

The main functions of the small intestine are mixing and propulsion of chyme and the absorption of fluid and nutrients. Peristaltic contractions move the chyme through the small intestine toward the ileocecal sphincter. At this point the chyme enters the cecum. When the cecum distends from the chyme, the sphincter closes. This closure slows the rate of movement of chyme from the small intestine into the large intestine. Closure also prevents material from returning to the ileum from the cecum.

CRITICAL THINKING

What might happen if the excretion of protective mucus in the small bowel was impaired?

LIVER

The liver is the largest internal organ. The liver serves a number of biochemical functions. It lies just under the diaphragm in the upper regions of the abdominal cavity. The liver is a vascular organ that gets a blood supply from two sources: the hepatic artery and the portal vein. The liver plays a major role in iron metabolism, plasma-protein production, detoxification of drugs and other matters circulating in plasma, and many other biochemical pathways.

▶NOTE A milliliter is equal to 0.5 tsp volume. One tablespoon volume is equal to 15 mL.

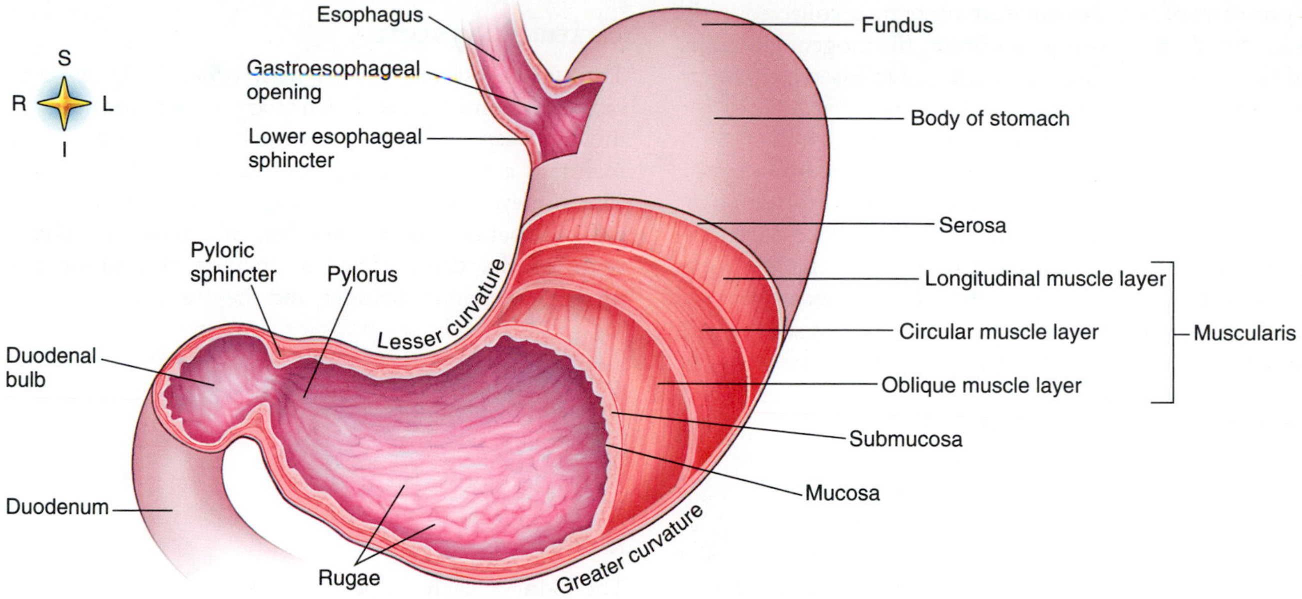

FIGURE 6-52 ■ Muscle layers of the stomach wall.

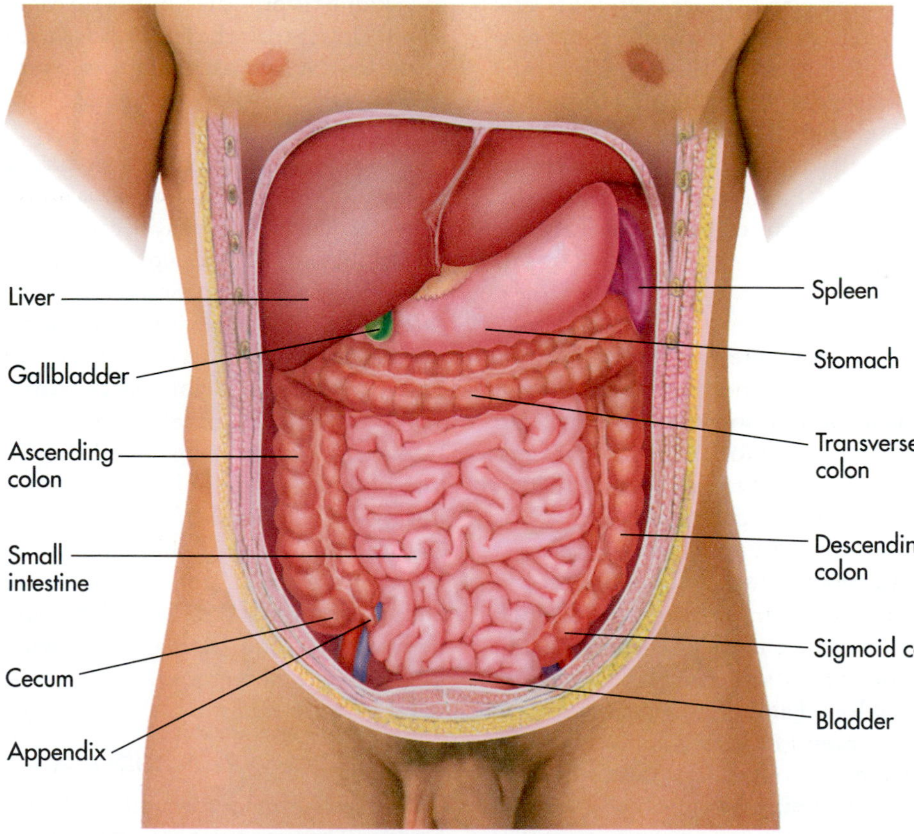

FIGURE 6-53 ■ Digestive organs.

The liver secretes about 600 to 1000 mL of bile each day. Bile contains no digestive enzymes, but it dilutes stomach acid and emulsifies fats. Most bile salts are reabsorbed in the ileum and are carried back to the liver in the blood. Other bile salts are lost through feces.

In addition to secreting bile, the liver has other functions. These functions are needed for healthy survival. The liver plays a major role in the metabolism of certain foods. The liver also helps maintain a normal blood glucose concentration. The liver also is a line of defense against many by-products of metabolism that are toxic if collected in the body. Blood proteins (e.g., albumin, fibrinogen, globulins, and clotting factors) also are made and released into the circulation by the liver.

GALLBLADDER

Bile is secreted regularly by the liver and is stored in the gallbladder. When chyme containing lipid or fat enters the duodenum, the gallbladder is stimulated by the hormones cholecystokinin and secretin. These hormones are secreted by the intestinal mucosa. The stimulation causes the gallbladder to contract, forcing concentrated bile into the small intestine. The only role of the gallbladder is to concentrate and store the bile made by the liver.

> **CRITICAL THINKING**
> When is the person who suffers from gallstones (cholelithiasis) most likely to have pain? Why?

PANCREAS

The pancreas is an exocrine gland. It secretes pancreatic juice. In addition, the pancreas is an endocrine gland that secretes hormones (e.g., insulin) into the blood. Pancreatic juice is the most critical digestive juice. The juice consists of digestive enzymes, sodium bicarbonate, and alkaline substances that neutralize the hydrochloric acid in the chyme entering the small intestine. Pancreatic juice also holds amylase. The amylase continues the digestion that began in the oral cavity.

LARGE INTESTINE

Chyme moves through the small intestine in 3 to 5 hours. Passage through the large intestine, however, takes 18 to 24 hours. Processes involving the absorption of water and salts, the secretion of mucus, the action of microorganisms, and the conversion of chyme produce feces. Feces remain in the colon until eliminated through defecation.

The contents of the large intestine are forced toward the anus by peristaltic contractions. These contractions occur 3 to 4 times each day. During movement of chyme through the large intestine, bacteria act on material that escaped digestion in the small intestine. As a result of this action, more nutrients may be released and absorbed. Some of the bacteria also synthesize vitamin K. This vitamin is needed for normal blood clotting to produce the vitamin B complex. Once formed, these vitamins are absorbed from the large intestine and enter the blood.

Distention of the rectal wall by feces starts the defecation reflex. This reflex causes weak contractions and relaxations of the internal anal sphincter. The external anal sphincter (under conscious cerebral control) stops the passage of feces out of the rectum until it is relaxed. During defecation, pressure in the abdominal cavity increases. This pressure forces the contents of the colon through the anal canal and out of the anus.

Urinary System

The urinary system works with other body systems to maintain homeostasis. The urinary system does this by removing waste products from the blood and by helping to maintain a constant body fluid volume and composition. The kidneys also are involved in the control of red blood cell production and metabolism of vitamin D. The contents of the urinary system include two kidneys, two ureters, the urinary bladder, and the urethra.

> **CRITICAL THINKING**
> Think about patients with renal failure. Why should you anticipate anemia and decreased calcium levels?

KIDNEYS

The kidneys, each shaped much like a kidney bean, lie on the posterior abdominal wall behind the peritoneum. The kidneys are on either side of the vertebral column near the lateral border of the psoas muscles. The superior pole of each kidney is protected by the rib cage. The right kidney is slightly lower than the left because of the superior position of the liver. A fibrous renal capsule surrounds each kidney, as does a dense deposit of adipose tissue that protects the kidney from injury.

The kidney is divided into an outer cortex and an inner medulla. The medulla consists of a number of triangular divisions. These divisions are called the *renal pyramids.* They extend into the cortex (Fig. 6-54). The papilla is the innermost end of a pyramid. Several large urinary tubes (calyces) extend to the renal pelvis from the kidney tissue.

The basic functional unit of the kidney is the nephron. The nephron is made of a large terminal end (called a *renal corpuscle*), a proximal convoluted tubule, the loop of Henle, and a distal convoluted tubule. The distal convoluted tubule empties into a collecting duct. This duct carries the urine from the cortex of the kidney to the calyces. The terminal end of the nephron is enlarged to form Bowman's capsule. The wall of Bowman's capsule is indented to form a double-walled chamber occupied by a network of blood capillaries known as the glomerulus. Together, the glomerulus and Bowman's capsule form the renal corpuscle.

URETERS, URINARY BLADDER, AND URETHRA

The ureters extend from the renal pelvis to the urinary bladder. The triangular area of the bladder wall between the two ureters and the urethra is called the *trigone.* (Figure 6-55 depicts the male urinary bladder.) This region differs from the rest of the bladder wall in that it does not expand during bladder filling.

The urinary bladder is a hollow, muscular organ. The bladder lies in the pelvic cavity just posterior to the pubic symphysis. The size of the bladder depends on the volume of urine.

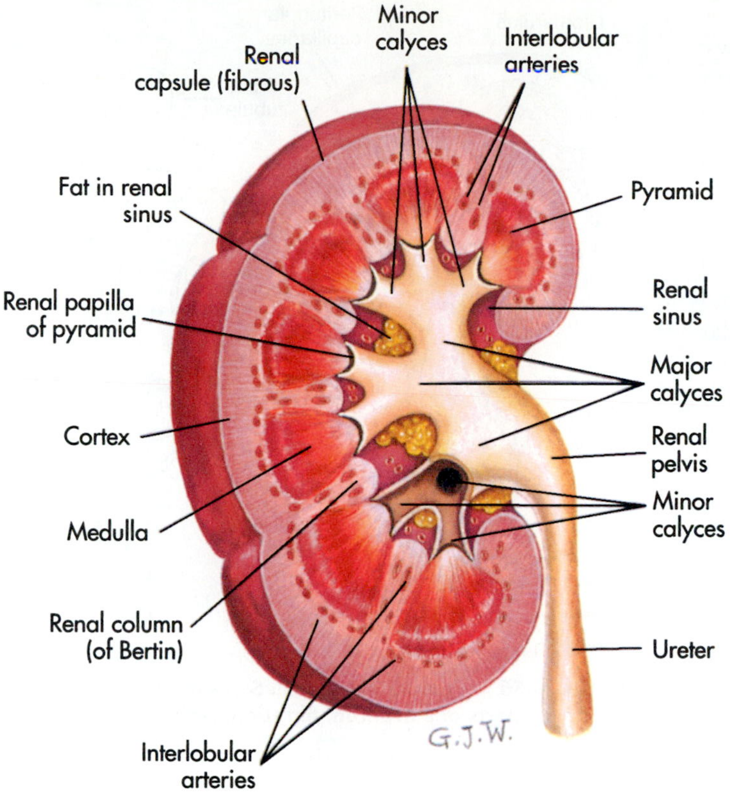

FIGURE 6-54 ■ Magnified wedge cut from a renal pyramid.

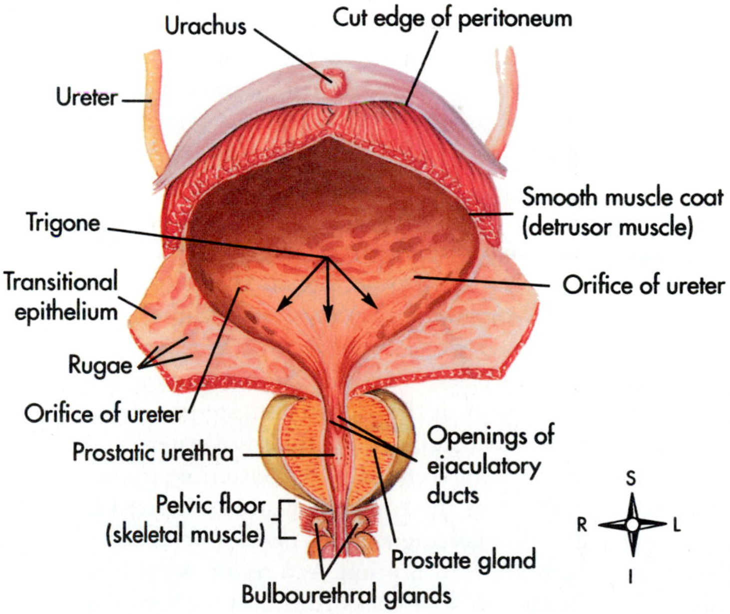

FIGURE 6-55 ■ Male urinary bladder.

> **CRITICAL THINKING**
> Why is the bladder more susceptible to injury when full versus empty?

At the junction of the urethra and the urinary bladder, smooth muscle of the bladder forms the internal urinary sphincter. The external urinary sphincter surrounds the urethra as the urethra extends through the pelvic floor. These sphincters control the flow of urine through the urethra. In the male the urethra extends to the end of the penis, where it opens to the outside (Fig. 6-55). The female urethra is much shorter than the male urethra. It opens into the vestibule anterior to the vaginal opening.

URINE PRODUCTION

Nephrons are the structural parts of the kidney and are where urine is produced. The more than 2 million nephrons form urine in a three-step process that includes filtration, reabsorption, and secretion.

1. The first step of urine formation is the passage of fluid from the glomerular capillaries. This fluid passes into Bowman's capsule. Blood flowing through the glomeruli exerts pressure. This pressure pushes water and small molecular dissolved substances out of the glomeruli and into the Bowman's capsule. Simply stated, glomerular blood pressure causes filtration through the glomerular capillaries. Glomerular filtration normally occurs at the rate of 125 mL/min or 180 L/day (glomerular filtration rate). Ninety percent of this filtrate is reabsorbed. Healthy persons produce 1 to 2 L of urine each day.
2. The filtrate leaves the renal capsule. The filtrate then flows through the proximal convoluted tubule, the loop of Henle, the distal convoluted tubule, and into the collecting duct. During this process, many substances in the filtrate are reabsorbed by the blood capillaries around the tubules. These substances reenter the general circulation. Substances reabsorbed include water, glucose and other nutrients, and most of the sodium and other ions.
3. Secretion is the process by which substances move into urine in the distal convoluted tubule and collecting duct from blood in the capillaries around these structures. Reabsorption moves substances out of the urine and into the blood. Secretion, however, moves substances out of the blood and into the urine. Secreted substances include hydrogen and potassium ions, ammonia, and certain drugs. (Figure 6-56 depicts the formation of urine.)

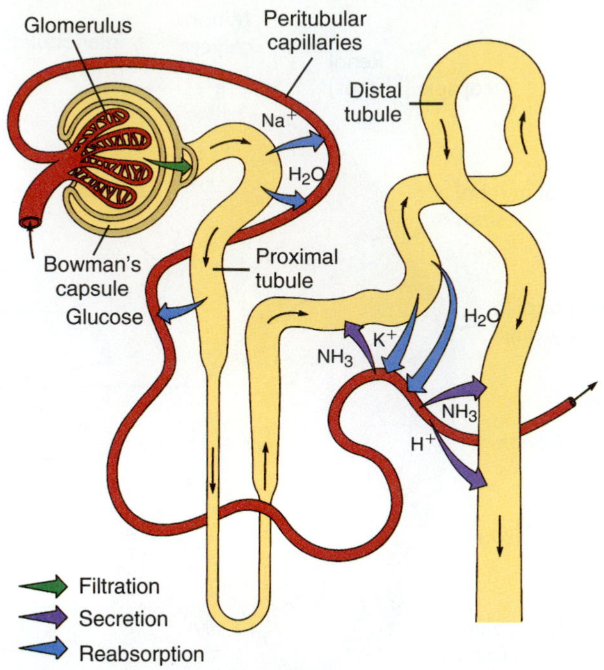

FIGURE 6-56 ■ Formation of urine. Steps in urine formation in successive parts of a nephron: filtration, reabsorption, and secretion.

URINE REGULATION

The body usually can control the amount and makeup of the urine it secretes. This involves hormonal mechanisms, autoregulation, and sympathetic nervous system stimulation.

Aldosterone is a steroid hormone secreted by the adrenal gland. This hormone passes through the circulatory system from the adrenal gland to the kidney. Aldosterone stimulates the tubules to reabsorb sodium salts and water.

Antidiuretic hormone secreted by the posterior pituitary gland tends to decrease the amount of urine produced by making distal and collecting tubules permeable to water, thus increasing water reabsorption. As a result, water is retained by the body in the presence of antidiuretic hormone.

Atrial natriuretic factor is a hormone secreted from the cells in the right atrium of the heart when the pressure in the right atrium increases. This hormone inhibits antidiuretic hormone secretion. The hormone also reduces the ability of the kidney to concentrate urine. As a result, the body produces a large volume of dilute urine.

Prostaglandins and kinins are substances formed in the kidneys. They affect kidney function. These substances are believed to influence the rate of filtrate formation and sodium ion reabsorption.

Autoregulation is the ability of the kidneys to regulate a stable glomerular filtration rate over a wide range of systemic blood pressures. When small increases in glomerular capillary pressure occur, the rate of filtrate formation increases substantially. Therefore large increases in arterial blood pressure increase the rate of urine production. Conversely, when arterial blood pressure decreases, urine production decreases. Through autoregulation the kidneys change the degree of constriction or dilation of the arterioles in the renal capsule to maintain glomerular capillary pressure and urine production within normal limits over a wide range of arterial blood pressures.

Sympathetic neurons innervate the blood vessels of the kidney. The sympathetic stimulation in response to severe stress, intense exercise, or circulatory shock constricts the small arteries and the afferent arterioles. This decreases renal blood flow.

Reproductive System

Most organs and systems of the human body are the same in the male and female. However, the reproductive systems are different. The purpose of the male reproductive system is to make spermatozoa. The purpose also is to transfer spermatozoa to the female. The purpose of the female reproductive system is to make oocytes. Others purposes include receiving the spermatozoa for fertilization, conception, gestation, and birth.

MALE REPRODUCTIVE SYSTEM

The male reproductive system consists of the testes, epididymis, ductus deferens, urethra, seminal vesicles, prostate gland, bulbourethral glands, scrotum, and penis (Fig. 6-57).

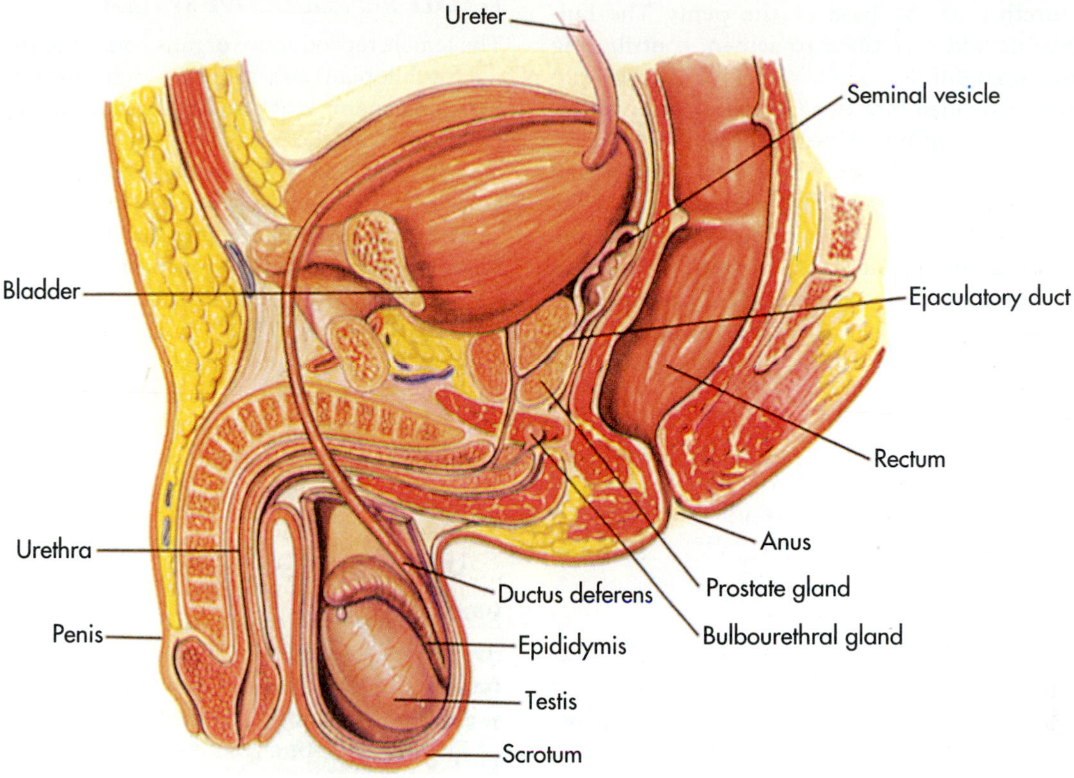

FIGURE 6-57 ■ Sagittal section of the male pelvis.

The testes are ovoid organs within the scrotum that develop as retroperitoneal organs in the abdominopelvic cavity. The testes move from the abdominal cavity to the scrotum by way of the inguinal canal. This canal is common to men and women. Normally the inguinal canal is closed, but it persists as a weak spot in the abdominal wall where the testes pass through it. If the inguinal canal weakens or ruptures, an inguinal hernia may result. Interstitial cells of the testes secrete the male hormone testosterone. Before puberty (12 to 14 years of age), the testes remain relatively simple and unchanged. At the time of puberty, however, the interstitial cells increase in number and size. At this time, spermatozoa production begins. The testes contribute about 5% of the seminal fluid (semen).

The final maturation of spermatozoa occurs within the epididymis. This is a convoluted comma-shaped structure. The epididymis is on the posterior side of the testis. Infection or injury can block one epididymis or both. This in turn can result in infertility.

The ductus deferens, or vas deferens, emerges from the tail of the epididymis. This duct ascends to the seminal vesicle, finally associating with the blood vessels and nerves that supply the testis. These structures and their coverings constitute the spermatic cord. The ductus deferens and the spermatic cord structures ascend and pass through the inguinal canal to enter the abdominal cavity. The ductus deferens crosses the lateral wall of the cavity. The duct then travels over the ureter, and loops over the posterior surface of the urinary bladder to approach the prostate gland. The ductus deferens is surrounded by smooth muscle. This muscle helps to propel sperm through the duct.

The urethra is a passageway for urine and male reproductive fluids. The urethra can be divided into three portions. The first portion is the prostatic portion (the part of the urethra that passes through the prostate gland). The second is the membranous portion (extending from the prostatic urethra through the muscular floor of the pelvis). Finally, the third portion is the spongy portion (extending the length of the penis).

The seminal vesicle is a sac-shaped gland that lies adjacent to each ductus deferens. A short duct from the seminal vesicle joins the ductus deferens to form the ejaculatory duct. These ducts project into the prostate gland and end by opening into the urethra. Seminal vesicles produce about 60% of seminal fluid.

The prostate gland consists of glandular and muscular tissue. The gland is about the size and shape of a walnut. The gland is located dorsal to the symphysis pubis at the base of the bladder, surrounding the prostatic urethra and the two ejaculatory ducts. Twenty to 30 small prostatic ducts secrete prostatic fluid into the prostatic urethra. The prostate gland contributes about 30% of seminal fluid.

The bulbourethral glands are a pair of small glands located near the membranous portion of the urethra. In young adults these glands are each about the size of a pea, but they decrease in size with age. The gland is a compound mucous gland with small ducts that unite to form a single duct from each gland. The two bulbourethral glands enter the spongy urethra at the base of the penis. The bulbourethral glands add secretions to semen, contributing about 5% of seminal fluid.

The scrotum is divided into two internal compartments by a connective tissue septum. Beneath the skin of the scrotum is a layer of superficial fascia (loose connective tissue) and a layer of cutaneous muscle. This muscle is called the *dartos muscle.* The dartos and the cremaster muscles of the abdomen are crucial for regulating temperature in the testes (required for spermatogenesis). They pull the testes near the body in cold temperatures. They also allow the testes to descend away from the body in warm temperatures and during exercise.

> **CRITICAL THINKING**
>
> **Patients may exhibit prostate glands greatly enlarged by benign or malignant disease. What symptoms would you expect?**

The penis consists of three columns of erectile tissue. Engorgement of this tissue with blood causes the penis to enlarge and become firm, producing an erection. The penis is the male organ of copulation and functions in the transfer of spermatozoa from the male to the female.

FEMALE REPRODUCTIVE SYSTEM

The female reproductive organs consist of the ovaries, uterine (or fallopian) tubes, uterus, vagina, external genital organs, and mammary glands. The internal reproductive organs lie within the pelvis between the urinary bladder and the rectum. These organs are held in place by a group of ligaments (Fig. 6-58).

The small ovaries are attached to the posterior of the broad ligament called the *mesovarium.* Two other ligaments associated with the ovary are the suspensory ligament and the ovarian ligament. The ovarian arteries, veins, and nerves traverse the suspensory ligament. They enter the ovary through the mesovarium. Each ovary has a dense outer portion called the *cortex.* Each ovary also has a looser inner portion called the *medulla.* Many small vesicles, called ovarian follicles (each of which contains an oocyte), are distributed throughout the cortex.

The uterine tubes are ducts for the ovaries. Each tube is located along the superior margin of the broad ligament. Each one opens right into the peritoneal cavity to receive the oocyte. Once inside the uterine tube, the oocyte is transported by cilia and peristaltic contractions of the smooth muscle within the uterine tube.

The uterus is the size and shape of a medium-sized pear. The uterus is oriented in the pelvic cavity with the larger

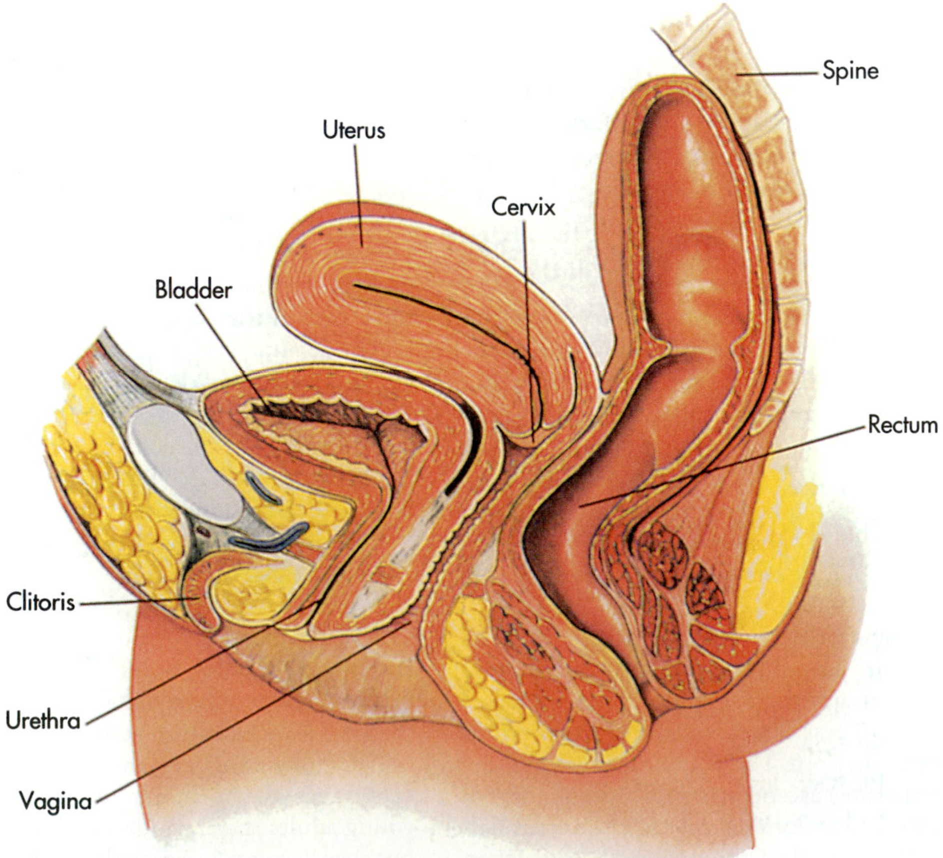

FIGURE 6-58 ■ Sagittal section of the female pelvis.

rounded portion (the fundus) directed superiorly. The narrower portion is the cervix, which is directed inferiorly. The main portion of the uterus (the body) is positioned between the fundus and the cervix. The major ligaments that hold the uterus in place are the broad ligament, round ligaments, and uterosacral ligaments (Fig. 6-59).

The vagina is the female organ of copulation. The vagina functions to receive the penis during intercourse. The vagina extends from the uterus to the outside of the body. The vagina provides a passage for menstrual flow and childbirth as well. The smooth muscle layer of the vagina allows the organ to increase in size to accommodate the penis during intercourse and to stretch greatly during delivery. The vaginal orifice is covered by a thin mucous membrane called the *hymen.* The openings in the hymen usually are enlarged during the first sexual intercourse but also may be perforated or torn during strenuous exercise.

The external genitalia is referred to as the vulva. The vulva consists of the vestibule and its surrounding structures (Fig. 6-60). The vestibule is the space into which the vagina and urethra open. The vestibule is bordered by a pair of thin, longitudinal skin folds called the *labia minora.* A small erectile structure, called the *clitoris,* is located in the anterior margin of the vestibule. The two labia minora unite over the clitoris to form a fold of skin known as the *prepuce.* Lateral to the labia minora are two prominent folds of skin called the *labia majora.* These folds unite anteriorly in an elevation over the pubic symphysis to form the mons pubis. Most of the time, the labia majora are in contact with each other. They conceal the deeper structures within the vestibule.

The perineum is divided into triangles by perineal muscles. The urogenital triangle contains the external genitalia. The posterior anal triangle contains the anal opening. The region between the vagina and the anus is called the *clinical perineum.* This area sometimes tears during childbirth.

The mammary glands are the organs of milk production. They are located within the breasts or *mammae.* Externally, the breasts of males and females have a raised nipple surrounded by a circular pigmented areola. Nipples are sensitive to tactile stimulation. They may become erect in response to sexual arousal. The areolae normally have a slightly bumpy surface. This is due to the presence of areolar glands just below their surface. Secretions from these glands protect the nipple and areola from chafing during nursing.

The female breasts begin to enlarge during puberty (usually between ages 12 and 13) under the effect of estrogen and progesterone. Each adult female mammary gland is made up of 15 to 20 glandular lobes covered by adipose tissue. Each lobe has a single lactiferous duct. This duct subdivides to form smaller ducts, each of which supplies a lobule. These ducts expand at their ends to form secretory sacs called *alveoli.* The alveoli secrete milk during nursing (Fig. 6-61).

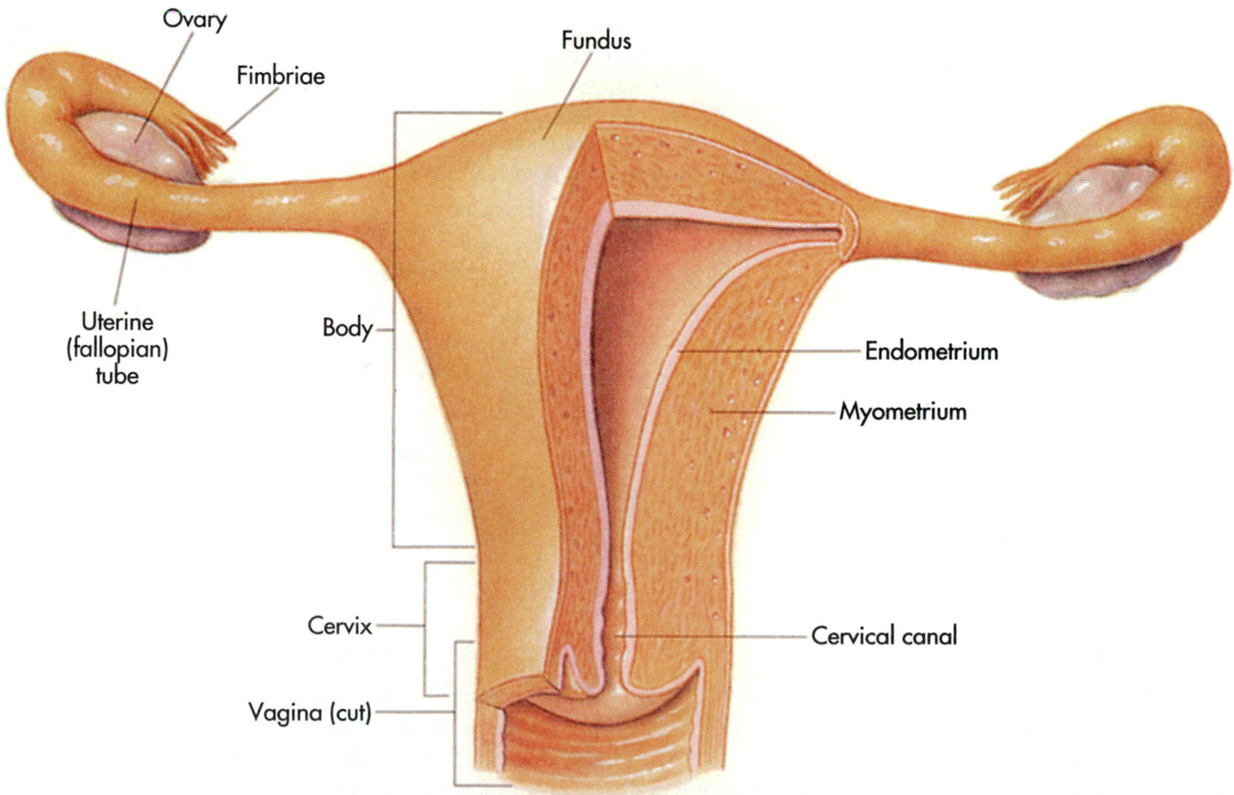

FIGURE 6-59 ■ Internal anatomy of the female pelvis.

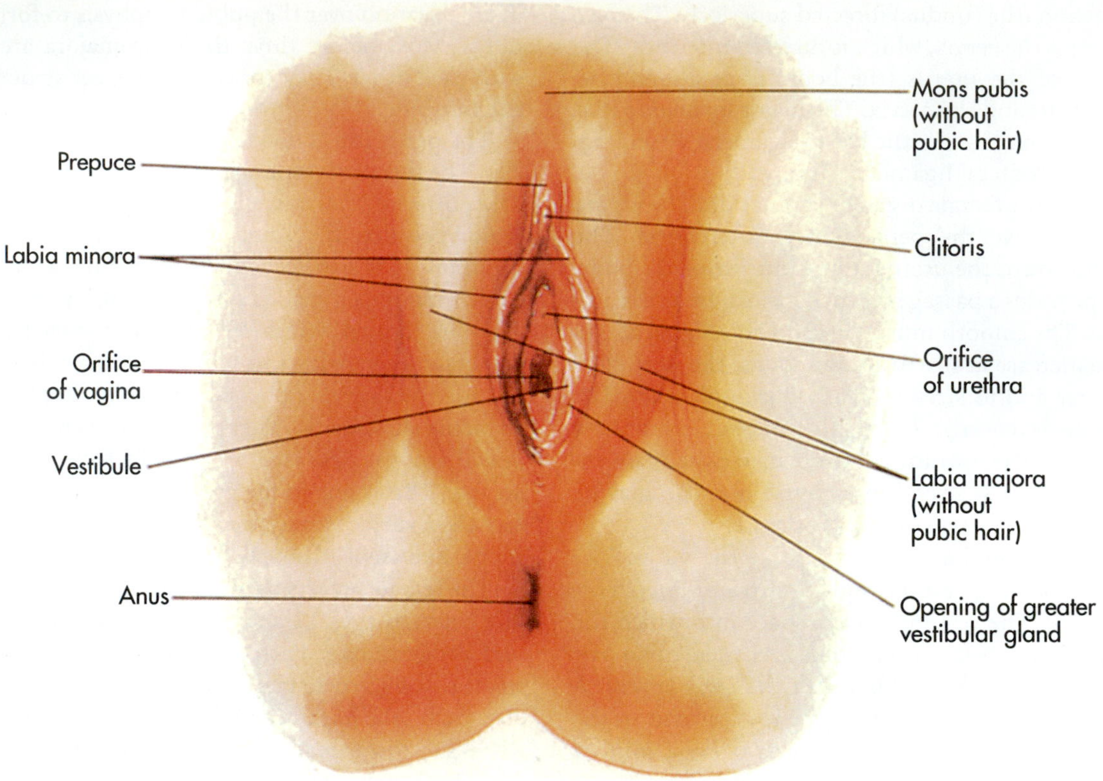

FIGURE 6-60 ■ Female external genitalia.

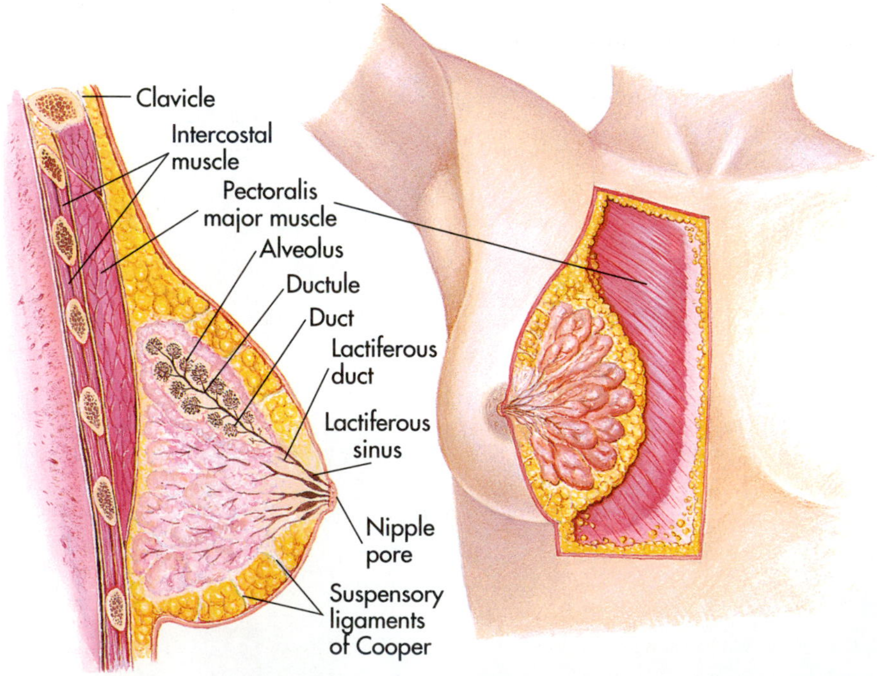

FIGURE 6-61 ■ Blood supply, mammary glands, and duct system of the right mamma.

SPECIAL SENSES

Senses provide the brain with information about the outside world. Four senses are recognized as special senses: smell, taste, sight, and hearing and balance. (The sense of touch now is considered to be a general sense, which consists of several types of nerve endings scattered throughout the body and not localized to a specific area.)

Olfactory Sense Organs

The receptors for the fibers of the olfactory or first cranial nerves lie in the mucosa of the upper part of the nasal cavity (Fig. 6-62). Most of the nasal cavity is involved with respiration. Only a small part is devoted to olfaction.

The dendrites of olfactory neurons extend to the epithelial surface of the nasal cavity, where they form vesicles.

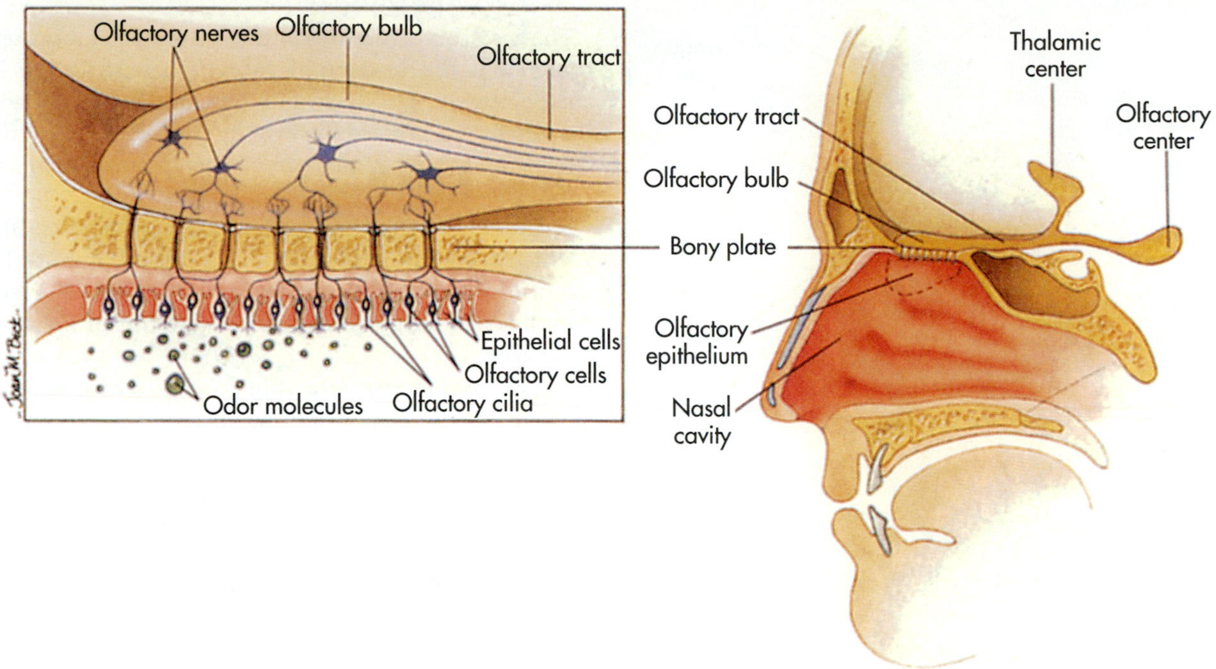

FIGURE 6-62 ■ Olfactory structures. Gas molecules stimulate olfactory cells in the nasal epithelium. Sensory information then is conducted along nerves in the olfactory bulb and olfactory tract to sensory processing centers in the brain.

These vesicles have long cilia. The cilia lie in a thin, mucous film on the epithelial surface. Olfactory cells are stimulated by molecules in the air. The resulting nerve impulses travel through the olfactory nerves in the olfactory bulb and olfactory tract. In the olfactory tract the impulses enter the thalamic and olfactory centers of the brain. In the brain the nervous impulses are interpreted as specific odors.

The exact mechanism of olfactory stimulation is not understood clearly. The range of smells are thought to be actually just a combination of seven main odors. These odors include (1) camphoraceous, (2) musky, (3) floral, (4) pepperminty, (5) ethereal, (6) pungent, and (7) putrid. Olfactory receptors are sensitive (even to slight odors). However, they also are fatigued easily. The olfactory system quickly adapts to ongoing stimulation. In fact, a certain odor may cease to be noticed in a short time. This is a key factor to consider when dealing with hazardous materials incidents (see Chapter 53).

Taste

The sensory structures that detect taste stimuli are called the *taste buds,* and the receptors for the taste nerve fibers are in the seventh and ninth cranial nerves. Most taste buds are associated with specialized portions of the tongue. However, taste buds also are located on other areas of the tongue, palate, lips, and throat.

Taste detected by taste buds can be divided into four basic types: bitter, sour, salty, and sweet. The tip of the tongue reacts more strongly to sweet and salty tastes, the back of the tongue to bitter taste, and the sides of the tongue to sour taste (Fig. 6-63). All the other taste sensations result from a combination of taste bud and olfactory receptor stimulation.

Visual System

The visual system includes the eyes, the accessory structures (eyelids, eyebrows, eyelashes, and tear glands), and the optic nerve, tracts, and pathways. The second cranial nerve (optic nerve) conducts impulses from the eye to the brain. In the brain these impulses create the sensation of vision. The third cranial nerve (oculomotor nerve) conducts impulses from the brain to the muscles of the eye, where they cause contractions that move the eye.

> **CRITICAL THINKING**
>
> Consider the neurological evaluation. Why is an examination of the eyes a key part of this?

ANATOMY OF THE EYE

The eye is composed of three layers: the fibrous tunic, consisting of the sclera and cornea; the vascular tunic, consisting of the choroid, ciliary body, and iris; and the nervous tunic, consisting of the retina (Fig. 6-64).

1. The sclera is the firm, opaque, white outer layer of the eye. The sclera helps to maintain the shape of the eye, protects the internal structures of the eye, and provides an attachment point for the muscles that move the eye. The sclera is continuous with the meningeal layers of the brain that extend along the optic nerve. The cornea is

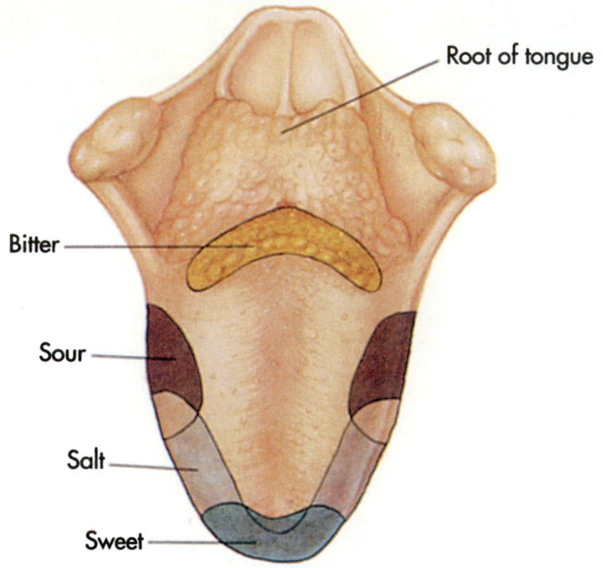

FIGURE 6-63 ■ **Tongue. Dorsal surface and regions sensitive to various tastes.**

continuous with the sclera. The cornea is an avascular and transparent structure that permits light to enter the eye. The cornea also bends and refracts entering light.

2. The vascular tunic contains most of the blood vessels of the eyeball. The part of this layer associated with the sclera is the choroid. Anteriorly, the vascular tunic consists of the ciliary body and the iris. The ciliary body consists of ciliary muscles that can change the shape of the lens and of complex capillaries involved in producing aqueous humor. The iris is the colored part of the eye. The iris consists mainly of smooth muscle that surrounds the pupil. Light enters through the pupil, and the iris regulates the amount of light by controlling the size of the pupil.
3. The retina consists of an outer pigmented retina and an inner sensory layer, which responds to light. The sensory retina contains photoreceptor cells, called *rods* and *cones,* and numerous relay neurons. (Rods are the receptors for night vision. Cones are the receptors for daytime and color vision.)

COMPARTMENTS OF THE EYE

The two compartments of the eye are separated by a lens. The lens is suspended between the two eye compartments by ligaments. These two compartments are known as the *anterior* and *posterior chambers.* The anterior chamber is filled with aqueous humor. This helps maintain intraocular pressure (pressure within the eye that keeps the eye expanded), refract light, and provide nutrition for the anterior chamber.

The posterior chamber of the eye is surrounded almost completely by the retina. The chamber is filled with a transparent, jellylike substance called vitreous humor. Like aqueous humor, the vitreous humor helps maintain intraocular pressure. In addition, the fluid helps to hold the retina in place and functions in the refraction of light in the eye.

ACCESSORY STRUCTURES

The accessory structures of the eye protect, lubricate, move, and aid in the function of the eye. These structures include the eyebrows, eyelids, conjunctiva, and lacrimal gland.

Eyebrows protect the eyes by providing shade from direct sunlight. They also prevent perspiration from running into the eyes.

Eyelids protect the eyes from foreign objects. Blinking, which normally occurs about 25 times per minute, helps to lubricate the eyes by spreading tears over their surfaces. Eyelids also help to regulate the amount of light entering the eyes.

The conjunctiva is a thin, transparent mucous membrane. It covers the inner surface of the eyelids and the outer surface of the sclera.

The lacrimal gland makes lacrimal fluid (tears) that leaves the gland through several ducts, passing over the anterior surface of the eyeball. The gland is in the superolateral corner of the orbit. The gland makes tears to moisten the surface of the eye, lubricate the eyelids, and wash away foreign objects. Tears also contain lysosomes that destroy some forms of bacteria.

Most tears evaporate from the surface of the eye. Excess fluid is collected in the medial corner of the eye by the lacrimal canals through a punctum (the opening of each canal). The lacrimal canals open into a lacrimal sac. This sac in turn continues into the nasolacrimal duct (Fig. 6-65).

Hearing and Balance

The organs of hearing can be divided into three portions: external, middle, and inner ear (Fig. 6-66). The external and middle ear are involved in hearing only. However, the inner ear functions in hearing and balance. The special senses of hearing and balance are transmitted by the vestibulocochlear nerve (eighth cranial nerve).

The external ear includes the auricle, or pinna. It also includes the external auditory meatus, which opens into the external auditory canal. The external auditory canal is lined by hairs and ceruminous glands. These glands make cerumen. This canal terminates medially at the eardrum, or tympanic membrane. The middle ear is an air-filled space within the temporal bone. The middle ear contains the auditory ossicles.

The inner ear holds the sensory organs for hearing and balance. The inner ear consists of interconnecting tunnels and chambers within the *bony labyrinth.*

Inside the bony labyrinth is another set of membranous tunnels and chambers called the *membranous labyrinth.* This labyrinth is filled with a clear fluid called *endolymph.* The space between the membranous and bony labyrinth is filled with a fluid called *perilymph.* These fluids are similar to cerebrospinal fluid.

The auricle is shaped to collect sound waves. It directs sound waves toward the external auditory meatus. From the meatus, sound waves travel through the auditory canal to the tympanic membrane, causing the membrane to vibrate.

The middle ear is connected to the inner ear by two membrane-covered openings. These are the round and oval windows. Two other openings that are not covered by

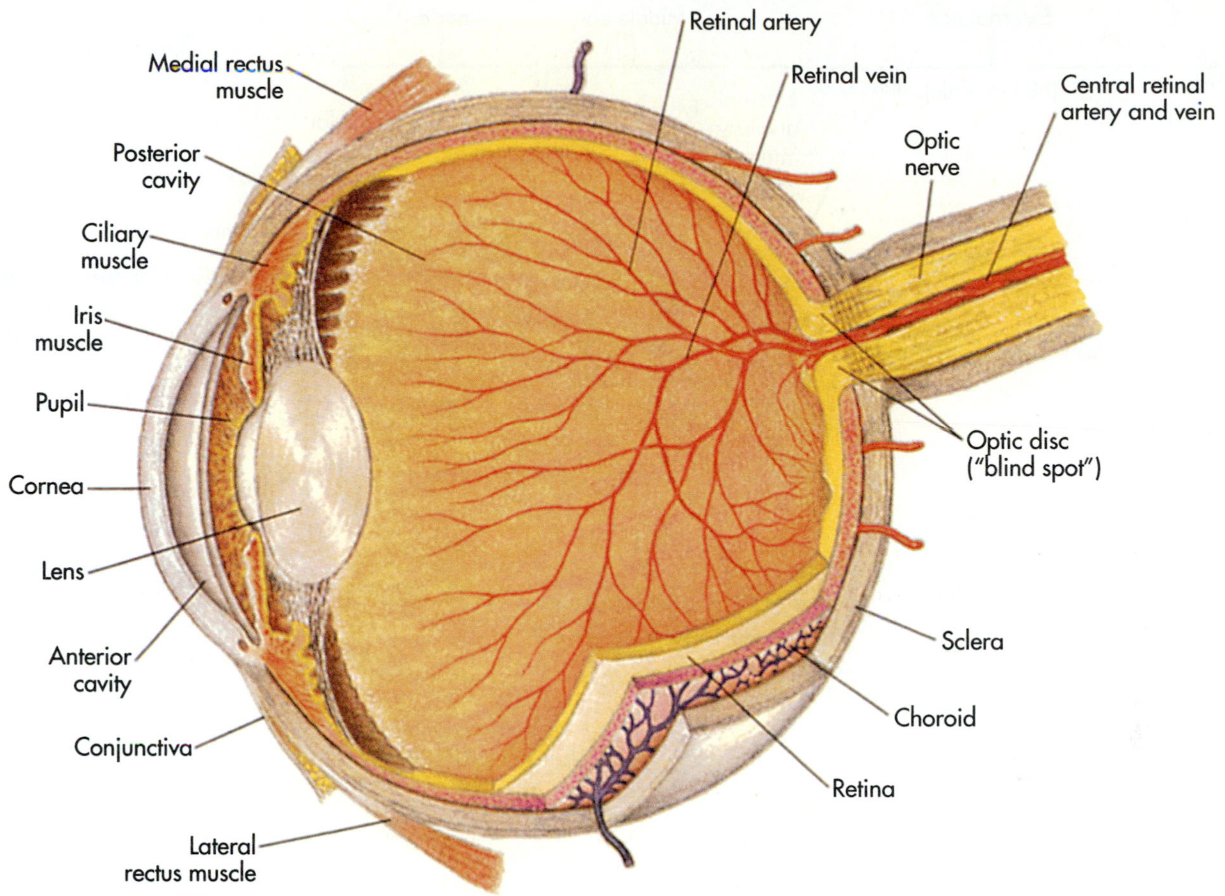

FIGURE 6-64 ■ Horizontal section through the left eyeball. The eye is viewed from above.

membranes offer a passage for air from the middle ear. One opens into the mastoid air cells. The second opening, the auditory (or eustachian) tube, opens into the pharynx. The eustachian tube allows the equalization of air pressure between the outside air and middle ear cavity. (Children have shorter eustachian tubes. This makes it easier for bacteria to travel from infected areas in the throat to the middle ear. This difference between children and adults is responsible for the increased frequency of earaches and ear infections in children.) The auditory ossicles of the middle ear (called the *malleus, incus,* and *stapes*) transmit vibrations from the tympanic membrane to the oval window.

CRITICAL THINKING

Besides pain and impaired hearing, what other symptom would you look for in a patient with an inner ear problem?

The bony labyrinth of the inner ear is divided into three regions. These are called the *vestibule, cochlea,* and *semicircular canals.* The vestibule and semicircular canals are involved primarily in balance. The cochlea is involved in hearing. The hearing sense organ, which lies inside the cochlea, is called the *organ of Corti.* In young, healthy persons, the frequencies that can be detected by the ear range (over octaves) from 20 to 20,000 cycles per second.

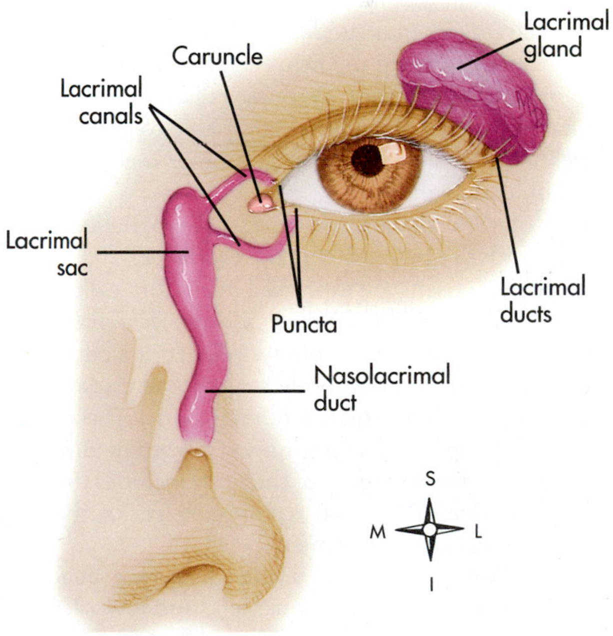

FIGURE 6-65 ■ Lacrimal structures of the eye.

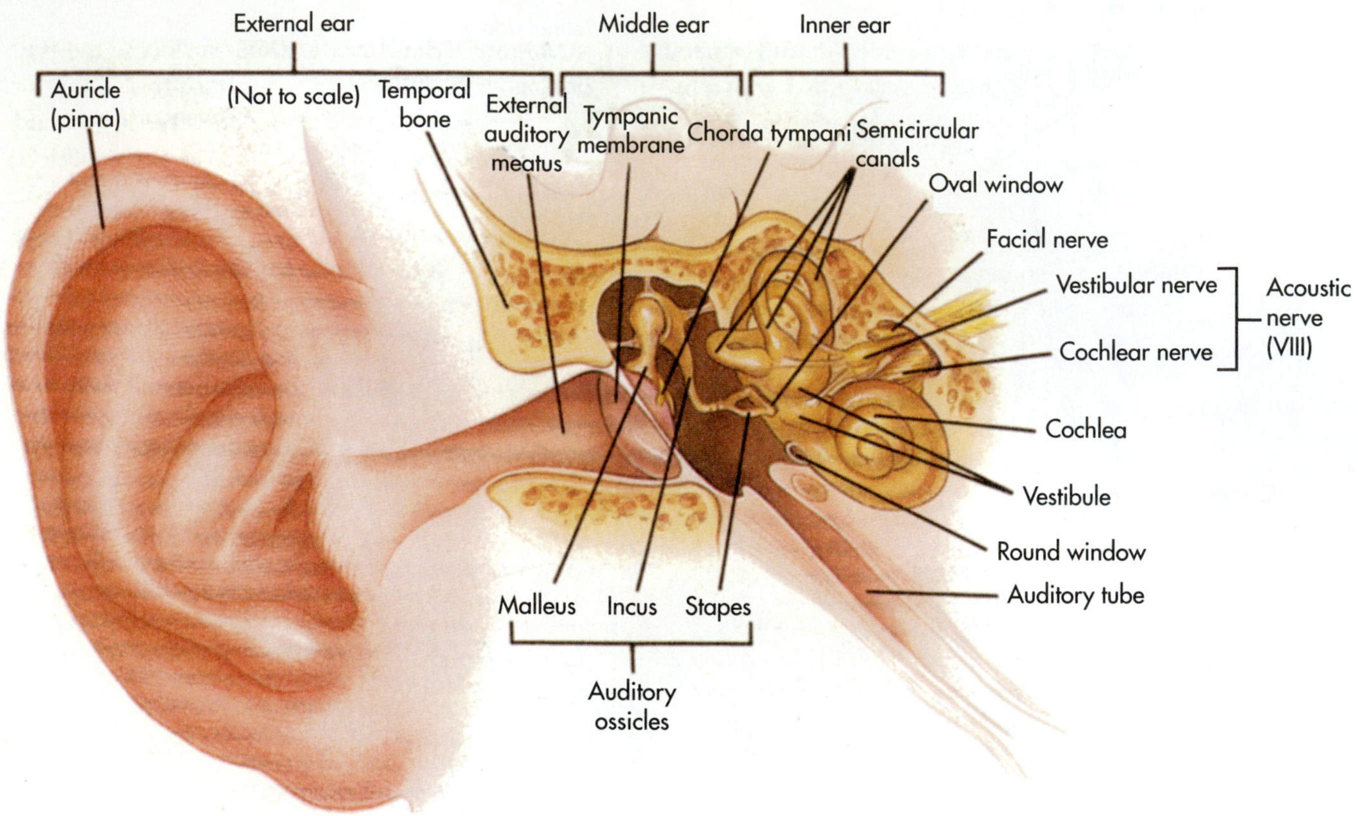

Figure 6-66 ■ External, middle, and inner ear.

SUMMARY

- The paramedic must understand human anatomy fully. This understanding will help the paramedic to organize a patient assessment by body region. Knowledge of anatomy also will help the paramedic to communicate well with medical direction and other members of the health care team.
- The anatomical position refers to a patient standing erect with the palms facing the examiner.
- Directional terms are expressed in anatomical terminology. Examples of these are *up* or *down, front* or *back,* and *right* or *left.* These terms always refer to the patient, not the examiner. Internal body structure is classified into anatomical planes of the human body. These planes can be thought of as imaginary straight-line divisions.
- The appendicular region of the body includes the limbs, or extremities. The axial region consists of the head, neck, thorax, and abdomen.
- The abdomen usually is divided into four quadrants: upper right, lower right, upper left, and lower left.
- The three major cavities of the human body are the thoracic cavity, the abdominal cavity, and the pelvic cavity.
- The thoracic cavity contains the trachea, esophagus, thymus, heart, great vessels, lungs, and the cavities and membranes that surround them. The abdominopelvic cavity is surrounded by membranes and contains organs and blood vessels.
- The cytoplasmic membrane encloses the cytoplasm. The membrane forms the outer boundary of the cell.
- Cytoplasm lies between the cytoplasmic membrane and the nucleus. Specialized structures in the cell (organelles) are located in the cytoplasm. These organelles perform functions key to the survival of the cell. The nucleus is a large, membrane-bound organelle. It ultimately controls all other organelles in the cytoplasm.
- All human cells, with the exception of the reproductive (sex) cells, reproduce by a process known as mitosis. In this process, cells divide to multiply.

- Four main types of tissue make up the many organs of the body. These are epithelial, connective, muscle, and nervous. Epithelial tissue covers surfaces and forms structures. Connective tissue is made of cells separated from each other by intercellular material. This material is known as the extracellular matrix. Muscle tissue is contractile tissue and is responsible for movement. The nervous tissue has the ability to conduct electrical signals. These signals are known as action potentials.
- A system is a group of organs arranged to perform a more complex function than any one organ can perform alone. The eleven major organ systems in the body are the integumentary, skeletal, muscular, nervous, endocrine, circulatory, lymphatic, respiratory, digestive, urinary, and reproductive.
- The integumentary system consists of the skin and accessory structures such as hair, nails, and a variety of glands. The functions of the integumentary system include protecting the body against injury and dehydration, defense against infection, and temperature regulation.
- The skeletal system consists of bone and associated connective tissues, including cartilage, tendons, and ligaments. The skeletal system provides a rigid framework for support and protection. It also provides a system of levers on which muscles act to produce body movements.
- The three primary functions of the muscular system are movement, postural maintenance, and heat production.
- The nervous and the endocrine systems are the major regulatory and coordinating systems of the body. The nervous system rapidly sends information. It does this by means of nerve impulses conducted from one area of the body to another. The endocrine system sends information more slowly. It does this by means of chemicals secreted by ductless glands into the bloodstream.
- The heart and cardiovascular system are responsible for circulating blood throughout the body. Blood transports nutrients and oxygen to tissues. Blood carries carbon dioxide and waste products away from tissues. In addition, blood carries hormones produced in endocrine glands to their target tissues. Blood also plays a key role in temperature regulation and fluid balance. Blood also protects the body from bacteria and foreign substances.
- The lymphatic system includes lymph, lymphocytes, lymph nodes, tonsils, spleen, and thymus gland. The lymphatic system has three basic functions. The first is to help maintain fluid balance in tissues. The second is to absorb fats and other substances from the digestive tract. The third is to play a role in the immune defense system of the body.
- The organs of the respiratory system and the cardiovascular system move oxygen to cells. They move carbon dioxide from cells to where it is released into the air. The entrance to the respiratory tract begins at the nasal cavity and includes the nasopharynx, oropharynx, laryngopharynx, and larynx. Below the glottis are the structures of the lower airway and lungs. These structures include the trachea, the bronchial tree, the alveoli, and the lungs.
- The digestive system provides the body with water, electrolytes, and other nutrients used by cells. The gastrointestinal tract is an irregularly shaped tube. Associated accessory organs (mainly glands) secrete fluid into the digestive tract.
- The urinary system works with other body systems to maintain homeostasis. It does this by removing waste products from the blood. It also does this by helping to maintain a constant body fluid volume and composition. The contents of the urinary system include two kidneys, two ureters, the urinary bladder, and the urethra.
- The purpose of the male reproductive system is to make and transfer spermatozoa to the female. The purpose of the female reproductive system is to make oocytes and to receive the spermatozoa for fertilization, conception, gestation, and birth. The male reproductive system consists of the testes, epididymis, ductus deferens, urethra, seminal vesicles, prostate gland, bulbourethral glands, scrotum, and penis. The female reproductive organs consist of the ovaries, uterine (or fallopian) tubes, uterus, vagina, external genital organs, and mammary glands.
- Senses provide the brain with information about the outside world. Four senses are recognized as special senses: smell, taste, sight, and hearing and balance.

REFERENCES

1. McCance K, Huether S: *Pathophysiology: the biologic basis for disease in adults and children,* ed 4, St Louis, 2002, Mosby.

SUGGESTED READINGS

Epstein O et al: *Clinical examination,* ed 2, St Louis, 1997, Mosby.
Seeley R et al: *Anatomy and physiology,* ed 6, 2002, McGraw-Hill.
Siedel H et al: *Mosby's guide to physical examination,* ed 5, St Louis, 2002, Mosby.
Thibodeau G, Patton K: *Anatomy and physiology,* ed 5, St Louis, 2003, Mosby.

CHAPTER 7

General Principles of Pathophysiology

OBJECTIVES

Upon completion of this chapter, the paramedic student will be able to:

1. Describe the normal characteristics of the cellular environment and the key homeostatic mechanisms that strive to maintain an optimal fluid and electrolyte balance.
2. Outline pathophysiological alterations in water and electrolyte balance and list their effects on body functions.
3. Describe the treatment of patients with particular fluid or electrolyte imbalances.
4. Describe the mechanisms in the body that maintain normal acid-base balance.
5. Outline pathophysiological alterations in acid-base balance.
6. Describe the management of a patient with an acid-base imbalance.
7. Describe the changes in cells and tissues that occur with cellular adaptation, injury, neoplasia, aging, or death.
8. Outline the effects of cellular injury on local and systemic body functions.
9. Describe changes in body functions that can occur as a result of genetic and familial disease factors.
10. Outline the causes, adverse systemic effects, and compensatory mechanisms associated with hypoperfusion.
11. Describe the ways in which the inflammatory and immune mechanisms respond to cellular injury or antigenic stimulation.
12. Explain how changes in immune status and the presence of inflammation can adversely affect body functions.
13. Describe the impact of stress on the body's response to illness or injury.

KEY TERMS

acidosis: A condition marked by a high concentration of hydrogen ions (i.e., a pH below 7.35).
active transport: A carrier-mediated process that can move substances against a concentration gradient.
aerobic: Of or pertaining to the presence of air or oxygen.
afterload: The total resistance against which blood must be pumped; also known as peripheral vascular resistance.
alkalosis: A condition marked by a low concentration of hydrogen ions (i.e., a pH above 7.45).
allergens: Substances that can produce hypersensitivity reactions in the body.
anaerobic: Of or pertaining to the absence of oxygen.
anion: An ion with a negative charge.

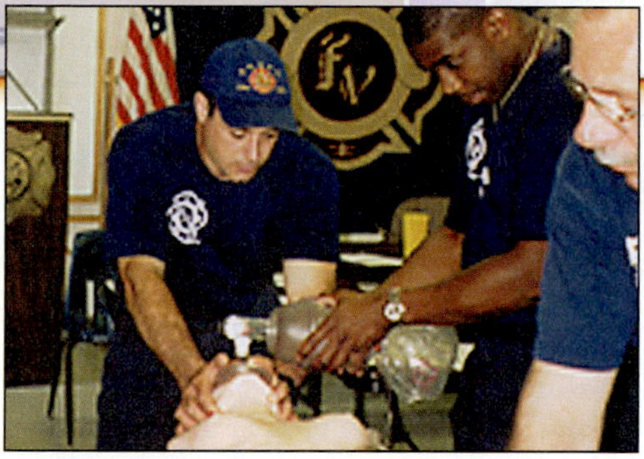

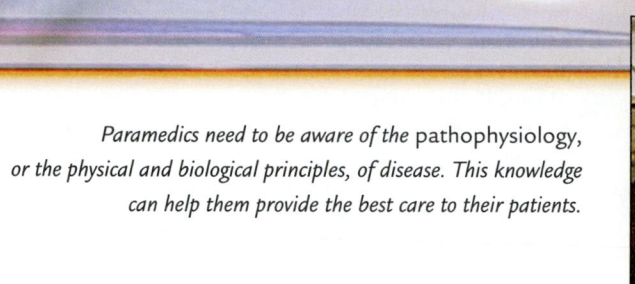

Paramedics need to be aware of the pathophysiology, *or the physical and biological principles, of disease. This knowledge can help them provide the best care to their patients.*

antigens: Substances (usually proteins) that cause the formation of an antibody and that react specifically with that antibody.
atrophy: Decrease in the size (shrinkage) of a cell, which adversely affects cell function.
B lymphocytes: The lymphocytes responsible for antibody-mediated immunity.
cardiac output: The volume of blood pumped each minute by the ventricle.
cation: An ion with a positive charge.
complement system: A group of proteins that coat bacteria; the proteins then either help kill the bacteria directly, or they assist neutrophils (in the blood) and macrophages (in the tissues) to engulf and destroy the bacteria.
diffusion: The process by which solid, particulate matter in a fluid moves from an area of higher concentration to an area of lower concentration, resulting in an even distribution of the particles in the fluid.
dysplasia: Abnormal cellular growth.
edema: The accumulation of fluid in the interstitial spaces.
extracellular fluid: The water found outside the cells, including that in the intravascular and interstitial compartments.
facilitated diffusion: A carrier-mediated process that moves substances into or out of cells from a high to a low concentration.
hypercalcemia: A higher than normal concentration of calcium in the blood.
hyperkalemia: A higher than normal concentration of potassium in the blood.
hypermagnesemia: A higher than normal concentration of magnesium in the blood.
hypernatremic: A term describing a higher than normal concentration of sodium in the blood.
hyperplasia: An excessive increase in the number of cells.
hypersensitivity reaction: An altered immunological response to an antigen that results in a pathological immune response upon reexposure.
hypertonic: A term used to describe a solution that causes cells to shrink.
hypertrophy: An increase in the size of a cell.
hypokalemia: A lower than normal concentration of potassium in the blood.
hypomagnesemia: A lower than normal concentration of magnesium in the blood plasma.
hyponatremic: A term describing a lower than normal concentration of sodium in the blood.
hypoperfusion: Severely inadequate circulation that results in insufficient delivery of oxygen and nutrients necessary for normal tissue and cellular function; also known as shock.
hypotonic: A term used to describe a solution that causes cells to swell.
hypoxemia: A lower than normal oxygen content of the blood as measured in an arterial blood sample.
immune response: A defense function of the body that produces antibodies to destroy invading antigens and malignancies.
inflammatory response: A tissue reaction to injury or to an antigen; it may include pain, swelling, itching, redness, heat, and loss of function.
interstitial fluid: Fluid that occupies the space outside the blood vessels and/or outside the cells of an organ or tissue.
intracellular fluid: The fluid found in all body cells.
ischemia: A state of insufficient perfusion of oxygenated blood to a body organ or part.
isotonic: A term used to describe a solution that causes cells neither to shrink nor to swell.

lactic acidosis: A disorder characterized by an accumulation of lactic acid in the blood, resulting in a lowered pH in muscle and serum.
mediated transport mechanisms: Mechanisms that use carrier molecules to move large, water-soluble molecules or electrically charged molecules across cell membranes.
metaplasia: A change from one cell type to another that is better able to tolerate adverse conditions; a conversion into a form that is not normal for that cell.
multiple organ dysfunction syndrome: The progressive failure of two or more organ systems after a severe illness or injury.
necrosis: Death of a cell or group of cells as the result of disease or injury.
negative feedback mechanisms: Mechanisms that tend to produce a response that balances a change in a system.
neoplasia: New and abnormal development of cells, which may be benign or malignant.
osmolality: The osmotic pressure of a solution.
osmosis: The diffusion of solvent (water) through a membrane from a less concentrated solution to a more concentrated solution.
partial pressure: The pressure exerted by a single gas.
peripheral vascular resistance: The total resistance against which blood must be pumped; also known as afterload.
pH: An inverse logarithm of the hydrogen ion concentration.
preload: The amount of blood returning to the ventricle.
semipermeable membrane: A membrane that allows some fluids and substances to pass through them but not others, usually depending on size, shape, electrical charge, or other chemical properties.
shock: A condition of severely inadequate blood flow to the body's peripheral tissues that is associated with life-threatening cellular dysfunction; also known as hypoperfusion.
solutes: Substances dissolved in solution.
Starling hypothesis: The concept that describes the movement of fluid back and forth across the capillary wall (net filtration).
stroke volume: The volume of blood ejected from one ventricle in a single heartbeat.
T lymphocytes: The lymphocytes responsible for cell-mediated immunity.
virulence: The relative strength of a pathogen.

SECTION ONE Cellular Physiology

BASIC CELLULAR REVIEW

As discussed in Chapter 6, the cell is the basic unit of higher life forms. All cells have various key components. The *cell membrane* separates the internal environment from the external environment. *Enzymes* help to carry out biochemical processes. The *internal membranes* encapsulate chemicals. Cells also contain genetic material for replication. In addition to all this, cells form the four basic types of tissue:

- Epithelial tissue
- Connective tissue (including hematological tissue)
- Muscle tissue
- Nervous tissue

Refer to Chapter 6 to review basic cellular function and tissue types. See the chapter appendix for an overview of medical terminology used in the health sciences.

CELLULAR ENVIRONMENT

The cells of the human body live in a fluid environment that consists mainly of water. Body water is essential for two reasons. First, it is the medium in which all metabolic reactions occur. Second, the body's health depends on precise regulation of the volume and composition of this fluid. The body has two fluid compartments: the intracellular fluid and the extracellular fluid (Fig. 7-1).

Intracellular and Extracellular Fluid

Intracellular fluid (ICF) is the fluid found inside all body cells. It accounts for 40% of total body weight. **Extracellular fluid** (ECF) is the fluid found outside the cells. This includes the intravascular and interstitial compartments. ECF accounts for about 20% of total body weight, with the intravascular component (blood plasma) composing about one third. The extracellular fluid between the cells and outside the vascular bed (i.e., connective tissue, cartilage, and bone) is known as **interstitial fluid** (IF). This category also includes special fluids, such as cerebrospinal fluid and intraocular fluid. The IF accounts for about 15% to 16% of total body weight.

Aging and the Distribution of Body Fluids

Body mass consists mainly of water. In fact, water accounts for 50% to 60% of total body weight in adults. With age, the distribution and amount of the total body water (TBW) change. For example, about 80% of a newborn infant's body weight is TBW. During childhood, TBW decreases to 60% to 65% of body weight, and it declines further with age (Table 7-1). TBW in the elderly decreases to 45% to 55%, increasing

NOTE In older adults, the normal reduction in total body water (TBW) becomes a significant factor if fever or dehydration is present. With illness or injury, loss of body fluids can be severe or life threatening.

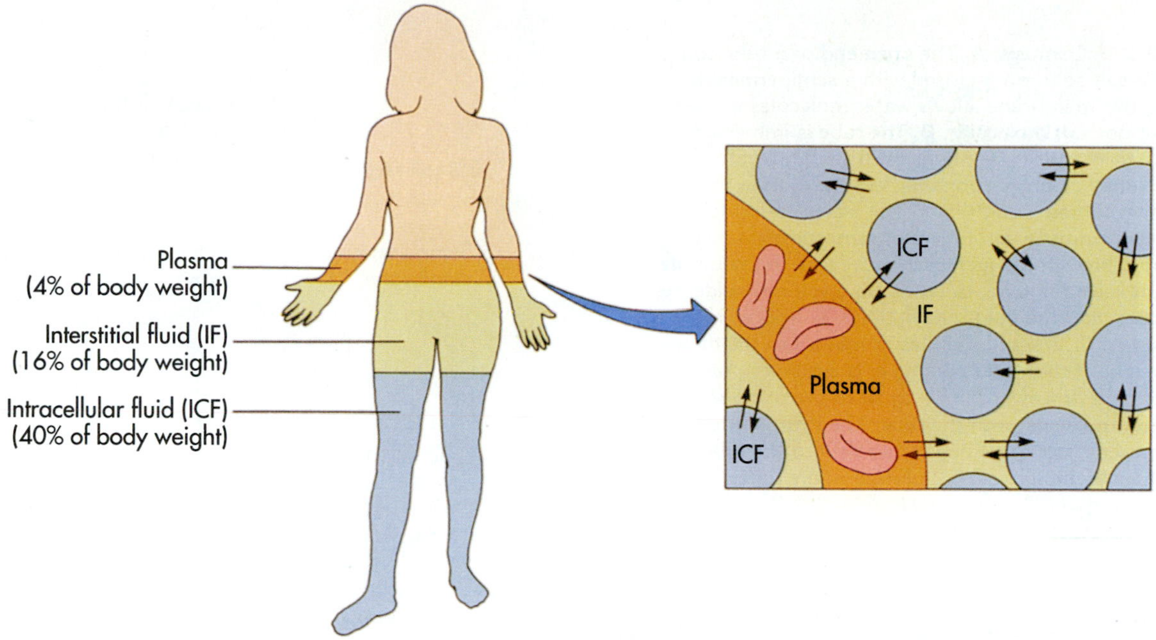

FIGURE 7-1 ■ Fluid compartments of the body.

TABLE 7-1 Total Body Water (TBW) Relative to Body Type

BODY BUILD	ADULT MALE (% TBW)	ADULT FEMALE (% TBW)	INFANT (% TBW)
Normal	60	50	70
Lean	70	60	80
Obese	50	42	60

From McCance KL, Huether SE: *Pathophysiology: the biologic basis for disease in adults and children*, ed 3, St Louis, 1998, Mosby.

the risk of dehydration and electrolyte abnormalities (see Chapter 45).

Water Movement between Intracellular Fluid and Extracellular Fluid

Body fluids constantly move from one compartment to another. In healthy individuals, the volume in each compartment remains about the same. To keep the volume stable, the body uses osmosis, diffusion, and mediated transport mechanisms. To understand illness and disease, the paramedic first must understand how fluids in the body move and how changes in these fluids can occur.

OSMOSIS

For the body to function well, molecules must be able to move within a cell or across cell membranes. Membranes separate fluid compartments. Most of these membranes allow water to pass freely. They also regulate the flow of **solutes** (substances dissolved in solution) on the basis of size, shape, electrical charge, or other chemical properties. These membranes are referred to as **semipermeable membranes.** Channels in these membranes permit the passage of solutes. The channels may be open at all times to specific solutes, or they may be closed at times, depending on the cell's makeup. Because the cell membrane can regulate the flow of solutes, the cell can maintain *homeostasis* (stability in the body's internal environment).

Osmosis is the flow of fluid across a semipermeable membrane. The fluid moves into a higher solute concentration from a lower one (Fig. 7-2). With gases, the driving force of osmosis is produced by the **partial pressure** of the dissolved gases. This is the *osmotic pressure.* These gases include oxygen, nitrogen, carbon dioxide, and water. With nongaseous particles (e.g., electrolytes), the osmotic pressure depends on two factors: (1) the number and molecular weight of particles on each side of the cell membrane and (2) the membrane's permeability to these particles.

> **NOTE** In any mixture of gases, the combination of the pressures exerted by all the gases is the *total pressure.* The pressure exerted by a single gas is the *partial pressure.* The partial pressure of a gas in a mixture is denoted by a *P* preceding the gas (e.g., the partial pressure of oxygen [Po_2] or the partial pressure of carbon dioxide [Pco_2]) (see Chapter 19).

When a living cell is placed in a solution that has a higher solute concentration (and a lower water concentration) than that inside the cell, the solution is called a **hypertonic** solution. When the cell is placed in this solution, the osmotic pressure exerted on it produces a net movement of water out of the cell. This causes the cell to dehydrate, shrink, and possibly die.

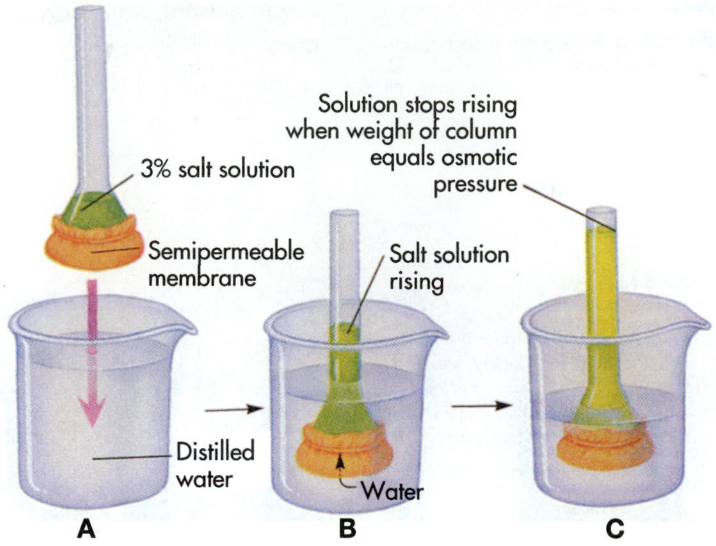

FIGURE 7-2 ■ Osmosis. **A,** The open end of a tube containing a 3% salt solution is closed with a semipermeable membrane; this membrane allows water molecules to pass through but not salt molecules. **B,** The tube is immersed in distilled water. Because it contains both salt and water molecules, the tube has proportionately less water than the beaker, which contains only water. The water molecules from the beaker diffuse with their concentration gradient into the tube through the membrane. Because the salt molecules cannot leave the tube, the total fluid volume inside the tube increases, and the fluid level in the tube rises as a result of osmosis. **C,** Water continues to move into the tube until the weight of the water column in the tube *(hydrostatic pressure)* exerts a downward force equal to the osmotic force moving water molecules into the tube. The hydrostatic pressure that prevents net movement of water into the tube is called the *osmotic pressure* of the solution in the tube.

NOTE Electrolytes are salt substances whose molecules dissociate into charged components when in water, producing positively and negatively charged ions. An ion with a positive charge is called a **cation.** An ion with a negative charge is called an **anion.** Sodium is the most abundant cation in the extracellular fluid (ECF). It is responsible for the osmotic balance of the ECF space. Potassium is the most abundant cation in the intracellular fluid (ICF). It maintains the osmotic balance of the ICF space. The body also has nonelectrolytes (substances with no electrical charge), such as glucose and urea.

Likewise, when a living cell is placed in a solution that has a lower solute concentration (and a higher water concentration) than that inside the cell, the solution is called a **hypotonic** solution. Osmotic pressure draws water from the solution into the cell. The net movement of water into the cell causes it to swell and possibly burst *(lyse).*

A cell may be placed in a solution that has the same solute and water concentration as the solution inside the cell. This solution is called **isotonic**. Isotonic solutions have no net movement of water molecules (Fig. 7-3 and Box 7-1).

DIFFUSION

Diffusion is a result of the constant motion of all the atoms, molecules, or ions in a solution. It is a passive process in which molecules or ions move from an area of higher concentration to an area of lower concentration (Fig. 7-4). An area of high concentration has more solute particles than an area of low concentration. Plus, the particles move randomly. Therefore more solute particles move from the higher concentration to the lower one than travel in the opposite direction. At *equilibrium* the net movement of solute stops. The random motion continues. However, the movement of solutes in one direction is balanced by equal movement in the opposite direction.

The concentration of a solute may be greater at one point in the solvent than it is at another point. This means that a *concentration gradient* exists. Solutes diffuse down their concentration gradients from high to low concentration until equilibrium is achieved. Some nutrients enter and some waste products leave the cell by diffusion. Maintenance of the proper intracellular concentrations of certain substances depends on this process.

CRITICAL THINKING

What happens to a raisin that is put into a cup of water and left there for an hour? Why does this change occur? Is the water hypotonic, hypertonic, or isotonic relative to the inside of the raisin? Does a concentration gradient exist?

MEDIATED TRANSPORT MECHANISMS

A number of vital molecules (e.g., glucose) cannot enter most cells by diffusion. Also, a number of products (e.g., some proteins) cannot exit most cells by diffusion. **Mediated transport mechanisms** are required to move large, water-soluble molecules or electrically charged molecules across the cell membranes. These mechanisms use carrier molecules. *Carrier molecules* are proteins that combine with solute molecules on one side of a membrane. They then change shape, pass through the membrane, and release the solute molecule on the other side (Fig. 7-5).

Carrier-mediated transport can be divided into two types: active transport and facilitated diffusion. **Active transport** moves substances *against* a concentration gradient, from areas of lower concentration to areas of higher concentration. The cell must expend energy to work against this concentration gradient. Active transport occurs at a faster rate than diffusion.

Facilitated diffusion moves substances into and out of cells from an area of higher concentration to an area of lower concentration. For these materials, the direction of movement is *with* the concentration gradient. As with active transport, this movement occurs more quickly than in nor-

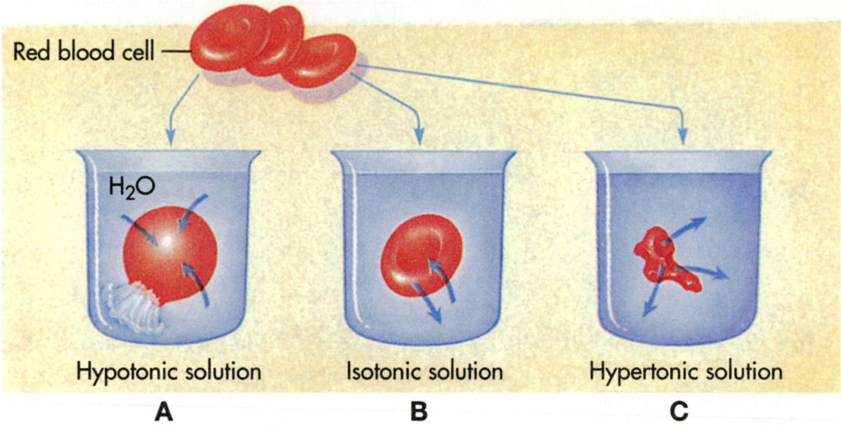

FIGURE 7-3 ■ Effects of hypotonic, isotonic, and hypertonic solutions on red blood cells. **A,** The *hypotonic solution,* which has a low ion concentration, causes swelling and lysis of the cells. **B,** In the *isotonic solution,* which has a normal ion concentration, the cells keep their normal shape. **C,** The *hypertonic solution,* which has a high ion concentration, causes shrinkage *(crenation)* of the cells.

BOX 7-1 Fluid Replacement Therapy

Intravenous therapy is based on hypertonic, hypotonic, and isotonic properties.

Hypertonic Solutions

A *hypertonic solution* has a higher concentration of solute molecules than that found in normal cells. When a hypertonic solution is infused into a normally hydrated patient, it draws water from the cells into the vascular space. Examples of hypertonic solutions are mannitol (Osmitrol), sodium bicarbonate, and 50% dextrose (D_{50}).

These solutions are often used to treat cerebral edema (mannitol), metabolic acidosis (bicarbonate), and profound hypoglycemia (50% dextrose). In addition, recent studies have suggested that some hypertonic solutions (e.g., Dextran, hetastarch, and sodium chloride [3%, 5%, and 7.5%]) should be used for volume restoration after trauma.[3] By drawing tissue fluid into the vascular space, hypertonic solutions may reduce both the volume of the infusion and the occurrence of pulmonary problems after resuscitation.

Hypotonic Solutions

A *hypotonic solution* has a lower solute concentration than that of normal cells. When a hypotonic solution is infused into a normally hydrated patient, water is drawn from the solution into the cells. Hypotonic solutions supply the patient with calories. They also replenish salt and water. They are used to hydrate patients. They are used to prevent dehydration as well. An example of a hypotonic solution is 2.5% dextrose in water. Another is 0.45% normal saline (½NS). Although technically isotonic (see below), 5% dextrose in water (D_5W) acts physiologically as a hypotonic solution. This is because the solute (glucose) is actively transported into cells, leaving excess free water behind.

Isotonic Solutions

In an *isotonic solution,* the concentration of solute molecules is the same as that found in most normal cells. When an isotonic solution is infused into a normally hydrated patient, water is neither drawn out of the cells nor moved into them. Rather, water stays in the vascular space. Isotonic solutions are usually given to replace extracellular fluid. This fluid may have been depleted as a result of blood loss or severe vomiting. In fact, an isotonic solution may be prescribed for any patient in whom the chloride loss equals or exceeds the sodium loss. An example of an isotonic solution is 0.9% normal saline. Another is lactated Ringer solution.

mal diffusion. However, unlike in active transport, facilitated diffusion does not require the cell to expend energy. The moving force in facilitated diffusion is a downhill concentration gradient.

Water Movement Between Plasma and Interstitial Fluid

Fluid is transferred between the circulating blood and the interstitial fluid as a result of pressure changes. These changes occur at the arterial and venous ends of the capillary. The human body has about 10 billion capillaries. Few of the body's functional cells are farther than $^5/_{1000}$ inch (20 to 30 microns) from one.

ANATOMY OF THE CAPILLARY NETWORK

A *capillary* is a thin-walled tube of endothelial cells. Capillaries do not have elastic or connective tissue or smooth muscle that would slow down the transfer of water and solutes. Blood comes into the capillary network from the arterioles. It flows through the capillary network and into the venules. The ends of the capillaries closest to the

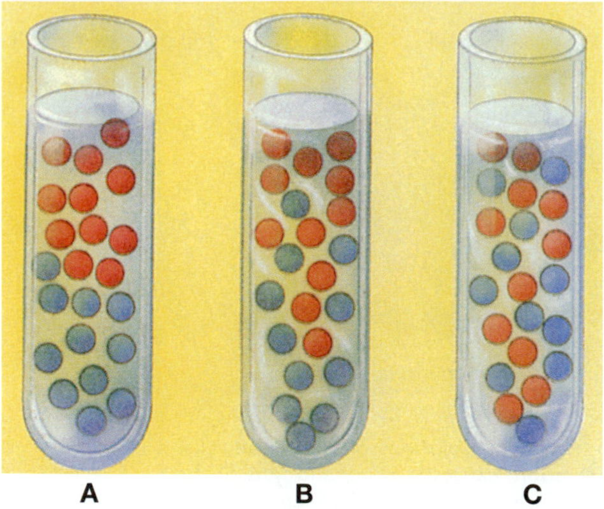

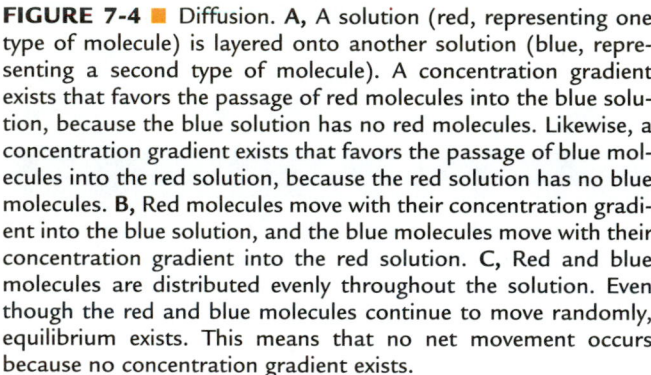

FIGURE 7-4 ■ Diffusion. **A,** A solution (red, representing one type of molecule) is layered onto another solution (blue, representing a second type of molecule). A concentration gradient exists that favors the passage of red molecules into the blue solution, because the blue solution has no red molecules. Likewise, a concentration gradient exists that favors the passage of blue molecules into the red solution, because the red solution has no blue molecules. **B,** Red molecules move with their concentration gradient into the blue solution, and the blue molecules move with their concentration gradient into the red solution. **C,** Red and blue molecules are distributed evenly throughout the solution. Even though the red and blue molecules continue to move randomly, equilibrium exists. This means that no net movement occurs because no concentration gradient exists.

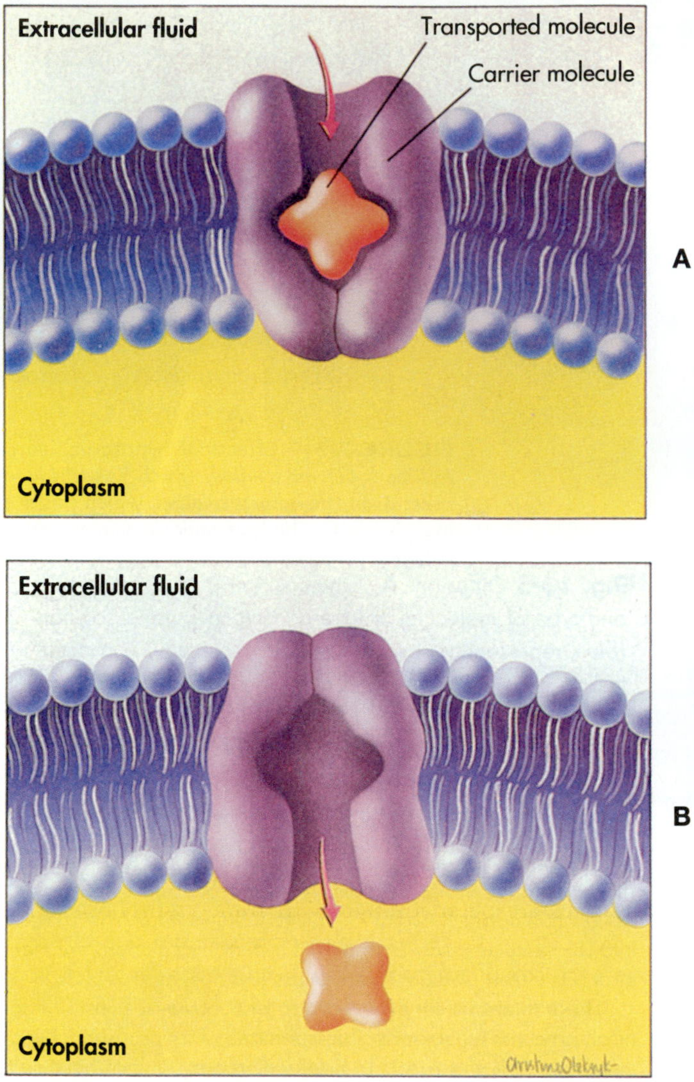

FIGURE 7-5 ■ Mediated transport by a carrier molecule. **A,** The carrier molecule binds with a molecule on one side of the plasma membrane and changes shape. **B,** The molecule is released on the other side of the plasma membrane.

arterioles are *arteriolar capillaries*. The ends closest to the venules are *venous capillaries*. The exchange of nutrients and metabolic end products takes place in the capillaries.

In some tissues the arterioles give rise to metarterioles. The metarterioles then give rise to capillaries. As described in Chapter 6, most tissues appear to have two distinct types of capillaries: true capillaries and thoroughfare channels. From a metarteriole, blood may flow into a thoroughfare channel. A thoroughfare channel connects arterioles and venules directly, bypassing the true capillaries. Blood flow through thoroughfare channels is relatively constant. From the thoroughfare channels, fluid commonly exits and reenters the network of true capillaries.

The capillaries of some tissues have small cuffs of smooth muscle. These cuffs, which encircle the proximal and distal portions of the capillary, are known as *capillary sphincters*. The sphincter at the arterial end is known as the *precapillary sphincter*. The sphincter at the venous end is known as the *postcapillary sphincter*. These sphincters control capillary blood flow. They open and close the entrance and exit of the capillary. Blood flow in true capillaries is not uniform. It depends on the contractile state of the arterioles and the precapillary and postcapillary sphincters (if present).

The blood flows through the capillaries to provide the exchange of gases and solutes between blood and tissue. This is referred to as *nutritional flow*. Blood also bypasses the capillaries in traveling from the arterial to the venous side of the circulation. This is known as *nonnutritional* or *shunt flow*. True arteriovenous anastomoses (AV shunts) occur naturally in the sole of the foot, the palm of the hand, the terminal phalanges, and the nail bed. These shunts are crucial to the regulation of body temperature. Some evidence suggests the presence of AV shunts upstream from the capillary sphincters.

Sympathetic fibers innervate almost all blood vessels of the body, except for the capillaries, the capillary sphincters, and most metarterioles. This innervation of blood vessels includes both vasoconstrictor and vasodilator (vasomotor) fibers. However, the vasoconstrictor fibers are the most critical in regulating blood flow. During normal circulation in the healthy body when arterial blood pressure is adequate,

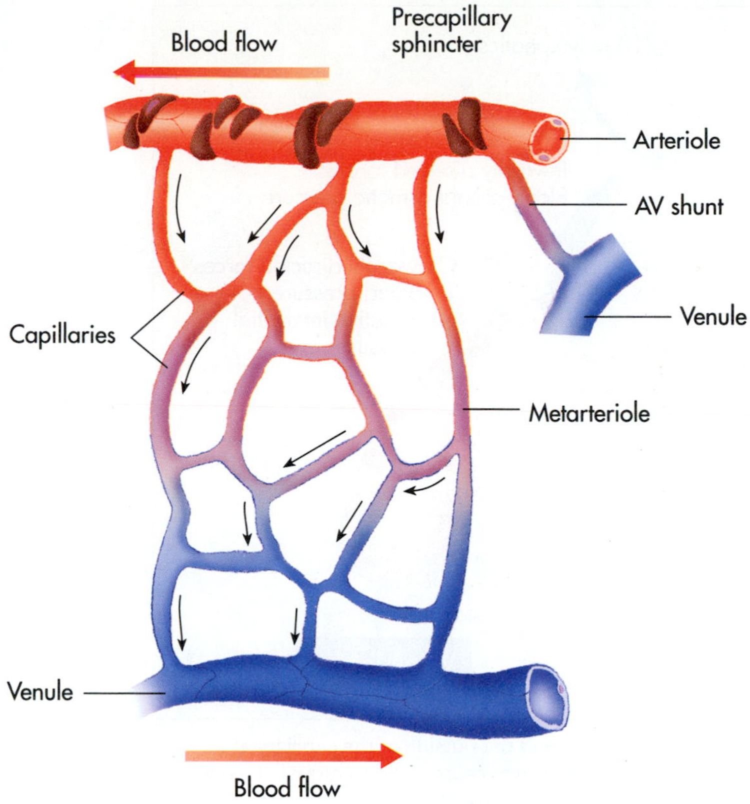

FIGURE 7-6 ■ Microcirculation. The circular structures on the arteriole and venule represent smooth muscle fibers; branching solid lines represent sympathetic nerve fibers. The arrows indicate the direction of blood flow.

arterioles are open (though with some vasomotor tone). Plus, AV shunts are closed. Moreover, about 20% of the capillaries are open at any given time (Fig. 7-6).

Diffusion Across the Capillary Wall. Tissue cells do not exchange material directly with blood. The interstitial fluid always acts as a "middle man." Nutrients must diffuse across the capillary wall into the interstitial fluid to enter cells. Metabolic end products first must move across cell membranes into interstitial fluid to diffuse into the plasma.

At the arteriole end of the capillary, the forces moving fluid out of the capillary are greater than the forces attracting fluid into it. At the venous end, these forces are reversed. Thus more fluid is attracted into the capillary. Hydrostatic and osmotic pressure are the two forces responsible for this movement of fluid. The osmotic pressure results from the presence of plasma proteins (mostly albumin), which are too large to pass through the wall of the capillary; this pressure is referred to as *blood colloid osmotic pressure* or *oncotic pressure.*

At the venous end of the capillary, the hydrostatic pressure is lower. The concentration of proteins in the capillary increases slightly. This occurs because of the movement of fluid out of the arteriolar end. The result is a higher plasma protein concentration and a higher colloid osmotic pressure. Consequently, nearly all the fluid that leaves the capillary at its arteriolar end reenters the capillary at its venous end. The remaining fluid enters the lymphatic capillaries. Eventually it is returned to the general circulation. The movement of fluid back and forth across the capillary wall is called *net filtration.* It is best described by the **Starling hypothesis:**

Net filtration =
Forces favoring filtration − Forces opposing filtration

The forces favoring filtration include capillary hydrostatic pressure and the interstitial oncotic pressure. The forces opposing filtration are the plasma oncotic pressure and the interstitial hydrostatic pressure.

Fluid also may be exchanged across the capillary wall as a result of the cyclic dilation and constriction of the precapillary sphincter. When this sphincter dilates, the pressure rises in the capillary. This forces fluid to move into the interstitial spaces. When the precapillary sphincter constricts, the pressure in the capillary drops. Thus, fluid moves into the capillary (Fig. 7-7).

CAPILLARY AND MEMBRANE PERMEABILITY

A key factor in the passage of fluid back and forth across the capillary wall is the integrity of the membrane. Changes in membrane permeability may allow plasma proteins to escape. The proteins then move into the interstitial space. The ensuing increase in interstitial oncotic pressure changes the relationship defined by the Starling hypothesis. It leads to osmotic movement of water into the interstitial space. This, in turn, results in tissue edema.

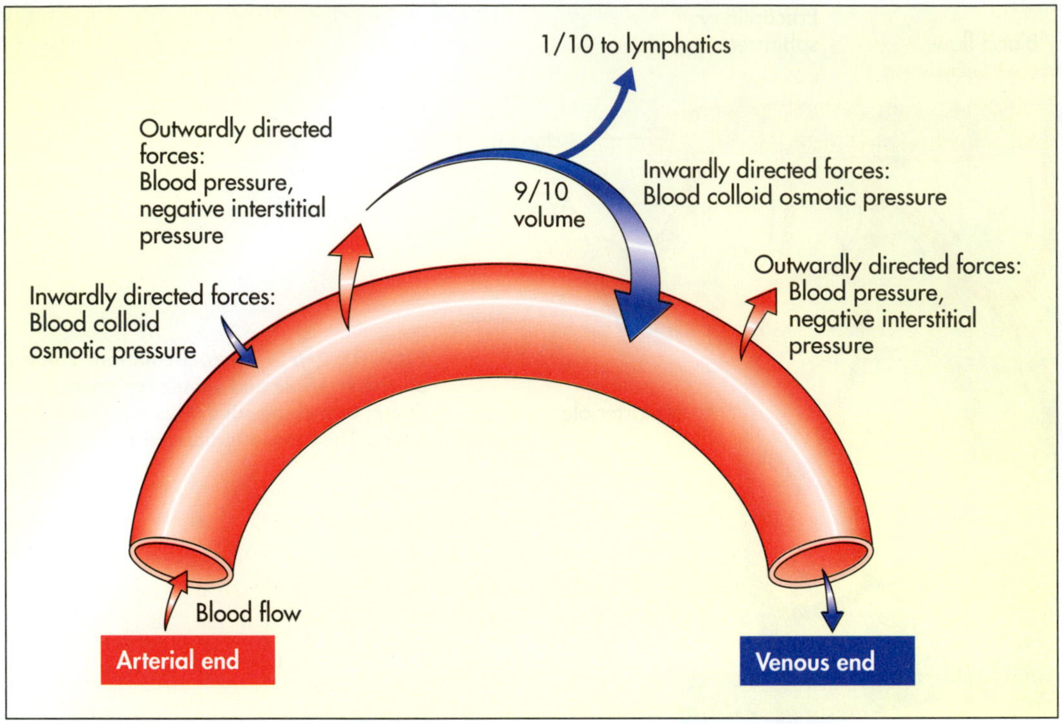

FIGURE 7-7 ■ Total pressure differences between the inside and the outside of the capillary at its arteriolar and venous ends. At the arteriolar end, the sum of the forces causes fluid to move from the capillaries into the tissues. At the venous end, the sum of the forces attracts fluid into the capillary.

Alterations in Water Movement

Edema is the accumulation of fluid in the interstitial spaces. It can be caused by any condition that leads to a net movement of fluid out of capillaries and into the interstitial tissues. Edema is a problem of fluid *distribution.* It does not always indicate a fluid excess.

PATHOPHYSIOLOGY OF EDEMA

Normal flow of fluid through the interstitial spaces depends on four factors:

1. The capillary hydrostatic pressure that filters fluid from the blood through the capillary wall
2. The oncotic pressure exerted by the proteins in the blood plasma, which attracts fluid from the interstitial space back into the vascular compartment
3. The permeability of the capillaries, which determines how easily fluid can pass through the capillary wall
4. The presence of open lymphatic channels, which collect some of the fluid forced out of the capillaries by the hydrostatic pressure of the blood and return the fluid to the circulation

When any of these four factors is altered, changes in water movement can occur. The mechanisms most often responsible for edema are (1) an increase in the hydrostatic pressure, (2) a decrease in the plasma oncotic pressure, (3) an increase in capillary permeability, and (4) lymphatic obstruction.

Increased Capillary Hydrostatic Pressure. An increase in hydrostatic pressure can be caused by venous obstruction. It also can be caused by sodium and water retention. With venous obstruction, the hydrostatic pressure of fluid in the capillaries can become great enough to push fluid out into the interstitial spaces. Conditions that can lead to venous obstruction and edema include thrombophlebitis (the formation of a blood clot and inflammation in a vein), chronic venous disease, hepatic obstruction (blockage of hepatic veins or common bile duct), tight clothing around an extremity, and prolonged standing.

Sodium and water retention can cause an increase in circulating fluid volume (volume overload). It also can cause edema. Congestive heart failure (CHF) and renal failure are two conditions associated with sodium and water retention.

Decreased Plasma Oncotic Pressure. Decreases in plasma albumin lead to a decrease in the plasma oncotic pressure. As a result, fluid moves into the interstitial space. This condition most often results from liver disease or protein malnutrition.

Increased Capillary Permeability. An increase in capillary permeability results in greater than normal filtration of fluid into the interstitial space. This condition often is associated with allergic reactions. It also is linked to inflammation and the immune response triggered by trauma. (The immune response is described later in this chapter.) Examples of such trauma are burns or crushing injuries. In such cases, proteins escape from the vascular bed. As a consequence, the capillary oncotic pressure decreases, and the fluid oncotic pressure increases. The result is edema.

Lymphatic Obstruction. An infection can cause blockage of the lymphatic channels, allowing proteins and fluid to amass in the interstitial space. This obstruction blocks the normal pathway. Thus, fluid is returned from the interstitial space into the circulation. This leads to edema in the region that normally is drained by the channels. Conditions that can cause obstruction in the channels include certain malignancies and parasitic infections. Surgical removal of lymphatics also can block the normal pathways. Surgical removal may occur after a radical mastectomy, which requires removal of the axillary lymph nodes.

CLINICAL MANIFESTATIONS OF EDEMA

Edema may be localized or generalized. Localized edema usually is limited to an injury site or an organ system. For example, an injury site may be a sprained ankle. An affected organ system may be the brain (cerebral edema) or the lungs (pulmonary edema). Edema of specific organs such as the brain, lungs, or larynx can threaten life.

Generalized edema is more widespread. It is most obvious in dependent parts of the body. It usually is noted first in the legs and ankles when the individual is standing or sitting. It is noted in the sacrum and buttocks when the person is lying down. Generalized edema usually causes weight gain, swelling, and puffiness. It often is linked to other symptoms caused by an underlying illness. In industrialized countries, the diseases that most often cause generalized edema are heart disease, kidney disease, and liver disease. In developing countries, the most common causes are malnutrition and parasitic disease. When edematous tissue is compressed with a finger (e.g., over the ankle or tibia), the fluid is pushed aside, leaving a "pit" or indentation that gradually refills with fluid. This condition is called *pitting edema* (Box 7-2). The accumulation of fluid in the peritoneal cavity is a condition called *ascites.*

BOX 7-2 Pitting Edema Scale

+1	Minor pitting of the skin without visible deformation; depression disappears quickly.
+2	No obvious distortion of the skin; depression typically normalizes within 10 to 15 seconds.
+3	Noted deformity of the skin; depression produces a definite pit that persists longer than 1 minute.
+4	Obvious gross deformity of the skin; depression produces a very deep pit that persists longer than 2 minutes.

CRITICAL THINKING

The rest, ice, compression, and elevation (RICE) treatment is used for swelling from a sprained ankle. Why does this treatment reduce tissue edema?

Water Balance, Sodium, and Chloride

Water follows the osmotic gradient established by changes in the sodium concentration. Hence sodium and water balance are closely related.

WATER BALANCE

Water balance is mainly regulated by antidiuretic hormone (ADH) (see Chapter 6). The secretion of ADH and the perception of thirst help regulate water balance. Release of ADH is triggered by an increase in the plasma **osmolality** (the osmotic pressure of a solution). It also may be triggered by a decrease in the circulating blood volume and a decline in venous and arterial pressure. An increase in the plasma osmolality stimulates hypothalamic neurons (called *osmoreceptors*). This causes the individual to feel thirsty. It also increases the release of ADH from the posterior pituitary gland.

In response to the release of ADH, water is reabsorbed into the plasma from the distal renal tubules and collecting ducts of the kidneys. This reduces the amount of water lost in the urine. Also, as the water is reabsorbed, the plasma osmolality decreases, returning to normal. Volume-sensitive receptors, as well as pressure-sensitive receptors (baroreceptors, which are found in the heart and great vessels), also can stimulate the release of ADH when body fluids are depleted. These fluids may be lost from conditions such as vomiting, diarrhea, or excess sweating.

NOTE Volume-sensitive receptors and baroreceptors are nerve endings. They are sensitive to changes in volume or pressure. Volume-sensitive receptors are located in the right and left atria and the thoracic vessels. Baroreceptors are found in the aorta, pulmonary arteries, and carotid sinus.

SODIUM AND CHLORIDE BALANCE

As mentioned before, sodium is the major ECF cation. Sodium balance is regulated by aldosterone. (Aldosterone is a hormone secreted by the adrenal cortex.) Along with chloride and bicarbonate, sodium regulates osmotic forces. Hence, it regulates water balance. (Chloride is the major ECF anion. It provides electroneutrality in relation to sodium. Increases or decreases in chloride occur in proportion to changes in sodium.)

Secretion of aldosterone is triggered by a decrease in sodium levels. It also is triggered by an increase in potassium levels. Aldosterone causes the distal tubules of the kidneys to increase both the reabsorption of sodium and the secretion of potassium.

The enzyme renin also is secreted by the kidneys. This occurs when the circulating blood volume is reduced or the sodium-water balance is disrupted. Renin stimulates the formation of angiotensin I. This is then changed to angiotensin II. Angiotensin II is a potent vasoconstrictor. It acts to stimulate the secretion of ADH, which results in the reabsorption of sodium and water. It also results in an increase in the systemic blood pressure. (This is described later in the chapter.) This mechanism for regulating sodium and water is known as the *renin-angiotensin-aldosterone system* (Fig. 7-8).

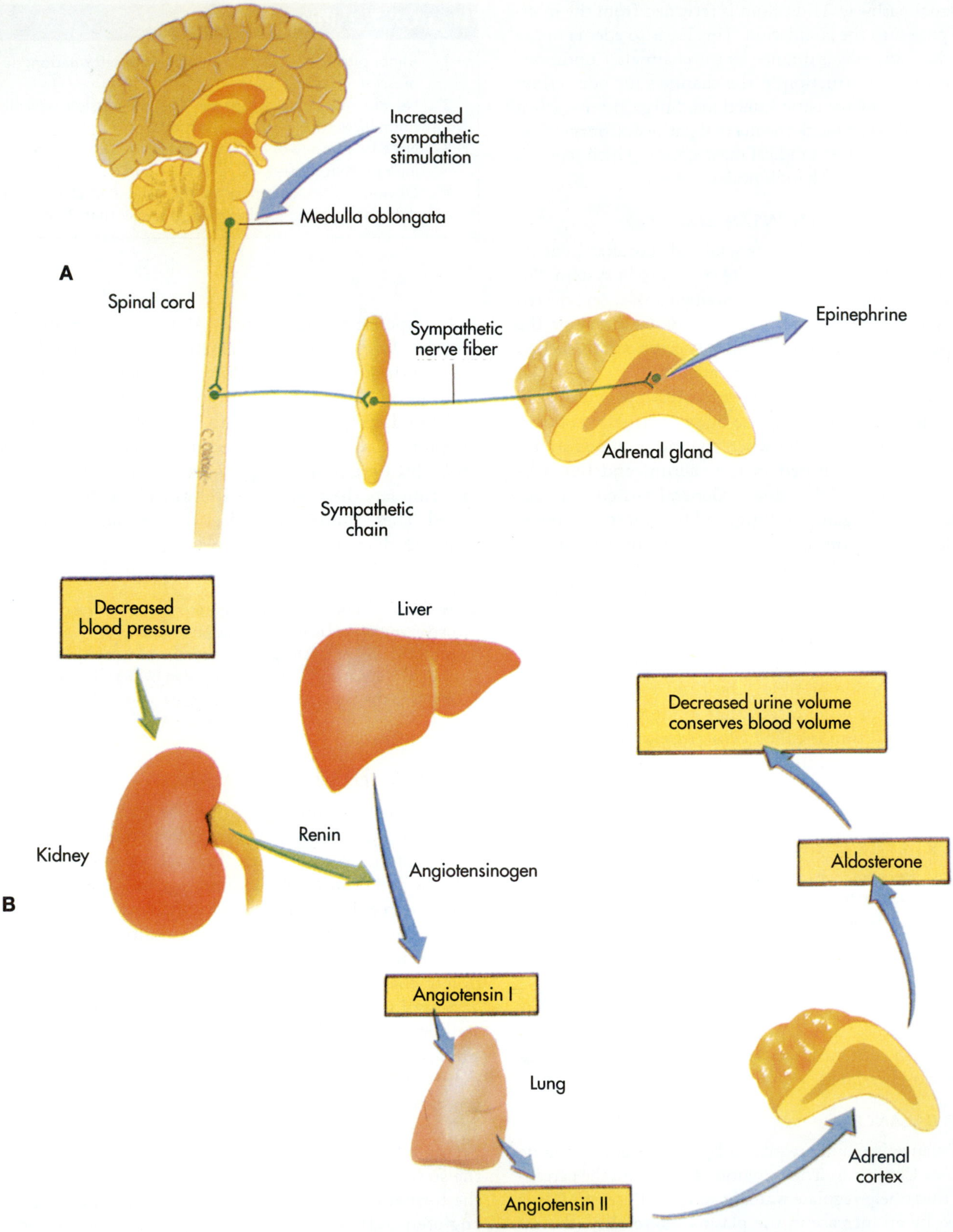

FIGURE 7-8 ■ The roles of the adrenal medulla **(A)**, the renin-angiotensin-aldosterone mechanism **(B)**, and the vasopressin (ADH) mechanism.

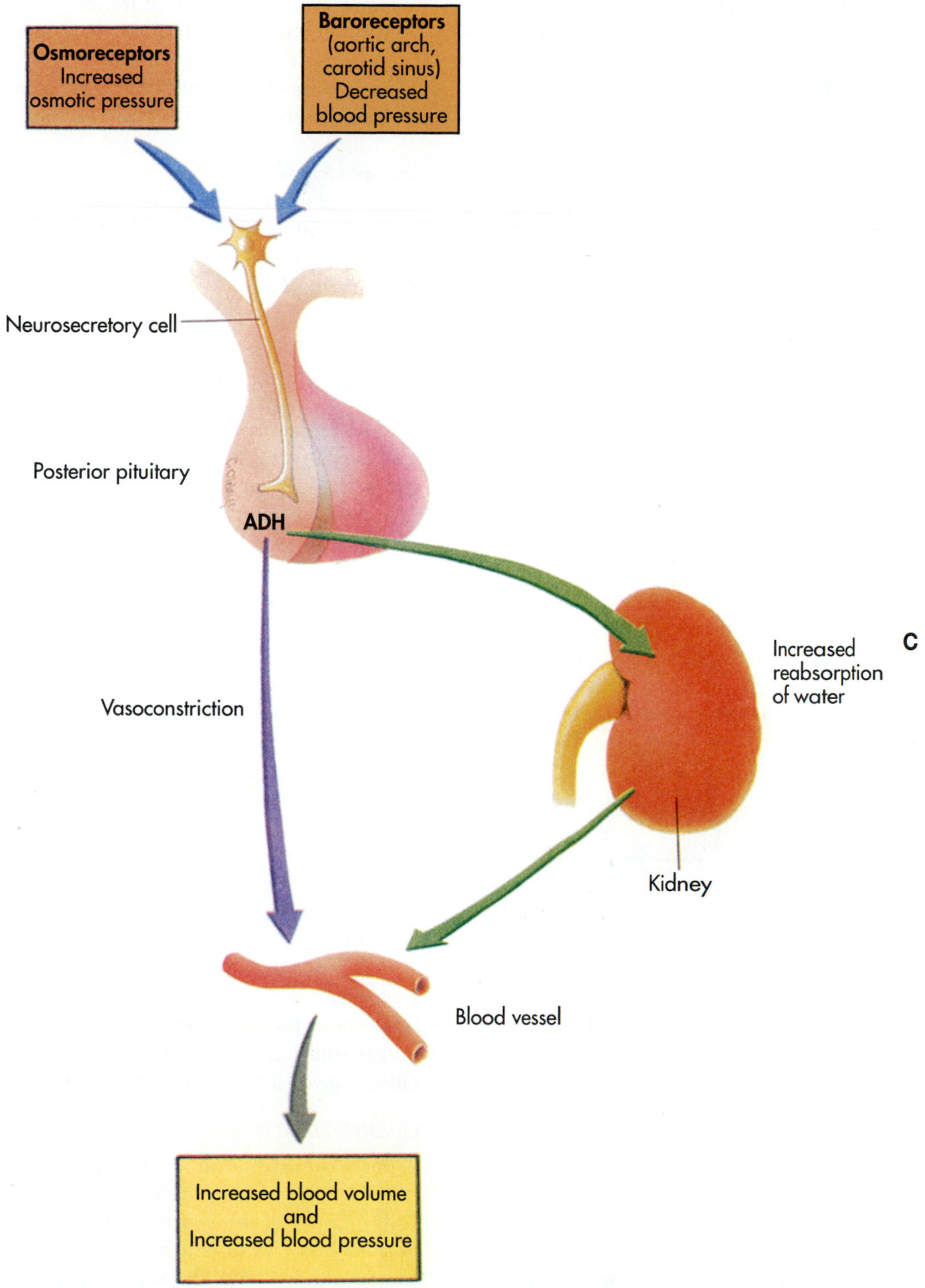

FIGURE 7-8, cont'd ■ (C) The role of the adrenal medulla in regulating blood pressure.

Natriuretic hormone also helps to regulate sodium. It does this by promoting the secretion of sodium in the urine. One result is a decrease in tubular reabsorption of sodium. Another result is a subsequent loss of sodium and water. *Atrial natriuretic factor* is a substance released from the atrial cells of the heart. (It is described in Chapter 6 and later in this chapter.) This substance also helps control the balance of sodium and water. It does this by promoting renal elimination of sodium.

ALTERATIONS IN SODIUM, CHLORIDE, AND WATER BALANCE

In the healthy body, homeostatic mechanisms maintain a constant balance between the intake and excretion of water. The water gained each day basically equals the water lost. The body gains water mainly in two ways: (1) when a person drinks fluids and eats moist foods and (2) when water is formed through the oxidation of hydrogen in food during the metabolic process. The body loses water through the kidneys as urine, through the bowel as feces, through the skin as perspiration, through exhaled air as vapor, and by the excretion of tears and saliva. Two abnormal states of body-fluid balance can occur. If the water lost exceeds the water gained, a water deficit occurs. This is *dehydration.* If the water gained exceeds the water lost, a water excess occurs. This is *overhydration.*

DEHYDRATION

Dehydration may be described in three ways. **Isotonic** dehydration is excessive loss of sodium and water in equal amounts. **Hypernatremic** dehydration is the loss of more water than sodium. **Hyponatremic** dehydration is the loss of more sodium than water.

> **CRITICAL THINKING**
>
> Consider the causes of dehydration and your knowledge of anatomy and physiology. What two age groups do you think are at highest risk for dehydration? Why?

Isotonic Dehydration

Possible Causes

Usually severe or long-term vomiting or diarrhea
Systemic infection
Intestinal obstruction

Signs and Symptoms

Dry skin and mucous membranes
Poor skin turgor
Longitudinal wrinkles or furrows of the tongue
Oliguria (decreased urinary output)
Anuria (essentially no urinary output [100 mL or less in 24 hours])
Acute weight loss
Depressed or sunken fontanelles in infants

Treatment

An intravenous infusion of an isotonic solution is administered. The solution has a solute concentration equal to that of blood (0.9% sodium chloride or normal saline typically is used).

Hypernatremic Dehydration

Possible Causes

Excessive use or misuse of diuretics
Continued intake of sodium in the absence of water consumption
Excessive loss of water with little loss of sodium
Profuse, watery diarrhea

Signs and Symptoms

Dry, sticky mucous membranes
Flushed, doughy skin
Intense thirst
Oliguria or anuria
Increased body temperature
Altered mental status

Treatment

Volume replacement is administered. This usually begins with isotonic fluids, because the patient often is both salt and water depleted, with the water supply being more depleted. (Isotonic fluids are relatively hypotonic in these patients.)

Hyponatremic Dehydration

Possible Causes

Use of diuretics
Excessive perspiration (heat-related illness)
Salt-losing renal disorders
Increased water intake (e.g., excessive use of water enemas)

Signs and Symptoms

Abdominal or muscle cramps
Seizures
Rapid, thready pulse
Diaphoresis (profuse sweating)
Cyanosis

Treatment

Intravenous fluid replacement (i.e., normal saline or lactated Ringer solution) is administered. Occasionally, hypertonic saline is given (e.g., in seizures caused by hyponatremia).

OVERHYDRATION

Because overhydration is an increase in body water, it results in a decrease in the solute concentration. (The total body amount of solute actually may be increased. However, because body water is increased more, the solute concentration is decreased.) This water excess may result from parenteral administration of excessive fluids, impaired cardiac function, impaired renal function, or some endocrine dysfunctions. Signs and symptoms of overhydration may include the following:

- Shortness of breath
- Puffy eyelids
- Edema

TABLE 7-2 Electrolyte Concentrations of Intracellular and Extracellular Fluid

Predominant Cations	Predominant Anions
Intracellular	*Intracellular*
Potassium (K^+)	Phosphate (PO_4^{3-})
Calcium (Ca^{++})	
Magnesium (Mg^{++})	*Extracellular*
	Chloride (Cl-)
Extracellular	Bicarbonate (HCO_3^-)
Sodium (Na^+)	

- Polyuria (voiding of a large volume of urine within a given time)
- Moist crackles (on pulmonary examination)
- Acute weight gain

Treatment for overhydration depends on the cause. Water restriction is the main treatment for excessive water administration. It also is the main treatment for certain endocrine problems. A diuretic may be indicated for patients with cardiac impairment. It also may be the treatment for renal impairment. When profound hyponatremia is associated with overhydration (a low serum sodium level and associated seizures or altered consciousness), administration of saline may be indicated.

ELECTROLYTE IMBALANCES

In addition to water and sodium imbalances, disturbances may occur in the balance of electrolytes other than sodium. These electrolytes include potassium, calcium, and magnesium (Table 7-2).

Potassium. Potassium is the major positively charged ion in ICF. The body must keep potassium levels within a narrow range. This allows normal function of the nerves, cardiac system, and skeletal muscle. *Obligate* potassium losses are losses that cannot be avoided. These usually are minimal. In addition, they normally can be replenished through the diet. Excess potassium usually is excreted by the kidneys. Potassium plays a key role in muscle contraction, enzyme action, nerve impulses, and cell membrane function. Potassium imbalances interfere with neuromuscular function. They may cause cardiac rhythm disturbances *(dysrhythmias)*. These may even include sudden cardiac death.

Hypokalemia is an abnormally *low* level of *potassium* in the blood. It can be caused by reduced dietary intake (rare), poor potassium absorption, increased gastrointestinal losses from vomiting or diarrhea, renal disease, infusion of solutions low in potassium, or the use of some medications (most commonly diuretics, but steroids, theophylline, and others have also been implicated). The most common cause of hypokalemia in the United States is the use of diuretics. Signs and symptoms of hypokalemia may include the following:

- Malaise
- Skeletal muscle weakness
- Cardiac dysrhythmias
- Decreased reflexes
- Weak pulse
- Faint or distant heart sounds
- Shallow respiration
- Low blood pressure
- Anorexia
- Vomiting
- Gaseous distention
- Excessive thirst (rare)

In-hospital treatment of hypokalemia involves intravenous or oral administration of potassium.

CRITICAL THINKING

What common illness mimics many of the signs and symptoms of fluid and electrolyte imbalance?

Hyperkalemia is an abnormally *high* level of *potassium* in the blood. This condition may be caused by acute or chronic renal failure, burns, crush injuries, severe infections or other conditions in which large amounts of potassium are released, excessive use of potassium salts, and a shift of potassium from the cells into the extracellular fluid (such as occurs in acidosis). Signs and symptoms of hyperkalemia may include the following:

- Cardiac conduction disturbances
- Irritability
- Abdominal distention
- Nausea
- Diarrhea
- Oliguria
- Weakness (an early sign) and paralysis (a late sign) of severe hyperkalemia

In-hospital treatment for hyperkalemia involves restriction of potassium. It also involves giving a cation exchange resin. This can be done orally or through a nasogastric tube. In an emergency, administration of ***calcium*** intravenously can save a patient's life. This is especially true with cardiac dysrhythmias, which are life-threatening. Other critical efforts include intravenous administration of glucose and ***insulin.*** This helps to lower the serum potassium level. It forces potassium intracellularly along with the glucose. ***Sodium bicarbonate*** also causes potassium to shift back into the cells.

Calcium. Calcium is a *bivalent cation* (an ion with two positive charges). It is essential for a variety of body functions. These include neuromuscular transmission, cell membrane permeability, hormone secretion, growth and ossification of bones, and muscle contraction (including smooth, cardiac, and skeletal muscle). Calcium intake in a balanced diet usually is sufficient for normal body needs. However, growing evidence suggests that certain groups (e.g., pregnant and lactating women) may have a shortage of calcium in their diets. Calcium is excreted through urine, feces, and perspiration.

Hypocalcemia is an abnormally *low* level of *calcium* in the blood. It may result from endocrine dysfunction (mostly underactivity of the parathyroid gland); renal insufficiency; a decreased intake or malabsorption of calcium; or a deficiency of, malabsorption of, or inability to activate vitamin D (which is responsible for calcium absorption). Signs and symptoms of hypocalcemia may include the following:

- Paresthesia (numbness or tingling sensation)
- Tetany (muscle twitching)
- Abdominal cramps
- Muscle cramps
- Neural excitability
- Personality changes
- Abnormal behavior
- Convulsions

In-hospital treatment for hypocalcemia involves intravenous administration of calcium ions. Calcium salt and vitamin D may be given orally for maintenance.

Hypercalcemia is an abnormally *high* level of *calcium* in the blood. It may be caused by various tumors. Other common causes include parathyroid overactivity, thyroid dysfunction, diuretic therapy, and excessive administration of vitamin D (as in the treatment of osteoporosis). Calcium can be deposited in various body tissues. These include many organ systems. Examples include the gastrointestinal system, central nervous system, renal system, neuromuscular system, and cardiovascular system. Signs and symptoms of hypercalcemia include the following:

- Hypotonicity of the muscles (decreased muscle tone or tension)
- Renal stones
- Altered mental status
- Deep bone pain

The treatment of hypercalcemia aims to control the underlying disease. It may include hydration. At times it also may include drug therapy to decrease the calcium level. In-hospital therapy for severe hypercalcemia may include forced diuresis with normal saline and ***furosemide.*** The patient also may be given calcium-lowering drugs. Examples of these are thyrocalcitonin, steroids (glucocorticoids), and plicamycin (a cytotoxic drug that inhibits bone reabsorption of calcium).

> **NOTE** Changes in the level of phosphate in the blood also can occur. This can result in hypophosphatemia or hyperphosphatemia. *Hypophosphatemia,* an abnormally low serum phosphate level, may be caused by intestinal malabsorption or increased excretion of phosphate by the kidneys. *Hyperphosphatemia,* an abnormally high serum phosphate level, is associated with acute or chronic renal failure or diminished activity of the parathyroid gland.

Magnesium. Like calcium, magnesium is a bivalent cation. It activates many enzymes. Magnesium is distributed throughout the body roughly as follows: 50% in an insoluble state in bone; 45% as an intracellular cation; and 5% in extracellular solution. Magnesium is excreted by the kidneys. Its physiological effects on the nervous system resemble those of calcium.

Hypomagnesemia is an abnormally *low* level of *magnesium* in the blood. It may be encountered in conditions involving alcoholism, diabetes, malabsorption, starvation, diarrhea, diuresis, and diseases that cause hypocalcemia and hypokalemia. The condition is characterized by increased irritability of the central nervous system. Signs and symptoms of hypomagnesemia include the following:

- Tremors
- Nausea or vomiting
- Diarrhea
- Hyperactive deep reflexes
- Confusion (including hallucinations)
- Seizures or myoclonus (muscle spasms)
- Cardiac dysrhythmias (which may lead to cardiac arrest)

In-hospital treatment for significant, symptomatic hypomagnesemia involves intravenous administration of a solution that contains magnesium. Most commonly this would be magnesium sulfate.

Hypermagnesemia is an abnormally *high* level of *magnesium* in the blood. It occurs mainly in patients with chronic renal insufficiency. It also can occur in patients who take large amounts of magnesium-containing compounds. Examples of such compounds are cathartics (e.g., magnesium citrate, magnesium sulfate) and antacids (e.g., magnesium hydroxide). Hypermagnesemia causes central nervous system depression, profound muscular weakness, and areflexia (absence of reflexes). It also causes cardiac rhythm disturbances, which may lead to sudden death. Signs and symptoms of hypermagnesemia include the following:

- Sedation
- Confusion
- Muscle weakness
- Respiratory paralysis

The most effective treatment for hypermagnesemia is hemodialysis. It can return blood levels to normal in about 4 hours. Calcium salts may be given parenterally as well. These act as an antagonist to magnesium. Administration of intravenous glucose and ***insulin*** also drives magnesium back into the cells. This treatment can be used in emergencies when respiratory depression or cardiac conduction defects are present.

Acid-Base Balance

Acids are produced by the body through normal metabolism. Two types of acids are produced: *respiratory acids* (culminating in carbon dioxide [CO_2]) and *nonrespiratory (metabolic) acids.* Bases are used in metabolic disturbances to return the body's plasma to normal. For physiologic functioning, the balance between acids and bases must be kept in a narrow range. The body's main regulators of acid-base balance are the lungs and the kidneys. The lungs secrete respiratory acids. The kidneys secrete metabolic acids.

pH

Hydrogen ions are protons with a positive charge. In chemistry, a hydrogen ion that loses its charge is marked with a positive sign (H+). Likewise, a hydrogen ion that gains a

BOX 7-3 pH Values

A solution of pH 1 is 1 million times as acidic as a solution of pH 7.
pH 2 is 100,000 times as acidic as pH 7.
pH 3 is 10,000 times as acidic as pH 7.
pH 4 is 1000 times as acidic as pH 7.
pH 5 is 100 times as acidic as pH 7.
pH 6 is 10 times as acidic as pH 7.
pH 7 is neutral (distilled water).
pH 8 is 1⁄10 as acidic as pH 7, or 10 times as alkaline.
pH 9 is 1⁄100 as acidic as pH7, or 100 times as alkaline.

charge is marked with a negative sign (H−). *Acids* are materials that release or donate hydrogen ions. *Bases* (alkaline substances) receive, or absorb, hydrogen ions. Thus, they neutralize positive charged ions. The concentration of hydrogen ions is expressed as the **pH.** This stands for the *potential for hydrogen.* The pH is the negative logarithm (base 10) of the hydrogen ion concentration. It is measured as activity in moles per liter. A mole (in chemistry) is 6.023 multiplied by 10^{23} molecules (the Avogadro number). Paramedics do not need to grasp the meaning of a number this large in real terms. However, they must understand the importance of a small change in pH: *The strength of an acid or a base changes by 10 times with **each** unit change of pH.* For example, a pH that changes by 0.3 unit (e.g., from 7.4 to 7.1) doubles the concentration of hydrogen ions (Box 7-3). The pH is neutral (6.8 to 7) when equal numbers of positive and negative ions are present. A solution increases in acidity as the pH increases. It increases in alkalinity (basicity) as the pH falls (Fig. 7-9).

BUFFER SYSTEMS

The healthy body is sensitive to changes in the concentration of hydrogen ions. In fact, it tries to maintain the pH of extracellular fluid at 7.4. This is carried out through three related compensatory mechanisms. These are carbonic acid–bicarbonate buffering, protein buffering, and renal buffering. These mechanisms are stimulated by changes in the pH. They require normal organ function to be effective in maintaining acid-base balance.

Carbonic Acid–Bicarbonate Buffering. Bicarbonate, carbon dioxide, and carbonic acid are always present in a dynamic balance in the blood. Bicarbonate (HCO_3^-) arises from the transport of carbon dioxide in the blood. Under the influence of the enzyme carbonic anhydrase, carbon dioxide dissolves in the water of blood. It reacts with water in red blood cells to form carbonic acid (H_2CO_3). Carbonic acid breaks down into hydrogen and bicarbonate ions. At a physiological pH of 7.4, the normal ratio of carbonic acid to bicarbonate is 1:20 and is summarized by the chemical equation:

$$CO_2 + H_2O \rightarrow H_2CO_3 \rightarrow H^+ + HCO_3^-$$

Bicarbonate may link up with a cation to form base bicarbonate (e.g., $NaHCO_3$). The ratio of carbonic acid to base bicarbonate determines the pH. As long as there is 1 millequivalent (mEq) of carbonic acid for each 20 mEq of base bicarbonate in the extracellular fluid, the pH stays within normal limits.

NOTE A millequivalent (see Chapter 18) is the number of grams of solute dissolved in 1 mL of a normal solution.

The carbonic acid-bicarbonate compensatory mechanism is triggered immediately by changes in pH. The respiratory rate helps maintain this balance (Fig. 7-10).

Protein Buffering. Both intracellular and extracellular proteins have negative charges. Both also can serve as buffers for changes in the pH. However, most proteins are inside cells. Protein buffering, therefore, is mainly an intracellular buffer system. Hemoglobin (Hb) is an excellent intracellular buffer, because it can bind with hydrogen ions (forming a weak acid) and carbon dioxide.

After oxygen is released in the peripheral tissues, hemoglobin binds with carbon dioxide and hydrogen ions. As the blood reaches the lungs, these actions reverse themselves. Hemoglobin binds with oxygen, releasing carbon dioxide and hydrogen ions. The hydrogen ions released combine with bicarbonate ions, forming carbonic acid. The carbonic acid breaks down into carbon dioxide and water. Then the lungs exhale the carbon dioxide. Therefore, in normal circumstances, respirations help maintain pH. The respiratory centers are more responsive to pH changes than to changes in the oxygen level of the tissues. For this reason, the amount of carbon dioxide in the blood (and hence the pH), rather than the need for oxygen in the tissues, controls the rate of breathing in healthy individuals. Within minutes of a decrease in the pH, alveolar ventilation increases in an effort to lower the carbon dioxide concentration.

Renal Buffering. The kidneys help maintain an acid-base balance through three mechanisms. One is the recovery of bicarbonate, which is filtered into the tubules. Another is the excretion of hydrogen ions against a gradient to acidify the urine. The third is the excretion of ammonium ions (NH_4), each of which carries a hydrogen ion with it. The renal system makes up for acid-base imbalances slowly compared with the protein and bicarbonate buffer systems. The kidneys can take several hours to days to restore the pH to the normal physiological range.

NOTE The concentration of carbonic acid is controlled by the lungs. (Carbonic acid is dissolved carbon dioxide.) The concentration of bicarbonate is controlled by the kidneys.

ACID-BASE IMBALANCE

As stated before, acid-base balance is maintained mainly through two factors: a respiratory element and a metabolic element. Any condition that increases the carbonic acid or

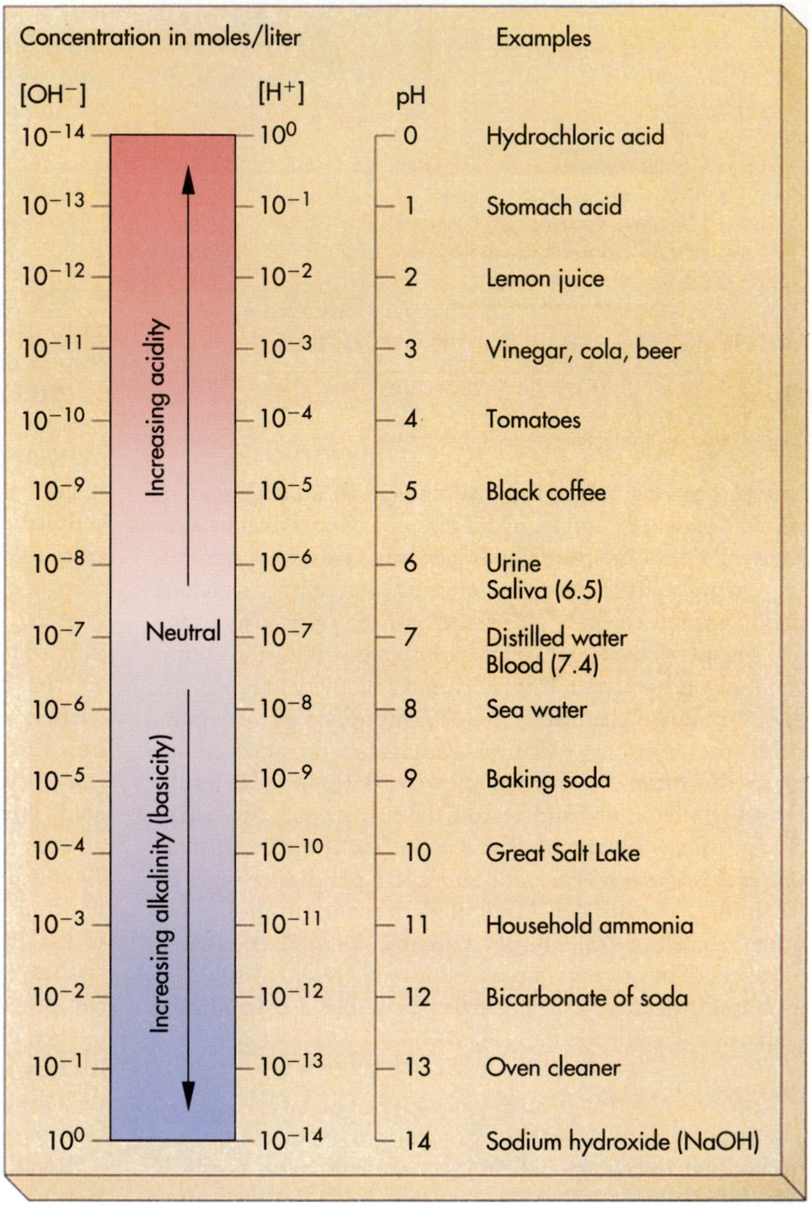

Concentration in moles/liter
Examples
[OH⁻]
[H⁺]
pH
10^-14 — 10^0 — 0 Hydrochloric acid
10^-13 — 10^-1 — 1 Stomach acid
10^-12 — 10^-2 — 2 Lemon juice
10^-11 — 10^-3 — 3 Vinegar, cola, beer
10^-10 — 10^-4 — 4 Tomatoes
10^-9 — 10^-5 — 5 Black coffee
10^-8 — 10^-6 — 6 Urine, Saliva (6.5)
10^-7 — Neutral — 10^-7 — 7 Distilled water, Blood (7.4)
10^-6 — 10^-8 — 8 Sea water
10^-5 — 10^-9 — 9 Baking soda
10^-4 — 10^-10 — 10 Great Salt Lake
10^-3 — 10^-11 — 11 Household ammonia
10^-2 — 10^-12 — 12 Bicarbonate of soda
10^-1 — 10^-13 — 13 Oven cleaner
10^0 — 10^-14 — 14 Sodium hydroxide (NaOH)
Increasing acidity
Increasing alkalinity (basicity)

FIGURE 7-9 ■ The pH scale. A pH of 7 is considered neutral. Values less than 7 are acidic (the lower the number, the more acidic the substance). Values greater than 7 are basic (the higher the number, the more basic the substance). Representative fluids and their approximate pH values are listed.

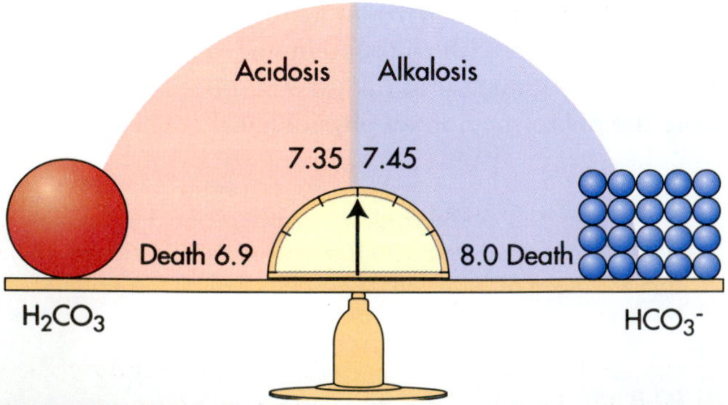

FIGURE 7-10 ■ Bicarbonate buffer system. When body fluids are in acid-base balance, the ratio of bicarbonate (HCO_3) to carbonic acid ($H_2CO_3^-$) normally is 20:1, and the pH is between 7.35 and 7.45.

decreases the base bicarbonate causes **acidosis.** Any condition that increases base bicarbonate or decreases carbonic acid causes **alkalosis.** In discussing acid-base imbalance, it is important to remember that acidosis makes the pH more acidic than normal. Alkalosis makes the pH less acidic than normal. Also, a patient can have both disorders at the same time (e.g., respiratory acidosis *and* metabolic alkalosis). When two disturbances are present, one usually dominates. The other attempts to compensate.

ACIDOSIS

The accumulation of acid and the resulting acidosis cause the pH to be more acidic compared to the normal pH of 7.4. (A decrease in pH means an increase acidity.) A discussion of respiratory and metabolic acidosis follows.

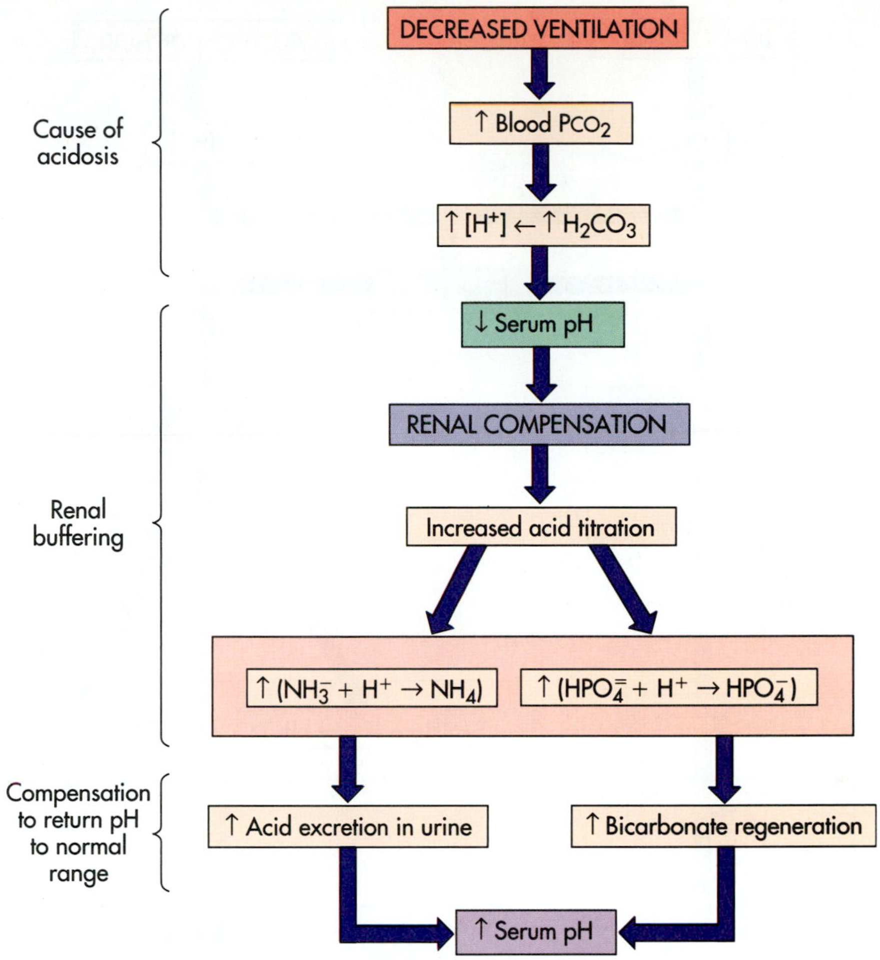

FIGURE 7-11 ■ Respiratory acidosis. An excess of carbon dioxide in the body results in acidosis.

Respiratory Acidosis. Respiratory acidosis is caused by the retention of carbon dioxide. This leads to an increase in the partial pressure of carbon dioxide (Pco_2). This state usually is caused by an imbalance in the production of carbon dioxide and its elimination through alveolar ventilation (Fig. 7-11). Respiratory acidosis can be summarized by the following chemical equation:

$$\downarrow \text{Respiration} = \uparrow CO_2 + H_2O \rightarrow \uparrow H_2CO_3 \rightarrow \uparrow H^+ + HCO_3^-$$

Reductions in alveolar ventilation may occur as a result of the following:

- Respiratory depression
- Respiratory arrest
- Cardiac arrest
- Neuromuscular impairment
- Medications (sedatives, hypnotics)
- Chest wall injury (e.g., flail chest, pneumothorax)
- Pulmonary disorders (e.g., airway obstruction, chronic obstructive pulmonary disease, pulmonary edema)

▶NOTE In respiratory acidosis, the primary abnormality is failure of the lungs to excrete carbon dioxide efficiently.

When the respiratory system cannot continue as a compensatory mechanism to correct the acidosis, the body's renal system must conserve bicarbonate and excrete more hydrogen ions to help bring the pH into normal limits. The kidneys take some time to restore pH. Thus, the patient in respiratory acidosis should be treated by improving ventilation to quickly eliminate carbon dioxide. This may be done by assisting ventilations to decrease the Pco_2. Supplemental oxygen also should be given to help correct any accompanying hypoxemia (which itself can lead to acidosis).

CRITICAL THINKING

What kind of acid-base imbalance exists in a patient you have just defibrillated and resuscitated from cardiac arrest? How are you going to treat that imbalance?

Metabolic Acidosis. Metabolic acidosis results from a buildup of acid or a loss of base. When excessive acid is produced by the body, the acid spills into the extracellular fluid. This, in turn, consumes some bicarbonate buffers. The result is an increase in acid and a decrease in available

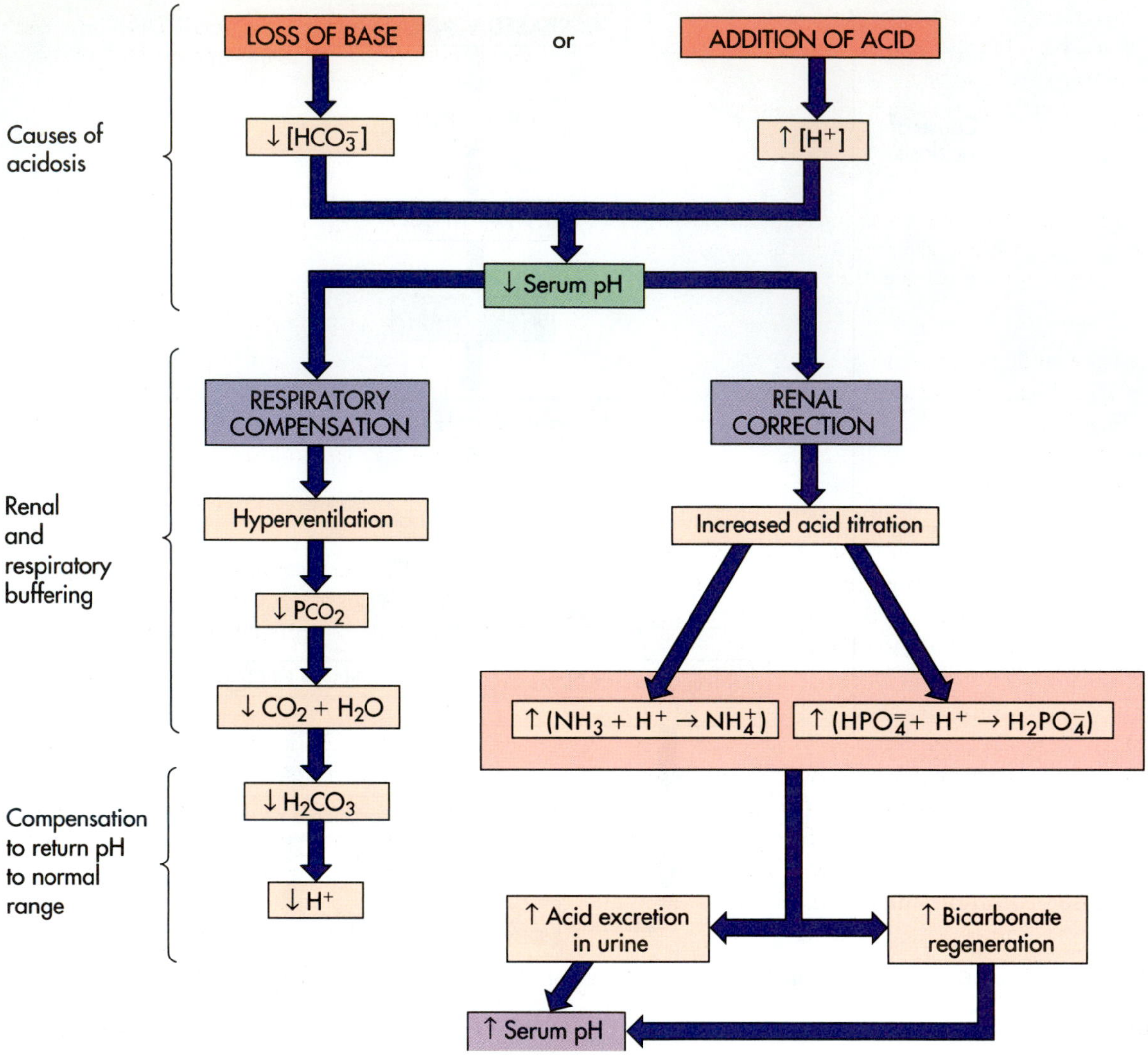

FIGURE 7-12 ■ Metabolic acidosis. With an excess of metabolic acids, bicarbonate is consumed and hydrogen ions are liberated, resulting in acidosis.

base (Fig. 7-12). Metabolic acidosis can be summarized by the following equation:

$$\uparrow H^+ + HCO_3^- \rightarrow \uparrow H_2CO_3 \rightarrow H_2O + \uparrow CO_2$$

The increase in available hydrogen ions forces the reaction to the right. This decreases the amount of base bicarbonate.

> **NOTE** Metabolic acidosis occurs when the amount of acid generated by the body exceeds the body's buffering capacity.

The healthy respiratory system instantly tries to make up for the acidosis. It does this by increasing the rate and depth of breathing to reduce carbon dioxide. As the carbon dioxide level falls, so does the concentration of carbonic acid. This moves the pH toward normal. In addition, the kidneys excrete more hydrogen ion to equilibrate the excess acid in the extracellular fluid.

The four most common forms of metabolic acidosis encountered in the prehospital setting are lactic acidosis, diabetic ketoacidosis, acidosis caused by renal failure, and acidosis caused by ingestion of toxins (poisons).

Lactic Acidosis. Lactic acid is made when a large number of cells are inadequately perfused. This results in a shift from **aerobic** (with oxygen) to **anaerobic** (without oxygen) metabolism. The end product of anaerobic metabolism is lactic acid. The lactic acid releases hydrogen ions and becomes lactate. This creates systemic acidosis. Normally, the liver changes lactate back into glucose, or lactate is oxidized to carbon dioxide and water. When lactic acid is produced faster than it is metabolized, **lactic acidosis** occurs. The most common causes of systemic lactic acidosis are extreme exertional states (e.g., seizures), **ischemia** (reduced blood supply) in large muscles or organs (e.g., mesenteric ischemia), circulatory failure, and shock. Specific complications associated with lactic acidosis are thought to include the following:

- Decreased force of cardiac contraction
- Decreased peripheral response to catecholamines
- Hypotension and shock
- Cardiac muscle that is refractory to defibrillation

CRITICAL THINKING

Think about the last time you ran so fast you had a muscle cramp. What acid-base changes were going on inside your body? How did your body compensate for those changes?

Treatment of lactic acidosis involves reestablishing tissue perfusion and cardiac output. This allows the liver to regenerate bicarbonate by metabolizing lactate to carbon dioxide and water. Medical direction may advise paramedics to use hyperventilation to induce respiratory alkalosis, vigorous rehydration to support circulation, and perhaps intravenous administration of ***sodium bicarbonate*** for immediate compensation (if the patient is in cardiac arrest). Correction of lactic acidosis often depends on identification and correction of the underlying cause.

Diabetic Ketoacidosis. Ketoacidosis usually is a complication of diabetes mellitus. It also may be seen in alcoholics (alcoholic ketoacidosis). Diabetic ketoacidosis usually results when a patient fails to take adequate ***insulin.*** It also may develop when the need for insulin increases. This may occur, for example, in cases of infection or trauma. Insulin is required for many cells to absorb glucose. With impaired glucose utilization, fatty acids are metabolized, producing ketone bodies and releasing hydrogen ions. Large amounts of ketone bodies exceed the ability of the body's buffering system to compensate. This results in acidosis and a decrease in blood pH. Prehospital care for patients with diabetic ketoacidosis involves administration of normal saline for volume repletion. (The pathophysiology of this disorder is further addressed in Chapter 32.)

Acidosis Caused by Renal Failure. The kidneys help maintain acid-base balance. They do this by reabsorbing or secreting either bicarbonate or hydrogen ions as needed. This keeps the pH constant. Renal failure affects the compensatory mechanisms of the kidneys to varying degrees. Patients with moderate to severe renal failure often have mild to moderate acidosis. Acidosis results because the failing kidneys are unable to excrete the acid waste products efficiently. These waste products are the result of normal metabolic processes.

Acidosis Caused by Ingestion of Toxins. Ingestion of some toxins can cause metabolic acidosis. Examples of such toxins are ethylene glycol, methanol, and salicylate, a component of aspirin. These and other toxins lead to the production of toxic metabolites. They may result in acid-base disorders. These disorders are characterized by metabolic acidosis and compensatory respiratory alkalosis. Treatment for various toxic ingestions frequently includes gastrointestinal evacuation but also may require hemodialysis, diuresis, hydration to promote excretion, and specific antagonistic or antidotal therapy.

NOTE In a patient with renal failure, administration of intravenous (IV) fluids may rapidly lead to overhydration.

ALKALOSIS

Alkalosis causes the blood and body fluids to be less acidic compared to the normal pH of 7.4. (An increase in pH means a decrease in acidity.)

Respiratory Alkalosis. Hyperventilation may produce respiratory alkalosis by decreasing the Pco_2 (Fig. 7-13). Hyperventilation is common in patients who are acutely ill. It is often seen in the early stages of sepsis, peritonitis, shock, and respiratory ailments. Respiratory alkalosis can be summarized by the following chemical equation:

$$\uparrow \text{Respiration} = \downarrow CO_2 + H_2O \rightarrow \downarrow H_2CO_3 \rightarrow \downarrow H^+ + HCO_3^-$$

NOTE Respiratory alkalosis is caused by hyperventilation. This lowers the partial pressure of carbon dioxide (Pco_2) in the *alveoli* (the air cells in the lungs) and subsequently the Pco_2 in the blood.

When carbonic acid is lacking because of excessive elimination of carbon dioxide, the blood pH rises. Thus, the kidneys must excrete bicarbonate ions and retain hydrogen ions. They do this in an effort to return the pH to normal. Treatment of respiratory alkalosis is directed at correcting the underlying cause of the hyperventilation. An initial approach is to place the patient on low-concentration oxygen. Another is to provide calming measures to assist the patient with slow, controlled breathing.

Metabolic Alkalosis. Metabolic alkalosis (rare) most often results from loss of hydrogen ions (primarily from the stomach), ingestion of large amounts of absorbable base sodium bicarbonate (baking soda) or calcium carbonate (Tums, other antacids), or excessive intravenous administration of alkali (e.g., intravenous injection of ***sodium bicarbonate***). The use of diuretics also may be a factor (Fig. 7-14). Metabolic alkalosis can be summarized by the following chemical equation:

$$\downarrow H^+ + HCO_3^- \rightarrow \downarrow H_2CO_3^- \rightarrow H_2O + \downarrow CO_2$$

The loss of hydrogen ions is the initial cause of metabolic alkalosis. This may result from vomiting (loss of hydrochloric acid), gastric suction, or increased renal excretion of hydrogen ions in the urine. When vomiting occurs, gastric acid is lost, but volume also is depleted.

Chronic use of diuretics can result in volume depletion. The loss of sodium chloride and potassium causes a relative increase in bicarbonate. (The kidneys defend against volume depletion. They increase reabsorption of sodium and thus water.) When sodium is reabsorbed, either potassium or hydrogen ions must be excreted. This action helps to maintain electrical neutrality. The excretion of hydrogen ions can lead to a net increase in bicarbonate. This, in turn, can lead to metabolic alkalosis.

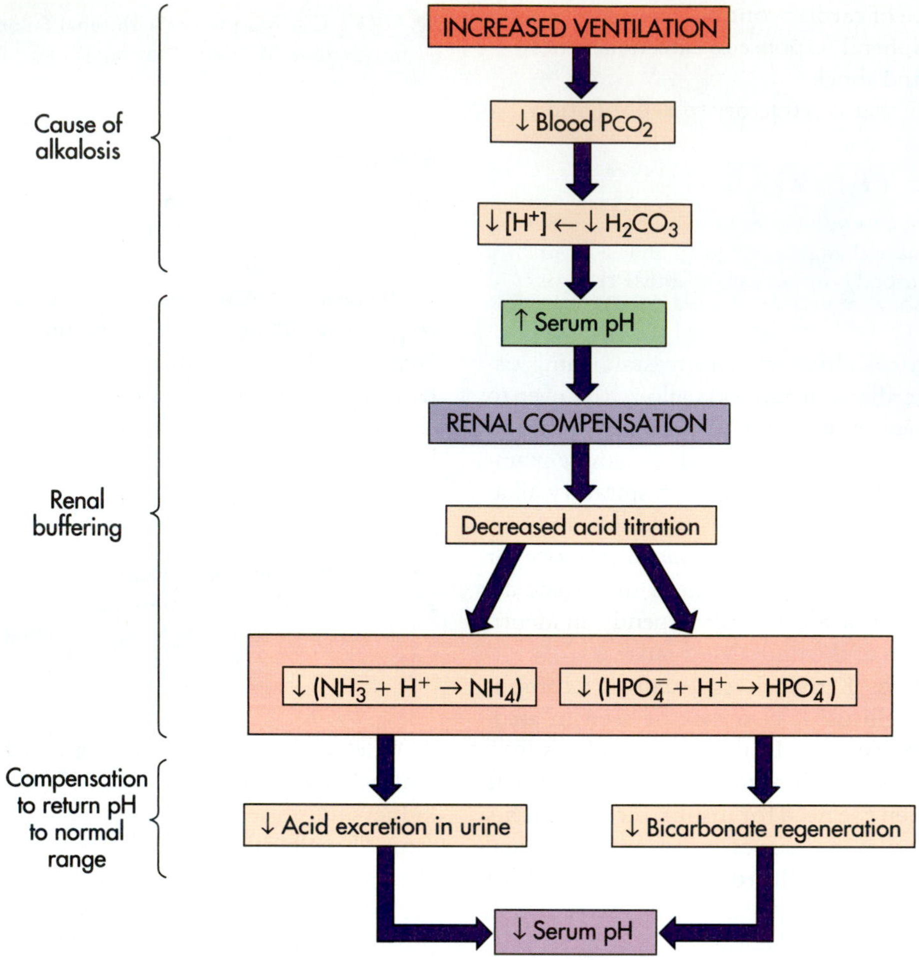

FIGURE 7-13 ■ Respiratory alkalosis. A deficit of carbon dioxide results in respiratory alkalosis.

At first, the respiratory system tries to compensate. It does so by retaining carbon dioxide. However, this mechanism is limited by the development of **hypoxemia.** (Hypoventilation causes a rise in the Pco_2 and a decrease in the partial pressure of oxygen [Po_2]. This, in turn, stimulates respiration.)

Treatment of metabolic alkalosis is aimed at correcting the underlying condition. Volume depletion, if present, should be corrected. This should be done with isotonic solutions. Hypokalemia may require correction with potassium replacement.

MIXED ACID-BASE DISTURBANCES

Many conditions may cause mixed abnormalities of acid-base regulation. These conditions include various forms of shock. In patients in shock, simultaneous respiratory and metabolic alterations are commonly seen. These develop because pathophysiological changes occur in both the respiratory and metabolic components of the acid-base system (Box 7-4; also see Table 7-3). Examples of mixed acid-base disturbances include the following:

- Combined respiratory and metabolic acidosis
- Metabolic acidosis and respiratory alkalosis
- Respiratory acidosis and metabolic alkalosis
- Combined respiratory and metabolic alkalosis

Acid-base balance can be a difficult concept to master. In providing emergency care, the paramedic should remember the following primary points:

1. Acid-base balance has two components: a respiratory (CO_2) factor and a nonrespiratory (metabolic) factor.
2. Respiratory acidosis is caused by an increase in the CO_2 level of the blood and body fluids as a result of inadequate breathing. The treatment of respiratory acidosis involves improving ventilation to lower the CO_2 level. Respiratory alkalosis results from hyperventilation.
3. Metabolic acidosis is caused by anaerobic metabolism and lactic acidosis. The treatment of metabolic acidosis involves neutralizing the acid by reestablishing tissue perfusion and cardiac output. Metabolic alkalosis is rare.
4. A patient may have two acid-base disturbances at the same time. One usually dominates, and the other attempts to compensate.
5. The patient's pH is always a product of *both* respiratory and metabolic components. Neutral pH is 6.8 to 7. The normal pH of blood is 7.4. A decrease in pH indicates an increase in acidity (more acid than normal); an increase in pH indicates a decrease in acidity (less acid than normal).

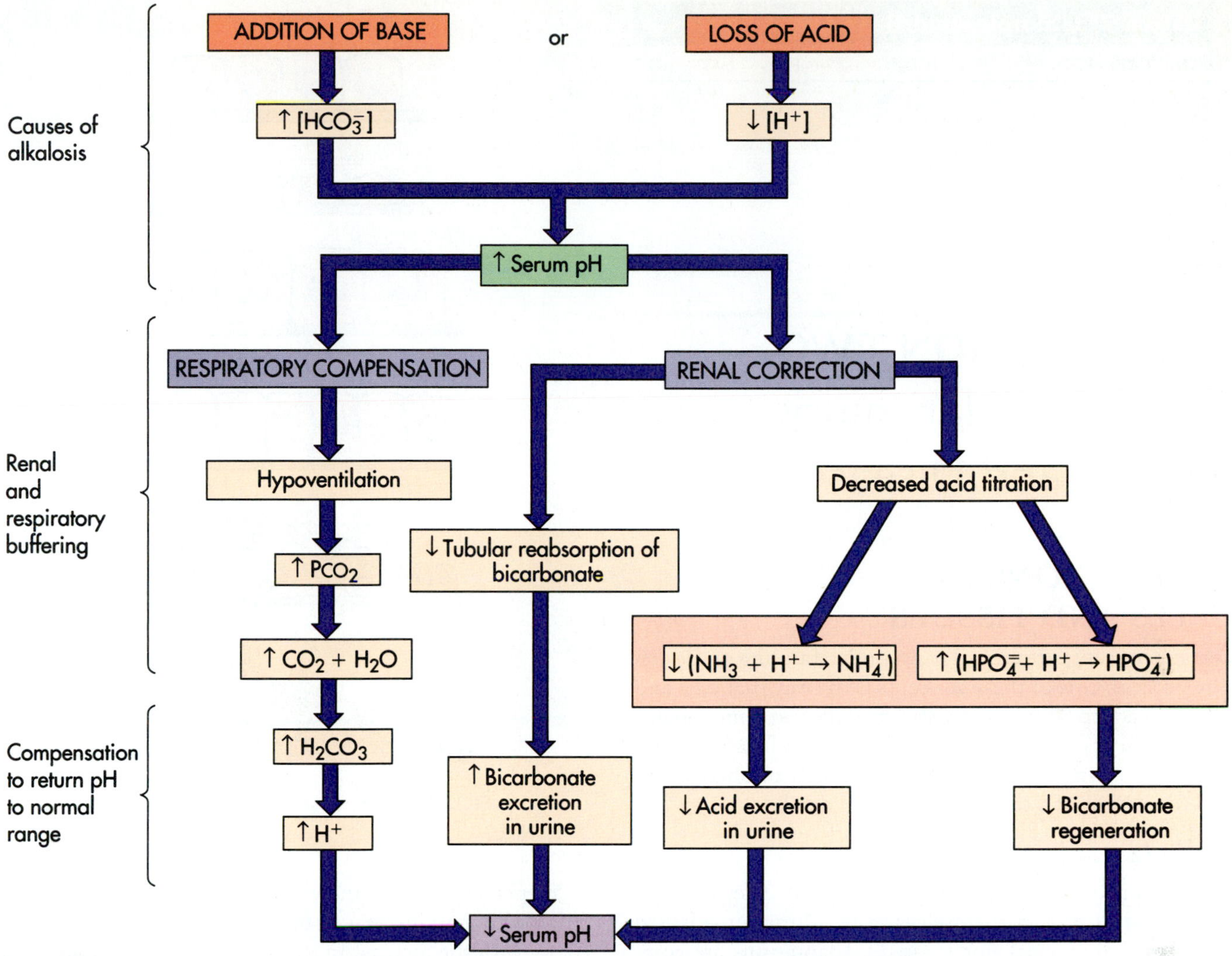

FIGURE 7-14 ■ Metabolic alkalosis. An excess of bicarbonate results in metabolic alkalosis.

BOX 7-4 Acid-Base Determination and Other Laboratory Studies

Blood Gas Analysis

Blood gas values are measured for two reasons. One reason is to determine whether the patient is well oxygenated. The second reason is to determine the patient's acid-base status. Most often, blood gas values are measured in a sample of arterial blood obtained in a heparinized syringe. Arterial samples are used for this test more often than venous samples for a good reason. Arterial samples give more direct information about the lungs' ability to oxygenate blood and remove carbon dioxide.

Acid-Base Determination

The patient's acid-base status is assessed by measuring the partial pressure of carbon dioxide (P_{CO_2}) and the hydrogen ion concentration (pH) of the arterial blood. The pH level indicates whether an acid or a base state is present. The P_{CO_2} value indicates whether a respiratory component is a factor in the acidosis or alkalosis. (For instance, it may show whether alveolar hypoventilation or hyperventilation is present.) Table 7-3 sums up the abnormalities that occur in mixed acid-base disturbances.

Currently, paramedics are not expected to determine the pH by blood gas analysis in the prehospital setting. Pulse oximetry allows continual assessment of the arterial oxygen saturation without invasive procedures. (Under normal circumstances, a saturation of 90% correlates with a partial pressure of oxygen [P_{O_2}] in arterial blood of 60 mm Hg.)

TABLE 7-3 Simple Acid-Base Disturbances

DISTURBANCE	HCO_3^2	Pco_2	pH
Metabolic acidosis	↓	↓	↓
Respiratory acidosis	↓	↑	↓
Metabolic alkalosis	↑	↑	↑

SECTION TWO
Cellular Injury and Disease

ALTERATIONS IN CELLS AND TISSUES

Certain concepts are crucial to an understanding of the disease process. One of these concepts is the way that cells and tissues react to injury, both structurally and functionally. Changes in the structure and function of cells and tissues can result from cellular adaptation, injury, **neoplasia** (actual formation of a tumor), aging, and death.

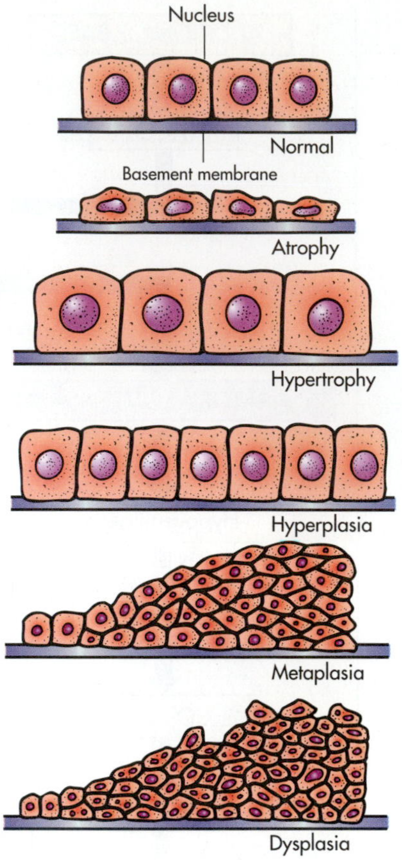

FIGURE 7-15 ■ Adaptive changes in cells.

Cellular Adaptation

Cells adapt to their environment (Fig. 7-15). They do so to escape and to protect themselves from injury. (An adapted cell is neither normal nor injured.) Adaptations are common. They are a central part of the response to changes in the physiological condition. In many instances the adaptation allows the cell to function more efficiently. For this reason, it can be difficult to distinguish between a pathological response and an extreme adaptation to changing conditions. The five most significant adaptive changes in cells are:

1. Atrophy (a decrease in cell size)
2. Hypertrophy (an increase in cell size)
3. Hyperplasia (an excessive increase in the number of cells)
4. Metaplasia (a change from one cell type to another that is better able to tolerate adverse conditions; a conversion into a form that is not normal for that cell)
5. Dysplasia (abnormal changes in mature cells)

Atrophy is a decrease in cellular size that adversely affects cell function. It can affect any organ. However, it is seen most often in skeletal muscle, the heart, the secondary sex organs, and the brain. Causes include decreased use, chronic inflammation, poor nutrition or starvation, inadequate hormonal or nervous stimulation, and reduced blood supply. An example of atrophy is a skeletal muscle that is reduced in size because of prolonged wearing of a cast. Atrophy may be reversed (in some cases) when normal function is restored.

Hypertrophy is an increase in the size of cells. (This occurs without an increase in the number of that type of cell.) Along with the increase in the size of the cells comes an increase in the size of the affected organ. Hypertrophy results when cells are required to do more work to achieve a task. Examples of "normal" or physiological hypertrophy are a weight lifter's large muscles, increased growth of the uterus during pregnancy, and the development of sexual organs in adolescence (initiated by sex hormones). Examples of pathological hypertrophy are enlargement of the heart (myocardial hypertrophy) and of the kidneys (which also can be physiological).

> **CRITICAL THINKING**
> What happens to muscle strength when the muscle cells are affected by each of these conditions: atrophy, hypertrophy, and hyperplasia?

Hyperplasia is an excessive increase in the number of cells. This results in an increase in the size of a tissue or an organ. Hyperplasia occurs in response to increased demand. It may be a pathological event. It also may be a normal adaptive mechanism that allows certain organs to regenerate *(compensatory hyperplasia)*. The formation of a callus is an example of compensatory hyperplasia. Another example is the increased formation of red blood cells that occurs at high altitudes. An example of pathological hyperplasia is endometrial hyperplasia. This condition can cause excessive menstrual bleeding. Hyperplasia and hypertrophy often occur together.

Metaplasia is a change into a form that is not normal for that cell. It also can be seen as the reversible replacement of normal tissue cells by other cells that may be better able to tolerate poor environmental conditions. An example of metaplasia is the change that occurs in the bronchial lining as a result of smoking. The normal ciliated epithelial cells are replaced by nonciliated squamous epithelial cells. The latter cells are more resistant to irritation. (Bronchial metaplasia can be reversed if the individual quits smoking.) Chronic inflammation of the cervix also can result in metaplasia.

Dysplasia is the development of abnormal changes in mature cells. The cells vary in size, shape, and color, and their relationship to one another also is abnormal. Dysplastic changes frequently are seen as precancerous. They occur most often in epithelial tissue. These changes often result from chronic irritation or inflammation. They frequently are found in cells near cancerous cells. Dysplasia is not considered a true cellular adaptation. Rather, it is seen as an atypical hyperplasia.

Cellular Injury

Many processes can injure a cell. The mechanisms involved in cellular injury are complex. The specific site of injury often is characteristic of a certain pathological process. As a rule, cellular injury occurs if the cell is unable to maintain homeostasis as a result of the following factors:

1. Hypoxic injury
2. Chemical injury
3. Infectious injury (i.e., bacteria, viruses)
4. Immunological and inflammatory injury
5. Genetic factors
6. Nutritional imbalances
7. Physical agents

HYPOXIC INJURY

Hypoxic injury is the most common cause of damage to a cell. It may result from a decrease in the amount of oxygen in the air, loss of hemoglobin or altered hemoglobin function, a decrease in the number of red blood cells, diseases of the respiratory or cardiovascular system, external compression (e.g., in trauma), or poisoning and loss of cytochromes. Hypoxic injury commonly is a result of atherosclerosis (narrowing of the arteries) and thrombosis (complete blockage of an artery or a vein by a blood clot). Prolonged ischemia leads to *infarction,* or cell death (see Chapter 29). Atherosclerosis and thrombosis are leading causes of myocardial infarction and stroke.[1]

> **NOTE** Cells need an adequate supply of oxygen. Without this, they cannot generate enough energy to maintain the mechanisms (ion pumps) that move some substances across the cell membrane. It also results in cellular swelling.

CHEMICAL INJURY

Many chemical agents can damage a cell. Examples include heavy metals (e.g., lead), carbon monoxide, ethanol, drugs, and complex toxins. Some of these chemicals injure cells directly (e.g., curare and cyanide). Others, when metabolized, produce a toxin that affects the cells (e.g., carbon tetrachloride [CCl_4]).

The injury begins with a biochemical interaction. The interaction occurs between a toxic substance and an integral part of the cell's structure. Some drugs and toxins (e.g., salicylate, certain venoms) affect the cellular membrane. This interaction can damage the plasma membrane. It can lead to increased permeability, cellular swelling, and irreversible cellular injury (see Chapter 36). Other toxins, such as carbon monoxide, mainly affect the cytochrome system found in the mitochondria. This leads to a halt in oxidative metabolism. Still other toxins affect the genetic material (a primary target for chemotherapeutic drugs).

INFECTIOUS INJURY

The **virulence** of microorganisms such as bacteria and viruses depends on their ability to survive and reproduce in the human body. The disease-producing potential of microorganisms depends on their ability to do the following:

- Invade and destroy cells
- Overcome the organism's defense system
- Produce toxins
- Produce hypersensitivity reactions

Bacteria. The survival and growth of bacteria are determined by the success of the body's defenses. They also depend on the bacteria's ability to resist these mechanisms (see Chapter 39). Many bacteria that survive and multiply in the body produce toxins. These can injure or destroy cells and tissues. The toxins take two forms: exotoxins and endotoxins.

Bacteria make exotoxins when they have been identified by viruslike particles called *bacteriophages.* These particles carry the genetic material needed to make the toxin. Exotoxins are produced by a microorganism. Then they are excreted into the medium surrounding it. Exotoxins have highly specific effects. These effects are produced by the release of exotoxins as metabolic products during bacterial growth. Several of the streptococci (bacteria that cause sore throats and rheumatic fever) produce an exotoxin. The bacterium *Clostridium botulinum,* which causes the severe food poisoning known as botulism, also produces an exotoxin.

> **NOTE** Toxoids are modified (harmless) toxins. They are used as vaccines so that the body can develop specific antibodies to them. The best-known toxoid is tetanus toxoid, which is made from tetanus toxin.

Endotoxins are complex molecules. They are contained in the cell walls of some bacteria. Endotoxins are released during treatment with antibiotics or when the cell walls disintegrate. Examples of bacteria that produce endotoxins are gonococci and meningococci. (These are the bacteria that cause gonorrhea and meningitis.) Endotoxins do not stimulate the production of strong antibodies. For this reason, it has not been possible to develop vaccines against endotoxin-bearing bacteria. Instead, to fight these bacteria, the body uses a group of proteins collectively called the **complement system.** These proteins coat the bacteria. Then, they help kill the microorganisms directly, or they help destroy them by assisting in having the bacteria taken up by neutrophils (in the blood) or macrophages (in the tissues). The *reticuloendothelial system* (composed of cells in the spleen, lymph nodes, liver, bone marrow, lungs, and intestines) works with the lymphatic system to dispose of the debris produced by the immune system's attack on invading organisms.

Bacteria that make endotoxins are also called *pyrogenic bacteria.* They are called this because they activate the inflammatory process. They also produce fever directly through the release of cell membrane toxins. As part of the inflammatory process, white blood cells are released from the bone marrow. This is the cause of the increased white blood cell count that is commonly found with infection. Inflammation also increases capillary permeability. This allows substances that destroy bacteria to migrate from the capillaries to the site of infection (see Chapter 39). Fever is caused by the release of *endogenous pyrogens* (proteins that act on the thermoregulatory centers of the hypothalamus). These proteins are released by macrophages or by circulating white blood cells that are attracted to the injury site (Fig. 7-16).

CRITICAL THINKING

Will treating a fever with antipyretic drugs cause the body to rid itself of the toxin that caused the fever?

A **hypersensitivity reaction** is a life-threatening pathogenic mechanism of bacterial toxins. Few toxins are capable of producing this type of reaction. An immunological response occurs with the first exposure to the toxin. Hypersensitivity develops the next time the individual is exposed to the toxin. The result is an inflammatory response. At times, the response is so extreme that the person is killed instead of the bacteria. For example, the complement system can activate blood clotting and can cause white blood cells to aggregate and form "clumps," which block blood vessels.

The net effect of overactivation of the complement system by endotoxins is the blockage of small blood vessels in the lungs (with the clumps) and the formation of tiny blood clots in small arteries elsewhere in the body. Luckily, this life-threatening reaction is rare. Moreover, the complement system normally acts as an efficient defense against most bacterial toxins without causing any damage. (Hypersensitivity reactions are further described later in this chapter and in Chapter 33.)

NOTE When the body's defenses fail and microorganisms multiply in the blood, bacteremia develops. This may lead to septicemia, a severe systemic infection in which pathogens are present in the bloodstream. The endotoxins (along with a number of proteins involved in the inflammatory response) cause vasodilation. This reduces blood pressure and oxygen delivery. The result is shock. Other signs of an inflammatory response to bacteremia may include chills, fever, and an altered level of consciousness. Rashes or red streaks also may be associated with bacteremia. (The red streaks are called *lymphangitis.*)

CRITICAL THINKING

In septic shock, toxins damage the cell membrane, making it more permeable. This allows fluids to leak out of the blood vessels more freely. How could that affect cardiac output?

Viruses. Viruses cause many human diseases. These include the common cold, influenza, chickenpox, smallpox, hepatitis, herpes, and acquired immunodeficiency syndrome (AIDS). Viruses are intracellular parasites that work very differently from bacteria (Fig. 7-17). Viruses lack much of the machinery that allows bacterial cells and other types of cells to grow rapidly and multiply. They can reproduce only by infecting the living cells of host tissue. (They often

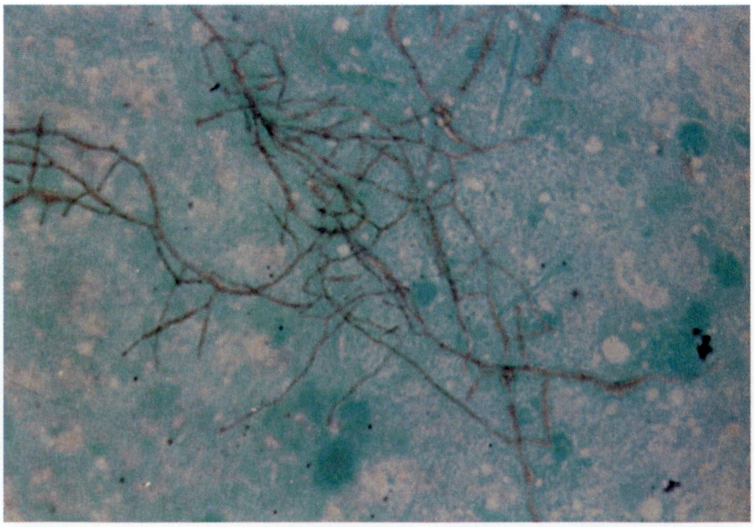

FIGURE 7-16 ■ *Nocardia* organisms, stained with Gomori methenamine silver stain, in a wound on the lower leg.

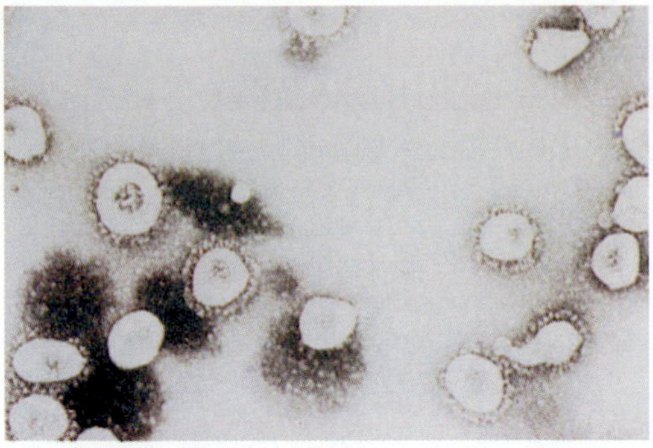

FIGURE 7-17 ■ *Coronavirus* particles.

destroy the host cell). Viruses usually consist of a protein coat *(capsid)* that encloses a core of nucleic acid. They have no organelles and therefore have no metabolism. They do not produce endotoxins or exotoxins.

Viruses need nucleic acid (either deoxyribonucleic acid [DNA] or ribonucleic acid [RNA]) to replicate. (Unlike all other cellular forms of life, viruses never have both DNA and RNA.) Cells are thought to engulf the virus particles by surrounding them with part of the cell membrane. Once inside the cell, the virus loses the capsid and begins to replicate the viral nucleic acids. Some viruses cause the cell to burst. Others replicate without destroying the cell.

The capsid enables the virus particle to resist phagocytosis, even though viruses often trigger a very strong immune response. Viruses can rapidly cause permanent and lethal injury in hosts, whether they are immunosuppressed or not. Rabies, smallpox, and influenza are examples of viral diseases that are highly infectious and that have high rates of illness (morbidity) and death (mortality).

Viral infections are easier to prevent than to treat. Vaccines have proven to be the best guard against viral disease (Box 7-5). Viral infections usually cause active illness. The signs and symptoms are based on the type and location of the cells infected. For this reason, certain viruses tend to cause respiratory illness (e.g., influenza). Others cause gastroenteritis (enteroviruses), central nervous system disease (e.g., St. Louis B encephalitis, rabies), or liver disease (hepatitis).

> **BOX 7-5 Influenza Vaccines**
>
> Influenza viruses are categorized into three major types: A, B, and C.
>
> Type A mutates every 2 to 3 years. (Type A influenza viruses have caused worldwide epidemics, killing tens of thousands of people.) Type B mutates every 3 to 6 years. Type C apparently does not mutate. The mutations allow the virus to escape containment by the immune system. This is true even if a person has had a previous influenza infection. Each year, virologists and epidemiologists analyze cultures from the southern hemisphere (where the flu season occurs during the northern hemisphere's summer). They try to determine which strains are likely to appear in the upcoming flu season and use this information to prepare effective vaccines. If the expected strain strikes, the vaccine can protect about 75% of those who have been vaccinated. It takes about 2 weeks after the shot to build antibodies.

IMMUNOLOGICAL AND INFLAMMATORY INJURY

Cellular membranes are damaged by direct contact with cellular and chemical components of the immune and inflammatory responses. These components include phagocytic cells (monocytes, neutrophils, and macrophages) and substances such as antibodies, lymphokines, complements, and proteases (see Chapters 37 and 39). If the cell membrane is injured or if the transport mechanism (which moves potassium into the cell and sodium out of it) begins to fail, intracellular water increases. This causes the cell to swell. If the swelling continues, the cell eventually may rupture.

INJURIOUS GENETIC FACTORS

Genetic disease results from a chromosomal abnormality or a defective gene. These genetic defects may be inherited. (An example of such a disease is sickle cell anemia.) They also may result from spontaneous mutations. (An example is Down syndrome.) Some genetic disorders can alter the cell's structure and function. Genetic disorders can cause changes in the structural or metabolic component of the specific target cells. Huntington disease and muscular dystrophy are examples of conditions caused by such disorders (see Chapter 37).

> **NOTE** The term *congenital* refers to any abnormality that is present at birth. This is the case even though the abnormality may not be detected until much later.

INJURIOUS NUTRITIONAL IMBALANCES

Cells need adequate amounts of essential nutrients to function normally. If the needed nutrients are not gained through the diet and taken to the cells, pathophysiological effects on the cells can occur. Damaging effects also can occur if excessive amounts of nutrients are consumed and taken to the cells. Examples of conditions caused by injurious nutritional imbalances include protein-calorie malnutrition, obesity, hyperglycemia, scurvy, and rickets.

INJURIOUS PHYSICAL AGENTS

Many physical agents can damage cells and tissues. Examples of physical agents (including environmental agents) that can cause cellular or tissue injury include the following:

- Temperature extremes (hypothermic and hyperthermic injury)
- Changes in atmospheric pressure (blast injury, decompression sickness)
- Ionizing radiation (radiation injury)
- Nonionizing radiation (radio waves, microwaves)
- Illumination (light injury, [e.g., vision injury, skin cancer])
- Mechanical stresses (e.g., noise-induced hearing loss, overuse syndromes)

Manifestations of Cellular Injury

An injured cell may show various types of abnormalities in its form and structure. These are known as *morphological abnormalities.* The two most common abnormalities of this type are cellular swelling and fatty change. Cellular injury is indicated by both local and systemic signs.

CELLULAR MANIFESTATIONS

In injured cells (and in some healthy cells), several substances accumulate. They include fluids and electrolytes, triglycerides (lipids), glucose, calcium, uric acid, protein, melanin, and bilirubin. These substances normally are present in certain cells of the body. However, abnormal intracellular accumulation may lead to cellular damage. Also, injured cells may be unable to get rid of excessive amounts of water, sodium, or calcium. This leads to increased injury. If water, sodium, or calcium continues to accumulate, the cells become permanently damaged.

Macrophages ingest debris from injured cells. Some macrophages circulate throughout the body. Others remain fixed in tissues (e.g., the liver and the spleen). Phagocytes migrate to injured tissue. They engulf dying cells and abnormal extracellular substances. As more phagocytes migrate to injured tissue to engulf the metabolites, the affected tissue begins to swell. Phagocytosis by the fixed macrophages of the reticuloendothelial system causes enlargement of the liver *(hepatomegaly)* or the spleen *(splenomegaly)*. This is seen with many diseases that are associated with abnormal accumulation of various metabolic products (amyloidosis) or abnormal cells (hemolytic disease).

Cellular Swelling. As described before, the swelling in injured cells results from membrane changes that allow potassium to leak rapidly out of the cell and sodium and water to enter the cell. The increase in intracellular sodium increases the osmotic pressure. This draws more water into the cell. If the swelling affects all cells in an organ, the organ increases in weight and becomes distended. Cellular swelling usually is reversible.

▶NOTE Inflammation is associated with cellular swelling. This is true whether the cause is infection, trauma, or an autoimmune reaction. Inflammation is often accompanied by fever.

Fatty Change. Fatty change occurs when the enzyme systems that metabolize fat are impaired or overwhelmed. When this happens, lipids accumulate inside the cell. This is common in liver cells (fatty liver), because these cells are actively involved in the metabolism of fat. Hepatic metabolism and secretion of lipids are crucial to proper body function. For this reason, deficiencies in these processes lead to major pathological changes. Alcohol abuse is a common cause of fatty liver. It usually is a precursor to cirrhosis.

Systemic Manifestations. Cellular injury produces many systemic manifestations. These include fever, malaise, loss of well-being, change in appetite, altered heart rate, an abnormal rise in WBCs, leukocytosis, and pain. In addition, testing of extracellular fluid may reveal the presence of cellular enzymes released by injured cells or tissue.

▶BOX 7-6 Normal Cellular Aging and Death

Cellular aging and death are common processes. They are natural functions of the cell cycle. As the cell ages, it becomes less efficient in carrying out its functions. It also is more at risk of damage from harmful environmental agents. With progressive damage, cells lose their ability to repair themselves. In time, they begin to malfunction. Changes in immunological cells slowly lead to decreased immunity and an increased risk of infectious disease. Malignancies increase with age as a result of decreased immunity. This also is due to an increased incidence of malignant transformation of various cells. Other examples of the manifestations of aging cells include gray hair, reduced muscle mass, menopause, arteriosclerosis, memory and vision impairment, and arthritis.

Cellular Death and Necrosis

A cell dies if it has been irreparably damaged. Shortly after cell death, structural changes begin to occur in the nucleus and cytoplasm. The *lysosome* (a membranous sac of digestive enzymes found in many cells) begins to undergo membrane breakdown. This releases the lysosomal enzymes, which begin to digest the cell. The nucleus shrinks and dissolves or breaks into fragments (Box 7-6).

Necrosis is the death of cells or tissues caused by injury or disease. It also can occur by cellular self-destruction *(autolysis)*. Different types of necrosis tend to occur in different organs or tissues. The type may indicate the cause of cellular injury. Necrotic changes take several hours to develop. They are easy to recognize on histological examination by their structure and staining characteristics.

HYPOPERFUSION

The term **hypoperfusion** is used to describe poor circulation of blood and nutrients to tissues. It can be caused by a number of medical and traumatic conditions.

Pathogenesis

Hypoperfusion often is the result of a decrease in cardiac output. Decreased cardiac output, if prolonged, leads to **shock** (a continued state of hypoperfusion), multiple organ dysfunction syndrome, and other disease states associated with impaired cellular metabolism.

DECREASED CARDIAC OUTPUT

Cardiac output (also known as the *minute volume*) is the total amount of blood pumped by the ventricles each minute. It is usually expressed in liters per minute (L/min). Cardiac output is a crucial determinant of organ perfusion. It depends on several factors. These include the strength of contraction, the rate of contraction, and the amount of blood returning through the veins *(venous return)* available to the ventricle **(preload).**

NOTE Cardiac output is determined by multiplying the heart rate by the volume of blood ejected by the ventricles during each beat (**stroke volume**). For example, if the ventricle contracts 72 times per minute and ejects 42 mL of blood with each contraction, the cardiac output would be 72 beats per minute multiplied by 42 mL per beat, or 3.02 L/min. Decreased cardiac output usually is associated with a decrease in blood pressure and tissue perfusion and impaired cellular metabolism.

COMPENSATORY MECHANISMS

The body uses compensatory mechanisms to manage blood pressure and cardiac output. These include a number of **negative feedback mechanisms.** A negative feedback mechanism is any mechanism that tends to balance a change in a system. A number of negative feedback mechanisms are crucial to the process of maintaining cardiac output and tissue perfusion. These include baroreceptor reflexes, chemoreceptor reflexes, the central nervous system ischemic response, hormonal mechanisms, reabsorption of tissue fluids, and splenic discharge of stored blood (seen in animals but minimal in humans).

Baroreceptor Reflexes. As mentioned before, baroreceptors (Fig. 7-18, *A*) are pressure-sensitive nerve endings found in the heart and great vessels. They keep blood pressure and cardiac output within a normal range. Normal blood pressure produces a constant, low-level stimulation of the baroreceptors. When the blood pressure moves out of the normal range, either up or down, stimulation of the baroreceptors increases (Box 7-7). The baroreceptor reflexes then act to correct the condition. If the arterial blood pressure increases, the baroreceptor reflexes act to lower blood pressure. Likewise, if the arterial blood pressure decreases, the baroreceptor reflexes act to increase blood pressure. Baroreceptors (Fig. 7-18, *A*) are not stimulated when the blood pressure is less than 60 mm Hg. When baroreceptor stimulation ceases because of a fall in arterial pressure, the negative feedback mechanism evokes several cardiovascular responses (Box 7-7). Vagal (parasympathetic) stimulation is reduced, and sympathetic response is increased. The increase in sympathetic impulses results in increased **peripheral vascular resistance** (PVR). It also results in an increase in the heart rate and stroke volume. Sympathetic responses also cause generalized arteriolar vasoconstriction. This reduces the size of the vascular compartment. As the veins constrict, blood is shifted into the central circulation. This, coupled with the constriction of blood vessels in the skin, muscles, and viscera, helps maintain perfusion of the central organs. The vasoconstriction in these peripheral vascular beds results in the characteristic pale, cool skin seen in patients suffering from hypovolemic shock.

NOTE Peripheral vascular resistance is the resistance to blood flow in the systemic circulation (small arteries, arterioles, venules, veins). **Afterload** is the systemic vascular resistance on the left side of the heart. It is the pressure against which the ventricle must contract to eject its contents.

BOX 7-7 Baroreceptor Responses to Changes in Blood Pressure: Sympathetic Nervous System

Baroreceptors (Fig. 7-18, *A*) help maintain blood pressure and cardiac output in two ways. Both of these are negative feedback mechanisms. Baroreceptors lower blood pressure in response to increased arterial pressure. They also increase blood pressure in response to decreased arterial pressure. Normal blood pressure partially stretches the arterial walls so that the baroreceptors produce a constant, low-level frequency stimulation. This stimulation increases progressively from a lower pressure limit of 60 mm Hg to a maximum at 180 to 200 mm Hg. Impulses from the baroreceptors travel through the vagus and the Hering nerve to the glossopharyngeal nerve. There, they inhibit the vasoconstrictor center of the medulla. They also excite the vagal center. These impulses result in vasodilation in the peripheral circulatory system. They also cause a decrease in the heart rate and strength of contraction. The combined effect is a decrease in arterial pressure. Baroreceptors adapt within 1 to 3 days to the ambient pressure in the immediate locale. They therefore are not responsible for modulating the average blood pressure on a long-term basis.

When low blood pressure stimulates a response in the baroreceptors, the effects on the heart include increases in the strength and rate of contraction. Peripheral effects include arteriolar constriction, a decrease in blood vessel size, and increased peripheral vascular resistance.

Chemoreceptor Reflexes. Low arterial pressure (if it leads to hypoxemia, acidosis, or both) also may stimulate peripheral chemoreceptor cells. These are found in the carotid and aortic bodies. Because of the location of these bodies, the chemoreceptor cells have a vast blood supply. When the Po_2 or pH decreases, chemoreceptor cells stimulate the vasomotor center of the medulla. At the same time, the rate and depth of ventilation are increased. This helps to eliminate excess carbon dioxide. It also helps to maintain acid-base balance. Chemoreceptors (Fig. 7-18, *B*) are more involved in the regulation of respiration than in regulation of the cardiovascular rate and rhythm or blood pressure. However, during profound hypotension or acidosis, though, chemoreceptors can and do produce vasoconstriction. This vasomotor stimulation results in enhanced peripheral vasoconstriction, which is initiated by the baroreceptors.

Central Nervous System Ischemic Response. Blood flow to the vasomotor center of the medulla can be reduced enough to cause ischemia. When this occurs, the neurons in the vasomotor center become excited. This raises the arterial blood pressure. This effect is known as the *central nervous system ischemic response.* The degree of sympathetic vasoconstriction can be intense. It can be so intense that it elevates the arterial pressure for as long as 10 minutes, sometimes to more than 200 mm Hg. If the ischemia lasts longer than a few minutes, the vagal centers are activated. This results in vasodilation in the periphery and bradycardia (a slowed heart rate). Like the chemoreceptor reflex, the central nervous system ischemic response functions only in

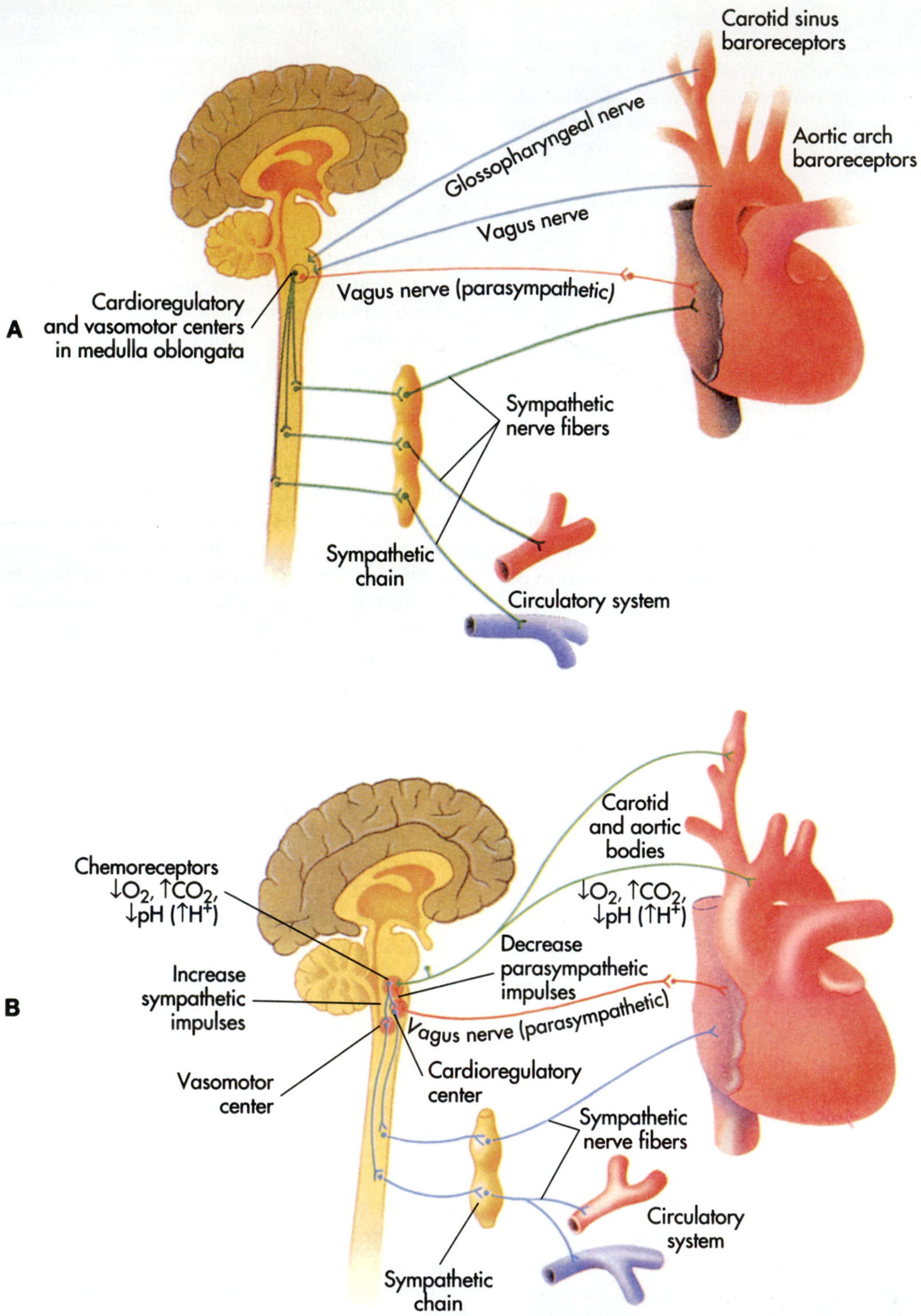

FIGURE 7-18 ■ **A,** Baroreceptor reflexes. Baroreceptors in the carotid sinuses and the aortic arch detect changes in blood pressure. Impulses are conducted to the cardioregulatory and vasomotor centers. The heart rate can be decreased by the parasympathetic system; the heart rate and stroke volume can be increased by the sympathetic system. The sympathetic system can also constrict or dilate blood vessels. **B,** Chemoreceptor reflexes. Chemoreceptors in the medulla and carotid and aortic bodies detect changes in blood oxygen, carbon dioxide, or pH levels. Impulses are conducted to the medulla. In response, the vasomotor center can cause constriction or dilation of blood vessels through the sympathetic system, and the cardioregulatory center can cause changes in the pumping activity of the heart through the parasympathetic and sympathetic systems.

emergency situations. Moreover, it does not become active until the blood pressure falls below 50 mm Hg.

Hormonal Mechanisms. Several hormonal mechanisms also help to control arterial pressure through negative feedback. These include the adrenal medullary mechanism, the renin-angiotensin-aldosterone mechanism, and the vasopressin mechanism.

Adrenal Medullary Mechanism. When sympathetic stimulation of the heart and blood vessels increases, stimulation of the adrenal medulla also increases. The hormones secreted by the adrenal medulla are epinephrine and norepinephrine. The effect of these hormones on the cardiovascular system is very similar to that produced by the sympathetic nervous system. As a result, the heart rate, the stroke volume, and vasoconstriction increase.

Renin-Angiotensin-Aldosterone Mechanism. As described before, renin is an enzyme. It is released by the kidneys into the circulatory system. Renin changes the structure of the plasma protein angiotensinogen, thereby producing angiotensin I. This, in turn, is converted by angiotensin-converting enzyme (mostly in the lungs), creating angiotensin II (active angiotensin).

> **NOTE** Angiotensin-converting enzyme (ACE) inhibitors are drugs that block the conversion of the precursor, angiotensin I, to the active molecule, angiotensin II. As a result, blood pressure is lowered, and less stress is put on the heart. Examples of ACE inhibitors include captopril (Capoten), enalapril (Vasotec), and lisinopril (Prinivil).

Angiotensin II causes vasoconstriction in the arterioles and to a lesser degree in the veins. This vasoconstriction results in increased peripheral vascular resistance, increased venous return to the heart, and a resultant increase in blood pressure. Angiotensin II also stimulates the release of aldosterone. Aldosterone acts on the kidneys to conserve sodium and water.

The renin-angiotensin-aldosterone mechanism is an important regulatory loop for increasing the blood pressure in circulatory shock. It takes about 20 minutes to become effective in hypovolemia caused by hemorrhagic shock. It remains active for about 1 hour.

> **CRITICAL THINKING**
> You are assessing your patient's radial pulse. What compensatory changes can you evaluate while doing this?

Vasopressin Mechanism. When the blood pressure drops or the concentration of solutes in the plasma increases (increased serum osmolality), the hypothalamic neurons are stimulated. This causes the anterior pituitary to increase secretion of vasopressin, or antidiuretic hormone (ADH). ADH acts directly on the blood vessels. It causes vasoconstriction within minutes after a rapid fall in the blood pressure. ADH also reduces the rate of urine production by enhancing reabsorption of water. This helps to maintain blood volume and blood pressure.

> **NOTE** Atrial natriuretic factor (ANF) also helps to control arterial pressure through a negative feedback mechanism. Its release is triggered by a rise in atrial pressure. (This is usually a sign of volume overload.) ANF increases the rate of urine production. Loss of water through the urine decreases blood volume. The result is a decrease in the atrial pressure. This is the only hormonal system actively used to decrease volume and pressure.

Reabsorption of Tissue Fluids. Arterial hypotension, arteriolar constriction, and reduced venous pressure during hypovolemia lower the blood pressure in the capillaries *(hydrostatic pressure).* This decrease promotes reabsorption of interstitial fluid into the vascular compartment. Large amounts of fluid may be drawn into the circulation during hemorrhage. It has been estimated that about 0.25 mL/min/kg of body weight, or 1 L/hr in the adult male, can be autoinfused from the interstitial spaces after acute blood loss.

Splenic Discharge of Blood. Some of the blood that circulates through the spleen continues through the microcirculation. It is stored in an area called the *venous sinuses.* The venous sinuses can store more than 300 mL of blood. Sudden reductions in blood pressure cause the sympathetic nervous system to stimulate constriction of these sinuses. Constriction can expel as much as 200 mL of this blood into the venous circulation to help restore blood volume or pressure in the circulation.

> **NOTE** An increase in preload or afterload or a decrease in stroke volume can lead to volume overload and pulmonary edema. This, in turn, can reduce tissue perfusion and impair cellular metabolism (see Chapter 29).

Types of Shock

Shock is classified according to the primary cause (Box 7-8). Although these classifications are separate and distinct, two or more types may be combined. Brief descriptions of the five types of shock are given below. A more detailed discussion of shock is presented in Chapter 21.

- *Hypovolemic shock* is most often caused by hemorrhage. It also may be caused by severe dehydration. In either case, circulating volume is lost.
- *Cardiogenic shock* results when the heart's pumping action cannot deliver adequate circulation for tissue perfusion.
- *Neurogenic shock* results most often from spinal cord injury that is accompanied by loss of sympathetic vasomotor tone.
- *Anaphylactic shock* occurs when the body is exposed to a substance that produces a severe allergic reaction.

BOX 7-8 Common Etiological Classifications of Shock

Hypovolemic shock	Anaphylactic shock
Cardiogenic shock	Septic shock
Neurogenic shock	

- *Septic shock* most often results from a serious systemic bacterial infection.

Regardless of the classification, the underlying defect in shock is inadequate tissue perfusion.

Multiple Organ Dysfunction Syndrome

Multiple organ dysfunction syndrome (MODS) is the progressive failure of two or more organ systems. This occurs after a very severe illness or injury. Sepsis and septic shock are common causes of MODS. However, it may follow any period of prolonged shock, regardless of the cause (see Chapter 21).

NOTE Multiple organ dysfunction syndrome (MODS) was first described in 1975. The mortality rate is 60% to 90%. The rate nears 100% if three or more organs are involved; if sepsis is present; and if the patient is over 65 years of age.[3]

PATHOPHYSIOLOGY

Any process that triggers the body's inflammatory response may initiate MODS. (This includes traumatic, septic, and burn injury.) The syndrome begins with vascular endothelial damage. This damage is caused by the release of endotoxins and inflammatory mediators into the circulation. When the vascular endothelium is damaged, it becomes permeable. It allows fluid and cells to leak into the interstitial spaces. This, in turn, contributes to hypotension and hypoperfusion. The release of mediators activates three major plasma enzyme cascades, or processes: complement, coagulation, and kallikrein/kinin.

The plasma protein cascade systems are responsible for mediating the inflammatory response. Each system consists of a series of inactive enzymes *(proenzymes)*. These are converted to active enzymes. This, in turn, initiates a cascade in which the substrate (a substance changed by an enzyme in a chemical reaction) of the activated enzyme is the next component of the system.

Complement activates phagocytes and induces further inflammation and damage to the endothelium. As a result of the endothelial damage, coagulation becomes uncontrolled. This results in the formation of microvascular thrombi and tissue ischemia. Activation of the kallikrein/kinin system releases bradykinin (a potent vasodilator), which contributes to low systemic vascular resistance. The overall effect of these three systems is a hyperinflammatory and hypercoagulable state that leads to edema formation, cardiovascular instability (hypotension), and clotting abnormalities. These inflammatory processes alter the normal pathways both of systemic blood flow and of blood flow in the individual organs. The result is a hyperdynamic circulation where the cardiovascular system responds to a decrease in PVR by an elevation in cardiac output that is above normal marked by an increase in the amount of blood returning to the heart through the veins. Blood is shunted past some regional capillary beds. Changes in capillary permeability allow the formation of interstitial edema. As a result, the delivery of oxygen to the tissues is decreased. In addition, the capillaries become blocked by tiny blood clots and by clumps of inflammatory cells. The resultant ischemia contributes to MODS.

BOX 7-9 Clinical Manifestations of Multiple Organ Dysfunction Syndrome

After resuscitation (within 24 hours), a patient with multiple organ dysfunction syndrome (MODS) develops a low-grade fever, tachycardia (rapid heart beat), dyspnea (difficulty breathing), and altered mental status (confusion, level of consciousness). The lungs also begin to fail. This results in adult respiratory distress syndrome (ARDS). After 7 to 10 days, bacteremia commonly develops. Signs of kidney and liver failure appear as well. During days 14 to 21, renal and liver failure become severe, and the gastrointestinal (GI) and immune systems fail, followed by cardiovascular collapse. If the patient does not improve by the end of the third week, survival is unlikely. Death usually occurs between day 21 and day 28.

The same hormonal responses that help conserve volume in shock cause the body to enter into a hypermetabolic (catabolic) state, altering carbohydrate, fat, and lipid metabolism to meet the increased demand for energy. In time, the sympathetic drive and the hyperdynamic circulation place great demands on the heart. The net result is depletion of oxygen and fuel supplies. The decrease in oxygen delivery to the cells, the hypermetabolism, and the associated myocardial depression create an imbalance in oxygen supply and demand. This is soon followed by tissue hypoxia with cellular acidosis and impaired cellular function. Finally, multiple organ failure begins (Box 7-9 and Fig. 7-19). No specific therapy exists for MODS. However, early detection is critical, because it allows supportive measures to be started at once.

Impairment of Cellular Metabolism

Energy is required for nearly all of the cellular activities that support life. The active transport pumps in the cell membrane use up a large portion of the cell's energy. They use this energy to maintain a normal fluid and electrolyte composition inside the cell. Adenosine triphosphate (ATP) and other high-energy phosphate molecules provide the fuel for all the energy-related functions of the cell. In the healthy body, most cellular metabolism is aerobic metabolism. Anaerobic metabolism occurs when the metabolic need for energy outstrips the oxygen supply. However, anaerobic metabolism can supply only a small fraction of the energy

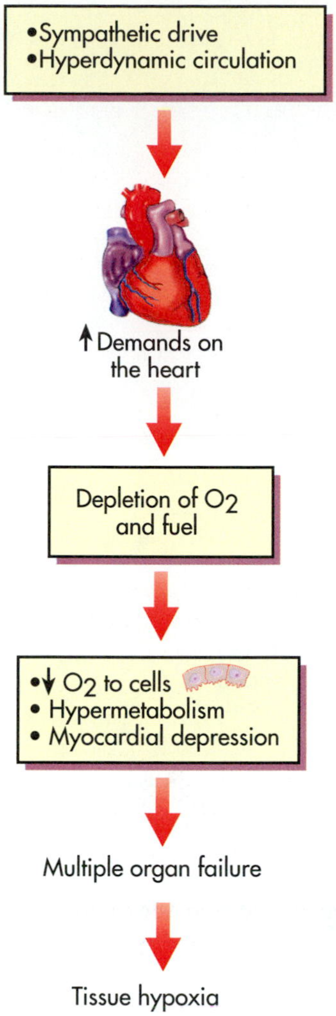

FIGURE 7-19 ■ Multiple organ dysfunction syndrome.

produced by aerobic metabolism. (Anaerobic metabolism generates 2 ATP molecules for every molecule of glucose. Aerobic metabolism generates 36 ATP molecules for every molecule of glucose). By itself, anaerobic metabolism cannot meet the body's energy needs.

Glucose is a key fuel for the production of energy. It is really the only fuel that can be used anaerobically under conditions of cellular hypoxia (as occurs in a state of shock). Under these conditions, glucose is metabolized to lactate and pyruvate. This produces a net sum of 2 ATP molecules. If oxygen is present (aerobic metabolism), pyruvate enters the *Krebs cycle.* This is a sequence of reactions that breaks down a molecule of pyruvic acid into molecules of carbon dioxide and water (Fig. 7-20). The Krebs cycle is 18 times more efficient at producing ATP than is glycolysis. (Glycolysis is the breakdown of glucose to lactate.) The Krebs cycle cannot occur in the absence of oxygen. Anaerobic production of ATP is inefficient. Thus, with anaerobic metabolism, the rate of glycolysis must be greatly increased to meet the body's energy demands. This leads to an increase in the production of lactic acid and resultant metabolic acidosis.

As tissue metabolites (and hydrogen ions) continue to accumulate, they stimulate vasodilation. This vasodilation opposes the previously described hormonally regulated constriction of the precapillary sphincters, thereby reducing the body's ability to continue vital tissue perfusion by maintaining the proper size of the vascular compartment. (The postcapillary sphincters are more resistant to the vasodilative effects of tissue metabolites. They stay constricted long after the precapillary sphincters dilate.) This in turn increases the capillary hydrostatic pressure. The result is fluid loss from the vascular space into the interstitial space. In addition, the insufficient energy production of anaerobic metabolism affects the cells' ability to maintain a normal sodium-potassium differential across the cell membrane. Intracellular potassium leaks out of the cell; sodium leaks into the cell. This creates cellular swelling and a decreased transmembrane potential. Energy production is further impaired. Finally, the cells are irreversibly damaged.

SELF-DEFENSE MECHANISMS

The body's first lines of defense against illness and injury are the external barriers. These include the skin and the mucous membranes of the digestive, respiratory, and genitourinary tracts. These structures form a barrier between the internal organs and the environment (see Chapter 39). When they are breached, chemicals, foreign bodies, or microorganisms are allowed to enter cells and tissues. The second and third lines of defense then are activated. These are the **inflammatory response** and the **immune response.**

Inflammatory Response

Inflammation is a local reaction to cellular injury. The response may be triggered by physical, thermal, or chemical damage. It also may be caused by microbial infection. When a microbial invasion occurs, this line of defense is activated. It prevents further invasion of the pathogen by isolating, destroying, or neutralizing the microorganism. As a rule, the response is protective. It is considered beneficial. However, if the response is sustained or directed toward the host's own **antigens,** healthy tissue may be destroyed.

> **NOTE** An *antigen* is a substance (usually a protein) that causes the formation of an antibody. The antigen reacts specifically with that antibody. Specific antibodies bind to specific antigens when the two fit together. The attachment of antibodies aids in the neutralization of antigens. It also aids in their removal from the body.

STAGES OF THE INFLAMMATORY RESPONSE

The inflammatory response may be divided into three separate stages. These are the cellular response to injury, the vascular response to injury, and phagocytosis.

Cellular Response to Injury. Metabolic changes occur with any type of cellular injury. The most common primary effect of cellular injury is damage to the cell's aerobic metabolism and ATP-generating process (oxidative phosphorylation). This leads to a decrease in energy reserves. When the energy sources are depleted, the sodium-

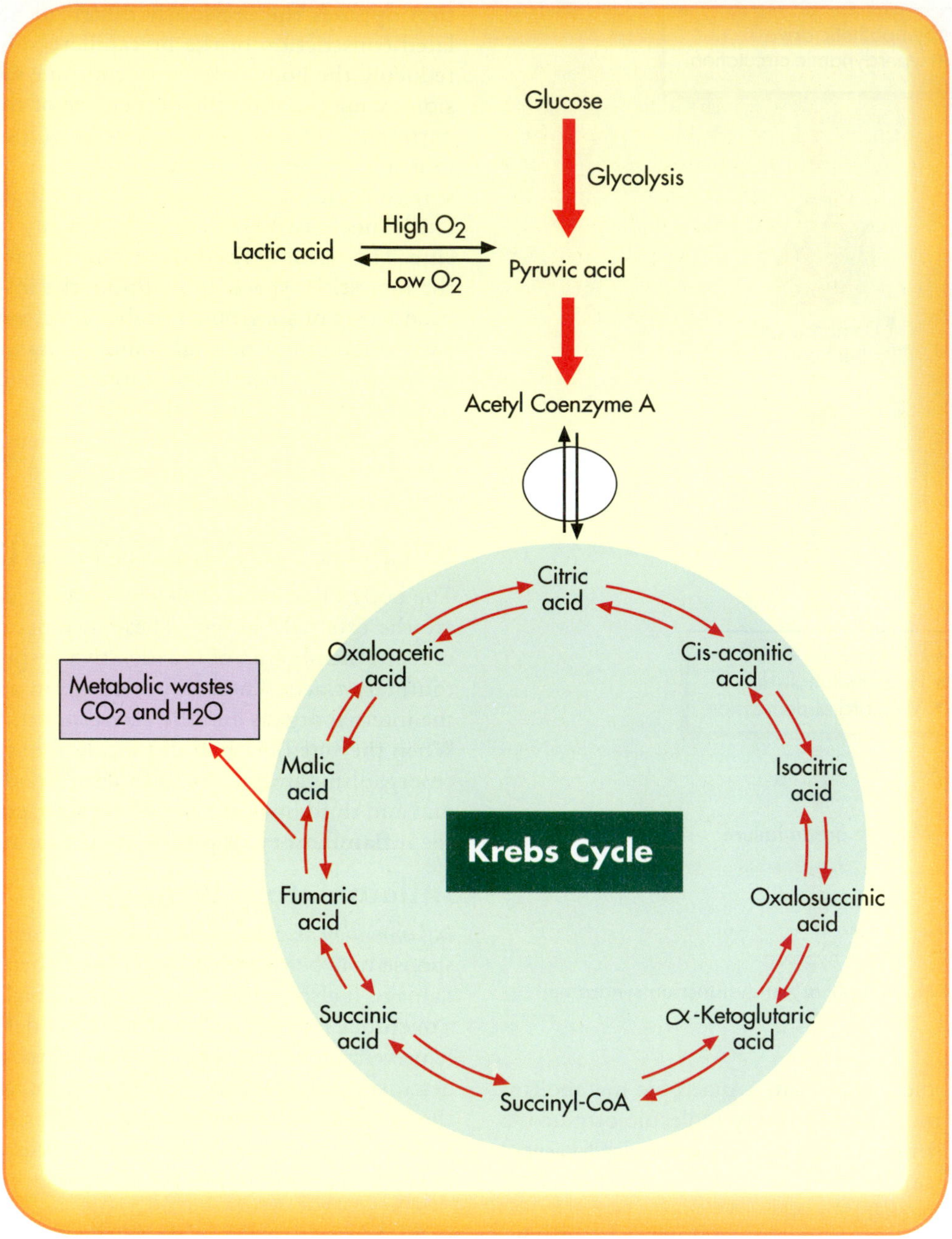

FIGURE 7-20 ■ Krebs cycle.

potassium pump can no longer work effectively. The cell begins to swell as sodium ions accumulate. The organelles in the cell also swell. This swelling, along with increasing acidosis, leads to further impairment of enzyme function. It also leads to further deterioration of the cell's membranes. In time, the membranes of the cellular organelles begin to leak. The release of hydrolytic enzymes by the lysosomes contributes further to cellular destruction and autolysis. As the cellular contents are dissolved by enzymes, the inflammatory response is stimulated in surrounding tissues.

Vascular Response to Injury. After cellular injury, localized hyperemia (an increase in organ blood flow) develops as the surrounding arterioles, venules, and capillaries dilate. The associated increase in filtration pressure and capillary permeability causes fluid to leak from the vessels. It leaks into the interstitial space. This creates edema. Leukocytes (particularly neutrophils and monocytes) begin to collect along the vascular endothelium. As a result of the release of *chemotactic factors* (chemicals that attract white cells to the site of inflammation), they soon migrate to the injured tissue.

Phagocytosis. *Phagocytosis* is the process by which leukocytes engulf, digest, and destroy pathogens. The circulating macrophages are also responsible for clearing the injured area of dead cells and other debris. *Intracellular* *phagocytosis* is the ingestion of bacteria and dead cell fragments. It occurs at the site of tissue invasion. It may extend into the general circulation if the infection becomes systemic. Intracellular phagocytosis stimulates the release of chemicals that induce lysis of the leukocytes. These leukocytes combine with dead organisms, proteins, and fluid to form an inflammatory exudate (commonly known as *pus*). This exudate is a by-product of the inflammatory process associated with bacterial infection. Exudate may be watery (***serous*** exudate), as is seen with blisters; thick and clotted (***fibrinous*** exudate), as is seen with lobar pneumonia; or pus filled (***purulent*** exudate), as is seen with cysts or abscesses. If bleeding occurs, the exudate is described as ***hemorrhagic*** exudate.

CRITICAL THINKING

Consider these signs or symptoms: heat, redness, pain, and swelling. What pathophysiological inflammatory response causes each of these?

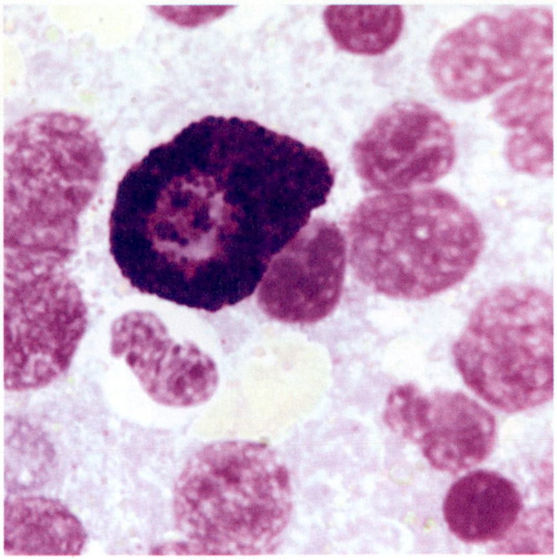

FIGURE 7-21 ■ Mast cell in bone marrow.

MAST CELLS

Mast cells are specialized cells (Fig. 7-21). They are widely distributed throughout connective tissues. Their cytoplasm is filled with granules containing *vasoactive amines* (histamine, serotonin) and chemotactic factors. When tissue is injured, the mast cells discharge their granules *(degranulation)* as part of the inflammatory response. Mast cell degranulation is stimulated by physical injury (e.g., thermal or mechanical trauma), chemical agents (e.g., toxins, snake and bee venoms), or hypersensitivity reactions. It also may be a direct result of the activity of complement components.

LOCAL AND SYSTEMIC RESPONSE TO ACUTE INFLAMMATION

Acute inflammation may be characterized by both local and systemic effects (Fig. 7-22). Local responses include vascular changes (vasodilation and increased vascular permeability) and the formation of exudate. Systemic responses include fever, leukocytosis, and an increase in circulating plasma proteins. The characteristic signs of localized inflammation are heat, redness, tenderness, swelling, and pain.

RESPONSES TO CHRONIC INFLAMMATION

Chronic inflammation lasts 2 weeks or longer. It can result from a persistent acute inflammatory response. This type of response may be caused by bacterial contamination by a foreign body (e.g., wood splinter, glass), persistent infection, or continued exposure to an antigen. If the inflammatory process is severe or prolonged, the body attempts to repair or replace tissue that has been damaged. To perform this repair, the body produces connective tissue fibers and new blood vessels. If the area of tissue destruction is large, scar tissue forms.

Immune Response

The skin and the inflammatory response are first to defend the body from injurious agents. They respond to every agent using the identical nonspecific mechanism. The immune response, however, is specific to each individual pathogen. Immunity may be natural, present at birth, or acquired. *Acquired immunity* develops through exposure to a specific antigenic agent or pathogen. It can be induced through vaccination (immunization) against certain infectious diseases. An example of such a disease is measles.

Acquired immunity is further classified as humoral immunity and cell-mediated immunity. *Humoral immunity* is associated with the production of antibodies that combine with and eliminate foreign material. *Cell-mediated immunity* is characterized by the formation of a group of lymphocytes that attack and destroy foreign material (see Chapter 39). Cell-mediated immunity is the body's best defense against viruses, fungi, parasites, and some bacteria. It also is the mechanism the body uses to reject transplanted organs.

CRITICAL THINKING

Consider hepatitis, feline leukemia, and chickenpox. What kind of immunity protects you from each of these?

NOTE The immune response is affected by age. Most infants are born with enough natural immunity to protect them from disease until they have made their own antibodies. However, the cells of the immune system become less efficient with age. Older people become more susceptible to disease. The aging immune system also becomes less able to eliminate abnormal cells that may develop.

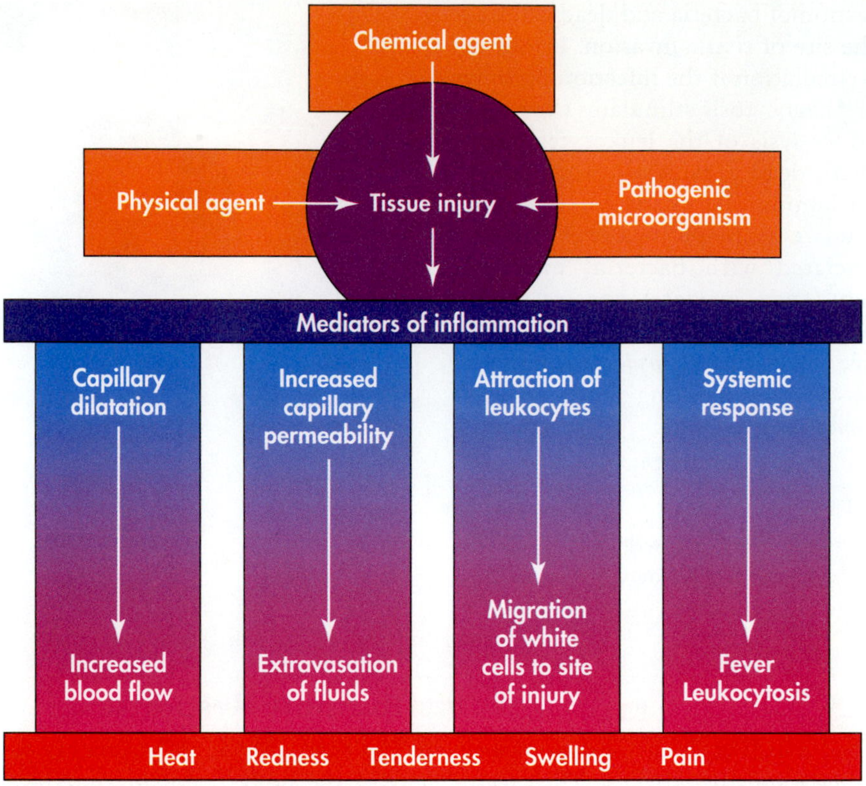

FIGURE 7-22 ■ Inflammation. (Modified from Crowley L: *Introduction to human disease,* ed 3, Boston, 1992, Jones & Bartlett.)

INDUCTION OF THE IMMUNE RESPONSE

As defined before, an antigen is a substance that *reacts* with preformed components of the immune system. For example, it may react with lymphocytes and antibodies. An antigen may be a molecule or a molecular complex. An immunogen is a specific type of antigen, one that also can bring about, or *induce,* the formation of antibodies. (Some antigens, therefore, are not immunogens because they are unable to induce the immune response.) To be immunogenic, the antigenic molecule must be:

- Sufficiently foreign to the host
- Sufficiently large
- Sufficiently complex
- Present in sufficient amounts

The immune response is triggered after foreign materials have been cleared from the area of inflammation. After phagocytes digest the pathogens, antigenic material appears on their surface. The antigen is recognized by receptors on lymphocytes as foreign, or "non-self." Then, a chain of events is put into motion to destroy or neutralize the antigen. Briefly, this involves two primary changes that occur among the lymphocytes. Some mature into plasma cells (derived from **B lymphocytes**), which produce antibody. Others mature into sensitized lymphocytes **(T lymphocytes).** These are capable of interacting directly with the foreign antigen to neutralize or destroy it. (The immune response is presented in more detail in Chapter 39.)

> **NOTE** *Immune tolerance* refers to the immune system's ability to allow self-antigens (versus non-self-antigens) to exist by preventing their recognition by lymphocytes and antibodies.

BLOOD GROUP ANTIGENS

In the early 1900s, researchers discovered that human blood had individual variations. A donor's blood was separated into plasma and red blood cell components and mixed with separated blood samples from another donor. Two reactions were noted. When combined with foreign plasma, the red cells either clumped together *(agglutinated)* or did not. Scientists also found that two distinct *agglutinins* (substances on red blood cells that act as antigens) were responsible for the clumping. Based on possible combinations of these antigens, four types of human blood were identified: A, B, AB, and O (Fig. 7-23).

Type A blood has anti-B antibodies in the plasma. It therefore clumps type B blood. Type B blood has anti-A antibodies. It therefore clumps type A blood. Type AB blood has neither antibody. Therefore people with this blood type can be given any of the four types of blood (*universal recipient*). Type O blood has both anti-A and anti-B antibodies but no antigens. It can therefore be given to patients with any blood type. Type O blood has become known as the *universal donor.*

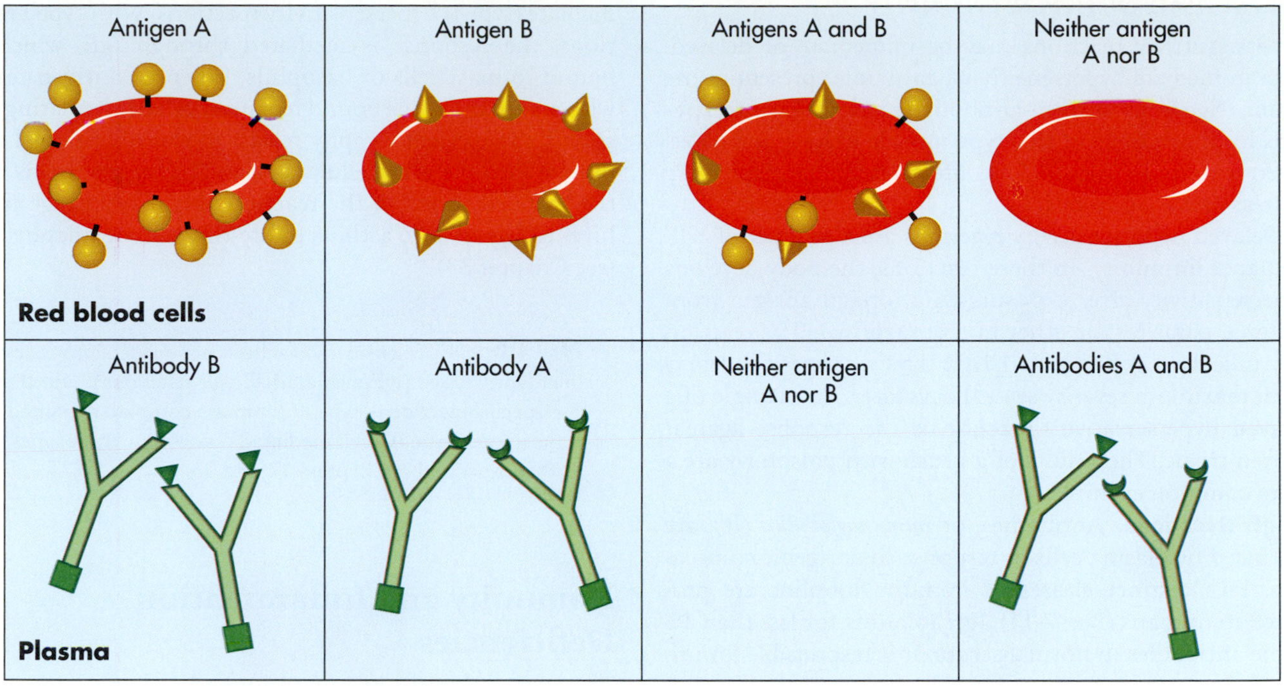

FIGURE 7-23 ■ ABO blood groups. In type A blood, the red blood cells have type A surface antigens and the plasma has type B antibodies. In type B blood, the red cells have type B surface antigens and the plasma has type A antibodies. In type AB blood, the red cells have both type A and type B surface antigens but no plasma antibodies. In type O blood, the red cells have no ABO surface antigens but the plasma has A and B antibodies.

RH FACTOR

In the late 1940s, another determinant in human blood was discovered: the Rh factor. (The acronym Rh was taken from the word *rhesus,* the species of monkey used in the research.) Researchers found that when the blood of a rhesus monkey was injected into a rabbit, the rabbit's immune system developed antibodies. When a sample of the rabbit's plasma was mixed with a sample of human red blood cells, the human cells usually clumped (Rh positive). About 85% of Americans have Rh-positive blood. Incompatibility between Rh^+ and Rh^- blood can cause a harmful immune response (e.g., through transfusion or during childbirth). The percentages of ABO and Rh blood groups in the general population are as follows:

O positive	38.4%
O negative	7.7%
A positive	32.3%
A negative	6.5%
B positive	9.4%
B negative	1.7%
AB positive	3.2%
AB negative	0.7%

VARIANCES IN IMMUNITY AND INFLAMMATION

The immune responses usually are protective. They help to protect the body from harmful microorganisms and other injurious agents. At times, however, these responses may be inappropriate. They may even have undesirable effects.

BOX 7-10 Autoimmune and Isoimmune Diseases

Graves disease
Rheumatoid arthritis
Myasthenia gravis
Immune thrombocytopenic purpura
Isoimmune neutropenia
Systemic lupus erythematosus (SLE)
Rh and ABO isoimmunization

Hypersensitivity: Allergy, Autoimmunity, and Isoimmunity

Hypersensitivity is an altered immunological reactivity to an antigen. It results in a pathological immune response upon reexposure. These abnormal responses include allergy, autoimmunity, and isoimmunity (Box 7-10). *Allergy* refers to an exaggerated immune response. This response is provoked by environmental **allergens.** *Autoimmunity* is an immune response against the host's own cells. (These are self-antigens.) *Isoimmunity* is an immune response directed against beneficial foreign tissues. (Examples of these are blood transfusions and transplanted organs.) Of these three responses, allergy is the most common. It also is the least life-threatening (see Chapter 33).

MECHANISMS OF HYPERSENSITIVITY

Hypersensitivity reactions may be immediate or delayed. With immediate hypersensitivity, antibodies present in the serum trigger an antigen-antibody reaction upon reexposure. Mild reactions of this type include itching and hives. Severe reactions may include life-threatening respiratory distress and anaphylaxis.

Delayed hypersensitivity reactions are a product of cell-mediated immunity. In these reactions, the body develops hypersensitivity after exposure to a foreign antigen from bacteria, parasites, or other microorganisms. The reaction may take several hours to 1 to 2 days to appear and may reach maximum severity several days later. An example of a delayed hypersensitivity reaction is the response against grafted tissue. The results of a brush with poison ivy are a more common example.

IgE Reactions. Antibodies, or *immunoglobulins (Ig),* are produced by plasma cells in response to antigenic stimulation. Five distinct classes of immunoglobulins are produced in humans (Box 7-11). IgE accounts for less than 1% of the antibodies in normal serum. It is responsible for immediate (type I) hypersensitivity reactions. With type I reactions, the response is mediated through IgE, which is bound to mast cells or basophils. When an antigen reacts with an IgE molecule bound to a mast cell or circulating basophil, these cells promptly release a host of chemical mediators into the extracellular space. The target organs and the manifestations of the reaction vary. They range from hives to hay fever to asthma to life-threatening anaphylaxis (see Chapter 33).

BOX 7-11 Classes of Immunoglobulins

IgG Immunoglobulins

IgG immunoglobulins account for 70% to 75% of the antibodies in normal serum. IgG is most abundant in blood. However, it also is found in lymph, cerebrospinal, synovial, and peritoneal fluid and breast milk. It is the main antibody involved in secondary immune responses. IgG is the only immunoglobulin that crosses the placenta. It provides temporary immunity in neonates.

IgM Immunoglobulins

IgM immunoglobulins account for about 5% to 10% of the antibodies in normal serum. Most anti A or anti B antibodies are of the IgM class. IgM triggers the increased production of IgG in acute infections and the complement fixation required for an effective antibody response.

IgA Immunoglobulins

IgA immunoglobulins account for about 15% of the antibodies in normal serum. This immunoglobulin is found in blood, secretions such as tears and saliva, and the respiratory tract, stomach, and accessory organs. IgA combines with a protein in the mucosa and defends body surfaces against invading microorganisms.

IgE Immunoglobulins

IgE immunoglobulins account for less than 1% of the antibodies in normal serum. IgE is found in some tissues and on the surface membranes of basophils and mast cells. IgE is responsible for immediate hypersensitivity reactions.

IgD Immunoglobulins

IgD immunoglobulins account for less than 1% of the antibodies in normal serum. The precise biological function of IgD is unknown.

NOTE Hypersensitivity reactions are divided into four distinct types: type I (IgE-mediated allergic reactions), type II (tissue-specific reactions), type III (immune complex–mediated reactions), and type IV (cell-mediated reactions). These types are further described in Chapters 17 and 33.

Immunity and Inflammation Deficiencies

The term *deficiencies* in immunity and inflammation indicates a failure of these mechanisms of self-defense. That is, they fail to function at normal capacity. The source of the deficiency may be congenital. (This means that it was caused by an anomaly present at birth.) The source also may be acquired. Examples include infection (e.g., the human immunodeficiency virus [HIV]), cancer (in particular the leukemias), immunosuppressive drugs, and aging. Whether the source is congenital or acquired, the deficiency usually is caused by a disruption in the function of the lymphocytes, although neutrophil dysfunction also has been described.

ACQUIRED DEFICIENCIES

Acquired immune deficiencies are far more common than congenital forms (Box 7-12). They may be classified into the following groups:

- Nutritional deficiencies (e.g., severe deficits in calorie or protein intake)
- Iatrogenic deficiencies (deficiencies caused by some form of medical treatment)
- Deficiencies caused by trauma (e.g., bacterial infection, burns)
- Deficiencies caused by stress (depressed immune function)
- Acquired immunodeficiency syndrome (AIDS)

NOTE Acquired immunodeficiency syndrome (AIDS) currently is the best known example of acquired dysfunction of the immune system. The human immunodeficiency virus (HIV) causes AIDS. It results in a debilitating illness that is manifested by various opportunistic infections and malignancies. Until recently, these were almost always fatal. The disease was first identified in 1981. Since then it has become a global health problem. It affects 5 million to 10 million people worldwide (see Chapter 39).

CRITICAL THINKING

Think about a time when you or someone close to you became ill because of an acquired immune deficiency. What kind of deficiency caused it? Was it preventable?

STRESS AND DISEASE

Prolonged emotional or psychological stress can result in physical illness. This type of illness can produce disturbances in three important areas: cognition, emotion, and behavior. The growing evidence of the link between stress and disease has created a new field of science called psychoneuroimmunology. *Psychoneuroimmunology* is the study of the three-way interaction of the emotional state, the central nervous system, and the body's defense against external infection and abnormal cell division (Fig. 7-24).

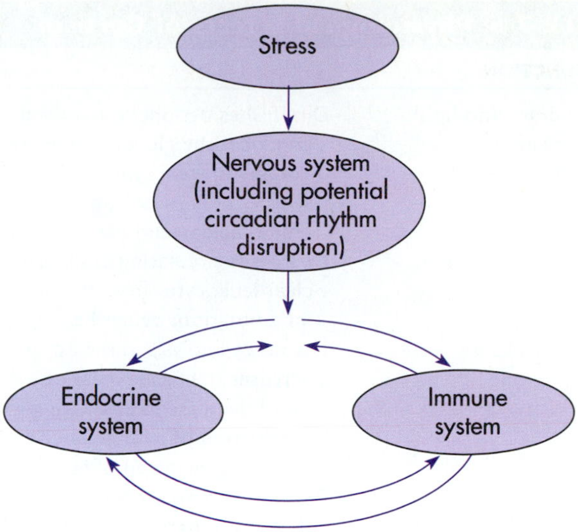

FIGURE 7-24 ■ Interaction of the emotional state, the central nervous system, and the body's defense against infection and abnormal cell division.

Neuroendocrine Regulation of Stress

As described in Chapter 2, the sympathetic nervous system is activated during the stress response. Stress causes the adrenal glands to release catecholamines (epinephrine, norepinephrine, and dopamine) into the bloodstream (Table 7-4). At the same time, the hypothalamus stimulates the pituitary gland to release the hormones ADH, prolactin, growth hormone, and adrenocorticotropic hormone (ACTH). ACTH, in turn, stimulates the cortex of the adrenal gland to release cortisol (Table 7-5).

CATECHOLAMINES

Catecholamines act by stimulating two major classes of receptors. These are alpha adrenergic receptors and beta adrenergic receptors. These two classes are further subcategorized into alpha-1 receptors, alpha-2 receptors, beta-1 receptors, and beta-2 receptors.

TABLE 7-4 Physiological Effects of the Catecholamines*

ORGAN	PROCESS OR RESULT
Brain	Increased blood flow Increased glucose metabolism
Cardiovascular system	Increased rate and force of contraction Peripheral vasoconstriction
Pulmonary system	Increased oxygen supply Bronchodilation Increased ventilation
Muscle	Increased glycogenolysis Increased contraction Increased dilation of skeletal muscle vasculature
Liver	Increased glucose production Increased gluconeogenesis Increased glycogenolysis Decreased glycogen synthesis
Adipose tissue	Increased lipolysis Increased fatty acids and glycerol
Skin	Decreased blood flow
Skeleton	Decreased glucose uptake and utilization (decreases insulin release)
Gastrointestinal and genitourinary tracts	Decreased protein synthesis
Lymphoid tissue	Increased protein breakdown (lymphoid tissue shrinks)

From McCance K, Heuther S: *Pathophysiology: the biologic basis for disease in adults and children,* ed 4, St Louis, 2002, Mosby.
*Some of these responses require the presence of glucocorticoids (e.g., cortisol) for maximal activity.

BOX 7-12 Acquired Immune Deficiencies

The following are associated with acquired immune deficiencies:
- Pregnancy
- Infancy
- Infection (e.g., maternal rubella during pregnancy [congenital], maternal *Cytomegalovirus* infection [during pregnancy], measles, leprosy, tuberculosis)
- Down syndrome
- Malignancies (e.g., Hodgkin disease, leukemia, myeloma)
- Stress caused by surgery or emotional trauma
- Malnutrition
- Aging
- Diabetes
- Alcoholic cirrhosis
- Sickle cell anemia
- Immunosuppressive treatment
- Anesthesia

From McCance K, Heuther S: *Pathophysiology: the biologic basis for disease in adults and children,* ed 4, St Louis, 2002, Mosby.

TABLE 7-5 Physiological Effects of Cortisol

FUNCTION	EFFECTS
Carbohydrate and lipid metabolism	Diminishes peripheral uptake and utilization of glucose; promotes gluconeogenesis in liver cells; enhances the gluconeogenic response to other hormones; promotes lipolysis in adipose tissue
Protein metabolism	Increases protein synthesis in the liver and depresses protein synthesis (including immunoglobulin synthesis) in muscle, lymphoid tissue, adipose tissue, skin, and bone; increases plasma level of amino acids; stimulates deamination (an oxidative reaction) in the liver
Inflammatory function	Decreases circulating eosinophils, lymphocytes, and monocytes; increases release of polymorphonuclear leukocytes from the bone marrow; decreases accumulation of leukocytes at the site of inflammation; delays healing; permissive for vasoconstrictive action of norepinephrine
Lipid metabolism	Promotes lipolysis in the extremities and lipogenesis in the face and trunk
Immune reserve	Decreases the tissue mass of all lymphoid tissues (e.g., decreases protein synthesis); promotes a rapid decrease in circulating lymphocytes, eosinophils, basophils, and macrophages; inhibits the production of interleukin-1 and interleukin-2 and consequently blocks cell-mediated immunity and the generation of fever
Digestive function	Promotes gastric secretion
Urinary function	Enhances urinary excretion
Connective tissue	Decreases proliferation of fibroblasts in connective tissue (thereby delaying healing)
Muscle	Maintains normal contractility and maximal work output for skeletal and cardiac muscle
Bone	Decreases bone formation
Vascular system and myocardial function	Maintains normal blood pressure; increases responsiveness of arterioles to the constrictive action of adrenergic stimulation; optimizes myocardial performance
Central nervous system	Modulates perceptual and emotional functioning (although the mechanism for this is unknown), which are essential for normal arousal and initiation of daytime activity

Modified from McCance KL, Huether SE: *Pathophysiology: the biologic basis for disease in adults and children,* ed 4, St Louis, 2002, Mosby.

TABLE 7-6 Physiological Actions of the Alpha and Beta Receptors

RECEPTOR	PHYSIOLOGICAL ACTIONS
Alpha-1 receptor	Increased glycogenolysis; smooth muscle contraction (blood vessels, genitourinary tract)
Alpha-2 receptor	Smooth muscle relaxation (gastrointestinal tract); smooth muscle contraction (some vascular beds); inhibition of lipolysis, renin release, platelet aggregation, and insulin secretion
Beta-1 receptor	Stimulation of lipolysis, myocardial contraction (increased rate, increased force of contraction)
Beta-2 receptor	Increased hepatic gluconeogenesis; increased hepatic glycogenolysis; increased muscle glycogenolysis; increased release of insulin, glucagon, and renin; smooth muscle relaxation (bronchi, blood vessels, genitourinary tract, gastrointestinal tract)

Modified from McCance KL, Huether SE: *Pathophysiology: the biologic basis for disease in adults and children,* ed 4, St Louis, 2002, Mosby.

- Alpha-1 receptors are postsynaptic. They are located on the effector organs (e.g., blood vessels, skeletal muscle). The main role of the alpha-1 receptors is to stimulate the contraction of smooth muscle. The alpha-2 receptors are found on the presynaptic nerve endings. Stimulation of the alpha-2 receptors serves as a negative feedback mechanism by inhibiting further release of norepinephrine.
- The beta-1 receptors are located mainly in the heart. Beta-2 receptors are located primarily in the bronchiolar and arterial smooth muscle. The beta receptors perform a number of functions. They stimulate the heart; dilate the bronchioles and the blood vessels in the skeletal muscle, brain, and heart; and aid in glycogenolysis.

Epinephrine activates both the alpha and beta receptors (Table 7-6); norepinephrine mainly excites the alpha receptors. (Alpha and beta receptors are discussed in more detail in Chapter 17.)

CORTISOL

Cortisol (hydrocortisone) circulates in the plasma. It mobilizes substances that are needed for cellular metabolism. The main metabolic effect of cortisol is the stimulation of gluconeogenesis. It also enhances the elevation of blood glucose. It does this by reducing glucose utilization. Cortisol also acts as an immunosuppressant; it reduces the reproduction of lymphocytes, particularly among the T lymphocytes. This, in turn, leads to a decrease in cellular immunity.

Cortisol also reduces the migration of macrophages into an inflamed area. It reduces phagocytosis, partly by stabilizing the lysosomal membranes. This decrease in immune cell activity may be beneficial, because it prevents immune-mediated

TABLE 7-7 Examples of Stress-Related Diseases and Conditions

TARGET ORGAN OR SYSTEM	DISEASE OR CONDITION
Cardiovascular system	Coronary artery disease Hypertension Stroke Disturbances of heart rhythm
Muscles	Tension headaches Muscle contraction backache
Connective tissues	Rheumatoid arthritis (autoimmune disease) Related inflammatory diseases of connective tissue
Pulmonary system	Asthma (hypersensitivity reaction) Hay fever (hypersensitivity reaction)
Immune system	Immunosuppression or deficiency Autoimmune diseases
Gastrointestinal system	Ulcer Irritable bowel syndrome Diarrhea Nausea and vomiting Ulcerative colitis
Genitourinary system	Diuresis Impotence Frigidity
Skin	Eczema Neurodermatitis Acne
Endocrine system	Diabetes mellitus Amenorrhea
Central nervous system	Fatigue and lethargy Type A behavior (impatience, competitive/aggressive attitude) Overeating Depression Insomnia

From McCance KL, Huether SE: *Pathophysiology: the biologic basis for disease in adults and children,* ed 4, St Louis, 2002, Mosby.

tissue damage. Two factors determine whether cortisol's effects are adaptive or destructive. These factors are the type of stress event and the length of exposure to the stressor.

Role of the Immune System

Many immunological conditions and diseases seem to be triggered by stress (Table 7-7). However, the exact mechanisms that link stress to these diseases and conditions have not yet been clearly defined. It is believed that the immune, nervous, and endocrine systems communicate through complex pathways. Also, they may be affected by factors involved in the stress reaction.

BOX 7-13 Example of Environmental Influence in Genetic Selection

The gene that causes sickle cell anemia was recognized to be much more common in environments in which malaria was prevalent. People with sickle cell disease have sickle-shaped red blood corpuscles, which clog the capillaries. This condition often proves fatal. However, in people who are carriers of the sickle cell trait, fewer than 1% of the red corpuscles are abnormal. These individuals do not die of sickle cell anemia, and they are more resistant to malaria than those who do not carry the sickle cell trait. Thus the trait proved protective, and its prevalence increased as a result of natural selection.

Interrelationship of Stress, Coping, and Illness

As noted above and in Chapter 2, the damage caused by stress is determined by the nature, intensity, and duration of the stressors. It also is affected by the way in which a person perceives the stressors and how well the individual is able to cope with them. The ability to spot the signs and symptoms of stress and to use stress management tactics is crucial to good health. Stress reduction techniques include meditation and imagery. In healthy individuals, such methods can help prevent harmful physiological and psychological illness arising from stress.

GENETICS AND FAMILIAL DISEASES

People are born with a predisposition to certain diseases. This predisposition is genetic. The genetics of some diseases are well known. Examples of such diseases are hemophilia or sickle cell anemia. With these, patients have no genetic predisposition, are carriers of the disease, or have the disease. Other disease processes certainly are linked to genetics. However, they also are strongly linked to environmental factors. Examples of such diseases are arthritis, diabetes, and hypertension. Medical researchers continue to try to reduce the incidence or severity of these inherited diseases. They are doing this through environmental manipulation.

Factors that Cause Disease

Certain factors can be said to cause disease. In general, these factors may be classified as *genetic* or *environmental.* Yet a strong interaction occurs between the two (Box 7-13). For example, genes cannot exert their effects without an environment in which to operate. Plus, environmental factors act differently on different people. On the other hand, the environment may be the same for a large number of people, but each individual has a unique genetic makeup. Thus, the interplay between genetics and the environment is very complex.

GENETIC FACTORS

Heredity is governed by the laws of chance and probability. This is so because each pair of chromosomes is sorted at random when packaged into eggs and sperm. More than 100,000 genes are involved in a person's genetic makeup. Thus, the range of variation is huge. Different types of genetic diseases can arise. These can occur because of individual genetic changes or because of abnormalities involving an entire chromosome.

Sometimes mistakes occur when chromosomes are packaged. This results in rearrangement of the chromosomes. Entire chromosomal abnormalities lead to diseases such as Down syndrome or Turner syndrome. More often, only a single gene on the chromosome is passed on, resulting in an abnormal protein. This is the type of genetic defect responsible for sickle cell anemia and hemophilia. Some conditions may involve more than one gene (i.e., they are *polygenic*) and a number of factors, but they still may have a strong inherited component. These diseases include coronary artery disease (CAD), hypertension, and cancer.

> ▶ **NOTE** Genes are not unchangeable units of inheritance. Under some circumstances, they can be affected by environmental influences (see Box 7-13).

ENVIRONMENTAL FACTORS

Many common chronic diseases may occur because of a mismatch between genetic and environmental factors (Tables 7-8 and 7-9). Important environmental factors include the following:

- Microorganisms and immunological exposure
- Personal habits and lifestyle
- Chemical substances
- Physical environment
- Psychosocial environment

The goal in preventing disease is to find the genetic and environmental influences that lead to major diseases. This knowledge will help individuals who have specific susceptibilities. They will be able to change certain environmental factors. This, in turn, may lessen their risk of developing the illness.

AGE AND GENDER

Age and gender also seem to play a role in the incidence of hereditary diseases. (These also are known as *familial diseases.*) This is especially true for diseases that are not caused by a single genetic defect. In the polygenic disorders, the combined effects of genes and environment over time play a role. These combined influences may result in diseases linked to age-related changes in metabolism. This may explain why heart disease, hypertension, and cancer are seen more often in people over age 40 than in people under that age.

Gender is associated with sex-specific diseases that arise from hormonal and anatomical differences. Two examples are breast cancer in women and testicular cancer in men.

TABLE 7-8 Environmental Factors that Affect the Occurrence of Disease

FACTORS	EXAMPLES
Microorganisms and immunological exposure	Bacteria Viruses Fungi Protozoa Vectors (e.g., insects and animals) Allergens
Personal habits and lifestyle	Smoking Physical exercise Dietary intake
Chemical substances	Toxins Pollutants Medications Solvents, fumes Contaminants
Physical environment	Climate Radiation Physical trauma Geographic location (e.g., sun exposure, altitude) Community (e.g., water and food supplies)
Psychosocial milieu	Family status (e.g., bereavement, loss, status change) Stress Coping skills Social isolation Ethnic and racial customs Religious customs

Lifestyle and environmental differences in gender-related activities also may play a role. These differences may be responsible for the predisposition to some diseases. Examples of gender, lifestyle, and environmental combinations include the higher rate of lung cancer and coronary artery disease in men who smoke cigarettes.

Analyzing the Risk of Disease

Epidemiologists are researchers who study disease. They use disease "rates" in their studies. They also use risk factor analysis. Disease rates help to describe the occurrence of disease. Risk factors are indicators of a person's predisposition to development of a disease.

DISEASE RATES

Three statistics are commonly used to assess the impact of a disease on a society. These are the incidence rate, the prevalence rate, and the mortality rate. The *incidence rate* refers to the number of new cases detected during a given period per the number of people in the population [surveyed.] The time period is usually 1 year. The *prevalence rate* refers to the number of people *living* with the disease per the number of people in the population surveyed. The *mortality rate* refers to the number of people who died from the disease during a

TABLE 7-9 Populations with Shared Disease Tendencies*

DISEASE	RATE AMONG POPULATIONS	SUGGESTED ENVIRONMENTAL FACTORS	SHARED GENE POOL
Early coronary artery disease	Very high in Finland (very low in Japan)	Animal fat intake	Genes for high blood cholesterol
Colon cancer	Low in developing countries (e.g., Africa); high in "westernized" countries (e.g., United States, Europe)	Dietary fiber and fat intake	None
Thalassemia (a type of anemia)	High in individuals of Mediterranean descent; low in other areas	None	Major dominant gene for thalassemia
Malaria (and many other infectious diseases)	High in some parts of Africa and Asia; low in United States and Europe	Trypanosomes, mosquitoes, disease control measures	None
Early non-insulin-dependent diabetes and obesity	Native Americans	Change from scarce food supply to plenty	Apparent shared gene pool among various Native American tribes
Lung cancer	Low in Mormons and Seventh Day Adventists	Health code forbids use of tobacco	None
Skin cancers	Higher among Caucasians than African Americans; higher in the Sun Belt	Ultraviolet light	Inherited level of skin pigmentation

From McCance KL, Huether SE: *Pathophysiology: the biologic basis for disease in adults and children,* ed 2, St Louis, 1994, Mosby.
*These tendencies are the result of shared environmental factors, a common gene pool, or both.

given period per the number of people in the population surveyed. The given period, again, is often 1 year.

The use of these disease rates can be shown in a study done to evaluate coronary artery disease in American men 50 to 64 years of age. The study found an incidence rate of 2.2%, a prevalence rate of 9.7%, and an annual mortality rate of 0.92% in this group.[2]

RISK FACTOR ANALYSIS

The presence of certain risk factors in any group of people is linked to an increased disease rate in that group. Diseases may have causal and noncausal risk factors. With *causal risk factors,* removal or elimination of the risk factors delays or prevents the disease. *Noncausal risk factors* can help predict a person's chances of developing the disease, but they have no direct effect on the underlying cause (Fig. 7-25). Risk factors cannot precisely predict whether a person will develop a disease. However, they can provide clues about the individual's likelihood of developing the disease.

Combined Effects and Interaction of Risk Factors

When one or more risk factors interact, the individual effects of risk factors may be greatly magnified. For example, some risk factors alone may pose little or no danger of disease. However, if another risk factor is added, the danger increases substantially.

FAMILIAL DISEASE TENDENCY

In some cases the members of a family (brothers and sisters, parents with children, spouse pairs, twins) are more prone to some diseases than are the people of the general population. Often the familial risk factors are genetic or shared factors in the environment. Examples include illnesses such as heart disease and pulmonary disease. These result from choices such as smoking and intake of dietary fat.

CRITICAL THINKING

Think about how many risk factors you have for heart disease. Which of these factors are genetic and which ones could you eliminate by modifying your habits or environment?

AGING AND AGE-RELATED DISORDERS

Advanced age is a risk factor for many diseases, such as heart attack, stroke, and cancer. This likely represents the cumulative effects of genetics and environmental factors. Disorders related to age occur throughout life (Table 7-10). Some disorders, such as dental cavities and "strep throat," are more common in younger age groups. The degenerative disorders (e.g., arthritis) are more common in older age groups.

Common Familial Diseases and Associated Risk Factors

Individuals who are high risk can take steps to avoid many familial diseases (Table 7-11). Examples of such diseases include coronary artery disease and colorectal cancer. These conditions are described in detail throughout this text.

TABLE 7-10 Age-Related Disorders

AGE	DISORDERS
Birth to 14 years	Congenital disorders Allergy Infection Cancer (leukemia, Wilms' tumor, medulloblastoma, retinoblastoma) Trauma or injury Diabetes (early onset)
15 to 30 years	Allergy (asthma) Endocrine disorders Trauma or injury (suicide) Venereal disease
30 to 40 years	Ulcer Hypertension Breast cancer Homicide Suicide Complications of pregnancy Alcoholism
40 to 60 years	Heart disease (hypertension, rheumatic disorder, infarction) Kidney disease (glomerular nephritis) Liver disease (cirrhosis) Cancer (lung, colon, breast, ovary)
60 to 80 years	Cardiovascular disease Cancer (lung, colon, prostate)
80 to 100 years	Cancer (leukemia, lymphoma, prostate cancer) Dementia (Alzheimer, Parkinson disease) Osteoporosis Infection Cardiovascular disease Trauma or injury (fracture)

Modified from King DW, Fenoglio CM, Lefkowitch JH: General pathology: principles and dynamics, Philadelphia, 1988, Lea & Febiger.

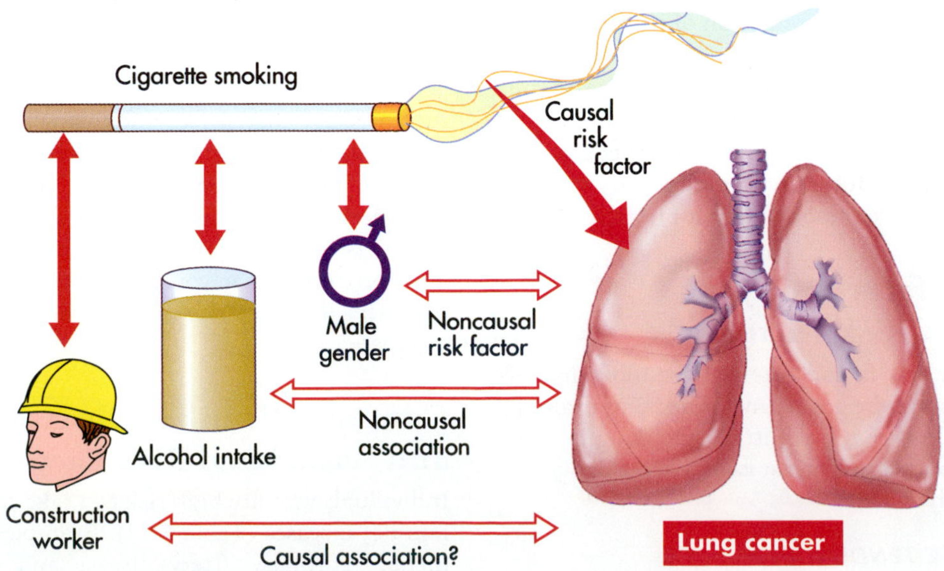

FIGURE 7-25 ■ Causal and noncausal risk factors and associations.

TABLE 7-11 Common Familial Diseases and Associated Environmental Risk Factors

DISEASE	ENVIRONMENTAL RISK FACTORS
Immunological Disorders	
Asthma and other allergies	Fur, dust, pollen, mold (other allergens)
Rheumatic fever	Group A *Streptococcus* bacterial infection
Cancer	
Breast cancer	Obesity, high dietary fat intake, alcohol ingestion, hormones
Colorectal cancer	Inadequate fiber intake, high dietary fat intake
Lung cancer	Cigarette smoke, environmental pollutants
Endocrine Disorders	
Diabetes mellitus (insulin dependent)	Viral infection, longstanding difficulty (years) controlling blood sugar
Diabetes mellitus (non-insulin dependent)	Obesity; high-sugar, low-fiber dietary intake; longstanding difficulty (years) controlling blood sugar
Hypertension	Diet, obesity, inadequate exercise (sedentary lifestyle)
Hematological Disorders	
Drug-induced hemolytic anemia	Aspirin, antibiotics, infection
Sickle cell anemia	Precipitated by cold weather, infection
Hemochromatosis	Ingestions (iron), transfusions
Cardiovascular Disorders	
Coronary artery disease	Exercise, alcohol ingestion, diet high in fat and salt, smoking, obesity, stress
Cardiomyopathies	Infection, ingestion of alcohol or use of other drugs
Mitral valve prolapse	Infection
Hypertension and stroke	Diet high in fat and salt, obesity
Renal Disorders	
Gout	Poor diet, injury, stress
Kidney stones	Decreased water intake
Gastrointestinal Disorders	
Malabsorption Disorders	
Lactose intolerance	Ingestion of milk products
Ulcerative colitis	Stress, consumption of trigger foods
Crohn disease	Stress, consumption of trigger foods
Peptic ulcers	Stress, diet that causes gastric irritation, infection
Gallstones	High dietary fat intake, obesity
Obesity	Diet high in fat, sugar, and total calories; stress that affects the appetite; cultural perceptions
Neuromuscular Disorders	
Multiple sclerosis	Virus, warm environment (heat-producing exercise, warm ambient temperature), stress
Alzheimer disease	Decreased mental stimulation later in life
Psychiatric Disorders	
Schizophrenia	Uncertain influence; dramatic success with drug treatment
Manic depression	Uncertain influence; dramatic success with drug treatment

SUMMARY

- Two facts illustrate the importance of body water. First, body water is the medium in which all metabolic reactions occur. Second, the precise regulation of the volume and composition of body fluids is essential to health. Water follows osmotic gradients established by changes in sodium concentrations. Thus, sodium and water balance are closely related.
- Two abnormal states of body-fluid balance can occur. If the water gained exceeds the water lost, a state of water excess, or overhydration, exists. If the water lost exceeds the water gained, a state of water deficit, or dehydration, exists.
- In addition to fluid imbalances, disturbances in the balance of electrolytes (other than sodium) may occur. These electrolytes include potassium, calcium, and magnesium. Imbalances of these electrolytes can interfere with neuromuscular function. They may even cause cardiac rhythm disturbances.
- The treatment of isotonic dehydration may include volume replacement with isotonic or occasionally hypotonic solutions. The treatment of hypotonic dehydration may involve intravenous replacement with normal saline or lactated Ringer solution. Occasionally hypertonic saline (e.g., in seizures caused by hyponatremia) is used. Interventions for overhydration depend on the cause. These interventions may include water restriction, administration of a diuretic, or, if hyponatremia is present, administration of saline.
- In-hospital treatment of hypokalemia involves intravenous or oral potassium replacement. Management of hyperkalemia may involve potassium restriction, enteral administration of a cation exchange resin, or intravenous administration of glucose and insulin, sodium bicarbonate, or calcium.
- Treatment of hypocalcemia involves intravenous administration of calcium ions. The management of hypercalcemia may include controlling the underlying disease, hydration, and, occasionally, drug therapy such as with furosemide and other calcium-lowering drugs.
- Hypomagnesemia typically is corrected by the administration of intravenous magnesium sulfate. The most effective treatment for hypermagnesemia is hemodialysis. Calcium salts that antagonize magnesium may also be given.
- The healthy body is sensitive to changes in the concentration of hydrogen ions (pH). It tries to maintain the pH of extracellular fluid at 7.4. This is accomplished through three interrelated compensatory mechanisms: carbonic acid–bicarbonate buffering, protein buffering, and renal buffering.
- Metabolic acidosis occurs when the amount of acid generated exceeds the body's buffering capacity. The four most common forms of metabolic acidosis encountered in the prehospital setting are lactic acidosis, diabetic ketoacidosis, acidosis resulting from renal failure, and acidosis caused by ingestion of toxins. Treatment for metabolic acidosis is aimed at correcting the underlying cause.
- Loss of hydrogen is the initial cause of metabolic alkalosis. This may be caused by vomiting (hydrochloric acid loss), gastric suction, or increased renal excretion of hydrogen ion in the urine. Treatment is directed at correcting the underlying condition. Volume depletion, if present, should be corrected with isotonic solutions.
- Respiratory acidosis is caused by the retention of carbon dioxide. This leads to an increase in the Pco_2. This condition usually is caused by an imbalance in the production of carbon dioxide and its elimination through alveolar ventilation. Treatment for respiratory acidosis involves improving ventilation quickly to eliminate carbon dioxide.
- Hyperventilation may produce respiratory alkalosis by decreasing the Pco_2. Treatment of respiratory alkalosis is directed at correcting the underlying cause of the hyperventilation. An initial approach is to place the patient on low-concentration oxygen. Another is to provide calming measures to assist the patient with slow, controlled breathing.
- An understanding of the processes of disease is crucial. This requires a knowledge of the structural and functional reactions of cells and tissues to injurious agents. Changes in cells and tissues can be caused by adaptation, injury, neoplasia, aging, or death.
- An injured cell may have an abnormal physical shape or size. Cell injury has both cellular and systemic indications.
- Certain factors cause disease. For the most part, these factors may be classified as genetic or environmental. However, a strong interaction occurs between the two.
- The term *hypoperfusion* is used to describe inadequate tissue circulation. Hypoperfusion may result from decreased cardiac output. Decreased cardiac output can lead to shock, multiple organ dysfunction syndrome, and other disease states associated with impaired cellular metabolism. Negative feedback mechanisms important in maintaining cardiac output and tissue perfusion are baroreceptor reflexes, chemoreceptor reflexes, the central nervous system ischemia response, hormonal mechanisms, reabsorption of tissue fluids, and splenic discharge of stored blood.

- The external barriers are the body's first line of defense against illness and injury. These barriers include the skin and the mucous membranes of the digestive, respiratory, and gastrointestinal tracts. When these barriers are breached, chemicals, foreign bodies, or microorganisms are allowed to penetrate cells and tissues. Then the second and third lines of defense are activated. These are the inflammatory response and the immune response. Both the external barriers and the inflammatory response respond to all organisms using the identical nonspecific mechanism. The immune response is specific to individual pathogens.
- Immune responses usually are protective. They help to protect the body from harmful microorganisms and other injurious agents. At times these responses may be inappropriate. They may even have undesirable effects. Examples of inappropriate responses include hypersensitivity and immunity or inflammation deficiencies.
- Many immune-related conditions and diseases are associated with stress. However, the exact mechanisms causing these illnesses have not yet been clearly defined. It is believed that the immune, nervous, and endocrine systems communicate through complex pathways and that they may be affected by factions involved in the stress reaction.

REFERENCES

1. American Heart Association: *Guidelines 2000 for cardiopulmonary circulation and emergency cardiovascular care,* International Consensus on Science, Dallas 2000, The Association.
2. National Highway Traffic Safety Administration: *EMT-paramedic national standard curriculum*, Washington, DC, 1998, US Department of Transportation, National Highway Traffic Safety Administration.
3. McCance K, Heuther S: *Pathophysiology: the biologic basis for disease in adults and children,* ed 2, St Louis, 1994, Mosby.

SUGGESTED READINGS

Alberts B et al: *Molecular biology of the cell,* ed 4, New York, 2001, Garland.

Berne RM, Levy MN, editors: *Physiology,* ed 4, St Louis, 1998, Mosby.

Halperin ML, Goldstein MB: *Fluid, electrolyte, and acid-base physiology,* ed 3, Philadelphia, 1999, WB Saunders.

Vander AJ et al: *Human physiology: the mechanisms of body function,* ed 6, New York, 1994, McGraw-Hill.

CHAPTER 8

Life Span Development

OBJECTIVES

Upon completion of this chapter, the paramedic student will be able to:

1. Describe the normal vital signs and body system characteristics of the newborn, neonate, infant, toddler, preschooler, school-aged child, adolescent, young adult, middle-aged adult, and older adult.
2. Identify the psychosocial features of the infant, toddler, preschooler, school-aged child, adolescent, young adult, middle-aged adult, and older adult.
3. Explain the effect of parenting styles, sibling rivalry, peer relationships, and other factors on a child's psychosocial development.
4. Discuss the physical and emotional challenges faced by the older adult.

KEY TERMS

Babinski reflex: A reflex movement in which the great toe bends upward when the outer edge of the sole is scratched.

menarche: The first menstruation and the commencement of the cyclic menstrual function.

menopause: The cessation of menses.

Moro reflex: A normal infant response elicited by a sudden loud noise. The infant flexes the legs, makes an embracing gesture with the arms, and usually gives a brief cry.

palmar grasp: A normal infant response. The infant curls the fingers in response to a touch on the palm of the hand.

puberty: The period of life when the ability to reproduce begins.

reciprocal socialization: A term that refers to a child's temperament and the responses it obtains from adults and family members. This interaction forms the basis for early social interactions with others and with the child's environment.

rooting reflex: A normal infant response elicited by touching or stroking the side of the cheek or mouth; this causes the infant to turn the head toward that side and to begin to suck.

sucking reflex: A normal infant response in which touching the infant's lips with the nipple of a breast or bottle causes involuntary sucking movements.

temperament: A person's style of behavior; the way the person interacts with the environment. It is the basis on which children develop relationships.

terminal drop: A theory that a decline in intelligence in older adulthood may be caused by the person's conscious or unconscious perception of coming death.

Paramedics care for patients from all age groups. Often, a patient's complaints are directly related to developmental characteristics common for that person's age group. Therefore it is important that paramedics study and understand the physiological and psychosocial development of human beings at different stages in life.

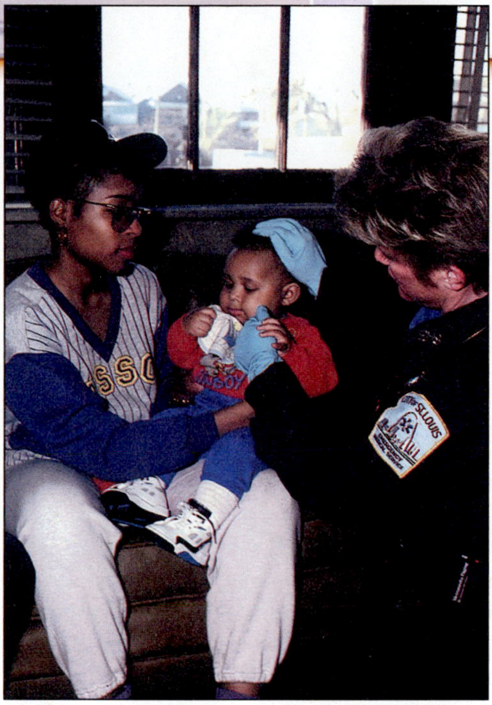

NOTE Age groups and development characteristics are defined in the *EMT-Paramedic National Standard Curriculum.*[1] These are general descriptions of development across the life span. They may differ slightly from other references in this and other textbooks. The age groups presented in this chapter are infants (birth to 1 year of age), toddlers (1 to 3 years of age) and preschoolers (3 to 5 years of age), school-aged children (6 to 12 years of age), adolescents (13 to 18 years of age), early adulthood (20 to 40 years of age), middle adulthood (41 to 60 years of age), and late adulthood (61 years of age or older).

NEWBORN

The term *newborn* is used for infants in the first few hours of life (Fig. 8-1). Children younger than 28 days of age are known as *neonates.* The term *infant* is used for a child 28 days to 1 year of age.

Vital Signs

During the first 30 minutes of life, the infant's heart rate is 100 to 200 beats per minute (bpm). By 1 year of age, the heart rate averages 120 bpm. At birth, the respiratory rate usually is 40 to 60 breaths/minute. This rate drops to 30 to 40 breaths/minute within a few minutes after delivery. By 1 year of age, 25 breaths/minute is considered normal. The average systolic blood pressure increases from 70 mm Hg at birth to 90 mm Hg at 1 year. Body temperature during infancy ranges from 98° to 100° F (36.7° to 37.8° C).

CRITICAL THINKING

Why are newborn, infant, and neonate considered distinct stages?

Weight

The full-term newborn normally weighs 3 to 3.5 kg (7 to 8 pounds). The baby's head accounts for about 25% of the total body weight. For the first few days of life, the total body weight may decrease 5% to 10% as a result of excretion of extracellular fluid. By the second week of life, birth weight is regained, and the child's weight exceeds the newborn weight. Although some babies gain weight faster than others, most gain an average of 140 to 168 g (5 to 6 ounces) per week. The increase in an infant's body weight should follow

CRITICAL THINKING

What considerations for patient care are necessary based on the size of the infant's head?

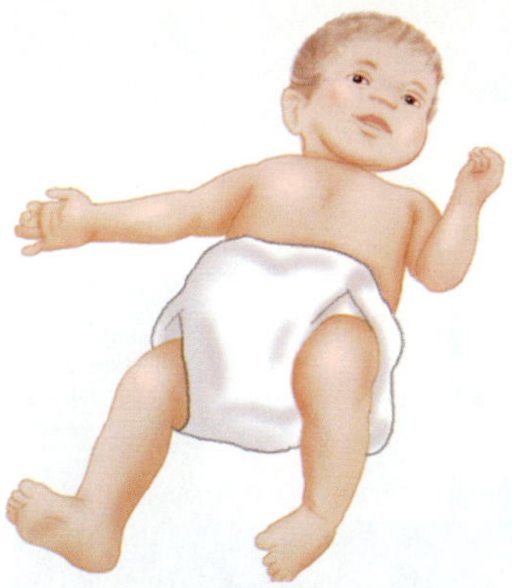

FIGURE 8-1 ■ Newborn.

a steady upward curve at about 30 g (1 ounce) per day during the first month of life (doubling the birth weight within 4 to 6 months and tripling it within 9 to 12 months). Monitoring the infant's weight every few weeks is a good way to keep track of development.

Cardiovascular System

At birth the infant's body must make some physiological changes to survive outside the womb. For example, the cardiovascular system must begin to work apart from the maternal circulation. Shortly after birth, the ductus venosus, ductus arteriosus, and foramen ovale (structures unique to fetal circulation) constrict. They close permanently within the first year of life. This results in an increase in systemic vascular resistance. It also results in an increase in aortic, left ventricular, and left atrial pressures. In addition, pulmonary vascular resistance decreases. This occurs because the lungs expand as the baby begins to breathe, which reduces the pulmonary arterial, right ventricular, and right atrial pressures (see Chapters 42 and 43). The left ventricle of the newborn's heart becomes stronger during the first year of life.

Respiratory System

Fetal lungs are filled with fluid. During delivery, the thorax is compressed, and the lung fluid is drained as the newborn gasps for air. Once the newborn gasps, the lung fluid that is left is absorbed via the lymphatic and pulmonary circulations. These strong first breaths open the alveoli. This allows additional respirations to occur more easily. The principal support for the chest wall comes from muscles rather than bones. These accessory muscles are immature and tire easily. The normal practice of using these muscles for breathing increases the infant's susceptibility to the accumulation of lactic acid in the blood *(lactic acidosis)*. In addition, collateral ventilation is decreased because newborns have fewer alveoli.

The infant's short, narrow airways are less stable than those of adults. Breathing occurs primarily through the nose during the first month of life. With infection or stress, the infant breathes more rapidly and may quickly lose body heat and fluids.

Nervous System

A healthy newborn can respond to a wide variety of stimuli and has a range of *reflexes* (Table 8-1). A number of these reflexes are essential for life outside the womb. These include the reflexes associated with breathing and eating. Other important reflexes are those that result from stress or discomfort. For example, obstruction of the airways may trigger a sneeze or a cough. Facial stimulation causes the baby to make sucking movements with the lips **(sucking reflex)** and to turn the head and move the lips toward the touch **(rooting reflex).** Crying may indicate hunger, pain, or discomfort from heat or cold. Some reflexes appear to have no useful purpose and gradually disappear during the first few months of life. These include the Babinski reflex, the Moro reflex, and the palmar grasp.

> **NOTE** The Babinski reflex is a normal response in infants and young children. However, in an older child or adult, it may indicate damage to the spinal cord (see Chapter 25).

Sleep may be very important to normal functioning of the brain. Newborns sleep an average of 16 to 18 hours per day. Sleep and wakefulness are evenly distributed over 24 hours. This sleep pattern gradually decreases to 14 to 16 hours per day with a 9- to 10-hour concentration of sleep at night. By 4 months of age an infant generally sleeps through the night but can be easily roused.

During the first year of life a newborn will make major advances in physical and mental skills. The brain and nervous system gradually mature during this period. To make room for brain growth, the posterior fontanel (unclosed joints between the bones of the skull) remains open until about 3 months of age. The anterior fontanel remains open for 9 to 18 months after birth. The anterior fontanel is usually level with or slightly below the surface of the skull. It is a good indicator of adequate hydration (with dehydration, the anterior fontanel may fall below the level of the skull and appear sunken). By the end of the first year, the development of mature nerves is virtually complete. The muscles have matured to the point where many infants can stand and walk with little or no assistance (Fig. 8-2).

Musculoskeletal System

At birth the only hard bones are in the fingers. As long bones mature, hormones act on the cartilage in the epiphyses of growing bones. This results in the deposition of calcium salts and the replacement of soft cartilage with hard bone. The epiphyseal plate lengthens, and bones thicken as new layers of bone are deposited on existing bone. Factors that influence bone growth include genetics, the production of growth hormone and thyroid hormone, nutrition, and the child's general health status. In infants, muscle weight accounts for about 25% of the entire musculoskeletal system.

TABLE 8-1 Reflexes Associated with Infancy

REFLEX	TEST	NORMAL FINDING
Babinski reflex	The examiner gently strokes the sole of the infant's foot.	The toes spread outward and upward.
Babkin reflex	The examiner presses on the palms of an infant who is lying on the back (supine).	The mouth opens, and the eyes close.
Moro reflex	A loud or startling noise is made near the infant.	The infant stretches the arms and legs, spreads the fingers, and then hugs self.
Palmar grasp reflex	The examiner puts an object or a finger in the infant's palm.	The fingers curl around the object or finger.
Rooting reflex	The examiner gently touches the infant's cheek or an area near the lips.	The infant's head turns toward the stimulation, and the mouth puckers.
Stepping reflex	The examiner holds the infant upright with the feet touching a solid surface.	The infant makes stepping movements that resemble walking.
Sucking reflex	The infant's mouth comes in contact with the nipple of a breast or bottle.	The infant's lips begin to pucker and suck.
Tonic neck reflex	The infant is placed in the supine position.	The infant turns the head and then extends the arm and leg on the side of the body toward which the head is turned.

Immune System

Babies are born with enough natural immunity from disease to protect them until they can make their own antibodies. This is known as *passive immunity*. Passive immunity arises from the mother's antibodies. These are passed through the blood to the fetus. If the baby is breast-fed, they also are passed through the mother's milk. Passive immunity lasts only for about 6 months after birth. After that interval, childhood immunizations against disease (e.g., pertussis, diphtheria, and tetanus) are usually recommended (see Chapter 44).

Other Developmental Milestones

Development during infancy depends on the interaction of heredity and the environment. Growth and development should be compared with standard growth charts showing norms. Box 8-1 lists some milestones from birth to 12 months of age.

Psychosocial Development

A baby's relationship with the caregiver (usually the mother) is a major factor in the infant's psychosocial development. This person is the baby's main source of comfort. The caregiver also represents the baby's main means of coping with stresses in the environment. Such stresses can include fear, pain, and anxiety. Erik Erikson[2] (a proponent of psychosocial theory) saw human development as the interaction between a person's genes and the environment. He theorized that life moves through a series of overlapping stages. Each stage is marked by a crisis that must be resolved. According to Erikson, the most critical stage, which occurs in infancy (up to $1^1/_2$ years of age), is the trust versus mistrust stage.[2] This stage is based on the infant's knowledge of two things: (1) that the surroundings are safe and predictable and (2) that causes and effects can be anticipated. For example, parental care is warm and loving, but punishment may result from not following rules. Consistency—or lack of it—in this type of care is the basis for trust versus mistrust issues.

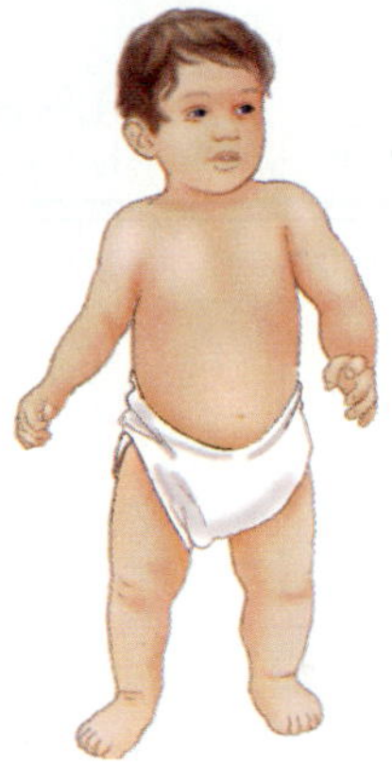

FIGURE 8-2 ■ Infant.

Continued

TEMPERAMENT

Temperament is a person's style of behavior. It also is the way a person interacts with the environment. Moreover, it is the basis on which children form relationships. Behavioral traits seen in children by 2 to 3 months of age can be used to define three general types of temperament.[3] About 35% of children do not fit any of these categories, instead demonstrating blends of these characteristics.

- *Easy children.* Easy children are characterized by regularity of bodily functions and low or moderate intensity of reaction. They accept new situations rather than withdraw from them. About 40% of children are easy children.
- *Difficult children.* Difficult children are characterized by irregularity in bodily functions and intense reactions. They withdraw from new situations. About 10% of children are difficult children.
- *Slow to warm up children.* Slow to warm up children are characterized by a low intensity of reaction and a

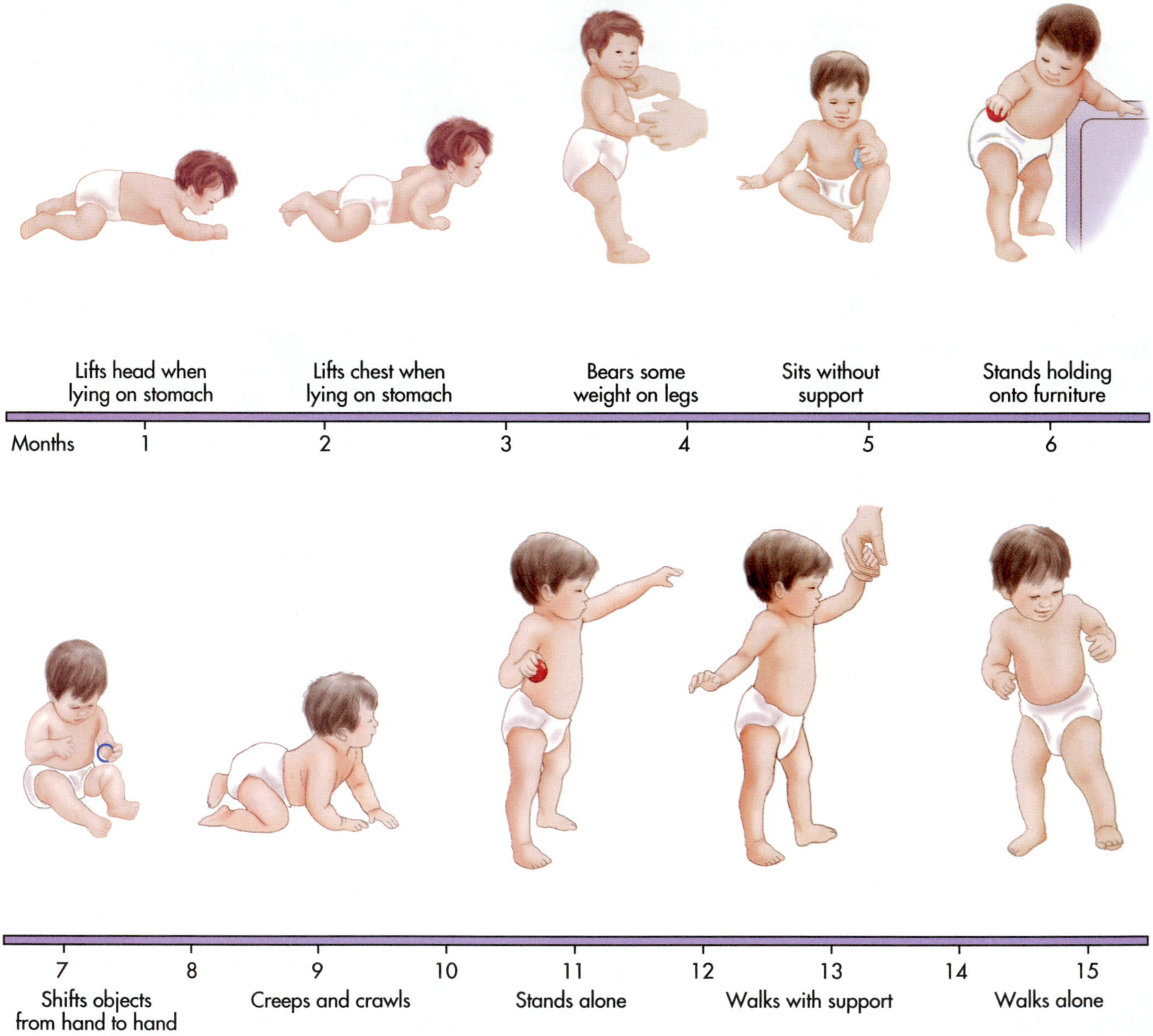
Lifts head when lying on stomach
Lifts chest when lying on stomach
Bears some weight on legs
Sits without support
Stands holding onto furniture
Months
1
2
3
4
5
6
7
8
9
10
11
12
13
14
15
Shifts objects from hand to hand
Creeps and crawls
Stands alone
Walks with support
Walks alone

FIGURE 8-2, cont'd ■ Infant.

BOX 8-1 Developmental Milestones (Birth through 12 Months)

Growth and development should be compared with standard growth charts showing established norms. It is important to remember that infants move through these stages at different rates.

2 months
- Tracks objects with eyes
- Recognizes familiar faces

3 months
- Moves objects to mouth with hands

4 months
- Drools without swallowing
- Reaches out to people

5 months
- Sleeps through the night without food
- Gains weight to twice birth weight
- Eruption of teeth may begin

6 months
- Sits upright in high chair
- Makes one-syllable sounds (ma, mu, da, di)

7 months
- Fears strangers
- Quickly changes from crying to laughing

8 months
- Responds to "No"
- Sits without assistance

9 months
- Responds to adult anger
- Pulls self to standing position
- Explores objects by sucking, chewing, and biting

10 months
- Recognizes own name
- Crawls well

11 months
- Attempts to walk unaided
- Shows frustration at restrictions

12 months
- Walks with assistance
- Gains weight to three times birth weight

somewhat negative mood. They adjust slowly to new situations. About 15% of children fall into this category.

A child's temperament and the responses this temperament obtains from adults form the basis for early social interactions. (Early social interactions are the child's interactions with others and with the child's environment.) This is known as **reciprocal socialization.** A baby's first interactions, combined with developmental changes, lead to specific relationships as follows[4]:

- During the first few weeks of life, infants are not much affected by an adult's appearance. The only exception is when the infant is fed.
- From about the start of the fourth week, infants begin to direct actions at the adults. Emotional reactions also appear at this time. The baby shows obvious signs of pleasure at the sight and sound of adults, especially females.
- During the second month, more complex and sensitive reactions emerge. These include smiling and vocal sounds aimed at the mother. Animated behavior is shown during interactions.
- By 3 months of age, the infant has formed a need for social interactions. That need continues to grow and is nourished by adults until the end of the second or the beginning of the third year. At that time, a need for peer interaction develops.

As the infant grows, the child's interactions become more complex. Bonding develops between the infant and family members. These bonds are considered *attachments.* For example, at 4 months of age, an infant shows *perceptual discrimination.* This means the child visually tracks the mother. At 9 months of age, an infant cries when the mother leaves. This is known as *separation anxiety* or *stranger anxiety.*

Separation from true attachments (e.g., separation from a parent) may result in a series of behaviors. The first is *protest* (loud crying, extreme restlessness, and rejection of all adults). Second is *despair* (nonstop crying, inactivity, and withdrawal). Third is *detachment* (a renewed but distant interest in surroundings, even if the mother comes backs). Some psychologists believe that attachments continue through a person's life span.

TODDLER AND PRESCHOOL YEARS

Children 1 to 3 years of age generally are considered toddlers. Those 3 to 5 years of age are considered preschoolers (Fig. 8-3).

Vital Signs

The heart rate in toddlers is usually 80 to 130 bpm. In preschoolers it is 80 to 100 bpm. Respirations for toddlers and preschoolers average 20 to 30 breaths/minute. A normal systolic blood pressure for toddlers is 70 to 100 mm Hg. For preschoolers it is 80 to 100 mm Hg. The normal body temperature for both age groups is 96.8° to 99.6° F (36° to 37.6° C).

Review of Body Systems

As children enter the toddler and preschool age groups, changes occur in some body systems.

Cardiovascular System. The capillary beds become better developed. They therefore are better able to assist in the body's thermoregulation. Hemoglobin approaches adult levels.

Respiratory System. The ear, nose, and throat structures in toddlers and preschoolers are similar to those in in-

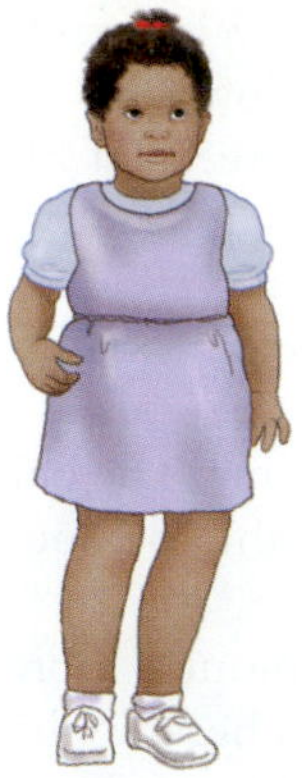

FIGURE 8-3 ■ Toddler and preschooler.

fants. Infants are at greatest risk for serious respiratory illness. Nevertheless, toddlers and preschoolers may acquire such infections in nursery school or preschool. Repeated upper respiratory tract infections may occur. However, they are rarely an indication of underlying disease in toddlers and preschoolers.

Nervous System. By age 2, much of the nervous system is completely developed. The myelination (the development of covering of the nerves) increases cognitive development. The brain weight is about 90% that of the adult brain. Visual acuity averages 20/30. Hearing is essentially mature by 3 to 4 years of age.

Musculoskeletal System. Muscle mass and bone density increase. Most children walk well with a normal gait by 2 years of age. Fine motor skills (e.g., scribbling with a pencil, stacking building blocks) become evident in toddlers and preschooler.

Immune System. Passive immunity no longer protects the children in these two age groups. They become more susceptible to minor respiratory and gastrointestinal infections.

Endocrine System. The endocrine organs mature and increase production of growth hormone, insulin, and corticosteroid. Children in the toddler and preschool age groups gain an average of 2.9 kg (6½ pounds) a year.

Renal System. The kidneys are well developed by age 2. At this time, many children begin to gain control of bladder and bowel functions. *Specific gravity* is a measure of the concentrating ability of the kidneys. This value and other measurements of urinary function are similar to those in adults.

Psychosocial Development

By 2 years of age, children have developed unique personality traits and moods, as well as specific likes and dislikes. Basic language skills are mastered by age 3. Refinement of these skills continues through childhood. Toddlers and preschoolers also begin to recognize the difference between men and women. They start to model themselves after people of their own gender. Box 8-2 lists other social milestones in the development of toddlers and preschoolers.

BOX 8-2 Social Milestones in Children 1 to 5 Years of Age

1 to 3 Years

- Can combine two different words
- Can complete some word phrases
- Follows directions
- Can point to a named part of the body
- Shows symbolic play when playing with toys
- Can remove some clothing

3 to 5 Years

- Can give first and last name
- Recognizes colors
- Speech is understandable to strangers.
- Completes short sentences and questions
- Can state name of a friend
- Begins to accept temporary absence of primary caregiver
- Plays independently in the presence of other children
- Shows increased level of confidence
- Shows sympathy at appropriate times (e.g., when another child is injured)
- Likes to hear and tell stories

CRITICAL THINKING

Reassuring and nonthreatening language should be used when treating toddlers and preschoolers. Consider how a 3-year-old child might interpret statements such as, "I'm going to give you a shot" or "You'll feel a stick in your arm."

PATTERNS OF PARENTING

Patterns of parenting begin to have an effect on children in the toddler and preschool years (Table 8-2). Most parenting styles fall into one of three categories[5]:

- *Authoritarian:* Authoritarian parents see obedience as a virtue. Conflicts with parents result in the child being punished. Children of authoritarian parents are not given much freedom or independence. Traits seen in these children may include low motivation to achieve, shyness, and hostility. These children also may have low self-esteem.
- *Authoritative:* Like authoritarian parents, authoritative parents think that rules must be followed. In this style of parenting, however, the child is given reasons for the rules. The child also is allowed to express a viewpoint, even though the parent has the final say. Authoritative parenting encourages a child to be independent. This style of parenting produces the most successful children. They tend to be responsible, assertive, self-reliant, and have high self-esteem.
- *Permissive:* Permissive parents give their children a lot of freedom. They are tolerant and accepting of the child's behavior, including both aggressive and sexual urges. These parents demand very little from their children. In

TABLE 8-2 Parenting Styles and Associated Traits in Children

AUTHORITARIAN STYLE	AUTHORITATIVE STYLE	PERMISSIVE STYLE
Low motivation to achieve	High motivation to achieve	Low motivation to achieve
Low self-esteem	Self-assertive	Low self-esteem
Shyness (girls)	Self-reliant	Lack of responsibility
Hostility (boys)	Friendliness, cooperativeness	Aggressiveness

fact, they tend to view their role as one of helping or serving the child. This style is the opposite of the other two parenting patterns. Traits seen in children raised by permissive parents are similar to those seen in children raised by authoritarian parents. These children are not especially independent, cooperative, or assertive. They often are discontented, distrustful, self-centered, and have low self-esteem.

SIBLING RIVALRY

First-born children often have a special relationship with their parents. They usually are expected to show self-control and responsibility when interacting with younger children. Parents are likely to be stricter with their first-born child, more demanding, and less consistent. They often spend more time with that child than with children who are born later. Because of these and other factors, sibling rivalry often becomes evident in the toddler and preschool age groups.

The characteristics of each child are one factor that influences how sibling conflicts occur. For example, a child may be fussy or easily bored or frustrated. A second factor is *family function.* This is how the family deals with daily problems and conflicts, and whether this is done in a respectful, productive, and nonaggressive way. Sibling rivalry can also be useful in child development. For example, disputes with brothers and sisters can promote crucial skills. These can include learning to value another person's point of view, learning to compromise and negotiate, and learning to control aggressive impulses.

PEER RELATIONSHIPS

Peer relationships offer a source of information about the child's world outside the family. They also expose the child to other types of families. In the toddler and preschool age groups, peer bonds are formed with others near the same age and maturity. These relationships often begin during play. Play may involve exploring a new toy, acting out fantasies, or using the imagination for new situations. Play also allows children to develop the ability to play simple games and competitive games with rules. This can lead to problem-solving skills and cognitive development. Play that involves others fosters interpersonal relationships. Toward the end of the preschool period, children begin to form lasting friendships. The importance of peer bonds and peer-group functions increases throughout childhood.

OTHER FACTORS THAT CAN AFFECT PSYCHOSOCIAL DEVELOPMENT

Two other key factors can have a significant impact on psychosocial development in the toddler and preschool age groups. These factors are divorce and exposure to aggression or violence.

About half of American marriages end in divorce. Several factors determine the effect divorce will have on toddlers and preschoolers. These include the child's age, cognition, and social competencies, and the child's sense of dependence on or independence from the parents. Children of divorced parents tend to have a higher rate of behavior problems as a result of family conflicts and stress than do children who live in a two-parent home. These problems may arise from a number of factors, including (1) social, economic, and emotional turmoil (including loyalty conflicts); (2) the child's reaction to the loss of the parent who leaves; (3) a change in the custodial parent's behavior toward the child; and (4) the type of day care the child attends as a result of the divorce. Common reactions to divorce in young children include depression, withdrawal, a fear of abandonment, and fear that their parents no longer love them. The parents' ability to recognize and respond to the child's needs is important to helping the child deal with the effects of divorce.

Exposure to violence may increase a child's acceptance of this type of behavior. For example, some children may regularly watch television shows or see video games with aggressive overtones. These children may model their behavior on these activities. It is particularly important that parents screen shows and play activities for children in the toddler and preschool age groups.

SCHOOL-AGE YEARS

Children are considered school age from 6 to 12 years of age. The heart rate in this age group is 70 to 110 bpm, the respiratory rate is 20 to 30 breaths/minute, the systolic blood pressure is 80 to 120 mm Hg, and body temperature averages 98.6° F (37° C) (Fig. 8-4).

Review of Body Systems

The growth of children in the school-aged years is slower and steadier than during infancy and the toddler and preschool years. School-aged children gain an average 6.6 cm (2½ inches) in height per year. Most bodily functions reach adult levels in this age group. Box 8-3 presents several important development milestones for school-aged children.

Nervous System. About 95% of the skull's growth is complete by age 10. In addition, children's skills and abilities become more varied as their nervous and musculoskeletal systems develop. Brain function increases in both hemispheres. The child's ability to concentrate and learn develops rapidly in this age group.

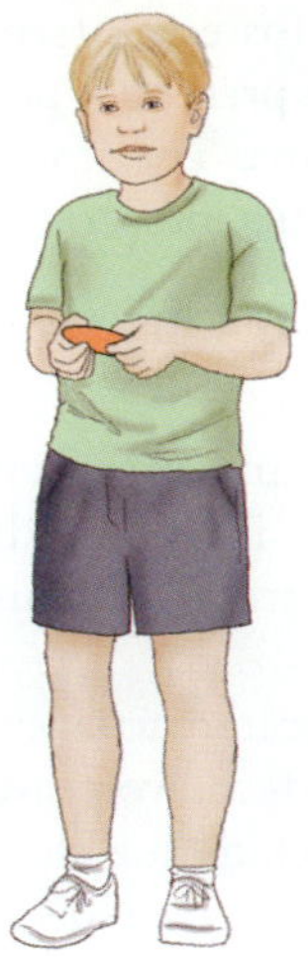

FIGURE 8-4 ■ School-aged child.

Reproductive System. The reproductive system becomes active when a child reaches **puberty.** Puberty is brought about by increasing levels of sex hormones in the body. For both genders, these hormone levels begin increasing before any external signs appear. The timing of puberty varies greatly. In girls it starts on average 2 years earlier (between ages 8 and 13) than in boys (between ages 13 and 15).

Lymphatic System. The lymphatic system plays a key role in fighting disease and infection. This system undergoes many changes throughout a child's growth until puberty, when growth slows. Until that time, the lymphatic tissues in school-aged children are proportionally larger than in adults.

Psychosocial Development

Between the ages of 6 and 12, the child's world expands outward from the family. At this time, relationships are formed with friends, teachers, coaches, caregivers, and others. As interactions with others increase, the school-aged child begins to compare himself or herself with others, thus developing a self-concept. Some situations can create stress and affect self-esteem. Self-esteem is often based on external factors (e.g., popularity with peers, experience of rejection, emotional support from family and friends). It seems to be higher in the early years of school age. Low self-esteem can have damaging effects in later development.

Psychosocial development varies by individual. Some children seem very mature. Others seem very immature. During this stage, behavior may depend on the child's mood and experience with various types of people. It may even be determined simply by what happened on a certain day. In addition, school-aged children begin to face the normal challenges of daily life. Fear of new situations (e.g., attending school) and peer pressure are predictable stressors for this age group.

Moral development occurs over time through experience. For school-aged children, control of behavior begins to shift from external sources (e.g., what parents believe is right or wrong) to more internal self-control. With this internal control, these children justify the morality of their choices.

BOX 8-3 Developmental Milestones in School-Aged Children

Physical Development

- Weight gain begins to consist more of muscle than fat; physical strength increases.
- Psychomotor skills (e.g., throwing, jumping, running) improve.
- Boys experience a "growth spurt" around age 12.
- Body changes indicate approaching puberty.
- Proportions of face and body become closer to those of adults.
- Eyes reach maturity in size and function.
- Permanent teeth begin to develop.
- Right- or left-handedness becomes well established.

Cognitive, Social, and Emotional Development

- Child is permitted more self-regulation with less supervision in the family setting.
- Parents usually spend less time with the child.
- Child's moral reasoning capabilities develop.
- Child gradually gains an understanding of the concept of death.
- Sexual interest grows rapidly with onset of puberty.
- Friendships become based on loyalty and mutual support.
- Social skills of giving, receiving, and sharing are learned.

Many theories attempt to explain moral development. Kohlberg's theory proposes six stages, extending from about 4 years of age through adulthood. The stages occur at three age-related levels of development: preconventional reasoning, conventional reasoning, and postconventional reasoning (Box 8-4).[6] Most experts agree that loving, caring, and positive bonds play key roles in moral education.

ADOLESCENCE

Individuals 13 to 19 years of age are adolescents (Fig. 8-5). Normal vital signs for this age group are a heart rate of 55 to 105 bpm, respirations of 12 to 20 breaths/minute, a systolic blood pressure of 100 to 120 mm Hg, and a body temperature of 98.6° F (37° C). Adolescence is the final phase of change in growth and development. Organs rapidly increase in size, including the heart, kidneys, spleen, and liver. Blood chemistry values are nearly the same as those in adults. Activity of the sebaceous glands causes the skin to toughen. Growth of bone and muscle mass is nearly completed during the 2- to 3-year adolescent growth spurt.

During adolescence an individual reaches reproductive maturity. In girls, the first external sign of puberty is a change in one or both nipples. The nipples change into what is known as a *breast bud.* A few months later, pubic hair and underarm hair begin to grow, and the breasts enlarge. Within about 2 years after the appearance of the breast bud and after body fat reaches 18% to 20% of body weight, **menarche** (first menstruation) usually occurs. Changes in the endocrine system cause the release of gonadotropin,

BOX 8-4 Kohlberg's Stages of Moral Development

Preconventional Reasoning (about 4 to 10 Years)

From 4 to 10 years of age, children respond to cultural control mainly to avoid punishment and attain satisfaction. The first two stages occur at this level:

- Stage 1: Punishment and obedience. Children obey rules and orders to avoid punishment; the child has no concern about moral rectitude.
- Stage 2: Naïve instrumental behaviorism. Children obey rules but only out of pure self-interest. They are vaguely away of fairness to others but only for their own satisfaction. The concept of *reciprocity* comes into play (i.e., "You scratch my back, I'll scratch yours.")

Conventional Reasoning (about 10 to 13 years)

From 10 to 13 years of age, children desire approval both from individuals and society. They not only conform, they actively seek to support society's standards. The next two stages occur at this level:

- Stage 3: Good boy–good girl mentality. Children seek the approval of others. They begin to judge behavior by intention (e.g., "She meant to do well.")
- Stage 4: Law and order mentality. Children are concerned with authority and with maintaining the social order. Correct behavior is "doing one's duty."

Postconventional Reasoning (13 years and older)

If true morality (an internal moral code) is to develop, it appears during these years. The person does not appeal to other people for moral decisions. Such decisions are made by an "enlightened conscience." The final two stages occur at this level:

- Stage 5: The person makes moral decisions legalistically or contractually. This means that the best values are those supported by law because they have been accepted by society as a whole. If a conflict arises between human need and the law, people work to change the law.
- Stage 6: An informed conscience defines what is right. An individual's actions are not based on fear, a need for approval, or legal demands, but on the person's own internalized standards of right and wrong.

Modified from Kohlberg L: A cognitive-developmental analysis of children's sex-role concepts and attitudes. In MacCoby E, editor: *The development of sex differences,* Stanford, Calif, 1996, Stanford University Press.

luteinizing hormone, and follicle-stimulating hormone. These hormonal substances promote estrogen and progesterone production. Progesterone affects breast development and the menstrual cycle. Estrogen causes the development of the female secondary sex characteristics, such as disposition of subcutaneous fat in the breast, thighs, and buttocks and the development of axial and pubic hair. Estrogen also promotes the buildup of endometrium in the uterus.

In boys, gonadotropin promotes testosterone production. Testosterone is a hormone produced by the testes. It causes the development of the male secondary sex characteristics. These include color and texture changes in the

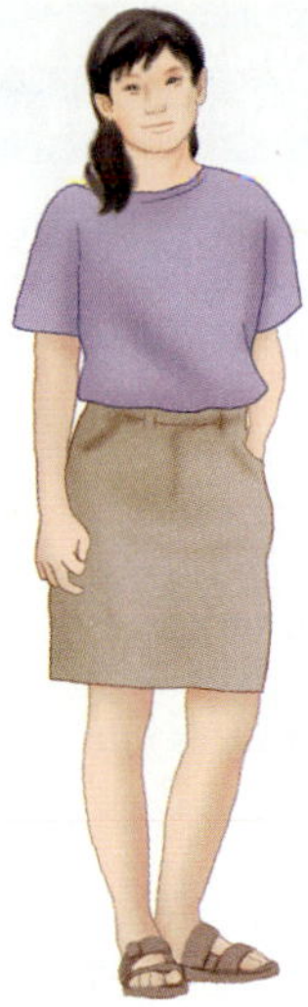

FIGURE 8-5 ■ Adolescent.

scrotum and an increase in the size of the testes. With these changes, the penis begins to enlarge and assume an adult shape, and pubic hair grows. At about age 14, a boy's first ejaculation of semen occurs during masturbation or sleep. Other male secondary sex characteristics that occur during late adolescence and early adulthood include a deepened voice, facial hair, underarm hair, and sometimes the growth of chest hair.

The development of secondary sex characteristics in both genders coincides with the last period of rapid growth in adolescence. Rapid growth is usually preceded by an increase in body fat. This body fat decreases during the period of growth and increases again in later years. Girls retain more fat than boys in the subcutaneous tissue in the areas of the breasts, thighs, and buttocks. Boys gain an average of 20 cm (8 inches) in height before age 21, when growth usually stops. Growth in girls is less dramatic. It usually is complete by age 18. During the period of rapid growth in adolescence, the hands and feet grow first. The arms and legs then begin to lengthen, and the shoulders become broader. Finally, the trunk of the body grows. The bones of the upper and lower jaw also grow. As a result, the face can change dramatically in appearance within a short time, especially in boys.

Psychosocial Development

In addition to physical changes, adolescence usually involves some emotional turmoil (Box 8-5). Adolescents may "try on" identities. These young people also begin to develop their adult personality. Conflicts with parents over school, manners, dress, hygiene, curfews, and other topics are common, because the adolescent has begun to express independence. As a result of these conflicts, most adolescents draw away from their parents. At the same time, they may emotionally move more toward their peers. Friendships with others who are also trying on various identities may result in the use of alcohol and other drugs, sexual experimentation,

BOX 8-5 Psychosocial Development of Adolescents

Some variations from the following descriptions are to be expected. Also, some characteristics and traits may be affected by other developmental issues.

13 to 14 Years
- Struggles with identity issues
- Displays moodiness
- Develops close friendships
- Pays less attention to parents
- Interests and clothing styles influenced by peer groups
- Shows ability to work
- Has same-sex friends
- Develops need for privacy
- Experiments with body (masturbation)
- May experiment with cigarettes, alcohol, and marijuana
- Has capacity for abstract thought

14 to 17 Years
- Becomes self-involved
- Shows extreme concern with body image and sexual attractiveness
- Examines personal and inner experiences
- Channels sexual and aggressive energies into creative activities (e.g., poetry, writing, music)
- Develops feelings of sexual love and passion
- Selects role models
- Shows greater capacity for setting goals

17 to 18 Years
- Develops secure personal identity
- Shows greater emotional stability
- Has heightened sense of humor
- Shows pride in work
- Shows stable interests and concern for others
- Has higher level of concern for the future
- Develops clear sexual identity and ability for sensual love
- Shows gradual interest in adult behavior
- Accepts social norms and cultural traditions
- Can set goals and follow through with plans

and extreme forms of behavior or dress. Antisocial behavior tends to peak at about the eighth or ninth grade level.

In the teenage years, both boys and girls are very concerned about their appearance. Comparisons are continually made among peers. Concerns about body image are common in this age group. These include weight issues, body odor, acne, and dandruff. All these conditions can arise from the hormonal changes associated with adolescence. During adolescence many teenagers, especially girls, become obsessed with weight loss. They may try fad diets to control their figures. Eating disorders are common in this age group. Obsession with weight loss may lead to bulimia, anorexia nervosa, and severe depression. In fact, depression and suicide are more common among adolescents than in any other age group.[1]

CRITICAL THINKING

It may be best to interview the adolescent and the parents separately. Why might this be important?

EARLY ADULTHOOD

Early adulthood spans the period from 20 to 40 years of age (Fig. 8-6). Average vital signs for this age group are a heart rate of 70 bpm, respirations of 16 to 20 breaths/minute, a blood pressure of 120/80 mm Hg, and a body temperature of 98.6° F (37° C). At the onset of early adulthood, individuals are reaching their physical peak. This is achieved between 19 and 26 years of age. Lifelong habits and routines develop. Body systems are at their optimal performance. This also is the age group in which pregnancy is most likely to occur. However, the aging process has begun. Some of the effects of aging (e.g., slowed reaction times, hearing loss, vision deficiencies) gradually become evident during this stage of life. Good health in early adulthood tends to be centered on lifestyle and physical fitness. Unintentional injury is the leading cause of death in this age group.

Psychosocial Development

The ability to love usually is well developed by early adulthood. This includes both romantic and affectionate love. Also, newly formed families bring on new challenges and stresses during this period. The highest levels of job stress are felt in this age group. Even so, fewer psychological issues related to well-being arise during early adulthood than during any other phase of life. Most individuals in this age group focus their attention on career and family as part of their psychosocial development. Their pursuits include the following:

- Selecting a mate
- Learning to live with a marriage partner
- Raising children
- Managing a home
- Finding a congenial social group
- Developing adult leisure-time activities
- Selecting a secure and stable occupation
- Establishing and maintaining an economic standard of living

MIDDLE ADULTHOOD

Middle adulthood extends from 41 to 60 years of age (Fig. 8-7). The average vital signs are the same as those for early adulthood. Also, body systems continue to work at a high level. However, the physiological aspects of aging may become more obvious during this stage. For example, cardiovascular health becomes a concern. Hearing and vision changes occur. Periodontal disease may develop. Weight control becomes more difficult. Cancer tends to strike often. For women, **menopause** normally occurs between age 45 and 55. This marks the end of reproductive capacity.

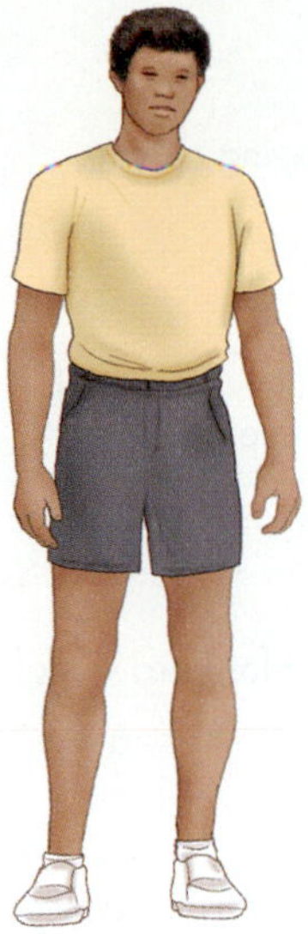

FIGURE 8-6 ■ Early adulthood.

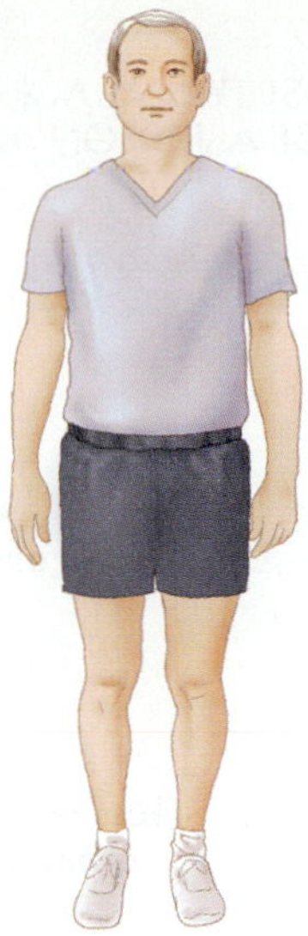

FIGURE 8-7 ■ Middle adulthood.

Psychosocial Development

Middle adulthood generally is a productive time for social and professional recognition. It often is a period of financial security. However, because of the physical changes just described, the person in middle adulthood often becomes concerned with the "social clock." The individual may feel a sense of time pressure to meet lifelong goals. Common causes of stress in this age group include financial commitments and responsibility for the care of elderly parents. Another stress is concern for young adult children who have moved out and are on their own. As the last child leaves home, a depression or sense of loss is not unusual for many parents *(empty nest syndrome)*. Others feel a sense of freedom and enjoy a greater chance for self-fulfillment.

Some adults in middle age experience a "mid-life crisis." They may make sudden and sometimes irrational changes in their life (similar to the identity issues seen in the teenage years). This may occur because of health worries, a change in physical appearance as a result of aging, or a change in the level of sexual activity with a spouse. However, most middle-aged adults tend to approach problems in their lives more as challenges than as threats. Important goals, for example, often are (1) to help their children to be responsible and happy adults; (2) to accept and adjust to aging parents; and (3) to accept the physiological changes of middle age.

LATE ADULTHOOD

People reach late adulthood at 61 years of age (Fig. 8-8). Vital signs in this age group depend on the individual's health status. Moreover, they are affected by the physiological changes in body systems that normally occur during this stage of life. A person's life span is determined by health, genetics, and other factors. The theoretical maximum life span for human beings is 120 years.[1]

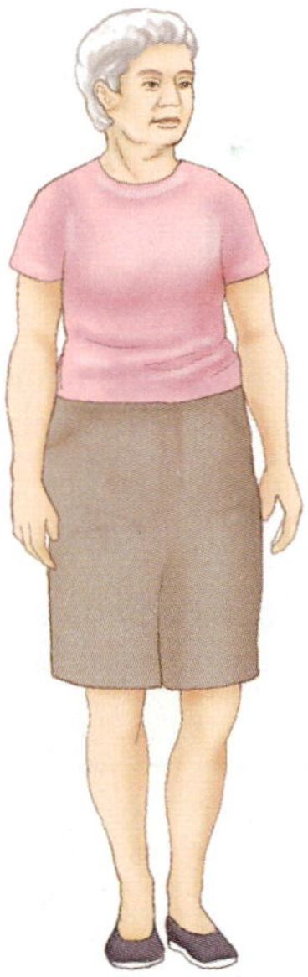

FIGURE 8-8 ■ Late adulthood.

Review of Body Systems

Body system changes associated with late adulthood vary from person to person (Fig. 8-9 and Box 8-6). They also vary from organ to organ and from function to function (see Chapter 45). Some occur dramatically. Others occur gradually. Some functions even remain constant well into old age. This variation can be seen in a number of systems. For example, a decrease in cardiac output and the ability to metabolize carbohydrates becomes evident early on. Changes in skin texture and hair color occur throughout late adulthood. The speed of nerve conduction and the manufacture of red blood cells do not decline until late old age.

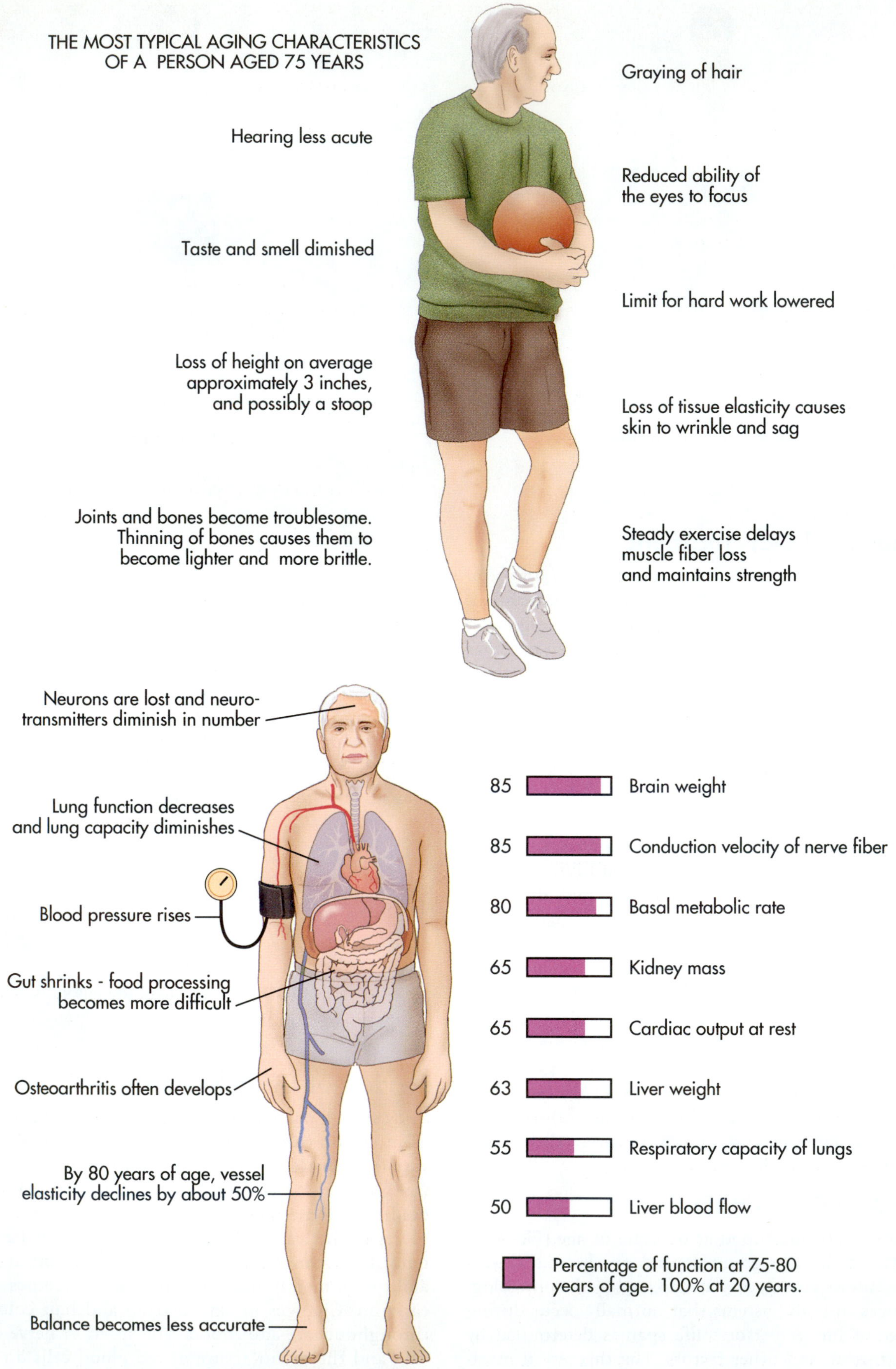
THE MOST TYPICAL AGING CHARACTERISTICS OF A PERSON AGED 75 YEARS
Hearing less acute
Taste and smell dimished
Loss of height on average approximately 3 inches, and possibly a stoop
Joints and bones become troublesome. Thinning of bones causes them to become lighter and more brittle.
Graying of hair
Reduced ability of the eyes to focus
Limit for hard work lowered
Loss of tissue elasticity causes skin to wrinkle and sag
Steady exercise delays muscle fiber loss and maintains strength
Neurons are lost and neuro-transmitters diminish in number
Lung function decreases and lung capacity diminishes
Blood pressure rises
Gut shrinks - food processing becomes more difficult
Osteoarthritis often develops
By 80 years of age, vessel elasticity declines by about 50%
Balance becomes less accurate
85 Brain weight
85 Conduction velocity of nerve fiber
80 Basal metabolic rate
65 Kidney mass
65 Cardiac output at rest
63 Liver weight
55 Respiratory capacity of lungs
50 Liver blood flow
Percentage of function at 75-80 years of age. 100% at 20 years.

FIGURE 8-9 ■ Body changes that occur in late adulthood.

BOX 8-6 Physiological Changes Associated with Late Adulthood

Cardiovascular System
- Functional changes occur as blood vessels thicken and peripheral resistance increases.
- By 80 years of age, vessel elasticity declines by about 50%.
- Blood flow to organs decreases.
- Baroreceptor sensitivity is reduced, and blood pressure tends to rise.
- Increased workload of the heart causes cardiomegaly, changes in the mitral and aortic valves, and decreased myocardial elasticity.
- The heart becomes less able to respond to exercise.
- The number of pacemaker cells in the heart diminishes, resulting in dysrhythmias (tachycardias are not well tolerated).
- The functional blood volume and platelet count decrease.
- The number of red blood cells decreases in late old age.
- Iron levels are poor.

Respiratory System
- Functional changes occur in the mouth, nose, and lungs.
- Lung function decreases, and lung capacity diminishes.
- The elasticity of the diaphragm declines, and the chest wall weakens.
- Diffusion through the alveoli diminishes from lifelong exposure to pollutants.
- Less oxygen becomes available for uptake by the blood.
- Coughing becomes ineffective because of weakened chest wall function and bone structure.

Nervous System
- Neurons are lost, and neurotransmitters diminish in number.
- Some taste buds are lost, and the olfactory sense diminishes.
- Pain perception decreases.
- The kinesthetic sense (sense of body movement) is lessened.
- Visual acuity diminishes.
- Reaction time declines.
- Hearing changes occur.
- The sleep-wake cycle is disrupted.

Musculoskeletal System
- Muscle mass is replaced by fibrous tissue.
- Progressive bone loss occurs, and changes in bones and joints become troublesome.
- Balance becomes less accurate.
- Osteoarthritis often develops.
- Shrinking of vertebral disks leads to loss of height and stooping posture.

Gastrointestinal System
- Secretion of saliva and gastric juices is reduced.
- Peristalsis and gastrointestinal secretions decrease.
- The esophageal sphincter becomes less effective, and internal intestinal sphincters lose tone.
- Vitamin and mineral deficiencies occur.
- Changes in the liver affect the metabolism of some drugs and foods.

Endocrine System
- Glucose metabolism and the production of insulin decrease.
- Production of triiodothyronine (T_3) by the thyroid gland declines.
- Production of cortisol decreases by about 25%.
- The pituitary gland becomes about 20% less effective.
- Women's reproductive glands begin to atrophy.

Renal System
- About 50% of the nephrons in the kidneys are lost.
- The filtration surface in the kidneys is reduced.
- Salt and water balance is compromised.
- Abnormal glomeruli become more common.
- The frequency of urination and the amount of urine eliminated decrease.

Psychosocial Development

Society's attitude toward age can either enhance or detract from an older person's sense of self-worth. Some cultures credit wisdom to age; others consider the elderly to be more of a burden. For those who enjoy good health and retirement, late adulthood is a time of happiness and personal fulfillment. For others, this period is marked by financial burdens and physical and emotional challenges.

FINANCIAL BURDENS

Most people in late age begin to accept and adjust to retirement. They also adjust to having a reduced income. However, they face new issues. For example, some must pay for health care, and they may need to establish new living arrangements. About 95% of older adults live in their homes. These individuals choose not to reside in home care facilities such as nursing homes and assisted care communities. The financial requirements for either type of living arrangement can be a burden for the older adult and the family. For example, an older person living at home may require in-home health and home care services to assist with tasks of daily living. An older person who lives in a home care facility may need constant nursing care and other types of supervision. These situations, plus the cost of health insurance, prescription medicines, and other health care needs, can create financial burdens, even for those who plan well for their retirement. In 2003, about 3.6 million older adults in the United States were living below the poverty level, and 2.2 million were considered to be "near-poor."[7]

CRITICAL THINKING

In an older patient's home, what clues may indicate that the person is under a financial strain or burden?

PHYSICAL AND EMOTIONAL CHALLENGES

In addition to the physical challenges linked to aging and the related health consequences, older adults face emotional challenges. Two emotional dilemmas are commonly faced in advancing years. One is accepting a decline in cognition. The other is dealing with the dying or death of a companion.

Aging does not always produce a decline in brain function. However, some conditions can cause a loss of mental faculties. Such conditions include circulatory disorders and some diseases common in older adults (e.g., Parkinson disease). Problems with short-term memory, learning, attention, and judgment may develop. This decline in mental capability is an important concern and a cause of depression in older adults. The term **terminal drop** refers to the theory that a decline in intelligence in later years may be caused by a person's conscious or unconscious perception of coming death.[8] (This decline is measured by a change in IQ tests.) Such a perception may cause the person to begin withdrawing from the world anywhere from a few weeks up to 5 years before death. Terminal drop may become evident by changes in mood or mental functioning or by the way the body responds. It also may be linked to the presence of a disease (e.g., cancer). According to the terminal drop theory, the higher a person's IQ in old age, the longer the person is likely to live after the IQ test.

The dying or death of a partner can be one of the most stressful events in life. The ways in which a person deals with the death or imminent death of a partner are based on a number of factors. These include the person's cultural or religious views, the cause and timing of death, the length and type of relationship, the person's quality of life before death, and the support of friends, family, and organizations. Most people experience a variety of emotions in dealing with death and dying. These range from initial denial to final acceptance (see Chapter 2).

SUMMARY

- The newborn is a baby in the first hours of life. A neonate is a baby younger than 28 days. An infant is a child 28 days to 1 year of age.
- The newborn normally weighs 3 to 3.5 kg (7 to 8 pounds). This weight typically triples in 9 to 12 months. The infant's head accounts for about 25% of the total body weight.
- At birth, structures unique to fetal circulation constrict and normally close within the first year of life. Fluid is expelled from the lungs during the first few breaths. Respiratory muscles and alveoli are not fully developed.
- Infants are born with protective reflexes related to breathing, eating, and stress or discomfort.
- At birth the anterior and posterior fontanels are open. Bone growth occurs at the epiphysis of the bones.
- Some passive immunity is conferred at birth and through the mother's breast milk.
- The caregiver is the major factor in the infant's psychosocial development.
- Temperament is a person's behavioral style. It is the way the person interacts with the environment.
- Toddlers are children 1 to 3 years of age. Preschoolers are 3 to 5 years of age.
- The hemoglobin level in toddlers and preschoolers approaches that of adults. The brain in this age group is about 90% of the adult brain weight. Muscle mass and bone density increase. Walking occurs by age 2, and fine motor skills develop. Control of bowel and bladder are achieved.
- Parenting styles can be described as authoritarian, authoritative, or permissive.
- Sibling rivalry, peer relationships, divorce, and exposure to aggression and violence affect a child's development.
- School-aged children range from 6 to 12 years of age. Physical growth slows, but brain function and the ability to learn quickly develop in this age group. Many children reach puberty during this time. Self-esteem and moral development are critical at this age.
- Adolescents are 13 to 19 years of age. The growth of bone and muscle mass is nearly complete in this age group. Reproductive maturity has been reached. Adolescence often involves some emotional turmoil, and antisocial behavior may be seen.
- Early adulthood spans the period from 20 to 40 years of age. Lifelong habits and routines develop. Body systems are at their optimal performance.
- Middle adulthood extends from 41 to 60 years of age. The physiological aspects of aging become more apparent in this age group. Menopause in women occurs during this stage.
- People reach late adulthood at 61 years of age. Body system changes vary widely from person to person, but the systemic changes of aging become apparent. Some adults in this age group face financial, physical, and emotional challenges.

REFERENCES

1. US Department of Transportation, National Highway Traffic Safety Administration: *EMT-paramedic national standard curriculum,* Washington, DC, 1998, The Department.
2. Erikson E: *Childhood and society,* ed 2, New York, 1963, WW Norton.
3. Dacey J, Travers J: *Human development,* ed 2, Madison, Wis, 1994, William C Brown Communications.
4. Hartup WW: Peer relations. In Mussen PH, Hetherington EM, editors: *Handbook of child psychology, vol 4, socialization, personality, and social development*, ed 4, New York, 1983, Wiley.
5. Baumrind D: *Early socialization and the discipline controversy,* Morristown, NJ, 1975, General Learning Press.
6. Kohlberg L: A cognitive-developmental analysis of children's sex-role concepts and attitudes. In MacCoby E, editor: *The development of sex differences,* Stanford, Calif, 1996, Stanford University Press.
7. Based on data from Current Population Reports, "Poverty in the United States: 2000," P60-214, Issued September, 2001 and related Internet releases of the U.S. Bureau of the Census.
8. Birren J: *The psychology of aging,* Englewood Cliffs, NJ, 1964, Prentice Hall.

PART THREE

IN THIS PART

CHAPTER 9 Therapeutic Communications

CHAPTER 10 History Taking

CHAPTER 11 Techniques of Physical Examination

CHAPTER 12 Patient Assessment

CHAPTER 13 Clinical Decision Making

CHAPTER 14 Assessment-Based Management

CHAPTER 15 Communications

CHAPTER 16 Documentation

CHAPTER 9

Therapeutic Communications

OBJECTIVES

Upon completion of this chapter, the paramedic student will be able to:

1. Define therapeutic communication.
2. List the elements of effective therapeutic communication.
3. Identify internal factors that influence effective communication.
4. Identify external factors that influence effective communication.
5. Explain the elements of an effective patient interview.
6. Summarize strategies for gathering appropriate patient information.
7. Discuss methods of assessing the individual's mental status during the patient interview.
8. Describe ways the paramedic can improve communication with a variety of patients. Such patients include (1) those who are unmotivated to talk; (2) hostile patients; (3) children; (4) older adults; (5) hearing-impaired patients; (6) blind patients; (7) patients under the influence of drugs or alcohol; (8) sexually aggressive patients; and (9) patients whose cultural traditions are different from those of the paramedic.

KEY TERMS

decoding: The act of interpreting symbols and format.
encoding: The act of placing a message in an understandable format (either written or verbal).

therapeutic communication: A planned, deliberate, professional act that involves the use of communications techniques to achieve two purposes: (1) a positive relationship with the patient and (2) a shared understanding of information between the patient and the paramedic. These two factors aid in the attainment of the desired patient care goals.

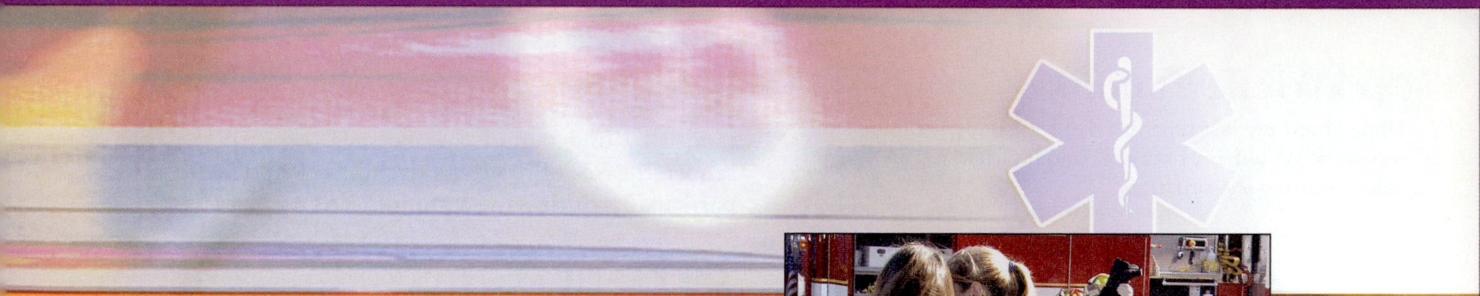

Therapeutic communication *can have several important effects. It can improve the paramedic's interaction with the patient, ensure better patient care, defuse potentially violent situations or prevent them from escalating, and reduce the risk of lawsuits.*

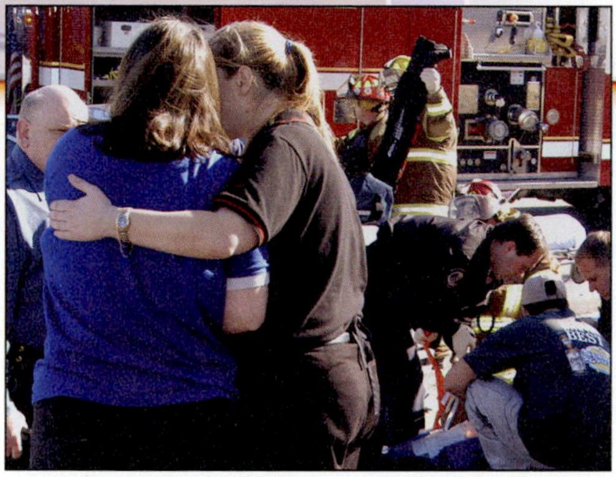

COMMUNICATION

Communication is the main element of human interaction. It involves both verbal and nonverbal behavior. Moreover, it includes all the symbols and clues people use to convey and receive meaning.[1] The process of communication has several elements. The paramedic must be aware of each element to interact well with a patient. Every element is crucial. In fact, information and meaning can be gained or lost if any one element is changed (Fig. 9-1). To achieve good communication, all participants must take equal responsibility for their part in the process. Communication is successful only when each person clearly gets the message.

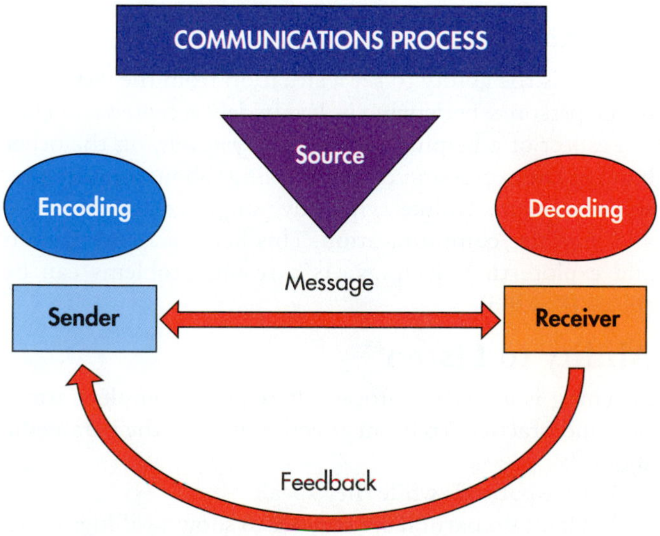

FIGURE 9-1 ■ The process of communication.

NOTE This chapter deals with communication between paramedics and their patients. However, these suggestions and techniques also can be used to improve communication between health care providers. This may include crew members. It also may include nurses, physicians, dispatchers, and other emergency providers.

Elements of the Communication Process

Communication is a dynamic process. It has six elements: the source, encoding, the message, decoding, the receiver, and feedback.

SOURCE

Verbal communication uses spoken or written words (common symbols) to express ideas or feelings. These common symbols should be simple, short, and direct. That way, confusion can be avoided (Box 9-1).

BOX 9-1 Techniques for Verbal Communication

- Use fewer words to avoid confusion.
- Use words that express an idea simply.
- Do not use vague phrases.
- Use examples (including demonstrations) if they will make the message easier to understand.
- Repeat the important parts of a message.
- Do not use technical jargon.
- Speak at an appropriate speed or pace.
- Do not pause for long periods or quickly change the subject.

CRITICAL THINKING
Think about the last time you had a misunderstanding with someone. Would any of the techniques listed in Box 9-1 have improved the situation?

ENCODING

Encoding involves putting a message in a format that, when translated, is understood by both the sender and the receiver. The format may be either written or verbal. Encoding is the responsibility of the sender *(encoder)*, because the sender defines the content and emotional tone of the message. In the process of communication, the sender role may pass from one person to another as information is exchanged. For example, at first the paramedic may act as the sender of the message by asking a patient for information. When the patient responds, that person assumes the role of the sender.

MESSAGE

The *message* is the information that is sent or expressed by the sender. It should be clear and organized. It should be communicated in a manner familiar to the person receiving it. The message may include verbal and nonverbal symbols (e.g., spoken words, facial expressions, gestures). As a rule, the more ways (or formats) in which a message is communicated, the more likely the receiver is to understand it. For example, combining soothing words and a reassuring touch for a patient in pain communicates the message of compassion better than spoken words alone.

Not all symbols have universal meaning. For example, a reassuring touch might be welcome to persons of certain cultures, while those of other cultures may find it offensive. Paramedics must take into account the cultural differences of people. They should also consider how they will deal with a language barrier before attempting to send a message.

DECODING

Decoding is the interpretation of symbols and formats. It prompts the receiver to respond to the sender's message. The decoding process can fail if symbols or words sent in the message are unfamiliar to both parties. It also can fail if interpretation of the message is based on different understandings of symbols or format. For example, the word *pain* may mean horrific discomfort to one person. However, it may mean a mild annoyance to another. Therefore, when communicating with a patient, the paramedic must carefully select words that cannot easily be misinterpreted.

NOTE Some medical conditions, such as a stroke, can make it more difficult for a person to encode or decode a message.

RECEIVER

The receiver is essentially the *decoder*. This is the person intended to understand the message. As with the role of sender, the role of receiver switches back and forth between participants during the communication process.

CRITICAL THINKING
Have you ever attended a class in which nothing made sense? Think back on the reason you didn't understand the content. Was it an encoding problem or a decoding problem?

FEEDBACK

Feedback is the receiver's response to the sender's message. The quality of the feedback reveals whether the message's intended meaning was received. If the intended meaning was not received, the sender must clarify the message by changing its content. The sender then assesses the new feedback. Like the message, feedback may be verbal or nonverbal.

INTERNAL FACTORS IN EFFECTIVE COMMUNICATION

To communicate well with patients, paramedics must genuinely like people. They must be able to empathize with others. They also must have the ability to listen (Box 9-2). Each of these internal factors plays an important role in therapeutic communication.

Liking Others

As a helping profession, health care depends on the relationships forged between patients and health care providers. These relationships are based on trust and caring. In fact, they cannot be achieved without a genuine concern for others and an understanding of human strengths and weaknesses. Patients must trust and believe that a paramedic *wants* to care for their needs. Paramedics can convey this trust to patients by accepting them as individuals.

Empathy

Empathy is the ability to see a situation from the viewpoint of the person experiencing it. It is widely accepted as a clinical aspect of a helping profession. *Sympathy,* on the other hand, is the expression of one's feelings about another person's problem. Unlike sympathy, empathy uses sensitive and objective communication. This helps patients explain and explore their feelings. As a result, problems can be solved (Box 9-3).

Ability to Listen

Listening is an active process. It requires complete attention and practice. To be an effective listener, the paramedic should[2]:

1. Face patients while they speak.
2. Maintain natural eye contact to show a willingness to listen.

BOX 9-2 Active Listening Attitudes and Guidelines

1. Listen to understand, not to ready yourself to reply, contradict, or argue back. This attitude is extremely important.
2. Remember that *understanding* involves more than simply knowing the dictionary meaning of the words used. It involves paying attention to the patient's tone of voice, facial expressions, and overall behavior.
3. Look for clues to what the individual is trying to say. As best you can, put yourself in the patient's shoes. Try to see the world as the patient sees it. Accept the patient's feelings as facts that must be taken into account, whether you share them or not.
4. Put aside your own views and opinions for the time being. Realize that you cannot listen to yourself inwardly and at the same time truly listen to the patient.
5. Control your impatience. Listening is faster than talking. The average person speaks about 120 words a minute. People can listen to about 400 words a minute. Do not jump ahead of the patient. Give the person time to tell the story. A patient doesn't always say what the paramedic expects to hear.
6. Do not prepare an answer while you listen. Get the whole message before deciding what to say. The patient's last sentence may put a whole new slant on what was said before.
7. Show the patient that you are alert and interested. This encourages the patient and improves communication.
8. Do not interrupt. Ask questions only to obtain more information. Do not try to trap the patient or force the individual into a corner.
9. Expect the patient's use of words to differ from yours. Do not quibble about terms—try to get at what was meant.
10. Your purpose is the opposite of a debater's goal. Look for areas of agreement, not for weak spots to attack with a barrage of counterarguments.
11. Before giving an answer in a particularly difficult discussion, summarize what you understand the patient to have said. If the patient disagrees with this version, clear up the contested points before giving your own views.
12. Let patients describe themselves and their interests, position, and opinions.

Adapted with permission from Legal Advocates for Abused Women, St. Louis.

BOX 9-3 Empathy versus Sympathy

The case below shows the difference between empathy and sympathy. It also shows how empathy can help the paramedic soothe the patient and gain his trust.

Your emergency medical services (EMS) crew is sent to the home of a 60-year-old man with substernal chest pain. When you arrive, the patient is sitting on the living room sofa with his wife. They are upset and afraid that he might die. Your crew begins standard procedures for a possible heart attack and prepares to transport the patient to the emergency department. On the way to the hospital, the paramedic and the patient, who is accompanied by his wife, have the following conversation:

Paramedic: Even though you're feeling better, I can tell you're worried and afraid.

Patient: Yes, I am. I'm afraid I'm going to die.

Paramedic: Would you like me to explain to you and your wife what will happen after we arrive in the emergency department? I can also explain what the doctors and nurses will do to make sure you get the best possible care.

Patient: Yes, we would like that very much.

The use of empathy, shown in this conversation, allows the paramedic to accomplish three things: (1) calm the patient and his wife; (2) provide the couple with useful information; and (3) partly address their concerns. If the paramedic had used sympathy alone (e.g., "I understand how you feel, but don't worry, everything will be okay"), the patient's fears would have been ignored. Also, the problem of the couple's agitation would not have been solved.

3. Assume an attentive posture (avoid crossing the legs and arms, because this may convey a defensive attitude).
4. Avoid distracting body movements (e.g., wringing the hands, tapping the feet, or fidgeting with an object).
5. Nod in acknowledgment when patients talk about important points or look for feedback.
6. Lean toward the speaker to communicate involvement.

One device for remembering ways to improve communication is the listening ladder (Fig. 9-2). This device has six steps to listening. They can easily be remembered from the acronym LADDER.[3]

EXTERNAL FACTORS IN EFFECTIVE COMMUNICATION

Good communication requires a suitable setting. The paramedic has control over a number of the external factors that affect the setting. Some of these are privacy, interruptions, eye contact, and personal dress. Control of these factors results in a better interaction between the paramedic and the patient.

Privacy, Interruptions, and the Physical Environment

When possible, the paramedic should ensure privacy during the encounter. This helps to eliminate distractions and to reduce any inhibitions the patient may feel. Interruptions should be kept to a minimum. Obviously, this is impossible if the paramedic is receiving critical patient care information from crew members. When possible, the lighting should be adequate. Noise and interference should be minimized. In addition, the patient interview should be started away from distracting equipment.

The paramedic should be aware of the patient's *private space.* This is a comfortable distance from the patient's body. It is about 4 to 5 feet[4] or twice the patient's arm length away. Private space is a form of subconscious personal protection

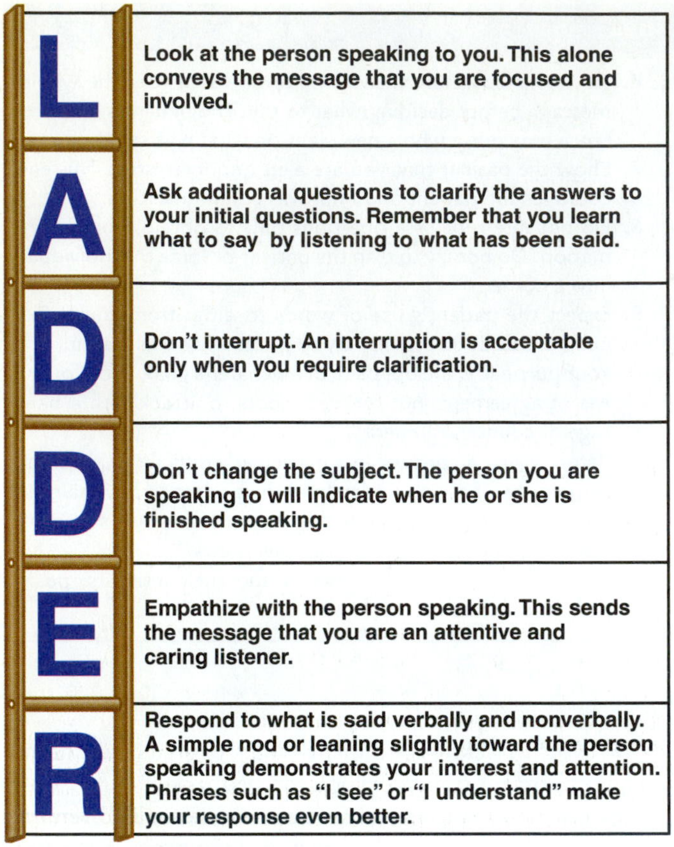
L
Look at the person speaking to you. This alone conveys the message that you are focused and involved.
A
Ask additional questions to clarify the answers to your initial questions. Remember that you learn what to say by listening to what has been said.
D
Don't interrupt. An interruption is acceptable only when you require clarification.
D
Don't change the subject. The person you are speaking to will indicate when he or she is finished speaking.
E
Empathize with the person speaking. This sends the message that you are an attentive and caring listener.
R
Respond to what is said verbally and nonverbally. A simple nod or leaning slightly toward the person speaking demonstrates your interest and attention. Phrases such as "I see" or "I understand" make your response even better.

FIGURE 9-2 ■ The ladder of listening.

that varies by individual and by culture. Some patients may become defensive if this space is invaded. Entering this space usually causes the patient to back away.

Eye Contact

The paramedic should maintain eye contact with the patient as much as possible, even when taking notes. Eye contact is a type of nonverbal communication. It can help express gentleness, sincerity, and authority and can help make the patient feel safe and secure. If possible, the paramedic should be positioned at eye level (equal seating) with the patient.

Personal Dress

Communication with a patient begins with first impressions. Paramedics' appearance should be professional. Their clothing should be clean and should meet professional standards (e.g., uniforms provided by the EMS agency). These standards help the patient instantly identify an emergency medical services (EMS) provider. They also help to set the tone of the paramedic-patient encounter.

PATIENT INTERVIEW

The ability to conduct a successful patient interview may be as important as physical assessment skills. The information gathered often helps to decide the direction of the physical examination. The patient interview should be started early. It should continue throughout the patient encounter.

Because of the emergency nature of their work, paramedics often think in terms of specific illnesses and injuries. They often must categorize patients into general groups, such as trauma or medical cases. However, good emergency care requires the paramedic to view each patient as an individual. Moreover, it requires paramedics to attend to a patient's needs in a caring, concerned, and receptive manner.

Communication Techniques

The paramedic should approach the conscious patient and make a personal introduction by name and title: "Hello. My name is [name], and I am a paramedic with [name of EMS agency]. What's your name?" Talking with the patient allows the paramedic to evaluate the person's level of consciousness and sensorium. It also may provide information on any hearing or speech impediments and language barriers. During the introduction, the paramedic should maintain eye contact with the patient.

Nonverbal communication can send a message of negative feelings. It also can convey the insecurities of both the patient and the paramedic. Voice inflection, facial expression, and body position are examples of these nonverbal cues. They may reflect anger, fear, or impatience. Similarly, starting intravenous therapy with trembling, sweaty hands may make the patient question the paramedic's skills. Nonverbal cues should be used to gain the patient's trust and cooperation. These can help the paramedic provide the best care for the patient.

Touch is a form of communication. It shows compassion and reassurance. Small gestures can help comfort a person in distress. A few examples are holding a patient's hand, squeezing a shoulder, or wiping tears from a patient's eyes. Experience and familiarity with patient care activities help determine the appropriateness of these gestures.

In talking with patients, the paramedic must listen to what is said and interpret what is said. Patients may say they feel fine. Yet their appearance and tone of voice may indicate that they are ill and afraid. If paramedics are unsure of the message in a patient's response, they should ask additional questions that will help them better understand what the patient is trying to communicate.

Most patients do not understand medical terminology. In addition, many have only a vague understanding of the way their bodies work. For these reasons, the paramedic should use common words and phrases that are easy to understand. The paramedic should guide and direct the patient interview without manipulating the patient's response. In other words, the paramedic should avoid asking leading questions (questions that can be answered with only "Yes" or "No"). Open-ended questions encourage a free-form response. For example, the paramedic should ask, "When did this pain begin?" rather than "Did the pain begin this morning?"

▶NOTE Open-ended questions:
Are asked in a narrative form
Encourage the patient to talk
Do not restrict the areas of response

The paramedic should ask only one question at a time. The patient should be given ample time to answer the question before the paramedic asks another question. If the patient's response does not seem relevant to the question, the response should be clarified. Paramedics should be flexible. They should not discount the patient's experiences or information.

Paramedics should try to answer all the patient's questions. However, this does not mean that they must provide a full explanation for each inquiry. Rather, a sensitive response that addresses the question is adequate. Paramedics should choose an answer carefully and should try to make sure that their answer does not upset the patient further.

Responses

The paramedic can use a number of tactics or responses to conduct a successful patient interview (Box 9-4). For example, the paramedic may use silence. This gives a patient more time to gather his or her thoughts. The paramedic also may *echo* a patient's words. This means that the paramedic paraphrases the patient's words. Echoing allows the paramedic to clear up or expand on the information provided. Empathy can be used to get a patient to talk more openly. Other tactics include asking a patient to clarify confusing statements and forcing the patient to focus on one factor of the interview (confrontation). At times the paramedic may need to interpret information by linking events, making associations, or inferring a cause based on what can be seen or concluded. The paramedic also can give the patient information to persuade the person to share facts or objective information. Finally, paramedics can summarize information by asking the patient open-ended questions that can be used to review and to clear up key details.

Traps in Interviewing

Paramedics must be aware of some traps that can be damaging to the patient interview. These include the following:

- Providing false reassurance
- Offering poor or unwanted advice
- Showing approval or disapproval
- Giving an opinion that takes away the patient's part in decision making
- Changing the subject inappropriately
- Stereotyping the patient or complaint
- Using professional jargon
- Talking too much
- Asking leading or biased questions
- Interrupting the patient
- Asking the patient "Why" questions (these can be viewed as accusations)
- Being defensive in response to criticism

BOX 9-4 Helpful Techniques for the Patient Interview

- Silence—Gives patients more time to gather their thoughts.
- Reflection—Echoing (i.e., paraphrasing) patients' words allows them to clarify or expand on the information provided.
- Empathy—Encourages patients to talk more openly.
- Clarification—Lets patients rephrase a word or thought that is confusing to the paramedic.
- Confrontation—Focuses patients' attention on one specific factor of the interview.
- Interpretation—Links events; makes associations or implies a cause; is based on observation or conclusion.
- Explanation—Provides information to patients; encourages sharing of facts or objective information.
- Summary—Provides a review of the interview; the paramedic can ask open-ended questions that allow patients to clarify details.

Developing a Good Rapport with the Patient

Skill in developing good rapport with a patient takes experience and practice. In most patient encounters, paramedics can follow some general guidelines to help establish good rapport:

1. Put patients at ease by letting them know you are "on their side"; that is, that you respect their comments, and you are there to help them.
2. Be alert for and respond to visual clues that a patient needs help.
3. Show compassion.
4. Assess the patient's level of understanding and insight. Use words and explanations at their level.
5. Show expertise.

CRITICAL THINKING
A suicidal patient keeps telling you that you don't care about him. What communications techniques could you use to persuade this patient that you are concerned about him?

STRATEGIES FOR OBTAINING INFORMATION

For the most part, patients communicate with health care providers in three ways. The first is by pouring out the information in the form of complaints. The second is by revealing some problems while hiding others they think are embarrassing. The third is by hiding the most embarrassing parts of their problem from the paramedic (and personally denying the issue). The best way to obtain information from the patient is to use techniques for open-ended and closed (direct) questions. These techniques include resistance, shifting focus, recognizing defense mechanisms, and distraction.

▶ **NOTE** Closed questions allow the paramedic to obtain specific information that focuses on a certain aspect of the patient's condition. "What part of your back hurts?" and "When was your last meal?" are two examples of closed questions.

Resistance

Often a patient is reluctant to give information for one of two reasons. First, the patient may want to maintain a personal image and is afraid of losing that image. Second, the patient may fear that the paramedic will respond with rejection and ridicule. Paramedics, therefore, should be nonjudgmental. This helps them to obtain information from patients (Box 9-5). To develop a trusting relationship, the paramedic must be willing to talk to the patient about *any* condition in a professional manner.

Shifting Focus

A patient may seem unwilling to discuss an obvious problem. In this situation, the paramedic may have to shift the focus of the questions away from that problem. For example, a man with groin pain at first may describe the pain (especially to a female paramedic) as being in his "lower back." By shifting the focus of questioning to low back pain, the paramedic can use another angle. The questions can focus on the presence or absence of radiating pain. This new line of questioning can make patients feel more comfortable when describing their condition.

Defense Mechanisms

Paramedics should recognize common defense mechanisms (see Chapter 2). If possible, they should try to anticipate them. For example, an upset parent with a seriously ill child may show regression or denial. The parent may be unable to provide needed information at the emergency scene. Confrontation may be required in these and similar situations to force the parent to deal with key issues. Confrontation can clarify roles. It also can help others identify problems and goals. However, this technique should be used only to obtain information critical for medical care. Confrontation must be performed in a professional way. This allows the patient to become aware of inconsistencies in interfering behavior or thoughts.

BOX 9-5 Approaching Sensitive Issues

Discussing sensitive issues can be awkward for both the patient and the paramedic. Such issues might include alcohol use, sexual subjects, and suicide risk. Still, these issues must not be avoided when the information is needed to ensure good patient care. The paramedic should use the following guidelines when sensitive issues are discussed with patients:

- Make sure privacy is maintained.
- Be confident, direct, and firm with your questions.
- Do not apologize for asking a sensitive question.
- Do not be judgmental.
- Use words that are understandable, but do not be patronizing.
- Be patient and proceed slowly.

Distraction

Paramedics may use distraction to help patients recognize irrational thoughts or behavior. This type of behavior may be seen in hostile situations in which patients "act out." In such cases, paramedics need to point out the unacceptable behavior. They also need to let patients know the self-defeating nature of the behavior. Often, this distraction prompts patients to let the paramedic handle the situation until they can gain self-control. When dealing with an angry or hostile patient, paramedics should:

- Avoid raising their voices to match the angry person's tone
- Have the person identify and describe the cause of anger
- Restate the cause of the anger
- Offer a solution (if possible) or empathize and acknowledge the person's feelings

METHODS OF ASSESSING MENTAL STATUS DURING THE INTERVIEW

Three methods can be used to assess a patient's mental status: observation, conversation, and exploration. (Assessment of the level of consciousness is discussed in more detail in other chapters.)

Observation

The first step in assessing mental status is to observe the patient. Paramedics should note the patient's appearance, level of consciousness, and body movements. Physical characteristics, dress, and grooming can provide clues. These may even indicate the patient's well-being, social status, religion, culture, and self-concept. Conscious patients for the most part are alert and able to speak intelligently. Body movements (e.g., gestures, facial expressions) should be appropriate for the situation. Abnormal body movements may indicate an unstable situation. Such movements may include unusual posture or gait or clenched fists.

Conversation

Conversation with patients should reveal whether they know who they are, where they are, and the day or date (i.e., whether they are oriented to person, place, and time). If the patient knows these things, the remote, recent, and intermediate facets of memory probably are intact. The patient should be able to speak at a normal pace and with even flow. Responses should not have long pauses or rapid shifts. (However, such nuances vary by geographical location.) During normal conversation, the patient should be able to show clear thinking, a normal attention span, and the ability to concentrate on and understand the discussion.

A patient's responses to the setting *(affect)* should match the situation. Normal reactions to stress may include autonomic responses. Some of these are sweating and trembling and odd facial movements (e.g., muscle twitching around the mouth, nose, and eyes). Reactive movements, such as not holding eye contact during conversation, should be noted. Other actions may indicate that a patient is uncomfortable or anxious. These include grooming movements, such as fixing the hair and straightening the clothes.

Exploration

Exploration offers a way to assess the patient's emotions. For example, by observing that the patient's mood is anxious, excited, or depressed and by noting the individual's energy level, the paramedic can gauge the mental status. Exploration can be done simply by interacting with the patient. This allows the paramedic to see whether actions and ideas are appropriate. An objective assessment must weigh the patient's culture and education as well. It also must take into account the person's values, beliefs, and previous experiences.

CRITICAL THINKING

The mental status examination is critical, both for medical reasons and for legal reasons. Why do you think this is so?

SPECIAL INTERVIEW SITUATIONS

At times paramedics may have to use special skills to interact successfully with a patient who is uncooperative or frightened or who has a disability (also see Chapter 10).

Patients Who Don't Want to Talk

Although most patients are more than willing to talk, some need more time and varying techniques to participate in a successful interview. Tough interviews generally stem from four factors[5]:

1. The patient's condition may affect the ability to speak.
2. The patient may fear talking because of psychological problems, cultural differences, or age.
3. The patient may have a cognitive impairment.
4. The patient may want to deceive the paramedic.

HELPFUL TECHNIQUES

The following techniques may be useful for communicating with a patient who is unmotivated to talk:

- Start the interview in the normal way. If the patient does not talk, review the nature of the call as received from the dispatch center. Take time to develop a rapport with the patient.
- Use open-ended questions to get a response. If this is unsuccessful, try direct questions.
- Provide positive feedback to appropriate responses from the patient.
- Make sure the patient understands the question. (Consider whether a language barrier or a hearing difficulty is a factor.)
- Continue asking questions to obtain critical information needed to provide treatment. (Unessential information may be difficult to obtain.)
- Question family members or others at the scene. If the patient has been uncommunicative for a long period, try to rule out a disease or disorder as the reason.
- Use summary and interpretation of events or conditions. Also, ask the patient if your summary and version are correct.
- Try to start a conversation by asking the patient questions about your care, equipment, or profession. If the patient responds, answer all questions fully (not with one-word answers).
- Realize that all the information needed may not be obtained.
- Observe the patient's responses to the setting and surroundings and record what you see. This sets a mental status baseline for later evaluations.
- Consider asking questions for which answers are known. This helps to gauge the patient's credibility.

NOTE Patients who are unconscious or unresponsive may be able to receive stimuli. Hearing is thought to be the last sensation lost with unconsciousness. It also is thought to be the first regained with consciousness.[4] The paramedic must not say anything near an unconscious patient that would not be said if the patient were fully conscious.

Hostile Patients

Paramedics should be alert for signs that a situation may turn violent. This is part of ensuring personal safety. Such signs may include clenched fists, a rising voice level, a threatening facial expression, or a history of violence toward others. If such a situation exists or is expected, the EMS crew should leave the scene. They also should request the help of law enforcement personnel. If safe retreat is not an option, the paramedics should stay far enough away from the patient to ensure their personal safety (see Chapter 40). Some guidelines that can be used in interviewing a hostile patient are:

- Try to use normal interviewing techniques.
- Never leave the patient alone without adequate assistance.
- Set limits and boundaries with the patient.
- Explain the advantages of cooperation to the patient.
- Follow local protocol for dealing with hostile patients, including the use of physical and chemical restraints.

Patients with Age-Related Factors

Communicating with children and older adults should not be difficult or a challenge. It works best when the paramedic takes into account the common developmental characteristics of a particular age group (see Chapter 8).

COMMUNICATING WITH CHILDREN

When communicating with children, the paramedic often must establish rapport with two people—the child and the parent. With children 1 to 6 years old, most conversation should be directed first to the parent. (Offering a toy may distract the child while the parent is interviewed.) The para-

BOX 9-6 Tips for Communicating with Children of Various Ages

- Infants respond best to firm, gentle handling and a quiet, calm voice. Older infants may have stranger anxiety. If possible, the parent should remain in view of the child.
- Preschoolers see the world only from their perspective and base everything on past experience. Use short sentences and give concrete explanations (e.g., you will need to hold still so that I can splint your arm and make you feel better).
- Adolescents want to be adults. Treat them with respect and use age-appropriate words. Do not talk to or treat them as if they were small children.

medic should be aware that information from the parent is that person's point of view, and the parent might be feeling defensive. Paramedics should not be judgmental if the parents had not provided proper care or safety for the child before the EMS arrived. (Paramedics should be observant but not confrontational.)

The paramedic should gradually begin to make contact with the child during the parent interview. This can be done by moving to eye level to speak with the child and by using a quiet, calm voice. The paramedic should keep in mind that children are especially responsive to nonverbal cues. Box 9-6 lists special considerations for communicating with children of various ages (also see Chapter 44).

COMMUNICATING WITH OLDER ADULTS

Many older adults are dealing with age-related diseases and the inevitability of death. Interviewing older adults may take longer than interviewing younger persons. Older patients may tire easily. They also may have physical disabilities that distort speech. Touch is generally important to most older adults. When interviewing an older person, the paramedic should always use the individual's last name and Mr., Mrs., or Ms. unless the patient says otherwise. In addition, the patient should be able to see the paramedic's face easily. The paramedic should keep eye contact and speak clearly and slowly. He or she should be willing to take extra time to get the needed information. Using short, open-ended questions and talking with family members usually are the best approaches for the patient interview (also see Chapter 45).

Hearing-Impaired Patients

When dealing with a patient with a hearing impairment, the paramedic should determine the patient's preferred method of communicating. It may be lipreading, signing, or writing. Writing often is the best out-of-hospital method for communicating with a deaf patient. If the patient prefers lipreading, the paramedic should (1) face the patient squarely, (2) make sure the light is adequate, (3) speak slowly using short words and phrases, and (4) enunciate clearly. Because many deaf patients lip-read, paramedics must speak clearly in full view of these patients. They also must realize that some deaf patients may nod "Yes" even if they do not understand the question.

If a patient is thought to be hearing-impaired or deaf, the paramedic should try to gain the person's attention. This can be done by a gentle touch or by slowly waving the hands in front of the patient. The paramedic also may try speaking a little louder or speaking into the patient's ear if the person is not wearing a hearing aid. If a hearing-impaired patient needs to be taken to a medical facility, the paramedic should inform the emergency department staff as soon as possible about the impairment. This allows arrangements to be made for someone to help the staff members communicate with patient. (This is also a good practice with patients who do not speak English.)

Paramedics might consider learning finger spelling and simple sign language to aid them in their work. These are both easily learned.

Blind Patients

When communicating with a blind patient, paramedics should determine or ascertain whether the patient also has a hearing impairment. (It is unusual for sightless people also to be deaf.) Paramedics should identify themselves in a normal voice. They should answer all the patient's questions about the emergency scene and the surroundings. They also should explain all examination and treatment procedures in detail before they touch the patient.

Most patients who have disabilities are very independent. In fact, they may resent unsolicited help. If a sightless person has a guide dog and the situation permits, the two should not be separated. If the dog was injured during the emergency, the paramedic should quickly advise the dispatch center to make special arrangements for care for the dog.

Patients Under the Influence of Street Drugs or Alcohol

If street drugs or alcohol play a part in an emergency, paramedics should ensure their personal safety. They should also be ready for unpredictable patient behavior. (The help of law enforcement officers may be needed to ensure scene safety.) During the patient interview, paramedics should ask simple or direct questions. Also, they should avoid any action the patient might see as a threat or confrontation (see Chapters 36 and 52).

Sexually Aggressive Patients

Paramedics should confront male or female patients who make improper sexual advances. This ensures that the patient is aware of the professional role of the caregiver. Paramedics should document any unusual incidents. They also should record the observations of any witnesses to any of the actions. Sexually aggressive patients should be cared for by paramedics of the same gender. Also, a chaperone or witness should be present during the care and transportation of the patient. Some EMS services use tape recorders during transport to record all interactions with sexually ag-

BOX 9-7 General Guidelines for Working with an Interpreter

As a paramedic, you sometimes will be called to assist a patient who does not speak English. Often someone in the home or at the scene can help you communicate with the person. When working with an interpreter, use the following guidelines:

1. Explain to the interpreter the key information you are trying to get before you begin the interview.
2. Ask a child to interpret only if no adult interpreter is available.
3. Speak directly to the patient or to a family member when asking questions. This establishes the primary relationship with that individual (not the interpreter). It also allows you to observe nonverbal clues.
4. Ask questions that call for one response at a time. For example, ask, "Do you have pain?" rather than "Do you have any pain, trouble breathing, or nausea?"
5. Try not to interrupt the patient, family member, or interpreter when that person is speaking.
6. Do not make comments about the patient or family to the interpreter; the patient or family may know some English.
7. Use simple language. Do not use medical terms for which other languages may have no similar words.
8. After the interview, if time permits, ask for the interpreter's impressions and observations of the interview.

Modified from Wong D: *Whaley and Wong's nursing care of infants and children*, ed 5, St Louis, 1995, Mosby.

BOX 9-8 General Guidelines on Personal Space*

Intimate Zone
- 0 to 1½ feet
- Visual distortion occurs.
- Best for assessing breath and other body odors

Personal Distance
- 1½ to 4 feet
- Perceived as an extension of self
- Speaker's voice is moderate.
- Body odors are not apparent.
- Much of the physical assessment occurs at this distance.

Social Distance
- 4 to 12 feet
- Used for impersonal business transactions
- Perceptual information is much less detailed.
- Much of the patient interview occurs at this distance.

Public Distance
- 12 feet or farther
- Interaction with others is impersonal.
- Speaker's voice must be projected.
- Subtle facial expressions are imperceptible.

*These are only general guidelines. Some cultures are more comfortable at a variety of distances when communicating.

gressive patients. The patient's legal consent may be required before a tape recorder is used.

Transcultural Considerations

When speaking with a patient from another culture, paramedics should introduce themselves and then ask the patient to do the same. Paramedics must be aware that they may be seen as a stereotype by the patient and family. For this reason, the roles of everyone involved in the care (paramedics, patient, and family members) must be clear.

Two pitfalls that paramedics must avoid when speaking with patients of a different culture are ethnocentrism and cultural imposition. *Ethnocentrism* is seeing one's own life as the most acceptable or best. It includes acting in a superior manner toward another culture's way of life. *Cultural imposition* is forcing one's beliefs, values, and patterns of behavior on people from another culture. Paramedics do not fall into these pitfalls on purpose. Yet they must be sensitive to how their actions and words may be seen by those of another culture. Other factors to consider in communicating with patients of another culture are:

- Some cultures expect health care workers to have all the answers to their illness.
- Different cultures accept illness or injury in different ways.
- Nonverbal cues (e.g., handshaking and touching) are seen differently in different cultures.
- Some cultures consider direct eye contact impolite or aggressive; patients may avert their eyes during an interview.
- Paramedics should not use touch as a means of reassurance with members of different cultural groups because touch may be easily misunderstood.
- Language barriers may present difficulties (Box 9-7).
- Personal space is often defined by culture. It also varies by individual (Box 9-8).

CRITICAL THINKING

Do you know anyone whose personal space requirements are much greater or much less than those listed here? How would this affect your interview with that person?

SUMMARY

- Therapeutic communication is a planned act. It is also a professional act. The paramedic, working with the patient, obtains information that is used to meet patient care goals.
- Communication is a dynamic process. It has six elements: the source, encoding, the message, decoding, the receiver, and feedback.
- To effectively communicate with patients, paramedics must genuinely like people. They must be able to empathize with others. They also must have the ability to listen.
- Good communication calls for a favorable physical environment. Factors such as privacy, interruption, eye contact, and personal dress are external influences. These factors can be controlled. This allows the paramedic to better communicate with the patient.
- The patient interview often decides the direction of the physical examination. Good care means that the paramedic sees each patient as an individual. It also means that the patient's needs are met in a caring, concerned, and receptive way.
- Open-ended and closed (direct) questions can be used to get information from the patient. Techniques include resistance, shifting focus, recognizing defense mechanisms, and distraction.
- The first step with any patient is to assess mental status. This can be done by observing the patient's appearance and level of consciousness. The paramedic also can look for normal or abnormal body movements. During normal conversation, the patient should be able to show clear thinking, a normal attention span, and the ability to concentrate on and understand the discussion. The patient's responses to the environment (i.e., affect) should be appropriate to the situation.
- Difficult interviews generally arise from four situations: (1) the patient's condition may affect the ability to speak; (2) the patient may fear talking because of psychological disorders, cultural differences, or age; (3) a cognitive impairment may be present; or (4) the patient may want to deceive the paramedic.

REFERENCES

1. Satir V: *The new peoplemaking,* Palo Alto, Calif, 1988, Science & Behavior Books.
2. Potter PA, Perry AG: *Fundamentals of nursing: concepts, process, and practice,* ed 5, St Louis, 2001, Mosby.
3. Moore M: *Embracing the mystery,* Madison, Wisc., 1999, MJM Publishing.
4. Rathus S: *Psychology,* ed 3, New York, 1987, Holt, Rinehart & Winston.
5. US Department of Transportation, National Highway Traffic Safety Administration: *EMT-paramedic national standard curriculum,* Washington, DC, 1998, The Department.

CHAPTER

10

History Taking

OBJECTIVES

Upon completion of this chapter, the paramedic student will be able to:

1. Describe the purpose of effective history taking in prehospital patient care.
2. List components of the patient history as defined by the Department of Transportation.
3. Outline effective patient interviewing techniques to facilitate history taking.
4. Identify strategies to manage special challenges in obtaining a patient history.

KEY TERMS

chief complaint: A patient's primary complaint.

clinical reasoning: Use of the results of questions to think about associated problems and body system changes related to the patient's complaint.

current health status: A focus on the patient's current state of health, environmental conditions, and personal habits.

family history: Illness or disease in a patient's family or family's background that may be relevant to the patient complaint.

history taking: Information gathered during the patient interview.

present illness: Identification of the chief complaint and a full, clear, chronological account of the symptoms.

significant past medical history: A patient's medical background that may offer insight into the patient's current problem.

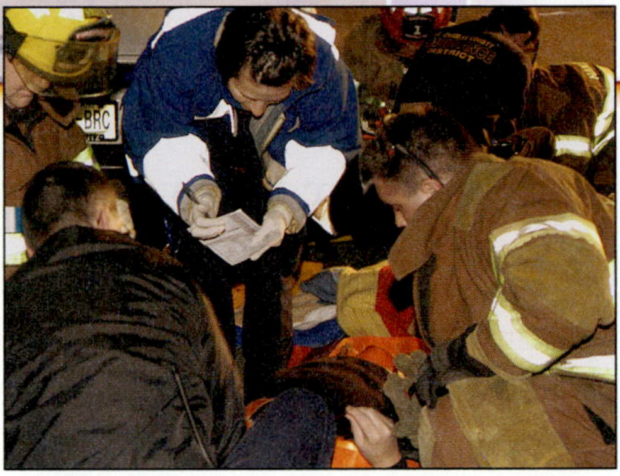

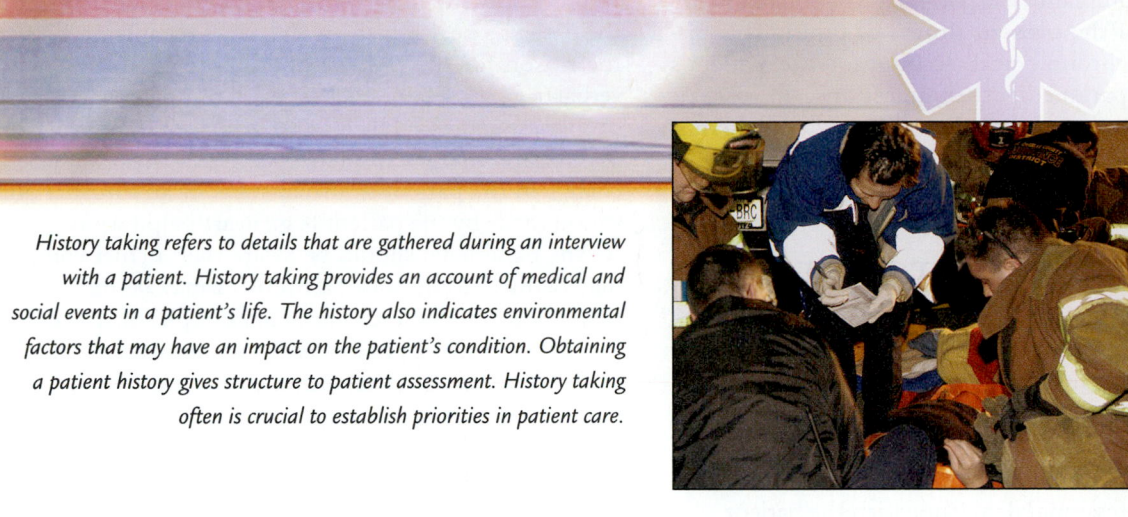

History taking refers to details that are gathered during an interview with a patient. History taking provides an account of medical and social events in a patient's life. The history also indicates environmental factors that may have an impact on the patient's condition. Obtaining a patient history gives structure to patient assessment. History taking often is crucial to establish priorities in patient care.

CONTENT OF THE PATIENT HISTORY

The patient history is made up of several parts. Each of these parts has a specific purpose, which offers a "snapshot" of patients and their condition. Box 10-1 lists the parts of a patient history. These parts are defined by the Department of Transportation in the *EMT-Paramedic National Standard Curriculum.*[1]

The patient history should include the date and time that the history was obtained. The history also should contain any identifying information of the patient (e.g., age, sex, race, birthplace, and occupation). Identifying information can be key, as illustrated in the following scenario: Your crew has been dispatched to a "sick case." On your arrival you find a woman who is ill with flulike symptoms. The symptoms include nausea, vomiting, and diarrhea. During your interview, she tells you that she is a 49-year-old businesswoman. In addition, she has just returned to the United States from an extended visit to her native home in Southeast Asia. In addition to the chance of gastrointestinal illness or food poisoning, you now suspect that she could be ill from an endemic disease (that is, a disease prevalent in a population or geographical region).

Documentation should include the source of the referral and patient history. For example, did the patient request emergency medical services (EMS) help, or did a family member, friend, law enforcement officer, or bystander initiate the EMS response? The paramedic also must decide whether the source of the referral and patient history is reliable, as illustrated in the following scenario: Your crew has been dispatched to a car crash. The driver of the car is a 17-year-old who has minor injuries. He is slurring his speech. In addition, his breath smells of alcohol. He denies alcohol or other drug use to you and the law enforcement officers at the scene. Is this patient history reliable?

BOX 10-1 Content of the Patient History

Date and Time

Identifying Data
- Age
- Sex
- Race
- Birthplace
- Occupation

Source of Referral
- Patient referral
- Referral by others

Source of History
- Patient
- Family
- Friends
- Police
- Others

Reliability
- Variable (memory, trust, motivation)
- Determined at the end of the evaluation

Chief Complaint
- Main part of history
- The one or more symptoms for which the patient is seeking medical care

Present Illness
- Identifies the chief complaint
- Provides a chronological account of the patient's symptoms

Medical History

Current Health Status

Review of Body Systems

The **chief complaint** (explained later in this chapter) is the main part of the patient history. The chief complaint is the reason why EMS assistance was summoned. After identifying the chief complaint, the paramedic obtains a history and description of the **present illness** or injury. This history provides a chronological account of the patient's symptoms. The paramedic then questions the patient about any **significant past medical history** and **current health status.** Also, the paramedic performs a review of body systems appropriate to the patient's symptoms or complaint. (See Chapter 12.)

TECHNIQUES OF HISTORY TAKING

As emphasized in Chapter 9, the paramedic should "set the stage" for a good paramedic-patient encounter. The paramedic can do this by making a good first impression. Also, the paramedic can make the environment conducive to free-flowing communication. The paramedic should do the following:

- Establish a professional demeanor with the patient.
- Ensure patient comfort and provide a safe environment.
- Greet the patient by name or surname and avoid demeaning terms (e.g., "Granny" or "Hon").
- Avoid entering the patient's personal space.
- Inquire about the patient's feelings.
- Be sensitive to the patient's feelings and experiences.
- Watch for signs of uneasiness.
- Use language that is appropriate and easily understood.
- Ask open-ended questions and direct questions (if needed).
- Use therapeutic communications techniques.

Opening questions may incorporate facilitation, reflection, clarification, empathetic responses, confrontation, interpretation, and asking patients about their feelings. These methods should use the techniques of communications described in Chapter 9:

Facilitation: Use positive actions or words to encourage the patient to say more. Maintain eye contact and use phrases such as "go on" and "I'm listening." These phrases encourage the patient to continue talking.

Reflection: Repeat or "echo" what the patient tells you. This encourages additional responses. Reflection usually will not bias the patient's story or interrupt the patient's train of thought.

Clarification: Ask questions to better grasp vague statements or words.

Empathy: Ask about the patient's feelings and show empathy to interpret the patient's feelings. This will help to gain your patient's trust.

Confrontation: Some issues may call for confronting patients about their feelings. For example, one may ask a patient who is severely depressed, "Have you ever thought about killing yourself?"

Interpretation: When appropriate, go beyond confrontation and make an inference from the patient's response. For example, draw an inference from the patient who says, "I think I'm going to die." One may infer that the patient may be gravely ill.

Chief Complaint

As previously stated, the chief complaint is the main part of the patient's health history. The chief complaint is usually the reason for the EMS response. The complaint may be verbal (e.g., complaint of chest pain) or nonverbal (e.g., pain or distress expressed by a facial grimace). Most chief complaints are characterized by pain, abnormal function, a change in the patient's normal state, or an unusual observation made by the patient (e.g., heart palpitations).

The paramedic should be aware that a chief complaint may be misleading. Also, a problem may be more serious than the complaint indicates. For example, the patient who has fallen down a flight of steps may complain of an injured ankle. However, physical examination may reveal possible internal injuries. In addition, patients often modify or substitute their chief complaint. They may do this to hide a problem they find embarrassing or hard to discuss. For example, a chief complaint of vaginal bleeding may be modified as "excessive menstruation." Actually, the bleeding was an abrupt hemorrhage that occurred during intercourse. Likewise, a chief complaint of "frequent headaches" may be substituted for feelings of depression with suicidal ideation. Thus determining the true reason for the patient's concern is one of the skills of **history taking,** and the true need may not be the stated chief complaint. First, the paramedic should determine the chief complaint. Then the paramedic should manage any life-threatening situations. Then the paramedic should get a history of the present illness and any relevant medical history.

CRITICAL THINKING

What illnesses or injuries could cause a chief complaint of confusion?

History of Present Illness

The present illness identifies the chief complaint. The present illness also provides a full, clear, and chronological account of the symptoms. Obtaining a full history of the present illness takes skill. It takes skill in asking proper questions related to the chief complaint and in interpreting the patient's response. For example, a patient's complaint of low back pain suggests a muscle strain. During direct questioning in the interview, however, the patient reveals a history of a burning sensation with urination and a low-grade fever for the past several days. This information suggests a urinary tract infection or renal stones. Thus the history of the present illness may be more crucial than the obvious chief complaint. The mnemonic *OPQRST* helps define the patient's complaint by focusing on essential elements of assessment (Box 10-2). Use of this or another memory device will help lead the paramedic through a thorough series of questions to better grasp the chief complaint. The paramedic should take notes while obtaining the health history. Most pa-

> **BOX 10-2 OPQRST Mnemonic**
>
> *O (onset/origin):* What were you doing when the pain started? Do you have a history of this problem?
> *P (provokes):* What provokes the symptoms? What makes the symptoms better? What makes them worse?
> *Q (quality):* What does the pain feel like? Is it sharp, dull, burning, or tearing?
> *R (region):* Where is the symptom? Where does it go? Is it in one or more areas?
> *S (severity):* On a scale of 1 to 10, with 1 being the least and 10 being the worst, what number would you give your pain or discomfort?
> *T (time):* How long have you had this symptom? When did it start? When did it end? How long did it last?

tients realize that it is hard to remember all details and accept note taking.

ONSET/ORIGIN

Onset and origin identify what the patient was doing when the pain began. The paramedic also notes whether there is any history of a similar episode. Questions to ask to obtain this information may include the following:

- "Did the pain or discomfort begin suddenly, or did it occur gradually over time?"
- "When did you last feel well?"
- "What were you doing when the pain started?"
- "Did the pain begin during a period of activity or while at rest?"
- "Have you ever had this type of pain or discomfort before? If so, is it the same or is it different than what you're experiencing now?"

PROVOKE/PALLIATION

Provoke and palliation refer to precipitating factors associated with the patient's complaints. Questions to ask to identify precipitating factors may include the following:

- "What makes your pain or discomfort better?"
- "What makes your pain or discomfort worse?"
- "Does the pain increase or decrease when you take a breath?"
- "Does lying down or sitting up affect your level of discomfort?"
- "Have you taken any medications for your symptoms? If so, did the medications make you feel better?"

QUALITY

Quality refers to how the patient perceives the pain or discomfort. Questions to ask to obtain quality of the pain include the following:

- "What does the pain feel like?"
- "Can you describe the pain to me?"
- "Is the pain sharp or dull?"
- "Is the pain constant, or does it come and go?"

REGION/RADIATION

Region and radiation refer to the location of the pain and whether it is localized or associated with pain elsewhere in the body. Questions to ask to identify region and radiation include the following:

- "Where is the pain?"
- "Can you point with one finger to the exact location of the pain?"
- "Does the pain stay in the same place or does it move?"
- "If the pain moves, where does it go? Does the pain go to more than one area?"

SEVERITY

Severity refers to how the patient rates the level of the pain or discomfort. Severity also provides a baseline for future evaluation of the patient's pain. Questions to ask the patient include the following:

- "On a scale of 1 to 10, with 1 being the least and 10 being the worst, how would you rate your pain or discomfort?"
- "How bad is the pain?"
- "Does the intensity of the pain vary or does it stay the same?"
- "Have you had this type of pain before? If so, how is this pain different, or is it exactly the same?"

TIME

Time refers to the duration of the pain or discomfort. Questions to ask to clarify the duration of the patient's pain or discomfort include the following:

- "Have long have you been feeling this way?"
- "Have you had this same type of pain before, and if so, how long did it last?"
- "When did the pain or discomfort start?"
- "How long did the pain or discomfort last?"
- "When did the pain or discomfort end?"

Significant Past Medical History

A key for history taking is for the paramedic to gather the significant past medical history. This step can occur after the paramedic gains a good grasp of the patient's chief complaint. The past medical history may include, for example, diabetes, cardiac, or respiratory disorders. This history may add insight into the patient's current state. Important past medical history information may include the following:

- General state of health
- Medications and allergies
- Childhood illnesses
- Adult illnesses
- Psychiatric illnesses
- Previous injuries
- Surgeries
- Hospitalizations

A variety of memory devices are used to recall key questions for gathering medical history. One example is the *SAMPLE Survey* (Box 10-3). The depth and focus of the pa-

BOX 10-3 Elements of the SAMPLE Survey

S: Signs and symptoms
A: Allergies
M: Medications
P: Past medical history
L: Last meal or oral intake
E: Events before the emergency

tient interview are based on the case at hand. However, the paramedic should gather as much information as possible at the scene and during transport to the hospital. The paramedic uses the answers to think about associated problems and body system changes related to the patient's complaint. This is known as **clinical reasoning.**

Current Health Status

A current health status focuses on a patient's current state of health. It also considers personal habits and environmental conditions (Box 10-4). Details regarding allergies, medications, last oral intake, and **family history** can be critical to the patient's current health status. Paramedics should ask female patients who have abdominal pain about their last menstrual period. (This is relevant for female patients of childbearing age.) The paramedic also should question these patients about their last bowel movement. Finally, the paramedic should identify events that occurred before the emergency.

BOX 10-4 Personal Habits and Environmental Conditions

Personal Habits

Tobacco use
Alcohol, other drugs and related substances
Diet
Screening tests
Immunizations
Sleep patterns
Exercise and leisure activities
Use of safety measures
Home situation, spouse, or significant other
Physical abuse or violence
Sexual history
Daily life
Important experiences
Religious beliefs
Patient outlook

Environmental Conditions

Home conditions: housing; cleanliness; temperature; economic condition; pets and their health

Occupation: description of past and present work; exposure to heat, cold, and industrial toxins; similar complaints of illness among co-workers

Travel: exposure to contagious diseases; residence in tropics; water and milk supply; and other possible sources of infection

Military record: geographical areas; exposure to chemicals

ALLERGIES

Few emergency medications cause an allergic reaction. Still, details regarding allergies can be critical. Such details also can be useful to others involved in the patient's care. For example, the patient may be sensitive to tetanus prophylaxis, antibiotics, radiographic contrast medium, and other drugs administered during treatment. Allergies to food and other substances may offer insight into the patient's state. If the patient is unconscious or unable to talk, the paramedic should look for medical alert information. The paramedic also should ask family members or friends about the patient's allergies. (Allergic reactions are addressed further in Chapter 17.)

NOTE Many persons have a life-threatening allergy to latex. Latex is a common substance found in emergency medical services care equipment.

MEDICATIONS

The paramedic should ask whether the patient takes any medications regularly. The paramedic also should ask whether the patient has used any medications that the patient does not take regularly. In addition to information about prescribed medicines, information about the use of over-the-counter medicines is key. The paramedic also should ask about the use of herbs, naturopathic, and homeopathic medicines. This line of questioning should include the reason and frequency of use. If possible, the paramedic should determine whether the patient adheres to a medication regimen. The medication history may offer clues to the chief complaint. For example, a diabetic patient may have taken insulin but may have eaten at odd intervals. Other examples include a patient with chest pain who takes various cardiac drugs, an irrational patient who takes prescribed sedatives, and a trauma patient who takes blood-thinning drugs. The patient's medication history may not always be relevant to the problem at hand. However, the history can point to potential problems that may be seen during the patient care episode.

CRITICAL THINKING

What would you do if you could not recognize the names or indications for the patient's home medicines?

LAST ORAL INTAKE

The time of the last meal or fluid intake is key when considering potential airway problems in a patient who loses consciousness or whose condition begins to deteriorate. Determining the patient's last oral intake also may help rule out some problems. These problems include food poisoning and food allergies. For example, symptoms of certain types of food poisoning do not usually appear for several hours. In contrast, patients who are sensitive to certain foods would develop an allergic reaction immediately after eating the foods. Some of these foods are peanut oil and shellfish.

> **NOTE** The time of the patient's last oral intake is crucial. The time can help to determine the appropriateness of surgery. Generally, if a patient has eaten or drunk within the previous 6 to 8 hours, surgery is delayed if possible. The delay is to prevent the patient from aspirating the stomach contents. This may occur during the induction of anesthesia. However, immediate surgery may be indicated after recent oral intake. If so, a nasogastric tube is inserted to evacuate the stomach.

FAMILY HISTORY

A family history of illness or disease may be relevant to the chief complaint. The paramedic should establish whether a family history of heart disease, high blood pressure, cancer, tuberculosis, stroke, diabetes, kidney disease, current contagious illness, or other ailments exists. The paramedic also should note the presence of hereditary diseases during the interview. Examples of these diseases include hemophilia or sickle cell anemia. The absence of such diseases should be noted as well. In time, the paramedic will develop a "personal line" of questioning. This will help the paramedic to analyze a patient's symptoms further.

LAST MENSTRUAL PERIOD

The paramedic should obtain a menstrual history when interviewing female patients between the ages of 12 and 55 years who have abdominal pain. This questioning may prompt the patient to discuss other significant symptoms. These symptoms may include vaginal discharge, bleeding, and pregnancy history. The patient's response should determine the need to pursue additional questions regarding contraceptive use, venereal disease, urinary tract infections, and ectopic pregnancy (see Chapter 41.)

LAST BOWEL MOVEMENT

The paramedic should ask a patient about his or her bowel habits. This information is key to see whether bowel movements have been normal or abnormal. A patient with abdominal pain may describe a recent history of diarrhea, constipation, or bloody bowel movements. This information will be helpful to the receiving physician to assess the patient for bowel obstruction, dehydration, or lower gastrointestinal bleeding. At this time, the paramedic also should ask the patient about any symptoms of abnormal urinary function. These symptoms may include blood in the urine, urethral discharge, pain or burning with urination, frequent urination, or the inability to void.

EVENTS BEFORE THE EMERGENCY

The paramedic should ask the patient and bystanders about events or actions that occurred before the emergency. For example, was a fainting episode preceded by exertion or straining? Did a loss of consciousness occur before or after a fall? The paramedic should attempt to correlate any event with the progression of an illness or injury.

Getting More Information

With experience, paramedics learn to communicate with more skill. They learn to get a fuller picture of a patient's illness or injury. They are able to obtain more information about a symptom or complaint. Thus they are able to use clinical reasoning to evaluate associated problems and possible effects on body systems. With this skill the paramedic is better able to ask direct questions. The paramedic also may have to obtain a history on sensitive topics. Such topics may include alcohol or other drug use, physical abuse or violence, and sexual issues. When questioning a patient about sensitive issues, the paramedic should follow these guidelines:

1. Remember that privacy is essential with all patients, regardless of age or sex.
2. Be direct and firm and do not apologize for asking a question.
3. Avoid confrontation.
4. Be nonjudgmental.
5. Use language that is easily understood but not patronizing.
6. Encourage the patient to ask any relevant questions.
7. Document carefully and use the patient's words (noted by quotation marks) when possible.

SPECIAL CHALLENGES

History taking often presents special challenges. Each patient is unique. Thus each patient encounter is slightly different from all others. The paramedic must be able to adapt quickly to the special requirements of each encounter. That way the paramedic can obtain the needed information quickly. Some challenges that commonly affect history taking follow.

Silence

Silence is often uncomfortable. Silence has many meanings and uses. For example, patients may use silence to collect thoughts, recall details, or decide whether they trust the paramedic. Silence also can defuse an emotionally tense event effectively. The paramedic should stay alert for nonverbal clues of distress or anxiety. These clues may include a worried expression or loss of eye contact. These clues often precede a silent period during the patient encounter. As a rule, when patients are ready to talk again, they will express feelings more clearly. A patient's silence also may result from a paramedic's lack of sensitivity, understanding, or compassion. An appropriate and caring "bedside manner" is key to good patient care.

Overly Talkative Patients

Interviewing talkative patients can be frustrating. This is especially the case when the paramedic has a limited amount of time to obtain a health history. Although there are no perfect solutions in these situations, the following techniques may be helpful:

- Accept a less comprehensive history.
- Give the patient free rein for the first several minutes.
- Ask questions that invite brief "yes" or "no" answers when appropriate.
- Summarize the patient's comments frequently.
- Refocus the discussion as needed.

Patients with Multiple Symptoms

Some patients (often older patients) have a longer medical history because of age, chronic illness, and medication use. In addition, many older patients are likely to suffer from more than one illness. The paramedic should expect a longer interview. The paramedic also should use the techniques presented in Chapter 9. These techniques will help patients with multiple symptoms focus on the most relevant aspects of the chief complaint.

> **CRITICAL THINKING**
>
> Often patients give you a list of multiple problems. You have to identify the chief complaint. What single question would you ask?

Anxious Patients

For the patient, family, and bystanders to be anxious in an emergency is normal. The paramedic must be sensitive to the nonverbal clues of anxiety. The paramedic also should be supportive in a calm and confident way. The professional and caring attitude of the paramedic often helps to reduce the patient's anxiety. The paramedic should be aware that the anxiety may not be related directly to the illness or injury. For example, an older patient on a fixed income may worry about the cost of a hospital stay. A victim of a car crash may worry about liability and losing car insurance.

False Reassurance

The paramedic may be tempted to provide false reassurance in certain cases. Examples of this are saying "it's all right" or "everything's going to be okay." This may be tempting as a way to comfort an ill or injured patient. The paramedic should avoid early reassurance or over-reassurance until such can be given with confidence. False reassurances may block open dialogue between the paramedic and the patient. The paramedic should reassure the patient that the patient's medical condition is understood and that good patient care is available. Patients also will be comforted to know that the outcome is hopeful (if appropriate) and that they will be treated with dignity and respect during their care. These verbal reassurances generally work well in most patient care situations.

Anger and Hostility

Anger and hostility are not too different from anxious behavior. They are similar in that they are natural responses in some emergency situations. The paramedic should expect these reactions at times to be displaced toward the EMS crew. The paramedics always must ensure personal and scene safety. However, anger and hostility toward the patient is never appropriate. A much more effective approach includes maintaining a calm, confident manner. This approach also includes setting limits on acceptable behavior. The paramedic should try to calm the patient as well.

Intoxication

The paramedic should manage patients who are intoxicated with alcohol or other drugs with caution. Their behavior may be difficult to predict. The paramedic should not challenge or aggravate intoxicated patients. As with managing patients who are angry or hostile, the paramedic must ensure personal and scene safety. The paramedic also must set limits for acceptable behavior. To ensure scene safety, the paramedic should call for assistance from law enforcement personnel when needed.

Crying

Crying can reduce tension. Crying also may help reestablish the patient's emotional stability during an emergency. If crying is excessive or uncontrollable, the paramedic should be patient. The paramedic should show compassion and use direct eye contact to help control the crying. Reducing exhaustive crying conserves energy and promotes comfort.

Depression

Communicating with a depressed patient can be difficult. The types and causes of depression are many (see Chapter 40). The depression seen in an emergency often is due to moderate to high anxiety. Depression also may be enhanced by alcohol or substance use. The paramedic should use the communication techniques described previously for anxious patients. If possible, the paramedic should identify the seriousness of the patient's state. A physician's evaluation is encouraged.

Sexually Attractive or Seductive Patients

Paramedics and patients may be sexually attracted to each other. The paramedic should accept these feelings as normal. However, the feelings should not affect the paramedic's behavior. If a patient becomes seductive or makes sexual advances, the paramedic should firmly set limits of what is acceptable. The paramedic also must make it clear that the relationship is a professional one. As discussed in Chapter 9, providing same-sex care often is the best practice. If this is not possible, an extra caregiver (or a chaperone) should stay with the patient.

Confusing Behavior or Histories

Emergency situations are often intense. In these situations, emotions can run high. Thus the paramedic should expect to find confusing histories. The paramedic also must expect to see abnormal behavior. Factors that may contribute to these situations include mental illness, delirium, dementia, drug use, illness, and injury. Identifying a pattern of patient behavior may be difficult. Still the paramedic should try to identify one (e.g., signs and symptoms consistent with a certain disorder). In addition, the paramedic should attempt to lead the patient in an appropriate line of questioning.

Developmental Disabilities

The paramedic should not overlook the aptitude of patients with developmental disabilities. These persons often are able to offer adequate information. The paramedic should interview them just like other patients; the paramedic should use easily understood words and phrases. An obvious omission in the patient's answers reveals the need for more questioning. Questions may need to be stated more clearly. If the patient has severe mental retardation, the paramedic should try to get information from family or friends (see Chapter 47).

Communication Barriers

As discussed in Chapter 9, barriers to communication may result from social or cultural differences. These barriers also may occur because of sight, speech, or hearing impairments. The paramedic should seek assistance if possible. Family members, translators, and those with special training in communicating with the blind or the deaf may be helpful in these situations.

Talking with Family and Friends

Friends and family are often at the scene of an emergency. Therefore the paramedic should consider them a good source of information. This is especially the case when the patient cannot provide all of the necessary information because of illness or injury. Sometimes family or friends are unavailable and more patient information is needed. In these cases, the paramedic should try to locate a third party (e.g., a neighbor) who can help supply the missing details.

SUMMARY

- Obtaining a patient history offers structure to the patient assessment. The history often sets priorities in patient care as well.
- Content of the patient history includes date and time, identifying data, source of referral, history, reliability, chief complaint, present illness, past medical history, and review of body systems.
- The paramedic should ensure patient comfort. Several methods are available to accomplish this. The paramedic should avoid entering the patient's personal space. Sensitivity to the patient's feelings and watching for signs of uneasiness also are important. The paramedic should use appropriate language and ask open-ended and direct questions. The paramedic should use therapeutic communications techniques as well.
- Many challenges can affect history taking. One of these challenges is silent or talkative patients. Another is patients with multiple symptoms. Then there are anxious, angry, or hostile patients. The paramedic also may see intoxication, crying, depression, and sexually attractive or seductive patients. False reassurance is a major issue to consider. Patient may present confusing behaviors and histories. Two other issues are developmental disabilities and communication barriers. With these last two, the issue of talking with family and friends can be complex as well.

REFERENCE

1. US Department of Transportation, National Highway Traffic Safety Administration: *EMT-Paramedic national standard curriculum,* Washington, DC, 1998, The Department.

SUGGESTED READINGS

Carpenito L, editor: *Nursing diagnosis: application to clinical practice,* ed 9, Philadelphia, 2002, Lippincott Williams and Wilkins.

Monahan F, et al: *Nursing care of adults,* Philadelphia, 1994, WB Saunders.

Seidel H, et al: *Mosby's guide to physical examination,* ed 5, St Louis, 2003, Mosby.

CHAPTER 11

Techniques of Physical Examination

OBJECTIVES

Upon completion of this chapter, the paramedic student will be able to:

1. Describe physical examination techniques commonly used in the prehospital setting.
2. Describe the examination equipment commonly used in the prehospital setting.
3. Describe the general approach to physical examination.
4. Outline the steps of a comprehensive physical examination.
5. Detail the components of the mental status examination.
6. Distinguish between normal and abnormal findings in the mental status examination.
7. Outline the steps in the general patient survey.
8. Distinguish between normal and abnormal findings in the general patient survey.
9. Describe physical examination techniques used for assessment of specific body regions.
10. Distinguish between normal and abnormal findings when assessing specific body regions.
11. State modifications to the physical examination that are necessary when assessing children.
12. State modifications to the physical examination that are necessary when assessing the older adult.

KEY TERMS

auscultation: A technique that requires the use of a stethoscope and is used to assess body sounds produced by the movement of various fluids or gases in organs or tissues.

inspection: A visual assessment of the patient and surroundings.

palpation: A technique in which an examiner uses the hands and fingers to gather information from a patient by touch.

percussion: A technique used to evaluate the presence of air or fluid in body tissues.

physical examination: An assessment of a patient that includes examination techniques, measurement of vital signs, an assessment of height and weight, and the skillful use of examination equipment.

tidal volume: The volume of gas inhaled or exhaled during a normal breath.

The paramedic must have a wide range of knowledge and skills to perform a comprehensive physical examination. This knowledge and skill also will aid the paramedic in making good clinical care decisions. This chapter presents the techniques of the basic physical examination. In addition, this chapter reviews the relevant pathophysiological significance of the physical findings. Some of the techniques presented are not used routinely with patients in the prehospital setting. Some apply to the examinations performed in the field. However, other techniques more likely will be performed in the expanded scope of practice activities.

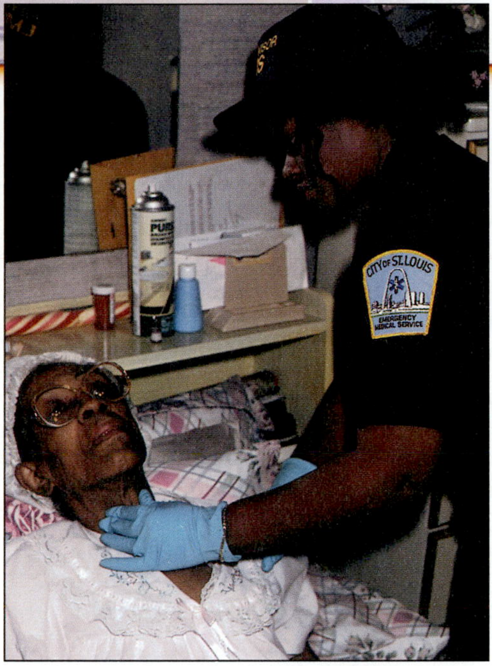

PHYSICAL EXAMINATION: APPROACH AND OVERVIEW

The **physical examination** consists of examination techniques, measurement of vital signs, an assessment of height and weight, and the skillful use of examination equipment (Box 11-1).

Examination Techniques

Four techniques commonly are used in the physical examination. These are **inspection, palpation, percussion,** and **auscultation.** These terms are referred to often in this text because they relate to the evaluation of specific body systems. Depending on the situation, these techniques may be the sole method for evaluating a patient. For example, this may be the case with an unconscious trauma patient. In other cases, these techniques may be integrated with history taking and other care procedures. If time permits, the paramedic should explain each technique that requires touch to the patient before performing it.

CRITICAL THINKING

You arrive at the scene of a motor vehicle crash. What will you look for during your initial patient inspection?

BOX 11-1 Components of the Physical Examination

Examination Techniques
Inspection
Palpation
Percussion
Auscultation

Measurement of Vital Signs
Pulse
Respirations
Blood pressure
Temperature (especially in children)

Assessment of Height and Weight

Equipment
Blood pressure cuff
Ophthalmoscope
Otoscope
Stethoscope

INSPECTION

Inspection is the visual assessment of the patient and the surroundings. This technique can alert the paramedic to the patient's mental status. Inspection also can alert the paramedic to possible injury or underlying illness. Patient hygiene, clothing, eye gaze, body language and position, skin color, and odor are significant inspection findings. The emergency medical services response may be to the patient's home. In this case, the paramedic should make a vi-

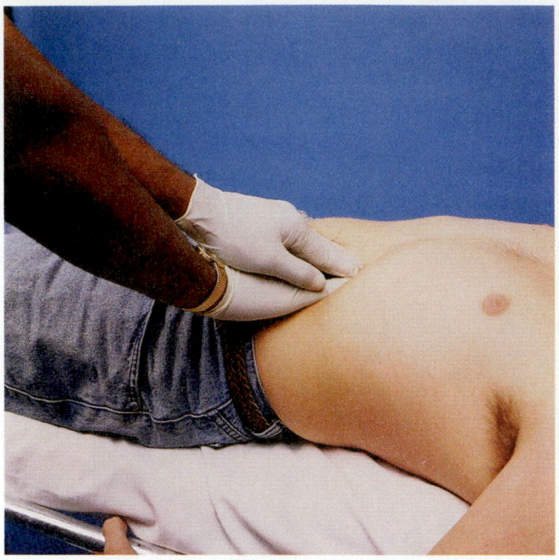

FIGURE 11-1 ■ Deep bimanual palpation.

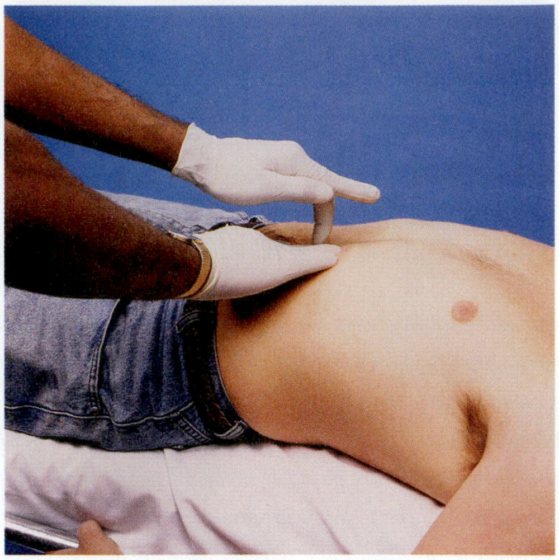

FIGURE 11-2 ■ Percussion technique.

sual inspection for cleanliness, prescription medicines, illegal drug paraphernalia, weapons, and signs of alcohol use. These and other items one sees can play a key role in determining the patient care activities.

PALPATION

Palpation is a technique in which the paramedic uses the hands and fingers to gather information by touch. Generally, the paramedic uses the palmar surface of the fingers and the finger pads to palpate for texture, masses, fluid, and crepitus and to assess skin temperature (Fig. 11-1). Palpation may be either superficial or deep; *the applications for each are addressed throughout this chapter*. Examining a patient by palpation is a form of invasion of the patient's body. Therefore the approach should be gentle and should be initiated with respect.

PERCUSSION

Percussion is used to evaluate the presence of air or fluid in body tissues. This technique is performed by the paramedic striking one finger against another to produce vibrations and sound waves of underlying tissue. Sound waves are heard as percussion tones (resonance). They are determined by the density of the tissue being examined. The denser the body area, the lower the pitch of the percussion tone. To percuss, the paramedic places the first joint of the middle finger of the nondominant hand on the patient, keeping the rest of the hand poised above the skin. The fingers of the other hand should be flexed and the wrist action loose. The paramedic then snaps the wrist of the dominant hand downward with the tip of the middle finger tapping the joint of the finger that is on the body surface. The tap should be sharp and rigid, percussing the same area several times to interpret the tone (Fig. 11-2). Box 11-2 describes percussion tones and examples of each. As with any other examination technique, percussion requires practice to obtain the skill needed for the physical examination.

BOX 11-2 Percussion Tones and Examples

Percussion Tone	Example
Tympany (the loudest)	Gastric bubble
Hyperresonance	Air-filled lungs (e.g., chronic obstructive pulmonary disease and pneumothorax)
Resonance	Healthy lungs
Dullness	Liver
Flat (the quietest)	Muscle

AUSCULTATION

Auscultation calls for the use of a stethoscope. This technique is used to assess body sounds made by the movement of various fluids or gases in the patient's organs or tissues. Auscultation is best performed in a quiet environment. Then the paramedic can focus on each body sound being assessed. The paramedic should isolate a particular area to note characteristics of intensity, pitch, duration, and quality. In the prehospital setting, auscultation most often is used to assess blood pressure and to evaluate breath sounds, heart sounds, and bowel sounds. To auscultate, the paramedic should place the diaphragm of the stethoscope firmly against the patient's skin for stabilization (Fig. 11-3). If a bell end piece is used, it should be positioned lightly on the body surface. This prevents the damping of vibrations.

NOTE The bell and diaphragm end pieces of a stethoscope selectively emphasize sounds of different frequencies. The bell is central for listening to low-pitched sounds (e.g., certain heart sounds). In contrast, the diaphragm filters out low-pitched sounds and therefore emphasizes high-pitched ones. Examples of high-pitched sounds include breath sounds and bowel sounds.

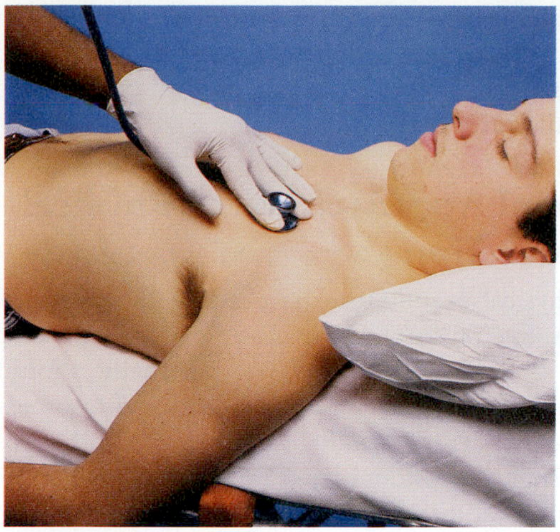

FIGURE 11-3 ■ Position of the stethoscope between the index and middle fingers.

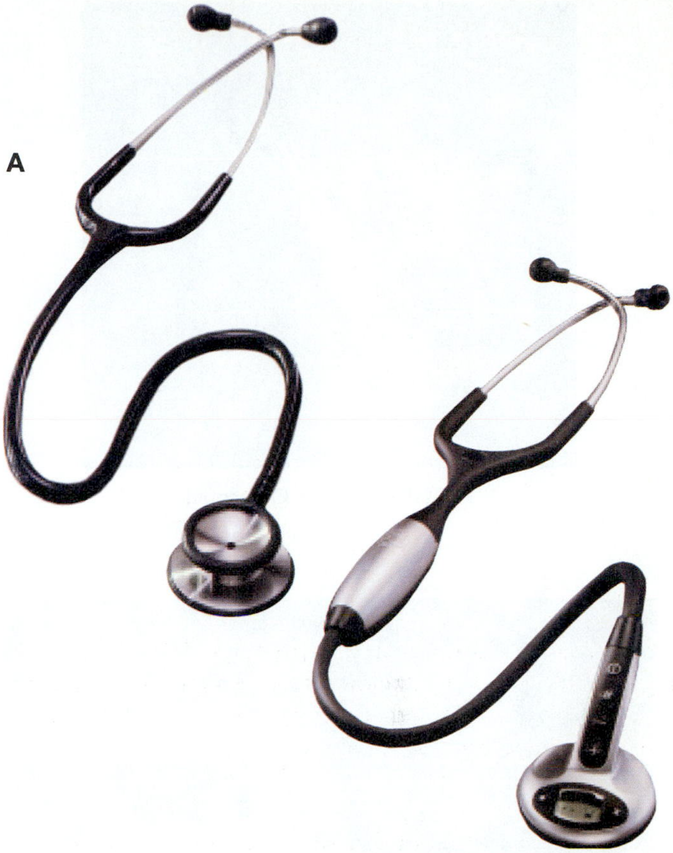

FIGURE 11-4 ■ Stethoscope types. A, Acoustic. B, Electronic.

Examination Equipment

Equipment used during the comprehensive physical examination includes the stethoscope, ophthalmoscope, otoscope, and blood pressure cuff. The ophthalmoscope and otoscope are nontraditional emergency medical services tools. They are being introduced to the paramedic with expanded scope of practice. These devices will not be used routinely with patients in the prehospital setting.

STETHOSCOPE

The stethoscope is used to evaluate sounds created by the cardiovascular, respiratory, and gastrointestinal systems. The three major types of stethoscopes are acoustic stethoscopes, magnetic stethoscopes, and electronic stethoscopes (Fig. 11-4).

Acoustic stethoscopes transmit sound waves from the source to the paramedic's ears. Most have a rigid diaphragm. This diaphragm transmits high-pitched sounds. The bell end piece transmits low-pitched sounds.

Magnetic stethoscopes have a single diaphragm end piece. The end piece contains an iron disk and a permanent magnet. The air column of the diaphragm is activated as magnetic attraction established between the iron disk and the magnet. A frequency dial adjusts for high-, low-, and full-frequency sounds.

Electronic stethoscopes convert sound vibrations into electrical impulses. These impulses are amplified. The impulses are transmitted to a speaker where they are converted to sound. These devices can compensate for environmental noise. Thus they may be beneficial for use in the prehospital setting.

OPHTHALMOSCOPE

The ophthalmoscope is used to inspect structures of the eye, including the retina, choroid, optic nerve disk, macula (an oval, yellow spot at the center of the retina), and retinal vessels. This device has a battery light source, two dials, and a viewer (Fig. 11-5). The dial at the top of the battery changes the light image. The dial at the top of the viewer allows for the selection of lenses. (Five lenses are available, but the large white light generally is used.)

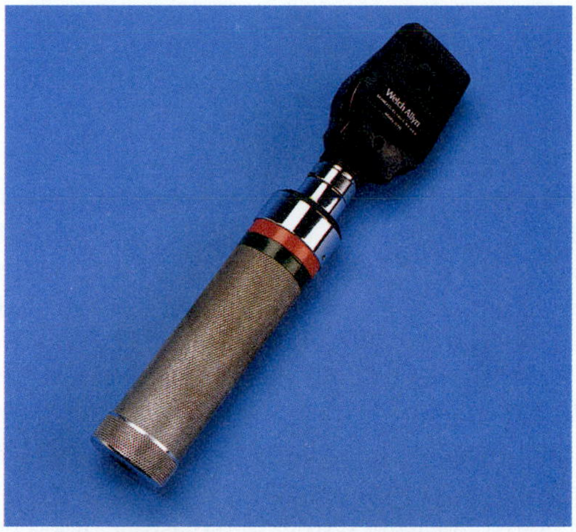

FIGURE 11-5 ■ Ophthalmoscope.

OTOSCOPE

The otoscope is used to examine deep structures of the external and middle ear. This device is basically an ophthalmoscope with a special ear speculum attached to the bat-

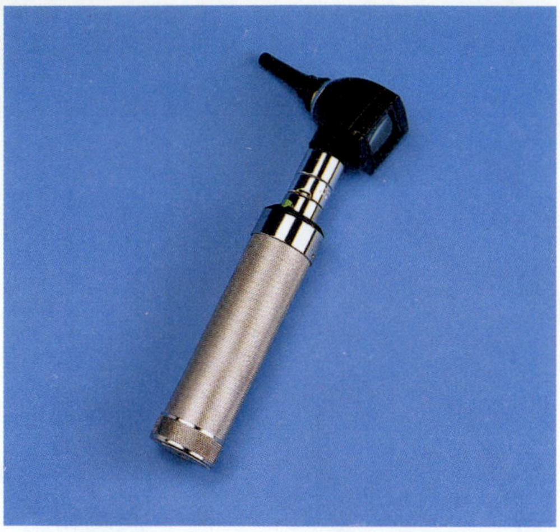

FIGURE 11-6 ■ Otoscope.

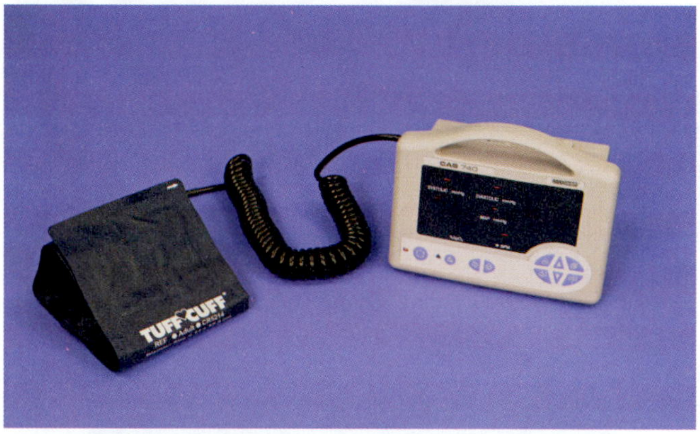

FIGURE 11-7 ■ Electronic blood pressure device.

tery tube (Fig. 11-6). Ear specula come in a number of sizes to conform to various ear canals. (The paramedic should choose the largest one that fits comfortably in the patient's ear.) The light from the otoscope allows one to visualize the tympanic membrane.

BLOOD PRESSURE CUFF

The blood pressure cuff is the sphygmomanometer. The blood pressure cuff most commonly is used (along with the stethoscope) to measure systolic and diastolic blood pressure. The common blood pressure cuff used in the prehospital setting consists of a pressure gauge that registers millimeter calibrations, a synthetic cuff with Velcro closures that encloses an inflatable rubber bladder, and a pressure bulb with a release valve. Blood pressure cuffs are available in a number of sizes. Adult widths should be one third to one half the circumference of the limb. For children, the width should cover about two thirds of the upper arm or thigh. (Blood pressure cuffs that are too large give a falsely low reading; cuffs that are too small give a falsely high reading.)

Electronic devices that automatically measure a patient's vital signs are available (Fig. 11-7). They are used by hospitals and some emergency medical services agencies to monitor the patient's blood pressure, pulse rate, body temperature, end-tidal carbon dioxide, and oxygen saturation at regular intervals.

General Approach to the Physical Examination

The physical examination is performed as a step-by-step process. Special emphasis is placed on the patient's present illness and chief complaint. The paramedic should know that most patients view a physical exam with some anxiety.

Often, patients initially feel vulnerable and exposed. To establish a professional trust early in the encounter is important. In addition, to ensure the patient's privacy when possible is key.

Overview of a Comprehensive Physical Examination

The physical examination is a systematic assessment of the body that includes the following components:

- Mental status
- General survey
- Vital signs
- Skin
- Head, eyes, ears, nose, and throat
- Chest
- Abdomen
- Posterior body
- Extremities (peripheral vascular and musculoskeletal)
- Neurological exam

NOTE The Centers for Disease Control and Prevention and the Occupational Safety and Health Administration have recommended that health care workers wear gloves "when handling blood-soiled items, body fluids, excretions and secretions, as well as surfaces, materials, and objects exposed to them."[1] This text assumes that all paramedics are gloved for certain care activities. Personal protective measures are listed on the inside cover of this book. These measures are dealt with further in Chapter 39.

MENTAL STATUS

The first step in any encounter with a patient is to note the patient's appearance and behavior. With this step, one also should assess for level of consciousness. A healthy patient is expected to be alert and responsive to touch, verbal instruction, and painful stimuli.

Appearance and Behavior

As mentioned before, a visual assessment of the patient can yield key information. Abnormal findings may include drowsiness, obtundation (inability to respond), stupor, or coma. A patient who is obtunded is insensitive to unpleasant or painful stimuli because of a reduced level of consciousness. This reduced level usually is produced by anesthetics or analgesics. Stupor is a state of lethargy and unresponsiveness. Stuporous patients usually are unaware of their surroundings. Coma is a state of profound unconsciousness. A patient in coma has no spontaneous eye movements. This patient does not respond to verbal or painful stimuli. In addition, the patient cannot be aroused.

▶NOTE Some medical direction agencies discourage the use of these terms to describe a patient's mental status. Because these terms are vague, they may be open to interpretation. Instead, one may describe the patient's reactions and verbal and motor responses with indexes such as the AVPU (alert, verbal, painful, unresponsive) scale or Glasgow Coma Scale (described in Chapters 12 and 24). These measurements often are considered better patient information.

POSTURE, GAIT, AND MOTOR ACTIVITY

The paramedic should observe the patient's posture, gait, and motor activity. The paramedic can do this by assessing pace, range, character, and appropriateness of movement. For example, most patients without physical disabilities can walk with good balance and without a limp, discomfort, or fear of falling. Abnormal findings may include ataxia (uncoordinated movement), paralysis, restlessness, agitation, bizarre body posture, immobility, and involuntary movements.

DRESS, GROOMING, PERSONAL HYGIENE, AND BREATH OR BODY ODORS

Dress, grooming, and personal hygiene should be appropriate for the patient's age, lifestyle, occupation, and socioeconomic group. A person's dress should match the temperature and weather conditions. (Older adults and children who are improperly dressed for temperatures or who have poor hygiene may be victims of neglect.) Medical jewelry (e.g., copper bracelets for arthritis, medical insignias) should be noted. Hair, fingernails, and cosmetics may reflect the patient's lifestyle, mood, and personality. These findings can point to a decreased interest in appearance (e.g., grown-out hair or faded nail polish). This may help to estimate the length of an illness.

Breath or body odors can point to underlying conditions or illness. Examples of breath odors include alcohol, acetone (seen with some diabetic conditions), feces (seen with bowel obstruction), and halitosis from throat infections and poor dental and oral hygiene. Renal and liver disease and poor hygiene also may result in body odor.

FACIAL EXPRESSION

Facial expressions may reveal anxiety, depression, elation, anger, or withdrawal. The paramedic should be alert to changes in facial expression. The paramedic should observe these while the patient is at rest, during conversation, during the examination, and when asking questions. Facial expressions should match the situation.

MOOD, AFFECT, AND RELATION TO PERSON AND THINGS

The patient's mood and affect also should match the situation. Mood and affect describe the patient's emotional state and the outward display of feelings and emotions; they are expressed verbally and nonverbally. Examples of abnormal findings include an unusual happiness in the presence of major illness, indifference, responses to imaginary persons or objects, and unpredictable mood swings.

CRITICAL THINKING

What physical clues do you look for in your friends or your partner that tell you about their mood?

Speech and Language

The patient's speech should be understandable and of a moderate pace. The paramedic should assess the quantity, rate, loudness, and fluency of the patient's speech patterns. Abnormal findings include aphasia (loss of speech), dysphonia (abnormal speaking voice), dysarthria (poorly articulated speech), and speech and language that changes with mood.

Thought and Perceptions

A healthy person's thoughts and perceptions are logical, relevant, organized, and coherent. Patients should have an insight into their illness or injury. They also should be able to show a level of judgment in making decisions or plans about their situation and their care. Although accurately assessing a person's thoughts and perceptions is difficult, the following usually are considered abnormal findings:

- Abnormal thought processes
  - Flight of ideas
  - Incoherence
  - Confabulation
- Abnormal thought content
  - Obsessions
  - Compulsions
  - Delusions
  - Feelings of unreality
- Abnormal perceptions
  - Illusions
  - Hallucinations

Memory and Attention

Healthy persons normally are oriented to person, place, and time ("oriented times 3"). The paramedic can use several other methods to assess a patient's memory and attention. One method is to ask the patient to count from 1 to 10 using only even or odd numbers (digit span). Another is to multiply by sevens (serial sevens). A third method is to spell simple words backward. The paramedic also should assess the patient's remote memory (e.g., birthdays), recent memory (e.g., events of the day), and the patient's new learning ability. New learning ability can be evaluated by giving the patient new information (e.g., the year and model of the ambulance). Later the paramedic would ask the patient to recall that information.

GENERAL SURVEY

The paramedic assesses the patient's level of consciousness and mental status first. Then the paramedic performs a general survey of the patient. In addition to the assessments described previously, the paramedic should evaluate the patient for signs of distress, apparent state of health, skin color and obvious lesions, height and build, sexual development, and weight. The paramedic also should assess vital signs during the general survey.

Signs of Distress

Obvious signs of distress include those that result from cardiorespiratory insufficiency, pain, and anxiety. Examples of these signs and symptoms are as follows:

- Cardiorespiratory insufficiency
  - Labored breathing
  - Wheezing
  - Cough
- Pain
  - Wincing
  - Sweating
  - Protectiveness of a painful body part or area
- Anxiety
  - Restlessness
  - Anxious expression
  - Fidgety movement
  - Cold, moist palms

CRITICAL THINKING

Combine one symptom from each of the groups of distress, and imagine how a patient with these symptoms might look and act.

Apparent State of Health

A patient's apparent state of health can be assessed by observation. The paramedic should note the patient's basic appearance as being acutely or chronically ill, frail, feeble, robust, or vigorous.

Skin Color and Obvious Lesions

Skin color can vary by body part and from person to person. A patient's normal skin color depends of course on race and can range from pink or ivory to deep brown, yellow, or olive. Skin color is best assessed by evaluating skin that usually is not exposed to the sun (e.g., the palms) or skin that has less pigmentation (e.g., lips and nail beds). Box 11-3 describes abnormal skin colors and their possible causes. Obvious skin lesions that can indicate illness or injury include rashes, bruises, scars, and discoloration (Fig. 11-8; Tables 11-1 and 11-2).

BOX 11-3 Abnormal Skin Color and Possible Causes

Color	Possible Causes
Pallor (decrease in color)	Shock, dehydration, fright
Cyanosis (bluish color)	Cardiorespiratory insufficiency, cold environment
Jaundice (yellow-orange color)	Liver disease, red blood cell destruction
Red	Fever, inflammation, carbon monoxide poisoning

Height and Build

Patients generally can be described as average, tall, or short, with a slender, lanky, muscular, or stocky build. All of these factors can reflect overall health. For example, a patient can be excessively thin (as seen with some eating disorders) or trim and muscular. Age and lifestyle also may affect height and body build.

Sexual Development

The paramedic will assess sexual development. The paramedic should decide whether the sexual characteristics are appropriate for the patient's age and sex. Normal changes associated with puberty include facial hair and deepening of the voice in men, increased breast size in women, and hair growth in the axillary and groin areas in both sexes.

Weight

Ideally a patient's body weight should be proportionate to height (Fig. 11-9). Weight conditions that are easily observed in the general survey include patients who are emaciated (extremely lean from lack of nutrition), plump, or obese (body weight that is 20% greater than desirable body weight for a person's age, sex, height, and body fluid). A recent gain or loss is a key finding and may be clinically important. Like body height and build, body weight can reflect the patient's health, age, and lifestyle.

CRITICAL THINKING

Think about three medical conditions that might result in significant weight loss. Now, think about three that might cause a significant weight gain.

Vital Signs

Vital signs are pulse, blood pressure, respirations, skin condition, and pupil size and reactivity.

Text continued on p. 248

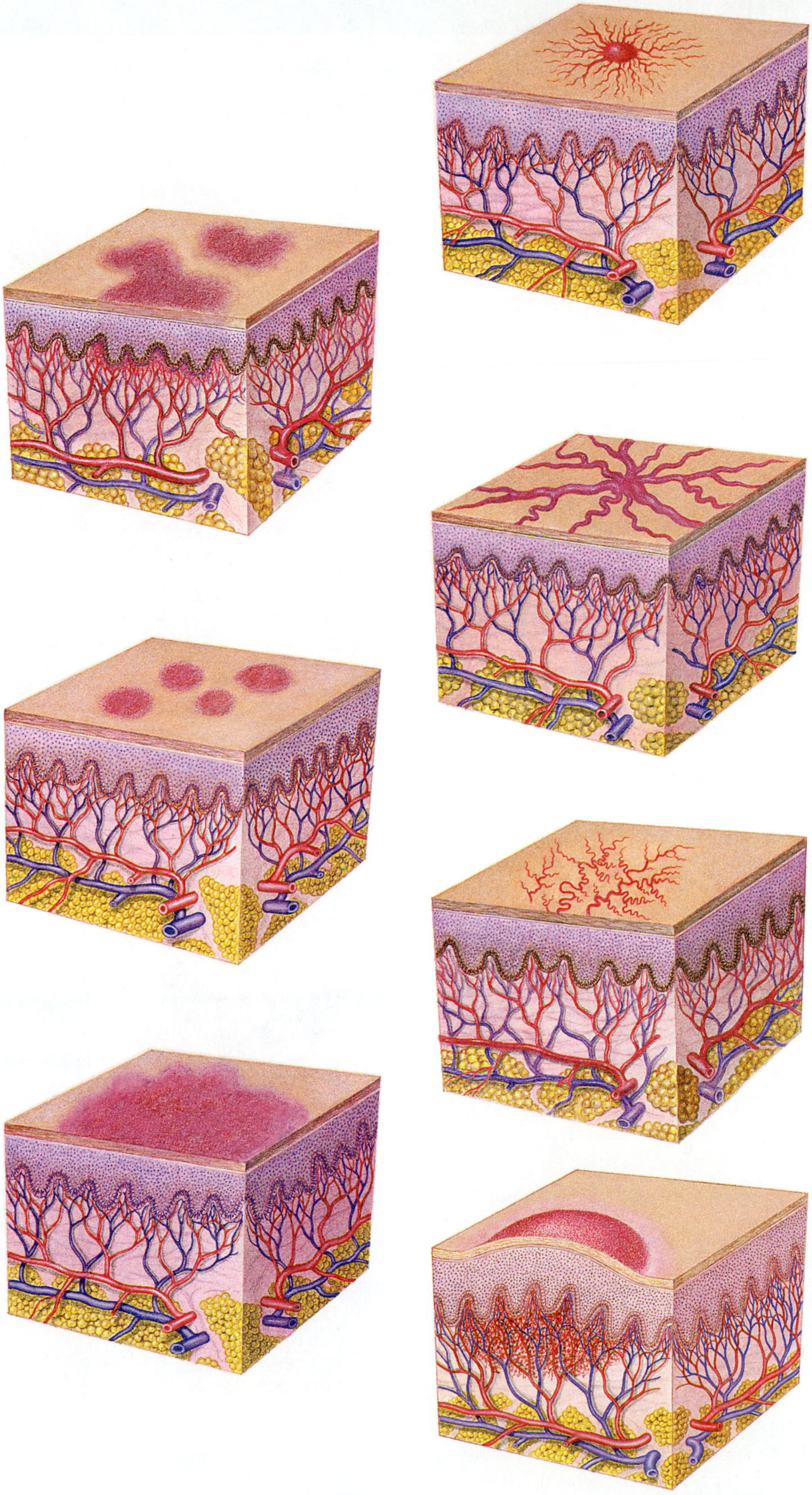
Spider angioma—red central body with radiating spiderlike legs that blanch with pressure to the central body
Cause: Liver disease, vitamin B deficiency, idiopathic
Purpura—red-purple nonblanchable discoloration greater than 0.5 cm diameter.
Cause: Intravascular defects, infection
Venous star—bluish spider, linear or irregularly shaped; does not blanch with pressure
Cause: Increased pressure in superficial veins
Petechiae—red-purple nonblanchable discoloration less than 0.5 cm diameter
Cause: Intravascular defects, infection
Telangiectasia—fine, irregular red line
Cause: Dilation of capillaries
Ecchymoses—red-purple nonblanchable discoloration of variable size
Cause: Vascular wall destruction, trauma, vasculitis
Capillary hemangioma (nevus flammeus)—red irregular macular patches
Cause: Dilation of dermal capillaries

FIGURE 11-8 ■ Characteristics and causes of vascular skin lesions.

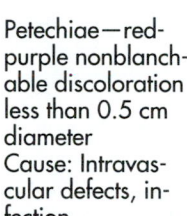

TABLE 11-1 Primary Skin Lesions

DESCRIPTION	EXAMPLES		
Macule A flat, circumscribed area that is a change in the color of the skin; less than 1 cm in diameter	Freckles, flat moles (nevi), petechiae, measles, scarlet fever	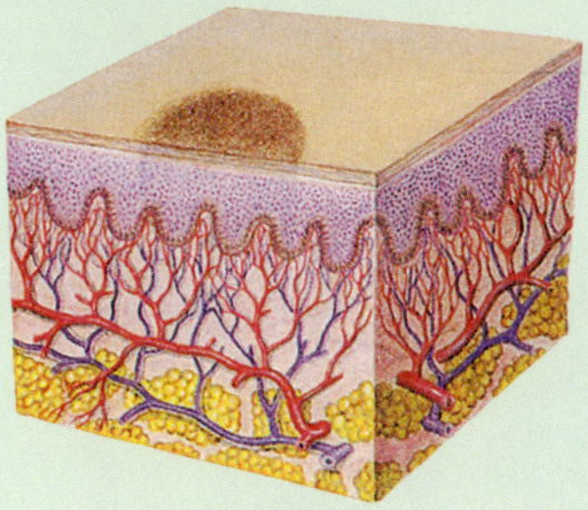	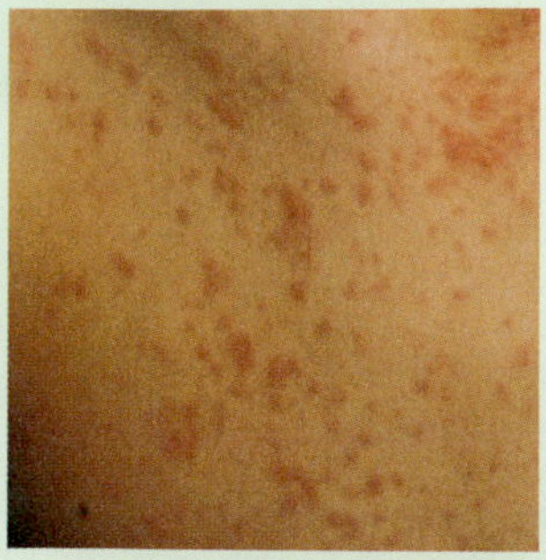 Measles. (From Habif, 1996.)
Papule An elevated, firm, circumscribed area; less than 1 cm in diameter	Wart (verruca), elevated moles, lichen planus	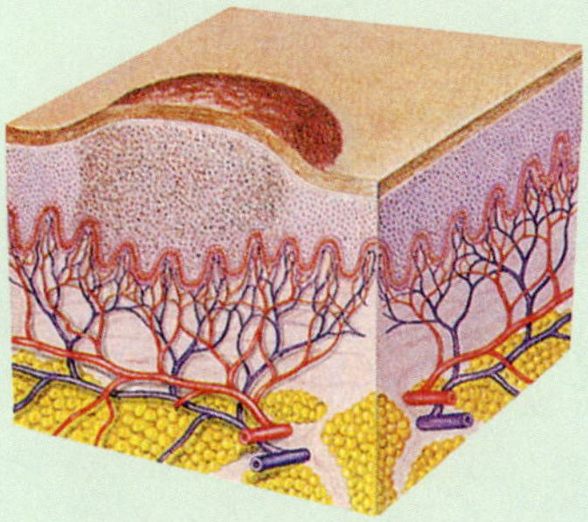	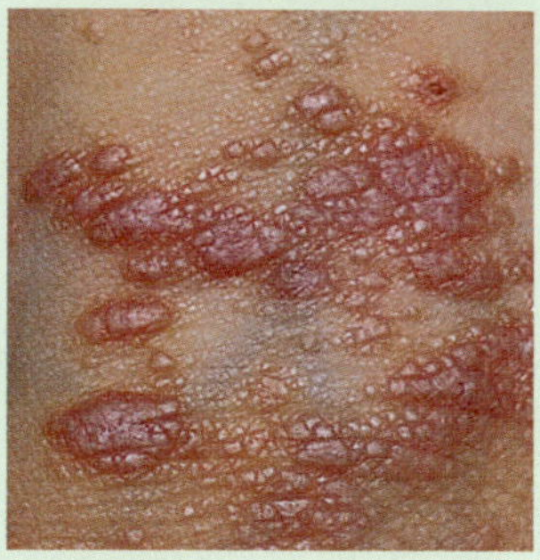 Lichen planus. (From Weston, Lane, Morelli, 1996.)
Patch A flat, nonpalpable, irregular-shaped macule greater than 1 cm in diameter	Vitiligo, port-wine stains, Mongolian spots, café au lait patch	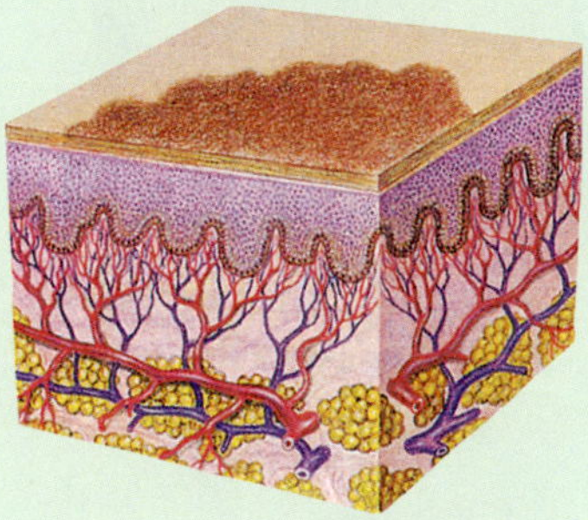	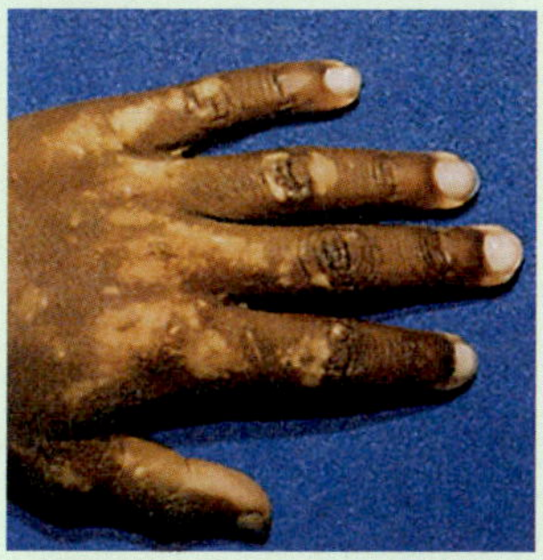 Vitiligo. (From Weston, Lane, Morelli, 1991.)
Plaque Elevated, firm, and rough lesion with flat top surface greater than 1 cm in diameter	Psoriasis, seborrheic and actinic keratoses	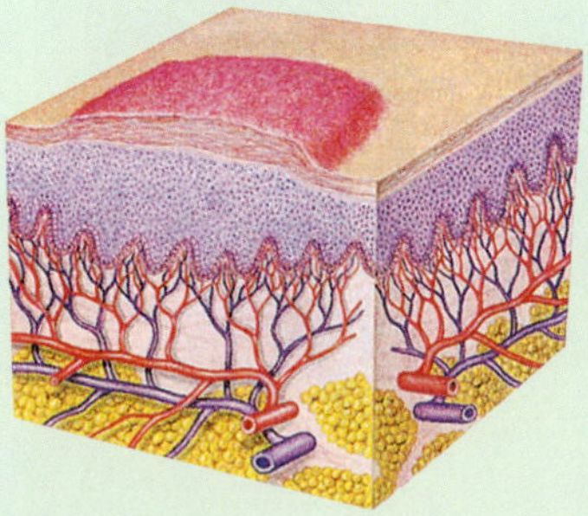	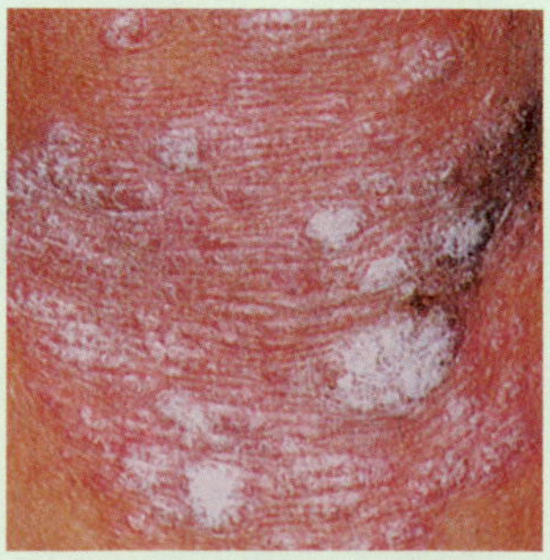 Plaque. (From Habif, 1996.)

Modified from Thompson, Wilson, 1995.

TABLE 11-1 Primary Skin Lesions—cont'd

DESCRIPTION	EXAMPLES		
Wheal Elevated, irregular-shaped area of cutaneous edema; solid, transient, variable diameter	Insect bites, urticaria, allergic reaction	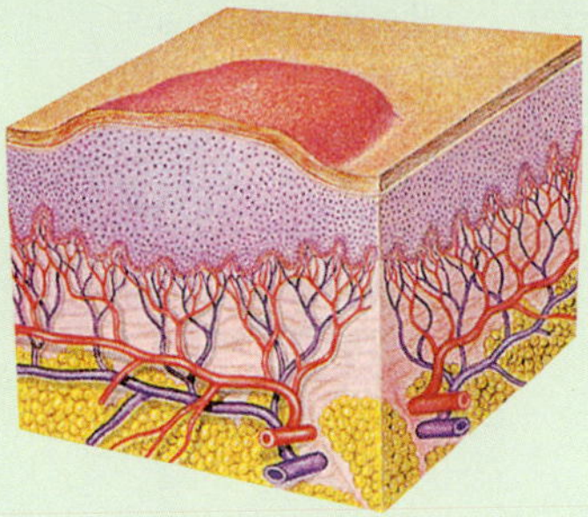	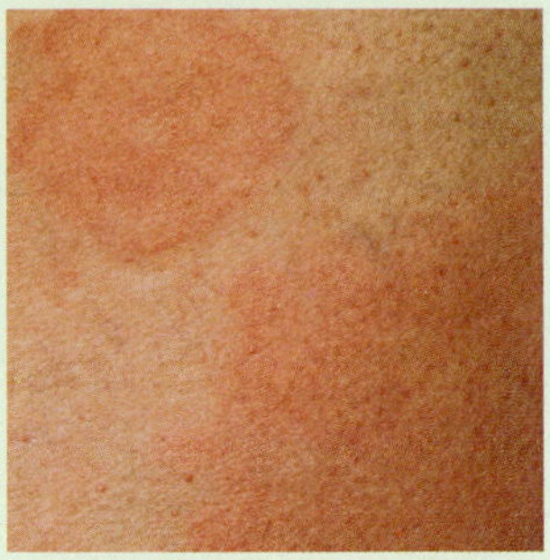 Wheal. (From Farrar et al, 1992.)
Nodule Elevated, firm, circumscribed lesion; deeper in dermis than a papule; 1 to 2 cm in diameter	Erythema nodosum, lipomas	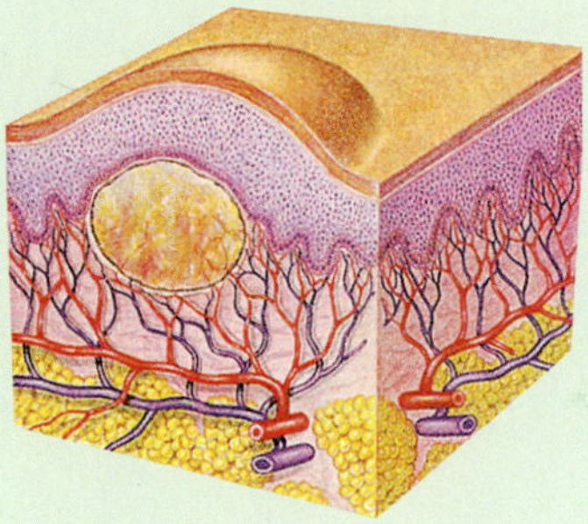	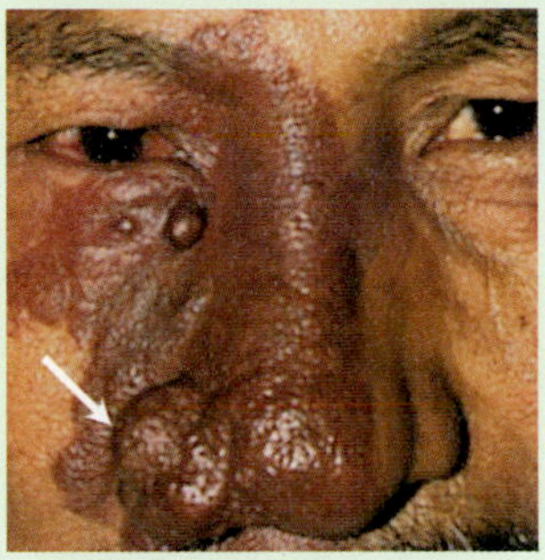 Hypertrophic nodule. (From Goldman, Fitzpatrick, 1994.)
Tumor Elevated and solid lesion; may or may not be clearly demarcated; deeper in dermis; greater than 2 cm in diameter	Neoplasms, benign tumor, lipoma, hemangioma	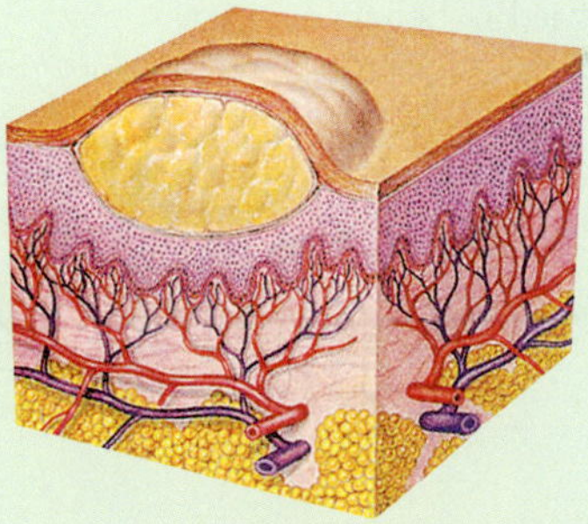	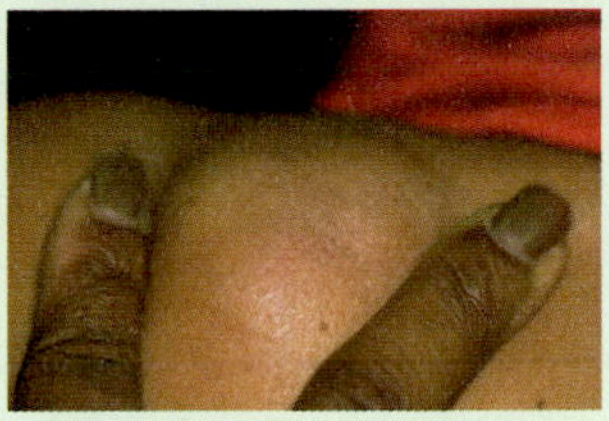 Lipoma. (From Lemmi, Lemmi, 2000).
Vesicle Elevated, circumscribed, superficial, not into dermis; filled with serous fluid; less than 1 cm in diameter	Varicella (chicken pox), herpes zoster (shingles)	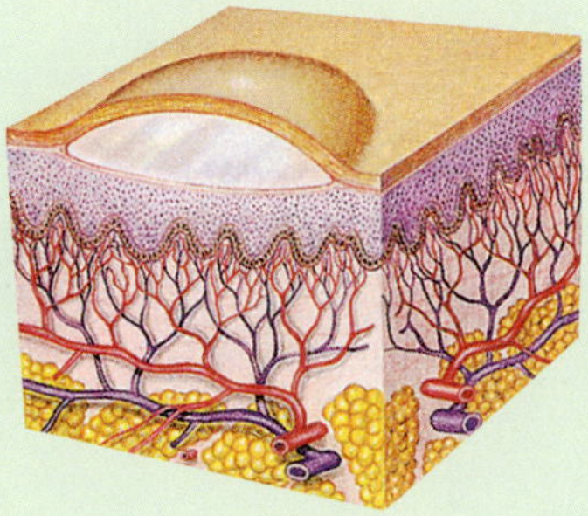	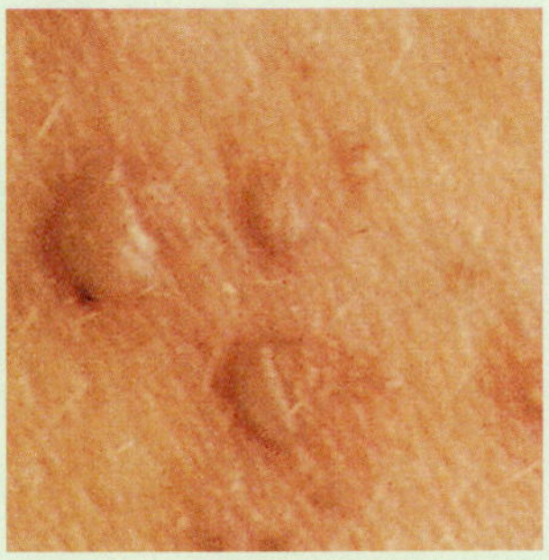 Vesicles caused by varicella. (From Farrar et al, 1992.)

Continued

TABLE 11-1 Primary Skin Lesions—cont'd

DESCRIPTION	EXAMPLES		
Bulla Vesicle greater than 1 cm in diameter	Blister, pemphigus vulgaris	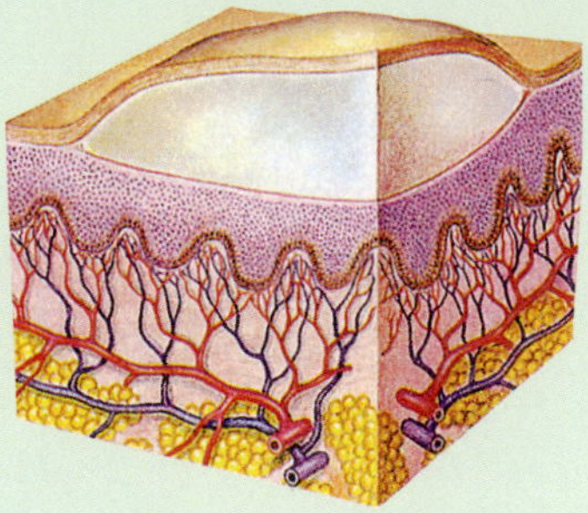	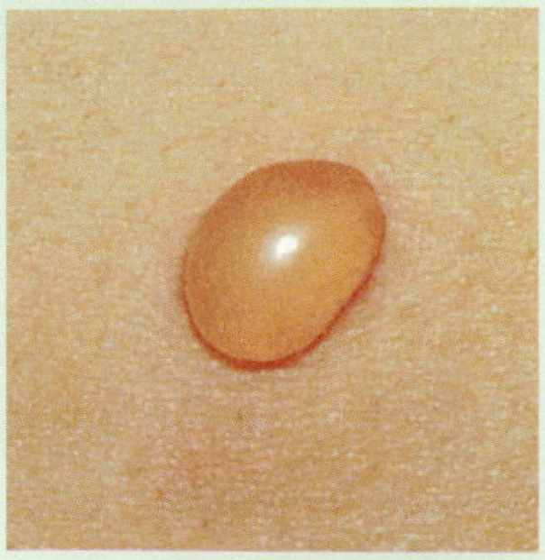 Blister. (From White, 1994.)
Pustule Elevated, superficial lesion; similar to a vesicle but filled with purulent fluid	Impetigo, acne	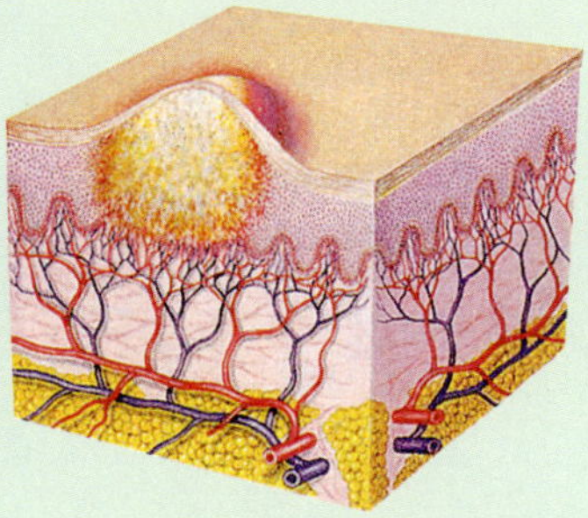	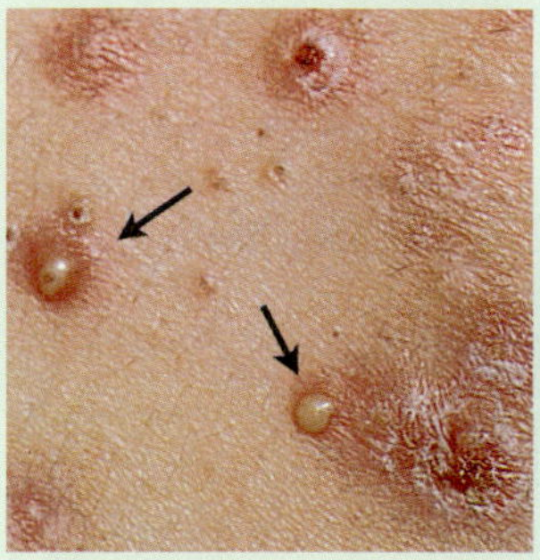 Acne. (From Weston, Lane, Morelli, 1996.)
Cyst Elevated, circumscribed, encapsulated lesion; in dermis or subcutaneous layer; filled with liquid or semi-solid material	Sebaceous cyst, cystic acne	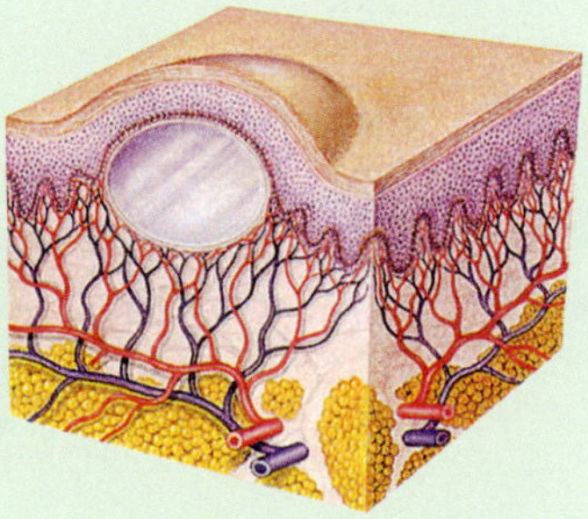	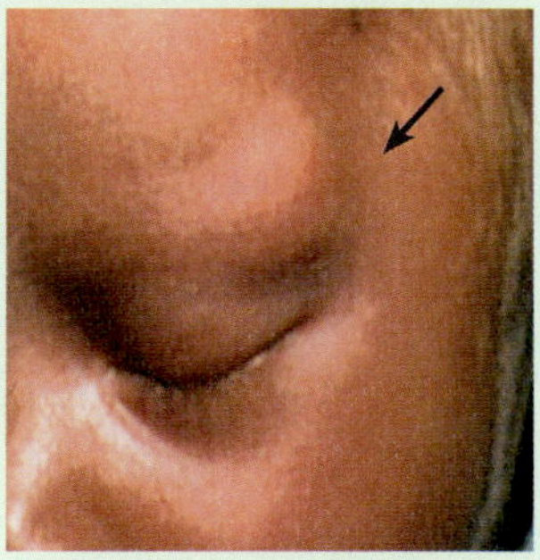 Sebaceous cyst. (From Weston, Lane, Morelli, 1996.)
Telangiectasia Fine, irregular, red lines produced by capillary dilation	Telangiectasia in rosacea	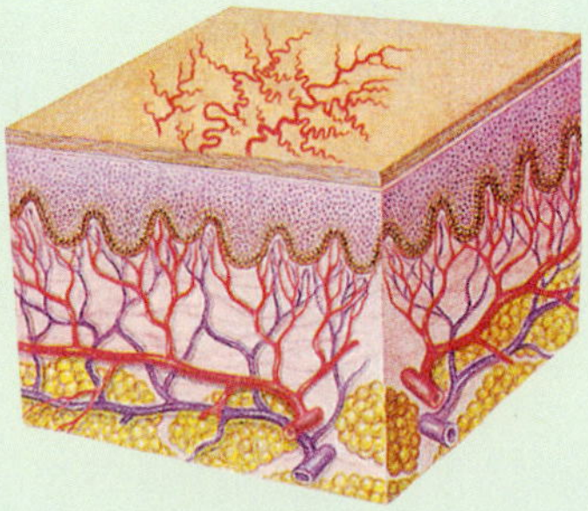	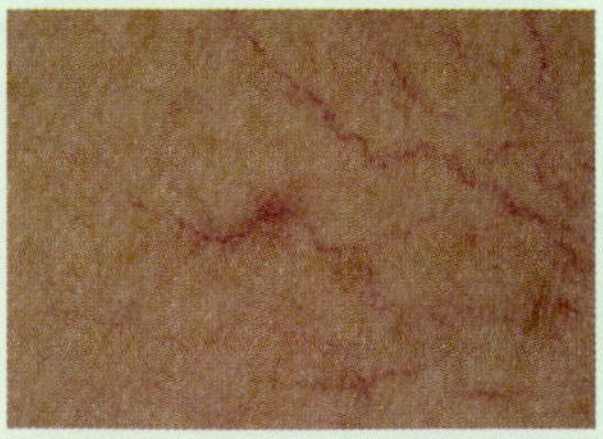 Telangiectasia. (From Lemmi, Lemmi, 2000.)

Modified from Thompson, Wilson, 1995.

TABLE 11-2 Secondary Skin Lesions

DESCRIPTION	EXAMPLES		
Scale Heaped-up, keratinized cells, flaky skin; irregular; thick or thin; dry or oily; variation in size	Flaking of skin with seborrheic dermatitis following scarlet fever, or flaking of skin following a drug reaction; dry skin	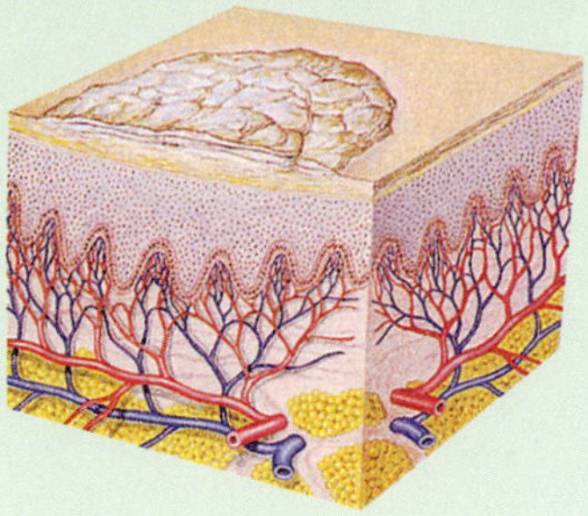	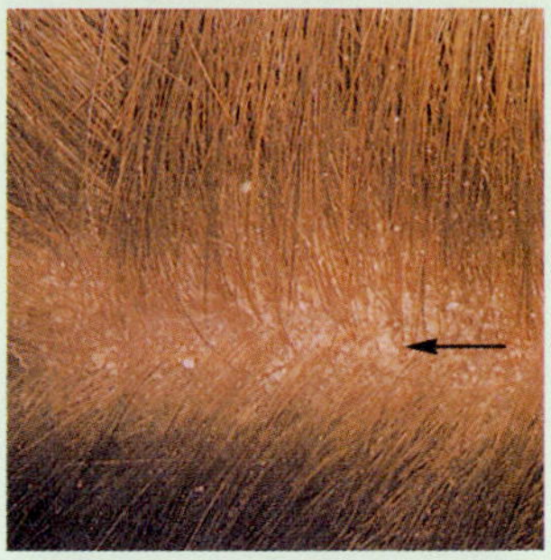 Fine scaling. (From Baran, Dawher, Levene, 1991.)
Lichenification Rough, thickened epidermis secondary to persistent rubbing, itching, or skin irritation; often involves flexor surface of extremity	Chronic dermatitis	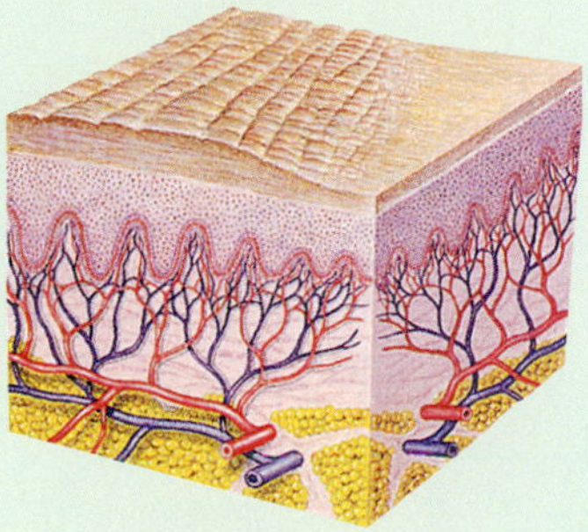	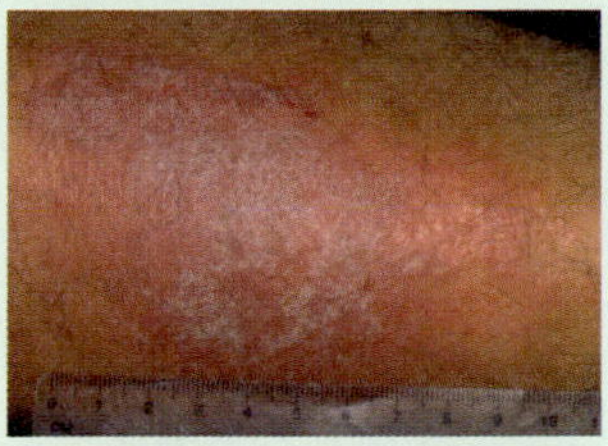 Lichenification. (From Lemmi, Lemmi, 2000.)
Keloid Irregular-shaped, elevated, progressively enlarging scar; grows beyond the boundaries of the wound; caused by excessive collagen formation during healing	Keloid formation following surgery	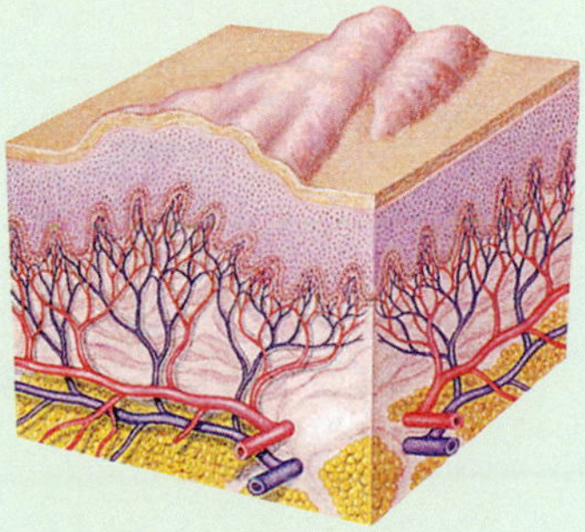	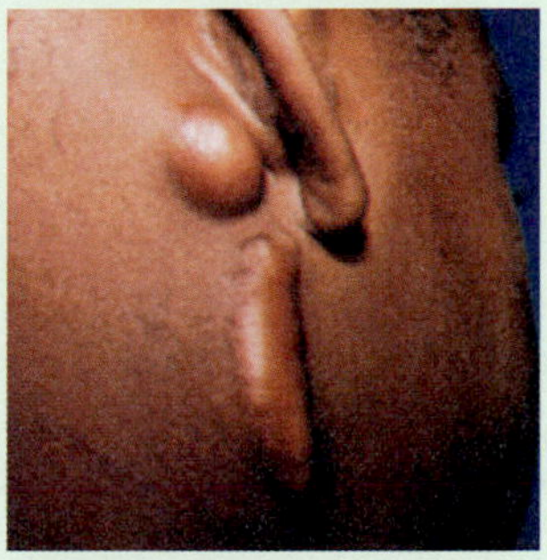 Keloid. (From Weston, Lane, Morelli, 1996.)
Scar Thin to thick fibrous tissue that replaces normal skin following injury or laceration to the dermis	Healed wound or surgical incision	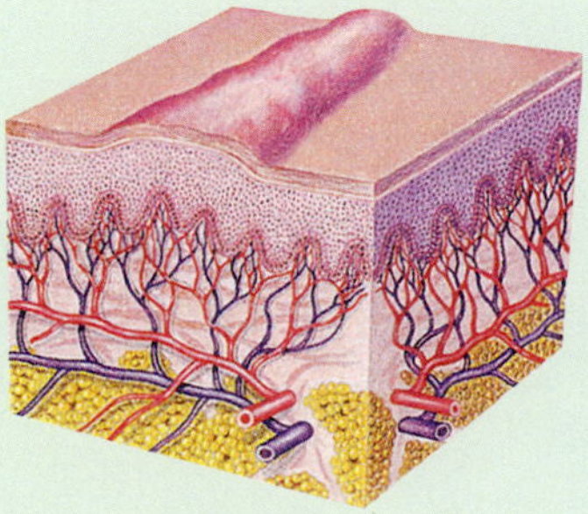	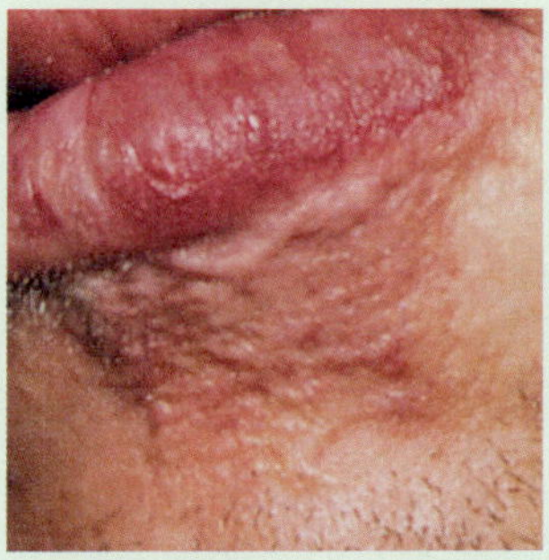 Hypertrophic scar. (From Goldman, Fitzpatrick, 1994.)

Modified from Wilson, Giddens, 2001.

Continued

TABLE 11-2 Secondary Skin Lesions—cont'd

DESCRIPTION	EXAMPLES		
Excoriation Loss of the epidermis; linear hollowed-out, crusted area	Abrasion or scratch, scabies	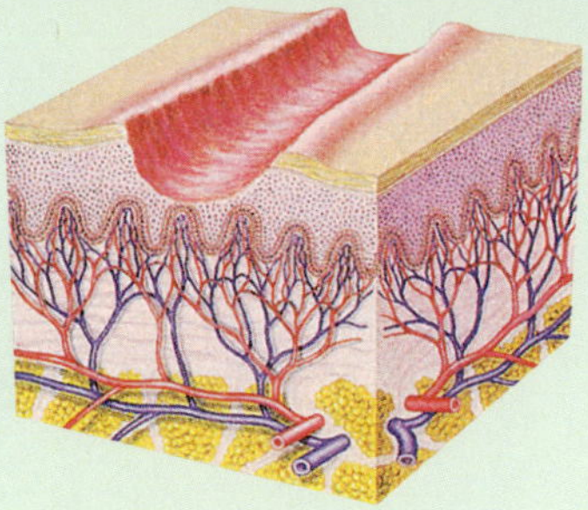	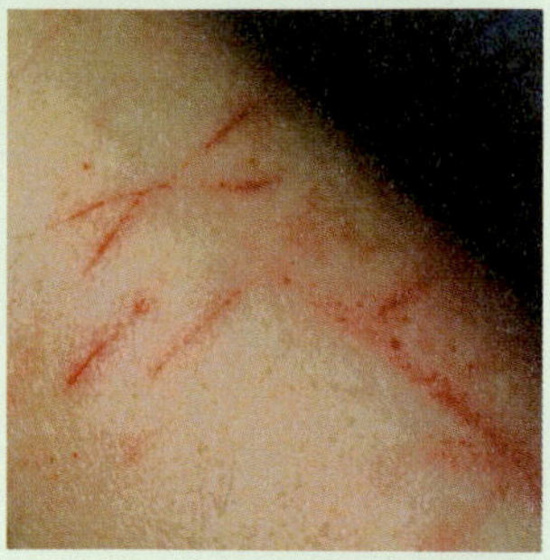 Excoriation from a tree branch. (From Lemmi, Lemmi, 2000.)
Fissure Linear crack or break from the epidermis to the dermis; may be moist or dry	Athlete's foot, cracks at the corner of the mouth	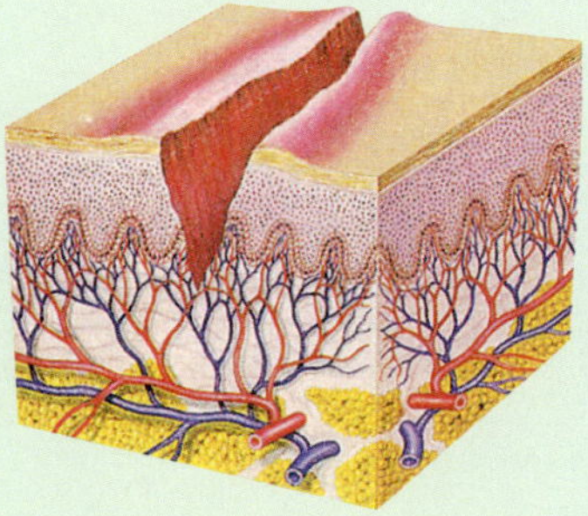	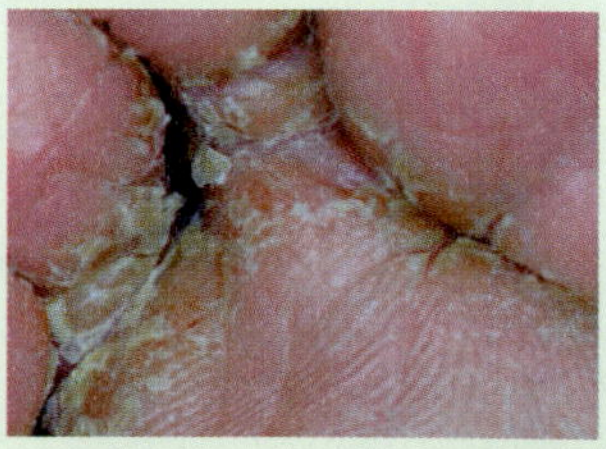 Scaling and fissures of tinea pedis. (From Lemmi, Lemmi, 2000.)
Erosion Loss of part of the epidermis; depressed, moist, glistening; follows rupture of a vesicle or bulla	Varicella, variola after rupture	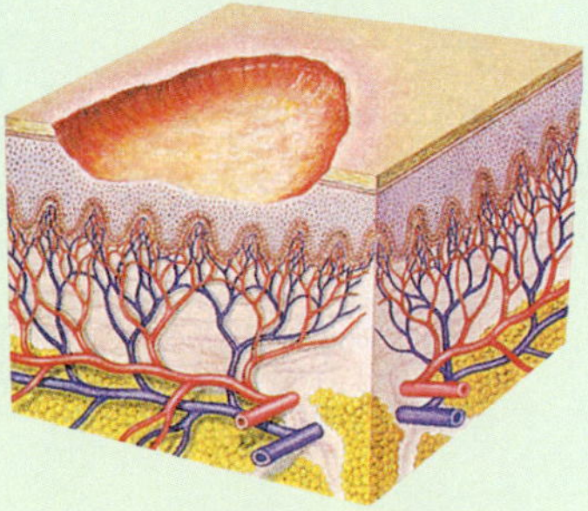	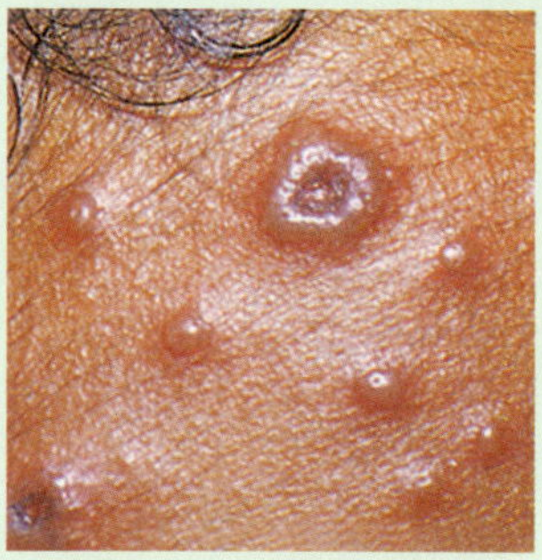 Erosion. (From Cohen, 1993.)
Ulcer Loss of epidermis and dermis; concave; varies in size	Decubiti, stasis ulcers	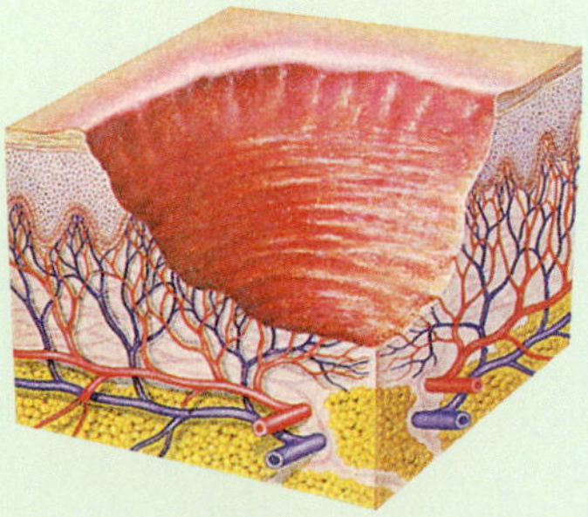	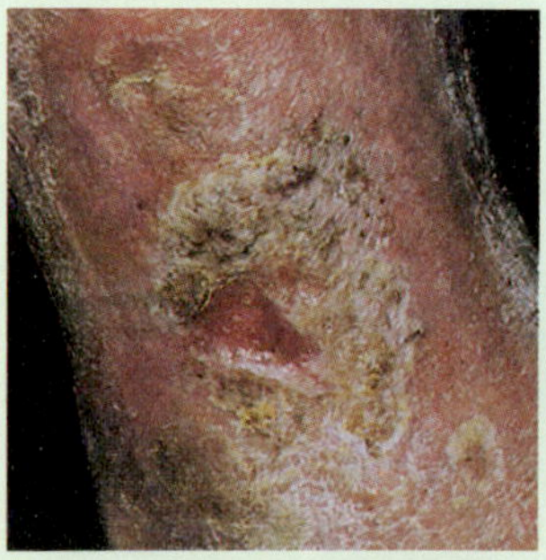 Statis ulcer. (From Habif, 1996.)

Modified from Wilson, Giddens, 2001.

TABLE 11-2 Secondary Skin Lesions—cont'd

DESCRIPTION	EXAMPLES		
Crust Dried serum, blood, or purulent exudates; slightly elevated; size varies; brown, red, tan, or straw-colored	Scab on abrasion, eczema	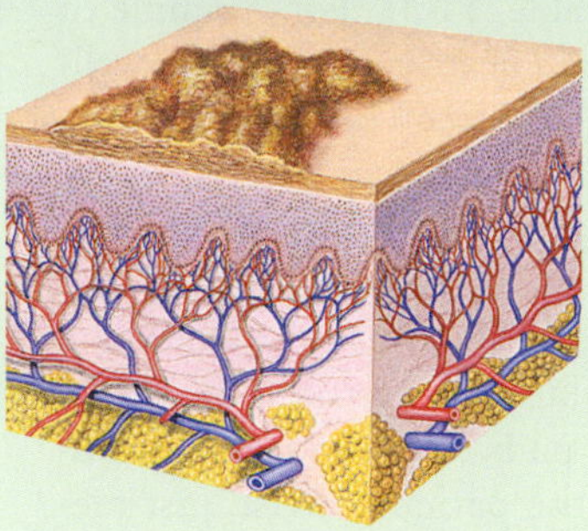	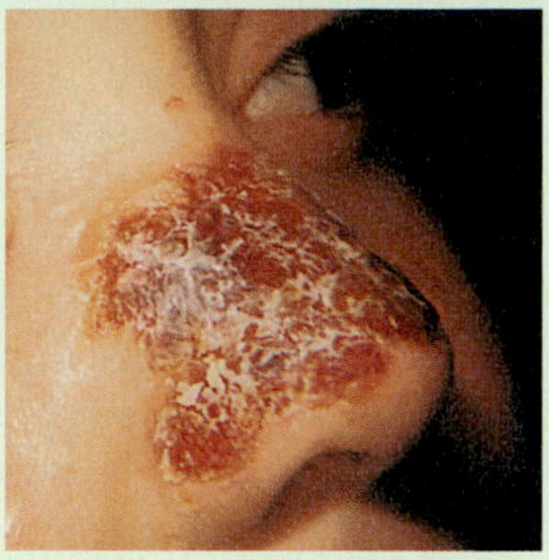 Scab.
Atrophy Thinning of skin surface and loss of skin markings; skin translucent and paperlike	Striae; aged skin	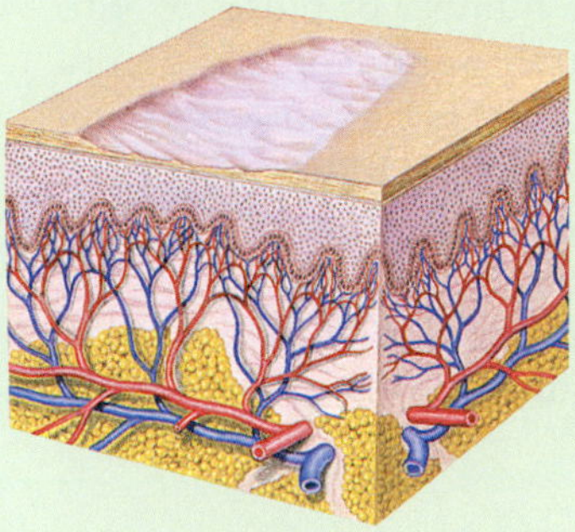	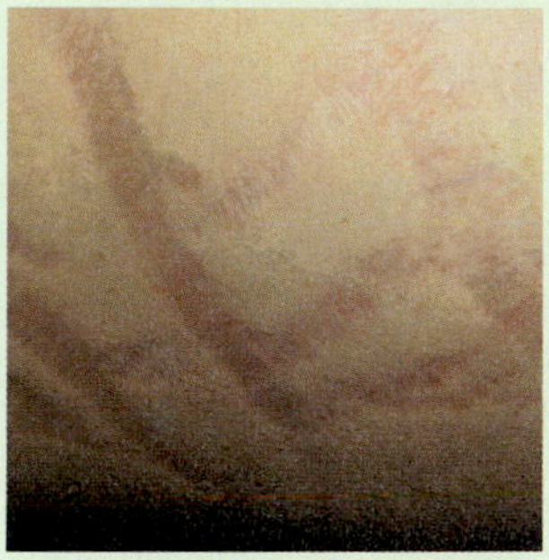 Striae.

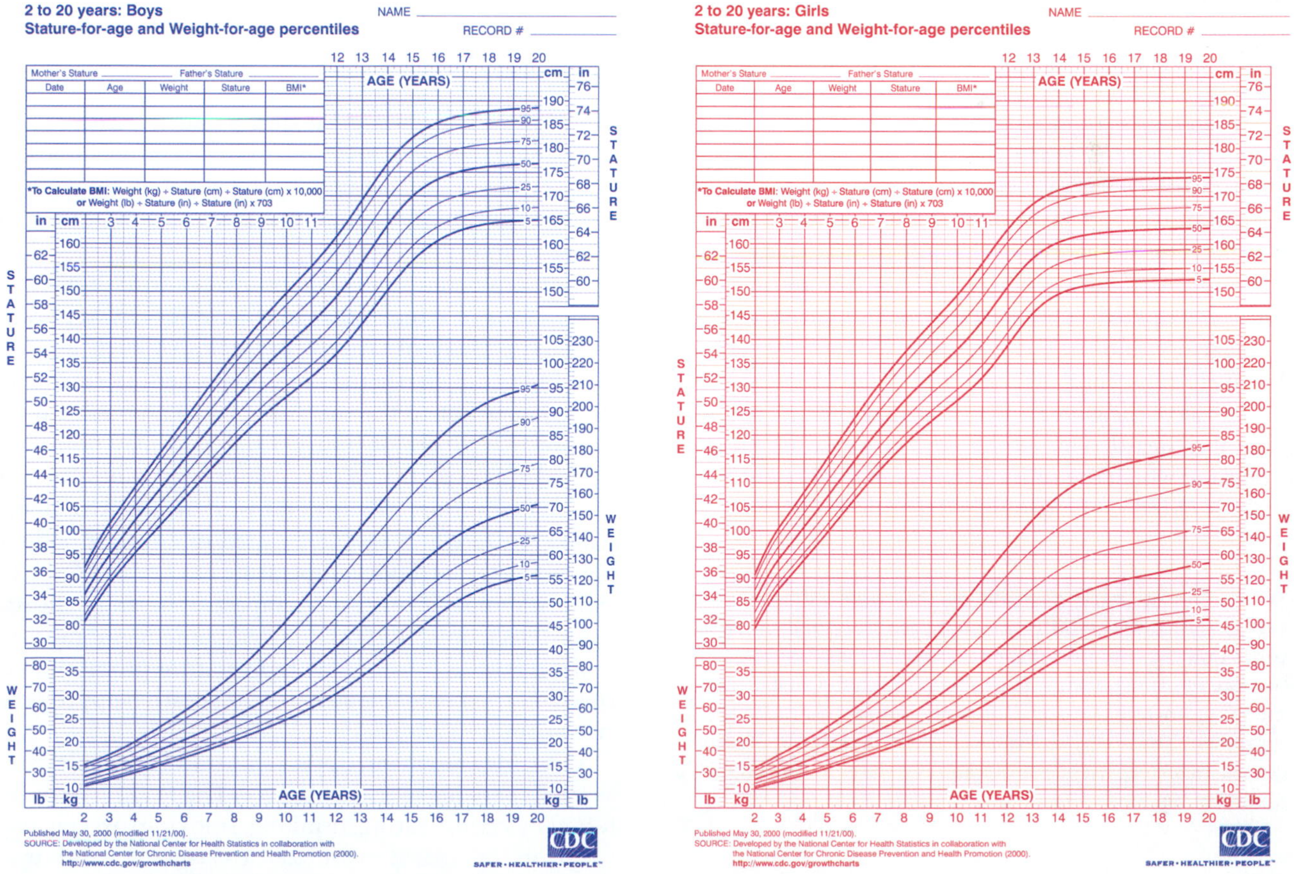

FIGURE 11-9 ■ Physical growth curves and National Center for Health Statistics percentiles for children, age 2 through 18 years, for height and weight. **A,** Boys. **B,** Girls.

PULSE

A normal resting pulse rate for an adult is usually between 60 and 100 beats per minute; it may be affected by the patient's age and physical condition (Table 11-3). For example, a child's pulse rate may be 80 to 100 beats per minute. A well-trained athlete's pulse rate may be 50 to 60 beats per minute. Factors such as pregnancy, anxiety, and fear also may produce a higher-than-normal pulse rate in healthy individuals.

Pulse rates may be obtained at the carotid artery in the neck. They also may be obtained at any pulse site where the artery lies close to the skin surface. To evaluate the radial pulse, the paramedic places the pads of the index and middle fingers at the distal end of the patient's wrist, just medial to the radial styloid. If pulsations are regular, the paramedic should count them for 15 seconds. Then the paramedic should multiply the number of pulses by 4 to determine the number of beats per minute. In addition to the number of times the heart beats per minute, the paramedic should assess the regularity and strength of the pulse. For example, the pulse can be regular or irregular, weak or strong. Application of an electrocardiogram monitor also may be useful in evaluating cardiovascular status after initial assessment of the pulse.

BLOOD PRESSURE

The systolic blood pressure is the pressure against the arterial walls when the heart contracts. The diastolic blood pressure is the pressure against the arterial walls when the heart relaxes. For both, the pressure is the amount of this pressure exerted. For all age groups,[2] systolic blood pressure ideally should be less than 120 mm Hg; diastolic pressure should be less than 80 mm Hg.

Blood pressure is best measured by auscultation. The blood pressure cuff is placed on the patient's arm with the lower end of the cuff positioned 1 to 2 inches (2 to 5 cm) above the antecubital space. The cuff is inflated to a point about 30 mm Hg above where the brachial pulse can no longer be palpated. The stethoscope is placed over the brachial artery, and the cuff is slowly deflated at a rate of 2 to 3 mm Hg per second. As the pressure falls, the paramedic should observe the gauge and note where the first sound or pulsation is heard. This is the patient's systolic pressure. The point at which the sounds change in quality or become muffled is noted as the patient's diastolic pressure.

> **NOTE** At times, determining the correct diastolic pressure is difficult. The difference between the point of muffled tones and the complete disappearance of pulsations varies by person. In some persons, the difference is a few millimeters of mercury; however, in some persons, pulsations never totally disappear. The ability to measure accurate diastolic pressures comes from experience and requires careful listening in a quiet setting.

Blood pressure may be estimated by palpation when vascular sounds are hard to hear with a stethoscope because of environmental noise. However, this method is less accurate than auscultation. Moreover, this method can only estimate systolic pressure. To estimate blood pressure by palpation, the paramedic should locate the brachial or radial pulse and apply the blood pressure cuff as described before. The paramedic maintains finger contact at the pulse site as the cuff slowly deflates. When the pulse becomes palpable, the gauge reading denotes the systolic pressure. Like pulse rates, a patient's blood pressure may be unusually high because of fear or anxiety. Other factors, such as a patient's age and normal level of physical activity, may be the cause of unusual blood pressure readings.

Alternate sites may be used to assess blood pressure when use of the patient's upper arm is not possible. Blood pressure readings in these alternate sites vary from those taken in the arm (Fig. 11-10).

RESPIRATIONS

The normal respiratory rate for adults is between 12 and 24 breaths per minute. The respiratory rate is found by watching the patient breathe, by feeling for chest movement, or by auscultating the lungs. The paramedic counts the respirations for 30 seconds. Then the paramedic multiplies by 2 to get breaths per minute. Rhythm and depth of respirations are assessed by visualization and auscultation of the thorax. Abnormal findings include shallow, rapid, noisy, or deep breathing; asymmetrical chest wall movement; use of accessory muscles of respiration; or congested, unequal, or diminished breath sounds.

SKIN

The skin can reveal a great deal about a patient's status. Skin color, temperature, and moisture provide good details. As discussed before, a patient's skin color and the presence of bruises, lesions, or rashes may indicate serious illness or injury.

Skin temperature may be normal (warm), hot, or cold. Evaluations of temperature may have specific applications in some patient situations. Examples of such are febrile seizures and hyperthermic and hypothermic emergencies. Skin that is hot to the touch points to a possible fever or heat-related illness or injury. Cold skin may point to decreased tissue perfusion and cold-related illness or injury. The dorsal surface of the hand is more sensitive than the palmar surface and should be used to estimate body temperature. Normal body temperature is 37° C (98.6° F). Oral, axillary, tympanic, or rectal temperatures can be measured using electronic, digital, or tympanic-membrane thermometers (Fig. 11-11). The temperature probe should be covered by a disposable sheath. The sheath helps to prevent cross-contamination.

Oral Measurement. Oral temperature usually is measured in patients over the age of 6. The readings may be affected by crying, eating, drinking, smoking, oxygen administration by mask, nebulizer treatments, and by the position of the thermometer in the patient's mouth. When using a traditional glass thermometer to assess oral tem-

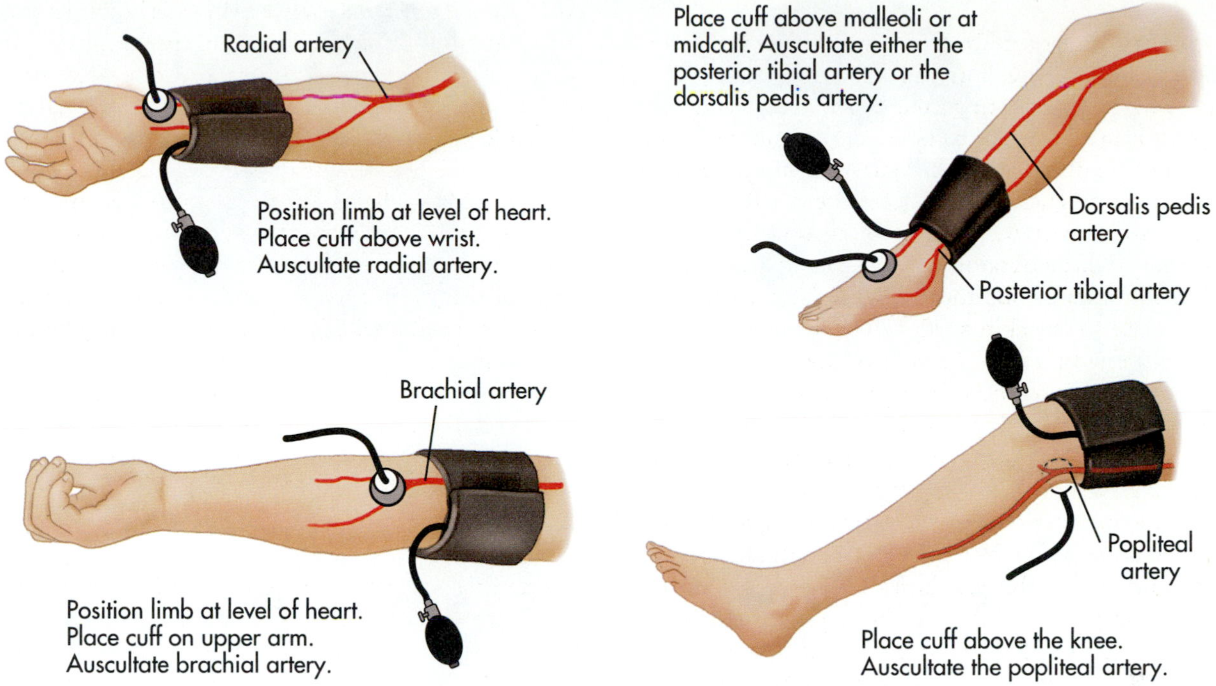
Radial artery
Position limb at level of heart.
Place cuff above wrist.
Auscultate radial artery.
Place cuff above malleoli or at midcalf. Auscultate either the posterior tibial artery or the dorsalis pedis artery.
Dorsalis pedis artery
Posterior tibial artery
Brachial artery
Position limb at level of heart.
Place cuff on upper arm.
Auscultate brachial artery.
Popliteal artery
Place cuff above the knee.
Auscultate the popliteal artery.

FIGURE 11-10 ■ Blood pressure measurement sites.

TABLE 11-3 Average Vital Signs by Age

AGE	PULSE (BEATS/MIN)	RESPIRATIONS (BREATHS/MIN)	BLOOD PRESSURE (MM HG)
Newborn	120-160	40-60	80/40
1 year	80-140	30-40	82/44
3 years	80-120	25-30	86/50
5 years	70-115	20-25	90/52
7 years	70-115	20-25	94/54
10 years	70-115	15-20	100/60
15 years	70-90	15-20	110/64
Adult	60-100	12-24	120/80

perature, the bulb of the thermometer should be placed in the sublingual area of the patient's mouth and should be left in place for 5 to 7 minutes. (Electronic device times are much shorter. A brief tone will alert the paramedic when the measurement is complete.) The paramedic should tell the patient to keep the mouth closed tightly around the thermometer. The paramedic can tell children to hold the thermometer in a "kiss" position. The paramedic should caution children not to bite on the probe.

Axillary Measurement. The axillary site often is used to take the temperature in children. The axilla frequently is used in children less than 6 years of age. The axilla also is used in children who are uncooperative, have diseases that suppress the immune system, and in those who have an altered level of consciousness. The paramedic measures axillary temperature by placing the thermometer probe firmly in the center of the patient's axillary space. The patient's arm should be held against the side of the chest. The paramedic should read the temperature in 5 minutes. This is the case when using a glass thermometer. If an electronic device is used, the paramedic should read it when the alert indicates. The temperature assessed at this site is usually 1° F (0.6° C) lower than the core temperature of the body.

Tympanic Measurement. The tympanic membrane is close to the hypothalamus. This position makes the tympanic membrane an ideal place to measure core temperature. The paramedic takes this measurement by placing the tip of the probe into the patient's ear canal. The paramedic then straightens the ear canal by gently pulling the pinna of the ear down and back in children less than 3 years of age or up and back in patients 3 years of age or older. When the thermometer is in the correct position and is activated per the manufacturer's instructions, a temperature reading is obtained within seconds.

Rectal Measurement. Measuring a patient's temperature by the rectal route poses a risk of perforation. In addition, the method can be distressing for the patient. This route generally is reserved for young children and patients who have an altered level of consciousness. When measuring rectal temperature, the paramedic should place the patient in the supine position (infants). The patient also can be placed in the left lateral recumbent position with the

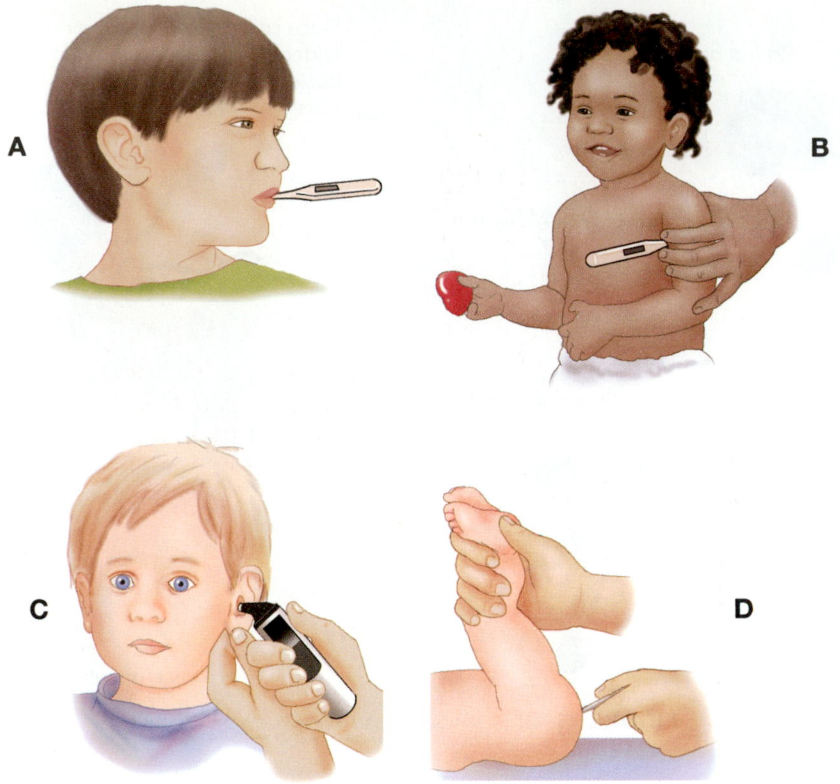

FIGURE 11-11 ■ Temperature assessment. **A,** Oral temperature measurement. **B,** Axillary temperature measurement. **C,** Tympanic temperature measurement. **D,** Rectal temperature measurement.

legs raised. This position exposes the anus. The paramedic inserts a lubricated probe no more than 2.5 cm (½ to 1 inch) into the rectum. The paramedic holds the probe securely in place for 5 minutes when using a glass thermometer or until the electronic device sounds the alert. Rectal readings provide the most accurate assessment. However, they may be impractical for prehospital use.

Skin moisture usually is classified as dry or wet. Dry skin is normal. Wet skin is clammy or diaphoretic. Diaphoretic skin may point to a drop in circulating blood volume called a hemodynamic deficit. An example of this type of deficit is hypovolemia. Diaphoretic skin also may point to another illness or injury that results in decreased tissue perfusion or increased sweat gland activity. Examples are cardiovascular and heat-related emergencies, respectively.

PUPILS

Examining the pupils for response to light may yield information on the neurological status of some patients. Unequal pupils (anisocoria) may be a normal finding in some patients. However, the pupils usually are equal and constrict when exposed to light. (The acronym *PERRL* indicates that the *p*upils are *e*qual, *r*ound, and *r*eact to *l*ight.) When testing the pupils for light response, the paramedic shines a penlight directly into one eye. The normal reaction is for the pupil exposed to the light to constrict. This occurs with a consensual constriction of the opposite eye. Table 11-4 lists abnormal pupillary reactions and possible causes.

ANATOMICAL REGIONS

The rest of this chapter deals with techniques of the physical examination as they relate to anatomical regions of the body. The paramedic should recall that anatomical and physiological aspects of the human body are age-related. They vary by person as well. An examination of the anatomical regions should be guided by a patient's chief complaint. A full examination of all regions often is called for in the emergency setting.

Skin

The general assessment of the skin was described previously. In addition, the comprehensive physical examination should include an evaluation of the texture and turgor of the skin, hair, and fingernails and toenails. (All of these are part of the integumentary system.)

TABLE 11-4 Abnormal Pupil Reactions

PUPIL SIZE	POSSIBLE CAUSES
Equal	
Dilated or unresponsive	Cardiac arrest, central nervous system injury, hypoxia or anoxia, drug use (LSD [lysergic acid diethylamide], atropine, amphetamines)
Constricted or unresponsive	Central nervous system injury or disease, narcotic drug use (heroin, morphine), eye medications
Unequal	
One dilated or unresponsive	Cerebrovascular accident, head injury, direct trauma to the eye, eye medications

TEXTURE AND TURGOR

The texture of the skin normally is smooth, soft, and flexible. In older adults, though, the skin may be wrinkled and leathery from decreases in collagen, subcutaneous fat, and sweat glands. Abnormal skin texture may result from lesions, rashes, tumors, and localized trauma.

Turgor refers to the elasticity of the skin (which normally decreases with age). To test skin turgor, the paramedic should pinch ("tent") a fold of skin and assess the ease and speed at which the skin returns to its normal position. (Skin on the back of the patient's hand or over the sternum is good for testing for turgor.) Tented skin that does not quickly return to its normal position may indicate dehydration.

HAIR

As part of the examination, the paramedic should inspect and palpate the patient's hair. The paramedic should note quantity, distribution, and texture. Key findings include a recent change in the growth or loss of hair. These may result from chemotherapy or hormone and endocrine disorders (e.g., menopause and diabetes). Thinning hair is common in older men and women.

FINGERNAILS AND TOENAILS

The paramedic should note the color, shape, and the presence or absence of lesions when assessing the patient's fingernails and toenails. Uncolored nails usually are transparent. Healthy nails are smooth and firm on palpation. Box 11-4 describes abnormal findings in the nails. With age, nails often develop longitudinal striations and may have a yellow tint because of insufficient calcium.

BOX 11-4 Abnormal Nail Findings

Beau's lines: Transverse depressions in the nail that inhibit nail growth; associated with systemic illness, severe infection, and nail injury.

Clubbing: A change in the angle between the nail and nail base that approaches or exceeds 180 degrees; associated with flattening and often enlargement of the fingertips; may indicate chronic cardiac or respiratory disease.

Onycholysis: The separation of a nail from its bed; associated with psoriasis, dermatitis, fungal infection, and other conditions.

Paronychia: Inflammation of the skin at the base of the nail; may result from local infection or trauma.

Psoriasis: Pitting, discoloration, and subungual thickening of the nail plate; may lead to splinter hemorrhages.

Splinter hemorrhages: Red or brown linear streaks in the nail bed; associated with minor nail trauma, bacterial endocarditis, and trichinosis.

Terry's nails: The presence of transverse white bands that cover the nail except for a narrow zone at the distal tip; associated with cirrhosis.

Transverse white lines: Longitudinal white streaks in the nail plate; may indicate a systemic disorder.

White spots: The presence of white spots that appear in the nail plate; usually result from minor injury or cuticle manipulation.

Head, Ears, Eyes, Nose, and Throat

An examination of the structures of the head and neck involves inspection, palpation, and auscultation.

HEAD AND FACE

To examine the head, the paramedic should inspect the skull for shape and symmetry. The paramedic should keep in mind that hair can hide abnormalities. The paramedic should part the hair in several places to assess for scaliness, lumps, or other lesions. The assessment should use a systematic palpation, moving from front to back, noting any swelling, tenderness, indentations, or depressions. The scalp should move freely over the skull, and the patient should not complain of pain or discomfort during the examination.

The paramedic should inspect the face for symmetry, expression, and contour. The paramedic should note any asymmetry, involuntary movements, masses, or edema. The paramedic should evaluate facial skin for color, pigmentation, texture, thickness, hair distribution, and any lesions.

EYES

The paramedic should verify that both eyes can see. The paramedic can do this by first soliciting the patient's history regarding visual disturbances. The paramedic then can ask the patient to demonstrate visual acuity. The paramedic can assess visual acuity by asking the patient to read printed material, count fingers at a distance, and demonstrate the ability to distinguish light from dark and through the use of various eye charts (e.g., a *Snellen chart*) (Fig. 11-12).

Both eyes should move equally well in the six cardinal fields of gaze (Fig. 11-13). To evaluate a patient's gaze, the paramedic should hold the patient's chin. Then the paramedic should watch the eyes as they track a penlight or finger (or a toy, in the case of a child) when it moves through

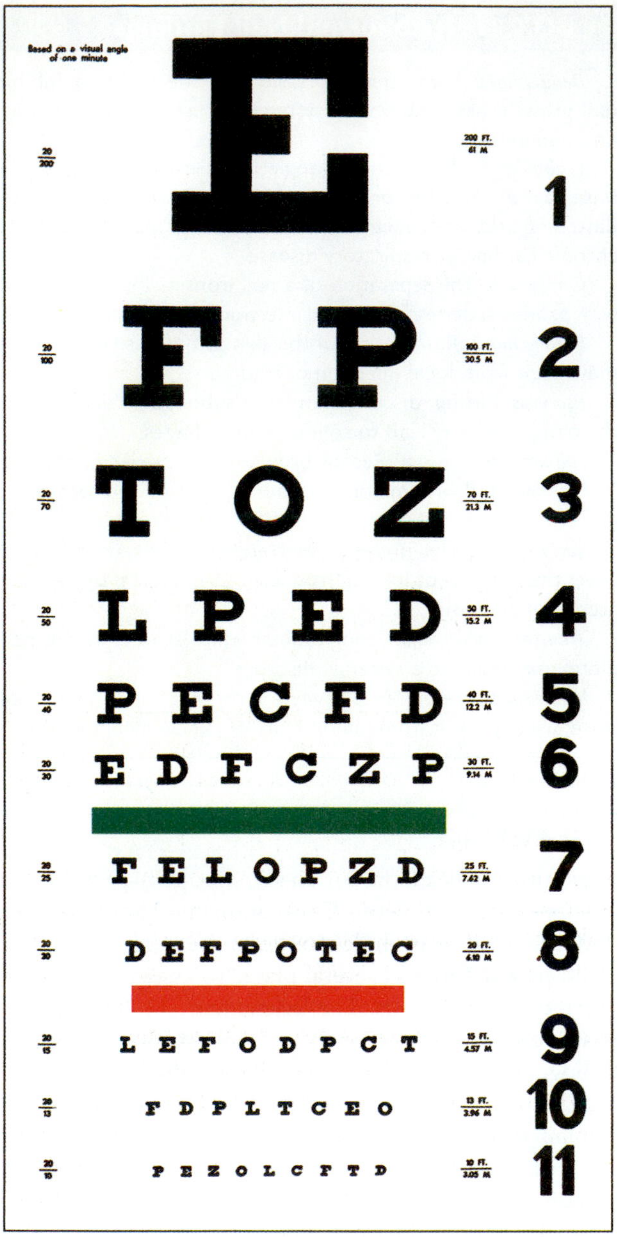

FIGURE 11-12 ■ Snellen chart.

the six visual fields in an H pattern. The paramedic should note any nystagmus (involuntary jerking movements of the eyes). Another method to check visual fields is to ask the patient to look at his or her nose. The paramedic then extends his or her arms with elbows at right angles and wiggles both index fingers at the same time to test peripheral vision. By asking the patient to identify finger movement and to track a moving object (e.g., a pencil, finger, or penlight), the paramedic can decide whether visual fields are grossly normal. This test should be done in four quadrants (up, down, right, and left). The paramedic also should check the eyes for normal position and alignment.

> **CRITICAL THINKING**
> When you perform an examination of the eyes, you are evaluating components of at least four body systems. What are they?

The paramedic should inspect the orbital area for edema and puffiness. The eyebrows should be free of scaliness. Inspection of the eyelids consists of noting the width of palpebral fissures (the elliptical opening between the upper and lower lids), edema, color, lesions, condition and direction of the eyelashes, adequacy of lid closure, and drainage. The paramedic also briefly should inspect the regions of the lacrimal gland and lacrimal sac for swelling. The paramedic should note excessive tearing or dryness of the eye.

The paramedic examines the conjunctiva and sclera by asking the patient to look up while the paramedic depresses both lower lids with the thumbs (Fig. 11-14). The sclera should be white; the cornea and the iris should be clearly visible; and the pupils should be of equal size, round, and reactive to light. The paramedic should palpate the lower orbital rim to determine structural integrity. The paramedic should be alert to the presence of contact lenses and ocular prostheses when examining a patient's eyes.

Ophthalmoscope Examination. The ophthalmoscope is used to assess the cornea for foreign bodies, lacerations, abrasions, and infection; the anterior chamber for hyphema (accumulation of blood) or hypopyon (accumulation of pus); the fundus to assess retinal vessels, the optic nerve, and retina; the vitreous; and to assess for foreign bodies under the eyelid. Ophthalmoscopic examinations should be done in a dark room. That way, the pupils are dilated. The patient does not need to remove contact lenses.

To perform an examination with an ophthalmoscope, the paramedic should follow these steps for each eye:

1. Ask the patient to fixate on a distant object.
2. Sit facing the patient at same seat height.
3. Turn on the ophthalmoscope light and select the 0 lens setting.
4. Use the right hand and eye to examine the patient's right eye and the left hand and eye to examine the patient's left eye.
5. Direct the patient to look over your shoulder, keeping both eyes open.
6. Hold the scope against your face and shine the light on the patient's pupil at a distance of about 10 inches from the face and at a 45-degree angle. A bright orange glow in the pupil ("red reflex") normally is visible (Fig. 11-15).
7. Move the light slowly toward the pupil to see the structures of the fundus. Rotate the lens to improve focus as needed.
8. Inspect the size, color, and clarity of the disk and integrity of vessels; assess for retinal lesions and appearance of the macula. A normal examination will reveal the following[3] (Fig. 11-16):
   - A clear, yellow optic nerve disk
   - Reddish pink (European American) or darkened (African American) retina

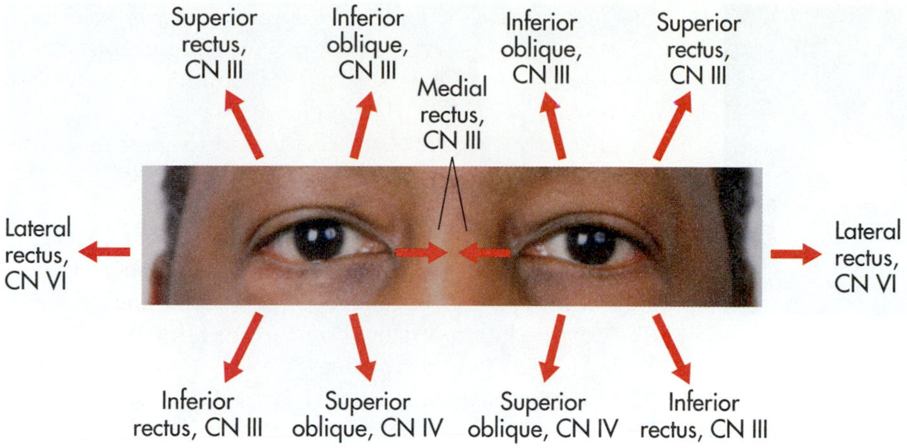

FIGURE 11-13 ■ Six cardinal fields of gaze. Cranial nerves and extraocular muscles associated with the six cardinal fields of gaze.

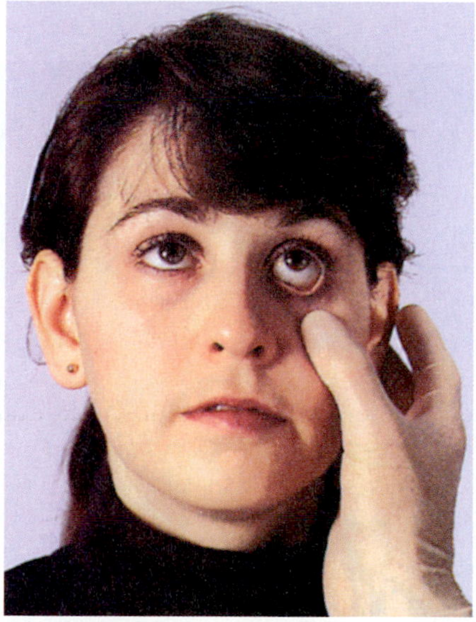

FIGURE 11-14 ■ Examining the cornea and sclera.

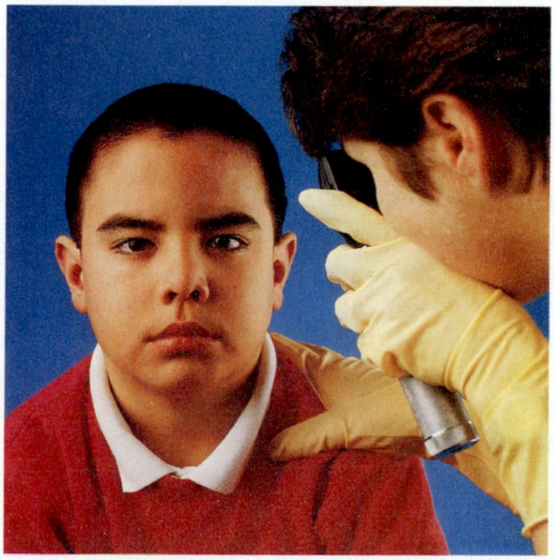

FIGURE 11-15 ■ Paramedic using an ophthalmoscope.

- Light red arteries and dark red veins
- A 3:2 vein-to-artery ratio in size proportion
- The avascular macula

EARS

The paramedic should inspect the external ear and surrounding tissues for signs of bruising, deformity, or discoloration. No discharge should come from either ear canal. Pulling gently on the ear lobes (lobules) should not produce pain or discomfort. The paramedic should palpate the skull and facial bones surrounding the ear and inspect the mastoid area for tenderness or discoloration. An alert, hearing patient who speaks the same language as the paramedic should be able to respond to questions without many requests for repetition. The paramedic should note hearing aids. An assessment of gross auditory keenness can be made by covering one ear at a time. The paramedic should ask the patient to repeat short test words spoken by the paramedic in soft and loud tones.

Otoscopic Examination. An otoscope is used to evaluate the inner ear for discharge and foreign bodies and to assess the eardrum. The paramedic performs an otoscopic exam using the following steps for each ear (Fig. 11-17):

1. Select the appropriate size of speculum.
2. Check the ear for foreign bodies before inserting the speculum.
3. Instruct the patient not to move during the examination to avoid injury to the canal and tympanic membrane. (Infants and young children may need to be restrained.)
4. Turn on the otoscope and insert the speculum into the ear canal, slightly down and forward. To ease insertion, pull the auricle up and backward in adults; back and downward in infants.
5. Identify cerumen and look for foreign bodies, lesions, or discharge.
6. Visualize and inspect the tympanic membrane for tears or breaks. A normal examination will reveal the following:
   - Cerumen will be dry (tan or light yellow) or moist (dark yellow or brown).
   - The ear canal should not be inflamed (a sign of infection).

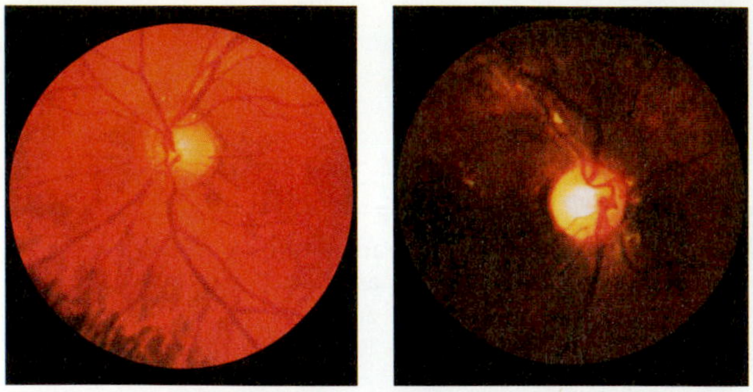

FIGURE 11-16 ■ Normal fundus examination.

- The tympanic membrane should be translucent or pearly gray (pink or red indicates inflammation).

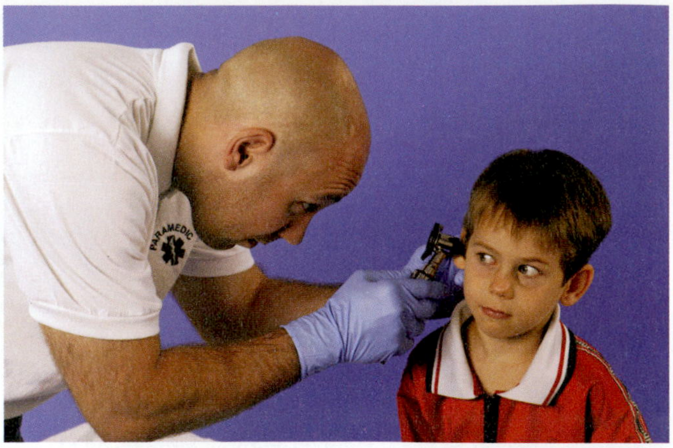

FIGURE 11-17 ■ Paramedic performing an otoscopic exam.

NOSE

The paramedic should inspect the nose for shape, size, color, and stability. The column of the nose should be midline with the face. The nares should be positioned symmetrically. (Slight asymmetry of nares is considered normal.) The paramedic should palpate the column of the nose and surrounding soft tissues for pain, tenderness, or deformity. The paramedic should inspect the frontal and maxillary sinuses for the presence of swelling and should palpate for tenderness along the bony brow on each side of the nose and the zygomatic processes.

Discharge from the nose can have a number of causes. For example, cerebrospinal fluid may be present as a result of head trauma; a bloody discharge (epistaxis) may result from trauma or from mucosal erosions involving blood vessels, hypertension, or bleeding disorders. A mucous discharge commonly results from allergy, upper respiratory tract infection, sinusitis, or cold exposure.

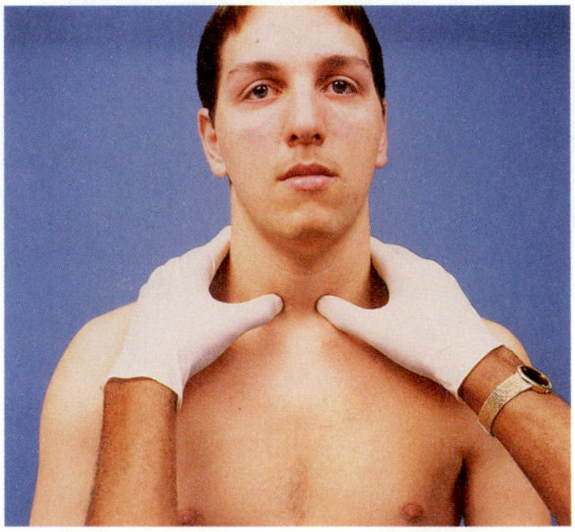

FIGURE 11-18 ■ Position of the thumbs to evaluate the midline position of the trachea.

MOUTH AND PHARYNX

The paramedic should inspect the lips for symmetry, color, edema, and skin surface irregularities. The lips should be pink. Pallor of the lips is linked with anemia; cyanosis is linked with cardiorespiratory insufficiency; red lips sometimes are a late finding in carbon monoxide poisoning. The lips should show no swelling, deformity, or pain on palpation.

Healthy gums in the oral cavity are pink and free of lesions and swelling. Patchy areas of pigmentation in the mouths of African Americans are not uncommon. Enlarged gums may indicate pregnancy, leukemia, poor oral hygiene, puberty, or use of some medications (e.g., ***phenytoin***). The mouth should be free of loose or broken teeth. Dental appliances may be present.

The paramedic should inspect the tongue for size and color. The tongue should be positioned in the midline of the oral cavity and should appear nonswollen, dull red, moist, and glistening. To inspect the oropharynx, the paramedic can use a tongue blade to depress the tongue. The normal palate is white or pink. If the oral cavity is inflamed or covered with exudate, an infection may be present. (Specific breath odors may indicate alcohol or other drug consumption or illness.) The tonsils normally are pink and smooth without edema, ulceration, or inflammation. A patient with a typical sore throat often has a reddened and edematous uvula and tonsillar pillars. A yellow exudate sometimes is present.

NECK

The paramedic should inspect the neck in the patient's normal anatomical position. If the paramedic suspects trauma, the paramedic should use spinal precautions. The trachea should be midline. No use of accessory muscles or tracheal tugging should occur during respiration. To palpate the neck, the paramedic places both thumbs along the sides of the distal trachea and systematically moves the hands toward the head (Fig. 11-18). The paramedic should take care not to apply bilateral pressure to the carotid arteries. Syncope or bradycardia may result.

The lymph nodes should not be tender. (Tender or swollen lymph nodes usually are the result of inflamma-

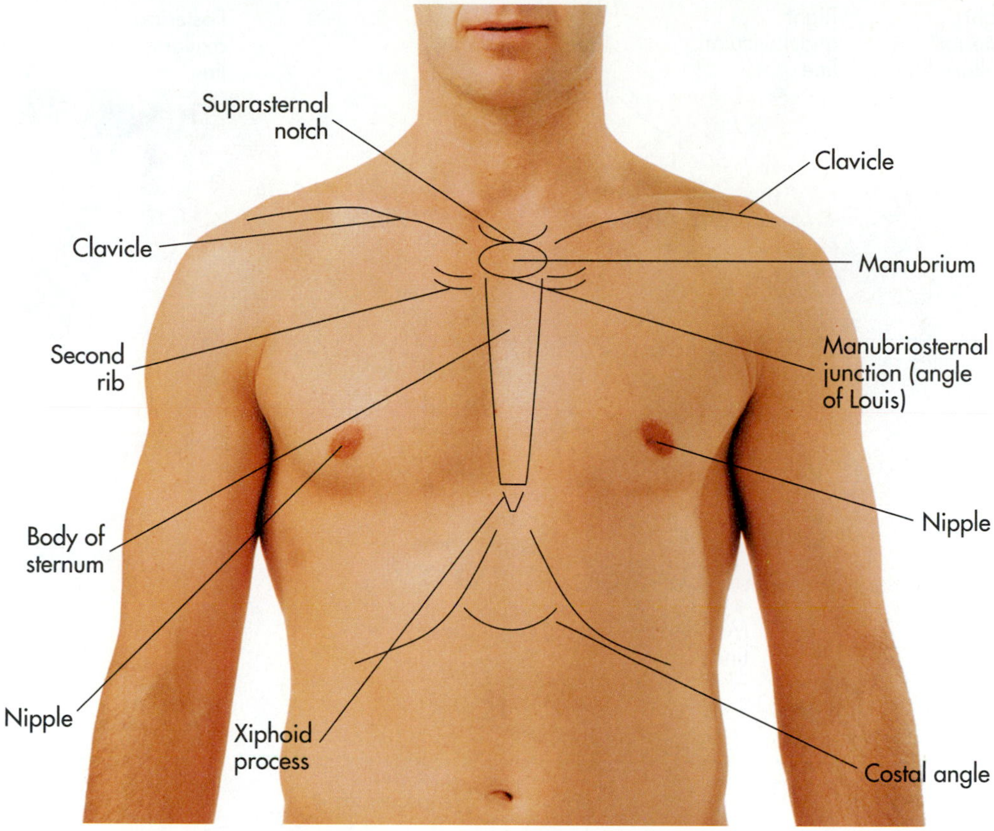

FIGURE 11-19 ■ Topographical landmarks of the chest.

tion.) The thyroid and cricoid cartilages should be free of pain and should move when the patient swallows. Bubbling or crackling sensations that can be palpated in the soft tissues of the neck may indicate the presence of subcutaneous emphysema. The paramedic should note distended neck veins or prominent carotid arteries (see Chapter 29).

HEAD AND CERVICAL SPINE

The temporomandibular joint connects the mandible of the jaw to the temporal bone of the skull. The joint sometimes can become painful or dislocated. Normally the patient should be able to open and close the mouth without pain or limitation in movement. Temporomandibular joint dysfunction is a common complaint.

For the patient who has not undergone trauma, the paramedic should inspect the cervical spine. The paramedic should palpate for tenderness or deformities. Range of motion can be tested in the following manner:

- Flexion: touching the chin to the chest
- Rotation: touching the chin to each shoulder
- Lateral bending: touching each ear to each shoulder
- Extension: tilting the head backward

The neck of a trauma patient may need to be moved for a general or neurological examination. Any such movement must be accompanied by the application of continuous manual protection and stabilization techniques for suspected cervical spine injury (see Chapter 25).

Chest

A paramedic must have a full knowledge of the structure of the thoracic cage. This knowledge is needed to perform a good respiratory and cardiac assessment. The ribs protect the vital organs within the thorax. The ribs also offer support for respiratory movements of the diaphragm and intercostal muscles (see Chapter 6). Damage to the actual bony structure of the thoracic cavity, such as a flail chest, can prevent or limit respiratory function. The ribs of the thorax also are used as anatomical landmarks. They help in finding certain areas for examination. Fig. 11-19 shows the landmarks of the chest. The paramedic can evaluate the thorax by using imaginary lines to note examination findings (Fig. 11-20). The paramedic should evaluate the chest using inspection, palpation, percussion, and auscultation.

INSPECTION

The paramedic should inspect the chest wall for symmetry on the anterior and posterior surfaces. The thorax is not completely symmetrical. However, a visual inspection of one side should offer a reasonable comparison to the other. Chest wall diameter often is increased in patients with obstructive pulmonary disease. This results in a barrel-shaped appearance of the thorax. Other chest wall deformities or asymmetry include a *funnel chest* (an indentation of the lower sternum above the xiphoid process),

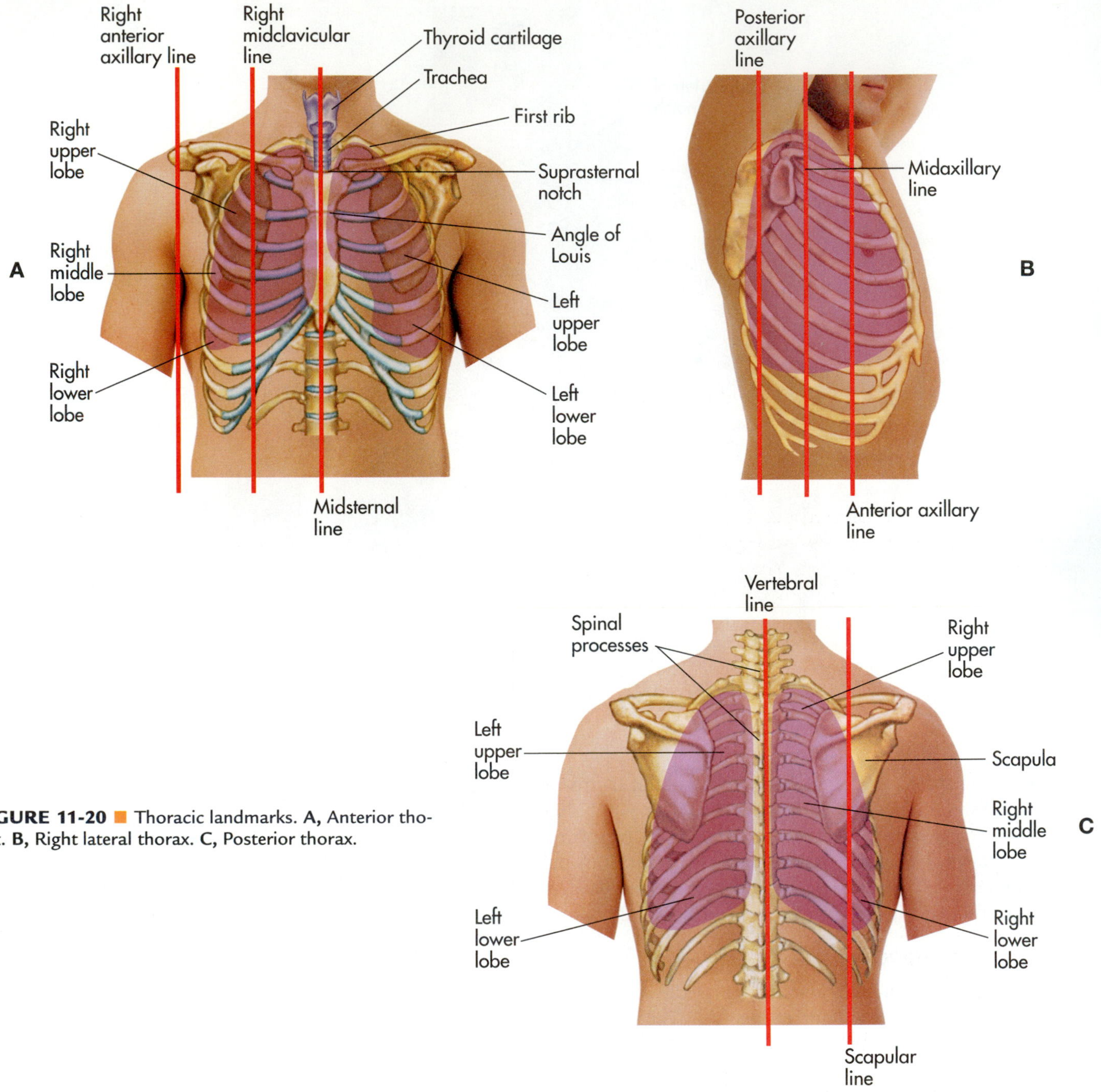

FIGURE 11-20 ■ Thoracic landmarks. **A,** Anterior thorax. **B,** Right lateral thorax. **C,** Posterior thorax.

pigeon chest (a prominent sternal protrusion), *thoracic kyphosis* (a posterior deviation of the spine that results in increased convexity of the chest), and *scoliosis* (a lateral deviation of the spine that results in an abnormal curvature) (Fig. 11-21).

> **CRITICAL THINKING**
>
> Evaluate breathing in a supine patient or friend while standing to the person's side, then at the head, and finally at the feet. Which position provides the best view of the symmetry of the thorax?

The paramedic should inspect the skin and nipples for cyanosis and pallor. Moreover, the paramedic should be alert to the presence of suture lines from chest wall surgery, skin pockets enclosing implanted pacemaker devices, implanted central venous lines, and dermal medication patches (e.g., ***nitroglycerin*** and contraceptives). The paramedic should note the pattern or rhythm of respirations. The paramedic also should note any use of accessory respiratory muscles (e.g., in-

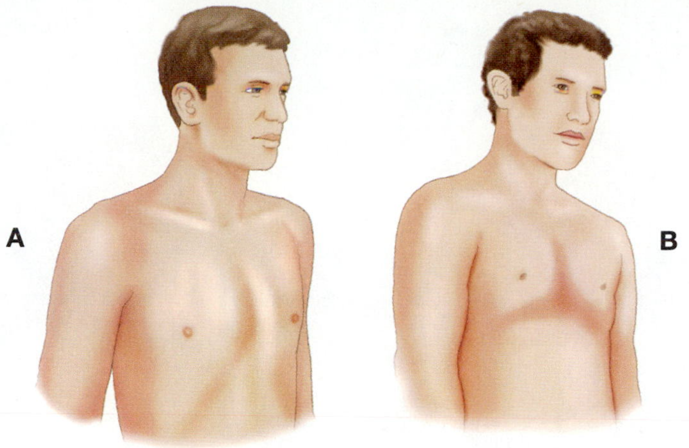

FIGURE 11-21 ■ **A,** Pigeon chest. **B,** Funnel chest.

tercostal or supraclavicular retractions or both). In addition, **tidal volume** is the volume of gas inhaled or exhaled during a normal breath. The paramedic should assess this by observing the rise and fall of the patient's chest. (See Chapter 19.)

PALPATION

The paramedic should palpate the thorax for pulsations, tenderness, bulges, depressions, crepitus, subcutaneous emphysema, and unusual movement and position. The examination begins with the paramedic noting the position of the trachea. The trachea should be midline and directly above the sternal notch. Starting with the patient's clavicles, the paramedic firmly palpates both sides of the patient's chest wall at the same time, front to back and right side to left side. The examination should proceed systematically. The patient should have no pain or discomfort.

To evaluate the anterior chest wall for equal expansion during inspiration, the paramedic places both thumbs along the patient's costal margin and the xiphoid process. The palms should be lying flat on the chest wall. The paramedic should note equal movement as the patient inhales and exhales. The paramedic checks the posterior chest wall for symmetrical respiratory movement by placing the thumbs along the spinous processes at the level of the tenth rib (Fig. 11-22).

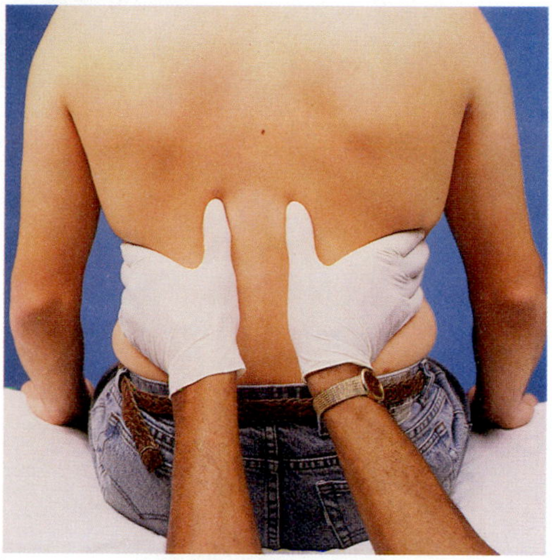

FIGURE 11-22 ■ Palpating the thoracic expansion. The thumbs are at the level of the tenth ribs.

PERCUSSION

The paramedic should perform percussion in symmetrical locations from side to side to compare the percussion note (Fig. 11-23). Resonance usually is heard over all areas of healthy lungs. Hyperresonance is associated with overinflation, or hyperinflation, of the lungs. Hyperresonance may indicate pulmonary disease, pneumothorax, or asthma. Dullness or flatness suggests the presence of fluid or pulmonary congestion. The level and movement of the diaphragm during breathing (diaphragmatic excursion) may be limited by disease or pain. Examples of such disease may be emphysema or tumor. An example of pain is from rib fracture.

AUSCULTATION

The thorax is auscultated best with the patient sitting upright (if possible). The patient should breathe deeply and slowly through an open mouth during the examination. The paramedic should be alert to the chance of resulting hyperventilation and fatigue. These may occur in ill and older patients.

The paramedic uses the diaphragm of the stethoscope to auscultate the high-pitched sounds of the patient's lungs. The paramedic holds the stethoscope firmly on the patient's skin. The paramedic should listen carefully as

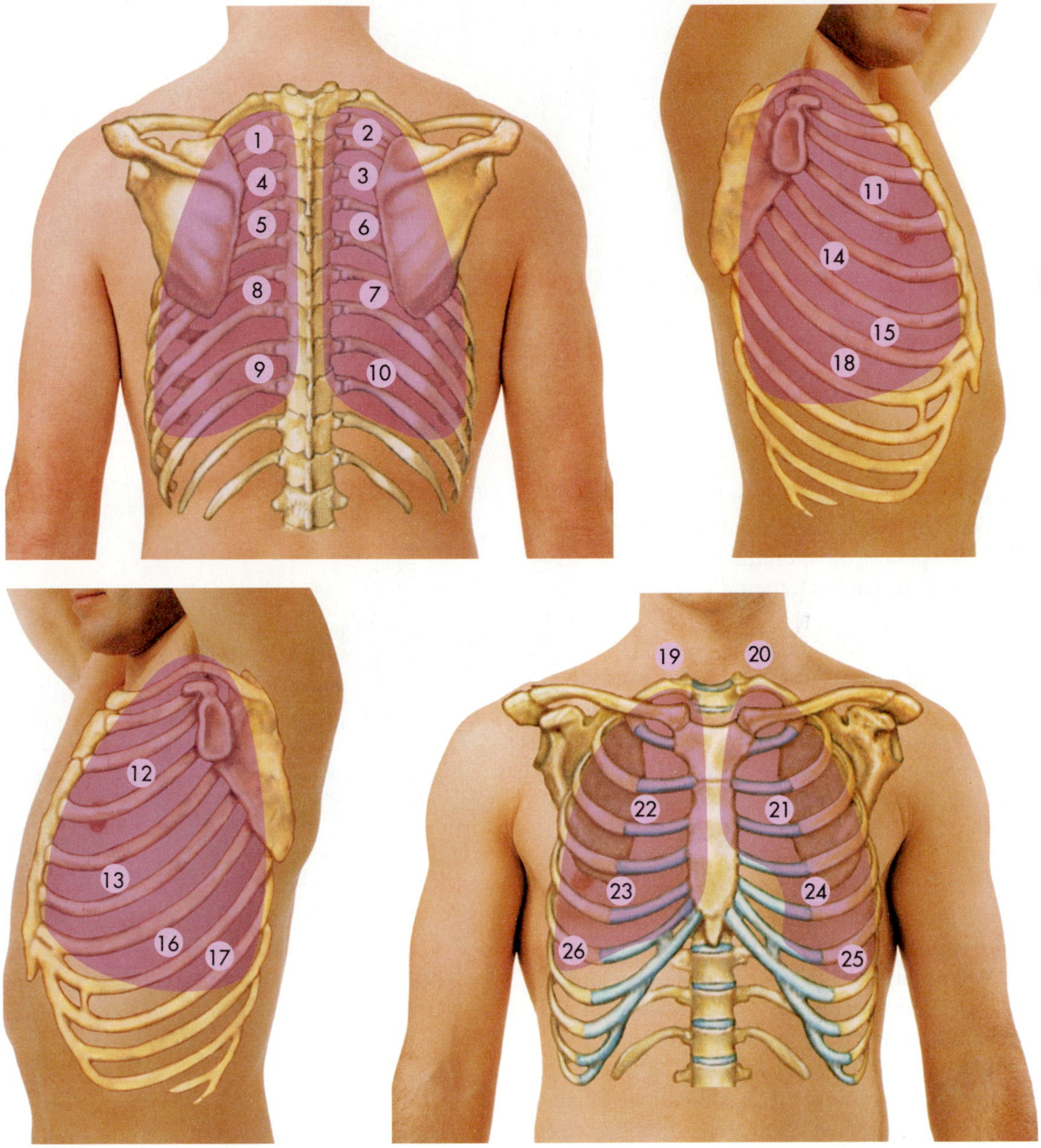

FIGURE 11-23 ■ Suggested sequence for systematic percussion and auscultation of the thorax. A, Posterior thorax. B, Right lateral thorax. C, Left lateral thorax. D, Anterior thorax.

the patient inhales and exhales. The chest auscultation should be systematic and thorough. Auscultation should allow evaluation of the anterior and the posterior lung fields.

Breath Sounds. Air movement creates turbulence as it passes through the respiratory tree. Air produces breath sounds during inhalation and exhalation. During inhalation, air moves first into the trachea and major bronchi. Then air moves into progressively smaller airways. Next, air moves to its final destination, the alveoli. During exhalation, the air flows from small airways to larger ones. This creates less turbulence. Therefore normal breath sounds generally are louder during inspiration.

Normal Breath Sounds. Normal breath sounds are classified as *vesicular, bronchovesicular,* and *bronchial* (Fig. 11-24). Vesicular breath sounds are heard over most of the lung fields and are the major normal breath sound. Lungs considered "clear" make normal vesicular breath sounds. These sounds are low pitched and soft and have a long inspiratory phase and a shorter expiratory phase.

Vesicular breath sounds are classified further as *harsh* or *diminished.* Harsh vesicular sounds may result from vigor-

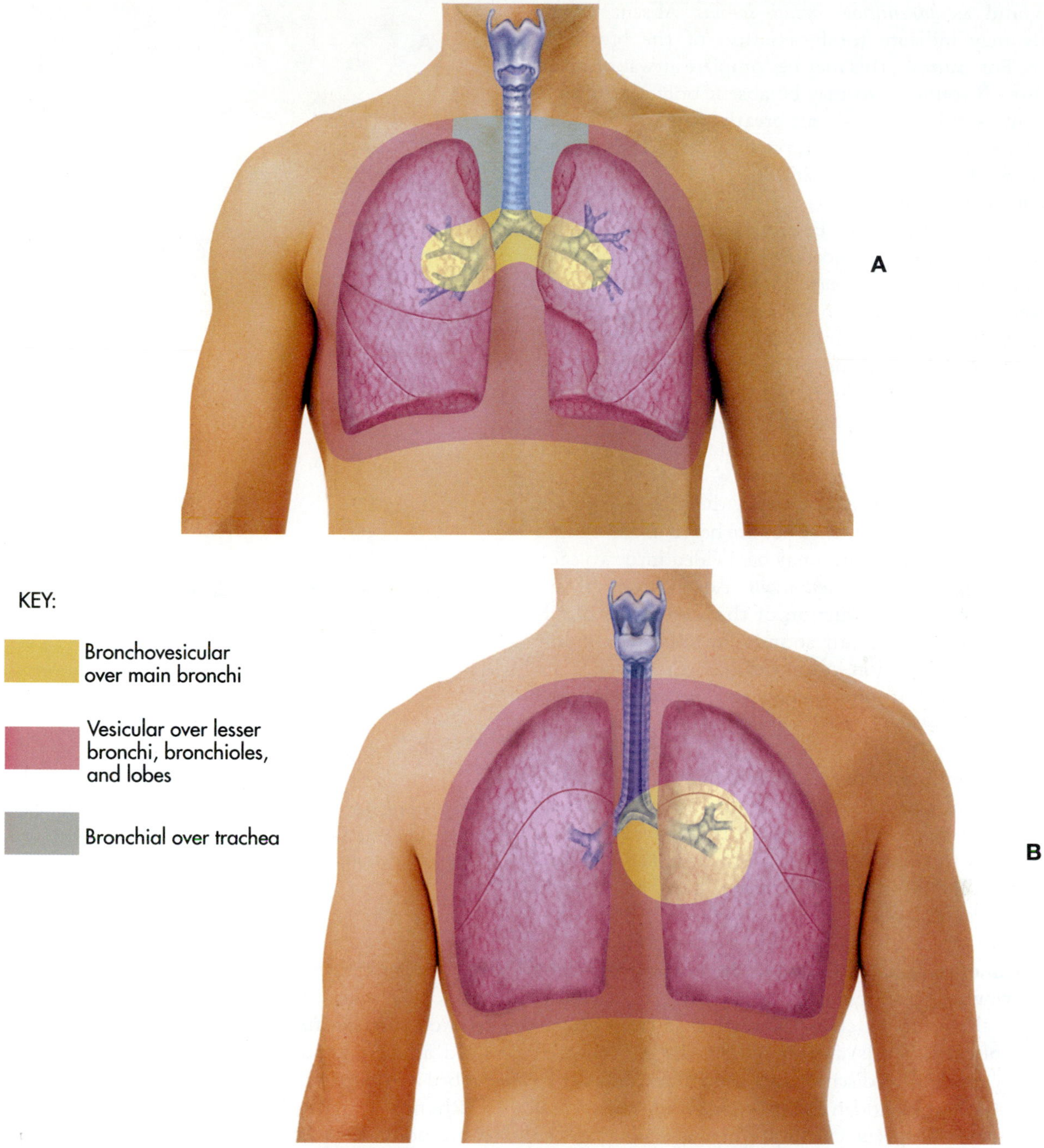

FIGURE 11-24 ■ Expected auscultatory sounds. **A,** Anterior view. **B,** Posterior view.

ous exercise. With vigorous exercise, ventilations are rapid and deep. These harsh sounds also occur in children who have thin and elastic chest walls in which breath sounds are more easily audible. Vesicular breath sounds may be diminished in older persons. These persons have less ventilation volume. Vesicular breath sounds also may be diminished in obese or muscular persons, whose additional overlying tissue muffles the sound.

Bronchovesicular breath sounds are heard over the major bronchi and over the upper right posterior lung field. These sounds are louder and harsher than vesicular breath sounds. Bronchovesicular breath sounds are considered to be of medium pitch. Bronchovesicular breath sounds have equal inspiration and expiration phases. They are heard throughout respiration.

Bronchial breath sounds are heard only over the trachea and are the highest in pitch. They are coarse, harsh, loud sounds with a short inspiratory phase and a long expiration. A bronchial sound heard anywhere but over the trachea is considered an abnormal breath sound.

Abnormal Breath Sounds. Abnormal breath sounds are classified as *absent, diminished,* and *incorrectly located bronchial* *sounds* and as *adventitious breath sounds.* Absent breath sounds may indicate total cessation of the breathing process. For example, this may be complete airway obstruction. Breath sounds also may be absent only in a specific area. Causes of localized absent breath sounds include endotracheal tube misplacement, pneumothorax, and hemothorax. (See Chapters 19 and 26.)

Diminished breath sounds may result from any condition that lessens the airflow. Examples include endotracheal tube misplacement, pneumothorax, partial airway obstruction, and pulmonary disease. Some airflow is present. However, diminished breath sounds usually indicate that some portion of the alveolar tissue is not being ventilated.

Bronchial breath sounds auscultated in the peripheral lung field indicate the presence of fluid or exudate in the alveoli. Either of these problems may block airflow. Diseases that contribute to this condition are tumors, pneumonia, and pulmonary edema.

Adventitious Breath Sounds. Adventitious breath sounds are abnormal sounds. They are heard in addition to normal breath sounds. They may be divided into two categories: *discontinuous* and *continuous.* Adventitious breath sounds result from obstruction of the large or small airways. Adventitious breath sounds are most commonly heard during inspiration. Adventitious breath sounds are classified as *crackles* (formerly known as *rales*), wheezes, and rhonchi (Fig. 11-25).

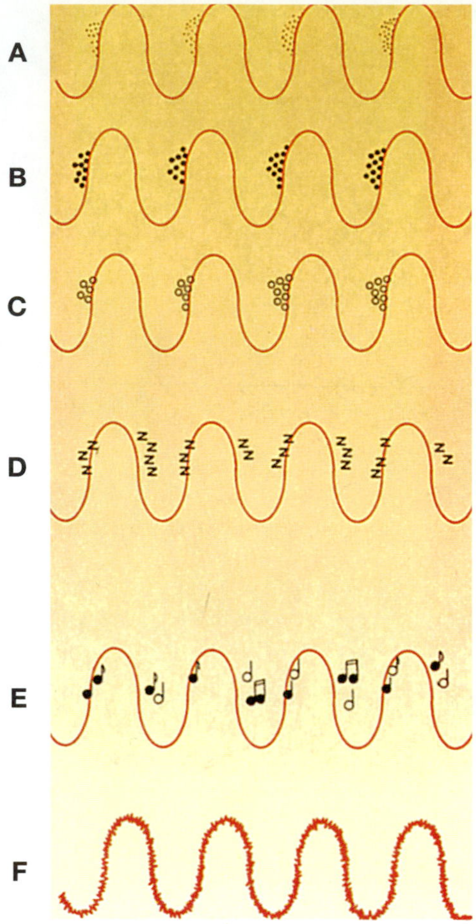

FIGURE 11-25 ■ Adventitious breath sounds. A, Fine crackles. B, Medium crackles. C, Coarse crackles. D, Rhonchi. E, Wheeze. F, Pleural friction rub.

Discontinuous Breath Sounds. Crackles are the high-pitched, discontinuous sounds that usually are heard during the end of inspiration. The sound is similar to the sound of hair being rubbed between the fingers. Crackles are caused by the disruptive passage of air in the small airways or alveoli or both. Crackles may be heard anywhere in the peripheral lung field.

The most typical causes of crackles are pulmonary edema and pneumonia in its early stages. Because gravity draws fluid downward, crackles often start in the bases of the lungs. Crackles may be classified further as *coarse crackles* (wet, low-pitched sounds) and *fine crackles* (dry, high-pitched sounds). Crackles are discrete and sometimes difficult to hear and may be overridden by louder respiratory sounds. If the paramedic suspects crackles when auscultating the chest, the paramedic should ask the patient to cough. A cough may clear secretions and make crackles more audible.

Continuous Breath Sounds. Wheezes are also known as sibilant wheezes. They are high-pitched musical noises. They are usually louder during expiration. Wheezes are caused by high-velocity air traveling through narrowed airways. Wheezes may occur because of asthma and other constrictive diseases and congestive heart failure. When wheezing occurs in a localized area, the paramedic should suspect a foreign body obstruction, tumor, or mucous plug. Wheezes are classified as mild, moderate, and severe. They should be described as occurring on inspiration or expiration or both.

Rhonchi are also known as *sonorous wheezes.* They are continuous, low-pitched, rumbling sounds. They are usually heard on expiration. Although rhonchi sound similar to wheezes, they do not involve the small airways. Rhonchi are less discrete than crackles and are auscultated easily. Rhonchi are caused by the passage of air through an airway obstructed by thick secretions, muscular spasm, new tissue growth, or external pressure collapsing the airway lumen. Ronchi may result from any condition that increases secretions. Examples are pneumonia, drug overdose, and long-term postoperative recovery.

Stridor usually is an inspiratory, crowing-type sound. Stidor can be heard without the aid of a stethoscope. Stridor indicates significant narrowing or obstruction of the larynx or trachea. Stridor may be caused by epiglottitis, viral croup, foreign body aspiration, or more than one of these factors. Stridor is heard best over the site of origin.

CRITICAL THINKING

Breathe in and out through an open mouth. Gradually purse your lips until only a small opening is present while you continue to inhale and exhale. How do the sounds change? As you narrow the opening, is the noise louder on inspiration or expiration?

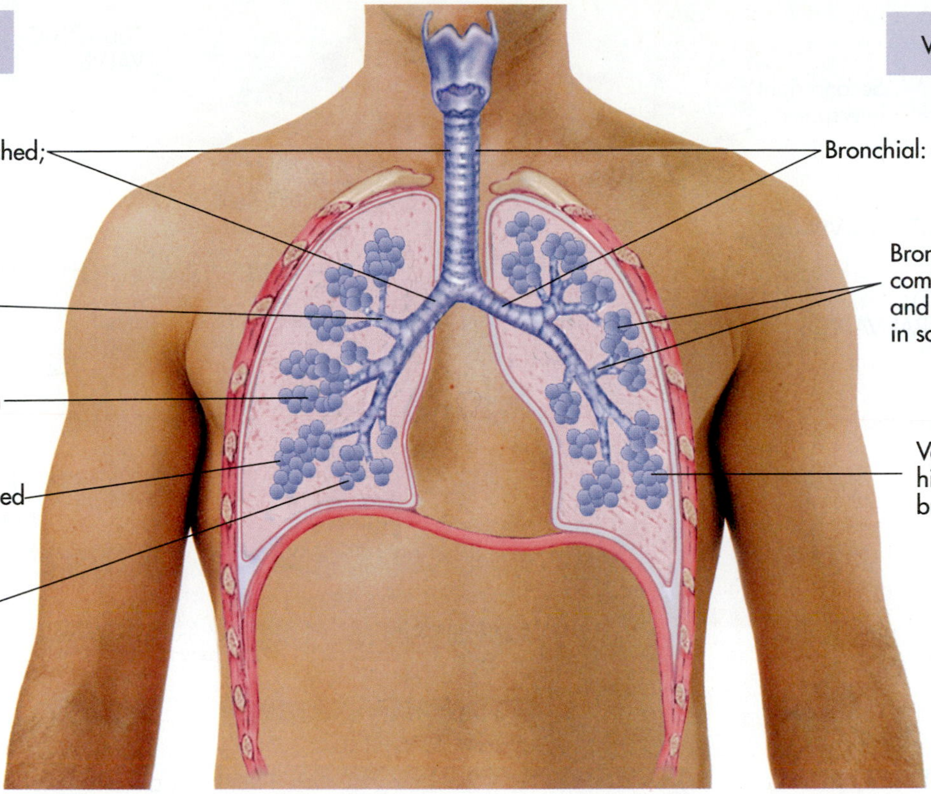

FIGURE 11-26 ■ Schema of breath sounds in ill and well patients

This is usually the larynx or trachea. Stridor often points to a problem that is life-threatening, especially in children. Its presence calls for careful observation for ventilatory failure and hypoxia.

Pleural Friction Rub. Although occurring outside the respiratory tree, a pleural friction rub also may be considered an adventitious breath sound. Pleural friction rub is a low-pitched, dry, rubbing or grating sound. The friction rub is caused by the movement of inflamed pleural surfaces as they slide on one another during breathing. The friction rub may be auscultated on inspiration and expiration. Pleural friction rub usually is loudest over the lower lateral anterior surface of the chest wall. Presence of a pleural friction rub may indicate pleurisy, viral infection, tuberculosis, or pulmonary embolism. (See Chapter 30.) Figure 11-26 shows a schema of breath sounds in ill and well patients.

Heart

In the prehospital setting one must examine the heart indirectly. In spite of this, certain information can be obtained. Details about the size and effectiveness of pumping action are obtained through a skilled assessment. This assessment includes palpation and auscultation.

PALPATION

The apical impulse is a visible and palpable force. The impulse is produced by the contraction of the left ventricle. Palpation of this impulse may be useful to compare the relationship of peripheral pulses with the pulse produced by ventricular contraction. The hearts of some patients with cardiac irregularities, for example, do not always produce a peripheral pulse with every ventricular contraction. By palpating or auscultating the apical impulse and the carotid pulse at the same time, the paramedic can note these pulse deficits (Fig. 11-27). Factors such as obesity, large breasts, and muscularity may make this landmark hard to see or palpate.

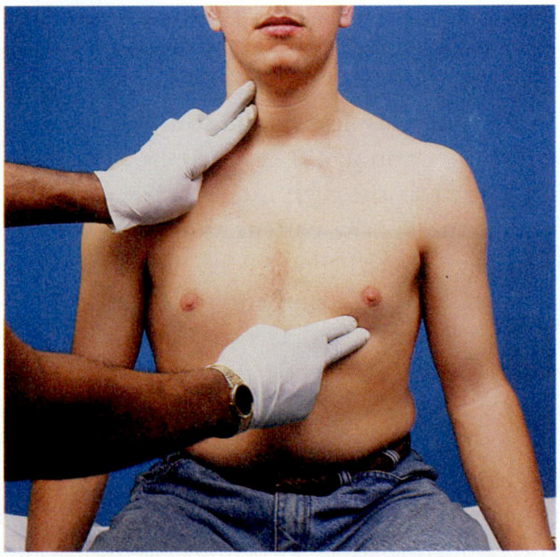

FIGURE 11-27 ■ Simultaneous palpation of the carotid artery and apical impulse.

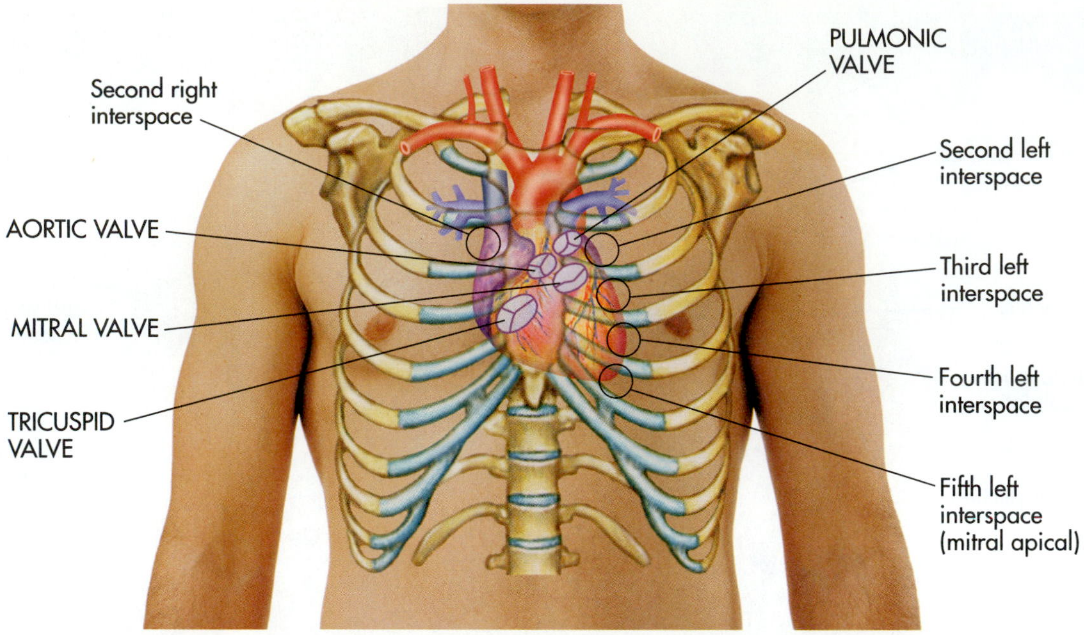

FIGURE 11-28 ■ Areas for auscultaton of the heart.

AUSCULTATION

Heart sounds may be auscultated for frequency (pitch), intensity (loudness), duration, and timing in the cardiac cycle (Fig. 11-28). A full evaluation of heart sounds calls for a high level of skill and experience, a quiet environment, and ample time to listen closely. However, the paramedic may assess two basic heart sounds quickly. These sounds may help to improve understanding of the patient's condition. The basic heart sounds S_1 and S_2 are normal sounds that occur when the myocardium contracts. They are best heard toward the apex of the heart at the fifth intercostal space. For evaluation of heart sounds, the patient should be sitting up and leaning slightly forward (Fig. 11-29, *A*), supine (Fig. 11-29, *B*), or in a left lateral recumbent position (Fig. 11-29, *C*). These positions bring the heart closer to the left anterior chest wall. To listen for S_1, the paramedic should ask the patient to breathe normally and hold the breath in expiration. To listen for S_2, the paramedic should ask the patient to breathe normally again and hold the breath in inspiration.

Heart sounds may be muffled or diminished by obesity or obstructive lung disease. Muffling also may occur as a result of the presence of fluid in the pericardial sac surrounding the heart muscle. Fluid buildup usually is the result of penetrating or severe blunt chest trauma, cardiac tamponade, or cardiac rupture and is considered a true emergency. Other causes of muffled or diminished heart sounds include infectious uremic pericarditis and malignancy. (See Chapters 26 and 29 for further discussion of abnormal heart sounds.)

Inflammation of the pericardial sac may cause a rubbing sound that is audible with a stethoscope. This is a pericardial friction rub. The rub may result from infectious pericarditis, myocardial infarction, uremia, trauma, and autoimmune pericarditis. These rubs have a scratching, grating, or squeaking quality. They tend to be louder on inspiration. They can be differentiated from pleural friction rubs by their continued presence when the patient holds the breath.

EXTRA SOUNDS

Extra sounds that sometimes can be heard during auscultation or can be felt by palpation include heart murmurs, bruits, and thrills. Heart murmurs are prolonged sounds caused by a disruption in the flow of blood into, through, or out of the heart. Most murmurs are caused by valvular defects. Some heart murmurs are serious. Others (e.g., some that occur in children and adolescents), though, are benign and have no apparent cause. Heart murmurs can be detected during auscultation of the heart.

A bruit is an abnormal sound or murmur that may be heard during auscultation of the carotid artery or another organ or gland. A bruit may indicate local obstruction. Bruits usually are low pitched and hard to hear. To assess blood flow in the carotid artery, the paramedic should place the bell of the stethoscope over the carotid artery at the medial end of the clavicle. Then the paramedic should ask the patient to hold his or her breath (Fig. 11-30).

Thrills are similar to bruits but are described as fine vibrations or tremors that may indicate blood flow obstruction. Thrills may be palpable over the site of an aneurysm or on the precordium (the area of the chest wall that overlays the heart and epigastrium). Like murmurs and bruits, thrills may be serious or benign.

Abdomen

The abdomen is divided by two imaginary lines. These lines separate the abdominal region into four quadrants. The quadrants are the upper right, lower right, upper left, and lower left (Fig. 11-31). These quadrants and their contents

A

B

C

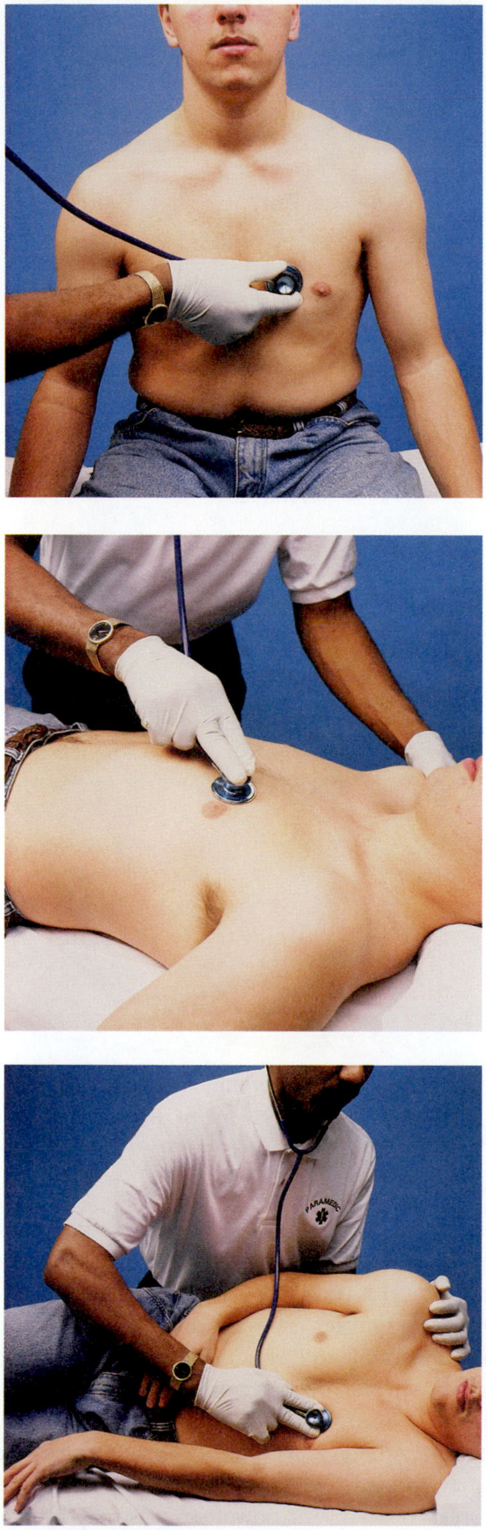

FIGURE 11-29 ■ Patient positions for auscultation. **A,** Sitting up, leaning slightly forward. **B,** Supine. **C,** Left lateral recumbent.

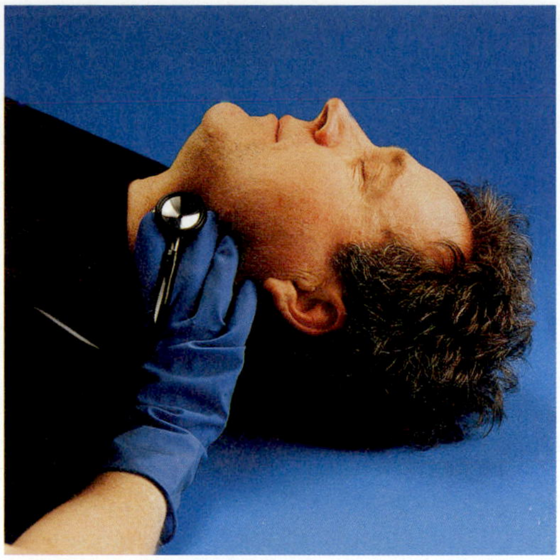

FIGURE 11-30 ■ Evaluation of carotid bruit.

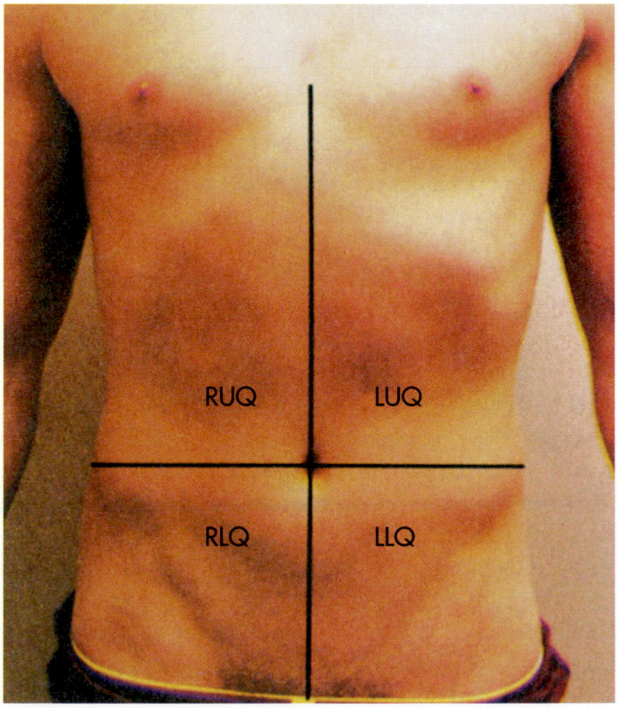

FIGURE 11-31 ■ Four quadrants of the abdomen. ***RUQ,*** Right upper quadrant; ***LUQ,*** left upper quadrant; ***RLQ,*** right lower quadrant; ***LLQ,*** left lower quadrant.

(Chapter 6) provide the basis for inspection, auscultation, percussion, and palpation (Box 11-5).

When examining a patient's abdomen, the paramedic should make sure that the patient is comfortable (with an empty bladder, if possible). The paramedic also should make sure the patient is in a supine position. The paramedic's hands and stethoscope should be warm. The paramedic should approach the patient slowly and respectfully. Any painful area should be examined last. Discoloration found in the flank, called Grey Turner's sign, may indicate possible kidney injury.

INSPECTION

The paramedic should inspect the abdomen visually for signs of cyanosis, pallor, jaundice, bruising, discoloration, swelling (ascites), masses, and aortic pulsations. The paramedic also should note surgical scars and implanted de-

BOX 11-5 Abdominal Quadrants

Right Upper Quadrant
Liver and gallbladder
Pylorus
Duodenum
Head of pancreas
Right adrenal gland
Portion of right kidney
Hepatic flexure of colon
Portions of ascending and transverse colon

Left Upper Quadrant
Left lobe of liver
Spleen
Stomach
Body of pancreas
Left adrenal gland
Portion of left kidney
Splenic flexure of colon
Portions of transverse and descending colon

Right Lower Quadrant
Lower pole of right kidney
Cecum and appendix
Portion of ascending colon
Appendix
Bladder (if distended)
Ovary and salpinx
Uterus (if enlarged)
Right ureter

Left Lower Quadrant
Lower pole of left kidney
Sigmoid colon
Portion of descending colon
Bladder (if distended)
Ovary and salpinx
Uterus (if enlarged)
Left ureter

vices such as automatic implanted cardioverter defibrillators. (See Chapter 29.) The abdomen should be evenly round and symmetrical (Fig. 11-32). Symmetrical distention of the abdomen may result from obesity, enlarged organs, fluid, or gas. Asymmetrical distention may result from hernias, tumor, bowel obstruction, or enlarged abdominal organs. A flat abdomen is common in adults who are athletic. Convex abdomens are common in children and in adults who have poor exercise habits. The umbilicus should be free of swelling, bulges, and signs of inflammation. The normal umbilicus usually is inverted, or it may protrude slightly. Discoloration around the umbilicus is called Cullen's sign. This may indicate peritoneal bleeding.

Abdominal movement during respiration should be smooth and even. As a rule, males have more abdominal involvement than females during respiration, so limited abdominal movement in the male patients with symptoms may indicate a pathological abdominal condition. Visible pulsations produced by blood flow through the aorta in the upper abdomen may be normal in thin adults. However, marked pulsations may indicate an abdominal aortic aneurysm.

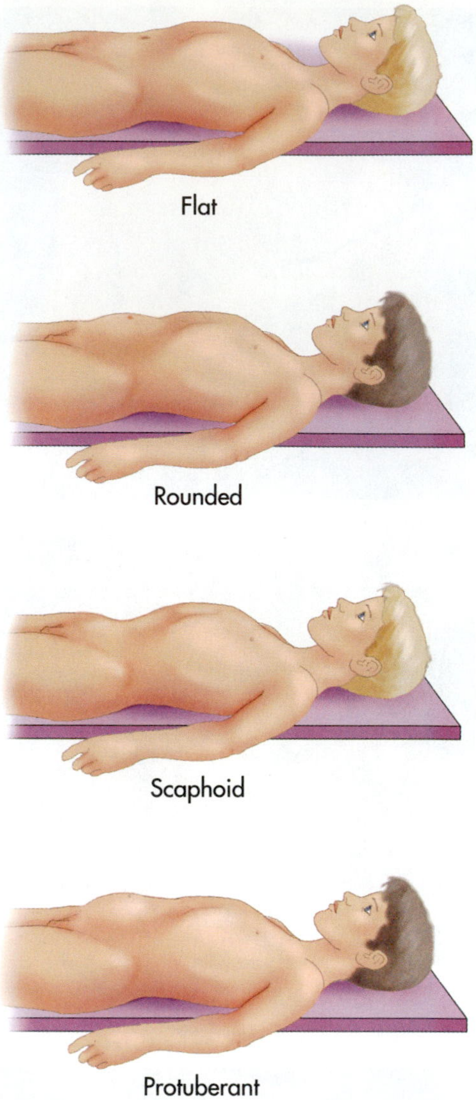

FIGURE 11-32 ■ Shape of the abdomen.

AUSCULTATION

Noting the presence or absence of bowel sounds to assess motility and to discover vascular sounds has limited value in the prehospital setting. Such findings do not affect or determine the approach to patient care. Moreover, the time needed for complete bowel sound assessment (about 5 minutes per quadrant) far exceeds the justifiable scene time for most patients. If auscultation is to be performed, though, it should always come before palpation because palpation may alter the intensity of bowel sounds.

To auscultate bowel sounds, the paramedic holds the diaphragm of the stethoscope on the abdomen with light pressure. If bowel sounds are present, they usually are heard as rumblings or gurgles. These sounds should occur irregularly. They may range in frequency from 5 to 35 per minute. Auscultation should be performed in all four quadrants. A minimum of 5 minutes per quadrant is needed to determine that normal bowel sounds are absent. Increased bowel sounds may indicate gastroenteritis or intestinal obstruction. Decreased or absent bowel sounds may indicate peritonitis (inflammation of the lining of the abdominal cavity) or ileus (inactive peristaltic activity resulting from one of several causes). (See Chapter 34.)

PERCUSSION AND PALPATION

Percussion and palpation of the abdomen may help to detect the presence of fluid, air, and solid masses. The paramedic should use a systematic approach, moving from side to side or clockwise. The paramedic should note any rigidity, tenderness, or abnormal skin temperature or color. The paramedic should observe the patient's face for signs of pain or discomfort. If the patient is complaining of abdominal pain, the paramedic should examine the painful quadrant last so that the patient will not unnecessarily tighten or "guard" the abdominal area. The abdominal assessment should begin with a light palpation, using an even pressing motion. As stated before, the paramedic's hands should be warm, and the paramedic should avoid sharp and quick jabs. Palpation may be done at the same time as percussion.

The paramedic begins percussion by evaluating all four quadrants of the abdomen in turn for tympany and dullness. (Tympany is the major sound that should be noted during percussion because of the normal presence of air in the stomach and intestines. Dullness should be heard over organs and solid masses.) When percussing the abdomen, proceeding from an area of tympany to an area of dullness is best. That way, the change in sound is easier to detect. Individual assessments of the liver and spleen (described in the following paragraphs) may be done if indicated by patient complaint or mechanism of injury. Patients who may require surgery for abdominal illness or injury are best served by rapid assessment, stabilization, and transport to an appropriate medical facility.

Percussion and Palpation of the Liver. The paramedic percusses the liver by starting just above the umbilicus in the right midclavicular line in an area of tympany. Percussion should continue in an upward direction until the change from tympany to dullness occurs. This change usually occurs slightly below the costal margin. It indicates the lower border of the liver. To determine the upper border of the liver, the percussion should begin in the same midclavicular line at the midsternal level, proceeding downward until the tympany from the lung area changes to dullness (usually between the fifth and seventh intercostal spaces). Liver size is related to age and sex. The liver usually is proportionately larger in adults than in children. The liver also is larger in males than in females.

For palpation of the liver, the patient should be supine and comfortable and should have a relaxed abdomen. The paramedic should perform the examination from the patient's right side and should begin by placing the left hand under the patient in the area of the eleventh and twelfth ribs (Fig. 11-33). The right hand should be placed on the abdomen, with the fingers pointing toward the patient's head and extended, resting just below the edge of the costal margin. The conscious patient should be instructed to breathe deeply through the mouth. During exhalation, the paramedic presses upward with the hand under the patient and gently pushes in and up with the right hand. If the paramedic feels the liver, it should be firm and nontender. (A healthy liver usually cannot be palpated unless the patient is thin.)

Percussion and Palpation of the Spleen. For percussion of the spleen, the patient must be lying supine or in a right lateral recumbent position. Percussion should begin at the area of lung tympany, just posterior to the midaxillary line on the left side. When percussing downward, a change from tympany to dullness should be audible between the sixth and tenth ribs. Large areas of dullness suggest an enlarged spleen. Stomach contents and air-filled or feces-filled intestines make splenic assessment by percussion difficult. These and other factors may affect percussion tones of dullness and tympany.

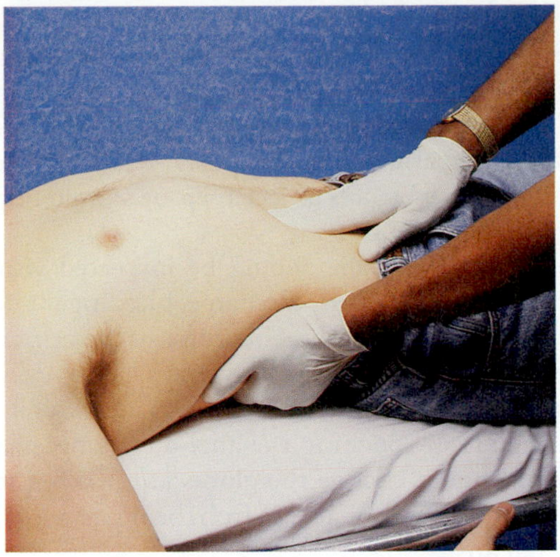

FIGURE 11-33 ■ Palpation of the liver.

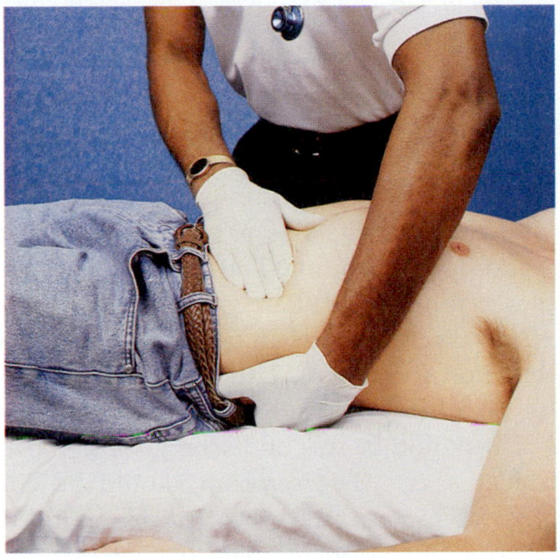

FIGURE 11-34 ■ Palpation of the spleen.

Palpation is a more useful assessment technique for evaluating the spleen. The patient should be lying supine with the paramedic positioned at the patient's left side. The paramedic places the left hand under the patient, supporting the lower left rib cage. The paramedic places the right hand just below the patient's lower left costal margin (Fig. 11-34). The paramedic should palpate the area gently by lifting up the left hand and pressing down with the right hand. (A normal spleen usually cannot be palpated in an adult. A palpable spleen is probably enlarged 3 times its normal size.) Palpation of the spleen can produce rupture of the organ. Palpation should be performed with caution.

Female Genitalia

Examination of the genitalia of either sex of patient can be awkward. The patient and the paramedic may feel uncomfortable. When possible, paramedics of the same sex as the patient should perform these exams. If that is not possible, a second person who acts as a chaperone should be present during the examination.

The external genitalia should be inspected visually to note any swelling, redness, discharge, bleeding, or evidence of trauma. Discoloration or tenderness of the genital tissue may be the result of traumatic bruising. Ulcers, vesicles, and discharges (with or without pain) indicate sexually transmitted disease. If touching the anal area is necessary, the paramedic should change the gloves afterward. Changing gloves helps to prevent bacteria from being introduced into the vaginal area.

CRITICAL THINKING

Examination of a patient's genitalia in the presence of another care provider is advisable. Why might this be important?

MALE GENITALIA

When examining the male genitalia, the paramedic should inspect the area visually. The paramedic should look for bleeding and signs of trauma. The shaft of the penis should be nontender and flaccid. Rarely, patients with leukemia, sickle cell disease, or spinal injury may have a persistent painful erection (priapism). The urethral opening should be free of blood (a possible result of pelvic trauma). The opening also should be free of discharge (a sign of sexually transmitted disease). The scrotum should be nontender and slightly asymmetrical. A swollen or painful scrotum may result from infection, herniation, testicular torsion, or trauma. Discoloration of the genitals is called Coopernail's sign and may indicate peritoneal bleeding.

ANUS

Examination of the anus is indicated in the presence of rectal bleeding or trauma to the area. Examination can be done with the patient in one of several positions. Most patients will find the side-lying position to be most comfortable. (The paramedic should protect the patient's privacy and use proper drapes.) Inspection of the sacrococcygeal and perineal areas should consider abnormal findings. These findings may include lumps, ulcers, inflammation, rashes, and excoriations. Excoriations are surface injuries caused by scratching or abrasions. Inflamed external hemorrhoids are common in adults and pregnant women.

METHOD OF TESTING FOR OCCULT BLOOD

A sample of feces can be tested for occult (microscopic) blood with guaiac test supplies (Fig. 11-35). To test for occult blood, the paramedic should follow these steps:

1. Explain the procedure to the patient. If possible, ask the patient to produce a stool specimen that is not mixed with urine or water. If necessary, the paramedic can collect a specimen by inserting a lubricated, gloved finger into the rectum.
2. Use clean disposable gloves and a wooden applicator to collect a small sample of fecal material.
3. Apply a thin smear of stool to each of the specimen papers in the test card. Close the slide cover.
4. Turn the test card over and open the flap. Apply two drops of guaiac developing solution on each paper sample and control strip in the test card. Test results are visible in 30 to 60 seconds. Blue indicates occult blood. No change in color indicates negative results.

6\. Properly dispose of all materials.

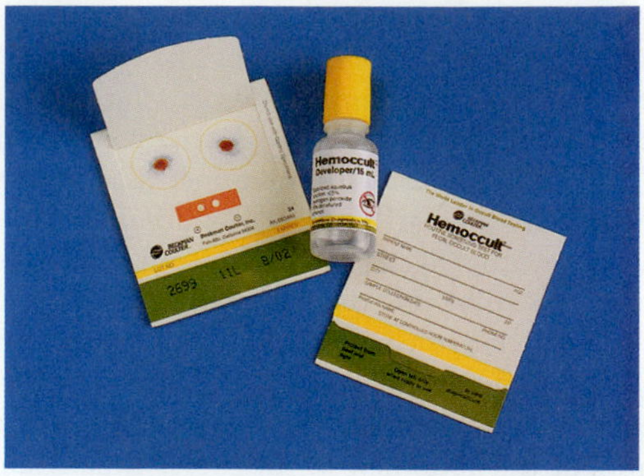

FIGURE 11-35 ■ Hemoccult kit.

EXTREMITIES

When examining the upper and lower extremities, a paramedic should pay attention to function. The paramedic also should pay attention to structure (see Chapter 6). The patient's general appearance, body proportions, and ease of movement are key. In particular, the paramedic should note any limitation in the range of motion. The paramedic should note an unusual increase in the mobility of a joint as well. Abnormal findings include the following:

- Signs of inflammation
  - Swelling
  - Tenderness
  - Increased heat
  - Redness
  - Decreased function
- Asymmetry
- Crepitus
- Deformities
- Decreased muscular strength
- Atrophy

EXAMINING UPPER AND LOWER EXTREMITIES

A full assessment of the upper and lower extremities includes an evaluation of the skin and tissue overlying the muscles, cartilage, and bones and of the joints for soft tissue injury, discoloration, swelling, and masses. The upper and lower extremities should be symmetrical in structure and muscularity. The paramedic should assess the circulatory status of each

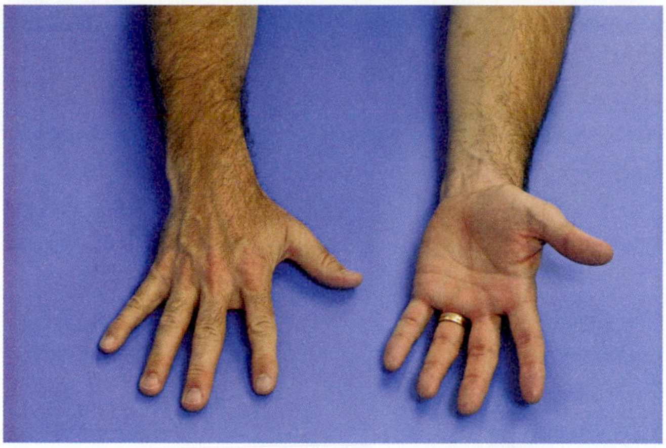

FIGURE 11-36 ■ Hands and wrists

extremity by determining skin color, temperature, sensation, and the presence of distal pulses. The paramedic should assess bones, joints, and surrounding tissues of the extremities for structural integrity and continuity. Muscle tone should be firm and nontender. The paramedic assesses joints for function by moving each joint through its full range of motion (described in Chapter 6). A normal range of motion occurs without pain, deformity, limitation, or instability.

Hands and Wrists. The paramedic should inspect both hands and wrists for contour and positional alignment (Fig. 11-36). The paramedic palpates the wrists, hands, and joints of each finger for tenderness, swelling, or deformity. To determine range of motion, the paramedic requests the patient to flex and extend the wrists, make a fist, and touch the thumb to each fingertip. All movements should be performed without pain or discomfort.

Elbows. The paramedic should inspect and palpate the elbows in the flexed and extended positions (Fig. 11-37). To determine the range of motion of the elbow, the paramedic should ask the patient to rotate the hands from palm up to palm down. The paramedic should inspect the grooves between the epicondyle and olecranon by palpation. Pain and tenderness should not be present when pressing on the lateral and medial epicondyle.

Shoulders and Related Structures. The paramedic should inspect and palpate the shoulders for symmetry and integrity of the clavicles, scapulae, and humeri. Pain, tenderness, or asymmetrical contour may indicate a fracture or dislocation. The patient should be able to shrug the shoulders. The patient should also be able to raise and extend both arms without pain or discomfort. The paramedic should palpate the following regions, noting any tenderness or swelling (Fig. 11-38):

- Sternoclavicular joint
- Acromioclavicular joint
- Subacromial area
- Bicipital groove

Ankles and Feet. The paramedic should inspect the patient's feet and ankles for contour, position, and size. Tenderness, swelling, and deformity are abnormal findings

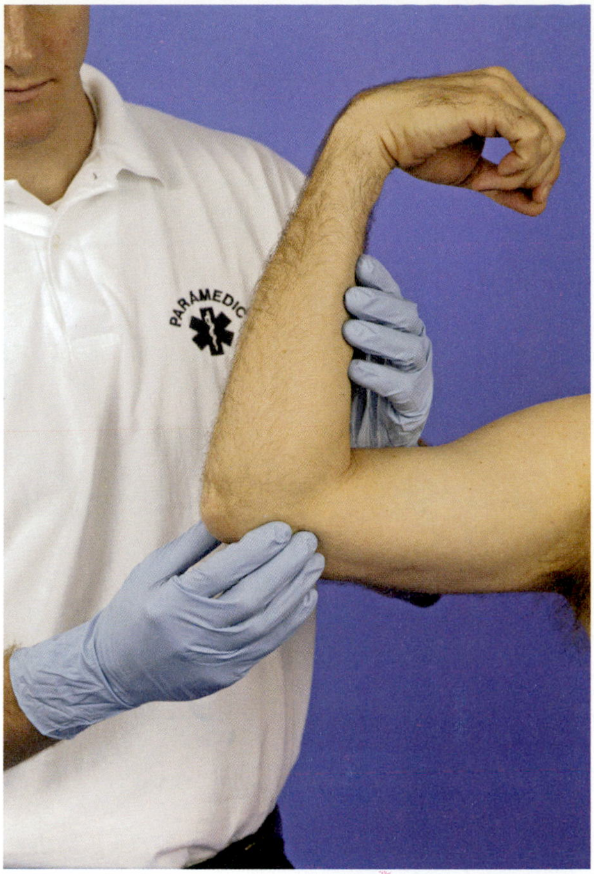

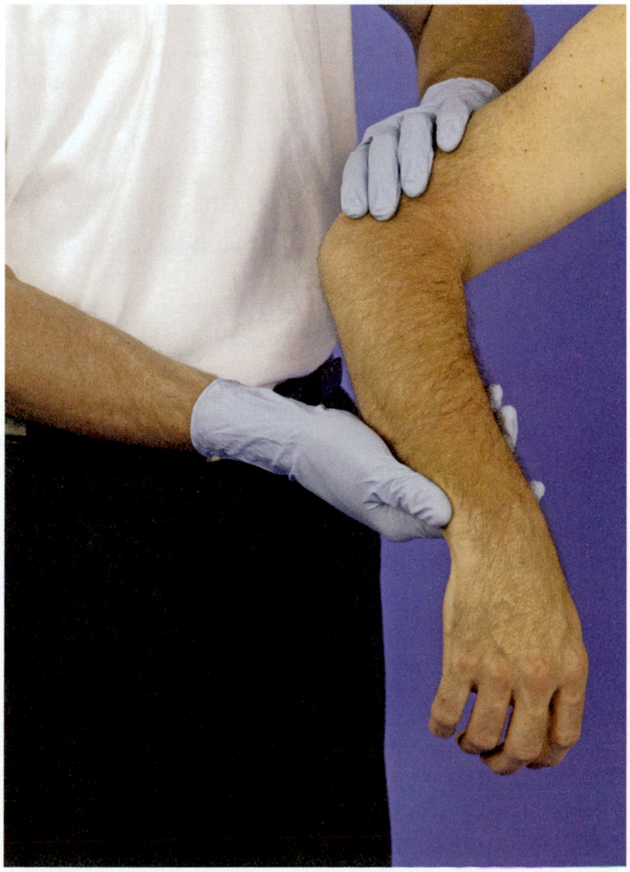

FIGURE 11-37 ■ Palpation of the lateral and medial epicondyle.

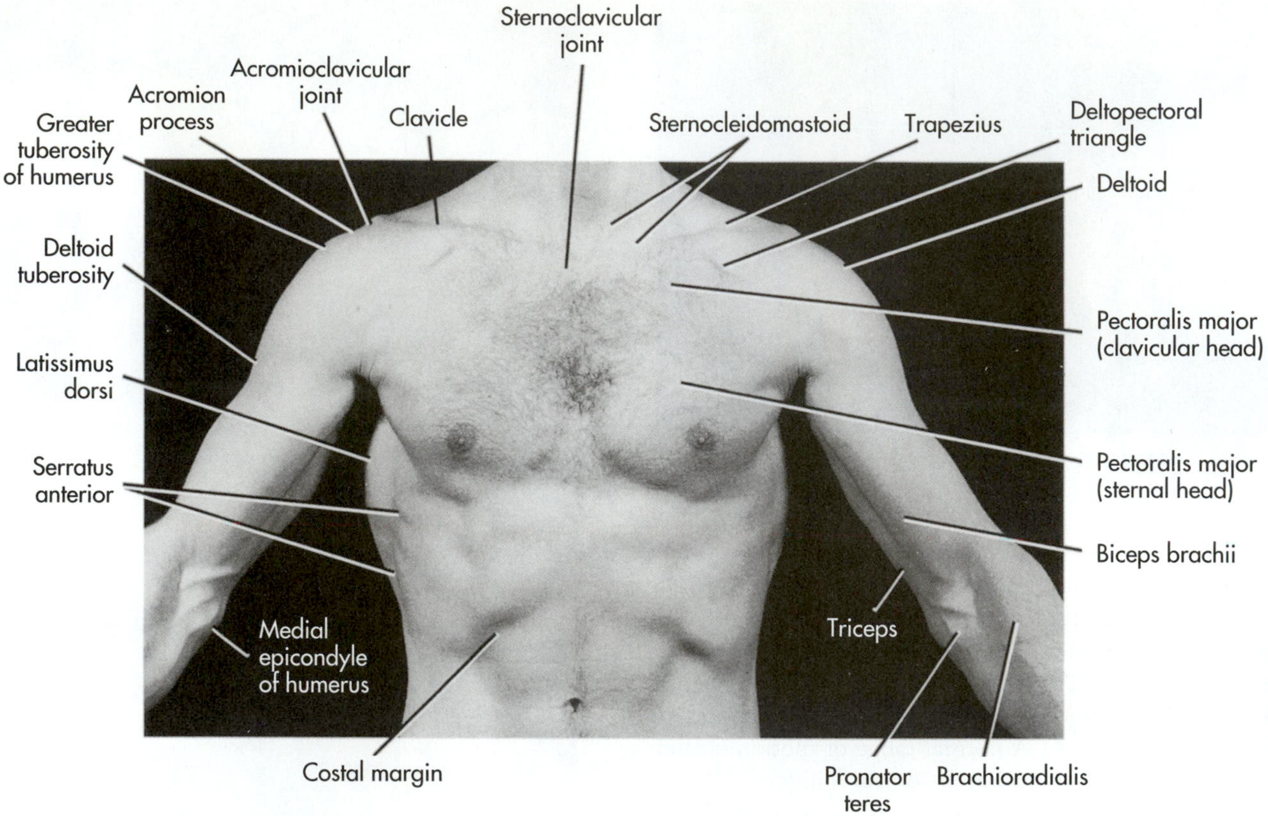

FIGURE 11-38 ■ Evaluation of shoulder and related structures.

on palpation. The toes should be straight and aligned with each other. The paramedic can determine range of motion by requesting the patient to bend the toes, point the toes, and rotate the feet inward and outward from the ankle (Fig. 11-39). These movements should be possible without pain or discomfort. The paramedic should inspect all surfaces of the ankles and feet for deformities, nodules, swelling, calluses, corns, and skin integrity.

Pelvis, Hips, and Knees. The paramedic should check the structural integrity of the pelvis. To palpate the iliac crest and the symphysis pubis, the paramedic places both hands on each anterior iliac crest. Then the paramedic presses downward and outward (Fig. 11-40). To determine stability, the paramedic places the heel of the hand on the symphysis pubis and presses downward. Deformity and point tenderness of the pelvis may be signs of fracture. These signs may mask major structural and vascular injury.

The paramedic should inspect and palpate the hips for instability, tenderness, and crepitus. The paramedic can examine the supine or unconscious patient by assessing the structural integrity of the iliac crest. A mobile patient should be able to walk without discomfort. A supine patient should be able to raise the legs and knees and rotate the legs inward and outward.

The paramedic should inspect and palpate the knees for swelling and tenderness. The patella should be smooth, firm, nontender, and midline in position. The patient should be able to bend and straighten each knee without pain.

PERIPHERAL VASCULAR SYSTEM

The peripheral vascular system includes arteries, veins, the lymphatic system and lymph nodes, and the fluids exchanged in the capillary bed. These can be evaluated during the physical examination of the upper and lower extremities.

Arms. When evaluating the arms, the paramedic should inspect from fingertips to shoulders. The paramedic should note size and symmetry. The paramedic also should note swelling, venous pattern, color of the skin and nail beds, and texture of the skin. If the paramedic notes arterial insufficiency because of a weak radial pulse, the paramedic should palpate the brachial pulse. Epitrochlear nodes and brachial nodes should be nonswollen and nontender (Fig. 11-41). A fine venous network on upper and lower extremities often is visible. The paramedic should be alert for enlargement of superficial veins during the exam.

Legs. During examination of the lower extremities, the patient should be supine. The patient also should be draped properly. (Shoes, socks, and hosiery should be removed for a full examination.) The paramedic should inspect visually from the groin and buttocks to the feet, noting the following:

- Size and symmetry
- Swelling
- Venous pattern and venous enlargement
- Pigmentation

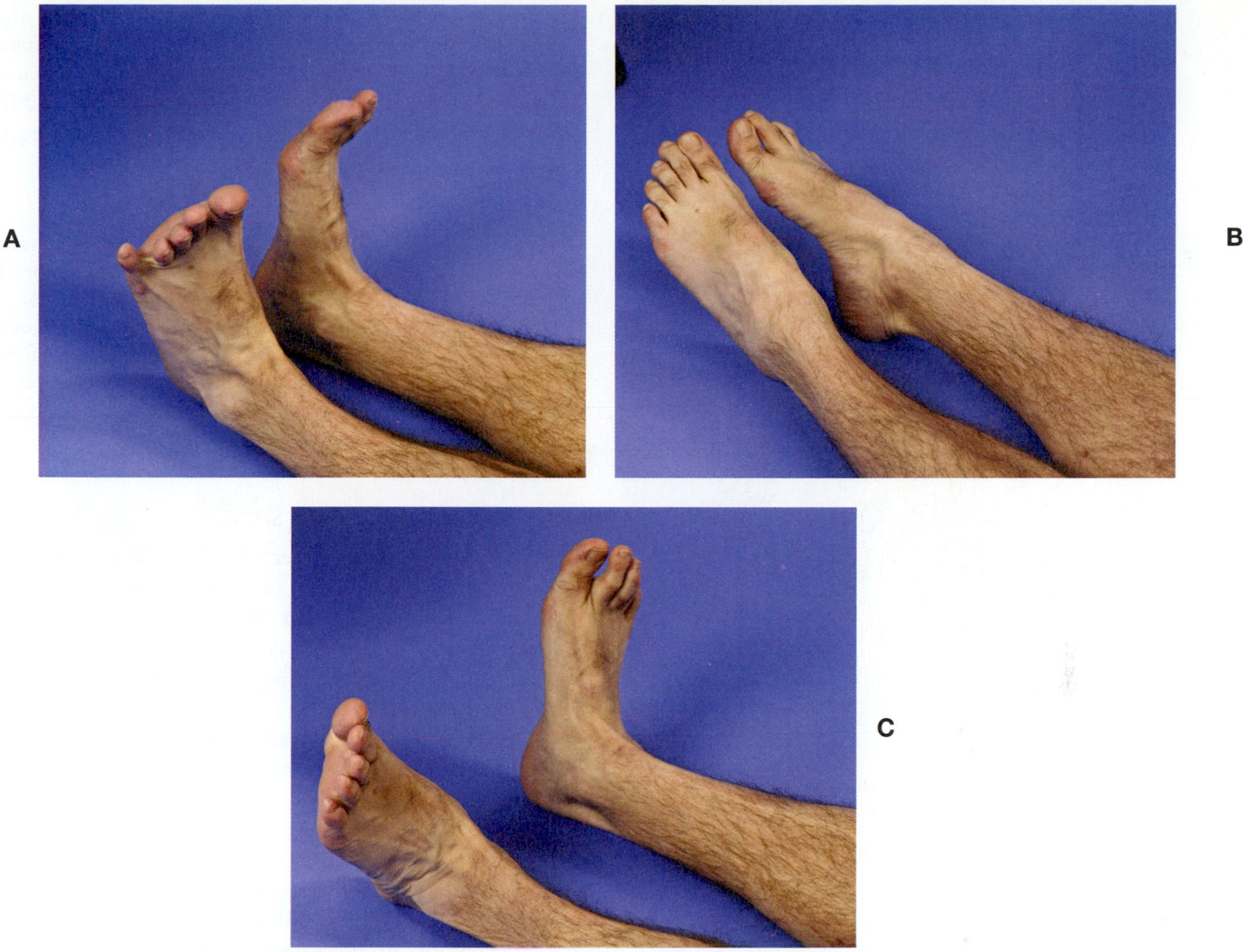

FIGURE 11-39 ■ Motor function of the foot and ankle. A, Bend toes. B, Point toes. C, Rotate feet in and out.

- Rashes, scars, or ulcers
- Color and texture of the skin
- Presence or absence of hair growth (indicating compromised arterial circulation)

The paramedic should palpate the superficial inguinal nodes in the groin to assess for swelling and tenderness. The paramedic should assess all lower extremity pulse sites for circulation, strength, and regularity. These sites include the femoral pulse, the popliteal pulse, the dorsalis pedis pulse, and the posterior tibial pulse (see Chapter 6). The temperature of the feet and legs should be warm. This indicates adequate circulation. The paramedic can evaluate for pitting edema over the dorsum of each foot, behind each medial malleolus, and over the shins. This can be done by pressing firmly on the skin with the thumb for at least 5 seconds. Edema is said to be pitting when depression of the tissue remains after removal of pressure.

Abnormal Findings. Findings that are considered abnormal during a peripheral vascular assessment include the following:

- Swollen or asymmetrical extremities
- Pale or cyanotic skin
- Weak or diminished pulses
- Skin that is cold to the touch
- Absence of hair growth
- Pitting edema

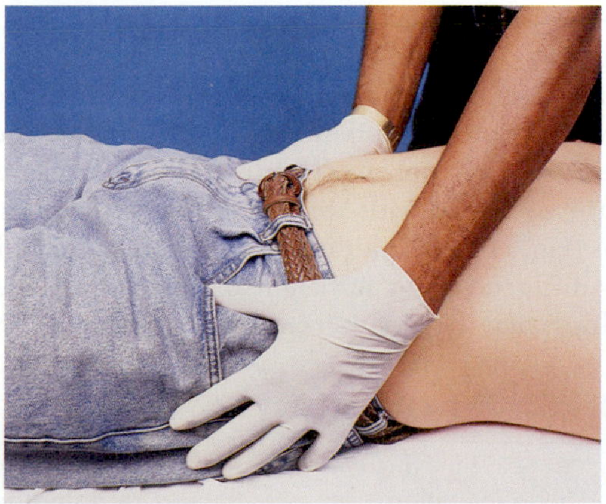

FIGURE 11-40 ■ Palpating the pelvis for stability.

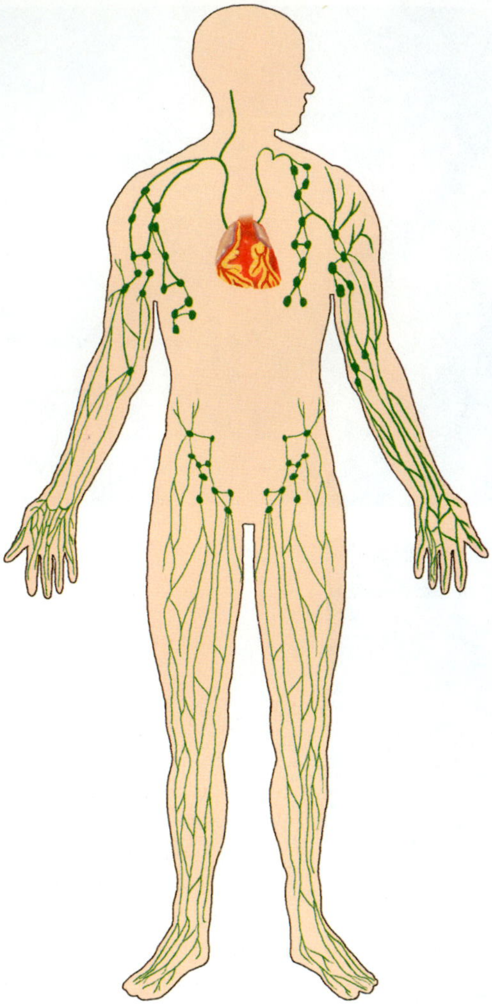

FIGURE 11-41 ■ Nodes of upper and lower extremities.

Spine

A full physical examination includes an assessment of the spine. This begins with a visual assessment of the cervical, thoracic, and lumbar curves. From the patient's side, the paramedic should note any curvature of the spine, including curvature associated with abnormal lordosis, kyphosis, and scoliosis (Fig. 11-42). In addition, the paramedic should look for any differences in the height of the shoulders or iliac crests (hips) that may result from abnormal spinal curvature.

CRITICAL THINKING

Consider a case in which no deformity of the spine is found during an examination. Can spine fracture or dislocation be ruled out?

CERVICAL SPINE

The patient's neck should be in a midline position. If the patient is alert and denies neck pain, the paramedic should palpate the posterior aspect for point tenderness and swelling. The only palpable landmark should be the spinous process of the seventh cervical vertebra at the base of the neck (Fig. 11-43). In the absence of suspected injury, the paramedic tests range of motion by directing the patient to bend the head forward, backward, and from side to side. These movements should not cause pain or discomfort.

NOTE The paramedic will need to test range of motion. However, the paramedic should never attempt to move the neck of a person who is unconscious. The paramedic also should never attempt this with a person who is unable or unwilling to do so on his or her own. Spontaneous cervical muscle spasm frequently is associated with significant cervical spine injury in the trauma victim.

THORACIC AND LUMBAR SPINE

The paramedic should inspect the thoracic and lumbar areas for signs of injury, swelling, and discoloration. Palpation should begin at the first thoracic vertebra. Palpation should move downward to the sacrum. Under normal conditions, the spine is nontender to palpation. The paramedic can evaluate range of motion by requesting the patient to bend at the waist forward and backward and to each side and also to rotate the upper trunk from side to side in a circular motion.

Nervous System

The details of an appropriate neurological examination vary greatly. The exam usually depends on the origin of the patient's complaint. For example, the exam may depend on whether the complaint refers to the peripheral nervous system or the central nervous system. The assessment and examination of the nervous system may be performed separately. However, neurological assessment often is completed during other assessments. A neurological examination may be organized into five categories:

- Mental status and speech
- Cranial nerves
- Motor system
- Sensory system
- Reflexes

MENTAL STATUS AND SPEECH

As discussed before, a healthy patient should be oriented to person, time, and place. Patients also should be able to organize their thoughts. They should be able to speak freely (provided they have no hearing or speech impediments). Abnormal findings include unconsciousness, confusion, slurred speech, aphasia, dysphonia, and dysarthria.

CRANIAL NERVES

The 12 cranial nerves can be categorized as sensory, somatomotor and proprioceptive, and parasympathetic (see Chapter 6). The following methods can be used to assess each of the cranial nerves:

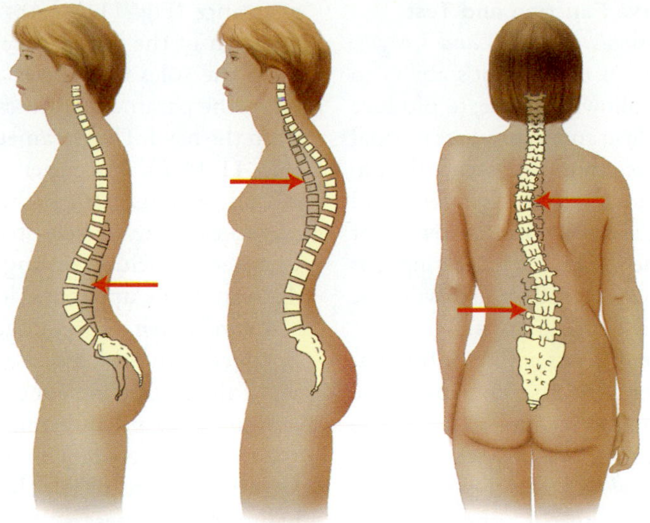

FIGURE 11-42 ■ Lordosis, kyphosis, scoliosis.

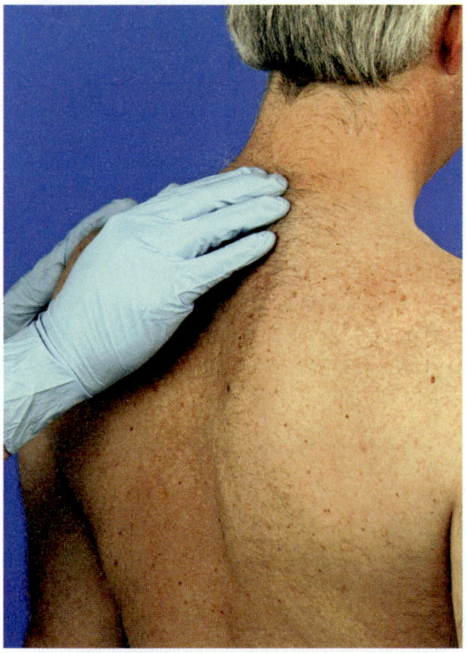

FIGURE 11-43 ■ Palpation of the seventh cervical spinous process.

Nerve	Nerve Function and Test
Cranial nerve I	*Olfactory:* Test sense of smell with spirits of ammonia.
Cranial nerve II	*Optic:* Test for visual acuity (previously described).
Cranial nerves II and III	*Optic and oculomotor:* Inspect the size and shape of the pupils; test the pupil response to light.
Cranial nerves III, IV, and VI	*Oculomotor, trochlear, abducens:* Test extraocular movements by asking the patient to look up and down, to the left and right, and diagonally up and down to the left and right (the six cardinal directions of gaze).
Cranial nerve V	*Trigeminal:* Test motor movement by asking the patient to clench the teeth while you palpate the temporal and masseter muscles. Test sensation by touching the forehead, cheeks, and jaw on each side.
Cranial nerve VII	*Facial*: Inspect the face at rest and during conversation, noting symmetry, involuntary muscle movements (tics), or abnormal movements. Ask the patient to raise the eyebrows, frown, show upper and lower teeth, smile, and puff out both cheeks. The paramedic can assess strength of the facial muscles by asking the patient to close eyes tightly so they cannot be opened and gently attempting to raise the eyelids. Observe for weakness or asymmetry.
Cranial nerve VIII	*Acoustic:* Assess hearing acuity (previously described).

Nerve	Nerve Function and Test
Cranial nerves IX and X	*Glossopharyngeal and vagus:* Assess the patient's ability to swallow with ease; to produce saliva; and to produce normal voice sounds. Instruct the patient to hold the breath, and assess for normal slowing of the heart rate. Testing for the gag reflex also will test the cranial nerves.
Cranial nerve XI	*Spinal accessory:* Ask the patient to raise and lower the shoulders and to turn the head.
Cranial nerve XII	*Hypoglossal:* Ask the patient to stick out the tongue and to move it in several directions.

CRITICAL THINKING

Why should abnormal findings in examination of one or more of the cranial nerves concern you?

MOTOR SYSTEM

An evaluation of a patient's motor system includes observing the patient during movement. The evaluation also includes observing the patient at rest. The paramedic should evaluate abnormal involuntary movements for quality, rate, rhythm, and fullness of range. Other body movement assessments include posture, level of activity, fatigue, and emotion.

Muscle Strength. Muscle strength should be bilaterally symmetrical. In addition, the patient should be able to provide reasonable resistance to opposition. One way to evaluate muscle strength in the upper extremities is to ask the patient to extend the elbow. Then the paramedic tells the patient to pull the arm toward the chest against opposing resistance (Fig. 11-44, *A*). The paramedic assesses muscle strength in the lower extremities by asking the patient to push the soles of the feet against the paramedic's palms. Next, the paramedic directs the patient to pull the toes toward the head. The paramedic provides opposing resistance (Fig. 11-44, *B*). The patient should be able to perform both of these actions easily without evident fatigue. Other methods to evaluate muscle strength and agility (illustrated in Chapter 6) include testing for flexion, extension, and abduction of the upper and lower extremities.

Coordination. To evaluate a patient's coordination, the paramedic should assess the patient's ability to perform rapid alternating movements. These include point-to-point movements, gait, and stance.

One point-to-point movement that the patient can perform easily is to touch the finger to the nose, alternating hands. Another test is to ask the patient to touch each heel to the opposite shin. Both movements should be done numerous times and quickly to assess coordination, which should be smooth, rapid, and accurate.

Gait can be evaluated in many ways. A healthy patient should be able to perform each of the following tasks without discomfort or losing balance:

- Walk heel to toe
- Walk on the toes
- Walk on the heels
- Hop in place
- Do a shallow knee bend
- Rise from a sitting position without assistance

Stance and balance can be evaluated by using Romberg's test and the pronator drift test. To perform Romberg's test, the paramedic asks the patient to stand erect with the feet together and arms at the sides (Fig. 11-45). The patient's eyes initially should be open and then closed. Although slight swaying is normal, a loss of balance is abnormal (a positive Romberg's sign). A patient should be able to stand in this position with one foot raised for 5 seconds without losing balance.

A

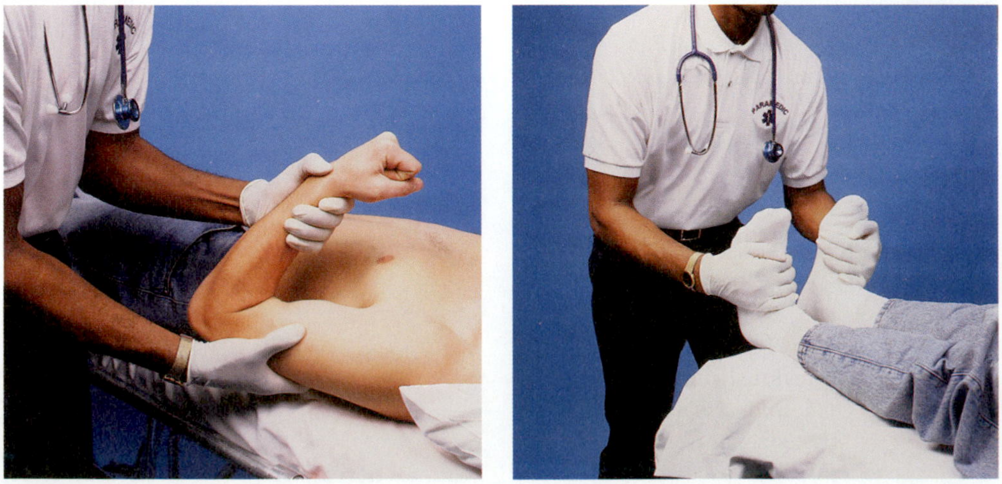

B

FIGURE 11-44 ■ Evaluating muscle strength of the upper (A) and lower (B) extremities.

▶ **NOTE** The paramedic should stay close to the patient being tested for gait, stance, and balance. That way, the paramedic can help to prevent injury from a fall or loss of balance. The paramedic also should consider the patient's age and physical condition in deciding the appropriateness of these examinations.

The pronator drift test (also known as an *arm drift test*) is performed by having the patient close the eyes and hold both arms out from the body (Fig. 11-46). A normal test will reveal that both arms move the same or both arms do not move at all. Abnormal findings include one arm that does not move in concert with the other or one arm that drifts down compared with the other.

SENSORY SYSTEM

The sensory pathways of the nervous system conduct sensations of pain, temperature, position, vibration, and touch. A healthy patient is expected to be responsive to each of these stimuli. Common assessments of the sensory system include evaluating the patient's response to pain and light touch. Each of the responses should be considered in relation to dermatomes (see Chapter 6).

In conscious patients the paramedic should perform a sensory examination with light touch on each hand and each foot. If the patient cannot feel light touch or is unconscious, the paramedic may evaluate sensation by gently pricking the hands and soles of the feet with a sharp object. The paramedic should make sure the object will not penetrate the skin (e.g., a paper clip or cotton swab). The sensory examination should proceed from head to toe. The exam should compare symmetrical areas on each side of the body and the distal and proximal areas of the body. A lack of sensory response may indicate spinal cord damage (see Chapter 25).

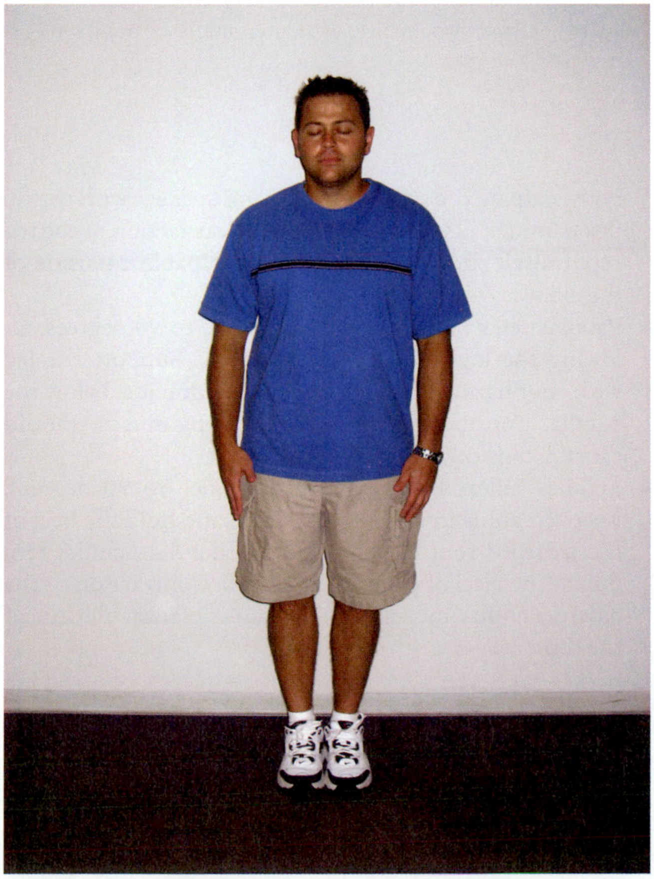

FIGURE 11-45 ■ Romberg's test.

REFLEXES

Testing a patient's reflexes can evaluate the function of certain areas of the nervous system as they relate to sensory impulses and motor neurons. Reflexes may be categorized as superficial reflexes and deep tendon reflexes (Table 11-5). Both types of reflexes should be tested as part of a thorough neurological examination.

SUPERFICIAL REFLEXES

Superficial reflexes are elicited by sensory afferents from skin. These include the upper abdominal, lower abdominal, cremasteric (for males), and plantar reflexes. All superficial reflexes are tested using the edge of a tongue blade (or similar object) or the end of a reflex hammer. An absent reflex may indicate an upper or lower motor neuron disorder.

- Upper and lower abdominal reflex: Place the patient supine. Gently stroke each quadrant of the abdomen with the tongue blade. A normal reflex is a slight movement of the umbilicus toward each area that is stroked.
- Cremasteric reflex: Place the patient supine. Gently stroke the inner thigh (proximal to distal). The testicle and scrotum should rise on the side that is stroked.

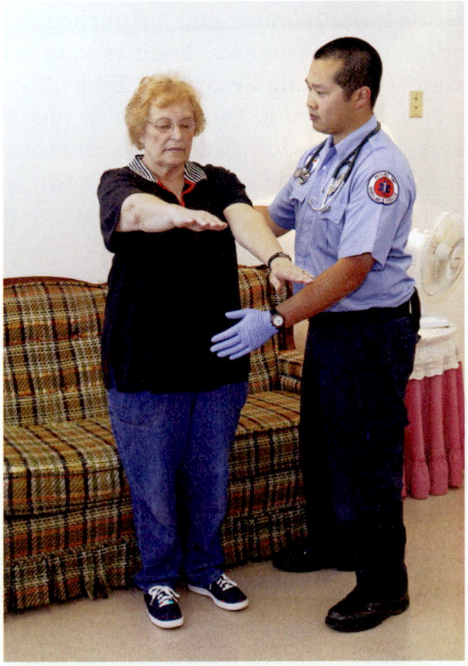

FIGURE 11-46 ■ Pronator drift test.

TABLE 11-5 Superficial and Deep Tendon Reflexes

REFLEX	SPINAL LEVEL EVALUATED
Superficial	
Upper abdominal	T7, T8, and T9
Lower abdominal	T10 and T11
Cremasteric	T12, L1, and L2
Plantar	L4, L5, S1, and S2
Deep Tendon	
Biceps	C5 and C6
Brachioradial	C5 and C6
Triceps	C6, C7, and C8
Patellar	L2, L3, and L4
Achilles	S1 and S2

Modified from Rudy, 1984.

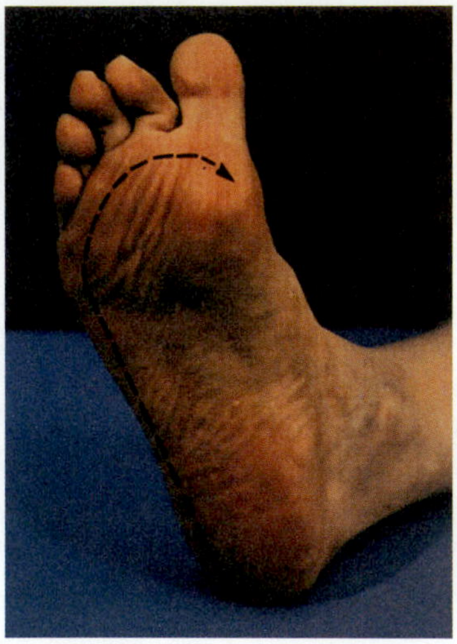

FIGURE 11-47 ■ Plantar reflex indicating the direction of the stroke and the Babinski sign—dorsiflexion of the great toe with or without fanning of the toes.

- Plantar reflex: Place the patient with legs extended. Gently stroke the lateral side of the foot from heel to the ball and then across the foot to the medial side. Fanning of all the toes should occur with the direction of the stroke (Fig. 11-47). The Babinski sign is present when there is dorsiflexion of the great toe with or without fanning of the other toes. (An abnormal finding in older children and adults, but a normal response in children less than 2 years of age.)

TABLE 11-6 Scoring Deep Tendon Reflexes

GRADE	DEEP TENDON REFLEX RESPONSE
0	No response
1+	Sluggish or diminished
2+	Active or expected response
3+	More brisk than expected, slightly hyperactive
4+	Brisk, hyperactive, with intermittent or transient clonus

DEEP TENDON REFLEXES

Deep tendon reflexes are elicited by sensory afferents from muscle rather than bone. They include the biceps reflex, brachioradial reflex, triceps reflex, patellar reflex, and the Achilles reflex. These reflexes should be tested on each extremity with a reflex hammer and a comparison made for visible and palpable responses. Deep tendon reflexes are graded using the scoring system in Table 11-6 and are recorded on a stick figure. Diminished or absent reflexes may indicate damage to lower motor neurons or the spinal cord. Hyperactive reflexes may suggest a motor neuron disorder. All reflexes are tested with the patient in a sitting position in the following manner (Fig. 11-48).

- Biceps reflex: Flex the patient's arm to 45 degrees at the elbow. Palpate the biceps tendon in the antecubital fossa. Place your thumb over the tendon and your fingers under the elbow. Strike your thumb with the reflex hammer. Contraction of the biceps muscle should cause visible or palpable flexion of the elbow.
- Brachioradial reflex: Flex the patient's arm up to 45 degrees. Rest the patient's forearm on your arm with the hand slightly pronated. Strike the brachioradial tendon (about 1 to 2 inches above the wrist) with the reflex hammer. Pronation of the forearm and flexion of the elbow should occur.
- Triceps reflex: Flex the patient's arm at the elbow up to 90 degrees and rest the patient's hand against the side of the body. Palpate the triceps tendon and strike it with the reflex hammer, just above the elbow. Contraction of the triceps muscle should cause visible or palpable extension of the elbow.
- Patellar reflex: Flex the patient's knee to 90 degrees, allowing the lower leg to hang loosely. Support the leg with your hand. Strike the patellar tendon just below the patella. Contraction of the quadriceps muscle should cause extension of the lower leg.
- Achilles reflex: Flex the patient's knee to 90 degrees. Keep the ankle in a neutral position and hold the heel of the patient's foot in your hand. Strike the Achilles tendon at the level of the ankle malleoli. Contraction of the gastrocnemius muscle should cause plantar flexion of the foot.

PHYSICAL EXAMINATION OF INFANTS AND CHILDREN

Examining the ill or injured child calls for special assessment skills. Children differ physiologically, psychologically, and anatomically from adults. Thus a pediatric patient assessment must take age and development into account.

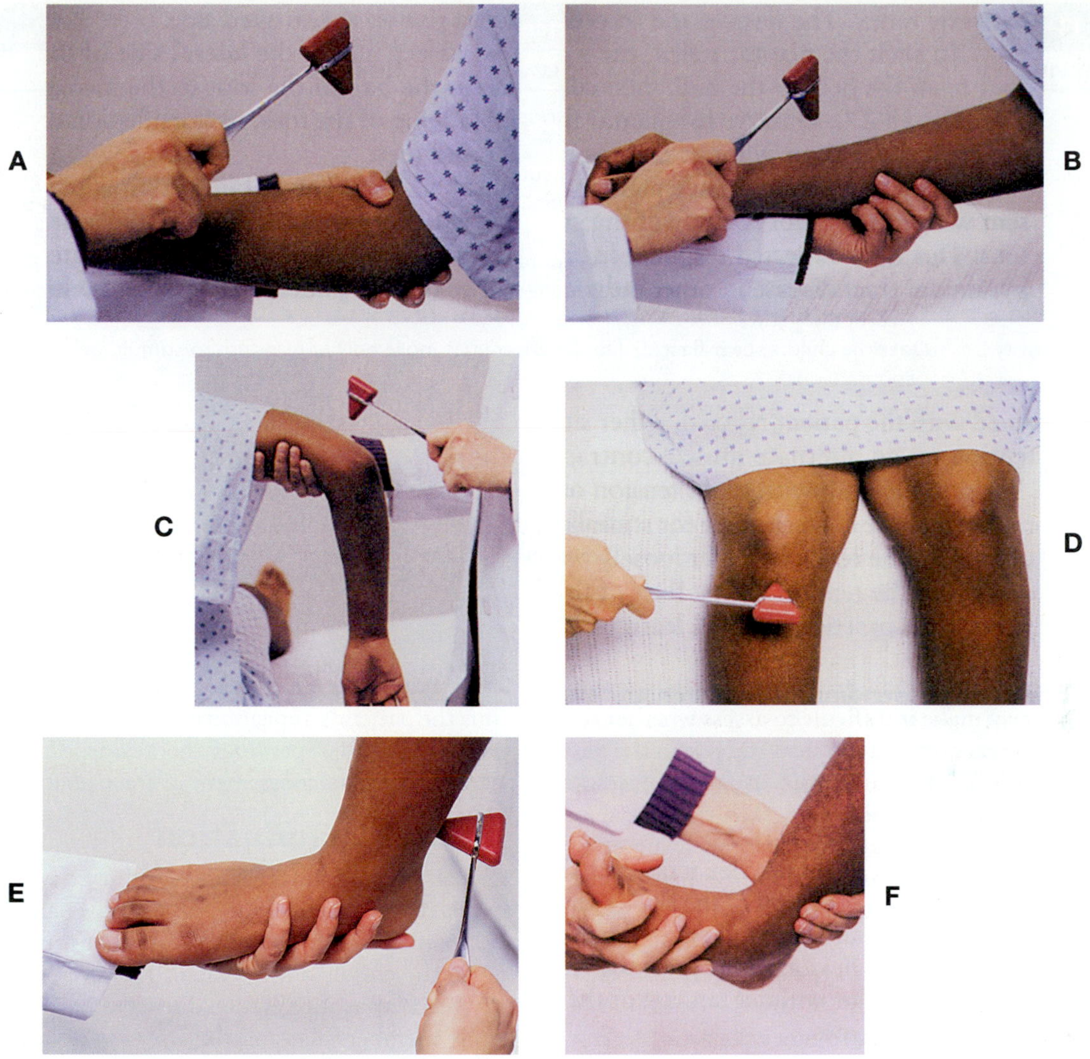

FIGURE 11-48 ■ Location of tendons for evaluation of deep tendon reflexes. **A,** Biceps. **B,** Brachioradial. **C,** Triceps. **D,** Patellar. **E,** Achilles. **F,** Evaluation of ankle clonus.

Approaching the Pediatric Patient

The assessment and management objectives in caring for critically ill or injured children are similar to those for any other patient. The approach to the pediatric patient must differ, though. The initial encounter with the sick or injured child sets the tone for the entire patient care episode. Thus the paramedic must consider the patient's age. The paramedic also must be sensitive to how the child perceives the emergency environment. The paramedic should consider the following six guidelines when approaching the pediatric patient[4]:

1. Remain calm and confident. The parent's anxiety is infectious. Stay under control and take charge of the situation in a gentle but firm manner.
2. Do not separate the child from the parent unless absolutely necessary. In fact, once parents are reassured, encourage them to touch, hold, or cuddle the child when such actions are practical. This comforts the parents and the child.
3. Establish rapport with the parents and the child. Much of a child's fear and anxiety reflects the parent's behavior. When the family is calm, the child is reassured and is less fearful.
4. Be honest with the child and parent. In simple, direct, nonmedical language, explain to the parent and the child what is happening as it occurs. When a procedure is going to hurt, inform the child. Never lie. Do not give the impression that there are options when none exist. For example, do not say, "Would you like to go for a ride in the ambulance?" The child may answer "No."
5. Whenever possible, assign one emergency caregiver to stay with the child. This person should obtain the history and be the primary person to initiate therapy. Even in a few moments, one person who remains on the child's level can establish a trusting relationship.
6. Observe the patient before the physical examination. If possible, the paramedic should at first assess the alert child with no touching. After the physical exam-

TABLE 11-7 Components of General Appearance for Assessment

ASSESSMENT FINDING	EVALUATION CONSIDERATIONS
Alertness	How perceptive is the child, and how responsive is the child to the presence of a stranger or to other aspects of the environment?
Distractibility	How readily does a person, object, or sound draw the child's attention? For example, drawing a child's attention to a toy when the child initially appeared disinterested in the surroundings is a positive sign
Consolability	Can a distressed child be comforted? For example, stopping a child from crying by speaking softly or offering a pacifier or a toy is an encouraging sign.
Speech or cry	Is the speech or cry strong and spontaneous? Weak and muffled? Hoarse? Absent unless stimulated? Absent altogether?
Spontaneous activity	Does the child appear flaccid? Do the extremities move only in response to stimuli, or are movements spontaneous?
Color	Is there pallor, a flushed appearance, cyanosis, or mottling? Does the skin coloring of the trunk differ from that of the extremities?
Respiratory efforts	Are there intercostal, supraclavicular, or suprasternal retractions in the resting state? Nasal flaring also indicates respiratory difficulty.
Eye contact	Does the child appear to gaze aimlessly, or does the child maintain eye contact with objects or persons? Even small infants, when well, preferentially fix their gaze on a face rather than other objects.

ination begins, the child's behavior may change radically. This may make it difficult to assess whether the behavior is a reaction to a physical state or to the perceived intrusion. The paramedic usually can assess the patient's general appearance, skin signs, level of consciousness, respiratory rate, and behavior easily before approaching the patient. During this observation, the paramedic also should note any area of the body that looks painful. The paramedic should avoid manipulating this area until the end of the examination. The paramedic should inform the child that he will give warning before he touches the area.

CRITICAL THINKING

The next time you are in a room with an infant or small child, try this "across the room" assessment technique. What can you tell about the level of distress and cardiopulmonary function by doing this?

General Appearance

A child's general appearance is assessed best at a distance. While the patient is in safe, familiar surroundings (e.g., a parent's arms), the paramedic visually should assess the child's level of consciousness, spontaneous movement, respiratory effort, and skin color. The child's body position also can offer helpful information. For example, the child may be lying limp or sitting upright to aid breathing. Other clues may help determine the child's willingness to cooperate during the examination. These clues may include crying, eye contact, concentration, and distractibility.

A visual inspection of the child's general appearance can be helpful. Appearance is a fairly reliable indicator of the patient's need for emergency care. Children who are seriously ill or injured usually do not attempt to hide their state. Their actions generally reflect the severity of the situation. Thus the patient's appearance is a valuable tool for the paramedic. Table 11-7 provides the key aspects of general appearance in initial assessment of the pediatric patient.

Physical Examination

A physical examination is best conducted with a knowledge of the development of children and changes that occur within age groups. The guidelines that follow vary according to the child's development. However, these guidelines may be used as a reference during the exam. Parents and family members also may be a source of information. The paramedic may direct questions regarding "normal" behavior and activity levels to the parents.

BIRTH TO 6 MONTHS

Children under 6 months of age typically are not frightened by the approach of a stranger. Thus the physical examination is fairly easy. During the examination, the paramedic should maintain the child's body temperature.

Healthy and alert infants usually are in constant motion. They may have a lusty cry. If the patient is under 3 months of age, poor head control is normal. Infants are "abdominal breathers." This causes the stomach to protrude and the infant's chest wall to retract during inspiration. This diaphragmatic involvement may give the impression of labored breathing. Skin color, nasal flaring, and intercostal muscle retraction are the best indicators of respiratory insufficiency.

In the infant, assessing the fontanelles is particularly important (Fig. 11-49). These sutures between the flat bones of the skull are fairly wide to allow a "give" in the skull during the birth process. (The anterior fontanelle, known as the *soft spot,* usually is present up to the age of 18 months.) The anterior fontanelle should be level with the skull or slightly depressed and soft. The fontanelle usually bulges

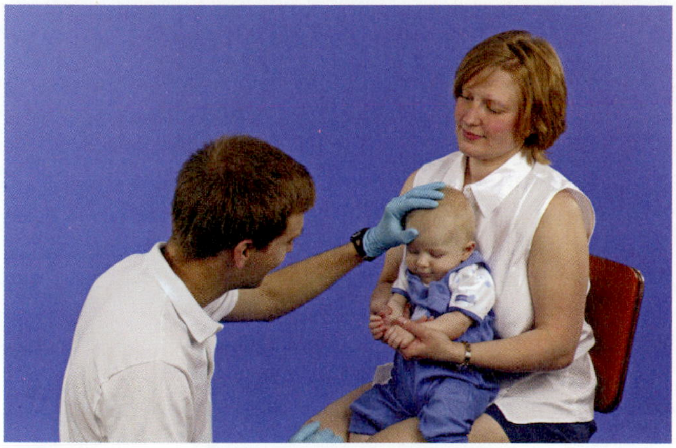

FIGURE 11-49 ■ Palpation of the anterior fontanelle.

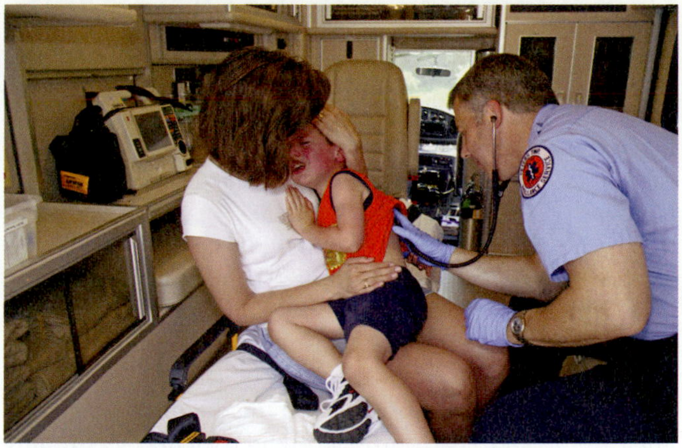

FIGURE 11-50 ■ Examining a child.

during crying and may feel firm if the child is lying down. In the absence of injury, the fontanelle is best examined with the child in an upright position. A sunken fontanelle may indicate dehydration, and a bulging fontanelle in the noncrying upright infant may indicate an increase in intracranial pressure.

7 MONTHS TO 3 YEARS

Patients from 7 months to 3 years of age often are difficult to evaluate. They have little capacity to understand the emergency event. In addition, they are likely to experience emotional problems as a result of illness, injury, or hospitalization. Children of this age fear strangers and may show separation anxiety. If possible, parents should be present and should be allowed to hold the child during the examination (Fig. 11-50). The paramedic should approach the child with a quiet, reassuring voice. If time permits, the paramedic should allow the patient to become accustomed to the examination environment.

During the physical assessment, the paramedic should explain each activity in short, simple sentences. The paramedic should give this explanation even though it may not improve cooperation. The best approach is to be gentle and firm. Another good idea is to complete the examination as quickly as possible. If physical restraint is necessary and if patient care activities will not be hindered, the paramedic should restrain the child with hands rather than mechanical devices (e.g., backboards).

4 TO 10 YEARS

Children in the 4- to 10-year age group are developing a capacity for rational thought. They may be cooperative during the physical examination. Depending on the child's age and the emergency scenario, the child may be able to provide a limited history of the event. These children also may experience separation anxiety. Moreover, they may view their illness or injury as punishment. Therefore the paramedic should approach the child slowly and speak in quiet and reassuring tones. Questions should be simple and direct.

During the examination, the paramedic should allow the child to take part by holding the stethoscope, penlight, or other pieces of equipment. This "helping" activity may lessen the child's fear. Helping also may improve the paramedic-patient relationship. Children of this age group have a limited understanding of their bodies. They also are reluctant to allow the paramedic to see or touch their "private parts" (seldom necessary in the prehospital setting). The paramedic should explain all examination procedures simply and completely. The paramedic should advise the child of any expected pain or discomfort.

ADOLESCENTS (11 TO 18 YEARS OF AGE)

Adolescents generally understand what is happening. They usually are calm, mature, and helpful. These patients are more adult than child. Thus the paramedic should treat them as such. Adolescents are preoccupied with their bodies. Usually they are concerned about modesty, disfigurement, pain, disability, and death. If appropriate, the paramedic should give reassurance about these concerns during the examination.

During the patient interview, the paramedic should respect the patient's need for privacy. Some adolescents may hesitate to reveal relevant history. This hesitancy may be even more obvious in the presence of family and friends. If the adolescent gives vague answers or seems uncomfortable, the paramedic should interview the parents and patient privately. The paramedic should consider the possibility of alcohol or other drug use, as well as the possibility of pregnancy.

PHYSICAL EXAMINATION OF OLDER ADULTS

As with pediatric patients, age-related physiological and psychological variations may create special challenges in patient assessment of older adults. The paramedic should not assume that all older adults are victims of age-related disorders. Individual differences in knowledge, mental reasoning, experience, and personality influence how these patients respond to examination.

Communicating with the Older Adult

Some older adults have sensory losses. This may make communications more difficult. Hearing and visual impairments, for example, are not uncommon. In addition, some older adults experience some memory loss and may become easily confused. Extra time may be needed to communicate effectively with these patients.

The paramedic should remain close to the patient during the interview. The older adult generally perceives a reassuring voice and gentle touch as comforting. Short and simple questions are best. The paramedic may need to speak louder than usual. In addition, the paramedic may need to repeat questions. The paramedic must be patient and careful not to patronize or offend patients by assuming that they have a hearing impairment or cannot understand a particular line of questioning.

Patient History

Older patients often have multiple health problems present at the same time. Patients may be vague and nonspecific when describing their chief complaint. This makes it hard to isolate a nonapparent injury or illness. Moreover, normal signs and symptoms of illness or injury may be absent because of decreased sensory function in some older adult patients.

Older patients with many health problems often take several medications. These medications increase the risk of illness from use and misuse. The paramedic should try to gather a full medication history. The paramedic must be alert to the relationship among drug interactions, disease, and the aging process (see Chapter 45).

As part of the history, the paramedic should assess the patient's functional abilities and any recent changes in daily activities. Many older adults attribute these changes to age. They may not mention them unless asked. These details may help indicate patient conditions that are not readily observable. Moreover, they may reveal the need for other pertinent lines of questioning. Examples of functional activities to be discussed with the patient include the following:

- Walking
- Getting out of bed
- Dressing
- Driving a car
- Using public transportation
- Preparing meals
- Taking medications
- Sleeping habits
- Bathroom habits

Physical Examination

During examination, the paramedic should ensure the older adult patient's comfort. The paramedic should explain procedures clearly and answer all questions sensitively. Many older patients with chronic illness may have lived with pain or discomfort for a long time. Thus their perception of what is painful may be different from that of other patients. The paramedic should observe for signs such as grimacing or wincing during the examination. These signs may indicate pain or a possible injury site. If the situation permits, the paramedic should perform the examination slowly and gently with consideration to the patient's feelings and needs.

Many older adults believe they will die in a hospital. If transportation is needed, patients may become fearful and anxious. The paramedic should be sensitive to these concerns. If appropriate, the paramedic can reassure patients that their condition is not serious. The paramedic should attempt to calm these patients and advise them that they will be well cared for in the hospital. The paramedic should record all examination findings carefully (see Chapter 16).

SUMMARY

- The examination techniques commonly used in the physical examination are inspection, palpation, percussion, and auscultation.
- Equipment used during the comprehensive physical examination includes the stethoscope, ophthalmoscope, otoscope, and blood pressure cuff.
- The physical examination is performed in a systematic manner. The exam is a step-by-step process. Emphasis is placed on the patient's present illness and chief complaint.
- The physical examination is a systematic assessment of the body that includes mental status, general survey, vital signs, skin, head, eyes, ears, nose and throat, chest, abdomen, posterior body, extremities, and neurological examination.
- The first step in any patient care encounter is to note the patient's appearance and behavior. This includes assessing for level of consciousness. This may include assessment of posture, gait and motor activity; dress, grooming, hygiene, and breath or body odors; facial expression; mood, affect, and relation to person and things; speech and language; thought and perceptions; and memory and attention.
- During the general survey, the paramedic should evaluate the patient for signs of distress, apparent state of health, skin color and obvious lesions, height and build, sexual development, and weight. The paramedic also should assess vital signs.
- The comprehensive physical examination should include an evaluation of the texture and turgor of the skin, hair, and fingernails and toenails.

- Examination of the structures of the head and neck involves inspection, palpation, and auscultation.
- A full knowledge of the structure of the thoracic cage is needed. This knowledge aids in performing a good respiratory and cardiac assessment. Air movement creates turbulence as it passes through the respiratory tree. Air movement produces breath sounds during inhalation and exhalation. In the prehospital setting the paramedic must examine the heart indirectly. However, the paramedic can obtain details about the size and effectiveness of pumping action through a skilled assessment that includes palpation and auscultation.
- The four quadrants of the abdomen and their contents provide the basis for inspection, auscultation, percussion, and palpation of this body region.
- An examination of the genitalia of either sex can be awkward for the patient and the paramedic. The paramedic should inspect the genitalia for bleeding and signs of trauma (if indicated).
- Examination of the anus is indicated in the presence of rectal bleeding or trauma to the area.
- When examining the upper and lower extremities, the paramedic should direct his or her attention to function. The paramedic also should pay attention to structure.
- Assessment of the spine begins with a visual assessment of the cervical, thoracic, and lumbar curves. The assessment continues with a region-by-region examination for pain, swelling, and range of motion.
- A neurological examination may be organized into five categories: mental status and speech, cranial nerves, motor system, sensory system, and reflexes.
- When approaching the pediatric patient, the paramedic should remain calm and confident. The paramedic should observe the child before beginning the physical examination. The paramedic also should make sure to avoid separation of the child and parent. Moreover, the paramedic must establish a rapport with parents and child and must be honest. One caregiver should be assigned to the child.
- The paramedic should not assume that all older adults are victims of disorders related to aging. Individual differences in knowledge, mental reasoning, experience, and personality influence how these patients respond to examination.

REFERENCES

1. Centers for Disease Control and Prevention: *Curriculum guide for public-safety and emergency-response workers: prevention of transmission of human immunodeficiency virus and hepatitis B virus,* Atlanta, 1989, US Government Printing Office.
2. US Department of Health and Human Services; National Institutes of Health; National Heart, Lung, and Blood Institute: *The Seventh Report of the Joint National Committee on Prevention, Detection, Evaluation, and Treatment of High Blood Pressure,* NIH Pub No 03-5233, Washington, DC, 2003, National Institutes of Health.
3. Potter P, Perry A: *Fundamentals of nursing: concepts, process, and practice,* ed 5, St Louis, 2001, Mosby.
4. Seidel J, Henderson D, editors: *Prehospital care of pediatric patients,* California EMSC Project, Los Angeles, 1987, American Academy of Pediatrics.

SUGGESTED READINGS

Epistein O et al: *Clinical examination,* London, 1992, Gower.

Seidel H et al: *Mosby's guide to physical examination,* ed 5, St Louis, 2003, Mosby.

Snell R, Smith M: *Clinical anatomy for emergency medicine,* St Louis, 1993, Mosby.

CHAPTER 12

Patient Assessment

OBJECTIVES

Upon completion of this chapter, the paramedic student will be able to:

1. Identify the components of the scene size-up.
2. Identify the priorities in each component of patient assessment.
3. Outline the critical steps in initial patient assessment.
4. Describe findings in the initial assessment that may indicate a life-threatening condition.
5. Discuss interventions for life-threatening conditions that are identified in the initial assessment.
6. Identify the components of the focused history and physical examination for medical patients.
7. Identify the components of the focused history and physical examination for trauma patients.
8. List the components of the detailed physical examination.
9. Describe the ongoing assessment.
10. Distinguish priorities in the care of the medical versus trauma patient.

KEY TERMS

focused history: A component of patient assessment to ascertain the patient's chief complaint, history of present illness, medical history, and current health status.

general impression: An immediate assessment of the environment and the patient's chief complaint used to determine whether the patient is ill or injured and the nature of the illness or the mechanism of injury.

initial assessment: A component of the patient assessment to recognize and manage all immediate life-threatening conditions.

ongoing assessment: A repeat of the initial assessment that is performed throughout the paramedic-patient encounter.

priority patients: Patients who need immediate care and transport.

scene size-up: An assessment of the scene to ensure scene safety for the paramedic crew, patient(s), and bystanders; a quick assessment to determine the resources needed to manage the scene adequately.

The prehospital setting usually lacks emergency physicians on the scene and diagnostic services. Because of this, priorities of care must be set based on patient assessment. These priorities include scene safety, recognition and management of life-threatening conditions, and identification of patients who require rapid stabilization and transport for definitive care. This chapter provides an overview of patient assessment. More in-depth assessment strategies are presented in this text by subject matter.

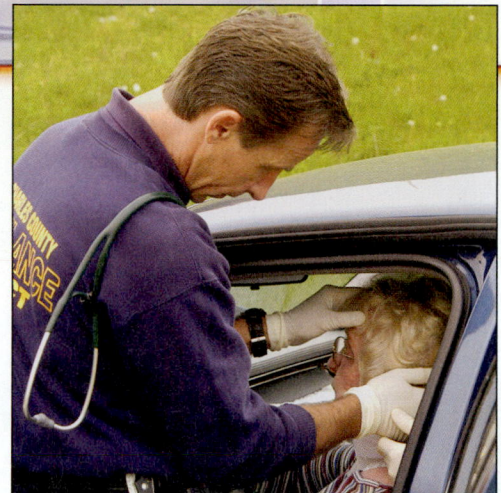

SCENE SIZE-UP AND ASSESSMENT

Scene size-up and assessment are the first steps taken during every emergency medical services response. These steps ensure scene safety for the paramedic crew, patient(s), and bystanders. The assessment of the scene and setting offer key information to the paramedic. The priorities in scene size-up and assessment include the following:

- Determine the nature of the incident.
- Determine the maximum potential number of persons already ill or injured and needing care.
- Assess for hazards at the scene.
- Initiate a mass casualty plan if called for (see Chapter 50).
- Notify the dispatch center to request more resources (e.g., law enforcement, fire, rescue, utility companies) and to alert area hospitals (as needed).
- Determine the best access routes and staging areas for responders.
- Secure the area as rapidly as possible, clearing unneeded persons from the scene.
- Begin triage (if needed).

Even scenes that seem safe may not be. Paramedics should never enter a potentially unsafe scene until they know it is safe to approach the patient. Examples of unsafe scenes include crash-and-rescue scenes, areas with toxic substances and low oxygen, crime scenes where violence is likely, and scenes that have unstable surfaces (e.g., slope, ice, or water). Personal safety is the first priority of the paramedic.

CRITICAL THINKING

Do you know a paramedic who has been injured on a scene? What caused the injury? Could the injury have been prevented?

Protective Clothing

The National Fire Protection Association[1] and Occupational Safety and Health Administration[2,3] standards for protective clothing and personal protective equipment have been adopted by many emergency response agencies. At a minimum, paramedics should have access to the following personal protective equipment (Fig. 12-1):

- Impact-resistant protective helmet with ear protection and chinstrap
- Safety goggles with vents to prevent fogging
- Lightweight, puncture-resistant turnout coat
- Slip-resistant waterproof gloves
- Boots with steel insoles and steel toe protection
- Self-contained breathing apparatus

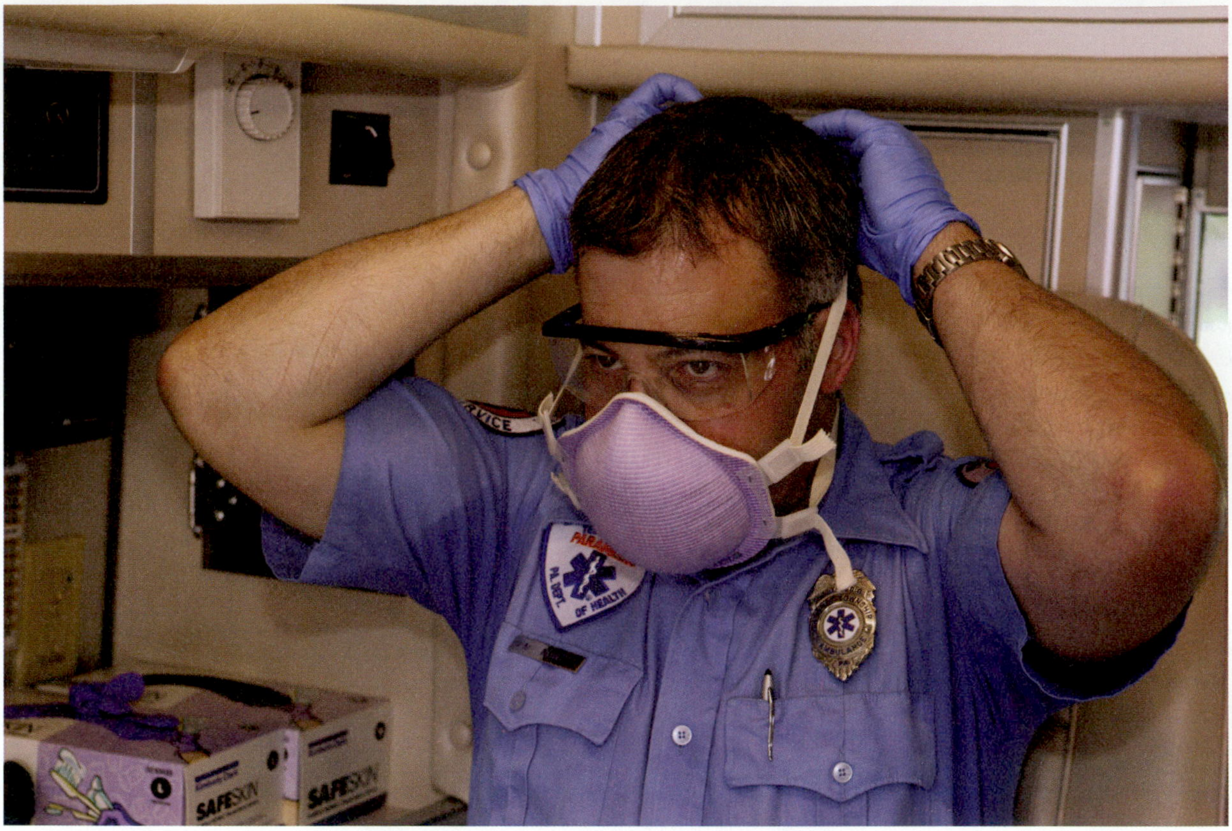

FIGURE 12-1 ■ Personal protective equipment.

Personal Protection from Blood-Borne Pathogens

The Occupational Safety and Health Act of 1991 adopted the recommendations established by the Centers for Disease Control and Prevention for personal protection from blood-borne pathogens. These universal precautions have been adopted by most states and public service entities. Now universal precautions are the minimum standard of practice recommended by the Occupational Safety and Health Administration (OSHA 29 CFR Part 1910.120). These precautions are intended to be used in the case of *all* patients in which the risk of exposure to blood or body fluids is increased. They also are intended to be used when the infection status of the patient is unknown. The paramedic should wash his or her hands before and after patient contact to reduce the risk of communicable disease infection. In addition, items of personal protection from blood-borne pathogens should include disposable gloves and masks, eye protection, and gowns when necessary. Personal protection from blood-borne pathogens is addressed further in Chapters 18 and 39. Table 12-1 summarizes the patient care activities and the recommended level of protection for these activities. These recommendations also are on the inside cover of this textbook.

PATIENT ASSESSMENT PRIORITIES

First, the emergency team must determine that the scene is safe. The team also must ensure that the needed resources are available or have been requested (Fig. 12-2). Then the emergency team can begin patient assessment (Fig. 12-3). Patient assessment involves the following four priorities[4]:

1. **Initial assessment:** to recognize and manage all immediate life-threatening conditions. Resuscitation may be necessary for critical patients (Box 12-1).
2. **Focused history** *and physical examination:* to obtain vital signs, reassess changes in the patient's condition, and perform appropriate physical examination for trauma and medical patients.
3. *Detailed physical examination:* to gather additional patient information.
4. **Ongoing assessment:** to continue monitoring the patient's status en route to the hospital and to provide treatment as necessary.

INITIAL ASSESSMENT

An initial assessment is performed on all patients. This assessment establishes priorities of care. The initial assessment consists of the paramedic's **general impression** of the patient. The assessment also includes finding condi-

TABLE 12-1 Examples of Recommended Personal Protective Equipment for Worker Protection against HIV and HBV Transmission* in Prehospital† Settings

TASK OR ACTIVITY	GLOVES	GOWN	PROTECTIVE MASK‡	EYEWEAR
Bleeding control with spurting blood	Yes	Yes	Yes	Yes
Bleeding control with minimal bleeding	Yes	No	No	No
Emergency childbirth	Yes	Yes	Yes, if splashing is likely	Yes, if splashing is likely
Blood drawing	Yes	No	No	No
Starting an intravenous line	Yes	No	No	No
Endotracheal intubation, esophageal obturator use	Yes	No	No, unless splashing is likely	No, unless splashing is likely
Oral/nasal suctioning, manually cleaning airway	Yes¶	No	No, unless splashing is likely	No, unless splashing is likely
Handling and cleaning of instruments	Yes	No, unless soiling is likely	No	No, unless microbial contamination is likely
Measuring blood pressure	No	No	No	No
Measuring temperature	No	No	No	No
Giving an injection	No	No	No	No

* The examples provided in this table are based on application of universal precautions. Universal precautions are intended to supplement rather than replace recommendations for routine infection control, such as handwashing and using gloves to prevent gross microbial contamination of hands (e.g., contact with urine or feces). *HIV,* Human immunodeficiency virus; *HBV,* hepatitis B virus.
† Defined as setting where delivery of emergency health care takes place away from a hospital or other health care facility.
‡ Refers to protective masks to prevent exposure of mucous membranes to blood or other potentially contaminated body fluids.
§ For clarification, see Appendix A.
¶ Although not clearly necessary to prevent HIV or HBV transmission unless blood is present, gloves are recommended to prevent transmission of other agents (e.g., herpes simplex).

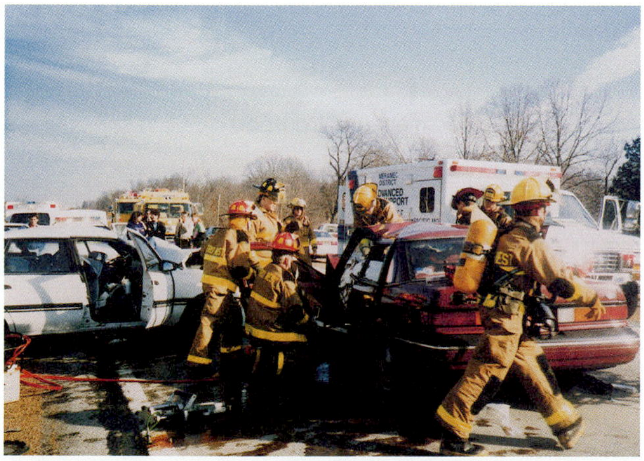

FIGURE 12-2 ■ Many resources may be needed at an emergency scene.

tions that threaten life and identifying **priority patients.** These patients need immediate care and transport.

General Impression of the Patient

The general impression is the paramedic's immediate assessment of the setting and the patient's chief complaint. The paramedic uses the general impression to determine whether the patient is ill or injured. The paramedic also uses the general impression to decide the nature of the illness or the mechanism of injury. As part of the general impression, the paramedic should identify the patient's general age, sex, and race.

Assessment for Life-Threatening Conditions

To assess for life-threatening conditions, the paramedic should conduct a systematic evaluation of the patient's level of consciousness, airway, breathing, and circulation.

LEVEL OF CONSCIOUSNESS

A priority with any patient is to assess the level of consciousness. This assessment usually can be done with a warm exchange with the patient. An example of such is "I'm a paramedic. How can I help you?" If the patient appears unconscious, gentle tactile stimulation (e.g., rubbing the patient's shoulder), along with questions such as "Are you okay?" and "Can you hear me?" may get a response. If the patient is unconscious or if spinal injury is suspected, the paramedic should immobilize the patient's cervical spine (see Chapter 25). The paramedic can assess the patient's level of consciousness quickly using the mnemonic evaluation *AVPU* (alert, verbal, painful, unresponsive).

CRITICAL THINKING

What does a patient's level of consciousness tell you about the patient's oxygenation and circulation?

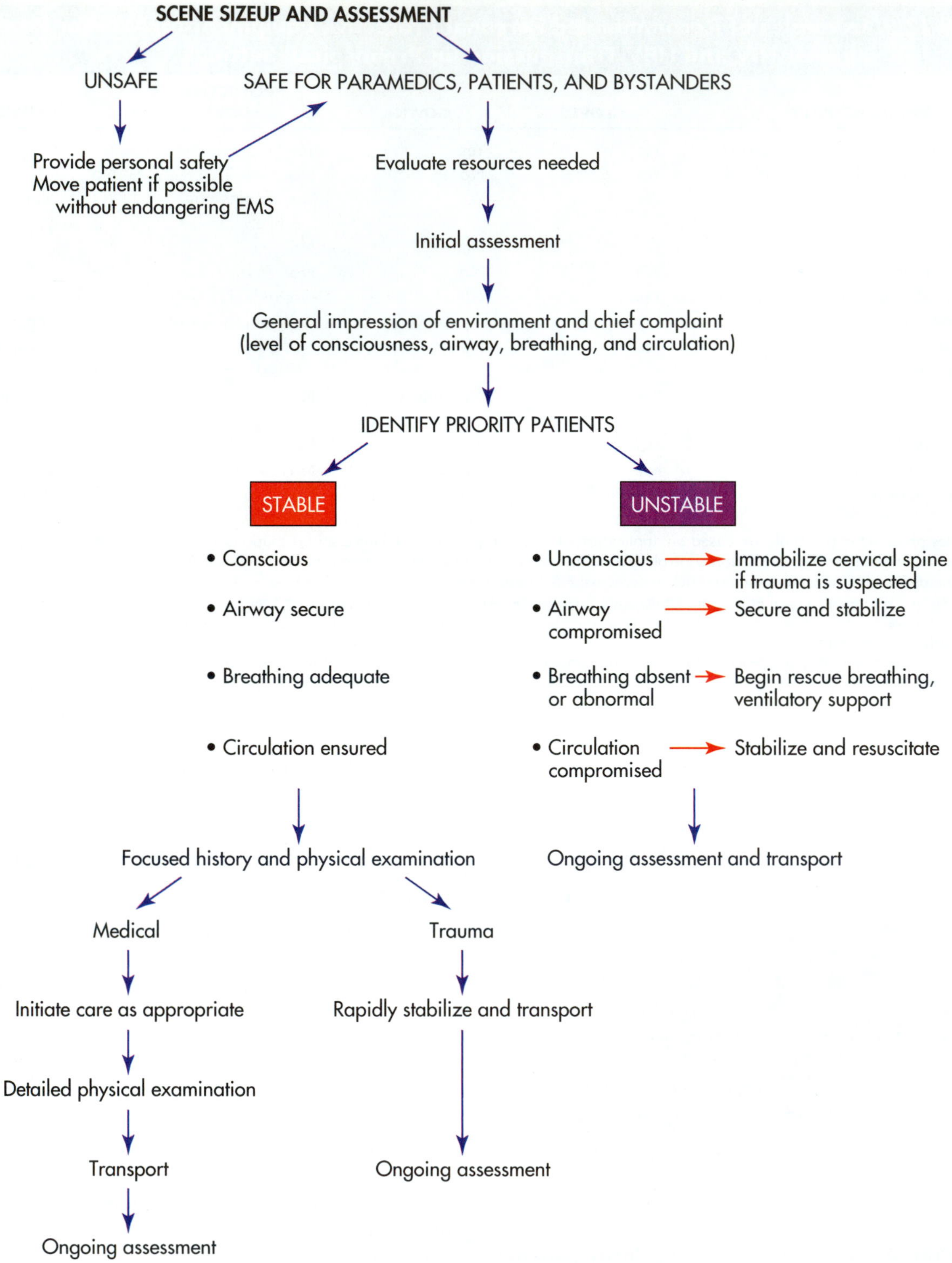
SCENE SIZEUP AND ASSESSMENT
UNSAFE
SAFE FOR PARAMEDICS, PATIENTS, AND BYSTANDERS
Provide personal safety
Move patient if possible without endangering EMS
Evaluate resources needed
Initial assessment
General impression of environment and chief complaint (level of consciousness, airway, breathing, and circulation)
IDENTIFY PRIORITY PATIENTS
STABLE
UNSTABLE
• Conscious
• Airway secure
• Breathing adequate
• Circulation ensured
• Unconscious
Immobilize cervical spine if trauma is suspected
• Airway compromised
Secure and stabilize
• Breathing absent or abnormal
Begin rescue breathing, ventilatory support
• Circulation compromised
Stabilize and resuscitate
Focused history and physical examination
Ongoing assessment and transport
Medical
Trauma
Initiate care as appropriate
Rapidly stabilize and transport
Detailed physical examination
Transport
Ongoing assessment
Ongoing assessment

FIGURE 12-3 ■ Components of patient assessment.

BOX 12-1 Resuscitation

Resuscitation may be called for during the initial assessment. The paramedic begins resuscitative measures such as airway maintenance, ventilatory assistance, and cardiopulmonary resuscitation immediately as needed after recognizing a life-threatening condition. Several emergency care procedures generally are required in situations involving seriously ill or injured patients. Nearly all medical and trauma patients, for example, need some form of supplemental oxygen. Other resuscitation procedures for medical and trauma patients are as follows:

Resuscitation Procedures for Medical Patients

- Oxygen and airway control
- Insertion of an intravenous line to administer drugs or volume-expanding fluid
- Administration of resuscitation medications
- Administration of electrical therapy (defibrillation, cardioversion, external pacing)

Resuscitation Procedures for Trauma Patients

- Oxygen and airway control
- Cervical spine immobilization
- Insertion of intravenous lines for volume-expanding fluid
- Administration of resuscitation medications
- Application of a pneumatic antishock garment if appropriate

AIRWAY

The paramedic should assess the airway for patency and can use one of three methods. The paramedic can see whether the patient can speak and can note signs of airway obstruction or respiratory insufficiency. These signs could include stridor or gurgling. Moreover, the paramedic can assess for patency by inspecting the oral cavity for foreign objects. Any condition that compromises the delivery of oxygen to body tissues is potentially life threatening. The paramedic must manage such a condition immediately. Factors that may compromise the airway include the following:

- Tongue obstructing the airway in an unconscious patient
- Loose teeth or foreign objects in the patient's airway
- Epiglottitis
- Upper airway obstruction from any cause
- Facial and oral bleeding
- Vomitus
- Soft-tissue trauma to the patient's face and neck
- Facial fractures

The paramedic must secure a compromised airway manually or with adjunct equipment (e.g., using modified jaw thrust, chin lift, oral or nasal airways, suction, or endotracheal or esophageal intubation with multilumen airways described in Chapter 19). When performing an airway procedure for patients who may have a cervical spine injury, the paramedic must keep manipulation of the cervical spine to a minimum. The paramedic must stabilize the head and neck in a neutral position. All patients must have an airway established and maintained during the initial assessment.

CRITICAL THINKING

Securing a patent airway should always receive priority over spinal immobilization. However, both are crucial tasks in the initial assessment.

The patient whose airway is obstructed by a foreign object should be managed using the guidelines currently recommended by the American Heart Association and the American Red Cross. If these maneuvers fail, medical direction may recommend direct laryngoscopy or cricothyrotomy (see Chapter 19).

BREATHING

The paramedic can assess breathing by evaluating the rate, depth, tidal volume, and symmetry of chest movement. He or she should expose the chest wall and palpate it for structural integrity, tenderness, and crepitus, observing for use of accessory muscles of respiration in the neck, chest, and abdomen. The paramedic should auscultate for the presence of bilateral breath sounds and should also listen to the patient's speech. A patient who has difficulty speaking without pain or who cannot talk without gasping for air may need ventilatory support. Respiratory abnormalities discovered during the physical examination that may indicate a potentially life-threatening condition include the following:

- Cyanosis
- Respiratory distress with dyspnea or hypoxia
- Asymmetrical chest wall movement
- Chest injury (e.g., tension pneumothorax, flail segment, open chest wound)
- Tracheal deviation
- Distended neck veins

Ill or injured patients with ineffective respirations need ventilatory support. These patients require supplemental high-concentration oxygen. If the respiratory rate of a critically ill or injured patient is less than 10 or more than 28 respirations per minute, ventilatory assistance may be needed. The paramedic may coordinate assisted ventilation with the patient's respiratory efforts. Or the paramedic may intersperse assisted ventilation between the patient's own respiratory efforts as needed to maintain adequate oxygenation.

CRITICAL THINKING

Some patients with respirations between 10 and 28 per minute may require assisted ventilation. Can you think of any such situations?

If respirations are absent, the paramedic should initiate rescue breathing with the patient. The paramedic can provide rescue breathing via a pocket mask. Positive-pressure ventilation, which can be provided via a bag-valve device, should follow. Endotracheal intubation may be indicated. The paramedic also should consider spinal precautions and barrier protection. The paramedic must take these precautions into account during all airway procedures (see Chapter 19).

CIRCULATION

The paramedic evaluates the patient's circulatory status after assessing airway and breathing. For trauma patients, this assessment includes a quick head-to-toe survey to spot and control severe bleeding. The paramedic should assess the patient's skin color, moisture, and temperature quickly. The paramedic also should evaluate the pulse for quality, rate, and regularity.

Pulse. A quick evaluation of the patient's pulse may reveal a normal heart rate, tachycardia, bradycardia, asystole, or an irregular heart rate. The site of an obtainable pulse also may offer critical details about a patient's systolic blood pressure and tissue perfusion. For example, a radial pulse may not be palpable in an uninjured extremity. Thus the patient is likely to be in a decompensated state of shock (hypoperfusion). A patient may lack a palpable femoral or carotid pulse. Thus the patient is in cardiopulmonary arrest.

Capillary refill. The capillary filling time may offer crucial details about the patient's cardiovascular status. The capillary refill test is thought to be most reliable in children younger than 12 years of age. The paramedic performs this test by blanching the patient's nail bed or the fleshy eminence at the base of the thumb. Then the paramedic observes the time it takes for normal color to return. A filling time of more than 2 seconds is caused by shunting and capillary closure to peripheral capillary beds. This indicates inadequate circulation and impaired cardiovascular function. Factors such as the patient's age, gender, and environment may affect the filling time. Thus the paramedic should use this test only as a possible indicator of circulatory status. Other signs and symptoms of inadequate circulation and impaired cardiovascular function include the following:

- Altered or decreased level of consciousness
- Distended neck veins
- Increased respiratory rate
- Pale, cool, diaphoretic skin
- Distant heart sounds
- Restlessness
- Thirst

> **CRITICAL THINKING**
>
> How do age, gender, and the environment affect capillary refill?

An unconscious person may lack a palpable femoral or carotid pulse. If this is the case, the paramedic should implement chest compressions and cardiac arrest protocols (see Chapter 29). In cases of severe external hemorrhage, the paramedic should control the bleeding using direct pressure, elevation, and pressure points (see Chapter 22). In most cases, these procedures to control bleeding also are effective during transport. Regardless of the cause, all patients with circulatory compromise need rapid stabilization. This may include intravenous administration of fluids, medications, and rapid transportation to an appropriate medical facility.

IDENTIFICATION OF PRIORITY PATIENTS

The paramedic uses the findings from the initial assessment to identify priority patients. These are patients who need stabilization and rapid transport. Examples of priority patients include those who have the following:

- Poor general impression
- Decreased level of consciousness (depressed or absent gag or cough reflex)
- No response to commands (unresponsiveness)
- Difficulty breathing
- Shock (hypoperfusion)
- Complicated childbirth
- Chest pain with a systolic pressure less than 100 mm Hg
- Uncontrolled bleeding
- Severe pain anywhere
- Multiple injuries

FOCUSED HISTORY AND PHYSICAL EXAMINATION: MEDICAL PATIENTS

For medical patients, their overall condition is crucial. The level of consciousness also is key. These two details dictate the focused history and physical examination. If the patient is responsive, the paramedic should assess the patient's history. The paramedic can do this by identifying the chief complaint, history of present illness, medical history, and current health status. The paramedic then performs a proper physical examination using the methods from Chapter 11. The paramedic should obtain a baseline set of vital signs. In addition, the paramedic should base emergency care on the signs and symptoms. The paramedic should provide this care in consultation with medical direction.

If the patient is unconscious, the paramedic should perform a rapid head-to-toe assessment. This assessment will help to identify any life-threatening conditions. The paramedic should give close attention to the airway of any patient with a decreased level of consciousness. The paramedic should assess baseline vital signs and if possible should obtain a patient history. The patient history may come from family, friends, bystanders, and/or medical identification devices (e.g., a medical alert bracelet or necklace).

FOCUSED HISTORY AND PHYSICAL EXAMINATION: TRAUMA PATIENTS

For a trauma patient, a focused history is used to identify and permit reconstruction of the mechanism of injury. Significant mechanisms of injury that identify priority patients include the following:

- Ejection from a vehicle
- Death in same passenger compartment

- Falls from greater than 20 feet
- Vehicle rollover
- High-speed vehicle collision
- Vehicle-pedestrian collision
- Motorcycle crash
- Injuries that cause unresponsive or altered mental status
- Penetration of the head, chest, or abdomen
- Hidden injuries (e.g., those caused by seat belts and air bags)

> **CRITICAL THINKING**
> A patient may have a mechanism of injury other than those listed here. Does that mean the patient has no life-threatening injuries?

Mechanisms of injury considered significant with infants and children include falls greater than 10 feet, bicycle collision, and medium-speed vehicle collision (see Chapter 20).

RAPID TRAUMA PHYSICAL EXAMINATION

The paramedic should perform a rapid trauma examination to identify life-threatening conditions on all patients with a significant mechanism of injury. In responsive patients the paramedic should seek symptoms before and during the trauma assessment. The rapid trauma physical examination is composed of the following:

- Continued spinal immobilization
- Mental status assessment
- Inspection and palpation of the head, neck, chest, abdomen, pelvis, and extremities for injuries or signs of injuries
- Inspection of the posterior surfaces of the body
- Baseline vital signs
- Patient history (chief complaint, history of present illness, medical history, current health status)

A patient without any significant mechanism of injury (e.g., a cut finger) should receive a proper assessment focused on the injury site. The paramedic should obtain baseline vital signs and a patient history.

DETAILED PHYSICAL EXAMINATION

The detailed physical examination should be specific to the patient and injury. A patient with a minor injury should not require a complete physical examination. A minor injury is a sprained ankle. However, an older patient who is having a hard time breathing is different. This patient should receive a detailed physical examination. A comprehensive and detailed physical examination (described in Chapter 11) includes the following:

- Mental status assessment
    - Appearance and behavior
    - Posture and motor activity
    - Speech and language
    - Mood
    - Thought and perceptions
    - Insight and judgment
    - Memory and attention
- General survey
    - Level of consciousness
    - Signs of distress
    - Apparent state of health
    - Skin color and obvious lesions
    - Height and build
    - Sexual development
    - Weight
    - Posture, gait, and motor activity
    - Dress, grooming, and personal hygiene
    - Odors on breath or body
    - Facial expression
- Examination of the following:
    - Skin
    - Head
    - Eyes
    - Ears
    - Nose and sinuses
    - Mouth and pharynx
    - Neck
    - Thorax and lungs
    - Cardiovascular system
    - Abdomen
    - Genitalia
    - Anus and rectum
    - Peripheral vascular system
    - Musculoskeletal system
    - Nervous system
- Baseline vital signs

ONGOING ASSESSMENT

The ongoing assessment is a repeat of the initial assessment. As the name implies, this assessment should be performed throughout the encounter with the patient. Stable patients are nonpriority patients. For these patients the paramedic should repeat the ongoing assessment and record it every 15 minutes. Unstable patients are priority patients. For these patients, the paramedic should perform the ongoing assessment every 5 minutes (at a minimum). The purpose of the ongoing assessment is as follows:

- To reassess mental status
- To reassess airway
- To monitor breathing for rate and quality
- To reassess circulation
- To reestablish patient priorities

> **CRITICAL THINKING**
> The ongoing assessment can identify trends in the patient's condition. What does that mean?

During the ongoing assessment, the paramedic also should reassess and record vital signs. The paramedic should investigate the patient complaint or injury further. In addition, the paramedic should assess the success of any interventions. This entails assessing the patient's response to patient care activities and determining the need to maintain or alter the care plan.

An ongoing assessment of the patient may help the paramedic to notice a trend. Full documentation of findings also may help the paramedic to see this trend in the assessment components. For example, a patient may have been cyanotic, hypotensive, and disoriented at the scene. After administering intravenous fluid therapy and high-concentration oxygen, this patient may have improved color and blood pressure. The patient also may appear to be more alert during transport. The documenting and reporting of trends in the assessment is crucial. Documentation helps other health care workers who are to assume care of the patient on arrival at the hospital.

CARE OF MEDICAL VERSUS TRAUMA PATIENTS

Much of the definitive care for medical patients often can be initiated in the prehospital setting. For some patients with heart problems and patients with respiratory difficulties and other medical emergencies, paramedic crews can institute proper care. Because of this, the time spent on scene with these medical patients may be slightly longer.

In contrast, most trauma patients require rapid transport. These patients should be taken to a proper medical facility for definitive care. Patients with internal bleeding, major fractures, head injury, and multiple-system trauma need life-saving care. This care can be provided only by specially trained physicians and support staff. Minimal time should be spent at the scene with these patients. Most trauma life-support training programs (e.g., basic trauma life support, prehospital trauma life support, and advanced trauma life support) recommend that patients needing immediate transport be stabilized and prepared for transport ("packaged") within 10 minutes after arrival of emergency medical services. Field management should be limited to airway control and ventilatory support, spinal immobilization, and major fracture stabilization. Intravenous fluid therapy should be initiated en route to the hospital. (Trauma management is addressed further in Part 6.)

SUMMARY

- Sizing up the scene consists of the initial steps performed on every emergency medical services response. These steps help to ensure scene safety. They also provide valuable information to the paramedic.
- Patient assessment comprises five priorities: initial assessment, resuscitation, focused history and physical examination, detailed physical examination, and ongoing assessment.
- The initial assessment includes the paramedic's general impression of the patient, the assessment for life-threatening conditions, and the identification of priority patients requiring immediate care and transport.
- Assessment of life-threatening conditions entails a systematic evaluation of the patient's level of consciousness, airway, breathing, and circulation.
- The paramedic begins resuscitative measures such as airway maintenance, ventilatory assistance, and cardiopulmonary resuscitation immediately after recognizing the life-threatening condition that necessitates each respective maneuver.
- The focused history and physical examination for medical patients are dictated by the patient's overall condition and level of consciousness.
- The paramedic performs a focused history for a trauma patient to reconstruct the mechanism of injury. The paramedic should perform a rapid trauma examination on all patients with a significant mechanism of injury to identify life-threatening conditions.
- The detailed physical examination should be specific to the patient. The exam also should be specific to the injury. The exam should include an assessment of mental status, general survey, a head-to-toe examination, and baseline vital signs.
- The ongoing assessment is a repeat of the initial assessment.

REFERENCES

1. National Fire Protection Association: *Standards on protective clothing for structural fire fighting; NFPA 1999,* Quincy, Mass, 1999, The Association.
2. Occupational Safety and Health Administration: *Fire brigade regulation,* 29 CFR 1910.156, Washington, DC, 1980, The Administration.
3. Occupational Safety and Health Administration: *Hazardous waste operations and emergency response (HAZWOPER),* Standard 1910.120, Washington, DC, 1990, The Administration.
4. US Department of Transportation, National Highway Traffic Safety Administration: *EMT-Paramedic national standard curriculum,* Washington, DC, 1998, US Government Printing Office.

CHAPTER

13

Clinical Decision Making

OBJECTIVES

Upon completion of this chapter, the paramedic student will be able to:

1. List the key elements of paramedic practice.
2. Discuss the limitations of protocols, standing orders, and patient care algorithms.
3. Outline the key components of the critical thinking process for paramedics.
4. Identify elements necessary for an effective critical thinking process.
5. Describe situations that may necessitate the use of the critical thinking process while delivering prehospital patient care.
6. Describe the six elements required for effective clinical decision making in the prehospital setting.

KEY TERMS

application of principle: A component of critical thinking in which the examiner makes patient care decisions based on conceptual understanding of the situation and interpretation of data gathered from the patient.

concept formation: A component of critical thinking that refers to all elements that are gathered to form a general impression of the patient.

data interpretation: A component of critical thinking in which the examiner gathers the necessary data to form a field impression and working diagnosis.

evaluation: A component of critical thinking in which the examiner assesses the patient's response to care.

reflection on action: A component of critical thinking (usually performed after the event) in which the examiner evaluates a patient care episode for possible improvement in similar future responses.

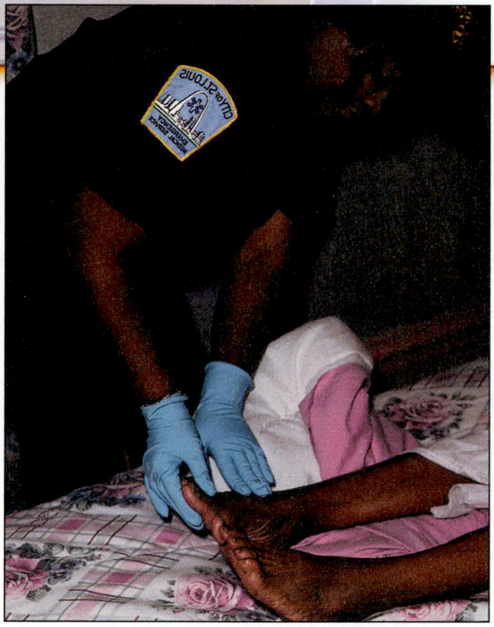

Unique to the emergency medical services profession is the uncertainty of the prehospital environment. The uncertainty is influenced heavily by factors that do not exist in other medical settings. Paramedics must be able to gather, weigh, and synthesize information. They also must be able to develop and apply proper patient care plans. In addition, they must apply judgment and exercise decision making. They must think and work well under pressure. These are the cornerstones of effective paramedic practice.

THE SPECTRUM OF PREHOSPITAL CARE

As described in Chapters 11 and 12, the paramedic must have a wide base of knowledge and skills to make good patient care decisions in the prehospital setting. On any given workday, the paramedic may be exposed to obvious critical life threats, potential life threats, and non–life-threatening situations (Box 13-1). On each call the emergency medical services provider also is expected to provide proper care and treatment.

BOX 13-1 Spectrum of Prehospital Care

Obvious Critical Life Threats
Major multisystem trauma
Devastating single-system trauma
End-stage disease presentations
Acute presentations of chronic conditions

Potential Life Threats
Serious multisystem trauma
Multiple disease etiologies

Non–Life-Threatening Presentations
Minor illness or injury
Emergency medical services system misuse

Protocols, standing orders, and patient care algorithms help to promote a standardized approach to patient care for classic presentations. These presentations clearly define and outline performance parameters. However, these standards have some limitations. First, they may not apply to nonspecific patient complaints. These complaints are ones that do not fit the model. Second, these standards do not take into account multiple disease etiologies or multiple treatment modalities. Third, they promote linear thinking ("cookbook medicine"). The paramedic must develop critical thinking skills. These skills will assist in unique patient care situations.

CRITICAL THINKING PROCESS FOR PARAMEDICS

Specific aspects, stages, and sequences are linked with the critical thinking process.[1] These include **concept formation, data interpretation, application of principle, evaluation,** and **reflection on action** (Fig. 13-1).

Concept Formation

Concept formation refers to all elements gathered to form a general impression of the patient. Concept formation is the "what" of the patient story. These elements are described in Chapters 11 and 12 and include the following:

- Scene assessment (mechanism of injury, social setting)
- Chief complaint

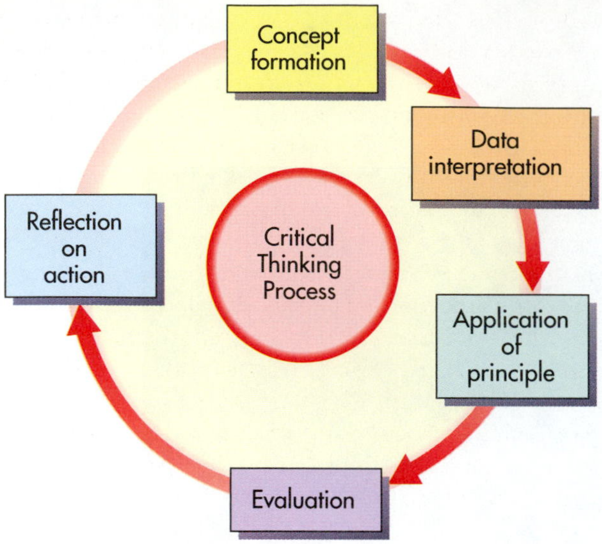

FIGURE 13-1 ■ Critical thinking process.

- Patient history
- Patient affect
- Initial assessment and physical examination
- Diagnostic tests

SCENARIO PART ONE

Your crew has been dispatched to a local park for a person with "difficulty breathing." On your arrival at the scene, you find an 18-year-old female sitting on a park bench surrounded by her friends. The scene is safe. She is crying and tells you that she cannot catch her breath. You attempt to calm the patient and provide her with supplemental oxygen. You obtain a history from the patient and her friends that she and her boyfriend had quarreled recently and that she became emotional during the argument. Her lung sounds are clear. She has no allergies and no significant medical history other than a recent sinus infection and denies any injury or pain. Aside from her increased respiratory rate, her vital signs are within normal range. Consider your concept formation for this patient.

> **CRITICAL THINKING**
> What effect would wrong or incomplete concept formation have on your critical thinking process during patient care? How can you enhance your concept formation skills while in your paramedic program?

Data Interpretation

Following concept formation, the paramedic must gather the needed data to form a field impression. This process also helps the paramedic to form a working diagnosis. This is the "working phase" of patient care. The quality of data interpretation rests on a few elements: the paramedic's knowledge of anatomy and physiology and of pathophysiology and previous experience in providing patient care. During the interpretation of data, the paramedic tries to get a full picture of the patient's situation. The paramedic's attitude can affect the success of this phase. The interaction between the paramedic and patient also can affect data interpretation (see Chapter 9). In some cases, the paramedic must condense and convey these data to the online physician. This physician can help the paramedic to decide on the right actions to take.

SCENARIO PART TWO

While assessing this patient, you recall a similar emergency response. In that response, you provided care to a young male with difficulty breathing. He had just lost a big tennis match. At first you assumed that the patient was having breathing difficulty because of emotions that resulted from his loss. Like the female patient you are caring for now, this male patient had no allergies and no significant medical history and denied any recent injury. His vital signs were within normal range. However, lung sounds were diminished slightly on the patient's left side. The patient also complained of mild pain on inspiration. You administered supplemental oxygen. Then you rapidly transported the patient to the emergency department. After obtaining a chest x-ray film, the emergency physician confirmed your suspicion of a spontaneous pneumothorax (which resolved during the patient's hospitalization). Compare this interpretation of data to that of the female patient you are caring for now.

Application of Principle

The next step in the critical thinking process is the application of principles of proper patient care. These principles are based on the paramedic's conceptual understanding of the situation. They also are based on the interpretation of the data gathered from the patient. Once the paramedic establishes the field impression and working diagnosis, the paramedic initiates treatment and intervention through protocols and standing orders or direct/online medical direction.

SCENARIO PART THREE

Based on your experience, your knowledge of patient care, and your interpretation of the data gathered from your patient, you decide that she is hyperventilating. You initiate proper treatment with calming measures. You encourage her to slow her respiratory rate. Although the female patient you are caring for presented much like the male patient you recall, your working diagnosis is different. You reach this conclusion because the female patient had clear, bilateral lung sounds. She also denied any pain on respiration.

Evaluation

The paramedic must evaluate the patient's response to the care on an ongoing basis. Evaluation includes the following:

- Reassessment of the patient (ongoing assessment)
- Reflection of action (effectiveness of the intervention)
- Revision of field impression (a change in the working diagnosis)

- Review of the appropriateness of the protocol, standing orders, or direct orders for the patient
- Revision of the treatment or intervention as needed

SCENARIO PART FOUR

After you have provided calming measures and oxygen to your patient, she has slowed her breathing. She also appears to be more relaxed. You reassess the patient. You find that her vital signs remain normal and her lung sounds remain clear. Based on these findings, you know that your field impression of hyperventilation was correct and that there is no need to change your working diagnosis or to revise your treatment. After consulting with medical direction, the decision is made that the patient's condition does not warrant transportation for physician evaluation.

Reflection on Action

Reflection on action occurs after the event. Reflection usually occurs through a run critique. In this the paramedic evaluates the care episode for improvement in similar future reponses. Reflection on action provides paramedics with an avenue to add to or alter their experience base.

SCENARIO PART FIVE

En route back to quarters, you discuss the call with a paramedic student. This student has just begun her field internship. Like you, she instantly thought that the patient was hyperventilating because of the fight that she had with her boyfriend. The paramedic student admitted that she had read about a spontaneous pneumothorax in her emergency medical technician training. However, she had never seen a patient who had one. Moreover, she would not have considered this possibility when caring for this patient. You discuss the pathology of a tension pneumothorax with her and the importance of assessing bilateral lung sounds in a patient who is having trouble breathing. This reflection on action reinforces your data interpretation skills and adds to the student's experience base.

FUNDAMENTAL ELEMENTS OF CRITICAL THINKING FOR PARAMEDICS

For an effective critical thinking process, some basic elements must be present. These elements include adequate knowledge and the ability to do the following:

- Focus on specific and multiple elements of data at the same time.
- Gather and organize data and form concepts.
- Identify and deal with medical ambiguity. This may include patients who do not fit the model.
- Differentiate between relevant and irrelevant data.
- Analyze and compare similar situations from past experience.
- Recall cases in which the working diagnosis was wrong.
- Articulate decision-making reasoning and construct arguments to support or discount the decision.

All of these elements were present in the previous scenario. At the scene the paramedic dealt with the patient's symptoms. He dealt with the input of friends as well. In addition, he focused on assessment and history findings. At the same time, he offered initial emergency care. The paramedic did this all within moments of arriving at the patient's side. He gathered and organized the data. He then concluded that the patient fit the model for hyperventilation syndrome. The paramedic also decided that the patient's sinus infection was not likely related to her present respiratory troubles. He recalled a certain case. In that case, his initial working diagnosis of hyperventilation syndrome was wrong. The paramedic used clinical decision making to support his diagnosis of hyperventilation syndrome. His decision making was based on his experience and on his assessment findings.

FIELD APPLICATION OF ASSESSMENT-BASED PATIENT MANAGEMENT

Assessment-based patient management places huge responsibility on the paramedic. (This is described further in Chapter 14.) The paramedic must have a systematic means of analyzing a patient's problems, determining how to solve them, carrying out a plan of action, and evaluating effectiveness of the treatment. The success of assessment-based patient management in the prehospital setting depends on an integration of interpersonal skills, scientific knowledge, and physical activities (skills).

The Patient Crisis Severity Spectrum

Emergency medical services is set into action daily for many reasons. Yet few prehospital calls present true threats to life. Minor medical and trauma events call for little critical thinking. They result in fairly easy decision making for the paramedic. Likewise, patients with clear life threats pose limited critical thinking challenges because they often fit the model for standardized treatment (e.g., cardiac arrest). However, some patients fall in the spectrum between minor and life-threatening events. These patients pose the most critical thinking challenges for the paramedic. An example is patients with mild to moderate respiratory distress. Another is patients with diffuse abdominal pain. Either of these situations could be minor or could have life-threatening elements.

Thinking under Pressure

Hormonal influences from the fight-or-flight response (described in Chapter 2) can have positive and negative effects on critical decision making. The response may offer greater visual acuity and auditory keenness. The response also allows for improved reflexes and strength. These can be helpful when one must make decisions and act on them. The negative aspects of the response may include reduced critical thinking skills. This can result from a decrease in the ability to concentrate and assess. The key to strong performance under pressure is mental conditioning. This results in instinctive performance and automatic responses for technical procedures.

Mental Checklist for Thinking under Pressure

Mental conditioning takes a good deal of practice. A checklist for thinking under pressure may help the paramedic to concentrate during stressful events. The mental checklist the paramedic should use is as follows:

- Stop and think.
- Scan the situation.
- Decide and act.
- Maintain clear and effective control.
- Regularly and continually reevaluate the patient.

CRITICAL THINKING

Do you think you can improve your performance under pressure by practicing imaginary critical situations in your head? Why or why not?

Practicing this checklist when under pressure will result in behaviors that refine clinical decision making. One of these positive behaviors is staying calm (not panicking). Another is assuming a plan for the worst case (erring on the side of the patient). A third is maintaining a systematic assessment pattern. In addition, the paramedic can learn to balance the various styles of situation analysis, data processing, and decision making. Applying the styles of situational analysis (reflective versus impulsive), data processing (divergent versus convergent), and decision making (anticipatory versus reactive) allows the paramedic to provide the best possible care in most situations. In time, paramedics are able to apply all of these approaches with skill.

SITUATIONAL ANALYSIS: REFLECTIVE VERSUS IMPULSIVE

In most patient care situations, paramedics should avoid closing off the pursuit of data too quickly. One may do this to try to reach a correct working diagnosis. For example, consider a patient who has abdominal pain in his lower right quadrant. This patient should not be assigned automatically a working diagnosis of appendicitis. (This is an impulsive decision because the patient fits the model.) Rather the paramedic should take time to reflect on other conditions. A condition such as food poisoning could be the cause of the patient's pain. In other situations (e.g., a patient with foreign body airway obstruction), the impulsive decision to clear the patient's airway with chest thrusts and back blows would be the most prudent course of action to follow.

DATA PROCESSING: DIVERGENT VERSUS CONVERGENT

Paramedics should avoid the trap of gathering only partial data. This may lead them down the wrong diagnostic or therapeutic path (a result of impulsive situational analysis). This is known as convergent data processing. The convergent approach may be best in some cases (e.g., giving a standard drug dose to a patient in cardiac arrest). However, the convergent approach can hinder care in complex cases (e.g., an elderly patient with multiple complaints). A divergent approach in data processing looks at all sides of a case. The paramedic does this before arriving at a solution (e.g., multiple illnesses and polydrug use in the elderly patient).

DECISION MAKING: ANTICIPATORY VERSUS REACTIVE

A paramedic's decision making can be seen as anticipatory or reactive. With reactive decision making, one waits until a problem occurs before starting treatment. This can affect patient care negatively. An example of this is waiting to address respiratory compromise in a patient with an allergic reaction until the patient has trouble breathing. The process that health care workers should use is anticipatory decision making. Anticipatory decision making is based on ongoing data collection and evaluation of the patient's condition. Using the same example, the paramedic applying this kind of decision making would treat early signs and symptoms of an allergic reaction. The paramedic would administer oxygen and medications. The paramedic also would have intubation equipment ready to manage the patient's airway. This would be in anticipation of respiratory compromise.

PUTTING IT ALL TOGETHER: THE SIX R'S

To put all components required for effective clinical decision making into action, the paramedic can think in terms of the six *R*'s listed next (Fig. 13-2):

1. *Read the patient.* The paramedic should observe the patient's level of consciousness and skin color. The paramedic should note the patient's position along with any obvious deformity or asymmetry. The paramedic can determine the chief complaint by talking to the patient. The paramedic also can identify the presence of a worsening or preexisting condition. The paramedic should evaluate skin temperature and moisture and assess the pulse for rate, strength, and regularity. Auscultation of the lungs will reveal upper or lower airway problems. The paramedic should identify all life threats and obtain an accurate set of vital signs.

NOTE Vital signs can be used as a triage tool. The paramedic can use vital signs to estimate severity. Vital signs also can help the paramedic identify the majority of life-threatening conditions. The paramedic should remember that the patient's age and physical and medical conditions can affect vital signs. Currently used medication also can affect vital signs.

2. *Read the scene.* As a part of the scene size-up, the paramedic should assess general environmental conditions. The paramedic should evaluate the immediate sur-

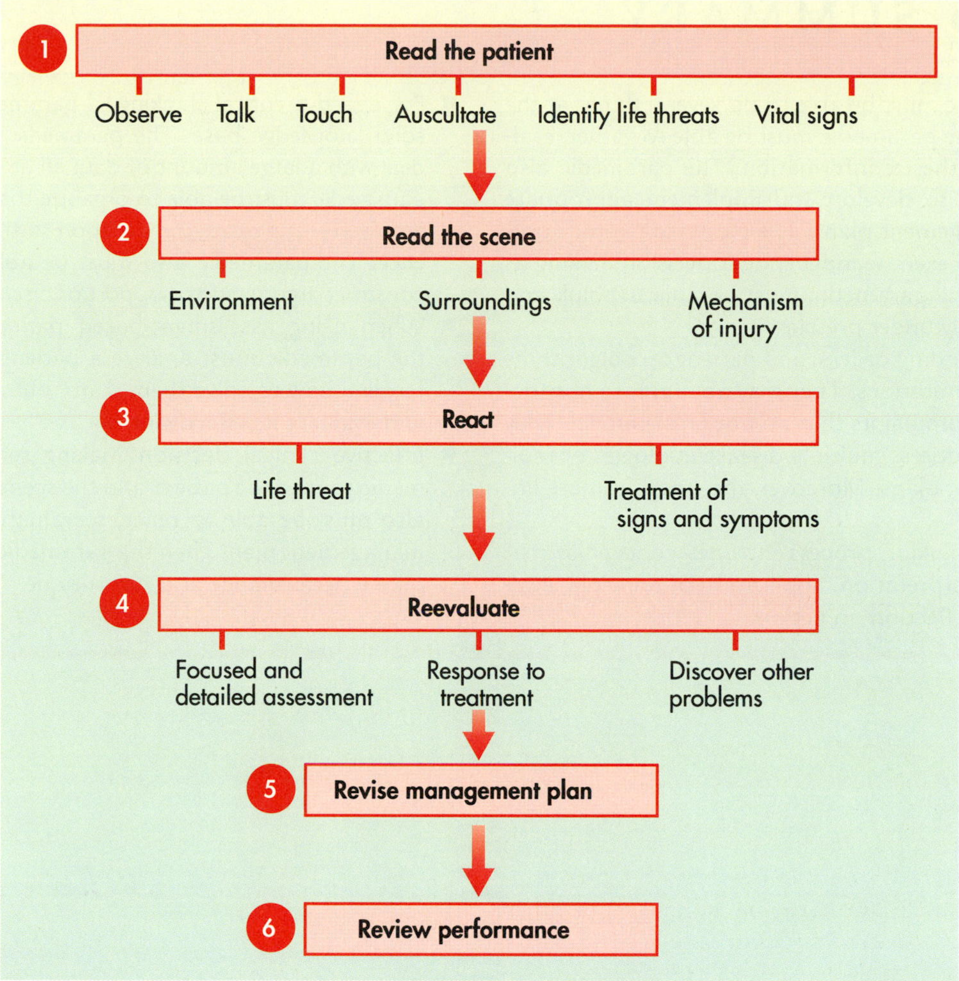

FIGURE 13-2 ■ The six *R*'s.

roundings and should attempt to identify any mechanism of injury.

3. *React.* The paramedic should manage all life threats in the order in which they are found. The paramedic should decide on the most common and likely cause of the life threat that fits the patient's initial presentation. The paramedic may not identify a clearly defined and recognizable presentation of medical illness in a priority patient. Thus treatment should be based on presenting signs and symptoms.
4. *Reevaluate.* Reevaluation includes a focused and detailed assessment. This assessment analyzes the patient's response to management and interventions and may lead the paramedic to find other problems. These problems may not have been evident during the initial assessment.
5. *Revise management plan.* Findings obtained during reevaluation may require the paramedic to revise the management plan. This revision will address more clearly the needs of the patient. The facts that patient conditions change and that patients do not respond in the same way to identical treatment intervention highlight the importance of ongoing assessment.
6. *Review performance at run critique.* A paramedic can review the details of the call through a run critique. This allows for the identification of areas that can be improved on similar calls in the future. The interest and investment of paramedics in the outcome of their personal cases often is the strongest stimulus to change their practice patterns favorably. This process also enhances the paramedic's experience base and in turn leads to improvement of data interpretation skills.

CRITICAL THINKING

Consider a negative or punitive run critique. How do you think this would influence your ability to perform under a similar circumstance in the future?

SUMMARY

- The paramedic must be able to do several things at the same time. The paramedic must be able to gather, evaluate, and synthesize information. The paramedic also must be able to develop and implement appropriate patient management plans. The paramedic must apply judgment and exercise independent decision making as well. Lastly, the paramedic must be able to think and work effectively under pressure.
- Protocols, standing orders, and patient care algorithms have several limitations. They may not apply to nonspecific patient complaints that do not fit the model. They also do not address multiple disease etiologies or multiple treatment plans. Moreover, they may promote linear thinking.
- The critical thinking process includes concept formation, data interpretation, application of principle, evaluation, and reflection on action.
- For effective critical thinking, a paramedic must have a solid knowledge base. The paramedic must be able to deal with a large amount of data all at once as well. The paramedic must be able to organize that data, deal with ambiguity, and relate the situation to similar past experience. The paramedic also must be able to reason and construct arguments to support or discount the decision.
- When using assessment-based patient management, the paramedic must analyze a patient's problems, determine how to solve them, carry out a plan of action, and evaluate its effectiveness.
- Effective clinical decision making requires the paramedic to read the patient and the scene. The paramedic also must be able to react, reevaluate, and revise the management plan. Then the paramedic must be able to review performance at a run critique.

REFERENCE

1. US Department of Transportation, National Highway Traffic Safety Administration: *EMT-Paramedic national standard curriculum*, Washington, DC, 1998, The Department.

SUGGESTED READINGS

Alfaro-Lefevre R: *Critical thinking in nursing: a practical approach,* Philadelphia, 1999, WB Saunders.

Benner P et al: *Clinical wisdom and interventions in critical care: a thinking-in-action approach,* Philadelphia, 1999, WB Saunders.

Pesut D, Herman J: *Clinical reasoning: the art and science of critical and creative thinking,* Albany, NY, 1999, Delmar Learning.

Potter P: *Virtual clinical excursions to accompany basic nursing: a critical thinking approach,* ed 5, St Louis, 2000, Mosby.

CHAPTER

14

Assessment-Based Management

OBJECTIVES

Upon completion of this chapter, the paramedic student will be able to:

1. Discuss how assessment-based management contributes to effective patient and scene assessment.
2. Describe factors that affect assessment and decision making in the prehospital setting.
3. Outline effective techniques for scene and patient assessment and choreography.
4. Identify essential take-in equipment for general and selected patient situations.
5. Outline strategies for patient approach that promote an effective patient encounter.
6. Describe techniques to permit efficient and accurate presentation of the patient.

KEY TERMS

action plan: A plan of action based on the patient's condition and the environment.

field impression: An impression of the patient's condition that the paramedic makes from pattern recognition and gut instinct that results from experience.

pattern recognition: The process of comparing gathered information with the paramedic's knowledge base of medical illness and disease.

presenting the patient: The effective communication and transfer of patient information in the course of out-of-hospital and hospital care.

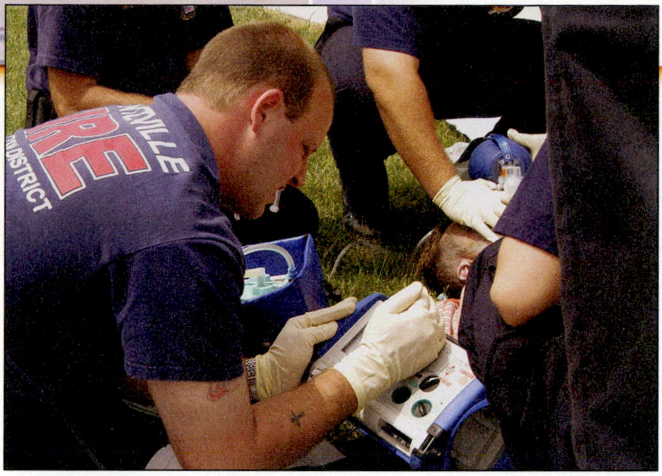

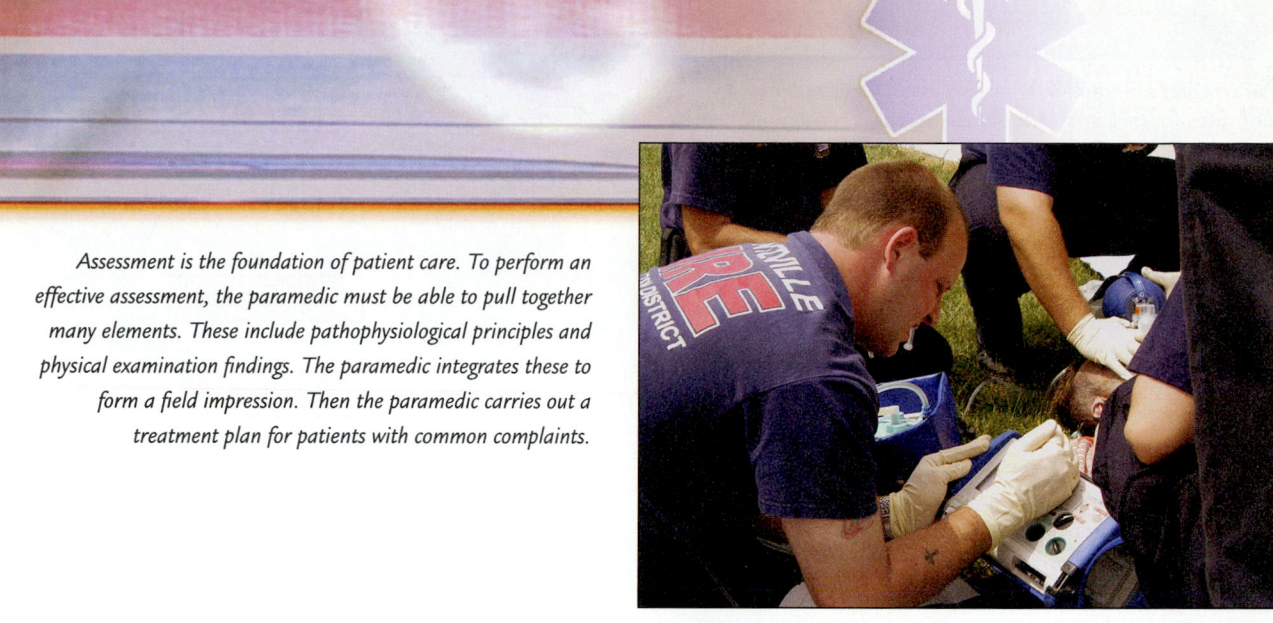

Assessment is the foundation of patient care. To perform an effective assessment, the paramedic must be able to pull together many elements. These include pathophysiological principles and physical examination findings. The paramedic integrates these to form a field impression. Then the paramedic carries out a treatment plan for patients with common complaints.

EFFECTIVE ASSESSMENT

Assessment-based management "puts it all together." The paramedic gathers, weighs, and synthesizes the information. The paramedic makes decisions based on this information. Then the paramedic takes appropriate actions required for the patient's care.

As described throughout this text, effective assessment depends on two things: the patient's history and the physical examination. Often as much as 80% of a medical diagnosis is based on the patient's history.[1] The paramedic's knowledge of disease helps him or her to hold a high degree of suspicion for possible illness. This knowledge also helps the paramedic to focus the history toward the complaint and associated problems. The paramedic must focus the exam toward body systems associated with the complaint as well. Some field situations may impair the thoroughness of the examination. For example, unsafe scenes or entrapment may hinder this process. Still, the paramedic must not overlook the value of the physical examination. The paramedic also must not perform the exam hastily.

Pattern Recognition

Paramedics first need to obtain the patient's history and perform the physical examination. Next, they can compare the details gathered with their knowledge base of illness and disease. They must ask whether the history and physical examination match a pattern of illness. For example, consider a 55-year-old man with chest pain and shortness of breath. This person matches a pattern for acute myocardial infarction. However, a 20-year-old woman with similar complaints would not match this pattern. Another example is a 4-year-old who is in respiratory distress and drooling. This patient matches a pattern for epiglottitis. Consider an older woman with distended neck veins and respiratory congestion who produces a pink, frothy sputum when she coughs. This person matches a pattern for congestive heart failure. **Pattern recognition** makes it possible for the paramedic to form a **field impression** and to begin a treatment plan (Box 14-1). Thus the greater the paramedic's knowledge, the better. Likewise, the greater the quality of the assessment details, the greater the chance for a correct assessment and good decision making.

CRITICAL THINKING

How can pattern recognition lead you down the wrong path?

Field Impression and Action Plan

The paramedic forms a field impression of the patient's condition from pattern recognition and gut instinct that comes from experience (Fig. 14-1). Once the paramedic forms a field impression, the paramedic can form an **action plan.** This plan is based on the patient's condition and the environment. Using the previous example of the two patients with

BOX 14-1 Pattern Recognition for Various Patient Presentations

Paramedics are trained in patient assessment and management priorities for patients with the following:

- Acute abdominal pain
- Allergic reactions
- Altered mental status
- Behavioral problems
- Chest pain
- Dyspnea
- Environmental or thermal problem
- Gastrointestinal bleeding
- Hazardous material or toxic exposure
- Medical and traumatic cardiac arrest
- Obstetrical or gynecological problems
- Seizures
- Syncope
- Trauma or multitrauma

chest pain, the field impression of the 55-year-old patient most likely leads to an action plan that includes the administration of oxygen, electrocardiograph monitoring, intravenous therapy, administration of ***aspirin***, pain relief, and perhaps drug therapy for cardiac rhythm disturbances. The 20-year-old patient's action plan most likely includes administration of oxygen, electrocardiograph monitoring to evaluate cardiac rhythm, and a more thorough assessment to detect a recent respiratory illness to rule out the possibility of pleurisy or pneumonia. (See Chapter 30.)

NOTE The paramedic should not ignore a gut instinct. If something seems wrong, the paramedic should keep looking. Gut instincts often help the paramedic to identify subtle physical findings. These findings are hard to quantify (e.g., patient affect or dull and lackluster eyes).

Following the field impression and the action plan, the paramedic provides basic life support and advanced life support treatment (Fig. 14-2). The paramedic bases this treatment on knowledge of the protocols and on judgment, that is, knowing when and how to apply the protocols. Judgment also involves knowing when it is appropriate to deviate from the protocols. For example, consider the administration of concentrated glucose to an unconscious diabetic patient. This patient is over 50 years of age and may have had a stroke. The administration can exacerbate cerebral damage. (See Chapter 32.) The cause of altered mental status indicates the need for the paramedic to deviate from a common protocol used to manage patients with suspected hypoglycemia.

CRITICAL THINKING

How can you continue to improve your patient care judgment?

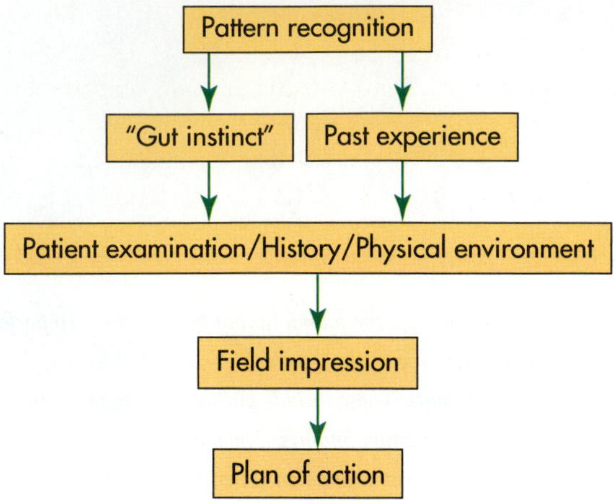

FIGURE 14-1 ■ Matrix pattern.

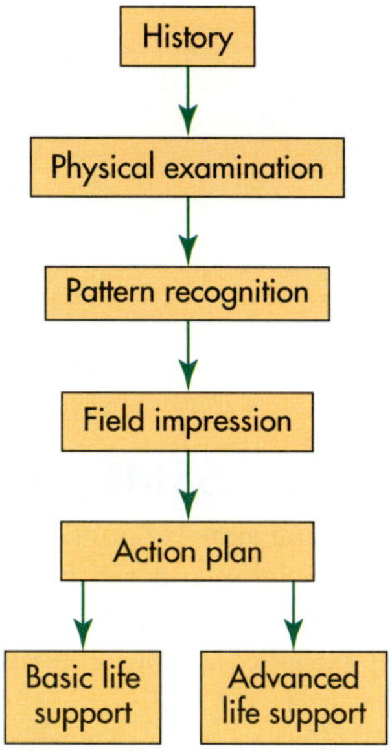

FIGURE 14-2 ■ Effective assessment.

Factors That Affect Assessment and Decision Making

Many factors can affect the quality of assessment and decision making by the paramedic. The following factors are discussed in this section:

- Paramedic's attitude
- Patient's willingness to cooperate
- Distracting injuries
- Labeling and tunnel vision
- Environment
- Patient compliance
- Considerations of personnel availability

CRITICAL THINKING

Have you ever seen any of these factors affect patient care?

PARAMEDIC'S ATTITUDE

The paramedic must be professional in all actions. Professionalism will help the paramedic to perform an effective assessment. The paramedic also must be nonjudgmental. A biased attitude can short circuit the information gathering process. This in turn can cause the paramedic to overlook key patient data. For example, a paramedic may assume that an indigent patient is intoxicated. Thus the paramedic may not consider complications from diabetes. The paramedic also may not consider hypoxia and hypovolemia that may have resulted from an internal injury.

PATIENT'S WILLINGNESS TO COOPERATE

Patients who do not cooperate can complicate the patient assessment. The assessment is required for the paramedic to formulate an action plan. As is discussed in later chapters, the paramedic should evaluate patients who are uncooperative, restless, or belligerent for the following conditions:

- Alcohol or other drug intoxication
- Head injury or concussion
- Hypoglycemia
- Hypothermia
- Hypovolemia
- Hypoxia
- Psychiatric illness
- Stroke

DISTRACTING INJURIES

Obvious but non-life-threatening injuries can distract the paramedic. These injuries may prevent the paramedic from doing a thorough assessment for more serious problems. Examples include open fractures and facial bleeding that is profuse. If needed, the paramedic should cover these wounds with dressings during the assessment. This will help the paramedic to focus on the more serious problems.

LABELING AND TUNNEL VISION

Labeling and tunnel vision can lead to an incorrect assessment and field impression. For example, labeling a patient as "just another drunk" can lead to a biased assessment. The same can happen by labeling someone who has been transported by ambulance many times for imagined illness as a "frequent flyer." Likewise, tunnel vision is assuming an incorrect field impression based on gut instinct. Tunnel vision also can be thought of as focusing on a portion of the presenting illness and thereby missing the big picture. This can result in a rushed judgment early in the patient assessment and in turn can result in an improper action plan.

ENVIRONMENT

Factors in the environment can have a significant impact. In fact, such factors can affect assessment techniques and decision making at the scene adversely. Examples include scene chaos, violent or dangerous situations, crowds of bystanders or other emergency workers, severe weather, and high noise levels. First, the paramedic must ensure personal safety. Then the paramedic should establish control of the environment quickly. This can include requesting the help of law officers. Law enforcement personnel can work to control the scene. That way, the paramedic can deliver appropriate assessment and care without distraction.

PATIENT COMPLIANCE

The patient is not always cooperative. The patient's willingness to comply with the assessment may depend on his or her trust in the paramedic crew. For example, the patient who sees the paramedic as competent and professional often provides a full history. The patient also often will agree to a full physical examination. Other factors that can affect compliance are cultural and ethnic barriers (see Chapter 47).

CONSIDERATIONS OF PERSONNEL AVAILABILITY

Depending on the emergency medical services (EMS) agency, crews may consist of a single paramedic and an emergency medical technician–Basic (EMT-B) or EMT-Intermediate (EMT-I), two paramedics, or several types or groups of responders (e.g., EMS, fire and rescue, and police). In cases in which only EMS is involved and only one paramedic is at the scene, the paramedic will work with the EMT-B. They will work to develop a proper sequence for gathering information and providing care. If two paramedics are available, the information gathering and treatment often can occur at the same time. Each paramedic can take on specific duties. If multiple responders and agencies are at the scene, roles and duties should be defined ahead of time. For example, one paramedic may be in charge of history taking and conferring with medical direction. Another paramedic may be in charge of treatment. The fire-rescue members may be in charge of extrication and gathering equipment. Finally, the law enforcement officers may be in charge of securing the scene.

> **CRITICAL THINKING**
>
> How can too many paramedics on the scene have a negative influence on patient assessment and care?

Assessment and Management Choreography

In cases where many responders are at the scene of an emergency, a coherent assessment can be difficult. A large emergency response may occur with multiple-tier response systems (e.g., EMS, fire, and police). The situation often is made more complex if the responders are trained at the same level (e.g., paramedic) without a clear direction for individual duties. Therefore members of the response team must have a preplan for deciding roles. The team can assign these predesignated roles by shift or crew or can rotate them among team members.

An example of a preplan for two paramedics is to assign one as the team leader and one as the patient care person. This type of plan must be flexible in rapidly changing field situations. However, the basic game plan allows others to participate and is important in preventing confusion at the scene. The following are sample responsibilities for each of the paramedics in this type of preplan:

1. Team leader responsibilities
   a. Accompanies the patient through to definitive care
   b. Establishes contact and a dialogue with the patient
   c. Obtains the history
   d. Performs the physical examination
   e. Presents the patient and gives verbal reports over the radio or at definitive care
   f. Completes all documentation
   g. Tries to maintain the overall patient perspective and provides leadership to the team by designating tasks and coordinating transportation
   h. Designates and actively participates in critical interventions during the resuscitative phase of initial assessment
   i. Acts as initial EMS command in multiple-casualty situations (see Chapter 50)
   j. Interprets the electrocardiogram, communicates with medical direction and relays drug orders, controls access to the drug box, and documents drug administration and effects during advanced cardiac life support
2. Patient care person responsibilities
   a. Provides scene cover (watches the team leader's back)
   b. Gathers scene information and talks to family members and bystanders
   c. Obtains vital signs
   d. Performs skills and interventions as requested by the team leader (e.g., attaches monitor leads, provides oxygen, initiates intravenous access, administers drugs, and obtains transportation equipment)
   e. Acts as triage group leader in multiple-casualty situations
   f. Administers drugs, monitors endotracheal tube placement, and monitors basic life support interventions during advanced cardiac life support

THE RIGHT STUFF

Having the "right stuff" means carrying the right equipment to the patient's side. Not having the right stuff can compromise care and also can cause confusion. The paramedic crew should always be prepared for the worst event. They should carry essential equipment to manage every aspect of patient care, including cardiac monitoring and defibrillation (Box 14-2).

NOTE The concept of having the right stuff can be compared with backpacking. A person who is backpacking must have essential items that are downsized to facilitate rapid movement with minimum weight and bulk.

BOX 14-2 Essential Items for All Aspects of Patient Care

Personal Protection
Eye shields
Gowns
Gloves
Masks

Airway Control
Endotracheal tubes, stylettes, and tape
Laryngoscope and blades
Nasal airways
Oral airways
Rigid Yankauer and flexible suction catheters
Suction (electrical or manual)

Breathing
Large-bore intravenous catheter for thoracic decompression
Manual ventilation bag-valve-mask
Mouth-powered ventilation device (pocket mask)
Occlusive dressings
Oxygen masks, cannulae, and extension tubing
Oxygen tank and regulator
Spare masks

Circulation
Bandages and tape
Blood pressure cuff and stethoscope
Dressings
Infection-control supplies (gloves and eye shields)
Intravenous fluids, catheters, and tubing
Note pad and pen or pencil

Disability and Dysrhythmia
Cardiac monitor and defibrillator
Flashlight
Rigid collar

Exposure
Scissors
Space blanket or other device to cover and protect the patient

OPTIONAL TAKE-IN EQUIPMENT

In addition to essential equipment for the EMS crew, the paramedic also can carry other equipment to the patient's side. For example, most EMS systems require that the paramedic carry drug boxes and kits for venous access supplies. This includes those agencies that have nontransporting emergency vehicles staffed by paramedic personnel as well. Most EMS systems require that paramedics carry these supplies even though they are not appropriate for every patient contact. Other factors that can affect what equipment the paramedic carries to the patient's side depend on the following:

- Local protocol
- Standing order flexibility
- Number of paramedic responders
- Difficulty in accessing patients

Other items that are essential on every call include patient care reports or worksheets, pens or pencils, personal wristwatches, flashlights, and portable radios or cellular telephones. Personal protective equipment also should be readily available.

CRITICAL THINKING
Have you been on ambulance calls when you did not have the right stuff? How did it affect patient care?

GENERAL APPROACH TO THE PATIENT

A calm and orderly manner is important for the paramedic when approaching a patient. To gain the patient's trust and cooperation, the paramedic must look and act the part of a professional. The paramedic also must show a caring and confident bedside manner. (See Chapter 9.) Patients may not be able to rate medical performance; however, they generally rate people skills and service.

As described before, a preplan should be in effect. This plan will help to prevent confusion at the scene and will improve the accuracy of the assessment. Ideally, one team member should be in charge of talking to the patient. This member should use an active and concerned dialogue that allows for careful listening. Taking notes when acquiring the history demonstrates a thorough assessment to the patient and prevents the paramedic from asking repetitive questions. All essential equipment should be at the patient's side. The EMS crew should be ready to provide resuscitative care if needed. An initial survey of the scene can offer important clues to help the paramedic formulate an impression. Initial size-up information that is useful in trauma situations includes hazards and potential hazards, mechanism of injury, and the number of patients at the scene.

Setting the Tone for the Patient Encounter

Two approaches in the initial assessment set the tone for the patient encounter. The first is the resuscitative approach. The second is the contemplative approach. The resuscitative approach recognizes the need for immediate intervention for patients who have life-threatening problems such as the following:

- Cardiorespiratory arrest
- Coma or altered level of consciousness
- Major trauma
- Possible cervical spine injury
- Respiratory distress or failure
- Seizures
- Shock or hypotension
- Unstable cardiac rhythms

A life-threatening problem may be present. In that case, the paramedic crew must take resuscitative action. The paramedic should delay history taking and other details. These must wait until the paramedic has performed immediate resuscitation measures.

Immediate intervention is not always needed to manage life threats. If immediate intervention is not needed, the paramedic can use the contemplative approach. With this approach, the paramedic obtains a patient history and performs a physical examination before providing patient care.

In any patient care encounter, the paramedic may need to move the patient immediately to the emergency vehicle if any of the following occur:

- The paramedic cannot provide lifesaving interventions at the patient's side
- The scene is too unstable or unsafe
- The scene is too chaotic to allow for thorough assessment
- Inclement weather hinders assessment and care

Looking to Find

Paramedics must find something before they can treat or report it. To find something, the paramedic must suspect it. Therefore during the initial assessment, the paramedic must look actively for any problems that pose a threat to life. The paramedic must be systematic in the assessment, rapidly determining the patient's chief complaint. Then the paramedic must assess the degree of distress. Next the paramedic must obtain baseline vital signs. The paramedic must stay focused on the patient's history and physical findings. A mental rule-out list often is a good approach in looking to find. This is a list that considers the most serious problems that could cause the patient's signs and symptoms *first.*

Experience assists the paramedic in developing the ability for multitasking. This is being able to ask questions, take notes, and perform tasks while listening to the patient's answers. In time the paramedic will gain the level of experience for multitasking. Until then the paramedic would do better to ask questions and then carefully listen to the patient's response. The paramedic can lose crucial clues by not listening. If a particular task is called for while the paramedic is obtaining a patient history, a partner should provide the patient care measure. The patient's ability to describe symptoms and the paramedic's ability to listen may influence the assessment greatly. The paramedic should remember that the severity and location of the patient's pain may not always correlate well with some potentially life-threatening conditions. For example, a patient with myocardial infarction may at first complain of pain only in the arm or shoulder. The paramedic's role is to assess and treat rapidly for the worst-case scenario.

PRESENTING THE PATIENT

Presenting the patient in the course of out-of-hospital and hospital care is twofold. It refers to the skills of effective communication. It also refers to the effective transfer of patient information. The paramedic routinely provides patient presentation. The paramedic may do this face to face, over the telephone or radio, and in writing. These communication skills are essential and help the paramedic to establish trust and credibility with co-workers and other health care team members. Good presentations suggest effective patient assessment and care to the listener, and vice versa. Poor presentation can compromise patient care. This may occur when the paramedic does not convey patient needs and status effectively to medical direction. (See Chapter 15.) The following are characteristics of an effective patient presentation:

- The presentation is concise, usually lasting less than 1 minute.
- The presentation is usually free of extensive medical jargon.

- The presentation follows the same basic information pattern.
- The presentation generally follows a standard format.
- The presentation includes pertinent findings and pertinent negatives.

When communicating a patient presentation, the paramedic should begin the report with the end in mind. For instance, the paramedic should anticipate discrete areas of information that others will ask for (Box 14-3). Moreover, the paramedic should be ready to provide those details. The paramedic will gain experience in presenting patients. Until then, the paramedic may elect to use a preprinted card or other memory device. These aids will help the paramedic to organize information and assessment findings.

CRITICAL THINKING

Can you think of any areas for improvement for your skills in "presenting the patient"?

BOX 14-3 Discrete Areas of Information

1. Patient identification, age, sex, and degree of distress
2. Chief complaint
3. Present illness or injury
   a. Pertinent details about the present problem
   b. Pertinent negatives (expected findings that are absent)
4. Medical history, including allergies and medications
5. Physical findings
   a. Vital signs
   b. Pertinent positive findings
   c. Pertinent negative findings
6. Assessment, including paramedic impression
7. Plan
   a. What has been done
   b. Orders requested

SUMMARY

- Assessment-based management "puts it all together." This means that the paramedic gathers, evaluates, and synthesizes information. The paramedic makes proper decisions based on the information. Then the paramedic takes the appropriate actions required for the patient's care.
- Factors that can affect the quality of assessment and decision making include the paramedic's attitude, the patient's willingness to cooperate, distracting injuries, labeling and tunnel vision, the environment, patient compliance, and considerations of personnel availability.
- Promoting a coherent assessment is the goal. Thus members of the response team should have a preplan for determining roles and responsibilities.
- The paramedic crew should always be prepared for the worst event. They should carry essential equipment to manage every aspect of patient care.
- A calm and orderly manner is essential for the paramedic. This is especially the case when approaching a patient. During the initial assessment the paramedic must look actively for problems that pose a threat to life.
- Presenting the patient in the course of prehospital and hospital care is twofold. Presentation refers to the skills of effective communication. Presentation also refers to the effective transfer of patient information.

REFERENCE

1. US Department of Transportation, National Highway Traffic Safety Administration: *EMT-Paramedic national standard curriculum,* Washington, DC, 1998, The Department.

SUGGESTED READINGS

Bell R, Krivich M: *How to use patient satisfaction data to improve healthcare quality,* Milwaukee, 2000, American Society of Quality/Quality Press.

Elling B, Elling K: *Principles of patient assessment in EMS,* Clifton Park, NY, 2002, Delmar Learning.

Gilles A: *Improving the quality of patient care,* New York, 1997, John Wiley & Son.

CHAPTER 15

Communications

OBJECTIVES

Upon completion of this chapter, the paramedic student will be able to:

1. Outline the phases of communications that occur during a typical emergency medical services (EMS) event.
2. Describe the role of communications in EMS.
3. Define common EMS communications terms.
4. Describe the primary modes of EMS communications.
5. Describe how EMS communications are regulated.
6. Describe the role of dispatching as it applies to prehospital emergency medical care.
7. Outline techniques for relaying EMS communications clearly and effectively.

KEY TERMS

duplex mode: A communications mode with the ability to transmit and receive traffic simultaneously through two different frequencies, one to transmit and one to receive.

EMS communications: The delivery of patient and scene information (either in person, in writing, or through communications technology) to other members of the emergency response team.

Federal Communications Commission: A federal agency with jurisdiction over interstate and international telephone and telegraph services and satellite communications.

multiplex mode: A communications mode with the ability to transmit two or more different types of information simultaneously, in either or both directions, over the same frequency.

simplex mode: A communications mode with the ability to transmit or receive in one direction at a time. Simultaneous transmission cannot occur.

SOAP format: A memory aid used to organize written and verbal patient reports; it includes subjective data, objective data, assessment data, and plan of patient management.

telemedicine: Technological communications that allow for the transmission of photographs, video, and other information to be sent directly from the scene to a hospital for physician evaluation and consultation.

Emergency medical services (EMS) communications refers to the delivery of information. This information relates to the patient and the scene. The information may be delivered in person, in writing, or through various devices. The information is delivered to other members of the emergency response team. These members include telecommunicators, EMS providers, emergency response workers, EMS system control and administration staff, and medical direction. This chapter focuses on the complexities of communications that are vital aspects of the EMS system.

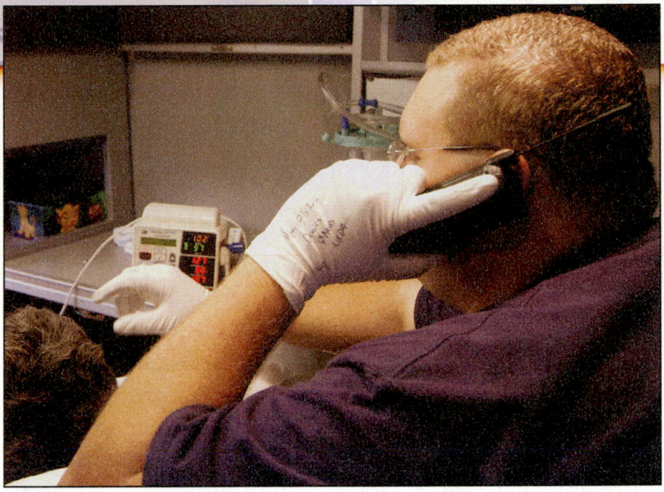

PHASES OF COMMUNICATIONS DURING A TYPICAL EMERGENCY MEDICAL SERVICES EVENT

Five phases of communications occur during a typical emergency medical services (EMS) event.[1] The first phase is the occurrence of the event. The second phase is the detection of the need for emergency services. The third phase is the notification and emergency response. The fourth phase is the EMS arrival, treatment, and preparation for transport. (The treatment includes consultation with medical direction.) The fifth phase is preparation of EMS for the next response.

In many urban areas the public requests help via a phone call. This call goes to a communications center or public safety answering point. Communications specialists receive the call. In the most modern systems, details about the origin of the call and history of the response to that locale are displayed automatically on a console (Fig. 15-1). The call taker then sends these details via digital technology to the telecommunicator. This person sends a response unit to the scene. In some public safety answering point systems, prearrival instructions are given to the caller. Emergency medical dispatchers or other qualified personnel give these instructions. The communication with the caller continues until the first EMS unit arrives at the scene.

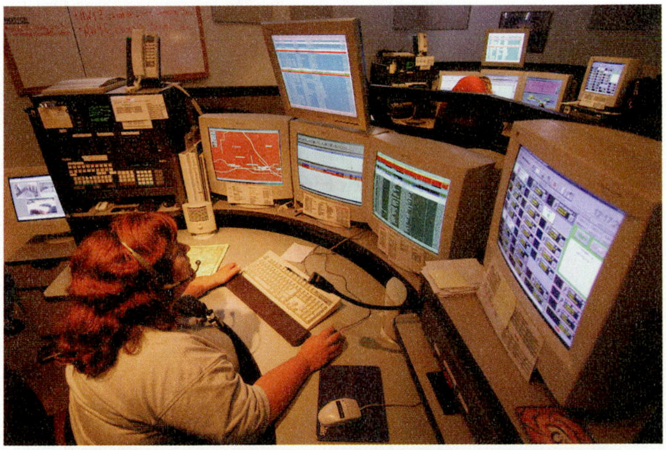

FIGURE 15-1 ■ Communication console (dispatch).

NOTE As described in Chapter 1, a telecommunicator is a person trained in public safety telecommunications. The term applies to call takers, dispatchers, radio operators, data terminal operators, or any combination of such functions in a public safety answering point located in a fire, police, or emergency medical services communications center.

The EMS unit is dispatched to the scene. Then the paramedic crew advises the communications center of response and arrival status via radio or cellular phone. The crew contacts medical direction for consultation and to give status reports. The paramedics render care at the emergency scene and packages the patient for transport. Then the patient is delivered to the receiving facility. Following the completion of the reporting, the paramedics make the EMS vehicle ready for the next emergency call.

ROLE OF COMMUNICATIONS IN EMERGENCY MEDICAL SERVICES

Verbal, written, and electronic communications allow the delivery of information between the person requesting help and the telecommunicator and between the telecommunicator and the paramedic. Communications occur between the paramedic, patient, hospital, and direct/online medical direction and between the paramedic and hospital personnel who receive the patient on arrival at the emergency department (Fig. 15-2). Good communications can occur only when key elements are in place. These elements make up the basic model of communications.

Basic Model of Communications

Communications can be verbal, nonverbal, or written. Communications serves a vital information function for decision making. Communications is the process by which one individual or group transmits meaning to others. The basic model of communications describes the relationships between an idea, encoding, a sender, a medium or channel, a receiver, decoding, and feedback (Fig. 15-3).

The *idea* is the meaning that is intended in the communications. Conveying the idea requires two things. First, it requires the sender to organize the intended meaning through a medium or channel. This is called encoding. (The medium or channel may be, for example, written or oral, facial or body expression, or voice modulation.) Second, it requires interpretation by the receiver. This is called decoding.

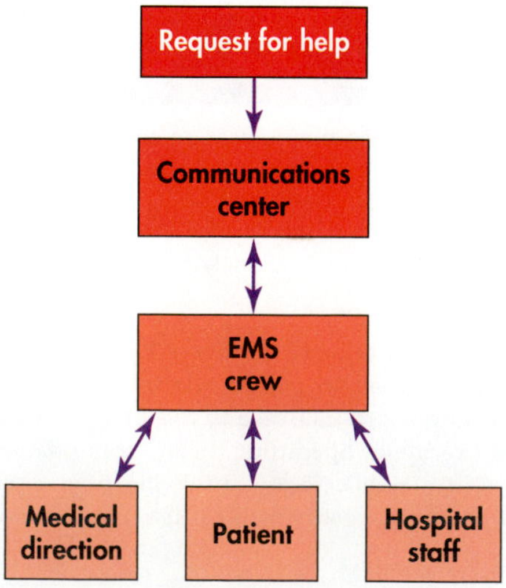

FIGURE 15-2 ■ Emergency medical services communications.

The receiver provides feedback that the initial idea was received. If communications are fully successful, there will be an overlap between the idea intended by the sender and the feedback provided by the receiver. (For instance, the receiver would interpret the decoding of the idea in a way identical to that intended by the sender.) Four common barriers to successful communications are as follows[2]:

1. *Attributes of the receiver.* Different persons react in different ways to the same message or idea. A variety of personal reasons may affect the interpretations of the message. These reasons may include cultural differences or language barriers. For example, a patient from one culture may find personal touch to be comforting, but a patient from another culture may be offended by touch.
2. *Selective perception.* Persons tend to listen to only part of an idea or message. They block out other information. They do this for a variety of reasons (e.g., values, mood, and motives of the sender). They may block out an idea when new information conflicts with established values, beliefs, or expectations. For example, the input of a newly licensed paramedic is not welcomed or respected by a paramedic supervisor.

> **CRITICAL THINKING**
> What tends to happen to you when you are talking with someone who continually interrupts you?

3. *Semantic problems.* Words that are used commonly may carry different meanings for different persons. One common issue is the use of vague or abstract words or phases. These words invite varying interpretation. Another is the use of medical terms and technical language ("lingo"). The receiver may not be able to understand these. For example, a paramedic refers to a patient as "comatose" during a radio report to the hospital. Medical direction asks for further clarification using the AVPU (alert, verbal, painful, unresponsive) scale.
4. *Time pressures.* Time pressures can lead to distortions in communications. A major temptation when pressed for time is to short circuit channels. In these cases the immediate demands of the situation are met. However, a number of unintended consequences can result. For example, the paramedic did not document medications administered in the field to a patient with cardiac arrest. This causes confusion about the next appropriate drug. It also causes billing problems after the event.

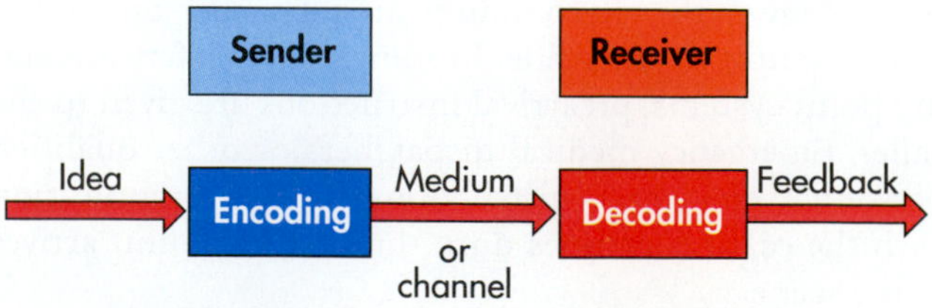

FIGURE 15-3 ■ Basic model of communications.

The paramedic should consider this basic model. The paramedic also should take into account the common barriers. These barriers block good communications. These are key to recall when conveying information to or receiving information from telecommunicators, co-workers, patients, bystanders, medical direction, and hospital personnel.

Proper Verbal Communications during an Emergency Medical Services Event

The role of proper verbal communications during an EMS event is to exchange system and patient information. This information is exchanged with other members of the response team. Communications must be done according to local protocol and patient privacy standards and regulations. (See Chapter 16.)

The terms used in **EMS communications** should be clear. The message should be conveyed in short narrative form. Technical or semantic jargon that cannot be understood clearly by all parties should be avoided. Some EMS services use a code to shorten radio transmissions. However, the English language usually is preferred for written and verbal messages. The paramedic should recall that many radio and phone communications are recorded. They may be replayed for patient care audits, media broadcasts, disciplinary hearings, and during legal proceedings. Professional conduct is important in all communications. The use of scanners by the general public to monitor emergency services is common in many communities. The paramedic should be aware of this. The paramedic should preserve patient confidentiality. In fact, the paramedic should not speak the name of the patient or provide descriptive phrases over unsecured airwaves.

Proper Written Communications during an Emergency Medical Services Event

Written documentation during an EMS event serves several key roles. It provides a written and legal record of the event. It conveys key clinical information from one component of the medical chain (EMS) to the next (emergency department). In addition, documentation is expected as part of professional work. Written documentation of patient care activities also becomes part of the patient's medical record (see Chapter 16). Other important ways in which written data can be used within the EMS system include the following:

1. Medical audit
2. Quality improvement/quality management
3. Billing
4. Data collection
5. Research

> **NOTE** Verbal communications can be affected by the terms used. Likewise, the effectiveness of written documentation can be impeded by the use of technical terms. Semantic jargon also can hinder the message. These types of terms often cannot be understood clearly by all parties.

In addition to the patient care report, other types of documentation that may be required by an EMS agency include the following:

- Personnel records documenting training and work assignments
- Call records that list or log dates, times, and other specifics of a call
- Vehicle maintenance records documenting vehicle service at regular intervals
- Vehicle and equipment cleaning records documenting procedures used to disinfect vehicle and emergency equipment
- Drug and equipment inventory records verifying daily checks of drug and fluid expiration, security measures of controlled substances as required by state and federal drug enforcement agencies, and monitor-defibrillator, radio, and telemetry checks
- Incident reports that document problem calls or unusual circumstances
- Records of significant exposures to communicable disease or biological hazard
- Records of any possible hazardous substances to which the patient or EMS provider may have been exposed

Technological Advances in the Collection and Exchange of Information

As technology evolves, it alters the way EMS gathers information. Technology also affects the way in which EMS exchanges information. Technology reduces the reliance on more traditional means of verbal and written communications. Examples of such advances include portable wireless voice and data devices, satellite terminals, global positioning systems for tracking emergency vehicles, diagnostic devices, and handheld tablet computers (Fig. 15-4). These and other devices can allow for real-time capture of EMS events

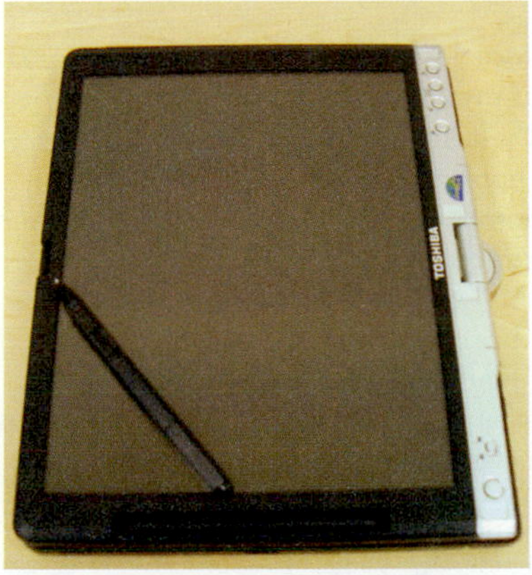

FIGURE 15-4 ■ Pen-based computer.

and data. They also may affect the role of medical direction in delivering patient care. They can provide for advanced notification and reduce the time to in-hospital diagnosis and therapy.

> **NOTE** Tablet computers are also known as electronic clipboards. These computers can send out patient information from a scene to a receiving hospital or a host computer. Then the data can be transferred electronically into a final report and patient record. This electronic information has the same legal status as a written document. The data take the place of the paper record of the incident.

COMMUNICATIONS SYSTEMS

The terms used to describe emergency communications technology are specific to the industry (Box 15-1). The following is an overview of the simple and complex communications systems.

Simple Systems

The minimum requirements for radio equipment used by an ambulance service include a self-contained desktop transceiver with a speaker, microphone, antenna, and mobile unit, and a two-way radio with multiple-frequency capability in the vehicle. Most EMS services also use handheld portable radios. (These often are called *portables.*)

BOX 15-1 Communications Terminology

911: A three-digit telephone number to facilitate the reporting of an emergency requiring response by a public safety agency

911 service area: The geographical area that has been granted authority by a state or local governmental body to provide 911 service

Abandoned call: A call placed to 911 in which the caller disconnects before the call can be answered by the public safety answering point (PSAP) telecommunicator

Advanced mobile phone service: The analog or digital radio interface used in wireless telephone systems

Alternate PSAP: A PSAP designated to receive calls when the primary PSAP is unable to do so

Alternate routing: The capability of routing 911 calls to a designated alternate location(s) if all 911 trunks to a primary PSAP are busy or out of service. Alternate routing may be activated upon request or automatically, if detectable, when 911 equipment fails or the PSAP itself is disabled.

Amplitude modulated: The encoding of a carrier wave by variation of its amplitude in accordance with an input signal

Attendant position: The customer premises equipment at which the telecommunicator answers and responds to calls

Automatic alarm and automatic alerting device: Any automated device that will access the 911 system for emergency services upon activation and does not provide for two-way communication. Many states prohibit the dialing of 911 by an automated device.

Automatic call distributor: Equipment that automatically distributes incoming calls to available PSAP call takers in the order the calls are received or queues calls until a call taker becomes available

Automatic location identification: The automatic display at the PSAP of the caller's telephone number, the address or location of the telephone, and supplementary emergency services information

Automatic number identification (ANI): Telephone number associated with the access line from which a call originates

Backup PSAP: Typically a disaster recovery answering point that serves as a backup to the primary PSAP and is not co-located with the primary PSAP

Basic 911: An emergency telephone system that automatically connects 911 callers to a designated answering point. Call routing is determined by originating central office only. Basic 911 typically does not support ANI or automatic location identification.

Call relay: Forwarding of pertinent information by a PSAP telecommunicator to the appropriate response agency; not to be confused with telephone relay service

Calling party hold: The capability of the PSAP to maintain control of a 911 caller's access line, even if the caller hangs up

Calling party's number: The callback number associated with a wireless telephone; similar to ANI for wireline telephones (Ref. NENA [National Emergency Number Association] 03-002)

Cell: The wireless telecommunications (cellular or PCS) antenna serving a specific geographical area

Circuit route: The physical path between two terminal locations

Computer-aided dispatch: A computer-based system that aids PSAP telecommunicators by automating selected dispatching and record-keeping activities

Consolidated PSAP: A facility where one or more public safety agencies choose to operate as a single 911 entity

Dedicated trunk: A telephone circuit used for a single purpose, such as transmission of 911 calls

Direct dispatch: The performance of 911 call answering and dispatching by personnel at the primary PSAP

Diverse routing: The practice of routing circuits along different physical paths to prevent total loss of 911 service in the event of a facility failure

Emergency call: A telephone request for public safety agency emergency services that requires immediate action to save a life, report a fire, or stop a crime; it may include other situations as determined locally

Emergency ring back: The capability of a PSAP telecommunicator to ring the telephone on a held circuit (a basic 911 feature); requires calling party hold; also known as *re-ring*

Emergency service trunks: Message trunks capable of providing ANI, connecting the serving central office of the 911 calling party and the designated enhanced 911 control office

Enhanced 911 (E911): An emergency telephone system that includes network switching, database and customer premises equipment elements capable of providing selective routing, selective transfer, fixed transfer, ANI, and automatic location identification

Adapted from National Emergency Number Association Technical Committee and PSAP Operational Standards Committee: *NENA master glossary of 911 terminology,* Arlington, Va, 1998, The Association.

BOX 15-1 Communications Terminology—cont'd

Forced disconnect: The capability of a PSAP attendant to disconnect a 911 call even if the calling party remains off hook; used to prevent overloading of 911 trunks

Global positioning system: A satellite-based location determination technology

Highway call box: A telephone enclosed in a box and placed along a highway that allows a motorist to summon emergency and nonemergency assistance

Management information system: A program that collects, stores, and collates data into reports to enable interpretation and evaluation of information such as performance, trends, and traffic capacities

Master street address guide: A database of street names and house number ranges within their associated communities defining emergency service zones and their associated emergency service numbers to enable proper routing of 911 calls.

National Emergency Number Association: A not-for-profit corporation established in 1982 to further the goal of "One Nation–One Number." The National Emergency Number Association is a networking source and promotes research, planning, and training. The National Emergency Number Association strives to educate, set standards, and provide certification programs, legislative representation, and technical assistance for implementing and managing 911 systems.

Primary PSAP: A PSAP to which 911 calls are routed directly from the 911 control office

Public safety answering point: A facility equipped and staffed to receive 911 calls. A primary PSAP receives the calls directly. If the call is relayed or transferred, the next receiving PSAP is designated a secondary PSAP.

Selective routing: The routing of a 911 call to the proper PSAP based on the location of the caller. Selective routing is controlled by the emergency service number, which is derived from the customer location.

Telecommunicator: As used in 911, a person who is trained and employed in public safety telecommunications. The term applies to call takers, dispatchers, radio operators, data terminal operators, or any combination of such functions in a PSAP.

Trunk: Typically, a communication path between central office switches or between the 911 control office and the PSAP.

These radios are capable of communications contact with the base station and data recording. The portable radio protects the crew and aids in optimal patient care. The radio does this by allowing continued contact with the communications center and medical direction. The data-recording part of the device offers medical and legal protection for the service and can verify the transmissions when contact is disrupted.

Complex Systems

More advanced radio communications systems exist. These include remote consoles, high-power transmitters, repeaters, satellite receivers, and high-power multifrequency vehicle radios. Some services also use mobile transmitter steering, vehicular repeaters, mobile encode-decode capabilities, mobile data terminals, microwave links, and other sophisticated communications devices.

BASE STATIONS

Base stations usually are located on a high spot such as a hill, mountain, or tall building. This location ensures optimal transmission and reception. Base stations generally are connected via telephone lines to dispatch centers. These centers are where all elements of the EMS response are coordinated. Depending on locale, one dispatch center may be responsible for all fire, police, and EMS communications activities. Base station transmitters usually are equipped with an antenna to boost their signal.

MOBILE TRANSCEIVERS

Vehicle-mounted transmitters usually operate at lower outputs than base stations. They provide a range of 10 to 15 miles over average terrain. Transmission over flat land or water increases this range. However, transmission over mountainous terrain, dense foliage, or urban areas with tall buildings decreases the range. Transmitters with higher outputs are available. These transmitters may offer greater ranges for transmission. Multichannel units are preferred over single-channel radios because of the many channels used in an EMS system.

PORTABLE TRANSCEIVERS

Portable transceivers are handheld or hand-carried devices. A paramedic uses these when working away from the emergency vehicle. These devices usually have a limited range. Many systems boost the signal through a mobile or vehicular repeater. Portable transceivers may be single-channel or multichannel units.

REPEATERS

Repeaters act as a special type of long-range transceiver. They receive transmissions from a low-power portable or mobile radio on one frequency. At the same time, they retransmit it at a higher power on another frequency. Repeaters may be fixed or vehicle mounted; EMS systems often use both. Repeaters are needed for large geographical areas. They are used to increase coverage from portable/mobile to portable/mobile units. They allow low-power units to receive other radio messages. They also allow two or more low-power units to communicate with each other when distances or obstructions normally would hinder this.

REMOTE CONSOLE

Most EMS systems use dispatch services located away from base stations. These remote centers control all base station functions. They are connected via dedicated telephone lines, microwave, or other radio means. Hospitals also often are equipped with a terminal that receives and displays telemetry transmissions. The console also provides contact with paramedic crews in the field. Consoles for these systems include an amplifier, a speaker, a telemetry oscilloscope, a microphone, receiving capabilities, and remote control circuits.

SATELLITE RECEIVERS AND TERMINALS

Satellite receivers sometimes are used depending on the area and the terrain. They are used to ensure that low-power units are always within coverage. The satellite receivers are strategically located. They are connected to the base station or repeater by dedicated phone lines, radio, or microwave relay. "Voting systems" automatically select the best audio signal. These systems pick up the signal from among multiple satellite receivers and the main base station receiver. (These also are used in other types of communications systems.)

Commonly available satellite terminals incorporate ground stations and transportable stations. They provide voice, data, and video communications. Portable satellite terminals are useful when other systems are not available. For example, they may be used during major disasters.

ENCODERS AND DECODERS

Selective call encoders are devices that look like a phone dial or the buttons of a push-button phone. When activated, the encoder transmits tone pulses or pairs of tones over the air. Receivers with decoders recognize the specific codes. This in turn opens the audio circuits of the receivers. Two-tone sequential paging alerts personnel using two pairs of specific frequency tones to address pagers and alert monitors selectively. A selective-address system usually has a code for calling all units within radio range (all call).

Hospitals in certain regions throughout the United States are tied together by radio systems known as Hospital Emergency Administrative Radio (HEAR by Motorola) or Emergency Administrative Communications (EACOM by Ericson). These radios use 1500-Hz rotary pulse dialing to transmit specific groups of rotary tone pulses to designated hospital-based receivers. Most ambulance services have access to this system.

CELLULAR TELEPHONES

Many EMS services use cellular phones (analog and digital). Cellular phones are an alternative to dedicated EMS communications systems. One benefit is that they have more channels. In addition, a cell phone offers a fairly secure link between EMS workers and area hospitals. The cell phone also allows the online physician to speak directly with the patient. Cell phone use for emergency services has disadvantages, however. One includes network usage that might limit channel access. High network usage might create problems in maintaining continuous communications in some areas. Another issue is lack of priority access. Yet another issue is the inability of calls to be monitored by other members of an emergency response team. Thus many EMS agencies that use cell phones have a backup option. They often have backup radio communications capabilities (Box 15-2).

BOX 15-2 Cellular Phone Technology

An analog cell phone is really a radio that allows two persons to communicate on one frequency. The analog signal fluctuates with the rise and fall of the caller's voice. This produces a wildly oscillating electrical wave (a "copy" of speech). The signal can be heard at the receiver's end. Digital cell phones use the same radio technology. They, however, use different frequencies. Moreover, they compress the caller's voice into digital 1s and 0s that remain stable for the length of their travel. Then the digital information is converted back to voice at the receiver's end. The digital signal generally is thought to provide better sound quality. A digital signal also is thought to provide a more secure method of transmission than using analog. Finally, digital technology provides the platform for wireless services such as data transmission and interactive computers.

DIGITAL

Digital modes of communications include digital phones, telemetry, fax transmissions, and digital signals used in some wireless phone, paging, and alerting systems. Telemetry and facsimiles are transmitted using electronic signals. These signals are converted into audio tones. These tones then are converted back into electronic signals by the receiver decoder. Then the signals can be displayed or printed. An example of telemetry is the transmission of a patient's electrocardiogram.

COMPUTER

Computer technology (e.g., that used with automated external defibrillators and other devices) has the potential to "save" at every step of data entry. Computers allow for (1) documentation in near real time; (2) sorting information in many categories; (3) creation of multiple reporting formats; and (4) quick online and retrieval system data access. Computer terminals also are used by some communications centers to dispatch units automatically to a scene. As with most technologies, computer devices are subject to human error. They also are subject to limitations. Thus they need regular upgrades. Moreover, the users have to obtain the proper education.

NOTE Advances in emergency medical services communications technology and **telemedicine** continue to evolve at a rapid pace. Video cameras, fax machines, cellular networks, and the Internet now allow photographs, videos (including movie-type imaging), and other information to be sent directly from the scene to a hospital for physician evaluation and consultation.

Operation Modes Used for Emergency Medical Services Communications

The operation modes commonly used in EMS communications include simplex, multiplex, duplex, and trunked.

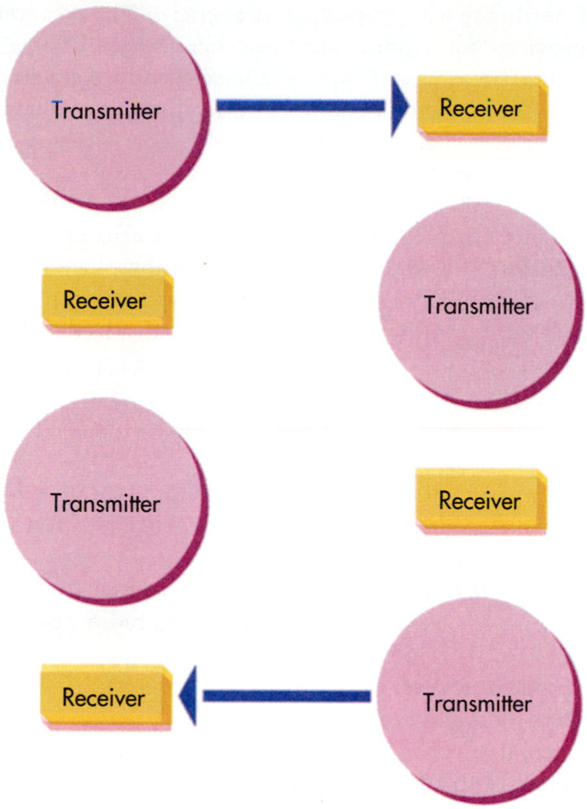

FIGURE 15-5 ■ Required equipment for simplex mode includes a transmitter and a receiver at each end of the communications path, both operating on the same frequency. In the simplex mode, only one end may operate at a time.

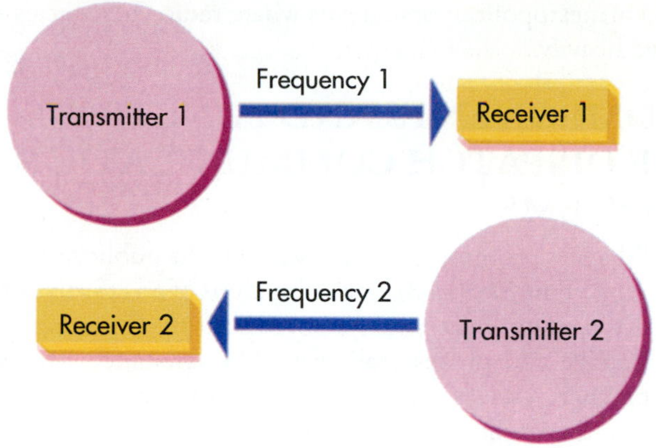

FIG. 15-6 ■ Duplex mode requires two frequencies so that both ends can communicate simultaneously.

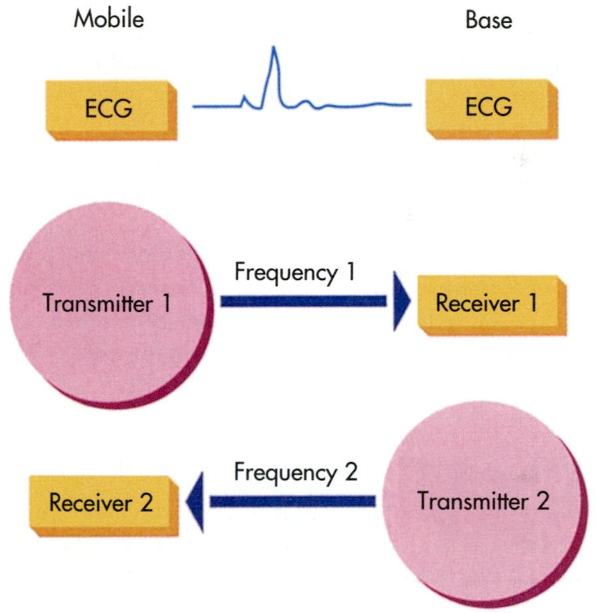

FIG. 15-7 ■ Multiplex mode operates similarly to duplex mode with added capabilities, such as simultaneous electrocardiogram and voice transmission.

SIMPLEX MODE

The **simplex mode** (Fig. 15-5) requires a transmitter and receiver at each end of the communications path. Both elements operate on the same frequency. However, only one end may operate at a time. This mode allows speakers to send a message without interruption, although it slows the communications process and takes away the ability to discuss a case.

DUPLEX MODE

The **duplex mode** (Fig. 15-6) uses two frequencies that allow both parties to communicate at the same time. The advantage of this mode is that either party can interrupt the other to facilitate discussion. However, a tendency exists for each end to interrupt the other.

MULTIPLEX MODE

The **multiplex mode** (Fig. 15-7) has the advantage of transmitting telemetry and voice simultaneously from a field unit. With this mode, either party can interrupt as needed, thereby facilitating discussion. As with the duplex mode, each party tends to interrupt the other. In addition, voice transmission may interfere with the transmission of data. Multiplex is the most common mode in use today with most EMS services.

TRUNKED SYSTEM

Trunking refers to systems that have five or more repeaters that work as a group. Each repeater is on a different channel. The trunking system may belong to a single user (e.g., a specific EMS agency or police department) or may be shared by a number of different public service agencies. When radio transmissions originate, computerized scanning automatically finds an available repeater in the system. Then the computer switches that transmission to the chosen repeater. As one fleet captures an open channel, it locks out all other users who share the system. This bars interference from other agencies. The trunked system is advantageous in major metropolitan operations where radio frequencies are used heavily.

COMPONENTS AND FUNCTIONS OF DISPATCH COMMUNICATIONS SYSTEMS

The dispatch communications system is the public safety answering point (Box 15-3). Some functions of an effective EMS dispatch communications system include the following[3]:

1. Receive and process calls for EMS assistance. The dispatcher receives and records calls for EMS assistance. The dispatcher selects an appropriate course of action for each call. This function involves obtaining as much information as possible about the emergency event, including name, callback number, and address, and it may include dealing with distraught callers. Emergency care instructions also may be provided while the incident is being dispatched.
2. Dispatch and coordinate the EMS resources. The dispatcher directs the proper emergency vehicles to the correct address. In addition, the dispatcher coordinates the movements of emergency vehicles while en route to the scene, to the medical facility, and back to the operations base.
3. Relay medical information. The dispatcher may provide a telecommunications channel between appropriate medical facilities and EMS personnel, fire, police, rescue workers, and private citizens. The channel may consist of telephone, radio, or biomedical telemetry.

> **BOX 15-3 911, Enhanced 911, and Computer-Aided Dispatch Systems**
>
> As described in Chapter 1, 911 was designated in 1988 as the universal emergency phone number. The number was chosen by the American Telephone and Telegraph Company. The number is meant to offer the public a toll-free number to reach a public safety answering point. (This service is still not available everywhere.) Since 1988, enhanced 911 has been created. Enhanced 911 is used in many areas of the country. This system allows for automatic caller location and identification. The system shows the caller's number and address on a terminal at the communications center.
>
> The most advanced centers use a computer-aided dispatch system. This monitors the available resources. The system makes an assignment based on access and routes for the ambulance closest to the map grid shown on the terminal. Global positioning systems tell the telecommunicator or system status controller which unit is closest to the origin of the call by air miles, or road miles if an intelligent map is used automatically to route the unit that is closest to the scene. That unit then is sent to the scene. The telecommunicator monitors the call from beginning to end. The telecommunicator records status changes by digital media (e.g., tapes, CDs, or DVDs).

4. Coordinate with public safety agencies. The dispatcher provides for communications between public safety units (fire, law enforcement, rescue) and elements of the EMS system. This helps to facilitate coordination of services such as traffic control, escort, fire suppression, and extrication. The dispatcher ensures an integrated, well-coordinated system. To do so, the dispatcher must know the location and status of all EMS vehicles. The dispatcher also must know the availability of support services. In larger systems, computer-aided dispatching may be used. This advanced technology allows one or more of the following capabilities or functions:

- Automatic emergency medical dispatch
- Automatic entry of 911
- Automatic call notification/request for assistance
- Automatic interface to automatic vehicle location with or without map display
- Automatic interface to mobile data terminal
- Computer messaging among multiple radio operators, call takers, or both
- Dispatch note taking, reminder aid, or both
- Emergency medical dispatch review
- Manual or automatic updates of unit status
- Manual entry of call information
- Radio control and display of channel status
- Standard operating procedure review
- Telephone control and display of circuit status

Dispatcher Training

Many EMS and public safety agencies require specialized medical training for their dispatch personnel. This training may include the Association of Public Communications Officials and Emergency Medical Dispatch Program (based on the National Highway Traffic Safety Administration National Standard Curriculum for Emergency Medical Dispatch). Emergency medical dispatchers are trained to do the following[4]:

- Use locally approved emergency medical dispatch guide cards (customized to local protocols and EMS response priorities)
- Quickly and properly determine the nature of the call
- Determine the priority of the call
- Dispatch the appropriate response
- Provide the caller with instructions to help treat the patient until the responding EMS unit arrives

A base of training in EMS helps the telecommunicator understand functions of the EMS system, personnel capabilities, and equipment limitations. The training also arms the dispatcher with the protocols to give prearrival instructions. These protocols might mitigate the event before the arrival of an EMS unit. A variety of dispatching systems and procedures are in place across the United States. Some of these are the simple call received–ambulance dispatched types. Then again others are the more advanced call prioritization–prearrival instructions systems.

Call Prioritization–Prearrival Instructions Systems

In a call screening–prearrival instructions system, an emergency medical dispatcher, paramedic, or nurse determines what type of assistance is needed for an emergency call. This may include referring the caller to other services, choosing basic life support or advanced life support response, selecting private or public EMS service, and determining use of audible and visual warning devices. While dispatching the proper unit, dispatchers can give the caller prearrival instructions. These instructions are crucial for these reasons:

- They provide instant help to the caller.
- They complement the call prioritization process.
- They allow the dispatchers to give updated information to responding units.
- They may be lifesaving in critical incidents.
- They provide emotional support for the caller, bystander, or victim.

CRITICAL THINKING

What are some potential consequences of a dispatching error?

REGULATION

Radio communications in the United States are regulated by the **Federal Communications Commission** (FCC). This commission develops rules and regulations for the use of all radio equipment and frequencies. In addition to the FCC, state and local governments may have rules and regulations for radio operations. The paramedic must be knowledgeable about these agencies. The paramedic also must follow their guidelines. The primary functions of the FCC include the following:

- Licensing and frequency allocation
- Establishing technical standards for radio equipment
- Establishing and enforcing rules and regulations for equipment operation, including monitoring frequencies for appropriate usage and spot-checking for appropriate licenses and records

CRITICAL THINKING

Why are these rules and regulations needed for good emergency medical services communications?

PROCEDURES FOR EMERGENCY MEDICAL SERVICES COMMUNICATIONS

Most EMS systems use a standard radio communications protocol. This protocol includes the desired format for message transmission and key words and phrases. Following this format aids in professional and efficient radio communications within the system. General guidelines for radio communications include the following:

- Think before you speak (formulate the message) to ensure that communications will be effective.
- Speak at close range (2 to 3 inches) when talking into a microphone.
- Speak slowly and clearly. Enunciate each word distinctly and avoid words that are difficult to hear.
- Speak in a normal pitch without emotion.
- Be brief and concise. Break up long messages into shorter ones.
- Avoid codes unless they are systems approved. Avoid dialect or slang.
- Advise the receiving party when the transmission has been completed.
- Confirm the receiving party has received the message.
- Always be professional, polite, and calm.

CRITICAL THINKING

Can you think of three reasons why a concise emergency medical services radio report is essential?

Relaying Patient Information

A standard format of transmission may be developed as a protocol for some EMS services. This format allows the best use of communications systems; it limits radio air time. In addition, physicians can receive details quickly regarding the patient's condition. Moreover, the chance of omitting any critical details is lessened.

Patient information can be reported to the hospital or dispatcher by radio or phone. Although the order of information delivery may vary by EMS system and scenario, the radio report should be brief and concise and should contain the following[1]:

- Unit and provider identification
- Description of the scene or incident
- Patient's age, sex, and approximate weight (for drug orders)
- Patient's chief complaint
- Associated symptoms
- Brief, pertinent history of present illness or injury
- Pertinent medical history, medications, and allergies
- Pertinent physical examination findings
  - Level of consciousness
  - Vital signs
  - Neurological examination
  - General appearance and degree of distress
  - Electrocardiogram results (if applicable)
  - Trauma index or Glasgow Coma Scale (if applicable)
  - Other pertinent observations and significant findings
- Any treatment given
- Estimated time of arrival
- Request for orders from or further questions for medical direction physician

> **NOTE** The use of telemetry to transmit a patient's electrocardiogram usually is reserved for the patient who requires diagnosis of a 12-lead electrocardiogram before the administration of some drugs. Telemetry transmission uses excessive air time. If warranted, 15 to 30 seconds of electrocardiogram transmission are usually adequate.

The SOAP Format

The **SOAP format** (or a similar method) is used by many paramedics as a memory aid to organize written and verbal patient reports. *SOAP* is an acronym for the following:

- *S*ubjective data: All patient symptoms including chief complaint, associated symptoms, history, current medications and allergies, and information provided by bystanders and family
- *O*bjective data: Pertinent physical examination information including vital signs, level of consciousness, physical examination findings, electrocardiogram, pulse oximetry readings, and blood glucose determinations
- *A*ssessment data: The paramedic's clinical impression of the patient based on subjective and objective data
- *P*lan of patient management: Treatment that has been provided and any requests for additional treatment

General Procedures for the Exchange of Information

When communicating with medical direction, the paramedic should repeat all orders received from the physician. The paramedic should confirm any orders that are unclear. The paramedic also should repeat those orders if they seem inappropriate. The paramedic should inform the receiving hospital of any significant changes in the patient's status before and during transport. General procedures of the exchange of information include the following:

- Protect the patient's privacy. (See Chapter 17.)
- Use proper unit numbers, hospital numbers, names, and titles.
- Avoid slang or profanity.
- Use the echo procedure (repeating what was heard) when receiving directions from the dispatcher or physician.
- Obtain confirmation that the message was received.

SUMMARY

- Communications regarding EMS refers to the delivery of information. The patient and scene information is delivered to other key members of the emergency response team.
- Verbal, written, and electronic communications allow the delivery of information between the party requesting help and the dispatcher, between the dispatcher and paramedic, and between the paramedic, hospital, and direct/online medical direction.
- Emergency communications technology has industry-specific terminology.
- The primary modes of EMS communications include simplex mode, duplex mode, multiplex mode, trunking system, digital, and computer.
- In the United States, the FCC regulates communications over the radio. The paramedic must be familiar with the regulatory agencies. The paramedic must follow their guidelines as well.
- The functions of an effective dispatch communications system include receiving and processing calls for EMS assistance, dispatching and coordinating EMS resources, relaying medical information, and coordinating with public safety agencies.
- A standard format of transmission of patient information is a wise idea. The standard allows for the best use of communications systems. The standard also allows physicians to receive details quickly about the patient. In addition, the standard decreases the chance of omitting any critical details.

REFERENCES

1. US Department of Transportation, National Highway Traffic Safety Administration: *Paramedic national standard curriculum,* Washington, DC, 1998, The Department.
2. Szilagyi A, Wallace M: *Organizational behavior and performance,* ed 5, Glenview, Ill, 1990, Addison-Wesley.
3. US Department of Transportation, National Highway Traffic Safety Administration: *Emergency medical dispatch: national standard curriculum,* Washington, DC, 1996, US Government Printing Office.
4. APCO Institute: *Emergency medical dispatch services,* South Daytona, Fla, 1998, The Institute. (www.apcointl.org/institute/pages/emd/htm)

CHAPTER 16

Documentation

OBJECTIVES

Upon completion of this chapter, the paramedic student will be able to:

1. Identify the purpose of the patient care report.
2. Describe the uses of the patient care report.
3. Outline the components of an accurate, thorough patient care report.
4. Describe the elements of a properly written emergency medical services document.
5. Describe an effective system for documentation of prehospital patient care.
6. Identify differences necessary when documenting special situations.
7. Describe the appropriate method to make revisions or corrections to the patient care report.
8. Recognize consequences that may result from inappropriate documentation.

KEY TERMS

narrative: The portion of the patient care report that allows for a chronological description of the call.

pertinent negative findings: Findings that warrant no medical care or intervention but that, by seeking them, show evidence of the thoroughness of the examination and history of the event.

pertinent oral statements: Statements made by the patient and other on-scene persons.

The patient care report is used effectively to document the essential elements of patient assessment, care, and transport.[1] The report is a legal document. Most importantly, the report helps to ensure that the patient is provided good care. Moreover, the report is the paramedic's best protection from liability action.

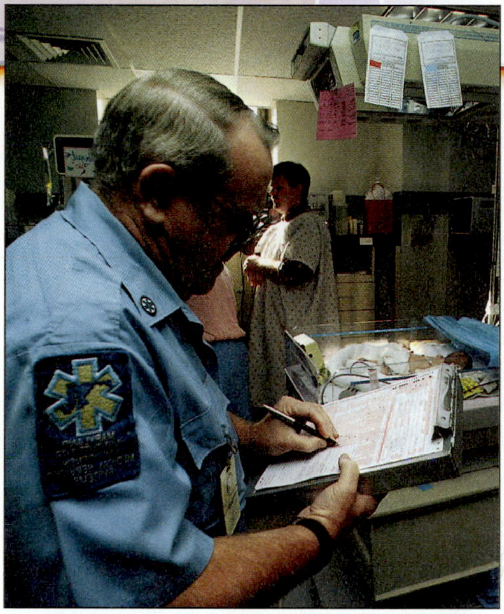

NOTE The requirements for record keeping vary throughout the United States. Most emergency medical services records are maintained a minimum of 10 years. (This includes patient care reports.) These records are maintained as a safety measure to guard against statute-of-limitation issues. *Accurate documentation is essential. It leads to accurate recall if litigation occurs.*

IMPORTANCE OF DOCUMENTATION

There are many reasons for creating thorough written documentation. Written documentation provides a tangible and legal record of an incident. Written documentation often is used by physicians, nurses, and others involved in the patient's care. Such documentation is used to understand better the patient's initial condition and the type of care given before hospital treatment. The emergency medical services (EMS) agency and medical direction also may use the report to monitor care in the field, evaluate individual performance, and conduct review conferences and other educational forums. These reports may be used to identify system issues regarding quality improvement. Examples of quality improvement issues that may be identified through the patient care report (PCR) and may result in policy changes to improve patient care include the following:

- Minimizing time spent on the scene for critical trauma patients
- Adding new medications to manage some medical emergencies better
- Changing the placement of emergency vehicles during peak response times in certain demographic areas

The PCR also offers a means of documenting any unique scene situations. These situations may have affected patient care. For example, traffic may have caused a long response time. An entrapped patient may have required prolonged extrication. The PCR also aids in tracking certain patient care skills of the paramedic (e.g., intravenous lines, intubations, and defibrillations). These skills may be required for relicensure or recertification. The PCR data are a main source for administrative and billing information as well. This information often is necessary for the economic survival of many EMS agencies (Box 16-1).

BOX 16-1 Importance of Documentation

Written documentation provides for the following:

- A tangible record of the incident
- A legal record of the incident
- Professionalism
- Medical audit
- Quality improvement
- Billing and administration
- Data collection

GENERAL CONSIDERATIONS

The PCR (Fig. 6-1) should be carefully detailed and should be legible. The PCR is viewed as a legal document and is part of the patient's medical record. Thus the use of slang terms or medical abbreviations that are not universally accepted should be avoided (Box 16-3). Many EMS systems develop agency-approved medical abbreviations.

The report should include all dates and response times. The PCR also should describe any difficulties that were encountered. (This should include while en route and during patient treatment, extrication, or transport.) In addition, the report should include observations at the scene, any previous medical care provided (and by whom), and time of patient extrication, if appropriate (Box 16-2). The times of all significant occurrences and interventions are useful to the receiving physician. The paramedic should record these as well. In particular, the PCR provides a legal and accurate recording of the following incident times:

- Time of call
- Time of dispatch
- Time of arrival at the scene
- Time at patient's side
- Time of vital sign assessments
- Time(s) of medication administration and certain medical procedures as defined by local protocol
- Time of departure from the scene
- Time of arrival at the medical facility (when transporting a patient)
- Time back in service

The PCR may be the only way for a paramedic to recall events of an emergency call accurately during testimony that occurs years after the incident. The paramedic must include as much detail as possible in the PCR. This level of detail will be useful for present and future use. (See Chapter 4.)

CRITICAL THINKING

Documentation of specific times on the patient care report is important. How can this information be useful?

THE NARRATIVE

The **narrative** portion of the PCR allows for a chronological account of the call. The narrative should be written concisely and clearly, using simple words. The paramedic should avoid uncommon abbreviations, unnecessary terms, and duplicate information. The paramedic should use a standard format established by medical direction. This format helps ensure completeness. The format also assists in quality improvement reviews. Components of the narrative portion of the PCR include the following:

- Initial contact
- All patient care activities (including medications and treatments)
- Initial assessment and vital signs
- Chief complaint
- Pertinent significant medical history
- Clock time of hospital contact
- Time of physician orders and advice (name of physician)
- **Pertinent negative findings**
- **Pertinent oral statements**
- Changes in patient status
- Patient response to treatment
- Vital sign reassessment
- Electrocardiogram interpretation
- Use of support services
- Time and condition of patient on delivery
- Name of receiving health care worker
- Signature of paramedic

BOX 16-2 Prehospital Care Report Data

The prehospital care report data include the following:

- Dates
- Response times
- Difficulties en route
- Communication difficulties
- Scene observations
- Reasons for extended on-scene time
- Previous care provided
- Time of extrication
- Time of patient transport
- Reason for hospital selection (trauma center designation, patient choice, or other concerns)

NOTE Documentation should never be used by the paramedic to construct patient care creatively. If the paramedic did not document the care, it was not done. Conversely, if the care was not done, the paramedic should not document it.

Pertinent negative findings may help to determine the course of treatment. These are findings that warrant no medical care or intervention. By seeking them, though, the paramedic shows evidence of the thoroughness of the examination and history of the event. The paramedic should record these findings. Examples of negative findings include the absence of diminished breath sounds, the absence of skin rashes, and the absence of abdominal tenderness. Pertinent oral statements are those made by the patient and other on-scene persons. The paramedic also should record these. Statements that may have an impact on patient care or resolution of the situation include the following:

- Mechanism of injury
- Patient's behavior
- First-aid interventions before EMS arrival
- Safety-related information (including disposition of weapons)
- Information of interest to crime scene investigators
- Disposal of valuable personal property (e.g., jewelry and wallets)

Text continued on p. 325

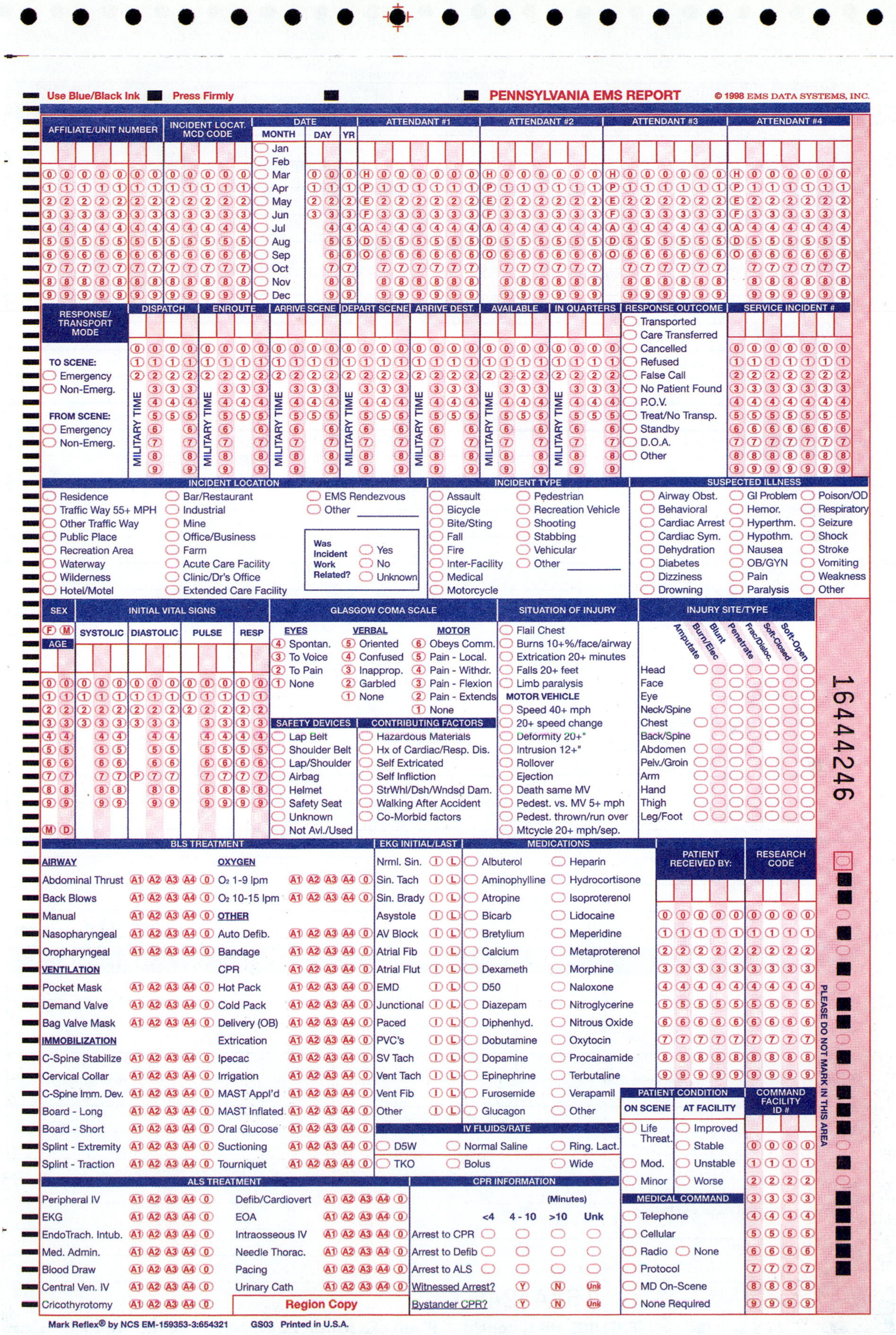
Use Blue/Black Ink ■ Press Firmly ■ ■ PENNSYLVANIA EMS REPORT © 1998 EMS DATA SYSTEMS, INC.

AFFILIATE/UNIT NUMBER | INCIDENT LOCAT. MCD CODE | DATE: MONTH, DAY, YR | ATTENDANT #1 | ATTENDANT #2 | ATTENDANT #3 | ATTENDANT #4

Jan, Feb, Mar, Apr, May, Jun, Jul, Aug, Sep, Oct, Nov, Dec

RESPONSE/TRANSPORT MODE
TO SCENE: Emergency, Non-Emerg.
FROM SCENE: Emergency, Non-Emerg.

DISPATCH | ENROUTE | ARRIVE SCENE | DEPART SCENE | ARRIVE DEST. | AVAILABLE | IN QUARTERS (MILITARY TIME)

RESPONSE OUTCOME: Transported, Care Transferred, Cancelled, Refused, False Call, No Patient Found, P.O.V., Treat/No Transp., Standby, D.O.A., Other

SERVICE INCIDENT #

INCIDENT LOCATION: Residence, Traffic Way 55+ MPH, Other Traffic Way, Public Place, Recreation Area, Waterway, Wilderness, Hotel/Motel, Bar/Restaurant, Industrial, Mine, Office/Business, Farm, Acute Care Facility, Clinic/Dr's Office, Extended Care Facility, EMS Rendezvous, Other

Was Incident Work Related? Yes, No, Unknown

INCIDENT TYPE: Assault, Bicycle, Bite/Sting, Fall, Fire, Inter-Facility, Medical, Motorcycle, Pedestrian, Recreation Vehicle, Shooting, Stabbing, Vehicular, Other

SUSPECTED ILLNESS: Airway Obst., Behavioral, Cardiac Arrest, Cardiac Sym., Dehydration, Diabetes, Dizziness, Drowning, GI Problem, Hemor., Hyperthm., Hypothm., Nausea, OB/GYN, Pain, Paralysis, Poison/OD, Respiratory, Seizure, Shock, Stroke, Vomiting, Weakness, Other

SEX: F M | AGE | M D

INITIAL VITAL SIGNS: SYSTOLIC, DIASTOLIC, PULSE, RESP

GLASGOW COMA SCALE
EYES: 4 Spontan., 3 To Voice, 2 To Pain, 1 None
VERBAL: 5 Oriented, 4 Confused, 3 Inapprop., 2 Garbled, 1 None
MOTOR: 6 Obeys Comm., 5 Pain - Local., 4 Pain - Withdr., 3 Pain - Flexion, 2 Pain - Extends, 1 None

SAFETY DEVICES: Lap Belt, Shoulder Belt, Lap/Shoulder, Airbag, Helmet, Safety Seat, Unknown, Not Avl./Used

CONTRIBUTING FACTORS: Hazardous Materials, Hx of Cardiac/Resp. Dis., Self Extricated, Self Infliction, StrWhl/Dsh/Wndsd Dam., Walking After Accident, Co-Morbid factors

SITUATION OF INJURY: Flail Chest, Burns 10+%/face/airway, Extrication 20+ minutes, Falls 20+ feet, Limb paralysis
MOTOR VEHICLE: Speed 40+ mph, 20+ speed change, Deformity 20+", Intrusion 12+", Rollover, Ejection, Death same MV, Pedest. vs. MV 5+ mph, Pedest. thrown/run over, Mtcycle 20+ mph/sep.

INJURY SITE/TYPE: Amputate, Burn/Elec, Blunt, Penetrate, Frac/Disloc., Soft-Closed, Soft-Open
Head, Face, Eye, Neck/Spine, Chest, Back/Spine, Abdomen, Pelv./Groin, Arm, Hand, Thigh, Leg/Foot

16444246

BLS TREATMENT
AIRWAY: Abdominal Thrust, Back Blows, Manual, Nasopharyngeal, Oropharyngeal
VENTILATION: Pocket Mask, Demand Valve, Bag Valve Mask
IMMOBILIZATION: C-Spine Stabilize, Cervical Collar, C-Spine Imm. Dev., Board - Long, Board - Short, Splint - Extremity, Splint - Traction
OXYGEN: O_2 1-9 lpm, O_2 10-15 lpm
OTHER: Auto Defib., Bandage, CPR, Hot Pack, Cold Pack, Delivery (OB), Extrication, Ipecac, Irrigation, MAST Appl'd, MAST Inflated, Oral Glucose, Suctioning, Tourniquet
(A1 A2 A3 A4 O)

EKG INITIAL/LAST: Nrml. Sin., Sin. Tach, Sin. Brady, Asystole, AV Block, Atrial Fib, Atrial Flut, EMD, Junctional, Paced, PVC's, SV Tach, Vent Tach, Vent Fib, Other (I L)

MEDICATIONS: Albuterol, Aminophylline, Atropine, Bicarb, Bretylium, Calcium, Dexameth, D50, Diazepam, Diphenhyd., Dobutamine, Dopamine, Epinephrine, Furosemide, Glucagon, Heparin, Hydrocortisone, Isoproterenol, Lidocaine, Meperidine, Metaproterenol, Morphine, Naloxone, Nitroglycerine, Nitrous Oxide, Oxytocin, Procainamide, Terbutaline, Verapamil, Other

PATIENT RECEIVED BY: | RESEARCH CODE

IV FLUIDS/RATE: D5W, Normal Saline, Ring. Lact., TKO, Bolus, Wide

PATIENT CONDITION: ON SCENE: Life Threat., Mod., Minor | AT FACILITY: Improved, Stable, Unstable, Worse

COMMAND FACILITY ID #

ALS TREATMENT: Peripheral IV, EKG, EndoTrach. Intub., Med. Admin., Blood Draw, Central Ven. IV, Cricothyrotomy, Defib/Cardiovert, EOA, Intraosseous IV, Needle Thorac., Pacing, Urinary Cath (A1 A2 A3 A4 O)

CPR INFORMATION (Minutes): <4, 4 - 10, >10, Unk
Arrest to CPR, Arrest to Defib, Arrest to ALS
Witnessed Arrest? Y N Unk
Bystander CPR? Y N Unk

MEDICAL COMMAND: Telephone, Cellular, Radio, None, Protocol, MD On-Scene, None Required

Region Copy

PLEASE DO NOT MARK IN THIS AREA

Mark Reflex® by NCS EM-159353-3:654321 GS03 Printed in U.S.A.

FIGURE 16-1 ■ Photo of a patient care report.

Continued

Use Blue/Black Ink - Press Firmly

SERVICE NAME	SERVICE #	INCIDENT #	TODAY'S DATE
INCIDENT LOCATION			

PATIENT INFO

PATIENT LAST NAME	FIRST	M.I.	PHONE	AGE	DATE OF BIRTH	SEX
STREET ADDRESS			SOCIAL SECURITY NUMBER	MEMBERSHIP (Y) Yes (N) No		
CITY	STATE	ZIP CODE	INSURANCE CODE #	MILEAGE		
PRIVATE PHYSICIAN			MEDICAID #	OUT		
○ BILL TO (COMPANY or NAME)		PHONE	MEDICARE #	SCENE		
ADDRESS	STREET		GROUP INSURANCE #	DEST		
CITY	STATE	ZIP CODE	OTHER INSURANCE #	IN		

CHIEF COMPLAINT	
CURRENT MEDICATIONS	○ NONE KNOWN
ALLERGIES (MEDS)	○ NONE KNOWN
PAST MEDICAL HISTORY	○ MI ○ CHF ○ COPD ○ ↑ BP ○ DIABETES ○ CANCER ○ NONE KNOWN ○ OTHER

NARRATIVE

○ Narrative 1 of ______

TIME	P	R	B/P	RHYTHM	TREATMENT	PROVIDER ID #	RESPONSE/COMMENTS
			/				
			/				
			/				
			/				
			/				
			/				
			/				

Crew Signatures:

A#1 ______

Signature of Person Receiving Patient ______ Time ______

A#2 ______

Command Physician ______ ID# ______

A#3 ______

A#4 ______

Service Copy

16444246

FIGURE 16-1, cont'd ■ Photo of a patient care report.

BOX 16-3 Common Abbreviations*

°C	degrees centigrade	CO_2	carbon dioxide
°F	degrees Fahrenheit	COPD	chronic obstructive pulmonary disease
μg	microgram	CPK	creatine phosphokinase
μm	micrometer	CPR	cardiopulmonary resuscitation
∞	dram	CSF	cerebrospinal fluid
@	at	CT	computed tomography
aa	of each	CVA	cerebrovascular accident; costovertebral angle
ABG	arterial blood gas	CVP	central venous pressure
ac	before meals	D&C	dilation and curettage
ad lib	freely as desired	D5W	5% dextrose in water
ADL	activities of daily living	db, dB	decibels
Ag	silver; antigen	dc	discontinue
AIDS	acquired immunodeficiency syndrome	DIC	disseminated intravascular coagulation
ALS	amyotrophic lateral sclerosis	diff	differential blood count
am	morning	dil	dilute
a.m.a.	against medical advice	DJD	degenerative joint disease
AMI	acute myocardial infarction	dL	deciliter
amp	ampule	DM	diastolic murmur
ARC	AIDS-related complex	DNR	do not resuscitate
ARDS	acute respiratory distress syndrome	DOE	dyspnea on exertion
AS	aortic stenosis	dx, DX	diagnosis
ASD	atrial septal defect	EBV	Epstein-Barr virus
Ba	barium	ECF	extracellular fluid
BE	barium enema	ECG	electrocardiogram
bid	2 times a day	ECT	electroconvulsive therapy
BM, bm	bowel movement	EDC	estimated date of confinement
BMR	basal metabolic rate	EDD	estimated date of delivery
BP	blood pressure	EEG	electroencephalogram
BPH	benign prostatic hypertrophy	EKG	electrocardiogram
BRP	bathroom privileges	elix	elixir
BSA	body surface area	EMG	electromyogram
BUN	blood urea nitrogen	ENG	electronystagmography
$\bar{c}$	with	ER	emergency room
c/o	complains of	ERG	electroretinogram
Ca	calcium, cancer, carcinoma	ESR	erythrocyte sedimentation rate
CAD	coronary artery disease	ESRD	end-stage renal disease
cap	capsule	EST	electroshock therapy
CAT	computed axial tomography	f∞	fluid ounce
cath.	catheter, catheterize	FANA	fluorescent antinuclear antibody test
CBC	complete blood count	Fe	iron
CBR	complete bed rest	FEV	forced expiratory volume
CC	chief complaint	FHR	fetal heart rate
cc	cubic centimeter	FRC	functional residual capacity
CCU	coronary care unit; critical care unit	FUO	fever of unknown origin
CDC	Centers for Disease Control and Prevention	Fx, fx	fracture, fractional urine test
CEA	carcinoembryonic antigen	g, gm, Gm	gram
CFT	complement-fixation test	Gc,GC	gonococcus
cg	centigram	GI	gastrointestinal
CHF	congestive heart failure	gr	grain
CHO	carbohydrate	grav I, II, III, etc.	pregnancy one, two, three, etc.
Cl	chlorine	gt, gtt	drop, drops
cm	centimeter	GTT	glucose tolerance test
cm^3	cubic centimeter	GU	genitourinary
CNS	central nervous system	GYN, Gyn	gynecological
CO	carbon monoxide		

From Potter PA, Perry AG: *Fundamentals of nursing: concepts, process, and practice,* ed 4, St Louis, 1997, Mosby.

*Note: The abbreviations in common use can vary widely from place to place. Each institution has a list of acceptable abbreviations that is the best authority for its records.

Continued

BOX 16-3 Common Abbreviations*—cont'd

H_2O	water	Mg	magnesium
h	hour	MG	myasthenia gravis
H+	hydrogen ion	MI	myocardial infarction
h/o	history of	MICU	medical intensive care unit
H&P	history and physical examination	mL	milliliter
HAV	hepatitis A virus	mm	millimeter
Hb	hemoglobin	mm^3	cubic millimeter
HBAg	hepatitis B antigen	mm Hg	millimeters of mercury
HBV	hepatitis B virus	MRI	magnetic resonance imaging
Hct, HCT	hematocrit	MS	multiple sclerosis
Hg	mercury	MW	molecular weight
Hgb	hemoglobin	N	nitrogen
HIV	human immunodeficiency (AIDS) virus	Na	sodium
HLA	human lymphocyte antigen	NICU	neonatal intensive care unit
hs	at bedtime	NIH	National Institutes of Health
HSV	herpes simplex virus	nm	nanometer
I&O	intake and output	NMR	nuclear magnetic resonance
IC	inspiratory capacity	NPO	nothing by mouth
ICP	intracranial pressure	NS	normal saline
ICU	intensive care unit	O_2	oxygen
IDDM	insulin-dependent diabetes mellitus	OD	right eye; optical density; overdose
IE	immunoelectrophoresis	OL	left eye
Ig	immunoglobulin	OOB	out of bed
IgA, etc.	immunoglobulin A, etc.	ORIF	open reduction and internal fixation
IM	intramuscular	OS	left eye
IOP	intraocular pressure	OT	occupational therapy
IPPB	intermittent positive pressure breathing	OTC	over-the-counter
IV	intravenous	oz, ∞	ounce
IVP	intravenous push; intravenous pyelogram	P&A	percussion and auscultation
IVU	intravenous urogram	$Pa{CO_2}$	partial pressure of carbon dioxide (arterial blood)
JRA	juvenile rheumatoid arthritis		
K	potassium	$Pa{O_2}$	partial pressure of oxygen (arterial blood)
kg	kilogram	para I, II, etc.	unipara, bipara, etc.
KUB	kidney, ureters, and bladder (radiograph)	PAT	paroxysmal atrial tachycardia
KVO	keep vein open	pc	after meals
L	liter	PCG	phonocardiogram
L&A	light and accommodation	$P{CO_2}$	partial pressure of carbon dioxide
LBBB	left bundle branch block	PCP	pulmonary capillary pressure; phencyclidine
LE	lupus erythematosus	PCV	packed cell volume
LGV	lymphogranuloma venereum	PCWP	pulmonary capillary wedge pressure
LLL	left lower lobe	PD	interpupillary distance; postural drainage
LLQ	left lower quadrant	PE	pulmonary embolism; physical examination
LMP	last menstrual period	PEEP	positive end-expiratory pressure
LNMP	last normal menstrual period	PEG	pneumoencephalography
LP	lumbar puncture	per	through; by way of
LUL	left upper lobe	PERRLA	pupils equal, round, and reactive to light and accommodation
LUQ	left upper quadrant		
LVH	left ventricular hypertrophy	PET	positron emission tomography
m	meter	PG	prostaglandin
m, min, ♏	minim	pH	hydrogen ion concentration (acidity and alkalinity)
MAP	mean arterial pressure		
mcg	microgram	PID	pelvic inflammatory disease
MCH	mean corpuscular hemoglobin	PKU	phenylketonuria
MCHC	mean corpuscular hemoglobin concentration	PM	postmortem
MCV	mean cell volume; mean corpuscular volume	pm	evening
mg	milligram	PMS	premenstrual syndrome

From Potter PA, Perry AG: *Fundamentals of nursing: concepts, process, and practice,* ed 4, St Louis, 1997, Mosby.

*Note: The abbreviations in common use can vary widely from place to place. Each institution has a list of acceptable abbreviations that is the best authority for its records.

BOX 16-3 Common Abbreviations*—cont'd

PND	paroxysmal nocturnal dyspnea; postnasal drip	sos	if necessary
Po_2	partial pressure of oxygen	sp. gr., SG, sg	specific gravity
PO, po	orally	SQ, subq	subcutaneous
PPD	purified protein derivative	SR	sedimentation rate
ppm	parts per million	ss	half
p.r.n.	when required; as often as necessary	SSS	sick sinus syndrome; specific soluble substance; short-stay surgery
PT	physical therapy; prothrombin time	stat	immediately
PTT	partial thromboplastin time	STD	sexually transmitted disease
PUO	pyrexia of unknown origin	STS	serological test for syphilis
PVC	premature ventricular contraction	susp	suspension
q	every	T_3	triiodothyronine
q2h	every 2 hours	T_4	tetraiodothyronine
q3h	every 3 hours	T&A	tonsillectomy and adenoidectomy
q4h	every 4 hours	TAB	typhoid and paratyphoid A and B
qd	every day	TAH	total abdominal hysterectomy
qh	every hour	TAT	tetanus antitoxin; thematic apperception test
qid	4 times a day		
qn	every night	TB, TBC	tuberculosis
qod	every other day	TBG	thyroxin-binding globulin
qns	quantity not sufficient	TG	triglyceride
R/O	rule out	TIA	transient ischemic attack
RA	rheumatoid arthritis	TIBC	total iron-binding capacity
RBBB	right bundle branch block	tid	3 times a day
RDA	recommended daily (dietary) allowance	TKO	to keep open
RDS	respiratory distress syndrome	TLC	total lung capacity; thin layer chromatography
Rh^+	positive Rh factor		
Rh^-	negative Rh factor	TPN	total parenteral nutrition
RHD	rheumatic heart disease	TPR	temperature, pulse, and respirations
RLL	right lower lobe	tr, tinct	tincture
RLQ	right lower quadrant	TST	triple sugar iron test
RML	right middle lobe	UIBC	unsaturated iron-binding capacity
ROM	range of motion	URI	upper respiratory infection
ROS	review of systems	UTI	urinary tract infection
RS	Reiter's syndrome	V&T	volume and tension
RSV	Rous sarcoma virus	VC	vital capacity
RUL	right upper lobe	VD	venereal disease
RUQ	right upper quadrant	VDA	visual discriminatory acuity
Rx	take, treatment	VDH	valvular disease of the heart
$\bar{s}$	without	VDRL	Venereal Disease Research Laboratory (test for syphilis)
SB	sternal border		
SC	subcutaneous	VS	vital signs
sib.	sibling	VSD	ventricular septal defect
SICU	surgical intensive care unit	VT	tidal volume
SIDS	sudden infant death syndrome	W/V	weight/volume
Sig	write on label	WBC	white blood cell; white blood count
SLE	systemic lupus erythematosus	WNL	within normal limits
sol	solution, dissolved	WR	Wasserman reaction

The paramedic should put into quotation marks certain statements. The paramedic should quote any statements made directly by patients or others that relate to possible criminal activity. The paramedic should quote admission of suicidal intention as well. In addition, the paramedic should document failed skills on the PCR. (Examples include unsuccessful attempts to start an intravenous line or to perform endotracheal intubation.)

CRITICAL THINKING

Why should you note the previous care given by bystanders in your report?

The narrative also should include the use of support services and mutual aid assistance. Such services might include helicopter, coroner, and rescue/extrication. Finally, the paramedic should sign the PCR. The PCR should list everyone who took part in the patient's care before delivery to the emergency department. Because a copy of the report is placed in the patient's hospital medical record, leaving a finished copy at the receiving hospital may be necessary. This requires completing the report in a timely fashion at the receiving hospital so that the EMS crew can be available for another call.

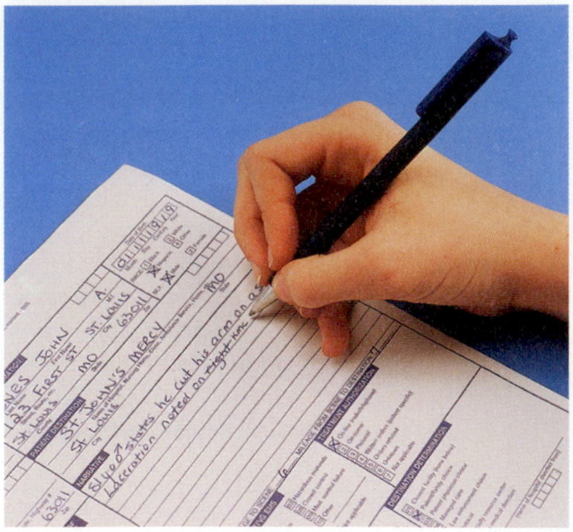

FIGURE 16-2 ■ Correction of a patient care report.

> **NOTE** The patient care report is valuable. The report provides the attending physician and emergency department staff the advantage of understanding the events and the care rendered in the prehospital setting. If possible, the paramedic should leave the report with the patient at the hospital.

ELEMENTS OF A PROPERLY WRITTEN EMERGENCY MEDICAL SERVICES DOCUMENT

A properly written EMS document is accurate, legible, timely, unaltered, and free of nonprofessional or extraneous information. A brief description of each of these elements is listed as follows:

1. *Accurate and complete.* All relevant information must be provided in the narrative and check-box sections of the report. This ensures accuracy. Completing all areas of the report shows a precise and full document. The paramedic should do this even if a section was unused. The paramedic should ensure that medical terms, abbreviations, and acronyms are used properly and are spelled correctly.
2. *Legible.* Legible means that all writing, especially in the narrative part of the report, can be read easily by others. Check-box markings should be clear and consistent from the top page of the report to all underlying pages.
3. *Timely.* Ideally, the documentation should be completed immediately after the paramedic completes the patient care. Delays in recording can result in serious omissions, which may be interpreted as negligent patient care.
4. *Unaltered.* If the paramedic makes errors while writing the report, the paramedic should draw a single line through the error. Then the paramedic should date and initial the error (Fig. 16-2). Any changes to a completed report should be accompanied by a proper "revision/correction" supplement with the date and time of revision.
5. *Free of nonprofessional/extraneous information.* The PCR must be free of jargon, slang, personal bias, libelous or slanderous remarks, and irrelevant opinion or impression.

> **NOTE** An emergency medical services report should be considered confidential. Moreover, the paramedic should respect this privacy. The paramedic should comply with patient privacy provisions. These provisions are outlined by agency policy and by the Health Insurance Portability and Accountability Act (2001) as described in Chapter 4.

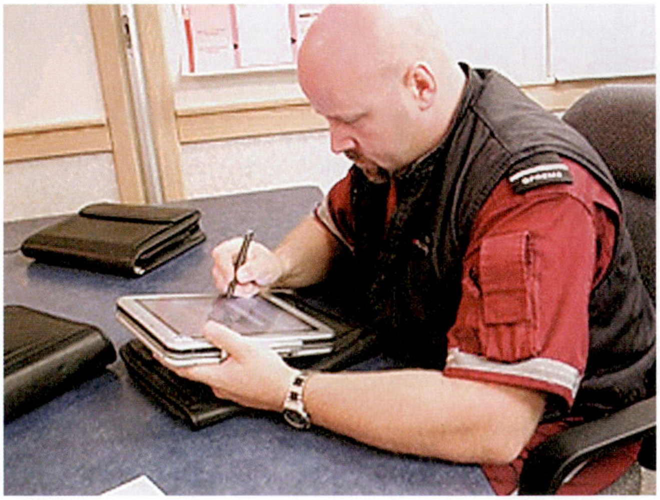

FIGURE 16-3 ■ Paramedic completing an electronic patient care report.

The paramedic also should apply these principles of documentation to computer-generated PCRs (Fig. 16-3).

SYSTEMS OF NARRATIVE WRITING

As with all other aspects of emergency care, the paramedic should develop a systematic approach for writing the narrative portion of the patient care report. Many approaches for writing the narrative can be used; however, the paramedic should adopt only *one* approach and use it consistently to avoid omissions in report writing. Examples of systems used to write the narrative include the SAMPLE history; SOAP format; CHART format; a physical approach from head to toe; a review of primary body systems; a chronological, call-incident approach; a patient management approach; and others. Regardless of the system used to organize the narrative, the paramedic must ensure that objective (versus subjective) elements of documentation make up the report.

▶NOTE Some information is viewed as objective. This information can be supported by facts and direct observation. Other information is viewed as subjective. This information cannot be supported by facts. An example of the latter is "the patient appears depressed." The paramedic generally should omit such information from the narrative. Or the paramedic should enter the information in the patient's own words using quotes. Some subjective observations should be documented carefully and reported to medical direction. An example is a child's behavior that is suspicious for possible physical or sexual abuse in the home.

The *SAMPLE history* (described in Chapter 10) can be used to organize the narrative part of a written report. To review, the SAMPLE history is comprised of *(S)* signs and symptoms, *(A)* allergies, *(M)* medications, *(P)* past medical history, *(L)* last meal or oral intake, and *(E)* events before the emergency.

The *SOAP format* is a method one can use to organize a patient report for most patient care encounters. SOAP is an acronym for the following:

Subjective data: All patient symptoms including chief complaint, associated symptoms, history, current medications and allergies, and information provided by bystanders and family

Objective data: Pertinent physical examination information, including vital signs, level of consciousness, physical examination findings, electrocardiogram, pulse oximetry readings, and blood glucose determinations

Assessment data: The paramedic's clinical impression of the patient based on subjective and objective data

Plan of patient management: Treatment that has been provided and any requests for additional treatment

The *CHART format* is an alternative to the SAMPLE and SOAP formats. The CHART format includes the following:

Chief complaint: The patient's primary complaint

History: History of present illness; significant medical history; current health status; review of systems

Assessment: General impression; vital signs; physical examination; diagnostic tests; field diagnosis

Rx (treatment): Standing orders or protocols; direct orders from online medical direction

Transport: Effects of interventions; mode of transportation; ongoing assessment findings

The *physical approach from head-to-toe* often is used to organize the narrative. The paramedic may use the physical approach after performing a full head-to-toe physical examination. Findings noted in the narrative are in the same order as they were in the exam. For example, the paramedic would begin by noting findings from examining the patient's head. Such findings, for example, may include pupillary response. The paramedic would end by noting circulatory findings. The paramedic would note the character of a pedal pulse or capillary refill when examining the patient's extremities.

A *review of primary body systems* also can be used in the narrative. The paramedic may use the review when the examination is performed for a chief complaint focused on one body system. For example, this may be chest pain with suspected myocardial infarction. With this approach, the paramedic limits findings to the cardiorespiratory system. Findings may include a description of the patient's pain, vital signs, electrocardiogram findings, associated breathing difficulties, significant medical history, allergies, and medication use.

The *chronological, call-incident approach* for writing a narrative begins by noting the time of arrival at the patient's side and initial examination findings, the time of vital sign assessment and reassessment, and a chronological listing of all patient care interventions performed at the scene and en route to the emergency department. This type of report commonly is used to document the events of a patient with major trauma with extended on-scene time. The paramedic also may use this format during a cardiac arrest event when numerous medications and electrical therapy are administered to the patient.

The *patient management approach* is used to organize and record the complete patient management plan. The report covers from the start to the finish of an emergency response. This approach might describe in detail how the patient was found, what interventions were performed and why, and any important assessment findings. The patient management approach differs slightly from the others described. This approach provides a more complete picture of the events at the scene, during care, and during transport of the patient.

CRITICAL THINKING

How many meanings can you think of for the word *lethargic*? Look it up in the dictionary. Should you use this word to document a patient's mental status? Why?

SPECIAL CONSIDERATIONS OF DOCUMENTATION

Several considerations for documenting patient care deserve special mention. Three of these include a patient's refusal of care or transport, situations and events where transportation is not needed, and situations involving mass casualties. Other situations that require careful documentation (e.g., caring for intoxicated patients and cases of abuse and neglect) are described in Chapters 4 and 46, respectively.

Patient Refusal of Care or Transport

As described in Chapter 4, a patient's refusal of care or transport is a major area of potential liability for paramedics and EMS agencies. Thorough documentation of these situations is crucial and should include the following:

- The paramedic's advice to the patient regarding the benefits of treatment and the risks associated with refusing care
- The advice rendered by medical direction via telephone or radio

- Clinical information (e.g., the patient's level of consciousness) that suggests competency
- The signatures of any witnesses to the event, according to local protocol
- A complete narrative, including quotations or statements made by others

If the patient refuses care or transport, the paramedic should document the incident carefully. The paramedic also should make it clear that the patient may call again for help, despite the initial refusal. When possible, the paramedic should encourage friends or family to stay with the patient.

When Care and Transportation are Not Needed

At times, care and transportation of a patient are not warranted. This situation may be the result of the patient's condition or a canceled request for help. After evaluation of the patient or scene, the paramedic may determine that circumstances do not warrant EMS transport (for example, for a car crash without injuries or a patient who has left the scene). At this point, the paramedic should advise the dispatch center and document the event. If the EMS unit is canceled en route to the scene, the paramedic should make note of the canceling authority and time of the cancellation. The canceling authority, for example, may be the dispatch center or EMS supervisor. Like refusal of care, thorough documentation of these events can protect the paramedic from potential liability.

Situations Involving Mass Casualties

A major incident may involve a large number of patients. Thus comprehensive documentation may have to be postponed. Documentation may need to be delayed until patients are triaged and transported for definitive care (see Chapter 50). These are difficult and unusual situations. In these circumstances, the paramedic should know and follow local documentation procedures.

DOCUMENT REVISION/ CORRECTION

As stated before, revising or correcting a patient care report sometimes is necessary. Most EMS agencies provide separate report forms for this purpose. If a separate report is needed, the paramedic should do the following:

- Note the purpose of the revision or correction and why the information did not appear on the original document.
- Note the date and time the revision or correction was made.
- Ensure that the revision or correction was made by the original author of the document.
- Make the revision or correction as soon as the need for it is realized.

Acceptable methods for making revisions or adding information to a document vary by agency. Some include making the change to the original form. Included with this would be initials, date, and time. Other methods include writing the corrections in the narrative. Still other methods include attaching a new report to the original. Supplemental narratives can be written on a separate form. These should be attached to the original. The paramedic should follow the policies set by the EMS agency and medical direction for revising or correcting reports.

CRITICAL THINKING

Consider this situation. Your supervisor asks you to change your documentation so the insurance company will pay for the transport. What would you do?

CONSEQUENCES OF INAPPROPRIATE DOCUMENTATION

Documentation that is incorrect or incomplete may have serious consequences with medical and legal implications. An inaccurate, incomplete, or illegible PCR may cause caregivers to provide improper care to a patient. For example, consider that a paramedic fails to mention that a patient with a possible myocardial infarction has an allergy to ***lidocaine***. This patient later becomes unconscious in the emergency department as a result of a ventricular rhythm disturbance. A lethal medication for that patient could be administered inadvertently. A PCR that is thoroughly completed in a professional manner may influence greatly the decision of an attorney who is considering the merits of an impending lawsuit for negligence or malpractice. (The converse also is true if the documentation is not thorough and professional.)

Finally, documentation should never become routine to the paramedic (Box 16-4). Documentation also should never be superficial. Good documentation should be completed in a timely manner. Moreover, documentation should be completed with careful attention to detail. This will ensure that the PCR is medically and legally sound.

BOX 16-4 The Paramedic's Responsibility for Documentation

As part of professional responsibility, the paramedic should do the following:

- View the task of documentation as one of utmost importance.
- Assume responsibility for self-assessment of all documentation.
- Appreciate the importance of good documentation among peers.
- Strive to set a good example to others regarding the completion of the documentation task.
- Respect the confidential nature of an emergency medical services report.

SUMMARY

- The patient care report is used to document the key elements of patient assessment, care, and transport.
- The three primary reasons for written documentation are that the medical community involved in the patient's care uses it, it is a legal record, and it is essential to data collection.
- The PCR should include dates and response times, difficulties encountered, observations at the scene, previous medical care provided, a chronological description of the call, and significant times.
- A properly written EMS document is accurate, legible, timely, unaltered, and free of nonprofessional or extraneous information.
- Many approaches for writing the narrative can be used. The paramedic should adopt only one approach. The paramedic should use this approach consistently to avoid omissions in report writing.
- Special documentation is necessary when a patient refuses care or transport. Such documentation also is needed in those cases when care or transportation is not needed. Special documentation also is needed for mass casualty incidents.
- Most EMS agencies have separate forms for revisions or corrections to the patient care report.
- Documentation that is inappropriate may have medical and legal implications.

REFERENCE

1. US Department of Transportation, National Highway Traffic Safety Administration: *EMT-Paramedic national standard curriculum,* Washington, DC, 1998, The Department.

SUGGESTED READINGS

Angell L et al: *Documentation: the language of nursing,* Upper Saddle River, NJ, 2000, Prentice-Hall.

Marelli T, Harper S: *Nursing documentation handbook,* St Louis, 2000, Mosby.

Milewski R et al: *Documentation: field guide,* Boston, 2000, Jones and Bartlett.

PART FOUR

IN THIS PART

CHAPTER 17 Pharmacology

CHAPTER 18 Venous Access and Medication Administration

CHAPTER

17

Pharmacology

OBJECTIVES

Upon completion of this chapter, the paramedic student will be able to:

1. Explain what a drug is.
2. Identify the four types of drug names.
3. Outline drug standards and legislation and the enforcement agencies pertinent to the paramedic profession.
4. Describe the paramedic's responsibilities in drug administration.
5. Distinguish among drug forms.
6. Outline autonomic nervous system functions that may be changed with drug therapy.
7. Discuss factors that influence drug absorption, distribution, and elimination.
8. Describe how drugs react with receptors to produce their desired effects.
9. List variables that can influence drug interactions.
10. Identify special considerations for administering pharmacological agents to pregnant patients, pediatric patients, and older patients.
11. Outline drug actions and care considerations for a patient who is given drugs that affect the nervous, cardiovascular, respiratory, endocrine, and gastrointestinal systems.
12. Explain the meaning of drug terms that are necessary to interpret information in drug references safely.

KEY TERMS

absorption: The process by which drug molecules are moved from the site of entry into the body into the general circulation.

adrenergic: Of or pertaining to the sympathetic nerve fibers of the autonomic nervous system, which use epinephrine or epinephrine-like substances as neurotransmitters.

agonists: Drugs that combine with receptors and initiate the expected response.

antagonists: Agents designed to inhibit or counteract the effects of other drugs or undesired effects caused by normal or hyperactive physiological mechanisms.

anticholinergic: Of or pertaining to the blocking of acetylcholine receptors, resulting in inhibition of transmission of parasympathetic nerve impulses.

biological half-life: The time required to metabolize or eliminate half the total amount of a drug in the body.

biotransformation: The process by which a drug is converted chemically to a metabolite.

chemical name: The exact designation of a chemical structure as determined by the rules of chemical nomenclature.

cholinergic: Of or pertaining to the effects produced by the parasympathetic nervous system or drugs that stimulate or antagonize the parasympathetic nervous system.

contraindications: Medical or physiological factors that make it harmful to administer a medication that would otherwise have a therapeutic effect.

controlled substance: Any drug defined in the categories of the Comprehensive Drug Abuse Prevention and Control Act (also known as the Controlled Substances Act) of 1970.

cumulative action: The effect that occurs when several doses of a drug are administered or when absorption occurs more quickly than removal by excretion or metabolism or both.

distribution: The transport of a drug through the bloodstream to various tissues of the body and ultimately to its site of action.

drug: Any substance taken by mouth; injected into a muscle, blood vessel, or cavity of the body; or applied topically to treat or prevent a disease or condition.

drug interaction: Modification of the effects of one drug by the previous or concurrent administration of another drug, thereby increasing or diminishing the pharmacological or physiological action of one or both drugs.

drug receptors: Parts of a cell (usually an enzyme or large protein molecule) with which a drug molecule interacts to trigger its desired response or effect.

excretion: The elimination of toxic or inactive metabolites, primarily by the kidneys; the intestines, lungs, and mammary, sweat, and salivary glands also may be involved.

first-pass metabolism: The initial biotransformation of a drug during passage through the liver from the portal vein that occurs before the drug reaches the general circulation.

generic name: The official, established name assigned to a drug.

idiosyncrasy: An abnormal or peculiar response to a drug.

loading dose: A large quantity of drug that temporarily exceeds the capacity of the body to excrete the drug.

maintenance dose: The amount of a drug required to keep a desired steady state of drug concentration in tissues.

official name: The name of a drug that is followed by the initials USP (United States Pharmacopeia) or NF (National Formulary), denoting its listing in one of the official publications; usually the same as the generic name.

parenteral: Of or pertaining to any medication route other than the alimentary canal.

pharmaceutics: The science of dispensing drugs.

pharmacodynamics: The study of how a drug acts on a living organism.

pharmacokinetics: The study of how the body handles a drug over a period of time, including the processes of absorption, distribution, biotransformation, and excretion.

placental barrier: A protective biological membrane that separates the blood vessels of the mother and the fetus.

potentiation: Enhancement of the effect of a drug, caused by concurrent administration of two drugs in which one drug increases the effect of the other.

summation: The combined effects of two drugs that equal the sum of the individual effects of each agent.

synergism: The combined action of two drugs that is greater than the sum of each agent acting independently.

therapeutic action: The desired, intended action of a drug.

therapeutic index: A measurement of the relative safety of a drug.

tolerance: A physiological response that requires that a drug dosage be increased to produce the same effect formerly produced by a smaller dose.

trade name: The trademark name of a drug, designated by the drug company that sells the medication.

untoward effects: Side effects that prove harmful to the patient.

Pharmacology can be defined as the science of drugs used to prevent, diagnose, and treat disease. Pharmacology deals with the interactions between living systems and chemical molecules. The paramedic must have a thorough understanding of a drug and its actions before it is administered. This understanding will help to ensure maximum effectiveness and will reduce the potential for harm.

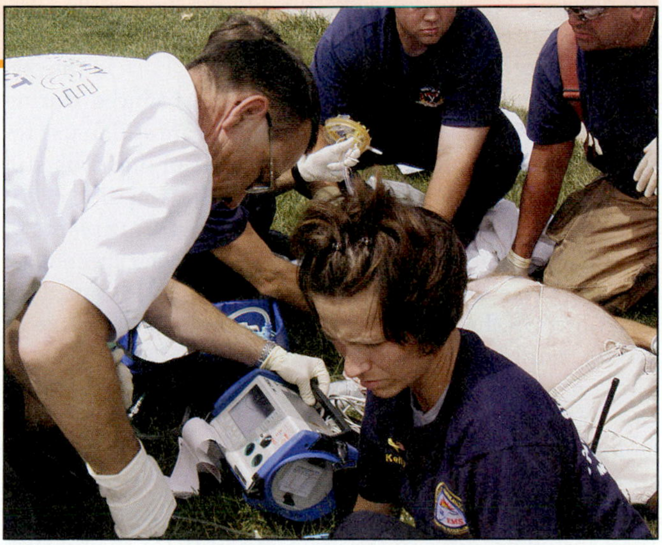

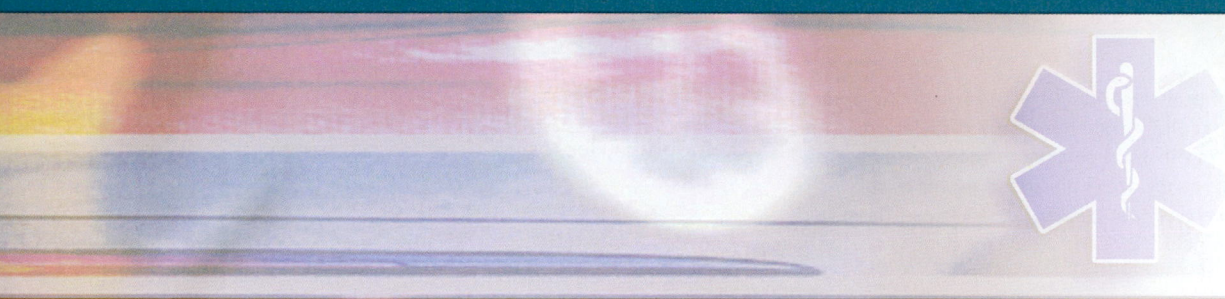

NOTE This chapter introduces the paramedic to general principles of pharmacology and emergency medications commonly used in the prehospital setting. A more complete description of the emergency drugs discussed in this chapter can be found in the *Emergency Drug Index.* Medications described in this text that are included in the index are denoted by bold italic type.

The drug information presented in this section conforms to current medical literature, to manufacturers' monographs, and to the clinical practice of the general medical community at the time of publication. Although every effort has been made to ensure accuracy and completeness, the authors, editors, medical advisers, and publisher disclaim liability for any discrepancies, incongruities, undetected errors, omissions in content, or reader misunderstanding. Local protocol for drug administration may vary from the information presented in this chapter. The paramedic should follow the guidelines established by medical direction.

SECTION ONE
Drug Information

HISTORICAL TRENDS IN PHARMACOLOGY

The science of pharmacology may date back as early as 10,000 to 7000 BC.[1] Medicinal herbs are thought to have been among the plants grown by human beings in the Neolithic period. Yet whether the herbs were thought to have healing properties is not known. A number of medicines are mentioned in the Bible. Some of these include gums, spices, oils, and maybe even narcotics. Drugs derived from plants were used heavily throughout the Middle Ages. They were used as digestives, laxatives, and diuretics.

The concept of "chemical medicine" was born in the seventeenth century. Some preparations introduced during the seventeenth and eighteenth centuries are still in use today. Opium ***(morphine)*** is a good example of one **drug** still in use. Accurate studies of drug dosage in the nineteenth century led to the development of manufacturing plants to produce drugs. In addition, knowledge of the expected actions of these drugs became more exact. Important drug discoveries in the twentieth and twenty-first centuries (e.g., ***insulin,*** antibiotics, and fibrinolytics) have had major effects on common illnesses such as diabetes, bacterial infections, and cardiovascular disease.

Modern health care and **pharmaceutics** are going through many changes due in large part to consumer awareness of disease prevention. Changes also come from the consumers' drive to take responsibility for their health and wellness. The health care and pharmaceutical industries actively seek to develop new drugs, treatments, cures, or other methods to prevent diseases that affect aging, everyday living, or life span. The federal government also provides incentives to pharmaceutical companies to research and develop less profitable drugs. These drugs are called *orphan drugs.* They treat rare, chronic diseases such as hemophilia, leprosy, Cushing's syndrome, and Tourette's syndrome.

Drug Names

A drug may be defined as "any substance taken by mouth, injected into a muscle, blood vessel, or cavity of the body, or applied topically to treat or prevent a disease or condition."[2] Drugs have been identified or derived from five major sources. These sources are plants (alkaloids, glycosides, gums, and oils), animals and human beings, minerals or mineral products, microorganisms, and chemical substances made in the laboratory (Box 17-1).

Drugs can be identified by the following four types of names:

1. **Chemical name:** The chemical name is an exact description. It describes the chemical composition of the drug. It also describes its molecular structure.
2. **Generic name** (nonproprietary name): This name often is an abbreviated form of the chemical name. The generic name is used more commonly than the chemical name. Generic drugs usually have the same therapeutic efficacy as nongeneric drugs. However, they generally are less expensive. This is the official name approved by the U.S. Food and Drug Administration (FDA).
3. **Trade name** (brand or proprietary name): The trade name is a trademark name designated by the drug company that sells the medication. Trade names are proper nouns, and the first letter is capitalized. This text shows the trade name in parentheses after the generic name of the drug. The trade name usually is suggested by the first manufacturer of the drug.
4. **Official name:** The official name of a drug is followed by the initials *USP (United States Pharmacopeia)* or *NF (National Formulary).* These initials denote the listing of the drug in one of the official publications. In most cases the official name is the same as the generic name.

BOX 17-1 Examples of Drugs and Their Sources

Plant Sources
Digoxin
Morphine sulfate
Atropine sulfate

Animal and Human Sources
Epinephrine
Insulin
Adrenocorticotropic hormone

Mineral or Mineral Product
Calcium chloride
Iodine
Iron
Sodium bicarbonate

Microorganism Sources
Penicillin
Streptomycin

Laboratory-Produced Chemicals
Diazepam (Valium)
Lidocaine (Xylocaine)
Midazolam (Versed)

An example of the four names for a drug would be as follows:

Chemical name:	ethyl 1-methyl-4-phenylisonipecotate hydrochloride
Generic name:	***meperidine hydrochloride***
Trade name:	Demerol
Official name:	meperidine hydrochloride USP

Sources of Drug Information

Several publications offer information on various drugs, their preparation, and recommended administration. These references include the *American Medical Association Drug Evaluation,* the *American Hospital Formulary Service Drug Information,* medication package inserts, the *Physician's Desk Reference,* and the *Nursing Drug Reference,* and *Mosby's Drug Consult* (Box 17-2). Paramedics should be familiar with these and with other emergency pharmacology manuals as well. This is crucial particularly regarding drugs that often are administered in the prehospital setting. The Internet also can be a good source of information about pharmacotherapeutics. Usually the Internet is the most current source. In addition, the findings of current research can be found on the Internet. This research provides details about certain drug studies and treatments.

BOX 17-2 Drug References

American Medical Association Drug Evaluation: The *Drug Evaluation* provides information on drug groups, dosages, prescribing information, and usage. It also covers valid clinical applications of drug use that differ from those approved by the Food and Drug Administration thus far.

Hospital Formulary: The *Hospital Formulary,* a manual published by the American Society of Hospital Pharmacists, provides an overview in monograph form of nearly every available (approved and unapproved) drug in the United States. The formulary is updated regularly and is available in all hospital pharmacies and in many emergency departments. The *Hospital Formulary* is considered by many to be the most reliable source of information on medications and drugs.

Medication package inserts: Most medications are packaged with written literature describing product use. These inserts provide valuable information as new drugs are introduced, and the health care professional should consult them to become familiar with the product.

Physician's Desk Reference: The *Physician's Desk Reference,* published yearly by the Medical Economics Company, is a concise compilation of drug information, including Food and Drug Administration–approved indications, contraindications, and adverse effects. In addition to providing product information through several cross-referenced indexes, the textbook serves as an identification guide by showing actual-size, color pictures of commonly prescribed medications. The *Physician's Desk Reference* also lists emergency telephone numbers for poison control centers throughout the United States.

Nursing Drug Reference: The *Nursing Drug Reference* is published yearly and includes nursing considerations, side effects, adverse reactions, precautions, interactions, and contraindications for drug and intravenous therapy. The textbook contains an alphabetical listing of commonly prescribed drugs and detailed monographs for drugs recently approved by the Food and Drug Administration.

Drug Standards and Legislation

Before 1906, little control was exercised over the use of medications. Drugs often were sold or distributed by traveling medicine men, drugstores, mail order companies, and legitimate and self-proclaimed physicians. The ingredients of drugs were not required to be listed. In fact, many drug products contained opium, heroin, and alcohol, which could be potentially harmful to the user.

In 1906 Congress passed the Pure Food and Drug Act. This act was meant to protect the public from mislabeled or adulterated drugs. The act prohibited the use of false and misleading claims for drugs. The act also restricted the sale of drugs with a potential for abuse (Table 17-1). The act designated the *United States Pharmacopeia* and the *National Formulary* as official standards. The act empowered the federal government to enforce these standards as well. In 1980 the United States Pharmacopeial Convention purchased the *National Formulary.* This made the *United States Pharmacopeia* the only official book of drug standards in the United States. In addition to the *United States Pharmacopeia,* other drug standards and legislation are listed in Box 17-3.

Standardization of drugs is necessary because drugs made by different manufacturers (name brand versus generic) may vary significantly in strength and activity. The strength, purity, or effectiveness of a drug can be measured through chemical analysis in a lab. This process is known as *assay.* A concentration of a drug can be determined by comparing its effect on an organism, animal, or isolated tissue to that of a drug that produces a known effect. This process is known as *bioassay* (biological assay). Bioassay is used to measure the bioequivalence, or relative therapeutic effectiveness, of two chemically equivalent drugs.

NOTE The Controlled Substances Act was passed in 1970. A controlled substance is any drug that is defined in the categories of the act. These categories include opium and its derivatives, hallucinogens, depressants, and stimulants. It is illegal for any person to possess a controlled substance. An exception is if the substance was obtained by a valid prescription or order. Another is if the possession of the drug is pursuant to actions in the course of professional practice. The authority for use of controlled substances and other prescription drugs is a function of state agencies. These agencies operate under restrictions of the government. The restrictions are provided by the federal Drug Enforcement Agency. Paramedics and other allied health workers who administer drugs should be familiar with state laws governing the administration and storage of drugs. They also should be familiar with the record-keeping requirements. Violations of the act are punishable by fine or imprisonment or both.

TABLE 17-1 Controlled Substances

CHARACTERISTICS	DISPENSING RESTRICTIONS	EXAMPLES
Schedule I		
Has high abuse potential Has no accepted medical use; for research, analysis, or instruction only May lead to severe dependence	Approved protocol is required.	Heroin, marijuana (cannabis), tetrahydrocannabinols, lysergic acid diethylamide (LSD), mescaline, peyote, psilocybin, methaqualone
Schedule II		
Has high abuse potential Has accepted medical uses May lead to severe physical or psychological dependence or both	Written prescription is necessary (signed by the practitioner); only emergency dispensing is permitted without written prescription (only required amount may be prescribed for emergency period). No prescription refills are allowed. Container must have warning label.*	Opium, morphine sulfate, hydromorphone, meperidine, codeine, oxycodone, methadone, secobarbital, pentobarbital, amphetamine, methylphenidate, cocaine, and others
Schedule III		
Has less abuse potential than drugs in Schedules I and II Has accepted medical uses May lead to moderate to low physical dependence or high psychological dependence	Written or oral prescription is required. Prescription expires in 6 months. No more than five refills are allowed in a 6-month period. Container must have warning label.*	Preparations containing limited quantities of or combined with one or more active ingredients that are noncontrolled substances (codeine, hydrocodone, morphine sulfate, dihydrocodeine, or ethylmorphine) and nonnarcotic drugs such as derivatives of barbituric acid, except those that are listed in another schedule, glutethimide, methyprylon, chlorphentermine, paregoric, and others
Schedule IV		
Has lower abuse potential compared with Schedule III drugs Has accepted medical uses May lead to limited physical or psychological dependence	Written or oral prescription is required. Prescription expires in 6 months, with no more than five refills allowed. Container must have warning label.*	Barbital, phenobarbital, chloral hydrate, meprobamate, fenfluramine, chlordiazepoxide, diazepam, oxazepam, clorazepate, flurazepam, lorazepam, dextropropoxyphene, pentazocine, mazindol, alprazolam, and others
Schedule V		
Has low abuse potential compared with Schedule IV drugs Has accepted medical uses May lead to limited physical or psychological dependence	Drug may require written prescription or may be sold without prescription (check state law).	Medications (generally for relief of coughs or diarrhea) that contain limited amounts of certain opioid controlled substances

*The warning must read "Caution: Federal law prohibits the transfer of this drug to any person other than the patient for whom it was prescribed."

Drug Regulatory Agencies

In July 1973 the Drug Enforcement Agency, an agency of the Department of Justice, became the sole legal drug enforcement body in the United States. Other regulatory bodies or services include the following:

CRITICAL THINKING

News stories often feature miracle drugs. These drugs are used in other countries but are not yet available in the United States. They are not available because they lack Food and Drug Administration approval. Why would the Food and Drug Administration not automatically approve drugs already known to be helpful in the international market?

- Food and Drug Administration: The FDA is responsible for enforcing the federal Food, Drug, and Cosmetic Act of 1937. The FDA may seize offending goods and criminally prosecute individuals involved.
- Public Health Service: The Public Health Service is an agency of the U.S. Department of Health and Human Services. One of the duties of the Public Health Service is to regulate biological products, which include viruses, therapeutic serums, antitoxins, or analogous products applicable in the prevention or cure of human diseases or injuries. The agency examines and licenses these products and inspects and licenses the establishments that produce them.
- Federal Trade Commission: The Federal Trade Commission is an agency of the federal government di-

BOX 17-3 Drug Standards and Legislation

1912: Congress passed the Sherley Amendment prohibiting fraudulent therapeutic claims.

1914: The Harrison Narcotic Act was passed to control the sale of narcotics and to help curb drug addiction or dependence. This was the first narcotic act to be passed by any nation, and it established the word *narcotic* as a legal term.

1938: Prompted by more than 100 deaths in 1937 from ingestion of a diethylene glycol solution of sulfanilamide, the federal Food, Drug, and Cosmetic Act was passed. This act contained a provision to prevent marketing of a new drug before it was tested properly. In addition, the act required that the label list all ingredients used in preparing the drug and the directions for drug use.

1952: The Durham-Humphrey Amendment changed the 1938 drug act, restricting the dispensing of legend (prescription) drugs.Legend drugs must bear the legend "Caution: Federal law prohibits dispensing without prescription."

1962: The Kefauver-Harris Amendment required that the safety and efficacy of a new drug be proved before the drug could be approved for use.

1970: The Comprehensive Drug Abuse Prevention and Control Act (also known as the Controlled Substances Act) superseded the Harrison Narcotic Act of 1914. The Controlled Substances Act classifies a controlled substance by its use and abuse potential. Drugs are classified into numbered schedules from schedule I (drugs with highest abuse potential) to schedule V (drugs with lowest abuse potential); see Table 17-1.

rectly responsible to the president of the United States. Its principal action with respect to drugs lies in its power to suppress false or misleading advertising aimed at the public.

- Canadian Drug Control: In Canada the Health Protection Branch of the Department of National Health and Welfare is responsible for administering and enforcing the Food and Drugs Act, the Proprietary or Patent Medicine Act, and the Narcotics Control Act.
- International Drug Control: International control of drugs began in 1912 when the first "Opium Conference" was held at The Hague. Various international treaties were adopted, obligating governments to control narcotic substances. These treaties were consolidated in 1961 into one document, known as the *Single Convention on Narcotic Drugs,* which became effective in 1964. Later the International Narcotics Control Board was established to enforce this law.

CRITICAL THINKING

Your patient is acutely ill. She reports taking only an herbal medicine, which is not found in standard drug reference materials. Where can you or the medical staff find information about these alternative therapies?

SECTION TWO Mechanisms of Drug Action

GENERAL PROPERTIES OF DRUGS

Drugs may act in the body in many ways. Some of these actions are desirable (a *therapeutic effect*). Others are considered undesirable or even harmful (a *side effect*). Drugs also may interact with other drugs. Interaction may produce uncommon and frequently unpredictable effects. (Allergic reactions to drugs are discussed in Chapter 33.) In addition, drugs generally exert several effects rather than a single one.

NOTE For the paramedic to perform a thorough patient assessment is critical. The paramedic also must obtain a pertinent medical (and drug) history from the patient. Being able to recognize and understand the reasons why certain drugs are prescribed for certain conditions or diseases is important for the paramedic. This knowledge can be important when forming a field impression of what is wrong with a patient based on the assessment and physical findings. With the knowledge of what drugs do, the paramedic would be able to use the right drug to manage the illness, disease, or condition.

One should note that *drugs do not confer any new functions on a tissue or organ; they only modify existing functions.* As is described later in this chapter, the actions of a drug are achieved by a biochemical interaction between the drug and certain tissue components in the body (usually receptors). A drug that interacts with a receptor to stimulate a response is known as an **agonist.** A drug that attaches to a receptor but does not stimulate a response is called an **antagonist.** Box 17-4 contains other pharmacological terms and their definitions.

To produce the desired effect, a drug first must enter the body. Then the drug must reach appropriate concentrations at its site of action. This process is influenced by three phases of drug activity: the pharmaceutical phase, the pharmacokinetic phase, and the pharmacodynamic phase.

Pharmaceutical Phase

Pharmaceutics is the science of dispensing drugs. One aspect of this field is the study of the ways in which the forms of drugs (solid or liquid) influence pharmacokinetic and pharmacodynamic activities (described in the following sections). All drugs must be in solution to cross the cell membranes to achieve absorption. The term *dissolution* refers to the rate at which a solid drug goes into solution

BOX 17-4 Pharmacological Terminology

Antagonism: the opposition of effects between two or more medications that occurs when the combined (conjoint) effect of two drugs is less than the sum of the drugs acting separately

Contraindications: medical or physiological factors that make it harmful to administer a medication that would otherwise have therapeutic value

Cumulative action: the tendency for repeated doses of a drug to accumulate in the blood and organs, causing increased and sometimes toxic effects; it occurs when several doses are administered or when absorption occurs more quickly than removal by excretion or metabolism

Depressant: a substance that decreases a body function or activity

Drug allergy: a systemic reaction to a drug resulting from previous sensitizing exposure and the development of an immunological mechanism

Drug dependence: a state in which withdrawal of a drug produces intense physical or emotional disturbance; previously known as habituation

Drug interaction: beneficial or detrimental modification of the effects of one drug by the prior or concurrent administration of another drug that increases or decreases the pharmacological or physiological action of one or both drugs

Idiosyncrasy: abnormal or peculiar responses to a drug (accounting for 25% to 30% of all drug reactions) thought to result from genetic enzymatic deficiencies or other unique physiological variables and leading to abnormal mechanisms of drug metabolism or altered physiological effects of the drug

Potentiation: the enhancement of effect caused by the concurrent administration of two drugs in which one drug increases the effect of the other drug

Side effect: undesirable and often unavoidable effect of using therapeutic doses of a drug; action or effect other than those for which the drug was originally given

Stimulant: a drug that enhances or increases body function or activity

Summation: the combined effect of two drugs such that the total effect equals the sum of the individual effects of each agent: (1 + 1 = 2)

Synergism: the combined action of two drugs such that the total effect exceeds the sum of the individual effects of each agent: (1 + 1 = 3 or more)

Therapeutic action: the desired, intended action of a drug

Tolerance: decreased physiological response to the repeated administration of a drug or chemically related substance, possibly necessitating an increase in dosage to maintain a therapeutic effect (tachyphylaxis)

Untoward effect: a side effect that proves harmful to the patient

after ingestion. The faster the rate of dissolution, the more quickly the drug is absorbed.

Pharmacokinetic Phase

Pharmacokinetics is the study of how the body handles a drug over a period of time. This includes the processes of **absorption, distribution, biotransformation,** and **excretion.** These factors affect a patient's response to drug therapy.

DRUG ABSORPTION

Absorption involves the movement of drug molecules from the entry site to the general circulation. The degree to which drugs attain pharmacological activity depends partly on the rate and extent to which they are absorbed. The rate and extent in turn depend on the ability of the drug to cross the cell membrane. The drug crosses the membrane through the processes of passive diffusion and active transport (described in Chapter 7). Most drugs enter the cell by passive diffusion. Yet some drugs require a carrier-mediated mechanism to assist them across the membrane.

Absorption begins at the site of administration. The rate and extent of absorption depend on the following factors[3]:

1. *The nature of the absorbing surface (cell membrane) the drug must traverse:* If a drug must pass through a single layer of cells such as the intestinal epithelium, transport is faster than if the drug must pass through several layers of cells (e.g., the skin). In addition, the greater the surface area of the absorbing site, the greater the absorption and the quicker the drug takes effect. For example, the small intestine offers a large absorption area, whereas the stomach has a relatively small absorption surface area.
2. *Blood flow to the site of administration:* A rich blood supply enhances absorption, and a poor blood supply delays it. For example, a patient with diminished blood flow may not respond to intramuscular administration of a drug because diminished circulation reduces absorption. In contrast, intravenous administration of a drug immediately places the drug in the circulatory system, where it is absorbed completely and delivered to its target tissue.
3. *The solubility of the drug:* The more soluble the drug, the more rapidly it is absorbed. For example, drugs that are prepared in oily solutions are absorbed more slowly than drugs dissolved in water or in isotonic sodium chloride.
4. *The pH of the drug environment:* In solution, many drugs exist in an ionized (electrically charged) and nonionized (uncharged) form. A nonionized drug is lipid (fat) soluble and readily diffuses across the cell membrane. An ionized drug is lipid insoluble and generally does not cross the cell membrane. Most drugs do not ionize fully following administration. Rather, they reach an equilibrium between their ionized and nonionized forms, allowing for the nonionized form to be absorbed. How and to what extent a drug ionizes depend on whether the drug is an acid or a base. An acidic drug such as ***aspirin*** is relatively nonionized and does not dissociate well in an acidic environment (e.g., the stomach) and therefore is absorbed easily there. A drug that is basic in the same acidic environment tends to ionize and is not absorbed easily through the gastric membrane. The reverse occurs when the drug is in an alkaline medium.
5. *The drug concentration:* Drugs administered in high concentrations tend to be absorbed more rapidly than those administered in low concentrations. In some situations, administration of a large dose **(loading dose)** first that temporarily exceeds the capacity for excretion of the drug is necessary. This rapidly establishes a therapeutic

drug level at the receptor site. A smaller dose **(maintenance dose)** then can be administered to replace the amount of drug excreted. Thus loading doses are based more on the volume of distribution (of which body size is an important component) and less on capacity for excretion (e.g., renal failure). Maintenance doses are exactly the opposite.

CRITICAL THINKING

Consider a common condition seen in the prehospital setting. This condition requires that drugs be given at higher than usual doses to achieve therapeutic levels. What is the condition?

6. *The form of the drug dosage:* Drug absorption can be manipulated by pharmaceutical processing. An example is a combination of an active drug with another substance that is slowly released or a drug that resists digestive action (enteric coatings).

ROUTES OF DRUG ADMINISTRATION

The mode of drug administration affects the rate at which onset of action occurs. Route of administration also may affect the therapeutic response that results. The routes of drug administration are categorized as follows:

- *Enteral* (administration along any portion of the gastrointestinal tract)
- **Parenteral** (administration by any route other than the gastrointestinal tract)
- *Pulmonary* (administration by inhalation or through an endotracheal tube)
- *Topical* (administration by application to the skin and mucous membranes)

The route of administration greatly influences drug absorption (Table 17-2). Chapter 18 describes the methods used to administer drugs by various routes.

Enteral Route. Drugs administered along any portion of the gastrointestinal tract are said to use the enteral route (Box 17-5). Administration may be orally, rectally, or through a nasogastric tube. The enteral method of giving drugs is the safest, most convenient route. This route also is the most economical route of administration. Yet the enteral route is the least reliable and slowest of the common routes because of the frequent changes in the gastrointestinal environment (e.g., with food contents, emotional state, and physical activity). This route allows for four types of absorption: oral absorption, gastric absorption, absorption from the small intestine, and rectal absorption.

Oral Absorption. The oral cavity has a rich blood supply. However, little absorption normally occurs in the mouth. Certain drugs, such as ***nitroglycerin*** (Nitrostat) tablets and some hormones, are prepared to be absorbed orally. When administered by sublingual or buccal routes, these drugs rapidly dissolve in the salivary secretions and are absorbed by the oral mucosa. Drugs that are absorbed in the upper gastrointestinal tract enter the systemic circulation. They initially bypass gastrointestinal fluids and the liver. Drugs absorbed in the stomach and intestines are absorbed into the portal vein system of the liver. They are subject to **first-pass metabolism** (described later) in the liver. In the sublingual route the medicine is placed under the tongue. The tablet or spray dissolves in the salivary secretions. The effects of sublingual medication usually are clear within a few minutes. With buccal administration the drug is placed between the teeth and mucous membrane of the cheek. As in the sublingual route, absorption by buccal administration usually is rapid.

TABLE 17-2 Comparison of Drug Absorption Rates by Common Routes of Administration

ROUTE	RATE OF ABSORPTION
Enteral	Slow
Sublingual	Rapid
Subcutaneous	Slow
Intramuscular	Moderate
Intravenous	Immediate (no absorption required)
Endotracheal	Rapid
Intraosseous	Immediate
Pulmonary	Rapid
Topical	Moderate

BOX 17-5 Some Emergency Drugs Administered Via the Enteral Route

Activated charcoal
Aspirin

CRITICAL THINKING

Nitroglycerin spray may be more effective in geriatric patients than the tablet form. Why do you think this is the case?

Gastric Absorption. The stomach also has a rich blood supply but is not considered an important site of drug absorption. The length of time a medication remains in the stomach varies, depending on the pH of the environment and gastric motility. As previously described, weakly acidic drugs tend to remain nonionized. These drugs are absorbed readily into the circulation. In comparison, basic drugs ionize in the stomach and are absorbed poorly. Altering the gastric emptying rate may alter the rate and extent of drug absorption. Many drugs are administered on an empty stomach with sufficient water (8 oz) to ensure rapid passage into the small intestine. Other drugs cause gastric irritation and usually are given with food.

Absorption from the Small Intestine. The small intestine has a rich blood supply. Thus it has a larger absorption area than the stomach. Most drug absorption occurs in the upper part of the small intestine. The pH of intestinal fluid is alkaline, which increases the rate of absorption of basic drugs. Prolonged exposure allows more time for drug absorption. An increase in intestinal motility (e.g., diarrhea) decreases exposure to the intestinal membrane and diminishes absorption.

Rectal Absorption. The surface area of the rectum is not large. However, the rectum is vascular and capable of drug absorption. Drugs administered rectally are subject to erratic absorption because of rectal contents, local drug irritation, and the uncertainty of drug retention. Fifty percent of a drug that has been administered rectally is estimated to bypass the liver after absorption. This makes first-pass metabolism by the liver less than that of an orally given dose.

CRITICAL THINKING

The drugs given rectally in emergencies usually are anticonvulsants. Why do you think this route would be chosen over the oral or intravenous route?

Parenteral Route. Drugs administered by injection are said to use the parenteral route (Box 17-6). The commonly used parenteral routes for administering medications include the following:

1. Subcutaneous route: A subcutaneous injection is given beneath the skin into the connective tissue or fat immediately beneath the dermis. This route is used only for small volumes of drugs (0.5 mL or less) that do not irritate tissue. The rate of absorption usually is slow and can provide a sustained effect.
2. Intramuscular route: An intramuscular injection is given into the skeletal muscle. Absorption generally occurs more rapidly than with a subcutaneous injection because of greater tissue blood flow.
3. Intravenous route: An intravenous injection is given directly into the bloodstream, bypassing the absorption process. This route produces an almost immediate pharmacological effect. Most intravenous drugs should be administered slowly to help prevent adverse reactions.
4. Intradermal route: An intradermal injection is made just below the epidermis. This route primarily is used for allergy testing and to administer local anesthetics.
5. Intraosseous route: An intraosseous injection is given directly into the bone marrow cavity of pediatric (and occasionally adult) patients through an established intraosseous infusion system. Agents infused by this method are thought to circulate via the medullary cavity of the bone. Through the numerous venous channels of long bones, fluids or drugs rapidly enter the central circulation. The length of time from injection to entry into the systemic circulation is thought to equal that of the intravenous route.[4] Emergency medications known to be effective when administered via the intraosseous route are ***epinephrine*** (Adrenalin), ***atropine, sodium bicarbonate, dexamethasone*** (Decadron), ***dopamine*** (Intropin), and ***dobutamine*** (Dobutrex).
6. Endotracheal route: Access to the endotracheal route generally is through an endotracheal tube, which allows drug delivery into the alveoli and systemic absorption via the capillaries of the lungs. Because of the large surface area of the alveolar sacs, the rate of absorption by this route is almost as rapid as that of the intravenous route. Administration of drugs via an endotracheal tube usually is reserved for situations in which an intravenous line cannot be established. Medications that can be administered by the endotracheal tube include ***lidocaine*** (Xylocaine), ***epinephrine*** (Adrenalin), ***atropine,*** and ***naloxone*** (Narcan). This route is erratic and may be less reliable than intravenous or intraosseous delivery and should therefore be used in adult patients only if these *first-line* methods are unavailable. Administration of 2 to 2½ times the recommended intravenous dose (diluted in 10 mL normal saline) is recommended when medication is given by this route.[5]

BOX 17-6 Examples of Emergency Drugs Administered Via the Parenteral Route

Adenosine (Adenocard)	Labetalol (Normodyne)
Amiodarone (Cordarone)	Lidocaine (Xylocaine)
Atropine	Midazolam (Versed)
Dextrose 50%	Morphine
Diazepam (Valium)	Naloxone (Narcan)
Diphenhydramine (Benadryl)	Oxytocin (Pitocin)
Epinephrine (Adrenalin)	Vasopressin (Pitressin)
Furosemide (Lasix)	Verapamil (Isoptin)

NOTE A mnemonic for the four medications that may be administered via the pulmonary route through an endotracheal tube is *L-E-A-N*, which stands for *l*idocaine, *e*pinephrine, *a*tropine, and *n*aloxone.

Pulmonary Route. Medication can be administered by inhalation. The medication can be in the form of gas or fine mist (aerosol). The most commonly used inhalation medications are bronchodilators (Box 17-7). However, the pulmonary circulation can absorb a number of other medications if necessary, such as drugs for endotracheal administration. Some vaccines are administered by nasal spray in select patient groups. Examples of these include live attenuated influenza vaccine (LAIV) and influenza virus vaccine live (Intranasal FluMist).

Because of the large surface area and the rich capillary network of the alveoli, drug absorption into the bloodstream is rapid. Bronchodilators and steroids can be given by inhalation devices, such as a nebulizer (described in Chapter 18). A nebulizer propels the drug into alveolar sacs.

BOX 17-7 Emergency Drugs Administered Via the Pulmonary Route

Albuterol (Proventil, Ventolin)	Metaproterenol (Alupent)
Amyl nitrite	Nitrous oxide/oxygen (Nitronox)
Epinephrine racemic (microNefrin)	Oxygen

BOX 17-8 Emergency Drugs Administered Via the Topical Route

Lidocaine (viscous solution)
Nitropaste (Nitro-Bid ointment)

Drugs that are given by a nebulizer device produce mainly local effects. Occasionally, nebulized drugs can produce unwanted systemic effects. An example of these effects is an elevated heart rate (tachycardia).

Topical Route. In most cases, drugs applied topically to the skin and mucous membranes are absorbed rapidly. They are intended to produce a local effect (Box 17-8). Only lipid-soluble compounds are absorbed through the skin. The skin acts as a barrier to most water-soluble compounds. To prevent adverse systemic effects, intact skin surfaces should be used as an administration site. Massaging the skin helps to promote drug absorption as the capillaries dilate and local blood flow increases.

DRUG DISTRIBUTION

Distribution is the transport of a drug through the bloodstream. The drug is transported to various tissues of the body and ultimately to its site of action. After a drug has entered the circulatory system, it is distributed rapidly throughout the body. The rate at which distribution occurs depends on the permeability of capillaries to the drug molecules.

To review, lipid-soluble drugs readily cross capillary membranes to enter most tissues and fluid compartments. Lipid-insoluble drugs require more time to arrive at their point of action. Cardiac output and regional blood flow also affect the rate and extent of distribution into body tissues. Generally, a drug is distributed first to organs that have a rich blood supply. These organs include the heart, liver, kidneys, and brain. Then, depending on its composition, the drug enters tissue with a lesser blood supply, such as muscle and fat.

Drug Reservoirs. Drugs may accumulate at certain locations that act as storage sites. At these sites the drugs form reservoirs by binding to specific tissues. As serum levels decline, tissue-bound drug is released from its storage site into the bloodstream. The released drug maintains the desired serum drug levels and may permit sustained release of the drug over time. This allows continued pharmacological effect at the receptor site. The two general processes that create drug reservoirs are plasma protein binding and tissue binding.

As drugs enter the circulatory system, they may attach to plasma proteins (mainly albumin), forming a drug-protein complex.

The extent to which this binding occurs affects the intensity and duration of the effect of the drug. The albumin molecule is too large to diffuse through the membrane of the blood vessel. Thus albumin traps the bound drug in the bloodstream. A drug bound to plasma protein is pharmacologically inactive. The protein becomes a circulating drug reservoir. The free drug (unbound drug) exists in proportion to the protein-bound fraction and is the only portion of the drug that is biologically active. As the free drug is eliminated from the body, the drug-protein complex dissociates, and more drug is released to replace the free drug that was metabolized or excreted. This process is summarized in the following equation:

$$\text{Free drug} + \text{Protein} \leftrightarrows \text{Drug-protein complex}$$

Albumin and other plasma proteins provide a number of binding sites. Yet two drugs can compete for the same site and displace each other. Certain combinations of drugs may be given at the same time. As a result, this competition can have serious consequences. For example, a patient taking the anticoagulant drug warfarin (Coumadin) may be given quinidine (e.g., Quinaglute Dura Tabs). The quinidine may displace some of the protein-bound warfarin. This may cause warfarin toxicity and in turn can lead to severe hemorrhage.

Other factors that influence the binding ability of a drug include the concentration of plasma proteins (especially albumin), the number of binding sites on the protein, the affinity of the drug for the protein, and the acid-base balance of the patient. Various disease states, such as liver disease, alter the ability of the body to handle many medications. These alterations result from a decrease in serum albumin levels (albumin is manufactured by the liver) and a decrease in hepatic metabolism. These and other factors may result in more free drug being available for distribution to tissue sites (increased free drug fraction and enhanced pharmacological response).

A second type of "drug pooling" occurs in fat tissue and bone. Lipid-soluble drugs have a high affinity for adipose tissue, where these drugs are stored. Because fat tissue has low blood flow, it serves as a stable reservoir for drugs. Some lipid-soluble drugs can remain in body fat for as long as 3 hours after administration. Other drugs (e.g., tetracycline) have an unusual affinity for bone. These drugs accumulate in bone after being absorbed onto the bone crystal surface.

CRITICAL THINKING

Tetracycline typically is not given to pregnant women because of the harmful effects it has on the development of the baby's teeth. Why would it affect the teeth?

Barriers to Drug Distribution. The blood-brain barrier and the **placental barrier** are protective membranes. These membranes prevent the passage of certain drugs into these body sites. The blood-brain barrier consists of a single layer of capillary endothelial cells. These cells line the blood vessels entering the central nervous system. The cells are tightly joined at common borders by continuous intercellular junctions. This special arrangement permits only lipid-soluble drugs to be distributed into the brain and cerebrospinal fluid. Examples of such drugs are general anesthetics and barbiturates. Drugs that are poorly soluble in fat (e.g., many antibiotics) have trouble passing this barrier. Thus they cannot enter the brain.

The placental barrier is made up of membrane layers. These layers separate the blood vessels of the mother and the fetus. Like the blood-brain barrier, the placental barrier is not permeable to many lipid-insoluble drugs. Thus the placenta offers some protection to the fetus. However, the placenta does allow the passage of certain non–lipid-soluble drugs. Examples of these are steroids, narcotics, anesthetics, and some antibiotics. If these drugs are given to the pregnant mother, they may affect the developing embryo or fetus or the neonate.

BIOTRANSFORMATION

After absorption and distribution, the body eliminates most drugs, first by biotransformation and then by excretion. Biotransformation (metabolism) is a process in which the drug is chemically converted to a metabolite. The purpose of biotransformation usually is to "detoxify" a drug and render it less active. The liver is the primary site of drug metabolism. However, other tissues also can be involved. Some of these include the plasma, kidneys, lungs, and the intestinal mucosa.

Orally administered drugs that are absorbed through the gastrointestinal tract normally travel to the liver before entering the general circulation. When this occurs, a large amount of the drug may be metabolized (first-pass metabolism) before reaching the systemic circulation. This reduces the amount of drug that is available for distribution in the body. Medications affected by this initial biotransformation in the liver may be given in higher dosages or administered parenterally (intravenously or intramuscularly) to bypass the liver.

Individuals metabolize drugs at variable rates. For example, patients with liver, renal, or cardiovascular disease are expected to have prolonged drug metabolism. Infants with immature metabolic capacity and older adults with degenerative metabolic function experience depressed biotransformation. If drug metabolism is delayed, drug accumulation and cumulative drug effects may occur. Therefore the paramedic may need to consider dosage reductions (particularly maintenance doses) for patients in these categories (Fig. 17-1).

EXCRETION

Excretion is the elimination of toxic or inactive metabolites. The kidney is the primary organ for excretion. However, the intestine, lungs, and mammary, sweat, and salivary glands also may be involved.

Excretion by the Kidneys. A drug can be excreted in the urine unchanged. Or a drug can be excreted as a chemical metabolite of its previous form. Renal excretion consists of three mechanisms: passive glomerular filtration, active tubular secretion, and partial reabsorption (Fig. 17-2).

Passive glomerular filtration is a simple filtration process. Filtration can be measured as the glomerular filtration rate (GFR) (described in Chapter 6). The GFR is the total quantity of glomerular filtrate formed each minute in all nephrons of both kidneys. (This measure is usually expressed in milliliters.) The availability of a drug for glomerular filtration depends on its free concentration in plasma. Unbound drugs and water-soluble metabolites are filtered by the glomeruli. Drugs highly bound to protein do not pass through this structure.

After filtration, lipid-soluble compounds are reabsorbed by the renal tubules. Thus they reenter the systemic circulation. Water-soluble compounds are not reabsorbed. Therefore they are eliminated from the body. Because of the proportional relationship between free and bound drug, as free drug is filtered from the blood, bound drug is released from its binding sites into the plasma. The rate of excretion and the **biological half-life** of the drug (described later in this chapter) depend on how quickly bound drug is released.

> **CRITICAL THINKING**
>
> You pick up your patient at the renal dialysis center. How will you know which medicines you can administer safely?

Active tubular secretion occurs in the renal tubules, where free drug can be transported or secreted from the blood across the structure called the proximal tubule and from there deposited in the urine. Drugs actively secreted by the renal tubules can compete with other drugs for the same active transport process. An example of competitive **drug interaction** is that between ***amiodarone*** (Cordarone) and ***digoxin*** (Lanoxin). The first drug reduces the removal or clearance of the second drug. (The term *clearance* refers to the complete removal of a drug by the kidneys.) The result of this competition for removal is an increase in the plasma concentration of the second drug.

Partial resorption is the resorption from the renal tubule by passive diffusion. Such resorption can be influenced greatly by the pH of the tubular urine. Weak acids are excreted more readily in alkaline urine. They are secreted more slowly in acidic urine. This is because they are ionized in alkaline urine but nonionized in acidic urine. The reverse is true for weak bases. For example, an increase in urinary pH decreases the resorption and increases the clearance of weak acids such as ***furosemide*** (Lasix) and ***aspirin.*** However, a decrease in urinary pH increases the clearance of weak bases such as amphetamine and tricyclic antidepressants.

As a rule, substances that are completely or almost completely excreted by the normal kidney can be removed by an artificial process that resembles glomerular filtration. This process is hemodialysis. (Chapter 34 describes hemodialysis further.) Hemodialysis can be used to remove a wide va-

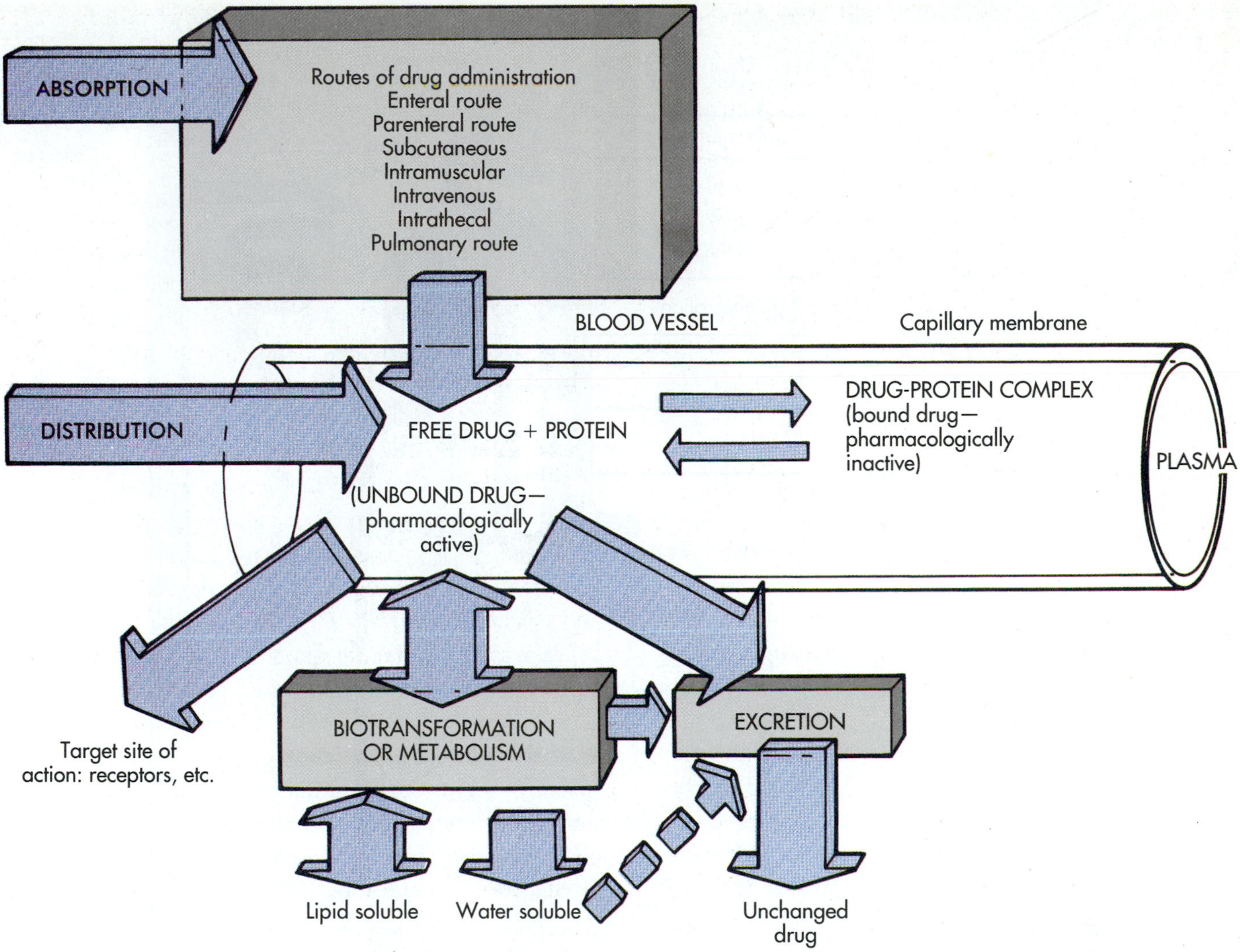

FIGURE 17-1 ■ Pharmacokinetic phase of drug action, showing absorption, distribution, biotransformation, and excretion of drugs. Only free drug is capable of movement for absorption, distribution to the target site of action, biotransformation, and excretion. The drug-protein complex represents bound drugs; because the molecule is large, it is trapped in the blood vessel and serves as a storage site for the drug.

riety of substances. Hemodialysis is not effective for drugs that are highly tissue or protein bound. Moreover, hemodialysis is of limited benefit for the removal of rapidly acting toxins.

Excretion by the Intestine. Drugs are eliminated through the intestine by biliary excretion. After liver metabolism the metabolites are carried in bile and passed into the duodenum. The metabolites then are eliminated with the feces. Some drugs are reabsorbed by the bloodstream. They are returned to the liver and then later excreted by the kidneys.

Excretion by the Lungs. Some drugs can be eliminated by the lungs. Examples are general anesthetics, volatile alcohols, and inhaled bronchodilators. Certain factors can alter drug elimination via the lungs. These factors include the rate and depth of respiration and cardiac output. Deep breathing and an increase in cardiac output (which increases pulmonary blood flow) promote excretion. However, respiratory compromise and decreased cardiac output may occur during illness or injury. This can prolong the period required to eliminate drugs through the lungs.

Excretion by the Sweat and Salivary Glands. Sweat is an unimportant means of drug excretion. However, this method can cause various skin reactions and can discolor the sweat. Drugs excreted in saliva usually are swallowed and are eliminated in the same manner as other orally administered medicines. Certain substances given intravenously can be excreted into saliva. This may cause the person to complain about the "taste of the drug," even though it was given intravenously.

Excretion by the Mammary Glands. Many drugs or their metabolites are excreted through the mammary glands in breast milk. Nursing mothers are advised not to take any medicine except under the supervision of a doctor. Mothers usually are advised to take prescribed medicines

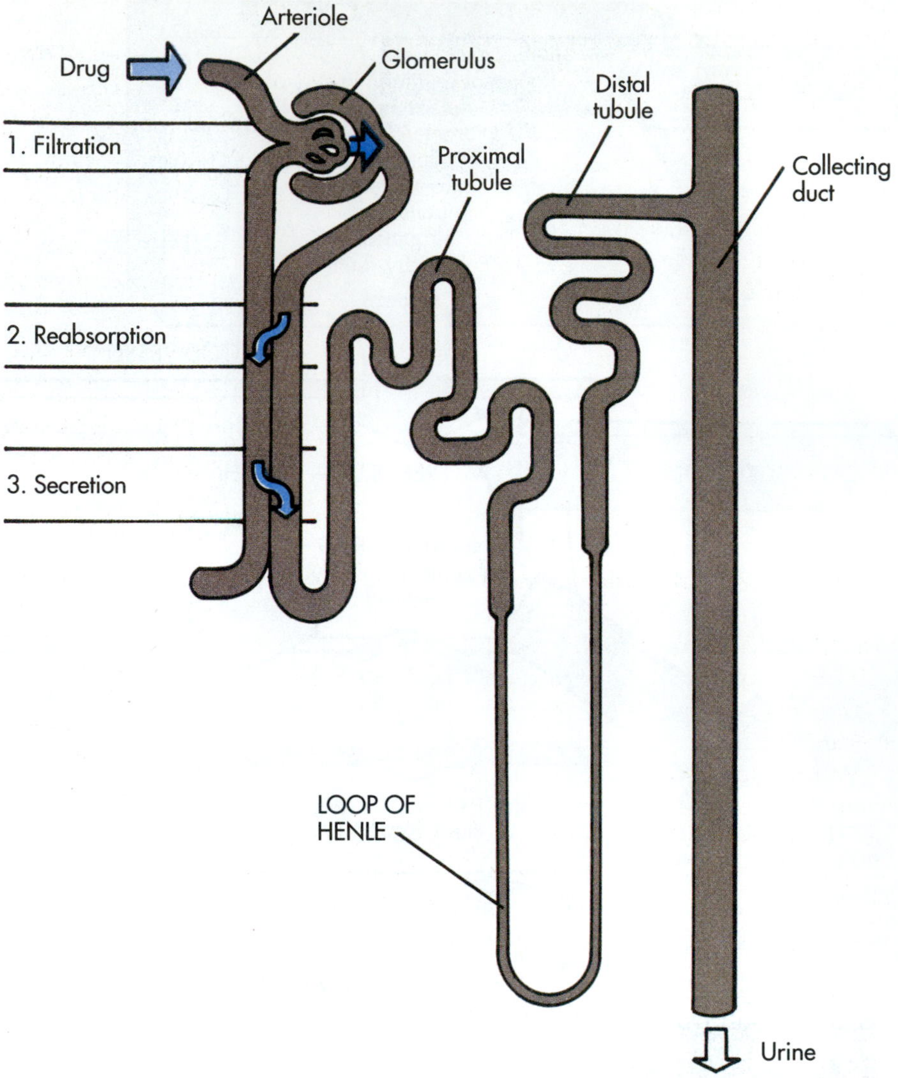

FIGURE 17-2 ■ Drug excretion process.

right after breast-feeding. This diminishes any risk to the infant.

FACTORS THAT INFLUENCE THE ACTION OF DRUGS

Many factors can alter the response to drug therapy, including age, body mass, gender, pathological state, genetic factors, psychological factors, environment, and time of administration. The paramedic should recognize these factors and should consider individual responses. The paramedic also must consider complications that may result from drug therapy.

Age. For the most part, pediatric and geriatric patients are known to be highly sensitive to drugs. In a child, this sensitivity results in part from the immature hepatic and renal systems. In an older adult, sensitivity results from the natural decline of these systems. These aspects of body function can reduce the efficiency of excretory and metabolic mechanisms. The older patient also may have underlying disease processes. This can create unexpected responses to drug therapy. Medication doses for children usually are modified based on body weight or surface area (see Chapter 44).

Body Mass. Many drugs are given according to body mass (kilograms). An indirect relationship exists between body mass and the final concentration of drug in a patient for any given dosage. (For instance, the larger the patient, the lower the concentration for any given dose of drug.) The average adult drug dose is determined by a process. The process determines what amount of a drug will be needed to produce a particular effect when administered to 50% of the population. This population includes only persons between the ages of 18 and 65 who weigh about 150 lb (68 kg). Therefore the appropriate drug doses for children who weigh less than 150 lb and are less than 18 years old is always based on body mass.

Gender. Drug effects differ in men and women. These differences result partly from size differences. Women usually are smaller in body mass than men are. Thus they may have higher concentrations of a drug when the standard dose is administered without consideration of size.

Differences in the relative proportions of fat and water in the bodies of men and women also can cause variations in drug distribution.

Environment. Drugs that affect mood and behavior may be susceptible to the individual's environment and the personality of the user. For example, sensory deprivation and sensory overload may affect a person's response to a drug. The physical environment also can affect the actions of some drugs for some persons. For example, temperature extremes and changes in altitude may increase sensitivity to some drugs.

CRITICAL THINKING

You can alter the environment in the ambulance. How might you do this to promote the action of pain-relieving drugs that you have given your patient?

Time of Administration. The presence or absence of food in the gastrointestinal tract affects the manner in which drugs are tolerated and absorbed. Other factors may influence drug activity and reactions to drug therapy. One of these is a person's biological rhythms (e.g., sleep-wake cycles and circadian rhythms).

Pathological State. Illness or injury and the severity of symptoms also can play a role in a person's sensitivity to drugs. Illness or injury can affect the type and amount of drug needed to achieve a desired effect. In addition, underlying disease processes such as circulatory, hepatic, or renal dysfunction can interfere with the physiological actions of the drug and drug elimination.

Genetic Factors. Genetics can alter the response of some persons to a number of drugs. For example, this can occur through inherited diseases or enzyme deficiencies or altered receptor site sensitivities. The results of genetic abnormalities may appear as idiosyncrasies or may be mistaken for drug allergies.

Psychological Factors. A patient's belief in the effects of a drug may strongly influence and potentiate drug effects. For example, a placebo can have the same result as a pharmacological agent if the patient thinks it will have the desired effect. In contrast, patient hostility and mistrust can lessen the perceived effects of a drug. The paramedic can enhance the action of a drug by telling the patient that the drug is going to work and when it will take effect.

Pharmacodynamic Phase

Pharmacodynamics is the study of how a drug acts on a living organism. This includes the pharmacological response observed relative to the concentration of the drug at an active site in the organism. As stated before, drugs do not confer any new function on a tissue or organ of the body; rather, they modify existing functions. Theories of drug action abound. However, most drug actions are thought to result from a chemical interaction between the drug and various receptors throughout the body. The most common form of drug action is the drug-receptor interaction.

BOX 17-9 Drug-Receptor Interaction Terms

Affinity: the propensity of a drug to bind or attach itself to a given receptor site

Efficacy (intrinsic activity): the ability of a drug to initiate biological activity as a result of binding to a receptor site

Agonist: a drug that combines with receptors and initiates the expected response

Antagonist: an agent that inhibits or counteracts effects produced by other drugs or undesired effects caused by normal or hyperactive physiological mechanisms

Competitive antagonist: an agent with an affinity for the same receptor site as an agonist (The competition with the agonist for the site inhibits the action of the agonist; increasing the concentration of the agonist tends to overcome the inhibition. Competitive inhibition responses are usually reversible.)

Noncompetitive antagonist: an agent that combines with different parts of the receptor mechanism and inactivates the receptor so that the agonist cannot be effective regardless of its concentration (Noncompetitive antagonist effects are considered to be irreversible or nearly so.)

Partial antagonist: an agent that binds to a receptor and stimulates some of its effects but may antagonize the action of other drugs with greater efficacy. (Antagonists frequently share some structural similarities with their agonists.)

DRUG-RECEPTOR INTERACTION

For the most part, most drugs are believed to bind to **drug receptors** to produce their desired effect (Box 17-9). According to this theory, a specific portion of the drug molecule (the active site) selectively combines or interacts with some molecular structure (the reactive site on the cell surface or within the cell). This interaction produces a biological effect. These reactive cellular sites are known as *receptors.*

The relationship of a drug to its receptor may be thought of as a key fitting into a lock (Fig. 17-3). The drug represents the key. The receptor represents the lock. The drug molecule with the best fit to a receptor produces the best response. After absorption a drug is believed to gain access to a receptor after it leaves the bloodstream and is distributed to tissues that contain receptor sites. To review, drugs that bind to a receptor and cause an expected physiological response are referred to as agonists. Conversely, drugs that bind to a receptor and the presence of which prevent a physiological response or other drugs from binding are referred to as **antagonists.**

DRUG-RESPONSE ASSESSMENT

In the prehospital setting the response to drug therapy often can be assessed by observing the effect of the drug on specific physical findings. Examples include monitoring blood pressure after administration of an antihypertensive medication and pain relief after administration of an analgesic.

Each drug has its own characteristic rate of absorption, distribution, biotransformation, and excretion. Thus the ef-

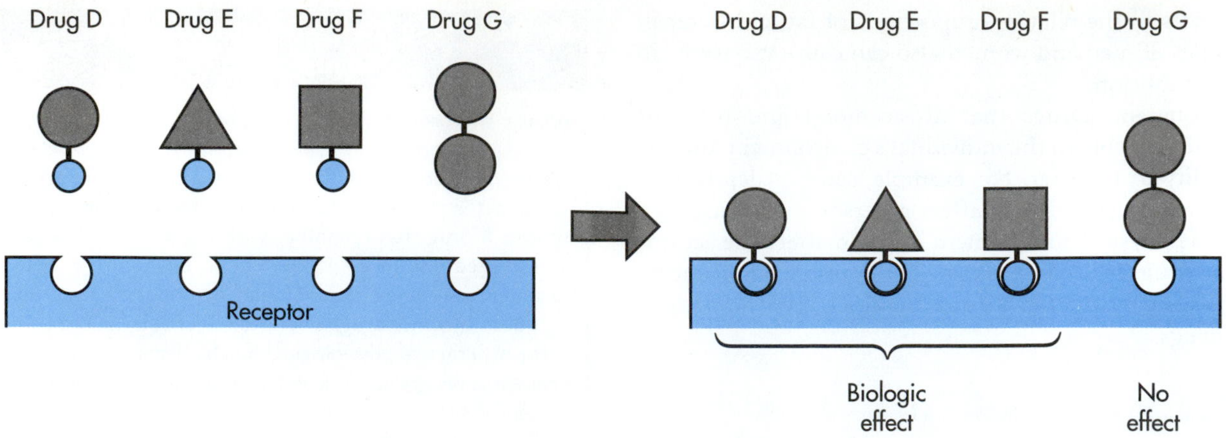

FIGURE 17-3 ■ Lock-and-key fit between a drug and the receptors through which it acts. The site on the receptor that interacts with a drug has a definite shape. A drug that conforms to that shape can bind and produce a biological response. In this example, only the shape along the lower surface of the drug molecule is important in determining whether the drug binds to the receptor.

BOX 17-10 Plasma-Level Profile Terms

Duration of action: the period from onset of drug action to the time when a drug effect is no longer seen

Loading dose: a bolus of a drug given initially to attain a therapeutic plasma concentration rapidly

Maintenance dose: the amount of drug necessary to maintain a steady therapeutic plasma concentration

Minimum effective concentration: the lowest plasma concentration that produces the desired drug effect

Onset of action or latent period: the interval between the time a drug is administered and the first sign of its effect

Peak plasma level: the highest plasma concentration attained from a doses

Termination of action: the point at which the effect of a drug is no longer seen

Therapeutic range: the range of plasma concentrations most likely to produce the desired drug effect with the least likelihood of toxicity (the range between minimum effective concentration and toxic level)

Toxic level: the plasma concentration at which a drug is likely to produce serious adverse effects

fectiveness of some drugs cannot be monitored solely by the patient's response. For example, medications such as theophylline, ***digoxin*** (Lanoxin), and ***phenytoin*** (Dilantin) must reach a certain concentration at the target site to achieve the desired effect. Tissue concentrations often are proportional to and can be estimated from drug levels in the blood determined by laboratory analysis. Therapeutic drug levels in the blood, or serum, generally indicate ranges in tissue drug concentration that produce the desired therapeutic response.

Plasma-level profiles (Box 17-10) demonstrate the relationship between the concentration of drug in the plasma and the effectiveness of the drug over time (Fig. 17-4). These profiles depend on the rate of absorption, distribution, biotransformation, and excretion after drug administration.

The therapeutic range for most drugs is based on the concentration that provides the highest probability of response with the least risk of toxicity.

The dosage (loading and maintenance) required to achieve a therapeutic concentration varies because of the previously described factors that influence the actions of drugs: age, body mass, gender, pathological state, and genetic and psychological factors. In most patients, doses in the therapeutic range have a high probability of producing the desired effect. Moreover, they have a low probability of toxicity. However, some patients fail to respond to doses in the therapeutic range. Still others may develop drug toxicity.

BIOLOGICAL HALF-LIFE

The rate of biotransformation and excretion of a drug determines its biological half-life. The biological half-life is defined as the time it takes to metabolize or eliminate 50% of a drug in the body. For example, a 100-mg injection of ***meperidine*** (Demerol) is given. Its half-life is 4 hours. Thus 50 mg will be eliminated in the first 4 hours, 25 mg (half of the remaining 50 mg) will be eliminated in the second 4 hours, and so on. A drug is considered to be eliminated from the body after five half-lives have passed.

CRITICAL THINKING

Adenosine (Adenocard) is an intravenous antidysrhythmic medicine. Adenosine has a half-life of only 1 to 3 seconds. How will this brief half-life influence the speed and frequency of administration of this drug?

The half-life of a drug is crucial when determining the rate of administration. A drug that has a short half-life (e.g., 2 to 3 hours) must be administered more often to maintain a therapeutic range than a drug with a long half-life, such as 12 hours. The half-life of a drug may be lengthened considerably in persons with liver dysfunction or renal disor-

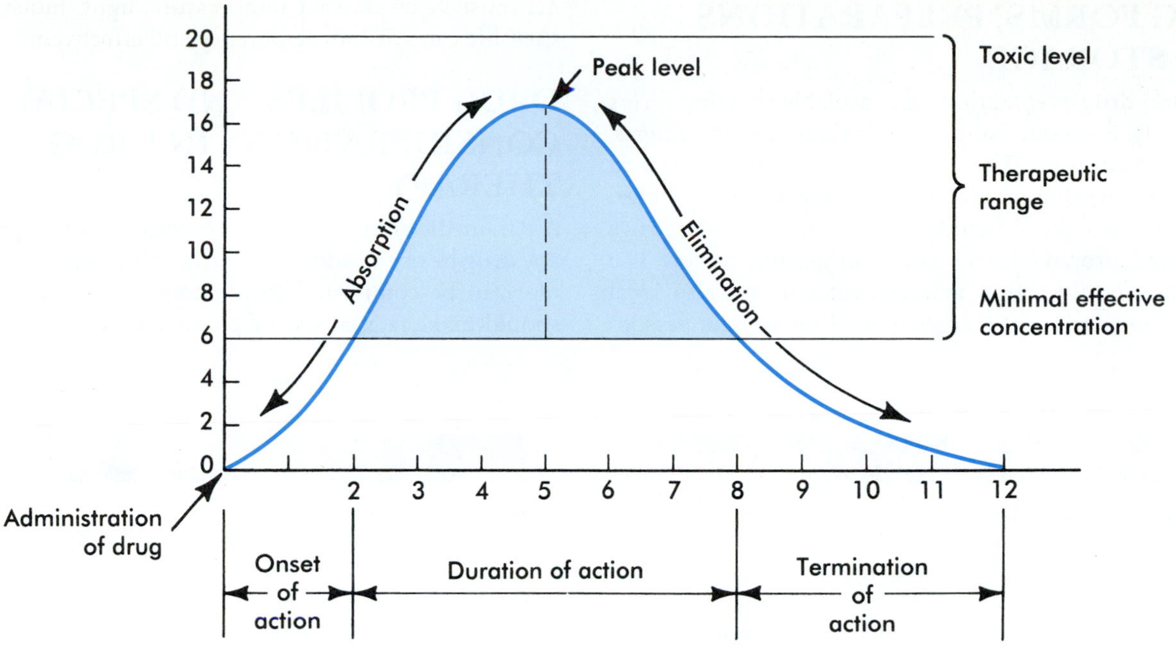

FIGURE 17-4 ■ Plasma-level profile of a drug.

ders. These and other disease processes may require a reduction in drug dosage, or the interval between doses may have to be lengthened.

THERAPEUTIC INDEX

The **therapeutic index** (TI) is a measurement of the relative safety of a drug. The index represents the ratio between two factors. The first factor is lethal dose 50 (LD_{50}). This is the dose of a drug that is lethal in 50% of laboratory animals tested. The second factor is effective dose 50 (ED_{50}). This is the dose that produces a therapeutic effect in 50% of a similar population. The therapeutic index is calculated as follows:

$$TI = \frac{LD_{50}}{ED_{50}}$$

The closer the ratio is to 1, the greater the danger in administering the drug to human beings. In certain drugs, such as ***digoxin*** (Lanoxin), the difference between the effective dose and the lethal dose is small. These drugs are said to have a low therapeutic index. In contrast, drugs such as ***naloxone*** (Narcan) have a wide margin between the effective dose and lethal dose (a high therapeutic index).

DRUG INTERACTIONS

Many variables can influence drug interactions, including intestinal absorption, competition for plasma-protein binding, biotransformation, action at the receptor site, renal excretion, and alteration of electrolyte balance. Not all drug interactions are dangerous; some may even be beneficial.

Some drug-drug interactions are clinically important. They can even be dangerous. The paramedic should be aware of common drug-drug interactions. In addition, the paramedic should seek medical direction before giving drugs concurrently. (See Mosby's Emergency Drug Index.*) The following drugs are associated with clinically significant drug-drug interactions:

- Blood thinners
- Tricyclic antidepressants
- Monoamine oxidase (MAO) inhibitors
- Amphetamines
- Digitalis glycosides
- Diuretics
- Antihypertensives

Other factors that can influence drug interactions include the following:

- Drug-induced malabsorption of food and nutrients
- Food-induced malabsorption of drugs
- Enzyme alterations that affect the metabolism of food or drugs
- Alcohol consumption
- Cigarette smoking that affects drug metabolism or excretion
- Food-initiated alteration of drug excretion

NOTE Grapefruit and its juice can boost blood levels of some drugs as much as 1000%. This occurs through liver enzyme inhibition. Emergency drugs that can be affected include verapamil (Isoptin) and midazolam (Versed).

Finally, some drugs are incompatible with each other. For example, ***epinephrine*** (Adrenalin) will precipitate (or crystallize) when mixed with ***sodium bicarbonate.***

* Sanders MJ: *Mosby's Emergency Drug Index,* Jensen Beach, Fla, Digital Objectives (www.digobj.com; PDA software).

DRUG FORMS, PREPARATIONS, AND STORAGE

Drugs and drug preparations are available in many forms (Box 17-11). Each one has specific indications, advantages, and disadvantages. These preparations are explained throughout the chapter and in the Emergency Drug Index.

Certain rules should guide the manner in which drugs are secured, stored, distributed, and accounted for. The paramedic should follow agency protocol and also local and state regulations. Emergency medical services personnel must be aware that temperature, light, moisture, and shelf-life can affect drug potency and effectiveness.

DRUG PROFILES AND SPECIAL CONSIDERATIONS IN DRUG THERAPY

A paramedic should be familiar with the drug profiles of any drug he or she administers. Not all aspects of drug profiles can be committed to memory. Thus the paramedic should make regular use of pharmacology references. The

BOX 17-11 Various Forms of Drug Preparations

Preparations for Oral Use

Liquids

Aqueous solution: substance dissolved in water and syrups
Aqueous suspension: solid particles suspended in liquid
Emulsion: fat or oil suspended in liquid with an emulsifier
Spirits: alcohol solution
Elixir: aromatic, sweetened alcohol and water solution
Tincture: alcohol extract of plant or vegetable substance
Fluid extract: concentrated alcoholic liquid extract of plant or vegetables
Extract: syrup or dried form of pharmacologically active drug, usually prepared by evaporating a solution

Solids

Capsule: soluble case (usually gelatin) that contains liquid, dry, or beaded drug particles
Tablet: compressed, powdered drugs in the form of a small disk
Troche or lozenge: medicated tablets that dissolve slowly in the mouth
Powder or granules: loose or molded drug substance for administration with or without liquids

Preparations for Parenteral Use

Ampule: sealed glass container for liquid injectable medication
Vial: glass container with rubber stopper for liquid or powdered medication
Cartridge or Tubex: single-dose unit of parenteral medication to be used with a specific injecting device

Intravenous infusions (suspended on hanger at bedside)

Flexible collapsible plastic bags (50 to 250 mL): used for continuous infusion of fluid replacement with or without medications
Intermittent intravenous infusions: usually secondary intravenous setup of a small plastic bag (50 to 250 mL) to which medication is added. The infusion runs as a "piggyback," hung separately from the primary intravenous infusion via a secondary administration tubing set usually for 20 to 120 minutes. The primary intravenous solution is run between medication doses.
Heparin lock: a port site for direct administration of intermittent intravenous medications without the need for primary intravenous solution

Preparations for Topical Use

Liniment: liquid suspension for lubrication that is applied by rubbing
Lotion: liquid suspension that can be protective, emollient, cooling, astringent, antipruritic, or cleansing
Ointment: semisolid medicine in a base for local protective, soothing, astringent, or transdermal application for systemic effects (nitroglycerin, scopolamine, estrogen)
Paste: thick ointment primarily used for skin protection
Plasters: solid preparations that are adhesive, protective, or soothing
Cream: emulsion that contains aqueous and oily bases
Aerosol: fine powder or solution in a volatile liquid that contains a propellant

Preparations for Use on Mucous Membranes

Drops for eyes, ears, or nose: aqueous solutions with or without gelling agent to increase retention time in the eye
Topical instillation of aqueous solution of medications: usually for topical action but occasionally for systemic effects (enema, douche, mouthwash, throat spray, gargle)
Aerosol sprays, nebulizers, and inhalers: aqueous solutions of medication delivered in droplet form to the target membrane, such as the bronchial tree (bronchodilators)
Nasal drugs: an alternative route for drugs with poor bioavailability and high molecular weight compounds such as peptides, steroids, and vaccines
Foam: powder or solution of medication in volatile liquid with propellant (vaginal foams for contraception)
Suppositories: usually medicinal substances mixed in a form but malleable base (coca butter to facilitate insertion into a body cavity [rectum or vagina])

Miscellaneous Drug Delivery Systems

Intradermal implants: pellets that contain a small deposit of medication that are inserted into a dermal pocket; they are designed to allow medication to leach slowly into tissue and usually are used to administer hormones such as testosterone or estradiol
Micropump system: small, external pump attached by belt or implanted that delivers medication via a needle in a continuous steady dose (insulin, anticancer chemotherapy, opioids)
Membrane delivery systems: drug-laden membranes are instilled into the eye to deliver a steady flow of medication (pilocarpine or corticosteroids)

paramedic also should seek medical direction as needed. One should note that paramedics are responsible for safe and effective drug administration. In addition, they are personally responsible for each drug they give. They are legally, morally, and ethically responsible. (See Chapter 18.) As part of the professional practice of patient management, paramedics must do the following:

- Use correct precautions and techniques when administering medications.
- Observe and document the effects of drugs.
- Maintain their knowledge base current regarding changes in trends in pharmacology.
- Establish and maintain professional relationships with other members of the health care team.
- Understand pharmacodynamics of the drugs they administer.
- Carefully evaluate patients to identify drug indications and **contraindications.**
- Take a drug history from patients that includes the following information:
  Prescribed medications (name, strength, daily dosage)
  Over-the-counter medications
  Vitamins
  Alternative drug therapies (e.g., homeopathic medicines and herbal medicines)
  Any drug allergies or adverse drug reactions
- Consult with medical direction as needed.

The components of a drug profile include the following:

Drug names: Usually the generic and trade names; may include chemical names.
Classification: The group to which the drug belongs
Mechanism of action: The pharmacodynamic properties of a drug; the way in which a drug causes its effects
Indications: Conditions for which the drug is administered as approved by the FDA
Pharmacokinetics: How the body handles the drug over time; includes absorption, distribution, biotransformation, excretion, and onset and duration
Side/adverse effects: Untoward or undesired effects that may be caused by the drug
Dosages: The amount of drug to be administered
Routes of administration: How the drug is given
Contraindications: Conditions in which it may be harmful to administer the drug
Special considerations: How the drug may affect pediatric patients, geriatric patients, pregnant patients, and other special groups (described next)
Storage requirements: How the drug should be stored

Special Considerations in Drug Therapy

Special considerations in drug therapy must be taken into account when one is caring for pregnant patients, pediatric patients, and older adult patients. These considerations are described next. They also are described throughout this text by subject matter and in the *Emergency Drug Index.*

PREGNANT PATIENTS

Before administering any drug to a pregnant patient, the paramedic should consider the expected benefits and the possible risks to the fetus. Drugs given to a pregnant patient may cross the placental barrier. In fact, they may harm the fetus or may be communicated to a newborn during breast-feeding. The FDA has established a scale to indicate drugs that may be harmful to a fetus during pregnancy (Box 17-12).

PEDIATRIC PATIENTS

Special considerations for administration of drugs to pediatric patients are presented here and throughout the text. Following is a summary of the pharmacokinetics that influence dosing principles in the neonate, infant, and pediatric populations.

Age. The effects of drugs are unpredictable among infants because of the variation in the development and maturation of the organ systems.

BOX 17-12 Pregnancy Category Ratings for Drugs

Drugs have been categorized by the Food and Drug Administration according to the level of risk to the fetus. These categories are listed for each drug herein under Pregnancy Safety and are interpreted as follows[1]:

Category A: Controlled studies in women fail to demonstrate a risk to the fetus in the first trimester, and there is no evidence of risk in later trimesters; the possibility of fetal harm appears to be remote.

Category B: Either (1) animal reproductive studies have not demonstrated a fetal risk but there are no controlled studies in pregnant women or (2) animal reproductive studies have shown an adverse effect (other than decreased fertility) that was not confirmed in controlled studies on women in the first trimester, and there is no evidence of risk in later trimesters.

Category C: Either (1) studies in animals have revealed adverse effects on the fetus and there are no controlled studies in women or (2) studies in women and animals are not available. Drugs in this category should be given only if the potential benefit justifies the risk to the fetus.

Category D: There is positive evidence of human fetal risk, but the benefits for pregnant women may be acceptable despite the risk, as in life-threatening diseases for which safer drugs cannot be used or are ineffective. An appropriate statement must appear in the "Warnings" section of the labeling of drugs in this category.

Category X: Studies in animals or human beings have demonstrated fetal abnormalities, there is evidence of fetal risk based on human experience, or both; the risk of using the drug in pregnant women clearly outweighs any possible benefit. The drug is contraindicated in women who are or may become pregnant. An appropriate statement must appear in the "Contraindications" section of the labeling of drugs in this category.

> **CRITICAL THINKING**
>
> Drug doses vary for pediatric and neonatal patients. They are almost always related to weight. How can you ensure accuracy of dosing for these patients in critical situations when seconds count, even though you know the wrong dose calculation could be lethal?

Absorption. Drug absorption in infants and children follows the same basic principles as it does in adults. A factor that influences drug absorption is blood flow at the site of intramuscular or subcutaneous administration. Blood flow usually is determined by the patient's cardiovascular function. Certain physiological conditions might reduce blood flow to the muscle and subcutaneous tissue. These conditions include shock, vasoconstriction, and heart failure. The smaller muscle mass of the infant further complicates drug absorption because of diminished peripheral perfusion to these areas. For orally administered drugs, underlying gastrointestinal function may influence drug absorption.

Liquids and suspensions disperse quickly in gastrointestinal fluids. Thus they are more readily absorbed than tablet or capsule forms. Increases in peristalsis (e.g., diarrheal conditions) and lowered gastrointestinal enzyme activities tend to decrease overall absorption of orally or rectally administered medications.

Distribution. Most drugs are distributed in body water. Thus increases in total body water and extracellular volume can increase the volume of the distribution. Compared with adults, infants have proportionately higher volumes of total body water (70% to 75% compared with 50% to 60%). Infants also have a higher ratio of extracellular to intracellular fluid (40% compared with 30%); higher dosages of water-soluble drugs may be needed to have effective blood levels in the newborn.

Another key factor that affects drug distribution is drug binding to plasma proteins. In general, protein binding of drugs is reduced in the infant; therefore the concentration of free drug in plasma is increased. This can result in a greater drug effect or toxicity. Regarding central nervous system effects, the blood-brain barrier in the infant is much less effective than in adults. This allows drugs greater access to this area.

Biotransformation. Various liver enzyme systems for metabolism generally mature unevenly. The infant therefore has a decreased ability to metabolize drugs. This predisposes the infant to developing toxicity from drugs metabolized by the liver. In addition, many drugs given to infants have slower renal clearance times and longer half-lives. Thus the paramedic must adjust dosages based on age and weight.

Elimination. The GFR is much lower in newborns than in older infants, children, and adults. Therefore drugs eliminated through renal function are cleared from the body slowly in the first few weeks of life. Renal excretory mechanisms progress to maturity after 1 year of age. Before that age, excretion of some substances through the renal system may be delayed because of immaturity. This may result in higher serum levels and a longer duration of action than intended.

OLDER ADULT PATIENTS

Key changes in drug responses occur with age in most individuals. Factors associated with aging that significantly affect pharmacokinetics include the likelihood of multiple diseases requiring the use of several drugs (also referred to as polydrug usage). In addition, nutritional problems, decreasing ability to metabolize drugs, and the possibility of decreased drug dosing compliance for a variety of reasons can influence the effects of drugs. This summary is meant to serve as a review of the pharmacokinetics that influence dosing principles in the older adult.

Age. Declines in the functional capacity of most major organ systems begin in young adulthood. These changes continue through life. Older adults do not lose specific function at a quicker rate than young and middle-aged adults; rather, they have less physiological reserves. Decreases in physiological function (GFR, cardiac function, maximal breathing capacity) generally are accepted as beginning no later than age 45. Decreased renal function has the greatest impact on medication administration and drug clearance.

Absorption. Little evidence exists of major changes in drug absorption with age. Yet conditions associated with age may alter the rate at which some drugs are absorbed. Examples of these conditions include altered nutritional habits, greater consumption of nonprescription drugs (e.g., antacids and laxatives), and changes in gastric emptying. The reduced production of gastric acid and slowed gastric motility may have an impact and may result in unpredictable rates of dissolution and absorption of weakly acidic drugs.

Distribution. Changes in body composition have been noted in the older adult. Such changes include reduced lean body mass, reduced total body water, and increased fat as a percentage of body mass. Levels of serum albumin—which binds many drugs, especially weak acids—also usually decline. This affects drug distribution; it decreases protein binding of drugs. This results in an increase in the amount of free drug in the circulation. Thus the ratio of bound to free drug in these patients may be significantly altered.

Biotransformation. The ability of the liver to metabolize drugs does not appear to decline consistently with age for all drugs. But disorders common with aging can impair liver function. One such example is congestive heart failure. Hepatic recovery from injury, such as that caused by alcohol or viral hepatitis, declines as well.

Certain drugs generally are believed to be metabolized more slowly in older adults. This is thought to be the case because of decreased liver blood flow. This decrease may lead to drug accumulation and toxicity. The paramedic must use caution when administering medication that is metabolized primarily in the liver to a patient with a history of liver disease. Older patients with severe nutritional deficiencies also may have impaired hepatic function.

Elimination. Renal function is the most critical factor for clearance of most drugs from the body. A natural reduction in renal function occurs with aging and usually is caused by loss of functioning nephrons and a decrease in blood flow. Both of these result in a decreased GFR. A decrease in renal function caused by decreases in renal blood flow also may occur because of congestive heart failure. The practical result of renal impairment is a prolongation of the half-life of many drugs and the possibility of accumulation to toxic levels. Other reversible conditions (e.g., dehydration) can cause further reduction in renal clearance of drugs.

Drug Administration Problems. Older adults commonly do not comply with their drug therapy. Noncompliance may be intentional or unintentional on their part but rarely affects the administration of emergency drugs. Still, the paramedic must be familiar with the most common factors that contribute to drug administration problems in older adults. This is crucial because noncompliance or errors may be a factor in the patient's condition. Following are some common causes of noncompliance and medication errors:

- The expense of drugs may lead to noncompliance in patients with fixed incomes. Older patients may not take prescribed medications routinely or may be unwilling to receive medications in emergency situations.
- Noncompliance in taking prescribed medications may result from forgetfulness or confusion, especially if the patient has several prescriptions and different dosing intervals.
- Older patients may forget instructions on the need to complete medication because symptoms have disappeared. Disappearance of symptoms often is regarded as the best reason to stop the therapy.
- Errors in self-administered medications may result from physical disabilities such as arthritis or visual impairment.
- Noncompliance may be deliberate. A patient may be opposed to taking a drug because of past experiences. A careful drug history is especially important when caring for older adults. The paramedic should remember that a patient has the right to refuse medication.

SECTION THREE
Drugs That Affect the Nervous System

REVIEW OF ANATOMY AND PHYSIOLOGY

The effects of many drugs depend on which branch of the autonomic nervous system they act. The effects also depend on whether the branch is stimulated or inhibited by drug therapy. The following is a discussion of the anatomy and physiology of the nervous system as they pertain to pharmacology (Box 17-13).

BOX 17-13 Emergency Drugs: Nervous System

Atropine (Atropine)	Morphine (Astramorph/PF)
Diazepam (Valium)	Naloxone (Narcan)
Dopamine (Intropin)	Norepinephrine (Levophed)
Epinephrine (Adrenalin)	Pancuronium (Pavulon)
Isoproterenol (Isuprel)	Phenytoin (Dilantin)
Labetalol (Normodyne)	Physostigmine (Antilirium)
Magnesium sulfate	Propranolol (Inderal)
Meperidine (Demerol)	Succinylcholine (Anectine)

As described in Chapter 6, the central nervous system (CNS) consists of the brain and spinal cord. The CNS serves as the collection point for nerve impulses. (Fig. 17-5) The peripheral nervous system consists of cranial and spinal nerves and all their branches (those nerves outside the CNS). The peripheral nervous system connects all parts of the body to the CNS. The somatic nervous system controls functions that are under conscious, voluntary control such as skeletal muscles and sensory neurons of the skin. The autonomic nervous system, mostly motor nerves, controls functions of involuntary smooth muscles, cardiac muscles, and glands. Four types of nerve fibers are found in most nerves:

1. *Visceral afferent* (sensory) *fibers,* which convey impulses from the internal organs to the CNS
2. *Visceral efferent* (motor) *fibers,* which convey impulses from the CNS to the internal organs, glands, and the smooth and cardiac (involuntary) muscles
3. *Somatic afferent* (sensory) *fibers,* which convey impulses from the head, body wall, and extremities to the CNS
4. *Somatic efferent* (motor) *fibers,* which convey impulses from the CNS to the striated (voluntary) muscles

Simply put, the peripheral (sensory) nervous system receives stimuli from the body. The CNS interprets these stimuli. The peripheral (motor) nervous system initiates responses to the stimuli. Together the visceral afferent and visceral efferent nerve fibers form the autonomic nervous system. In contrast, the somatic afferent and somatic efferent nerve fibers form the somatic nervous system. Thus the autonomic nervous system and the somatic nervous system can be regarded as subdivisions of the peripheral nervous system (Box 17-14).

Autonomic Division of the Peripheral Nervous System

The autonomic division of the peripheral nervous system provides almost every organ with a double set of nerve fibers: sympathetic (also known as **adrenergic**) and parasympathetic (also known as **cholinergic**). The cell bodies of the neurons in these two divisions are located in dif-

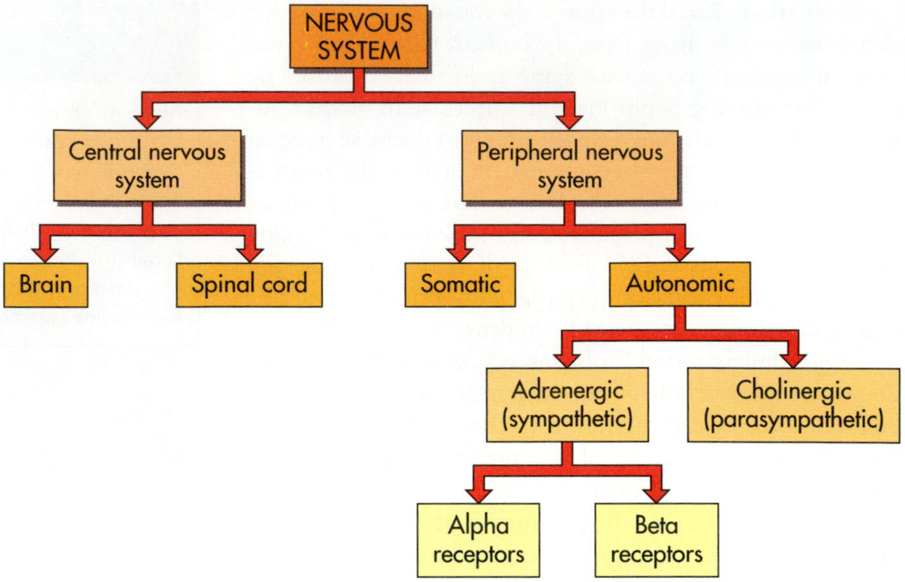

FIGURE 17-5 ■ Overview of the nervous system.

BOX 17-14 Organization of the Nervous System

Central Nervous System	Peripheral Nervous System
Brain	Cranial nerves
Spinal cord	Visceral afferent nerve fibers
	Visceral efferent nerve fibers
	Somatic afferent nerve fibers
	Somatic efferent nerve fibers
Spinal nerves	Visceral afferent nerve fibers
	Visceral efferent nerve fibers
	Somatic afferent nerve fibers
	Somatic efferent nerve fibers

ferent areas of the CNS. They also exit the spinal cord at different levels. The sympathetic fibers exit from the thoracic and lumbar regions of the spinal cord. The parasympathetic fibers exit from the cranial and sacral portions of the spinal cord.

The sympathetic and parasympathetic systems generally work as *physiological antagonists* on effector organs. That is, one division carries impulses that inhibit a certain function. The other division usually carries impulses that augment that function. As a rule, the sympathetic system prepares the body for vigorous muscular activity, stress, and emergencies (fight or flight). The sympathetic nervous system tends to affect widespread areas of the body for sustained periods of time. In contrast, the parasympathetic system lowers muscular activity, operates during nonemergency situations, conserves energy, and produces selective and localized responses of short duration. The sympathetic and parasympathetic systems operate at the same time. Yet one usually has more dominant effects at any given time.

Autonomic innervation by the sympathetic and parasympathetic nervous system may be viewed as involving a two-neuron chain. This chain exists in a series between the CNS and the effector organs. This two-neuron chain is composed of a preganglionic neuron, located in the CNS, and a postganglionic neuron, located in the periphery (Fig. 17-6). The area that serves as a functional junction between these two neurons is known as a *synapse*. The preganglionic fibers pass between the CNS and the nerve cell bodies in the peripheral nervous system (ganglia). The postganglionic fibers pass between the ganglia and the effector organ. Many of the sympathetic ganglia lie close to the spinal cord. Others lie about midway between the spinal cord and the effector organ. The parasympathetic ganglia lie close or within the walls of the effector organ. The difference in location of the ganglia in these two divisions is the anatomical reason for the widespread responses caused by the sympathetic division versus the localized responses caused by the parasympathetic division.

Neurochemical Transmission

Most neurons are insulated electrically from each other. Because of this insulation, the fibers communicate by way of neurotransmitters. These are chemicals that are released from one neuron at the presynaptic nerve fiber. These neurotransmitters then cross the synapse where they may be accepted by the next neuron at a specialized site called a *receptor.* (Neurotransmitters bind only to specific receptors on the postsynaptic membranes that recognize them.) The neurotransmitter then is deactivated or taken up into the presynaptic neuron.

In the sympathetic and parasympathetic divisions, the neurotransmitter for the preganglionic fiber at the junction between the preganglionic fiber and the synapse is acetylcholine. The neurotransmitter at the junction between the parasympathetic postganglionic fiber and the effector cell is also acetylcholine. Fibers that release acetylcholine are

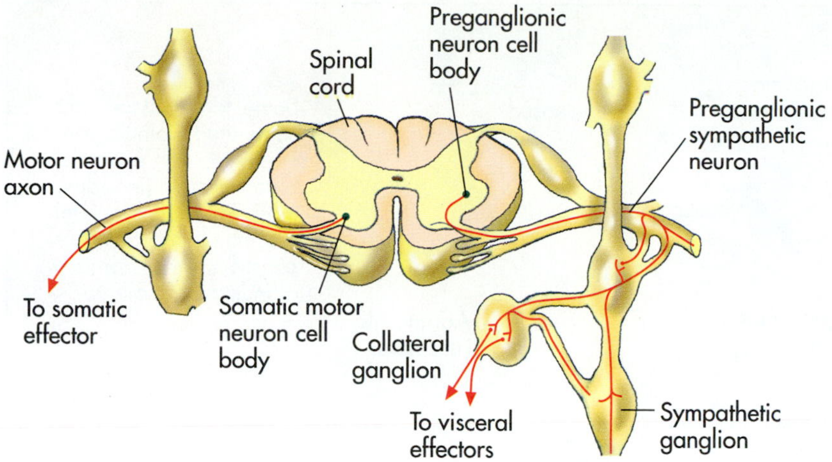

FIGURE 17-6 ■ Autonomic conduction pathways.

known as cholinergic fibers. All preganglionic neurons of the autonomic division and all postganglionic neurons of the parasympathetic division are cholinergic.

> **NOTE** All preganglionic nerves use the same neurotransmitter: acetylcholine.

The neurotransmitter between the sympathetic postganglionic fiber and the effector cell is norepinephrine. This chemical is a member of the catecholamine family. Fibers that release norepinephrine are known as adrenergic fibers. (This is a term derived from *noradrenalin,* the British name for norepinephrine.) Most postganglionic neurons of the sympathetic division are adrenergic; that is, they release norepinephrine. However, a few are cholinergic. The actions of the autonomic nervous system depend on the interaction between the neurotransmitter released by the ganglionic cells and the receptor effector cells. For example, stimulation of the sympathetic nerves causes excitatory effects in some organs and inhibitory effects in others. Likewise, parasympathetic stimulation causes excitation in some organs but inhibition in others.

> **NOTE** Two different neurotransmitters exist for postganglionic neurons. All parasympathetic postganglionic neurons release acetylcholine onto their target tissue. Most sympathetic postganglionic neurons release norepinephrine onto their target tissue.

The parasympathetic and sympathetic systems function continuously. They innervate many of the same organs at the same time. Thus the opposing actions of the two systems balance one another. (Most organs, however, are controlled predominantly by one or the other of the two systems.) As previously stated, the sympathetic system usually dominates during stressful events. The parasympathetic system is most active during periods of emotional and physical calm.

Transmission of Nerve Impulses in the Autonomic Nervous System

Both branches of the autonomic nervous system have multiple receptors. The variety among neurotransmitters and receptors accounts for the differences in response to stimulation of sympathetic and parasympathetic nerves (excitatory or inhibitory).

The parasympathetic nervous system has *nicotinic* and *muscarinic* receptors (Fig. 17-7). Nicotinic receptors (stimulated by nicotine) are found at the neuromuscular junctions of skeletal muscles. They also are found on the postganglionic neurons of the parasympathetic nervous system. Muscarinic receptors (stimulated by the mushroom poison, muscarine) are found at the neuromuscular junction of cardiac and smooth muscle. They also are found on glands and on the postganglionic neurons of the sympathetic nervous system. Drugs that can activate nicotinic receptors typically do not activate muscarinic receptors. The difference between nicotinic and muscarinic receptors is crucial in drug therapy. For example, when acetylcholine binds to nicotinic receptors, an excitatory response occurs. When acetylcholine binds with muscarinic receptors, it results in excitation or inhibition. This depends on the target tissue in which the receptors are found (Table 17-3). When acetylcholine binds to muscarinic receptors in cardiac muscle, the heart rate slows. When it binds to muscarinic receptors in smooth muscle cells of the gastrointestinal tract, the rate and amplitude of contraction increase. ***Atropine*** blocks muscarinic but not nicotinic receptor sites. (Thus ***atropine*** affects the heart rate but does not cause paralysis.) However, the nicotinic receptor blocker curare causes paralysis.

> **NOTE** The two types of cholinergic receptors are nicotinic receptors and muscarinic receptors. Nicotinic responses are of fast onset and short duration and are excitatory. Muscarinic receptors are of slow onset and long duration and may be excitatory or inhibitory.

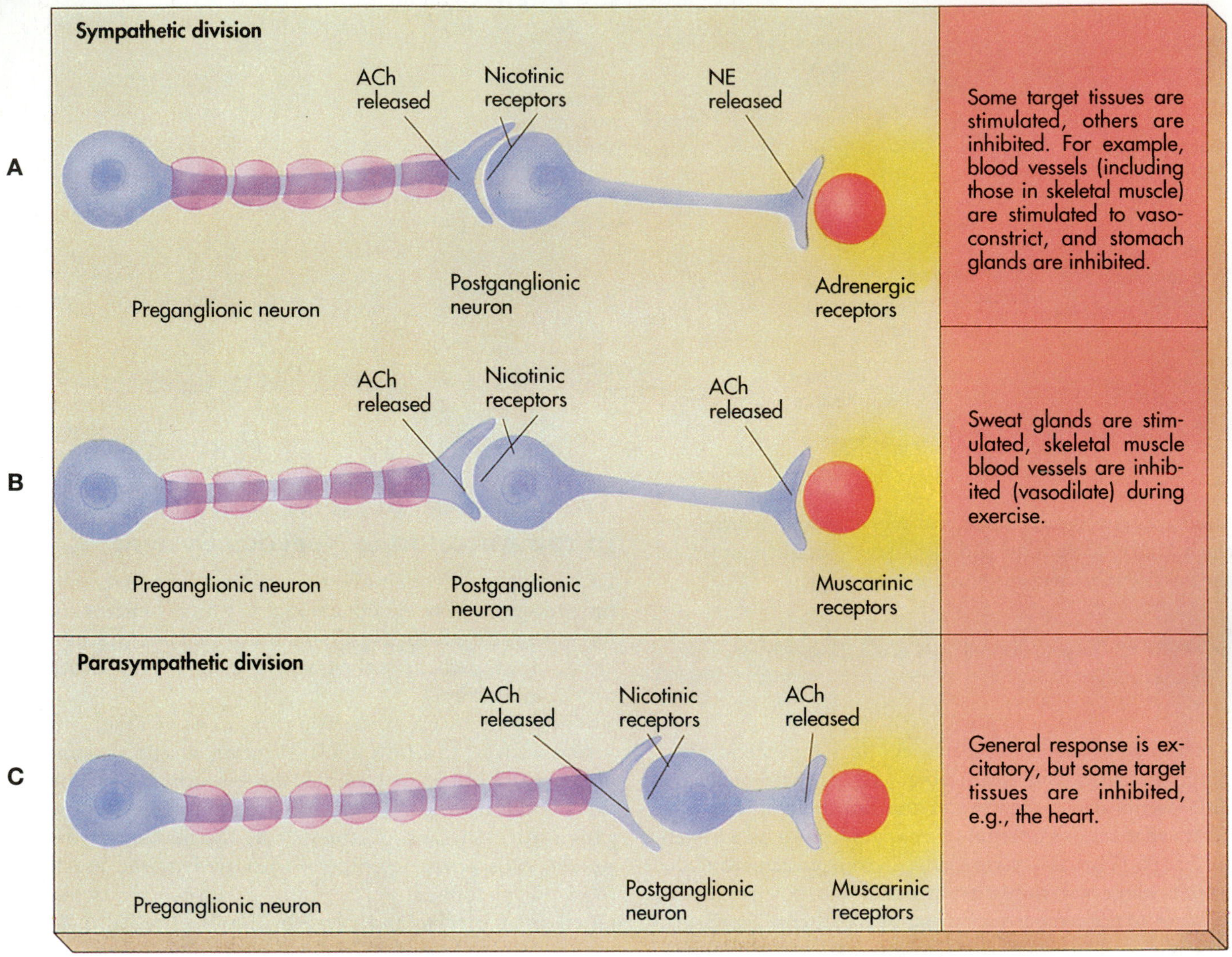

FIGURE 17-7 ■ Location of the nicotinic, muscarinic, and adrenergic receptors in the autonomic nervous system. Nicotinic receptors are found on the cell bodies of sympathetic and parasympathetic postganglionic cells in the autonomic ganglia. **A,** Adrenergic receptors are found in most target tissues innervated by the sympathetic division. **B,** Some sympathetic target tissues have muscarinic receptors. **C,** All parasympathetic target tissues have muscarinic receptors. *NE,* Norepinephrine; *ACh,* acetylcholine.

CRITICAL THINKING

Imagine that your patient has eaten some poisonous mushrooms containing muscarine. What signs or symptoms related to pulse rate would you expect? What signs or symptoms related to gastrointestinal tract activity? Lastly, what signs or symptoms related to pupil diameter?

For the sympathetic (adrenergic) nervous system, the major receptor types belong to two structural categories. These are the alpha receptors and beta receptors (and their subgroups, described in the following text). Norepinephrine binds to and activates both types of receptor molecules. Yet norepinephrine has more affinity for alpha receptors. The hormone epinephrine is produced by the adrenal medulla and is classified as an adrenergic substance. Epinephrine has nearly equal affinity for both receptors. In tissues containing alpha and beta receptor cells, one type is more abundant. As a result, that type has a predominant effect. Both receptors can be excitatory or inhibitory. For example, beta receptors are stimulatory in cardiac muscle. Yet they are inhibitory in intestinal smooth muscle (Table 17-4).

NOTE The two major types of adrenergic receptors are alpha and beta. Both receptors can be excitatory or inhibitory.

TABLE 17-3 Sites for Muscarinic and Nicotinic Actions of Acetylcholine

SITE	MUSCARINIC ACTIONS*	NICOTINIC ACTIONS
Cardiovascular		
Blood vessels	Dilation	Constriction
Heart rate	Slowed	Increased
Blood pressure	Decreased	Increased
Gastrointestinal		
Tone	Increased	Increased
Motility	Increased	Increased
Sphincters	Relaxed	—
Glandular secretions	Increased salivary, lacrimal, intestinal, and sweat secretion	Initial stimulation and then inhibition of salivary and bronchial secretions
Skeletal muscle	—	Stimulation
Autonomic ganglia	—	Stimulation
Eye	Pupil constriction	—
	Decreased accommodation	—
Blocking agent	Atropine	Tubocurarine
Remarks	Above effects increase as dosage increases.	Increased dosage inhibits effects and causes receptor blockade.

*Usual sites for therapeutic effects.

Drugs That Affect the Autonomic Nervous System

The nervous and endocrine systems are responsible for controlling and coordinating body functions. These two systems share three characteristics: a high level of integration in the brain, the ability to influence functions in distant regions of the body, and the extensive use of negative feedback mechanisms (described in Chapter 7). One main difference between the two systems is the mode of transmission of information.

The endocrine system transmission is chiefly chemical. The information moves via blood-borne hormones. The hormones are not targeted for a specific organ. Instead, they diffusely affect many cells and organs at the same time. In contrast, the nervous system mainly relies on rapid electrical transmission of information over nerve fibers. Chemical impulses carry signals only between nerve cells and their effector cells in a localized manner, perhaps affecting only a few cells. (Drugs that affect the endocrine system are presented later in this chapter.)

CLASSIFICATIONS

The autonomic drugs mimic or block the effects of the sympathetic and parasympathetic divisions of the autonomic nervous system (see Box 17-15). These drugs can be classified into four groups:

1. Cholinergic (parasympathomimetic) drugs, which mimic the actions of the parasympathetic nervous system
2. Cholinergic blocking (parasympatholytic) drugs, which block the actions of the parasympathetic nervous system
3. Adrenergic (sympathomimetic) drugs, which mimic the actions of the sympathetic nervous system or the adrenal medulla
4. Adrenergic blocking (sympatholytic) drugs, which block the actions of the sympathetic nervous system or adrenal medulla

Cholinergic Drugs. As described earlier, acetylcholine plays a key role in the parasympathetic and sympathetic divisions of the nervous system. Acetylcholine has two major effects in the nervous system: (1) a stimulant effect on the ganglia, adrenal medulla, and skeletal muscle (the nicotinic effect) and (2) stimulant effects at postganglionic nerve endings in cardiac muscle, smooth muscle, and glands (the muscarinic effect). Drugs that affect nicotinic or cholinergic receptor sites on autonomic ganglia are ganglionic-stimulating drugs (e.g., nicotine and nicotine gum) and ganglionic-blocking drugs (e.g., mecamylamine).

Cholinergic drugs (choline esters) act directly with cholinergic receptors on postsynaptic membranes, or they act indirectly by inhibiting the enzyme that normally destroys acetylcholine. This inhibition results in an accumulation of acetylcholine. This in turn causes a longer and more intense response at various effector sites. Cholinergic drugs have little therapeutic value. For the most part, they are not thought of as emergency drugs. The main exception to this is ***physostigmine*** (Antilirium), which is an indirect-acting cholinergic drug. ***Physostigmine*** may be used to manage extreme cases of poisoning resulting from atropine-type drugs. (See Chapter 36.) Indirect-acting cholinergic drugs are used to treat myasthenia gravis, a condition characterized by weakness of the skeletal muscles. These drugs work to elevate the concentration of acetylcholine at myoneural junctions. This in turn increases muscle strength and function.

Cholinergic blocking **(anticholinergic)** agents have many uses in emergency medicine. These drugs work by

TABLE 17-4 Autonomic Innervation of Target Tissues

ORGAN	EFFECT OF SYMPATHETIC STIMULATION	EFFECT OF PARASYMPATHETIC STIMULATION
Heart		
Muscle	Increased rate and force (b)	Slowed rate (c)
Coronary arteries	Dilation (b),* constriction (a)*	Dilation (c)
Systemic blood vessels		
Abdomen	Constriction (a)	None
Skin	Constriction (a)	None
Muscle	Dilation (b, c), constriction (a)	None
Lungs		
Bronchi	Dilation (b)	Constriction (c)
Liver	Release of glucose into blood (b)	None
Skeletal muscles	Breakdown of glycogen to glucose (b)	None
Metabolism	Increase of up to 100% (a, b)	None
Glands		
Adrenal glands	Release of epinephrine and norepinephrine (c)	None
Salivary glands	Constriction of blood vessels and slight production of thick, viscous secretion (a)	Dilation of blood vessels and thin, copious secretion (c)
Gastric glands	Inhibition (a)	Stimulation (c)
Pancreas	Inhibition (a)	Stimulation (c)
Lacrimal glands	None	Secretion (c)
Sweat glands		
Merocrine glands	Copious, watery secretion (c)	None
Apocrine glands	Thick, organic secretion (c)	None
Gut		
Wall	Decreased tone (b)	Increased motility (c)
Sphincter	Increased tone (a)	Decreased tone (c)
Gallbladder and bile ducts	Relaxation (b)	Contraction (c)
Urinary bladder		
Wall	Relaxation (b)	Contraction (c)
Sphincter	Contraction (a)	Relaxation (c)
Eye		
Ciliary muscle	Relaxation for far vision (b)	Contraction for near vision (c)
Pupil	Dilation	Constriction (c)
Erector pili muscles	Contraction (a)	None
Blood	Increased coagulation (a)	None
Sex organs	Ejaculation (a)	Erection (c)

a, Mediated by alpha receptors; *b*, mediated by beta receptors; *c*, mediated by cholinergic receptors.
*Normally blood flow through coronary arteries increases as a result of sympathetic stimulation of the heart because of increased demand by cardiac tissue for oxygen. In experiments that isolate the coronary arteries, however, sympathetic nerve stimulation, acting through alpha receptors, causes vasoconstriction. The beta receptors are relatively insensitive to sympathetic nerve stimulation but can be activated by drugs.

blocking the muscarinic effects of acetylcholine. Thus they decrease the action of acetylcholine on its effector organ.

The best known cholinergic blocking drug used in emergency care is ***atropine.*** Atropine is a belladonna alkaloid that acts as a competitive antagonist. Atropine works by occupying muscarinic receptor sites. This action prevents or reduces the muscarinic response to acetylcholine. Large doses dilate the pupils, inhibit accommodation of the eyes, and increase the heart rate by blocking the cholinergic effects of the heart. Synthetic substitutes for ***atropine*** have been created. These were created to obtain only the antispasmodic effects of the drug. (For example, they may be used to treat gastric and duodenal ulcers.) These synthetic drugs include dicyclomine (Bentyl) and glycopyrrolate (Robinul).

Adrenergic Drugs. Adrenergic drugs are designed to produce activities like those of neurotransmitters. The three types of adrenergic agents are direct acting, indirect acting, and dual acting (direct and indirect).

Direct-acting Drugs. Three naturally occurring catecholamines are present in the body: epinephrine, norepinephrine, and dopamine. Epinephrine acts mainly as an emergency hormone. Epinephrine is released by the adrenal medulla. Norepinephrine acts as a critical transmitter of nerve impulses. Dopamine is a precursor of epinephrine and norepinephrine. Dopamine has a transmitter role of its own in certain parts of the CNS. Examples of synthetic catecholamine drugs and the three endogenous catecholamines are ***epinephrine*** (Adrenalin), ***norepinephrine*** (Levophed), ***dopamine*** (Intropin), and ***dobutamine*** (Dobutrex).

BOX 17-15 Anatomical and Functional Terms for the Autonomic Nervous System

The anatomical names and functional terms for the autonomic nervous system often are used interchangeably: sympathetic or adrenergic, and parasympathetic or cholinergic. The terms *parasympathomimetic* and *sympathomimetic* mean to mimic or to produce an effect similar to activation of either system. The words *parasympatholytic* and *sympatholytic* mean to block the normal effects seen with activation of either system. The term *anticholinergic* is synonymous with *parasympatholytic.*

Anatomical Name	Functional Term	Primary Neurotransmitter
Sympathetic	Adrenergic	Norepinephrine
Parasympathetic	Cholinergic	Acetylcholine

Catecholamines depend on their ability to act directly with alpha and beta receptors. Two subgroups of alpha receptors have been identified. These are $alpha_1$ and $alpha_2$. $Alpha_1$ receptors are postsynaptic receptors. They are located on the effector organs. The chief role of the $alpha_1$ receptor is to stimulate contraction of smooth muscle. In the vasculature, this results in an increase in blood pressure. $Alpha_2$ receptors are found on presynaptic and postsynaptic nerve endings. When stimulated, presynaptic receptors inhibit the further release of norepinephrine. Like $alpha_1$ receptors, $alpha_2$ postsynaptic receptors produce vasoconstriction to increase resistance in blood vessels and thus increase blood pressure.

Beta receptors are subdivided into $beta_1$ and $beta_2$ receptors based on their response to drugs. However, the division also follows anatomical distinctions. $Beta_1$ receptors are located mainly in the heart. $Beta_2$ receptors are located mainly in the bronchiolar and arterial smooth muscle. Beta receptors stimulate the heart; dilate bronchioles; dilate blood vessels in the skeletal muscle, brain, and heart; and aid in glycogenolysis (Table 17-5).

NOTE Use of a memory aid to differentiate the physiological effects of beta receptors may be helpful: A person has one heart ($beta_1$ effects) and two lungs ($beta_2$ effects).

Norepinephrine acts mainly on alpha receptors. It causes almost pure vasoconstriction of the blood vessels. Epinephrine acts on alpha and beta receptors. It produces a mixture of vasodilation and vasoconstriction. This effect depends on the number of alpha and beta receptors present in the target tissue. The following are the most important alpha and beta activities in human beings:

1. Alpha activities
   - Vasoconstriction of arterioles in the skin and splanchnic area, resulting in a rise in blood pressure and peripheral shunting of blood to the heart and brain from the shifting of blood volume
   - Pupil dilation
   - Relaxation of the gut
2. Beta activities
   - Cardiac acceleration and increased contractility
   - Vasodilation of arterioles supplying the skeletal muscle
   - Bronchial relaxation
   - Uterine relaxation

Indirect-acting and dual-acting Drugs. Indirect-acting adrenergic drugs act indirectly on receptors. They do this by triggering the release of the catecholamines, norepinephrine, and epinephrine. These chemicals then activate the alpha and beta receptors. Dual-acting adrenergic drugs have indirect and direct effects. An example of a drug in this group is ephedrine (ephedrine sulfate).

Adrenergic blocking agents may be classified into alpha- and beta-blocking drugs. Alpha-blocking drugs block the vasoconstricting effect of catecholamines. They are used in certain cases of hypertension. They also are used to help prevent necrosis when ***norepinephrine*** (Levophed) or ***dopamine*** (Intropin) has leaked, or extravasated, into the tissues. They have limited clinical application in the prehospital setting.

NOTE All drugs with alpha effects should be administered through a secure intravenous line. This line should be well positioned in a large vein because of the possibility of extravasation and tissue necrosis.

Beta-blocking agents have greater clinical application. They often are used in emergency care. These drugs block beta receptors. They inhibit the action of beta receptors at the effector site. Beta-blocking agents are grouped into selective beta-blocking agents and nonselective beta-blocking agents. The selective blocking agents block $beta_1$ or $beta_2$ receptors. The nonselective beta-blocking agents block $beta_1$ and $beta_2$ receptor sites. Selective $beta_1$-blocking agents also are known as *cardioselective blockers* because they block the $beta_1$ receptors in the heart. Examples of important selective $beta_1$-blocking agents are ***metoprolol*** (Lopressor, Toprol-XL) and ***atenolol*** (Tenormin). These drugs are antihypertensives and antidysrhythmics. They are used in managing hypertension. They also are used in select patients with suspected myocardial infarction and high-risk unstable angina.

Nonselective beta-blocking agents inhibit both beta receptors in the smooth muscle of the bronchioles and blood vessels. Examples include the antianginal antihypertensives nadolol (Corgard) and ***propranolol*** (Inderal), and the antihypertensive ***labetalol*** (Normodyne, Trandate). (***Labetalol*** also has some alpha-blocking activity.)

CRITICAL THINKING

Doctors usually will not prescribe a nonselective beta-blocker such as propranolol (Inderal) for patients with a history of asthma. Why is that?

TABLE 17-5 Actions of Autonomic Nervous System Neuroreceptors

EFFECTOR ORGAN OR TISSUE	RECEPTOR	ADENERGIC EFFECT	CHOLINERGIC EFFECT
Eye, iris			
Radial muscle	α_1	Contraction (mydriasis)	—
Sphincter muscle		—	Contraction (miosis)
Eye, ciliary muscle	β_2	Relaxation for far vision	Contraction for near vision
Lacrimal glands	—	—	Secretion
Nasopharyngeal glands	—	—	Secretion
Salivary glands	α_1	Secretion of potassium and water	Secretion of potassium and water
	β	Secretion of amylase	—
Heart			
SA node	β_1	Increased heart rate	Decrease heart rate; vagus arrest
Atrial	β_1	Increased contractility and conduction velocity	Decrease contractility; shorten action potential duration
AV junction	β_1	Increased automaticity and propagation velocity	Decrease automaticity and propagation velocity
Purkinje system	β_1	Increased automaticity and propagation velocity	—
Ventricles	β_1	Increased contractility	—
Arterioles			
Coronary	α_1, β_2	Constriction, dilation	Dilation
Skin and mucosa	α_1, α_2	Constriction	Dilation
Skeletal muscle	α, β_2	Constriction, dilation	Dilation
Cerebral	α_1	Constriction (slight)	—
Pulmonary	α_1, β_2	Constriction, dilation	—
Mesenteric	α_1	Constriction	—
Renal	$\alpha_1, \beta_1, \beta_2$, D	Constriction, dilation	—
Salivary glands	α_1, α_2	Constriction	Dilation
Veins, systemic	α_1, β_2	Constriction, dilation	—
Lung			
Bronchial muscle	β_2	Relaxation	Contraction
Bronchial glands	α_1, β_2	Decreased secretion; increased secretion	Stimulation
Stomach			
Motility	α_1, β_2	Decrease (usually)	Increase
Sphincters	α_1	Contraction (usually)	Relaxation (usually)
Secretion	—	Inhibition (?)	Stimulation
Liver	α, β_2	Glycogenolysis and gluconeogenesis	Glycogen synthesis
Gallbladder and ducts	—	Relaxation	Contraction
Pancreas			
Acini	α	Decreased secretion	Secretion
Islet cells	α_2, β_2	Decreased secretion; increased secretion	—
Intestine			
Motility and tone	$\alpha_1, \beta_1, \beta_2$	Decrease	Increase
Sphincters	α_1	Contraction (usually)	Relaxation (usually)
Secretion	α_2	Inhibition (?)	Stimulation
Adrenal medulla	—	—	Secretion of epinephrine and norepinephrine (nicotinic effect)
Kidney			
Renin secretion	α_1, β_1	Decrease; increase	—
Ureter			
Motility and tone	α_1	Increase	Increase
Urinary bladder			
Detrusor	β_2	Relaxation (usually)	Contraction
Trigone and sphincter	α_1	Contraction	Relaxation
Sex organs, male	α_1	Ejaculation	Erection
Skin			
Pilomotor muscles	α_1	Contraction	—
Sweat glands	α_1	Localized secretion	Generalized secretion
Fat cells	$\alpha_2; \beta_1(\beta_3)$	Inhibition of lipolysis; stimulation of lipolysis	—
Pineal gland	β	Melatonin synthesis	—

BOX 17-16 Classifications of Pain

Acute pain: pain sudden in onset that usually subsides with treatment (e.g., pain associated with acute myocardial infarction, acute appendicitis, renal colic, or traumatic injuries)
Chronic pain: persistent or recurrent pain that is difficult to treat (e.g., pain that accompanies cancer and rheumatoid arthritis)
Referred pain: visceral pain felt at a site distant from its origin (e.g., pain from a myocardial infarction felt in the arm)
Somatic pain: pain arising from skeletal muscles, ligaments, vessels, or joints
Superficial pain: pain arising from the skin or mucous membrane
Visceral pain: "deep" pain arising from smooth musculature or organ systems that may be difficult to localize and is often described as dull or aching.

Narcotic Analgesics and Antagonists

Narcotic analgesics relieve pain. Narcotic antagonists reverse the effects of some narcotic analgesics. Pain has two components. The first is the sensation of pain. This involves the nerve pathways and the brain. The second is the emotional response to pain. This may be a result of the individual's anxiety level, previous pain experience, age, gender, and culture. Box 17-16 lists and defines classifications of pain.

Opiates are drugs that contain or are extracted from opium. The term *opioid* refers to synthetic drugs. These drugs have pharmacological properties that are similar to those of opium or ***morphine.*** Morphine is the chief alkaloid of opium. Opioids work by binding with opioid receptors in the brain and other body organs. This alters the patient's perception of pain and emotional response to a pain-causing stimulus. Opioid analgesics include ***morphine,*** codeine (methylmorphine), hydromorphone (Dilaudid, Dilaudid HP), ***meperidine*** (Demerol), methadone (Dolophine, Methadose), oxycodone (OxyContin, Percodan, Tylox, Percocet), hydrocodone (Lortab), and propoxyphene (Darvon, Dolene).

NOTE Endorphins serve as the body's own supply of opiates. They do this by binding to opiate receptors, thereby blocking pain.

Opioid analgesics may produce undesirable effects such as nausea and vomiting, constipation, urinary retention, cough reflex suppression, orthostatic hypotension, respiratory depression, and CNS depression (including respiratory depression). Most of these effects can be overcome by careful administration and close patient monitoring.

Opioid antagonists block the effects of opioid analgesics. (Examples of such effects are opioid-induced respiratory depression and sedation.) Opioid antagonists block the effects by displacing the analgesics from their receptor sites. ***Naloxone*** (Narcan), naltrexone (Trexan), and ***nalmefene*** (Revex) are opioid antagonists.

Opioid agonist-antagonist agents have analgesic and antagonist effects. The exact mechanism of action is unknown. These drugs, though, may have pharmacokinetic and adverse effects similar to those of ***morphine.*** They may antagonize some opioid receptors competitively. Yet they may have varying degrees of agonist effect at other opioid receptor sites. Examples of these drugs include pentazocine (Talwin), and nalbuphine (Nubain). These drugs generally have a lower potential for creating dependency than opioid analgesics. In addition, withdrawal symptoms are not as severe as those of the opioid agonist drugs. They may bring about withdrawal symptoms in addicts.

BOX 17-17 Examples of Anesthetics

Inhalation Anesthetics
Gases
Cyclopropane
Nitrous oxide; oxygen (Nitronox)

Volatile liquids
Halothane (Fluothane)
Methoxyflurane (Penthrane)
Enflurane (Ethrane)
Isoflurane (Forane)

Intravenous Anesthetics
Ultrashort-acting barbiturates
Thiopental sodium (Pentothal)
Thiamylal sodium (Surital)
Methohexital sodium (Brevital Sodium)

Nonbarbiturates
Etomidate (Amidate)
Fentanyl (Sublimaze)
Sufentanil (Sufenta)
Alfentanil (Alfenta)

Intravenous Anesthetics, cont'd
Dissociative anesthetics
Ketamine (Ketalar)

Neuroleptic anesthetics
Droperidol-fentanyl (Innovar injection)

Local Anesthetics
Topical
Benzocaine (Anbesol)
Ethyl chloride cocaine
Lidocaine (Xylocaine)
Tetracaine (Pontocaine)

Injectable
Lidocaine (Xylocaine)
Procaine (Novocain)

Nonnarcotic Analgesics

Nonnarcotic analgesics interfere with local mediators released when tissue is damaged in the periphery of the body. These mediators stimulate nerve endings and they cause pain. When nonnarcotic analgesics are present, the nerve endings in damaged tissues are stimulated less often. This differs from the mechanism of narcotic analgesics. Narcotic analgesics act at the level of the CNS. An example of a nonnarcotic analgesic is ***ketorolac*** (Toradol), a nonsteroidal antiinflammatory drug that exhibits analgesic activity.

CRITICAL THINKING
A nonnarcotic analgesic may be selected instead of a narcotic for a paramedic returning to work on the ambulance. Why?

Anesthetics

Anesthetic drugs are CNS depressants. They have a reversible action on nervous tissue. The three major types of anesthesia are general, regional, and local. General anesthesia is achieved by intravenous or inhalation routes and is the most common type of anesthesia used during surgery to induce uncon-

BOX 17-18 The Physiology of Sleep

Sleep can be viewed as a series of rhythms. Each has its own brain wave patterns. These rhythms can be divided into two major categories: rapid eye movement (REM) and non–rapid eye movement (non-REM). During sleep, a person moves through REM sleep. Then the person moves through four stages of non-REM sleep. Rapid eye movement, or active, sleep is the time of irregular body activity, vivid dreaming, and rapid eye movements. During REM sleep, the eyes move back and forth under the closed lids as they follow the action of a dream. The heart rate, blood pressure, and respirations may become irregular. During non-REM sleep, the person drifts out of wakeful awareness. The muscles relax, and the blood pressure, heartbeat, and breathing begin to decline. The brain sends signals to the arms, legs, and other large muscles to stop moving. At that point, "sleep paralysis" occurs. The first REM period lasts nearly 10 minutes. The whole cycle repeats itself usually four to five times each night. Each cycle lasts an average of 90 minutes. As the night wears on, REM periods lengthen, and non-REM periods grow shorter. The final REM period of the night may last as long as 1 hour.

sciousness. Regional anesthesia is obtained by injecting a local anesthetic drug. The drug is injected near a nerve trunk or at specific sites in a large region of the body (e.g., spinal block). Local anesthesia is achieved topically to produce a loss of sensation. Local anesthesia also can be achieved by injection to block an area surrounding an operative field, making it insensitive to pain (e.g., minor wound repair) (Box 17-17).

Antianxiety and Sedative-Hypnotic Agents and Alcohol

Antianxiety and sedative-hypnotic agents and alcohol are presented together because of their similarities in pharmacological action. Antianxiety agents are used to reduce feelings of apprehension, nervousness, worry, or fearfulness.

Sedatives and hypnotics are drugs that depress the CNS, produce a calming effect, and help induce sleep (Box 17-18). The major difference between a sedative and a hypnotic is the degree of CNS depression induced by the agent. For example, a small dose of an agent administered to calm a patient is called a *sedative;* a larger dose of the same agent sufficient to induce sleep is called a *hypnotic.* Thus an agent may be a sedative or a hypnotic, depending on the dose used.

As stated before, alcohol has actions that are characteristic of sedative-hypnotic or antianxiety drugs. Socially, alcohol is used mainly as a self-prescribed antianxiety agent. Alcohol is a major source of drug abuse and dependency.

Scattered throughout the brain stem is a group of nuclei. All together this group is called the *reticular formation.* The reticular formation and its neural pathways make up a system known as the *reticular activating system* (described in Chapter 6). This system is involved with the cycle of sleep and wake. Through these pathways, the reticular activating system collects incoming signals from the senses and viscera. The system then processes and passes these signals to the higher brain centers. The reticular activating system determines the level of awareness to the environment. Thus the reticular activating system also governs actions and responses to the environment. Antianxiety and sedative-hypnotic agents and alcohol act by depressing this system.

CLASSIFICATIONS

Two prototypical groups of drugs are used to treat anxiety or to induce sleep. These are the benzodiazepines and barbiturates, respectively. Benzodiazepines make up the drug class most often used today to treat anxiety and insomnia. Barbiturates make up an older drug class with many uses. These uses range from sedation to anesthesia.

Benzodiazepines. Benzodiazepines were introduced in the 1960s as antianxiety drugs. At present, they are among the most widely prescribed drugs in clinical medicine. This is partly because of their high therapeutic index. Overdoses of 1000 times the therapeutic dose have been reported not to result in death unless taken with other CNS depressants, such as alcohol.[6] Benzodiazepines are thought to work by binding to specific receptors in the cerebral cortex and limbic system. (These systems together govern emotional behavior.) These drugs are highly lipid soluble and are distributed widely in the body tissues. They also are highly bound to plasma protein, usually more than 80%. Benzodiazepines have four actions: anxiety reducing, sedative-hypnotic, muscle relaxing, and anticonvulsant. All benzodiazepines are Schedule IV drugs because of their potential for abuse. Commonly prescribed benzodiazepines are alprazolam (Xanax), clonazepam (Klonopin), ***diazepam*** (Valium), flurazepam (Dalmane), ***midazolam*** (Versed), ***lorazepam*** (Ativan), and temazepam (Restoril).

CRITICAL THINKING

Consider that you are preparing to reduce a dislocated shoulder. Why would a benzodiazepine be preferred over a narcotic?

NOTE Flumazenil (Romazicon) is a specific benzodiazepine receptor antagonist. Flumazenil has been shown to be effective in reversing benzodiazepine-induced sedation and coma[7] (see Chapter 36 and the Emergency Drug Index).

Barbiturates. Barbiturates were once the most commonly prescribed class of medications for sedative-hypnotic effects. However, they virtually have been replaced by the benzodiazepines. Barbiturates are divided into four classes according to their duration of action: ultrashort acting, short acting, intermediate acting, and long acting. The differences in onset and duration of action depend on their lipid solubility and protein-binding properties. Ultrashort-acting barbiturates commonly are used as intravenous anesthetics. These drugs act rapidly and can produce a state of anesthesia in a few seconds. An example of an ultrashort-acting barbiturate is thiopental sodium (Pentothal).

Short-acting barbiturates produce an effect in a short time (10 to 15 minutes). They also peak over a short period

(3 to 4 hours). This class of drugs rarely is used to treat insomnia; it more often is used for preanesthesia sedation and in combination with other drugs for psychosomatic disorders. Examples include pentobarbital (Nembutal) and secobarbital (Seconal).

Intermediate-acting barbiturates have an onset of 45 to 60 minutes. They peak in 6 to 8 hours. Short-acting and intermediate-acting barbiturates produce similar patient responses. Examples of intermediate-acting barbiturates include amobarbital (Amytal) and butabarbital (Butisol).

Long-acting barbiturates require more than 60 minutes for onset. They peak over 10 to 12 hours. These agents are used to treat epilepsy and other chronic neurological disorders. They also are used to sedate patients with severe anxiety. Examples of long-acting barbiturates include mephobarbital (Mebaral) and phenobarbital (Luminal).

Miscellaneous Sedative-hypnotic Drugs. The previously discussed drug classes do not include all of the antianxiety and sedative-hypnotic drugs. In fact, a number of other antianxiety and sedative-hypnotic drugs do not fall into these classes. These agents are more similar to barbiturates than benzodiazepines because they are generally shorter acting. Examples of miscellaneous drugs with antianxiety and sedative-hypnotic effects are chloral hydrate (Noctec), ***etomidate*** (Amidate), and zolpidem (Ambien). In addition to these drugs, antihistamines such as ***hydroxyzine*** (Vistaril, Atarax) have pronounced sedative effects.

Alcohol Intake and Behavioral Effects

Alcohol is a general CNS depressant that can produce sedation, sleep, and anesthesia. In addition, alcohol enhances the sedative-hypnotic effects of other drug classes, including all general CNS depressants, antihistamines, phenothiazines, narcotic analgesics, and tricyclic antidepressants. If alcohol is taken with other drugs, this enhancement could result in coma or death. Blood alcohol is measured in milligrams per deciliter. Characteristic behavioral effects can be predicted based on the amount of alcohol consumed and blood alcohol levels. Behavioral effects associated with alcohol intake are described further in Chapter 36.

Anticonvulsants

Anticonvulsant drugs are used to treat seizure disorders. The most notable of these disorders is epilepsy. Epilepsy is a neurological disorder characterized by a recurrent pattern of abnormal neuronal discharges within the brain. These discharges result in a sudden loss or disturbance of consciousness, sometimes associated with motor activity, sensory phenomena, or inappropriate behavior. Epilepsy is estimated to occur in 0.5% to 1% of the population. In 50% of these cases, the cause is unknown (primary or idiopathic epilepsy). Secondary epilepsy is epilepsy that can be traced to trauma, infection, a cerebrovascular disorder, or some other illness. (Epilepsy is discussed further in Chapter 31.)

The exact mode and site of action of anticonvulsant drugs are not understood. In general, these drugs depress the excitability of neurons that fire to initiate the seizure. These drugs also suppress the neurons responsible for generalization of the small focal depolarization, thus preventing the spread of seizure discharge. Anticonvulsants are presumed to modify the ionic movements of sodium, potassium, or calcium across the nerve membrane. Thus they reduce the response to incoming electrical or chemical stimulation. Benzodiazepines also stimulate major inhibitory neurotransmitters in the CNS. Many patients need drug therapy throughout their lives to control seizure disorders.

Several drugs are available for the control of seizure disorders. The choice of drug depends on the type of seizure disorder (generalized, partial, or status.) The choice of drug also depends on the patient's **tolerance** and response to the prescribed medication. Box 17-19 presents classes of anticonvulsant drugs.

BOX 17-19 Classes of Anticonvulsant Drugs

Barbiturates
Mephobarbital (Mebaral)
Phenobarbital (Luminal)

Benzodiazepines
Clonazepam (Klonopin)
Diazepam (Valium)
Lorazepam (Ativan)

Hydantoins
Ethotoin (Peganone)
Fosphenytoin (Cerebyx)
Mephenytoin (Mesantoin)
Phenytoin (Dilantin)

Succinimides
Ethosuximide (Zarontin)
Methsuximide (Celontin)
Phensuximide (Milontin)

Other
Carbamazepine (Tegretol)
Divalproex (Depakote)
Gabapentin (Neurontin)
Lamotrigine (Lamictal)
Magnesium sulfate
Topiramate (Topamax)
Valproic acid (Depakene)

Central Nervous System Stimulants

Central nervous system stimulants are classified by where they exert their major effects in the nervous system: on the cerebrum, the medulla and brainstem, or in the hypothalamic limbic regions. All CNS stimulants work to increase excitability by blocking activity of inhibitory neurons or their respective neurotransmitters or by enhancing the production of the excitatory neurotransmitters. Some of the more common CNS stimulant drugs are anorexiants and amphetamines.

ANOREXIANTS

Anorexiants are appetite suppressants. They are used to treat obesity. They work by producing a direct stimulant effect on the hypothalamic and limbic regions. They perhaps have this effect on other areas of the nervous system as well. Examples of anorexiants include phendimetrazine (Plegine) and mazindol (Mazanor, Sanorex).

A new class of drugs (gastrointestinal lipase inhibitors, or fat blockers) block the absorption of about 30% of dietary fat. These drugs sometimes are used to manage obesity along with a reduced-calorie diet. An example of a gastrointestinal lipase inhibitor is orlistat (Xenical).

▶**NOTE** At one time, a two-drug combination of fenfluramine and phentermine (fen-phen) was used to manage obesity. The combination was withdrawn from the market in 1997. It was found to have serious complications. These included potentially fatal primary pulmonary hypertension and valvular heart disease.

AMPHETAMINES

Amphetamines stimulate the cerebral cortex and reticular activating system. This stimulation increases alertness and responsiveness to environmental surroundings. Amphetamines mainly are used to treat attention deficit hyperactivity disorder (ADHD) and narcolepsy. For the most part, ADHD is seen in children and adolescents and is characterized by a short attention span and impulsive behavior. ADHD is described further in Chapter 40.

Individuals with narcolepsy experience excessive drowsiness, sudden sleep attacks during daytime hours, and sometimes sleep paralysis. Medications used to treat these disorders include methamphetamine (Desoxyn), amphetamine-mixed salts (Adderall), and dextroamphetamine tablets and elixir. Nonamphetamine CNS stimulants used to treat ADHD include methylphenidate (Ritalin, Concerta) and pemoline (Cylert). Paradoxically, amphetamines and other stimulants have a calming effect on children with ADHD. Likely, the drugs do this by increasing neurotransmitter levels of dopamine.

Psychotherapeutic Drugs

Psychotherapeutic drugs include antipsychotic agents, antidepressants, and lithium. These drugs are used to treat psychoses and affective disorders, especially schizophrenia, depression, and mania (see Chapter 40).

CENTRAL NERVOUS SYSTEM AND EMOTIONS

The neurotransmitters acetylcholine, norepinephrine, dopamine, serotonin, and MAO have a major effect on emotion (Fig. 17-8). Alterations in the levels of these chemicals are linked to changes in mood and behavior. Drug therapy alleviates symptoms by temporarily modifying unwanted behavior.

▶**NOTE** Acetylcholine is released from central neural tissue into the cerebrospinal fluid during activity. Norepinephrine and dopamine have widespread inhibitory effects. They affect functions such as sleep and arousal, affect, and memory. Serotonin levels affect mood and behavior. Monoamine oxidase is an enzyme that inactivates dopamine and serotonin, both of which are produced during intense emotional states.

ANTIPSYCHOTIC AGENTS

The main use of antipsychotic drugs is to treat schizophrenia. This class of drugs is the only clearly effective treatment for this condition. There are other psychiatric indications for the use of antipsychotic drugs. These drugs are used to treat Tourette's syndrome. They also are used to control disturbing behavior in patients with senile dementia associated with Alzheimer's disease. Effective antipsychotic (neuroleptic) drugs block dopamine receptors in specific areas of the CNS. These drugs can be classified into the following groups:

- Phenothiazine derivatives
  Chlorpromazine (Thorazine)
  Thioridazine (Mellaril)
  Fluphenazine (Prolixin)
- Butyrophenone derivatives
  Haloperidol (Haldol)
- Dihydroindolone derivatives
  Molindone (Moban)

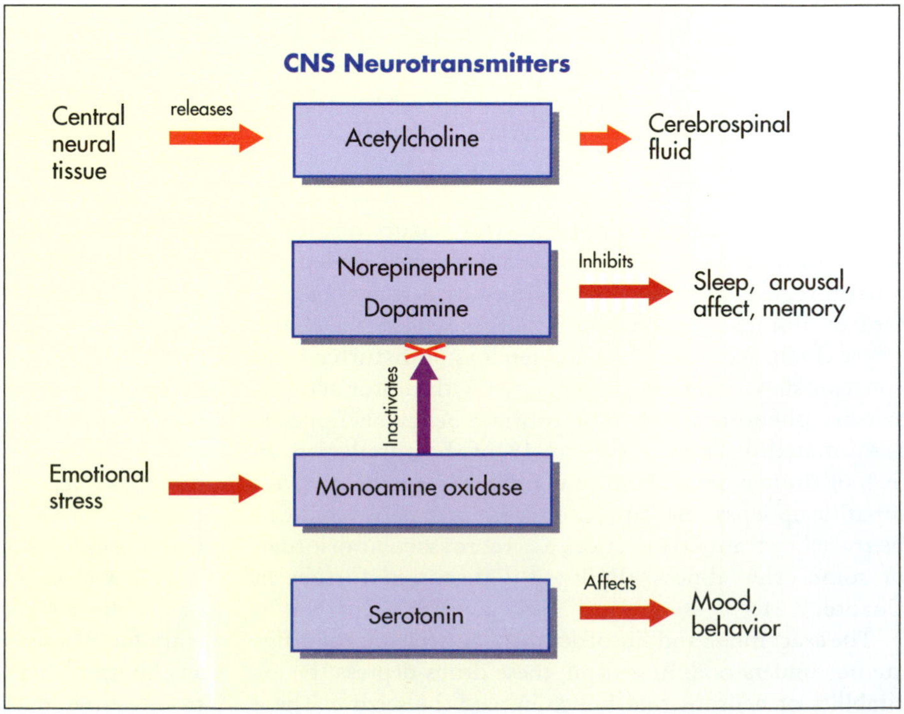

FIGURE 17-8 ■ Neurotransmitters in the brain and their effects on emotion.

- Dibenzoxazepine derivatives
  Loxapine (Loxitane)
- Thienbenzodiazepine derivatives
  Olanzapine (Zyprexa)
- Atypical agents
  Clozapine (Clozaril)
  Risperidone (Risperdal)

With continued use of antipsychotics, some patients develop supersensitivity of dopamine receptors. This leads to tardive dyskinesia. Tardive dyskinesia is a potentially irreversible neurological disorder characterized by involuntary repetitious movements of the muscles of the face, limbs, and trunk. Other identifying features include excessive blinking of the eyelids, lip smacking, tongue protrusion, foot tapping, and rocking side-to-side.

ANTIDEPRESSANTS

Antidepressants are used to treat affective disorders (mood disturbances) including depression, mania, and elation. Tricyclic antidepressants, selective serotonin reuptake inhibitors, and MAO inhibitors are prescribed for depression; lithium (an antimanic drug) is the preferred treatment for mania.

> **NOTE** Depression may be exogenous. That means depression results from a person's response to a loss or disappointment. (For example, depression may be thought of as "the blues.") Exogenous depression is considered normal. This depression usually is temporary and remits without the use of drug therapy. Endogenous depression, however, lasts 6 months or longer. Endogenous depression is characterized by the absence of external causes; it may be the result of genetic or biochemical alterations. Antidepressants often are needed to treat this disorder. Depression is discussed further in Chapter 40.

Tricyclic Antidepressants. Tricyclic antidepressants are thought to treat depression by increasing levels (blocking the reuptake) of the neurotransmitters norepinephrine and serotonin. Examples include mirtazapine (Remeron), nortriptyline (Pamelor), and amitriptyline (Elavil).

> **CRITICAL THINKING**
> You know that tricyclic antidepressants increase the levels of norepinephrine. Thus what side effects might you expect in an overdose?

Selective Serotonin Reuptake Inhibitors. Selective serotonin reuptake inhibitors work to block the reabsorption or reuptake of serotonin. This makes more of the chemical available to the brain. These drugs do have some side effects; for example, insomnia and difficulty reaching orgasm. However, these drugs often treat depression without the adverse effects of other antidepressants, such as the dry mouth caused by tricyclic antidepressants or the dietary restrictions mandated by MAO inhibitors. Examples of selective serotonin reuptake inhibitors are fluoxetine (Prozac), sertraline (Zoloft), paroxetine (Paxil), fluvoxamine (Luvox), and citalopram (Celexa).

Monoamine Oxidase Inhibitor Antidepressants. Central-acting monoamines, especially norepinephrine and serotonin, are thought to cause depression and mania. Monoamine oxidase is an enzyme found in nerve cells. The enzyme is thought to be produced during tense emotional states. The enzyme is responsible for metabolizing norepinephrine within the nerve. Monoamine oxidase inhibitors block this enzyme. This leads to increased levels of norepinephrine. Examples of MAO inhibitors used to treat depression include isocarboxazid (Marplan), phenelzine (Nardil), and tranylcypromine (Parnate). Monoamine oxidase inhibitors also are used as antihypertensive agents (described later in this chapter).

Lithium. Lithium is a cation that is closely related to sodium. Both cations are transported actively across cell membranes. However, lithium cannot be pumped as effectively out of the cell as sodium. Lithium therefore accumulates in the cells. This results in a decrease in intracellular sodium and perhaps an improvement in the symptoms of a manic state. In addition, lithium appears to enhance some of the actions of serotonin. Lithium may decrease levels of norepinephrine and dopamine. Lithium also appears to block the development of dopamine receptor supersensitivity that may accompany long-term therapy with antipsychotic agents. Lithium carbonate is used to treat manic disorders and comes in capsule, tablet, and syrup form (e.g., lithium citrate).

Drugs for Specific Central Nervous System–Peripheral Dysfunction

Several movement disorders result from an imbalance of dopamine and acetylcholine. Two of the most common are Parkinson's disease (including parkinsonism syndromes) and Huntington's disease.

PARKINSON'S DISEASE

Parkinson's disease is a chronic disabling disease characterized by rigidity of voluntary muscles. Parkinson's disease also is characterized by tremor of the fingers and extremities. The disease most often affects persons over age 60, although it may occur in younger persons. Parkinson's disease may occur especially after acute encephalitis or cases of carbon monoxide or metallic poisoning or from the use of some illicit drugs. The disease is thought to result from an abnormally low concentration of dopamine. Parkinsonism syndromes mimic the symptoms of Parkinson's disease. They usually are idiopathic but may result from treatment with antipsychotic drugs (drug-induced parkinsonism) that block dopaminergic receptors (e.g., ***haloperidol*** [Haldol], metoclopramide [Clopra, Emex], and phenothiazines [e.g., Thorazine, Mellaril]). Symptoms of Parkinson's disease include the following:

- Immobile facial expression (parkinsonism facies)
- Bobbing of the head
- Resting tremor
- Pill-rolling of the fingers
- Shuffling gait
- Forward flexion of the trunk
- Loss of postural reflexes

BOX 17-20 Drugs That Affect Dopamine in the Brain

Amantadine (Symmetrel)	Levodopa (Larodopa)
Bromocriptine (Parlodel)	Pergolide (Permax)
Carbidopa-levodopa (Sinemet)	

HUNTINGTON'S DISEASE

Huntington's disease is an inherited disorder characterized by progressive dementia and involuntary muscle twitching (chorea). Like Parkinson's disease, Huntington's disease is thought to be related to an imbalance of dopamine, acetylcholine, and perhaps other neurotransmitters.

Drugs with Central Anticholinergic Activity

Drugs that inhibit or block acetylcholine are referred to as anticholinergic. They work by restoring the normal dopamine-acetylcholine balance in the brain. Common anticholinergic agents include benztropine (tablets and injections) and ethopropazine hydrochloride.

Drugs That Affect Dopamine in the Brain

Three classifications of drugs affect dopamine in the brain: those that release dopamine, those that increase brain levels of dopamine, and dopaminergic agonists (Box 17-20). Levodopa (L-dopa) is a drug that increases brain levels of dopamine. Levodopa is the current drug of choice in the treatment of movement disorders associated with dopamine-acetylcholine imbalance.

MONOAMINE OXIDASE INHIBITORS

Two types of MAO have been identified. The first one is monoamine oxidase A. It metabolizes norepinephrine and serotonin. The second one is monoamine oxidase B. It metabolizes dopamine. Selegiline (Deprenyl) is a selective inhibitor of monoamine oxidase B. It retards the breakdown of dopamine Selegiline often is used along with levodopa because it enhances and prolongs the antiparkinsonism effects of levodopa. (Selegiline allows the dose of levodopa to be reduced.)

Skeletal Muscle Relaxants

Skeletal muscle contraction is evoked by a nicotinic cholinergic transmission process. Such contractions can be modified by drugs just as the autonomic ganglionic transmission can be. Skeletal muscle relaxants can be classified as central-acting, direct-acting, and neuromuscular blockers.

CENTRAL-ACTING MUSCLE RELAXANTS

Central-acting drugs are used to treat muscle spasms. They are thought to work by producing CNS depression in the brain and spinal cord. Antispastic agents include carisoprodol (Soma), cyclobenzaprine (Flexeril), and ***diazepam*** (Valium).

DIRECT-ACTING MUSCLE RELAXANTS

Direct-acting muscle relaxants work directly on skeletal muscles to produce muscle relaxation. This results in a decrease in muscle contraction. Dantrolene (Dantrium) is an example of a direct-acting muscle relaxant.

NEUROMUSCULAR BLOCKERS

Neuromuscular blocking drugs produce complete muscle relaxation and paralysis. They do this by binding to the nicotinic receptor for acetylcholine at the neuromuscular junction. Neuromuscular nerve transmission is thus blocked. Nerve transmission remains blocked for a variable period depending on the type and amount of neuromuscular blocker used.

Neuromuscular blockers sometimes are used to achieve total paralysis before endotracheal intubation (described in Chapter 19), to relieve muscle spasms of the larynx, to suppress tetany, during electroconvulsive therapy for depression, and to allow for breathing control by a respirator. These blocking agents produce complete paralysis. Thus a patient's breathing must be supported. The effectiveness of ventilation and oxygenation must be monitored closely. (These muscle relaxants do not inhibit pain or seizure activity.) Examples of neuromuscular blockers include ***pancuronium*** (Pavulon), vecuronium (Norcuron), and ***succinylcholine*** (Anectine).

SECTION FOUR
Drugs That Affect the Cardiovascular System

REVIEW OF ANATOMY AND PHYSIOLOGY

The heart is made up of many interconnected branching fibers or cells that form the walls of the two atria and two ventricles. Some of these cells are specialized to conduct electrical impulses. Others have contraction as their main role. All of these cells are nourished through a profuse network of blood vessels (coronary vasculature). Cardiac drugs are classified by their effects on these tissues. Boxes 17-21 and 17-22 list cardiac drugs and pharmacological terms that describe their actions.

BOX 17-21 Emergency Drugs: Cardiovascular System

Drugs Used to Treat Dysrhythmias	Drugs Used to Optimize Cardiac Output and Blood Pressure
Adenosine (Adenocard)	Calcium chloride
Amiodarone (Cordarone)	Digoxin (Lanoxin)
Atropine	Dobutamine (Dobutrex)
Beta-adrenergic blockers	Dopamine (Intropin)
Atenolol (Tenormin)	Epinephrine (Adrenalin)
Metoprolol (Lopressor, Toprol-XL)	Furosemide (Lasix)
Calcium channel blockers	Nitroglycerin (Nitrostat, Tridil)
Diltiazem (Cardizem)	Norepinephrine (Levophed)
Verapamil (Isoptin)	Sodium bicarbonate
Dopamine (Intropin)	Vasopressin (Pitressin)
Isoproterenol (Isuprel)	
Lidocaine (Xylocaine)	
Magnesium	
Procainamide (Pronestyl)	

BOX 17-22 Pharmacological Terms to Describe Actions of Cardiovascular Drugs

Chronotropic: Chronotropic drugs affect heart rate. If the drug accelerates the heart rate (e.g., isoproterenol [Isuprel]), it is said to have a positive chronotropic effect. A drug that decreases the heart rate (e.g., verapamil [Isoptin]) is said to have a negative chronotropic effect.

Dromotropic: Dromotropic drugs affect conduction velocity through the conducting tissues of the heart. If a drug speeds conduction, it is said to have a positive dromotropic effect. Examples of drugs with positive dromotropic effects include isoproterenol (Isuprel) and phenytoin (Dilantin). Drugs with negative dromotropic effects delay conduction (e.g., verapamil [Isoptin] and adenosine [Adenocard]).

Inotropic: Inotropic drugs strengthen or increase the force of cardiac contraction (a positive inotropic effect). Some examples include digoxin (Lanoxin), dobutamine (Dobutrex), epinephrine (Adrenalin), and isoproterenol (Isuprel). A drug that weakens or decreases the force of cardiac contraction has a negative inotropic effect. An example of such a drug is propranolol (Inderal).

Cardiac Glycosides

Cardiac glycosides are naturally occurring plant substances. They have characteristic effects on the heart. These compounds contain a carbohydrate molecule (sugar). When combined with water, the molecule is converted into a sugar plus one or more active substances. Glycosides may work by blocking certain ionic pumps in the cellular membrane. This indirectly increases the calcium concentration to the contractile proteins. A key cardiac glycoside is ***digoxin*** (Lanoxin). ***Digoxin*** is used to treat heart failure and to manage certain tachycardias.

Digitalis glycosides can affect the heart in two distinct ways. First, they increase the strength of contraction. This is a positive inotropic effect. Second, they have a dual effect on the electrophysiological properties of the heart. They have a modest negative chronotropic effect. (This causes slight slowing of the heart rate.) They also have a profound negative dromotropic effect, decreasing conduction velocity of impulses in the heart.

Many patients who take cardiac glycosides develop side effects at one time or another because of the small therapeutic index of the drugs. The symptoms may be neurological, visual, gastrointestinal, cardiac, or psychiatric. These symptoms often are vague and can be attributed easily by the patient to a viral illness. A high index of suspicion in patients taking cardiac glycosides who report experiencing flulike symptoms is important. The most common side effects of cardiac glycosides are anorexia, nausea or vomiting, visual disturbances (flashing lights, altered color vision), and cardiac rhythm disturbances (usually slowing with varying degrees of blocked conduction).

NOTE Proarrhythmias are serious dysrhythmias. They apparently are generated by antidysrhythmic agents. All antidysrhythmic drugs have some degree of proarrhythmic effects. The sequential use of two or more antidysrhythmic drugs compounds these effects. As a rule, use of no more than one agent is best to manage dysrhythmias. (That is, of course, unless use of more than one agent is absolutely necessary.)

The toxic effects of cardiac glycosides are dose related. These effects may be increased by the presence of other drugs, such as diuretics. These other drugs may predispose the patient to cardiac rhythm disturbances. Dysrhythmias may include bradycardias, tachycardias, and even ventricular fibrillation. For these reasons, patients taking these drugs require close monitoring. Treatment for digitalis toxicity may include correction of electrolyte imbalances, neutralization of the free drug, and use of antidysrhythmics.

Antidysrhythmics

Antidysrhythmic drugs are used to treat and prevent disorders of cardiac rhythm. The pharmacological agents that suppress dysrhythmias may do so by direct action on the cardiac cell membrane ***(lidocaine*** [xylocaine]*)*, by indirect action that affects the cells ***(propranolol*** [Inderal]*)*, or both.

Cardiac rhythm disturbances may be caused by ischemia, hypoxia, acidosis or alkalosis, electrolyte abnormalities, excessive catecholamine exposure, autonomic influences, drug toxicity, or scarred and diseased tissue. Dysrhythmias result from disturbances in impulse formation, disturbances in impulse conduction, or both.

CLASSIFICATIONS

Antidysrhythmic drugs have been classified into categories based on their fundamental mode of action on cardiac muscle.[8] Drugs that belong to the same class do not always produce identical actions. However, all antidysrhythmic drugs have some ability to suppress automaticity.

> **NOTE** Local protocols and standing orders are meant to assist and guide emergency medical services. These orders often are put into effect to allow paramedics to use certain drugs in certain cases. With these orders in place, the paramedics can act before seeking medical direction. One such example is antidysrhythmic drugs for a patient with specific cardiac conduction disturbances. Another is first-line cardiac life support drugs for a patient in cardiac arrest.

Class I. Class I drugs are sodium channel blockers. These work to slow conduction. They are divided further into subclasses (Ia, Ib, and Ic) based on the extent of sodium channel blockade. Examples of Class Ia drugs include quinidine (Quinaglute, Duraquin), disopyramide (Norpace), and ***procainamide*** (Pronestyl). Class Ib drugs decrease or have no effect on conduction velocity. Examples include ***lidocaine*** (Xylocaine) and ***phenytoin*** (Dilantin). Class Ic drugs profoundly slow conduction and are indicated only for control of life-threatening ventricular dysrhythmias. An example of a Class Ic drug is flecainide (Tambocor).

Class II. Class II drugs are beta-blocking agents. These drugs reduce adrenergic stimulation of the heart. An example is ***propranolol*** (Inderal).

> **CRITICAL THINKING**
> How might the signs of shock in a patient taking digoxin (Lanoxin) or propranolol (Inderal) vary from what might be expected normally?

Class III. Class III drugs produce potassium channel blockade. This increases the contractility. Unlike other antidysrhythmic agents, drugs in this class do not suppress automaticity. They also have no effect on conduction velocity. These drugs are thought to cease dysrhythmias that result from the reentry of blocked impulses. An example of such a drug is ***amiodarone*** (Cordarone).

Class IV. Class IV drugs are also known as *calcium channel blockers.* These drugs are thought to work by blocking the inflow of calcium through the cell membranes of the cardiac and smooth muscle cells. This action depresses the myocardial and smooth muscle contraction, decreases automaticity, and in some cases decreases conduction velocity. Examples of calcium channel blockers include ***verapamil*** (Isoptin) and ***diltiazem*** (Cardizem).

Antihypertensives

High blood pressure affects as many as 50 million adults and children in the United States[9] and has been related directly to an increased incidence of stroke, cerebral hemorrhage, heart and renal failure, and coronary heart disease. The exact mechanism of action of many antihypertensive drugs is unknown. The ideal antihypertensive drug should accomplish the following:

- Maintain blood pressure within normal limits for various body positions
- Maintain or improve blood flow without compromising tissue perfusion or blood supply to the brain
- Reduce the workload of the heart
- Have no undesirable side effects
- Permit long-term administration without intolerance

CLASSIFICATIONS

Certain drugs are used to reduce blood pressure in patients with chronic hypertension. These drugs usually are given in low-dose combinations and are titrated to effect. These drugs include diuretics, sympathetic blocking agents (sympatholytic drugs), vasodilators, angiotensin-converting enzyme (ACE) inhibitors, calcium channel blockers, and the newer class, angiotensin II receptor antagonists.[10]

Diuretics. Diuretics are the drugs of choice in managing hypertension. They often are used with other antihypertensive agents. Diuretics cause a loss of excess salt and water from the body by the kidneys. The decrease in plasma and extracellular fluid volume decreases preload and stroke volume. The decrease in fluid volume has a direct effect on size of the arterioles, resulting in lowered blood pressure. This response causes an initial decline of cardiac output. That is followed by a decrease in peripheral vascular resistance. These responses result in a lowering of the blood pressure.

Thiazides are diuretics that work well to lower blood pressure. Many antihypertensive agents cause retention of sodium and water. Yet thiazides may be given concomitantly to help prevent this side effect. An example of a thiazide diuretic is hydrochlorothiazide (HCTZ).

Loop diuretics are strong, short-acting agents. They inhibit sodium and chloride reabsorption in the loop of Henle. These drugs cause excessive loss of potassium. They also cause an increase in the excretion of sodium and water. Loop diuretics have fewer side effects than most other antihypertensives. However, hypokalemia and profound dehydration can be a result of their use. These agents are prescribed to patients who have renal insufficiency. They also may be given to patients who cannot take other diuretics. An example of a loop diuretic is ***furosemide*** (Lasix).

> **NOTE** Many drugs are excreted by the kidneys. Thus patients with renal system dysfunction (acute or chronic renal failure) may accumulate drugs in their systems. These patients often require modifications in drug doses and dosing intervals. These changes are in addition to diet modification and fluid restriction.

Potassium-sparing agents can be effective as an antihypertensive when they are used in combination with other diuretics. They promote sodium and water loss without a loss of potassium. These agents are used to treat hypertensive patients who become hypokalemic from other diuretics. They also can be used by patients who are apparently resistant to the antihypertensive effects of other diuretics. Potassium-sparing agents are also used to treat some edematous states. (An example of such is cirrhosis of the liver with ascites.) An example of a potassium-sparing agent is spironolactone (Aldactone).

Sympathetic blocking agents. Sympathetic blocking agents may be classified as beta-blocking agents and adrenergic-inhibiting agents. Beta-blocking agents are used to treat cardiovascular disorders, including patients with suspected myocardial infarction, high-risk unstable angina, and hypertension. These drugs work by decreasing cardiac output and inhibiting renin secretion from the kidneys. Both actions result in lower blood pressure. Beta-blocking drugs compete with epinephrine for available beta receptor sites as well. This inhibits tissue and organ response to beta stimulation. Examples of beta-blocking agents include the following:

- $Beta_1$-blocking agents (cardioselective)
  Acebutolol (Sectral)
  Atenolol (Tenormin)
  Metoprolol (Lopressor, Toprol-XL)
- $Beta_1$- and $beta_2$-blocking agents (nonselective)
  Labetalol (Normodyne, Trandate) (also has $alpha_1$-blocking properties)
  Nadolol (Corgard)
  Propranolol (Inderal)

Adrenergic-inhibiting agents work by modifying the actions of the sympathetic nervous system. They are effective antihypertensive drugs. Arterial pressure is influenced through various mechanisms of the heart, blood vessels, and kidneys. Sympathetic stimulation increases the heart rate and force of myocardial contraction, constricts arterioles and venules, and causes the release of renin from the kidneys. Blocking this sympathetic stimulation can reduce blood pressure.

Adrenergic-inhibiting agents are classified as centrally acting adrenergic inhibitors or peripheral adrenergic inhibitors. The mechanism by which many of these agents work is unknown. Generally, most of these agents are believed to have multiple sites of action. Examples include the following drugs:

- Centrally acting adrenergic inhibitors
  Clonidine hydrochloride (Catapres)
  Methyldopa (Aldomet)
  Prazosin hydrochloride (Minipress)
- Peripheral adrenergic inhibitors
  Doxazosin (Cardura)
  Guanethidine sulfate (Ismelin)
  Reserpine (Sandril, Serpasil)
  Phentolamine (Regitine)
  Phenoxybenzamine (Dibenzyline)
  Terazosin (Hytrin)

Vasodilator Drugs. Vasodilator drugs act directly on the smooth muscle walls of the arterioles, veins, or both. They lower peripheral resistance. Thus they lower blood pressure. This stimulates the sympathetic nervous system and also activates the baroreceptor reflexes. In turn this leads to an increase in heart rate, cardiac output, and renin release. Medications that inhibit the sympathetic response usually are given with vasodilator drugs.

In addition to their use as antihypertensives, some vasodilator drugs work to treat angina pectoris (ischemic chest pain). For example, nitrates dilate veins and arteries. Their dilating effects on veins lead to venous pooling of blood. They also reduce the amount of blood return to the heart. Thus these effects reduce left ventricular end-diastolic volume and pressure. The subsequent decrease in wall tension helps to reduce myocardial oxygen demand and also relieves the chest pain of myocardial ischemia. Vasodilator drugs are classified as arteriolar dilators and arteriolar and venous dilators. Examples of each include the following:

- Arteriolar dilator drugs
  Diazoxide (Hyperstat IV)
  Hydralazine (Apresoline)
  Minoxidil (Loniten)
- Arteriolar and venous dilator drugs
  Sodium nitroprusside (Nipride, Nitropress)
  Nitrates and nitrites
  Amyl nitrite inhalant
  Isosorbide dinitrate (Isordil, Sorbitrate)
  Nitroglycerin sublingual tablet (Nitrostat)
  Nitropaste (Nitro-Bid ointment, Nitrostat, Nitrol)
  Intravenous ***nitroglycerin*** (Tridil)

Angiotensin-converting Enzyme Inhibitor Drugs. As described in Chapter 7, the renin-angiotensin-aldosterone system plays a key role in maintaining blood pressure. This system also plays a key role in the sodium and fluid balance. A disturbance in this system can result in hypertension. In addition, kidney damage can result in an inability to regulate the release of renin through normal feedback mechanisms. This causes elevated blood pressure in some patients.

Angiotensin II is a strong vasoconstrictor that raises blood pressure. Angiotensin II also causes the release of aldosterone. Aldosterone contributes to sodium and water retention. By inhibiting conversion of the precursor angiotensin I to the active molecule angiotensin II (which is brought about through ACE), the renin-angiotensin-aldosterone system is suppressed and blood pressure is lowered. Examples of ACE inhibitors include captopril (Capoten), enalapril (Vasotec), benazepril (Lotensin), fosinopril (Monopril), lisinopril (Prinivil, Zestril), and quinapril (Accupril).

Calcium channel blockers. Calcium channel blocking agents such as ***verapamil*** (Isoptin), amlodipine (Norvasc), felodipine (Plendil), and ***diltiazem*** (Cardizem, Tiazac) reduce peripheral vascular resistance by inhibiting the contractility of vascular smooth muscle. They dilate coronary vessels through the same mechanism. The effects of these drugs are important in treating hypertension, decreasing the oxygen requirements of the heart (through decreased afterload), and increasing oxygen supply (by abolishing coronary artery spasm), thus relieving the causes of angina pectoris. The various drugs in this class differ in degree of selectivity for coronary (and peripheral) vasodilation or decreased cardiac contractility.

Angiotensin II Receptor Antagonists

Angiotensin II receptor antagonists are a new class of antihypertensive agent. They block the renin-angiotensin-aldosterone system more completely than ACE inhibitors. They lower blood pressure by selectively inhibiting the actions of angiotensin II receptors that include vasoconstriction, renal tubular sodium reabsorption, aldosterone release, and stimulation of central and peripheral sympathetic activity. These drugs are used to manage hypertension in those who cannot deal with the adverse effects of ACE inhibitors. (Some of these effects include cough and angioedema.) The drugs appear to be equally effective in lowering systolic and diastolic pressure. They also are being studied for their effectiveness in treating congestive heart failure, diabetic nephropathy, and vascular diseases such as atherosclerosis. Drugs in this classification include candesartan (Atacand), irbesartan (Avapro), losartan (Cozaar, Hyzaar), telmisartan (Micardis), and valsartan (Diovan).

Antihemorrheologic Agents

Antihemorrheologic agents are used to treat peripheral vascular disorders caused by pathological or physiological obstruction (e.g., arteriosclerosis). These drugs improve the blood flow (and the delivery of oxygen) to ischemic tissues. They do this by restoring red blood cell flexibility and lowering blood viscosity. An example of an antihemorrheologic agent is pentoxifylline (Trental).

SECTION FIVE
Drugs That Affect the Blood

ANTICOAGULANTS, FIBRINOLYTICS, AND BLOOD COMPONENTS

Bleeding and thrombosis are altered states of hemostasis. An understanding of the drugs that affect blood coagulation is crucial. An understanding of the use of fibrinolytic agents and blood components also is crucial. In the prehospital arena, these concepts will assist in the management of patients.

Anticoagulants

As described in Chapter 6, platelets are small cell fragments in the blood. They provide the initial step in normal repair of blood vessels. Blood coagulation is a process that results in the formation of a stable fibrin clot that entraps platelets, blood cells, and plasma. The end result of this process is called a blood clot or thrombus. Abnormal thrombus formation is the major cause of myocardial infarction (from coronary thrombosis) and stroke (from cerebral vascular thrombosis).

The coagulation process also occurs in the venous system, although the underlying mechanisms responsible for the thrombosis differ. Arterial thrombi commonly are associated with atherosclerotic plaques, hypertension, and turbulent blood flow that damages the endothelial lining of blood vessels. Damage to the endothelium causes platelets to stick and aggregate in the arterial system. Arterial thrombi are made up mostly of platelets, but they also involve the chemical substances that contribute to the coagulation process (in particular, fibrinogen and fibrin). Myocardial infarctions and strokes are often the result of arterial thrombi.

The three major risk factors for various thromboses are stasis, localized trauma, and hypercoagulable states. Stasis is reduced blood flow. Stasis results from immobilization or venous insufficiency. Stasis is responsible for the increased incidence of deep vein thrombosis in most bedridden patients. Localized trauma may initiate the clotting cascade and may cause arterial and venous thrombosis. Hypercoagulability of the blood is the cause of the increased incidence of deep vein thrombosis in women who take birth control pills. Hypercoagulability also is responsible for many of the familial thrombotic disorders (see Chapter 29).

AGENTS THAT AFFECT BLOOD COAGULATION

Drugs that affect blood coagulation may be classified as antiplatelet, anticoagulant, and fibrinolytic agents.

Antiplatelet Agents. Drugs that interfere with platelet aggregation are known as *antiplatelet* or *antithrombic* drugs. These drugs sometimes are prescribed as a prophylactic. They may be prescribed for patients at risk of developing arterial clots. They also are prescribed for those who have suffered myocardial infarction or stroke. Antiplatelet agents also are given to patients with certain valvular heart diseases, valvular prostheses, and various intracardiac shunts. Among the most common antiplatelet drugs are ***aspirin,*** dipyridamole (Persantine), clopidogrel (Plavix), ticlopidine (Ticlid), and abciximab (ReoPro).

Anticoagulant Agents. Anticoagulant drug therapy is used to prevent intravascular thrombosis. The therapy works by decreasing blood coagulability. Such therapy commonly is used to prevent postoperative thromboembolism. Anticoagulant agents also are used during hemodialysis and in reperfusion therapy for some patients with acute coronary syndromes. Anticoagulant therapy is a preventive measure against future clot formation. The therapy has no direct effect on a blood clot that has formed already or on ischemic tissue injured by inadequate blood supply as a result of a thrombus. The major side effect of anticoagulant therapy is hemorrhage and bleeding complications. Examples of anticoagulant agents include warfarin (Coumadin) and ***heparin*** (Liquaemin).

> **NOTE** Platelet adhesion, activation, and aggregation that result in the formation of an arterial thrombus are pivotal in the pathogenesis of acute coronary syndromes (acute myocardial infarctions). Recent studies indicate that the administration of a glycoprotein IIb/IIIa receptor antagonist may reduce ischemic complications after plaque fissure or rupture. (These drugs inhibit glycoprotein receptors in the membrane of platelets and help prevent platelet aggregation.) These drugs may be included along with aspirin, heparin, and beta-blockers during in-hospital reperfusion therapy for select patients. Examples of glycoprotein IIb/IIIa inhibitors include abciximab (ReoPro), eptifibatide (Integrilin), and tirofiban (Aggrastat).

Fibrinolytic Agents. Fibrinolytic drugs dissolve clots after their formation. They do so by promoting the digestion of fibrin. Fibrinolytic therapy has become the treatment of choice for treating acute myocardial infarction in certain groups of patients. Fibrinolytic therapy also has become the treatment of choice in managing some stroke patients. The goal is to reestablish blood flow and prevent ischemia and tissue death. Fibrinolytic therapy also has been used in acute pulmonary embolism, deep vein thrombosis, and peripheral arterial occlusion. Fibrinolytics are used in the prehospital setting in several areas of the United States. These drugs include ***streptokinase*** (Streptase), ***reteplase*** (Retavase), ***tissue plasminogen activator*** ([t-PA] Activase, recombinant Alteplase), anistreplase (APSAC, Eminase), and tenecteplase (TNKase) (see Chapter 29 and the Emergency Drug Index).

> **CRITICAL THINKING**
>
> Fibrinolytics have the potential to dissolve clots. This in turn may reverse the serious effects of myocardial infarction and stroke. So why are fibrinolytics not given to everyone who is suspected of having these conditions?

Antihemophilic Agents

Hemophilia (further described in Chapter 37) is a group of hereditary bleeding disorders. With these, a person lacks one of the factors needed for the coagulation of blood. These disorders are characterized by persistent and uncontrollable bleeding that can occur after even a minor injury. Bleeding may occur into joints, the urinary tract, and at times the CNS. Hemophilia A is the classic form of hemophilia and is caused by a deficiency of factor VIII. Hemophilia B is the Christmas disease and results from a deficiency in factor IX complex. Replacement therapy of the missing clotting factor can be effective in managing hemophilia. These include factor VIII (Factorate), factor IX (Konyne), and antiinhibitor coagulant complex (Autoplex).

> **NOTE** Coagulation factors refer to the 13 proteins contained in blood plasma. These proteins interact to produce a blood clot.

Hemostatic Agents

Hemostatic agents hasten clot formation. The formation of clots in turn reduces bleeding. Systemic hemostatic agents (e.g., Amicar and Cyklokapron) generally are used to control rapid blood loss after surgery by inhibiting fibrinolysis. Topical hemostatic agents (e.g., Gelfoam and Novacell) are used to control capillary bleeding during surgical and dental procedures.

Blood and Blood Components

The healthy body maintains a normal balance of blood and its components. However, illness and injury such as hemorrhage, burns, and dehydration may affect this balance. These conditions may impair this balance and require replacement therapy.

Knowledge of how to manage an imbalance of blood or blood components is crucial. The usual treatment of choice is to replace the sole blood component that is deficient. Replacement therapy may include transfusing the following:

- Whole blood (rarely used)
- Packed red blood cells
- Fresh-frozen plasma
- Plasma expanders (dextran)
- Platelets
- Coagulation factors
- Fibrinogen
- Albumin
- Gamma globulins

Antihyperlipidemic Drugs

Hyperlipidemia refers to an excess of lipids in the plasma. Several types of hyperlipidemia occur; all are associated with elevated levels of cholesterol and triglycerides. This condition is thought to play a role in the development of atherosclerosis. Thus antihyperlipidemic drugs sometimes are used along with diet and exercise to control serum lipid levels (Box 17-23). Antihyperlipidemic drugs do not reverse existing atherosclerosis.

BOX 17-23 Examples of Antihyperlipidemic Drugs

Atorvastatin (Lipitor)	Gemfibrozil (Lopid)
Fenofibrate (Tricor)	Pravastatin (Pravachol)
Fluvastatin (Lescol)	Simvastatin (Zocor)

SECTION SIX

Drugs That Affect the Respiratory System

REVIEW OF ANATOMY AND PHYSIOLOGY

The respiratory system includes all structures that are involved in the exchange of oxygen and carbon dioxide. Serious narrowing of any portion of the respiratory tract may be an indication for drug therapy (Box 17-24). Emergencies involving the respiratory system usually are caused by reversible conditions such as asthma, emphysema with infection, and foreign body airway obstruction (see Chapter 19).

Smooth muscle fibers line the tracheobronchial tree. They directly influence the diameter of the airways. The bronchial smooth muscle tone is maintained by impulses from the autonomic nervous system. Parasympathetic fibers from the vagus nerve stimulate bronchial smooth muscle through the release of acetylcholine. This neurotransmitter interacts with the muscarinic receptors on the membranes of the cell, producing bronchoconstriction.

Sympathetic fibers mainly affect beta$_2$ receptors in the lungs through the release of epinephrine from the adrenal medulla and the release of norepinephrine from the peripheral sympathetic nerves. The epinephrine reaches the lungs by way of the circulatory system. Epinephrine interacts with beta$_2$ receptors to produce smooth muscle relaxation and bronchodilation. Thus the beta$_2$ receptor plays the dominant role in bronchial muscle tone. (Although beta$_1$ receptors also are found on bronchial smooth muscle, their ratio to beta$_2$ receptors is 1:3.)

BOX 17-24 Emergency Drugs: Respiratory System

Albuterol (Proventil, Ventolin)	Epinephrine (Adrenalin) 1:1000
Dexamethasone (Decadron)	Racemic epinephrine (microNephrin)
Diphenhydramine (Benadryl)	

Bronchodilators

Bronchodilator drugs are the primary treatment for obstructive pulmonary disease such as asthma, chronic bronchitis, and emphysema. These drugs are classified as sympathomimetic drugs or xanthine derivatives. Many of these drugs are administered by inhalation via a nebulizer or pressure cartridge (see Chapter 30).

SYMPATHOMIMETIC DRUGS

Sympathomimetic drugs are grouped according to their effects on receptors. Nonselective adrenergic drugs have alpha, beta$_1$ (cardiac), and beta$_2$ (respiratory) activity. Nonselective beta adrenergic drugs have beta$_1$ and beta$_2$ effects. Selective beta$_2$ receptor drugs act primarily on beta$_2$ receptors in the lungs (bronchial smooth muscle). Box 17-25 summarizes the alpha, beta$_1$, and beta$_2$ activities of the adrenergic drugs used as bronchodilators.

Nonselective adrenergic drugs stimulate alpha and beta receptors. The alpha activity lessens vasoconstriction to reduce mucosal edema. Beta$_2$ activity produces bronchodilation and vasodilation. Undesirable beta$_1$ effects include an increase in heart rate and force of contraction.

BOX 17-25 Alpha, Beta$_1$, and Beta$_2$ Activities of Adrenergic Drugs Used as Bronchodilators

Alpha Effects (Vasoconstriction)

Systemic effects
Vasoconstriction
Increased blood pressure
Inhalation
Decreased bronchial congestion
Increased duration of action for coadministered beta$_2$ drugs

Beta$_1$ Effects

Systemic effects
Cardiac stimulation
Increased heart rate
Increased force of contraction
Possible palpitations and dysrhythmias
Relaxation of gastrointestinal tract
Inhalation
Some bronchodilation and increased heart rate
Fewer effects than with subcutaneous administration

Beta$_2$ Effects

Systemic effects
Bronchiole dilation
Stimulation of skeletal muscles (tremors)
Vasodilation (mainly in blood vessels supplying muscle)
Glycogenolysis

Central Nervous System Effects

Anxiety
Dizziness
Inhalation
Insomnia
Irritability
Nervousness
Sweating
Lower incidence of systemic effects than with subcutaneous administration

Undesirable $beta_2$ effects include muscle tremors and CNS stimulation. Examples of nonselective adrenergic drugs include epinephrine inhalation aerosol (Bronkaid Mist, Primatene Mist), epinephrine inhalation solution (Adrenalin), and ***racemic epinephrine*** inhalation solution (microNephrin).

Nonselective beta adrenergic drugs are not selective for $beta_2$ receptors. Thus they have a wide range of effects (described before). Examples of nonselective beta adrenergic drugs include ***epinephrine*** (Adrenalin, Asmolin, and others), ephedrine (Ephed II), and ethylnorepinephrine (Bronkephrine), which each have some alpha activity; isoproterenol inhalation solution (Aerolone, Vapo-Iso, Isuprel); and isoproterenol inhalation aerosol (Isuprel Mistometer, Norisodrine Aerotrol).

The action of $beta_2$ selective drugs lessens the incidence of unwanted cardiac effects caused by $beta_1$ adrenergic agents. Patients with hypertension, cardiac disease, or diabetes can better tolerate this group of bronchodilators. Examples of selective $beta_2$ receptor drugs include ***albuterol*** (Proventil, Ventolin), Levalbuterol (Xopenex) bitolterol (Tornalate), salmeterol (Serevent), and isoetharine (Bronkosol, others).

XANTHINE DERIVATIVES

The xanthine group of drugs includes caffeine, theophylline, and theobromine. These drugs relax smooth muscle (particularly bronchial smooth muscle), stimulate cardiac muscle and the CNS, increase diaphragmatic contractility, and promote diuresis through increased renal perfusion. The action of various theophylline compounds depends on the concentration of theophylline, which is the active ingredient. Theophylline products vary in their rate of absorption and therapeutic effects. Aminophylline (Amoline, Somophyllin, Theo-Dur, Aminophyllin), dyphylline (Dilor, Droxine, Lufyllin), and theophylline (Bronkodyl, Elixophyllin, Somophyllin-T, others) are some of the many theophylline-containing preparations. Theophylline preparations generally are not considered a first-line drug in the treatment of acute reactive airway disease such as asthma.

Other Respiratory Drugs

A number of other drugs can be used to treat asthma and other obstructive pulmonary diseases. These drugs include prophylactic asthmatic agents such as cromolyn sodium (Intal, sodium cromoglycate); aerosol corticosteroid agents such as beclomethasone dipropionate (Vanceril inhaler, Beclovent); ***dexamethasone*** (Decadron); antileukotrienes such as montelukast (Singulair) and zafirlukast (Accolate); and muscarinic antagonists (anticholinergics) such as ***ipratropium*** (Atrovent) and glycopyrrolate (Robinul). These drugs reduce the allergic or inflammatory response to a variety of stimuli. They also have an effect on bronchial smooth muscle. In the acute care setting, intravenously administered steroids (e.g., ***methylprednisolone*** [Solu-Medrol]) may be given in an attempt to decrease the inflammatory response and improve airflow.

Mucokinetic Drugs

Mucokinetic drugs are used to move respiratory secretions, excessive mucus, and sputum along the tracheobronchial tree. These agents work by altering the consistency of these secretions. Thus the secretions can be removed from the body more easily. Persons with chronic pulmonary disease often use mucokinetic drugs. These drugs help to clear their respiratory passages. They also improve ciliary activity in the airways.

Mucokinetic drugs include diluents (water, saline solution), aerosols, and mucolytic drugs or expectorants (Mucomyst).

> **NOTE** Mucus is a normal secretion produced by the surface cells in the mucous membranes. Sputum is an abnormal viscous secretion. Sputum consists mainly of mucus. Sputum originates in the lower respiratory tract.

Oxygen and Miscellaneous Respiratory Agents

Oxygen is mainly used to treat hypoxia and hypoxemia. Oxygen is a colorless, odorless, and tasteless gas. It is essential for sustaining life. (Oxygen and oxygen delivery are described in detail in Chapter 19.)

DIRECT RESPIRATORY STIMULANTS

Direct respiratory stimulants are known as analeptics. These act directly on the medullary center of the brain. They act to increase the rate and depth of respirations. These drugs are considered inferior to mechanical ventilatory measures to treat respiratory depression and to counteract drug-induced respiratory depression caused by anesthetics. An example of a direct respiratory stimulant is doxapram (Dopram).

REFLEX RESPIRATORY STIMULANTS

Spirits of ammonia is given by inhalation and acts as a reflex respiratory stimulant. The noxious vapor is used sometimes in cases of fainting. The vapor works by irritating sensory nerve receptors in the throat and stomach. These nerve receptors send afferent messages to the control centers of the brain to stimulate respiration.

RESPIRATORY DEPRESSANTS

Respiratory depressants include opiates and barbiturate drugs previously described. Respiratory depression is a common side effect of these drugs. However, they seldom are given to inhibit rate and depth of respiration intentionally.

COUGH SUPPRESSANTS

The cough is a protective reflex to expel harmful irritants. The cough may be productive when removing irritants or secretions from the airway. The cough also may be nonproductive (dry and irritating). The cough may be prolonged. The cough also can result from an underlying disorder.

BOX 17-26 Examples of Narcotic and Nonnarcotic Antitussive Agents

Narcotic Agent
Codeine

Nonnarcotic Agents
Benzonatate (Tessalon)
Dextromethorphan (Sucrets, Robitussin DM)

Thus treatment with antitussive drugs may be indicated. Box 17-26 presents a few narcotic and nonnarcotic antitussive agents.

ANTIHISTAMINES

Histamine is a chemical mediator found in almost all body tissues. The concentration is highest in the skin, lungs, and gastrointestinal tract. The body releases histamine when exposed to an antigen, such as pollen or insect stings. This results in increased localized blood flow, increased capillary permeability, and swelling of the tissues. In addition, histamine produces contractile action on bronchial smooth muscle.

Allergic responses involving histamines and other chemical mediators include local effects such as angioedema, eczema, rhinitis, urticaria, and asthma. Systemic effects from the release of histamine and certain other mediators may result in anaphylaxis (see Chapter 33).

Antihistamines compete with histamine for receptor sites. Thus they prevent the physiological action of histamine. Two types of histamine receptors are H_1 receptors (these act mainly on the blood vessels and the bronchioles) and H_2 receptors (these act mainly on the gastrointestinal tract). In addition to blocking some actions of histamine, antihistamines also have anticholinergic or atropine-like action. This may result in tachycardia, constipation, drowsiness, sedation, and inhibition of secretions. Most antihistamines have a local anesthetic effect as well. This effect may soothe the skin irritation caused by an allergic reaction. The chief clinical use of antihistamines is for allergic reactions. However, they also sometimes are prescribed to control motion sickness or as a sedative or antiemetic. Examples of antihistamines are dimenhydrinate (Dramamine), ***diphenhydramine*** (Benadryl), ***hydroxyzine*** (Vistaril), ***promethazine*** (Phenergan, others), and the newer H_1 receptor antagonists, loratadine (Claritin), cetirizine (Zyrtec), and fexofenadine (Allegra).

SEROTONIN

Serotonin is a naturally occurring vasoconstrictor material. Serotonin is found in platelets and in the cells of the brain and intestine. Serotonin has several pharmacological actions, which are exerted on various smooth muscles and nerves. Serotonin is not administered as a drug. However, serotonin has a major influence on other drugs and some disease states. Serotonin is helpful in repairing damaged blood vessels, stimulates smooth muscle contraction, and acts as a neurotransmitter in the CNS, where it has an effect on sleep, pain perception, and some mental illnesses.

ANTISEROTONINS

Antiserotonins are serotonin antagonists. They work to inhibit responses to serotonin and its influence on other drugs and disease states. Specific antiserotonins block smooth muscle contraction and vasoconstriction and inhibit the action of serotonin in the brain. Some antiserotonins are used to treat vascular headaches and allergic disorders. Examples of these drugs include cyproheptadine (Periactin), lysergic acid diethylamide (LSD), and methysergide maleate (Sansert).

SECTION SEVEN
Drugs That Affect the Gastrointestinal System

REVIEW OF ANATOMY AND PHYSIOLOGY

The gastrointestinal system is composed of the digestive tract, the biliary system, and the pancreas (see Chapter 6). The primary function of the gastrointestinal system is to provide the body with water, electrolytes, and other nutrients used by cells. Drug therapy for the gastrointestinal system can be divided into two groups: drugs that affect the stomach and drugs that affect the lower gastrointestinal tract. In emergency care, conditions of the stomach or gastrointestinal tract that may require drug therapy usually are limited to nausea and vomiting (Box 17-27.)

Drugs That Affect the Stomach

Conditions of the stomach that may require drug therapy include hyperacidity, hypoacidity, ulcer disease, nausea, vomiting, and hypermotility.

ANTACIDS

Antacids buffer or neutralize hydrochloric acid in the stomach. They are prescribed for the relief of symptoms associated with hyperacidity. These conditions include peptic ulcer, gastritis, esophagitis, heartburn, and hiatal hernia. Common over-the-counter antacids include Alka-Seltzer, Gaviscon, and Rolaids.

ANTIFLATULENTS

Antiflatulents prevent the formation of gas in the gastrointestinal tract. Gas retention is a common condition with diverticulitis, ulcer disease, and spastic or irritable colon. These drugs sometimes are used along with antacids. Simethicone (Mylicon) is an example of an antiflatulent.

BOX 17-27 Emergency Drugs: Gastrointestinal System

Activated charcoal	Prochlorperazine (Compazine)
Diphenhydramine (Benadryl)	Promethazine (Phenergan)
Hydroxyzine (Vistaril)	Syrup of ipecac

DIGESTANTS

Digestant drugs promote digestion in the gastrointestinal tract. They work by releasing small amounts of digestive enzymes in the small intestine. Examples of digestants include pancreatin (Creon) and pancrelipase (Pancrease).

EMETICS AND ANTIEMETICS

Vomiting is an action that is involuntary. Vomiting is coordinated by the emetic center of the medulla. Vomiting may be initiated through the CNS as a secondary reaction to emotion, pain, or disequilibrium (motion sickness); through irritation of the mucosa of the gastrointestinal tract or bowel; or through stimulation from the chemoreceptor trigger zone of the medulla by circulating drugs and toxins (e.g., opiates or digitalis).

Emetics. Emetics induce vomiting. They rarely are administered today as part of the treatment for drug overdoses and poisonings. These drugs include apomorphine and ***syrup of ipecac.*** The treatment of drug overdoses and poisoning is addressed further in Chapter 36.

Antiemetics. Drugs used to treat nausea and vomiting include antagonists of histamine, acetylcholine, and dopamine and other drugs the actions of which are not understood clearly. These drugs work best when they are given before rather than after nausea and vomiting have begun. For example, drugs used to treat motion sickness or vertigo should be taken 30 minutes before traveling. Common antiemetics include scopolamine (Transderm-Scōp), dimenhydrinate (Dramamine), ***diphenhydramine*** (Benadryl), ***hydroxyzine*** (Vistaril), meclizine (Antivert), ***promethazine*** (Phenergan), prochlorperazine (Compazine), and ondansetron (Zofran).

> **NOTE** Cannabinoids are drugs that are derived from hemp plants. They have been used experimentally to prevent vomiting in patients who receive cancer chemotherapy. Examples of these drugs include dronabinol (Marinol) and nabilone (Cesamet). These drugs use a synthetic derivative of the active ingredient in marijuana.

CYTOPROTECTIVE AGENTS

Cytoprotective agents are drugs that protect cells from damage. They are used along with other drugs to treat peptic ulcer disease by protecting the gastric mucosa. Examples of these drugs include sucralfate (Carafate) and misoprostol (Cytotec).

H_2 RECEPTOR ANTAGONISTS

As described before, the action of histamine is mediated through H_2 receptors. Histamine has been associated with gastric acid secretion. H_2 receptor antagonists block the H_2 receptors. They reduce the volume of gastric acid secretion and its acid content. Examples of H_2 receptor antagonists include cimetidine (Tagamet), ranitidine (Zantac), and famotidine (Pepcid).

PROTON PUMP INHIBITORS

Proton pump inhibitors are used to treat symptomatic gastroesophageal reflux disease, short-term treatment of erosive esophagitis, and maintenance of erosive esophagitis healing. Some agents also are approved for use with antibiotics to treat *Helicobacter pylori* infection (associated with duodenal ulcers). The proton pump (potassium adenosine triphosphate enzyme system) is the final pathway for secretion of hydrochloric acid by the parietal cells of the stomach. Proton pump inhibitors decrease hydrochloric acid secretion by inhibiting the actions of the parietal cells. In addition, the gastric pH of the stomach is altered. Examples of proton pump inhibitors include esomeprazole (Nexium), lansoprazole (Prevacid), omeprazole (Prilosec), pantoprazole (Protonix), and rabeprazole (AcipHex).

Drugs That Affect the Lower Gastrointestinal Tract

Constipation and diarrhea are two common conditions of the lower gastrointestinal tract. Both conditions may require drug therapy. Drugs used to manage these conditions include laxatives and antidiarrheals.

LAXATIVES

Laxatives produce defecation. They are used to evacuate the bowel and to soften hardened stool for easier passage. Situations that may indicate the need for laxative use include the following:

- Constipation
- Neurological diseases (e.g., multiple sclerosis or Parkinson's disease)
- Pregnancy
- Rectal disorders
- Drug poisoning
- Surgery and endoscopic examination

Numerous types of laxatives are available. Many can be bought without a prescription. Examples include saline laxatives (Epsom salt, Milk of Magnesia), stimulant laxatives (Dulcolax, castor oil, Ex-Lax), bulk-forming laxatives (Mitrolan, Metamucil), lubricant laxatives (mineral oil), fecal moistening agents (Colace, glycerin suppositories), and those used for bowel evacuation (GoLYTELY, Chronulac). Regular or excessive use of laxatives is common in older adults and in those with eating disorders. Laxative abuse may result in permanent bowel damage and electrolyte imbalance.

ANTIDIARRHEAL DRUGS

Antidiarrheal drugs are used to reduce an abnormal frequency of bowel evacuation. Common causes of acute and chronic diarrhea include bacterial or viral invasion, drugs, diet, and numerous disease states (e.g., diabetes insipidus and inflammatory bowel syndromes). Drugs used to treat diarrhea include the following:

- Adsorbents
  Bismuth subsalicylate (Pepto-Bismol)
- Anticholinergics
  Donnatal
- Opiates
  Paregoric
  Codeine
- Other agents
  Diphenoxylate (Lomotil)
  Loperamide (Imodium)

SECTION EIGHT
Drugs That Affect the Eye and Ear

TREATMENT OF EYE DISORDERS

Drugs That Affect the Eye

Drugs used to treat eye disorders include antiglaucoma agents, mydriatics and cycloplegics, antiinfective/antiinflammatory agents, and topical anesthetics.

ANTIGLAUCOMA AGENTS

Glaucoma is an eye disease. In this disease the pressure of the fluid in the eye is abnormally high. The pressure is so high that it causes compression or obstruction of the small internal blood vessels of the eye, the fibers of the optic nerve, or both. The result is nerve fiber destruction and partial or complete loss of vision. Glaucoma is a common eye disorder in persons over age 60 and is responsible for 15% of blindness in adults in the United States.[11] Agents used to reduce the pressure in chronic glaucoma include cholinergic and anticholinesterase drugs. Some of these drugs (e.g., pilocarpine) dilate the pupil of the eye, and some constrict the pupil; others (e.g., acetazolamide) slow the secretion of aqueous fluid. If these drug therapies fail, surgery may be indicated. If glaucoma is diagnosed early, drugs can control it for a lifetime. Most physicians recommend testing for glaucoma every 2 years after age 35.

MYDRIATIC AND CYCLOPLEGIC AGENTS

Mydriatic and cycloplegic agents are applied topically. They cause dilation of the pupils and paralysis of accommodation to light. They are used to treat inflammation. They also are used to relieve ocular pain by putting the eye to rest. These drugs are used during routine eye examinations and in ocular surgery as well. Examples of these drugs include atropine ophthalmic solution, cyclopentolate hydrochloride ophthalmic solution (Cyclogyl), homatropine ophthalmic solution (Isopto Homatropine), epinephrine, and oxymetazoline (OcuClear).

> **CRITICAL THINKING**
>
> You are caring for an older adult patient. This patient had mydriatic eye drops instilled by an ophthalmologist. If you did not know this history, what might you consider after your physical examination of this patient?

ANTIINFECTIVE/ANTIINFLAMMATORY AGENTS

Antiinfective and antiinflammatory agents are used to treat eye conditions such as conjunctivitis, sty, and keratitis (corneal inflammation caused by bacterial infection). Examples of these drugs include bacitracin (Baciquent), chloramphenicol (Chloroptic), erythromycin (Ilotycin), and natamycin (Natacyn).

TOPICAL ANESTHETIC AGENTS

Local anesthetics are used to prevent pain in surgical procedures and eye examinations. They also are used in the treatment of some eye injuries (e.g., a corneal abrasion). These drugs usually have a rapid onset (within 20 seconds) and last 15 to 20 minutes. Examples of these drugs include proparacaine (Ophthaine) and ***tetracaine*** (Pontocaine). Other eye medications include artificial tear solutions and lubricants to provide additional moisture, irrigation solutions, and antiallergic agents to relieve symptoms of itching, tearing, and redness. Many of these drugs and solutions are available without a prescription.

Drugs That Affect the Ear

Drugs used to treat disorders of the external ear canal include antibiotics, steroid/antibiotic combinations, and miscellaneous preparations. These drugs include the following:

- Antibiotics used to treat infections
  Chloramphenicol (Chloromycetin Otic)
  Gentamicin sulfate (Garamycin)
- Steroid/antibiotic combinations used to treat superficial bacterial infections
  Neomycin sulfate/polymyxin B sulfate/hydrocortisone (Cortisporin Otic)
  Neomycin/colistin/hydrocortisone (Coly-Mycin S Otic)
- Miscellaneous preparations used to treat ear wax accumulation, inflammation, pain, fungal infections, and other minor conditions
  Boric acid in isopropyl alcohol (Aurocaine 2)
  Triethanolamine with chlorobutanol in propylene glycol (Cerumenex)

Persons with inner ear infections or serious illness associated with hearing impairment may require antibiotics with systemic effect. Naturally, they will also require a thorough evaluation by a doctor. These actions will help to prevent complications.

SECTION NINE
Drugs That Affect the Endocrine System

REVIEW OF ANATOMY AND PHYSIOLOGY

The endocrine system works to control and integrate body functions. (Box 17-28 presents emergency drugs that affect the endocrine system.) Information from various parts of the body is carried via blood-borne hormones to distant sites. Hormones are natural chemical substances. They act after they have been secreted into the bloodstream from endocrine glands (ductless glands that secrete internally). These glands include the anterior and posterior pituitary, thyroid, parathyroid, and adrenal glands and the thymus, pancreas, testes, and ovaries. Hormones from the various endocrine glands work together to regulate vital processes, including the following:

- Secretory and motor activities of the digestive tract
- Energy production
- Composition and volume of extracellular fluid
- Adaptation (e.g., acclimatization and immunity)
- Growth and development
- Reproduction and lactation

Drugs That Affect the Pituitary Gland

The hormones of the anterior and posterior pituitary gland are important for regulating the secretion of other hormones in the body (see Chapter 6). Box 17-29 lists drugs that affect the anterior and posterior pituitary. (Disorders of the endocrine glands are described further in Chapter 32.)

Drugs That Affect the Thyroid and Parathyroid Glands

The thyroid hormone controls the rate of metabolic processes. Thyroid hormone is required for normal growth and development. Parathyroid hormone regulates the level of ionized calcium in the blood. Parathyroid hormone does this through the release of calcium from bone, the absorption of calcium from the intestine, and controlling the rate of calcium excretion by the kidneys.

Disorders of the thyroid gland include goiter (enlargement of the thyroid gland), hypothyroidism (thyroid hormone deficiency), and hyperthyroidism (thyroid hormone excess). Disorders of the parathyroid include hypoparathyroidism and hyperparathyroidism. Box 17-30 lists the drugs used to treat these disorders.

Drugs That Affect the Adrenal Cortex

The adrenal cortex secretes three major classes of steroid hormones: glucocorticoids (cortisol), mineralocorticoids (primarily aldosterone), and sex hormones. Glucocorticoids raise blood glucose, deplete tissue proteins, and suppress the inflammatory reaction. Mineralocorticoids regulate electrolyte and water balance. Sex hormones are estrogen, progesterone, and testosterone and are produced in small amounts by men and women. The sex hormones have little physiological effect under normal circumstances. Box 17-31 lists drugs that affect the adrenal cortex. Two disorders of the adrenal cortex are Addison's disease (adrenal cortical hypofunction) and Cushing's disease (adrenal cortical hyperfunction) (see Chapter 32).

BOX 17-28 Emergency Drugs: Endocrine System

Dexamethasone (Decadron)	Methylprednisolone (Solu-Medrol)
Dextrose 50%	Oxytocin (Pitocin, Syntocinon)
Glucagon	
Insulin	

BOX 17-29 Drugs That Affect the Anterior and Posterior Pituitary Gland

Anterior Pituitary Gland Drugs

Used to treat growth failure in children caused by growth hormone deficiency:
Somatrem (Protropin)
Somatropin (Humatrope)

Posterior Pituitary Gland Drugs

Used to treat the symptoms of diabetes insipidus resulting from antidiuretic hormone deficiency:
Vasopressin (Pitressin)

BOX 17-30 Drugs That Affect the Thyroid and Parathyroid Glands

Thyroid Drugs

Used to treat hypothyroidism and to prevent goiters:
Thyroid
Iodine products
Levothyroxine (Synthroid, Levoxyl)

Parathyroid Drugs

Used to treat hyperparathyroidism:
Vitamin D
Calcium supplements

BOX 17-31 Drugs That Affect The Adrenal Cortex

Glucocorticoids
Betamethasone (Celestone)
Dexamethasone (Decadron)
Methylprednisolone (Solu-Medrol)
Triamcinolone (Aristocort)

Mineralocorticoids
Desoxycorticosterone acetate (Doca)
Fludrocortisone (Florinef)

Adrenal Steroid Inhibitors
Aminoglutethimide (Cytadren)
Metyrapone (Metopirone)

BOX 17-32 Drugs That Affect the Pancreas

Insulin Preparations
Rapid acting
Humulin 70/30 (NPH/regular)
Regular insulin
Lispro
Semilente

Intermediate acting
Lente insulin
NPH insulin

Long acting
Ultralente
PZI

Oral Hypoglycemic Agents
Glimepiride (Amaryl)
Glipizide (Glucotrol)
Glyburide (Micronase)
Metformin (Glucophage)
Thiazolidinedione (Actos)

Hyperglycemic Agents
Dextrose
Diazoxide (Proglycem)
Glucagon
Oral glucose (Glutose, Insta-Glucose)

Drugs That Affect the Pancreas

The pancreas is an exocrine gland (providing digestive juices to the small intestine). However, the pancreas also is an endocrine gland. The endocrine portion of the pancreas consists of pancreatic islets (islets of Langerhans). These cells produce the hormones that enter the circulatory system.

Hormones of the Pancreas

The pancreatic hormones play a key role. They help to regulate the concentration of certain nutrients in the circulatory system. The pancreas secretes two major hormones: insulin and glucagon.

Insulin is the primary hormone that regulates glucose metabolism. In general, insulin increases the ability of the liver, adipose tissue, and muscle to take up and use glucose. Glucose not immediately needed for energy is stored in the skeletal muscle, liver, and other tissues. This stored form of glucose is called glycogen.

Glucagon mainly influences the liver. Yet glucagon has some effect on skeletal muscle and adipose tissue. In general, glucagon stimulates the liver to break down glycogen. Thus glucose is released into the blood. Glucagon also inhibits the uptake of glucose by muscle and fat cells. The balancing action of these two hormones protects the body from hyperglycemia and hypoglycemia.

This balance of hormonal actions is important when one considers the metabolic problems that can occur in diabetes mellitus. The relationship of glucagon and insulin to other hormones and substances such as ***dextrose 50%*** (D50) and ***thiamine*** (vitamin B_1) is addressed in Chapter 32. Box 17-32 lists drugs that affect the pancreas.

SECTION TEN
Drugs That Affect the Reproductive System

TREATMENT OF DISORDERS OF THE REPRODUCTIVE SYSTEM

Drugs That Affect the Female Reproductive System

Drugs that affect the female reproductive system include synthetic and natural substances such as hormones, oral contraceptives, ovulatory stimulants, and drugs used to treat infertility.

FEMALE SEX HORMONES

Two main types of hormones are secreted by the ovary: estrogen and progesterone. Supplemental estrogen is indicated for estrogen deficiency or replacement, treatment of breast cancer, and as prophylaxis for osteoporosis in postmenopausal women (controversial). Progesterone (and synthetic progestins) may be used to treat hormonal imbalance, endometriosis, and specific cancers and to prevent pregnancy when used properly.

ORAL CONTRACEPTIVES

Oral contraception is the most effective form of birth control and is known as "the pill." Oral contraception is a combination of estrogen and progesterone. This combination results in the suppression of ovulation (see Chapter 41). Several types of oral contraceptives and drug combinations are available. All are nearly 100% effective in preventing pregnancy.

OVULATORY STIMULANTS AND INFERTILITY DRUGS

The absence of ovulation in women is anovulation. The condition may be pathological in women with abnormal bleeding or infertility. The condition sometimes is treated with gonadotropins, thyroid preparations, estrogen, and synthetic agents. One example of a drug used to induce ovulation and increase fertility is clomiphene citrate (Clomid).

▶**NOTE** Certain drugs are used during labor and delivery. These drugs help to increase or decrease uterine contractility. Some of these drugs include oxytocin (Pitocin) and ritodrine (Yutopar), respectively. In prehospital care, oxytocin is used to control hemorrhages that occur after the delivery of the infant and placenta (see Chapter 42).

Drugs That Affect the Male Reproductive System

The male sex hormone is testosterone. Adequate amounts of this hormone are needed for normal development and for the maintenance of male sex characteristics.

Testosterone therapy is indicated for the treatment of hormone deficiency (e.g., testicular failure), impotence, delayed puberty, female breast cancer, and anemia. The choice of dosage and length of therapy depend on the diagnosis, age of the patient, and intensity of side effects/adverse reactions. An example of an oral testosterone drug is methyltestosterone (Metandren).

▶**NOTE** Impotence is the inability of a man to achieve or maintain an erection. This can lead to decreased sexual function. The condition afflicts as many as 20 million Americans on a continuing basis.[12]

Drugs That Affect Sexual Behavior

Sexual drive (libido) can be affected by psychological, social, and physiological factors or by a combination of these. Negative effects of these factors can result in a lack of interest in sexual activity in men and women and impotence in men.

DRUGS THAT IMPAIR LIBIDO AND SEXUAL GRATIFICATION

Some drugs interfere with sympathetic nervous stimulation. At times they may cause sexual dysfunction. Drugs may interfere with the nervous system mechanisms (directly and indirectly) that are responsible for sexual arousal. Some of these drugs include antihypertensives, antihistamines, antispasmodics, sedatives and tranquilizers, antidepressants, alcohol, and barbiturates.

DRUGS THAT ENHANCE LIBIDO AND SEXUAL GRATIFICATION

A patient may change medicines to avoid drug-induced sexual dysfunction. (The patient should do this under a doctor's supervision.) In addition, a patient may be prescribed drugs to enhance libido and sexual gratification. Drugs that enhance sexual function include levodopa (L-Dopa), tadalafil (Cialis), vardenifil (Levitra), and sildenafil citrate (Viagra).

▶**NOTE** The administration of nitroglycerin (Nitrostat) or nitrate/nitrite medications is contraindicated in patients who have taken Cialis, Levitra, and Viagra within the previous 24 to 48 hours because the combination can cause a lethal drop in blood pressure. Other drugs that may produce untoward effects in patients taking drugs to enhance sexual gratification include some antibiotics, cimetidine, and some blood pressure-lowering medications.[13] The paramedic should question the patient about the use of sexual enhancement drugs. The paramedic must do this before administering any of these medications.

SECTION ELEVEN
Drugs Used in Neoplastic Diseases

ANTINEOPLASTIC AGENTS

Antineoplastic agents are used in cancer chemotherapy. They are used to prevent the increase of malignant cells (Box 17-33). These drugs do not directly kill tumor cells. Rather they interfere with cell reproduction or replication through various mechanisms.

▶**NOTE** Any person who handles antineoplastic agents should be trained properly in the safety procedures. These drugs are considered cytotoxic. (They are toxic to human cells.)

Antineoplastic agents are nonselective. They are injurious to all cells in the body. Side effects from these drugs may include infection, hemorrhage, nausea and vomiting, and changes in bowel habits. Short-term toxicity from these agents may affect the pulmonary, cardiovascular, renal, and integumentary systems. Prehospital care for these patients mainly is supportive and is aimed at providing comfort measures and emotional support.

BOX 17-33 Examples of Antineoplastic Agents

Doxorubicin (Adriamycin)	Methotrexate (Amethopterin)
Fluorouracil (Adrucil)	Streptozocin (Zanosar)
Mechlorethamine (Mustargen)	

SECTION TWELVE

Drugs Used in Infectious Disease and Inflammation

TREATMENT OF INFECTIOUS DISEASE AND INFLAMMATION

Antibiotics

Antibiotics are used to treat local or systemic infection. Antibiotics kill or suppress the growth of microorganisms. They do this by disrupting the bacterial cell wall, by disturbing the functions of the cell membrane, or by interfering with the metabolic functions of the cell. This group of drugs includes penicillins, cephalosporins, and related products; macrolide antibiotics; tetracyclines; fluoroquinolones; and miscellaneous antibiotic agents (e.g., metronidazole [Flagyl] and spectinomycin [Trobicin]). Antibiotics are much more toxic to bacteria than they are to a patient. Some antibiotics, though, may produce hypersensitivity. This can lead to a fatal reaction if the drug later is given to a sensitized patient.

NOTE In time, some bacteria that are at first sensitive to antibiotics may become resistant to them. The bacteria develop ways to evade the effect of a drug. Widespread use and misuse of antibiotics leads to the development of resistant strains of bacteria. Bacterial resistance may even complicate treatment when a person is infected with an antibiotic-resistant organism.

PENICILLINS

Penicillins are active against gram-positive and some gram-negative bacteria (Box 17-34). Penicillins are used to treat many infections, including tonsillitis, pharyngitis, bronchitis, and pneumonia. Examples of penicillins include amoxicillin (Amoxil), ampicillin (Amcill), dicloxacillin (Dynapen), and penicillin V potassium (Pen-Vee K). Penicillin can produce severe anaphylactic reactions.

CEPHALOSPORINS

Cephalosporins (and related products) resemble penicillins. Yet they are active against gram-positive and gram-negative bacteria. Cephalosporins are used widely to treat ear, throat, and respiratory infections. They also are useful for treating urinary tract infections. Urinary tract infections often are caused by bacteria that are resistant to penicillin-type antibiotics. Examples of cephalosporins and related products include cefazolin (Ancef), cephalothin (Keflin), cephalexin (Keflex), and cefotaxime (Claforan). About 6% to 10% of those who are allergic to penicillins are also allergic to cephalosporins.

BOX 17-34 Gram's Stain

Gram's stain is an iodine-based stain used to differentiate various types of bacteria. Basically, a specimen is stained with gentian violet. This is followed by Gram's solution. Then the specimen is treated with a decolorizing agent such as acetone. The specimen then is counterstained with a red dye (safranin). Specimens that retain the dark violet stain are known as gram-positive; those that lose the violet stain after decolorization but take up the counterstain (causing them to appear pink) are gram-negative. Examples of gram-positive bacteria are staphylococci, streptococci, and pneumococci. Examples of gram-negative bacteria are gonococci and meningococci.

MACROLIDE ANTIBIOTICS

Macrolides (erythromycins) are used to treat infections of the skin, chest, throat, and ears. Macrolides are useful for treating pertussis (whooping cough) and legionnaires' disease. Examples of erythromycin drugs include Eryc, E-Mycin, E.E.S, and Erythrocin. Other antibacterial agents include azithromycin (Zithromax) and clarithromycin (Biaxin).

TETRACYCLINES

Tetracyclines are active against many gram-negative and gram-positive organisms (broad-spectrum). Tetracyclines commonly are used to treat conditions such as acne, bronchitis, syphilis, gonorrhea, and certain types of pneumonia. Examples of tetracyclines include demeclocycline (Declomycin), doxycycline (Vibramycin), and tetracycline (Achromycin). Tetracyclines may discolor developing teeth. Thus they usually are not prescribed for children under the age of 12 or for pregnant women.

CRITICAL THINKING

Explain how antibiotics and infectious organisms work like a lock and key.

FLUOROQUINOLONES

Fluoroquinolone antibiotics are the treatment of choice for some human gastrointestinal infections, particularly severe food-borne illness caused by *Campylobacter* or *Salmonellae* bacteria. They are also used to treat urinary tract infections, venereal disease, bone and joint infections, some types of pneumonia, and other human illness. Examples of fluoroquinolones include ciprofloxacin (Cipro), gatifloxacin (Tequin), and levofloxacin (Levaquin).

Antifungal and Antiviral Drugs

As discussed, persons can get an infection from bacterial organisms. In addition, they can be infected by fungi and viral diseases.

BOX 17-35 Categories of Fungal Infections

Examples of Superficial Infections

Candidiasis (thrush): Affects the genitals or inside of the mouth and vaginal and intertriginous areas

Tinea (including ring worm, athlete's foot, jock itch): Affects external areas of the body

Examples of Subcutaneous Infections (Rare)

Mycetoma (Madura foot): Occurs in tropical countries

Sporotrichosis: May follow inoculation of spores through a puncture or scratch

Examples of Deep Infections

Aspergillosis

Blastomycosis

Candidiasis (that spreads from its usual site to the esophagus, urinary tract, or other internal sites)

Cryptococcosis

Histoplasmosis

TABLE 17-6 Common Viruses and Viral Diseases or Conditions

VIRAL FAMILY	DISEASES OR CONDITIONS
Papovavirus	Warts
Adenovirus	Cold sores, genital herpes, chickenpox, herpes zoster (shingles), congenital abnormalities (cytomegalovirus)
Picornavirus	Poliomyelitis, viral hepatitis A and B, respiratory infections, myocarditis, rhinovirus (common cold)
Togavirus	Yellow fever, encephalitis
Orthomyxovirus	Influenza
Paramyxovirus	Mumps, measles, rubella
Coronavirus	Common cold
Rhabdovirus	Rabies
Retrovirus	Acquired immunodeficiency syndrome, degenerative brain disease, possibly cancer

ANTIFUNGAL DRUGS

Some fungi are harmlessly present at all times in areas of the body such as the mouth, skin, intestines, and vagina. These fungi are prevented from multiplying through competition from bacteria. The actions of the immune system also prevent them from multiplying. Fungal infections are more common and serious in persons taking antibiotics long term (antibiotics destroy the bacterial competition), in those who are immunosuppressed as a complication of illness (e.g., infection with the human immunodeficiency virus), and in those who are taking corticosteroids or immunosuppressant drugs (described later in this chapter). Fungal infections can be classified broadly into superficial infections, subcutaneous infections, and deep infections (Box 17-35). Examples of antifungal drugs include tolnaftate (Tinactin), fluconazole (Diflucan), and nystatin (Mycostatin). About 50 species of fungi can cause illness and sometimes fatal disease in human beings.

ANTIVIRAL DRUGS

To date, few effective drugs exist to treat minor viral infections such as colds. In fact, few drugs exist for use in any viral infections. This is due partly to the relative delay in the onset of symptoms that occurs in viral diseases. This delay in turn makes drug therapy difficult once the disease is established. Some viral infections are trivial and harmless (e.g., warts). Yet others are serious diseases such as influenza, rabies, acquired immunodeficiency syndrome, and probably some types of cancers (Table 17-6).

Many agents have been tested as antiviral drugs. However, few have been proved to work against specific virus-infected cells without toxic effects to uninfected cells. Examples of specific antiviral drugs include acyclovir (Zovirax) and valacyclovir (Valtrex), which is effective against herpes infection. Others are zidovudine (Retrovir, AZT, ZDV) and lamivudine (Epivir). At present, these drugs are used to treat human immunodeficiency infection.

NOTE A few drugs offer symptomatic relief from flu viruses. These drugs include oseltamivir (Tamiflu) and zanamivir (Relenza). These drugs are effective against A and B flu viruses. Others include amantadine (Symmetrel) and rimantadine (Flumadine). These drugs are effective against flu virus A (see Chapter 39).

PROTEASE INHIBITORS

The manner in which protease inhibitors work is not understood clearly. Yet they appear to inhibit the replication of retroviruses (e.g., human immunodeficiency virus) in acute and chronically infected cells. Side effects and adverse reactions of these drugs include nausea and vomiting, headache, malaise, fever, and flulike symptoms. Examples of protease inhibitors include indinavir (Crixivan), ritonavir (Norvir), and saquinavir (Invirase).

NOTE The administration of antiviral drugs and protease inhibitors for a health care worker who has been exposed to body fluids that may contain human immunodeficiency virus or another virus known or suspected to be resistant to antiviral drugs is important and is a postexposure prophylaxis recommendation by the Centers for Disease Control and Prevention.[14]

Other Antimicrobial Drugs and Antiparasitic Drugs

Various drugs are used to treat atypical microbial infection (e.g., *Mycobacterium tuberculosis* and *M. leprae*) and infection and disease caused by parasite and insect vector (e.g., trichomoniasis and malaria). Box 17-36 lists examples of these drugs and their classifications.

> **NOTE** Malaria is still a prevalent disease in tropical areas. Malaria may be carried into the United States by refugees and immigrants. Tuberculosis is on the rise in individuals with acquired immunodeficiency syndrome. Tuberculosis also is on the rise in the homeless, drug abusers, and those taking immunosuppressant drugs.

Antiinflammatory and Nonsteroidal Antiinflammatory Drugs

INFLAMMATION

Inflammation is a defense mechanism of body tissues in response to physical trauma, foreign biological and chemical substances, surgery, radiation, and electricity. Regardless of the event producing inflammation, the response is similar. For example, if bacterial infection or an injury to the tissues occurs, chemical mediators are released or activated. These mediators cause vasodilation and increased blood flow (localized warmth and redness at the site). This process brings phagocytes and other leukocytes to the area. The process prevents the spread of infection by limiting the infected site. Finally, phagocytes clean the area. The damaged tissues are repaired.

Inflammation can be localized or systemic. Local inflammation is confined to a specific area of the body. Symptoms include redness, heat, swelling, pain, and loss of function. Systemic inflammation occurs in many parts of the body. In addition to local symptoms at the inflammation site, red bone marrow produces and releases large numbers of neutrophils that promote phagocytosis, pyrogens stimulate fever production, and increased vascular permeability in severe cases may result in decreased blood volume. Drugs used to treat inflammation or its symptoms may be classified as analgesic-antipyretic drugs and nonsteroidal antiinflammatory drugs. A number of medications have both properties.

BOX 17-36 Examples of Antimicrobial and Antiparasitic Drugs

Antimalarial Agents
Pyrimethamine (Daraprim)
Quinacrine (Atabrine)
Quinine (Quinamm)

Antitubercular Agents
Aminosalicylate (Nemasol)
Capreomycin (Capastat)
Isoniazid (Izonid, INH)
Rifampin (Rifadin)
Streptomycin

Antiamebic Agents
Emetine
Iodoquinol (Yodoxin)
Paromomycin (Humatin)

Antihelminthic Agents
Diethylcarbamazine (Hetrazan)
Mebendazole (Vermox)

Antiprotozoal Agents
Metronidazole (Flagyl)

Leprostatic Agents
Clofazimine (Lamprene)
Dapsone (DDS)

Cephalosporins
Cefaclor (Ceclor)
Cefazolin (Ancef)
Cefprozil (Cefzil)
Ceftriaxone (Rocephin)
Cefuroxime (Ceftin)
Cephalexin (Keflex)

Fluoroquinolones
Ciprofloxacin (Cipro)
Levofloxacin (Levaquin)

Penicillins
Amoxicillin (Amoxil)
Ampicillin (Polycillin)
Dicloxacillin (Dynapen)
Penicillin G
Penicillin V

ANALGESIC-ANTIPYRETIC DRUGS

An antipyretic drug is one that reduces fever. The temperature regulating mechanism of the body is located in the anterior hypothalamus. (This is known as the thermostat of the body.) Normally, the set point of this hypothalamic center is about 98.6° F (37° C). When an inflammatory response occurs in the body, endogenous pyrogens are released by the phagocytic leukocytes. This produces fever. Analgesic-antipyretic drugs work by reversing the effect of the pyrogen on the hypothalamus. Thus the set point of the hypothalamus is returned to normal. The analgesic effects of these drugs act on peripheral pain receptors to block activation. Examples of these drugs include the following:

- Acetaminophen (Datril, Tylenol, Panadol, and others)
- ***Aspirin***/acetylsalicylic acid (A.S.A, Aspergum, Bayer Aspirin, and others)
- ***Aspirin*** (buffered) (Aluprin, Bufferin, Alka-Seltzer, and others)

NONSTEROIDAL ANTIINFLAMMATORY DRUGS

Aspirin is the oldest model of the nonsteroidal antiinflammatory drug. New drugs have been developed. Like ***aspirin,*** these drugs are analgesic, antipyretic, and antiinflammatory. These drugs often are prescribed for patients with various inflammatory conditions. (One such condition is rheumatoid arthritis.) The new drugs also often are prescribed for those who cannot tolerate ***aspirin.*** In addition, these drugs may be used to treat painful joint disorders (with or without inflammation) such as osteoarthritis, low back pain, and gout. One should note that like ***aspirin,*** the other nonsteroidal antiinflammatory agents may decrease platelet activity. This could result in gastrointestinal bleeding. Long-term use of some NSAIDs has been linked to an increased risk for heart attack and stroke.

> **NOTE** Gout is a metabolic disease associated with high levels of uric acid in the blood (hyperuricemia). Gout is characterized by attacks of acute pain, swelling, and tenderness of joints. The condition is treated with uricosuric drugs, colchicine, and nonsteroidal antiinflammatory drugs.

Nonsteroidal antiinflammatory drugs are thought to act by inhibiting specific enzymes so that prostaglandins (substances that promote inflammation and pain) are not formed. Examples of these drugs include the following:

- ***Aspirin*** (Bayer Timed-Release, Bufferin, and others)
- Diflunisal (Dolobid)
- Ibuprofen (Advil, Motrin, Nuprin, and others)
- Indomethacin (Indocin and others)
- Naproxen (Anaprox, Aleve, Naprosyn)
- Sulindac (Clinoril)
- ***Ketorolac*** (Toradol)
- Cyclooxygenase-2 inhibitors
  Celecoxib (Celebrex)
  Valdecoxib (Bextra)

SECTION THIRTEEN
Drugs That Affect the Immunological System

REVIEW OF ANATOMY AND PHYSIOLOGY

As described earlier in this chapter and in Chapter 6, the immunological system is composed of cells and organs. These cells and organs defend the body against invasion by foreign substances. Organs and tissues of the immune system include the spleen, tonsils, lymph nodes, and thymus (Fig. 17-9).

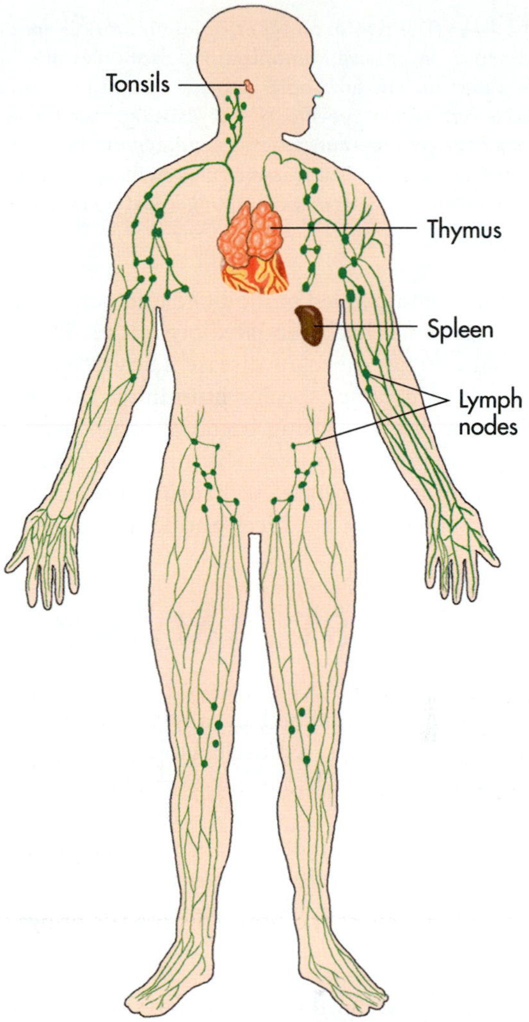

FIGURE 17-9 ■ Organs and tissues of the immune system.

Drugs Used to Treat the Immune System

IMMUNOSUPPRESSANTS

Immunosuppressant drugs reduce the activity of the immune system. They do this by suppressing the production and activity of lymphocytes. These drugs are given after transplant surgery. They help to prevent the rejection of foreign tissues. They also are given to halt the progress of autoimmune disorders when other treatments are ineffective. Examples of immunosuppressant drugs include antirejection drugs (used in organ transplantation), anticancer drugs, and corticosteroids.

> **CRITICAL THINKING**
>
> It would be important to know that a patient with altered level of consciousness is taking an immunosuppressant drug. Why is this?

IMMUNOMODULATING AGENTS

Immunomodulating agents are drugs that increase the efficiency of the immune system. These agents activate the immune defenses or modify a biological response to an unwanted stimulus. These drugs include vaccines that protect against specific infectious agents. One drug belonging to this group is the interferons. (They are used to treat viral infections such as hepatitis C and certain types of cancer.) Another drug in this group is zidovudine (AZT, Retrovir). (Zidovudine is used to treat acquired immunodeficiency syndrome.) Some immunomodulating agents enhance the ability of a vaccine to stimulate the immune system. Thus they are added to the vaccine for this reason.

SERUMS AND VACCINES

Serum is the clear fluid that separates from blood when blood clots. Serum contains salts, glucose, and other proteins. Serum also includes antibodies formed by the immune system. Antibodies are formed to fight against infection. Serum from the blood of a person (or in rare cases an animal) infected with a microorganism usually contains antibodies. Therefore that serum may protect against that microorganism if the serum is injected into someone else. This relationship forms the basis for passive immunization (see Chapter 39).

▶ **NOTE** The two main types of immunization are passive and active. In passive immunization, antibodies are injected into a person. The antibodies provide instant but short-lived protection against specific disease-causing bacteria, viruses, or toxins. Active immunization stimulates the body to make its own antibodies. These antibodies fight against such microorganisms. This type confers longer-lasting immunity.

Vaccines contain killed or modified microorganisms. The latter are known as live attenuated organisms. These organisms usually do not cause the disease. The vaccines are given to a person to produce specific immunity. This immunity may be for a disease-causing bacterial toxin, virus, or bacterium (active immunization). The infectious agent may invade the body at a later time. At that time, the sensitized immune system quickly produces antibodies to destroy the agent or the toxin it produces. Examples of live attenuated vaccines are those given to protect against measles, mumps, rubella, yellow fever, and polio. Diphtheria and tetanus vaccines contain inactivated bacterial toxins. Cholera, typhoid fever, pertussis, rabies, viral hepatitis B, influenza, and Salk injected polio vaccines contain killed organisms. (In the case of hepatitis B the vaccine contains only part of the hepatitis B virus.)

▶ **NOTE** Smallpox was declared extinct by the World Health Organization in 1980 because of near universal vaccination. With today's threat of bioterrorism, though, smallpox vaccinations are being considered for some health care workers, including emergency medical services. See Chapter 39 and Chapter 54.

SUMMARY

- A drug may be defined as any substance taken by mouth; injected into a muscle, blood vessel, or cavity of the body; or applied topically to treat or prevent a disease or condition.
- Drugs can be identified by four types of names. These include the chemical name; generic or nonproprietary name; trade, brand, or proprietary name; and official name.
- The Drug Enforcement Agency is the sole legal drug enforcement body in the United States. Other regulatory bodies or services include the FDA; the Public Health Service; the Federal Trade Commission; in Canada, the Health Protection Branch of the Department of National Health and Welfare; and for international drug control, the International Narcotics Control Board.
- Paramedics are held responsible for the safe and effective administration of drugs. In fact, they are responsible for each drug they provide to a patient. They are legally, morally, and ethically responsible.
- Drug allergies can be divided into four classifications based on the mechanism of the immune reaction. They are type I (anaphylactic), type II (cytotoxic), type III (serum sickness), and type IV (contact dermatitis) reactions.
- The parasympathetic and sympathetic nervous systems function continuously. They innervate many of the same organs at the same time. The opposing actions of the two systems balance each other. In general, the sympathetic system dominates during stressful events. The parasympathetic system is most active during times of emotional and physical calm.
- The degree to which drugs attain pharmacological activity depends partly on the rate and extent to which they are absorbed. Absorption in turn depends on the ability of the drug to cross the cell membrane. The rate and extent of absorption depend on the nature of the cell membrane the drug must cross, blood flow to the site of administration, solubility of the drug, pH of the drug environment, drug concentration, and drug dosage form.
- The route of drug administration influences drug absorption. These routes can be classified as enteral, parenteral, pulmonary, and topical.
- Distribution is the transport of a drug through the bloodstream to various tissues of the body and ultimately to its site of action. After absorption and distribution, the body eliminates most drugs. The body first biotransforms the drug and then excretes the drug. The kidney is the primary organ for excretion; however, the intestine, lungs, and mammary, sweat, and salivary glands also may be involved.
- Many factors can alter the response to drug therapy, including age, body mass, gender, pathological state, genetic factors, and psychological factors.
- Most drug actions are thought to result from a chemical interaction. This interaction is between the drug and various receptors throughout the body. The most common form of drug action is the drug-receptor interaction.
- Many variables can influence drug interactions, including intestinal absorption, competition for plasma-protein binding, biotransformation, action at the receptor site, renal excretion, and alteration of electrolyte balance.
- Narcotic analgesics relieve pain. Narcotic antagonists reverse the narcotic effects of some analgesics. Nonnarcotic analgesics interfere with local mediators released when tissue is damaged in the periphery of the body. These mediators stimulate nerve endings and cause pain.
- Anesthetic drugs are CNS depressants that have a reversible effect on nervous tissue. Antianxiety agents are

used to reduce feelings of apprehension, nervousness, worry, or fearfulness. Sedatives and hypnotics are drugs that depress the CNS. They produce a calming effect. They also help induce sleep. Alcohol is a general CNS depressant that can produce sedation, sleep, and anesthesia.

- Anticonvulsant drugs are used to treat seizure disorders. Most notably they treat epilepsy.
- All CNS stimulants work to increase excitability. They do this by blocking activity of inhibitory neurons or their respective neurotransmitters or by enhancing the production of the excitatory neurotransmitters.
- Psychotherapeutic drugs include antipsychotic agents, antidepressants, and lithium. These drugs are used to treat psychoses and affective disorders, especially schizophrenia, depression, and mania.
- Several movement disorders can result from an imbalance of dopamine and acetylcholine. Drugs that inhibit or block acetylcholine are referred to as anticholinergic. Three classes of drugs affect brain dopamine: those that release dopamine, those that increase brain levels of dopamine, and dopaminergic agonists.
- The autonomic drugs mimic or block the effects of the sympathetic and parasympathetic divisions of the autonomic nervous system. These drugs are classified into four groups: cholinergic (parasympathomimetic) drugs, cholinergic blocking (parasympatholytic) drugs, adrenergic (sympathomimetic) drugs, and adrenergic blocking (sympatholytic) drugs.
- Skeletal muscle relaxants can be classified as central acting, direct acting, and neuromuscular blockers.
- Cardiac drugs are classified by their effects on specialized cardiac tissues. Cardiac glycosides are used to treat congestive heart failure and certain tachycardias. Antidysrhythmic drugs are used to treat and prevent disorders of cardiac rhythm. The pharmacological agents that suppress dysrhythmias may do so by direct action on the cardiac cell membrane (lidocaine), by indirect action that affects the cell (propranolol), or both.
- Antihypertensive drugs used to reduce blood pressure are classified into four major categories: diuretics, sympathetic blocking agents (sympatholytic drugs), vasodilators, and ACE inhibitors. Calcium channel blockers also are used to treat persons with hypertension who do not respond to other drug therapies.
- Antihemorrheologic agents are used to treat peripheral vascular disorders. These disorders are caused by pathological or physiological obstruction (e.g., arteriosclerosis). These agents improve blood flow to ischemic tissues.
- Drugs that affect blood coagulation may be classified as antiplatelet, anticoagulant, or fibrinolytic agents. Drugs that interfere with platelet aggregation are known as antiplatelet or antithrombic drugs. Anticoagulant drug therapy is designed to prevent intravascular thrombosis. The therapy decreases blood coagulability. Fibrinolytic drugs dissolve clots after their formation. These drugs work by promoting the digestion of fibrin.
- Hemophilia is a group of hereditary bleeding disorders. These disorders involve a deficiency of one of the factors needed for the coagulation of blood. Replacing the missing clotting factor can help manage hemophilia.
- Hemostatic agents speed up clot formation, thus reducing bleeding. Systemic hemostatic agents are used to control blood loss after surgery. They work by inhibiting the breakdown of fibrin. Topical hemostatic agents are used to control capillary bleeding. They are used during surgical and dental procedures.
- The treatment of choice in managing a loss of blood or blood components is to replace the sole blood component that is deficient. Replacement therapy may include transfusing whole blood (rare), packed red blood cells, fresh-frozen plasma, plasma expanders, platelets, coagulation factors, fibrinogen, albumin, or gamma globulins.
- Hyperlipidemia refers to an excess of lipids in the plasma. Antihyperlipidemic drugs sometimes are used along with diet and exercise to control serum lipid levels.
- Bronchodilator drugs are the primary form of treatment for obstructive pulmonary disease such as asthma, chronic bronchitis, and emphysema. These drugs may be classified as sympathomimetic drugs and xanthine derivatives.
- Mucokinetic drugs are used to move respiratory secretions, excessive mucus, and sputum along the tracheobronchial tree.
- Oxygen is used chiefly to treat hypoxia and hypoxemia.
- Direct respiratory stimulant drugs act directly on the medullary center of the brain. These drugs are analeptics. They increase the rate and depth of respiration.
- Spirits of ammonia is a reflex respiratory stimulant. The drug is administered by inhalation.
- A cough may be prolonged or result from an underlying disorder. In such a case, treatment with antitussive drugs may be indicated.
- The main clinical use of antihistamines is for allergic reactions. They also are used to control motion sickness or as a sedative or antiemetic.
- Drug therapy for the gastrointestinal system can be divided into drugs that affect the stomach and drugs that affect the lower gastrointestinal tract. Antacids buffer or neutralize hydrochloric acid in the stomach. Antiflatulents prevent the formation of gas in the gastrointestinal tract. Digestant drugs promote digestion in the gastrointestinal tract. They do this by releasing small amounts of hydrochloric acid in the stomach. Drugs used to induce vomiting may be administered as part of the treatment of certain drug overdoses and poisonings. Drugs used to treat nausea and vomiting include antagonists of histamine, acetylcholine, and dopamine and other drugs the actions of which are not understood clearly.

Continued

- Cytoprotective agents and other drugs are used to treat peptic ulcer disease by protecting the gastric mucosa. H_2 receptor antagonists block the H_2 receptors. They also reduce the volume of gastric acid secretion and its acid content.
- Two common conditions of the lower gastrointestinal tract may require drug therapy: constipation and diarrhea. Drugs used to manage these conditions include laxatives and antidiarrheals.
- Drugs used to treat eye disorders include antiglaucoma agents, mydriatics, cycloplegics, antiinfective/antiinflammatory agents, and topical anesthetics.
- Drugs used to treat disorders of the ear include antibiotics, steroid/antibiotic combinations, and miscellaneous preparations.
- The endocrine system works to control and integrate body functions. A number of drugs are used to treat disorders of the anterior and posterior pituitary, the thyroid and parathyroid glands, and the adrenal cortex.
- The pancreatic hormones play a key role in regulating the amount of certain nutrients in the circulatory system. The two main hormones secreted by the pancreas are insulin and glucagon. Imbalances in either of these may call for drug therapy. This therapy is meant to correct metabolic derangements.
- Drugs that affect the female reproductive system include synthetic and natural substances such as hormones, oral contraceptives, ovulation stimulants, and drugs used to treat infertility.
- The male sex hormone is testosterone. Adequate amounts of this hormone are needed for normal development. Adequate amounts also are needed for the maintenance of male sex characteristics.
- Antineoplastic agents are used in cancer chemotherapy to prevent the increase of malignant cells.
- Antibiotics are used to treat local or systemic infection. This group includes penicillin, cephalosporins, and related products; macrolide antibiotics; tetracyclines; and miscellaneous antibiotic agents.
- Persons can be infected by bacterial organisms, fungi, and viruses. Examples of antifungal drugs include tolnaftate (Tinactin), fluconazole (Diflucan), and nystatin (Mycostatin).
- Few drugs exist for use in any viral infections. One antiviral drug is acyclovir (Zovirax). This drug is effective against herpes infection. Another one is zidovudine (Retrovir, AZT), which currently is used to treat human immunodeficiency virus infection.
- Drugs used to treat inflammation or its symptoms may be classified as analgesic-antipyretic drugs and nonsteroidal antiinflammatory drugs. A number of medications have both properties.
- Immunosuppressant drugs reduce the activity of the immune system. They do this by suppressing the production and activity of lymphocytes. These drugs are prescribed after transplant surgery. They can help to prevent the rejection of foreign tissues. They also are sometimes given to halt the progress of autoimmune disorders.
- Immunomodulating agents are drugs that help the immune system to be more efficient. They do this by activating the immune defenses and by modifying a biological response to an unwanted stimulus.
- Serum contains agents of immunity. These are antibodies. The antibodies can protect against an organism if the serum is injected into someone else. This forms the basis for passive immunization. Vaccines are composed of killed or altered microorganisms. These are administered to a person to produce specific immunity to a disease-causing bacterial toxin, virus, or bacterium (active immunization).

REFERENCES

1. Lyons A, Petrucelli R: *Medicine: an illustrated history,* New York, 1987, Abradale Press.
2. Glanze W, editor: *Mosby's medical, nursing, and allied health dictionary,* ed 4, St Louis, 1994, Mosby.
3. McKenry L, Salerno E: *Mosby's pharmacology in nursing,* ed 18, St Louis, 1992, Mosby.
4. Pratt J: Intraosseous infusion, *Int Pediatr* 4(1):19, 1989.
5. American Heart Association: *Guidelines 2000 for cardiopulmonary resuscitation and emergency cardiovascular care,* International Consensus on Science, Dallas, 2000, The Association.
6. Syverud S et al: Prehospital use of neuromuscular blocking agents in a helicopter ambulance program, *Ann Emerg Med* 17(3):237, 1988.
7. Rosen P, Barkin R: *Emergency medicine: concepts and clinical practice,* ed 4, St Louis, 1998, Mosby.
8. Gonzalez E et al: Intravenous amiodarone for ventricular arrhythmias: overview and clinical use, *Resuscitation* 39:33, 1998.
9. American Heart Association: *Basic life support for healthcare providers,* Dallas, 1997, The Association.
10. National Institutes of Health; National Heart, Blood, and Lung Institute: *The Sixth Report of the Joint National Committee on Prevention, Detection, Evaluation, and Treatment of High Blood Pressure,* NIH Pub No 98-480, Washington, DC, 1997, The Institutes.
11. American Medical Association: *The American Medical Association home medical encyclopedia,* New York, 1989, The Association.
12. *The medical advisor: the complete guide to alternative and conventional treatments,* Alexandria, Va, 1996, Time-Life Books.
13. Hazinski et al: *2000 handbook of emergency cardiovascular care for healthcare providers,* Dallas, 2000, American Heart Association.
14. US Department of Health and Human Services, Centers for Disease Control: Public Health Service guidelines for the management of health care worker exposures to HIV and recommendations for postexposure prophylaxis, No RR-7, *MMWR* 47, 1-46, 1998.

APPENDIX
Herbs

HERBAL PRODUCTS

The use of herbs and herbal products is common in the United States; it is estimated that nearly half of all Americans use herbs on a regular basis.[1, 2] Unlike prescription drugs and over-the-counter medications, herbal products used as supplements are not regulated by the Food and Drug Administration (FDA). Proof of product purity and accuracy in the amount of active ingredient in each pill is not required, and there are no standards on the accuracy and amount of information that must be provided on the label of herbal products. Some herbal products have been shown to be effective, while others have been shown to be ineffective. In addition, some herbs when taken internally can interact with prescription medications, producing untoward effects. Therefore, all persons should advise their physician and pharmacist if they are using herbal supplements. Although there are hundreds of herbal ingredients and thousands of herbal products that can be purchased without a prescription, the following section provides information about common herbal supplements used in the United States.

HERBAL SUPPLEMENTS

Bilberry

(Airelle, Bleaberry, Burren, Dyeberry, Huckleberry, Hurtleberry, Myrtle, Trackleberry, Whortleberry)

COMMON USES

Diarrhea, improving vision, mouth/throat inflammation

CONTRAINDICATIONS/INTERACTIONS

May inhibit platelet aggregation; should not be used before surgery or near maternal delivery; should not be used with other drugs or herbs that might affect clotting, including aspirin, nonsteroidal antiinflammatory agents, heparin, or warfarin.

Cranberry

(Arandano, Moosebeere, Mossberry)

COMMON USES

Urinary tract disorders; susceptibility to kidney stones

CONTRAINDICATIONS/INTERACTIONS

None noted

Echinacea

(Black Sampson, Hedgehog, Kansas Snakeroot, Red Sunflower, Purple Cone Flower)

COMMON USES

Preventing and treating infection (especially the cold or flu); low immune status

CONTRAINDICATIONS/INTERACTIONS

May boost certain areas of the immune system and exacerbate a person's systemic disease. Not recommended in patients with autoimmune diseases, multiple sclerosis, AIDS, HIV infection, tuberculosis, or in transplant patients or persons taking immunosuppressive drugs (e.g., anti-HIV drugs).

Evening Primrose

(Fever Plant, King's Cureall, Night Willow-Herb, Scabish, SunDrop)

COMMON USES

Premenstrual syndrome; hot flashes; inflammatory disorders; migraine headache

CONTRAINDICATIONS/INTERACTIONS

May cause uterine contraction in pregnant women; may lower seizure threshold (increasing drug dosage requirements) in patients with seizure disorders and in those taking phenothiazine (e.g., patients with schizophrenia).

Garlic

(Camphor of the Poor, Nectar of the Gods, Rust Treacle, Stinking Rose)

COMMON USES

Improving circulation; lowering blood lipid levels; hypertension; inflammatory disorders; menstrual disorders; childhood earaches; diarrhea; colds and flu symptoms; and numerous other ailments

CONTRAINDICATIONS/INTERACTIONS

May augment anticoagulant effect and may increase bleeding time; should not be used with other drugs or herbs that might affect clotting, including aspirin, nonsteroidal antiinflammatory agents, heparin, or warfarin; should not be used prior to surgery or near maternal delivery.

Ginger

COMMON USES

Nausea; motion sickness; morning sickness; inflammation; indigestion

CONTRAINDICATIONS/INTERACTIONS

May inhibit platelet aggregation (in large doses); should not be used with other drugs or herbs that might affect clotting, including aspirin, nonsteroidal antiinflammatory agents, heparin, or warfarin; should not be used prior to surgery or near maternal delivery.

Ginkgo Biloba

(Duck Foot, Kew, Madenhair, Silver Apricot)

COMMON USES

Memory improvement; altitude sickness; poor circulation; inflammatory disorders; impotence

CONTRAINDICATIONS/INTERACTIONS

Augments anticoagulant effect and may increase bleeding time; should not be used with other drugs or herbs that might affect clotting, including aspirin, nonsteroidal antiinflammatory agents, heparin, or warfarin; should not be used prior to surgery or near maternal delivery; may lower seizure threshold in patients with seizure disorders.

Ginseng

COMMON USES

Physical and mental exhaustion; stress; viral infection; diabetes; headache

CONTRAINDICATIONS/INTERACTIONS

May lower blood glucose levels; should not be used by persons with diabetes; may alter bleeding or clotting times; should not be used with other drugs or herbs that might affect clotting, including aspirin, nonsteroidal antiinflammatory agents, heparin, or warfarin; should not be used prior to surgery or near maternal delivery; may contain cardiac glycosides and should not be used by persons taking digoxin.

Grape Seed

(Activin, oligomeric proanthocyanidins [OPC's], Red Wine Extract)

COMMON USES

Antioxidant; chronic disease prevention; leg cramps; inflammation

CONTRAINDICATIONS/INTERACTIONS

None noted.

Kava Kava

(Ava Pepper, Awa, Intoxicating Pepper, Kawa, Kew, Sakau, Tonga)

COMMON USES

Nervous anxiety; insomnia; stress

CONTRAINDICATIONS/INTERACTIONS

May enhance the effects of alcohol or other sedating substances; should be avoided in persons taking antidepressants, pain medications, tranquilizers, antihistamines, and anticholinergic drugs; may antagonize the effect of dopamine and should be avoided in persons with Parkinson's disease; may increase the effects of anesthesia and should be avoided prior to surgery; extended use may cause discoloration of the skin, nails, and hair; chronic use may produce neurological symptoms; should be avoided in pregnant women and nursing mothers.

Milk Thistle

(Holy Thistle, Lady's Thistle, Marian Thistle, St. Mary Thistle, Silymarin)

COMMON USES

Liver disorders (alcohol or drug induced, hepatitis B, hepatitis C); breast and prostate cancer

CONTRAINDICATIONS/INTERACTIONS

Should be avoided in persons who have allergies to ragweed, marigolds, daisies, or chrysanthemums; safety during pregnancy has not been established.

Saw Palmetto

(American Dwarf Palm, Cabbage Palm, Sabal, Shrub Palmetto)

COMMON USES

Benign prostatic hypertrophy (BPH); urinary problems

CONTRAINDICATIONS/INTERACTIONS

May have antihormone effects; should be avoided in persons with hormone-dependent cancers and during pregnancy.

St. John's Wort

(Demon Chaser, Goatweed, Hypericum, Klamath Weed)

COMMON USES

Anxiety; depression; sleep disorders; viral infection

CONTRAINDICATIONS/INTERACTIONS

May potentiate the effects of MAO inhibitors, selective serotonin reuptake inhibitors (SSRIs), and tricyclics; should not be used in persons with serious depression or suicidal tendencies; may increase levels of dopamine and norepinephrine and should be avoided in persons with hypertension; may decrease serum levels of digoxin, theophylline, reserpine, and some HIV drugs; inhibits iron absorption; may cause stomach upset, sleep disturbance; photosensitivity.

Valerian Root

(All-Heal, Amantilla, Baldrian, Capon's Tail, Heliotrope, Setwall, Vandal Root)

COMMON USES

Anxiety; stress; depression; insomnia

CONTRAINDICATIONS/INTERACTIONS

May enhance the effects of alcohol or other sedating substances; should be avoided in persons taking antidepressants, pain medications, tranquilizers, antihistamines, anticholinergic drugs, and the herb Kava Kava; may increase the effects of anesthesia and should be avoided prior to surgery.

REFERENCES

1. Bennett J, Brown CM: Use of herbal remedies by patients in a health maintenance organization, *J Am Pharm Assoc* 40(3):353-358, 2000.
2. Anonymous: *Consumer use of dietary supplements.* A publication of Prevention Magazine, 2000.

SUGGESTED READING

Blumenthal M, Goldberg A, Brinckmann J: *Herbal medicine expanded commission E monographs,* Newton, Mass., 2000, Integrative Medicine Communications.

Gruenwald J, Brendler T, Jaenicke C: *PDR for herbal medicines,* ed 2, Montvale, N.J., 2000, Medical Economics Co.

Wichtl M: *Herbal drugs and pharmaceuticals,* ed 4, Boca Raton, Fla., 2004, CRC Press.

2003 Mosby's Nursing Drug Reference.

2003 Mosby's Drug Consult.

CHAPTER 18

Venous Access and Medication Administration

OBJECTIVES

Upon completion of this chapter, the paramedic student will be able to:

1. Convert selected units of measurement into the household, apothecary, and metric systems.
2. Identify the steps in the calculation of drug dosages.
3. Calculate the correct volume of drug to be administered in a given situation.
4. Compute the correct rate for an infusion of drugs or intravenous fluids.
5. List measures for ensuring the safe administration of medications.
6. Describe actions paramedics should take if a medication error occurs.
7. List measures for preserving asepsis during parenteral administration of a drug.
8. Explain drug administration techniques for the enteral and parenteral routes.
9. Describe the steps for safely initiating an intravenous infusion.
10. Identify complications and adverse effects associated with intravenous access.
11. Describe the steps for safely initiating intravenous access.
12. Describe the steps for safely initiating an intraosseous infusion.
13. Explain drug administration techniques for percutaneous routes.
14. Identify special considerations in the administration of pharmacological agents to pediatric patients.
15. Explain the technique for obtaining a venous blood sample.
16. Describe the safe disposal of contaminated items and sharps.

KEY TERMS

gram: A metric unit of mass equal to $^{1}/_{1000}$ of a kilogram.

kilogram: A metric unit of mass equal to 1000 grams, or 2.2046 pounds.

liter: A metric unit of capacity equal to 1 cubic decimeter, 61.025 cubic inches, or 1.0567 liquid quarts.

medical asepsis: The removal or destruction of disease-causing organisms or infected material.
meter: A metric unit of length equal to 1000 millimeters.
microgram: A metric unit of mass equal to $^1/_{1,000,000}$ of a gram.
milligram: A metric unit of mass equal to $^1/_{1000}$ of a gram.
milliliter: A metric unit of capacity equal to $^1/_{1000}$ of a liter.

Certain key skills are required of all paramedics. The ability to insert a needle or an intravenous catheter into a vein safely (i.e., gain venous access) is a crucial skill. A paramedic also must be able to administer prescribed medications. These skills, and the patient care they require, are critical to medication therapy.

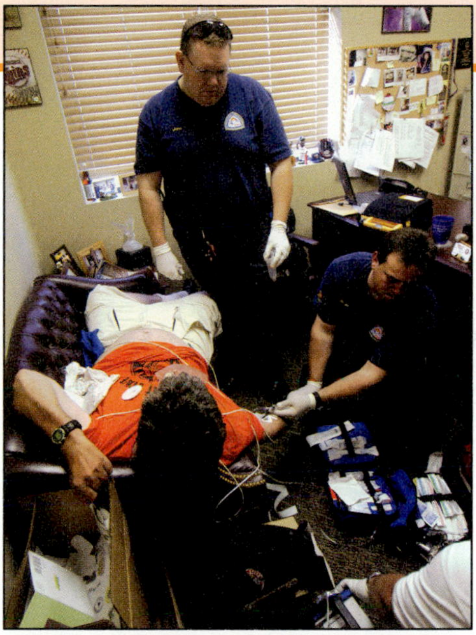

NOTE Mathematical skills are important in the administration of drugs. These skills include multiplication and division, figuring percentages, and working with Roman numerals, fractions, decimal fractions, and proportions. Paramedics must have a good working knowledge of these principles. They also must be adept at calculations.

MATHEMATICAL EQUIVALENTS USED IN PHARMACOLOGY

Three systems for measuring drug dosages are in common use today. These are the metric system, the apothecary system, and the common household system (Box 18-1). Each system deals with units of mass and volume. A physician may use any of these three systems in ordering drugs.

Metric System

The French developed the metric system of weights and measures in the latter part of the eighteenth century. Congress declared it to be the official measurement system in the United States in 1866.[1] Use of the metric system is not required in the United States. However, it has been adopted by the medical sciences and pharmacies. It also is

BOX 18-1 Systems of Equivalents

Metric System
1.0 g = 0.001 kg
1.0 g = 1000 mg
1.0 L = 1000 mL

Apothecary System
1.0 grain (gr) = $^1/_{60}$ dram (dr) or $^1/_{480}$ oz
60 gr = 1 dr
8 dr = 1 oz (or K)
1.0 minim (m) = $^1/_{60}$ fluid drams (f dr) or $^1/_{480}$ fluid ounces (f oz)
60 m = 1 f dr (or f l)
8 f dr = 1 f oz (or f K)

Household System
1.0 lb = 16 oz
1.0 pt = ½ quart (qt) = ⅛ gallon (gal)
1.0 pt = 16 f oz = 32 tablespoons (T)
1.0 T = 3 teaspoons (t)
1.0 t = 5 mL
1.0 T = 15 mL
1.0 pt = 480 mL
1.0 qt = 960 mL
1.0 gal = 3.84 L

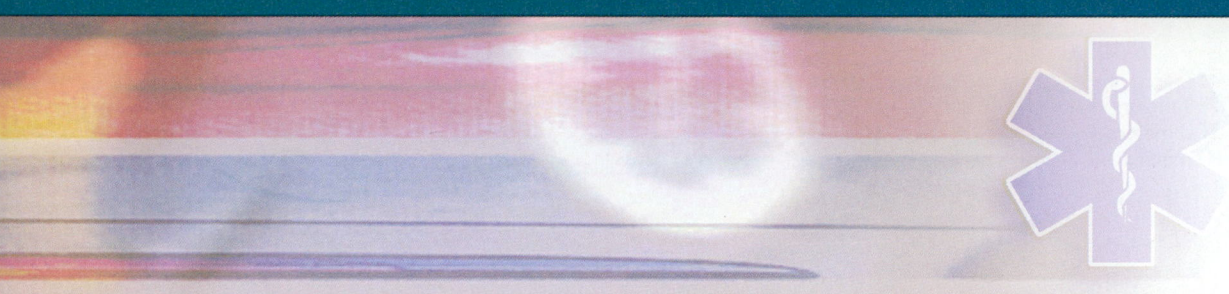

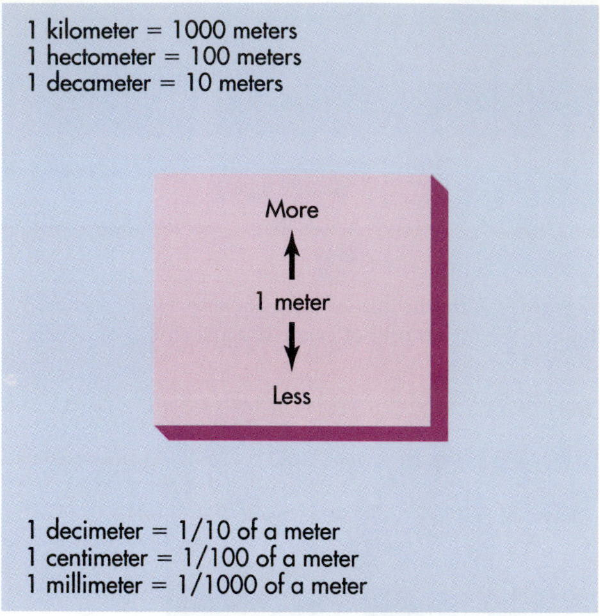

FIGURE 18-1 ■ The *meter* measures length.

TABLE 18-1 Common Metric Prefixes

PREFIX	MEANING
kilo-	1000 times greater
deci-	10 times less
centi-	100 times less
milli-	1000 times less
micro-	1 million times less

used in weighing currency at the federal mints. The armed forces use it as well. About 92% of the countries of the world use the metric system.

DEFINITIONS OF UNITS

The basic metric units of measurement are the meter, the liter, and the gram. The **meter** is the unit for linear measurement. The **liter** is the unit for capacity or volume. The **gram** is the unit for weight. A meter is slightly longer than a yard. A liter is slightly more than a quart. A gram is slightly more than the weight of a metal paper clip.

The basic units of the metric system can be divided or multiplied by 10, 100, or 1000 parts to form secondary units. These secondary units differ from each other by 10 or some multiple of 10. Subdivisions of these basic units are made when the decimal is moved to the left. Multiples of the basic unit are made when the decimal is moved to the right. The names of the secondary units are formed by putting a Greek or Latin prefix on the primary unit (Table 18-1).

The meter (m) is the unit of length from which the other metric units of length are derived (Fig. 18-1). Centimeters (cm) and millimeters (mm) are the primary linear measurements used in medicine. For example, they are used to measure the size of body organs and to measure blood pressure.

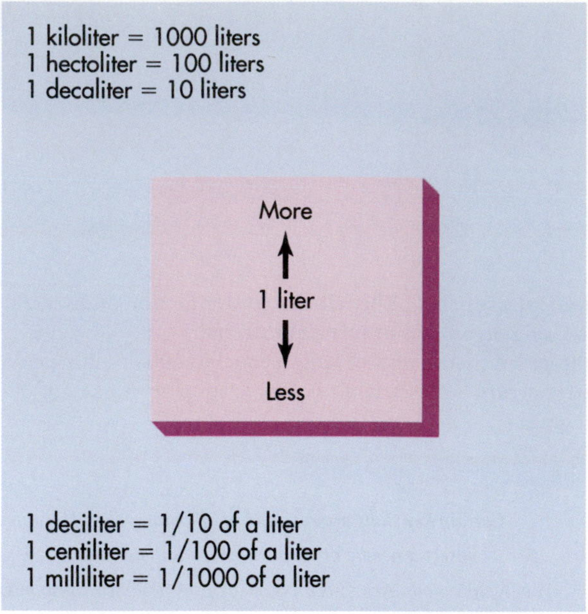

FIGURE 18-2 ■ The *liter* measures capacity.

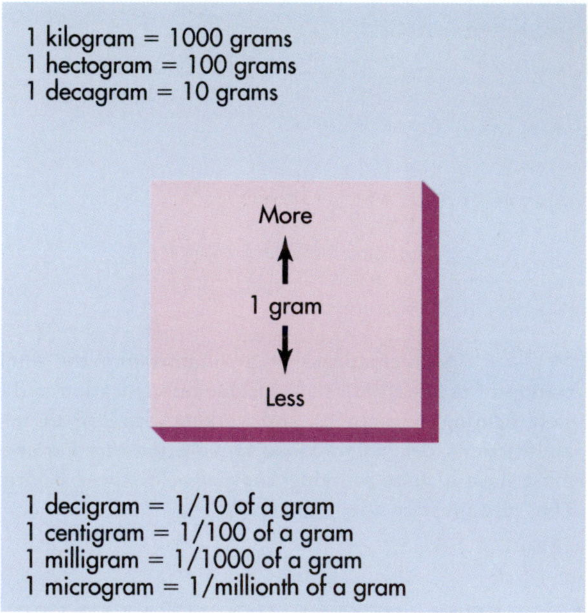

FIGURE 18-3 ■ The *gram* measures weight.

The liter (L) is the unit of capacity or volume (Fig. 18-2). A fractional part of a liter is expressed in milliliters (mL) or cubic centimeters (cc). The liter is equal to 1000 mL (1000 cc). A **milliliter,** therefore, is $\frac{1}{1000}$ of a liter. The National Bureau of Standards recommends that the unit of measure *ml* or *mL* be used to express fractional parts of a liter.

The gram (g) is the metric unit used in weighing drugs and various pharmaceutical preparations (Fig. 18-3). The gram equals the weight of 1 mL of distilled water at 4° C. A **kilogram** (kg) is equal to 1000 grams, or 2.2 pounds. A **milligram** (mg) is equal to $\frac{1}{1000}$ of a gram. A **microgram** (μg) is equal to $\frac{1}{1,000,000}$ of a gram.

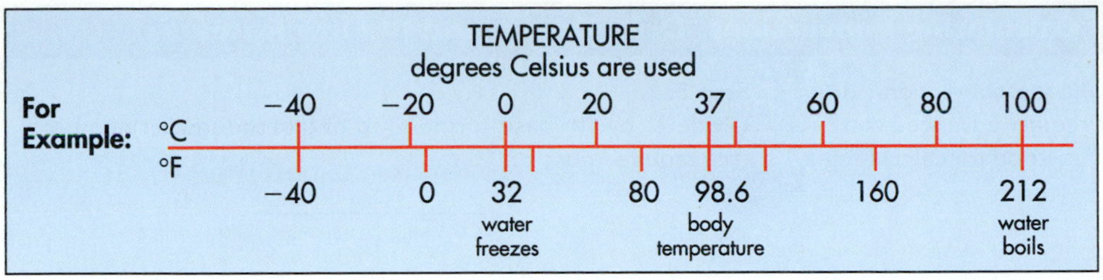

FIGURE 18-4 ■ Temperature conversions.

METRIC STYLE OF NOTATION

The National Bureau of Standards recommends the following style of metric notation except where it conflicts with the proper use of English[2]:

- Units are not capitalized (gram, not Gram).
- Unit abbreviations are not followed by a period (mL, not m.L. or mL.).
- A single space is left between the quantity and the symbol (24 kg, not 24kg).
- Unit abbreviations are not pluralized (kg, not kgs).
- As a rule, fractions are not used, only decimal notation (0.25 kg, not $\frac{1}{4}$ kg).
- For numerical quantities less than 1, a 0 is placed to the left of the decimal point (0.75 mg, not .75 mg).

CRITICAL THINKING

Placing a 0 to the left of the decimal point reduces the likelihood of a drug dosing error. Why?

Apothecary System

The apothecary system is thought to be less precise than the more widely adopted metric system. It also is thought to be less convenient. Only a few medications are now available in units of the apothecary system. ***Aspirin*** is an example of one.

The primary unit of mass in the apothecary system is the grain (gr). The grain was derived from the age-old standard of the weight of a single grain of wheat (about 60 to 65 mg). ***Aspirin*** (5 gr) contains 325 milligrams of medication (5 grain × 65 mg = 325 mg). Other units of mass used in the apothecary system are the dram (dr), ounce (oz), and pound (lb). Sixty grains equals 1 dram, and 8 drams equals 1 ounce.

The primary unit of volume in the apothecary system is the minim (m). The minim equals the volume of water that would weigh 1 gr (about 0.005 or 0.006 mL). The equivalent of 60 m is 1 fluid dram (f dr), and 8 f dr equals 1 fluid ounce (f oz).

In written prescriptions, the apothecary system puts the abbreviation before the numeral. Whole numerical amounts are usually set in lower case Roman numerals. For example, 10 grains would be grains x. Fractional amounts are usually given in Arabic numerals rather than decimal form. For example, $\frac{1}{4}$ grain would be grain $\frac{1}{4}$, not 0.25 grain.

NOTE The only apothecary conversion needed in emergency drug therapy is pounds to kilograms: 1 kilogram = 2.2 pounds. When the weight of an adult patient is converted from pounds to kilograms, the whole number can be rounded up when the number to the right of the decimal point is 5 or greater. For example, 70.90 kg could be rounded up to 71 kg.

Household System

Household measures include the glass, cup, tablespoon, teaspoon, drop, quart, and pint. Standard measures of the household system are not available in most homes. For example, the average coffee cup may hold 5 to 9 oz or more. The average household teaspoon may hold 4 to 6 mL of liquid. Household measurements are only approximations.

Temperature Conversions

Normal body temperature is 98.6° Fahrenheit, or 37° Celsius (centigrade). A simple formula can be used to convert temperatures. To convert a Celsius reading to Fahrenheit, multiply the Celsius reading by $\frac{9}{5}$. Then add 32. To convert a Fahrenheit reading to Celsius, subtract 32 from the Fahrenheit reading. Then multiply by $\frac{5}{9}$ (Fig. 18-4).

NOTE Remember these temperature conversion formulas:
Celsius to Fahrenheit: (°C $\frac{9}{5}$) + 32
Fahrenheit to Celsius: (°F − 32) ($\frac{5}{9}$)

DRUG CALCULATIONS

While providing emergency care, the paramedic must calculate adult and pediatric drug dosages and infusion rates, as well as the strength of drug solutions and diluted solutions. These tasks involve the use of basic math skills in a logical order. This requires a working knowledge of decimals, fractions, ratios, and proportions. This text offers common equations used for drug calculations. These equations are accepted in the medical community. Other drug calculation methods may work as well (Box 18-2).

Calculation Methods

Paramedics should choose a method of calculation that is precise and reliable. To perform drug calculations, paramedics should

- Convert all units of measure to the same unit and system.

BOX 18-2 "T" Method of Calculating Conversions, Drug Doses, and IV Flow Rates

The "T" method is a method for calculating conversions, drug doses, and IV flow rates that does not require advanced mathematical skills. Guidelines for using the T method for calculating a drug dose are listed below:

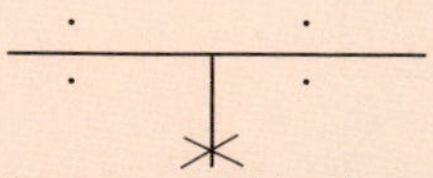

1. One T is required for every step in the calculation. (To use the T method, you must know two things: [1] the prescribed dose, and [2] the gram or milligram or microgram per mL concentration of the drug.)
2. The number entered on the lower right side of the T is always a "given in 1" (a known factor, such as known in 1 mL or known in 1 kg), or a multiple of 10 when converting within the metric system, that will never have to be solved for. The answer solved for in the equation will always be on top of the T or in the lower left side. The number on top of the T is always the larger number (either a known number or one to be solved for). The number in the lower left side is always the smaller number (either a known number or one to be solved for).

Larger Number	
Smaller Number	Given in 1

3. If a number is placed on top of the T, it will always be divided by the other number in the T to find the answer.

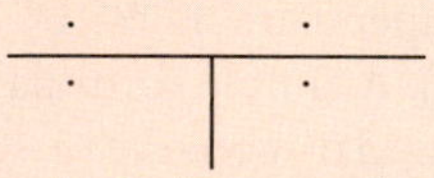

4. If both numbers are in the bottom of the T, multiplication must be performed to find the answer.

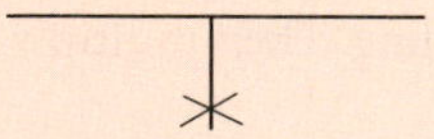

Example 1: You are to administer meperidine 25 mg IM. You have 50 mg of the drug in 1 mL of solution. How many milliliters will you give?

Step 1:
Place the "given" (50 mg/in 1 mL) in the lower right corner of the T.

	50 mg in 1 mL

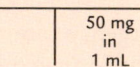

Step 2:
Place the larger number (the desired dose of 25 mg) on top of the T.

25 mg	
	50 mg in 1 mL

Step 3:
Divide 25 by 50 (basic formula) to obtain the smaller number (the required dose of 0.5 mL).

25 mg	
(0.5 mL)	50 mg

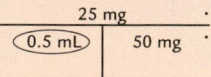

Example 2: You are to administer lidocaine 1 mg/kg IV to a 177-pound man. You have 100 mg in 5 mL of solution. How many milliliters will you give? This calculation will require four steps (four Ts).

Step 1:
Convert the patient's weight to kilograms:

177 lb	
(80 kg)	2.2 lb in 1 kg

Step 2:
Calculate the prescribed dose in milligrams:

80 mg	
1 mg	80 kg

Step 3:
Determine the mg/mL concentration of the drug. (Remember, in this example, there are 5 mL of solution, not 1 mL.)

100 mg	
(20 mg per mL)	5 mL

Step 4:
Use the basic formula to calculate the dose:

80 mg	
(4 mL)	20 mg in 1 mL

BOX 18-2 "T" Method of Calculating Conversions, Drug Doses, and IV Flow Rates, cont'd

Example 3: You are to administer atropine 0.02 mg/kg IV to a pediatric patient who weighs 30 pounds. You have 1 mg of the drug in 10 mL of solution. How many milliliters will you give? This calculation will require four steps (four Ts).

Step 1:
Convert the patient's weight to kilograms:

30 lb	
(13.6 kg)	2.2 lb in 1 kg

Step 2:
Calculate the prescribed dose in milligrams:

0.27 mg	
0.02 mg	13.6 kg

Step 3:
Determine the mg/mL concentration of the drug.

1 mg	
(0.1 mg/mL)	10 mL

Step 4:
Use the basic formula to calculate the dose:

0.27 mg	
(2.7 mL)	0.1 mg/ in 1 mL

- Check the computed dosage to determine whether it is reasonable.
- Use one dosage calculation method consistently.

CONVERSION OF UNITS OF MEASURE

Most emergency drug preparations do not require conversion. Most drugs are packaged in milligrams and administered in milligrams. However, some drugs, such as ***dopamine,*** are packaged in milligrams but administered in micrograms (μg). These drugs must be converted to like units. When conversion to like units is required, the conversion must be done before the drug dose is calculated.

Example

You are to administer ***dopamine*** at a rate of 800 μg per minute. You have 200 mg of the drug in 250 mL of solution. Convert 800 μg to 0.8 mg so that both measures of weight are in the same units:

$$800\ \mu g \div 1000 = 0.8\ mg$$

CRITICAL THINKING

Imagine that you failed to convert the 800 μg of dopamine to 0.8 mg in this example. Would you overdose or underdose your patient?

NOTE *Math tip:* Move the decimal point to the right when multiplying (converting the measurement to smaller units). Move it to the left when dividing (converting the measurement to larger units).

When the dose is given per unit of weight (kg), the patient's weight must be converted from pounds to kilograms. This should be done before the total dose to be given is calculated.

Example

You are to give 1 mg/kg of ***lidocaine*** to a patient who weighs 132 lb. Divide 132 by 2.2 to convert pounds to kilograms (132 lb = 60 kg). The total dose equals 1 mg/kg multiplied by 60 kg. This equals 60 mg.

$$132\ lb \div 2.2 = 60\ kg$$
$$1\ mg/kg \times 60\ kg = 60\ mg$$

ASSESSMENT OF COMPUTED DOSES

Many emergency drugs are packaged in units that contain enough drug for a normal adult dose. After doing the math, the paramedic should decide whether the answer is reasonable.

Example

You are to administer 8 mg of ***diazepam.*** It is supplied in a 2 mL ampule that contains 10 mg of the drug. Therefore, a reasonable calculation of volume would be less than 2 mL.

Methods of Calculation

Many drug calculations can be performed almost intuitively. This is because many drugs are packaged to supply one adult dose. However, a paramedic should never rely on intuitive calculations, no matter how simple the drug dose may seem. The three methods of calculation discussed below are in common use.

METHOD 1: BASIC FORMULA ("DESIRE OVER HAVE")

For method 1, information must be substituted in the following formula:

$$\frac{D}{H} \times Q = X$$

In this formula, *D* is the desired dose to be given. *H* is the known dose on hand. *Q* is the unit of measure or volume on hand. *X* is the unit of measure to be given. Many consider "desire over have" to be the easiest formula to use. It works for nearly all emergency drug calculations.

Example

You are to administer 25 mg of ***diphenhydramine.*** You have a 10 mL vial that contains 50 mg of the drug. How many milliliters will you give? Using the desire over have formula, calculate the dose.

$$\frac{25 \text{ mg}}{50 \text{ mg}} \times 10 \text{ mL} = \text{X}$$

$$\frac{25}{5} \times 1 \text{ mL} = \text{X}$$

$$5 \times 1 \text{ mL} = \text{X}$$

$$\text{X} = 5 \text{ mL}$$

▶**NOTE** *Math tip:* When using the basic formula, always divide the bottom number into the top number.

METHOD 2: RATIOS AND PROPORTIONS

Method 2 uses ratios and proportions to calculate the drug dosage. A *ratio* compares two numbers and is the same as a fraction. When used to calculate drug doses, a ratio refers to the weight or quantity of a drug in solution. For example, the ratio of 10 mg of ***morphine*** in 1 mL of solution is 10 mg to 1 mL. A *proportion* is an equation made up of two ratios; it states that the two ratios are equal. For example, $^2/_3$ is equal to $^4/_6$ (2 : 3 :: 4 : 6); therefore the ratios are equivalent and the proportions are true.

To use method 2, the equation must be set up to ensure that the same units of measure are stated in the same sequence (e.g., mg : mL = mg : *x* mL). *x* is the quantity (e.g., mL) to be solved. The formula can be expressed as

Dose on Hand : Volume on Hand :: Desired Dose : Desired Volume

Example

You are to administer 40 mg of ***furosemide.*** You have 100 mg of the drug in 10 mL of solution. How many milliliters will you give? Calculate the dose using ratios and proportions:

100 mg : 10 mL :: 40 mg : *x* mL

Multiply inside numbers (means) and outside numbers (extremes). Drop the unit of measurement terms.

Means

100 mg : 10 mL :: 40 mg : *x* mL

Extremes

▶**NOTE** *Math tip:* Remember the phrases *middle for means* and *end for extremes.* In a proportion, the product of the means is always equal to the product of the extremes.

Solve the proportion by dividing both sides of the equation by the number before x (100).

$$\frac{100x}{100} \times \frac{400}{100} = 4 \text{ mL}$$

To check your answer, multiply the means and then multiply the extremes. The sum product will be equal if the proportion is true.

$$\left.\begin{array}{l}100 \times 4 = 400 \\ 10 \times 40 = 400\end{array}\right\} \text{Sum parts are equal}$$

METHOD 3: DIMENSIONAL ANALYSIS

Dimensional analysis works well for complex drug calculations. These may call for several conversions of a similar basic dimensional unit so that all units of measure are changed to like units (e.g., milligrams). Dimensional analysis is based on the same tenet as the basic formula. However, it does not require memorization of the desire over have equation. All conversion factors are set up in one equation. They are separated by multiplication signs.

▶**NOTE** *Math tip:* When using dimensional analysis, convert all units to the easiest math operation. This reduces the chance of error.

Example

You are to administer 0.8 mg of ***naloxone.*** The drug is packaged in 1 mL of solution containing 0.4 mg of the drug.

Step 1: Set up the equation, placing the desired unit of measure in the answer to the left of the equal sign. Place the first factor to the right of the equal sign. Make sure it is the same unit as the answer.

$$\text{mL} = \frac{1 \text{ mL}}{0.4 \text{ mg}} \times \frac{0.8 \text{ mg}}{1}$$

Step 2: Cancel like units of measure in the numerator and denominator, and reduce the fraction, if needed:

$$\text{mL} = \frac{1 \text{ mL}}{0.4 \cancel{\text{mg}}} \times \frac{0.8 \cancel{\text{mg}}}{1}$$

▶**NOTE** *Math tip:* The only unit remaining after canceling the like units should be the unit of the answer. If this is not the case, the equation is set up incorrectly.

Step 3: Multiply the numerators and then the denominators.

$$\text{mL} = \frac{1 \text{ mL}}{0.4} \times \frac{0.8}{1}$$

Step 4: Divide the numerator by the denominator to solve the equation.

$$\text{mL} = \frac{0.8 \text{ mL}}{0.4} = 2 \text{ mL}$$

Calculating Intravenous Flow Rates

To calculate intravenous (IV) flow rates, paramedics must know three factors. First, they must know the volume to be infused. Second, they must know the period of time, in minutes, over which the fluid is to be infused. Third, they must know the number of drops (gtt) per milliliter the infusion set delivers *(drop factor)*. The flow rate can then be calculated using the following equation:

$$\text{gtt/min} = \frac{\text{Volume to be infused} \times \text{Drop factor}}{\text{Duration of infusion (minutes)}}$$

Example

You are to give 250 mL of normal saline over 90 minutes. Your infusion set delivers 10 gtt/mL. Calculate the drops per minute using the above formula.

$$\text{gtt/min} = \frac{250\ \cancel{\text{mL}} \times 10\ \text{gtt}/\cancel{\text{mL}}}{90\ \text{minutes}} = \frac{2500\ \text{gtt}}{90\ \text{min}} =$$

27.7 or 28 gtt/min

▶**NOTE** The two intravenous (IV) infusion sets most often used in emergency care are microdrip tubing and macrodrip tubing. Microdrip tubing delivers 60 gtt/mL. Macrodrip tubing delivers 10, 15, or 20 gtt/mL. *Math tip:* When a drop factor of 60 is used, the gtt/min always equals the mL/hr infusion.

CRITICAL THINKING

When would it be best to use microdrip tubing? When would it be better to use macrodrip tubing?

Calculating Infusion Rates

Paramedics may need to administer medications via a continuous IV infusion. Calculating the correct drip rate is crucial (Box 18-3 and Box 18-4). This helps to avoid overdosing or underdosing the patient. To properly calculate and give a prescribed drug by continuous infusion, paramedics must know three things. First, they must know the prescribed dose. Second, they must know the concentration of the drug in 1 mL of solution. Third, they must know the drop factor of the IV infusion set. The calculation is then made using the following IV drip formula:

$$\text{gtt/min} = \frac{\text{Prescribed dose} \times \text{Drop factor}}{\text{Concentration of drug in 1 mL}}$$

Example

You are to administer a ***procainamide*** infusion at 3 mg/min. You have 1 g of the drug in 250 mL of 5% dextrose in water (D_5W). The infusion set delivers 60 gtt/mL. How many drops per minute will you deliver?

Convert all units to like measurements and calculate the concentration of the drug in 1 mL.

$$1\ \text{g} \times 1000 = 1000\ \text{mg}$$
$$1000\ \text{mg} \div 250\ \text{mL} = 4\ \text{mg/mL}$$

Calculate the drops per minute using the IV drip formula:

$$\text{gtt/min} = \frac{3\ \text{mg/min} \times 60\ \text{gtt/mL}}{4\ \text{mg in 1 mL}} = \frac{180}{4} = 45\ \text{gtt/min}$$

BOX 18-3 "Clock" Method of Calculating Flow Rates

Visualize a clock to calculate flow rates of IV medications. For example, if the concentration of a drug in solution is 4 mg/mL and microdrip tubing is used that delivers 1 mL in 60 drops, and 60 drops are delivered in 1 minute, then 4 mg will be delivered with every 60 drops of solution. Picturing a clock where 4 mg and 60 drops are at the 12:00 position, you can calculate that 15 drops/minute will deliver 1 mg/minute; 30 drops will deliver 2 mg/min; and 45 drops will deliver 3 mg/min. You can use this same method with any drug in solution when microdrip is being used.

LIDOCAINE INFUSION CLOCK

- Mix 2 g of lidocaine in 500 mL D_5W or NS (or 1 g in 250 mL) = 4 mg/mL
- Infusion dose range = 2-4 mg / min
- When administered with a minidrip (60 gtt / mL) intravenous administration set, lidocaine drip rates resemble a seconds "clock"

60 gtts / min = 4 mg / min

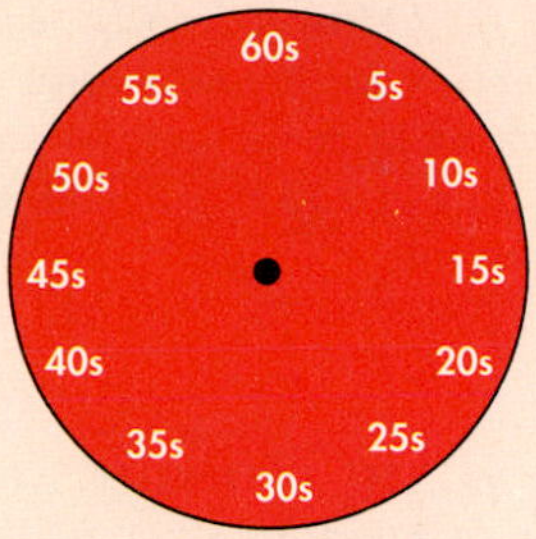

30 gtts / min = 2 mg / min

BOX 18-4 Shortcut for Calculating Dopamine Drips

Dopamine is a very strong drug. Calculating the correct dose can daunt the best mathematician. The following is a shortcut for calculating dopamine infusions using 60 drop/minute intravenous (IV) tubing and a standard mixture of drug in solution (e.g., 400 mg in 250 mL; 800 mg in 500 mL).

Formula:

$$\frac{\text{Dose} \times \text{Weight (kg)} \times 60\ \text{Drops/min}}{1600} = \text{Drops per minute}$$

Example:

You are to administer 5 µg/kg of dopamine per minute to a 75 kg patient.

$$\frac{5\ \mu\text{g} \times 75\ \text{kg} \times 60\ \text{Drops/min}}{1600} = 14\ \text{Drops per minute}$$

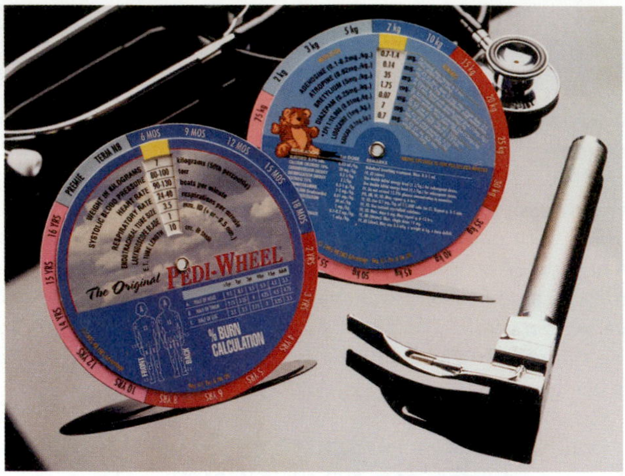

FIGURE 18-5 ■ PediWheel.

▶**NOTE** *Math tip:* Most advanced cardiac life support (ACLS) drugs (except for ***dopamine*** and ***magnesium sulfate***) that are administered by continuous IV infusion are mixed "1 in 250" (1 g of drug in 250 mL of solution) to yield a concentration of 4 mg/mL.

Calculating Drug Dosages for Infants and Children

The doses of some medications for infants and children are administered in the same proportion to body weight as the doses for adults. Others are given in very reduced doses. This is due to differences in the child's ability to metabolize the drug. Pediatric drug doses are often calculated in the prehospital setting by using memory aids or with the advice of medical direction. Some of the memory aids are charts, tapes, dosage books, and dosage wheels (Fig. 18-5). The most precise way to calculate a pediatric drug dose is based on the child's body surface area. Body surface area as a function of weight is described in Chapter 44.

▶**NOTE** Paramedics are authorized to administer a medication. This authorization is given through an on-line or off-line process either by phone, cell phone, or radio. The paramedics must follow all care protocols, policies, and procedures. This is their legal duty. These policies specify the regulations of administration. This includes policies on the stocking and supply of drugs.

DRUG ADMINISTRATION

During the administration of any drug, safety should always be a high priority.

Safety Considerations and Procedures

Paramedics should follow these guidelines when administering drugs to patients:

- Focus on the procedure and avoid distractions (including when preparing the medicines).
- In the prehospital setting, make sure you clearly understand medication orders received from medical direction. Repeat all orders back to medical direction for confirmation. Do this before administering a drug. In the emergency department or other patient care areas, make sure you have a written order for every medication you administer. Verify the patient's name on the person's armband or identification tag. Also, verify that the patient is not allergic to the medication. Strictly follow these *five patient rights* of drug administration: Make sure the *right* patient receives the *right* dose of the *right* drug via the *right* route at the *right* time. Also make sure to document the drug administration accurately and thoroughly. This is the sixth patient right of drug administration.
- Make a habit of reading the label of the medicine and comparing it to the medication order at least three times before administration:

  First—When removing the drug from the drug kit or supply area

  Second—When preparing the medication for administration

  Third—Just before administering the drug to the patient (before the container is discarded).
- Always check the correct route of administration. Some medications can be prepared for administration by several routes. For instance, the route could be intramuscular or intravenous.
- Make sure the information on the label matches the prescriber's order.
- Never give a medicine from an unlabeled container. Also, never give a medicine from a container on which the label is not legible.
- If you are unsure of your drug calculation, have a coworker check it. You also can contact medical direction for verification.
- Handle multidose vials carefully. Use aseptic technique. This way, medicines are not wasted or contaminated.
- When preparing more than one injection, always label the syringe immediately. Keep the medication container with the syringe. Do not rely on your memory to recall which solution is in which syringe.
- Never administer a medicine that is unlabeled and that was prepared by someone else. In doing so, you accept the blame. You will be responsible for accuracy, dose, and correct medication.
- Never administer a medication that is outdated. Likewise, never give one that looks discolored, cloudy, or in any other way unusual, or as if someone has tampered with it.
- If the patient or your co-workers express doubt or concern about a medication or dose, recheck it. Do not administer

it until you are sure no error has been made. Remember that the patient has the right to refuse a medication.

- Carefully monitor the patient for any adverse effects. Monitor for at least 5 minutes after you give the medication. (Intramuscular and oral medicines may require longer monitoring.)
- Document all medications given. This includes the name of the drug, the dosage, and the time and route of administration. When documenting parenteral medications, note the site of injection. The patient's response, adverse as well as intended, also is recorded.
- It is critical to return and dispose of any unused medication. Follow all guidelines set by the government and the local emergency medical services (EMS) agency.

CRITICAL THINKING

Your clinical preceptor hands you an unlabeled syringe of medication and tells you to give it by means of intramuscular injection. What do you do?

Medication Errors

Medication errors occur with some frequency. More than 700,000 patients receive the wrong medicine or the incorrect dose of medicine in U.S. hospitals each year.[3] About 7000 people die from medication errors each year.[4] Common causes of medication errors include the following:

- The prescriber ordered the wrong dose of medication.
- Drug calculations were incorrect.
- Drugs were administered via the wrong route.
- The drug was given to the wrong patient.

If a medication error occurs, paramedics should do the following:

- Accept responsibility for the error.
- Advise medical direction or the prescriber right away.
- Assess and monitor the patient. Monitor for effects of the drug.
- Document the error. Make sure to follow local and state drug administration policies and those of the medical direction institution.
- Make changes in their personal practice technique to helps prevent such an error in the future.
- Follow EMS agency procedures to document the incident. Follow activities for quality improvement as identified by your EMS agency.

MEDICAL ASEPSIS

Medical asepsis is the removal or destruction of disease-causing organisms or infected material. Medical asepsis is performed by using clean technique (rather than sterile technique). *Clean technique* requires hygienic measures, cleaning agents, antiseptics, disinfectants, and barrier fields.

NOTE *Sterile technique* means using sterile equipment and sterile fields that are free of all forms and types of life. This is also known as *surgical asepsis. Clean technique* focuses on destroying or inhibiting only pathogens (not all forms and types of life).

BOX 18-5 Examples of Antiseptics and Disinfectants

Antiseptics	Disinfectants
Hexachlorophene	Cresol
Silver nitrate	Carbolic acid
Benzoyl peroxide	Lysol

Antiseptics and Disinfectants

Antiseptics and disinfectants are chemical agents. They are used to kill specific groups of microorganisms. They generally do not work very well against spores of bacteria and fungi, many viruses, and some resistant bacterial strains. Disinfectants are used only on nonliving objects. They are toxic to living tissue. Antiseptics are applied only to living tissue. They are more dilute, to prevent cell damage. Some chemical agents have both antiseptic and disinfectant properties. Examples of these are alcohol and some chlorine compounds (Box 18-5 and Table 18-2).

UNIVERSAL PRECAUTIONS IN MEDICATION ADMINISTRATION

Universal precautions should be a crucial part of an encounter with a patient. (These are described in the chapter appendix.) When administering drugs, paramedics should follow handwashing procedures. They should also follow gloving procedures if indicated. Face shields should be used during administration of endotracheal drugs.

NOTE Many consider handwashing the most crucial step in reducing the risk of transmission of organisms from one person to another or from one site to another on a patient.[4] Handwashing protects both the paramedic and the patient. If soap and water are not available, a sanitizing gel or wipe should be used.

ENTERAL ADMINISTRATION OF MEDICATIONS

Enteral medications are drugs that are administered and absorbed through the gastrointestinal tract (see Chapter 17). Enteral drugs are given by means of oral, gastric, or rectal administration.

Oral Route

The oral route is the most frequently used method of drug administration. The patient should be in an upright or sitting position. The pill, tablet, or capsule should be placed

TABLE 18-2 Sterilization and Disinfection Methods for Equipment Used by Paramedics

ORGANISMS DESTROYED	METHODS	USES
Sterilization		
All forms of microbial life, including high numbers of bacterial spores	Steam under pressure (autoclave), gas (ethylene oxide), dry heat, or immersion in an EPA-approved chemical sterilant for a prolonged period (e.g., 6 to 10 hours or according to the manufacturer's instructions). *Note:* Liquid chemical sterilants should be used only on instruments that cannot be sterilized or disinfected with heat.	Instruments or devices that penetrate the skin or come into contact with normally sterile areas of the body (e.g., scalpels, needles). Use of disposable invasive equipment eliminates the need to reprocess these items. When indicated, however, arrangements should be made with a health care facility for reprocessing of reusable invasive instruments.
High-Level Disinfection		
All forms of microbial life except high numbers of bacterial spores	Hot water pasteurization (176° to 212° F [80° to 100° C] for 30 minutes), or exposure to an EPA-registered chemical sterilant, except for a short exposure time (10 to 45 minutes or as directed by the manufacturer).	Reusable instruments or devices that come into contact with mucous membranes (e.g., laryngoscope blades, endotracheal tubes).
Intermediate-Level Disinfection		
Mycobacterium tuberculosis, vegetative bacteria, most viruses, and most fungi, but not bacterial spores	EPA-registered hospital disinfectant chemical germicides with a label claim of tuberculocidal activity; commercially available hard surface germicides; or solutions with at least 500 parts per million (ppm) free available chlorine (a 1:100 dilution of common household bleach—approximately 1 cup of bleach per gallon of tap water).	Instruments and equipment that come into contact only with intact skin (e.g., stethoscopes, blood pressure cuffs, splints) and that have been visibly contaminated with blood or bloody body fluids. Surfaces must be cleaned of visible material before the germicide is applied.
Low-Level Disinfection		
Most bacteria, some viruses, some fungi, but not *Mycobacterium tuberculosis* or bacterial spores	EPA-registered hospital disinfectants (no label claim for tuberculocidal activity).	Routine housekeeping or removal of soiling in the absence of visible blood contamination.
Environmental Disinfection		
	Any cleaner or disinfectant agent intended for environmental use.	Environmental surfaces that have become soiled and that should be cleaned and disinfected (e.g., floors, woodwork, ambulance seats, countertops).

*To ensure the effectiveness of any sterilization or disinfection process, equipment and instruments must first be thoroughly cleaned of all visible soiling.
EPA, Environmental Protection Agency.

in the patient's mouth and swallowed with enough fluid (4 to 8 ounces) to make sure the drug reaches the stomach.

CRITICAL THINKING

Think of some clinical situations in which oral administration of a drug would not be the best technique. Why is this so?

Many oral drugs come in solid and liquid forms (Box 18-6). If the medication is in a suspension, the stock bottle or unit dose should be shaken thoroughly before the drug is poured for administration. A drug not packaged as a unit dose should be measured in a medicine cup or a medicine dropper or by syringe.

Administration of Medications by Gastric Tube

Most drugs that can be given orally can also be given via a gastric tube (orogastric tube, nasogastric tube). Before giving a drug by this route, the paramedic must make sure the tube has been inserted correctly (see Chapter 34). This can be done by injecting 30 mL to 50 mL of air into the tube and auscultating the epigastric region for the sound of air movement. Once correct insertion has been verified, the drug is administered through the tube, followed by a small amount of water (about 30 mL). The water flushes the drug and helps to maintain the patency of the tube. An emergency drug that is given by gastric tube is ***activated charcoal.***

BOX 18-6 Forms of Solid and Liquid Oral Medications

- Caplets
- Capsules
- Time-released capsules
- Lozenges
- Pills
- Tablets
- Elixirs
- Emulsions
- Suspensions
- Syrups

BOX 18-7 Procedure for Administering Rectal Drugs*

1. Carefully restrain the child. If possible, place the child in a knee-chest or lateral recumbent position with the legs flexed at the hips and the knees.
2. Draw the drug dose into a syringe and remove the needle. (A slightly higher dose may be required because absorption is incomplete. Consult medical direction.)
3. Insert the lubricated syringe just beyond the external sphincter (aiming just above the junction of the skin and mucous membranes and toward the rectal wall).
4. Inject the solution into the rectum.
5. Aid drug retention by squeezing the buttocks together with manual pressure.

*Although the procedure is described for a child, it also is appropriate for adults.

Rectal Administration of Medications

Some drugs, such as suppositories, are made for rectal administration (Box 18-7). Other drugs can be given by the rectal route when vascular access cannot be established. Emergency drugs that can be given rectally include ***diazepam*** and ***lorazepam.***

PARENTERAL ADMINISTRATION OF MEDICATIONS

Parenteral drugs are administered outside the gastrointestinal tract. This term usually refers to injections. Drugs are administered parenterally by the intradermal, subcutaneous, intramuscular, intravenous, and intraosseous routes. (Percutaneous medications also are discussed in this section.)

NOTE Parenteral administration of drugs can be very hazardous. This is because drugs given by injection are usually thought to be irretrievable. Also, a slight risk of infection exists because the skin is broken. Other possible hazards associated with parenteral administration include cellulitis or abscess formation, necrosis, skin sloughing, nerve injury, prolonged pain, and periostitis (inflammation of connective tissue covering bones). The use of aseptic technique, ensuring an accurate drug dosage, finding the proper site for the injection, and administering the injection at the proper rate are essential to minimize the risk of harm.

Equipment Used for Injections

SYRINGES AND NEEDLES

The choice of syringe and needle depends on three factors: (1) the route of administration, (2) the characteristics of the fluid (e.g., aqueous or oil based), and (3) the volume of medication. Syringes in common use today are made of disposable plastic. Sizes range from 1 mL tuberculin and insulin syringes to 60 mL irrigation syringes.

Tuberculin syringes are marked in 0.01 mL gradients. They should be used when the volume to be given is small. Insulin syringes are available in 0.5 and 1 mL volumes. They are marked in 1-unit increments. When used with the specified strength of insulin, this syringe allows the patient to draw up the correct dose easily without doing any calculations. Tuberculin and insulin syringes should not be substituted for each other. Fig. 18-6 shows syringes used to accurately measure varying amounts of liquids and liquid medications.

Needles vary in length and gauge. Length ranges from ⅜ inch to 3 inches or longer. Gauge ranges from 12 gauge (large lumen) to 30 gauge (small lumen). Smaller lumen (larger gauge) needles are usually used for intradermal injections. Subcutaneous injections are usually given with a ⅝-inch, 23- or 25-gauge needle. Intramuscular injections are usually given with a 1- to 2-inch, 19- or 21-gauge needle; occasionally a 16- or 18-gauge needle is used.

In 2000 Congress passed the Healthcare Worker Needlestick Prevention Act. The following year, the Occupational Safety and Health Administration (OSHA) amended its Bloodborne Pathogens Standard to recommend needleless systems or "needle safe" devices (sharps with engineered sharps protection). These devices collect body fluids or deliver medications without the use of a needle. Thus, they help prevent blood exposure and needlestick injury (Box 18-8). Examples of these devices include self-sheathing hypodermic syringes, self-blunting phlebotomy needles, retracting lancets, and disposable retracting scalpels.

CONTAINERS USED FOR PARENTERAL MEDICATIONS

Medications given by injection are usually supplied in three forms. They come in single-dose ampules, multidose vials, or prefilled syringes. Single-dose ampules are glass containers that hold one dose of a medication for injection. After use, the ampule is thrown away. Multidose vials are glass containers that come with rubber stoppers. These permit several medication doses to be withdrawn for injection.

Paramedics must prepare a medication for injection. To do this, they must pick the right needle and syringe. The size of the syringe must be in proportion to the volume of solution to be given. To withdraw medication from an ampule or vial, the paramedic should follow these steps:

1. Assemble the equipment (alcohol swab or gauze, syringe, 18-gauge needle to withdraw medication if using an ampule, and appropriate-gauge needle for injection).
2. Compute the volume of medication to be given.

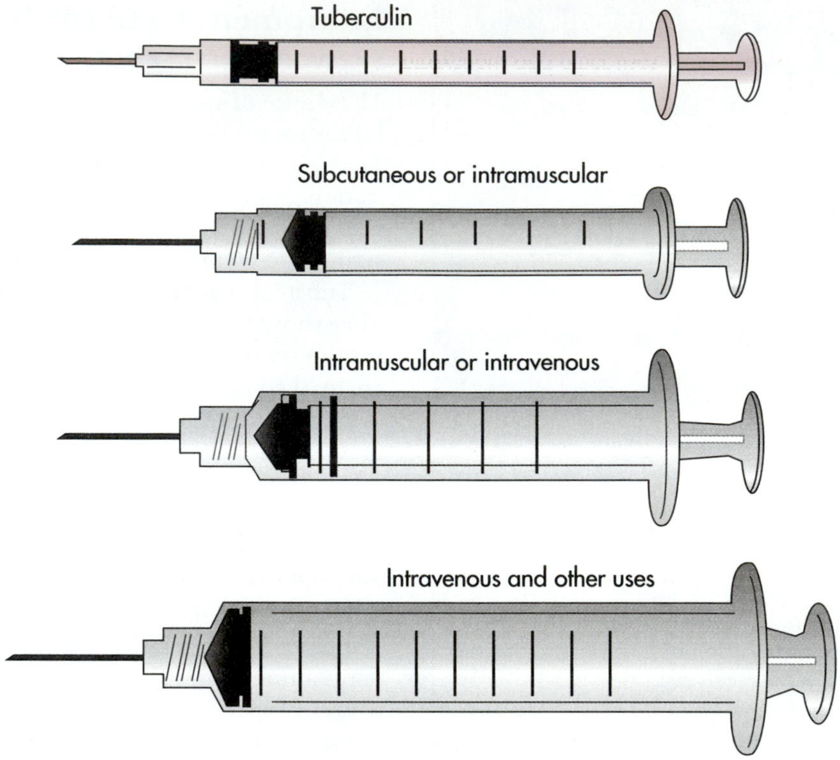

FIGURE 18-6 ■ Syringes.

> **BOX 18-8 Prevention of Needle and Sharps Injuries**
>
> Each year, health care workers suffer 600,000 to 1 million injuries from conventional needles and sharps.* Infection with the hepatitis C virus (HCV) is the most common infection caused by needle-stick and sharps injury.† However, the transmission of other diseases also is possible. These diseases include human immunodeficiency virus (HIV) infection, hepatitis B, syphilis, herpes simplex, herpes zoster, Rocky Mountain spotted fever, and tuberculosis. The following precautions can help prevent exposure to these pathogens:
>
> - Paramedics should get help when administering infusion therapy or injections to uncooperative patients.
> - Needles should not be recapped, purposely bent or broken by hand, removed from disposable syringes, or otherwise manipulated by hand. If a needle must be recapped or removed because there is no alternative or because a specific medical procedure requires it, the paramedic should use a mechanical device or a one-handed technique. Needleless products should be used when available.
> - Disposable syringes and needles, scalpel blades, and other sharp items should be placed in puncture-resistant containers for disposal.

*Evaluation of safety devices for preventing percutaneous injuries among healthcare workers during phlebotomy procedures, *Morbidity and Mortality Weekly Report* 46 (02): 21-25, 1997.

†Recommendations for prevention and control of hepatitis C virus (HCV) infection and HCV-related chronic disease, *Morbidity and Mortality Weekly Report* 47 (RR-19), 1-39, 1998.

3. If using a vial (Fig. 18-7):
   (a) Clean the rubber stopper with alcohol.
   (b) Using the needle chosen for the injection, inject a volume of air into the vial equivalent to the amount of solution to be withdrawn. (This prevents the formation of a vacuum in the vial. A vacuum can make the solution hard to withdraw.) Withdraw the volume required and remove the syringe from the vial.
   (c) Gently push in the plunger of the syringe to expel air from the solution.
4. If using an ampule (Fig. 18-8):
   (a) Lightly tap or shake the ampule to dislodge any solution from the neck of the container.
   (b) Wrap the neck of the glass ampule with an alcohol swab or gauze dressing to protect the fingers.
   (c) Grasp the ampule, snap off the top, and discard the top in an appropriate medication disposal container. (The ampule is designed to break easily when pressure is exerted at the neck.)
   (d) Carefully insert an 18-gauge needle (a filter needle, if recommended by the drug manufacturer to retain particles in the solution) into the solution without allowing it to touch the edges of the ampule and draw the solution into the syringe.
   (e) Carefully remove the 18-gauge needle and discard it in the appropriate container. Attach the needle to be used for injection.
   (f) Gently push in the plunger of the syringe to expel air.

Some hospitals and EMS services require the use of a filter needle. This is a precaution against the inclusion of

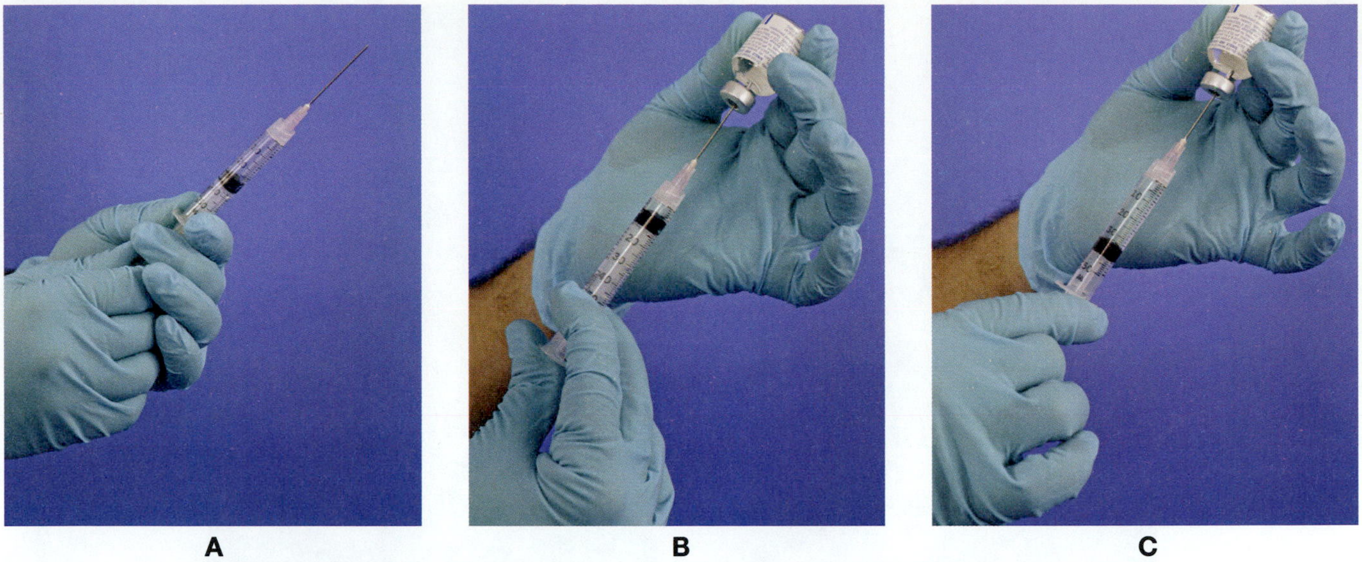

FIGURE 18-7 ■ Withdrawing medication from a vial. **A,** An amount of air equal to the volume to be given is drawn into the syringe. **B,** The air is injected into the drug vial. **C,** The drug is drawn into the syringe.

glass particles when medications are withdrawn from an ampule. A further precaution is the use of in-line tubing filters for intravenous injections.

Mixing Medications. Two compatible drugs can be mixed into one injection if the total volume of the dosage is within accepted limits. For example, this technique can be used with ***meperidine*** and ***hydroxyzine.*** When mixing medications, it is crucial not to contaminate one with the other. It also is crucial to maintain aseptic technique. Any doubt about compatibility should be discussed with medical direction. It also can be verified by consulting a proper reference, such as a drug compatibility chart. To mix medications, the paramedic should follow these steps:

> **NOTE** Some medications are dry powders that must be reconstituted before administration. An example is ***glucagon.*** Carefully read the manufacturer's information. Use the correct amount of the diluent prescribed for this purpose. Always mix the diluent and powder in the closed vial before withdrawing the dose. Some drugs are packaged in a vial that contains the diluent and powder in two compartments (Mix-o-Vial).

Mixing Medications from Two Vials

1. Use only one syringe to mix the drugs.
2. Aspirate a volume of air equivalent to the dose of the first drug. Inject the air into vial A, making sure the needle does not touch the solution. Withdraw the needle.
3. Aspirate a volume of air equivalent to the dose of the second drug. Inject the air into vial B. Withdraw the required medication from vial B.
4. Put a new sterile needle on the syringe and insert it into vial A. Be careful not to push in the plunger or expel the drug from the syringe into the vial. This would pose a risk of infection and result in mixing of the drugs.
5. Withdraw the desired amount of the drug from vial A into the syringe.
6. Put a new sterile needle on the syringe and administer the injection.

Mixing Medications from One Vial and One Ampule

1. Withdraw the desired drug dose from the vial first.
2. Use the same syringe and needle to withdraw medication from the ampule.
3. Put a new sterile needle on the syringe and administer the injection.

Prefilled Syringes. Several manufacturers make prefilled syringes (Fig. 18-9). The techniques for activating and using the products vary. Paramedics should be familiar with the devices used by particular EMS systems. The technique for activating a common type of prefilled syringe is as follows:

1. Calculate the volume of medication to be administered.
2. Remove the protective caps from the syringe barrel and medication cartridge.
3. Screw the cartridge into the syringe barrel.
4. Gently push in the plunger of the syringe to expel air.

PREPARING THE INJECTION SITE

The injection site is prepared by cleansing the area using aseptic technique. The *Guidelines for Prevention of Intravascular Catheter-Related Infections,*[5] published by the Centers for Disease Control and Prevention (CDC), state that "although 2% chlorhexidine-based preparation is preferred, tincture of iodine, an iodophor, or 70% alcohol can be used."

The steps in preparing the injection site are as follows:

1. Thoroughly scrub the site with the appropriate cleanser to remove dirt, dead skin, and other surface contaminants.
2. Clean the site, using overlapping, concentric circles and moving outward from the site.
3. Allow the site to dry.

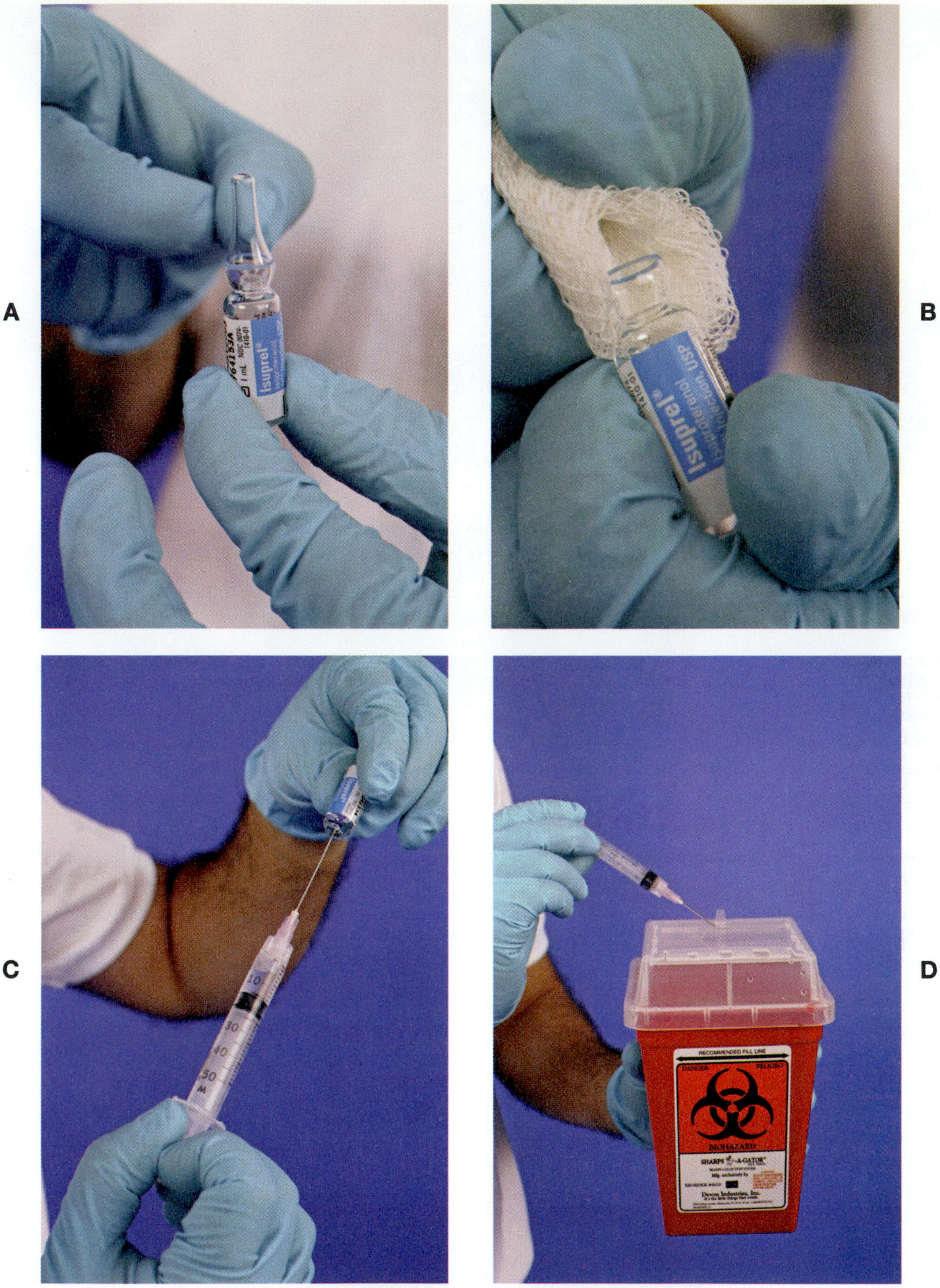

FIGURE 18-8 ■ Withdrawing medication from an ampule. **A,** The ampule is tapped to remove drug from the neck. **B,** The top of the ampule is broken off with a gauze pad. **C,** The drug is withdrawn from ampule. Care must be taken to make sure the needle does not touch the sides of the ampule. **D,** Sharps are discarded in an appropriate container.

A

B

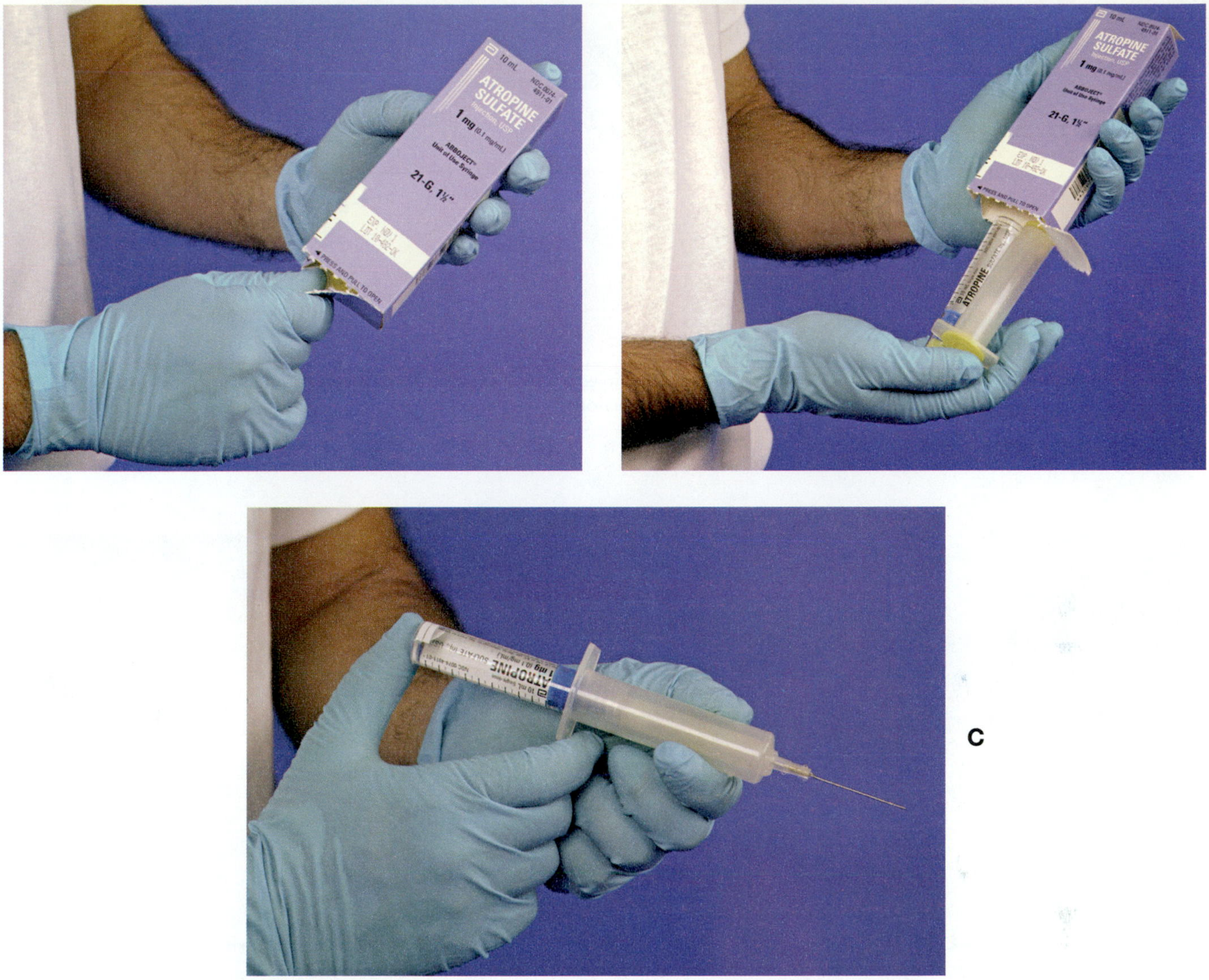

C

FIGURE 18-9 ■ Prefilled medication syringe. **A,** Drug in packaging. **B,** Components in box. C, Assembled syringe with needle.

Intradermal Injections

An intradermal injection is made just below the *epidermis,* or outer layer of skin (Figs. 18-10 and 18-11). This site is commonly used for allergy testing. It also is commonly used for administration of local anesthetics. A tuberculin syringe usually is used for intradermal injections. The volume injected is usually less than 0.5 mL. Common sites for intradermal injections are the medial surface of the forearm and the back. The steps for administering an intradermal injection are as follows:

1. Choose the injection site and cleanse the skin surface.
2. Hold the skin taut with one hand.
3. With the other hand, hold the syringe (with the needle bevel up) at a 10- to 15-degree angle to the injection site.
4. Gently puncture the skin. Insert the needle until the bevel is completely under the skin surface. Inject the medication. (Intradermal injections usually produce a raised wheal that resembles a mosquito bite.)
5. Withdraw the needle and dispose of the equipment appropriately.

Subcutaneous Injections

Subcutaneous injections are given to place medication below the skin into the subcutaneous layer (Fig. 18-12). The volume of such an injection is usually less than 0.5 mL. It is administered through a $\frac{1}{2}$- or $\frac{5}{8}$-inch, 23- or 25-gauge needle. In the prehospital setting, the drug most often given by

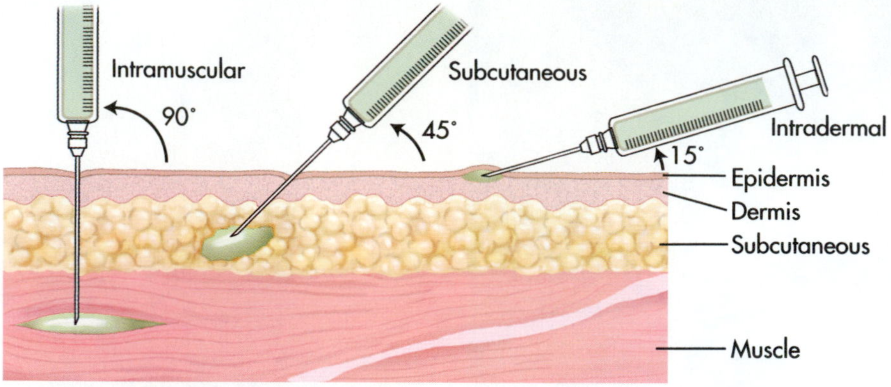

FIGURE 18-10 ■ Comparison of angle of injection and deposition of medication for intramuscular, subcutaneous, and intradermal injections.

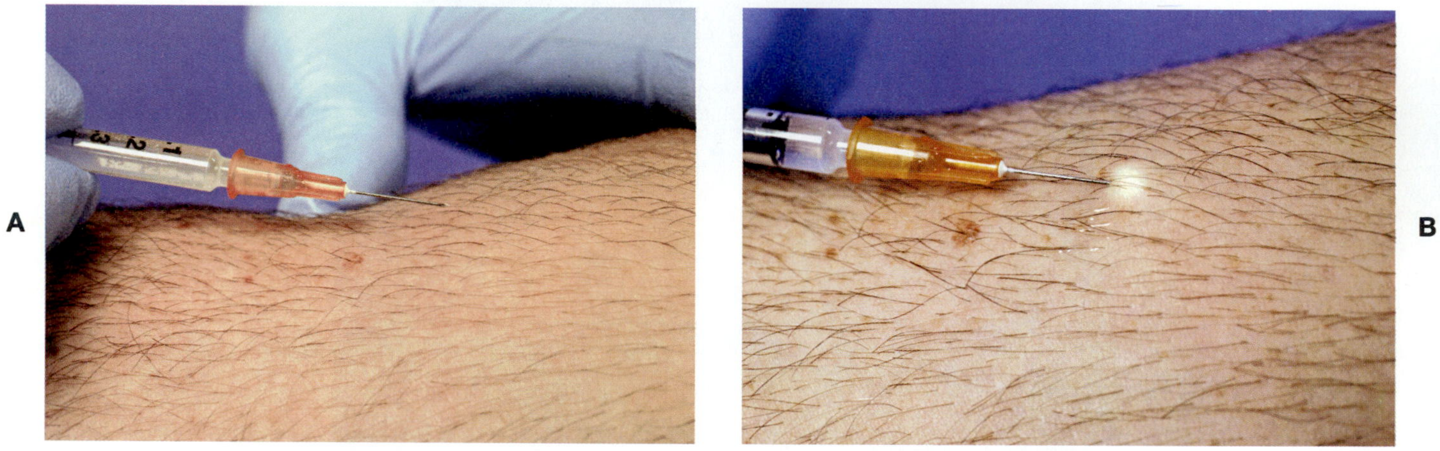

FIGURE 18-11 ■ Intradermal injection. **A,** Choose the site and cleanse the skin. Then, with the bevel up, insert the needle at a 15-degree angle. **B,** Wheal produced by the injection.

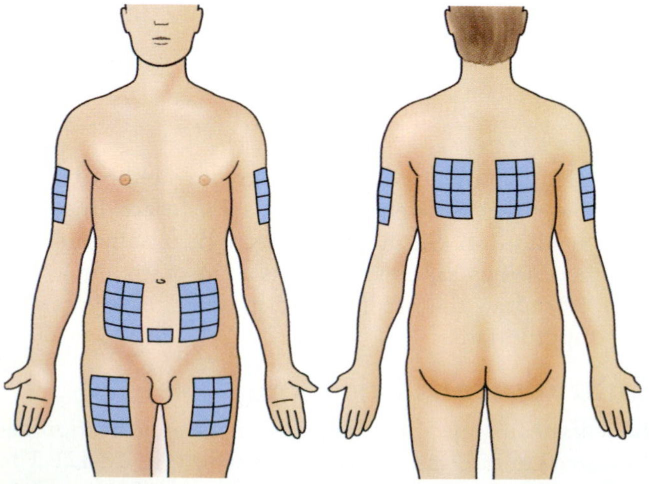

FIGURE 18-12 ■ Sites commonly used for subcutaneous injections.

this route is ***epinephrine.*** The steps for subcutaneous injections are as follows (Fig. 18-13):

1. Choose the injection site and cleanse the area.
2. Elevate the subcutaneous tissue by gently pinching the injection site.
3. With the needle bevel up, insert the needle at a 45-degree angle in one quick motion.
4. Pull back slightly on the plunger (aspirate) to ensure needle placement. If no blood is aspirated, gently but smoothly inject the medication. If blood is present on aspiration, withdraw the needle, discard the medication and equipment, and begin again.
5. After the injection, withdraw the needle at the same angle at which it was inserted. Use an alcohol swab to massage the site. This helps distribute medication and promote absorption by dilating blood vessels in the area and increasing blood flow.

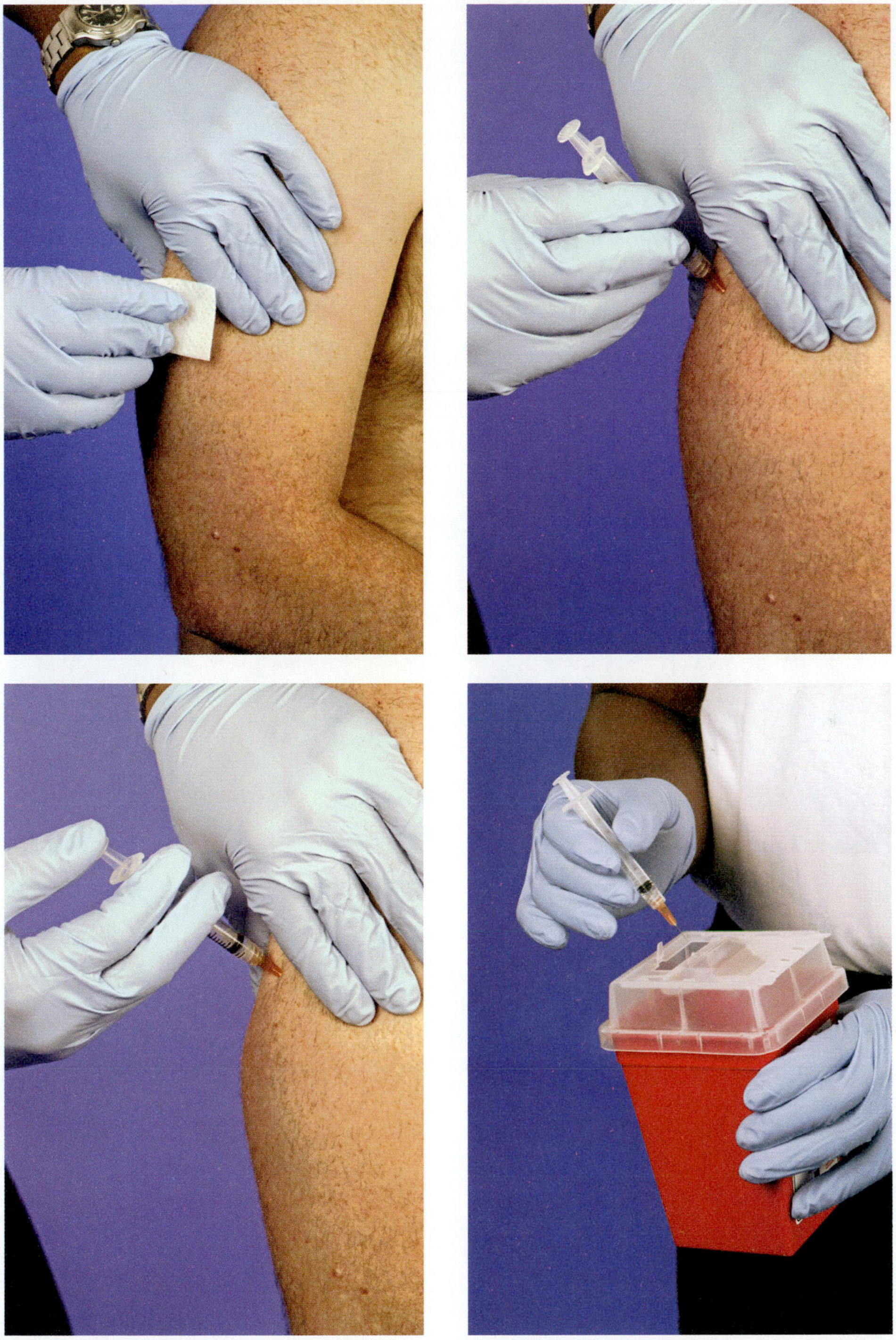

A B C D

FIGURE 18-13 ■ Subcutaneous injection. **A,** Cleanse the skin. Then, grasp it to maximize the amount of subcutaneous tissue available. **B,** Insert the needle. Pull back on the plunger to aspirate (to check needle placement). **C,** Slowly push in the plunger to deliver the medication. **D,** Remove the needle. Discard it in an appropriate container.

Intramuscular Injections

Deeper injections are made into muscle tissue. These pass through the skin and subcutaneous tissue. They are given when a drug is too irritating to be injected subcutaneously or when a greater volume or faster absorption is desired. (Irritation still may occur via this route.) A maximum volume of 5 mL may be given by intramuscular injection in a large muscle mass (e.g., gluteal muscle).

The type of needle used depends on four factors: (1) the site of the injection; (2) the condition of the tissue; (3) the size of the patient; and (4) the type of drug to be injected (i.e., small-lumen needles are used for thin solu-

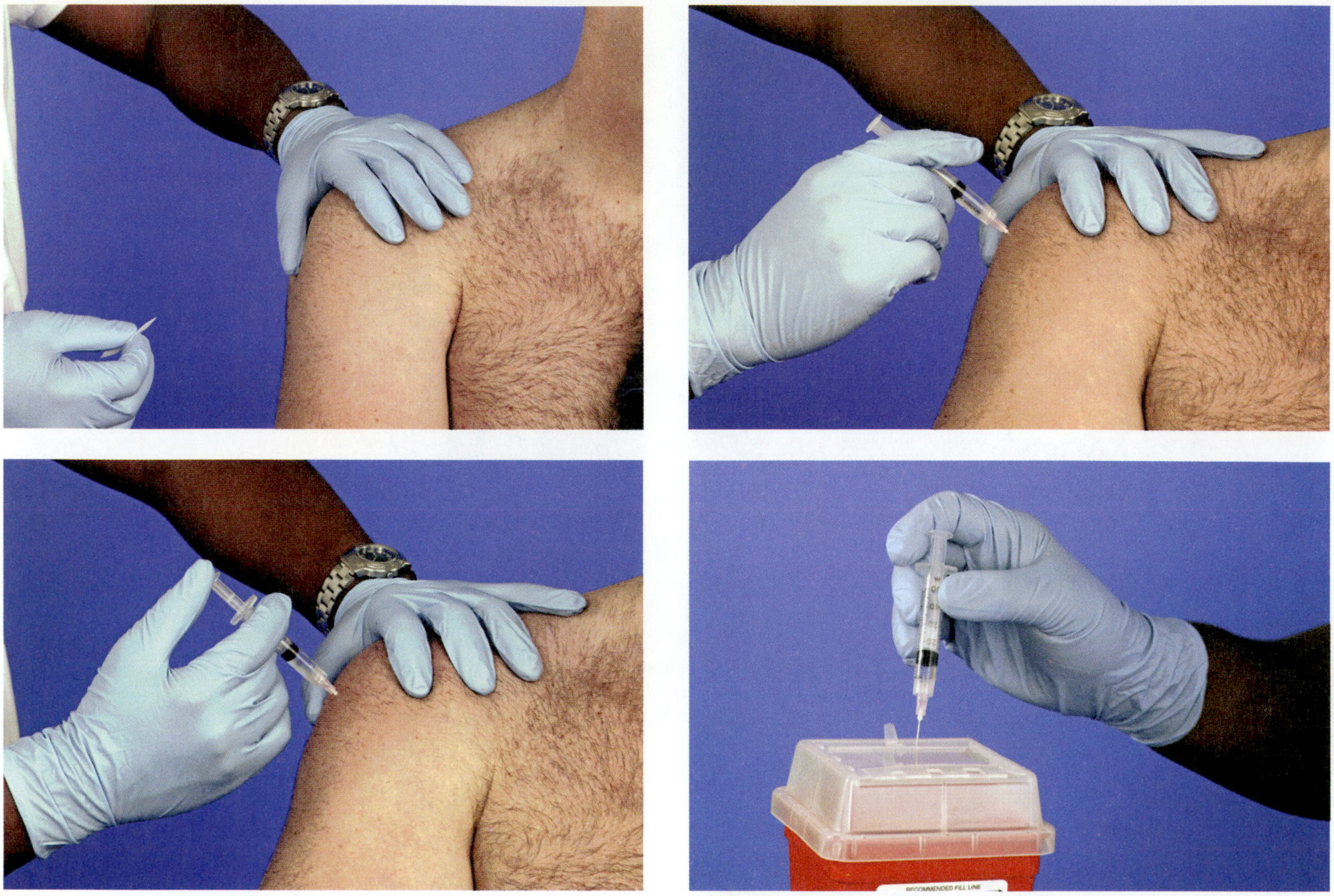

A B C D

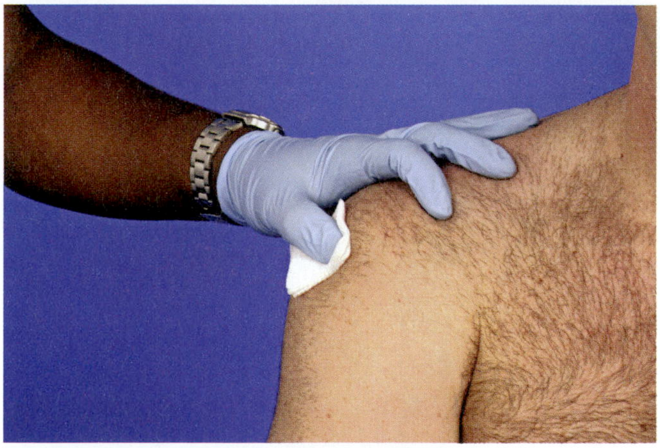

FIGURE 18-14 ■ Intramuscular injection. **A,** Choose the site. Cleanse the skin and pull it tight. **B,** Insert the needle. Pull back on the plunger to aspirate (to check needle placement). **C,** Slowly push in the plunger to deliver the medication. **D,** Remove the needle. Discard it in an appropriate container. Then, massage the skin over the injection site.

tions, and larger lumen needles are used for suspensions and oils). Because the muscle layer is below the subcutaneous layer, a longer needle generally is used (usually 1½ inches and 19 or 21 gauge). The procedures for intramuscular injections are mostly the same as those described before (Fig. 18-14). However, the needle is inserted at a 90-degree angle. Also, the skin is held taut, not pinched.

Several muscles are commonly used for intramuscular injections. These are the deltoid muscle, several gluteal muscles (dorsogluteal site), the vastus lateralis muscle, the rectus femoris muscle, and the ventrogluteal muscle. The deltoid muscle is located in the upper arm. It forms a triangular shape, with the base of the triangle along the acromion process and the peak of the triangle ending approximately one third of the way down the lateral aspect of the upper arm (Fig. 18-15). This muscle is used primarily for vaccinations involving only a small volume of drug. This is because the muscle is small and can accommodate only small doses of injection (1 mL or less). When injections are made in this location, care must be taken to avoid hitting the radial nerve. The patient should be sitting up-

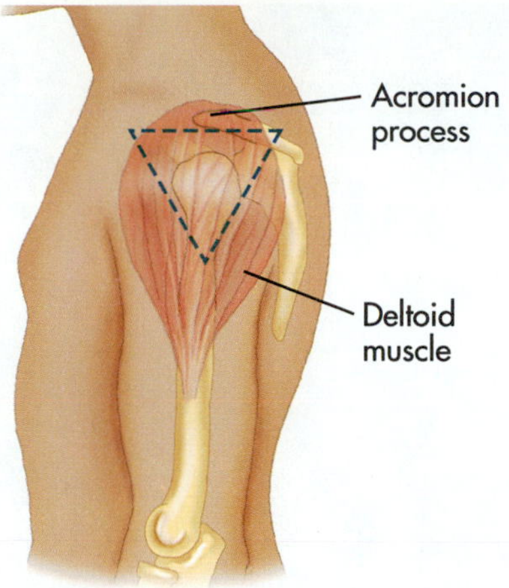

FIGURE 18-15 ■ The injection site for the deltoid muscle roughly forms an inverted triangle, with the acromion process as the base. The muscle may be visible in well-developed patients.

right or lying flat. The person should be told to relax the arm muscles.

The dorsogluteal site consists of several gluteal muscles. The gluteus medius muscle is most often used for injections. The dorsogluteal site can be defined in two ways. The first method is to divide the buttocks on one side into imaginary quadrants; the medication is administered into the upper outer quadrant. The second method is to locate the posterior-superior iliac spine and the greater trochanter of the femur. An imaginary line is drawn between the two landmarks; the injection is given up and out from this line (Fig. 18-16). This site should not be used for children under 3 years of age. In that age group, the muscles are not yet well developed and the proximity of the sciatic nerve (the largest nerve in the body) poses a risk. Large, well-developed muscles can accommodate an injection of up to 5 mL. However, volumes over 3 mL may be uncomfortable for the patient. When an injection is administered at the dorsogluteal site, the patient should be lying prone. The toes should be pointing inward to promote muscle relaxation. Another complication of gluteal injections is inadvertent injection into the hip joint. The paramedic can minimize this risk by paying attention to anatomical landmarks.

The vastus lateralis and the rectus femoris muscles lie side by side in the thigh. To identify the necessary landmarks, the paramedic should place one hand on the patient's upper thigh and one hand on the lower thigh. The area between the hands is the middle third of the thigh and the middle third of the underlying muscle (Fig. 18-17). The vastus lateralis lies lateral to the midline and is the preferred injection site for children. It is well developed in all patients and has few major blood vessels and nerves that can be injured. The rectus femoris is most often used for self-injection because of its accessibility. Acceptable volumes for injection vary with the age of the patient and the size of the muscle. Up to 5 mL may be injected into a well-developed adult. The patient should be sitting upright or lying supine and should be advised to relax the muscles.

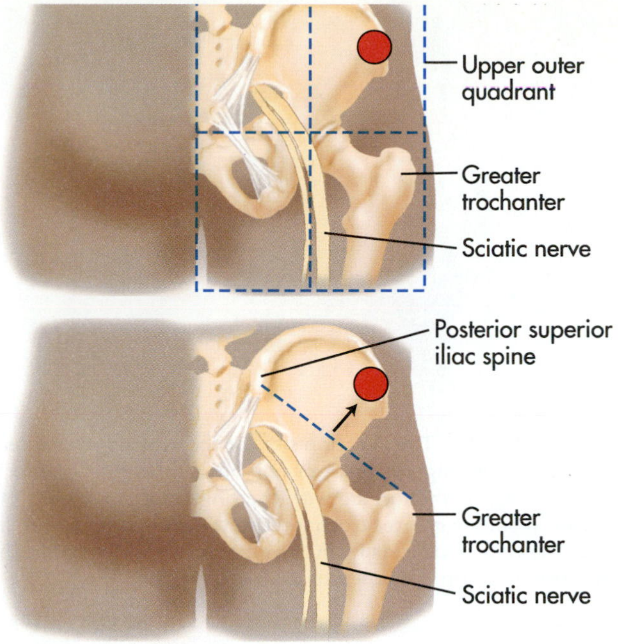

FIGURE 18-16 ■ The injection area for the dorsogluteal site can be defined in two ways. **A,** The buttocks can be divided on one side into imaginary quadrants. The center of the upper outer quadrant should be used as the injection site. **B,** The posterior-superior iliac spine and the greater trochanter are located by palpation. An imaginary line is drawn between the two. The injection site should be above and out from that line.

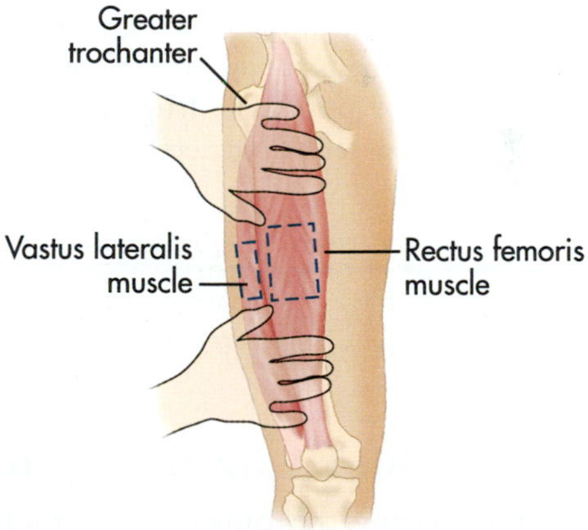

FIGURE 18-17 ■ The injection sites for the vastus lateralis muscle and the rectus femoris muscle can be defined through landmarks. One hand is placed below the greater trochanter. The other hand is placed above the knee. The space between the two hands defines the middle third of the underlying muscle. The rectus femoris is on the anterior thigh. The vastus lateralis is on the lateral side.

The ventrogluteal muscle is accessible when the patient lies in a supine or lateral recumbent position. The paramedic should palpate the greater trochanter using the palm, with the index finger pointing to the anterior-superior iliac spine. The paramedic's remaining three fingers should extend toward the iliac crest. The injection is made into the

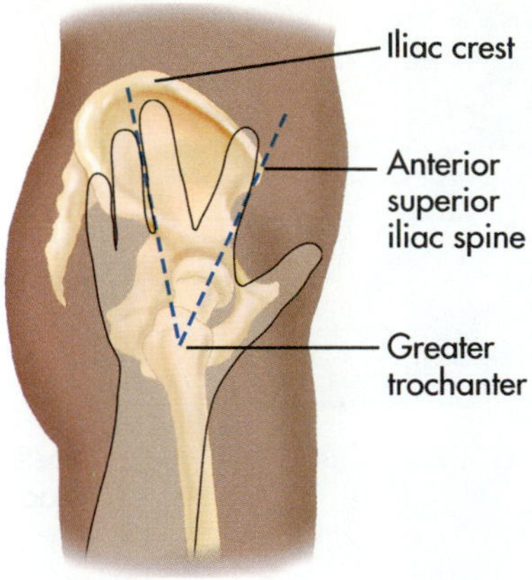

FIGURE 18-18 ■ The injection site for the ventrogluteal muscle is defined by placing the palm of one hand on the trochanter of the femur. A V is then made with the fingers of that hand. One side runs from the greater trochanter to the anterior-superior iliac spine. The other side runs from the greater trochanter to the iliac crest. The injection is made into the center of the V.

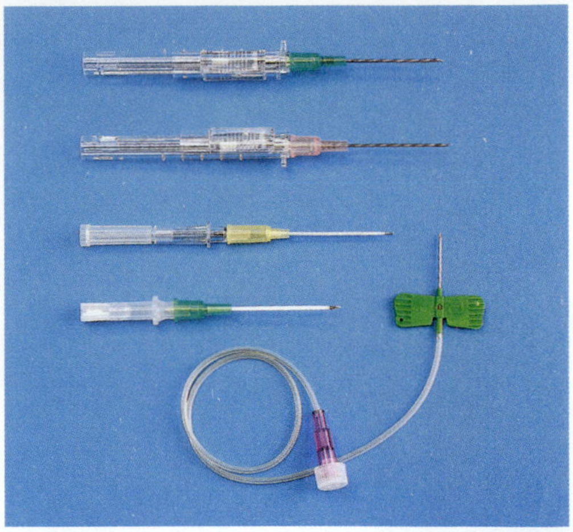

FIGURE 18-19 ■ Various types of intravenous (IV) catheters.

center of the V formed by the fingers (Fig. 18-18). This injection site may be used for all patients. It is a desirable site because it has no large nerves or fat tissue. In the adult, this muscle may accommodate up to 5 mL of drug.

Intravenous Therapy

Intravenous cannulation is used to gain access to the body's circulation. It is indicated for three reasons. The first is to administer fluids. The second is to administer drugs. The third is to obtain specimens for laboratory determinations. The intravenous route puts the drug directly into the bloodstream. This bypasses all barriers to drug absorption.

> **CRITICAL THINKING**
>
> There are benefits to choosing the upper extremity for intravenous access in an adult. What are they?

Intravenous Fluid Administration

In the prehospital setting, the route of choice for fluid therapy is through a peripheral vein in an extremity. If the arms have no major injury, upper extremity veins should be used. (Some EMS agencies advise against using upper extremity sites if a major injury to the neck or upper thorax has occurred on that side.) If upper extremity sites are not available, lower extremity sites may be used. IV fluids often used in the prehospital setting include normal saline, lactated Ringer solution, and mixtures of glucose and water (see Chapter 17). For the most part, normal saline and lactated Ringer solution are used for fluid replacement. They also are used as a means of administering a drug.

TYPES OF INTRAVENOUS CATHETERS

The three main types of intravenous catheters are (1) the hollow needle (butterfly) type; (2) the indwelling plastic catheter over a hollow needle (e.g., Angiocath or Jelco); and (3) the indwelling plastic catheter inserted *through* a hollow needle (e.g., Intracath; this type is seldom used in the prehospital setting) (Fig. 18-19).

Hollow needles are not advised for IV fluid replacement in the prehospital setting. It is very difficult to stabilize the needle. In some cases a butterfly catheter may be used for a pediatric patient if it can be stabilized adequately. This sometimes can be achieved by using armboards or other immobilization devices. In the prehospital setting, use of the over-the-needle catheter is preferred. This type of catheter is easily secured. Also, it is more comfortable for the patient.

PERIPHERAL INTRAVENOUS INSERTION

An area commonly used for peripheral intravenous therapy is the hands. Another is the arms. This includes the antecubital fossae (AC space). Other sites are the long saphenous veins and the external jugular veins. However, the incidences of embolism and infection are higher at the latter two sites. Figs. 18-20 through 18-22 show sites and techniques for peripheral cannulation.

Another factor in the selection of a puncture site for intravenous therapy is the patient's clinical status. Injuries or diseases involving an extremity interfere with the use of veins in that extremity for venipuncture or venous cannulation. Examples of such conditions include trauma, dialysis fistula, and a history of mastectomy.

Steps

1. If the patient is conscious, explain the procedure. Give the reason intravenous therapy is necessary and describe the procedure.
2. Assemble the equipment (Fig. 18-23).
   (a) Inspect the prescribed fluid for contamination, appearance, and expiration date. Never use fluids that are cloudy, outdated, or in any way suspect for contamination.
   (b) Prepare the microdrip or macrodrip infusion set. Attach the infusion set to the bag of solution.
3. Clamp the tubing and squeeze the reservoir on the infusion set until it fills halfway. Then open the clamp and flush the air from the tubing. Close the clamp.

A

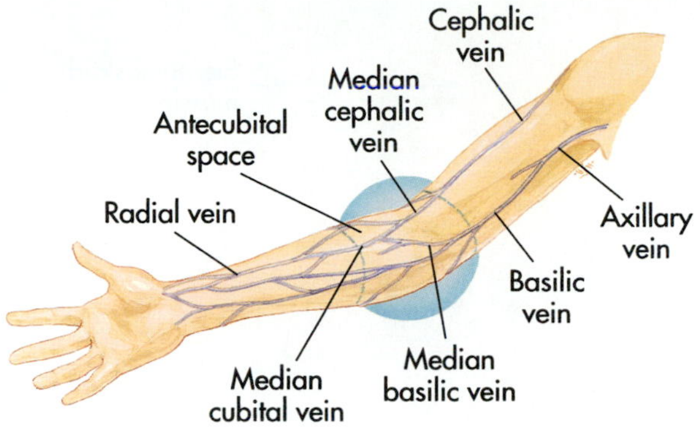

B

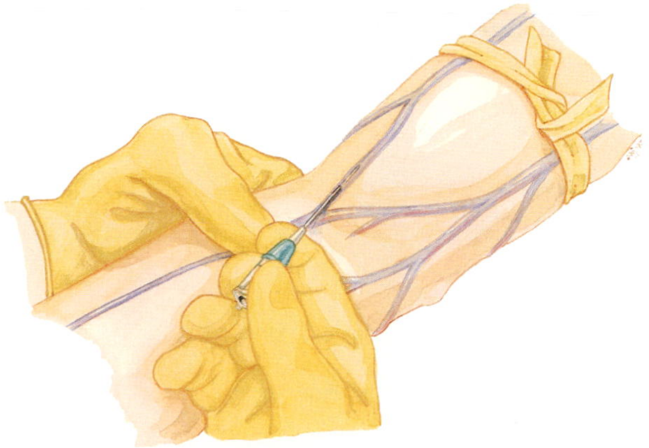

C

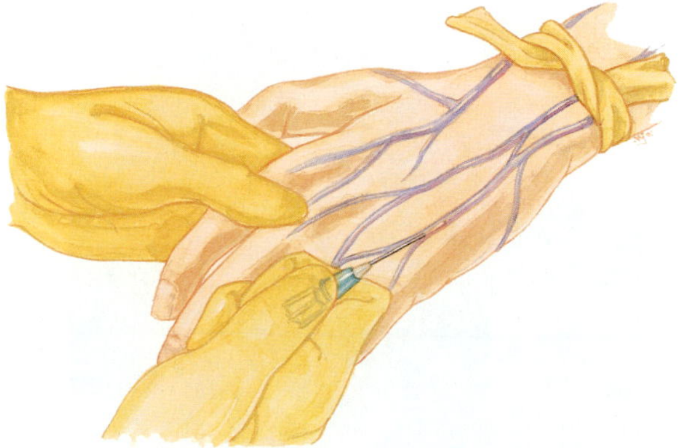

FIGURE 18-20 ■ **A,** Veins of the upper extremity. **B,** Antecubital venipuncture. **C,** Dorsal hand venipuncture.

A

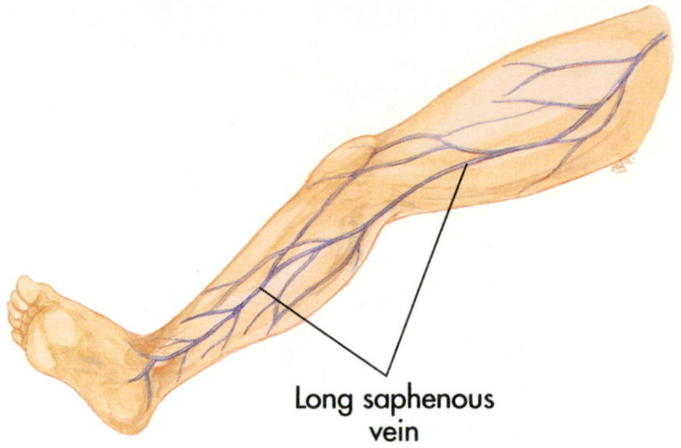

B

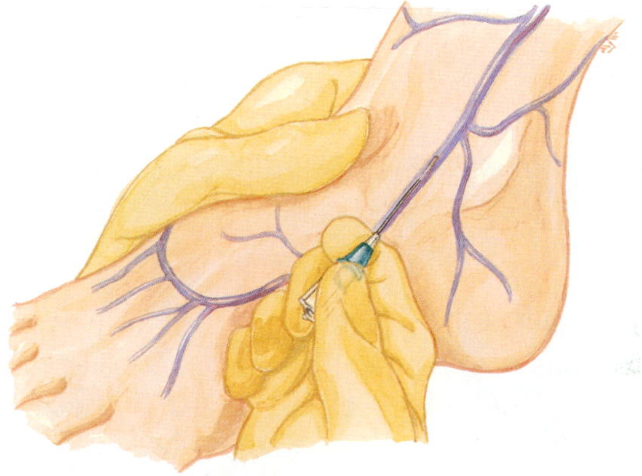

FIGURE 18-21 ■ **A,** Long saphenous vein. **B,** Venipuncture of the long saphenous vein.

4. Select the catheter. A large-bore catheter (14 to 16 gauge) should be used for fluid replacement. A smaller bore catheter (18 to 20 gauge) should be used for "keep open" lines. "Keep open" lines are used to maintain hydration and to establish a channel for IV medication if needed.
5. Prepare other equipment:
   - Alcohol, chlorhexidine/alcohol, or iodine wipes to cleanse the skin
   - Sterile dressings or 4 × 4 gauze pads
   - Adhesive tape, torn or cut into several strips
   - Syringes and Vacutainers for blood samples
   - Tourniquet (rubber drain tubing or blood pressure cuff may be used)
6. Put on gloves for personal and patient protection.
7. Select the puncture site. If using an upper extremity, allow the patient's arm to hang dependent, and apply the tourniquet several inches above the antecubital space. (The tourniquet should be just tight enough to tamponade venous vessels but not occlude arterial flow.) When selecting a suitable vein, begin by looking at the dorsum of the hand and forearm. Choose a vein that is fairly straight and easily accessible. The forearm is better than the hand because it allows hand movement and is more easily secured after cannulation. If a second puncture attempt is necessary, the second puncture should always be *proximal* to the first puncture. Therefore the vein selected for initial cannulation should be the most suitable distal vein. Avoid veins near joints, where immobilization is difficult, and veins near injured areas. If the long saphenous vein is chosen, begin site selection near the medial malleolus of the foot. To locate the external jugular vein, place the patient in a supine head-down position and turn the patient's head toward the opposite side.
8. Prepare the puncture site and cleanse the area:
   (a) Thoroughly clean the site with alcohol to remove dirt, dead skin, blood, and other surface contaminants. Allow the area to dry.
   (b) Clean the site using overlapping, concentric circles and moving outward.
9. Stabilize the vein by applying distal pressure and tension to the point of entry (Fig. 18-24, *A*). With the bevel up, pass the needle through the skin and into the vein from the side or directly on top (Fig. 18-24, *B*). (Using a "bevel down" technique in infants and children may facilitate

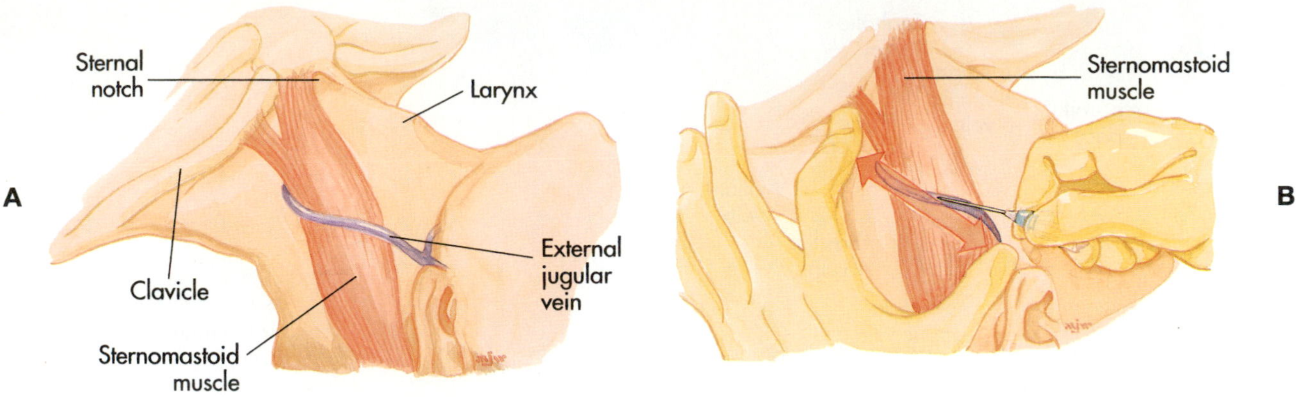

FIGURE 18-22 ■ **A,** Anatomy of the external jugular vein. **B,** External jugular venipuncture.

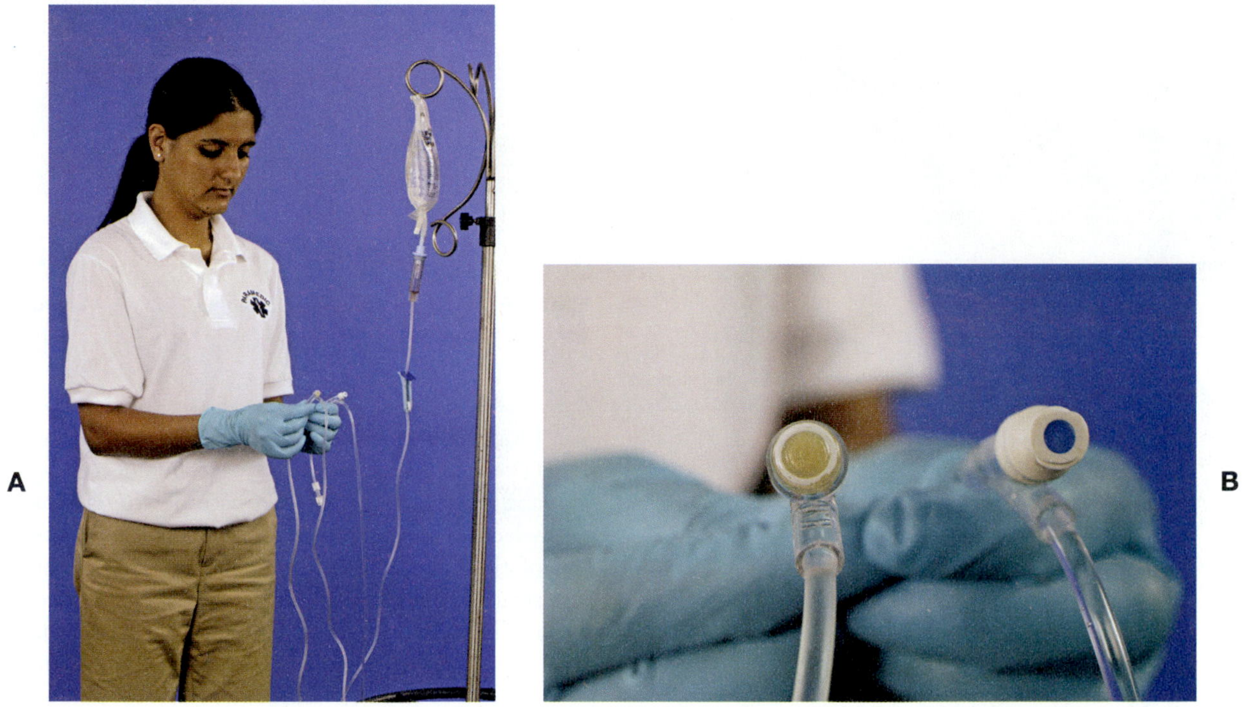

FIGURE 18-23 ■ **A,** Intravenous infusion setup. **B,** Needle and needleless ports.

entry into constricted peripheral veins.[6]) Advance the needle and catheter about 2 mm beyond the point where blood return in the hub of the needle was first encountered. Slide the catheter over the needle and into the vein. While stabilizing the catheter, withdraw the needle (Fig. 18-24, *C*). Apply pressure on the proximal end of the catheter to stop escaping blood. Obtain blood samples, if needed, with a syringe or Vacutainer.

10. Release the tourniquet and attach the IV tubing (Fig. 18-24, *D*). Open the tubing clamp and allow fluid infusion to begin at the prescribed flow rate (Fig. 18-24, *E*).
11. Cover the puncture site with a dressing to ensure asepsis and to secure the line. Anchor the tubing and secure the catheter. Catheter movement can increase the risk of phlebitis and cause migration of pathogens along the cannula into the vein.
12. Document the infusion procedure.

CENTRAL VENOUS CANNULATION

Central venous cannulation may be within the scope of paramedic practice in some EMS systems. However, central venous infusion should never be used for rapid fluid replacement in the prehospital setting. Sites for central venous cannulation include the femoral vein, internal jugular vein, and subclavian vein (Figs. 18-25 to 18-27).

Steps. The preparation for cannulation of the central vessels is the same as that for the peripheral veins. Certain

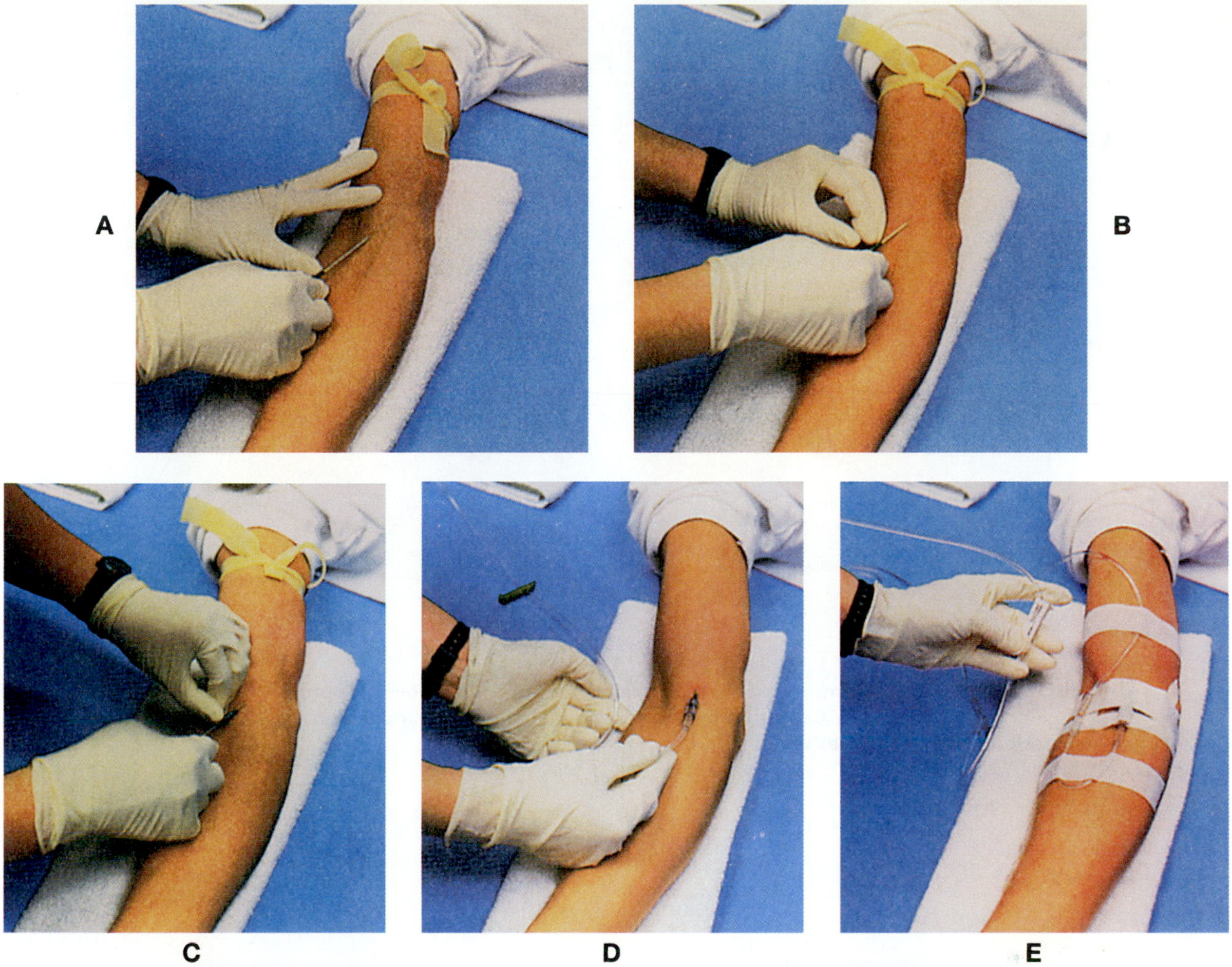

FIGURE 18-24 ■ Technique for intravenous catheterization. **A,** Stabilize the vein by applying distal pressure and tension to the point of entry. **B,** With the bevel up, pass the needle into the vein from the side or directly on top. **C,** Slide the catheter over the needle and into the vein. While stabilizing the catheter, withdraw the needle. **D,** Release the tourniquet and attach the intravenous tubing. **E,** Open the tubing clamp. Adjust the infusion to begin at the prescribed flow rate.

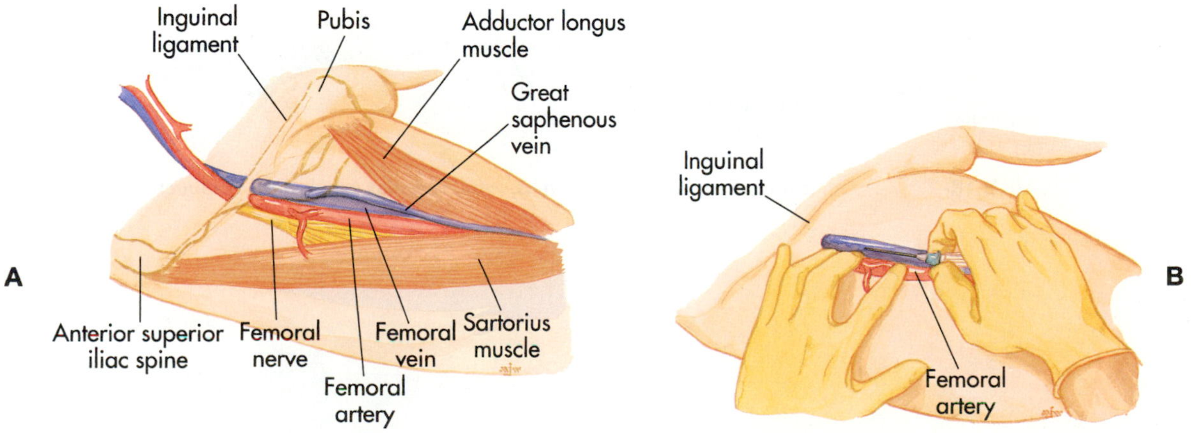

FIGURE 18-25 ■ **A,** Anatomy of the femoral vein. **B,** Femoral venipuncture.

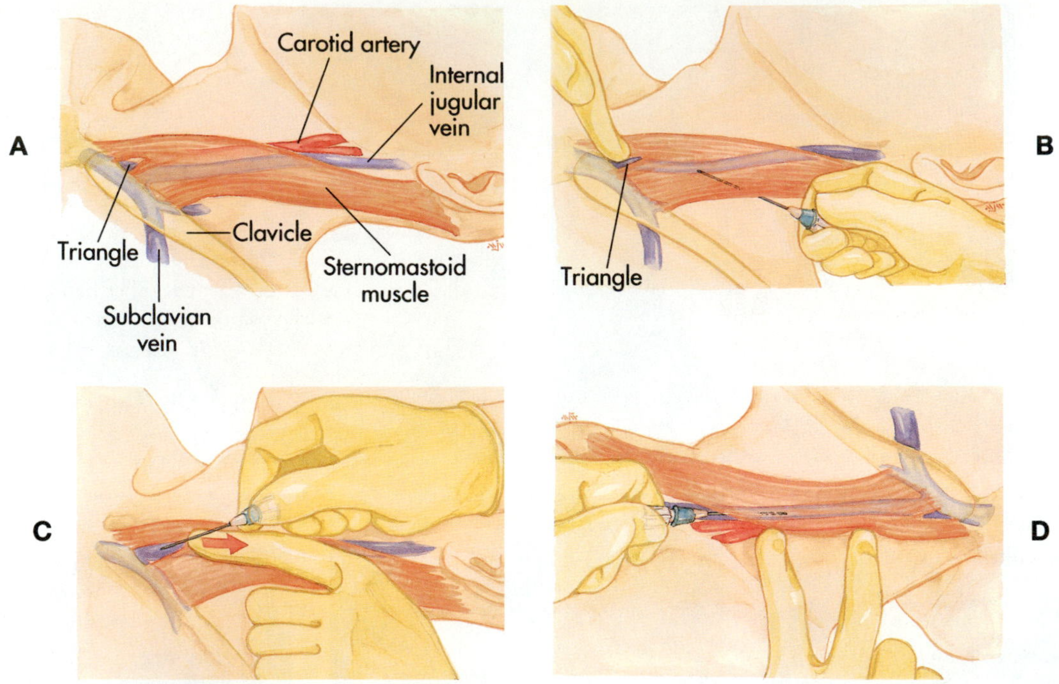

FIGURE 18-26 ■ **A,** Anatomy of the internal jugular vein. **B,** Posterior approach for internal jugular venipuncture. **C,** Central approach for internal jugular venipuncture. **D,** Anterior approach for internal jugular venipuncture.

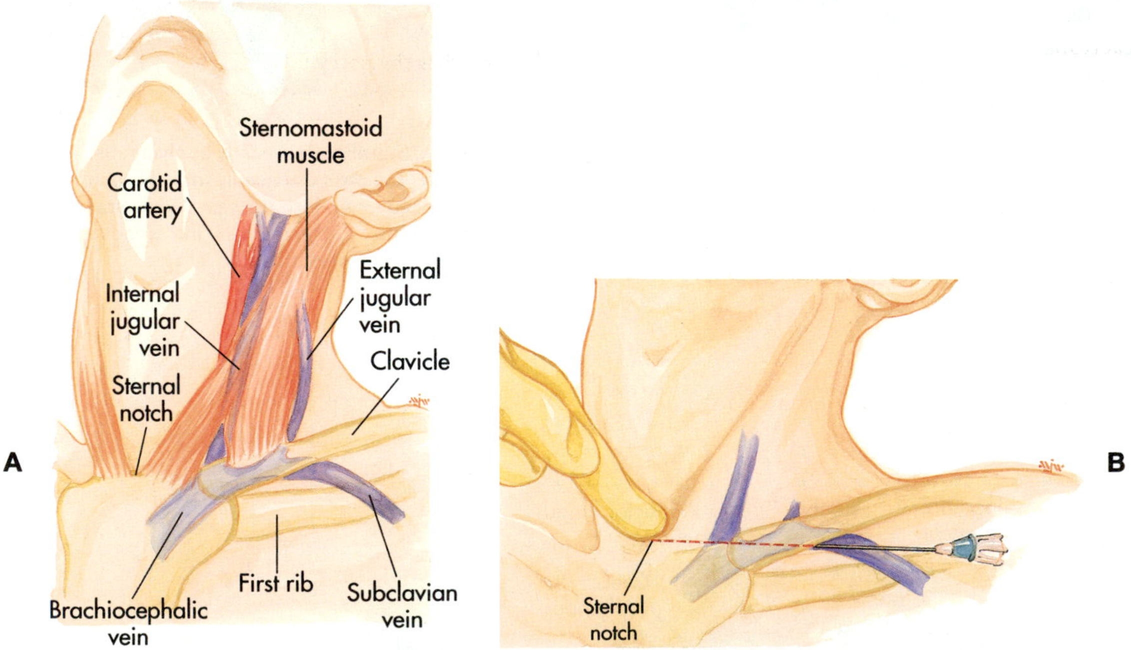

FIGURE 18-27 ■ **A,** Anatomy of the subclavian vein. **B,** Infraclavicular subclavian venipuncture.

factors affect the success of central venous cannulation. Two of these are the position of the patient's body and the paramedic's knowledge of anatomy. The paramedic's familiarity with the procedure also is a key factor. Central venous cannulation calls for special training and authorization from medical direction.

NOTE Central line placement is not considered useful in the prehospital setting. Complications include pneumothorax, arterial injury, and abnormal placement.

Complications of Intravenous Techniques

Several possible complications are associated with all intravenous techniques. These include local complications, systemic complications, infiltration, and air embolism.

LOCAL AND SYSTEMIC COMPLICATIONS

Local complications may involve hematoma formation, thrombosis, cellulitis, and phlebitis. Systemic complications include the following:

- Sepsis
- Pulmonary embolism
- Catheter fragment embolism
- Fiber embolism originating from cotton or paper fibers in the catheter irrigation solution, leading to foreign body reactions
- Arterial puncture

INFILTRATION

Infiltration may occur when the needle or catheter has been displaced. It may occur when blood or fluid leaks from around the catheter and escapes into the tissues *(extravasation)*. It also can occur if a vein is punctured more than once during initiation of IV access. Signs and symptoms include the following:

- Coolness of the skin at the puncture site
- Swelling at the puncture site, with or without pain
- Sluggish or absent flow rate

If infiltration is suspected, the paramedic should lower the fluid reservoir to a dependent position to check for backflow of blood into the tubing. (The absence of backflow suggests infiltration.) If any of the signs and symptoms are present, the intravenous flow should be discontinued (Box 18-9). The needle or catheter should be removed immediately. Moreover, a pressure dressing should be applied to the site. An alternative puncture site should be chosen and the infusion restarted with new equipment. In addition, the incident should be documented.

AIR EMBOLISM

Air embolism is uncommon. However, it can be fatal. The volume of air that the human bloodstream can tolerate has not been firmly established. However, fatalities have been reported after 100 mL of air entering the cardiovascular system.[8] A total of 10 mL of air can be fatal in a critically ill patient.

The embolism is caused by air entering the bloodstream via the catheter tubing. The risk of air embolism is greatest when a catheter is passed into the central circulation, where negative pressure may actually pull in air. Air can enter the circulation either on insertion of the catheter or when the tubing is disconnected to replace solutions or add new extension tubing (Box 18-10). With subsequent pumping, blood foaming occurs in the heart. If enough air enters the heart chamber, it can impede the flow of blood. This, in turn, can lead to shock.

Signs and symptoms of air embolism include hypotension, cyanosis, weak, rapid pulse, and loss of consciousness. If air embolism is suspected, the following steps should be taken:

1. Close the tubing.
2. Turn the patient on the left side with the head down. (If air has entered the heart chambers, this position may keep the air in the right side of the heart and away from the cardiac valves. The pulmonary artery may absorb small air bubbles.)

BOX 18-9 Discontinuation of an Intravenous Infusion

To discontinue an intravenous (IV) infusion and remove the intravenous catheter, follow these steps:

1. Put on gloves.
2. Carefully remove any securing tapes and dressings.
3. Close the drip chamber to stop the flow of fluid.
4. Place sterile gauze over the insertion site and apply gentle pressure with one hand. With the other hand, quickly withdraw the catheter, pulling straight back from the angle of insertion.
5. Apply firm pressure to the insertion site for 2 to 5 minutes to prevent bleeding or bruising.
6. Cover the insertion site with a bandage.
7. Appropriately dispose of all equipment.

BOX 18-10 Replacement of Intravenous Solutions

At times a bag of intravenous (IV) fluids must be replaced during an infusion. To do this, prepare all equipment in advance and follow these steps:

1. Hold the infusing bag upside down in one hand and remove the spike chamber. Discard the old bag.
2. Quickly insert the spike chamber into the new bag and squeeze the chamber.
3. Insert an 18-gauge needle into an injection port in the IV tubing to allow air to be expelled from the tubing before it reaches the patient.
4. After the air has been expelled, remove the needle and adjust the flow rate of the infusion.
5. Document the time the IV fluids were replaced.

3. Check tubing for leaks.
4. Administer high-concentration oxygen.
5. Notify medical direction.

Accidental disconnection of the IV tubing can cause an air embolism. This may occur during patient movement. The chance of an air embolism can be minimized by making sure that all tubing connections are secure. Also, fluid containers should be changed before they are empty.

Complications Specific to Central Venous Cannulation

Cannulation of the central veins presents specific dangers. These are in addition to the complications common to all intravenous techniques. The paramedic must be alert to these dangers. They can be fatal if unrecognized. (Although the femoral vein is not truly a central vein, because the catheter is inserted in an area below the diaphragm, it is included in this section.)

COMPLICATIONS OF FEMORAL VEIN CANNULATION

Local Complications

- Hematoma may occur, either from the vein itself or from the adjacent femoral artery.
- Thrombosis may extend to the deep veins and lead to edema of the leg.
- Phlebitis may extend to the deep veins.
- Use of the femoral vein frequently precludes subsequent use of the saphenous vein.

Systemic Complications

- Thrombosis or phlebitis may occur and extend to the iliac veins or even the inferior vena cava.

COMPLICATIONS OF INTERNAL JUGULAR AND SUBCLAVIAN VEIN CANNULATION

Local Complications

- Hematoma may occur, either from the vein itself or from an adjacent artery.
- Damage may occur to an adjacent artery, nerve, or lymphatic duct. Inadvertent puncture of the carotid artery is not uncommon when jugular vein cannulation is attempted. If a hematoma occurs on one side of the neck, it is hazardous to attempt puncture on the opposite side. This could result in bilateral hematomas that severely compromise the airway.

Systemic Complications

- Pneumothorax is common.
- Hemothorax can occur.
- Air embolism can occur.
- Fluid may infiltrate into the mediastinum or the pleural cavity from an extruded catheter.

Intravenous Medications

Medications can be administered directly into the circulating blood via the vascular system. This is referred to as administering medications via the intravenous route. Intravenous medications can be given by injection or infusion. An intravenous injection can be given through a previously established intravenous infusion line, heparin or saline lock, or implantable port (e.g., Port-A-Cath, Hickman catheter). It also can be administered directly into the vein with a sterile needle or butterfly device. An intravenous infusion is given by adding a drug to an infusing intravenous solution. (An example of such a solution is normal saline.) Another method is to dilute the drug in a larger volume of fluid and administer the medication through a volume control, in-line device (e.g., burette, Volutrol, infusion pump). Sometimes the medication is given by intermittent infusion through an existing infusion site (*intravenous piggyback* or *secondary set*).

Intravenous injections normally involve a small amount of medication (usually less than 5 mL). These are called *intravenous push* or *intravenous bolus* medications. To give such an injection (Fig. 18-28), the paramedic should clean the injection port of the IV line with alcohol or remove the cap from the needleless port. The prescribed medication is then injected slowly (usually over 1 to 3 minutes). The rate of injection depends on the type of medication and the patient's response. Most intravenous tubing has one-way valves to prevent backflow of medication. If such a valve is not present or cannot be identified, the tubing above the injection site should be clamped during drug administration. After the injection, the infusion of fluids is continued.

Intravenous infusions for drug administration can take several forms. To add a medication to the fluid reservoir of an established intravenous line, the paramedic should follow these steps (Fig. 18-29):

1. Compute the volume of the drug to be added to the fluid reservoir.
2. Draw up the prescribed dose into a syringe. If prefilled syringes are used, note the volume of medication in the syringe and the dose to be used.
3. Cleanse the rubber sleeve of the fluid reservoir with an alcohol swab.
4. Puncture the rubber sleeve (if a needle is used) and inject the prescribed medication into the fluid reservoir.
5. Withdraw the needle (if a needleless system is not used) and discard the needle and syringe. Gently mix the medication with the fluid by agitating the reservoir.
6. Label the fluid reservoir with (1) the name of the medication added, (2) the amount of the medication added, (3) the resultant concentration of the medication in the reservoir, (4) the date and time the infusion was prepared, and (5) the name of the paramedic who prepared the infusion.
7. Calculate the rate of administration in drops per minute as prescribed.

A number of in-line, volume control devices allow more accurate delivery of medication diluted in precise amounts of fluids than is possible by simply setting the drip rate manually. These devices are often used to give intravenous medications to children and adults who need precise doses. Medications that can readily cause toxicity when given too rapidly (e.g., antidysrhythmics, vasopressors) are well suited to this delivery method. In-line devices include electronic

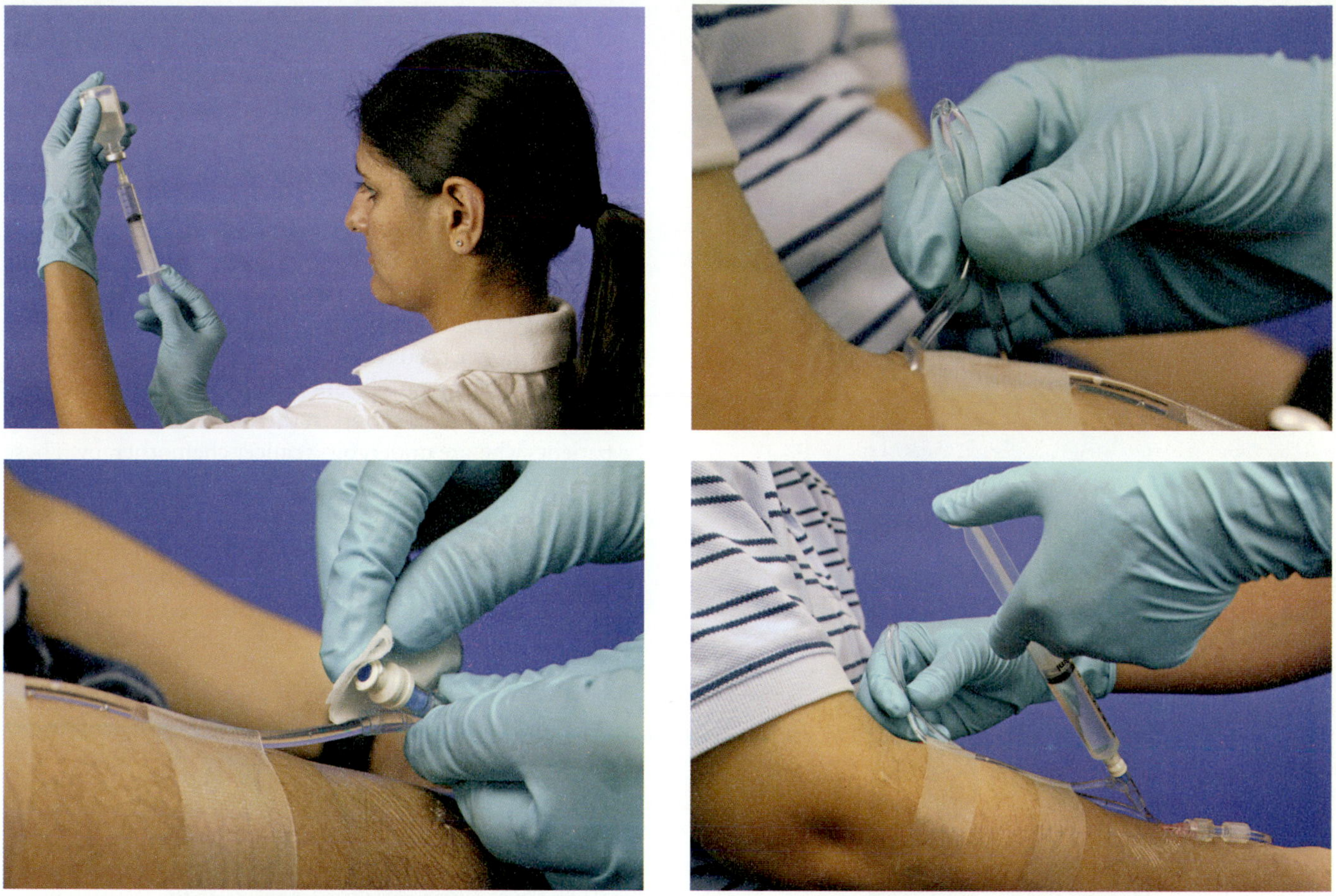

A B C

FIGURE 18-28 ■ Administration of a drug by intravenous (IV) route. **A,** Prepare the correct volume of the drug. Cleanse the injection port. **B,** If the tubing does not have a one-way valve, pinch the line to clamp it. **C,** Inject the drug at the recommended rate. Resume IV flow (with a small flush if indicated) and monitor the patient.

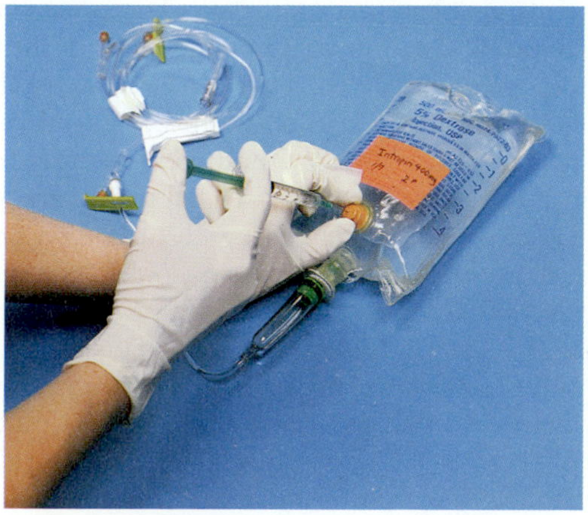

FIGURE 18-29 ■ Adding medication to an intravenous reservoir.

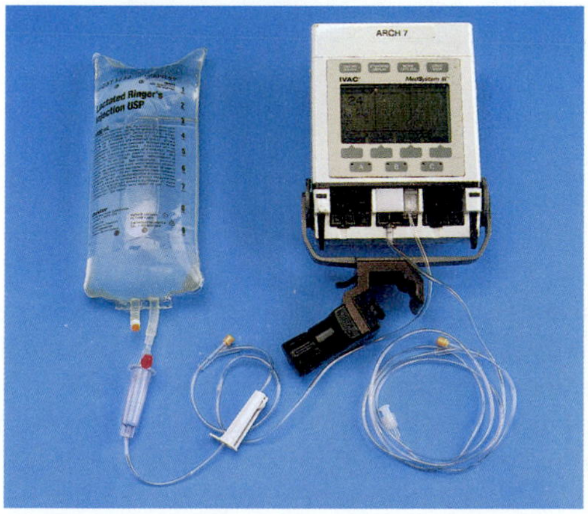

FIGURE 18-30 ■ Intravenous infusion pump.

flow rate regulators that regulate fluid passage by means of a magnetically activated metal ball valve. They also include infusion pumps that exert pressure on tubing or fluid by pumping against pressure gradients. Paramedics should follow the instructions of the equipment's manufacturer. They also should become familiar with these devices before using them (Fig. 18-30). Other mechanical (nonelectric) devices are available. (Dial-A-Flow is one such device.) These devices are used by some EMS agencies to closely regulate flow rate.

Intermittent infusions are given via a setup that is secondary to the primary intravenous infusion. The piggyback

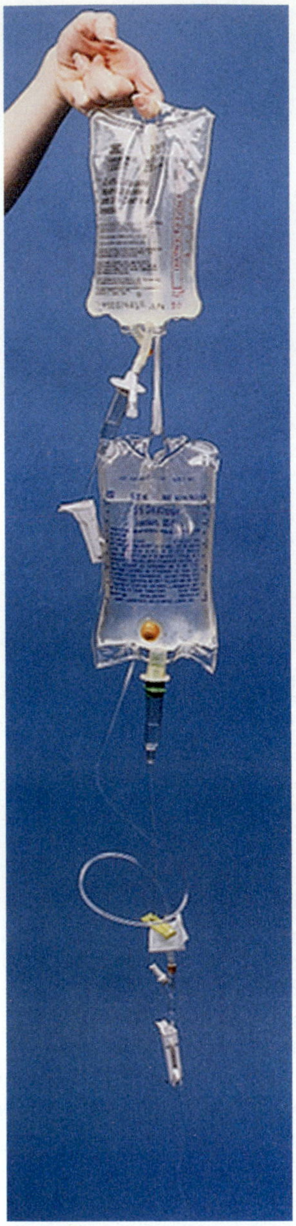

FIGURE 18-31 ■ Intravenous piggyback setup.

medication is hung in tandem and connected to the primary setup (Fig. 18-31). Most intermittent diluted drug infusions are meant to have a total infusion time of 20 or 30 minutes to 1 hour. The time depends on the drug and the patient's response. To prepare an intermittent infusion, the paramedic should follow these steps:

1. Prepare the prescribed medication. Add it to the secondary fluid as described here.
2. Bleed the air out of the secondary administration set. Attach a 1 inch, 18-gauge needle.
3. Cleanse the medication port of the primary infusion tubing. Insert the needle or access pin of the piggyback medication.
4. Tape the needle (if present) to the medication port securely.
5. Calculate the flow rate of the secondary infusion in drops per minute.
6. Lower the primary infusion reservoir so that its center of gravity is lower than the secondary infusion reservoir.
7. Clamp the tubing of the primary infusion to allow the piggyback medication to infuse. Open the piggyback line flow clamp. Adjust the flow rate to the desired dose. After administration of the piggyback medication, restart the primary infusion. Discard the piggyback equipment.
8. Always label the bag with the medication.

Another device used to administer a drug intravenously is a drug pump. Drug pumps are used by patients who need a slow injection of medication in the home. An example may be patients who are undergoing cancer chemotherapy. These devices usually consist of a syringe with a battery attachment that regulates the injection of medication. Drug pumps are used to give medication subcutaneously. They also can be attached to indwelling vascular devices (Box 18-11). Such devices include the Port-A-Cath or Hickman catheter.

NOTE To prevent damage to central venous catheters, the paramedic should:

Use the clamp on the clamping sleeve provided on silicone catheters

Avoid using scissors or any other sharp object around the device

Use only small-gauge needles (22 to 25 gauge) with a needle length of 1 inch or less when accessing the injection port

Administer fluids or medications gently (never force them)

Intraosseous Medications

Studies have shown that intraosseous (IO) infusion is relatively safe and effective in children. The procedure currently is used by EMS agencies in many areas of the United States for vascular access. It is used in critically ill children (and less commonly in adults) when peripheral cannulation is unavailable. (Other methods of obtaining vascular access in children are discussed in Chapters 43 and 44.)

Fluids and drugs infused through IO access pass quickly from the marrow cavities into the sinusoids. Then they pass to large venous channels and emissary veins. Next, they pass into the systemic circulation. Normal saline, lactated Ringer solution, D_5W, plasma, blood, and most advanced life saving (ALS) medications may be infused quickly by this route (Fig. 18-35). Drugs administered by the IO route must be followed by a saline flush of at least 5 mL. This ensures that the drug is delivered into the central circulation.[6]

IO infusion generally should be considered only for unconscious children. Moreover, it should be considered *only* when peripheral cannulation is unobtainable. Example scenarios include cardiopulmonary arrest and peripheral vascular collapse (as in shock, major trauma, or burns). In addition, IO infusion is recommended in critically ill children in whom vascular access is impaired by obesity or edema, and in children with life-threatening status asthmaticus.

BOX 18-11 Indwelling Vascular Devices

Heparin or Saline Lock

A heparin or saline lock is a peripheral intravenous cannula. It has no attached intravenous tubing (Fig. 18-32). These devices allow ready access to peripheral veins. They are used for brief administration of medications. They also are used for intravenous (IV) therapy that is administered frequently on an outpatient basis (e.g., chemotherapy). The cannula is filled with 0.5 to 1 mL of a heparin or saline solution. This prevents clotting when the device is not in use.

To gain access to the peripheral vein, 4 mL of normal saline is drawn into a syringe. Aseptic technique is used; 2 mL of the normal saline is used to flush the heparin lock reservoir before and after infusion of the prescribed medication or IV fluid. After intravenous therapy, 0.5 to 1 mL of heparin or 3 mL of 0.9% normal saline should be injected into the reservoir. This keeps the lock patent.

Atrial Catheters

An atrial catheter (Fig. 18-33) is a long, Silastic indwelling catheter. These are sometimes used by patients with cancer, gastrointestinal dysfunction, or debilitating diseases. They also are used by patients who need intermittent IV administration of antibiotics, nutritional supplements, or other intravenous medications. Patients are sometimes discharged from the hospital with the catheter in place. They are taught to maintain it and to administer various medications and fluids through the device.

The atrial catheter is about 90 mm long and 1.6 mm in diameter. It is surgically placed in the right atrium using local anesthesia and under fluoroscopic guidance. On the patient's chest, the catheter looks like a thin, white cord with a Luer plug attached to the end. It protrudes from a small incision near the clavicle. This is usually covered with a dressing. Atrial catheters should be used for venous access only in emergency situations such as acute fluid loss, pulmonary edema, or cardiac arrest. Connecting intravenous lines to the catheter increases the risk of infection and embolism. For this reason, the catheter should not be used in patients in stable condition. When access to an atrial catheter is necessary, the following steps should be taken[3]:

1. Gather the equipment:
   - 20 mL, 5 mL, and 3 mL syringes
   - 18-gauge needle
   - 30 mL multidose vial of bacteriostatic 0.9% normal saline solution; povidone-iodine (Betadine); and intravenous administration set
2. Draw up 3 mL of normal saline and set it aside.
3. Put on gloves for patient and personal protection.
   Note: Most patients with an atrial catheter are immunosuppressed or severely debilitated. They therefore are susceptible to routine pathogens. Paramedics should take special care to prevent contamination.
4. Explain the procedure to the patient.
5. Clamp the catheter with a padded, smooth shunt clamp to avoid nicking or severing the catheter.
   Note: The atrial catheter is a central line catheter. Thus an air embolism is possible when the tubing or syringes are changed.
6. Remove and discard the intermittent infusion device. (Connections are usually taped to prevent disconnection and air embolism.)
7. Wipe the connection site with povidone-iodine and allow it to dry.
8. Connect the 5 mL syringe. Remove the clamp and withdraw 5 mL of blood. (Do not use heparinized blood for the specimen.)
9. Replace the clamp.
10. Attach the 3 mL syringe of normal saline to the catheter. Remove the clamp and flush to prevent clot formation in the catheter.
11. Replace the clamp and remove the syringe.
12. Connect the intravenous tubing to the catheter. Make sure the tubing is free of air.
13. Remove the clamp and begin the infusion.
14. Tape the connection site between the intravenous tubing and the catheter. Use as with any other peripheral intravenous line.

Implantable Ports

Implantable ports are venous access devices. They are surgically implanted, with the distal end of the catheter inserted into a large central vein. An example of such a device is the Port-A-Cath

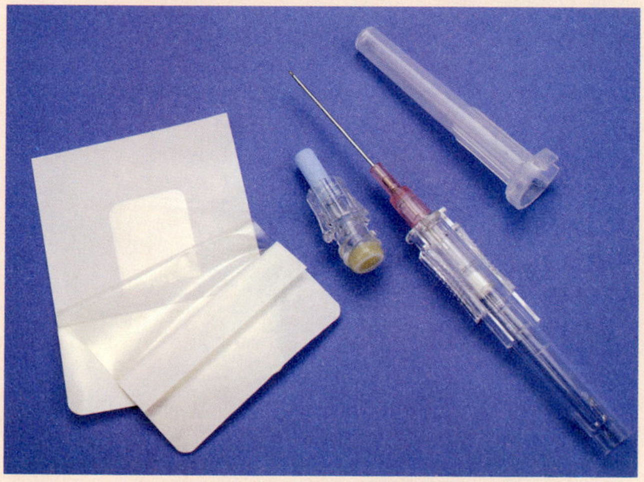

FIGURE 18-32 ■ Saline lock.

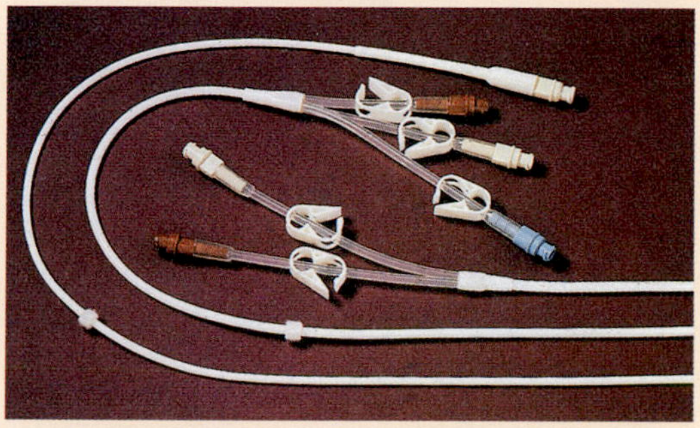

FIGURE 18-33 ■ Single-lumen, dual-lumen, and triple-lumen right atrial catheters.

Continued

BOX 18-11 Indwelling Vascular Devices, cont'd

(Fig. 18-34). The injection end of the catheter is implanted subcutaneously, often on the chest wall. It has a self-sealing septum over a small chamber or reservoir. The tubing extends from the side of the reservoir to the venous insertion point. Each time the implantable port is accessed, the skin must be punctured with a needle. However, no daily cleansing is required, as it is with partially implanted ports such as the Hickman catheter. Implantable ports should not be used in patients in stable condition. When an implantable port must be used, the following steps should be taken:

1. Locate the device and stabilize it with one hand.
2. Puncture the skin and septum with a Huber needle attached to a 3 mL syringe containing sterile saline. (Huber needles are noncoring, stainless steel needles that allow the port to close after puncture. They may be straight for injections or angled 90 degrees for intravenous infusion.)
3. Aspirate blood to determine patency. Then inject the saline to flush the system.
4. Connect intravenous tubing to the reservoir. Make sure the tubing is free of air.
5. Tape the connection site between the intravenous tubing and the reservoir.
6. After use, flush the device with a heparinized solution.

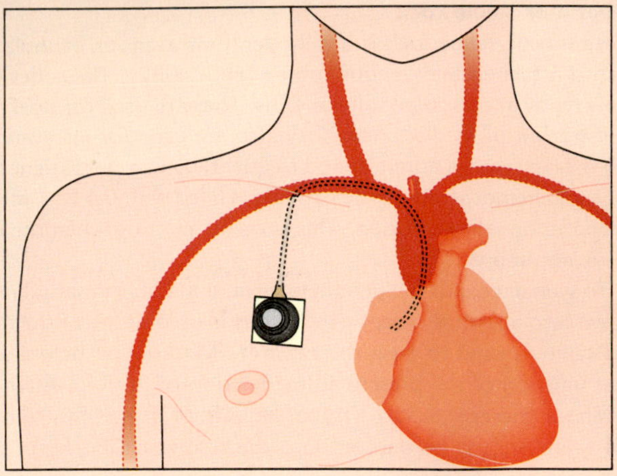

FIGURE 18-34 ■ Port-A-Cath.

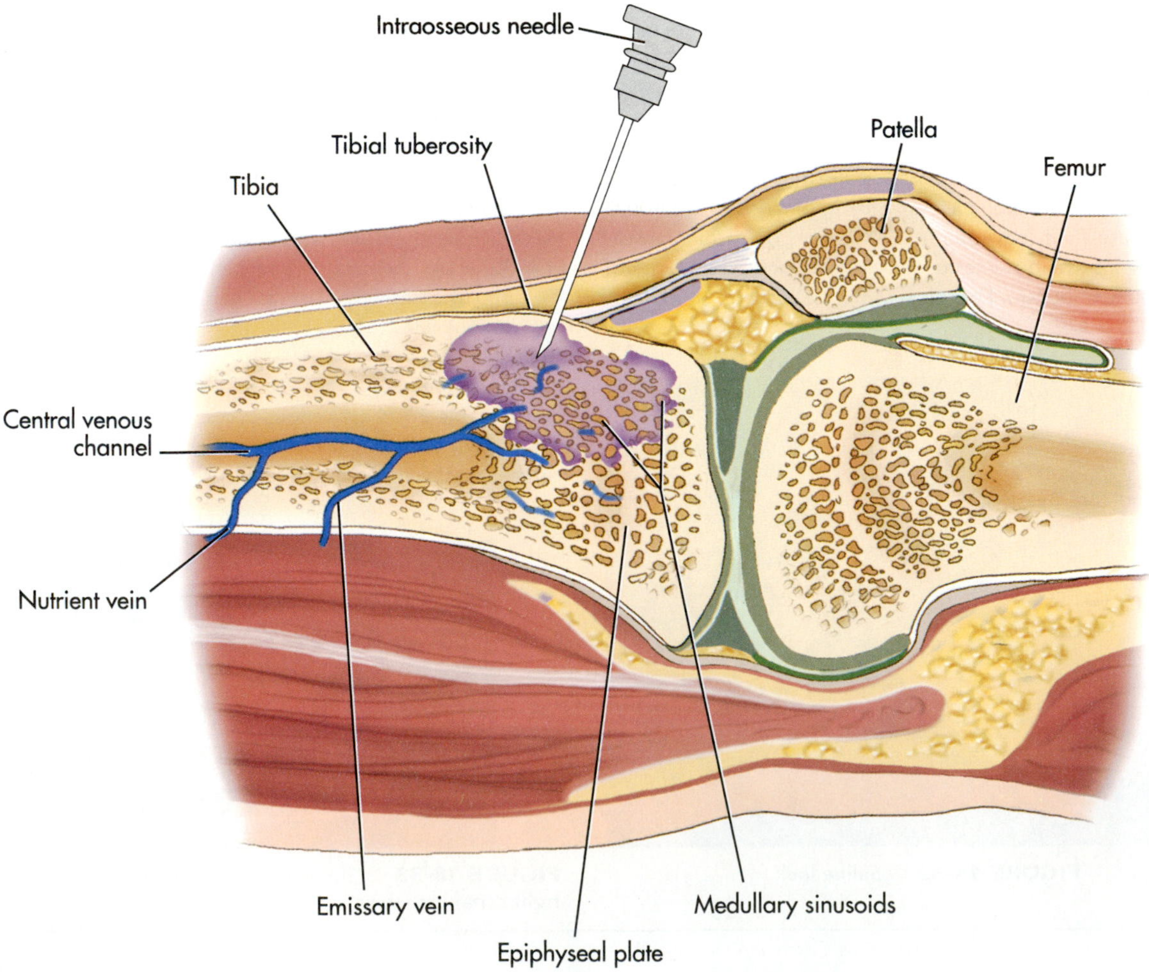

FIGURE 18-35 ■ Obtaining intraosseous access.

Special training and authorization for this procedure must be provided by medical direction.

The site of choice for initiation of this procedure in children is the tibia, one to two fingerbreadths below the tubercle on the anteromedial surface. An alternative choice is the femur, two to three fingerbreadths above the lateral condyles in the midline.

NECESSARY EQUIPMENT

Alcohol wipes
Povidone-iodine (Betadine) wipes
Tape
Bone marrow needle or commercial intraosseous needle
IV tubing (pediatric infusion set)
IV fluids (specified by medical direction): normal saline, lactated Ringer solution, or special pediatric fluids

INSERTION TECHNIQUE (FIG. 18-36)

1. Put on gloves for personal and patient protection.
2. Cleanse the site as previously described for peripheral and central cannulation.
3. Prepare the needle for insertion. Insert the needle pointing away from the epiphyseal plate. Advance it to the periosteum.

A B C D

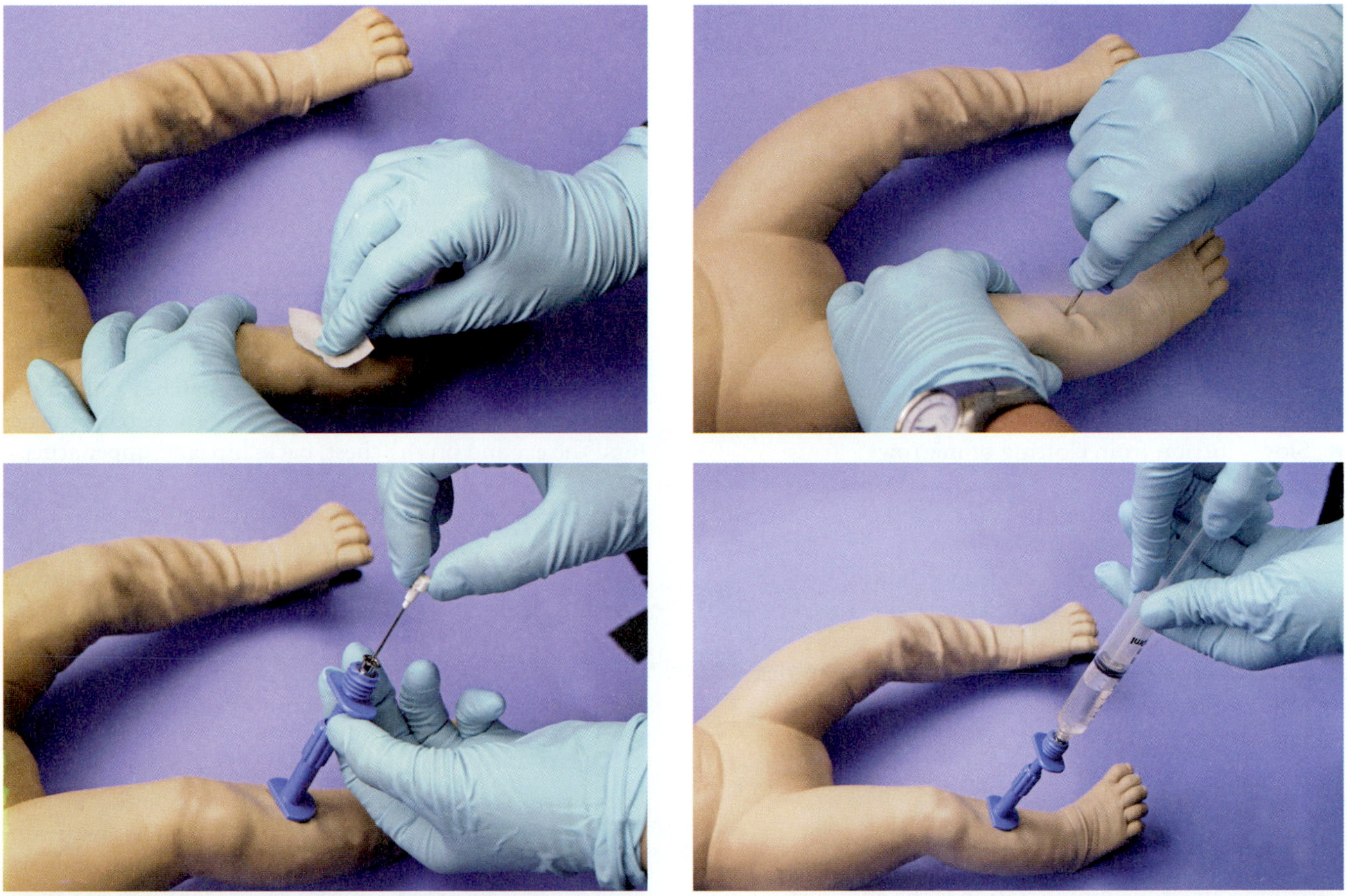

E

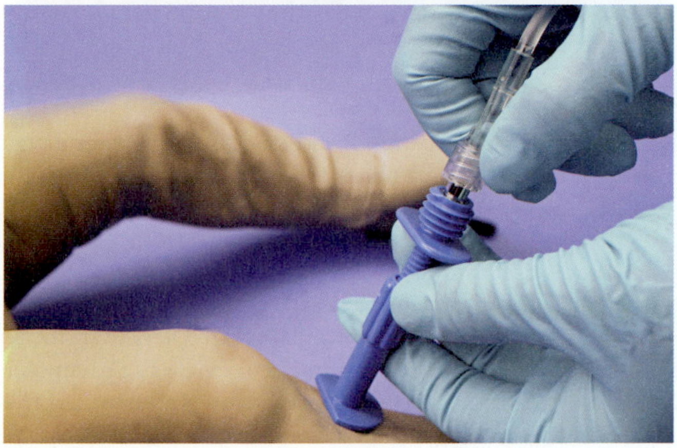

FIGURE 18-36 ■ Intraosseous infusion. **A,** Cleanse the site. **B,** Using a screwing motion, insert the bone marrow needle away from the epiphyseal plate. Advance the needle until a pop is felt (this occurs when the needle penetrates the marrow). **C,** Remove the stylet. **D,** Aspirate for marrow and then flush with saline. **E,** Attach the intravenous tubing, and adjust the infusion to the prescribed flow rate. Check for signs of infiltration.

4. Using a boring or screwing motion, advance the needle until it penetrates the bone marrow (usually noted by decreased resistance and a slight popping sound).
5. Remove the stylet.
6. Aspirate bone marrow into a saline-filled syringe. (Bone marrow may not always be aspirated.)
7. Infuse saline by syringe to ensure placement of the needle and to clear clots.
8. Secure the needle with tape and a securing screw if so equipped (although the needle is usually well stabilized by the bone).
9. Attach standard IV tubing and fluids to infuse under gravity or pressure as prescribed by medical direction
10. Apply a dressing to the site.
11. Document the procedure.

CONTRAINDICATIONS

- Fracture of the site or proximal to the site
- Traumatized extremity
- Cellulitis
- Burns that may be infected by the technique
- Congenital bone disease

POTENTIAL COMPLICATIONS

Technical

- Subperiosteal infusion from improper placement
- Penetration of posterior wall of medullary cavity, resulting in soft tissue infusion
- Slow infusion from clotting of marrow

Systemic

- Osteomyelitis (occurs in fewer than 0.6% of cases, usually with prolonged infusion)
- Fat embolism (not yet reported in children)
- Slight periostitis at the injection site (usually clears within 2 to 3 weeks)
- Infection (acceptably low rate, comparable to that with other infusion techniques)
- Fracture

ADMINISTRATION OF PERCUTANEOUS MEDICATIONS

Percutaneous drug administration is the administration of drugs that are absorbed through the mucous membranes or skin. These include topical drugs, sublingual drugs, buccal drugs, inhaled drugs, endotracheal drugs, and drugs for the eye, nose, and ear.

Topical Drugs

In addition to the various emollients and antibiotic ointments, the most commonly used transdermal emergency medication is ***nitroglycerin***. Two types of topical ***nitroglycerin*** preparations are available. These are ***nitropaste*** and transdermal ***nitroglycerin*** delivery patches. These can be applied to any clean, dry area of the upper arm or hair-free portion of the chest. ***Nitropaste*** has a lanolin-petrolatum base. It is applied in ½-inch increments with special papers to measure the dose. Transdermal ***nitroglycerin*** patches have an adhesive back (Fig. 18-37). They come in a solid or semisolid form (depending on the manufacturer.) Paramedics should always wear gloves when applying or removing these medications. This prevents inadvertent self-absorption of the drug. More information is available in the *Emergency Drug Index*.

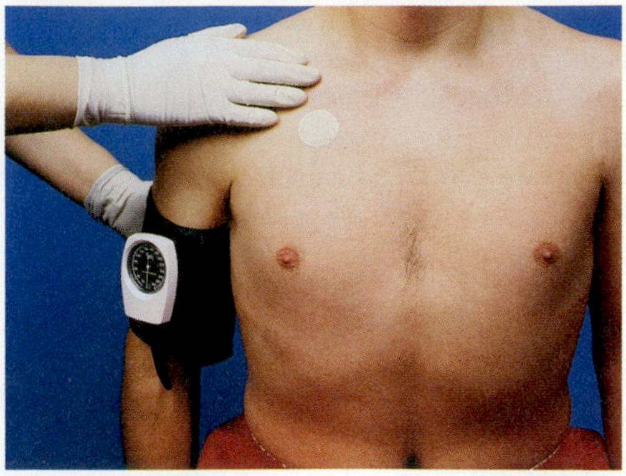

FIGURE 18-37 ■ Application of a nitroglycerin patch.

Drugs such as scopolamine, clonidine, and estrogen are also used in patch form. These drug patches can affect the patient unfavorably during illness. Paramedics should be able to recognize the different types of patches and should remove them if indicated. Usual sites for the patches are behind the ear and on the chest, back, hip, and upper arms.

Sublingual Drugs

The most frequently prescribed sublingual drugs are nitrates (e.g., ***nitroglycerin***), which are used to treat angina pectoris. The tablet should be placed under the tongue, where it dissolves. The patient should not drink fluids while the drug is being absorbed. If the patient inadvertently swallows the tablet, the effects are diminished and delayed.

Buccal Drugs

Buccal drugs are held between the patient's cheek and gum. They dissolve to achieve their desired effects. As with sublingual drugs, the patient should not drink fluids while the drug is being absorbed. Glucose gel preparations are an example of an emergency medication administered via the buccal route.

Inhaled Drugs

In addition to oxygen and ***nitrous oxide,*** several other drugs may be administered by means of inhalation. These include bronchodilators, corticosteroids, antibiotics, and mucokinetic agents delivered through aerosolization.

Aerosols are liquid or solid particles of a substance dispersed in gas or solution. The effectiveness of aerosolization therapy depends on the number of droplets that can be suspended in the gas or solution, the particle size (diameter in microns), output (cc/min), and the rate and depth of the patient's breathing. Rapid, shallow breathing reduces the

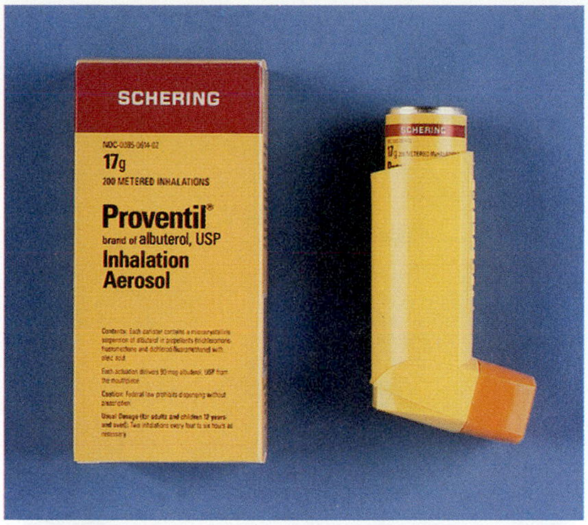

FIGURE 18-38 ■ Metered-dose inhaler (MDI).

number and retention of droplets that reach the deep bronchioles of the lungs. The delivery of drugs by this method has certain advantages over other routes. Specifically, these are rapid onset of the drug's effect and fewer or less intense systemic side effects.

Aerosols are made by devices called *nebulizers*. The most common nebulizers are intermittent positive pressure breathing (IPPB) devices (designed for in-hospital use). Out-of-hospital devices include metered-dose inhalers (pressure cartridges) and hand-held nebulizers. Hand-held nebulizers operate by means of a compressed air or oxygen source regulated by a flowmeter.

METERED-DOSE INHALER

The metered-dose inhaler (MDI) is now the most commonly used device in aerosol therapy (Fig. 18-38). It is convenient. Also, it delivers a measured dose with each push of the cartridge. MDIs are usually prescribed for self-treatment of asthma. Other medications prepared in MDIs are ***albuterol*** and ***isoetharine.*** Paramedics should follow these steps to administer a drug by this method:

1. Remove the mouthpiece and protective cap from the canister (the drug container).
2. Carefully snap off the cap and turn the mouthpiece sideways.
3. Insert the canister stem into the hole inside the mouthpiece.
4. Shake the canister and mouthpiece well.
5. Invert the MDI and hold it close to the patient's mouth. Instruct the patient to exhale, pushing as much air from the lungs as possible.
6. Place the mouthpiece in the patient's mouth. Instruct the patient to close the lips loosely around it, with the tongue underneath the mouthpiece. As the patient inhales deeply over 5 seconds, press down on the canister quickly and then release it.
7. Instruct the patient to hold his or her breath 5 to 10 seconds before exhaling.
8. Repeat the procedure in 5 to 10 minutes to take advantage of possibly deeper penetration by a second round of therapy (if required). Most MDI medications are administered using aero chambers (spacers). These are beneficial devices for children and for patients with problematic conditions. For example, some patients might need additional time to inhale the medication. Others may lack coordination. Still others may be hampered by a high level of anxiety or by a diminished ability to inhale for 5 seconds. Aero chambers allow the patient to receive the maximum benefit of the drug and do not require exact synchronization.

CRITICAL THINKING

What happens to the medication if the patient does not use the metered-dose inhaler (MDI) properly?

HAND-HELD NEBULIZERS

Hand-held nebulizers are another means of administering some medications via inhalation in the prehospital setting. Various manufacturers make disposable nebulizer kits. The kits usually include a mouthpiece or aerosol mask, oxygen tubing, and reservoir tubing (Fig. 18-39). These devices are attached to a nonhumidified portable or on-board oxygen source. They use the Bernoulli principle to create an aerosol mist (sometimes referred to as a *jet* or *pneumatic nebulizer*). Medications appropriate for nebulization therapy include ***albuterol, metaproterenol, isoetharine,*** and ***atropine.***

The specific procedure may vary slightly. It may depend on the patient's ability to tolerate the treatment by mouthpiece or mask. A tight seal around the mouthpiece is required. The patient therefore must be able to cooperate during treatment. Both mouthpiece and mask methods have advantages. With treatment by mouthpiece, less of the drug is wasted. However, patients with severe dyspnea who are mouth breathers tolerate mask administration much better.

To administer a medication via a hand-held nebulizer, paramedics should follow these steps:

1. Using aseptic technique, mix the prescribed drug with a specified amount of normal saline. Then instill it into the nebulizer. Some medications come in a packaged unit dose and have a fixed amount of diluent (usually 0.9% normal saline).
2. Attach the nebulizer to a T-piece and mouthpiece and connect it with tubing to the unit delivering nonhumidified oxygen (for the hypoxic patient) or compressed gas. (If the patient cannot use the mouthpiece, a simple face mask may be used in its place.)
3. Adjust the oxygen flowmeter to a rate of 4 to 6 L/min to create a steady, visible mist. (This rate usually offers a steady mist without too much wastage of medication. The higher the flow rate, the greater the use of medication.) If an aerosol mask is used, the oxygen flow rate should be kept at 6 to 10 L/min. This pre-

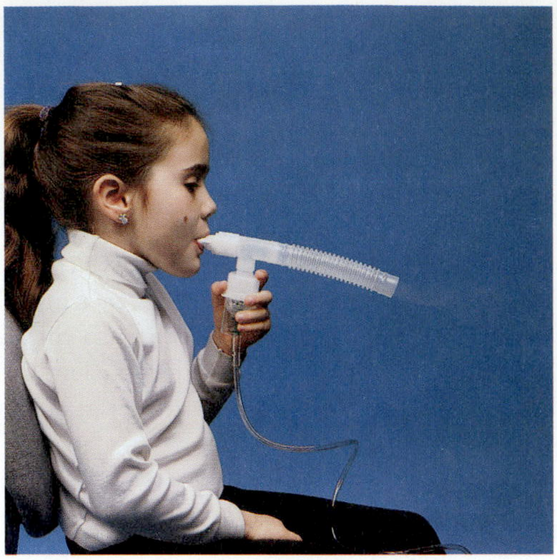

FIGURE 18-39 ■ Administration of medication with a hand-held nebulizer.

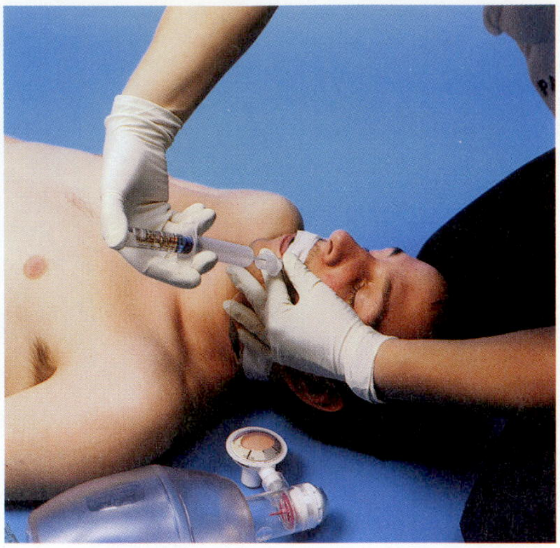

FIGURE 18-40 ■ Administration of a drug through an endotracheal (ET) tube.

vents the buildup of exhaled carbon dioxide in the mask.

4. When the mist is visible, begin treatment. Instruct the patient to inhale slowly and deeply by mouth. Have the person hold a breath for 3 to 5 seconds before exhaling. This results in topical deposition of the aerosol particles deep within the tracheobronchial tree. Inhalation and exhalation should be continued until the aerosol canister is depleted of the medication. Repeat treatments usually are not given more often than every 15 to 20 minutes (usually to a maximum of three). Treatment of severe asthma, however, may include continuous administration of nebulized beta agonists, tailored to the patient's response.

The patient must be cooperative to undergo nebulization therapy. The individual must be able to follow instructions to breathe deeply so that the drug can be absorbed. This therapy would be ineffective if the patient is unable to inhale the drug sufficiently or if bronchospasm is too severe. In such cases, administration via another route should be considered.

Notable changes in the heart rate or dysrhythmias may occur during nebulization therapy. If these occur, treatment should be stopped and medical direction should be contacted for further orders. Paramedics and ambulance crews should avoid the medication vapor stream during nebulization therapy.

Endotracheal Drugs

The endotracheal (ET) route of drug administration is an alternative. It may be used when intravenous access cannot be established. Emergency drugs typically administered by this route include ***lidocaine, epinephrine, atropine,*** and ***naloxone.*** When giving medication by this route, paramedics should follow these steps (Fig. 18-40):

1. Make sure the ET tube is in the correct position. This can be checked by direct visualization and by auscultation (see Chapter 19).
2. Make sure oxygenation and ventilation of the patient's lungs are adequate.
3. Prepare the medication (per medical direction) so that it is 2 to $2\frac{1}{2}$ times the intravenous dose. Dilute the dose to 10 mL with normal saline (or prepare a 10 mL normal saline flush, per protocol).
4. Hyperventilate the patient's lungs.
5. Remove the air source from the ET tube. Inject the medication through a catheter deep into the tube, or inject it directly into the tube and follow with a normal saline flush (per protocol). (Some ET tubes have a drug port; with these tubes, the air source need not be removed for drug administration.)
6. Resume ventilations with several large ventilations. This helps to ensure that the medication penetrates as deeply as possible into the pulmonary tree (which enhances absorption).
7. Monitor the patient for the desired therapeutic effect. Also monitor for any side effects.

Drugs for the Eye, Nose, and Ear

Eye medications are usually in the form of drops or ointments. To administer these drugs, the paramedic should have the patient lie down or sit with the head tilted back. Stabilizing the patient's head with one hand, the paramedic uses the thumb or fingers of the other hand to pull down the lower lid gently. The medication should be applied into the conjunctival sac of the lower lid, never onto the eyeball (Fig. 18-41).

Nose drops are best administered with the patient lying down with the head over the edge of a bed in a midline position. The drops are instilled into each nostril. The patient should be instructed not to blow the nose for several minutes to allow absorption of the drug. To administer a nasal spray, the paramedic should have the patient inhale through one nostril while blocking the other and squeezing the spray applicator. The patient's head should be upright or tilted back during administration of the drug (Fig. 18-42).

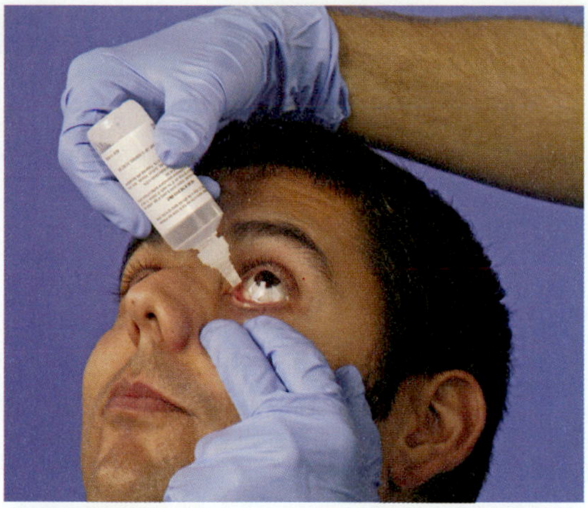

FIGURE 18-41 ■ Administration of eye medication.

Ear medications are usually in the form of drops. The patient should lie down with the affected ear up. With adults or children over age 3, the paramedic should gently pull the top of the ear up and back to straighten the ear canal. The prescribed number of drops is then instilled. In children under age 3, the ear is pulled down and straight back. The patient should remain in the ear-up position for about 10 minutes to allow the medicine to disperse. To prevent contamination of the drops, the paramedic should not allow the tip of the dropper to come into contact with the ear canal. Placing a cotton ball in the ear canal after administration of the drug may reduce seepage of the drops onto the face.

SPECIAL CONSIDERATIONS FOR PEDIATRIC PATIENTS

Administering drugs to infants and children can be quite difficult. This is especially true in emergency situations. The following guidelines may be helpful for this process:

- Try to establish a positive relationship with the child. Accept fearful or anxious behavior as a natural response.
- Be honest with the child when explaining a medication or procedure that will be unpleasant or painful.
- If appropriate, allow the child to help administer the medication (e.g., by holding the medicine cup or by placing a pill in the mouth).
- Use mild physical restraint only if it is required. Explain to the child why it is needed.
- Enlist the assistance of parents or other caregivers when possible.
- When parenteral medications are required, make sure to stabilize the injection site well and to give the injection quickly. Two or more individuals should be available to hold a child over 4 years of age, even if the child promises to "be still."
- Remember when administering medications that the younger and smaller the child, the smaller the margin for error.

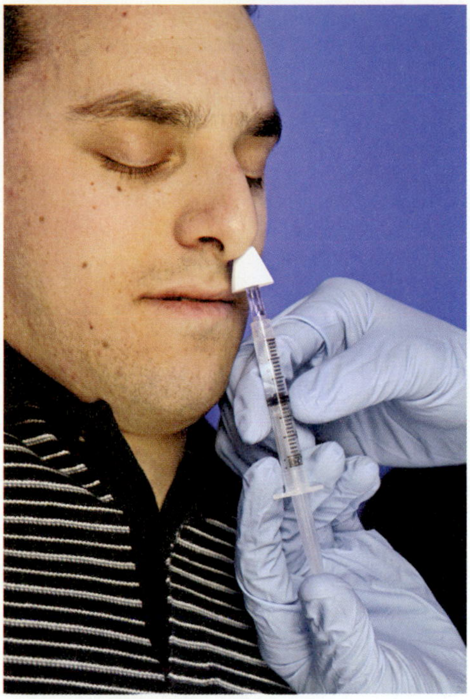

FIGURE 18-42 ■ Nasal administration of naloxone.

OBTAINING A BLOOD SAMPLE

Venous blood samples are often obtained in the prehospital setting for glucose testing and for laboratory determinations performed in the hospital. If possible, these samples should be obtained when an IV line is established. If they are to be obtained from the IV site, this should be done before any fluids are infused. When obtaining a blood sample from an IV site, the paramedic should follow these steps:

1. Prepare all equipment in advance.
2. After removing the needle from the IV catheter, exert manual pressure above the IV site to prevent the free flow of blood from the catheter.
3. While stabilizing the site, insert the Vacutainer into the hub of the IV catheter.
4. Push blood collection vacuum tubes (Table 18-3) into the barrel of the Vacutainer to draw blood from the IV catheter.
5. After obtaining the required specimens, attach the IV tubing and begin infusion.
6. Label the sample with the patient's name and the time and date it was obtained.

> **CRITICAL THINKING**
>
> Why should a venous blood sample never be drawn above an IV infusion site?

If no IV line is to be used, the paramedic must obtain the blood sample using a Vacutainer (Fig. 18-43) or a needle and syringe and then transfer the sample to an evacuation

TABLE 18-3 Types of Blood Sample Tubes

STOPPER COLOR	ADDITIVE/ PRESERVATIVE	TESTS DONE ON BLOOD SAMPLE	COMMENTS
Green 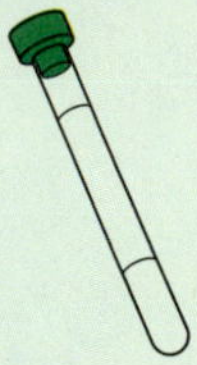	Heparin	Electrolytes, glucose; not enzymes	Invert tube several times. Heparin prevents blood from clotting without killing cells.
Lavender 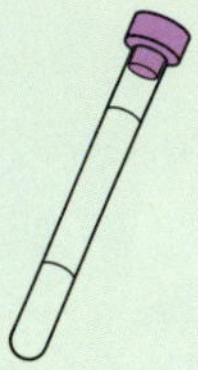	Ethylenediamine tetraacetic acid (EDTA) anticoagulant	Blood cell count, hemoglobin (Hb), hematocrit (Hct), erythrocyte sedimentation rate (ESR)	Invert tube several times to prevent clotting. EDTA tubes are used to collect samples for whole-blood hematology testing.
Light blue 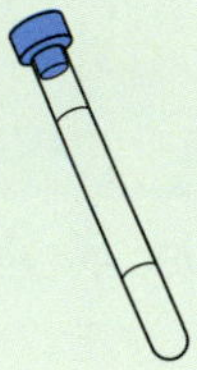	Sodium citrate	Prothrombin time (PT), activated partial thrombin time (aPTT), fibrinogen levels	Tube must be filled completely. Invert tube several times to prevent clotting. Sodium citrate tubes are used to collect samples primarily for coagulation studies. Such tests are often needed for patients with bleeding problems (e.g., in the abdomen, brain, or elsewhere).
Red 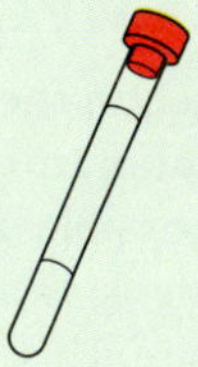	None	Serum electrolytes, liver and other enzymes, therapeutic drug levels, blood bank procedures	The tube need not be inverted, because the objective is to produce a clot. Some companies make tubes with clot activators, which hasten clotting to speed testing. Paramedics should make sure they know which kind of tube they have.

Modified from Miller CD:EMS Pocket Guide, Hong Kong, 1996, JEMS.

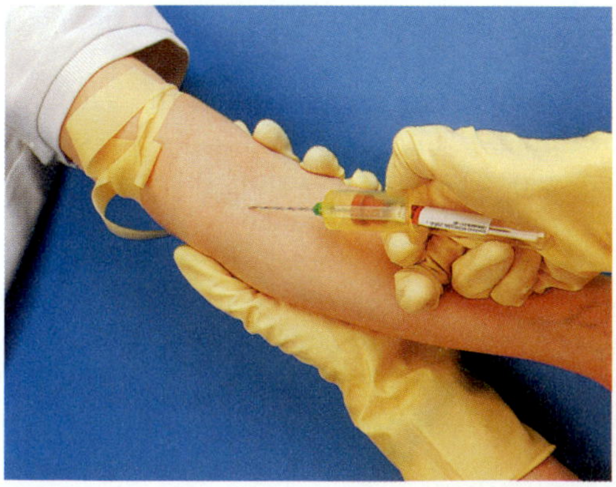

FIGURE 18-43 ■ Obtaining a blood sample with a Vacutainer.

tube. The steps for obtaining a blood sample using a needle and syringe are as follows:

1. Apply a tourniquet above the selected site.
2. Cleanse the site as previously described for venipuncture.
3. Using an 18- or 20-gauge needle attached to a 10- or 12-cc syringe, enter the vein.
4. With an even, steady motion, draw back on the plunger to obtain the sample.
5. After the sample has been obtained, release the tourniquet, withdraw the needle, and apply manual pressure to the site.
6. Immediately transfer the sample to the appropriate evacuation tube. Do not force additional blood into the tube; each tube has the correct amount of vacuum for the amount of blood required in the vial. Forcing blood into a vacuum tube can cause expulsion of contents and can lead to unnecessary injury or exposure to contents.
7. Label the sample with the patient's name and the time and date it was obtained.

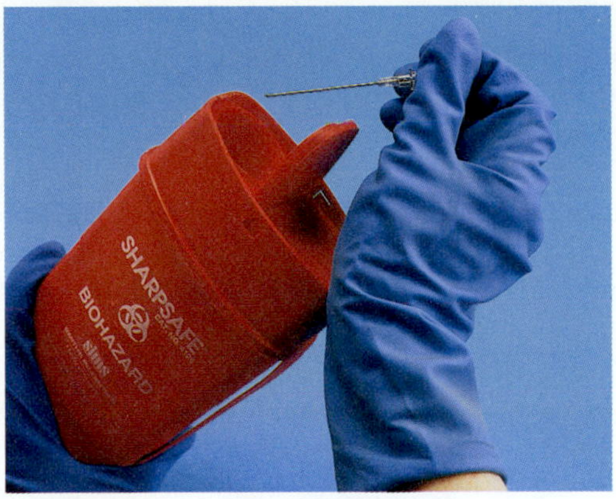

FIGURE 18-44 ■ Disposal of a needle and syringe in a sharps container.

DISPOSAL OF CONTAMINATED ITEMS AND SHARPS

Needles and other sharp objects can injure the patient, the paramedic, co-workers, and others. They also can be a source of infection with hepatitis or the human immunodeficiency virus (HIV). The CDC recommends that needles *not* be capped, bent, or broken before disposal. Rather, they should be discarded with the syringe intact in a special container (i.e., sharps container) that is clearly marked (Fig. 18-44). These containers should be puncture proof and leak proof. When full (as indicated by the "Full line," which is usually no more than three-fourths of the space), the container should be discarded according to established policies for disposition of contaminated items and sharps.

SUMMARY

- Three systems for measuring drug dosage are in common use today. These are the metric system, the apothecary system, and the common household system. Each system deals with units of mass and volume. Any of these three systems may be used by a physician when ordering drugs.
- Paramedics should choose a drug calculation method that is precise. It also should be reliable. Paramedics should
  (1) Convert all units of measure to the same size and system.
  (2) Assess the computed dosage to determine whether it is reasonable.
  (3) Use one method of dose calculation consistently.
- Many drug calculations can be performed almost intuitively. Nevertheless, paramedics should never rely on intuitive calculations. Methods of calculation include the basic formula (desire over have), ratios and proportions, and dimensional analysis.
- Intravenous flow rates can be calculated using the following formula:

$$\text{Drops/min} = \frac{\text{Volume to be infused} \times \text{Drops/mL of infusion set}}{\text{Total time of infusion (min)}}$$

- Safety procedures should be a high priority during the administration of any medication. The paramedic must make sure the *right* patient receives the *right* dose of the *right* drug via the *right* route at the *right* time.
- An incident involving a medication error may occur. In such a case, paramedics should take responsibility for their actions. They should quickly advise medical direction. They also should assess and monitor the patient for effects of the drug. They must document the error as required by local, state, and medical direction policies. In addition, they must change their personal practice to prevent a similar error in the future.
- Medical asepsis is accomplished by using clean technique, which involves hygienic measures, cleaning agents, antiseptics, disinfectants, and barrier fields.
- Enteral drugs are administered and absorbed through the gastrointestinal tract. They are given by the oral, gastric, and rectal routes. Parenteral drugs are administered outside the intestine. They are usually injected. Parenteral drugs are given by the intradermal, subcutaneous, intramuscular, intravenous, and intraosseous routes.
- In the prehospital setting, the route of choice for fluid replacement is through a peripheral vein in an extremity. The over-the-needle catheter generally is preferred in this setting.
- Several possible complications are associated with all intravenous techniques. These include local complications, systemic complications, infiltration, and air embolism.
- Cannulation of the central veins presents specific dangers. These are in addition to the complications common to all intravenous methods.
- Fluids and drugs that are infused by the intraosseous route pass from the marrow cavities into the sinusoids. Next, they pass into large venous channels and emissary veins. Then they pass into the systemic circulation. The site of choice for IO infusions in children is the tibia, one to two fingerbreadths below the tubercle on the anteromedial surface.
- Percutaneous drugs are absorbed through the mucous membranes or skin. These include topical drugs, sublingual drugs, buccal drugs, inhaled drugs, endotracheal drugs, and drugs for the eye, nose, and ear.

Continued

- Administering drugs to infants and children can be quite difficult. This often is especially true in emergency situations. Paramedics frequently calculate pediatric drug doses by using memory aids. Some of these aids include charts, tapes, and dosage books. Doses also are calculated with the advice of medical direction.
- If possible, venous blood samples should be obtained when intravenous access is established. They also should be obtained before any fluids are infused. If no IV line is to be used and a blood sample is still needed, it must be obtained with a needle and syringe (or a special vacuum needle and sleeve).
- The CDC recommends that needles not be capped, bent, or broken before disposal. Rather, they should be left on the syringe and discarded in an appropriate, clearly marked container that is puncture proof and leak proof.

REFERENCES

1. Moseley R: *Everything you always wanted to know about metrics,* Valdese, NC, 1978, R&R Enterprises.
2. Salerno E: Pharmacology for health professionals, St Louis, 1999, Mosby.
3. Institute for Healthcare Improvement: *Healthplan,* Boston, 1998, The Institute.
4. Institute of Medicine, National Academy of Sciences, The National Academy Press.
5. Centers for Disease Control and Prevention: *Morbidity and Mortality Weekly Report* 51(No RR-10), 2002.
6. American Heart Association: *Pediatric advanced life support,* Dallas, 1997, The Association.
7. Hospital Infection Control Practices Advisory Council: Part II. Recommendations for isolation precautions in hospitals. www.cdc.gov/ncidod/hip/isolat/ isopart2.htm. Accessed 1997.
8. *Needle and cannula technique,* Chicago, 1977, Abbott Laboratories.

APPENDIX
Universal Precautions: Measures to Prevent Transmission of the Human Immunodeficiency Virus (HIV)

Universal precautions (i.e., universal blood and body fluid precautions) were developed by the Centers for Disease Control and Prevention (CDC) in 1987. They are the minimum standard of practice recommended by the Occupational Safety and Health Act of 1991 and by all health care agencies.

Universal precautions should be used in the care of all patients. However, they are especially important for paramedics and others who work in emergency care. These health care professionals face a higher risk of exposure to blood. Also, the patient's infection status usually is unknown at this point.

Universal precautions include the following:

1. All health care workers should routinely use appropriate barrier precautions to prevent skin and mucous membrane exposure when contact with blood or other body fluids of any patient is anticipated. Gloves should be worn for touching blood and body fluids, mucous membranes, or nonintact skin of all patients; for handling items or surfaces soiled with blood or body fluids; and for performing venipuncture and other vascular access procedures. Gloves should be changed after contact with each patient. Masks and protective eyewear or face shields should be worn during procedures that are likely to generate droplets of blood or other body fluids, to prevent exposure of mucous membranes of the mouth, nose, and eyes. Gowns or aprons should be worn during procedures that are likely to generate splashes or a spray of blood or other body fluids.
2. The hands and other skin surfaces should be washed immediately and thoroughly if they become contaminated with blood or other body fluids. The hands should be washed immediately after gloves are removed.
3. All health care workers should take precautions to prevent injuries caused by needles, scalpels, and other sharp instruments or devices during procedures, when cleaning used instruments, during disposal of used needles, and when handling sharp instruments after procedures. Needles should not be recapped, purposely bent or broken by hand, removed from disposable syringes, or otherwise manipulated by hand. After use, disposable syringes and needles, scalpel blades, and other sharp items should be placed in puncture-resistant containers for disposal. The containers should be located as close as practical to the area where these items are used. Large-bore reusable needles should be placed in a puncture-resistant container for transport to the processing area.
4. Saliva has not been implicated in the transmission of HIV. However, to minimize the need for emergency mouth-to-mouth resuscitation, mouthpieces, resuscitation bags, or other ventilation devices should be available for use in areas where the need for resuscitation is predictable.
5. Health care workers who have exudative lesions or weeping dermatitis should refrain from all direct patient care and from handling patient care equipment until the condition resolves.
6. Pregnant health care workers are not known to be at greater risk of contracting HIV infection than health care workers who are not pregnant. However, if a health care worker becomes infected with HIV during pregnancy, the infant is at risk of infection as a result of perinatal transmission. Because of this risk, pregnant health care workers should be especially familiar with and strictly follow precautions for minimizing the risk of HIV transmission.

Implementation of universal precautions for all patients eliminates the need for the isolation category of blood and body fluid precautions, which was previously recommended by the CDC for patients known to be or suspected of being infected with blood-borne pathogens. Isolation precautions (e.g., against enteric, acid-fast bacillus [AFB]) should be used as necessary if associated conditions such as infectious diarrhea or tuberculosis are diagnosed or suspected.

Centers for Disease Control: Precautions to prevent transmission of HIV: universal precautions_recommendations for prevention of HIV transmission in health care settings. *Morbidity and Mortality Weekly Report* 36(suppl no 2S), 1987. Accessed on February 15, 2005 at http://aepo-xdv-www.epo.cdc.gov/wonder/prevguid/ poooo318/body0006.htm.

PART FIVE

IN THIS PART

CHAPTER 19 Airway Management and Ventilation

CHAPTER

19

Airway Management and Ventilation

OBJECTIVES

Upon completion of this chapter, the paramedic student will be able to:

1. Distinguish between respiration, pulmonary ventilation, and external and internal respiration.
2. Explain the mechanics of respiration.
3. Explain the relationship of the partial pressures of gases in the blood and lungs to atmospheric gas pressures.
4. Describe pulmonary circulation.
5. Explain the process of exchange and transport of gases in the body.
6. Describe voluntary, chemical, and nervous regulation of respiration.
7. Discuss the assessment and management of medical or traumatic obstruction of the airway.
8. Outline the causes and effects of and preventive measures for pulmonary aspiration.
9. Outline the essential parameters for evaluating the effectiveness of the airway and breathing.
10. Describe the indications, contraindications, and techniques for delivery of supplemental oxygen.
11. Discuss methods of patient ventilation based on the indications, contraindications, potential complications, and use of each method.
12. Describe the use of manual airway maneuvers and mechanical airway adjuncts based on the indications, contraindications, potential complications, and techniques for each.
13. Describe assessment techniques and devices used to ensure adequate oxygenation, correct placement of the endotracheal tube, and elimination of carbon dioxide.
14. Explain variations in assessment and management of airway and ventilation problems in pediatric patients.
15. Given a patient scenario, identify possible alterations in oxygenation and ventilation based on a knowledge of gas exchange and the mechanics of breathing.

KEY TERMS

anatomical dead space: The volume of the conducting airways from the external environment down to the terminal bronchioles.

atelectasis: An abnormal condition characterized by the collapse of lung tissue; it prevents the respiratory exchange of oxygen and carbon dioxide.

compliance: The ease with which the lungs and thorax expand during pressure changes. The greater the compliance, the easier the expansion.

Fick principle: The principle used to determine cardiac output. It assumes that the amount of oxygen delivered to an organ is equal to the amount of oxygen consumed by that organ plus the amount of oxygen carried away from that organ.

gag reflex: A normal neural response triggered by touching the soft palate or posterior pharynx.

hypocarbia: A state of diminished carbon dioxide in the blood; also known as hypocapnia.

hypoxemia: A state of decreased oxygen content of arterial blood.

hypoxia: A state of decreased oxygen content at the tissue level.

intrapulmonic pressure: The pressure of the gas in the alveoli.

intrathoracic pressure: The pressure in the pleural space; also known as intrapleural pressure.

minute volume: The amount of gas inhaled or exhaled in 1 minute. It is found by multiplying the tidal volume by the respiratory rate.

physiological dead space: The sum of the anatomical dead space plus the volume of any nonfunctional alveoli.

pulmonary ventilation: The movement of air into and out of the lungs. This process brings oxygen into the lungs and removes carbon dioxide.

respiration: The exchange of oxygen and carbon dioxide between an organism and the environment.

tidal volume: The volume of air inspired or expired in a single, resting breath.

The absence of an adequate airway and ineffective ventilation are major causes of preventable death and cardiopulmonary complications in all patients. A thorough understanding of the respiratory system and mastery of airway management and ventilation are important aspects of prehospital emergency care.

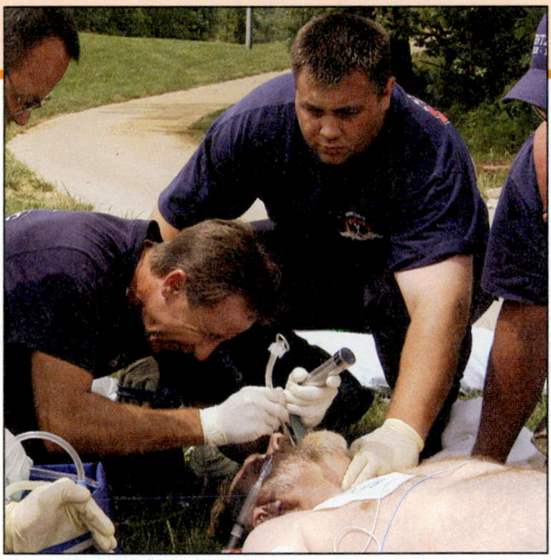

SECTION ONE RESPIRATORY PHYSIOLOGY

MECHANICS OF RESPIRATION

Respiration is the exchange of oxygen and carbon dioxide between an organism and the environment. For the gas exchange to occur, air must move freely into and out of the lungs. This brings oxygen into the lungs and removes carbon dioxide. The process is known as **pulmonary ventilation.**

The two phases of respiration are external respiration and internal respiration. *External respiration* is the transfer of oxygen and carbon dioxide between the inspired air and pulmonary capillaries. *Internal respiration* is the transfer of oxygen and carbon dioxide between the capillary red blood cells and the tissue cells.

Pressure Changes and Ventilation

Gas flows from an area of higher pressure or concentration to an area of lower pressure or concentration. For gas to flow into the lungs, a pressure gradient is required. This pressure

> **CRITICAL THINKING**
>
> Think of two medical conditions that could impair (1) external respiration and (2) internal respiration.

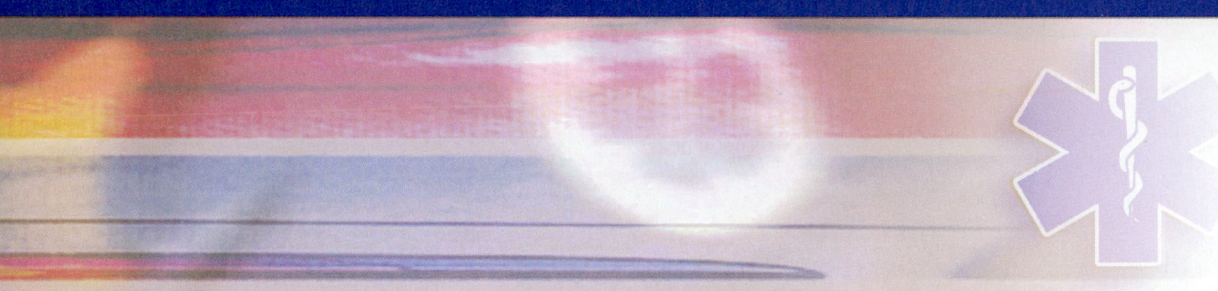

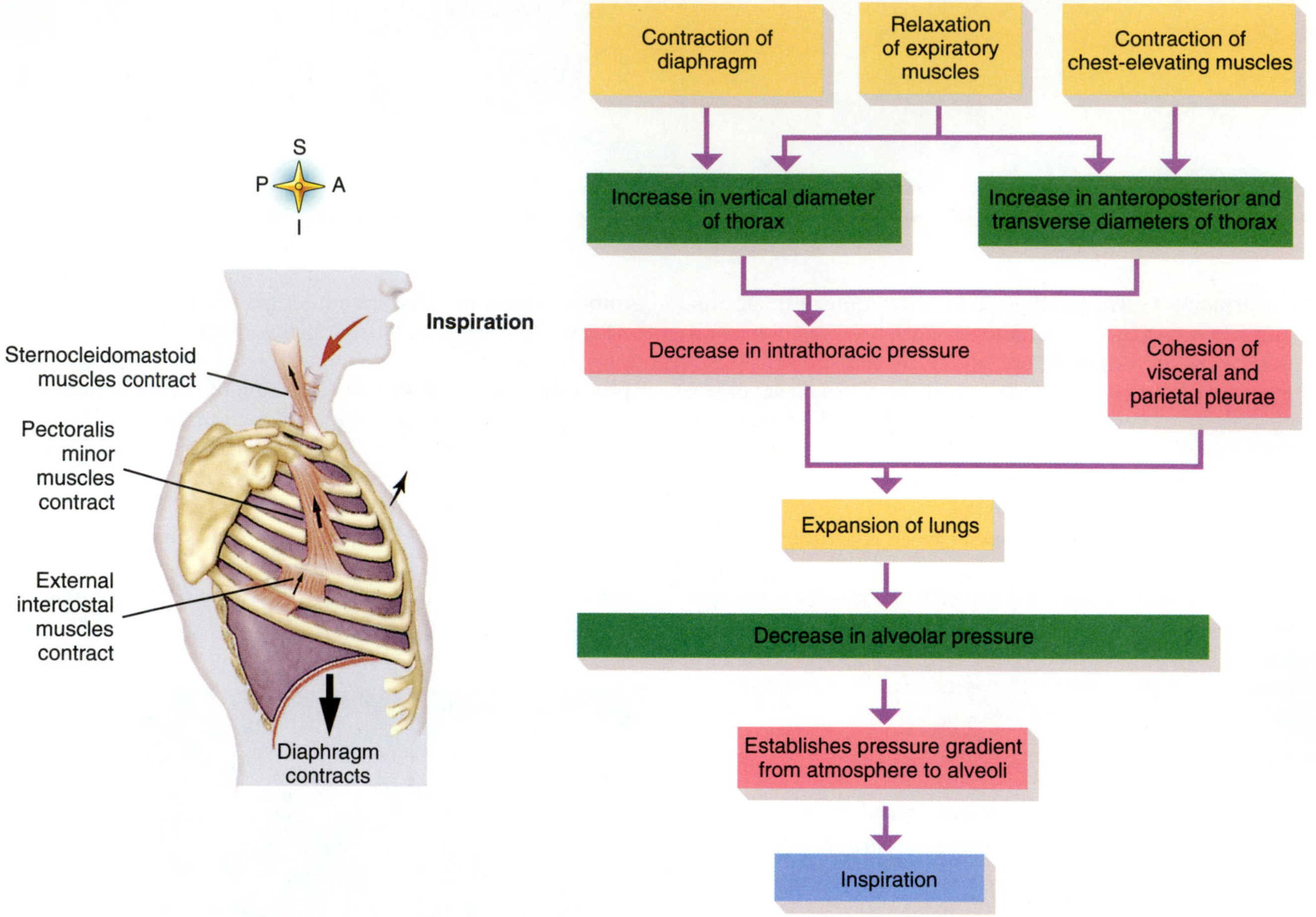

FIGURE 19-1 ■ Mechanics of inspiration.

gradient is produced by differences between atmospheric pressure, **intrapulmonic pressure,** and intrapleural pressure (also known as **intrathoracic pressure).**

Atmospheric pressure is the pressure of the gas around us. It varies with differences in altitude. At sea level, it is 760 mm Hg. *Intrapulmonic pressure* is the pressure of the gas in the alveoli. Depending on the size of the thorax, this pressure varies a little above and below 760 mm Hg. The intrapulmonic pressure also depends on whether it is measured during inspiration or expiration. *Intrathoracic pressure* is the pressure in the pleural space. It normally is less than the atmospheric pressure (usually 751 to 754 mm Hg). However, it may exceed the atmospheric pressure during coughing or straining during bowel movements.

During inspiration the chest wall expands. This increases the size of the thoracic cavity and expands the lungs. The expansion results from muscle movement and negative pressure in the pleural space. As the thorax expands, the lung space increases. This causes a drop in the intrapulmonic pressure of about 1 mm Hg below atmospheric pressure. The pressure gradient results in gas flow into the lungs. At end inspiration the thorax stops expanding and the alveoli stop expanding. The intrapulmonic pressure becomes equal to the atmospheric pressure, and gas no longer moves into the lungs (Fig. 19-1).

As the chest wall relaxes during expiration, the respiratory muscles are at rest. The process of inspiration reverses. Elastic recoil causes the thorax and lung space to decrease in size. This increases the intrapulmonic pressure. The pressure gradient created in the thoracic cavity produces a decrease in alveolar volume and increases the intrapulmonic pressure about 1 mm Hg over the atmospheric pressure. The pressure gradient results in gas flow out of the lungs. At the end of expiration the opposing forces and pressures become equal. The thoracic volume no longer decreases. The intrapulmonic pressure becomes equal to the atmospheric pressure, and gas movement out of the lungs stops (Fig. 19-2).

Muscles of Respiration

The expansion of the lungs and thorax is caused by the movement of the diaphragm and the internal and external intercostal muscles (Fig. 19-3). On inspiration, the diaphragm contracts and the dome of the diaphragm flattens. This increases the superior-inferior dimension of the chest cavity. The internal and external intercostal muscles

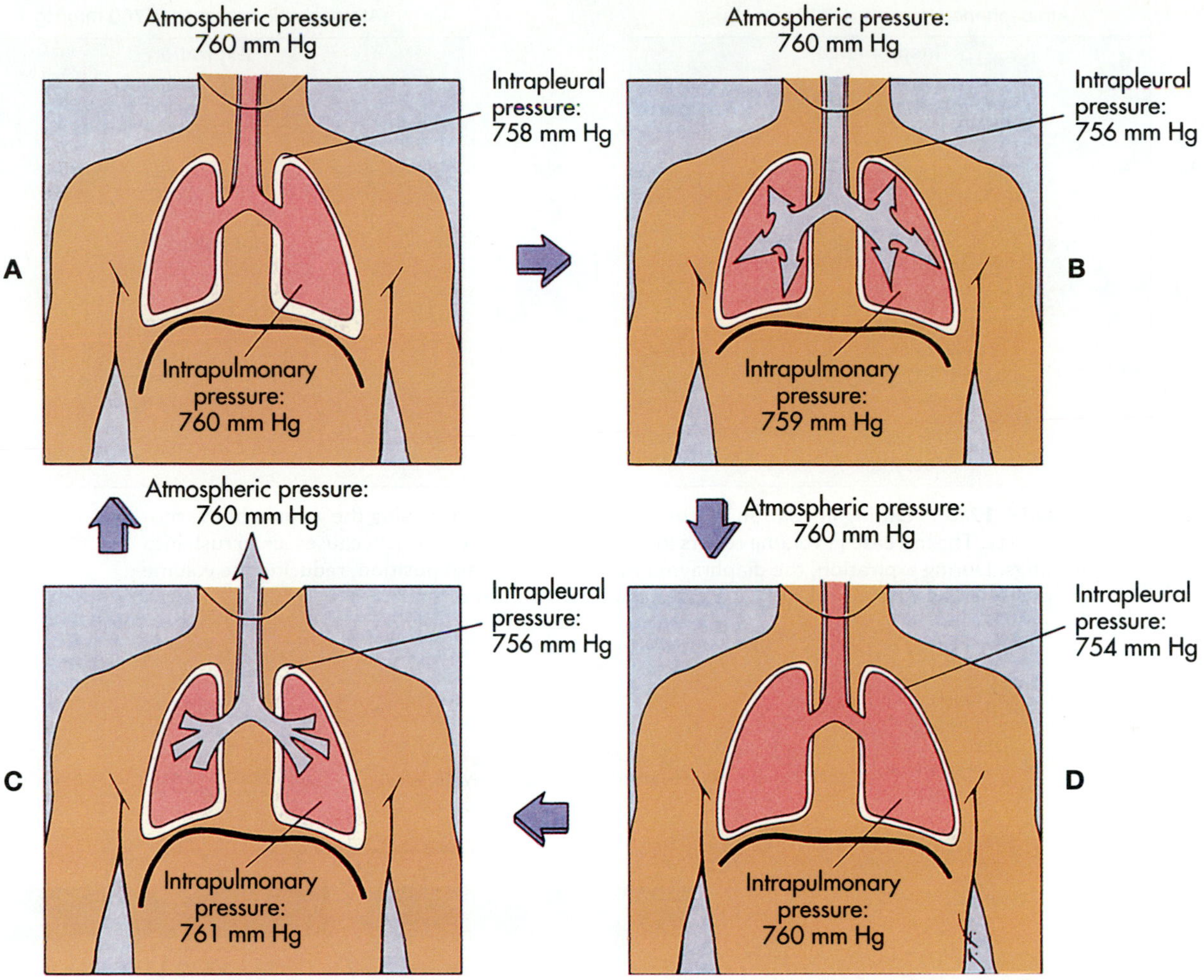

FIGURE 19-2 ■ Pressure changes during inspiration and expiration. **A,** At the end of expiration, intrapulmonary pressure equals atmospheric pressure, and no movement of air occurs. **B,** During inspiration, the volume of the pleural space increases, causing the pressure in the intrapulmonary spaces (alveoli) to decrease. Air then flows from the outside of the body, where the pressure is greater (760 mm Hg), into the alveoli, where it is lower (759 mm Hg). **C,** At the end of inspiration, intrapulmonary pressure again equals atmospheric pressure, and no movement of air occurs. **D,** During expiration, the volume of the pleural spaces decreases, causing the intrapulmonary pressure to increase. Because the intrapulmonary pressure exceeds the atmospheric pressure, air flows out of the lungs.

also contract. This raises the ribs. It also increases the front-to-back (anterior-posterior) and side-to-side dimensions of the chest cavity.

CRITICAL THINKING

How will interruption of the chest wall from a stab wound change the mechanics of breathing?

Expiration is a passive motion. During expiration, relaxation of the diaphragm and internal intercostal muscles allows the elastic recoil properties of the lungs to decrease the size (or volume) of the thoracic cavity (Fig. 19-4). The ease with which the lungs and thorax expand during pressure changes is known as **compliance.** The greater the compliance, the easier the expansion. Diseases that decrease compliance increase the energy required for breathing. Examples of such diseases are asthma, emphysema, bronchitis, and pulmonary edema.

Work of Breathing

In people who are healthy, the energy needed for normal, quiet breathing is about 3% of the total body expenditure. Factors that increase the amount of energy needed for ventilation include loss of pulmonary surfactant, an increase in airway resistance, or a decrease in pulmonary compliance. These factors can increase the energy requirement to as much as 33% of the total body expenditure.

The pulmonary alveoli have a tendency to collapse. This is the result of recoil caused by the elastic fibers and the surface tension of the alveolar walls. The surface tension is created because water molecules are attracted to each other in

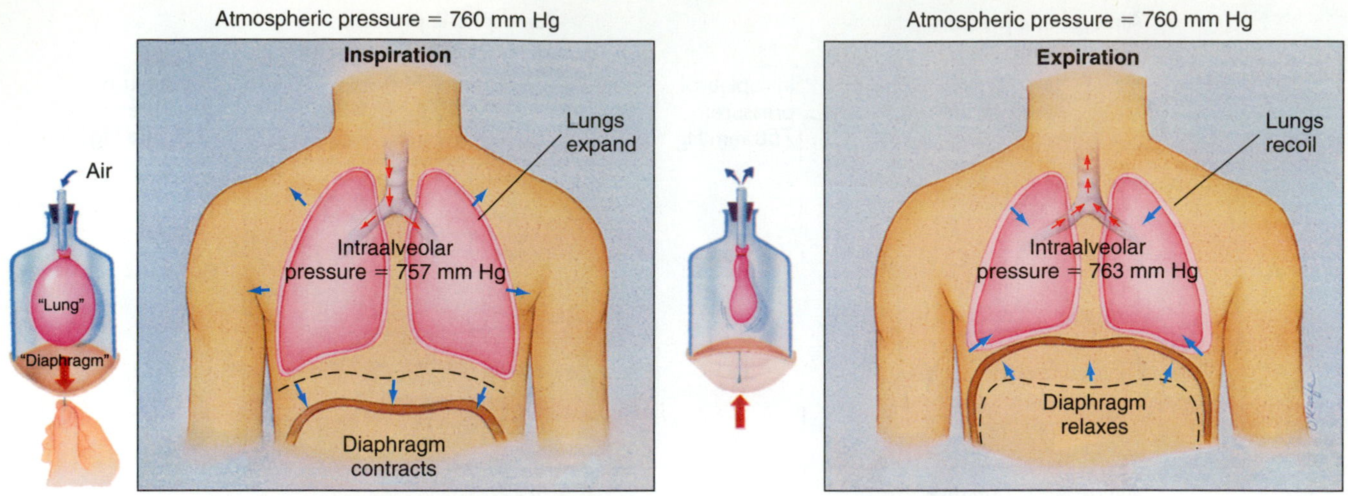

FIGURE 19-3 ■ During inhalation, the diaphragm contracts, increasing the volume of the thoracic cavity. The increase in volume results in a decrease in pressure, which causes air to rush into the lungs. During expiration, the diaphragm returns to an upward position, reducing the volume of the thoracic cavity. Air pressure increases and forces air out of the lungs.

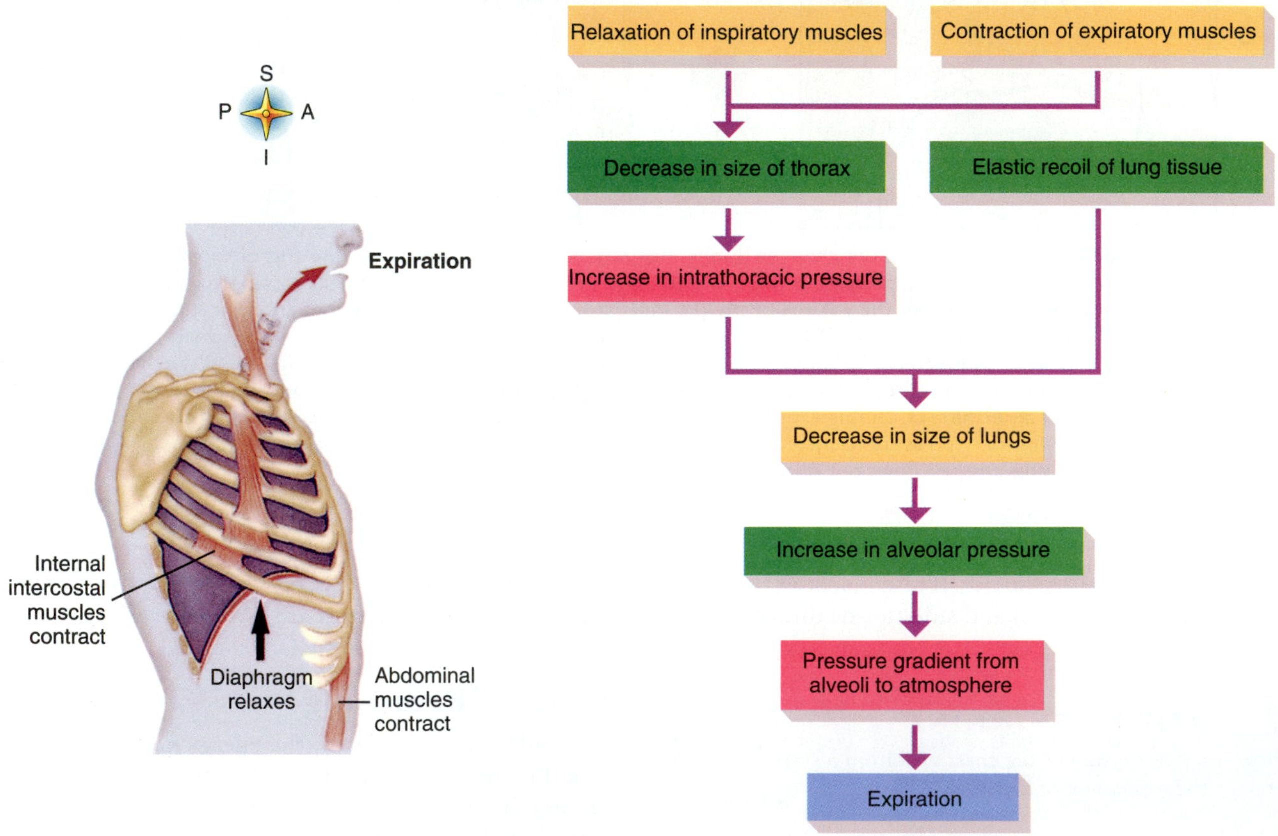

FIGURE 19-4 ■ Relaxation of the diaphragm and contraction of the chest-depressing muscles (the internal intercostal muscles) reduce the thoracic volume. This increases pressure in the lungs, pushing air out.

the alveolar membrane. Pulmonary surfactant lowers the surface tension. It does this by intermingling with the water molecules to reduce the cohesive force. This helps to prevent collapse of the alveolus at the end of expiration.

Surfactant is constantly being replenished by certain alveolar cells. Its production is thought to be stimulated by normal ventilation. If this production decreases, as occurs in pneumonia, very high ventilation pressures may be needed to produce lung expansion.

The elastic forces of the lung oppose lung expansion. Viscous and frictional forces often play the central role in impeding airflow into and out of the lungs. Much of the resistance to airflow is provided by the upper airways of the respiratory tract. The nasal passages cause about 50% of the total airway resistance during nose breathing. The mouth, pharynx, larynx, and trachea account for approximately 20% to 30% of airway resistance during quiet mouth breathing. This may increase to about 50% during times of increased ventilation (e.g., during vigorous exercise).

Airway resistance falls greatly as the bronchial tree continues to branch toward the alveoli. This happens because of the large increase in the total cross-sectional diameter of the airways. Still, the presence of airway secretions or bronchiolar constriction can lead to increased airway resistance. These factors may occur separately. More often, they occur at the same time (e.g., as in asthma). When resistance to airflow increases, the usual pressure gradient needed for ventilation is inadequate. Therefore muscular effort is needed to create a larger pressure gradient.

Structural changes in the lungs or thorax as a result of trauma or disease also may increase the amount of work needed for effective ventilation. This increased work usually is obvious from the use of *accessory muscles* during labored breathing. The accessory muscles include the scalenes and the sternocleidomastoid (deep muscles of the neck and thorax), posterior neck and back muscles, and the abdominal muscles (Fig. 19-5).

Lung Volumes and Capacities

At rest, the average adult breathes about 12 to 24 times per minute. One fifth of this inspired air never reaches the alveoli for gas exchange. Instead, it fills the upper respiratory tract and lower nonrespiratory bronchioles. This area is referred to as **anatomical dead space.** The term **physiological dead space** refers to the anatomical dead space plus the volume of any nonfunctional alveoli. Usually the anatomical and physiological dead spaces are nearly identical. However, this is not always the case. In patients with respiratory diseases, such as emphysema, the alveolar walls begin to degenerate. The destruction of these walls can increase the size of the physiological dead space up to 10 times that of the anatomical dead space (Fig. 19-6).

The lungs can hold about eight times the amount of air brought in by a normal resting inhalation. From the first breath of life, the lungs are never fully emptied. Even after forced expiration, a "residual volume" of air remains in the alveoli. This residual volume is replenished slowly. At least 16 breaths, and at times more, are needed to renew the residual volume of air in the lungs.

Tidal volume is the volume of gas inhaled or exhaled during a normal breath. The tidal volume of the average adult is about 500 to 600 mL. Of this, 150 mL remains in the anatomical dead space (the bronchi, bronchioles, and other prealveolar structures) until it is exhaled during the next respiratory cycle. Therefore 150 mL of the atmospheric gas inhaled during each inspiration never reaches the alveoli. It is merely moved into and out of the airways. A paramedic observing the rise and fall of a patient's chest is indirectly observing tidal volume.

The *inspiratory reserve volume* is the amount of gas that can be forcefully inhaled after inspiration of the normal tidal volume. This amount is usually 2000 to 3000 mL. The *expiratory reserve volume* is the amount of gas that can be forcefully exhaled after expiration of the normal tidal volume. This volume usually is less than the inspiratory reserve volume (about 1200 mL). The *residual volume* is the gas that remains in the respiratory system after forced expiration. The normal residual volume is 1000 to 1200 mL.

The combined measurements of tidal volume, inspiratory reserve volume, expiratory reserve volume, and residual volume constitute the maximum volume to which the lungs can be expanded.

Pulmonary capacities are the sum of two or more pulmonary volumes. The more common pulmonary capacities are as follows (Fig. 19-7):

- *Inspiratory capacity:* Inspiratory capacity is the tidal volume plus the inspiratory reserve volume. This capacity reflects the amount of gas a person can inspire maximally after a normal expiration (about 3500 mL).
- *Functional residual capacity:* Functional residual capacity is the expiratory reserve volume plus the residual volume. This capacity reflects the amount of gas remaining in the lungs at the end of a normal expiration (about 2300 mL).
- *Vital capacity:* Vital capacity is the volume of gas that can move on deepest inspiration and expiration or the sum of the inspiratory reserve volume, the tidal volume, and the expiratory reserve volume. This capacity is about 4600 mL.
- *Total lung capacity:* Total lung capacity is the sum of the vital capacity and the residual volume (about 5800 mL).

CRITICAL THINKING

Consider a severe burn that encircles the chest. Which respiratory volumes will be affected?

Minute Volume and Minute Alveolar Ventilation

The **minute volume** is the amount of gas inhaled or exhaled in 1 minute. It is found by multiplying the tidal volume by the respiratory rate. For example, a patient's respiratory rate may be 10 breaths per minute, and the resting

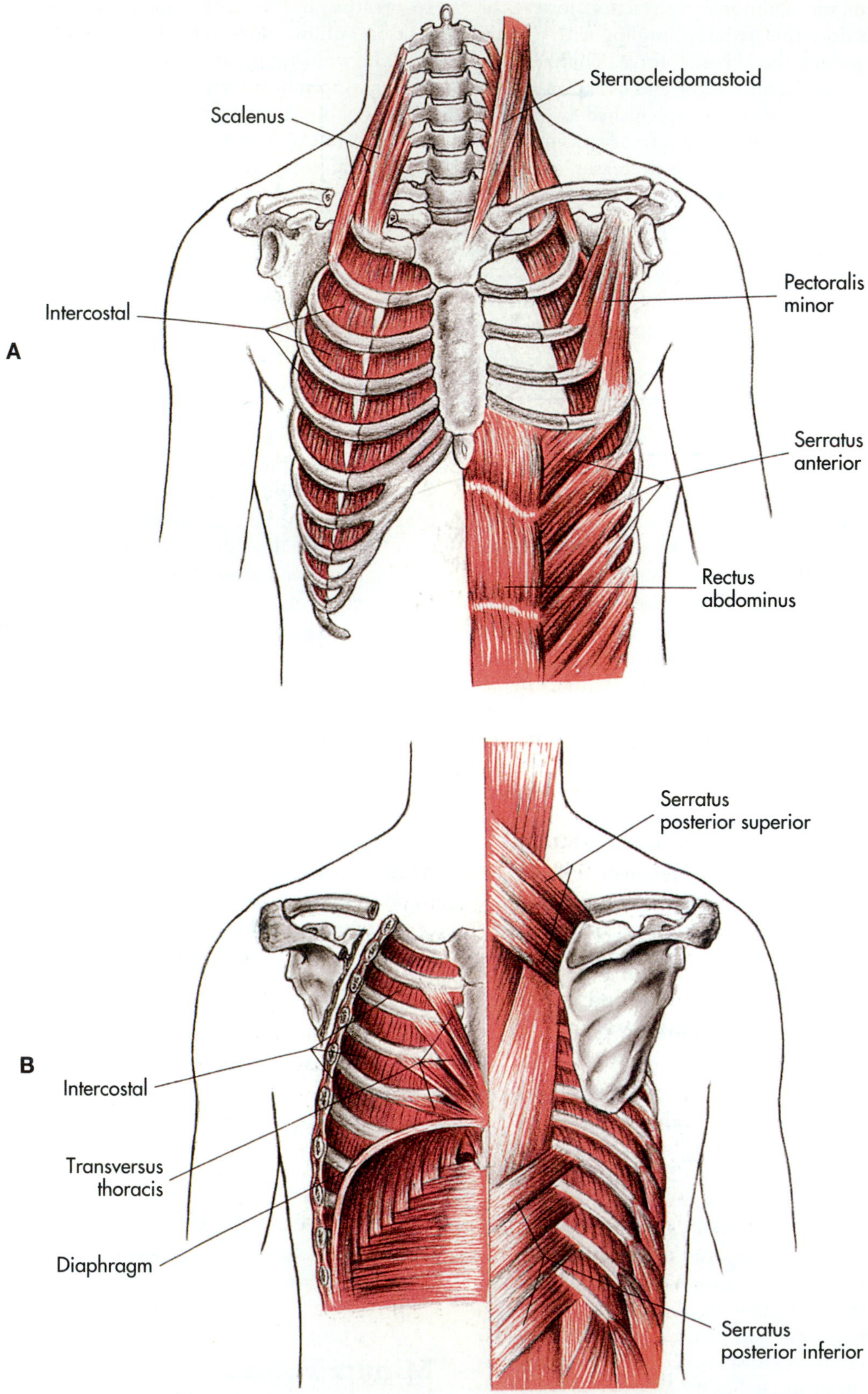

FIGURE 19-5 ■ Muscles of ventilation. **A,** Anterior view. **B,** Posterior view.

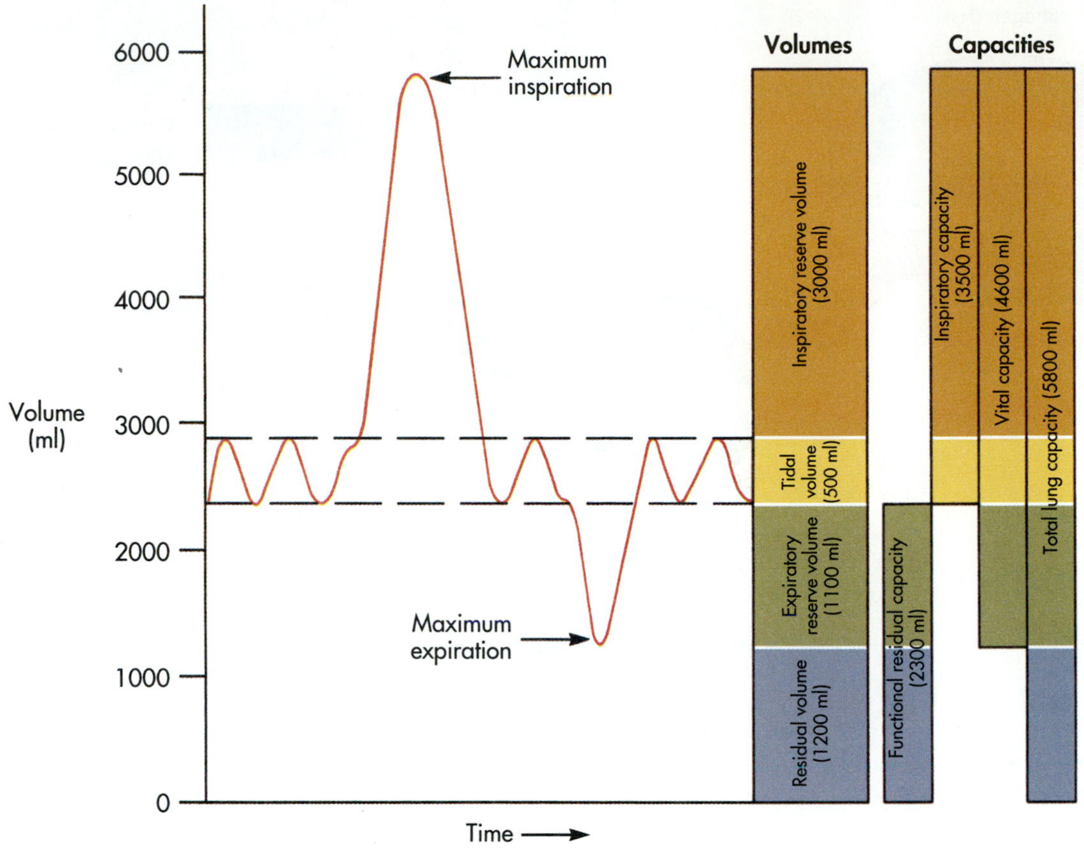

FIGURE 19-6 ■ Lung volumes and capacities. Tidal volume during resting conditions.

Pulmonary Capacities	
Tidal volume + Inspiratory reserve volume **Inspiratory capacity (3500 mL)**	Expiratory reserve volume + Residual volume **Functional residual capacity (2300 mL)**
Inspiratory reserve volume Tidal volume + Expiratory reserve volume **Vital capacity (4600 mL)**	Vital capacity + Residual volume **Total lung capacity (5800 mL)**

FIGURE 19-7 ■ Pulmonary capacities.

tidal volume may be 500 mL. Thus the average minute volume is 5 L/min.

Much of the gas that is inspired during respiration fills the anatomical dead space before reaching the alveoli. That air therefore is unavailable for gas exchange. The amount of inspired gas available for gas exchange during 1 minute is referred to as the *minute alveolar ventilation.* The minute alveolar ventilation is calculated by subtracting the amount of dead space from the tidal volume and then multiplying the result by the respiratory rate:

Minute alveolar ventilation = (Tidal volume − Dead space) × Respiratory rate

If the tidal volume or the respiratory rate, or both, increase, the minute volume also increases. Likewise, if the tidal volume or the respiratory rate, or both, decrease, the minute volume decreases. The paramedic must note the depth of respiration (tidal volume) and the respiratory rate to determine whether the patient's respiratory status is adequate.

MEASUREMENT OF GASES

The mixture of gases that make up the atmosphere exerts a combined partial pressure. This pressure is measured in millimeters of mercury, or torr (1 torr = 1 mm Hg), based on the percentage of a particular gas (Table 19-1). The atmospheric pressure at sea level (760 mm Hg) represents 100%. Nitrogen makes up about 78.62% of the volume of dry atmospheric gas at sea level. The partial pressure that results from nitrogen is calculated by multiplying 78.62% by 760 mm Hg. This equals 597 mm Hg, or a partial pressure of nitrogen (PN_2) of 597 torr. Oxygen accounts for 20.84% of the volume of atmospheric gas. The partial pres-

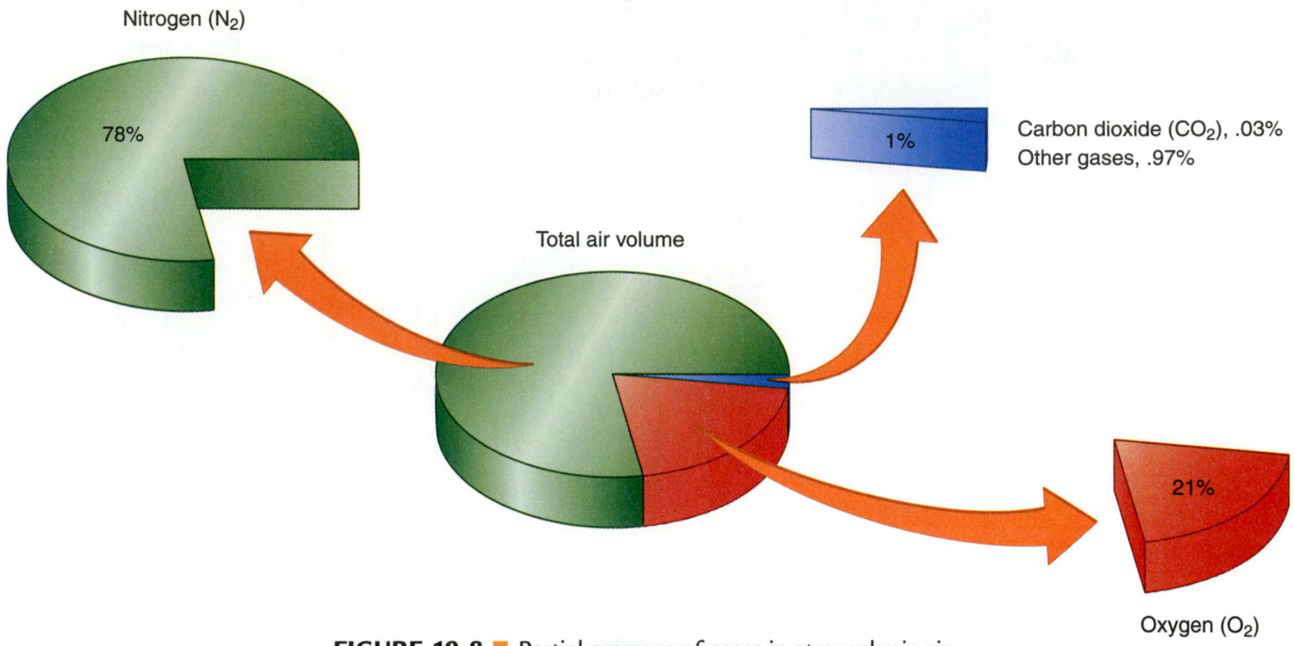

FIGURE 19-8 ■ Partial pressure of gases in atmospheric air.

TABLE 19-1 Concentration of Gases

GAS	CONCENTRATION
Atmospheric Gases	
Nitrogen	597 torr (78.62%)
Oxygen	159 torr (20.84%)
Carbon dioxide	0.3 torr (0.50%)
Water (vapor)	3.7 torr (6.2%)
Alveolar Gases	
Nitrogen	569 torr (74.9%)
Oxygen	104 torr (13.7%)
Carbon dioxide	40 torr (5.2%)
Water (vapor)	47 torr (6.2%)

sure of oxygen (Po_2), therefore, is found by multiplying 20.84% by 760 mm Hg. This equals 159 mm Hg, or a Po_2 of 159 torr (Fig. 19-8).

Another partial pressure can be measured when gas comes into contact with water. The water molecules convert into a gas, evaporate, and exert a partial pressure. This partial pressure is known as *water vapor pressure* (PH_2O).

The compositions of alveolar gas and dry atmospheric gas are not the same. This is a result of several factors: humidification of the air entering the respiratory system by the body, the exchange of oxygen and carbon dioxide between the alveoli and the blood, and incomplete emptying of the alveoli with expiration.

PULMONARY CIRCULATION

The process of gas exchange in the lungs is the opposite of that which occurs in the tissues throughout the rest of the body. As inspired gas enters the lungs, the respiratory system brings oxygen to the blood and removes carbon dioxide. Blood that is low in oxygen returns to the heart from all parts of the body. Passing through the right side of the heart, the blood flows into either lung through the pulmonary artery. From there it flows into the smaller pulmonary arterioles. Then it flows into capillaries that surround each of the hundreds of millions of alveoli inside the lungs (Fig. 19-9).

The alveoli are now filled with a high concentration of oxygen molecules and a low concentration of carbon dioxide molecules as a result of the inhaled air. They have the pressure gradient required for gas exchange. Oxygen molecules move into the surrounding capillaries at the same time that carbon dioxide molecules move into the alveoli to

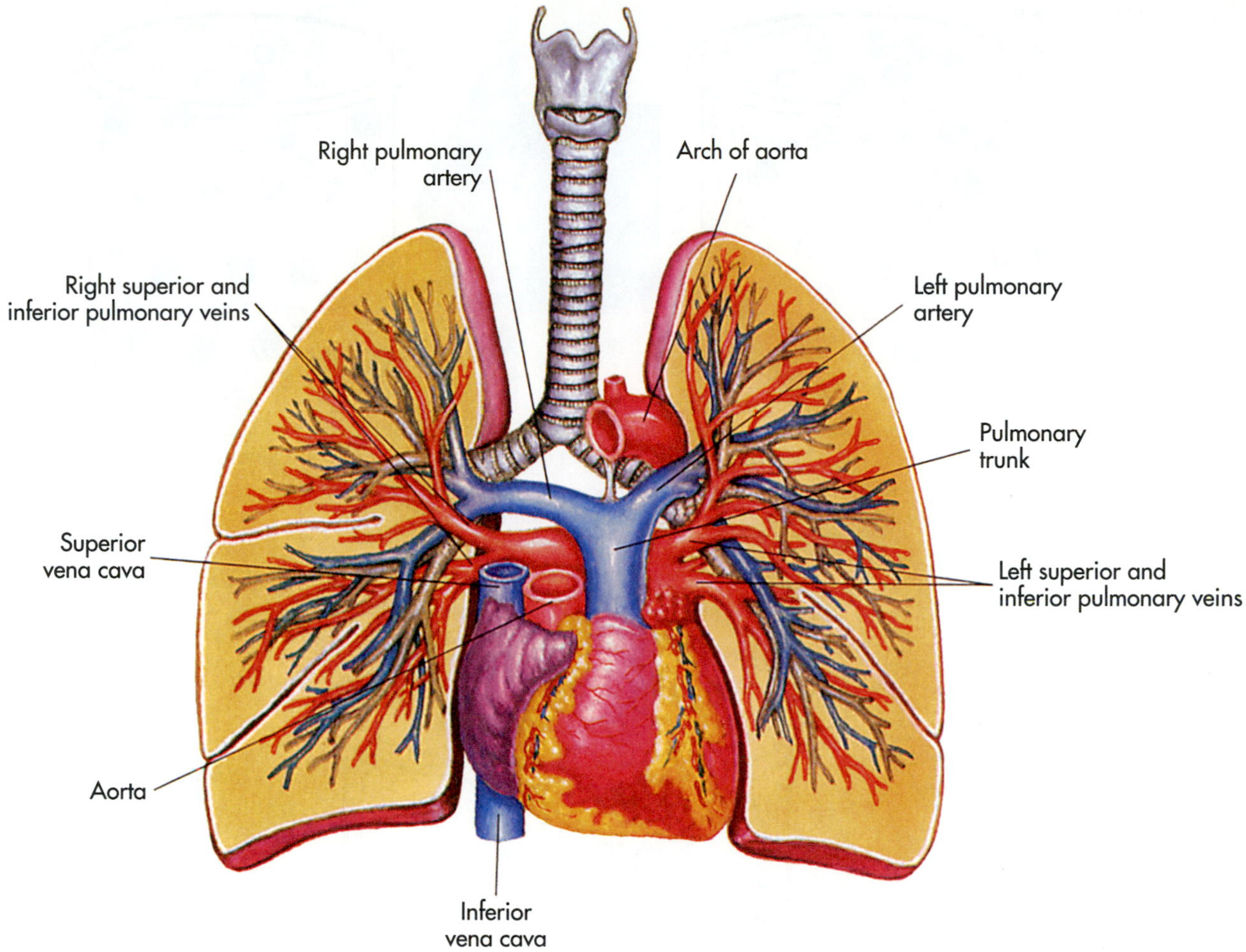

FIGURE 19-9 ■ Pulmonary circulation.

be exhaled. The blood is now rich in oxygen. It flows through the pulmonary venules into the pulmonary veins. From there it flows into the left atrium and then into the left ventricle. Next, it flows back out through the aorta to the body's tissues. To supply enough oxygen to the body tissues, an alveolus fills and empties more than 15,000 times in a day of normal breathing.

Exchange and Transport of Gases in the Body

The volume of oxygen taken up in the lungs can be measured. It can be calculated from the difference in the amount of oxygen in inspired and expired air. The volume of carbon dioxide that is eliminated can be determined in a similar way.

As noted in Chapter 6, *metabolism* is defined as all the chemical changes that occur in the body. In a healthy body with a constant metabolism, the relationship between tissue carbon dioxide production and oxygen consumption remains the same. In general, the amount of oxygen taken up by the capillary blood is greater than the amount of carbon dioxide released by the blood to the alveolar gas. Thus the expired volume is a little less than the inspired volume.

At rest, the combined consumption of oxygen by all the body cells is about 200 mL per minute. About the same amount of carbon dioxide is produced by the cells. About 20% of atmospheric gas is oxygen. Thus the total oxygen inspired is 20% multiplied by 5 L (the average amount of air inhaled in 1 minute). Of this, 200 mL crosses the alveoli into the pulmonary capillaries. The remaining 800 mL is exhaled. The 200 mL of oxygen is added to the amount of oxygen already in the pulmonary capillaries. It is then taken to the body tissues by the circulatory system. After the body cells use the oxygen, the oxygen that is left in the blood returns to the heart and lungs. This exchange of oxygen and carbon dioxide is carried out by the passive process of diffusion. *Diffusion* is the tendency for molecules in solution to move from an area of higher concentration to an area of lower concentration (see Chapter 7).

Diffusion

Molecules of gases are in constant, random motion. This motion is fueled by collisions with other molecules. If the blood is divided by a permeable barrier, such as a capillary wall or cell membrane, many gas molecules come into contact with and cross the barrier. The chance is much greater that highly concentrated molecules will strike and cross the

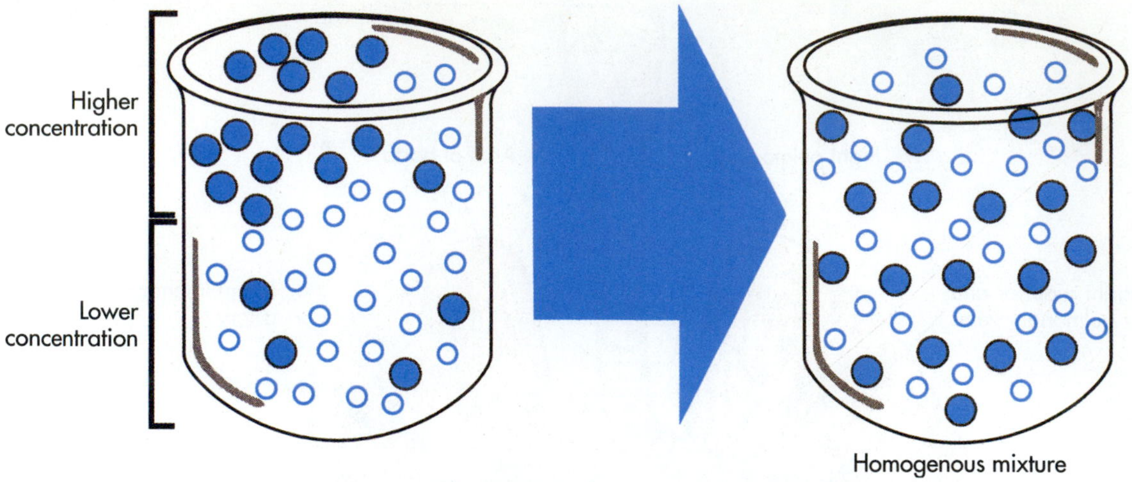

FIGURE 19-10 ■ Random movement of gas proceeds from a higher concentration to a lower concentration until a homogeneous mixture of gases is achieved.

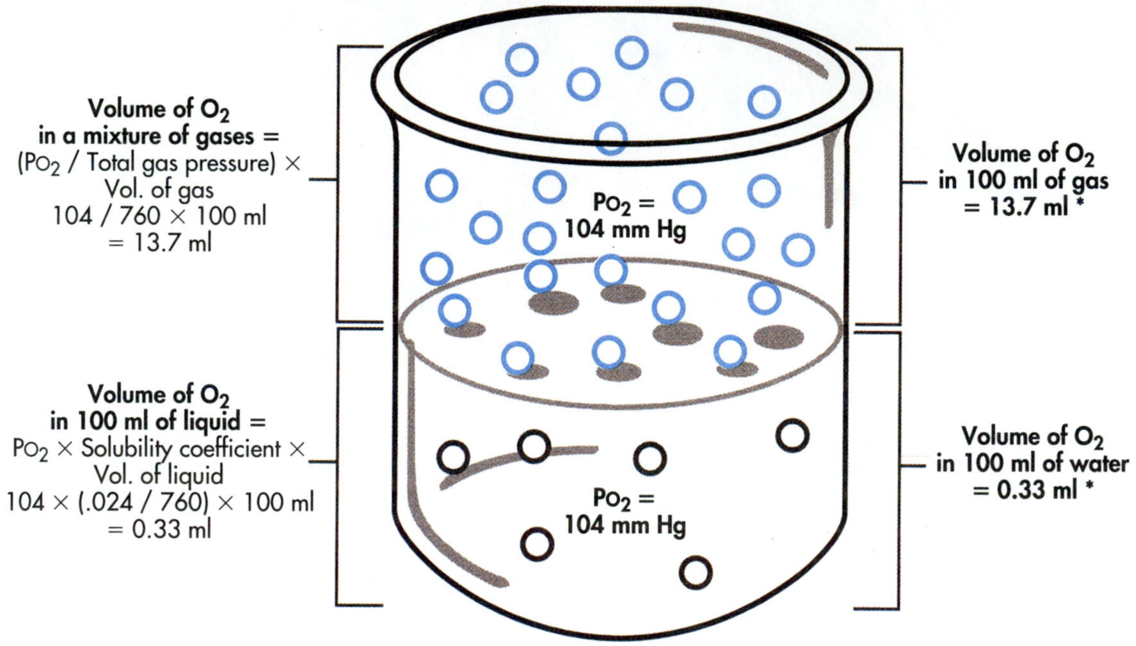

FIGURE 19-11 ■ At equilibrium, the concentration of a gas in liquid is determined by the partial pressure of the gas and by the solubility of the gas in the liquid. *At atmospheric pressure (760 mm Hg) and 98.6° F (37° C).

membrane than less concentrated molecules. Thus the concentration of molecules on either side of a permeable membrane tends to be equal (Fig.19-10).

The diffusion of gases through liquid is determined by the pressure of the gases. It also is determined by the solubility of the gases in liquid (Fig. 19-11). When a free gas comes into contact with liquid, the number of gas molecules that dissolve in the liquid is directly proportional to the pressure of the gas. When the free gas pressure is higher than the pressure of the gas in the liquid, enough molecules dissolve in the liquid to allow the free gas pressure to equal the dissolved gas pressure.

On the other hand, if a liquid containing a dissolved gas at a high pressure is exposed to a free gas at a lower pressure, gas molecules leave the liquid and enter the free gas until the pressures become equal (the general gas law). This is the underlying theme of the exchange of gases between the cells and the capillary blood throughout the body. The partial pressure of the free gas (PO_2) in the lungs is greater than the partial pressure of the dissolved oxygen in the bloodstream. Thus oxygen diffuses from the lungs to the blood. The partial pressure of oxygen in the blood is higher than that in the peripheral tissues. Thus oxygen diffuses from the blood into the tissues.

In addition to its pressure, the solubility of a gas also is a factor. The solubility of gases in a liquid affects the behavior

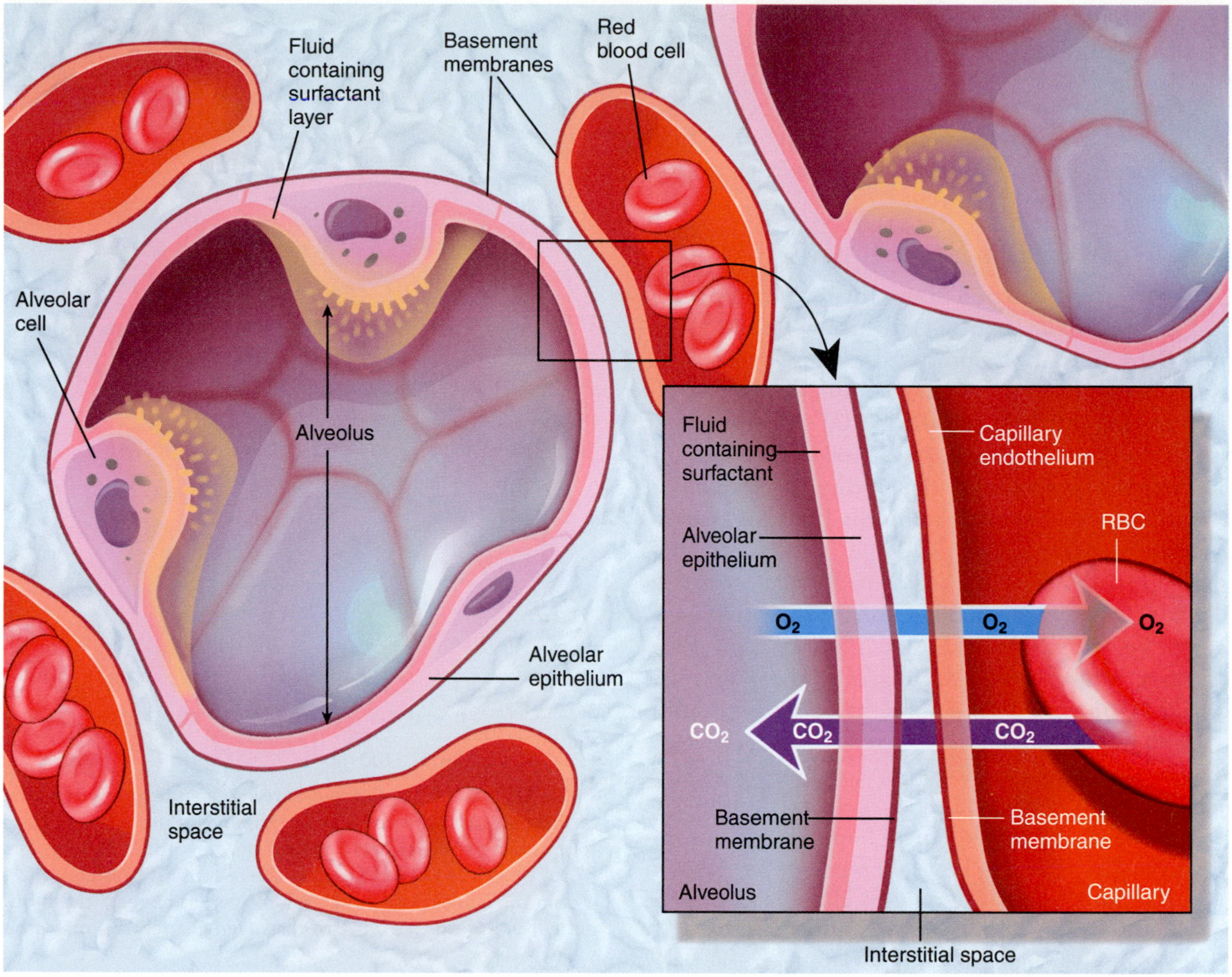

FIGURE 19-12 ■ Gas exchange structure of the lung. Each alveolus is continually ventilated with fresh air. The inset shows a magnified view of the respiratory membrane composed of the alveolar wall (fluid coating, epithelial cells, and basement membrane), interstitial fluid, and the wall of a pulmonary capillary (basement membrane and endothelial cells). The gases, carbon dioxide (CO_2) and oxygen (O_2), diffuse across the respiratory membrane.

of the gases. The ease with which gases dissolve determines the absolute number of gas molecules that diffuse through the liquid at a given pressure. For example, a liquid may be exposed to two different gases at the same pressure. The number of molecules of each gas that diffuse may not be the same because of the differing solubilities of the two gases.

Blood entering the pulmonary capillaries is systemic venous blood that has been circulated to the lungs via the pulmonary arteries. The partial pressure of carbon dioxide (Pco_2) is relatively high in this blood; the partial pressure of oxygen (Po_2) is low. The alveoli have a greater concentration of oxygen than the blood entering the pulmonary capillaries. Thus oxygen molecules diffuse from the alveoli into the blood. Carbon dioxide moves from the blood, where it is more concentrated, into the alveoli, where it is less concentrated (Fig. 19-12).

The blood flowing through the pulmonary capillaries is separated from the alveolar air by a thin layer of tissue. This layer is known as the respiratory membrane. The membrane is composed of the alveolar wall (surfactant, epithelial cells, and basement membrane), interstitial fluid, and the wall of the pulmonary capillary (basement membrane and endothelial cells). The differences in the partial pressures of oxygen and carbon dioxide on the two sides of the membrane result in diffusion. Oxygen moves into the blood and carbon dioxide into the alveoli. With this diffusion, the capillary blood Po_2 level rises. The capillary blood Pco_2 level falls. Diffusion of these gases stops when alveolar and capillary partial pressures equalize. In healthy people this gas exchange occurs so quickly that the blood leaving the lungs to be pumped through the arteries has nearly the same Po_2 (80 to 100 mm Hg) and Pco_2 (35 to 40 mm Hg) as alveolar air.

The diffusion of gases at the capillary-alveolar level can be affected in a number of ways. Some respiratory diseases (e.g., emphysema) destroy and collapse the alveolar walls. This results in the formation of fewer but larger alveoli. This condition is known as **atelectasis.** The degenerative process reduces the total area available for diffusion. In some diseases the alveolar-capillary membrane becomes thick or less permeable. This forces gas molecules to travel farther. Thus it decreases the rate of diffusion. An example of such a disease is pulmonary edema. With this condition, fluid collects in the alveoli and pulmonary interstitial space. This forces gases to diffuse through a thicker than normal layer of fluid and tissue.

Oxygen Content of Blood

Oxygen is present in the blood in two forms. It is physically dissolved in the blood. It also is chemically bound to hemoglobin (Hb) molecules. Compared with carbon dioxide and nitrogen, oxygen is relatively insoluble in water. Only 0.3 mL of oxygen can be dissolved in 100 mL of blood at the normal alveolar and arterial Po_2 of 100 mm Hg. In contrast, 197 mL of oxygen (about 98%) is carried in red blood cells. In red blood cells, it is chemically bound to hemoglobin (oxyhemoglobin) (Fig. 19-13).

Hemoglobin can unload carbon dioxide and absorb oxygen 60 times faster than blood plasma. When fully converted to oxyhemoglobin (HbO_2), each hemoglobin molecule can carry four molecules of oxygen. At this point, it is said to be *fully saturated.* Hemoglobin nears full saturation at a Po_2 of 80 to 100 mm Hg.

The degree to which hemoglobin combines with oxygen increases rapidly when the Po_2 is 10 to 60 mm Hg. This is because about 90% of total hemoglobin is combined with oxygen when the Po_2 is 60 mm Hg. Increases in Po_2 above 60 mm Hg produce only small increases in the amount of oxygen bound to hemoglobin. If the Po_2 falls slightly, the amount of oxyhemoglobin decreases only slightly. It still provides adequate oxygenation to tissues. The body adapts to higher Po_2 values. It is important that paramedics understand this in dealing with patient situations involving high altitudes, excessive exercise, or cardiac and pulmonary disease. The partial pressure of oxygen in the blood plasma is the main factor in determining the extent to which oxygen combines with hemoglobin. However, oxyhemoglobin does not contribute to the Po_2 of the blood. Only the physically dissolved oxygen molecules can create gas pressure. This oxygen uptake by hemoglobin molecules removes dissolved oxygen from blood plasma. It also maintains a low Po_2. This allows diffusion to continue (Fig. 19-14).

Venous blood entering the lungs has a Po_2 of 40 mm Hg and a hemoglobin saturation of 75%. Oxygen diffuses from the alveoli (because of its higher Po_2 of 100 mm Hg) into the plasma. This diffusion raises the plasma Po_2. This produces an increase in the uptake of oxygen by the hemoglobin molecules. In the tissue capillaries, this process is reversed. As the blood enters the capillaries, the plasma Po_2 is greater than the Po_2 in the fluid surrounding the capillaries. This causes diffusion across the capillary membranes to the cells of the tissues.

▶**NOTE** Diagnostic tests that can be used in the field to monitor the oxygen content of blood and the effectiveness of gas exchange include pulse oximetry monitoring, peak expiratory flow testing, end-tidal carbon dioxide monitoring, and esophageal detection device monitoring. These techniques are described later in this chapter and in Chapter 30.

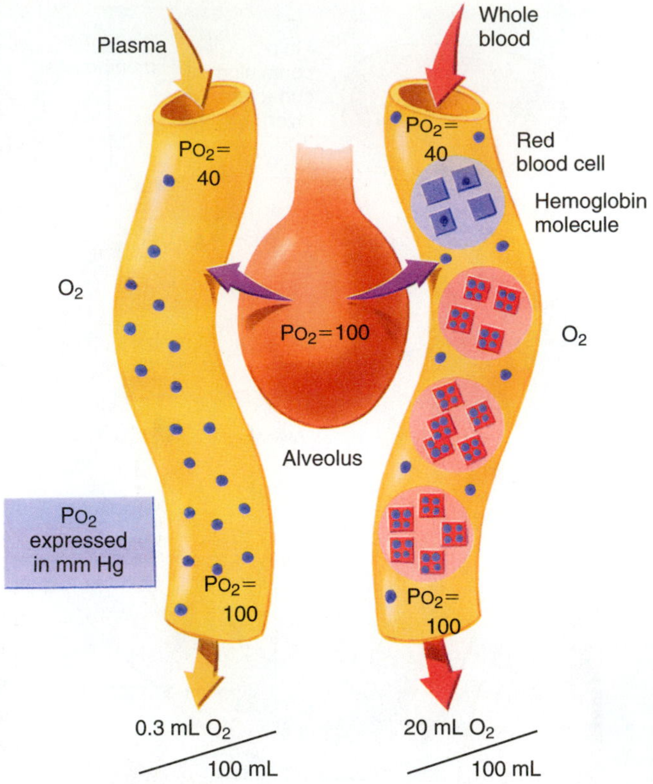

FIGURE 19-13 ■ Oxygen-carrying capacity of the blood. If blood consisted only of plasma, the maximum amount of oxygen that could be transported would be only about 0.3 mL per 100 mL of blood. However, because the red blood cells contain hemoglobin molecules, which act as "oxygen sponges," the blood can actually carry up to 20 mL of dissolved O_2 per 100 mL of blood.

Carbon Dioxide Content of Blood

The amount of carbon dioxide produced by the body is fairly constant. It is determined by the body's rate and type of metabolism. If the metabolic rate increases, more carbon dioxide is produced. For instance, this may occur during exercise. In contrast, as the metabolic rate decreases, less carbon dioxide is produced. This may occur during sleep. Certain types of metabolic processes also result in increased carbon dioxide production. An example is the metabolism that occurs in the absence of oxygen. (This is *anaerobic metabolism.*) Another example is the body's production of ketoacids when metabolism occurs in the absence of insulin.

Carbon dioxide is transported in the blood in three major forms: plasma, blood proteins, and bicarbonate ions. As with oxygen, the solubility of carbon dioxide in water is very minimal. It accounts for 8% of the carbon dioxide carried in plasma. About 20% of the carbon dioxide is present in blood proteins (including hemoglobin). About 72% is in

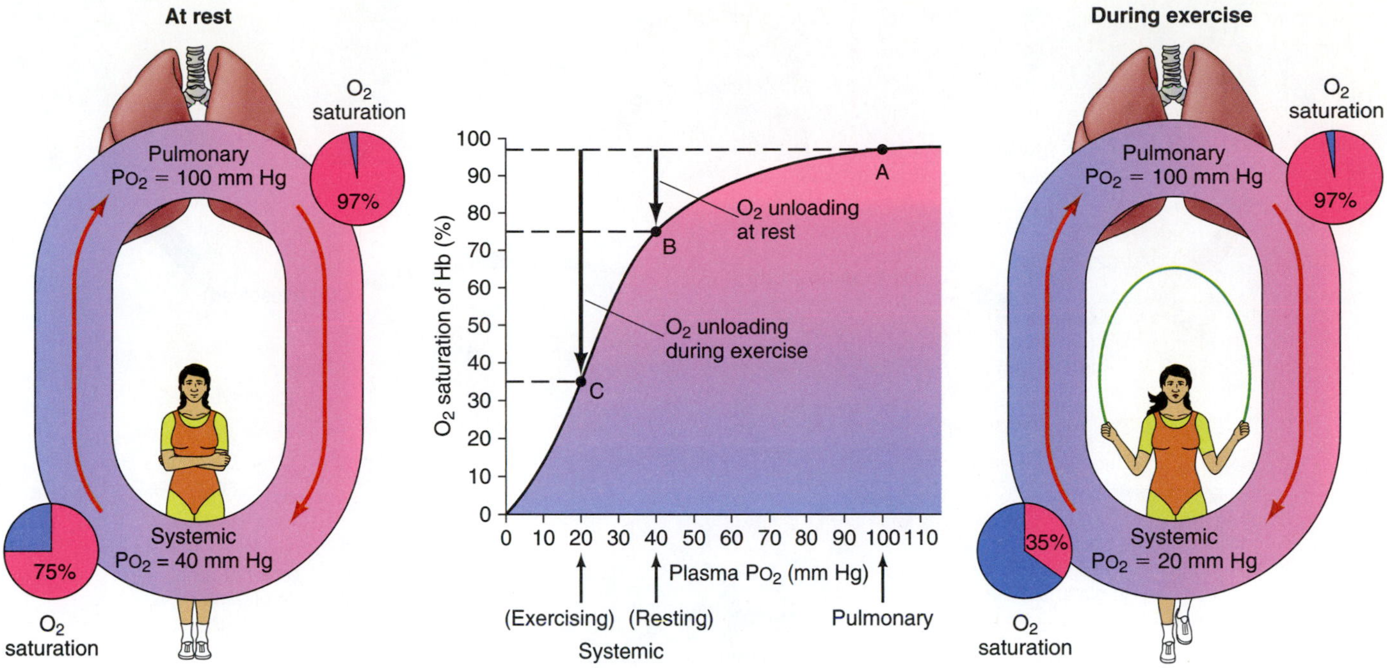

FIGURE 19-14 ■ Oxygen (O_2) unloading at rest and during exercise. At rest fully saturated hemoglobin (Hb) unloads almost 25% of its O_2 when it reaches the low partial pressure of oxygen (PO_2) environment (40 mm Hg) in systemic tissues *(left inset)*. During exercise the tissue PO_2 is even lower (20 mm Hg). Consequently, fully saturated Hb unloads about 70% of its O_2 *(right inset)*. As the graph shows, a slight drop in the tissue PO_2 (from *B* to *C*) greatly increases O_2 unloading.

the form of bicarbonate ions. When arterial blood flows through tissue capillaries, oxyhemoglobin gives up oxygen to the tissues. At the same time, carbon dioxide diffuses from the tissues into the blood. As a result, a small amount of the carbon dioxide dissolves in the plasma.

> **NOTE** The way in which a patient's lungs are ventilated can change the pH of blood. It also may enhance or hinder oxygenation at the tissue level. For example, carbon dioxide levels may be high (resulting in a drop in pH in capillary blood). Thus the oxygen affinity for hemoglobin is reduced. On the other hand, if carbon dioxide levels are low (resulting in a rise in pH in capillary blood), the oxygen affinity for hemoglobin is increased. The response of hemoglobin to changes in pH is called the *Bohr effect* (Fig. 19-15 and 19-16).

Oxygen-free hemoglobin binds more readily to carbon dioxide than hemoglobin binds with oxygen. Thus some of the carbon dioxide that diffuses into red blood cells binds to hemoglobin to form carbaminohemoglobin (HbNHCOOH). The remainder of the carbon dioxide reacts with water to form carbonic acid. Bicarbonate, in contrast to carbon dioxide, is very soluble in water. Venous blood rich in carbon dioxide is returned to the lungs. Because the blood PCO_2 is greater than that in the alveoli, carbon dioxide from the blood diffuses into the alveoli. From there it is exhaled and eliminated from the body (Fig. 19-16).

Factors That Influence Blood Oxygenation

In healthy people, the process of breathing fully oxygenates the blood at the alveolar-capillary level. It also allows carbon dioxide to be eliminated. The movement and utilization of oxygen in the body to perfuse tissues can be described by the Fick principle. (This is a method also used to measure cardiac output.) According to the **Fick principle,** the amount of oxygen that the lungs deliver to the blood is directly related to the amount of oxygen that the body consumes. The movement and utilization of oxygen is based on the following conditions:

1. An adequate amount of oxygen must be available to saturate the hemoglobin on red blood cells as they pass by alveolar membranes in the lungs. This requires adequate ventilation of the lungs through the patient's airway, a high partial pressure of oxygen in inspired air (FIO_2), and minimal obstruction to the diffusion of oxygen across the alveolar-capillary membrane.
2. The red blood cells must be circulated to the tissue cells. This requires adequate cardiac function, an adequate volume of blood flow, and proper routing of blood through the vascular channels.
3. The red blood cells must be able to load oxygen in the pulmonary capillaries. They also must be able to unload the oxygen at the site of peripheral tissue cells.

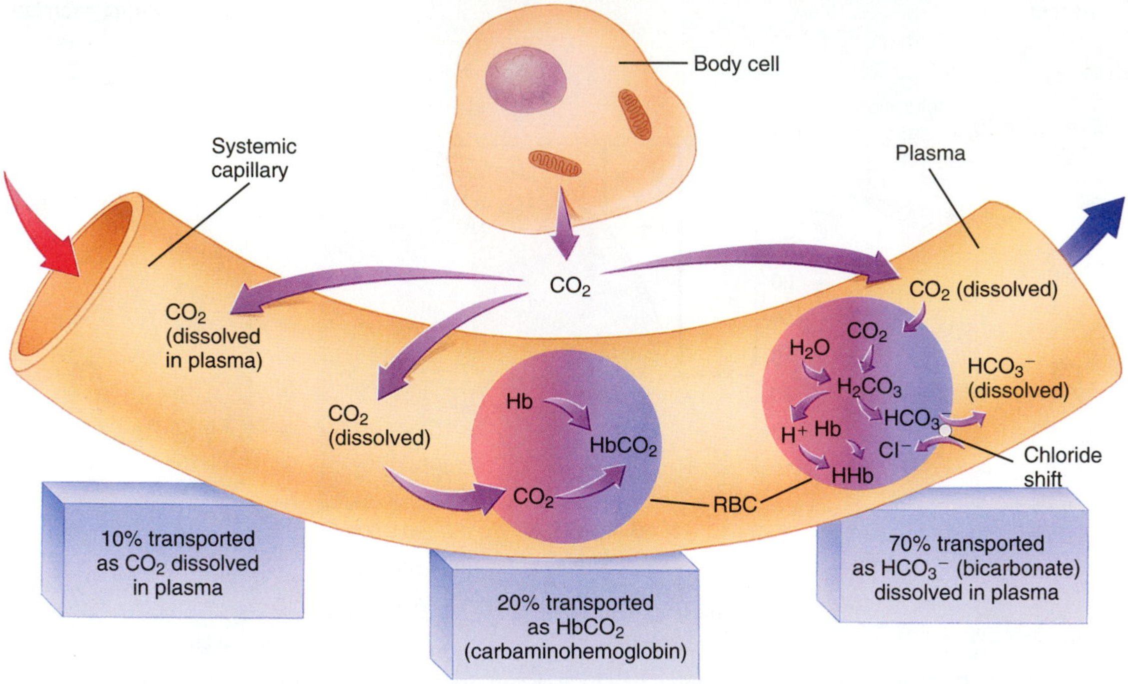

FIGURE 19-15 ■ Interaction of the partial pressure of oxygen (Po_2) and the partial pressure of carbon dioxide (Pco_2) on gas transport by the blood. An increase in the Pco_2 in systemic tissues decreases the affinity between hemoglobin (Hb) and oxygen (O_2). This appears as a right shift of the oxygen-hemoglobin dissociation curve. The phenomenon is known as the *Bohr effect.* A right shift can also be caused by a decrease in the plasma pH.

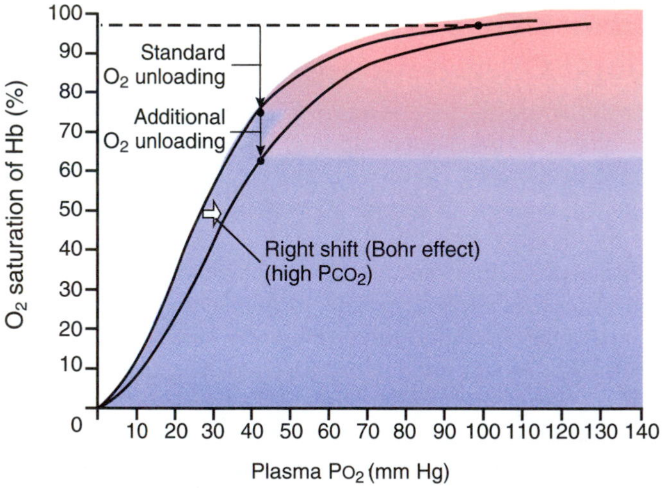

FIGURE 19-16 ■ Carbon dioxide transport in the blood. Carbon dioxide (CO_2) dissolves in the plasma. Some of the dissolved CO_2 enters red blood cells (RBCs) and combines with hemoglobin (Hb) to form carbaminohemoglobin ($HbCO_2$). Some of the CO_2 enters RBCs and combines with water (H_2O) to form carbonic acid (H_2CO_3); this process is facilitated by an enzyme (carbonic anhydrase) present inside each cell. Carbonic acid then dissociates to form hydrogen ion (H+) and bicarbonate (HCO_3^-). The H+ combines with the hemoglobin. The HCO_3^- diffuses down its concentration gradient into the plasma. As HCO_3^- leaves each red blood cell, chloride (Cl^-) enters. This phenomenon is known as the *chloride shift.* It prevents an imbalance in charge.

This requires normal hemoglobin levels, circulation of the oxygenated red blood cells to the tissues in need, close approximation of the cells to the capillaries to allow for diffusion of oxygen, and ideal conditions of pH, temperature, and other factors.

Hypoxemia is a state of decreased oxygen content of the arterial blood. It may lead to **hypoxia** (decreased oxygen content at the tissue level). Some abnormal conditions can result in inadequate blood oxygenation (Box 19-1).

Regulation of Respiration

Respiration is controlled by a number of factors. When paramedics evaluate a patient, key elements they must consider include the various mechanisms responsible for rhythmic ventilation. The rate and depth of breathing are also crucial factors.

Voluntary Control of Respiration

Breathing is mainly an involuntary process. Within limits, however, the pattern of respiration can be consciously altered. For example, voluntary hyperventilation can lead to a decrease in the blood Pco_2, vasodilation of the peripheral blood vessels, a decrease in blood pressure, or a combination of these effects. Hyperventilation causes excessive loss of exhaled carbon dioxide, which produces **hypocarbia,** resulting in cerebral vascular constriction, reduced cerebral perfusion, paresthesia (tingling sensation), dizziness, or even feelings of euphoria.

BOX 19-1 Abnormal Conditions That Can Affect Blood Oxygenation

Depressed Respiratory Drive
Head injury
Central nervous system depressants (anesthetics, narcotics, sedatives)

Paralysis of Respiratory Muscles
Spinal injury
Inhalation injury
Neuromuscular diseases

Increased Resistance in the Respiratory Airways
Asthma
Bronchitis
Emphysema
Congestion

Decreased Compliance of the Lungs and Thoracic Wall
Interstitial lung disease as a result of inhalation of toxic substances
Infection (pneumonia, tuberculosis)
Lung cancer
Connective tissue diseases
Chronic pulmonary hypertension

Chest Wall Abnormalities
Chest wall injury (flail chest)
Scoliosis
Eschar (full-thickness burn contractions)

Decreased Surface Area for Gas Exchange
Emphysema
Tuberculosis
Pneumonia
Pulmonary edema
Atelectasis

Increased Thickness of the Respiratory Membrane
Pulmonary edema (caused by heart failure, pneumonia, infections)
Interstitial fibrosis

Ventilation and Perfusion Mismatching*
Asthma
Pneumonia
Pulmonary embolus
Pulmonary edema
Myocardial infarction
Respiratory distress syndrome
Shock

Reduced Capacity of the Blood to Transport Oxygen
Anemias
Hemoglobin alterations
Carbon monoxide poisoning
Methemoglobinemia

*Ventilated alveoli that are not perfused or perfused alveoli that are not ventilated.

Breathing also can be affected by voluntary apnea. An example of this is when children hold their breath. In such cases the arterial blood Pco_2 increases, whereas the Po_2 decreases. As the apneic period continues, the abnormal levels of Pco_2 and Po_2 trigger the respiratory centers. These changes in the levels override the child's conscious control of breathing. If loss of consciousness occurs, the respiratory center resumes normal function.

CRITICAL THINKING

If a prolonged, deep breath is held, what vagal effects might the patient experience?

Nervous Control of Respiration

The inspiratory muscles are the diaphragm and intercostal muscles. These are composed of skeletal muscle. They cannot contract unless they are stimulated by nerve impulses. The two phrenic nerves responsible for moving the diaphragm originate from the third, fourth, and fifth cervical spinal nerves. The 11 pairs of intercostal nerves originate from the first through the eleventh thoracic spinal nerves. The nerve impulses that control these respiratory muscles originate in neurons of the medulla. The respiratory center in the medulla is bilateral. Each lateral area is made up of two groups of neurons. (These are the inspiratory and expiratory centers.) The two groups are responsible for the basic rhythm of respiration (Fig. 19-17).

The inspiratory center neurons are spontaneously active. They exhibit a pattern of activity followed by fatigue and then activity again. When active they send impulses along the spinal cord to the phrenic and intercostal nerves. This stimulates the muscles of inspiration.

The expiratory center is inactive during quiet respiration. The exact nervous system mechanisms that control the activity of this center are unknown. However, the expiratory center appears to be stimulated when the activity of the inspiratory center increases. (For example, this may occur during heavy or labored breathing.) When activated, the expiratory center counters the inspiratory center, responding to a forceful inspiration with a forceful expiration.

Two distinct neural mechanisms are responsible for the basic respiratory rhythm established by the inspiratory and expiratory centers: the vagal reflex *(Hering-Breuer reflex)* and the pneumotaxic center. The vagus nerve conveys sensory information from the thoracic and abdominal or-

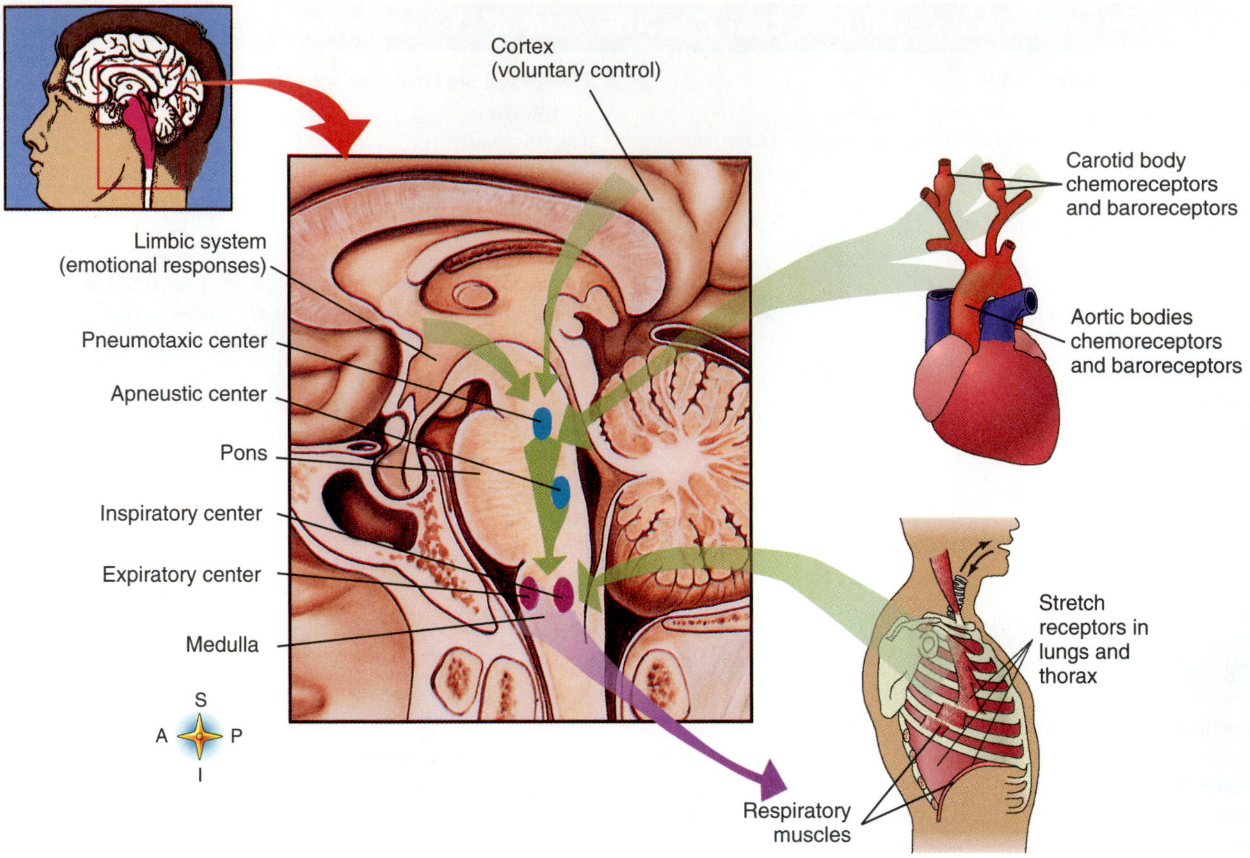

FIGURE 19-17 ■ Regulation of breathing. The inspiratory and expiratory areas of the medulla make up the medullary rhythmicity area. The pneumotaxic center and apneustic center of the pons influence the basic respiratory rhythm by means of neural inputs to the medullary rhythmicity area. The brainstem also receives input from other parts of the body. Information from chemoreceptors, baroreceptors, and stretch receptors can alter the basic breathing pattern, as can emotional (limbic) and sensory input. Despite these subconscious reflexes, the cerebral cortex can override the "automatic" control of breathing to some extent to allow such activities as singing or blowing up a balloon. Green arrows show the flow of information to the respiratory control centers. The purple arrow shows the flow of information from the control centers to the respiratory muscles that drive breathing.

gans. Some of the vagus nerve fibers end in stretch or inflation receptors in the walls of the bronchi, bronchioles, and lungs. When the stretch receptors are stimulated by expansion of the lungs, information is communicated by the vagus nerve to the medulla. The medulla produces discharges of inhibitory impulses. This, in turn, causes inspiration to stop. The cessation of inspiration is followed by expiration or deflation of the lungs. As expiration continues, the stretch receptors are no longer stimulated. This allows the inspiratory center to become active again. Thus the Hering-Breuer reflex limits inspiration. It also prevents overinflation of the lungs.

The pneumotaxic center is located in the pons above the respiratory center in the medulla. It has an inhibitory effect on the inspiratory center. When the activity of the inspiratory center stops, inhibitory impulses from the pneumotaxic center stop. When this occurs, the inspiratory center is free to send impulses to initiate inspiration again. The pneumotaxic center appears to be active only in labored breathing. In quiet breathing the stretch receptors are the main control mechanisms for rhythmic breathing.

The apneustic center is located in the lower portion of the pons. Nerve impulses from this area stimulate the inspiratory center. The apneustic center neurons are constantly active during normal respiratory rates. They are overridden, however, by the pneumotaxic center when the demand for increased ventilation arises.

CRITICAL THINKING
What change in breathing would you expect in a patient who has an injury affecting the pons?

Chemical Control of Respiration

The activities of the respiratory centers are determined by changes in oxygen and carbon dioxide concentrations. They also are determined by the hydrogen ion concentration (pH) of body fluids. (An example of such a fluid is cerebrospinal fluid.) The partial pressure of carbon dioxide is the major factor that controls respiration.

The chemoreceptive area in the medulla has neurons that are sensitive to changes in carbon dioxide and pH. An increase or decrease in the plasma Pco_2 is accompanied by changes in pH. An increase in the Pco_2 and the resulting decrease in pH adversely affect cellular metabolism. Excess carbon dioxide must be eliminated to return the pH to normal. For example, the body responds to an increase in Pco_2 of 5 mm Hg with an increase in ventilation of 100%. On the other hand, a decrease in Pco_2 inhibits ventilation. The carbon dioxide created by normal metabolism is allowed to build up and return the Pco_2 to normal. Through these adaptive measures, the Pco_2 is kept within a normal range of 35 to 45 mm Hg (Fig. 19-18).

Compared with the body's sensitivity to pH and carbon dioxide levels, oxygen plays a fairly small part in regulating respiration. However, if the Po_2 levels in the arterial blood fall and the pH and Pco_2 are held constant, ventilation increases.

Chemoreceptors monitor the arterial Po_2. They are located in the medulla and peripherally at the bifurcation of the common carotid arteries and in the arch of the aorta. These peripheral receptors are known as the *carotid* and *aortic bodies.* The carotid and aortic bodies are in intimate contact with the arterial blood of the great vessels. Thus their blood supply is greater than their use of oxygen. Moreover, the Po_2 of their tissues is very close to that of arterial blood. The nerve fibers from these bodies enter the brainstem. There they synapse with the neurons of the medulla and initiate a respiratory response.

Carbon dioxide and hydrogen ion concentrations are the major regulators of respiration. However, a reduced Po_2 in the arterial blood can play a part in regulating respiration. When a patient is hypotensive (e.g., in shock), the Po_2 in the arterial blood may fall to low levels. This stimulates the sensory receptors in the carotid and aortic bodies. This, in turn, leads to an increased rate and depth of ventilation. This can occur without a significant change in the blood Pco_2. However, it usually is accompanied by metabolic acidosis that occurs secondary to anaerobic metabolism (see Chapter 7).

Po_2 plays a role in respiratory regulation at high altitudes. At these altitudes, the barometric pressure is low. This causes the Po_2 in the arterial blood to drop. The low Po_2 levels stimulate the carotid and aortic bodies. Lowered barometric pressure does not affect the body's ability to eliminate carbon dioxide. The increase in ventilation (triggered by the lowered arterial Po_2) results in a drop in the carbon dioxide levels in the blood.

Patients with severe emphysema or chronic bronchitis have chronically elevated Pco_2 levels. These patients may rely on the low Po_2 as the stimulus for ventilation *(hypoxic drive).* In diseases with chronic elevation of Pco_2, the chemoreceptors become less sensitive to a high carbon dioxide level. They fail to be stimulated by it. Over time, hypoxia becomes the only remaining respiratory drive.

Control of Respiration by Other Factors

A number of other factors may play a role in the control of respiration. These include body temperature, drugs and medications, pain, emotion, and sleep.

An increase in body temperature can affect the respiratory center neurons. Such an increase may be caused by a febrile illness or an increase in physical activity. The increase can cause an increase in ventilation. On the other hand, major decreases in body temperature can lower the ventilation rate. An extreme example of this can occur during severe hypothermia. With this, patients can appear almost apneic.

Some drugs, such as ***epinephrine,*** stimulate respiration. The release of this specific drug increases ventilation. It does this by promoting cellular metabolism during stressful events and vigorous exercise. However, drugs such as ***diazepam*** and ***morphine*** may decrease respirations. A person who takes an overdose of narcotics or barbiturates can become apneic.

Pain anywhere in the body may produce a reflex stimulation of ventilation. Examples include performing a sternal rub on a patient or stepping into a cold shower. Also, certain emotions, such as laughing or crying, require an increase in the movement of air into and out of the lungs. Situations involving fear and anger cause rapid breathing.

As the body's activity and metabolism slow, so does the formation of impulses to stimulate the respiratory centers. During times of decreased activity, ventilation decreases also.

Modified Forms of Respiration

The cough reflex and the sneeze reflex are protective mechanisms. The function of each is to dislodge foreign matter or irritants from the respiratory passages. Coughing generally is preceded by an inspiration of greater than normal force (about 2.5 L of gas). The glottis then closes, and the muscles of the thorax contract forcibly. This causes an increase in intrapulmonic pressure. The pressure change in the lungs increases to about 100 mm Hg. When this pressure is reached, the vocal cords part, and air escapes from the lungs at high velocity. This air carries foreign materials and particles of mucus out of the lungs.

Sneezing is a violent expulsion of gas. The gas is forced or directed through the nasal cavity. It may occur as a result of nasal irritants, stimulation of the fifth cranial nerve (trigeminal nerve) in the nose, or exposure to bright lights. During the sneeze reflex, the uvula and the soft palate are depressed to direct air through both the nasal passages and the oral cavity.

Other forms of modified respiration include the sigh and the hiccough (in rare cases these are chronic disorders). Sighing is a slow, deep inspiration followed by a prolonged expiration. This modified respiratory effort is thought to be a protective reflex to hyperinflate the lungs and to reexpand alveoli that might have been collapsed (atelectasis).

The hiccough results from a spasmodic contraction of the diaphragm with the sudden inspiration cut short by the

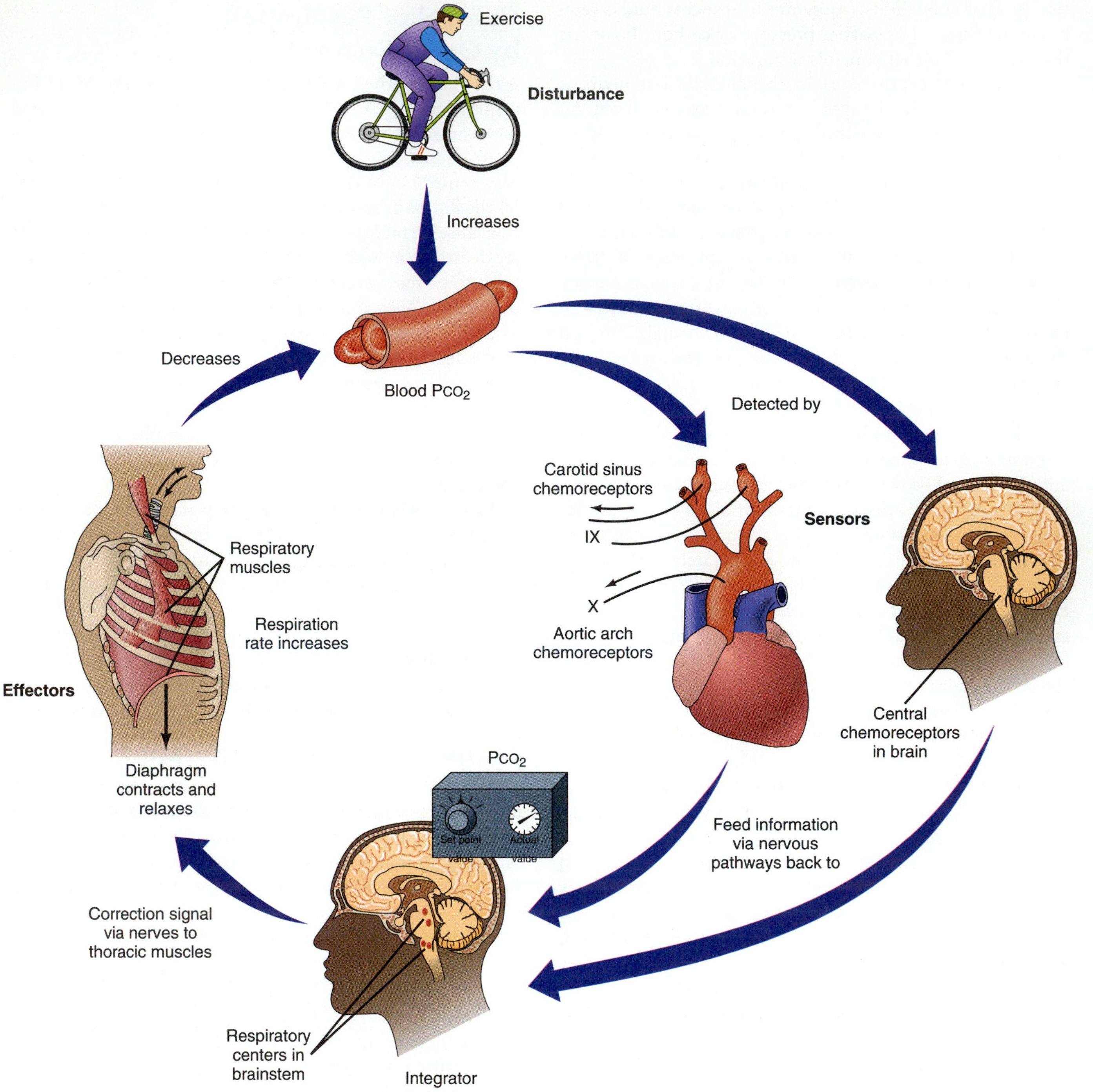

FIGURE 19-18 ■ Negative feedback control of respiration. The diagram summarizes the feedback loop by which the respiratory rate is increased in response to a high plasma partial pressure of carbon dioxide (P_{CO_2}). Increased cellular respiration during exercise causes a rise in the plasma P_{CO_2}. This is detected by central chemoreceptors in the brain and perhaps by peripheral chemoreceptors in the carotid sinus and aorta. Feedback information is relayed to integrators in the brainstem. These respond to the increase in P_{CO_2} above the set point by sending nervous correction signals to the respiratory muscles, which act as effectors. The effector muscles increase their alternating contraction and relaxation, thereby increasing the rate of respiration. As the respiration rate increases, the rate of CO_2 loss from the body increases and the P_{CO_2} drops accordingly. This brings the plasma P_{CO_2} back to its set point value.

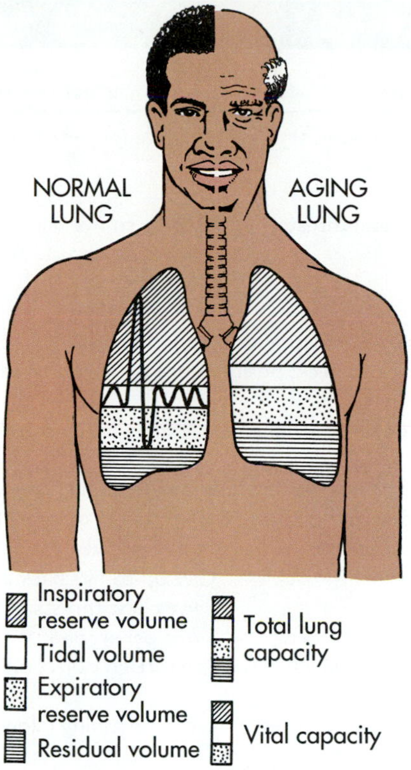

FIGURE 19-19 ■ Changes in lung volumes with aging. Note particularly the decrease in vital capacity and the increase in residual volume that occur with aging.

closure of the glottis. Hiccoughs serve no known useful physiological purpose. They usually cease with time. However, they may indicate a pathological condition.

Special Considerations in Older Patients

Respiratory disorders create distinctive problems for the older patient. As a result of aging, the respiratory function of older patients may be compromised. Pulmonary changes that occur as a result of aging decrease vital capacity (Fig. 19-19). They also increase the physiological dead space. Ventilation-perfusion mismatching also tends to increase. This leads to a gradually lowered Po_2. The changes in pulmonary physiology include the following:

1. Alterations in lung and chest wall compliance
   - Increased thoracic rigidity
   - Decreased elastic recoil (total lung capacity remains unchanged because of opposing loss of chest wall compliance and weakened respiratory muscles)
2. Enlarged alveolar ducts and sacs
   - Fewer alveoli
   - Less alveolar surface for gas exchange

The aging process also changes the body's ventilatory control mechanisms. As a person grows older, for example, the body's arterial Po_2 falls. Yet no significant change in arterial Pco_2 occurs. Several methods have been developed to calculate the expected Po_2 in older persons. One method is to keep in mind that a person who is 70 years old is expected to have a Po_2 of 70 mm Hg. Using this value as a baseline, the expected change is a 1 mm Hg decrease in Po_2 for every year over 70 or a 1 mm Hg increase in Po_2 for every year under 70. For example, a person who is 65 years old would be expected to have a Po_2 of 75 mm Hg. A person who is 75 years old would be expected to have a Po_2 of 65 mm Hg.

The functioning of the body's chemoreceptors also declines with age. This results in a diminished ventilatory response to hypoxia, hypercapnia, and similar conditions. It also may predispose the older individual to respiratory failure. It is important that older patients with respiratory compromise from any cause receive immediate intervention, oxygenation, and ventilatory support.

SECTION TWO
RESPIRATORY PATHOPHYSIOLOGY

A common cause of poor ventilation is upper airway obstruction. This type of obstruction is typically caused by inhalation of food, a foreign body, or fluid (vomitus, saliva, blood, neutral liquids). Establishing and maintaining a clear airway in any patient who has poor ventilation from any cause is the most critical lifesaving maneuver a paramedic can perform. It should always be a first-order priority of patient care. Early detection, early intervention, and education of the general public in basic life support measures are major factors in preventing unnecessary deaths from airway compromise.

> **NOTE** Brain damage may occur 4 to 6 minutes after interruption of breathing and circulation. After 6 minutes of circulatory arrest, brain damage almost always occurs. After 10 minutes of circulatory arrest, some portions of the brain have been irreversibly damaged to the point of death.[2]

FOREIGN BODY AIRWAY OBSTRUCTION

About 3000 deaths each year result from foreign body obstruction of the airway.[1] Immediate removal of the obstruction might have prevented the resulting hypoxemia, unconsciousness, or cardiopulmonary arrest that caused these deaths. The management of foreign body airway obstruction by health care providers, as recommended by AHA and ARC standards, is summarized in Table 19-2.

TABLE 19-2 Management of Foreign Body Airway Obstruction

<table>
<tr><th>PATIENT'S CONDITION</th><th>OBJECTIVES</th><th>ADULT (>8 YR)</th><th>CHILD (1–8 YR)</th><th>INFANT (<1 YR)</th></tr>
<tr><td>Conscious victim</td><td>1. Assessment: Check for airway obstruction.</td><td colspan="2">Ask, "Are you choking?" Determine whether victim can cough or speak.</td><td>Observe for breathing difficulty.</td></tr>
<tr><td></td><td>2. Act to relieve obstruction.</td><td colspan="2">Perform five subdiaphragmatic abdominal thrusts (Heimlich maneuver).</td><td>Give up to five back blows. Give five chest thrusts at the rate of one per second.</td></tr>
<tr><td></td><td>3. Be persistent.</td><td colspan="3">Repeat step 2 until obstruction is relieved or victim loses consciousness.</td></tr>
<tr><td>Victim who loses consciousness</td><td>4. Position victim.</td><td colspan="3">Turn on back as unit, supporting head and neck; position face up, arms by sides.</td></tr>
<tr><td></td><td>5. Check for foreign body.</td><td>Perform tongue-jaw lift and finger sweep.</td><td colspan="2">Perform tongue-jaw lift. Remove foreign object only if visible.</td></tr>
<tr><td></td><td>6. Give rescue breaths.</td><td colspan="3">Open airway with head-tilt chin-lift maneuver. Attempt rescue breathing (slow ventilations 1½-2 seconds [sec] each for adult and 1-1½ sec each for child or infant). If first ventilation attempt is unsuccessful, reposition head and reattempt ventilation.</td></tr>
<tr><td></td><td>7. Act to relieve obstruction.</td><td colspan="2">Perform five subdiaphragmatic abdominal thrusts (Heimlich maneuver).</td><td>Give up to five back blows. Give five chest thrusts at the rate of one per second.</td></tr>
<tr><td></td><td>8. Check for foreign body.</td><td>Perform tongue-jaw lift and finger sweep.</td><td colspan="2">Perform tongue-jaw lift. Remove foreign object only if visible.</td></tr>
<tr><td></td><td>9. Attempt rescue breathing.</td><td colspan="3">Open airway with head-tilt chin-lift maneuver. Attempt rescue breathing (slow ventilations 1½-2 sec each for adult and 1-1½ sec each for child or infant).</td></tr>
<tr><td></td><td>10. Be persistent.</td><td colspan="3">Repeat steps 6 through 8 until obstruction is relieved or until advanced procedures become possible (i.e., use of Kelly clamp or Magill forceps, or cricothyrotomy).</td></tr>
<tr><td>Unconscious victim</td><td>1. Assessment: Determine unresponsiveness.</td><td colspan="2">Tap or gently shake shoulder. Shout, "Are you okay?"</td><td>Tap or gently shake shoulder.</td></tr>
<tr><td></td><td>2. Position victim.</td><td colspan="3">Turn on back as unit, supporting head and neck; position face up, arms by sides.</td></tr>
<tr><td></td><td>3. Open airway.</td><td colspan="2">Open airway with head-tilt chin-lift maneuver.</td><td>Open airway with head-tilt chin-lift maneuver without hyperextension.</td></tr>
<tr><td></td><td>4. Assessment: Determine breathlessness.</td><td colspan="3">Maintain an open airway. Place ear over mouth; observe chest. Look, listen, and feel for breathing (3-5 sec).</td></tr>
<tr><td></td><td>5. Give rescue breaths.</td><td colspan="2">Seal mouth to mouth with barrier device or bag-valve device.</td><td>Seal mouth to nose/mouth with barrier device.</td></tr>
<tr><td></td><td></td><td colspan="3">Attempt rescue breathing (slow ventilations 1½-2 sec each for adult and 1-1½ sec each for child or infant). If first ventilation is unsuccessful, reposition head and reattempt ventilation.</td></tr>
<tr><td></td><td>6. Act to relieve obstruction.</td><td colspan="2">Perform five subdiaphragmatic abdominal thrusts (Heimlich maneuver).</td><td>Give up to five back blows. Give five chest thrusts at the rate of one per second.</td></tr>
<tr><td></td><td>7. Check for foreign body.</td><td colspan="2">Perform tongue-jaw lift and finger sweep.</td><td>Perform tongue-jaw lift. Remove foreign object only if visible.</td></tr>
<tr><td></td><td>8. Provide rescue breathing.</td><td colspan="3">Open airway with head-tilt chin-lift maneuver. Attempt rescue breathing (slow ventilations 1½-2 sec each for adult and 1-1½ sec each for child or infant).</td></tr>
<tr><td></td><td>9. Be persistent.</td><td colspan="3">Repeat steps 6 through 8 until obstruction is relieved or until advanced procedures become possible (i.e., use of Kelly clamp or Magill forceps, or cricothyrotomy).</td></tr>
</table>

Adapted from American Heart Association: *Basic life support for healthcare providers,* Dallas, 1997, The Association.

▶**NOTE** Methods to relieve foreign body airway obstruction (FBAO) in an unconscious victim of any age have been simplified for lay rescuers. Lay rescuers are to begin standard cardiopulmonary resuscitation (CPR) when an unrelieved, responsive choking victim becomes unresponsive, or when an unresponsive person suspected of having a foreign body airway obstruction is encountered, evaluated, and treated. The only difference from regular CPR is that the lay rescuer should open the airway widely whenever ventilations are attempted. This is to look for a foreign object and remove it if seen. Blind finger sweeps are not to be used by lay rescuers for victims of any age.

Airway Obstruction in a Conscious Patient

Meat is the most common cause of foreign body airway obstruction in conscious adults. (However, a variety of other foods and foreign objects are responsible for obstruction in children and in some adults.) Factors associated with choking include large, poorly chewed pieces of food, an elevated blood alcohol level, and poorly fitting dentures. The patient often is middle aged or older.

CRITICAL THINKING

How can you relieve a foreign body airway obstruction using only your hands?

Foreign bodies may cause partial or complete airway obstruction. A patient with a partly obstructed airway usually can speak. The person can usually cough forcefully in an effort to expel the object. If air exchange is adequate, the rescuer should not intervene.[2] A patient with a partial obstruction should be monitored closely. The person should be encouraged to persist with spontaneous coughing and breathing efforts. If the obstruction persists or air exchange becomes inadequate (evidenced by a weak, ineffective cough, also wheezing, increased respiratory difficulty, decreased air movement, and cyanosis), the patient should be managed as though a complete airway obstruction existed.

Patients with complete airway obstruction cannot speak *(aphonia),* exchange air, or cough. They often grasp the neck between the thumb and fingers. (This is a universal sign of choking.) These patients need immediate rescuer intervention. Complete airway obstruction causes hypoxemia. It can lead to an acute myocardial infarction in patients with atherosclerotic cardiovascular disease. Airway obstruction inevitably leads to cardiac arrest in all patients if not corrected within minutes.

Airway Obstruction in an Unconscious Patient

Although upper airway obstruction may lead to loss of consciousness and cardiopulmonary arrest, more often the obstruction is caused by unconsciousness and cardiopulmonary arrest.[2] The primary source of upper airway obstruction in an unconscious patient is the tongue.

The tongue is attached to the mandible by the muscles that form the floor of the mouth. The normal tone of these muscles allows for air exchange by keeping the posterior pharynx open. If a patient is unconscious or has neuromuscular dysfunction, relaxation of these muscles may cause the airway to be blocked by the tongue. Airway obstruction by the tongue is common in the following situations:

- Cardiac arrest
- Trauma
- Stroke
- Intoxication with alcohol, barbiturates, or psychotropic drugs
- Paralysis caused by muscle relaxants
- Myasthenia gravis
- Fractured facial and nasal bones

Laryngeal Spasm and Edema

Spasmodic closure of the vocal cords often is caused by an aggressive intubation technique. (Endotracheal intubation is discussed later in this chapter.) It also may occur during *extubation* (removal of the endotracheal tube). This may be the case especially if the patient is semiconscious. Laryngeal spasm is best managed with aggressive ventilation and a forceful upward pull on the jaw. At times it may require the use of muscle relaxants. Maintaining steady pressure against the cords with the endotracheal tube sometimes overcomes the spasmodic closure.

Swelling of the glottic and subglottic tissues of the airway can close off the larynx. The formation of edema may result from inflammatory or mechanical causes such as epiglottitis, croup, allergic reaction, thermal injuries, strangulation, blunt trauma, or drowning. Associated swelling may partly or completely obstruct the airway. Aggressive airway management is required for the patient's survival when this occurs.

Fractured Larynx

The most common cause of external trauma to the larynx is a motor vehicle crash. If a trauma patient has localized laryngeal pain on palpation or swallowing, stridor, hoarseness, difficulty with speech *(dysphonia),* or hemoptysis (coughing up blood), a fracture of the larynx should be suspected. Laryngeal injury can result in a lack of support for the vocal cords. This may cause them to collapse into the tracheal-laryngeal opening. They then would obstruct the airway. Subcutaneous emphysema, dysphagia (difficult swallowing), and throat discomfort that increases with coughing or swallowing indicate the possibility of an impending airway obstruction as a result of a fracture. The paramedic should remain alert to the possibility of laryngeal fracture. This is important because laryngeal edema can rapidly close off the airway.

Certain types of injury may cause laryngeal fracture. Examples include a clothesline injury and blunt trauma to the neck. A laryngeal fracture requires rapid intervention. The paramedic must secure an open airway before laryngeal edema and hemorrhage cause complete closure.

Tracheal Trauma

Trauma to the trachea is rare but serious. The most common site of tracheal injury is the area bordered by the cricoid cartilage and the third tracheal ring. This injury seldom occurs as an isolated event. More often it is associated with injuries to the surrounding esophagus and cervical spine. Central nervous system (CNS) injuries and abdominal and thoracic trauma also usually accompany tracheal injury. (Tracheal trauma is described in more detail in Chapter 24.)

ASPIRATION BY INHALATION

Aspiration is the active inhalation of food, a foreign body, or fluid (e.g., vomitus, saliva, blood, neutral liquids) into the airway. Depending on the type and degree of aspiration, the syndrome may cause spasm, mucus production, atelectasis, a change in pH (if the substance is acidic), or coughing. Prevention of aspiration is far superior to any known treatment. Aspiration is prevented mainly by controlling and maintaining the airway. Paramedics should always be prepared for the chance of aspiration in patients with a diminished level of consciousness.

About 80% of the approximately 3000 deaths each year from foreign body aspiration occur in children.[1] Running with food or other objects in the mouth, seizures, and forced feeding are among the risk factors in this age group. Hot dogs and peanuts are foods children commonly aspirate. In adults, obstruction may be caused by dental or nasal surgery, loss of consciousness, swallowing of poorly chewed food, and alcohol intoxication.

Large food particles and other foreign bodies can block the airway. This may cause hypoventilation of lower lung segments.

The size of the particle determines which airway is obstructed and to what extent. Approximately 60% of foreign bodies are found in the right mainstem bronchus, 19% in the left, and 21% at the larynx or vocal cords.[3] (The left mainstem bronchus branches from the trachea at a 45- to 60-degree angle. Thus foreign body occlusion of this bronchus is less likely than of the right mainstem bronchus, which is shorter, wider, and more vertical.) When the larynx or trachea is completely obstructed, the victim can die from asphyxiation within minutes.

The average adult stomach has a capacity of 1.4 L. It manufactures an additional 1.4 L of gastric juices in each 24-hour period. Hydrochloric acid is manufactured by special cells in the gastric mucosa. With the assistance of a protein-dissolving enzyme (pepsin), this acid helps break down large pieces of food into smaller ones.

Vomitus contains not only partly digested food particles but also acidic gastric fluid. Saliva is a watery, slightly acidic fluid. It is secreted in the mouth by the major salivary glands and the smaller salivary glands in the mucous membranes that line the mouth. Saliva contains the digestive enzyme amylase. This enzyme helps break down carbohydrates. Saliva also contains a number of other substances. These include minerals (e.g., sodium, calcium, and chloride); proteins; mucin (the principal constituent of mucus); urea; white blood cells; debris from the lining of the mouth; and bacteria.

The consequences of aspiration of neutral liquids (liquids that are neither acidic nor basic) are easier to reverse with supportive therapy than the consequences of aspiration of acids or bases. Nonetheless, aspiration of a large volume of neutral liquids also is associated with a high mortality rate.

Pathophysiology of Aspiration

Two conditions are associated with a high risk of aspiration: (1) a diminished level of consciousness and (2) mechanical disturbances of the airway and gastrointestinal (GI) tract.

A diminished level of consciousness may be caused by trauma, alcohol or other drug intoxication, a seizure disorder, cardiopulmonary arrest, a stroke, or a CNS dysfunction. The common element of these conditions is depression or loss of the gag reflex, with or without a full stomach. The **gag reflex** is a normal neural reflex triggered by touching the soft palate or posterior pharynx.

Iatrogenic obstructions (i.e., those caused by medical procedures) are a common type of mechanical obstruction. This type of obstruction results from the use of various devices to control upper airway problems. Examples include removal of certain airway devices (risk of vomiting on removal), placement of a nasogastric tube (the artificial opening through the esophageal sphincter increases the risk of regurgitation and aspiration), and intubation, which requires an adequate seal at the tracheal orifice to prevent aspiration. These mechanical airway devices are discussed later in this chapter.

Other mechanical or structural problems that may lead to a high risk of aspiration include tracheostomy and esophageal motility disorders such as hiatal hernia and esophageal reflux. Other individuals at risk include those with intestinal obstructions.

The chance of aspiration increases whenever vomiting occurs. Vomiting follows stimulation of the vomiting center of the medulla. This stimulation can result from irritation anywhere along the GI tract, from information passed to the medulla from the frontal lobes of the brain, or from disturbances in the balance mechanism of the inner ear. Once this center is stimulated, the following seven events occur:

1. A deep breath is taken.
2. The hyoid bone and larynx are elevated. This opens the pre-esophageal sphincter.
3. The opening of the larynx closes.
4. The soft palate is elevated, closing the posterior nares.
5. The diaphragm and the abdominal muscles contract forcefully. This compresses the stomach and increases the intragastric pressure.
6. The lower esophageal sphincter relaxes. The stomach contents are propelled into the lower esophagus.
7. If the patient is unconscious or unable to protect the airway, pulmonary aspiration may occur.

Effects of Pulmonary Aspiration

The severity of pulmonary aspiration depends on the pH of the aspirated material, the volume of the aspirate, and whether particulate matter (e.g., food) and bacterial contamination are present in the aspirate. It generally is accepted that when the pH level of an aspirated material is 2.5 or lower, severe pulmonary damage occurs. When the pH is below 1.5, the patient usually dies. The mortality rate among patients who aspirate material that is grossly contaminated (as occurs in bowel obstruction) approaches 100%.

The toxic effects on the lungs from gastric acid (which has a pH of less than 2.5) can be equated with those of chemical burns. These are severe injuries that produce pulmonary changes such as destruction of surfactant-producing alveolar cells, alveolar collapse and destruction, and destruction of pulmonary capillaries. The permeability of the capillaries increases with massive flooding of the alveoli and bronchi with fluid. The resulting pulmonary edema creates areas of hypoventilation, shunting, and severe hypoxemia. The massive fluid shift from the intravascular area to the lungs also may produce hypovolemia severe enough to require volume replacement.

> **NOTE** The risk of pulmonary aspiration can be minimized by continuously monitoring the patient's mental status, properly positioning the patient to allow for drainage of secretions, limiting ventilation pressures to avoid gastric distention, and using suction devices and esophageal or endotracheal (ET) intubation. Airway protection should be provided if the risk of aspiration exists. It also should be provided promptly after an occurrence of aspiration.

SECTION THREE
AIRWAY EVALUATION

ESSENTIAL PARAMETERS OF AIRWAY EVALUATION

Evaluation of the respiratory system is presented in depth in Chapter 12. This discussion is limited to essentials of airway evaluation that are used to identify immediate signs of life-threatening airway compromise. The essential parameters of airway evaluation are rate, regularity, and effort, in addition to recognition of airway problems that might indicate respiratory distress.

Rate, Regularity, and Effort

The normal respiratory rate in a resting adult is 12 to 24 breaths per minute. Regularity is defined as a steady inspiratory and expiratory pattern. Breathing at rest should be effortless. It also should be marked by only subtle changes in rate or regularity.

Patients in respiratory distress often compensate for their inability to breathe easily by sitting upright with the head tilted back (upright sniffing position), by leaning forward on the arms (tripod position), or by lying down with the head and thorax slightly elevated (semi-Fowler's position). These patients frequently avoid lying flat, or supine.

> **CRITICAL THINKING**
> Why would lying flat on the back (i.e., in the supine position) most likely worsen respiratory distress?

Recognition of Airway Problems

Respiratory distress may be caused by upper or lower airway obstruction, inadequate ventilation, impairment of the respiratory muscles, ventilation-perfusion mismatching, diffusion abnormalities, or impairment of the nervous system. Dyspnea often is associated with hypoxia.

> **NOTE** Recognition and management of respiratory failure are crucial to the patient's survival. The brain can survive only a few minutes of anoxia. All therapies will fail if the airway is not adequate.

OBSERVATION TECHNIQUES

Visual clues can aid the recognition of airway problems. Paramedics should note the patient's preferred position to facilitate breathing. They also should assess the rise and fall of the patient's chest. Other visual clues to respiratory distress include the following:

- Gasping for air
- Cyanosis
- Nasal flaring
- Pursed-lip breathing
- Retraction of the intercostal or subcostal muscles, suprasternal notch, and supraclavicular fossa during respirations (Fig. 19-20)

AUSCULTATION AND PALPATION TECHNIQUES

Air movement can be evaluated by listening to respirations without using a stethoscope (Fig. 19-21). A stethoscope is used to assess air movement in both lung fields. Palpation of

> **NOTE** *Pulsus paradoxus* is an exaggeration of the normal blood pressure variation that occurs with breathing. It is defined as a fall in systolic pressure of 10 mm Hg or more on spontaneous inspiration. At times it is associated with a change in the quality of the pulse. The condition is occasionally observed in patients with asthma or chronic obstructive pulmonary disease (COPD) and in victims of blunt or penetrating chest trauma (see Chapter 26). Pulsus paradoxus is difficult to measure. The paramedic should rely on more obvious signs and symptoms of respiratory distress.

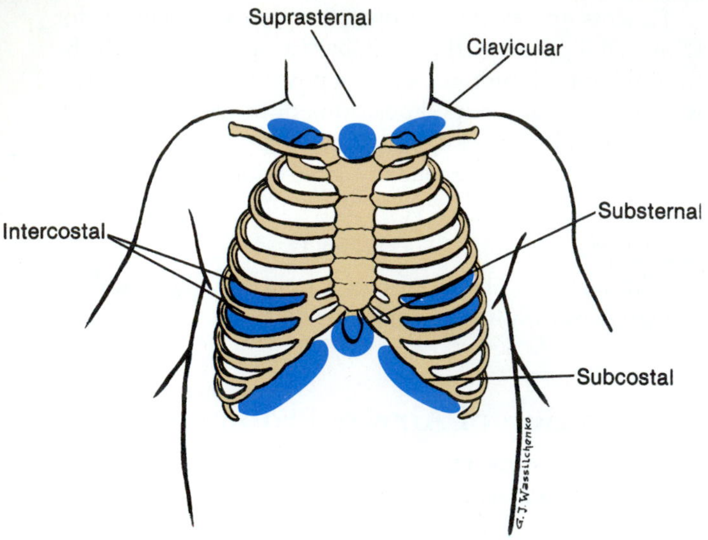

FIGURE 19-20 ■ Areas of chest muscle retractions.

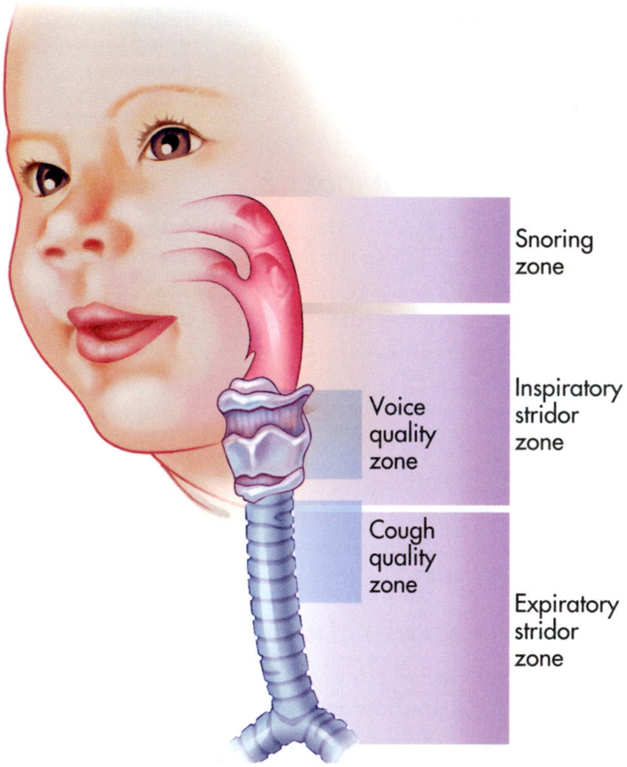

FIGURE 19-21 ■ A loud, gasping snore suggests enlarged tonsils or adenoids. With inspiratory stridor, the airway is compromised at the level of the supraglottic larynx, vocal cords, subglottic region, or upper trachea. Expiratory stridor, or central wheeze, results from narrowing or collapse of the lower trachea or bronchi. Airway noise during both inspiration and expiration often represents a fixed obstruction of the vocal cords or subglottic space. Hoarseness or a weak cry is a by-product of obstruction of the vocal cords. If a cough is croupy or low pitched, a tracheal disorder should be suspected.

the chest wall helps determine the presence or absence of paradoxical (contrary) motion of the chest wall, inspiration, expiration, and any retraction of accessory muscles.

OTHER SIGNS OF RESPIRATORY DISTRESS

Other signs that indicate possible causes of respiratory distress include resistance or changing compliance when assisting or delivering respirations with a bag-valve-mask (seen in asthma, chronic obstructive pulmonary disease [COPD], and tension pneumothorax), and the presence of pulsus paradoxus.

History

Obtaining a history to determine the progression and duration of the dyspneic event also helps guide the direction of patient care. For example, the paramedic should ask whether the event was sudden in onset or occurred over time. If it occurred over time, the length of that period should be determined. The paramedic also should ask whether any known causes or triggers initiated the difficulty breathing. The paramedic must know if the respiratory distress is continuous or recurring. Other questions that should be asked in obtaining a patient's history include the following:

- What makes it better?
- What makes it worse?
- Do any other symptoms occur at the same time (e.g., cough, chest pain, fever)?
- Has any treatment with drugs been attempted?
- Has the patient taken all medications and treatments as prescribed?

It also is crucial to determine whether the patient has been previously evaluated or hospitalized for this condition and whether the person has ever been intubated because of respiratory problems.

Changes in the Respiratory Pattern

As previously stated, the breathing process should be comfortable, regular, and performed without distress. Abnormal respiratory patterns are commonly seen in ill or injured patients (Fig. 19-22 and Box 19-2). Recognizing these patterns may help paramedics to determine the proper patient care.

Inadequate Ventilation

Inadequate ventilation is said to occur when the body cannot compensate for increased oxygen demand or cannot maintain a normal range of oxygen/carbon dioxide balance. Numerous factors can cause inadequate ventilation, including infection, trauma, brainstem injury, and a noxious or hypoxic atmosphere. A patient who has inadequate ventilation may have a number of symptoms. The person also may have various respiratory rates and breathing patterns. Some medical experts distinguish between inadequate ventilation caused by a problem in the mechanics of breathing (usually defined by the Pco_2) and inadequate oxygenation but normal ventilation, as seen in pulmonary embolus and often pneumonia.

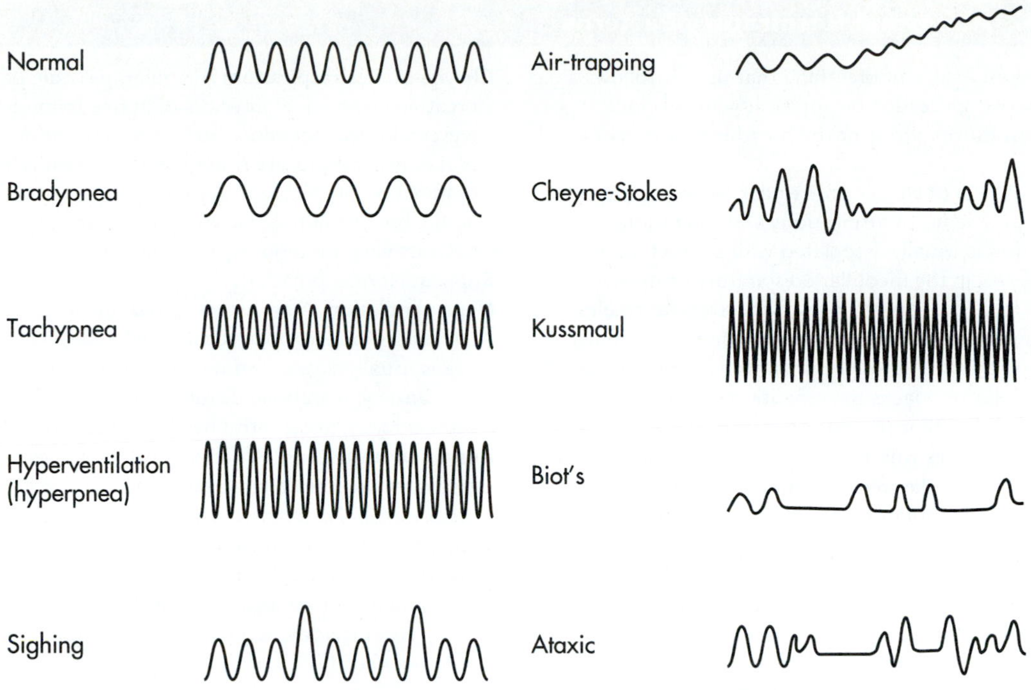

Some influences on the rate and depth of breathing

The rate and depth of breathing will

Increase with	*Decrease with*
Acidosis (metabolic)	Alkalosis (metabolic)
Anxiety	Central nervous system lesions (cerebrum)
Aspirin poisoning	Myasthenia gravis
Oxygen need (hypoxemia)	Narcotic overdoses
Pain	Obesity (extreme)
Central nervous system lesions (pons)	

FIGURE 19-22 ■ Patterns of respiration. The horizontal axis indicates the relative rate; the vertical swings indicate the relative depth.

SUPPLEMENTAL OXYGEN THERAPY

Supplemental oxygen therapy may be provided for two reasons: (1) enriched oxygen in the atmosphere increases the oxygen content in pulmonary capillary blood; and (2) increasing the available oxygen allows the patient to compensate without increasing the work of breathing.

Oxygen Sources

The most common form of oxygen used in the prehospital setting is pure oxygen gas, delivered in liters per minute (LPM). This gas is stored under pressure in stainless steel or lightweight alloy cylinders (Fig. 19-23). These cylinders have been color coded by the U.S. Pharmacopeia to distinguish various compressed gases. Steel green and white cylinders have been assigned to all grades of oxygen. Stainless steel and aluminum cylinders are not painted. Common sizes of oxygen cylinders (and their factors) that are used in emergency care include the following (Box 19-3):

Cylinder	Factor
D cylinder (425 L of oxygen)	0.16
Jumbo D cylinder (640 L of oxygen)	0.28
E cylinder (680 L of oxygen)	0.28
M cylinder (3450 L of oxygen)	1.56

Oxygen cylinders are filled under a pressure of 2000 to 2200 psi. Thus safety is critical when this equipment is handled. The paramedic should ensure that the correct regulator is firmly attached before moving an oxygen cylinder. Also, a cylinder should never be handled by the neck assembly alone. Most oxygen cylinders are considered "empty" at 200 psi. (This is the safe residual pressure.) As a rule, tanks with less than 500 psi are too low to keep in service.

LIQUID OXYGEN

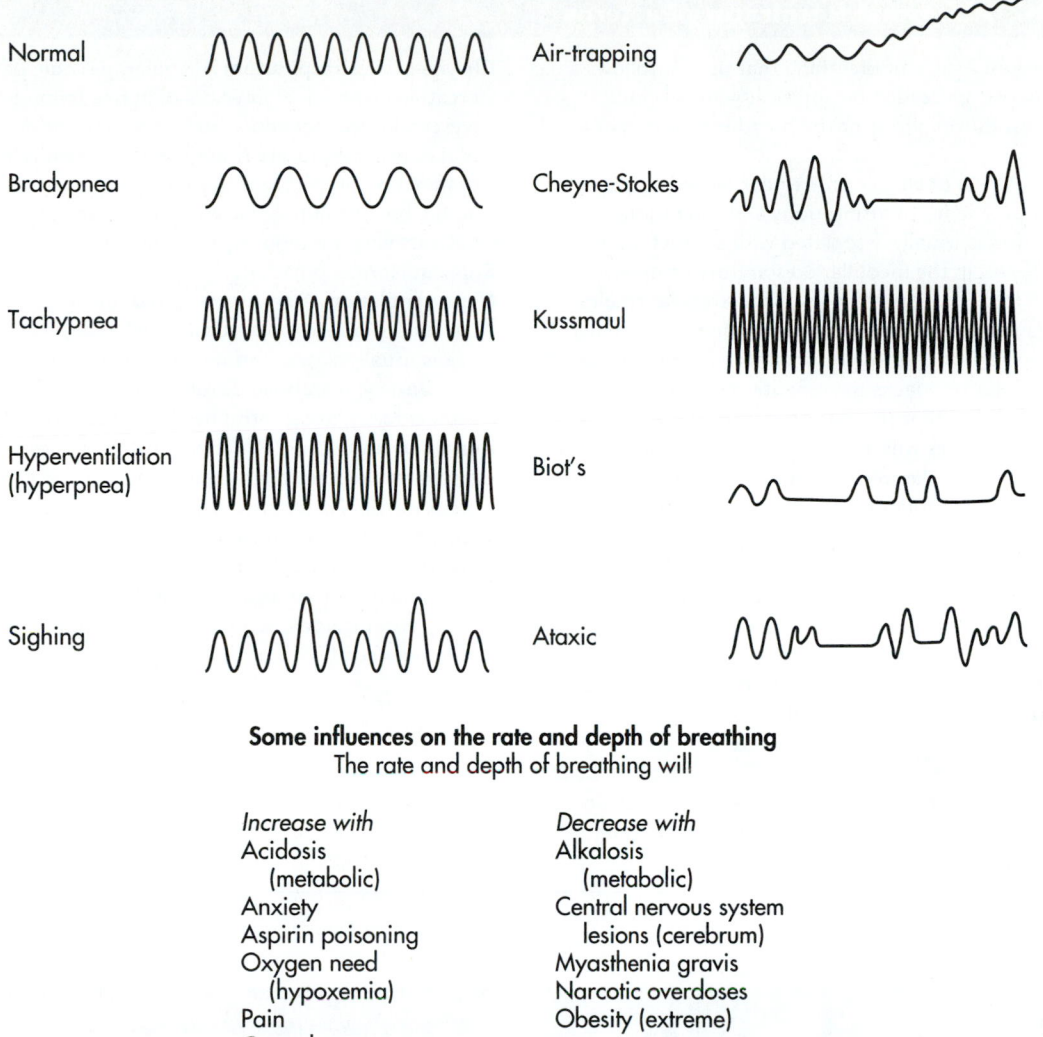

Liquid oxygen (LOX) has been cooled to its aqueous state. However, it converts to a gaseous state when warmed. The liquid form is used by some aeromedical services and by

BOX 19-2 Abnormal Respiratory Patterns

Agonal respiration: A type of breathing that usually follows a pattern of gasping succeeded by apnea. It generally indicates the onset of respiratory arrest or the breathing pattern of a dying person.

Ataxic pattern: A type of cluster or irregular breathing pattern characterized by a series of inspirations and expirations. Ataxic respiration is usually associated with a structural or compressive lesion in the medullary respiratory centers.

Biot pattern: A respiratory pattern involving irregular respirations varying in depth and interrupted by intervals of apnea (absence of breathing). Although similar to Cheyne-Stokes respiration, this pattern lacks the repetitiveness of that type and is often irregular. Biot respiration is usually seen in patients with head injuries who have increased intracranial pressure. Unlike Cheyne-Stokes respiration, the Biot ataxic pattern frequently produces ventilatory failure and may lead to apnea.

Bradypnea: A persistent respiratory rate slower than 12 breaths per minute. This abnormal rate may be a result of the patient guarding against respiratory discomfort caused by chest wall injury, respiratory failure, cerebral vascular accident (CVA), pulmonary infection, or narcotic poisoning. However, bradypnea is more commonly caused by respiratory drive depression that occurs secondary to neurological disturbances.

Central neurogenic hyperventilation: A pattern of breathing marked by rapid and regular ventilations at a rate of about 25 per minute. Increasing regularity, rather than rate, is an important diagnostic sign because it indicates an increasing depth of coma.

Cheyne-Stokes respiration: A regular, periodic pattern of breathing with equal intervals of apnea followed by a crescendo-decrescendo sequence of respirations. Cheyne-Stokes respirations are thought to represent a level of cortical dysfunction of the brain. Although some children and older adults breathe in this pattern during sleep, it is usually seen in patients who are seriously ill or injured.

Eupnea: Normal breathing.

Hyperventilation: A persistent, rapid, deep respiration that often results in hyperpnea. Compared with tachypnea, hyperpnea is usually slower and much deeper. Its causes include exercise, anxiety, metabolic disturbances (e.g., diabetic ketoacidosis), and central nervous system (CNS) illness.

Kussmaul respiration: An abnormally deep, very rapid sighing respiratory pattern characteristic of diabetic ketoacidosis or other metabolic acidosis.

Tachypnea: A persistent respiratory rate that exceeds 20 breaths per minute. It may be common in patients who are in pain, frightened, or anxious. The many other causes of tachypnea include fractured ribs, pneumonia, pneumothorax, pulmonary embolus, and pleurisy.

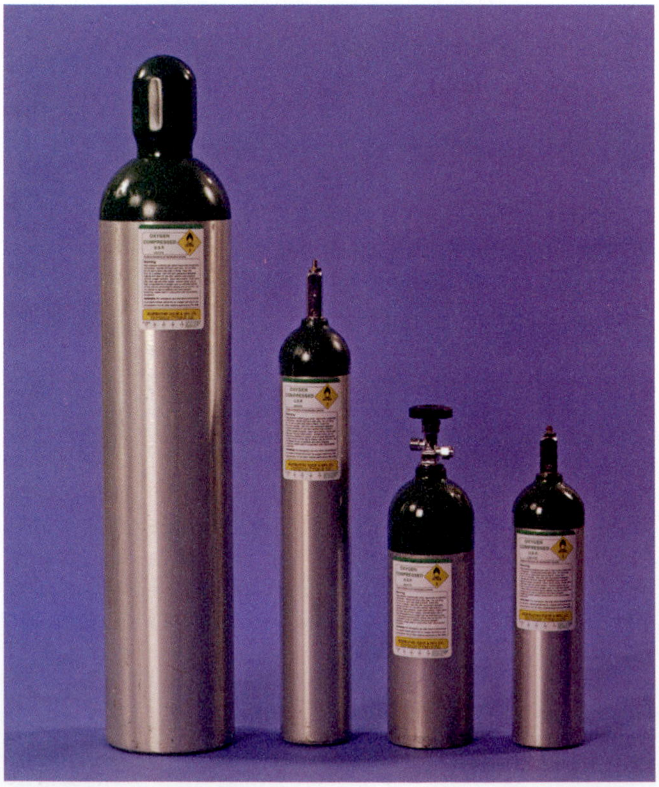

FIGURE 19-23 ■ Oxygen cylinders: D, jumbo D, E, and M.

BOX 19-3 Calculating Oxygen Tank Life

This method can be used to estimate the amount of oxygen available in an oxygen cylinder. First, subtract the safe residual pressure (200 psi) from the tank pressure. Second, multiply the result by the tank's factor (cylinder constant). This equals the volume of gas. Third, divide the volume of gas by the liters per minute (LPM) delivery. This equals the tank life in minutes.

Example

The tank pressure in an E cylinder is 650 psi. You are delivering 6 L/min of oxygen to the patient.

Step 1. Subtract the safe residual pressure from the tank's psi:

$$650 - 200 = 450$$

Step 2. Multiply the result by the E cylinder factor to obtain the volume of gas:

$$450 \times 0.28 = 126$$

Step 3. Divide the volume of gas by the LPM delivery to determine the tank life in minutes:

$$126 \div 6 = 21 \text{ minutes}$$

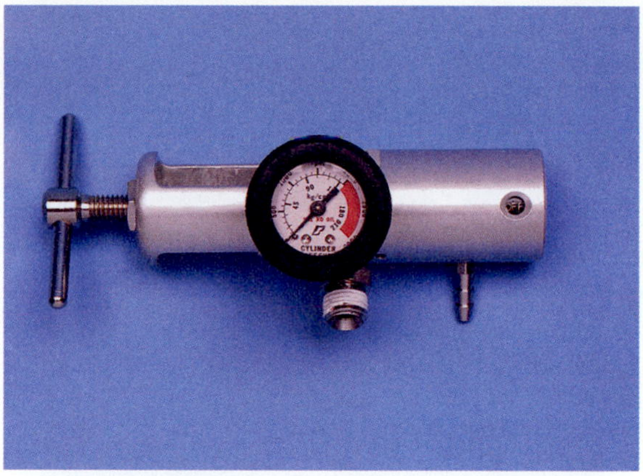

FIGURE 19-24 ■ Therapy regulator.

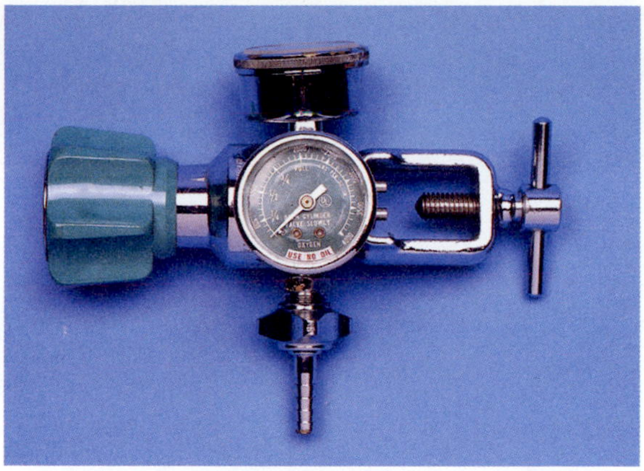

FIGURE 19-25 ■ Flowmeter.

other emergency medical services (EMS) agencies when the weight and space that a standard oxygen system occupies must be considered. The main advantage of liquid oxygen is that a much larger volume of gaseous oxygen can be stored in an aqueous state. One disadvantage of liquid oxygen is the cost. (LOX is more expensive than pressurized oxygen.) Another is the fact that the units generally require upright storage. Finally, special requirements are necessary for large-volume storage and cylinder transfer.

REGULATORS

High-pressure regulators are used to transfer cylinder gas from tank to tank. They are attached to cylinder stems and allow cylinder gas to be delivered under high pressure. *Therapy regulators* are used to deliver a safe pressure of oxygen to patients (Fig. 19-24). They are attached to the cylinder stem. Therapy regulators work through a regulator mechanism whereby 50 psi escape pressure is reduced ("stepped down") to 30 psi for safe delivery to the patient.

▶NOTE Therapy regulators (used for delivery of oxygen to patients) are attached to smaller oxygen cylinders by a yoke assembly with a pin index safety system. This system prevents the paramedic from using a regulator with the wrong type of gas. It requires that the yoke pins match the corresponding holes in the valve assembly for oxygen to be delivered. Larger oxygen cylinders have valve assemblies with a threaded outlet specific to medical oxygen.

FLOWMETERS

Flowmeters control the amount of oxygen that is delivered to the patient (Fig. 19-25). These devices are connected to the pressure regulator. They are adjusted to deliver oxygen at a set number of liters per minute. Some EMS agencies attach disposable humidifiers to the flowmeter. This provides moisture to the dry oxygen coming from the supply cylinder. Humidified oxygen is desirable for long-term oxygen administration and for patients with croup, epiglottitis, or bronchiolitis (see Chapter 30).

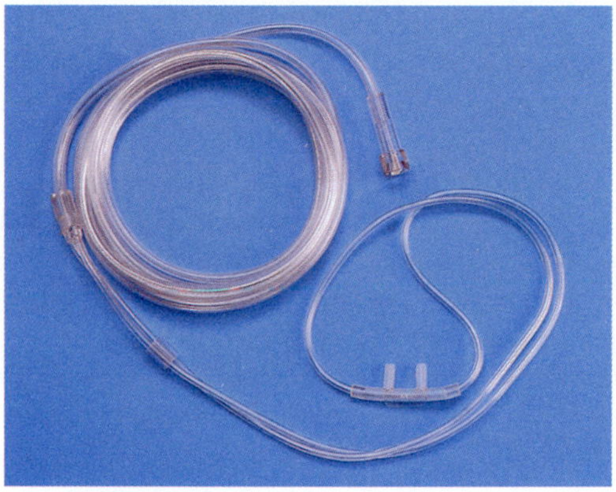

FIGURE 19-26 ■ Nasal cannula.

TABLE 19-3 Oxygen Delivery Devices

DEVICE	FLOW RATE (L/MIN)	OXYGEN (O_2)% DELIVERED
Nasal cannula	1-6	24-44
Simple face mask	6-10	35-60
Partial rebreather mask	6-10	35-60
Nonrebreather mask	10-15	80-95
Venturi mask	4-8	24-50

L/min, Liters per minute.

Oxygen Delivery Devices

Patients who have spontaneous respirations can receive supplemental oxygen through several different oxygen delivery devices. These are the nasal cannula, simple face mask, partial rebreather mask, nonrebreather mask, and Venturi mask (Table 19-3).

NASAL CANNULA

The nasal cannula (Fig. 19-26) delivers low-concentration oxygen. This is done by way of two small plastic prongs placed into the nostrils. Nasal cannulas should not be used

TABLE 19-4 Approximate Oxygen Concentration for Liters Per Minute Flow

LITERS PER MINUTE	OXYGEN CONCENTRATION
1	24%
2	28%
3	32%
4	36%
5	40%
6	44%

in patients with poor respiratory effort, severe hypoxia, or apnea. They also should not be used in patients who breathe primarily through the mouth. As a rule, the nasal cannula is well tolerated. However, it does not deliver high-volume/high-concentration oxygen. The relationship of approximate oxygen concentrations to liter per minute flow is listed in Table 19-4.

It is difficult to obtain oxygen concentrations greater than 30% to 35% with a nasal cannula. This is because the patient continues to mouth breathe during oxygen administration. The mouth breathing reduces the concentration of oxygen inspired through the nose. The device also is ineffective if the patient's nose is blocked by blood or mucus. For these reasons, use of the nasal cannula is limited to patients who would benefit from low-concentration oxygen delivery. This may include some patients with chest pain and patients who have chronic pulmonary disease. The maximum oxygen flow rate for a nasal cannula is 6 L/min.

SIMPLE FACE MASK

The simple face mask (Fig. 19-27) is a soft, clear plastic mask. It conforms to the patient's face. Small perforations in the mask allow atmospheric gas to be mixed with oxygen during inhalation. They also permit the patient's exhaled air to escape. Oxygen concentrations of 35% to 60% can be delivered through this device with a flow rate of 6 to 10 L/min. A flow rate of less than 6 L/min can produce an accumulation of carbon dioxide in the mask; therefore oxygen delivery through any face mask should always exceed this minimum. Flow rates above 10 L/min do not enhance oxygen concentration. All masks must be well fitted to the patient's face for optimal benefit. Leaks reduce the oxygen concentration.

PARTIAL REBREATHER MASK

The partial rebreather mask (Fig. 19-28) has an attached oxygen reservoir bag. The bag should be filled before the patient uses the mask. This device has vent ports covered by one-way disks. These allow a portion of the patient's exhaled gas to enter the reservoir bag and be reused. The remainder of the carbon dioxide–loaded gas escapes into the atmosphere. Oxygen concentrations of 35% to 60% can be delivered with a flow rate that prevents the reservoir bag from collapsing completely on inspiration. Partial rebreather masks should not be used in patients with apnea or poor respiratory effort. As with the simple face mask, delivery of volumes above 10 L/min with this device does not enhance oxygen concentration.

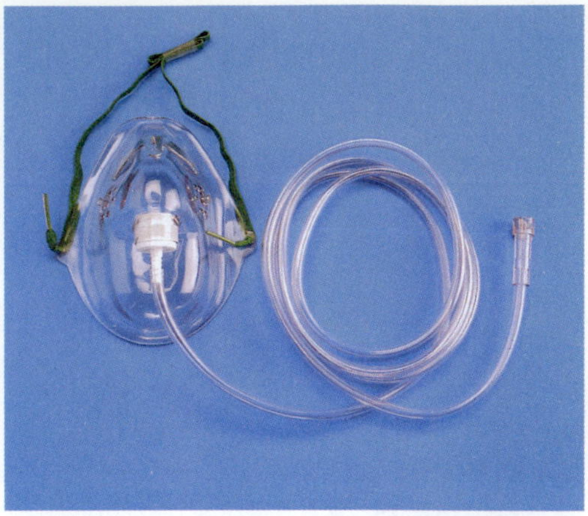

FIGURE 19-27 ■ Simple face mask.

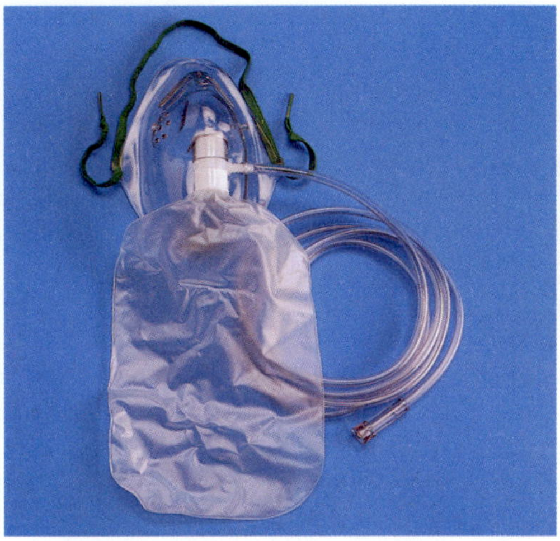

FIGURE 19-28 ■ Partial rebreather mask.

NONREBREATHER MASK

The nonrebreather mask (Fig. 19-29) is similar in design to the partial nonrebreather. However, a flutter valve assembly in the mask piece stops the patient's exhaled air from returning to the reservoir bag. This device delivers oxygen concentrations up to and above 95%. The flow rate must be adequate to keep the reservoir bag partly inflated during inspiration. (Patients with severe respiratory distress may need up to 20 L/min to maintain inflation of the reservoir bag.) Paramedics should ensure that the mask is seated firmly over the patient's mouth and nose. They also should ensure that the reservoir bag is never less than two thirds full. This device most often is used in patients who need high-concentration oxygen delivery (10 to 15 L/min). Like

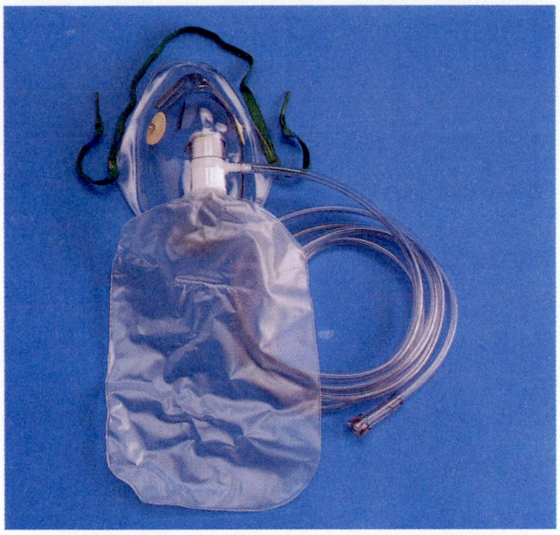

FIGURE 19-29 ■ Nonrebreather mask.

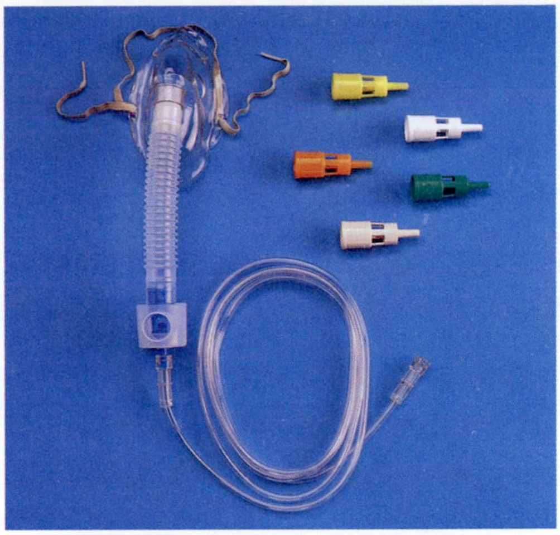

FIGURE 19-30 ■ Venturi mask.

other masks, it should not be used in patients with apnea or poor respiratory effort.

> **CRITICAL THINKING**
> What could happen if the oxygen source is disconnected from a nonrebreather mask?

VENTURI MASK

The Venturi mask (Fig. 19-30) is a high-airflow oxygen entrainment delivery device. It delivers a precise fraction of inspired oxygen (Fio_2) at typically low concentrations. The device was originally designed to deliver 30% to 40% concentrations. However, it has since been adapted to deliver higher oxygen percentages. The Venturi mask uses "jet mixing" of atmospheric gas and oxygen to achieve the desired mixture.

Color-coded adapters in various sizes are attached to the mask to control the oxygen flow rate. (Standard size adapters are 3, 4, and 6 L/min.) The color codes and adapters state the exact liter flow to use to obtain the precise Fio_2. Choosing a different liter flow greatly alters the Fio_2 delivered. The various Venturi masks deliver 24% to 50% oxygen. They are advised for patients who rely on a hypoxic respiratory drive. This includes, for example, patients with chronic obstructive pulmonary disease. The main benefit of the Venturi mask is that it allows precise regulation of the Fio_2. It also permits the paramedic to titrate oxygen for the patient with COPD so as not to exceed the patient's hypoxic drive while allowing enrichment of supplemental oxygen. Care must be taken to match the proper Fio_2 to the correct flow rate. Otherwise, the Venturi mask does not deliver the indicated Fio_2.

VENTILATION

Patient ventilation can be provided by several methods in the prehospital setting. These include rescue breathing (mouth to mouth, mouth to nose, mouth to stoma), mouth-to-mask breathing, bag-valve devices, and automatic transport ventilators.

Rescue Breathing

As discussed before, inspired air has an oxygen concentration of about 21%. Of this 21%, about 4% is used by the body. The remaining 17% is exhaled. Ventilation by rescue breathing can provide adequate oxygenation to a patient with respiratory insufficiency.

Rescue breathing has some advantages. First, no equipment is needed. Second, it is immediately available. However, it also has disadvantages. One disadvantage is the limitation of the vital capacity of the rescuer. (About 700 to 1000 mL is needed to ventilate an adult.) Another drawback is the low amount of oxygen delivered in expired air compared with other methods of ventilation with supplemental oxygen. Also, a rescuer may find it difficult to force air past any obstructions in the airway. The risk exists that a disease will be transmitted through direct body fluid contact. Another risk is the transmission of an unknown communicable disease at the time of the event. Complications common to all rescue breathing techniques include the following:

- Hyperinflation of the patient's lungs
- Gastric distention
- Blood/body fluid contact concerns
- Rescuer hyperventilation

> **CRITICAL THINKING**
> What are two harmful effects of gastric distention during artificial ventilation?

MOUTH-TO-MOUTH METHOD

Paramedics should use the following guidelines in delivering ventilations mouth to mouth:

1. If no spinal injury is suspected, position the patient with optimal head-tilt and chin-lift. (If spinal injury is

suspected, maintain in-line stabilization and maintain an open airway through the jaw-thrust without head-tilt technique, described later in this chapter.) If necessary, clear the airway of vomitus, body fluids, and foreign objects.
2. Pinch the patient's nostrils closed.
3. Inhale a deep breath.
4. Seal your mouth over the patient's mouth, which should be slightly open.
5. Exhale into the patient's mouth until the chest rises and resistance is produced by the patient's lung expansion.
6. Break contact with the patient's mouth to allow for passive exhalation.
7. Repeat the process, providing a full ventilation of 700 to 1000 mL (longer than 2 seconds in duration) every 5 to 6 seconds as needed.

Mouth-to-mouth breathing usually results in the exchange of saliva between the victim and the rescuer. Transmission of the hepatitis B virus (HBV) and the human immunodeficiency virus (HIV) during rescue breathing has not been documented. However, rare instances of herpes transmission during cardiopulmonary resuscitation (CPR) have been reported.[2] When possible, personal barrier protection devices should be used.

MOUTH-TO-NOSE METHOD

Mouth-to-nose ventilation is very similar to the technique described for mouth-to-mouth rescue breathing. The differences in the mouth-to-nose method are as follows:

- If no spinal injury is suspected, the rescuer must keep one hand on the patient's forehead to maintain an open airway while using the other hand to close the patient's mouth. (If a spinal injury is suspected, the jaw-thrust without head-tilt technique should be used. The rescuer's cheek is used to seal the patient's mouth.)
- The patient's nose is left open.
- The rescuer's mouth is placed over the patient's nose with as tight a seal as possible.
- During passive exhalation by the patient, the rescuer's mouth is removed from the patient's nose and the patient's mouth is opened for exhalation. The head-tilt or jaw-thrust position must be maintained to ensure an open airway.
- Mouth-to-nose ventilation may be appropriate for patients who have injuries to the mouth and lower jaw and for patients with missing teeth or dentures (which makes a tight seal around the mouth difficult). It also may overcome psychological barriers in having mouth-to-mouth contact with a patient.

VENTILATION OF INFANTS AND CHILDREN

To provide ventilations to infants and children, the paramedic should use the mouth-to-mouth-and-nose technique as described below:

1. Position the patient with a *slight* head-tilt and chin-lift sufficient to open the airway. Hyperextension of a pediatric patient's neck may block the airway. (Use spinal precautions as needed [See Chapter 25].)

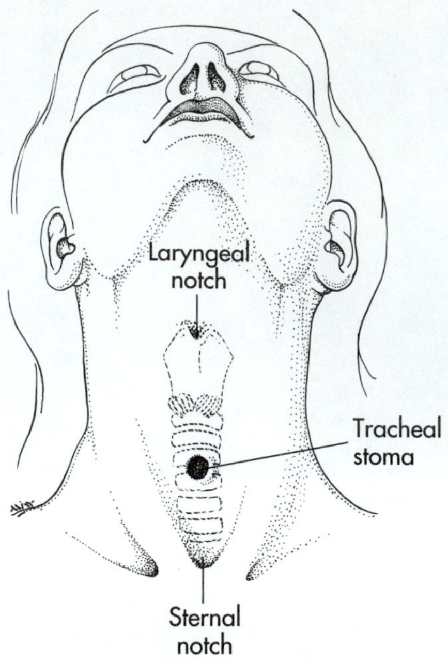

FIGURE 19-31 ■ Stoma.

2. During ventilation, the rescuer's mouth should cover both the mouth and the nose of the infant or small child up to 1 year of age.
3. Use smaller breaths than for an adult patient, but the breaths should be large enough to make the chest rise.
4. When allowing for passive exhalation, break contact with the patient's mouth and nose.
5. Provide slow ventilations (1 to 1½ seconds in duration) every 3 seconds.

MOUTH-TO-STOMA METHOD

A *stoma* is a temporary or permanent surgical opening in the neck of a patient who has had a laryngectomy or tracheostomy (Fig. 19-31). The airway of such a patient has been surgically interrupted. The larynx is no longer connected to the trachea (Box 19-4).

The stoma created by a laryngectomy is large and round; the edge of the tracheal lining can be seen attached to the skin. The stoma in tracheostomy patients is usually no more than several millimeters in diameter. It usually contains one or two concentric tubes (one fitting inside the other) made of plastic or metal. The method of ventilating these patients is the same, regardless of the type of stoma.

Stomas and breathing tubes may become clogged with secretions, encrusted mucus, and foreign matter, leading to inadequate ventilation. If cleaning is needed, wipe the neck opening with gauze. If the breathing tubes are clogged, they can be removed or suctioned. The tracheostomy tube or stoma is suctioned by passing a sterile suction catheter through the external opening into the trachea. *Do not insert the catheter more than 7 to 12 cm (3 to 5 inches) into the trachea.* Once the airway is partly open, begin ventilations by the mouth-to-stoma method (mouth-to-stoma ventilation is bacteriologically cleaner than the mouth-to-mouth

BOX 19-4 Special Considerations for Patients Who Have Had a Laryngectomy

When providing care for a patient who has had a laryngectomy, paramedics sometimes may need to suction the tracheostomy tube or remove, clean, and replace a tube that has become obstructed by mucus. (Patients who have had a laryngectomy have a less effective cough. As a result, mucus plugs often obstruct breathing tubes.)

The steps for suctioning a breathing tube are as follows:

1. Preoxygenate the patient.
2. Inject 3 mL of sterile saline down the trachea.
3. Step 2 usually results in coughing. If it does not, instruct the patient to exhale.
4. Insert the suction catheter into the trachea until resistance is met (without negative pressure).
5. Step 4 usually results in coughing. If it does not, instruct the patient to cough or exhale.
6. Suction while withdrawing the catheter.

If the breathing tube cannot be cleared and requires replacement, follow these steps:

1. Lubricate a same-size tracheostomy tube or endotracheal (ET) tube (5 mm or larger).
2. Instruct the patient to exhale.
3. Gently insert the tube 1 to 2 cm (about ½ to ¾ inch) beyond the balloon cuff.
4. Inflate the cuff.
5. Confirm the patient's comfort and verify the patency and proper placement of the tube.

Stenosis (spontaneous narrowing of a stoma) may be life threatening. It also makes replacing a tracheostomy tube difficult or impossible. When stenosis is a factor, an ET tube must be placed before total obstruction occurs.

method) by using a pediatric-size pocket mask over the top of the stoma or by securing the airway with an endotracheal (ET) tube placed through the stoma.

The technique for stoma ventilation is basically the same as that for other methods of artificial ventilation. However, the patient's head should be kept straight (rather than tilted back), with the patient's shoulders slightly elevated. This position allows more effective ventilation. If the patient's chest does not rise or if air is heard to escape through the patient's upper airway, the patient may be a "partial neck breather." These patients are able to inhale and exhale some air through their nose and mouth. If this occurs, the patient's nostrils must be pinched closed and the mouth sealed with the palm of one hand during ventilation.

Mouth-to-Mask Devices

Mouth-to-mask devices have become popular. They are used as an alternative to mouth-to-mouth methods of ventilation. These masks are constructed of a clear, flexible material. They are available with one-way valves, bacterial filters, and ports for supplemental oxygen delivery (Fig. 19-32). They are made by a number of manufacturers and

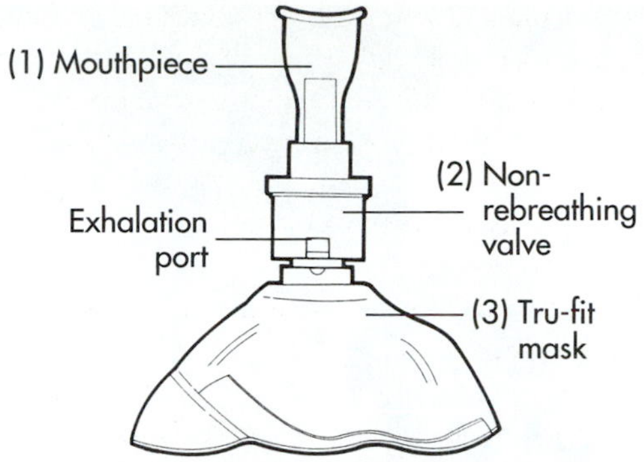

FIGURE 19-32 ■ Mouth-to-mask device.

are available in a variety of sizes. The mouth-to-mask technique offers several advantages:

- It eliminates direct contact with the patient's mouth and nose.
- It provides more effective ventilation than the mouth-to-mouth method or a bag-valve-mask device.
- It is aesthetically more acceptable than mouth-to-mouth ventilation.
- Supplemental oxygen delivery is possible.
- The one-way valve eliminates exposure to exhaled gases and sputum.
- The mask is easy to apply.

TECHNIQUE

The mask device can be used in patients with or without spontaneous respirations. If the device is immediately available, it is the preferred method of initial ventilation for the patient (Fig. 19-33). To apply the mask, the paramedic should follow these steps:

1. If no spinal injury is suspected, position the patient with optimal head-tilt and chin-lift. The use of an oropharyngeal or nasopharyngeal airway is indicated in an unconscious patient. (If a spinal injury is suspected, spinal precautions should be used.)
2. Connect the one-way valve to the mask. Oxygen tubing should be connected to the inlet port with an oxygen flow rate of 15 L/min. Using supplemental oxygen provides a higher concentration of oxygen in the inspired air. An oxygen flow rate of 10 L/min, combined with rescuer ventilations, can supply an oxygen concentration of 50%. An oxygen flow rate of 15 L/min provides an inspired oxygen concentration of about 80%.
3. Position yourself at the patient's head (cephalic technique) or side (lateral technique). Clear the airway of secretions, vomitus, and foreign objects. Place the mask on the patient's face and create an airtight seal. Using the thumb side of the palm with both hands, apply pressure to the sides of the mask. If using the cephalic technique, apply upward pressure to the mandible just in front of the ear lobes, using the index, middle, and ring fingers of both hands while maintaining head-tilt. If using the lateral technique, seal the mask by placing the index finger and thumb of the hand closer to the top of the patient's head along the border of the mask and place the thumb of the

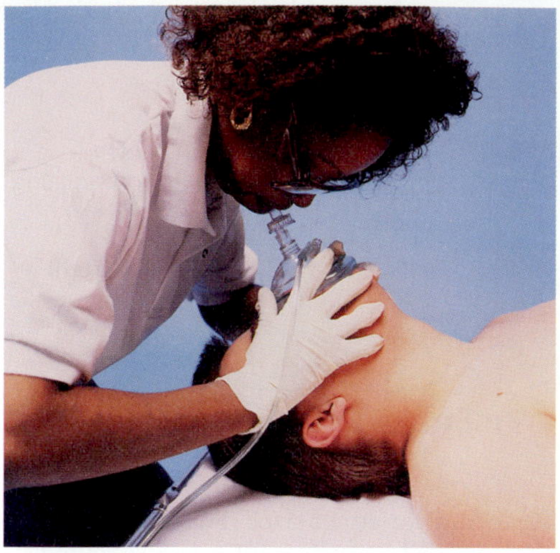

FIGURE 19-33 ■ Mouth-to-mask ventilation technique (cephalic technique).

▶ BOX 19-5 Application of Cricoid Pressure (Sellick Maneuver)

Applying pressure to the solid ring of the cricoid cartilage can occlude the esophagus. This reduces the risk of regurgitation and aspiration. This type of pressure can also help to minimize gastric distention during bag-valve-mask (BVM) ventilation. Cricoid pressure should be applied if vomiting is likely to occur. It also is indicated if the patient is unconscious while intubation or artificial ventilation is performed.

Cricoid pressure should be used with caution if cervical spine injury is suspected, because it may cause additional damage to the spine. Complications include laryngeal trauma with excessive force and esophageal rupture from unrelieved high gastric pressures.

other hand along the lower margin of the mask. Place the remaining fingers of the hand closer to the patient's feet and lift the jaw while performing a head-tilt chin-lift.

4. Blow into the opening of the mask, observing chest rise and fall. If available, a second rescuer should apply cricoid pressure (*Sellick maneuver;* Box 19-5). This helps prevent gastric inflation during positive pressure ventilation and reduces the chance of regurgitation and aspiration.
5. Remove the mask from the patient's face to allow for passive exhalation.

If oxygen is not available, the tidal volumes and inspiratory times for mouth-to-mask ventilation should be the same as for mouth-to-mouth breathing (10 mL/kg or 700 to 1000 mL delivered over longer than 2 seconds). If supplemental oxygen (minimum flow rate of 10 L/min) is used with the face mask, lower tidal volumes of 6 to 7 mL/kg (400 to 600 mL) should be provided over 1 to 2 seconds until the chest rises.[4]

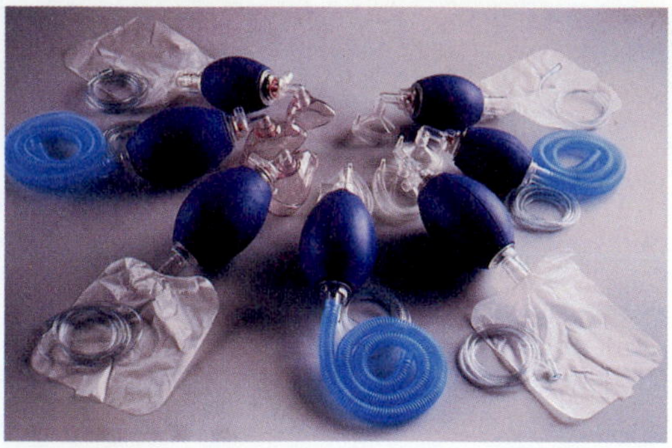

FIGURE 19-34 ■ Disposable and reusable adult and pediatric bag-valve devices.

Bag-Valve Devices

Bag-valve devices consist of a self-inflating bag and a nonrebreathing valve (Fig. 19-34). They can be used with a mask, an ET tube, or another invasive airway device. An adequate bag-valve unit should have (1) a self-refilling bag that is disposable or easily cleaned or sterilized, (2) a nonjam valve system that allows a minimum oxygen inlet flow of 15 L/min, (3) a non–pop-off valve, (4) standard 15 and 22 mm fittings, (5) a system for delivering high-concentration oxygen through an inlet port at the back of the bag or by an oxygen reservoir, and (6) a nonrebreathing valve.[5]

The device also should perform in all common environmental conditions and under extremes of temperature. It should be available in both adult and pediatric sizes.

▶ NOTE All paramedics should be proficient in delivering effective oxygenation and ventilation with a bag-valve device to adults, children, and infants. It is the preferred method of ventilatory support, particularly if the transport time is short.[6]

When the bag-valve device is compressed, air is delivered to the patient through a one-way valve. The air inlet to the bag is closed during delivery. When the bag is released, the patient's expired gas passes through an exhalation valve into the atmosphere. This prevents the patient's exhaled air from reentering the bag-valve device. As the patient exhales, atmospheric air and supplemental oxygen from the reservoir refill the bag.

Use of the bag-valve device with a mask is difficult. This is because of the problem of creating an effective seal between the mask and the patient's face while maintaining an open airway. For this reason, it has been recommended that two rescuers use the device. One should hold the mask and maintain the airway while the second compresses the bag with two hands. If three rescuers are available, one rescuer can be solely responsible for maintaining the mask seal while providing spinal precautions as indicated.

When properly used, the bag-valve device has many benefits. The rescuer can provide a wide range of inspiratory pressures and volumes to adequately ventilate patients of varying sizes and underlying pathological conditions. It can be used to assist patients with shallow respirations. It performs adequately in extremes of environmental temperatures. Oxygen concentrations ranging from 21% (room air concentration) to nearly 100% (using supplemental oxygen and a reservoir) can be achieved. In addition, manual compression of the bag can give the rescuer a sense of the patient's lung compliance, which is an advantage over mechanical methods of ventilation.

TECHNIQUE

Ventilation with the bag-valve device is best accomplished when the patient has been intubated. If the patient has not been intubated, the bag-valve device may be used with a mask. The following technique is recommended for use with the bag-valve-mask (BVM) device:

1. The rescuer is positioned at the top of the patient's head.
2. If no spinal injury is suspected, place the patient in the optimal head-tilt chin-lift position, with the patient's head elevated in extension. (If a spinal injury is suspected, spinal precautions should be used.)
3. Clear the airway of secretions, vomitus, and foreign objects. If the patient is unconscious, insert an oropharyngeal or nasopharyngeal airway. The patient's mouth should remain open under the mask.
4. Connect an oxygen source. Then flush the reservoir with high-concentration oxygen.
5. Place the mask on the patient's face, making a tight seal. This can be accomplished by placing the thumb on the nose area and an index finger on the chin, and then spreading the remaining fingers along the mandible. The anterior displacement of the mandible must be maintained. To compress the bag, the rescuer's other hand presses the bag against his or her body (e.g., the thigh), or another rescuer compresses the bag with two hands as recommended by the American Heart Association (AHA). The bag should be compressed smoothly, delivering 6 to 7 mL/kg of air (approximately 500 mL for the average adult) over 2 seconds. (A third rescuer may provide cricoid pressure.)

PEDIATRIC CONSIDERATIONS

Smaller bag-valve devices are needed for infants and children. This helps to reduce the chances of overinflation and barotrauma. Bag-valve devices are used mainly for pediatric patients who are in respiratory arrest. BVM devices equipped with a fish-mouth– or leaf-flap–operated outlet valve should not be used to provide supplemental oxygen to a spontaneously breathing infant or child. If the valve fails to open during inspiration, the child receives only the exhaled gases from within the mask itself. For this reason, bag-valve devices for ventilation of full-term neonates, infants, and children should have a minimum volume of 450 to 500 mL.[7] At least 10 to 15 L/min of oxygen flow is needed to maintain an adequate oxygen volume in the reservoir of a pediatric bag (Fig. 19-35).

> **▶NOTE** A child's flat nasal bridge makes achieving a mask seal difficult. In addition, compressing the mask against the face may result in obstruction. The mask seal is best achieved with jaw displacement using two rescuers to provide bag-valve-mask (BVM) ventilation.

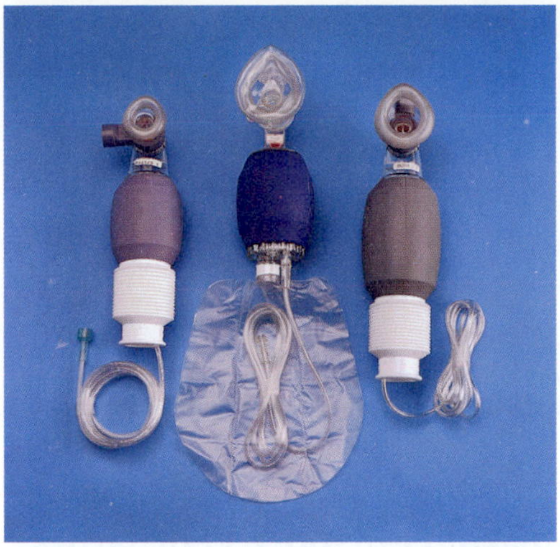

FIGURE 19-35 ■ Pediatric bag-valve-mask device.

Technique. The following procedure is used to artificially ventilate a pediatric patient with a bag-valve-mask device:

1. Ensure a proper mask fit by using a length-based resuscitation tape or by measuring from the bridge of the nose to the cleft of the chin.
2. Ensure a proper mask position and seal. Place the mask over the mouth and nose (avoid compressing the eyes). With one hand, place a thumb on the mask at the apex and place the index finger on the mouth at the chin (like a C clamp). With gentle pressure, push down on the mask to establish an adequate seal. Maintain the airway by lifting the bony prominence on the chin, with the remaining fingers placed on the mandible, forming an E. Avoid putting pressure on the soft area under the chin.
3. Provide ventilations at a rate of one breath every 3 seconds.
4. Obtain chest rise with each ventilation. Saying "squeeze" with each ventilation should provide adequate volume to initiate chest rise. Do not overinflate.
5. Allow adequate time for exhalation by releasing the bag and saying, "release, release."
6. Continue with ventilations using the "squeeze, release, release" method.
7. Assess BVM ventilation by observing adequate rise and fall of the chest, by listening for lung sounds at the third intercostal space and midaxillary line, and by checking for improvement in skin color or heart rate, or both (see Chapter 11).

> **CRITICAL THINKING**
> What should you do if you find that it is suddenly harder to ventilate a patient who is not intubated?

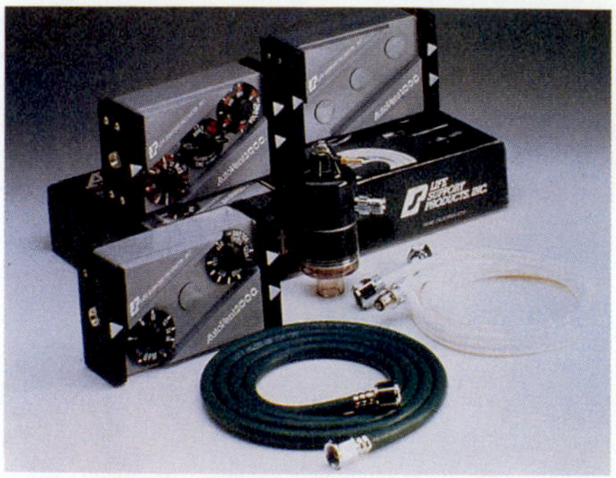

FIGURE 19-36 ■ Autovent 1000, 2000, and 3000.

Automatic Transport Ventilators

Several time-cycled, gas-powered, automatic transport ventilators (ATVs) are available for field use or intrahospital transport of patients who require ventilatory support (Fig. 19-36). Most of these ventilators consist of a plastic control module. This module is connected by tubing to any 50 psi gas source (e.g., air or different concentrations of oxygen, including 100% oxygen). The exit valve of the control module is connected by one or two tubes (based on the model) to the patient valve assembly to deliver selected tidal volumes (400 to 1200 mL for adults, 200 to 600 mL for children). Another control selects respiratory rates from 8 to 22 breaths per minute for adults. It selects rates from 8 to 30 breaths per minute for children. (Most ATVs are not to be used in children under 5 years of age.) Most units provide a 40 L/min flow of oxygen. This flow remains constant despite changes in the patient's airway or lung compliance.

NOTE Automatic transport ventilators (ATVs) should have a default rate of 10 breaths per minute for adults and 20 breaths per minute for children. The paramedic should be able to adjust the rate once the patient has been intubated with a tracheal tube or alternative airway.[8]

The volume of gas delivered by the automatic ventilator is determined by the length of time the manual trigger is depressed or by the inspiratory effort of the spontaneously breathing patient. Most units are designed to limit the inspiratory pressure to 60 to 80 cm of water. When this pressure is reached, an alarm sounds. At this time, excess gas flow is vented off, preventing possible lung damage. ATVs allow the paramedic to use both hands to obtain a tight face-to-mask seal on a patient who has not been intubated. Cricoid pressure also can be applied with one hand while the other hand seals the mask on the face. ATVs also allow the paramedic to perform other tasks when the ventilator is used on a patient who has been intubated. Most ATVs should not be used in patients who are awake, who have an obstructed airway, and/or who have increased airway resistance (e.g., pneumothorax, asthma, pulmonary edema).

BOX 19-6 Personal Protective Equipment

The Centers for Disease Control and Prevention (CDC) recommend that health care workers, in addition to taking the normal precautions for personal protection from communicable diseases, use masks, eyewear (e.g., safety glasses and face shields), and gowns when splashing of blood or other body fluids is likely. During airway management, certain patient reactions may occur. These may include vomiting and coughing. Exposure to blood and other body fluids also is possible. Because of these possibilities, the paramedic should observe barrier precautions.

AIRWAY MANAGEMENT

Science and technology have produced many devices for providing airway management. However, the paramedic must not neglect basic airway management procedures. A basic procedure that secures a safe and functional airway is better than a more technically difficult procedure. Airway management should progress rapidly from the least to the most invasive procedures and devices (see algorithm on next page). Paramedics also should make sure they are always equipped with the appropriate personal protective equipment for these procedures (Box 19-6).

NOTE Unconscious patients lack the muscular tone and control to maintain a patent airway. For this reason, an airway must be established and maintained in the initial assessment of all unconscious patients. Any injury severe enough to cause loss of consciousness is severe enough to cause spinal injury. Spinal precautions should be considered in all trauma patients who need airway management or ventilatory support until an x-ray film of the spine has been made.

Manual Techniques for Airway Management

Manual techniques for airway management have been described by the AHA and the American Red Cross (ARC). These include the head-tilt chin-lift method, the jaw-thrust, and the jaw-thrust without head-tilt. The paramedic should not use manual maneuvers to open the airway in patients who are responsive or when attempts to open the patient's mouth are met with resistance. All such maneuvers are hazardous if spinal injury is a factor. In addition, none of these maneuvers protects against aspiration.

The head-tilt chin-lift maneuver (Fig. 19-37) is preferred for opening the airway when a spinal injury is not suspected. The head-tilt is performed by placing one hand on the victim's forehead and applying firm backward pressure with the palm to tilt the head back. The fingers of the other hand then are placed under the bony part of the lower jaw (near the chin) and lifted to bring the chin forward. These fingers support the jaw and help to maintain the head-tilt position.

AIRWAY MANAGEMENT

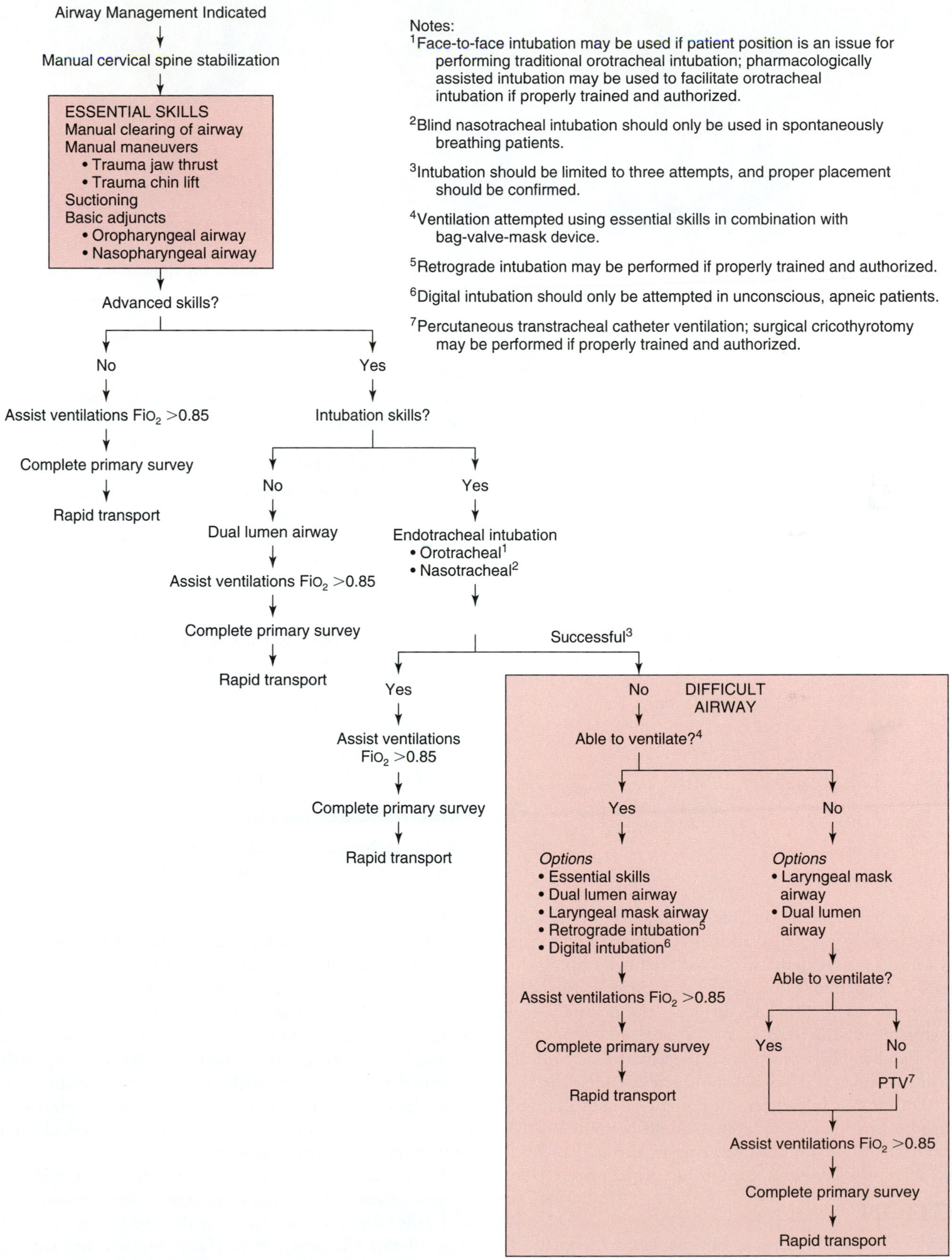

Notes:

[1]Face-to-face intubation may be used if patient position is an issue for performing traditional orotracheal intubation; pharmacologically assisted intubation may be used to facilitate orotracheal intubation if properly trained and authorized.

[2]Blind nasotracheal intubation should only be used in spontaneously breathing patients.

[3]Intubation should be limited to three attempts, and proper placement should be confirmed.

[4]Ventilation attempted using essential skills in combination with bag-valve-mask device.

[5]Retrograde intubation may be performed if properly trained and authorized.

[6]Digital intubation should only be attempted in unconscious, apneic patients.

[7]Percutaneous transtracheal catheter ventilation; surgical cricothyrotomy may be performed if properly trained and authorized.

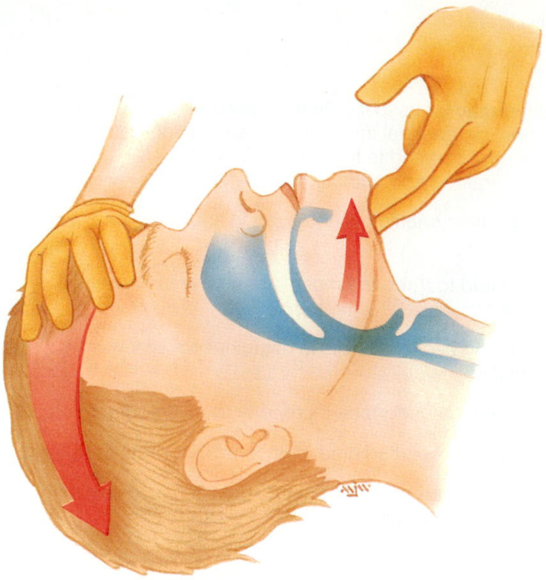

FIGURE 19-37 ■ Head-tilt chin-lift maneuver.

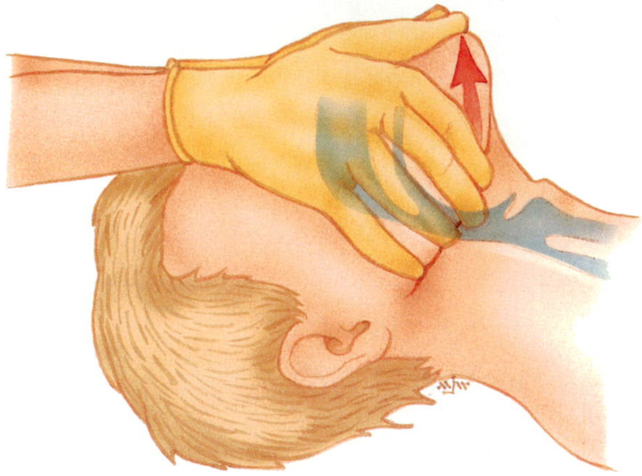

FIGURE 19-38 ■ Jaw-thrust maneuver.

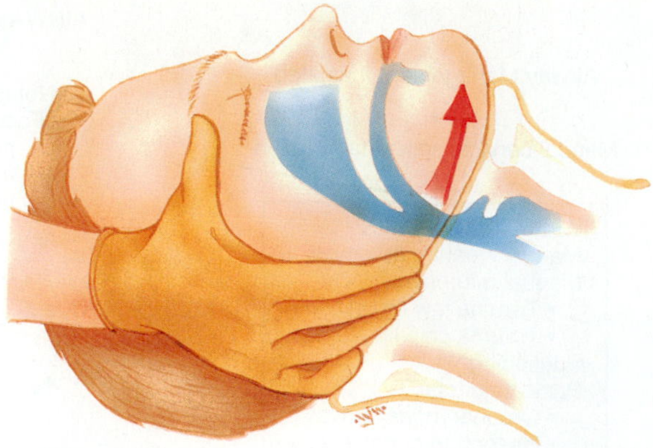

FIGURE 19-39 ■ Jaw-thrust without head-tilt maneuver.

The jaw-thrust maneuver (Fig. 19-38) may be used to gain additional forward displacement of the mandible if no spinal injury is suspected. This is achieved by grasping the angles of the patient's lower jaw and lifting with both hands, one on each side. This displaces the mandible forward while tilting the head back.

If a spinal injury is suspected, the jaw-thrust without head-tilt maneuver (Fig. 19-39) should be used to open the airway. During this maneuver, the patient's head should be stabilized. Also, the cervical spine should be immobilized with neutral, in-line stabilization. The jaw-thrust maneuver should then proceed without extension of the neck.

SUCTION

Suction can be used to remove vomitus, saliva, blood, food, and other foreign objects that might block the airway or increase the likelihood of pulmonary aspiration by inhalation. Many factors can predispose a person to aspiration. For this reason, every patient should be considered a possible aspiration victim.

Suction Devices

Fixed and portable mechanical suction devices are available through a number of manufacturers. Fixed suction devices (Fig. 19-40) are mounted in patient care areas of hospitals and nursing homes. They also are used in many emergency vehicles. These systems are electrically operated by vacuum pumps or powered by the vacuum produced by a vehicle engine manifold. Fixed suction devices furnish an air intake of at least 40 L/min. They provide a vacuum of more than 300 mm Hg when the tube is clamped.

Portable suction devices may be oxygen or air powered, electrically powered, or manually powered (Fig. 19-41). To operate effectively, these devices should furnish an air intake of no less than 20 L/min.

Suction Catheters

Suction catheters are used to clear secretions and debris from the oral cavity and airway passages. The two broad classifications of catheters are whistle-tip suction catheters and tonsil-tip suction catheters.

The whistle-tip catheter is a narrow, flexible tube. It is used primarily for tracheobronchial suctioning to clear secretions through either an ET tube or the nasopharynx (Fig. 19-42). This catheter is designed with molded ends and side holes to cause minimal trauma to the mucosa. It should be lubricated before insertion. A side opening in the proximal end is covered with the thumb to produce suction. Using sterile technique, the paramedic advances the catheter to the desired location. Suction is applied intermittently as the catheter is withdrawn.

The tonsil-tip (Yankauer) suction catheter is a rigid pharyngeal catheter. It is used to clear secretions, blood clots, and other foreign material from the mouth and pharynx (Fig. 19-43). The device is carefully inserted into the oral cavity under direct visualization. Then it is slowly withdrawn while suction is activated.

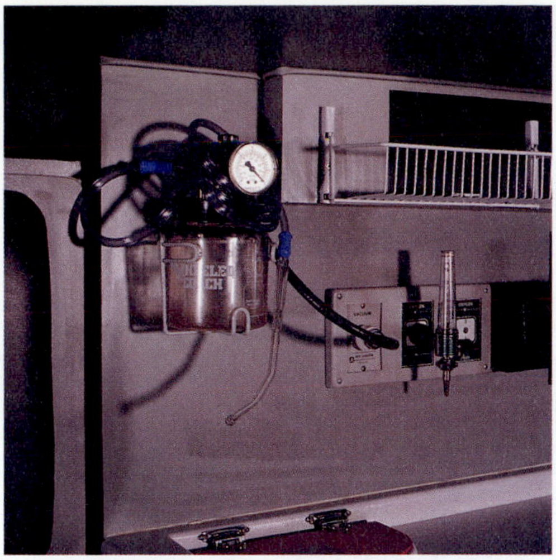

FIGURE 19-40 ■ Fixed suction unit.

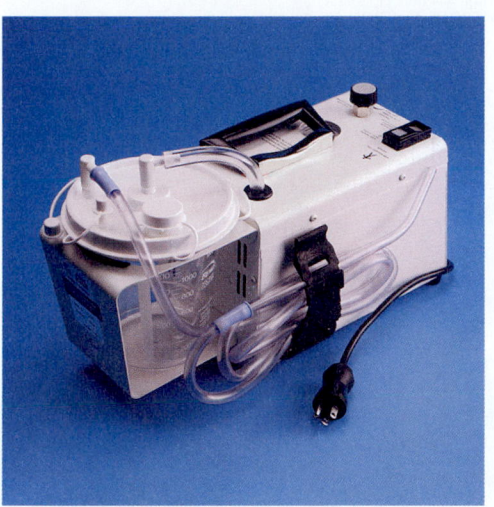

FIGURE 19-41 ■ Portable suction unit.

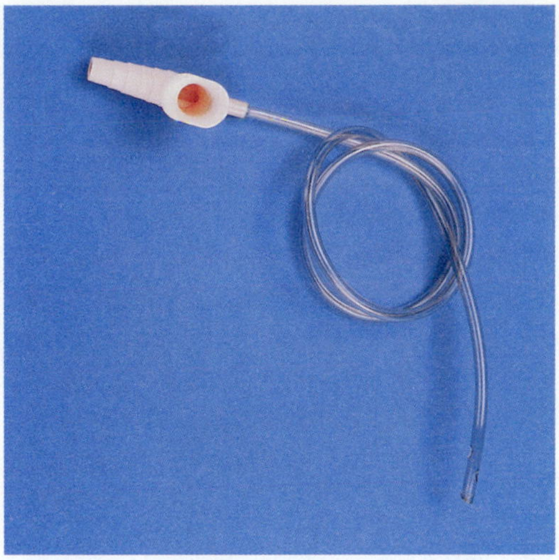

FIGURE 19-42 ■ Soft (whistle-tip) suction catheter.

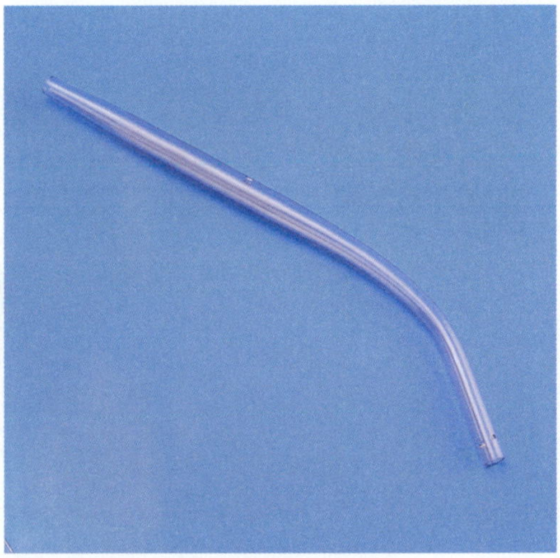

FIGURE 19-43 ■ Rigid (tonsil-tip [Yankauer]) suction catheter.

Before any suctioning is begun, all equipment should be checked. Also, the suction should be set between 80 and 120 mm Hg. (Higher suction is needed for tracheobronchial suctioning.) If possible the patient's lungs should be oxygenated with 100% oxygen for at least 2 minutes before suction is initiated. *Suction should never be applied for longer than 10 to 15 seconds in adult patients. It should never be applied for longer than 5 seconds in pediatric patients.* If more suctioning is needed, the patient's lungs should be reoxygenated first. Possible complications from suctioning include the following:

- Sudden hypoxemia that occurs secondary to decreased lung volume during the application of suction
- Severe hypoxemia that may lead to cardiac rhythm disturbances and cardiac arrest
- Airway stimulation that may increase arterial pressure and cardiac rhythm disturbances
- Coughing that may result in increased intracranial pressure with reduced blood flow to the brain and increased risk of herniation in patients with head injury
- Soft tissue damage to the respiratory tract

TRACHEOBRONCHIAL SUCTIONING

Before tracheobronchial suctioning is performed through an ET tube (Fig. 19-44), the patient must be oxygenated with 100% oxygen for 5 minutes.[7] For tracheal suctioning, a Y- or T-piece or a lateral opening should lie between the suction tube and the source of the on-off suction control. Using sterile technique, the paramedic advances the catheter to the desired location (about the level of the carina.) Suction is applied intermittently by closing the side opening as the catheter is withdrawn in a rotating motion. The patient's cardiac rhythm should be monitored throughout the procedure. If dysrhythmias or bradycardia develops,

STEP-BY-STEP SKILL

FIGURE 19-44 ■ Tracheobronchial suctioning.

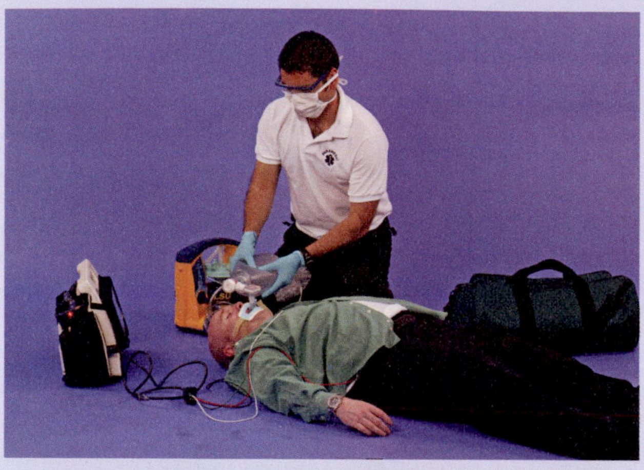

A ■ Bag the intubated patient with a bag-valve device.

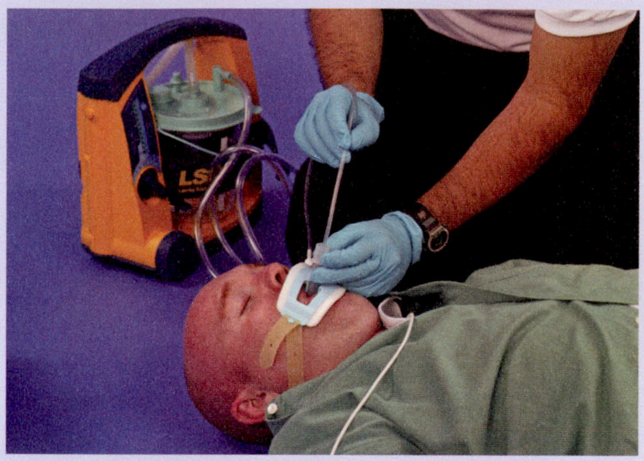

B ■ Introduce the suction catheter through the endotracheal tube without suction.

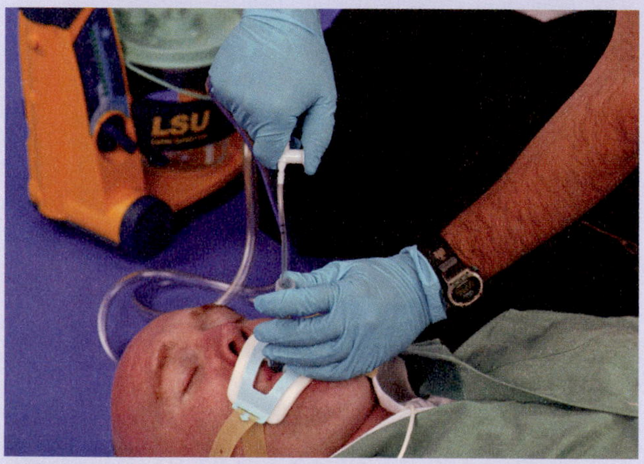

C ■ Withdraw the catheter with suction intermittently applied while observing the electrocardiographic (ECG) rhythm.

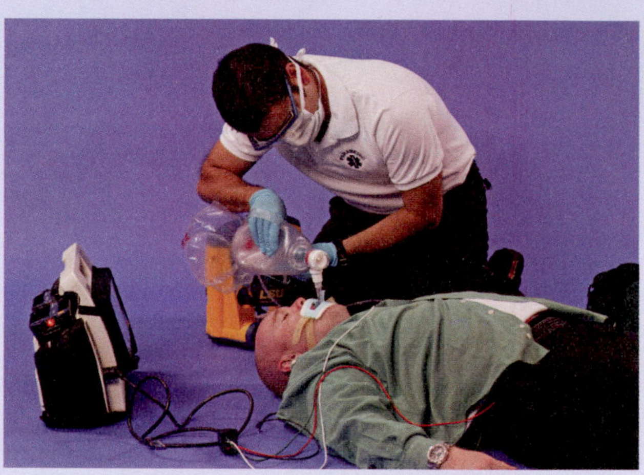

D ■ Ventilate the patient and reevaluate the respiratory status.

suctioning should stop. The patient then should be manually ventilated and oxygenated. Before suctioning is resumed, the patient should be ventilated with 100% oxygen for about 30 seconds.

> **NOTE** It may be necessary to inject 3 to 5 mL of sterile saline down the endotracheal (ET) tube to loosen secretions before suctioning.

GASTRIC DISTENTION

Gastric distention results from the trapping of air in the stomach. As the stomach enlarges, it pushes against the diaphragm and interferes with lung expansion. The abdomen becomes more and more distended (especially in small children). Resistance may be felt to BVM ventilation.

Management. Management of gastric distention begins by slightly increasing the BVM ventilation inspiratory time. (Large-volume suction should be readily available.) If possible the patient should be placed in a left lateral recumbent position. Manual pressure should be slowly applied to the upper stomach or epigastric region. Gastric distention that cannot be managed with these techniques may require insertion of a gastric tube (Fig. 19-45).

GASTRIC TUBES

Gastric distention is very common in patients who are ventilated but have not been intubated. Gastric decompression for gastric distention or vomiting control can be achieved

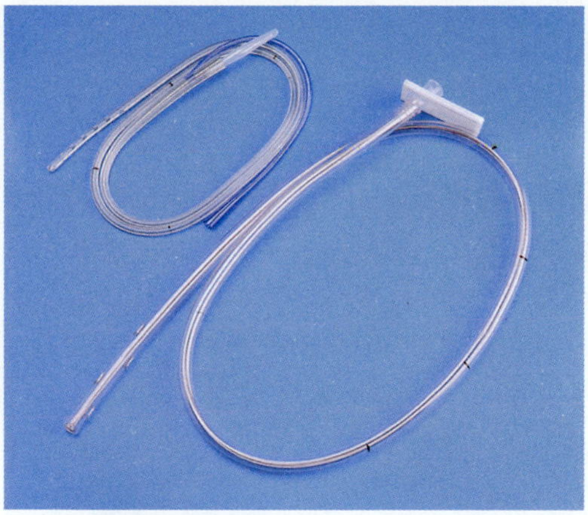

FIGURE 19-45 ■ *Top,* Nasogastric/orogastric tube. *Bottom,* Oral gastric lavage tube.

through nasogastric (NG) or orogastric emptying or decompression of the stomach. Gastric decompression is done with extreme caution in patients who have esophageal trauma or esophageal disease. Gastric decompression should not be performed if an esophageal obstruction is present. NG decompression should not be attempted in a patient with facial trauma or esophageal varices (large, swollen veins in the esophagus that are susceptible to hemorrhage).

Nasogastric Decompression

1. Prepare the patient.
   (a) Place the head in a neutral position.
   (b) Preoxygenate.
   (c) Instill a topical anesthetic or intravenous (IV) ***lidocaine*** (per medical direction or protocol).
   (d) Locate the larger nostril.
2. Measure the NG tube to the correct insertion length and lubricate it with viscous lidocaine or water-soluble lubricant per protocol (Fig. 19-46).
3. Advance the tube gently along the nasal floor and into the stomach. (Having the patient swallow during insertion may help advance the tube into the esophagus and prevent tracheal insertion.)
4. Confirm placement.
   (a) Auscultate the epigastric region while injecting 30 to 50 mL of air.
   (b) Note gastric contents in the NG tube.
   (c) Ensure that no reflux appears around the NG tube.
5. Secure the NG tube in place and attach to suction if indicated.

Orogastric Decompression

1. Prepare the patient and tube as described above for NG insertion.
2. Introduce the orogastric tube down the midline of the oropharynx and into the stomach.
3. Confirm placement. Secure the orogastric tube as described above for NG insertion.

Complications of Gastric Decompression. Whatever the method chosen, gastric decompression is uncomfortable for the patient. It may induce nausea and vomiting even when the gag reflex is suppressed. In addition, gastric tubes interfere with mask seals. They also interfere with visualization of airway structures during intubation. Complications of the procedures include nasal, esophageal, or gastric trauma, tracheal placement, and gastric tube obstruction.

MECHANICAL ADJUNCTS IN AIRWAY MANAGEMENT

The use of mechanical devices for airway management should never delay manual opening of the airway. These devices should be used only after efforts have been made to open the airway manually.

Nasopharyngeal Airway (Nasal Airway)

Nasal airways (Fig. 19-47) are used to maintain an open airway passage in unconscious patients or in patients who are responsive but not alert enough to control their own airway. Insertion of a nasal airway may be useful as a temporary airway maintenance maneuver. It may be used to control the airway in patients with seizures or possible cervical spine injury. It also may be used before nasotracheal intubation (described later in this chapter). In addition, it can serve as a guide for insertion of a nasogastric tube.

CRITICAL THINKING

Think about two or three specific patient conditions that would warrant the use of a nasal airway.

DESCRIPTION

Nasal airways are soft and pliable. They have a gentle curve, and the outer end is flared. Nasal airways are available in a variety of sizes to accommodate infants and adults. They range in length from 17 to 20 cm (about 7 to 8 inches) and in size from 12 to 36 French. (As with most other catheters, the French scale system is used to indicate internal diameter. Each unit of the scale equals about ⅓ mm. A 21 French catheter, for example, is 7 mm [about ⅓ inch] in diameter.)

To determine the correct size, the paramedic should choose an airway with a tube length equal to the distance from the tip of the patient's nose to the earlobe (Fig. 19-48). The following are the recommended sizes of nasopharyngeal airways:

- Large adult: 8 to 9 mm (0.3 to 0.35 inch) internal diameter (24 to 27 French)
- Medium adult: 7 to 8 mm (about ⅓ inch) internal diameter (21 to 24 French)
- Small adult: 6 to 7 mm (about ¼ inch) internal diameter (18 to 21 French)

INSERTION

The nasal airway should be lubricated with a water-soluble lubricant. This helps to ease the airway through the nasal cavity. The device is placed in the nostril with the beveled

STEP-BY-STEP SKILL

FIGURE 19-46 ■ **Insertion of a nasogastric tube.**

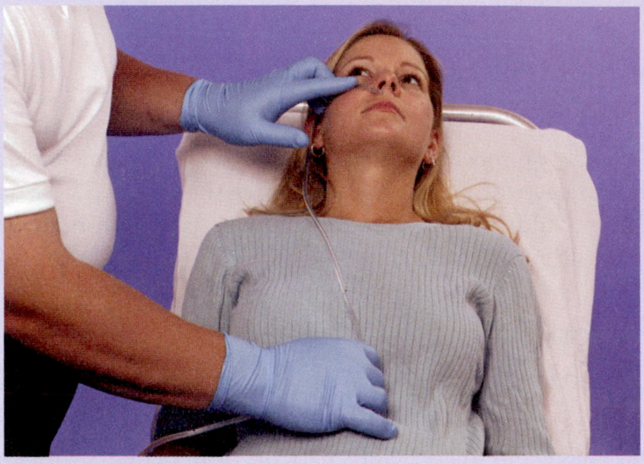

A ■ Position the patient. Measure the tube from the nose to the ear, and from the ear to the xiphoid process.

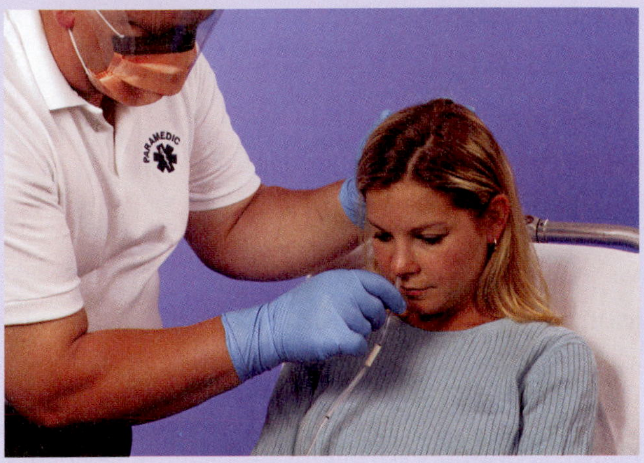

B ■ Lubricate the tube and insert it into the largest nostril. Advance the tube to the proper length.

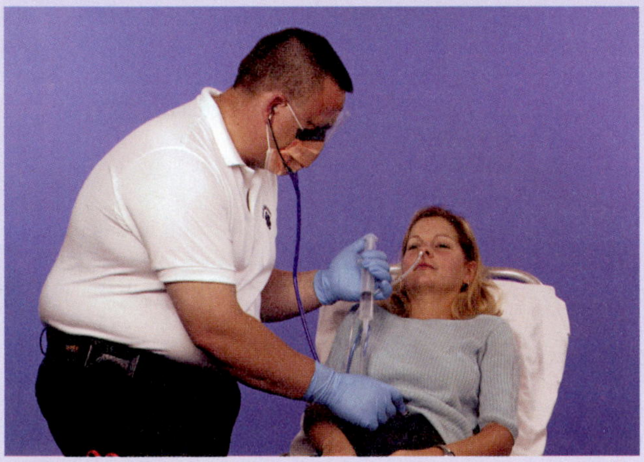

C ■ Verify correct placement of the tube by injecting 30 to 50 mL of air while auscultating over the epigastric area.

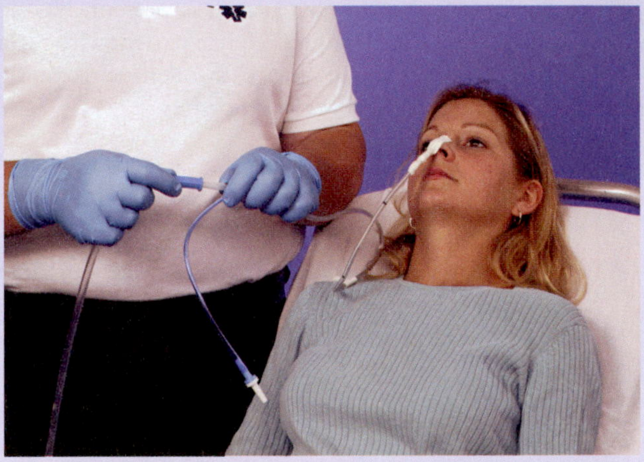

D ■ Secure the tube and attached the suction unit.

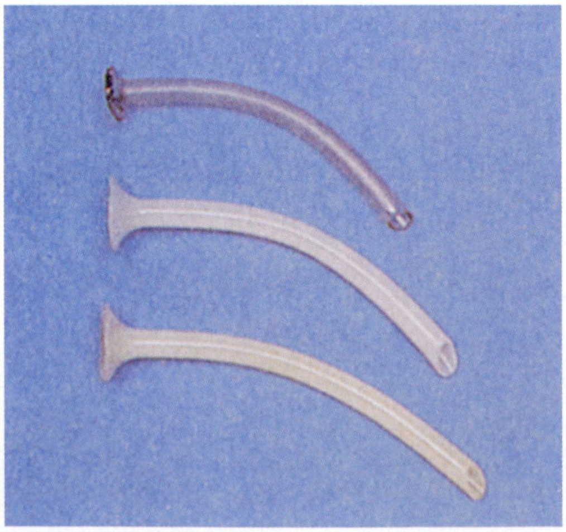

FIGURE 19-47 ■ Nasal airways.

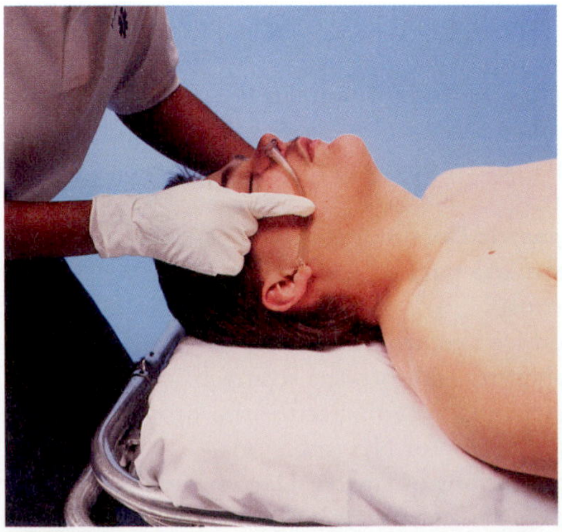

FIGURE 19-48 ■ Measuring a nasal airway.

tip (designed to protect nasal structures) directed toward the nasal septum. The airway is gently passed close to the midline, along the floor of the nostril, following the natural curve of the nasal passage. The airway should not be forced. If resistance is encountered, rotating the tube slightly may help, or insertion can be attempted through the other nostril (Fig. 19-49).

After insertion, the nasal airway rests in the posterior pharynx behind the tongue. If the patient begins to gag, the tube may be stimulating the posterior pharynx. It may be necessary to remove the airway or withdraw it 0.5 to 1 cm (¼ to ½ inch) and reinsert it. The paramedic should maintain displacement of the mandible with the head-tilt chin-lift or jaw-thrust without head-tilt maneuver when using this airway.

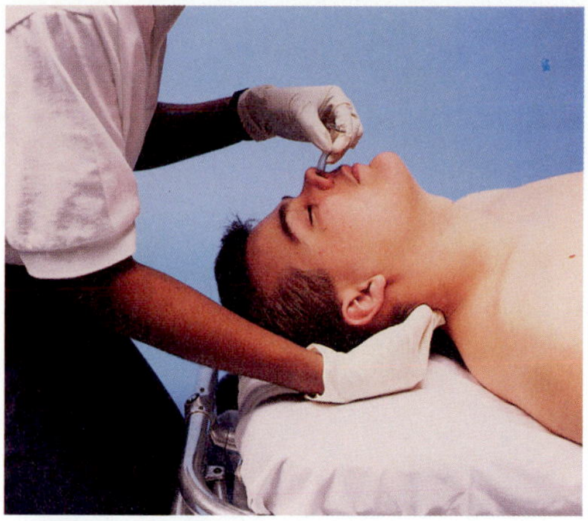

FIGURE 19-49 ■ Insertion of a nasal airway.

> ▶**NOTE** Nasal airways (and nasogastric [NG] tubes) should not be used in patients with a fracture of the basal skull or facial bones. These devices could be inadvertently inserted into the cranial cavity in these patients.

ADVANTAGES

- A nasal airway is well tolerated by conscious and semiconscious patients with an intact gag reflex.
- Insertion is a quick procedure.
- A nasal airway may be used when insertion of an oropharyngeal airway is contraindicated or difficult because of oral trauma or soft tissue injury.

POSSIBLE COMPLICATIONS

- Long nasal airways may enter the esophagus.
- The airway may precipitate laryngospasm and vomiting in patients with a gag reflex.
- The airway may injure the nasal mucosa, causing bleeding and possibly airway obstruction.
- Small-diameter airways may become obstructed by mucus, blood, vomitus, and the soft tissues of the pharynx.
- A nasal airway does not protect the lower airway from aspiration.
- Suctioning through a nasal airway is difficult.

Oropharyngeal Airway (Oral Airway)

Oral airways are designed to prevent the tongue from obstructing the glottis. They are indicated in unconscious or semiconscious patients who have no gag reflex and who are not intubated.

DESCRIPTION

The oral airway is a semicircular device designed to hold the tongue away from the posterior wall of the pharynx. Most oropharyngeal airways are made of disposable plastic. The two types of airways most often used are the Guedel airway and the Berman airway. The Guedel airway is distinguished by its tubular design. The Berman airway is distinguished by the airway channels along each side of the device (Fig. 19-50).

> ▶**NOTE** The cuffed oropharyngeal airway (COPA) is a modified oral airway. It has a distal inflatable cuff and proximal standard 15 mm connector. This allows attachment of a bag-valve device to the airway. The COPA may be a useful adjunct in airway management during resuscitation.

Like nasopharyngeal airways, oral airways are available in a variety of sizes. These range from infant to adult. The size is based on the distance in millimeters from the flange to the distal tip. The proper size for the patient may be determined by placing the airway next to the face so that the flange is at the level of the patient's central incisors and the bite block segment is parallel to the patient's hard palate. The airway should extend from the corner of the mouth to the tip of the ear lobe or the angle of the jaw (Fig. 19-51). The following sizes are recommended[7]:

- Large adult: 100 mm (about 4 inches) (Guedel size 5)
- Medium adult: 90 mm (about 3½ inches) (Guedel size 4)
- Small adult: 80 mm (about 3.1 inches) (Guedel size 3)

INSERTION

Before an oral airway is inserted, the mouth and pharynx should be cleared of all secretions, blood, or vomitus. In an adult or older child, the oral airway may be inserted upside down or at a 90-degree angle (Fig. 19-52, *A*). This helps the paramedic to avoid catching the tongue during insertion. As the oral airway passes the crest of the tongue, it is rotated into the proper position. It should be situated against the posterior wall of the oropharynx. Another method of insertion is recommended for pediatric patients (Fig. 19-52, *B*). (It also can be used in adults.) A tongue blade is used to displace the tongue inferiorly and anteriorly. The airway then is inserted and moved posteriorly toward the back of the oropharynx, following the normal curve of the oral cav-

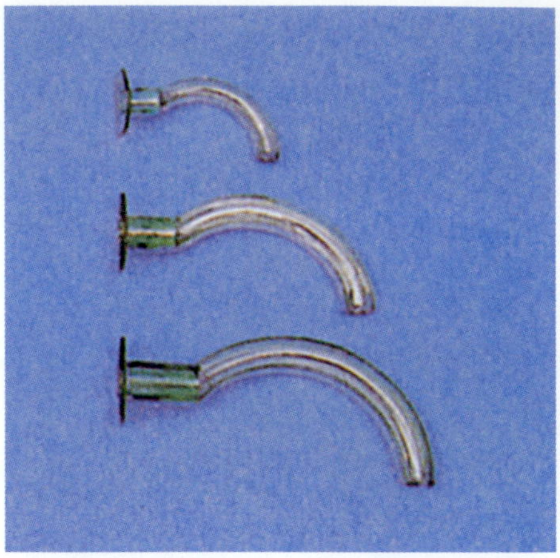

FIGURE 19-50 ■ Oral airways.

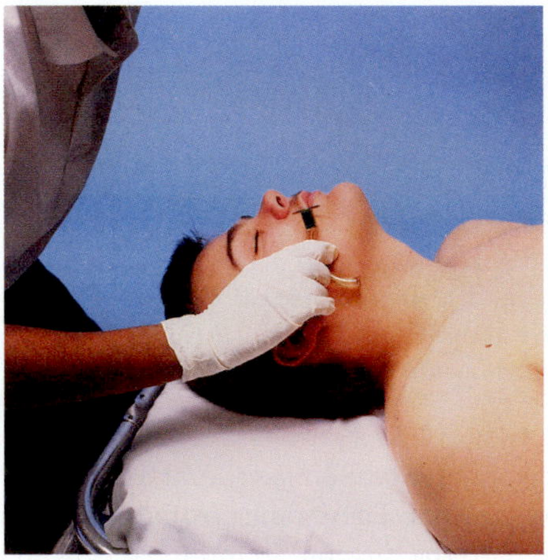

FIGURE 19-51 ■ Measuring an oral airway.

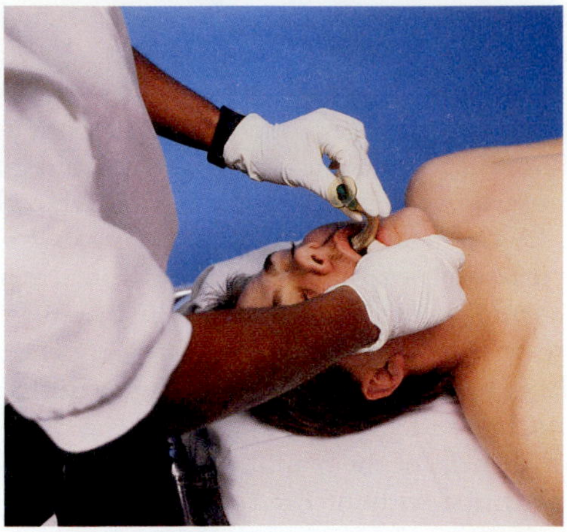

A

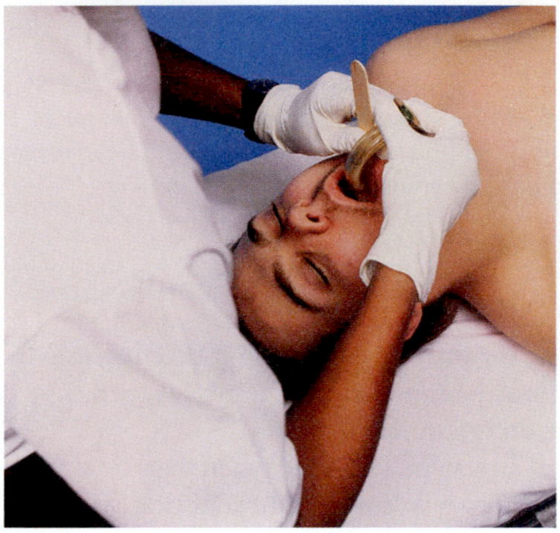

B

FIGURE 19-52 ■ **A**, Inserting an airway upside down. **B**, Alternative method of inserting an oral airway.

ity. Regardless of the method of insertion, trauma to the face and oral cavity should be avoided. In addition, the paramedic should be sure the patient's lips and tongue are not caught between the teeth and the airway.

CRITICAL THINKING

Why is this method of oral airway insertion used for infants and young children?

Proper placement of the airway is confirmed by observable chest wall expansion. It also is confirmed by good breath sounds on auscultation of the lungs during ventilation. The paramedic must remember that even with an oral airway in place, the patient's head must be kept in proper position. This helps to ensure a patent airway.

ADVANTAGES

- An oral airway secures the tongue forward and down, away from the posterior pharynx.
- It provides easy access for airway suction.
- It serves as a bite block to protect an ET tube and the airway in the event of convulsions.

POSSIBLE COMPLICATIONS

- Oral airways that are too small may fall back into the oral cavity, resulting in blockage of the airway.
- Long airways may press the epiglottis against the entrance of the trachea, producing a complete airway obstruction.
- The airway may stimulate vomiting and laryngospasm in a patient with a gag reflex.
- The airway does not protect the lower airway from aspiration.
- Improper insertion may push the tongue back, causing it to obstruct the airway.

ADVANCED AIRWAY PROCEDURES

Advanced airway procedures described in this text include endotracheal intubation, digital or blind intubation, nasotracheal intubation, the laryngeal mask airway (LMA), and multilumen airways. All these procedures require special training. Before performing advanced airway procedures, the paramedic must either receive authorization from medical direction or must be operating under written protocols. These written protocols are developed by medical direction and the EMS agency. The paramedic also should be aware that long-term complications may result from these procedures. This may be true even when the procedures are properly performed. Such complications include aspiration, tracheal stenosis, transient dysphagia, and voice changes.

Endotracheal Intubation

Tracheal intubation is the preferred technique for controlling the airway in patients who are unable to maintain an open airway. Indications for tracheal intubation include the following situations:

- The rescuer is unable to ventilate an unconscious patient with conventional methods (mouth-to-mask method, BVM).
- The patient cannot protect his or her own airway (coma, respiratory and cardiac arrest).
- Prolonged artificial ventilation is needed.

Tracheal intubation has the following advantages:

- The airway is isolated, which prevents aspiration of material into the lower airway.
- Ventilation and oxygenation are easier.
- Suctioning of the trachea and bronchi is easier.
- Wasted ventilation and gastric insufflation are prevented during positive-pressure ventilation.
- A route is provided for administration of some medications (e.g., ***lidocaine, epinephrine, atropine*** and ***naloxone***).

DESCRIPTION

The common ET tube is a flexible tube that is open at both ends (Fig. 19-53). The proximal end has a standard 15 mm (about 0.6 inch) adapter. This adapter connects to various oxygen delivery devices for positive-pressure ventilation. The end of the tube that is inserted into the trachea is beveled to aid placement between the vocal cords. The adult tube size (5 or larger) has a balloon cuff that closes off the remainder of the tracheal opening. This cuff prevents aspiration of fluids around the tube. It also minimizes air leakage during ventilation. The cuff is attached to a small tube. This tube has a one-way inflating valve with a port designed to fit a standard syringe. A properly positioned ET tube with the cuff inflated allows administration of high concentrations of oxygen at controlled pressures.

In addition to the common ET tube, specialized variations are available. They include the following:

- Armored or anode tubes, which have an inner spiral of flat metal to prevent kinking or compression.
- "Trigger" tubes, which have a thin cord running down the anterior wall of the tube, to which a ring is attached proximally. (Pulling on the ring with a finger or thumb increases the curvature of the tube. This may help the paramedic maneuver the tube anteriorly without using a stylet.)
- Tubes with medication ports for ET drug administration.

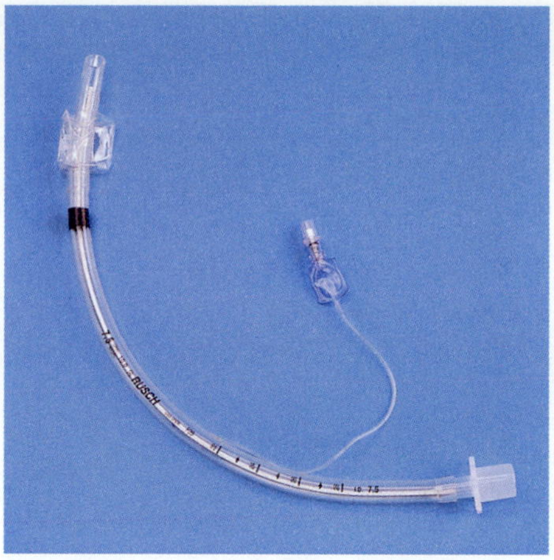

FIGURE 19-53 ■ Endotracheal (ET) tube.

ENDOTRACHEAL TUBE SIZES

The markings on the ET tube indicate the internal diameter of the tube in millimeters. (The tubes are available in graduated sizes from 2.5 to 10 mm.) The length of the tube from the distal end is indicated in centimeters at several levels. Recommended ET tube sizes are 7 to 8 mm (about ⅓ inch) internal diameter for men and 7 mm (about ¼ inch) internal diameter for women.[9] Tube sizes are expressed simply as "size 6" or "size 7," without the millimeter designation.

Infant and pediatric ET tubes are available with and without balloon cuffs. Cuffed ET tubes are indicated only for children over the age of 8 to 10 years. Children under 8 to 10 years of age have a circular narrowing at the level of the cricoid cartilages. This narrowing serves as a functional cuff. It minimizes air leakage at the cricoid ring. Accordingly, uncuffed ET tubes are recommended for this age group. Cuffed tracheal tubes for young children may be appropriate when high ventilatory pressures are indicated. This may occur with status asthmaticus and acute respiratory distress syndrome (ARDS) (see Chapter 30).

Various methods can be used to determine the correct ET tube size for infants and children. An estimate of tracheal tube size for children older than 1 year may be made using one of the following equations[9]:

Uncuffed tube:

$$\text{Tracheal tube size (mm)} = \left(\frac{\text{Age in years}}{4}\right) \div 4$$

Cuffed tube:

$$\text{Tracheal tube size (mm)} = \left(\frac{\text{Age in years}}{4}\right) \div 3$$

Another method for selecting a correct ET tube size is to use length-based resuscitation tapes (for children up to 35 kg) (see Chapter 44). Suggested sizes for ET tubes and suction catheters for adult and pediatric patients are listed in Table 19-5.[9]

TABLE 19-5 Pediatric and Adult Tracheal Tube and Suction Catheter Sizes*

APPROXIMATE AGE/SIZE (WEIGHT)	INTERNAL DIAMETER OF TRACHEAL TUBE (MM)	SUCTION CATHETER SIZE (FRENCH)
Premature infant (<1 kg)	2.5	5
Premature infant (1 to 2 kg)	3.0	5 or 6
Premature infant (2 to 3 kg)	3.0 to 3.5	6 or 8
0 month to 1 year/infant (3 to 10 kg)	3.5 to 4.0	8
1 year/small child (10 to 13 kg)	4.0	8
3 years/child (14 to 16 kg)	4.5	8 or 10
5 years/child (16 to 20 kg)	5.0	10
6 years/child (18 to 25 kg)	5.5	10
8 years/child to small adult (24 to 32 kg)	6.0 cuffed	10 or 12
12 years/adolescent (32 to 54 kg)	6.5 cuffed	12
16 years/adult (50+ kg)	7.0 cuffed	12
Adult female	7.0 cuffed	12 or 14
Adult male	7.0 to 8.0 cuffed	14

*These are approximations and should be adjusted on the basis of clinical experience. Tracheal tube selection for a child should be based on the child's size or age. One size larger and one size smaller should be allowed for individual variation. Color-coding based on length or the size of the child may facilitate approximation of the correct tracheal tube size.

NECESSARY EQUIPMENT

A laryngoscope is required for visualization of the glottis during tracheal intubation. Although various makes are available, all have a number of features in common. The standard laryngoscope includes a handle made of plastic or stainless steel. The handle contains the batteries for the light source and attaches to a plastic or stainless steel blade with a bulb placed in the distal third. The electrical contact between the blade and the handle is made at a connection point called the *fitting*. The indentation of the blade is attached to the bar of the handle. When the blade is elevated to a right angle with the laryngoscope handle, the blade snaps into place and the bulb lights (Fig. 19-54). (Failure of the bulb to light may be the result of a loose connection between the bulb and the bulb socket, a damaged bulb, or faulty batteries.) Other necessary equipment includes a 10 mL syringe for cuff inflation, water-soluble lubricant, and suction equipment.

Two types of blades (available in various sizes) are used with the laryngoscope: a straight blade, such as the Miller, Wisconsin, or Flagg blade (Fig. 19-55), and a curved blade, such as a MacIntosh blade (Fig. 19-56). The tip of a straight blade is applied directly to the epiglottis to expose the vocal cords. Advocates of the straight blade claim it provides more exposure of the glottis and less need for a stylet. A straight blade usually is recommended for infant intubation. This is because it provides greater displacement of the tongue into the floor of the mouth and better visualization of the glottic structures.

CRITICAL THINKING

Ask several paramedics and anesthesiologists which laryngoscope blade they prefer and why.

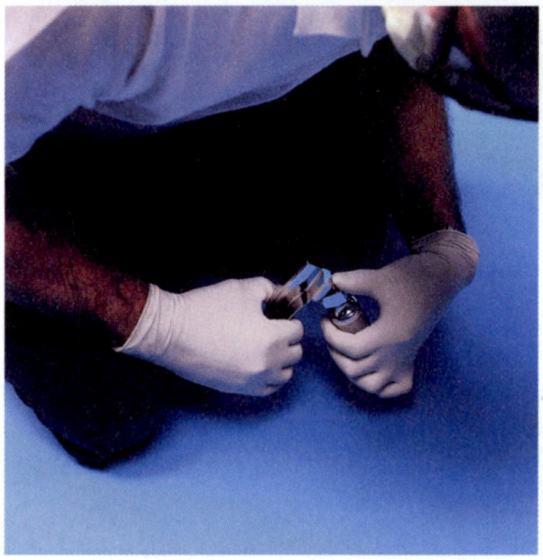

FIGURE 19-54 ■ Attaching a blade to the handle of a laryngoscope.

The curved blade design is intended to displace the tongue to the left and to elevate the epiglottis without touching it. Advocates of the curved blade claim it reduces the chance of dental trauma. They also claim it provides more room for passage of the ET tube. The choice of blade is a matter of personal preference and the patient's anatomy. Paramedics should acquire expertise in using both curved and straight blades; some patients can be intubated more easily with one type than the other. Occasions also may arise when only one type of blade is available. Versatility with both curved and straight blades may improve the patient's chances of survival.

A malleable stylet (preferably plastic coated) may be inserted through the ET tube before intubation (Fig. 19-57). The stylet conforms to any desired configuration and may

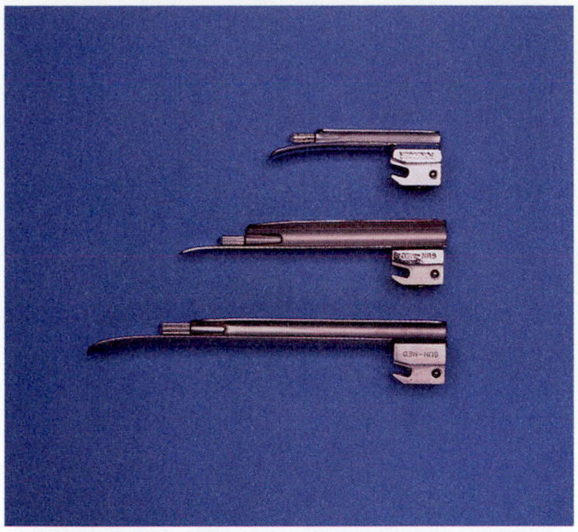

FIGURE 19-55 ■ Types of straight laryngoscopic blades.

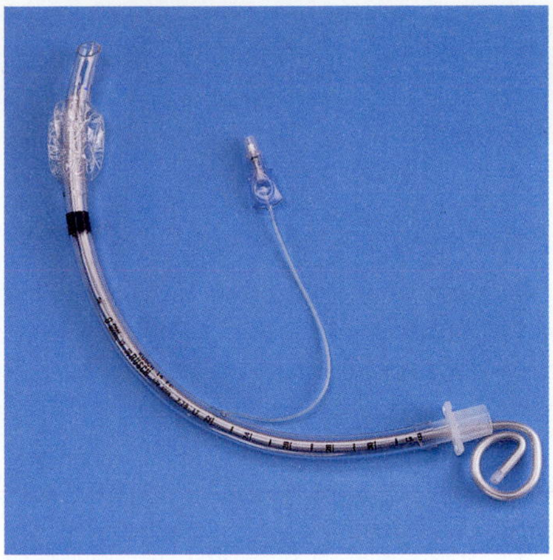

FIGURE 19-57 ■ Endotracheal (ET) tube with malleable stylet.

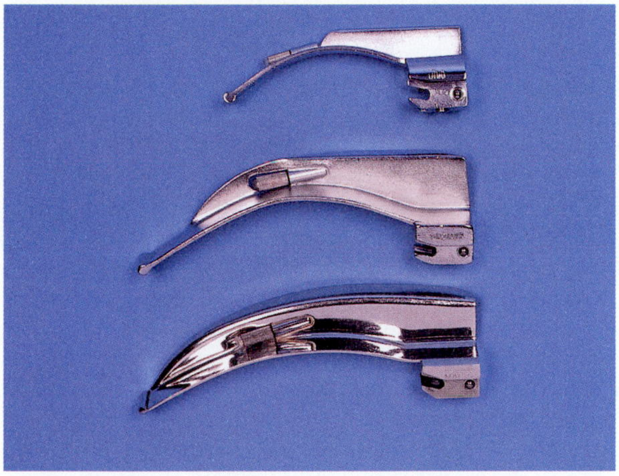

FIGURE 19-56 ■ Types of curved laryngoscopic blades.

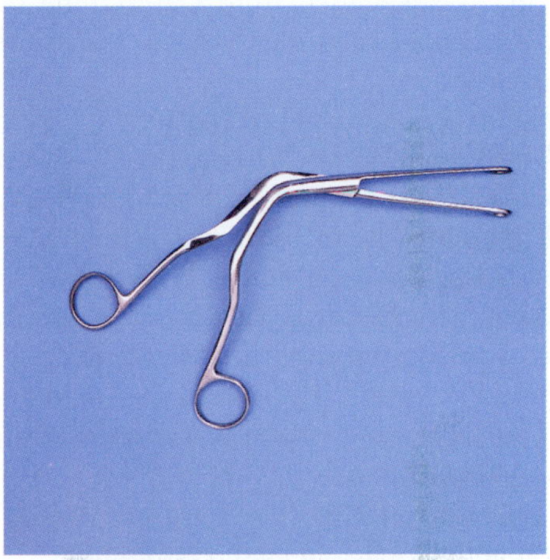

FIGURE 19-58 ■ Magill forceps.

facilitate proper placement of the ET tube. If used, the stylet must be recessed at least 1 to 2 cm ($^1/_2$ to $^3/_4$ inch) from the distal end of the ET tube to prevent injury to the patient. Recession of the stylet tip is maintained by bending the proximal end of the stylet over the proximal rim of the adapter so that it does not advance through the lumen with manipulation of the ET tube. If the stylet is allowed to extend beyond the distal end of the tube, the mucosal surface of the larynx or trachea or the vocal cords may be damaged. A gum elastic bougie can be used to assist with ET tube placement. This large flexible device is placed in the trachea, after which the tracheal tube is passed over the bougie and into position in the trachea.

Some doctors also authorize the use of Magill forceps (Fig. 19-58). This is a scissors-style clamp with circular tips. It may be used to help direct the tip of the ET tube into the larynx during intubation and to remove some foreign bodies. Use of this device requires special training and authorization from medical direction.

PREPARING FOR INTUBATION

The patient should be ventilated by other standard procedures before intubation (e.g., mouth-to-mask method, BVM). The paramedic should assess the adequacy of ventilation by observing the chest rise and fall during ventilation, by auscultating for breath sounds, and by noting the patient's skin color. Before intubation, the patient should be hyperventilated with 100% oxygen for 1 to 2 minutes. In addition, the time required for intubation when the patient is not being ventilated should not exceed 30 seconds. If intubation is not completed within this time, the procedure should be halted. The patient's lungs should then be well ventilated and oxygenated for 15 to 30 seconds by other means before intubation is attempted again. Pulse oximetry and the electrocardiogram (ECG) should be monitored continuously during intubation attempts.

Before intubation, all equipment should be examined and tested for defects. The paramedic should check the integrity of the cuff of the ET tube by inflating the balloon with 5 to 8 mL of air and checking for leaks in the cuff or inlet port. The blade of the laryngoscope should be snapped into place to examine the light bulb. The bulb should be secured in its socket and checked for brightness ("light, bright, and tight").

ANATOMICAL CONSIDERATIONS

The ET tube may be passed into the trachea through the mouth (orotracheal method) or through the nose (nasotracheal method). The orotracheal method is used most often. It is performed under direct visualization of the glottic opening. The nasotracheal route basically is a "blind" technique. The following anatomical structures are key landmarks during intubation:

- The trachea is in the midline of the neck and has its superior entry at the level of the glottic opening. With orotracheal intubation, the vocal cords should be visualized while the tube is passed to ensure entry into the trachea.
- The uvula is suspended from the midline of the soft palate. It is used as a guide for correct placement of the laryngoscope.
- The epiglottis is attached to the base of the tongue. It should be visualized and elevated to expose the glottis and vocal cords. Pressure on the solid ring of the cricoid (Sellick maneuver) can block the esophagus, reducing the risk of regurgitation during the intubation attempt. It also may help to better visualize the entrance of the trachea by pushing it slightly posteriorly.

The trachea extends to the level of the second intercostal space anteriorly, at which point it divides into the left and right mainstem bronchi. The right main bronchus branches off at a very slight angle to the trachea, whereas the left branches at a 45- to 60-degree angle.

NOTE An endotracheal (ET) tube that has been advanced too far most often enters the right main bronchus, bypassing and occluding the origin of the left main bronchus. If this occurs, atelectasis and pulmonary insufficiency of the left lung may result. Therefore it is crucial that the paramedic evaluate ET tube placement by auscultating both lungs. With proper ET tube placement, breath sounds should be of almost equal intensity over both lung fields. Certain pathological conditions (e.g., pneumothorax, hemothorax, surgical removal of a lung) may result in unequal breath sounds even when an ET tube is in the proper position.

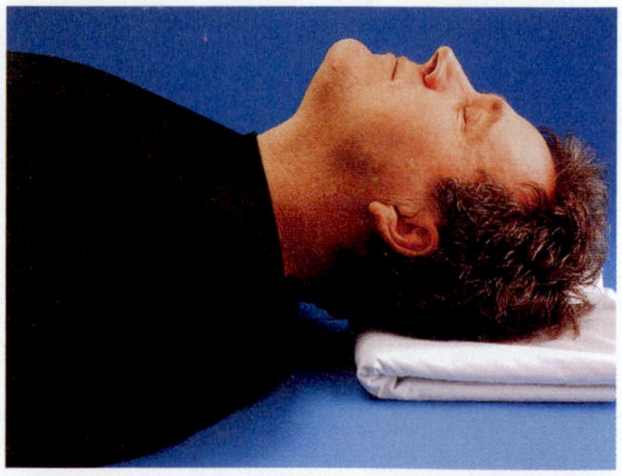

FIGURE 19-59 ■ Sniffing position.

BOX 19-7 Removal of Foreign Bodies by Direct Laryngoscopy

Direct laryngoscopy and use of Magill forceps to remove foreign bodies should be attempted only after manual techniques for clearing the airway have proved unsuccessful. The steps for removing a foreign body from the airway by direct laryngoscopy are as follows:

1. Assemble the necessary laryngoscopic equipment. (Have suction ready for immediate use in case of vomiting.)
2. Place the supine patient in the sniffing position (see Fig. 19-59) with the head extended.
3. Hyperventilate the patient with supplemental oxygen if possible.
4. Insert the laryngoscope, visualizing the glottic opening and surrounding structures.
5. If foreign matter is seen, grasp it with Magill forceps or a Kelly clamp and remove it from the airway.
   Note: Forceps removal of foreign matter should be attempted only with direct visualization of the obstruction. Even then, caution must be exercised to avoid soft tissue damage from the teeth of the forceps.
6. If spontaneous respirations resume within 5 seconds, remove the blade of the laryngoscope and monitor the patient.
7. If spontaneous respirations do not resume, insert an endotracheal (ET) tube, administer 100% oxygen, and assess the patient's circulatory status.

If complete foreign body obstruction of the upper airway cannot be relieved, needle cricothyrotomy or transtracheal jet insufflation may be warranted. These advanced airway procedures provide oxygenation until tracheal intubation or tracheostomy can be performed in a controlled setting.

Orotracheal Intubation

In preparation for orotracheal intubation, a patient who is not a trauma victim should be placed in the sniffing position (Fig. 19-59). In this position, the neck is flexed at the fifth and sixth cervical vertebrae. The head is extended at the first and second cervical vertebrae. This allows the three axes of the mouth, pharynx, and trachea (oropharyngeolaryngeal axis) to be aligned for direct visualization of the larynx. (When trauma is not a factor, it may help to place a few layers of towels under the patient's head to elevate it.)

The orotracheal tube should be lubricated. Also, a stethoscope, stylet, and suction equipment (with large-bore catheters) should be readily available. As in all advanced airway procedures, the patient's lungs should be hyperventilated with 100% oxygen for 1 to 2 minutes before intubation. The orotracheal intubation procedure is as follows (Fig. 19-60):

1. Position yourself at the patient's head.
2. Inspect the oral cavity for secretions and foreign material. Suction the mouth and pharynx if needed.

STEP-BY-STEP SKILL

FIGURE 19-60 ■ Orotracheal intubation.

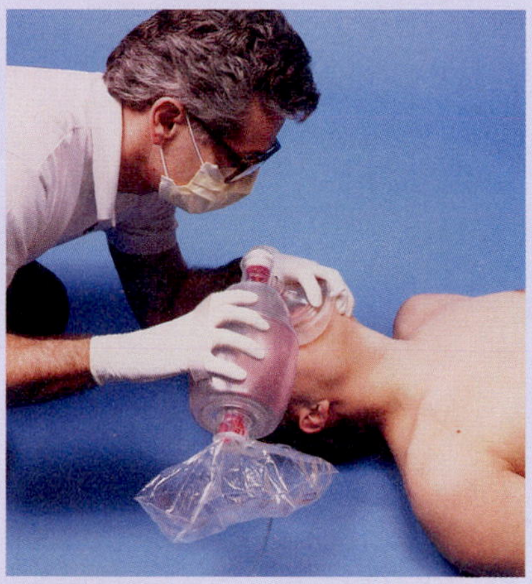

A ■ Before intubation, hyperventilate the patient's lungs with 100% oxygen for at least 1 to 2 minutes.

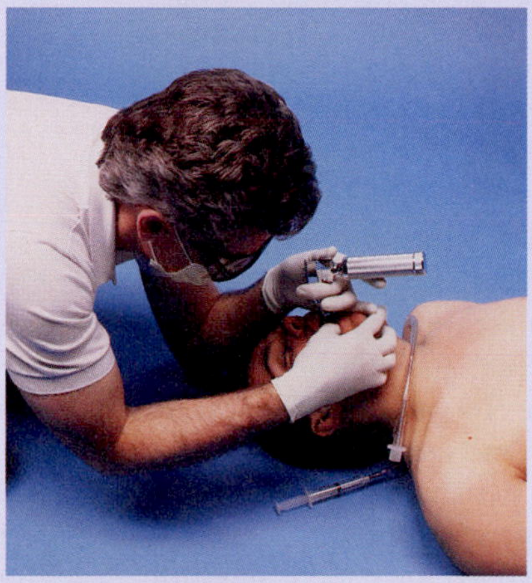

B ■ Holding the laryngoscope in the left hand, insert the blade into the right side of the patient's mouth, displacing the tongue to the left.

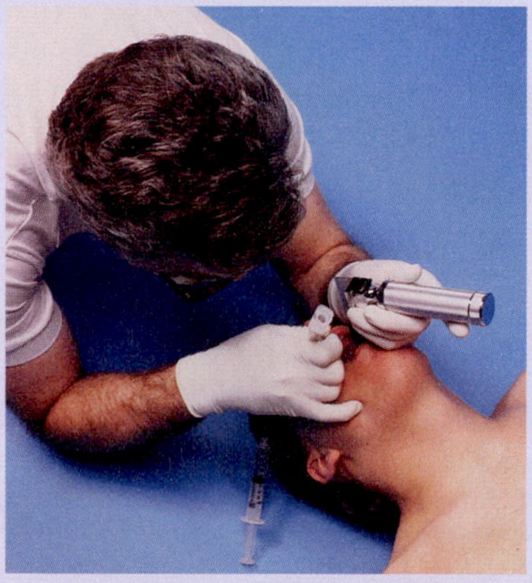

C ■ Advance the endotracheal (ET) tube through the right corner of the mouth and, under direct vision, through the vocal cords.

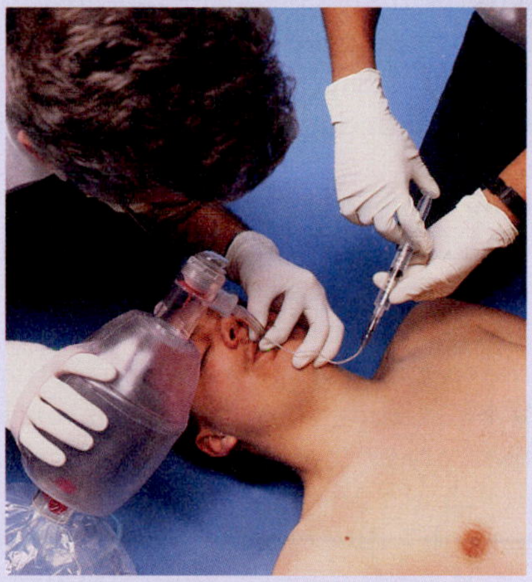

D ■ Inflate the cuff with about 10 mL of air. Ventilate the patient's lungs with a mechanical airway device.

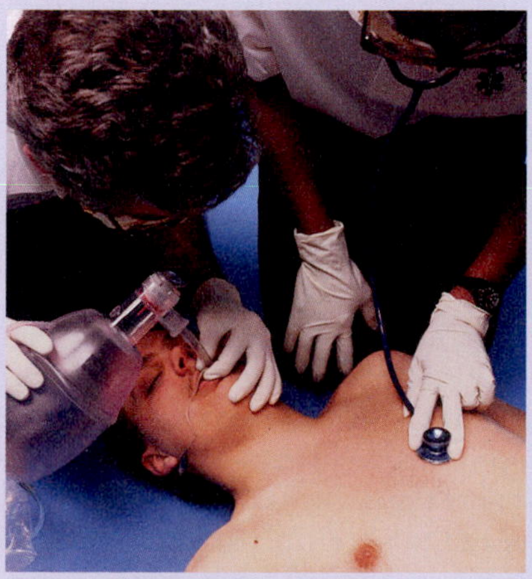

E ■ Confirm correct placement of the ET tube by primary and secondary confirmation methods.

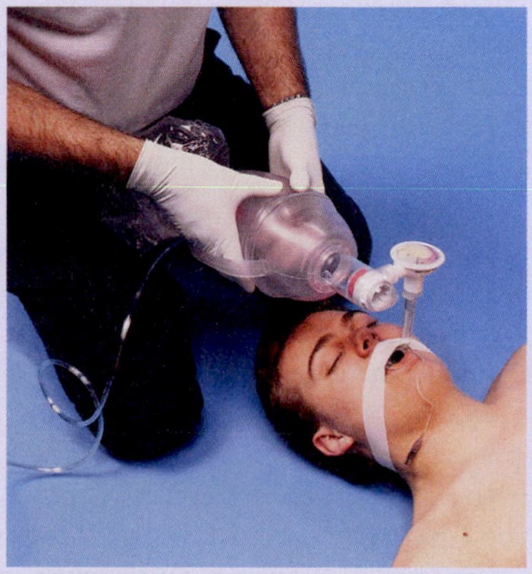

F ■ Secure the ET tube in place and provide ventilatory support with supplemental oxygen.

▶NOTE When possible, a second rescuer should apply cricoid pressure during tracheal intubation in adults. This helps to protect against regurgitation of gastric contents. It also aids in tube placement. The second rescuer should apply backward, upright, rightward pressure (BURP) to help bring the vocal cords into the field of vision of the paramedic doing the intubation.

3. Open the patient's mouth with the fingers of the right hand. Retract the patient's lips on the teeth or gums to avoid pinching them in the blade. The "crossed-finger technique" also may be useful in opening the patient's mouth. To perform this procedure, cross the right thumb and index finger to form an X. Place the thumb on the patient's lower incisors and the index finger on the patient's upper incisors; apply crossed-finger pressure to open the patient's mouth.
4. Grasp the lower jaw with the right hand and draw it forward and upward. Remove any dentures.
5. Holding the laryngoscope in the left hand, insert the blade into the right side of the mouth, displacing the tongue to the left. Move the blade toward the midline and the base of the tongue and identify the uvula. Working gently and avoiding pressure on the lips and teeth are essential.
6. When using a curved blade, advance the tip of the blade into the vallecula, the space between the base of the tongue and the pharyngeal surface of the epiglottis (Fig. 19-61). When using a straight blade, insert the tip under the epiglottis (Fig. 19-62). The glottic opening is exposed by exerting upward traction on the handle. Never use a prying motion with the handle and do not use the teeth as a fulcrum.
7. Advance the ET tube through the right corner of the mouth and, under direct vision, through the vocal cords (Fig. 19-63). If a stylet has been used, it should be removed from the tube after the tube passes through the cords into the trachea.
8. After viewing the vocal cords, ensure that the proximal end of the cuffed tube has advanced past the cords about 1 to 2.5 cm (½ to 1 inch) (Fig. 19-64). The tip of the tube should then be halfway between the vocal cords and the carina. This position allows some displacement of the tube tip during flexion or extension of the patient's neck without extubation or movement of the tip into the mainstem bronchus. (In the average adult, the distance from teeth to carina is 27 cm (about 11 inches). The paramedic should observe the depth markings on the ET tube during intubation. In the average adult, the tube is properly positioned when the patient's teeth are between the 19 and 23 cm marks on the tube. This places the tip of the tube 2 to 3 cm [¾ to 1½ inches] above the carina.) The average tube depth in men is 22 cm (about 9 inches) ("teeth and tube at 22"). The average tube depth in women is 21 cm (about 8½ inches).

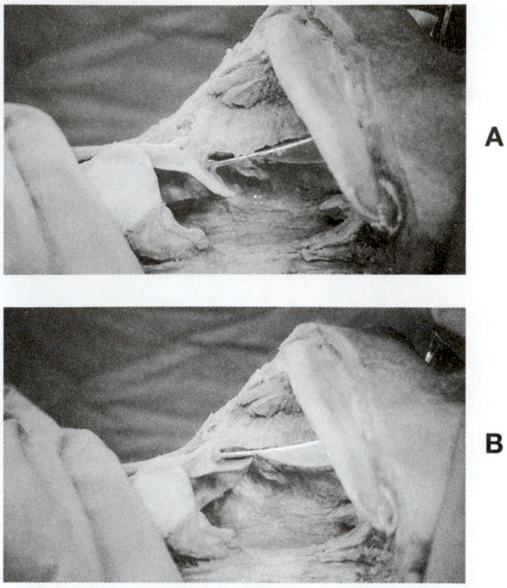

FIGURE 19-61 ■ **A,** When a curved laryngoscopic blade is used, the tip of the blade is inserted into the vallecula. **B,** Direct pressure is exerted on the blade upward and toward the feet, using a lifting motion to expose the vocal cords.

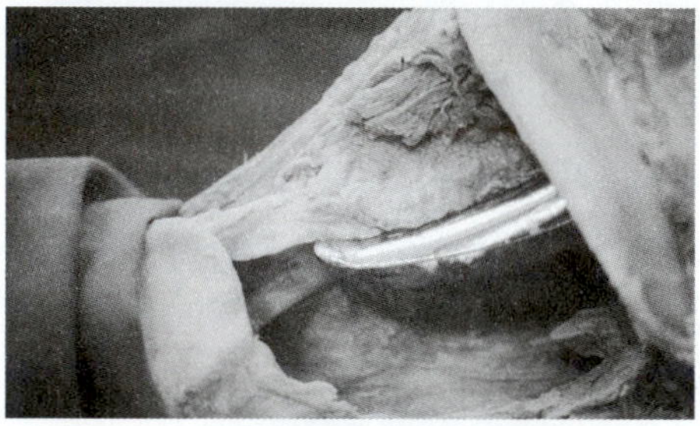

FIGURE 19-62 ■ A straight laryngoscopic blade is used to lift the epiglottis, directly exposing the vocal cords.

9. Inflate the cuff with about 10 mL of air to prevent any air leaks around the tracheal cuff seal.[5]
10. Attach the tube to a mechanical airway device and ventilate the patient's lungs.
11. During ventilation, confirm accurate tube placement using primary and secondary confirmation methods.[10]

Primary Confirmation Methods. Initially confirm proper tube placement by auscultating over the epigastrium, the midaxillary region, and the anterior chest line on the right and left sides of the chest. If stomach gurgling is present or chest expansion is absent, immediately remove the tracheal tube. Reattempt intubation after oxygenating the patient's lungs with 100% oxygen for 15 to 30 seconds. When appropriate tube placement has been confirmed, reconfirm and note the tube mark at the front of the patient's teeth. Secure the tube to the patient's head and face with tape or a commercially available device. Then reevaluate lung sounds to ensure that the tube was not inadvertently repositioned. Finally, insert an oral airway or bite block.

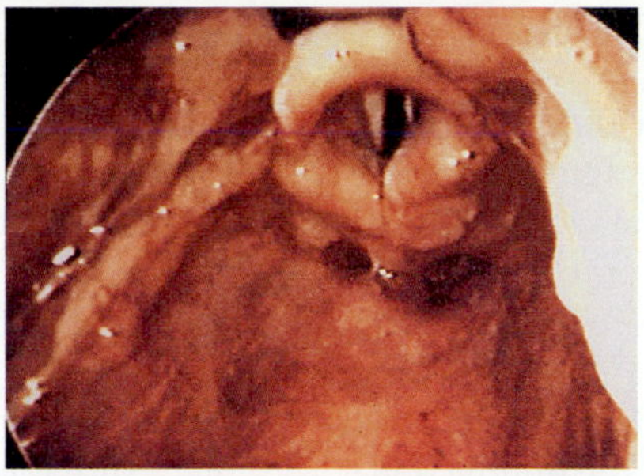

FIGURE 19-63 ■ View of the vocal cords.

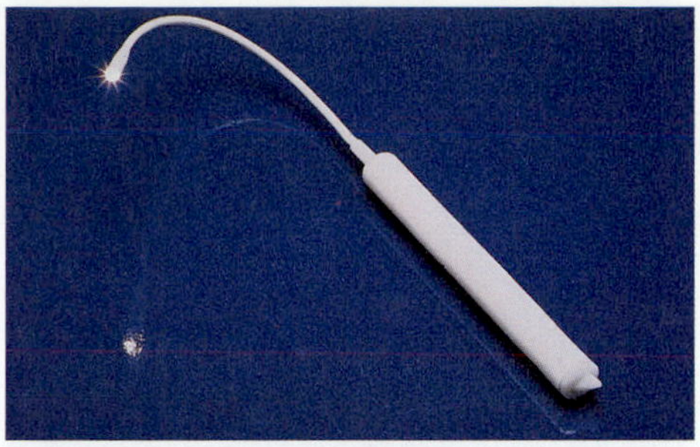

FIGURE 19-65 ■ Light wand for fiberoptic intubation.

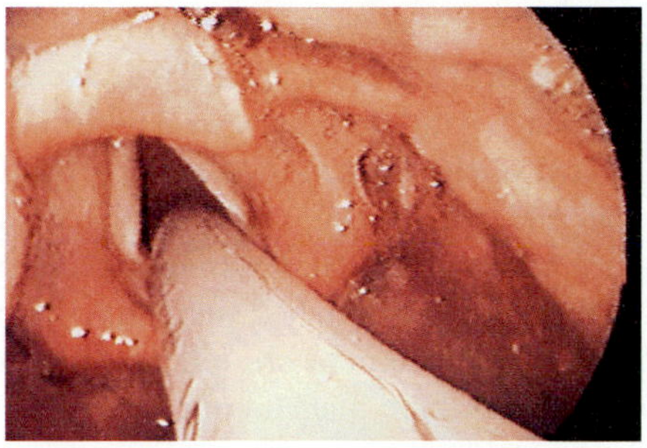

FIGURE 19-64 ■ Endotracheal (ET) tube passing through the vocal cords.

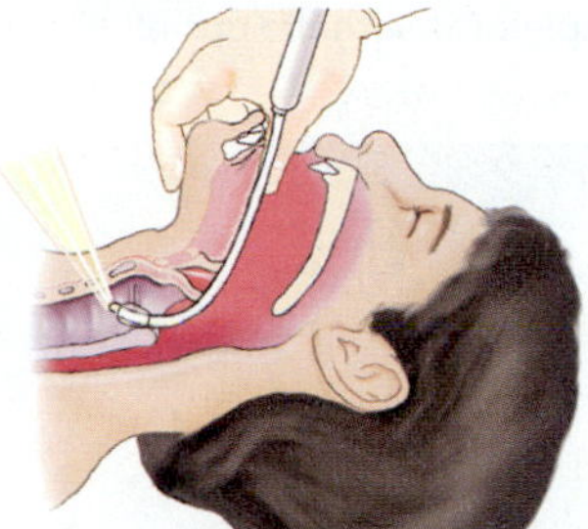

FIGURE 19-66 ■ Fiberoptic intubation. The endotracheal (ET) tube is inserted with the aid of a lighted stylet.

This prevents the patient from biting down and blocking the airway.

> **NOTE** If breath sounds are decreased or absent in the left lung, the orotracheal tube may have passed into the right mainstem bronchus, effectively bypassing the origin of the left main bronchus. If this is the case, the cuff should be deflated and the tube withdrawn 1 to 2 cm (about ½ to ¾ inch). The cuff then should be reinflated and tube placement should be verified as above.

Secondary Confirmation Methods. A second method of determining correct tube placement requires the use of mechanical devices. These include end-tidal carbon dioxide detectors, esophageal detectors, and pulse oximetry for patients who have a perfusing rhythm. These devices are described later in this chapter.

Transillumination Technique (Lighted Stylet). Malleable fiberoptic stylets, or "light wands" (Fig. 19-65), have a high-intensity light at the distal end. The light is powered by a small battery housing at the operator end. This method has the advantage of not requiring manipulation of the patient's head and neck. This is because visualization of the vocal cords is not required or attempted. Placement of the ET tube is facilitated by observation of the light from the end of the ET tube passing through the soft tissues of the neck. These stylets are 6 mm in diameter and are therefore too large for pediatric use. The procedure for fiberoptic intubation is as follows (Fig. 19-66):

1. Position yourself at the side of the patient's head. If a spinal injury is suspected, have a second rescuer maintain in-line spinal immobilization.
2. Hyperventilate the patient with 100% oxygen for 1 to 2 minutes before intubation.
3. Lift the patient's tongue and mandible anteriorly by hand to position the epiglottis.
4. Advance the ET tube in combination with the lighted stylet through the oropharynx and the glottis. Transillumination of the skin of the neck causes the airway structures to become more distinct. When the thyroid and cricoid cartilages are illuminated by a bright circle of light, the stylet should be held stationary. At this point, the ET tube advanced 1 to 2 cm (½ to ¾ inch).
5. Inflate the cuff and remove the stylet. Verify proper tube placement using primary and secondary methods.
6. Secure the tube as described before.

If the illumination creates a dim, indistinct light, the esophagus has probably been intubated. If this occurs, the ET tube should be removed. The patient's lungs should be hyperventilated with 100% oxygen before the intubation is attempted again. A disadvantage of this method is that ambient light may make it difficult to see illumination created by the stylet. This issue can be minimized by darkening the work area during intubation. A few layers of dark blankets also can be placed around the patient's neck during the procedure.

STEP-BY-STEP SKILL

FIGURE 19-67

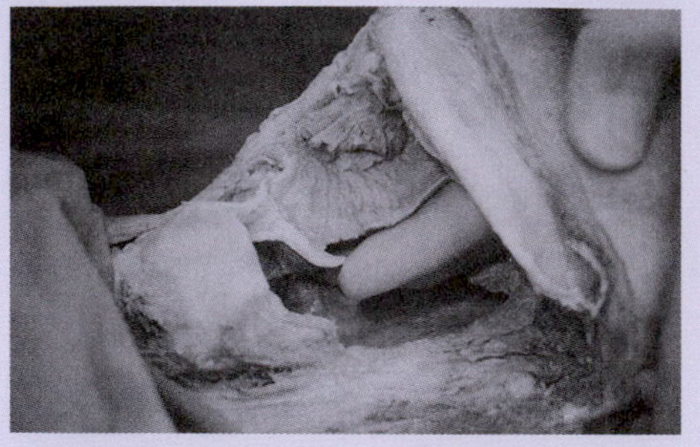

A ■ Locate the epiglottis with the tips of the fingers of one hand.

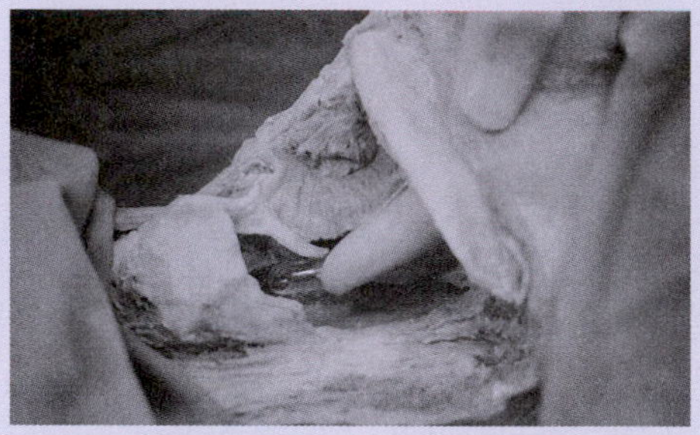

B ■ Using the palpated epiglottis as a landmark, guide the endotracheal (ET) tube into the larynx.

Lighted stylets also can be used to help verify placement after intubation by other methods. Once the cuff has been inflated and lung sounds auscultated, the stylet is advanced through the ET tube. A bright light below to the thyroid cartilage indicates proper placement. In addition, the list of indicators of proper ET placement should be used to assess placement.

Digital (Blind) Intubation

Before the advent of laryngoscopes, intubation was performed by inserting the intubator's fingers into the patient's mouth. The fingers would be used to guide the ET tube into the trachea. This is not a common prehospital procedure. However, digital intubation may be necessary in cases of patient entrapment, in patients whose airway is blocked from view by large amounts of blood or other secretions, or if equipment fails. Digital intubation also may be used in certain disaster situations in which victims are widespread and equipment is in short supply. The procedure for digital (blind) intubation is as follows:

1. Position yourself at the patient's left side. If a spinal injury is suspected, have a second rescuer maintain in-line spinal immobilization.
2. Hyperventilate the patient with 100% oxygen for 1 to 2 minutes before intubation.
3. Use a bite stick or other device to hold the patient's mouth open. This helps to protect the rescuer's fingers.
4. Bend the tube and stylet combination into a J or hockey stick configuration.
5. Insert the gloved left middle and index fingers into the patient's mouth. Alternating fingers, "walk" down the patient's tongue, pulling the tongue and epiglottis away from the glottic opening.
6. When a flap of cartilage covered by mucous membrane is felt with the middle finger, the epiglottis has been located (Fig. 19-67, *A*). Maintain contact and advance the ET tube with the right hand. Use the index finger of the left hand as a guide (Fig. 19-67, *B*). The index finger maintains the tube position against the middle finger, leading the tip of the tube into the glottic opening. It may be helpful for a second rescuer to perform the Sellick maneuver to close off the esophagus and help prevent aspiration.
7. Once the cuff of the ET tube passes the tips of the paramedic's fingers, inflate the cuff, remove the stylet, and verify placement in the usual manner.
8. Secure the tube as previously described.

Correct ET tube placement should be confirmed often. At a minimum, reconfirm placement each time a patient is moved or has a sudden change in condition.

Potential Complications from Intubation Procedures

- Lacerated lips or tongue (oral)
- Dental trauma from the laryngoscope (oral)
- Lacerated pharyngeal or tracheal mucosa
- Tracheal rupture
- Avulsion of an arytenoid cartilage
- Vocal cord injury
- Vomiting and aspiration of stomach contents
- Significant release of epinephrine and norepinephrine, leading to hypertension, tachycardia, or cardiac rhythm disturbances
- Vagal stimulation (particularly in infants and children), resulting in bradycardia and hypotension
- Increased intracranial pressure in patients with a head injury
- Accidental intubation of the esophagus
- Accidental intubation of a bronchus

In addition, rupture of the cuff, inflation port malfunction, or severance or kinking of the inflation tube may cause cuff malfunction and air leakage.

Nasotracheal Intubation

At times nasotracheal intubation may be the airway procedure of choice. This may be the case in patients who have spontaneous respirations, when laryngoscopy is difficult, or when the motion of the cervical spine must be limited. Examples of such conditions include the following:

- Medication overdose
- Asthma or anaphylaxis

- Chronic obstructive pulmonary disease
- Stroke
- Seizure (status epilepticus with constant seizure activity)
- Altered mental status

These and other situations may make it difficult to align the oropharyngeolaryngeal axis. This rules out successful orotracheal intubation. It should be noted that nasotracheal intubation is a blind procedure. It carries a high risk of improper tube placement. This is due to the fact that the paramedic cannot visualize the vocal cords.

In general, conscious patients tolerate a nasotracheal tube better than an orotracheal tube. Also, a nasotracheal tube often causes less trauma to the tracheal mucosa. This is because the tube moves less inside the trachea with head motion than does an orotracheal tube. If time allows, the paramedic should prepare the patient using a vasoconstrictor spray and topical anesthetic. (Examples of these are phenylephrine spray and lidocaine jelly.) These measures may make the patient more comfortable. They also reduce the risk of nasal hemorrhage, which may occur secondary to the procedure. If time allows, placement of a soft nasopharyngeal airway before the procedure may show which nostril is more passable. This also may compress the mucosa, allowing less traumatic placement of the ET tube (Fig. 19-68).

> **NOTE** Nasotracheal intubation generally is not recommended in patients who are apneic, who have midfacial fractures or nasal fractures, or who are suspected of having a basal skull fracture.

INSERTION

The procedure for inserting a nasotracheal tube is as follows:

1. Choose a cuffed ET that is 1 mm smaller than optimal for oral intubation. (Most ET tubes are designed for both orotracheal and nasotracheal intubation. Some longer ET tubes are designed specifically for this procedure. A ringed ET tube [Endotrol] is also available that controls the tip of the ET tube to aid entry into the trachea.) Prepare and check all needed equipment (balloon cuff, syringe, suction, stethoscope). Stylets are not used in nasotracheal intubation. This is because the stylet reduces flexibility and increases the risk of injury during blind insertion.
2. Make sure the patient's lungs have been well oxygenated and hyperventilated for 1 to 2 minutes before insertion.
3. Lubricate the ET tube with a water-soluble or lidocaine jelly.
4. Insert the tube with the flange facing the nasal septum. Advance the tube along the nasal floor of the nostril that is clearer and more direct. If both nostrils appear open, advance through the larger nostril first. If the chosen nostril is impassable, try the other nostril before selecting an ET tube that is 0.5 mm smaller in diameter.
5. Stand beside the patient with one hand on the tube and the thumb and index finger of the other hand palpating the larynx. The curve of the tube should follow the natural curve of the airway. Gently advance the tube while rotating it medially 15 to 30 degrees until maximal airflow is heard through the tube. Gently and swiftly advance the tube during early inspiration. Voluntary tongue extrusion in cooperative patients is helpful. Otherwise, the tongue can be wrapped with gauze and pulled forward. Flexion of the neck (if no spinal instability is suspected) and posterior pressure on the thyroid cartilage may help position the larynx.
6. Externally observe the advancement of the tube toward the carina. Misting or condensation on the tube should be evident as the tube approaches tracheal placement. This occurs because the patient's exhaled breath has a high concentration of water vapor. The water vapor promptly condenses on exposure to cooler room air. However, tube misting is not always a reliable indicator of proper tube position.
7. On completion of intubation, verify proper tube placement as described before. Inflate the cuff with about 10 mL of air and secure the tube in place. Ventilations may then be assisted with supplemental oxygen, or the patient's lungs can be ventilated by mechanical means.
8. If intubation fails, withdraw the tube and redirect it after ventilation and oxygenation of the patient. It may be possible to recognize tube misplacement by inspecting and palpating the neck for bulges.

POSSIBLE COMPLICATIONS

- Epistaxis (nosebleed)
- Vagal stimulation
- Injury to the nasal septum or turbinates
- Retropharyngeal laceration
- Vocal cord injury
- Avulsion of an arytenoid cartilage
- Esophageal intubation
- Intracranial tube placement if the patient has a basilar skull fracture

Intubation with Spinal Precautions

Nasal or oral intubation may be performed in patients suspected of having a spinal injury. The procedure is as follows:

1. Auscultate for bilateral breath sounds while manual or mechanical ventilations are in progress. This provides a baseline.
2. One rescuer should apply manual in-line stabilization from the patient's side. The rescuer places the hands over

> **NOTE** Intubation of patients suspected of having a spinal injury is controversial[11] and should be authorized by medical direction. Any type of airway manipulation may be dangerous. If the paramedic and medical direction elect to intubate the trachea of a patient suspected of having a spinal injury, in-line stabilization must be maintained. Two trained rescuers are required.

STEP-BY-STEP SKILL

FIGURE 19-68 ■ Nasotracheal intubation.

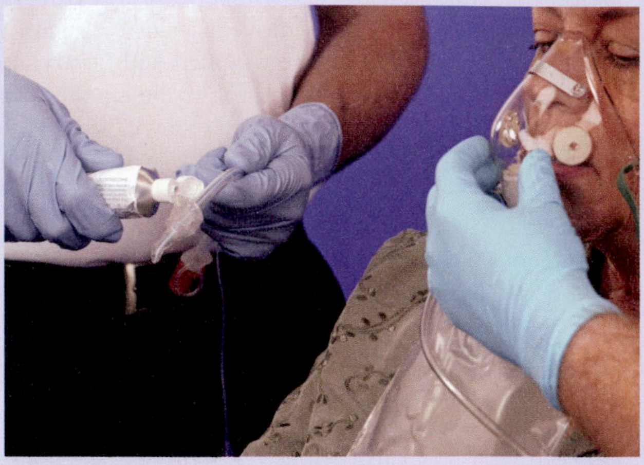

A ■ Oxygenate the patient while the nasotracheal tube is prepared and lubricated.

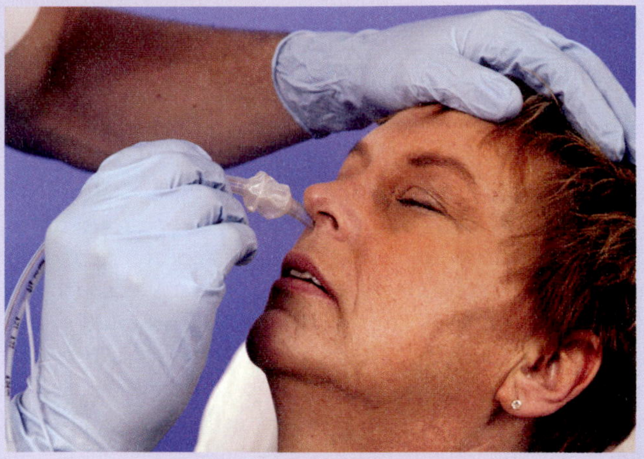

B ■ Insert the tube into the larger nostril.

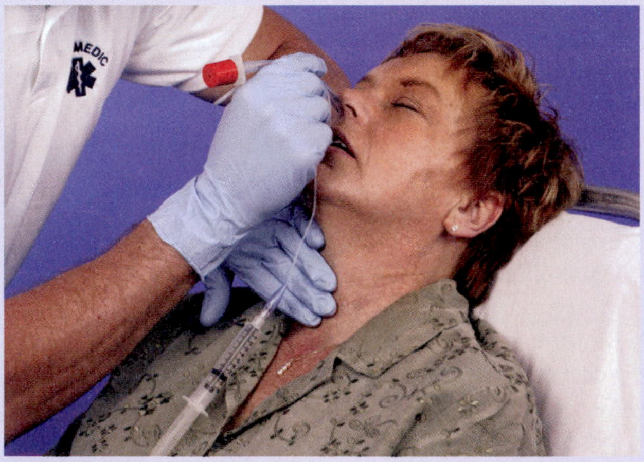

C ■ Palpate the larynx while listening for airflow over the tube as it is advanced.

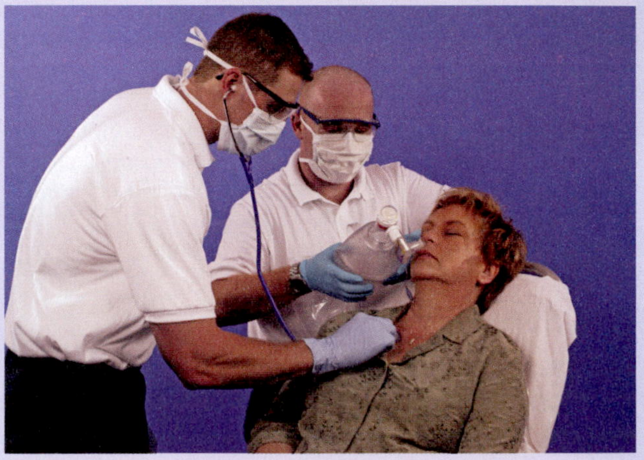

D ■ Ventilate the patient and confirm correct placement of the tube.

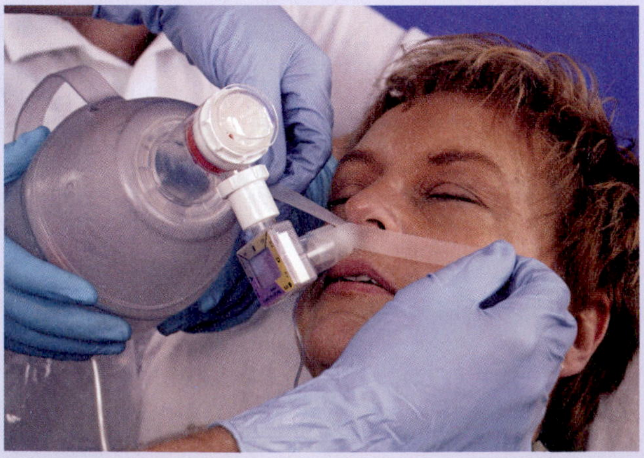

E ■ Secure the tube and monitor the patient.

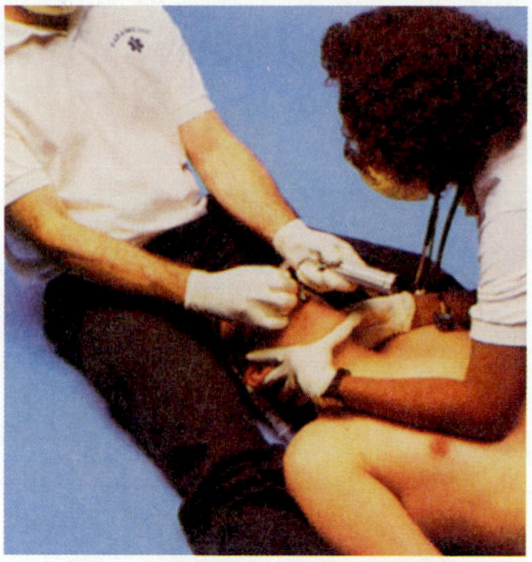

FIGURE 19-69 ■ Intubation in a sitting position.

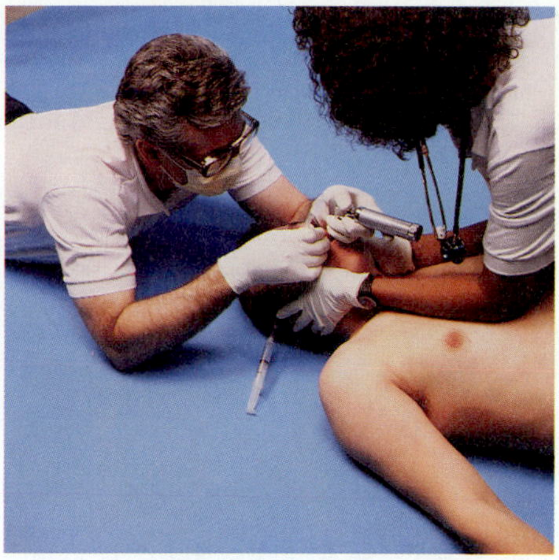

FIGURE 19-70 ■ Intubation in a prone position.

the patient's ears. The little fingers should be under the occipital skull. The thumbs should be on the face over the maxillary sinuses. Stabilization (without distraction) should be maintained in a neutral position throughout the procedure. Thin padding under the patient's head may be necessary to maintain neutral, in-line positioning.

3. In one method of intubation, the primary paramedic is positioned at the patient's head. The legs straddle the patient's shoulders and arms, and the patient's head is secured between the paramedic's thighs. The grip of the primary rescuer in this position and of the other rescuer (from the side) prevents the head from moving during the intubation. In this position, the primary paramedic may need to lean back to visualize the vocal cords (Fig. 19-69). With another method, the primary paramedic lies prone at the patient's head, and the other rescuer (at the patient's side) maintains the in-line position alone (Fig. 19-70).

FACE-TO-FACE OROTRACHEAL INTUBATION

Face-to-face orotracheal intubation (Fig. 19-71) may be used when the paramedic cannot take a position above the patient's head (e.g., the patient is in a sitting position). In this method of intubation, a second rescuer maintains in-line immobilization of the patient's neck and head from behind the patient. The primary rescuer takes a position facing the patient. The patient's mouth is opened with the left hand. The laryngoscope is held in the right hand, and the blade is inserted into the patient's mouth, following the normal curve of the tongue. After visualizing the vocal cords from a position above the patient's mouth, the primary rescuer passes an ET tube between the cords with the left hand. The cuff is inflated, and the syringe removed. The patient then is ventilated with a BVM. After proper placement has been confirmed as previously described, the ET tube is secured in place.

EXTUBATION

The ET tube is not usually removed in the prehospital setting. However, the patient may develop intolerance to the tube. Also, it may not be possible to sedate the patient to improve tolerance. In such cases medical direction may advise extubation. If time allows, the patient's lungs first should be hyperventilated with 100% oxygen. To remove the ET tube, the paramedic should tilt the patient or backboard to one side and proceed as follows:

1. Have suction available. (The oral cavity and the area above the cuff should be suctioned before the ET tube is removed.)
2. Deflate the cuff completely.
3. Swiftly withdraw the tube on cough or expiration.
4. Assess the patient's respiratory status.
5. Provide high-concentration oxygen; assist ventilations as needed.

> ▶**NOTE** Patients who are awake are at high risk of laryngospasm immediately after extubation. Also, they may be difficult to reintubate should respiratory distress or failure occur again.

Advantages of Endotracheal Intubation

- It provides complete airway control.
- It helps prevent aspiration.
- It prevents gastric distention.
- It may provide a route for administration of some drugs.
- Positive-pressure ventilation can be delivered.
- Tracheal suctioning is possible.
- High concentrations of oxygen and large volumes of ventilation can be delivered.

Special Considerations for Pediatric Intubations

In addition to the differences in airway and ventilation procedures for pediatric patients, the anatomical differences of the pediatric airway must be considered.[6] These anatomical differences include the following:

1. The infant's upper airway is relatively small; the tongue is disproportionately large. Therefore posterior displace-

STEP-BY-STEP SKILL

FIGURE 19-71 ■ Face-to-face orotracheal intubation.

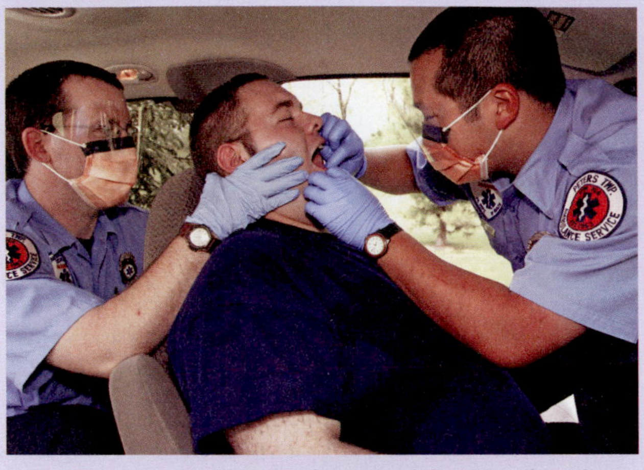

A ■ One rescuer maintains in-line immobilization. The primary rescuer takes a position facing the patient and opens the person's mouth. The primary rescuer then should follow these steps:

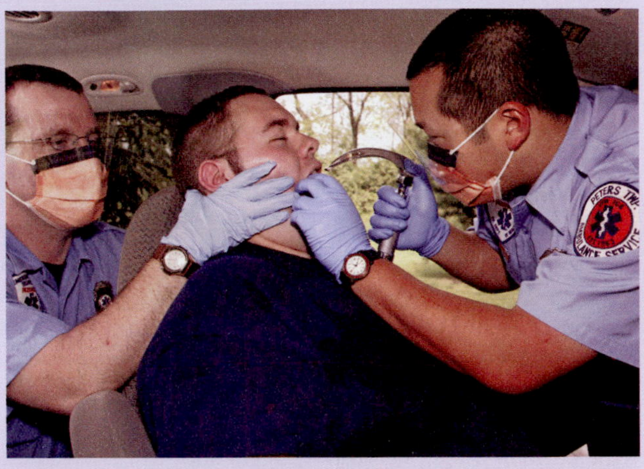

B ■ Holding the laryngoscope in the right hand, insert it into the patient's mouth.

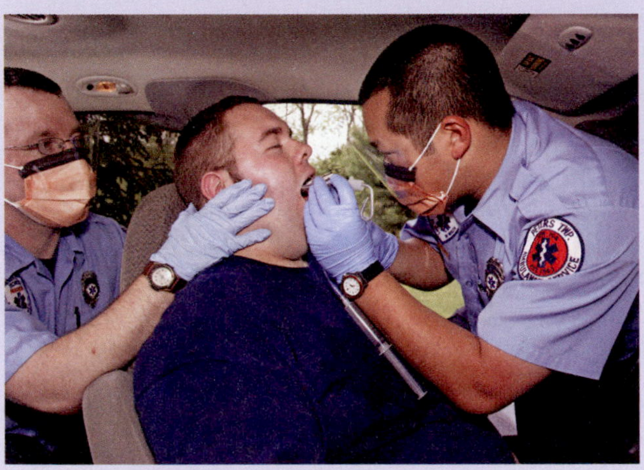

C ■ With the left hand, pass the endotracheal (ET) tube into the mouth and through the vocal cords.

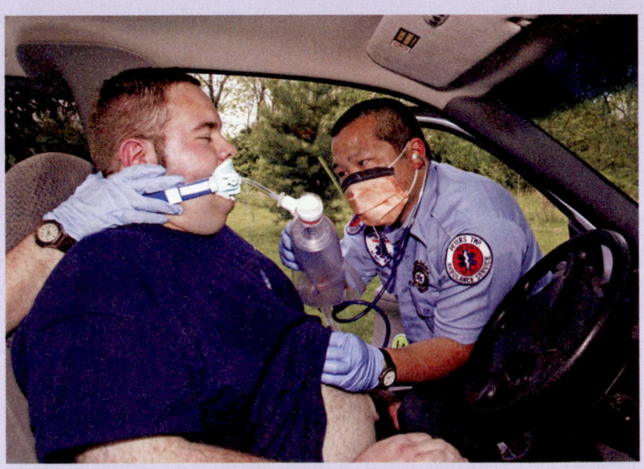

D ■ Inflate the cuff. Ventilate the patient and confirm correct placement of the tube. Secure the tube in place.

ment of the tongue easily obstructs the airway. In addition, the larger tongue of the pediatric patient tends to make laryngoscopy more difficult.

2. The epiglottis is shaped like the Greek letter omega (σ). It is narrower and longer in children than in the adult. Because of this, the epiglottis is more difficult to control with a laryngoscopic blade. The larynx lies more anteriorly in relation to the base of the tongue than in the adult. It also is elevated under the base of the tongue, making visualization more difficult. The glottic opening is at the third cervical vertebra in premature neonates, the third to fourth cervical vertebra in term neonates, and the fourth to fifth cervical vertebra in adults.
3. During the first few months of life, the infant's vocal cords slope from back to front. As a result, the ET tube frequently gets hung up in the angle formed by the cords. This problem can be minimized by rotating the ET tube or by having a second rescuer perform the Sellick maneuver during intubation.
4. The cricoid cartilage is the narrowest part of the airway in the infant and young child. As the child reaches 8 to 10 years of age, the vocal cords become the narrowest part. This remains the case into adulthood.
5. The distance from the vocal cords to the carina varies and can be correlated with the patient's height. This distance is about 4 to 5 cm (2 to 2½ inches) at birth and 6 to 7 cm (3 to 3½ inches) by 6 years of age. During placement of the ET tube, the tube should be advanced until breath sounds are lost unilaterally (usually on the left side). It should then be withdrawn slowly until breath sounds return, indicating that the tube tip is at the carina. After the return of breath sounds, the tube should be withdrawn 2 to 3 cm (¾ to 1½ inches) farther, placing it at a safe distance above the carina and below the cords. The tube should then be secured with tape or a commercial device.

> **NOTE** The correct depth of insertion of an endotracheal (ET) tube in children over age 2 can be approximated by adding one half the patient's age to 12.
>
> $$\text{Depth of insertion (cm)} = \frac{\text{Patient's age}}{2} + 12$$
>
> As an alternative, the depth of insertion can be estimated by multiplying the internal diameter of the tube by 3.[7]
>
> $$\text{Depth of insertion (cm)} = \text{ET tube internal diameter} \times 3$$

6. Children use the diaphragm as the major muscle for ventilation. They require full diaphragmatic excursion to breathe. Gastric distention caused by swallowing air or artificial ventilation can inhibit the child's respiratory efforts. Infants are nose breathers until 3 to 5 months of age.
7. Deciduous teeth begin to develop at about 6 months. These are lost between 6 and 8 years. They may become dislodged during airway procedures such as intubation and oral airway insertion and by the child biting on the airway.

During any airway procedure, the paramedic should remember that the airway structures of children are very fragile and easily damaged. Therefore great care must be taken not to injure these patients.

Adjuncts to Aid Confirmation of Endotracheal Tube Placement

Several adjuncts often can help to determine correct ET tube placement. These include end-tidal carbon dioxide detectors, bulb- or syringe-type esophageal detection devices, and pulse oximeters.

END-TIDAL CARBON DIOXIDE DETECTORS

Capnography is the measurement of carbon dioxide concentrations in exhaled air. This measurement is made possible by end-tidal carbon dioxide detectors. End-tidal carbon dioxide detectors are designed to help verify ET tube placement. They also are designed to reveal inadvertent esophageal intubation. These devices provide a noninvasive estimate of alveolar ventilation, carbon dioxide production, and arterial carbon dioxide content. Their use as an adjunct to assessment of ET tube placement is strongly encouraged.[7]

> **NOTE** The color indicators of colorimetric carbon dioxide (CO_2) detectors can be affected by vomitus. They also can be affected if the patient recently drank a carbonated beverage (if the endotracheal tube is placed in the esophagus).

The two types of carbon dioxide detectors are disposable colorimetric devices and the electronic monitor. Colorimetric devices are made of plastic and contain a chemical indicator in the upper part that is sensitive to carbon dioxide gas. When the detector is attached to an ET tube, the color of the indicator changes with elevated carbon dioxide concentrations, such as would be expected in the trachea but not in the esophagus (Fig. 19-72). Any color change indicates tracheal placement; no color change indicates esophageal intubation. A memory aid for colorimetric devices is as follows: *yellow* (yes, the tube is correctly placed); *tan* (think about it; the tube may not be properly placed); and *purple* (problem; the tube is not in the trachea).

> **NOTE** Cardiac output is very low during cardiopulmonary resuscitation. Consequently, the carbon dioxide detector may show no color change even when the endotracheal (ET) tube is in the trachea. In such cases a second method of confirming tube placement should be used, such as an esophageal detector.

Electronic devices can confirm successful tracheal tube placement within seconds of an intubation attempt, as well as subsequent tracheal dislodgement.[10] An infrared analyzer measures the percentage of carbon dioxide gas at each phase

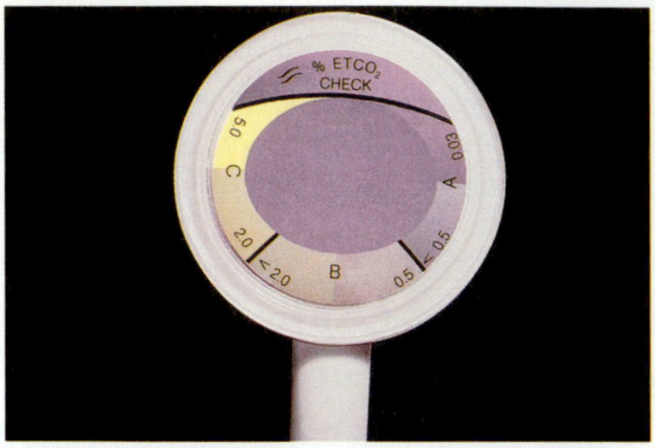

FIGURE 19-72 ■ Colorimetric end-tidal carbon dioxide (CO_2) detector.

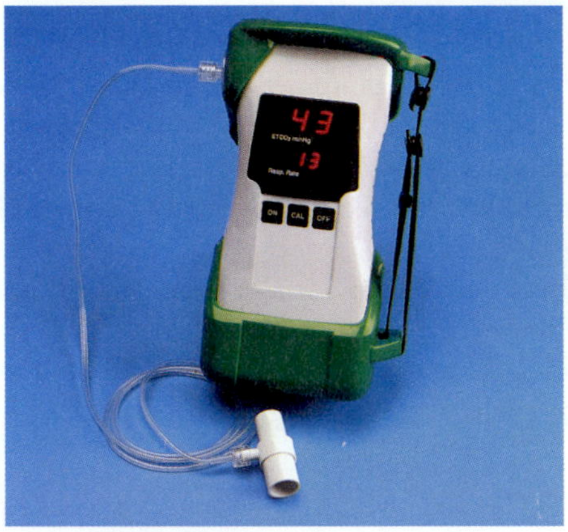

FIGURE 19-73 ■ Digital (or electronic) end-tidal carbon dioxide (CO_2) detector.

of respiration (Fig. 19-73). Capnometers provide a numerical reading of exhaled CO_2 levels. The information may also be displayed in a digital waveform using a capnograph with printout capability (similar to an ECG tracing) (Box 19-8). Both colorimetric and electronic devices may be useful as indicators of circulation during some cardiac arrest situations because an increase in end-tidal carbon dioxide concentrations seems to be related to effective perfusion during external chest compression.[12] Some capnometers can be used in patients who have not been intubated (i.e., those using nasal or oral airway adjuncts). They are helpful in determining the effectiveness of EMS treatments.

> **CRITICAL THINKING**
>
> Your patient is in full arrest, therefore the measurements from your end-tidal carbon dioxide ($ETCO_2$) detector are inconclusive. Also, you can't get the oxygen saturation monitor to work. You are not sure whether you hear breath sounds clearly. What should you do?

BULB- AND SYRINGE-TYPE ESOPHAGEAL DETECTORS

Esophageal detection devices (e.g., the Toomey syringe) are attached to the end of the ET tube (Fig. 19-74). They operate on the principle that the esophagus is a collapsible tube. As such, a vacuum is created when air is removed from the esophagus. This occurs with the bulb device after it is compressed or when air is withdrawn by the syringe device if the ET tube is in the esophagus. If the ET tube has been correctly placed in the trachea, the bulb device easily refills with air or the syringe device is easily aspirated when the plunger is pulled back. Esophageal detection devices also can be used to verify correct placement of multilumen airways (described later in this chapter).

PULSE OXIMETRY

Pulse oximeters (Fig. 19-75) help determine how well the patient is being oxygenated. They measure the transmission of red and near-infrared light through arterial beds. Hemoglobin absorbs red and infrared light waves differently when it is bound with oxygen (oxyhemoglobin) and when it is not (reduced hemoglobin). Oxyhemoglobin absorbs more infrared than red light. Reduced hemoglobin absorbs more red than infrared light. Pulse oximetry reveals arterial saturation by measuring this difference.

The oximeter probe is placed on an area of thin tissue, such as a finger, toe, or ear lobe. One side of the probe sends wavelengths of light through the arterial bed. The other side detects the presence of red or infrared light. Using this balance of red and infrared colors, the oximeter calculates the oxygen saturation of the blood and displays it on the monitor screen.

The percentage of hemoglobin saturated with oxygen is denoted as the Sao_2. It depends on a number of factors. These include the Pco_2, pH, temperature, and whether the hemoglobin is normal or altered. The lower range of normal for the Sao_2 is 93% to 95%. The upper range is 99% to 100%. Once the Sao_2 falls below 90% (corresponding to a Po_2 of 60 mm Hg), further decreases are associated with a marked decline in oxygen content (Box 19-9).

Difficulties and inaccuracies may result from the use of pulse oximeters. Therefore paramedics should consider them only as another tool to assist the monitoring of a patient's oxygenation levels. Circumstances that may produce false readings include the following[13]:

- Dyshemoglobinemia (hemoglobin saturation with compounds other than oxygen [e.g., carbon monoxide, methemoglobinemia])
- Excessive ambient light (sunlight, fluorescent lights) on the oximeter's sensor probe
- Patient movement
- Hypotension
- Hypothermia/vasoconstriction
- Patient use of vasoconstrictive drugs
- Patient use of nail polish
- Jaundice

Laryngeal Mask Airway

The laryngeal mask airway (LMA) is an advanced airway control device. It may be used in the prehospital setting when conventional ET intubation is unsuccessful, when access to the patient is limited, when an unstable neck injury

BOX 19-8 Capnography Waveforms

Capnography waveforms on the monitor screen are condensed to provide assessment information in a 4-second view. Printouts of waveforms provide the same information in "real time" and may differ in duration from that of the monitor screen. The following are example waveforms for both intubated and non-intubated patients.*

Normal Ranges:

Arterial $PaCO_2$	35–45 mm Hg
Capnography $EtCO_2$	35–45 mm Hg (4–6) Vol. %)

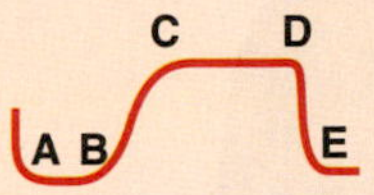

A–B Respiratory baseline
B–C Expiratory upslope
C–D Expiratory plateau
D End-tidal value—peak CO_2 concentration—normally at the end of exhalation
D–E Inspiratory downstroke

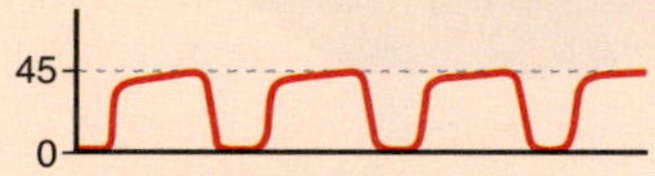

Normal capnography tracing

Capnography—Intubated Patients

May be used to:
- Verify ET tube placement
- Monitor or detect ET tube dislodgement
- Monitor loss of circulatory function
- Assess adequacy of CPR compressions
- Confirm return of spontaneous circulation

Examples:

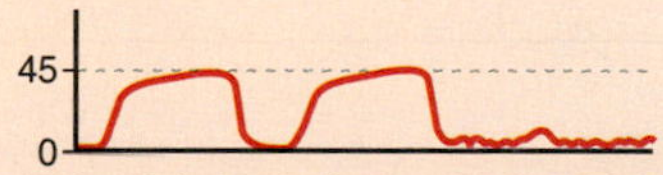

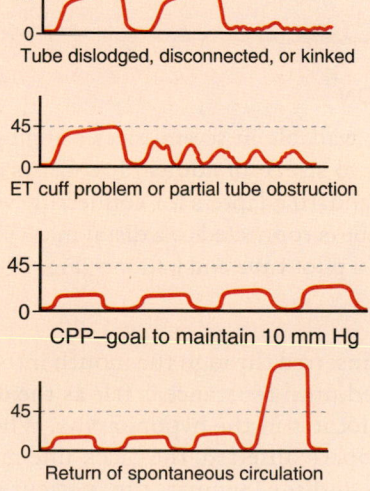

Tube dislodged, disconnected, or kinked

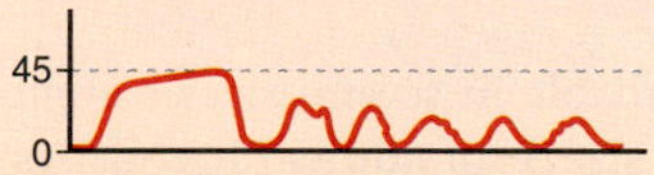

ET cuff problem or partial tube obstruction

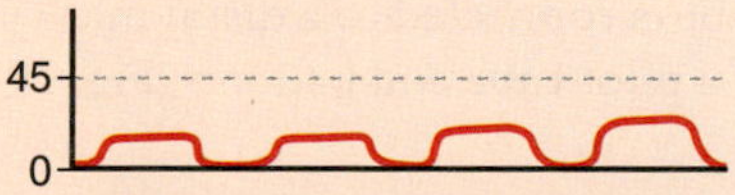

CPP–goal to maintain 10 mm Hg

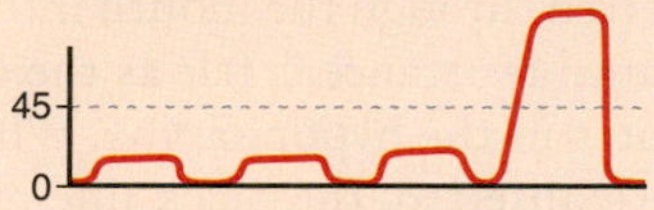

Return of spontaneous circulation

Capnography—Non-Intubated Patients

May be used to:
- Assess asthma and COPD
- Document and monitor procedural sedation
- Detect apnea or inadequate breathing
- Measure hypoventilation
- Evaluate hyperventilation

Examples:

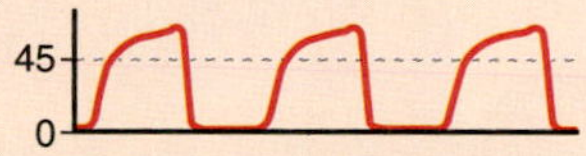

Waveform has a "shark fin" appearance during bronchospasm

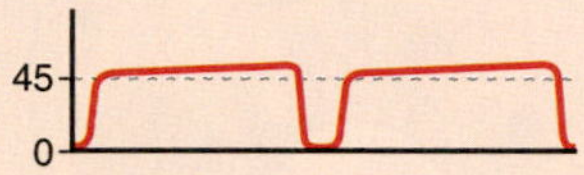

Hypoventilation

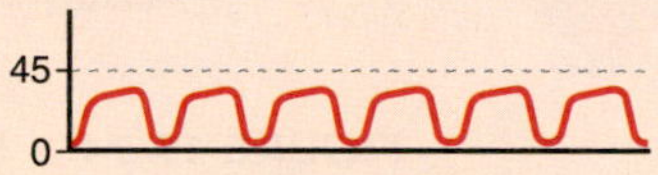

Hyperventilation

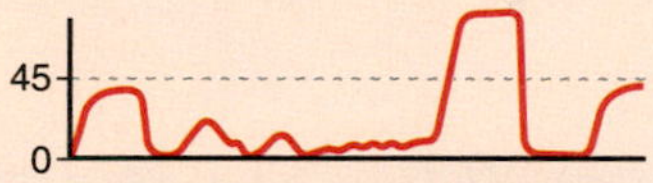

Irregular apneustic breathing

*Level of sedation and severity of conditions may affect respiratory rate and $EtCO_2$ level in patients.

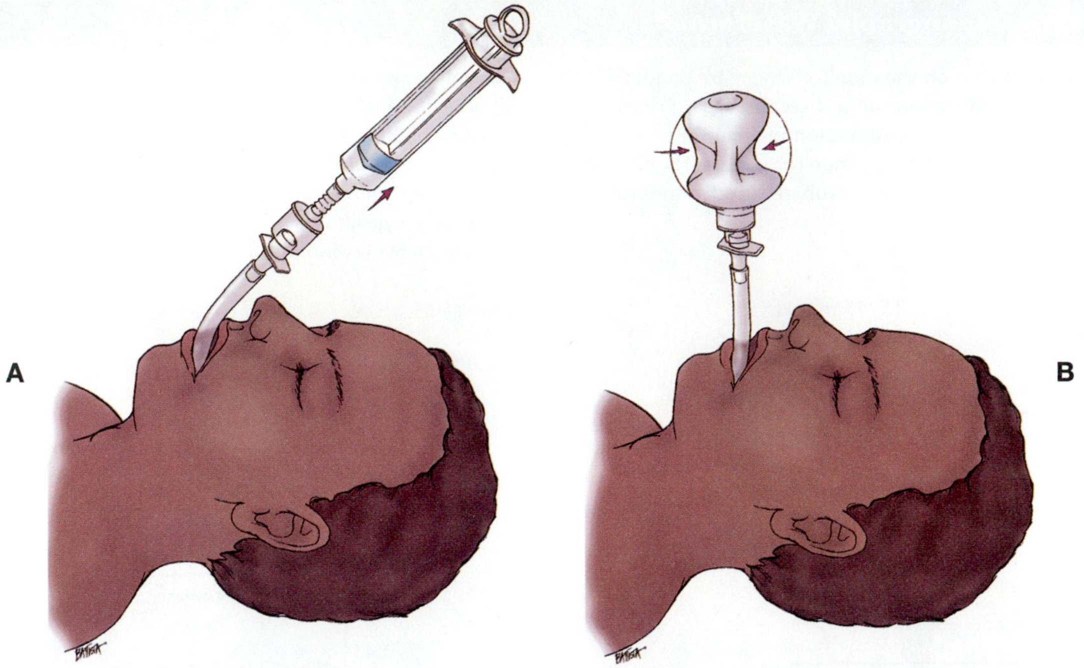

FIGURE 19-74 ■ Esophageal intubation detector. **A,** Syringe. **B,** Bulb.

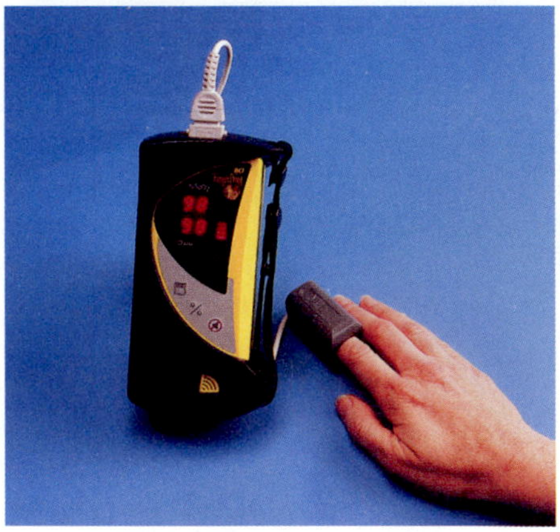

FIGURE 19-75 ■ Pulse oximeter.

may be present, or when appropriate positioning of the patient for tracheal intubation is impossible.[14] The LMA also allows ET intubation through the device. This allows easier placement of the tube.

NOTE The laryngeal mask airway (LMA) does not offer full protection against aspiration. However, aspiration is uncommon with this device. A small number of patients cannot be ventilated adequately with the LMA. Also, it is contraindicated in conscious patients and in those with an intact gag reflex.

BOX 19-9 Oxygen Saturation and Partial Pressure (Po_2)

With 90% saturation, Po_2 drops to 60 mm Hg
With 75% saturation, Po_2 drops to 40 mm Hg
With 50% saturation, Po_2 drops to 27 mm Hg

DESCRIPTION

The LMA is available in several sizes (ranging from size 1 for neonates to size 5 for adults.) It consists of a proximal tube with standard adapters for connecting ventilatory devices. The tube is connected to a distal mask that is inflated by means of a pilot tube and balloon (Fig. 19-76).

INSERTION

The LMA is inserted through the mouth into the pharynx. It is advanced until resistance is felt as the distal portion of the tube locates in the hypopharynx. When the device has been properly inserted, the black line marked on the LMA rests midline against the patient's upper lip. Inflating the cuff seals the larynx and leaves distal opening of the tube just above the glottis, providing a clear and secure airway. After the pilot cuff has been inflated, proper placement is confirmed by observing equal rise and fall of the chest, by ensuring bilateral breath sounds, and with end-tidal CO_2 detectors, esophageal detectors, and pulse oximetry monitoring (in a patient who has a

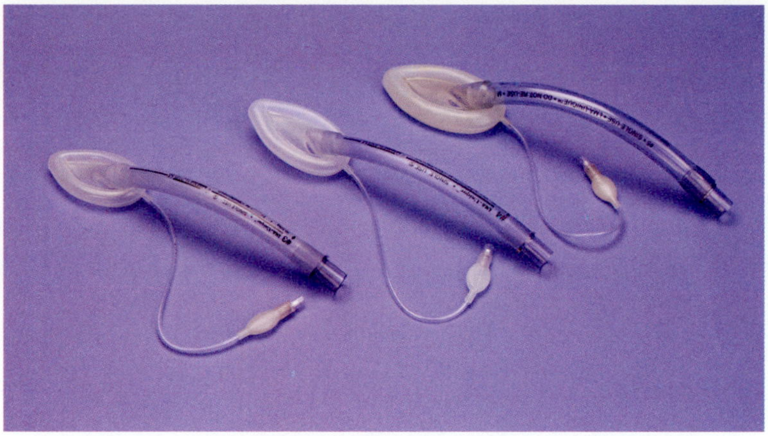

FIGURE 19-76 ■ Laryngeal mask airways.

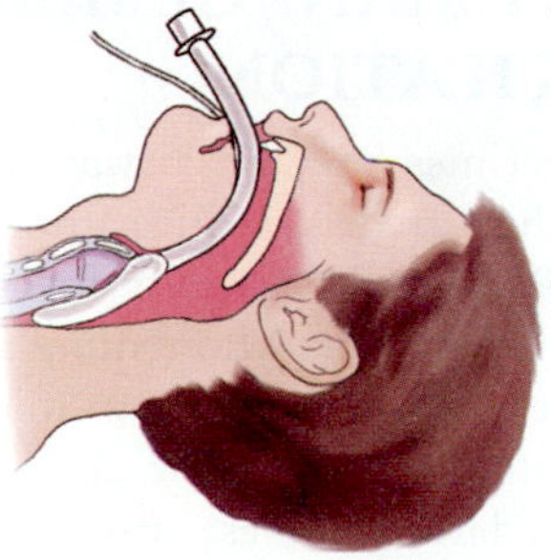

FIGURE 19-77 ■ Ventilation of a patient with a laryngeal mask airway (LMA).

perfusing rhythm) (Fig. 19-77). Use of the LMA requires special training and authorization from medical direction. The LMA may be hard to maintain during patient movement. This can make it difficult to use during patient transport.

NECESSARY EQUIPMENT

- Water-soluble lubricant
- Syringes
- Bag-valve device
- Oxygen source and connecting tubing
- Suction equipment
- Stethoscope

COMMON ADVANTAGES

- Less skilled training or maintenance is required than for ET intubation.
- Laryngoscopy and visualization of the vocal cords are not required.
- Minimal spinal movement is required for insertion.
- ET intubation can be achieved through the LMA.

COMMON DISADVANTAGES

- The patient must be unresponsive and have no gag reflex.
- Not all patients can be adequately ventilated with the LMA.
- The airway must be removed when the patient becomes responsive or agitated.
- The airway should be replaced with an ET tube as soon as possible.

COMMON CONTRAINDICATIONS

- Presence of a gag reflex
- Caustic ingestion
- Esophageal trauma or disease

Multilumen Airways

Multilumen airways (e.g., the esophageal-tracheal Combitube [ETC] and the pharyngeal-tracheal lumen [PtL]), allow for either esophageal or tracheal insertion. They use a plastic tube with twin lumens that are separated by a partition wall. One tube resembles an ET tube and has an open distal end. The other tube is blocked by an obturator at the distal end. Both tubes use low-pressure balloons that provide a seal for either the trachea or the esophagus, depending on placement. When inflated, the large pharyngeal balloon fills the space between the base of the tongue and the soft palate, anchoring the tube in position. The multilumen airway usually finds its way into the esophagus because of the stiffness and curve of the tube and the shape and the structure of the pharynx.

Multilumen airways are another option for airway control when endotracheal intubation is indicated but is unsuccessful or unavailable. The LMA and ETC (preferred over the PtL) provide superior ventilation compared with face masks in cardiac arrest.[14] Multilumen airways reduce but do not eliminate the risk of aspiration.

INSERTION

Multilumen airways are inserted by gently guiding the device into the esophagus or trachea. (This insertion is achieved without hyperextension or flexion of the patient's head. It also is done without visualization of the glottic opening.) The pharyngeal and distal balloons are then inflated. This isolates the oropharynx above the upper balloon. It isolates the esophagus (or trachea) below the lower balloon. Ventilation is at first provided through the

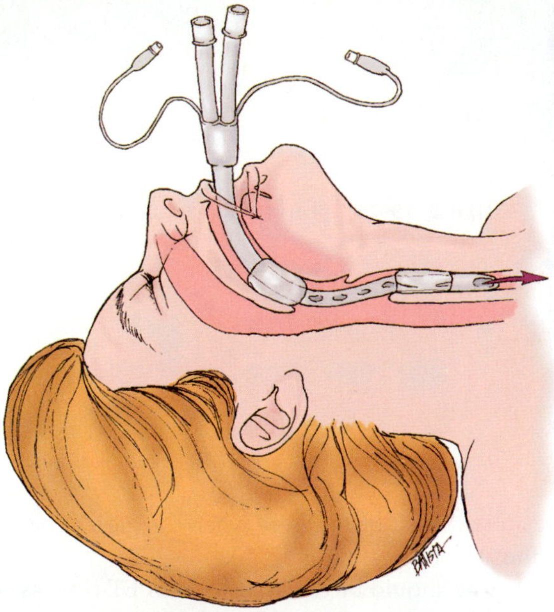

FIGURE 19-78 ■ Placement of the esophageal-tracheal Combitube (ETC) airway.

esophageal lumen. (This is due to the significant chance of esophageal placement with blind insertion.) In this position air passes into the pharynx and beyond the glottis into the trachea. The placement is confirmed by primary and secondary confirmation methods previously described. Fig. 19-78 shows placement of the ETC airway.

If breath sounds and chest movement are absent with ventilation through the esophageal lumen, ventilation should be performed through the tracheal lumen without changing the position of the airway. Air passes through this lumen directly into the trachea. Placement is confirmed in the usual manner.

NECESSARY EQUIPMENT

- Water-soluble lubricant
- Syringes
- BVM
- Oxygen source and connecting tubing
- Suction equipment
- Stethoscope

The various kinds of balloon-system devices share advantages, disadvantages, and contraindications.

COMMON ADVANTAGES

- Airways cannot be improperly placed.
- Less skill training or skill maintenance is needed than for endotracheal intubation.
- Minimal spinal movement is required for insertion.
- Suctioning is easily done.

COMMON DISADVANTAGES

- The patient must be unresponsive and without a gag reflex.
- The airway must be removed when the patient becomes responsive or agitated.
- Proper identification of the tube's location may be difficult, leading to ventilation through the wrong lumen.
- The trachea cannot be suctioned when the tube is in the esophagus.
- The airway should be replaced with an ET tube as soon as possible.

COMMON CONTRAINDICATIONS

- Patient height less than 5 feet or age under 14 years
- Caustic ingestion
- Esophageal trauma or disease
- Presence of a gag reflex

PHARMACOLOGICAL ADJUNCTS TO AIRWAY MANAGEMENT AND VENTILATION

Sedation is sometimes used in airway management and ventilation to reduce anxiety, induce amnesia, and decrease the gag reflex. Possible indications for sedation include combative patients, patients who require aggressive airway management but who are too alert to tolerate intubation, and agitated trauma patients. The classes of drugs commonly used for sedation in these situations are tranquilizers, barbiturates, benzodiazepines, and narcotics.

> **NOTE** Sedating a patient with a poor airway is risky. The patient may suffer respiratory arrest. The paramedic must always consult medical direction regarding these patients.

Paralytic Agents in Emergency Intubation

Paralysis may be used for emergency intubation. Paralysis involves the use of neuromuscular blocking drugs. These drugs are indicated for combative patients who need to be intubated. For instance, a patient suffering a head injury may be agitated and combative. These drugs should not be used in the following situations:

- Patients who will be difficult to ventilate (e.g., patients with facial hair)
- Patients who will be difficult to intubate (e.g., patients with short necks, obstructions)

PHARMACOLOGY

As described in Chapter 17, neuromuscular blockers produce skeletal muscle paralysis. They do this by binding to the nicotinic receptor for acetylcholine (ACh) at the neuromuscular junction. To review, this junction is the point of contact between the nerve ending and the muscle fiber (see Chapter 6). When nerve impulses pass through this junction, ACh and other chemicals are released. This release causes the muscle to contract. The two types of neuromuscular blocking drugs are depolarizing agents and nondepolarizing agents.

Depolarizing agents invade the neuromuscular junction and bind to the receptors for ACh. These drugs produce depolarization of the muscular membrane. Thus they often lead to fasciculations (uncontrollable muscle twitching). These drugs also may lead to some muscular contractions. An example of a depolarizing agent is ***succinylcholine.*** Succinylcholine has a rapid onset of action. Yet it has the briefest duration of action of all the neuromuscular blocking drugs. This makes it the drug of choice for emergency endotracheal intubation.

Nondepolarizing agents also bind to the receptors for ACh. However, they block the uptake of ACh at the neuromuscular junction without initiating depolarization of the muscle membrane. Examples of nondepolarizing drugs include ***vecuronium*** and ***pancuronium.*** These drugs have a longer onset and duration than depolarizing agents.

Neuromuscular blocking agents produce complete paralysis. Thus ventilatory support must be provided. Ventilation and oxygenation must be closely monitored to ensure that they are adequate. If the patient is conscious, the paramedic should explain the effects of the medication before administering it. Administration of ***atropine*** should be strongly considered, particularly in children, before a blocking agent is administered. ***Lidocaine*** given prior to administration of a blocking agent may blunt any increase in intracranial pressure associated with intubation. Finally, ***diazepam, etomidate, midazolam,*** or another sedative approved by medical direction should be used in any conscious patient to whom a blocking agent is administered; neuromuscular blocking agents do not inhibit pain or seizure activity.

Rapid Sequence Intubation

Rapid sequence intubation (RSI) involves the administration of a potent sedative and a neuromuscular blocking agent at the same time. These are administered for the purpose of ET intubation. The blocking agent most often used is ***succinylcholine*** (see the EDI). RSI provides optimal intubation conditions. It also minimizes the risk of aspiration of gastric contents. RSI is indicated in the following situations[15]:

- Emergency intubation is warranted.
- The patient has a "full" stomach.
- Intubation is predicted to be successful (Box 19-10).
- If intubation fails, ventilation is predicted to be successful.

RSI is not indicated for patients in cardiac arrest or deeply comatose patients when immediate intubation is required. Relative contraindications include concern that intubation or mask ventilation would be unsuccessful; significant facial or laryngeal edema, trauma, or distortion; or a spontaneously breathing patient who requires upper airway muscle tone and positioning (e.g., upper airway obstruction, epiglottitis).[16]

The purpose of RSI is to avoid positive-pressure ventilation until the ET tube is correctly placed in the trachea with the cuff inflated. This is especially true for the patient who needs intubation and who is at risk of aspiration. RSI requires special training and authorization from medical direction. The effectiveness of RSI performed in the field

BOX 19-10 Signs for Assessing the Difficulty of Intubation

The potential difficulty of an intubation can be judged by the accessibility of the oropharynx. Visibility of the oropharynx ranges from complete visualization, including the tonsillar pillars (indicating an easy intubation) to no visualization at all, with the uvula pressed against the tongue (indicating a difficult intubation).

Other situations that indicate a potentially difficult intubation include the following:

- An immobilized trauma patient
- Children
- A short neck that makes visualization of the cords more difficult
- Prominent upper incisors that limit working space
- Receding mandible that may limit the line of vision
- Limited jaw opening
- Limited cervical mobility
- Upper airway conditions (e.g., burns, neck injury, epiglottitis)
- Facial trauma
- Laryngeal trauma

Mallampati Signs as Indicators of Difficult Intubation

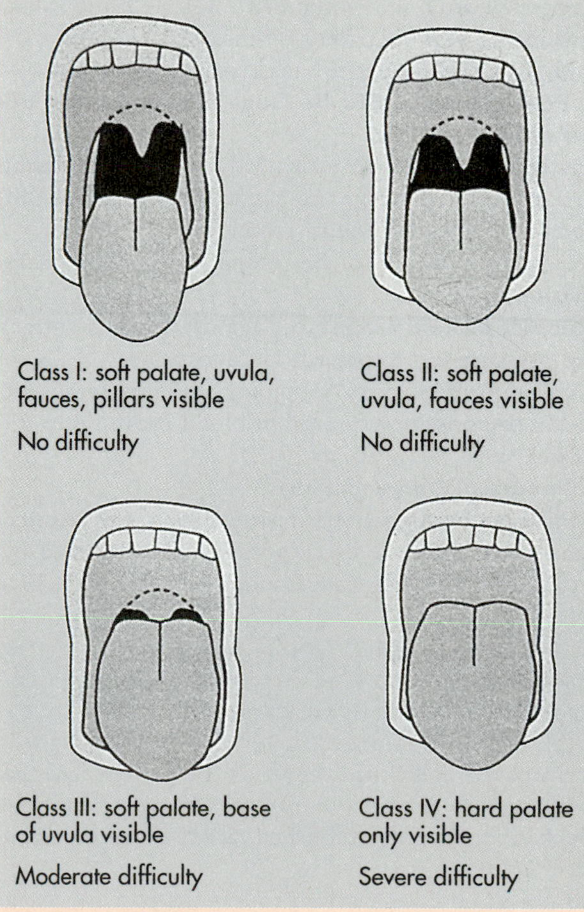

> **BOX 19-11 The Six "Ps" of Rapid Sequence Intubation**
>
> 1. Preparation
> 2. Preoxygenation
> 3. Pretreatment
> 4. Paralysis (with sedation)
> 5. Placement of the tube
> 6. Postintubation management

should be monitored through a quality improvement process. RSI is intended to take the patient from a conscious, breathing state to a state of unconsciousness. This is accomplished with complete neuromuscular paralysis. Intubation is performed without interposed mechanical ventilation. The six steps of RSI (the six "Ps") are preparation, preoxygenation, pretreatment, paralysis (with sedation), placement of the tube, and postintubation management (Box 19-11). Each step is described below.

TECHNIQUE

1. Preparation

- Assess the patient for difficulty of intubation (e.g., using the Mallampati score in Box 19-10).
- Prepare all drugs and equipment.
- Ensure one or more patent IV lines.
- Explain the procedure to the patient.

2. Preoxygenation (To Be Done Simultaneously With Preparation)

- Preoxygenate the patient with 100% oxygen for 5 minutes (an essential step of the "no-bagging" approach of RSI).
- Consider the use of a pulse oximeter.

3. Pretreatment (To Be Done 3 Minutes Before Intubation)

- Consider ***lidocaine*** to protect against a rise in intracranial pressure and to prevent laryngospasm.
- Consider beta blockers or opioids to reduce sympathoadrenal response (e.g., a drop in blood pressure) to intubation.

4. Paralysis (With Sedation)

- Administer a sedative (per protocol) to produce unconsciousness. This should be immediately followed by a rapid push of the neuromuscular blocker (see the EDI).

> **CRITICAL THINKING**
> How would you decide whether a patient needs more sedation after a paralytic has been given?

- Perform the Sellick maneuver as the patient loses consciousness to prevent vomiting. (Once neuromuscular blockade has been established, active vomiting cannot occur.)
- Do not initiate ventilations unless the patient's oxygen saturation falls below 90%.
- Within 45 seconds of administration of ***succinylcholine***, the patient will be relaxed enough for intubation.

5. Placement

- Perform orotracheal intubation and confirm placement.

6. Postintubation Management

- Secure the tube in place.
- Begin mechanical ventilation.
- Monitor the patient continuously.

If RSI is unsuccessful and the patient cannot be intubated, the patient's airway should be managed by other means (e.g., a multilumen airway, BVM, cricothyrotomy).

TRANSLARYNGEAL CANNULA VENTILATION

Translaryngeal cannula ventilation is also known as *percutaneous transtracheal ventilation* and *needle cricothyrotomy.* It may be valuable in the initial stabilization of a patient whose airway cannot be managed by the usual manual measures. It also may be valuable in patients who cannot be intubated by oral or nasal means. It is a temporary procedure. It provides oxygenation when the airway is obstructed as a result of edema of the glottis, fracture of the larynx, or severe oropharyngeal hemorrhage. Translaryngeal cannula ventilation requires special training and authorization from medical direction.

Description

Translaryngeal cannula ventilation provides high-volume, high-pressure oxygenation of the lungs. This occurs through cannulation of the trachea below the glottis. The procedure delivers a large volume of oxygen through a small port at high pressure to the lungs. This oxygen delivery (50 psi) is much greater than can be achieved with other methods (e.g., 1 psi with a therapy regulator).

Necessary Equipment

- A 12- or 14-gauge over-the-needle catheter with a 5 or 10 mL syringe
- Alcohol or povidone-iodine swabs
- Adhesive tape or appropriate ties
- Pressure-regulating valve and pressure gauge attached to a high-pressure (30 to 60 psi) oxygen supply. (Most oxygen tanks and regulators can provide 50 psi at 15 L/min or when opened to flush.)
- High-pressure tubing connecting the high-pressure regulating valve to a hand-operated release valve (5 foot tubing is recommended)
- A release valve connected by tubing to the catheter (this may be provided via a Y- or T-connector, through a three-way stopcock directly attached to the high-pressure tubing, or by cutting a hole in the oxygen line to provide a "whistle-stop" effect).

Technique

The steps in translaryngeal cannula ventilation are as follows (Fig. 19-79):

1. Make sure the patient is supine. Also make sure the cricothyroid membrane has been identified. (If a spinal

STEP-BY-STEP SKILL

FIGURE 19-79 ■ Translaryngeal cannula ventilation.

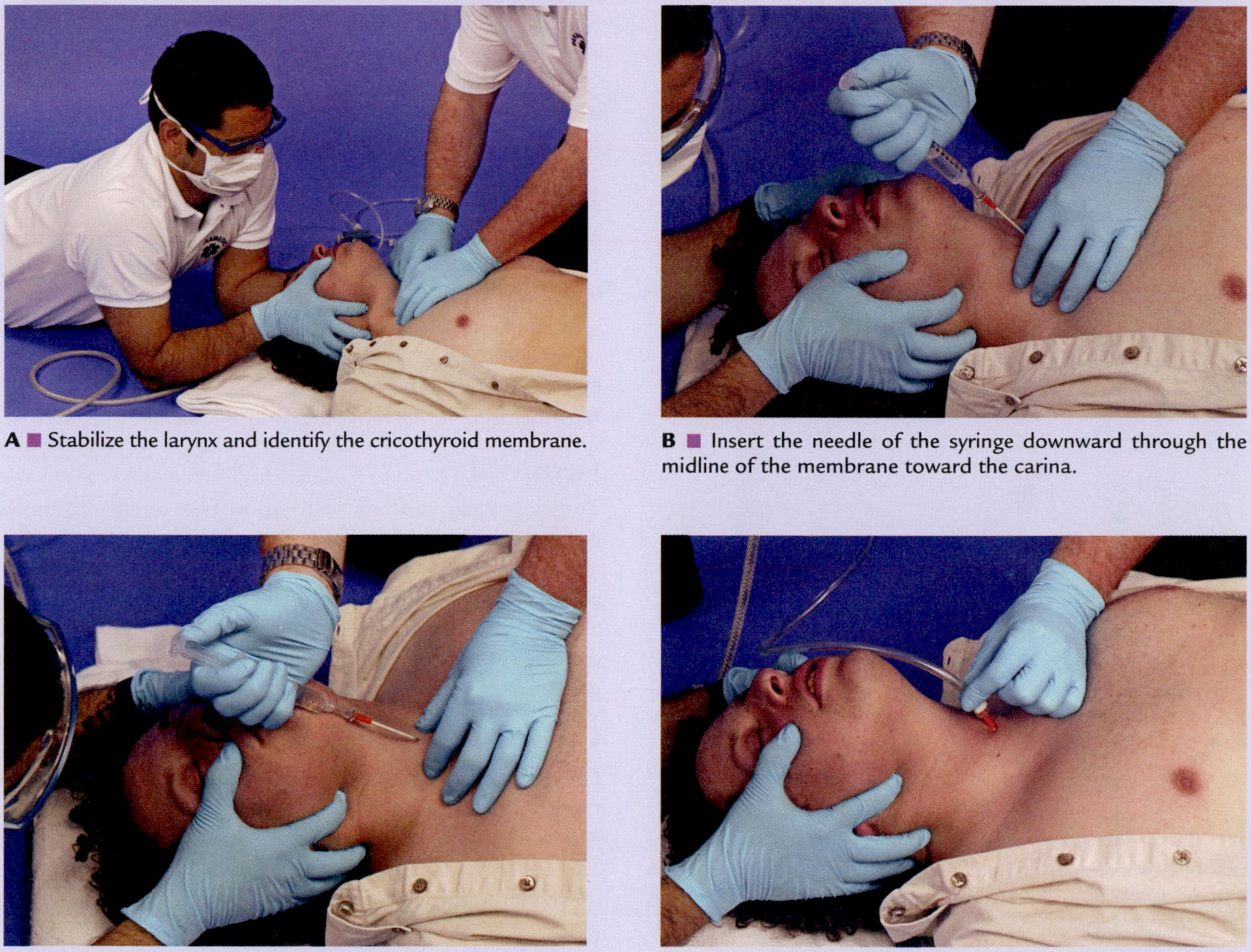

A ■ Stabilize the larynx and identify the cricothyroid membrane.

B ■ Insert the needle of the syringe downward through the midline of the membrane toward the carina.

C ■ While inserting the needle, draw back on the plunger of the syringe. If air enters the syringe, the needle is in the trachea.

D ■ After removing the needle and syringe, stabilize the catheter and connect the end of the oxygen tubing from the hub of the cannula to the oxygen regulator. Provide for a release valve.

injury is suspected, in-line stabilization may be provided as for nasal and tracheal intubation.)

2. Stabilize the larynx using the thumb and middle finger of one hand. With the other hand, palpate the small depression below the thyroid cartilage (the "Adam's apple"). Slide the index finger down to locate the cricothyroid membrane.
3. Insert the needle of the syringe downward through the midline of the membrane at a 45- to 60-degree angle toward the patient's carina. Apply negative pressure to the syringe during insertion. The entrance of air into the syringe indicates that the needle is in the trachea (Fig. 19-80, *A*).
4. Advance the catheter over the needle toward the carina and remove the needle and syringe (Fig. 19-80, *B*). Care must be taken not to kink the catheter when removing the needle and syringe.
5. Hold the hub of the catheter to prevent accidental dislodgement while providing ventilation. Remove the end of the oxygen tubing from the hub of the cannula and connect it to the oxygen regulator. Provide for a release valve as described before.

CRITICAL THINKING

What conditions could make it difficult to locate the anatomical landmarks for translaryngeal cannulation or cricothyrotomy?

When the release valve is closed, oxygen under pressure is introduced into the trachea. The pressure is adjusted to a level

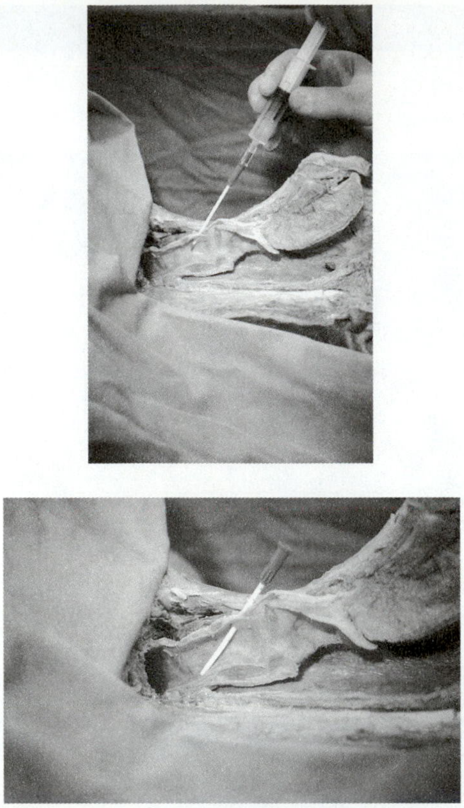

FIGURE 19-80 ■ **A,** Insert a large-bore catheter through the cricothyroid membrane, directing it toward the feet. While inserting the catheter, draw back on the plunger of the syringe; when air enters the syringe, the needle is in the airway. **B,** Slide the catheter off the stylet into the larynx.

that allows adequate lung expansion. The patient's chest must be observed closely. The release valve must be opened to allow for exhalation. The correct ratio of inflation to deflation varies. It depends on whether upper airway obstruction is present. For an open upper airway, an inspiratory to expiratory ratio of 1 to 4 seconds is adequate. Ratios of about 1 to 8 seconds are needed to prevent barotrauma (injuries caused by excessive pressures [e.g., pneumothorax]) when the upper airway is obstructed.[17]

▶NOTE If the chest remains inflated during exhalation, a complete upper airway obstruction may be present. In such cases a longer expiratory time should be allowed. If this does not produce adequate deflation, a second large-bore catheter may be inserted through the cricothyroid membrane next to the first one. If the chest remains distended, a cricothyrotomy should be performed.

Advantages

- It is the least invasive of surgical procedures.
- It can be initiated quickly.
- When performed by a trained paramedic, it is simple, inexpensive, and effective.
- Minimal spinal movement is needed for insertion.

Disadvantages

- The technique is an invasive procedure.
- Constant monitoring is required.
- Jet ventilation is required
- The airway is not protected.
- The procedure does not allow for efficient elimination of carbon dioxide.
- The patient's lungs may be adequately ventilated for only 30 to 45 minutes.

Possible Complications

- High pressure during ventilation and air entrapment may cause pneumothorax.
- Hemorrhage may occur at the insertion site. The thyroid and esophagus also may be perforated if the needle is advanced too far.
- Direct suctioning of secretions is impossible.
- Subcutaneous emphysema may occur.

Removal

Translaryngeal cannula ventilation is a temporary emergency procedure. It provides time for the use of other airway management techniques. Removal should follow only after successful orotracheal or nasotracheal intubation or after a cricothyrotomy or a tracheostomy has been performed. Removal involves withdrawing the catheter and dressing the wound.

CRICOTHYROTOMY

Cricothyrotomy is a surgical procedure. It allows rapid entrance to the airway through the cricothyroid membrane. The procedure can be performed quickly. It is much faster and easier than a tracheostomy. In addition, it does not require manipulation of the cervical spine.

Description

Cricothyrotomy can provide ventilation and oxygenation for patients in whom airway control is not possible by other means. It should not be performed on patients who can be orally or nasally intubated. Few situations require this surgical procedure. Relative indications for cricothyrotomy include severe facial or nasal injuries that preclude oral or nasal intubation, massive midfacial trauma, possible spinal trauma preventing adequate ventilation, anaphylaxis, and chemical inhalation injuries. Like translaryngeal cannula ventilation, cricothyrotomy requires special training and authorization from medical direction.

Necessary Equipment

Commercially prepared cricothyrotomy kits are available through a number of manufacturers (Fig. 19-81). If such a kit is not available, the following equipment is required:

- Scalpel blade
- Size 6 (preferred) or size 7 ET tube or tracheostomy tube
- Antiseptic solution

BOX 19-12 Retrograde Intubation

Retrograde, or guided, intubation (RI) is a less-invasive procedure than cricothyrotomy. It can be used in a patient whose cervical spine is properly stabilized when orotracheal or nasotracheal intubation attempts have failed. Like other surgical procedures, this advanced airway technique calls for special training and authorization from medical direction. Because of the time needed to perform RI, it generally is not recommended for patients who are apneic. The steps in the procedure are as follows:

1. Puncture the cricothyroid membrane with a needle that is large enough to accommodate the guide wire.
2. Pass the guide wire through the needle into the oropharynx. Aim the wire superiorly so that its distal end may be retrieved from the patient's mouth. Then withdraw the needle.
3. Advance the endotracheal (ET) tube over the distal end of the wire. Pass the wire into the ET tube through the side hole (Murphy's eye).
4. Pull the wire somewhat taut and straight.
5. Advance the ET tube over the wire into the trachea to the cricoid area. Relax the cricothyroid end of the wire. Then advance the ET tube to the desired intratracheal location.
6. Release the cricothyroid end of the wire. Withdraw the wire from the ET tube.
7. Secure the ET tube. Assist ventilations with a bag-valve-mask (BVM) device.

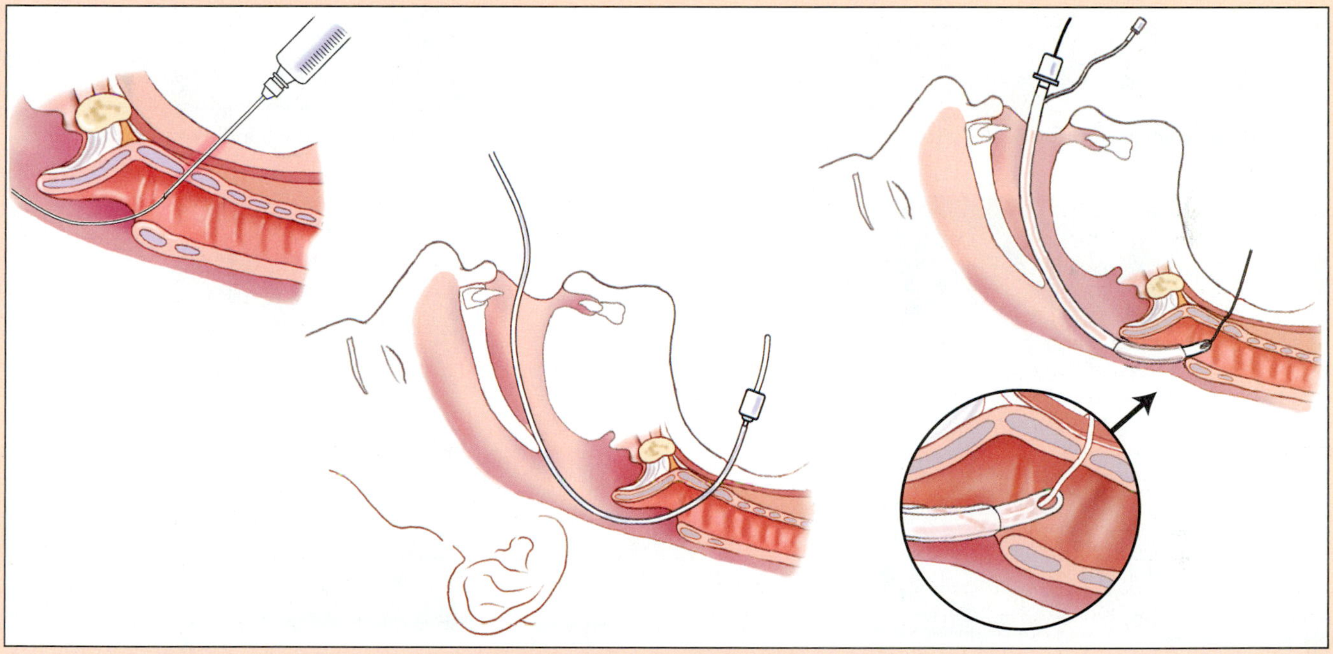

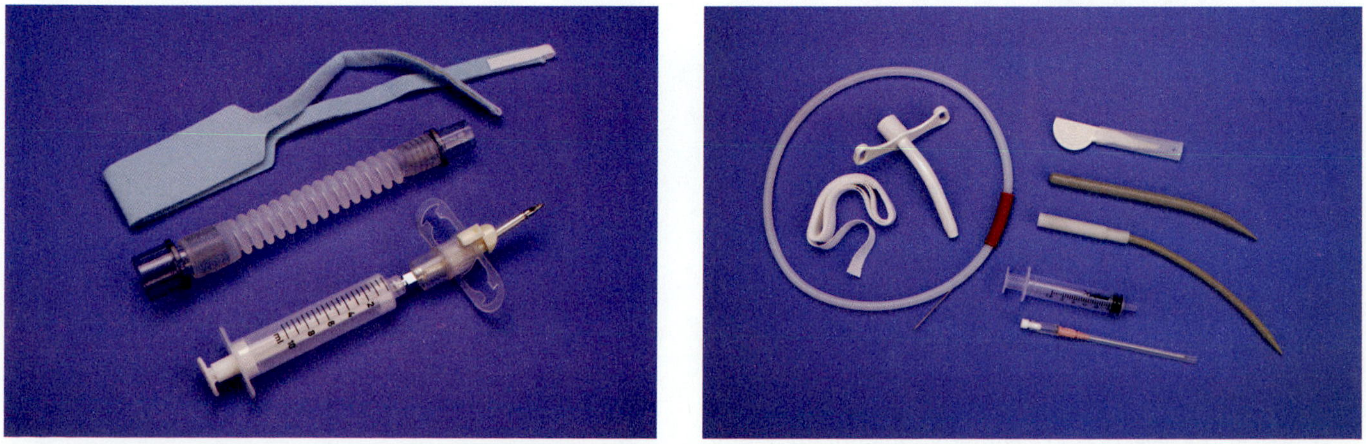

FIGURE 19-81 ■ Commercial cricothyrotomy kit.

STEP-BY-STEP SKILL

FIGURE 19-82 ■ **Surgical cricothyrotomy.**

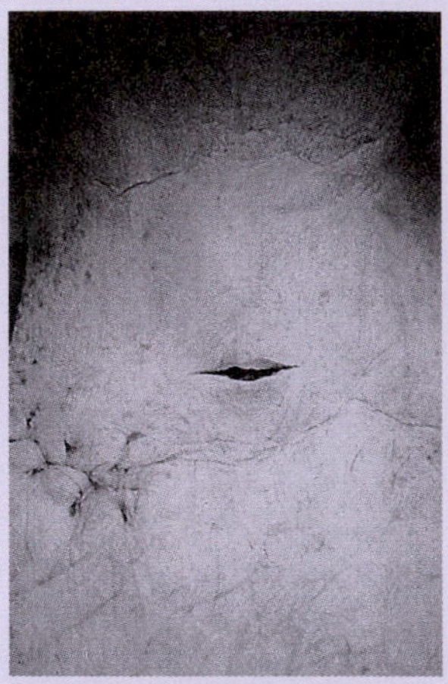

A ■ Make an incision through the cricothyroid membrane.

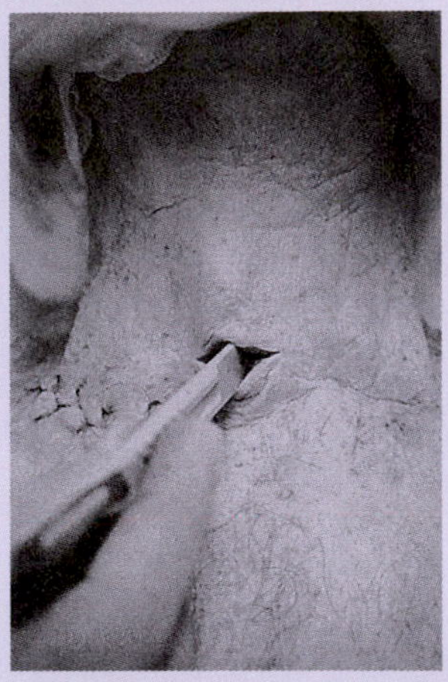

B ■ Open the hole by twisting the handle of a scalpel in it, *or*

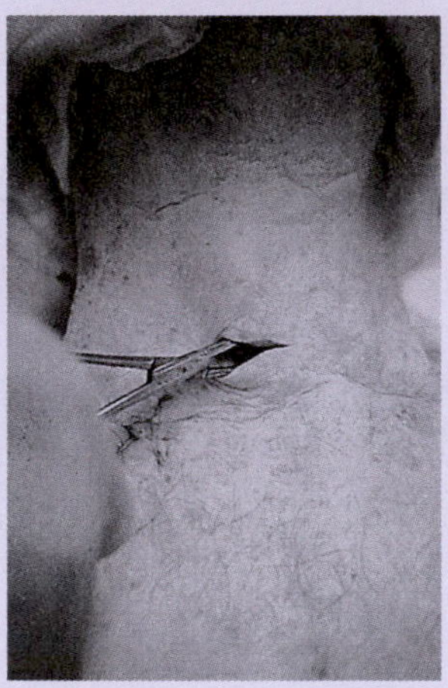

C ■ Open the hole with a clamp.

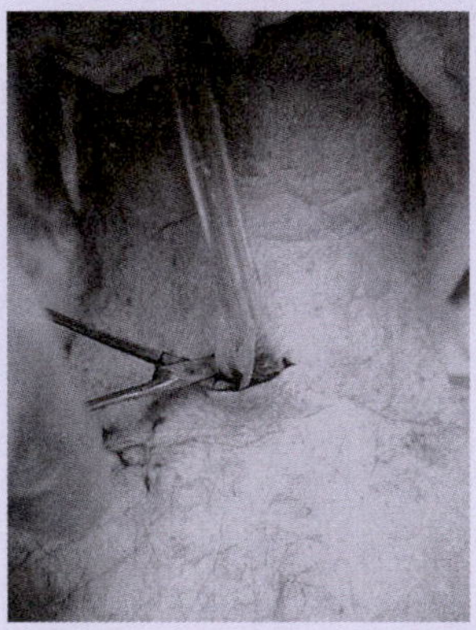

D ■ Insert the endotracheal (ET) tube.

- Oxygen source
- Suction device
- Bag-valve device

Technique

In patients suspected of having a spinal injury, in-line stabilization should be maintained throughout the procedure. If possible, the neck should be cleaned with alcohol or another antiseptic solution. The steps in the surgical procedure are as follows (Fig. 19-82):

1. Locate the anatomical landmarks of the neck. Identify the cricothyroid membrane.
2. Make a 2 cm (¾ inch) horizontal incision with the scalpel at the level of the cricothyroid membrane. (Some physicians may recommend a vertical skin incision instead of a horizontal one.)
3. Open the incision in the cricothyroid membrane by inserting the scalpel handle. Rotate it 90 degrees. This allows placement of a size 6 or size 7 ET tube or tracheostomy tube, which will not damage the larynx. The cuff should be inflated and the tube securely tied.
4. Provide ventilation by a bag-valve device with the highest available oxygen concentration.
5. Determine the adequacy of ventilation. This can be done through bilateral auscultation and observation of rise and fall of the chest.

▶**NOTE** Use of a smaller diameter endotracheal (ET) tube may aid in successful placement. Once the tube is in the airway, the paramedic should be careful not to advance it more than a few centimeters. This helps to avoid mainstem intubation.

Possible Complications

- Prolonged procedure time
- Hemorrhage
- Aspiration
- Possible misplacement
- False passage
- Perforation of the esophagus
- Injury to the vocal cords and carotid and jugular vessels lateral to the incision (the patient must be immobilized)
- Subcutaneous emphysema

Contraindications

- Inability to identify anatomical landmarks
- Underlying anatomical abnormality (e.g., tumor, subglottic stenosis)
- Tracheal transection
- Acute laryngeal disease caused by trauma or infection
- Small child under 10 years of age (in these patients, inserting a 12- to 14-gauge catheter over the needle may be safer than a cricothyrotomy)

Removal

In the prehospital setting, no attempt should be made to remove endotracheal tubes used during an emergency cricothyrotomy.

SUMMARY

- A key aspect of emergency care is a full understanding of the respiratory system. Another is mastery of airway management and ventilation techniques.
- The two phases of respiration are external respiration and internal respiration. External respiration is the transfer of oxygen and carbon dioxide between the inspired air and pulmonary capillaries. Internal respiration is the transfer of oxygen and carbon dioxide between the peripheral blood capillaries and the tissue cells.
- The mixture of gases that compose the atmosphere exerts a combined partial pressure of 100%, or 760 mm Hg at sea level. The composition of atmospheric gas is 21% oxygen; 0.03% carbon dioxide, and 78% nitrogen.
- The respiratory system delivers oxygen from inspired air to the blood and removes carbon dioxide.
- The 200 mL of oxygen that crosses the alveoli each minute is added to the oxygen already in the pulmonary capillaries. It is then transported to the body tissues by the circulatory system. After the body cells use the oxygen, the oxygen remaining in the blood returns to the heart and lungs. This exchange of oxygen and carbon dioxide is carried out by the passive process of diffusion.
- Respiration is controlled at any instant by a number of factors. Breathing is mainly an involuntary process. Within limits, however, the pattern of respiration can be consciously changed. The inspiratory muscles are made up of skeletal muscle. They cannot contract unless they are stimulated by nerve impulses. The activities of the respiratory centers are determined by changes in oxygen and carbon dioxide concentrations. They are also determined by the pH of the body fluids.
- The elderly cannot effectively make up for changes in airway and ventilation. Pulmonary changes that occur as a result of aging reduce vital capacity and increase physiological dead space. Po_2 also tends to decline gradually as a person ages.
- Causes of inadequate ventilation include upper airway obstruction and aspiration by inhalation. The most crucial lifesaving action for any patient who has respiratory problems from any cause is establishing and maintaining an open airway. This should always be the first priority of patient care.
- Essential parameters of airway evaluation include rate, regularity, effort, and recognition of airway problems that might indicate respiratory distress.
- The most common form of oxygen used in the prehospital setting is pure oxygen gas. This is delivered in liters per minute (LPM). Therapy regulators are used to deliver a safe pressure of oxygen to patients. Flowmeters control the amount of oxygen delivered to the patient. Several oxygen delivery devices provide supplemental oxygen to patients who have spontaneous respirations. They are the nasal cannula, simple face mask, partial rebreather mask, nonrebreather mask, and Venturi mask.
- In the prehospital setting, ventilation can be provided in several ways. These methods include rescue breathing (mouth-to-mouth, mouth-to-nose, mouth-to-stoma), mouth-to-mask breathing, use of bag-valve devices, and automatic transport ventilators.
- Emergency airway management should progress rapidly from the least to the most invasive techniques. Manual techniques for airway management include the head-tilt chin-lift method, the jaw-thrust, and the jaw-thrust without head-tilt.
- Suction catheters are used to clear the air passages of secretions and debris.

Continued

- Relief of gastric distention and/or emesis control can be accomplished through nasogastric or orogastric decompression.
- Mechanical devices for airway management include the nasal airway, oral airway, endotracheal intubation, digital intubation, nasotracheal intubation, laryngeal mask airway, multilumen airways, translaryngeal cannula ventilation, and cricothyrotomy.
- Rapid sequence intubation (RSI) involves administration of a potent sedative and a neuromuscular blocking drug at the same time. These are administered for the purpose of ET intubation.
- In the management of a child's airway, the differences in the pediatric airway must be considered. Compared to the adult airway, the child's upper airway structures have very different proportions. Their orientation to each other also differs. Smaller bag-valve devices are needed for infants and children. These reduce the chance of overinflation and barotrauma.
- End-tidal carbon dioxide detectors, pulse oximeters, and esophageal detectors can help the paramedic determine whether an ET tube has been placed correctly.

REFERENCES

1. National Safety Council: *Injury facts,* Chicago, 2002, The Council.
2. American Heart Association: *Basic life support for healthcare providers,* Dallas, 1997, The Association.
3. Tintinalli J et al: *Emergency medicine: a comprehensive study guide,* ed 2, New York, 1988, McGraw-Hill.
4. American Heart Association: Guidelines 2000 for cardiopulmonary resuscitation and emergency cardiovascular care, International Consensus on Science, *Circulation* 102(8):37, 2000.
5. American Heart Association: *ACLS provider manual,* Dallas, 2001, The Association.
6. American Heart Association: Guidelines 2000 for cardiopulmonary resuscitation and emergency cardiovascular care, International Consensus on Science, *Circulation* 102(8):267, 2000.
7. American Heart Association: *Pediatric advanced life support,* Dallas, 1997, American Heart Association.
8. American Heart Association: Guidelines 2000 for cardiopulmonary resuscitation and emergency cardiovascular care, International Consensus on Science, *Circulation* 102(8):96, 2000.
9. American Heart Association: Guidelines 2000 for cardiopulmonary resuscitation and emergency cardiovascular care, International Consensus on Science, *Circulation* 102(8):300, 2000.
10. American Heart Association: Guidelines 2000 for cardiopulmonary resuscitation and emergency cardiovascular care, International Consensus on Science, *Circulation* 102(8):101, 2000.
11. American College of Surgeons: *Upper airway management: advanced trauma life support,* Chicago, 1985, The College.
12. Garnet R et al: End-tidal carbon dioxide monitoring during cardiopulmonary resuscitation, *JAMA* 257(4):1379, 1987.
13. Mackreth B: Assessing pulse oximetry in the field, *JEMS* 15(6):56, 1990.
14. American Heart Association: Guidelines 2000 for cardiopulmonary resuscitation and emergency cardiovascular care, International Consensus on Science, *Circulation* 102(8):98, 2000.
15. Marx JA et al: *Emergency medicine: concepts and clinical practice,* ed 5, St Louis, 2002, Mosby.
16. American Heart Association: Guidelines 2000 for cardiopulmonary resuscitation and emergency cardiovascular care, International Consensus on Science, *Circulation* 102(8):302, 2000.
17. Stothert J et al: High pressure transtracheal ventilation: the use of large-gauge intravenous-type catheters in the totally obstructed airway, *Am J Emerg Med* 8:184, 1990.

PART SIX

IN THIS PART

CHAPTER 20 Trauma Systems and Mechanism of Injury

CHAPTER 21 Hemorrhage and Shock

CHAPTER 22 Soft Tissue Trauma

CHAPTER 23 Burns

CHAPTER 24 Head and Facial Trauma

CHAPTER 25 Spinal Trauma

CHAPTER 26 Thoracic Trauma

CHAPTER 27 Abdominal Trauma

CHAPTER 28 Musculoskeletal Trauma

CHAPTER

20

Trauma Systems and Mechanism of Injury

OBJECTIVES

Upon completion of this chapter, the paramedic student will be able to:

1. Describe the incidence and scope of traumatic injuries and deaths.
2. Identify the role of each component of the trauma system.
3. Predict injury patterns based on knowledge of the laws of physics related to forces involved in trauma.
4. Describe injury patterns that should be suspected when injury occurs related to a specific type of blunt trauma.
5. Describe the role of restraints in injury prevention and injury patterns.
6. Discuss how organ motion can contribute to injury in each body region depending on the forces applied.
7. Identify selected injury patterns associated with motorcycle and all-terrain vehicle collisions.
8. Describe injury patterns associated with pedestrian collisions.
9. Identify injury patterns associated with sports injuries, blast injuries, and vertical falls.
10. Describe factors that influence tissue damage related to penetrating injury.

KEY TERMS

blunt trauma: An injury produced by the wounding forces of compression and change of speed, both of which can disrupt tissue.

cavitation: A temporary or permanent opening produced by a force that pushes body tissues laterally away from the track of a projectile.

kinematics: The process of predicting injury patterns that can result from the forces and motions of energy.

penetrating trauma: An injury produced by crushing and stretching forces of a penetrating object that results in some form of tissue disruption.

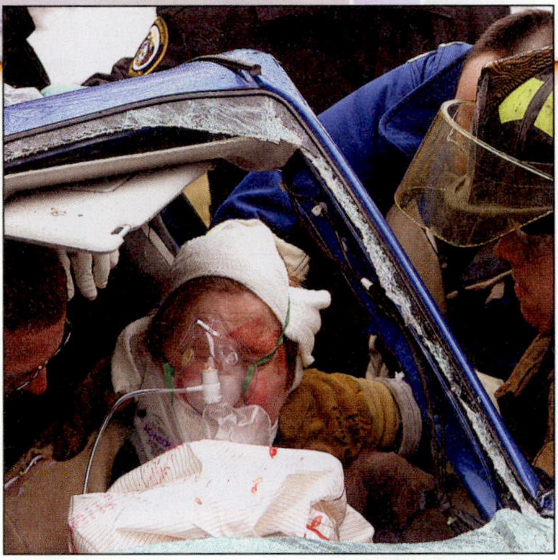

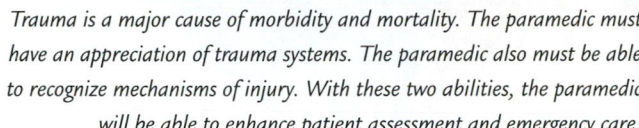

Trauma is a major cause of morbidity and mortality. The paramedic must have an appreciation of trauma systems. The paramedic also must be able to recognize mechanisms of injury. With these two abilities, the paramedic will be able to enhance patient assessment and emergency care.

EPIDEMIOLOGY OF TRAUMA

Unintentional injury is a devastating medical and social problem. Unintentional injury is the leading cause of death among persons 1 to 34 years of age and the fifth leading cause of death among all Americans.[1] Trauma deaths in 1999 were exceeded only by infection with the human immunodeficiency virus for persons 34 to 37 years of age and by heart disease, cancer, stroke, and chronic lower respiratory diseases among all other age groups. In 2001, about 98,000 unintentional injury deaths occurred in the United States. The National Safety Council estimates that the total number of unintentional injuries in the United States approaches 61 million annually. Of these injuries, 9 million are disabling, 350,000 result in permanent impairment, and 8.4 million result in permanent disabilities. The economic effect of unintentional injuries in the United States exceeds $500 billion each year.

▶**NOTE** In any given 10-minute period in the United States, 2 persons are killed. In that same time period, about 390 persons suffer a disabling injury. Costs amount to more than $9.8 million.

Trends in Trauma Deaths

Deaths from unintentional injury are increasing yearly. However, most deaths from trauma can be prevented. The increase in deaths points to the need for increased safety and health efforts to reverse the trend. Motor vehicle crashes, falls, poisoning by solids and liquids, fire and burns, and drowning have been the top five causes of trauma deaths since 1970 (Fig. 20-1).[2]

▶**NOTE** More than 3000 deaths resulted from the terrorist attacks of September 11, 2001. These deaths are not included in these statistics. They are not included because the acts were intentional.

Phases of Trauma Care

Trauma care is divided into three phases. The three phases are preincident, incident, and postincident.[3] The preincident phase refers to the prevention of intentional and unintentional trauma deaths. Paramedics and other health care professionals play a key role in this phase. A part of this phase includes taking part in public education. (For example, paramedics may educate the public on the use of personal restraint systems, motorcycle helmets, and the proper use of 911.) Paramedics also promote legislation that supports injury prevention programs. (See Chapter 3.)

The incident phase is the trauma event. The paramedic can prevent many of these events through education and by practicing personal safety. Thus the paramedic's role in this phase is to "practice what you preach" and to teach by example. The paramedic can achieve this by driving safely. The paramedic also should use personal restraint systems while on and off duty. During the incident phase, the application of active (e.g., seat belts) and passive (e.g., air bags) systems can alter the outcome of a trauma event significantly.

The postincident phase is when the paramedic uses his or her expertise and skills. (This is the delivery of emergency care to injured patients.) Important responsibilities for the paramedic in this phase include the following:

- Performing lifesaving maneuvers
- Properly preparing the patient for transportation to an appropriate medical facility
- Promptly transporting the patient to the appropriate medical facility (Box 20-1)

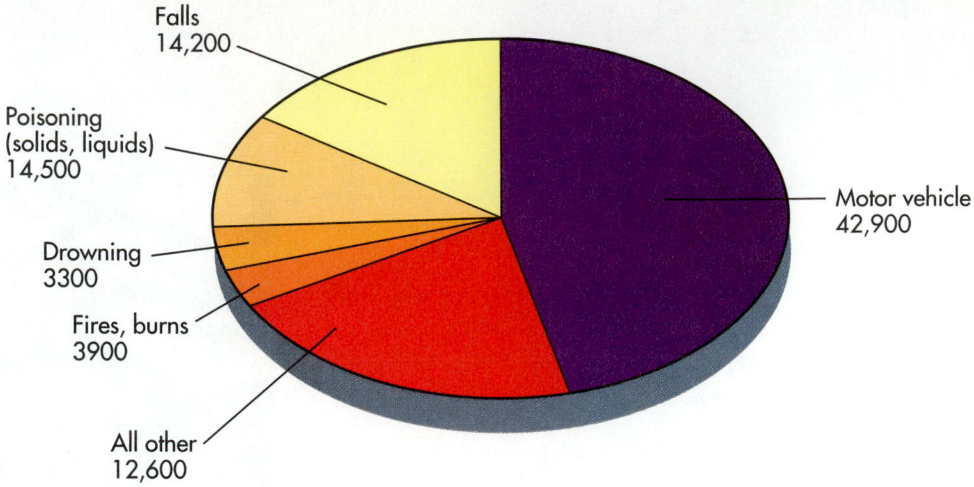

FIGURE 20-1 ■ Deaths from unintentional injury by event.

BOX 20-1 The Golden Hour

The first hour after severe injury is known as the golden hour and is a critical period. In this period, surgical intervention for the trauma patient can enhance survival and reduce complications. The paramedic must recognize patients who are in this group. The paramedic also must ensure that prehospital care does not delay patient transportation. The paramedic can best serve these patients through rapid assessment, stabilization of life-threatening injuries, and rapid transportation to an appropriate medical facility for definitive care.

The factor most critical to any severely injured patient's survival is the length of time that elapses between the incident and definitive care[3] (Box 20-2).

Trauma Systems

The eight components of a sophisticated trauma system are as follows[5]:

1. Injury prevention
2. Prehospital care, including management, transportation, and trauma triage guidelines
3. Emergency department care
4. Interfacility transportation if needed
5. Definitive care
6. Trauma critical care
7. Rehabilitation
8. Data collection and trauma registry

CRITICAL THINKING

How can you learn more about the components of the trauma system during your career as a paramedic?

The paramedic plays a crucial role in the trauma system. An aspect of this role is being involved in injury prevention programs. Another aspect includes entering appropriate patients into the trauma care system. Lastly, the paramedic fulfills this role by taking part in data collection and research. This research can influence health care improvements in caring for injured patients (Box 20-3).

Trauma Centers

As described in Chapter 1, the U.S. Department of Health and Human Services released the *Position Paper on Trauma Center Designation* in 1980. Since then, states have developed comprehensive trauma systems. More than 700 hospitals now have a designated specialty in trauma.[6]

The American Medical Association recommended categorization of hospital emergency services in the early 1970s.[7] In 1990 the Task Force of the American College of Surgeons (ACS) Committee on Trauma published *Resources for Optimal Care of the Injured Patient.* The paper described three levels of trauma centers. (The classification has since been expanded to four.) These levels are based on resources (essential and desired), admissions, staff, research, and education involvement.

A level I trauma center can provide total care for every aspect of injury. This center is qualified to care for the most severely injured patient, especially in the surgical critical care setting. The level I center is followed by level II, III, and IV facilities. Hospitals identified as trauma centers have resources needed to handle trauma patients. The assignment of category to a trauma center also enables emergency medical services providers to transport patients rapidly to the most appropriate facility. Based on ACS guidelines, some government agencies have designated certain institutions as trauma centers. Other specialized care facilities—such as pediatric trauma centers, burn centers, hyperbaric centers, and poison treatment centers—provide care for critically ill or injured patients with special needs. The ACS Committee on Trauma also established guidelines for field triage, interhospital triage to specialized care facilities, and mass casualty triage. These criteria are based on the patient's condition, mechanism of injury, injury severity indexes, and available patient care resources.

CRITICAL THINKING

Where can you find the trauma triage criteria for your area?

BOX 20-2 Prevention of Trauma Deaths

Deaths from trauma occur in three periods: immediate, early, and late. Each period presents its own unique problems.[4]

Immediate
Immediate death occurs within seconds or minutes of the injury. Lacerations of the brain, brainstem, upper spinal cord, heart, aorta, or other large vessels usually cause these deaths. Few if any patients in this category can be saved. Effective injury prevention programs are the only way to reduce the number of these deaths.

Early
The second peak of death occurs within the first 2 to 3 hours after injury. The causes of these deaths usually are major head injury, hemopneumothorax, ruptured spleen, lacerated liver, pelvic fracture, or multiple injuries associated with significant blood loss. Most of these injuries can be treated with available techniques. However, the time lapse between injury and definitive care is critical.

Late
The third peak of death occurs days or weeks after the injury. These deaths most often result from sepsis, infection, or multiple organ failure. Prehospital emergency care focused on early recognition and management of life-threatening injuries is critical to the prevention of late deaths from trauma.

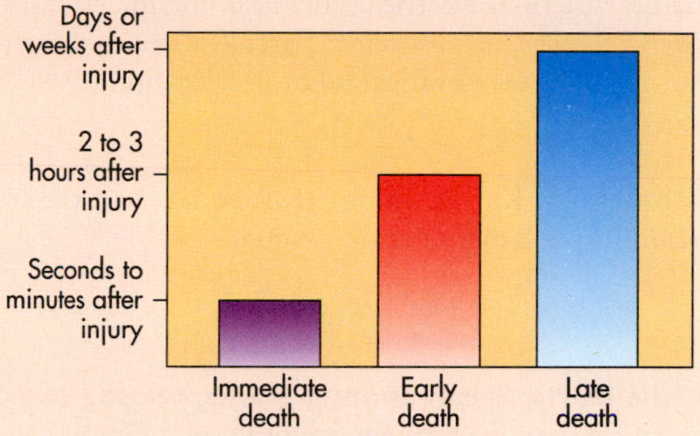

BOX 20-3 Trauma Registries

Trauma registries allow for the collection of injury data by individual hospitals or groups of hospitals on a local, regional, or state level. The American College of Surgeons funded these registries and the data collection software programs. (An example of a registry is the National Trauma Data Bank. An example of a software program is NATIONAL TRACS.) The registries and programs are meant to provide online data management. They also are intended to provide the exchange nationally of injury data for a variety of commercial registry programs. Trauma registries generate periodic standard reports. These reports offer statistical data. The data allow facilities to compare the trends and to compare other key details regarding trauma care.

Transportation Considerations

Determining the proper level of care and hospital destination is based on the patient's needs and condition. The determination also is based on the advice of medical direction. First, the paramedic determines the level of care needed and the destination facility. Then the paramedic can make decisions about the mode of transportation. (For example, the paramedic chooses between ground or air ambulance.)

GROUND TRANSPORTATION

As a rule the paramedic should use ground transportation by ambulance if the appropriate facility can be reached within a "reasonable time." Reasonable time is defined by national standards (e.g., definitive care within 60 minutes after the injury for severe trauma) and local protocol. Factors that affect the decision to use ground or air transportation include geographical location, topographical area, population, weather, availability of resources, traffic conditions, and time of day.

AEROMEDICAL TRANSPORTATION

The availability and use of aeromedical services varies throughout the United States. Aeromedical services can provide rapid response time, high-quality medical care, and rapid transportation to appropriate care facilities. Helicopters also can provide aerial surveillance of a medical scene. Helicopters also can provide transportation of additional personnel and equipment to the emergency scene. Paramedic crews should consult with medical direction and follow local protocol regarding the use of aeromedical services. (Use of aeromedical services is addressed further in Chapter 49.) The paramedic should consider air transportation in the following situations:

- The time needed to transport a patient by ground to an appropriate facility poses a threat to the patient's survival and recovery.
- Weather, road, or traffic conditions would seriously delay the patient's access to definitive care.
- Critical care personnel and equipment are needed to care for the patient adequately during transportation.

SECTION ONE
KINEMATICS

ENERGY

A transfer of energy from an external source to the human body causes injuries. The extent of injury is determined by three things: the type and amount of energy applied, how quickly the energy is applied, and the part of the body to which energy is applied.

Physical Laws

Knowledge of four basic laws of physics is required to understand the wounding forces of trauma:

1. *Newton's first law of motion.* An object, whether at rest or in motion, remains in that state unless acted upon by an outside force.
2. *Conservation of energy law.* Energy cannot be created or destroyed; it can only change form. (Energy can take mechanical, thermal, electrical, chemical, and nuclear forms.)
3. *Newton's second law of motion:* Force (F) equals mass (M) multiplied by acceleration (a) or deceleration (d).

$$F = M \times a \text{ or } F = M \times d$$

4. *Kinetic energy:* Kinetic energy (KE) equals half the mass (M) multiplied by the velocity squared (V^2).

$$KE = \frac{1}{2} m \times V^2$$

As the kinetic energy formula shows, velocity is much more critical than mass in determining total kinetic energy. For example, a car and its unrestrained 150-lb driver are traveling 60 miles per hour. According to Newton's first law of motion, the car remains in motion until acted upon by an outside force. If the driver gradually applies the brakes, the friction of the brakes slowly converts the mechanical energy of the car to thermal energy (conservation of energy law); the energy transfer occurs gradually through the slow deceleration. If the car strikes a tree, though, and is stopped instantly, the tree absorbs the mechanical energy, the car, and the driver. When the front of the car has stopped, the rear of the car continues forward until all of the energy of its motion is absorbed. The driver is traveling in the same direction and at the same speed as the car before impact. So, like the rear of the car, the driver continues forward. The driver suffers injuries in anatomical areas that strike the vehicle.

In this sequence the tree stops the motion of the front of the car. The steering column continues forward and stops against the dashboard. The driver's sternum stops against the steering column. The driver's chest cavity and its contents hit the sternum and are crushed from behind by the posterior thorax, deforming the entire chest. The kinetic energy in this example is calculated as follows:

KE = one half of the mass times the velocity squared, or

$$KE = \frac{1}{2} m \times V^2$$

$$KE = \frac{150}{2} \times 60^2$$

$$KE = 270{,}000 \text{ units of energy}$$

As shown in this calculation, the 150-lb driver traveling 60 miles per hour must change 270,000 units of kinetic energy (known as *foot-pounds,* calculated as pounds multiplied by miles per hour) into another form of energy when he or she stops. In addition, recall that force equals mass multiplied by acceleration. (That is Newton's second law of motion.) Thus the 150-lb driver is moving forward in the car with about 9000 ft-lb of force when stopped by the steering column. The energy of the motion of the body causes tissue destruction as this energy is absorbed into the body cells when the body stops. This example illustrates the principle. However, the actual total force also is determined by the true rate of deceleration, or "g" force, and several other factors. Lap and shoulder restraints and air bags increase the distance over which the body stops its movement. This can decrease the deceleration force a great deal.

> **CRITICAL THINKING**
>
> Can you apply these same four laws of physics to another traumatic situation, such as a fall onto concrete? What force is applied? What factors influence the kinetic energy?

Kinematics

Kinematics is the process of predicting injury patterns. Specific types and patterns of injuries are associated with certain mechanisms. In addition to individual factors (such as age) and protective factors (such as restraint systems, helmets, and air bags), the paramedic should consider the following when evaluating the trauma patient:

- Mechanism of injury
- Force of energy applied
- Anatomy
- Energy (for example, mass; velocity; distance; and thermal, electrical, and chemical forms)

SECTION TWO
BLUNT TRAUMA

BLUNT TRAUMA

Blunt trauma is an injury produced by the wounding forces of compression and change of speed (usually deceleration). These forces can disrupt tissue. Direct compression is the pressure on a structure and is the most common type of force applied in blunt trauma. The amount of injury depends on the length of time of compression, the force of compression, and the area compressed. For example, compression of the thorax can lead to rib fracture or pneumothorax. Other compression injuries include contusions and lacerations of solid organs and rupture of hollow (air-filled) organs.

Acceleration is an increase in the velocity of a moving object. Deceleration is a decrease in the velocity of a moving object. Both can produce major injury. For example, consider a car that comes to a stop abruptly. The occupant's body continues its constant velocity after the impact until it decelerates as a result of striking the steering wheel, restraint system, or dashboard. The external aspect of the body is stopped forcibly. However, the contents of the cranial, thoracic, and peritoneal cavities remain in motion because of inertia. As a result, tissues can be stretched, crushed, ruptured, lacerated, or sheared from their points of attachment. Examples of injuries caused by a change of speed include concussion, cardiac or pulmonary contusion, organ laceration, and aortic tear.

Motor Vehicle Collision

The various injuries produced by blunt trauma are illustrated best through examination of vehicle collisions. Forces that cause blunt trauma, however, can result from a variety of impacts. As described in the previous example, a vehicle collision involves three separate impacts as the energy is transferred. In the first impact, the vehicle strikes an object. In the second, the occupant collides with the inside of the car. In the third, the internal organs collide inside the body. The injuries that result depend on the type of collision and the position of the occupant inside the vehicle. The injuries also depend on the use or nonuse of active or passive restraint systems.

A vehicle collision is classified by the type of impact: head-on, lateral, rear-end, rotational, and rollover. The forces of compression and change of speed produce predictable injury patterns in each type of collision.

HEAD-ON (FRONTAL) IMPACT

Head-on collisions result when forward motion stops abruptly. (For example, one vehicle collides with another one traveling in the opposite direction.) The first collision occurs when the vehicle hits the second vehicle, resulting in damage to the front of the car. As the vehicle abruptly stops, the occupant continues to move at the speed of the vehicle before impact. The front seat occupant continues forward into the restraint system, steering column, or dashboard. This results in the second collision. The occupant who is not restrained usually travels in one of two pathways in relationship to the dashboard. The two pathways are down-and-under or up-and-over. The precise course of this pathway determines how the organs collide inside the body and the extent of tissue damaged.

In the down-and-under pathway the occupant travels downward into the vehicle seat and forward into the dashboard or steering column (Fig. 20-2). The knees become the leading part of the body, striking the dashboard. The upper legs absorb most of the impact. Predictable injuries include knee dislocation, patellar fracture, femoral fracture, fracture or posterior dislocation of the hip, fracture of the acetabulum, vascular injury, and hemorrhage. After the initial impact of the knees into the dashboard, the body rotates forward. As the chest wall hits the steering column or dashboard, the head and torso absorb energy as indicated in the description of the up-and-over pathway.

CRITICAL THINKING

How does the use of lap and shoulder restraints influence the patterns of injury described here?

In the up-and-over pathway the body in forward motion strikes the steering wheel. As this occurs, the ribs and underlying structures absorb the momentum of the thorax (Fig. 20-3). Predictable injuries from this transfer of energy include rib fracture, ruptured diaphragm, hemopneumothorax, pulmonary contusion, cardiac contusion, myocardial rupture, and vascular disruption (most notably aortic rupture).

If the abdomen is the point of impact, compression injuries can occur to the hollow abdominal organs, solid organs, and lumbar vertebrae. The kidneys, liver, and spleen are subject to vascular tears from supporting tissue. Such injuries may include the tearing of renal vessels from their points of attachment to the inferior vena cava and descending aorta. Predictable injuries include liver laceration, spleen rupture, internal hemorrhage, and abdominal organ incursion into the thorax (ruptured diaphragm).

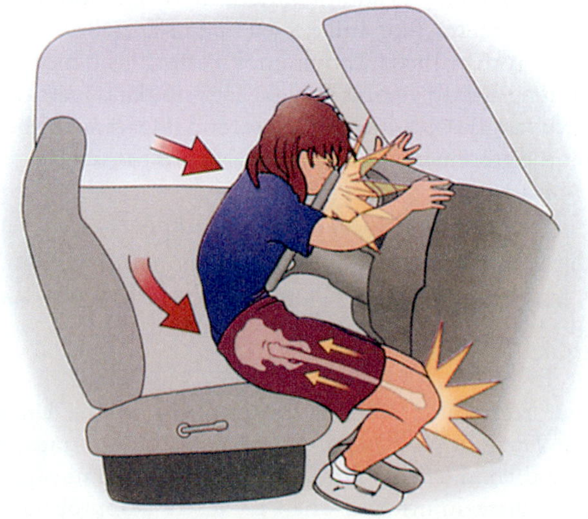

FIGURE 20-2 ■ Down-and-under pathway.

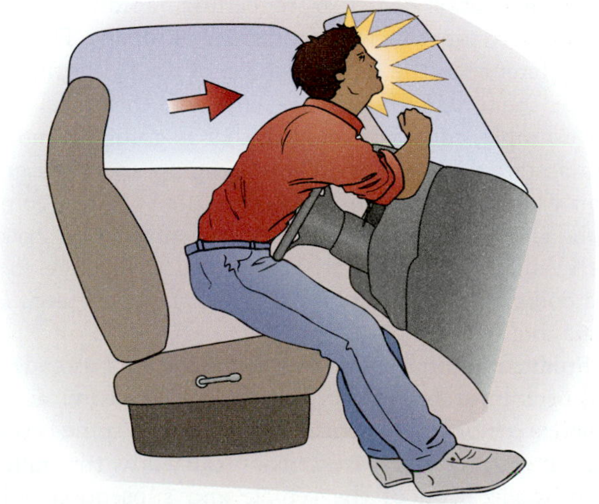

FIGURE 20-3 ■ Up-and-over pathway.

If the head absorbs most of the impact, the cervical vertebrae take up the continued momentum of the body. Cervical flexion, axial loading, and hyperextension (further described in Chapter 25) can result in fracture or dislocation of the cervical vertebrae. In addition, severe angulation of the cervical vertebrae can damage the soft tissues of the neck. This may cause spinal cord injury and spinal instability, even without fracture. Other predictable injuries include trauma to the brain (e.g., concussion, contusion, shearing injury, and edema) and disruption of vessels inside the head (intracranial vascular disruption), resulting in subdural or epidural hematoma.

LATERAL IMPACT

Lateral impact occurs when a vehicle is struck from the side. Injury patterns depend on whether the damaged vehicle remains in place or moves away from the point of impact. The external shell of a vehicle that remains in place after impact usually intrudes into the passenger compartment and usually directs force at the lateral aspect of the person's body. Predictable injuries result from compression to the torso, pelvis, and extremities. Examples of these injuries include fractured ribs, pulmonary contusion, ruptured liver or spleen (depending on the side involved), fractured clavicle, fractured pelvis, and head and neck injury. Vehicles that have side-impact air bags can guard against injury in some lateral impacts.

If the damaged vehicle moves away from the point of impact, the occupant accelerates away from the point of impact. The occupant moves laterally with the car. The effects of inertia on the head, neck, and thorax produce lateral flexion and rotation of the cervical spine. This movement can result in neurological injury. Such movement also can result in tears or strains of the lateral ligaments and supporting structures of the neck. Injuries also can occur on the side of the passenger opposite the impact as the occupant is propelled toward the other side of the car. If other occupants are in the vehicle, secondary collision with other passengers is likely.

REAR-END IMPACT

A vehicle that is struck from behind rapidly accelerates, causing it to move forward under the occupant. The greater the difference in the forward speed of the two vehicles, the greater the force and damaging energy of the initial impact. For example, consider a vehicle that is going 50 mph and hits a stationary vehicle. The damaging energy is greater than when a vehicle going 50 mph hits a vehicle going 30 mph. Thus in forward collisions, the sum of the speeds of both vehicles is the velocity that produces damage. In rear-end collisions the difference between the two speeds is the damaging velocity.

Predictable injuries in rear-end collisions include back and neck injuries and cervical strain or fracture caused by hyperextension. The cervical portion of the spine is susceptible to secondary hyperextension caused by the rapid forward acceleration of the vehicle and subsequent relative rearward movement of the occupant. If the vehicle collides with an object in front of it, the paramedic should suspect injuries associated with frontal impact.

ROTATIONAL IMPACT

Rotational impacts occur when an off-center portion of the vehicle (usually the front quarter) strikes an immovable object or one that is moving more slowly or in the opposite direction. The part of the vehicle striking the object stops during impact. The rest of the vehicle continues in forward motion until the energy is transformed completely. The occupant moves inside the vehicle with the forward motion. The occupant usually is struck by the side of the car as the vehicle rotates around the point of impact. A rotational impact results in injuries common to head-on and lateral collisions.

ROLLOVER ACCIDENTS

In rollover crashes or collisions the person tumbles inside the vehicle. The occupant is injured wherever his or her body strikes the vehicle. The various impacts occur at many different angles, which can cause multiple-system injuries. Predicting injury patterns from rollover collisions is difficult. These crashes can produce any of the injury patterns that are associated with other types of collisions.

RESTRAINTS

In recent years, public awareness programs and various state laws have increased the use of personal restraints. According to the National Safety Council, among passenger vehicle occupants over 4 years of age, seat belts saved an estimated 11,899 lives in 2000. Another 9238 lives could have been saved if *all* passengers over 4 years of age had worn seat belts. At this time, all states and the District of Columbia have child safety seat laws. Forty-nine states and the District of Columbia have mandatory seat belt use laws in effect (the one exception is New Hampshire).

A serious hazard to unrestrained occupants is ejection from the vehicle after impact. Among crashes in which a fatality occurred in 2000, only 10% of restrained passenger car occupants were ejected, compared with 22% of those who were unrestrained.[2,7] In addition, 1 of every 13 ejection victims suffers a spinal fracture, and ejected victims are killed 6 times more often than those who are not ejected.[3] The mortality rate among ejected victims is high. This results in part from the occupant being subjected to a second impact as the body strikes the ground or another object outside the vehicle.

> **CRITICAL THINKING**
>
> How can you apply this knowledge about ejection statistics to your practice in each of the phases of trauma care (preincident, incident, and postincident)?

Four restraining systems are available in the United States. These are lap belts, diagonal shoulder straps, air bags, and child safety seats. All of these restraints significantly reduce injuries. If they are used inappropriately, however, these protective devices also can produce injuries.

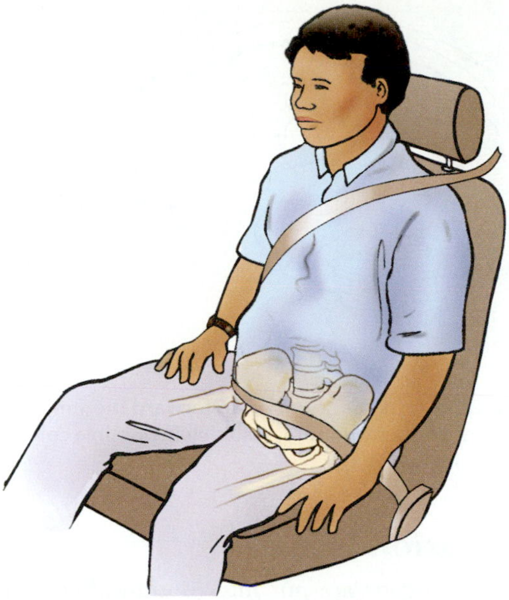

FIGURE 20-4 ■ Properly positioned seat belt.

Lap Belts

The lap belt, used alone or with a shoulder strap, is the most commonly used active restraint system. A person should direct the lap belt at a 45-degree angle to the floor between the anterior-superior iliac spine and the femur (Fig. 20-4). A lap belt worn tightly enough to stay in this position absorbs energy forces. The belt protects the abdominal cavity by transferring energy to the strong, bony pelvis.

However, the lap belt often is worn incorrectly. If the lap belt is worn above the anterior-iliac spine, the forward motion of the body during impact is absorbed by vertebrae T12, L1, and L2. As the thorax is propelled forward, the abdominal organs are compressed between the vertebral column and the lap belt. This compression can cause injury to the liver, spleen, duodenum, and pancreas. A sign of these abdominal injuries is abrasions or a lap belt imprint over the abdomen.

Major injury can result even when a person uses a lap belt correctly. These injuries occur from angulation of the lumbar spine, pelvis, thorax, and head around the restraint system. Injuries also occur from failure of the restraint system to decrease the impact forces. Injuries that can occur during high-speed impacts include sternal fractures, chest wall injuries, lumbar vertebral fractures, head injuries, and maxillofacial trauma.

Diagonal Shoulder Straps

Use of a shoulder strap helps absorb the forward motion of the thorax after impact. When a person wears the shoulder strap with the lap belt, the shoulder strap prevents the thorax, face, and head from striking the dashboard, windshield, or steering column. Clavicular fracture can result from the position of the shoulder strap. Organ collision inside the body with resultant internal organ injury, cervical fracture, and spinal cord injury still can occur during high-speed impacts, even when personal restraint systems are used.

Air Bags

Some vehicles are equipped with side-impact air bags to protect against lateral impacts. However, the more common air bag is a frontal air bag that inflates from the center of the steering wheel and from the dashboard during frontal impact. These devices cushion the forward motion of the occupant when used with a lap and shoulder belt. Frontal air bags deflate rapidly. They are effective only with initial frontal and near-frontal collisions. They are ineffective in multiple collisions, rear-impact collisions, and lateral or rollover impacts. These systems do not prevent movement in the down-and-under pathway. Thus the occupant's knees still may be the point of impact. This may result in leg, pelvis, and abdominal injuries.

An air bag can produce significant injury if it is deployed in proximity (10 inches or closer) to the occupant. Deployment in these situations can produce spinal fractures, hand and eye injury, and facial and forearm abrasions. The following groups are at higher risk of injury from air bag deployment[8]:

- Infants and children less than 12 years of age
- Adults of short stature (less than 5 ft 2 in)
- Older adults
- Persons with special medical conditions

Most air bag injuries are minor cuts, bruises, or abrasions. Most of these injuries are far less serious than the head, neck, and chest injuries that air bags prevent. However, 146 air bag–related deaths have been reported by the National Highway Traffic Safety Administration as of October 1999. Most of these deaths occurred as a result of the occupant being too close to the air bag when it deployed. This problem occurred more commonly from the child not being restrained adequately with lap/shoulder devices or child safety seats during precrash braking. To protect against injury from air bag deployment, the driver of the vehicle should be positioned at least 10 inches from the air bag cover; the front seat passenger should be positioned at least 18 inches away from the air bag cover; and children under 12 years of age should always ride in the back seat and be in the proper restraint device for their size.

Child Safety Seats

The leading cause of death in children under 4 years of age is injuries sustained in motor vehicle crashes. For each of these deaths, the U.S. Department of Health, Education, and Welfare estimates that thousands more suffer debilitating injury. The National Safety Council reports that an estimated 4816 lives have been saved by child restraints from 1975 through 2000, with 316 lives saved in 2000 alone.

Child safety seats come in several shapes and sizes. This variety accommodates the different stages of physical development. These seats include infant carriers, booster seats, and toddler seats. Child safety seats use a combination of lap belts, shoulder belts, full-body harnesses, and harness-and-shield apparatus to protect the child during vehicle collision. Predictable injuries likely to occur even with the appropriate use of child safety seats include blunt

BOX 20-4 Transportation of Children in an Ambulance

Although no formal regulations have been established, it is recommended that child safety seats be available in emergency vehicles. In addition to practicing safe driving in all patient transports, the paramedic should observe the following guidelines.*

The method or device used to secure children during transport must provide effective restraint without compromising the safety of others on board.

Younger children and infants who do not require spinal immobilization should be transported in child safety seats appropriate for their size. If an appropriate safety seat is not available, the paramedic should ask to borrow one from family members (preferably one that has not been in a motor vehicle collision).

Any time a child is secured to a device such as a safety seat or spine board, the paramedic must ensure that the device is secured to the stretcher.

For any patient where medically appropriate, position the patient on the stretcher with the back of the stretcher placed upright at least at a 45-degree angle. This angle optimizes transportation safety in the event of an impact or deceleration.

If the child is secured in a safety seat, the seat should be secured to the stretcher using at least two belts placed at a 90-degree angle to each other; that is, one strap oriented vertically the other strap oriented horizontally to secure the child seat to the upright stretcher. A child safety seat secured to the stretcher with the stretcher back in the upright position has performed well in the crash testing conducted to date.

Restraint systems applied to a flat stretcher are less secure in a crash. If a suboptimal restraint technique such as this must be used, the paramedic should notify the driver to exert additional caution during transport to minimize the risk.

Older children who do not require special positioning should be secured on a stretcher that has had the back elevated to an angle of at least 45 degrees.

The paramedic should use shoulder harnesses to restrain patients who must be immobilized in the supine position on a backboard and therefore cannot have the back of the stretcher elevated for protection. The paramedic should *never* secure the parent and child together on the stretcher. The paramedic also should *never* allow infants or young children to ride in the arms or lap of a parent or rescuer.

*The Center for Pediatric Emergency Medicine: Teaching resource for instructors in prehospital pediatrics for paramedics: safe transport of children. http://www.cpem.org/trippals/38TRANSP.PDF. Accessed March 16, 2004.

abdominal trauma, change-of-speed injuries from deceleration forces, and neck and spinal injury. A large amount of misuse of child safety seats occurs. (For example, common issues include location, installation, and strapping.) Public education on the correct use of child safety seats is a key prevention measure. For information on transporting children in an ambulance, see Box 20-4.

ORGAN COLLISION INJURIES

Organs can be injured as a result of movement caused by deceleration and compression forces. The paramedic must maintain a high degree of suspicion regarding injuries to organs based on the principles of kinematics.

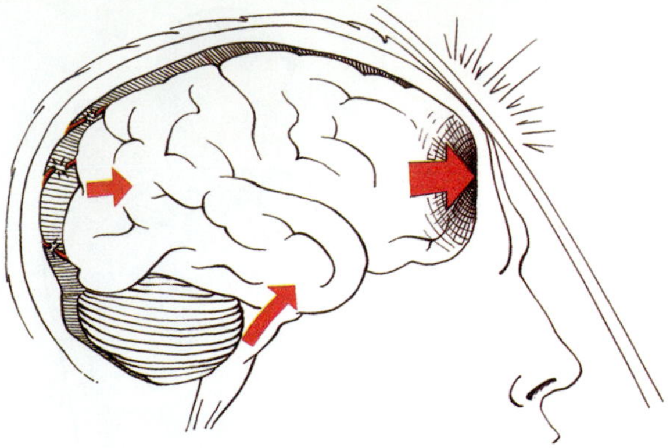

FIGURE 20-5 ■ After cessation of forward motion of the skull, the brain continues its motion, resulting in possible contusion and intracerebral hemorrhage.

Deceleration Injuries

When body organs are put into motion after an impact, they continue to move. They move in opposition to the structures that attach them to the body. Thus a risk exists of separation of body organs from their attachments. Injury to the vascular pedicle or mesenteric attachment can lead to brisk or exsanguinating hemorrhage.

HEAD INJURIES

When the head strikes a stationary object, the cranium comes to an abrupt stop. However, brain tissue inside the cranium continues to move. The brain moves until it is compressed against the skull (Fig. 20-5). This movement can cause brain tissue to be bruised, crushed, or lacerated. Such movement also can cause blood vessels attached to the brain and skull to be torn, producing intracranial hemorrhage. Other injuries associated with deceleration of the head include central nervous system injury, caused by stretching of the spinal cord and its attachments, and cervical fracture.

THORACIC INJURIES

The aorta often is injured by severe deceleration forces. The aorta is affixed at several points. Proximally the aorta is affixed by the aortic valve in the descending portion of the aorta arch by the ligamentum arteriosum. The descending aorta also is attached to the thoracic spine. As the thorax hits a stationary object, the heart and aorta continue in motion. This motion is in opposition to their attachment at the lower end of the aortic arch. The aorta usually is sheared at the level of its ligamentum arteriosum attachment (Fig. 20-6). Frank rupture of the aorta leads to rapid exsanguination. However, transection and dissection through to the internal lining (intima and media of the aorta) can tamponade. This can allow patients to arrive at an emergency department and survive the injury.

ABDOMINAL INJURIES

When deceleration forces are applied to the abdomen, intraabdominal organs and retroperitoneal structures (most commonly the kidneys) are affected. The forward motion of the kidneys can shear them away from their vascular

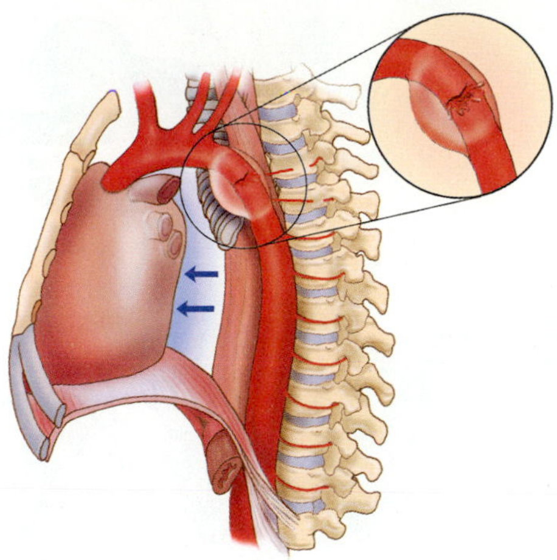

FIGURE 20-6 ■ Shearing forces along the descending aorta move in opposition to the attachments at the lower end of the aortic arch.

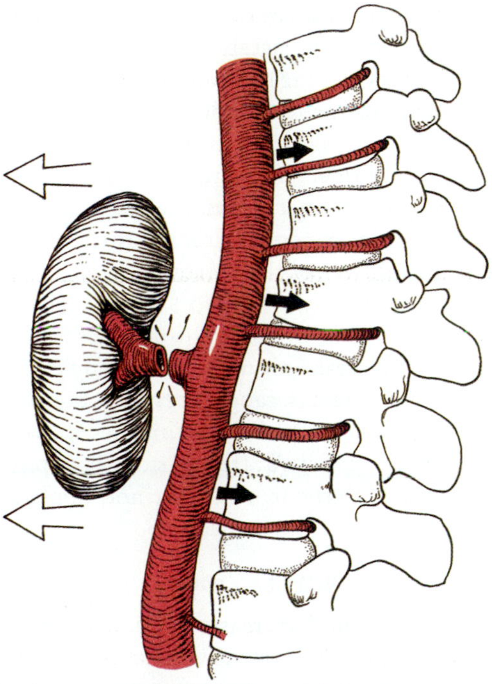

FIGURE 20-7 ■ Forward motion of the kidney can cause separation at its midpoint from its vascular pedicle.

pedicle attachments (Fig. 20-7). The forward motion of the small and large intestines can result in mesenteric tears. The downward and forward motion of the liver can cause separation at its midpoint from its vascular and hepatic duct pedicle. The spleen is restrained by the diaphragm and abdominal wall attachments. The forward motion of the spleen can result in a tear of the splenic capsule.

Compression Injuries

Compressive forces can injure any portion of the body. This discussion is limited to injuries of the head, thorax, and abdomen.

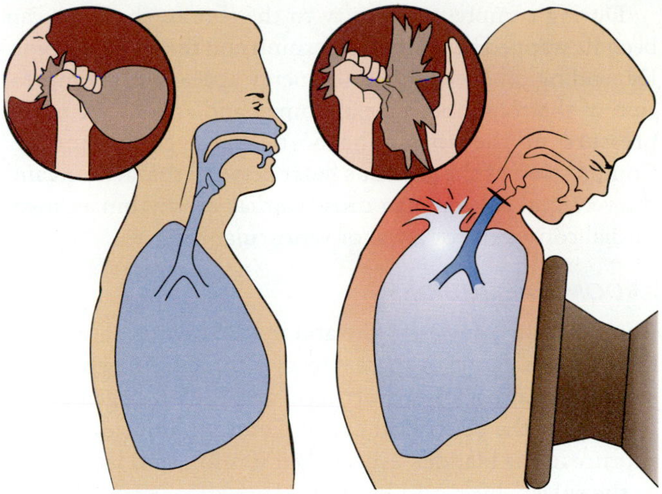

FIGURE 20-8 ■ In a crash or collision, the lungs are similar to an air-filled paper bag held tightly at the neck and compressed with the other hand. Thoracic compression against the closed glottis causes the lungs to pop.

HEAD INJURIES

Compression injuries to the head can result in open fractures, closed fractures, and bone fragment penetration (depressed skull fracture). Associated injuries include brain contusion and lacerations of brain tissue. Compression forces to the skull also can produce hemorrhage from fractured bone, meningeal vessels, or the brain itself. If facial structures are involved in the injury, soft tissue trauma and facial bone fractures can occur (see Chapter 24). The paramedic also should consider central nervous system injury. The paramedic should assume cervical fracture when evaluating injuries to the head. Compression injury to the vertebral bodies can result in compression fracture, hyperextension, and hyperflexion injury.

THORACIC INJURIES

Compression injury to the thorax often involves the lungs and heart. Associated injuries to external structures include fractured ribs and sternum, which can lead to an unstable chest wall, open pneumothorax, or both.

A serious lung injury that can occur from compression forces is called the paper bag effect. This injury occurs when increased intrathoracic pressure causes rupture of the lungs. For example, a driver of a car is threatened by an approaching vehicle. The driver notes the potential collision. Thus the driver instinctively takes a deep breath and holds it. This protective inhalation fills the lungs (paper bag) with air against the closed glottis and creates a closed container (Fig. 20-8). As the thorax strikes the steering column, the inward motion of the chest wall causes an increase in lung pressure. This increased pressure results in alveolar rupture (as when a hand strikes the paper bag). This phenomenon is thought to be the cause of most pneumothoraces after vehicle trauma.[9] Penetration of a fractured rib through the pleura and laceration of the lung also contribute to pneumothorax after blunt trauma to the chest.

During compression injury to the thorax, the heart can become trapped between the sternum and the thoracic spine. Depending on the amount of energy applied, the compression of the contents of the abdomen and an increase in the pressure in the aorta, the aortic valve could rupture. Compression of the patient's heart between the sternum and the vertebral column can cause cardiac dysrhythmias, myocardial contusion, or atrial or ventricular rupture.

ABDOMINAL INJURIES

Compression injuries to the abdominal cavity can have serious effects. Some of these effects include solid organ rupture, vascular organ hemorrhage, and hollow organ perforation into the peritoneal cavity. Common injuries include rupture of the bladder, especially if it is full, and lacerations to the spleen, liver, and kidneys.

Just as the paper bag effect produces a pneumothorax in thoracic injury, compression of the abdominal cavity can cause increases in intraabdominal pressure. This increase in pressure can exceed the tensile strength (resistance to lengthwise stretch) of the walls of hollow organs or the diaphragm. Predictable injuries include rupture or herniation of the diaphragm and rupture of hollow organs such as the gallbladder, urinary bladder, duodenum, colon, stomach, and small bowel.

OTHER MOTORIZED VEHICULAR COLLISIONS

Injuries from other motorized vehicular collisions include those involving motorcycles, all-terrain vehicles (ATVs), snowmobiles, motorboats, water bikes, jet skis, and farm machinery. This text deals with only motorcycles and ATVs because of their common recreational use and popularity. According to the National Highway Traffic Safety Administration, about 55,000 motorcycle riders and passengers are injured each year. More than 2000 die from their injuries.

Small motorized vehicles are thought to be more dangerous than other motor vehicles because they offer little protection to the rider. They offer minimum protection from the transfer of energy associated with collisions. The injuries from small motor vehicle crashes usually are more severe than those from car crashes. As with other types of motor vehicle collision, predictable injuries depend on the type of collision that occurs.

Motorcycle Collision

Common motorcycle collisions result from impact that is head-on or at an angle. They also result from laying the motorcycle down.

HEAD-ON IMPACT

The center of gravity of a motorcycle is above the front axle, forward of the rider's seat. When the motorcycle strikes an object that stops its forward motion, the rest of the bike and the rider continue forward until acted on by an outside force. Usually, the motorcycle tips forward. At that point, the rider is propelled over the handlebars. Secondary impacts with the handlebars or other objects stop the forward motion of the rider. Predictable injuries caused by these secondary impacts include head and neck trauma and compression injuries to the chest and abdomen. If the feet remain on the foot rests during impact, the midshaft of the femur absorbs the rider's forward motion (Fig. 20-9). This can result in bilateral fractures to the femur and lower leg. Severe perineal injuries can result if the rider's groin strikes the tank or handlebars of the motorcycle.

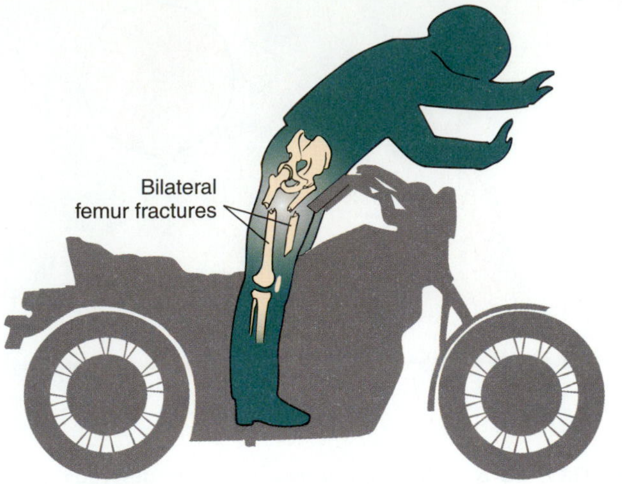

FIGURE 20-9 ■ Head-on impact motorcycle collision.

ANGULAR IMPACT

A motorcycle may strike an object at an angle. When this occurs, the rider often is caught between the motorcycle and the second object. Predictable injuries include crush-type injuries to the patient's affected side. Examples of such are open fractures to the femur, tibia, and fibula and fracture and dislocation of the malleolus.

LAYING THE MOTORCYCLE DOWN

Professional racers and recreational riders often use the strategy of laying the motorcycle down before striking an object. This protective maneuver separates the rider from the motorcycle and the object. The maneuver allows the rider to slide away from the bike. Predictable injuries include massive abrasions (road rash) and fractures to the affected side as the rider slides on the ground or pavement (Fig. 20-10). These injuries can be severe. However, they usually are less serious than those that occur from other types of impacts.

All-Terrain Vehicles

Injuries from crashes involving ATVs are different from those seen in motorcycle collisions. All-terrain vehicles have a higher center of gravity than motorcycles. They also have a large, flat front tire that makes them difficult to steer. A specific balance different than that required for riding motorcycles or bicycles is necessary to keep the ATV from overturning.

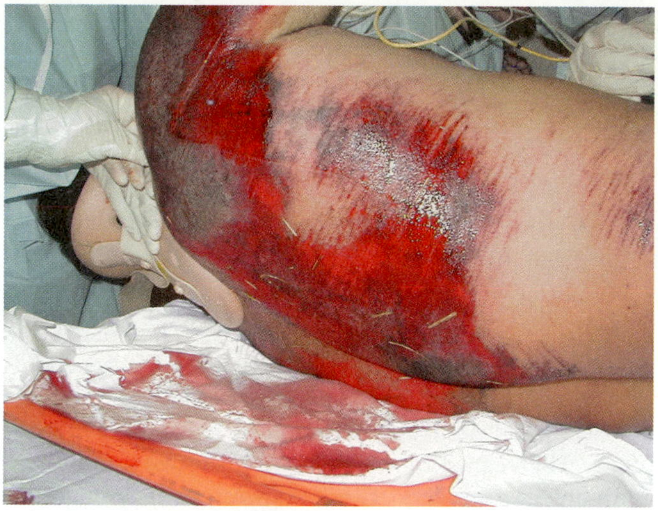

FIGURE 20-10 ■ Road rash (abrasions).

A natural tendency is for the rider to put a foot down to support the ATV when stopping. This can lead to the rear tire running over the rider's foot, catching the leg, and throwing the rider forward off the vehicle and onto his or her shoulder or crushing the rider. Predictable injuries from ATV collisions include extremity injury and fracture, clavicular fracture, and serious head and neck injuries.

Personal Protective Equipment

Protective equipment for riders of small motor vehicles includes boots, leather clothing, eye protection, and helmets. Helmets are structured to absorb the energy of an impact, thereby reducing injuries to the face, skull, and brain, and are estimated to be 29% effective in preventing fatal injuries.[1] Nonuse of helmets increases head injuries by more than 300%.[3]

PEDESTRIAN INJURIES

In 2001, 90,000 persons were injured in auto-pedestrian collisions in the United States. Of those injuries, 5800 were fatal.[1] All collisions of this nature can cause serious injuries. They require a high degree of suspicion for multiple-system trauma.

Three main mechanisms of injury (multiple impacts) exist in auto-pedestrian collisions. The first impact occurs when the bumper of the vehicle strikes the body. The second occurs as the pedestrian strikes the hood of the vehicle. The third occurs when the pedestrian strikes the ground or another object.

Predictable injuries depend on whether the pedestrian is an adult or a child. Variations in the height of the pedestrian in relation to the bumper and hood of the car affect the injury pattern. The velocity of the vehicle also is a major factor. However, even low speeds can result in serious trauma because of the mass of the vehicle and the transfer of energy. Another consideration in evaluating an auto-pedestrian collision is the possibility the patient may have been hit by another vehicle.

Adult Pedestrian

Most adult pedestrians who are threatened by an oncoming vehicle try to protect themselves by turning away from the vehicle. Therefore injuries often are a result of lateral or posterior impacts. During the initial impact, the adult usually is struck by the vehicle bumper in the lower legs. This often produces lower-extremity fractures.

The second impact occurs as the pedestrian falls toward the hood of the vehicle. This impact can result in fractures to the femur, pelvis, thorax, and spine. The impact also can produce intraabdominal or intrathoracic injury. In addition, the head and spine can be injured if the victim strikes the hood or windshield.

The third impact occurs as the victim strikes the ground or is thrown against another object. This can result in serious damage to the hip and shoulder of the affected side as the body makes contact with the landing surface. Sudden deceleration and compression forces are associated with this impact. These forces can cause fractures, internal hemorrhage, and head and spinal injury.

Child Pedestrian

As noted, adults try to protect themselves from auto-pedestrian injury. However, children tend to face the oncoming vehicle. Therefore their injuries often are the result of a frontal impact. Because children are smaller than most adults, the initial impact of the vehicle occurs higher on the body. Impact usually occurs above the knees or pelvis. Predictable injuries from the initial impact include fractures to the femur and pelvic girdle and internal hemorrhage.

The second impact occurs as the front of the hood of the vehicle continues forward, making contact with the victim's thorax. The victim instantly is thrown backward, forcing the head and neck to flex forward. Depending on the position of the patient in relation to the vehicle, the child's head and neck may contact the hood of the vehicle. Predictable injuries include abdominopelvic and thoracic trauma, facial trauma, and head and neck injury.

The third impact occurs as the child is thrown downward to the ground or another landing surface. Because of the child's smaller size and weight, the child can fall under the vehicle and be dragged for some distance. The child also can fall to the side of the vehicle and be run over by the front or rear wheels. Predictable injuries consist of those previously described and may include traumatic amputation.

OTHER CAUSES OF BLUNT TRAUMA

Other causes of blunt trauma include sports injuries, vertical falls, and blast injuries.

Sports Injuries

Persons of all ages take part in sports. Sports that often are associated with injuries include contact sports, such as football, basketball, hockey, and wrestling; high-velocity sports, such as downhill skiing, water skiing, bicycling, rollerblading, and skateboarding; racquet sports; and water sports, such as swimming and diving. Sports offer a range of health benefits. However, they also can produce severe injury.

Injuries related to sports are caused by forces of acceleration and deceleration, compression, twisting, hyperextension, and hyperflexion. The paramedic can use the general principles of kinematics to predict injuries by determining the following:

- What energy forces were transferred to the patient?
- To what part of the body was the energy transferred?
- What associated injuries should be considered as a result of the energy transfer?
- How sudden was the acceleration or deceleration?
- Was compression, twisting, hyperextension, or hyperflexion involved in the injury?

CRITICAL THINKING

Injuries related to sports often occur outside. What other considerations will you have for patient care based on the environment?

If the patient used protective equipment, the paramedic should evaluate it. This will help the paramedic determine the mechanism of injury. For example, the condition and structural stability of a helmet can provide clues as to the amount of energy transferred to the patient during the injury. Other examples include broken skis, broken hockey sticks, and structural deformities of bicycles.

Blast Injuries

Blast injury is damage to a patient who is exposed to a pressure field that is produced by an explosion of volatile substances. Explosions of this nature mainly have been a wartime concern. However, in recent years the number of blast injuries has increased. These result from homemade bombs used in social protests and terrorist activities. Other causes include exploding car batteries, industrial use of volatile substances, chemical reactions in clandestine drug laboratories, explosions in mining, and transportation incidents or crashes involving hazardous materials.

CRITICAL THINKING

In all incidents related to blast injury, what is your first consideration on the scene?

Blasts release large amounts of energy. This energy is in the form of pressure and heat. If this release of energy is confined in a casing (e.g., a bomb), the pressure ruptures the casing and ejects fragments of the housing at a high velocity. The remaining energy is transmitted to the surrounding environment. This energy can severely injure bystanders. Blast injuries are classified as *primary, secondary, tertiary,* and *miscellaneous* (Fig. 20-11).

PRIMARY BLAST INJURIES

Primary blast injuries result from sudden changes in environmental pressure. These injuries usually occur in gas-containing organs. The most severe damage occurs when poorly supported tissue is displaced beyond its elastic limit. The organs and tissues most vulnerable to primary blast injury are the ears, lungs, central nervous system, and gastrointestinal tract. Predictable damage to these areas includes hearing loss, pulmonary hemorrhage, cerebral air embolism, abdominal hemorrhage, and bowel perforation. Thermal burns also can result from the release of energy in the form of heat. These injuries are likely to occur on unprotected areas that are close to the source of explosion (see Chapter 23). (For example, thermal burns might occur on the face and hands.) In closed spaces, because of blast reflection, victims farther from the explosion may be injured as severely as those close to the explosion.

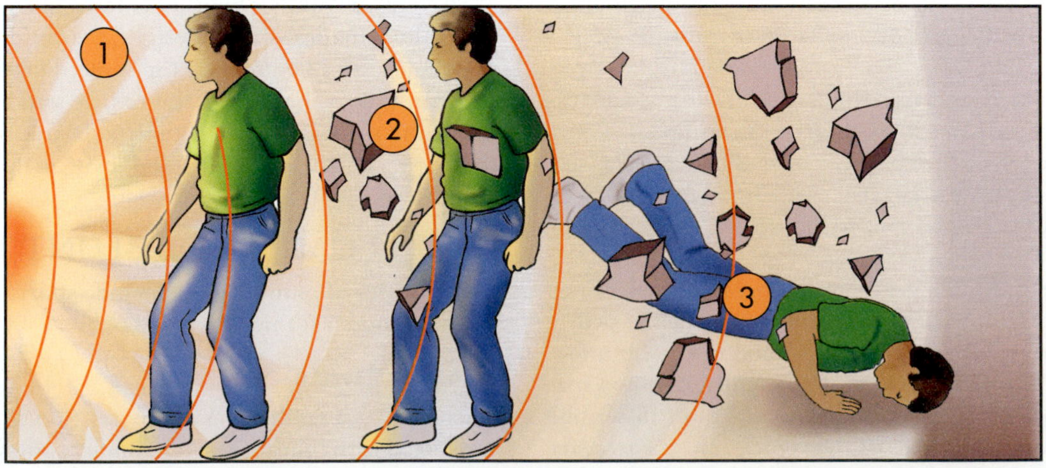

FIGURE 20-11 ■ Three phases of injury occur during a blast. First, the pressure wave strikes the patient. Then flying debris can produce injury. In the third phase, the patient is thrown and is injured after impact with the ground or other objects.

SECONDARY BLAST INJURIES

Secondary blast injuries usually result when bystanders are struck by flying debris. (Examples of such debris include glass, metal, or falling mortar.) Obvious injuries are lacerations and fractures. Flying debris also can cause high-velocity missile-type injuries. This type of injury can result if nails, screws, or casing fragments are part of the debris.

TERTIARY BLAST INJURIES

Tertiary blast injuries occur when victims are propelled through space by an explosion and strike a stationary object. These injuries are similar to those from vertical falls. They also are similar to those from ejections from cars or small motor vehicles. In most cases, the sudden deceleration from the impact causes more damage than the acceleration through space because the deceleration is more sudden. Injuries from these forces include damage to the abdominal viscera, central nervous system, and musculoskeletal system.

MISCELLANEOUS BLAST INJURIES

Miscellaneous blast injuries result from radiation exposure and inhalation of dust and toxic gases (further described in Chapter 53). Predictable injuries include those to the eyes, lungs, and soft tissues.

Vertical Falls

Falls accounted for 14,200 deaths in 2001 and were the second leading cause of accidental death in the United States.[1] In predicting injuries associated with falls, the paramedic should evaluate three things: the distance fallen, the body position of the patient on impact, and the type of landing surface struck. Injuries associated with vertical falls are a result of deceleration and compression. More than half of all falls occur in homes; nearly four out of five involve a person 65 years of age or older.

Falls from some levels rarely are associated with fatal injury. However, falls from distances greater than 3 times the height of an individual (15 to 20 feet) are more likely to be associated with severe injuries. As a point of reference for these distances, the roof of a one-story house is about 15 feet from the ground, and the roof of a two-story house is about 30 feet from the ground.

> **CRITICAL THINKING**
>
> What patients may be susceptible to serious injury from a fall that is from a low level?

Adults who have fallen more than 15 feet usually land on their feet. A predictable injury from this vertical fall is bilateral calcaneus fractures. As the energy dissipates from the initial impact, the head, torso, and pelvis push downward. The body is forced into flexion. When this occurs, hip dislocations and compression fractures of the spinal column in the thoracic and lumbar areas are seen. About 10% of patients with calcaneal fracture have associated spinal fractures. If the patient leans forward or tries to break the fall with outstretched hands, bilateral Colles' fractures to the wrists (clinically evident by the so-called silver fork deformity) are likely.

If the distance fallen is less than 15 feet, most adults land in the position in which they fell. For example, an adult who falls head first strikes the landing surface with the head, arms, or both. Predictable injuries depend on the body part that strikes the landing surface and the route of transfer of energy through the body. The paramedic should suspect internal injuries if the trunk of the body is the initial impact area. The ability of the landing surface to absorb energy influences the severity of injury. For example, less damage is expected from a fall on a soft, grassy surface than from a fall on asphalt or concrete.

Children tend to fall head first, regardless of distance fallen or body position during the fall. They fall head first because their heads are proportionally larger and heavier. For this reason, children who experience a vertical fall usually are victims of head injury. Older adult patients sustain a high number of low-distance falls, often resulting in hip fracture.

SECTION THREE
PENETRATING TRAUMA

PENETRATING TRAUMA

All penetrating objects, regardless of velocity, cause tissue disruption **(penetrating trauma).** This damage occurs as a result of two types of forces: crushing and stretching. The character of the penetrating object, its speed of penetration, and the type of body tissue it passes through or into determine which of the two mechanisms of injury predominates.

Cavitation

Cavitation is an opening produced by a force that pushes body tissues laterally away from the tract of a projectile. The amount of cavitation produced by a projectile is related directly to the density of tissue it strikes. Cavitation also is related directly to the ability of the body tissue to return to its original shape and position. For example, consider a person who receives a high-velocity blow to the abdomen. This person experiences abdominal cavitation at the moment of impact. However, because of the lower density of the abdominal musculature, the cavitation is temporary. (Cavitation lasts only a few microseconds.) Cavitation is temporary even in the presence of severe intraabdominal injury (Fig. 20-12).

Permanent cavities are produced by penetrating injuries in which the force of the projectile exceeds the tensile strength of the tissue. Tissues with high water density (e.g., liver, spleen, and muscle) or solid density (e.g., bone) are more prone to permanent cavitation. Certain injuries (e.g.,

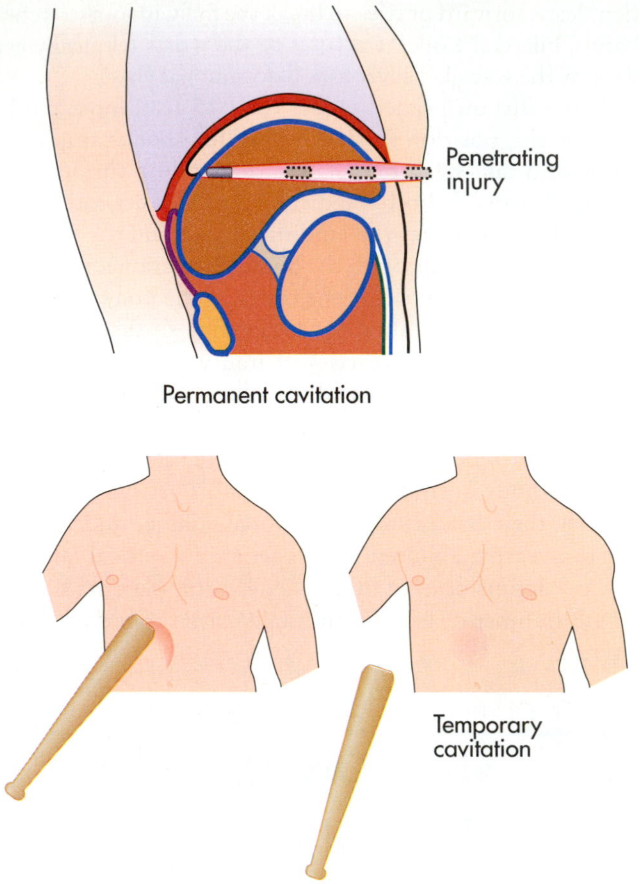

FIGURE 20-12 ■ Permanent and temporary cavitation.

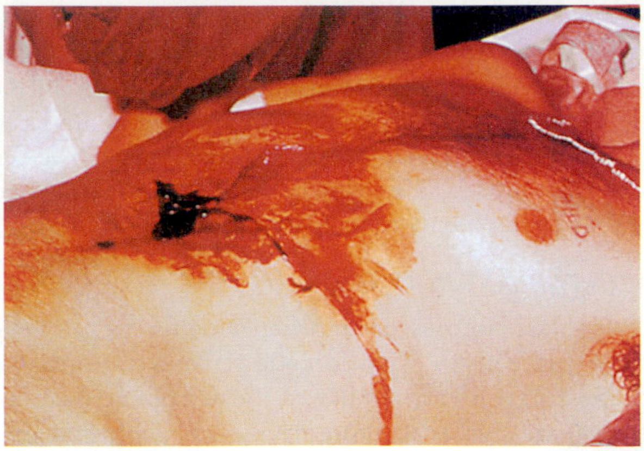

FIGURE 20-13 ■ Stab wound in which a knife has pierced the liver and pancreas and entered the splenic vein.

a stab wound to the abdomen) can produce cavitations as tissues are displaced in frontal and lateral directions.

Ballistics

The energy created and dissipated by the object into surrounding tissues determines the effect of a projectile on the body. The paramedic should consider the principles of kinematics when dealing with injuries from penetrating trauma. To review, kinetic energy equals half the mass of an object multiplied by the square of its velocity. With reference to ballistic trauma, doubling the mass doubles the energy. However, doubling the velocity quadruples the energy. Therefore a small-caliber bullet traveling at a high speed can produce more serious injury than a large-caliber bullet traveling at a lower speed. This is the case as long as the large-caliber bullet does not strike a major vessel or organ.

DAMAGE AND ENERGY LEVELS OF PROJECTILES

Injuries caused by penetrating trauma result from three energy levels. The levels are low, medium, and high. This discussion considers hand-driven weapons as low-energy projectiles and bullets as medium- and high-energy projectiles.

Low-energy projectiles such as knives, needles, and ice picks cause tissue damage by their sharp, cutting edges (Fig. 20-13). The amount of tissue crushed in these injuries usually is minimal because the amount of force applied in the wounding process is small. The more blunt the penetrating object, the more force that must be applied to cause penetration. The more force needed to cause penetration, the more tissue crushed. The damage of tissue from low-energy injuries usually is limited to the pathway of the projectile.

When evaluating a patient with a stab wound, the paramedic should attempt to identify the weapon used to cause the wound. The paramedic also should consider the possibility of multiple wounds, embedded weapons, and hidden yet extensive internal damage to organs of the thorax and abdomen, and penetration of multiple body cavities. A high degree of suspicion of serious injury is also indicated for stab wounds to areas of the back and flank. These wounds may be associated with penetrating injuries to hollow organs and injuries to retroperitoneal organs, specifically the kidneys. Penetrating injuries of the thorax can involve the abdomen, just as abdominal injuries can involve the thorax.

> **CRITICAL THINKING**
>
> Your patient has a stab wound in the midaxillary line, lateral to the left nipple. What organs may be affected by this mechanism? What else would you like to know about this injury?

Firearms can be labeled as medium- and high-energy weapons. Medium-energy weapons include handguns and some rifles. The injury tract produced by medium-energy weapons usually is 2 to 3 times the diameter of the projectile. Examples of high-energy weapons include military/assault rifles such as AR-15s, M-16s, and AK 47/74s and some hunting rifles. As with medium-energy injuries, the injury tract produced by high-energy weapons usually is 2 to 3 times the diameter of the projectile.

IMPLICATIONS OF SOFT BODY ARMOR

Some emergency medical services agencies have adopted soft body armor policies. The armor offers extra protection for paramedics against blunt and penetrating trauma. Most agencies follow U.S. Department of Justice guidelines to determine the type of body armor protection for the types of weapons most commonly found in their community. There are seven levels of body armor protection. Authorities generally recommend a type III or higher protection level for emergency medical services providers. These soft vests protect against low- and some medium- and high-velocity weapons (see Chapter 52).

WOUNDING FORCES OF MEDIUM- AND HIGH-ENERGY PROJECTILES

A firearm cartridge is composed of a bullet made of metal, gunpowder to propel the bullet, a primer to explode and ignite the gunpowder, and a cartridge case that surrounds these components. When the trigger is pulled, the metal hammer strikes the firing pin, which ignites the primer. The gunpowder ignites and forces the bullet to exit the cartridge case.

The mechanism of injury from firearms is related to the energy created and dissipated by the bullet into the surrounding tissues. When a firearm is discharged, several events affect this dissipation of energy and ultimately the wounding forces of the missile:

1. As the missile travels through air, it experiences wind resistance, or drag. The greater the drag, the greater the slowing effect on the missile. Therefore a firearm discharged at close range usually produces a more severe injury than the same firearm discharged at a greater distance.
2. As the missile travels through air, a sonic pressure wave spreads out behind the missile. Because the speed of sound in tissue is about 4 times the speed of sound in air, the sonic pressure wave jumps ahead and precedes the missile through the tissue. This pressure wave displaces tissue and sometimes stretches it dramatically.
3. The localized crush of tissue in the path of the missile and the momentary stretch of the surrounding tissue cause tissue disruption.

When a projectile strikes a body, tissue stretches at the point of impact to allow entry of the penetrating object (temporary cavitation). The energy of the projectile exceeds the tensile strength of the tissue. Thus tissue crush occurs, forcing surrounding tissues outward from the path of the projectile (permanent cavitation). The differences in wounds caused by projectiles vary with the amount and location of crushed and stretched tissue (Fig. 20-14). The wounding forces of a missile depend on the projectile mass, deformation, fragmentation, type of tissue struck, striking velocity, and range.[8]

Projectile Mass. Tissue crush is limited by the physical size or profile of the projectile. If the missile strikes point first, the crushed area is no larger than the diameter of the bullet. If the missile is tilted as it strikes the body, the amount of crushed tissue is no larger than the length and longitudinal cross section of the bullet.

Deformation. Some firearm missiles deform when striking tissue (e.g., expanding hollow- or soft-point hunting bullets). The points of these projectiles typically flatten on impact. The diameter of the bullet expands, creating a larger area of crushed tissue. Military use of these bullets in war is forbidden.

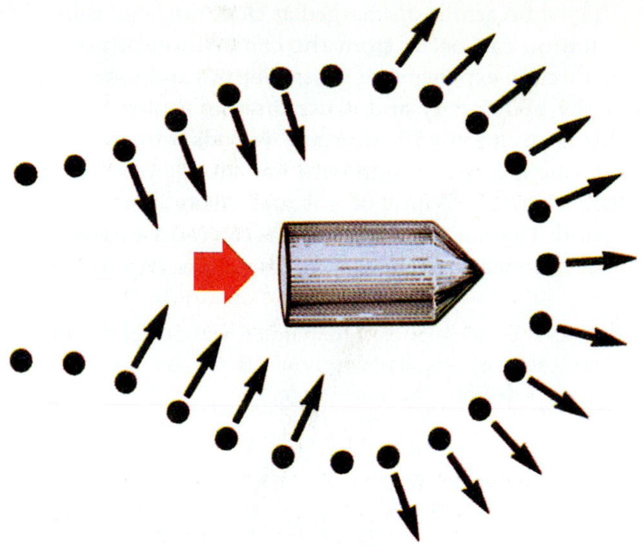

FIGURE 20-14 ■ Bullet passing through tissue. Outward stretching of the permanent cavity as the tissue particles move away from the penetrating missile cause the temporary cavity.

Fragmentation. Each piece of missile crushes its own path through tissue, causing extensive tissue damage. These fragments produce a larger frontal area than a single, solid bullet and disperse energy into the surrounding tissues rapidly. Tissues weaken from the multiple fragment tracts and increase the subsequent stretch of the temporary cavity. The higher the velocity, the more likely the bullet is to fragment. If a bullet fragments, there may be no exit wound.

Type of Tissue Struck. Tissue disruption varies greatly with tissue type. For example, elastic tissues such as the bowel wall, lung, and muscle tolerate stretch much better than nonelastic organs such as the liver.

Striking Velocity. The velocity of a missile determines the extent of cavitation and tissue damage. Low-velocity missiles localize injury to a small radius from the center of the injury tract. These missiles have little disruptive effect, pushing the tissue aside. High-velocity missiles produce more serious injuries because they lose more energy to the tissues and produce more cavitation.

Bullet yaw, or tumble, in tissue also contributes to cavitation and tissue damage. The center of gravity of a wedge-shaped bullet is nearer to the base than to the nose. As the missile strikes body tissue, it slows rapidly. Momentum carries the base of the bullet forward; the center of gravity becomes the leading part of the missile. This forward rotation around the center of mass causes an end-over-end motion. This movement in turn produces more energy exchange and more tissue damage.

Range. The distance of the weapon from the target is a key factor in the severity of ballistic trauma. Air resistance (drag) slows the missile significantly; therefore increasing the distance of the projectile from the target decreases the velocity at the time of impact.

If the firearm is discharged at close range (within 3 feet), cavitation can occur from the combustion of powder and the forceful expansion of gases. The gas and powder can enter the body cavity and cause internal explosion of tissue. This is common with shotgun wounds. Internal explosion of tissue is less common with handguns because they produce a small amount of gas and create a small entrance wound. The expansion of only gas can cause extensive tissue destruction, especially in an enclosed area (e.g., the skull).

▶NOTE Blanks are ammunition without projectiles. The explosion of gas explains how blanks can cause injury or death when fired at short range.

SHOTGUN WOUNDS

Shotguns are short-range, low-velocity weapons. They fire multiple lead pellets. These pellets are encased in a larger shell. Each pellet (there may be 9 to 400 or more, depending on pellet size and gauge of gun) is considered a missile capable of producing tissue damage. Each shell contains pellets, gunpowder, and a plastic or paper wad that separates the pellets from the gunpowder. This wad of unsterile material increases the potential for infection in shotgun wounds.

The energy transferred to body tissue and the tissue damage that results depends on several things: the gauge of the gun, size of the pellets, powder charge, and distance from the victim. For example, a 12-gauge, full-choke shotgun with number 6 shot (275 pellets) concentrates 95% of the pellets into a 7-inch circle at 10 yards. At close range a shotgun injury can create extensive tissue damage similar to that from a high-velocity missile weapon.

ENTRANCE AND EXIT WOUNDS

The presence of entrance and exit wounds is affected by several factors, including range, barrel length, caliber, powder, and weapon (Fig. 20-15). In general, an entrance wound over soft tissue is round or oval and may be surrounded by an abrasion rim or collar. If the firearm is discharged at intermediate or close range, powder burns (tattooing) may be present (Box 20-5).

Exit wounds, if present, are generally larger than entrance wounds because of the cavitational wave that occurs as the bullet passes through the tissues. As the bullet exits the body, the skin can explode, resulting in ragged and torn tissue. This splitting and tearing often produces a starburst or stellate wound.

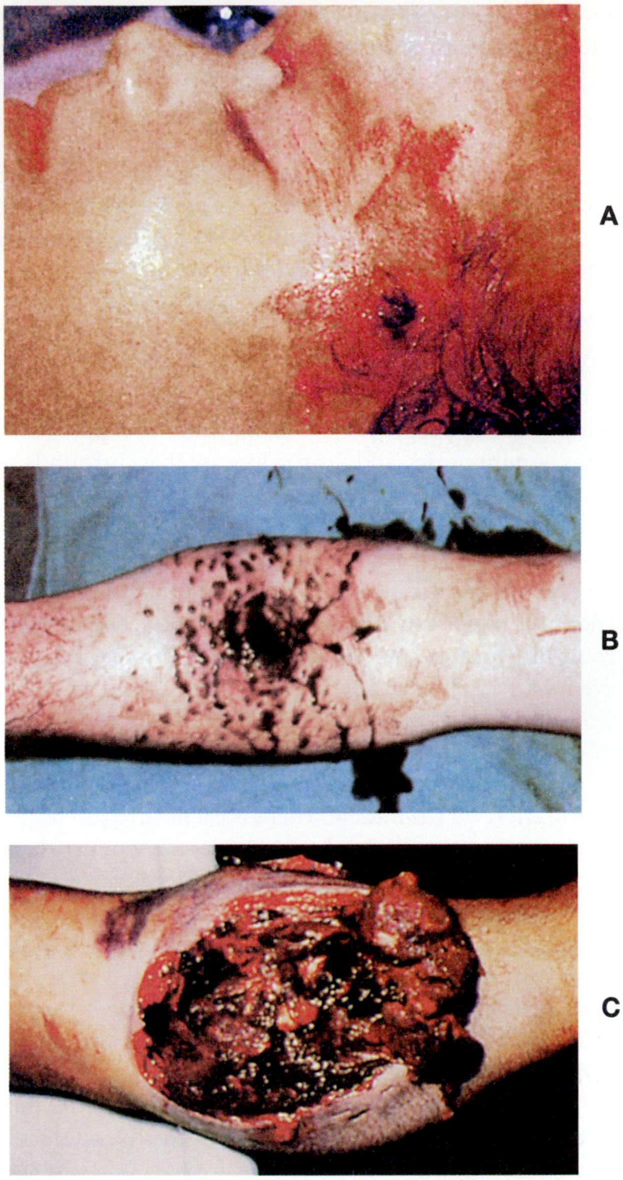

FIGURE 20-15 ■ **A,** The powder marks show that this .22-caliber bullet wound was inflicted at close range. **B,** A short-range shotgun wound to the forearm. **C,** Exit wound caused by a powerful shotgun fired at close range.

CRITICAL THINKING

You locate an entrance wound but no exit wound on a patient who was shot. Does this mean that the injury is not serious?

If the muzzle is in direct contact with the skin at the time of firearm discharge, expanding gases can enter the tissue. These gases can produce crepitus. The burning gases also can produce thermal injury at the entrance site and along the injury tract.

▶NOTE The paramedic should describe and document the appearance of all wounds. However, the paramedic should refrain from commenting or speculating on which is the entry or exit wound. Such speculation can result in the paramedic being served a subpoena. The paramedic may be subpoenaed to testify in court in an area that is beyond the scope of paramedic practice.

SPECIAL CONSIDERATIONS FOR SPECIFIC INJURIES

Locating ballistic injuries requires a thorough physical examination of the patient because the resulting trauma from high- and medium-velocity missiles is unpredictable.

BOX 20-5 Forensic Considerations in Managing Gunshot Wounds

Lifesaving procedures always take precedence over forensic considerations. However, the paramedic should not touch or move weapons or other environmental clues unless it is absolutely necessary for patient care. Other forensic considerations follow:

- Document the exact condition of the patient and wound appearance on arrival at the scene. This should include environment of the patient and body position in relation to objects and doorways.
- Disturb the scene as little as possible.
- If possible, cut or tear clothing along a seam to avoid altering tears made by a penetrating object.
- Avoid cutting through a bullet hole in the clothing.
- Do not shake clothing.
- Keep all clothing in a paper bag rather than a plastic bag that may alter evidence. Do not give clothing to the victim's family members.
- Save any avulsed tissue for forensic pathological examination.
- If the bullet is retrieved, place it in a padded container to prevent marring and secure the evidence until it is delivered to the authorities (obtain a receipt).

The impact of any projectile is critical in determining the type and severity of injury. Fractions of an inch can make a significant difference in the amount of trauma the patient suffers. These differences often are impossible to distinguish in the field.

Head Injuries. Gunshot wounds to the head typically are devastating because of the direct destruction of brain tissue and subsequent swelling. Patients with head wounds often sustain severe face and neck injuries as well. These can result in major blood loss, difficulty in maintaining airway control, and spinal instability.

As a medium-energy projectile penetrates the skull, the energy is absorbed within the closed space of the cranium. The force of the injury compresses brain tissue against the cranial cavity, often fracturing orbital plates and separating the dura from the bone. Depending on the qualities of the missile, the bullet may not have enough force to exit the skull after penetration. This is what occurs with .22- and .25-caliber handguns. In these injuries the bullet follows the curvature of the interior of the skull. As it follows this curvature, it produces significant damage.

High-velocity wounds to the skull produce massive destruction. Pieces of the skull and brain typically are destroyed. At close range, high-velocity wounds result in part from the large quantities of gas produced by combustion of the propellant. If the weapon is held in contact with the head, the gas follows the bullet into the cranial cavity, producing an explosive effect.

Thoracic Injuries. Gunshot wounds to the thorax can result in severe injury to the pulmonary and vascular systems. If the lungs are penetrated by a missile, the pleura and pulmonary parenchyma (the tissue of an organ, as distinguished from supporting and connective tissue) are likely to be disrupted, producing a pneumothorax. On occasion, the pulmonary defect allows air that cannot be expelled to continue to flow into the thoracic cavity. The subsequent increase in pressure eventually can cause collapse of the lung and a shift in the mediastinum to the unaffected side (tension pneumothorax).

Vascular trauma from penetrating injuries can result in massive internal and external hemorrhage. For example, if the pulmonary artery or vein, venae cavae, or aorta is injured, the patient can bleed to death within minutes. Other vascular injuries from penetrating trauma to the thorax can result in hemothorax and, if the heart is involved, myocardial rupture or pericardial tamponade.

Penetrating injury can cause thoracic trauma in the absence of visible chest wounds. For example, a bullet can enter the abdomen and travel upward through the diaphragm and into the thorax. The paramedic should evaluate all victims of abdominal gunshot wounds for thoracic injury. Likewise, the paramedic should evaluate all victims of thoracic gunshot wounds for abdominal injury.

Abdominal Injuries. Gunshot wounds to the abdomen usually require surgery to determine the extent of injury. Penetrating trauma can affect multiple organ systems, causing damage to air-filled and solid organs, vascular injury, trauma to the vertebral column, and spinal cord injury. The paramedic should assume a serious injury when managing victims of penetrating abdominal trauma. This should be the rule even if a patient appears to be stable.

Extremity Injuries. At times, gunshot wounds to the extremities are life threatening. Sometimes such wounds can result in lifelong disability. Special considerations with these injuries include vascular injury with bleeding into soft tissues and damage to nerves, muscles, and bones. The paramedic should evaluate any extremity that has sustained penetrating trauma for bone injury, motor and sensory integrity, and the presence of adequate blood flow (e.g., pulses and capillary refill).

Vessels can be injured by being struck by the bullet or by temporary cavitation. Either mechanism can damage the lining of the blood vessel, producing hemorrhage or thrombosis. Penetrating trauma can damage muscle tissue by stretching it as the muscle expands away from the path of the missile. Stretching that exceeds the tensile strength of the muscle produces hemorrhage.

Bone struck by a penetrating object can be deformed and fragmented. If this occurs, the transfer of energy causes pieces of bone to act as secondary missiles, crushing their way through surrounding tissue.

SUMMARY

- Trauma is the leading cause of death among persons 1 to 34 years of age and is the fifth leading cause of death among all Americans.
- Trauma care is divided into three phases: preincident, incident, and postincident.
- Components of the trauma system include injury prevention, prehospital care, emergency department care, interfacility transportation (if needed), definitive care, trauma critical care, rehabilitation, data collection, and trauma registry.
- Injuries are caused by a transfer of energy from some external source to the human body. The extent of injury is determined by the type of energy applied, by how quickly it is applied, and by the part of the body to which the energy is applied.
- Blunt trauma is an injury produced by the wounding forces of compression and change of speed, which can disrupt tissues.
- Four restraining systems are available in the United States. These are lap belts, diagonal shoulder straps, child safety seats, and air bags. All of these significantly reduce injuries. However, if they are used inappropriately, these protective devices also can produce injuries.
- Organ injuries can result from sudden movement caused by deceleration and compression forces. The recognition of these injuries requires a high degree of suspicion. The paramedic must use the principles of kinematics.
- Small motorized vehicles such as motorcycles, all-terrain vehicles, snowmobiles, motorboats, water bikes, and farm machinery are considered to be more dangerous than other motor vehicles. They are more dangerous because they offer little protection to the rider. They offer minimal protection from the transfer of energy associated with collisions.
- All auto-pedestrian collisions can produce serious injuries. They require a high degree of suspicion for multiple-system trauma.
- Sports provide a variety of health benefits. However, they also can produce severe injury.
- Blast injury is damage to a patient exposed to a pressure field that is produced by an explosion of volatile substances. Blasts release large amounts of energy in the form of pressure and heat.
- Falls from greater than 3 times the height of a person (15 to 20 feet) are associated with an increased incidence of severe injuries. In predicting injuries associated with falls, the paramedic should evaluate three things: the distance fallen, the body position of the patient on impact, and the type of landing surface struck.
- All penetrating objects, regardless of velocity, cause tissue disruption. The character of the penetrating object, its speed of penetration, and the type of body tissue it passes through or into determine whether crushing or stretching forces will cause injury.

REFERENCES

1. National Safety Council: *Injury facts,* Chicago, 1999, The Council.
2. National Safety Council: *Injury facts,* Chicago, 2002, The Council.
3. National Association of Emergency Medical Technicians: *PHTLS: basic and advanced prehospital life support,* ed 5, St Louis, 2003, Mosby.
4. Baker C et al: Epidemiology of trauma deaths, *Am J Surg* 140:144, 1980.
5. US Department of Transportation, National Highway Traffic Safety Administration: *Paramedic national standard curriculum,* Washington, DC, 1998, US Government Printing Office.
6. The National Foundation for Trauma Care. http://www.traumacare.com. Accessed Feb 11, 2003.
7. Kuehl A, editor: *EMS medical director's handbook,* St Louis, 1989, Mosby.
8. McSwain N, Kerstein M: *Evaluation and management of trauma,* Norwalk, Conn, 1987, Appleton-Century-Crofts.

CHAPTER 21

Hemorrhage and Shock

OBJECTIVES

Upon completion of this chapter, the paramedic student will be able to:

1. Describe how to recognize signs and symptoms of internal or external hemorrhage.
2. Define shock.
3. Outline the factors necessary to achieve adequate tissue oxygenation.
4. Describe how the diameter of resistance vessels influences preload.
5. Describe the function of the components of blood.
6. Outline the changes in the microcirculation during the progression of shock.
7. List the causes of hypovolemic, cardiogenic, neurogenic, anaphylactic, and septic shock.
8. Describe pathophysiology as a basis for signs and symptoms associated with the progression through the stages of shock.
9. Describe key assessment findings to distinguish the etiology of the shock state.
10. Outline the prehospital management of the patient in shock based on knowledge of the pathophysiology associated with each type of shock.
11. Discuss how to integrate the assessment and management of the patient in shock.

KEY TERMS

disseminated intravascular coagulation: A grave coagulopathy that results from the overstimulation of the clotting and anticlotting processes in response to disease or injury.

hemostasis: The cessation of bleeding by mechanical or chemical means or by substances that arrest the blood flow.

pulse pressure: The difference between systemic and pulmonic pressure.

Severe illnesses and trauma can threaten the normal internal environment of the body. During such events, the protective systems of the body try to compensate. They work to maintain cellular oxygenation. The paramedic must be able to integrate pathophysiological principles and assessment findings. This will help the paramedic to form a field impression and to implement a treatment plan for the patient with hemorrhage or shock.

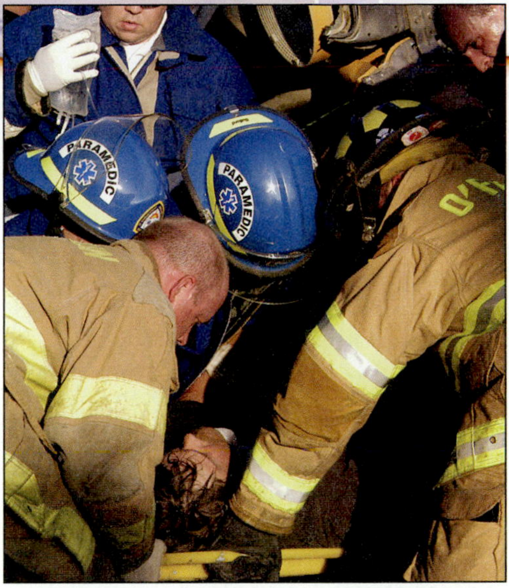

HEMORRHAGE

Hemorrhage occurs when there is a disruption, or "leak," in the vascular system. Sources of hemorrhage can be external or internal.

External Hemorrhage

External hemorrhage results from soft tissue injury (described in Chapter 22). External hemorrhage accounts for nearly 10 million emergency department visits in the United States each year.[1] Most soft tissue trauma is accompanied by mild hemorrhage. In addition, most soft tissue trauma does not pose a threat to life, yet it can carry major risks of morbidity and disfigurement. The seriousness of the injury depends on three factors: the anatomical source of the hemorrhage (arterial, venous, capillary), the degree of vascular disruption, and the amount of blood loss that the patient can tolerate.

▶**NOTE** Education and prevention before the event are the best ways to avoid significant trauma. One strategy to this effect is to educate the public. (For example, the use of personal restraint systems can be emphasized.) Another strategy is the enforcement of laws. (An example is the enactment of helmet laws.) A third strategy involves the environment and engineering. (For example, walk signals at busy intersections can be installed.) These and other strategies can help reduce the occurrence of significant injury (see Chapter 3).

Internal Hemorrhage

Internal hemorrhage can result from a blunt or penetrating trauma. Internal hemorrhage also can result from acute or chronic illnesses. Internal bleeding that leads to an insufficient amount of circulating blood can occur in one of four body cavities: the chest, abdomen, pelvis, or retroperitoneum. Intracranial hemorrhage also can cause grave hemodynamic instability from loss of blood. Internal hemorrhage is associated with higher morbidity and mortality rates than external hemorrhage. Signs and symptoms that can indicate significant internal hemorrhage include the following:

- Bright red blood from mouth, rectum, or other orifice
- Coffee-ground appearance of vomitus
- Melena (black, tarry stools)
- Hematochezia (passage of red blood through the rectum)
- Dizziness or syncope on sitting or standing
- Orthostatic hypotension (described later in this chapter)

CRITICAL THINKING
Internal hemorrhage is associated with an increase in morbidity and mortality rates. Why do you think this is the case?

Physiological Response to Hemorrhage

The cessation of bleeding by chemical means is **hemostasis.** Clotting of blood is the initial response of the body to hemorrhage. This vascular reaction (further described in

Chapter 22) involves local vasoconstriction, formation of a platelet plug, coagulation, and the growth of fibrous tissue into a blood clot that permanently closes and seals the injured vessel. If hemorrhage is severe, these mechanisms can fail. This failure results in shock (hypoperfusion).

DEFINITION OF SHOCK

Shock was defined by Gross in 1850 as a "rude unhinging of the machinery of life"[2] and since has been redefined by many others. Robert M. Hardaway, professor of surgery at Texas Tech University School of Medicine in El Paso, Texas, defines shock this way[3]:

> I believe that the best definition of shock is inadequate capillary perfusion. As a corollary of this broad definition, almost anyone who dies, except one who is instantly destroyed, must go through a stage of shock—a momentary pause in the act of death.

Shock is not a single event. It does not have one specific cause and treatment. Rather, it is a complex group of physiological abnormalities. Plus, it can result from a variety of disease states and injuries. There are many complexities involved in shock. Thus, it is not adequately defined by pulse rate, blood pressure, or cardiac function. Moreover, it cannot be reduced to loss of circulating blood (hypovolemia) or loss of pressure in the vascular system (systemic vascular resistance). Shock may affect the entire body, or it may occur at a tissue or cellular level, even with normal hemodynamics. An understanding of cellular physiology is needed to recognize the subtle aspects of shock. This also will aid in properly assessing the severity of various stages of shock.

TISSUE OXYGENATION

The adequate oxygenation of tissue cells is known as perfusion. To achieve adequate oxygenation, three parts of the cardiovascular system must work properly. These three parts are the heart, vasculature, and lungs. When any one of these does not work properly, a decrease in cellular oxygenation can occur.

Heart

The pumping action of the heart produces pressure changes that circulate blood through the body. This repetitive pumping action is known as the *cardiac cycle.*

Cardiac output (described in Chapter 7) is a crucial determinant of organ perfusion. Cardiac output depends on several factors, including strength of contraction, rate of contraction, and amount of venous return available to the ventricle (preload). The formula to determine cardiac output is as follows:

$$\text{Cardiac output (CO)} = \text{Heart rate (HR)} \times \text{Stroke volume (SV)}$$

In 1870 Adolph Fick came up with the first method for measuring cardiac output in healthy animals and human beings. The method is called the Fick principle (described in Chapter 19). To review, the Fick principle assumes that the quantity of oxygen delivered to an organ is equal to the amount of oxygen consumed by that organ plus the amount of oxygen carried away from that organ. The Fick principle often is used to estimate perfusion either to an organ or to the whole body. This estimate can be done only when oxygen content of the arterial and venous blood is known and oxygen consumption remains fixed.

Vasculature

The entire vascular system is lined with smooth, low-friction endothelial cells. All vessels larger than capillaries have layers of tissue surrounding the endothelium. These layers of tissue are known as tunicae. They provide supporting connective tissue to counter the pressure of blood contained in the vascular system. The layers have elastic properties to dampen pressure pulsations and minimize flow variations throughout the cardiac cycle. The layers also have muscle fibers to control the vessel diameter. The vascular system maintains blood flow by changes in pressure and peripheral vascular resistance.

Fluid flows through a tube in response to pressure gradients between the two ends of the tube. The difference in pressure between the two ends determines flow. The difference in pressure does not determine the absolute pressure in the tube. In many animals and human beings the two ends are the aorta and the venae cavae.

Systemic pressure is left-sided pressure and pulmonic pressure is right-sided pressure. These are the measurements of pressure in the vascular system. Systemic pressure, like pulmonic pressure, has two phases: systolic and diastolic. The difference between these two pressures is the **pulse pressure.** Pressure is greatest at its origin (the heart). Pressure is least at its terminating point (the venae cavae). This pressure gradient changes significantly at the arteriole as a result of peripheral vascular resistance. Pulse pressure reflects the tone of the arterial system. Pulse pressure is more sensitive to changes in perfusion than the systolic or diastolic pressures alone.

The peripheral vascular resistance is the afterload. Afterload is the total resistance against which blood must be pumped. Afterload is a measure of friction between the vessel walls and fluid and between the molecules of the fluid themselves (viscosity), both of which oppose flow. When the resistance to flow increases, blood pressure must increase for the flow to remain constant. Resistance to blood flow increases with increased fluid viscosity or vessel length and decreased vessel diameter.

Viscosity is the physical property of a liquid characterized by the degree of friction between its component molecules (e.g., between the blood cells and between the plasma proteins). Viscosity normally plays a minor role in blood flow regulation because it remains fairly constant in healthy persons. Vessel length in the human body also remains fairly constant. Vessel diameter is the main factor affecting the resistance to blood flow.

CRITICAL THINKING

How do firefighters use these principles of viscosity and vessel diameter when fighting a fire?

Major arteries are large. They offer little resistance to flow unless they have an abnormal narrowing. (An abnormal narrowing is known as stenosis.) Arterioles have a much smaller diameter than arteries. They offer the major resistance to blood flow. The smooth muscle in the arteriole walls can relax or contract. The smooth muscle can change the diameter of the inside of the arteriole as much as fivefold. Thus the vasoconstriction or vasodilation of these vessels primarily regulates arterial blood pressure.

Microcirculation

The microcirculation of the body is divided into pulmonary microcirculation and peripheral microcirculation. Separate pumps, the right side and left side of the heart, respectively, produce pressure in each of these divisions.

At any given moment, about 5% of the total circulating blood is flowing through the capillaries. This 5% is exchanging nutrients and picking up the waste from metabolism. The muscular arterioles are the major resistance vessels. They regulate regional blood flow to the capillary beds. The venules and veins serve as collecting channels and storage (capacitance) vessels. They normally contain 70% of the blood volume. The mechanisms that control blood flow to the tissues are described in Chapter 7 and include the following:

- Local control of blood flow by the tissues
- Nervous control of blood flow
- Baroreceptor reflexes
- Chemoreceptor reflexes
- Central nervous system ischemia response
- Hormonal mechanisms
- Adrenal-medullary mechanism
- Renin-angiotensin-aldosterone mechanism
- Vasopressin mechanism
- Reabsorption of tissue fluid

Lungs

Tissue cells require adequate oxygen to function. Adequate oxygen must be available to the red blood cells as they pass through the capillary membranes in the lungs. (This is the first component of the Fick principle.) The high partial pressure of oxygen in inspired air, adequate depth and rate of ventilation, and matching of pulmonary ventilation (described in Chapter 19) and perfusion make adequate oxygenation possible.

CRITICAL THINKING

Can you think of what might impair each of these components of adequate oxygenation?

THE BODY AS A CONTAINER

The healthy body is a smooth-flowing fluid delivery system inside a container. The container must be filled to achieve adequate preload and tissue oxygenation. The external size of the container of any human body is relatively constant, yet the volume of the vascular component in the container is related directly to the diameter of the resistance vessels. This diameter can change rapidly. Any change in the diameter of the vessels changes the volume of fluid that the container holds. Thus this affects preload.

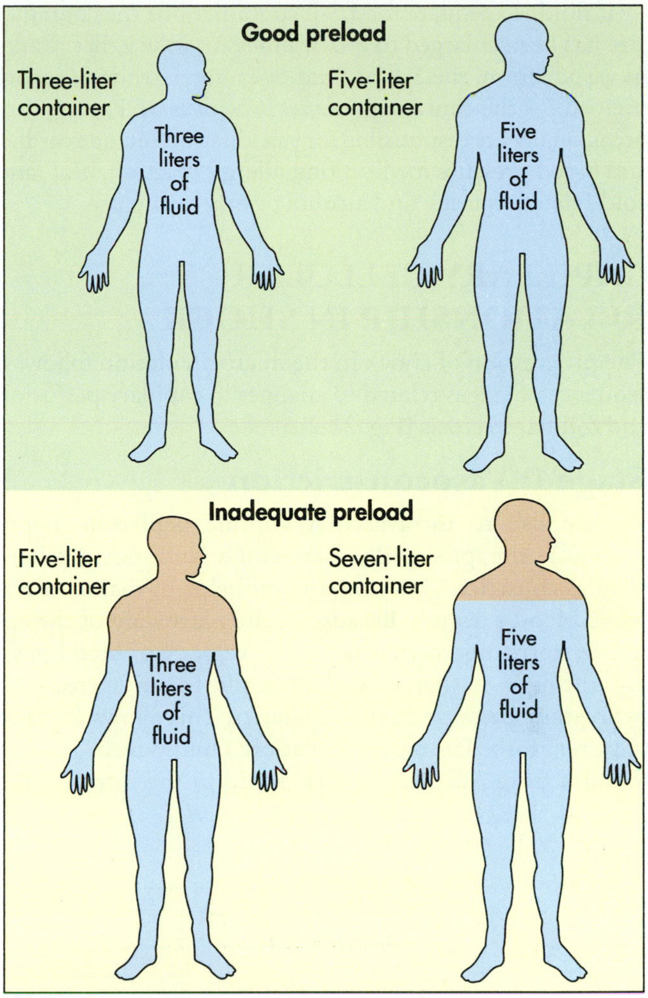

FIGURE 21-1 ■ Fluid volume versus container volume.

An example of this principle is a 5-L container. This is the normal container size for a 70-kg adult male (Fig. 21-1). If the fluid volume is 5 L, preload is adequate. With a strong myocardium, cardiac output and perfusion also are adequate. If 2 L of this fluid has been lost, externally or internally, the 3 L that remain are inadequate to supply an effective preload. Because cardiac output depends on preload, a decrease in preload notably decreases cardiac output.

If the patient is hypovolemic and the 5-L container has remained the same size despite the 3-L volume, the patient becomes hypotensive or loses pressure in the container because of decreased cardiac output. However, if the container is reduced to 3 L by compensatory mechanisms (e.g., vasoconstriction), the 3-L container can provide adequate preload to the heart with the 3 L of available fluid. This is at the expense of certain tissues that are not perfused in this constricted state.

If fluid is adequate for a 5-L container but the container size has been enlarged to 7 L by illness or injury that results in vasodilation, the 5 L of fluid does not provide adequate preload for the container *(relative hypovolemia)*. Factors that occasionally are responsible for vasodilation include cardiac and blood pressure medications, allergic reaction, heat- and cold-related injuries, and alcohol or other drug use.

CAPILLARY-CELLULAR RELATIONSHIP IN SHOCK

The progression of shock in the microcirculation follows a sequence of stages related to changes in capillary perfusion and cellular necrosis (Fig. 21-2).[2]

Stage 1: Vasoconstriction

In response to intravascular volume depletion (hypovolemia), the precapillary arterioles and postcapillary venules constrict. This constriction helps to maintain systemic blood pressure. Because of the narrowing of the entrance to the microcirculation, the velocity of blood passing through it increases. This leads to an increase in hydrostatic pressure in the capillaries. This allows for fluid to be reabsorbed into the circulation. Fluid is reabsorbed as it shifts from the extravascular space to the intravascular space *(transcapillary refill)*. As shock progresses, oxygen and nutrient delivery to the cells supplied by these capillaries decreases; anaerobic metabolism replaces aerobic metabolism; and production of lactate and hydrogen ions increases. Shortly thereafter, the lining of the capillaries can begin to lose the ability to hold large molecules within the capillary. Thus the capillary lining permits protein-containing fluid to leak into the interstitial spaces. This is known as the *leaky capillary syndrome.*

> **CRITICAL THINKING**
> If this leak persists, what effect will it have on preload and cardiac output?

Arteriovenous shunts open, particularly in the skin, kidneys, and gastrointestinal tract. The shunts cause less flow to the arterioles and thus less flow through the capillaries. Sympathetic stimulation produces pale, sweaty skin; a rapid, thready pulse (caused by hypovolemia and vasoconstriction); and an elevation in blood glucose level. The release of epinephrine dilates coronary, cerebral, and skeletal muscle arterioles and constricts other arterioles. As a result, blood is shunted to the heart, brain, and skeletal muscle. Moreover, capillary flow to the kidneys and abdominal or-

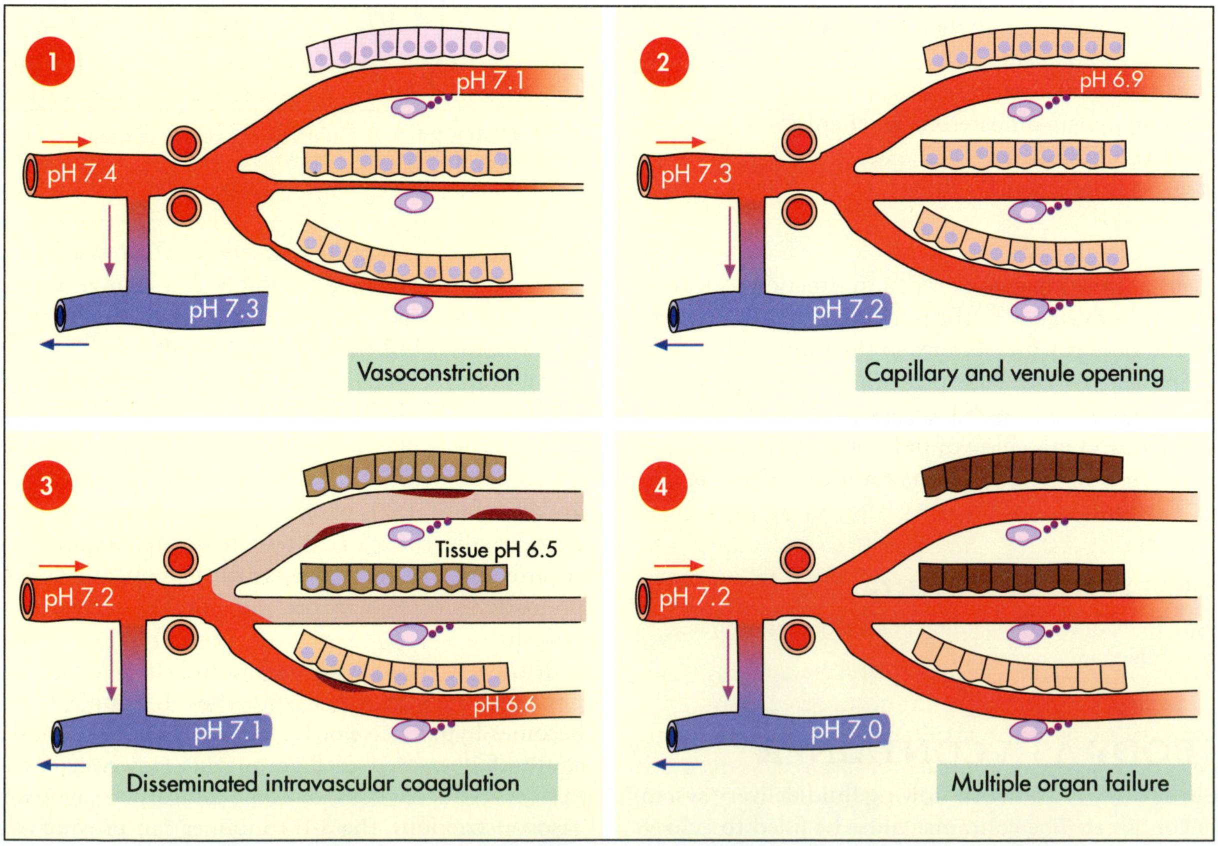

FIGURE 21-2 ■ Diagram of the microcirculation in shock, progressing from *(1)* vasoconstriction, *(2)* capillary and venule opening, *(3)* disseminated intravascular coagulation, and *(4)* multiple organ failure.

gans decreases. The vasoconstriction stage of shock must be treated by prompt restoration of circulatory fluid volume. Otherwise, shock progresses to the next stage.

> **NOTE** Stage one of shock occurs when intravascular blood volume is decreased by about 15%. Blood pressure and heart rate usually are normal at this stage of compensation. This stage is reversible if the hemorrhage is controlled.

Stage 2: Capillary and Venule Opening

As shock progresses, the precapillary sphincter relaxes. This results in some expansion of the vascular space. Postcapillary sphincters resist the relaxation effects. Thus they remain closed. This causes blood to pool or stagnate in the capillary system. The capillaries become engorged with fluid. Arterial hypotension, secondary arteriolar vasoconstriction, and opening of arteriovenous shunts result in less blood flow through arterioles. These conditions also contribute to the stagnation of blood flow in the capillaries.

The vascular space expands greatly as increasing hypoxemia (low oxygen in blood) and acidosis lead to the opening of more venules and capillaries. When this occurs, even normal blood volume may be inadequate to fill the container. The capillary and venule capacity can increase to the point that the volume of available blood returning to the great veins and venae cavae is reduced. This in turn results in decreased venous return and a fall in cardiac output. In addition, the viscera (lungs, liver, kidneys, and gastrointestinal mucosa) can become congested with fluid. The low arterial blood pressure, extremely constricted arterioles, presence of arteriovenous shunts, and many open capillaries result in stagnant capillary flow.

> **CRITICAL THINKING**
> What happens to the function of the heart as acidosis increases?

Sluggish blood flow and a decrease in the amount of oxygen delivered to the cell results in cell metabolism occurring without oxygen. This is called anaerobic metabolism. Anaerobic metabolism results in the production of lactic acid. The respiratory system tries to make up for the increase in acid production (acidosis) by increasing ventilation to release carbon dioxide. This produces a partially compensated metabolic acidosis. As the acidosis increases and pH falls, the red blood cells may cluster together. (This is known as *rouleaux formation.*) Rouleaux formation halts perfusion in the vital organ capillaries. In turn, this affects nutritional flow and prevents the removal of waste products of metabolism. Clotting mechanisms also are affected; this leads to hypercoagulability. This stage of shock often advances to the third stage if fluid resuscitation is inadequate or delayed. This stage also may progress if the shock state is complicated by trauma or infection (sepsis).

> **NOTE** Stage 2 of shock occurs with a 15% to 25% decrease in intravascular blood volume. Heart rate, respiratory rate, and capillary refill are increased, and pulse pressure is decreased at this stage. Blood pressure still may be normal.

Stage 3: Disseminated Intravascular Coagulation

Stage 3 of shock is resistant to treatment. (This is *refractory shock.*) However, stage 3 shock is still reversible. Blood begins to coagulate in the microcirculation. This coagulation clogs capillaries and is referred to as **disseminated intravascular coagulation.** Clumps of red blood cells may occlude the capillaries. This occlusion decreases capillary perfusion, prevents delivery of oxygenated substrates such as glucose, and prevents removal of metabolites. As a result, distal tissue cells switch to anaerobic metabolism, and lactic acid production increases.

As stage 3 of shock continues, lactic acid accumulates around the cell. The cell no longer has the energy needed to maintain homeostasis, or the balance to function normally. Water and sodium leak into the cell through the cellular membrane. Potassium leaks out. Lastly, the cells swell and die (also known as the *washout* phase). Microinfarcts (small areas of dead cells) develop in the organs. Microthrombi produce capillary congestion, fluid leaks, rupture of cells, and hemorrhage. The pulmonary capillaries become permeable to fluid, which leads to pulmonary edema. The edema decreases the absorption of oxygen and results in problems with carbon dioxide elimination. This can lead to acute respiratory failure or adult respiratory distress syndrome (further described in Chapter 30). If shock and disseminated intravascular coagulation continue, the patient progresses to multiple organ failure.

> **NOTE** Stage 3 of shock occurs with a 25% to 35% decrease in intravascular blood volume. At this stage, hypotension occurs. This stage of shock usually requires blood replacement.

Stage 4: Multiple Organ Failure

The amount of cellular necrosis (death) required to produce organ failure varies with each organ. Cellular necrosis also depends on the underlying condition of the organ. Usually hepatic failure occurs first and usually is followed by renal failure and heart failure. But if any given area of capillary occlusion persists for more than 1 to 2 hours, the cells nourished by that capillary undergo changes that rapidly become irreversible. In this stage of shock, blood pressure falls severely (to levels of 60 mm Hg or less). Even if blood pressure is returned to normal after a couple of hours, the ability of the cell to obtain energy from oxygen through anaerobic metabolism fails. Thus the cell dies from inadequate capillary perfusion (described in the beginning of this discussion). Inadequate tissue perfusion and cell death are the results of irreversible shock.

If cellular necrosis damages a critical amount of the vital organ, the organ soon fails. Failure of the liver and kidneys is common. This failure often presents early in this stage. Capillary blockage can cause heart failure. Gastrointestinal bleeding and sepsis can result from gastrointestinal mucosal necrosis. In addition, pancreatic necrosis can lead to further clotting disorders and severe pancreatitis. Pulmonary thrombosis can produce hemorrhage and fluid loss into the alveoli. This can lead to death from respiratory failure.

▶**NOTE** Stage 4 of shock occurs when intravascular blood volume is decreased by 35% to 40%.

CLASSIFICATIONS OF SHOCK

More than 100 types of shock have been discussed in the medical literature. In emergency care, shock commonly is classified based on the initiating cause. (For example, the cause may be hypovolemia.) Although these classifications are separate and distinct, two or more types often are combined. For example, hypovolemia may occur in septic shock. Elements of cardiogenic shock may occur in hypovolemic shock. Regardless of the classification, the underlying defect is inadequate tissue perfusion.

Hypovolemic Shock

In the United States, hypovolemic shock most often is caused by hemorrhage. Hypovolemic shock also can result from dehydration (commonly seen with severe diarrhea and vomiting). In either case, a loss of circulating volume occurs. Illnesses and injuries that can lead to hypovolemic shock include hemorrhage, burns, severe or prolonged diarrhea, vomiting, endocrine disorders, and internal third space loss, as in peritonitis. In addition to loss of circulating volume, tissue injury resulting from trauma can worsen shock. Tissue injury causes microemboli and further activates the inflammatory and coagulation systems.

▶**NOTE** Most patients with shock have hypovolemia. Thus shock is assumed to be hypovolemic in origin until it is proved otherwise. The paramedic at first should manage the patient with shock with a fluid bolus. The paramedic should do this unless the lungs are wet (identified by crackles). Crackles on physical examination indicate cardiogenic shock instead.

Cardiogenic Shock

Cardiogenic shock results when the cardiac pump cannot deliver adequate circulating blood volume for tissue perfusion. Cardiogenic shock can result from inadequate filling of the heart, poor contractility of the heart, and obstruction of blood flow from the heart to central circulation. The patient in cardiogenic shock usually suffers from an acute myocardial infarction, a serious cardiac rhythm disturbance, cardiac tamponade, tension pneumothorax, cardiac contusion, severe valvular heart disease, cardiomyopathy, pulmonary embolism, or dissecting aortic aneurysm. Shock that develops from cardiac tamponade, tension pneumothorax, or pulmonary embolism is known as *obstructive shock* because the common pathophysiology in these conditions is obstruction to blood flow. Cardiogenic shock occurs in 5% to 10% of patients hospitalized for myocardial infarction. The associated mortality rate in these patients approaches 80%.

CRITICAL THINKING
Why does cardiogenic shock develop in a patient who has had a severe myocardial infarction?

Neurogenic Shock

Neurogenic shock is also known as *spinal cord, distributive,* or *vasogenic shock.* Neurogenic shock results from vasomotor paralysis below the level of injury. Normal vasomotor tone through sympathetic nervous system control is lost. This results in a decrease in peripheral vascular resistance. The loss of sympathetic impulses causes vasodilation and increases the size of the container (so to speak). So even normal intravascular volume is inadequate to fill the enlarged vascular compartment and perfuse the tissues. Because of the mechanism of injuries responsible for this syndrome, respiratory insufficiency, head injury, or both also may be present.

▶**NOTE** Fainting may be due to mild, readily reversible vasogenic shock. This shock can occur in the absence of injury. This shock results from bradycardia that produces a drop in cardiac output.

Anaphylactic Shock

Anaphylactic shock occurs when the body is exposed to a substance that produces a severe allergic reaction. Common causes include antibiotic agents (especially penicillins), venoms, and insect stings. The body responds to the release of histamine and other mediators. Histamine and other mediators act on receptors in the systemic and pulmonary microcirculation. They also produce an effect on bronchial smooth muscle. Histamine causes arterioles and capillaries to dilate and increases capillary membrane permeability. Intravascular fluid leaks into the interstitial space and results in a decrease in intravascular volume. In addition, many of the mediators released cause constriction of the upper and lower airways. This creates the potential for complete airway obstruction (see Chapter 33).

Septic Shock

Septic shock most often results from a serious systemic bacterial infection. Septic shock is thought to be caused by toxins that are a part of the microorganism (endotoxin–gram-negative sepsis) or are released by the organism (exotoxin–gram-positive shock). These toxins stimulate the release of complex vasoactive agents. The agents affect arterioles, capillaries, and venules. They alter pressure in the microcirculation and increase capillary permeability. Septic shock can result from staphylococcal and streptococcal infections, pneumonia, postoperative infections, and infections from indwelling urinary catheters. Between 40,000 and 100,000 persons develop septic shock each year. Septic shock most often occurs in older adults (particularly nursing home residents), alcoholics, neonates, and patients who are immunosuppressed (e.g., patients with cancer, human immunodeficiency virus infection, or sickle cell disease).

STAGES OF SHOCK

The degree of hypoperfusion and anaerobic metabolism can be categorized by stages of the response of the body to the shock syndrome. The three stages are (1) compensated shock, (2) uncompensated (or decompensated) shock, and (3) irreversible shock.[4] Table 21-1 lists the stages of shock and the signs and symptoms of each.

Compensated Shock

Compensated shock (Fig. 21-3) is associated with some decreased blood flow and perfusion to the tissues. However, the compensatory responses of the body can overcome a decrease in available fluid. An increase in catecholamine production maintains cardiac output and a normal systolic blood pressure.

The decrease in perfusion and subsequent increase in acidosis lead to a chemoreceptor response. This response increases the rate and depth of ventilation. (This helps correct the acidosis by decreasing P_{CO_2}.) Sympathetic stimulation increases heart rate and contractility, causes bronchodilation, leads to increases in peripheral vascular resistance, and decreases capillary flow in some capillary beds, such as the gastrointestinal tract. The patient may exhibit delayed capillary refill and cool skin as the blood is shunted from the skin to the vital organs. In spite of maintaining normal blood pressure and urinary output, some patients may show signs of decreased perfusion to the brain (lethargy, confusion, combativeness), even at this stage. If the underlying cause of shock is untreated, the compensatory mechanisms collapse.

UNCOMPENSATED SHOCK

Uncompensated shock (Fig. 21-4) occurs when the body is no longer able to maintain systemic blood pressure. The systolic pressure usually drops before the diastolic pressure because the systolic pressure depends more on blood volume. Diastolic pressure may rise at first because of vasoconstriction. The decrease in systolic pressure, along with maintained or increased diastolic pressure, can lead to a narrow pulse pressure. The pulse pressure can be narrowed to such an extent that it is not detectable with a blood pressure cuff.

As the compensatory mechanisms of the body begin to fail, systolic and diastolic pressure drop. Cerebral blood flow decreases as well. P_{O_2} may drop; however, P_{CO_2} usually remains normal or low unless the patient has a head or chest injury that leads to hypoventilation. The clinical signs of uncompensated shock include hypotension, tachycardia, tachypnea, delayed capillary refill, and decreased urinary output. Shunting of blood and tissue hypoxia may cause the patient to have cold extremities and cyanosis. Effects on the cardiovascular system include a decreased preload and an increased rate of contraction caused by catecholamine stimulation. Although myocardial contractions initially can be stronger as a result of catecholamine release, in the latter phases of uncompensated shock, myocardial strength may decrease as a result of the following factors:

1. Ischemia can result from a reduction of circulating red blood cells, a lower oxygen saturation (P_{O_2}), and decreased coronary perfusion because of hypotension (especially diastolic hypotension).
2. Cardiodepressant substances (e.g., myocardial toxin released from the ischemic pancreas) can depress heart function in late shock.
3. Necrosis of myocardium (essentially simulating myocardial infarction) can result from associated ischemia.

TABLE 21-1 Stages of Shock

VITAL SIGNS	SIGNS AND SYMPTOMS		
	COMPENSATED SHOCK	UNCOMPENSATED SHOCK	IRREVERSIBLE SHOCK
Heart rate	Mild tachycardia	Moderate tachycardia	Bradycardia, severe dysrhythmias
Level of consciousness	Lethargy, confusion, combativeness	Confusion, unconsciousness	Coma
Skin	Delayed capillary refill, cool skin	Delayed capillary refill, cold extremities, cyanosis	Pale, cold, clammy skin
Blood pressure	Normal or slightly elevated measurement	Decreased systolic and diastolic pressure	Frank hypotension

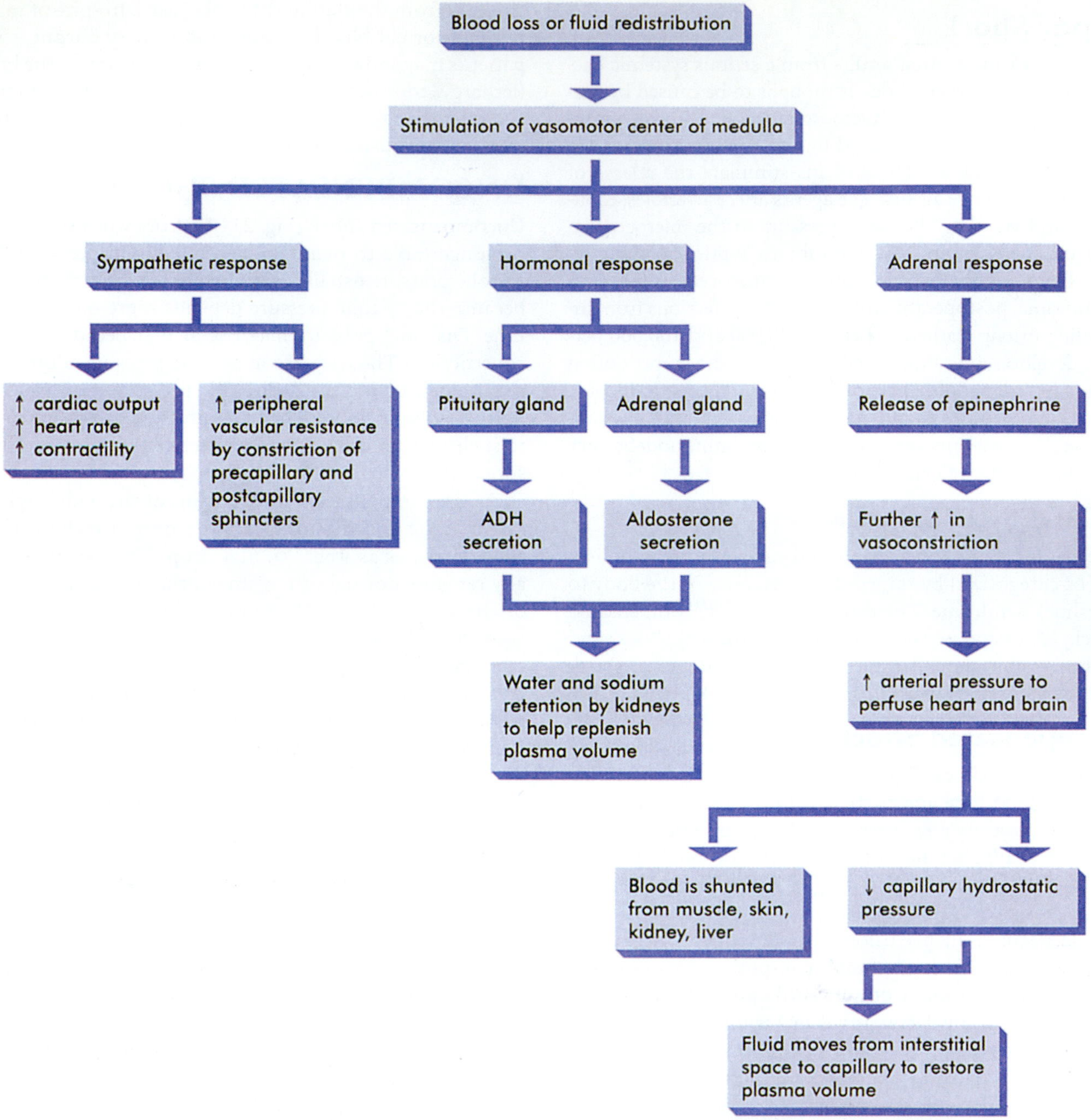

FIGURE 21-3 ■ Compensated shock. This stage of shock is reversible.

4. Decreased preload can lead to decreased contractility.
5. Acidosis can lead to decreased contractility.
6. Cardiac rhythm disturbances can result from hypoxia.

Irreversible Shock

The progression of cellular ischemia and necrosis and then organ death, even with oxygenation and perfusion restored, indicate the third stage of shock (Fig. 21-5). Despite a return to normal perfusion, patients with irreversible shock as a result of massive cellular damage do not survive. Cells and the vital organs begin to die from the lack of energy. The membrane pumps fail. The various organelles in the cells break down one after the other. Thus necrosis is inevitable even if cell perfusion is restored.

Decompensation may occur suddenly or may be delayed from 1 day to 3 weeks after the onset of shock. The clinical signs of irreversible shock include bradycardia; serious dysrhythmias; frank hypotension; evidence of multiple organ failure; and pale, cold, and clammy skin. Cardiopulmonary collapse usually is imminent in these patients.

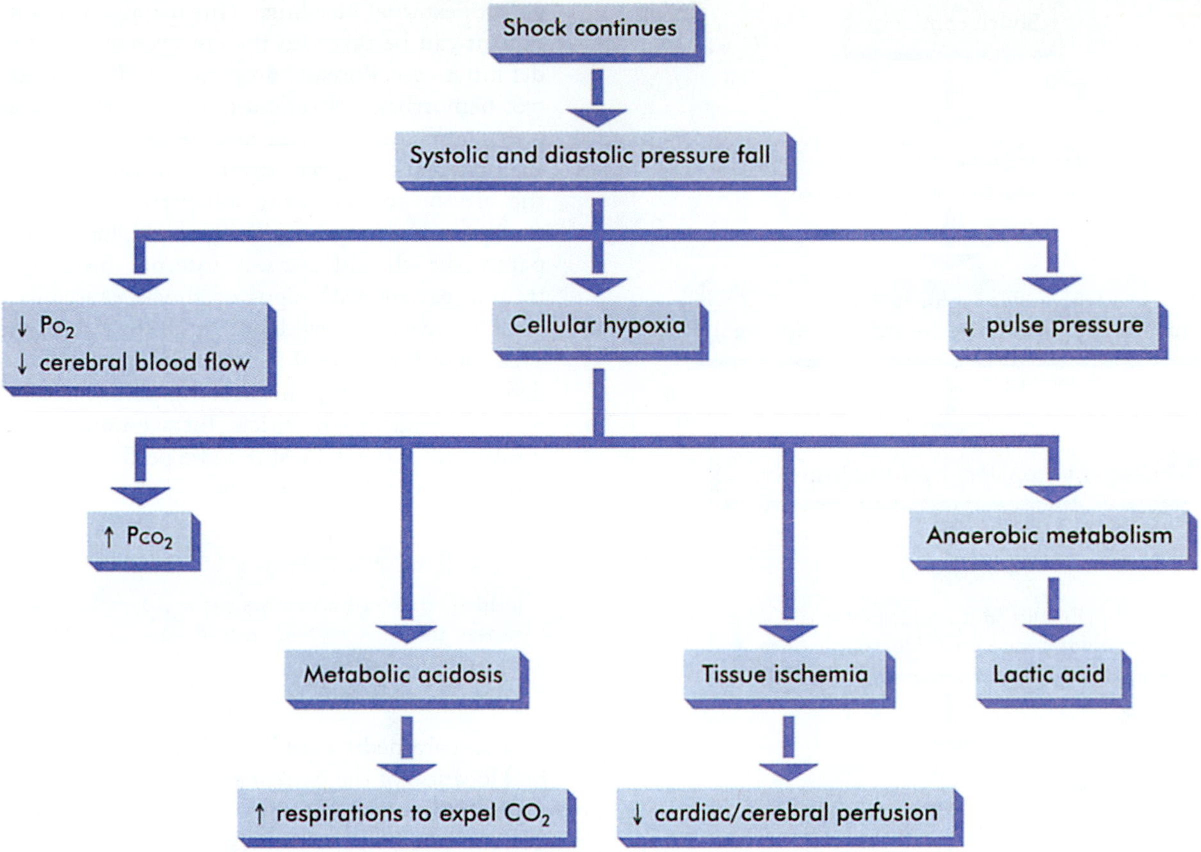

FIGURE 21-4 ■ Uncompensated shock. This stage of shock is reversible.

NOTE During the prehospital management of shock, it is impossible to tell uncompensated and irreversible shock apart. Therefore management of the shock victim should always focus on resuscitation. This is especially true because irreversible shock usually occurs over a longer period of time. Rapid resuscitation and transportation to an appropriate medical facility can prevent the development of irreversible shock. Fluid resuscitation in these patients should be guided by medical direction and established protocol.

Variations in Physiological Response to Shock

Many variations in physiological response occur among patients who are in shock. Determining factors include the following:

- Age and relative health
- Older adults, who are less able to compensate
- Children, who compensate longer and deteriorate faster
- General physical condition
- Preexisting disease
- Ability to activate compensatory mechanisms
- Medications, some of which can interfere with compensatory mechanisms
- Specific organ system affected

CRITICAL THINKING
What diseases can influence a patient's response to shock?

MANAGEMENT AND TREATMENT PLAN FOR THE PATIENT IN SHOCK

The management and treatment plan for the patient in shock focuses on assessment. The paramedic must assess oxygenation and perfusion of the body organs. The goals of the treatment plan are to ensure a patent airway, to provide adequate oxygenation and ventilation, and to restore perfusion.

Initial Assessment

The initial assessment can help to identify whether cell perfusion is adequate. The following five-step description of the initial assessment focuses on evaluating the shock victim, but the paramedic should be aware of common objectives in evaluating any patient with other types of serious illness or injury:

1. *Airway.* The airway must be opened and patency must be maintained to ensure adequate air movement.
2. *Breathing.* The respiratory pattern often reflects the adequacy of ventilation. Respiration can offer clues to the presence of shock. For example, if the patient is acidotic,

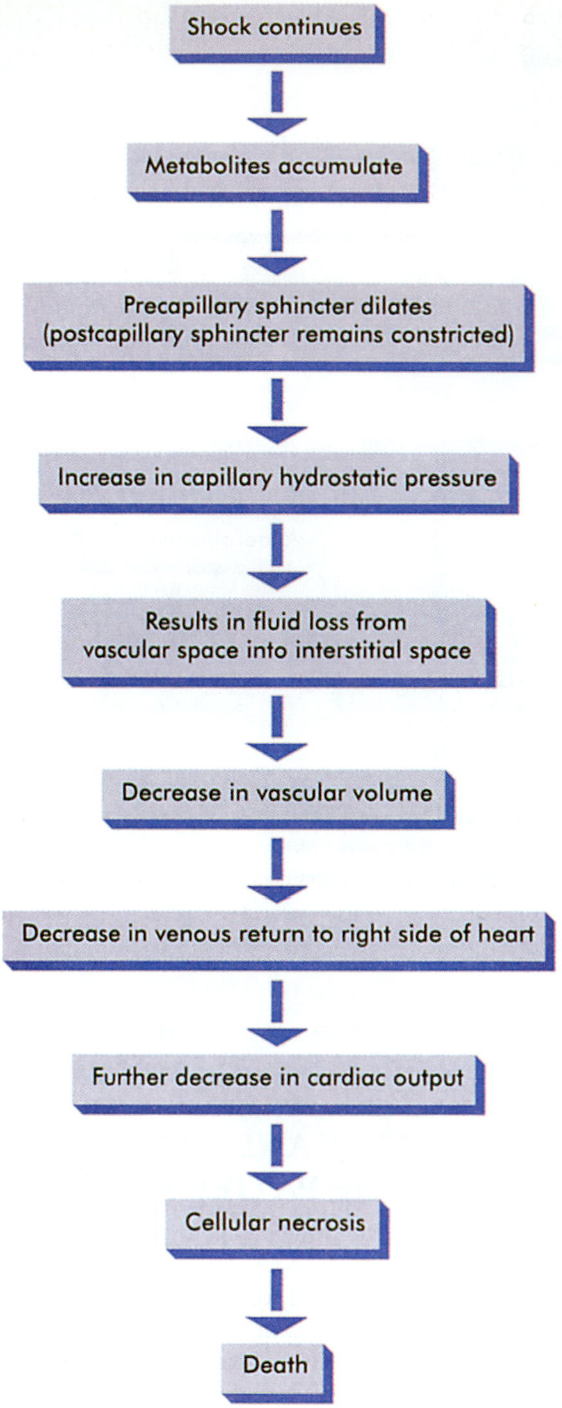

FIGURE 21-5 ■ Irreversible shock. Regardless of fluid replacement and an initial favorable response in blood pressure, death will ensue within 1 day to 3 weeks.

the rate and depth of ventilation increase in an attempt to reduce carbon dioxide content of the blood and compensate for the metabolic acidosis.

3. *Circulation.* The paramedic should assess the patient's circulatory status. The first step is to check the patient for any uncontrolled arterial bleeding. In cases of external hemorrhage, applying direct pressure can almost always help to gain control. (See Chapter 22 for ways to control external bleeding.) This usually works until the patient can be taken to the emergency department for definitive care. Pressure dressings can be applied to control hemorrhage. (Examples of such are bandages or a pneumatic antishock garment [PASG], per protocol.) If the paramedic suspects internal bleeding, after securing the airway and ensuring adequate ventilation, rapid transport to a proper facility is the highest priority. The paramedic should suspect internal bleeding in any trauma patient with signs of shock, especially trauma patients without evidence of external blood loss. Treatment for internal hemorrhage must be directed at definitive care to stop the bleeding. Thus rapid transport to a proper facility is critical. Intravenous fluid therapy, if initiated in the field, should be performed en route to avoid a delay of definitive care.

CRITICAL THINKING

Consider a patient with early signs and symptoms of shock. However, the patient's SaO_2 reading is normal. Should you administer oxygen?

The paramedic should evaluate the rate, character, and location of the patient's pulse as part of the circulatory assessment. Pulse rates increase fairly early in shock. The increase helps to maintain an adequate cardiac output. The contraction strength of the heart also may increase. However, both of these attempts to maintain cardiac output may be negated by the decrease in preload. Tachycardia usually will not occur until the patient has suffered a 10% to 15% volume depletion (relative to container size) as a result of blood loss or an increase in container size. The character of the pulse can be strong or weak. The strength of the pulse provides an estimate of the filling volume of the artery being palpated and an indirect measurement of systolic pressure.

Tissue perfusion sometimes can be estimated by evaluating the color, moisture, and temperature of the skin. These guidelines can be unreliable in patients who have been exposed to extremes of temperature. They also can be unreliable in those suffering from septicemia and shock caused by neurological injury. An evaluation of the fingers and toes (the most distal points of circulation) is crucial. These areas can be the first to show inadequate tissue perfusion. If ambient temperatures are moderate and tissue perfusion is adequate, these areas will be pink, warm, and dry.

The capillary refill test (described in Chapter 12) can offer useful details on the pediatric patient's tissue perfusion. These measurements should be used only as a guide. The accuracy of this test can be affected by the environment and by the patient's general health, age, and gender.

4. *Disability.* The evaluation of the patient's level of consciousness is crucial in assessing cerebral oxygenation. The patient can become restless, agitated, and confused

as cerebral ischemia develops. In addition to shock, cerebral edema and intracranial hemorrhage from head injury can compromise cerebral perfusion. Any significant change in the patient's behavior or responses should be considered an indicator of a critical perfusion deficit to the brain. This is true whether the decrease in cerebral circulation is from shock or from an increase in intracranial pressure. The paramedic can measure the patient's level of consciousness with the AVPU (alert, verbal, painful, unresponsive) scale. The paramedic also can measure consciousness with other evaluation methods (see Chapter 24).

NOTE Some authorities believe that the level of consciousness and other indicators of adequate brain functions are the best way to determine appropriate blood pressure for the trauma patient. They contend that the brain is the organ most sensitive to changes in physiological state. The goals of this patient-focused method of shock management are to ensure that systolic pressure is at least 90 mm Hg and that the patient has positive peripheral pulses and is awake or responsive to stimuli.[5]

5. *Exposure of the body surfaces.* The paramedic should expose the body surfaces in the initial assessment as indicated by situation or mechanism of injury. A visual inspection can reveal conditions that may be life-threatening. These conditions can be hidden by clothing.

Differential Shock Assessment Findings

Shock is assumed to be hypovolemic until it is proved otherwise. However, assessment findings that can help the paramedic to differentiate between hypovolemic shock and other causes of shock include the following:

1. *Cardiogenic shock.* The patient often has a chief complaint of chest pain, dyspnea, or extreme heart rates (tachycardia, bradycardia, other dysrhythmias). Some patients also show signs of congestive heart failure such as jugular vein distention (described in Chapters 26 and 29).
2. *Distributive shock* (neurogenic shock, anaphylactic shock, septic shock). The patient's history or situation may reveal a mechanism that suggests vasodilation is the cause of the shock state. Signs and symptoms of distributive shock that are unusual in the presence of hypovolemic shock include warm flushed skin (especially in dependent areas). Those of neurogenic shock include a normal pulse rate (relative bradycardia).
3. *Obstructive shock* (caused by obstruction to blood flow). These patients often are the victims of a major chest injury (usually a penetrating type of injury). Or they reveal a history that is consistent with pulmonary embolism. (For example, they have had a recent surgery or long bone fracture.) Patients with cardiac tamponade or tension pneumothorax often have jugular vein distention. Also, patients with tension pneumothorax almost always have decreased breath sounds on the affected side.

Detailed Physical Examination

As discussed, the first action is the initial assessment and management of any life-threatening conditions. Then the paramedic should evaluate the patient further. A systematic approach offers a way to evaluate potentially life-threatening conditions and allows the paramedic to assess the patient's perfusion status further. This assessment should begin with baseline measurements of the patient's vital signs and evaluation of the patient's electrocardiogram.

CRITICAL THINKING

Can blood donation cause a fluid deficit large enough to cause shock? If so, how is that fluid deficit managed?

The paramedic should expect the pulse rate to increase above normal limits after a fluid deficit of 10% to 15%. Some patients, though, continue to have normal pulse rates even though a volume deficit of this extent exists. Thus the patient's pulse rate should be only one factor in evaluating the patient's level of perfusion.

Bradycardia, which can result from hypoxemia, existing neurological injury, increased vagal tone, preexisting illness, or prior medication use, also can indicate severe myocardial ischemia, a primary cause of cardiogenic shock. Bradycardic rhythms often occur just before cardiac arrest. When the paramedic notes a bradycardic rhythm, the paramedic should optimize oxygenation by increasing the fraction of inspired oxygen and by assisting ventilations if needed.

The diastolic pressure at first rises as peripheral vascular resistance increases with increased vascular tone. These changes decrease the container size. Blood also is shunted away selectively from certain portions of the body. When the heart can no longer pump blood to keep the container full on the arterial side, the diastolic pressure begins to drop. The paramedic should expect this when blood loss is greater than 20% to 25% of normal circulating blood volume.

The systolic pressure falls when the heart can no longer pump enough blood to fill the container at the end of cardiac contraction. Systolic pressure usually is more sensitive to volume depletion than is diastolic pressure. Therefore systolic pressure drops first. However, as the fluid deficit approaches 25%, systolic and diastolic pressures both begin to drop.

The paramedic should consider evaluation of orthostatic vital signs in conscious patients suspected of having lost circulating blood volume. The paramedic should consider this, provided that the paramedic does not suspect spinal injury or another condition that rules out this procedure. A rise from a recumbent position to a sitting or standing position associated with a fall in systolic pressure (after 1 minute) of 10 to 15 mm Hg or a concurrent rise in pulse rate (after 1 minute) of 10 to 15 beats per minute indicates a significant (at least 10%) volume depletion (postural hypotension) and a decrease in perfusion status.

A fluid deficit still can exist even after the systolic pressure returns to normal following fluid replacement. Therefore fluid replacement initiated in the prehospital setting should continue until indicators of adequate tissue perfusion are present (e.g., improved skin color, capillary refill of less than 2 seconds in pediatric patients, and normal pulse oximetry readings).

Resuscitation

Resuscitation of the shock victim is aimed at restoring adequate peripheral tissue oxygenation as quickly as possible. As previously stated, the paramedic accomplishes this by ensuring adequate oxygenation, maintaining an effective ratio of volume to container size, and rapidly transporting the victim to an appropriate medical facility.

> **NOTE** The overresuscitation of trauma patients can occur. In patients with closed head injury or pulmonary or cardiac contusion, one must avoid fluid overload. As stated before, medical direction and protocol should guide fluid resuscitation for the shock patient.

RED BLOOD CELL OXYGENATION

Adequate oxygenation of red blood cells is required for adequate tissue oxygenation. For red blood cell oxygenation to be adequate, the patient must have a patent airway. Ventilation also must be supported with a high fraction of inspired oxygen. If needed, the paramedic can assist ventilation with positive pressure. In addition, the paramedic should correct any abnormality that interferes with adequate ventilation (e.g., obstructed airway, pneumothorax, hemothorax, open chest wound, or unstable chest wall) (see Chapter 26).

RATIO OF VOLUME TO CONTAINER SIZE

The second component necessary to maintain adequate oxygen-carrying capacity requires that the container be full of fluid. The paramedic can achieve this by decreasing the size of the container. This is especially the case in shock states not associated with hemorrhage. In addition, in some cases of distributive shock, vasoconstricting drugs can be used to manage the shock when reduction of container size is the main concern. Volume replacement also may be necessary in these patients. One should note that vasoconstricting drugs generally are not recommended to treat patients in hypovolemic shock until fluid volume replacement is complete. Complete volume replacement rarely occurs in the prehospital setting.

PNEUMATIC ANTISHOCK GARMENT

The PASG (Fig. 21-6) is thought by some to be effective in managing shock through the following mechanisms[6]:

- The PASG reduces vessel diameter and artificially increases peripheral resistance in the tissues beneath the PASG. This helps to maintain perfusion pressure to the patient's other vital organs.

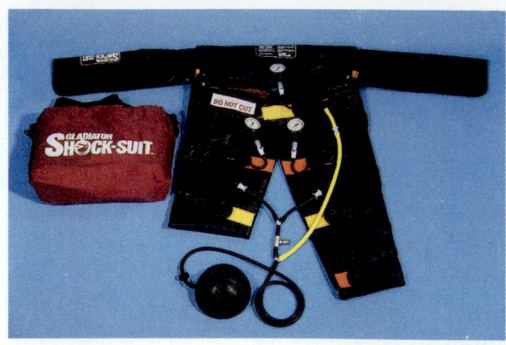

FIGURE 21-6 ■ JOBST Gladiator shock suit.

- The PASG can arrest hemorrhage by tamponading any bleeding vessels in the abdomen, pelvis, or lower extremities.
- The PASG can help to stabilize pelvic and lower-extremity fractures when it is inflated. Thus the PASG decreases movement and subsequent blood loss.

Although decisions on the use of the PASG are left to local protocol and medical direction, pulmonary edema, cardiogenic shock, ruptured diaphragm, and hemorrhage within the chest cavity generally are considered contraindications for the PASG.[2,6] Some medical direction authorities feel that use of a PASG also is contraindicated in the following situations:

- Impaled objects in the abdomen (precluding inflation of the abdominal section of the garment)
- Advanced pregnancy (third trimester pregnancy precludes inflation of the abdominal compartment)
- Evisceration (no inflation of the abdominal compartment)

GENERAL PNEUMATIC ANTISHOCK GARMENT GUIDELINES

The paramedic should apply the PASG when indicated after the lower extremities and abdomen have been inspected for major wounds. He or she must always position the garment below the level of the patient's lowest rib. The patient's blood pressure and lung sounds should be monitored before, during, and after inflation. He or she should stop inflation when an adequate blood pressure has been obtained. The paramedic must inflate the leg compartments before or with the abdominal compartment. *The paramedic should never inflate the abdominal section before inflating the leg sections.* Doing so can cause the abdominal compartment to act as a constrictive band that reduces venous return from the legs.

> **CRITICAL THINKING**
> Consider that the abdominal compartment of the pneumatic antishock garment is inflated mistakenly before the leg segments. What effect can this have on cardiac output?

After PASG inflation the garment should seldom if ever be deflated in the prehospital setting. The PASG should be deflated only with a physician's direction. The abdominal section is deflated before the leg sections. The patient should be monitored closely during the deflation process. Removal of the garment before fluid replacement commonly results in a rapid fall of blood pressure and cardiac output, which can lead to cardiac arrest.

Changes in temperature and atmospheric pressure can cause a notable change in the pressure within the PASG. The paramedic should monitor the patient constantly when the patient is moved from a cold environment to a warm one or when transported by air. The relationship among temperature, atmospheric pressure, and pressure within the PASG is as follows:

- A rise in temperature raises the pressure within the PASG; a fall in temperature decreases the pressure.
- A fall in atmospheric pressure causes an increase in PASG pressure; a rise in atmospheric pressure produces a decrease in garment pressure.

The PASG is not without complications even with appropriate use. Sustained inflation of the garment for more than 1 to 2 hours can lead to decreased tissue perfusion, ischemia of the underlying tissues, and loss of the limb, even without underlying fracture.

FLUID RESUSCITATION IN SHOCK

Almost every shock victim, except for patients in cardiogenic shock, requires volume expanders as part of resuscitation. The selection of intravenous (IV) fluids for initial volume replacement varies according to medical direction. In prehospital care the most common emergency requiring fluid replacement is loss of volume caused by hemorrhage or dehydration. The type of fluid replacement needed depends on the nature and extent of the volume loss. The two main categories of fluids used in resuscitation are crystalloids and colloids. The paramedic should follow the recommendations for fluid resuscitation provided by medical direction.

Crystalloids. Crystalloid solutions are created by dissolving crystals such as salts and sugars in water. These solutions do not have as much osmotic pressure as colloid solutions. They can be expected to equilibrate more quickly between the vascular and extravascular spaces. Two thirds of the infused crystalloid fluid leaves the vascular space within 1 hour. So 3 mL of a crystalloid solution is needed to replace 1 mL of blood. Examples of crystalloid solutions are lactated Ringer's solution, normal saline, and glucose solutions in water.

Hypertonic solutions have higher osmotic pressure than that of body cells. They include 5% dextrose in 0.9% sodium chloride, 7.5% saline, and 5% dextrose in 0.45% sodium chloride. Hypotonic solutions have a lower osmotic pressure than that of body cells (e.g., distilled water and 0.45% sodium chloride).

Lactated Ringer's solution is the fluid of choice for resuscitating patients in shock.[6] The solution is well balanced and contains many of the chemicals found in human blood. Lactated Ringer's solution contains sodium chloride, small amounts of potassium and calcium, and 28 mEq of lactate, which can act as a buffer to neutralize acidity when metabolized by the liver. One third of the infused solution remains in the vascular space after 1 hour.

Normal saline contains 154 mEq/L of sodium. Normal saline has no buffering capabilities. Although preferred by some physicians, the higher chloride content of normal saline is less desirable than the more balanced lactated Ringer's solution. As in lactated Ringer's solution, nearly one third of the infused normal saline remains in the vascular space after 1 hour. This makes it an equally effective volume expander. Studies have not shown superiority of one option over the other.

Glucose-containing solutions (e.g., 5% dextrose in water) have immediate volume expansion effects. However, the glucose leaves the intravascular compartment rapidly with a resultant free water increase. The volume-replacement benefits of glucose solutions only last 5 to 10 minutes while the glucose is metabolized. Thus use of 5% dextrose in water as a replacement fluid in volume deficits is inappropriate. Glucose solutions most often are used to maintain vascular access for administration of IV medications.

> **NOTE** Five percent dextrose in water is an isotonic solution. When administered, however, the dextrose molecules leave the circulation so rapidly that its effect is that of a hypotonic solution.

Colloids. Colloid solutions contain molecules (usually protein) that are too large to pass through the capillary membrane. These solutions exhibit osmotic pressure. They remain within the vascular compartment for a considerable time. Examples of colloid solutions are whole blood, packed red blood cells, blood plasma, and plasma substitutes. Colloids generally are reserved for in-hospital use and are not recommended for prehospital management of shock.[6]

Whole blood replacement sometimes is indicated after initial fluid resuscitation with a crystalloid solution in patients who have had a major loss of blood. Whole blood replacement rarely is given. Rather, packed red cells are transfused and other blood components are transfused as necessary. Whole blood is drawn in a citrate solution to prevent clotting. Whole blood can be refrigerated up to 3 weeks. A type and crossmatch should be obtained when possible before a patient is given blood to determine the patient's ABO group and Rh type (described in Chapter 7). Typing and crossmatching also will determine whether other antibodies are present that may cause a transfusion reaction. Several types of blood transfusion reactions may occur during or up to 96 hours after infusion. Symptoms may range from mild fever to life-threatening shock. If a reaction is suspected (e.g., during an interhospital transfer), the paramedic should stop the transfusion and contact medical direction.

Centrifugation, the process of spinning compartmentalized blood to separate particles from liquid, separates packed red blood cells from the plasma component of blood. Like whole blood, packed red cells must be typed and crossmatched and may be refrigerated for up to 3 weeks. The advantage of packed red blood cells over whole blood is that the volume of hemoglobin per unit is almost twice that of whole blood. In addition, because there is no plasma, circulatory overload is less likely and transfusion reactions are less frequent.

Blood plasma is procured by separating the blood cells from the whole citrated blood. Blood plasma may be given without concern for ABO compatibility. Blood plasma contains fibrinogen, albumin, gamma globulins, *hemoagglutinins* (an agglutinin that clumps red blood corpuscles), prothrombin (a chemical that is part of the clotting cascade, further described in Chapter 22), other clotting factors, sugar, and salts. Blood plasma sometimes is used to restore effective blood volume in circulatory failure associated with burns, traumatic shock, and hemorrhage. Blood plasma more commonly is used to correct clotting deficiencies.

Plasma substitutes do not increase oxygen-carrying capacity by replacing red blood cells. They also do not improve clotting by the addition of plasma protein. Yet at times they are used to restore circulating blood volume as an emergency treatment for hypovolemia caused by blood loss. Plasma substitutes such as dextran and hetastarch have osmotic properties similar to those of plasma. Thus they stay in the intravascular space longer than crystalloid solution. Plasma substitutes do not carry the human immunodeficiency virus or hepatitis viruses. They also do not require type and crossmatching before administration. They are readily available as well. Plasma substitutes do have some adverse effects, including increased bleeding tendencies and immune suppression. Emergency vehicles can carry plasma substitutes, but expense and storage issues make them impractical for general use in the prehospital setting.

▶NOTE **Oxygen-carrying blood substitutes (e.g., PolyHeme) are being studied. They may have future application in prehospital care for severely injured patients. These solutions contain hemoglobin from red blood cells (treated to destroy viruses). In addition, they are compatible with all blood types. They do not require refrigeration and can be stored up to several months.**

Theory of Fluid Flow. The flow of fluid through a catheter is related directly to its diameter (to the fourth power) and inversely related to its length. Therefore a catheter with a large diameter has a much greater flow than a catheter with a small diameter; short catheters provide faster flow rates than longer catheters of equal diameter. Other factors that affect the flow of fluid include the diameter and length of the tubing, the size of the vein, and the viscosity and temperature of the IV fluid. (Temperature affects viscosity; warm fluids generally flow better than cold ones.) Pressure bags are available that pressurize the IV system to 300 mm Hg to maximize the rate of fluid administration. Table 21-2 lists the maximum rate of fluid flow for various gauges of 2-inch Medicut catheters without pressure on the bag at a height of 1 m above the patient.[7] When aggressive fluid resuscitation is indicated, the paramedic should do the following:

- Use short, large-diameter catheters.
- Use warm fluids of low viscosity (if possible).
- Keep the tubing short, and pressurize the IV system.

TABLE 21-2 Needle Gauges and Maximum Fluid Flow

NEEDLE GAUGE*	MAXIMUM FLUID FLOW
18 gauge	4.81 L/hr or 80 mL/min
16 gauge	7.45 L/hr or 124 mL/min
14 gauge	9.67 L/hr or 161 mL/min

*Inside diameter.

CRITICAL THINKING

Aside from flow, what other benefits do warmed fluids offer for the patient in shock who needs a large-volume fluid bolus?

Key Principles in Managing Shock

The paramedic should follow these key principles as part of the plan for managing shock (Fig. 21-7):

1. Establish and maintain an open airway.
2. Administer high-concentration oxygen. Assist ventilation as needed.
3. Control external bleeding (if present).
4. By order of medical direction or per protocol, initiate IV fluid replacement if appropriate. Two large-bore IV lines of a volume-expanding fluid commonly are established in cases of hypovolemia. *The IV administration of fluids in the prehospital setting should not delay patient transportation because crystalloid solutions cannot restore the oxygen-carrying capacity of blood.* Generally, the patient is best served by rapid assessment, airway stabilization, immobilization, and rapid transportation to an appropriate medical facility. Many emergency medical services authorities recommend that IV therapy for shock resuscitation be initiated en route to the hospital.
5. Consider the use of a PASG (per protocol). The paramedic should consider use of the PASG especially if transportation time is long, pelvic fractures are suspected, or a patient is deteriorating despite IV therapy.
6. Maintain the patient's normal body temperature. Patients in shock often are unable to conserve body heat. They can become hypothermic easily.
7. In the absence of spinal or head injury and if hypovolemia is suspected and ventilation is adequate, consider

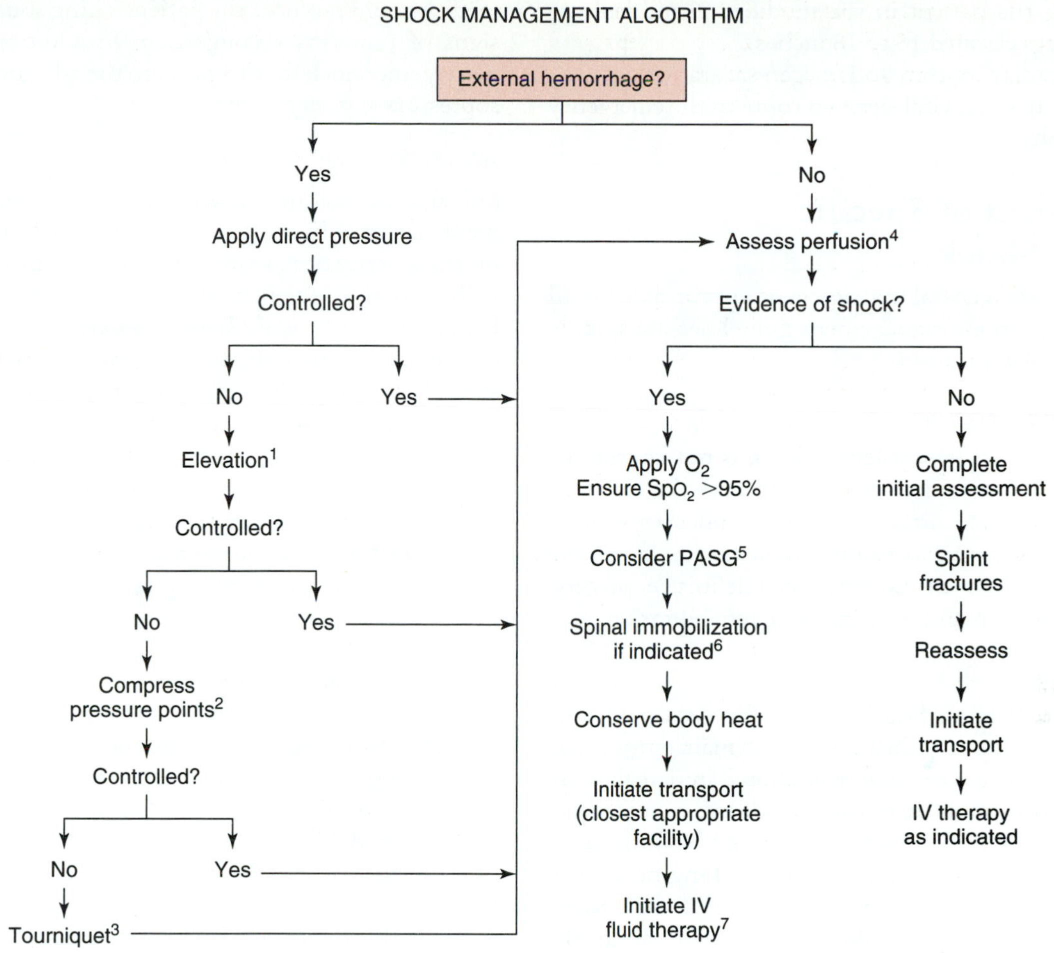

Notes:

1 Elevation should be considered unless contraindicated by fractures or inability to elevate a specific body part.

2 Compression should be applied proximal to the bleeding site in one of the following locations: axillary artery, brachial artery, femoral artery, or popliteal artery.

3 A wide material such as a cravat, belt, or blood pressure cuff should be used; a tourniquet should not be placed distal to the elbow or knee.

4 Assessment of perfusion includes presence quality, and location of pulses; skin color, temperature, and moisture; and capillary refilling time.

5 PASG should be considered for decompensated shock (SBP <90 mm Hg), and suspected pelvic, intraperitoneal, or retroperitoneal hemorrhage, and in patients with profound hypotension (SBP <60 mm Hg). PASG is contraindicated in penetrating thoracic trauma, abdominal evisceration, pregnancy, impaled object in the abdomen, and traumatic cardiopulmonary arrest, or for splinting the lower extremity fractures. Follow local protocol.

6 See Chapter 25 for spinal immobilization guidelines.

7 Initiate two large-bore (14- or 16-gauge) IV catheters. An initial bolus of 1 to 2 liters of warmed (102° F) lactated Ringer's solution or normal saline should be given rapidly. For pediatric patients, the initial fluid bolus should be 20 mL/kg. Check with medical directors regarding the volume of fluid bolus in shock.

FIGURE 21-7 ■ Shock management algorithm.

positioning the patient in the modified Trendelenburg position (legs elevated 15 to 18 inches).

8. Monitor cardiac rhythm and oxygen saturation.
9. Frequently reassess vital signs en route to the emergency department.

Management of Specific Forms of Shock

In addition to the general management appropriate for all shock victims, certain management guidelines are specific to each shock classification.

HYPOVOLEMIC SHOCK

The management of hypovolemic shock is not considered complete until the volume is replaced and the cause or causes of shock are corrected. This includes crystalloid fluid replacement in cases of simple dehydration or volume replacement because of hemorrhage, definitive surgery, critical care support, and postoperative rehabilitation.

CARDIOGENIC SHOCK

The management of cardiogenic shock focuses on improving the pumping action of the heart and on managing cardiac rhythm irregularities. The paramedic should initiate fluid resuscitation in the adult with 100 to 200 mL of a volume-expanding fluid. Fluid resuscitation should be initiated as long as the patient has no crackles in the lung fields. The crackles would indicate pulmonary edema. If the patient improves, fluid therapy should be continued cautiously. Fluid therapy should continue until the blood pressure stabilizes and the pulse rate decreases. The paramedic should assess lung sounds often. If the patient shows signs of increased lung congestion, the paramedic should adjust the rate of infusion to keep the vein open.

Drug therapy for cardiogenic shock varies according to cause. Drug therapy can include vasopressors, vasodilators, inotropic drugs, and antidysrhythmics (usually after fluid infusion) (see Chapter 29). Patients with cardiogenic shock caused by myocardial ischemia or infarction require reperfusion strategies (clot busting drugs or surgery) and possible circulatory support. The paramedic must manage obstructive causes of cardiogenic shock immediately, including tension pneumothorax and cardiac tamponade (see Chapter 26).

NEUROGENIC SHOCK

The management of neurogenic shock is similar to the management for hypovolemia. However, the paramedic must take care during fluid therapy to avoid circulatory overload. Throughout the resuscitation phase, the paramedic should monitor the patient's lung sounds closely for signs of pulmonary congestion. In addition, patients in neurogenic shock may respond to the administration of vasopressors (e.g., ***dopamine***).

ANAPHYLACTIC SHOCK

Subcutaneous administration of ***epinephrine*** is the treatment of choice in acute anaphylactic reactions. Depending on the severity of reaction, other treatment modalities can include oral, IV, or intramuscular administration of antihistamines such as ***diphenhydramine.*** The paramedic can administer bronchodilators to treat bronchospasm and steroids to reduce the inflammatory response.

Crystalloid volume replacement also is indicated. Crystalloids may compensate for the increased container size caused by vasodilation resulting from histamine release during an anaphylactic reaction. Paramedics should anticipate the need for aggressive airway management in any allergic reaction (see Chapter 33).

SEPTIC SHOCK

The management of septic shock in the prehospital setting can include the management of hypovolemia (if present) and the correction of metabolic acid-base imbalance. Depending on the patient's response to the infection, prehospital care may involve fluid resuscitation, respiratory support, and the administration of vasopressors to improve cardiac output. If possible, the paramedic should obtain a thorough patient history. The history will help to identify the cause of sepsis. Any immunocompromised group of patients has an increased risk of septic shock. Examples of such groups include those with human immunodeficiency virus infection, some cancer patients receiving chemotherapy, and patients with indwelling urinary or vascular catheters.

INTEGRATION OF PATIENT ASSESSMENT AND THE TREATMENT PLAN

The goals of prehospital care for the patient with severe hemorrhage or shock include rapid recognition of the event, initiation of treatment, prevention of additional injury, rapid transport to an appropriate medical facility by ground or air ambulance, and advanced notification of the receiving facility. The paramedic should follow guidelines established by local protocol and medical direction in determining the appropriate prehospital level of care for patients and in identifying the appropriate medical facility for patient transport.

SUMMARY

- The seriousness of external hemorrhage depends on the anatomical source of the hemorrhage, the degree of vascular disruption, and the amount of blood loss that can be tolerated by the patient. Internal bleeding that causes the patient to be unstable usually occurs in one of three body cavities: the chest, abdomen, or retroperitoneum.
- Shock is not a single entity. Shock does not have one specific cause and treatment. Rather, shock is a complex group of physiological abnormalities. Moreover, shock can result from a variety of disease states and injuries.
- To achieve adequate oxygenation of tissue cells (perfusion), three distinct components of the cardiovascular system must function properly: the heart, vasculature, and lungs.
- The healthy body is a smooth-flowing fluid delivery system inside a container. The volume of the container is related directly to the diameter of the resistance vessels. This diameter can change rapidly.
- Normal adult blood volume is 4.5 to 5 L.
- The progression of shock affects the microcirculation. This progression follows a sequence of stages related to changes in capillary perfusion and cellular necrosis. These stages include vasoconstriction, capillary and venule opening, disseminated intravascular coagulation, and multiple organ failure.
- In emergency care, shock commonly is classified based on the cause. (For example, the cause may be hypovolemic, cardiogenic, neurogenic, anaphylactic, or septic.)
- The response of the body to the shock syndrome (hypoperfusion and its associated anaerobic metabolism) can be categorized into stages: compensated shock, uncompensated (or decompensated) shock, and irreversible shock.
- Variations in the physiological response to shock can occur based on a number of factors. The patient's age and health are factors. The patient's ability to activate compensatory mechanisms plays a role. The specific organ affected is a factor as well.
- The management and treatment plan for the patient in shock focuses on assessment. The paramedic must assess oxygenation and perfusion of the body organs. The goals of the treatment plan are to ensure a patent airway, to provide adequate oxygenation and ventilation, and to restore perfusion. The initial survey can help to identify the adequacy of cellular perfusion.

REFERENCES

1. Rosen P, Barkin R: *Emergency medicine: concepts and clinical practice,* ed 5, St Louis, 2003, Mosby.
2. Mann FC: Systems of surgery, *Bull Johns Hopkins Hosp* 25:205, 1914.
3. Hardaway R, editor: *Shock: the reversible stage of dying,* Littleton, Mass, 1988, PSG Publishing.
4. US Department of Transportation, National Highway Traffic Safety Administration: *EMT-Paramedic national standard curriculum,* Washington, DC, 1998, The Department.
5. Criss E: Trauma management in the new millennium, *J Emerg Med Serv JEMS* 24(12):34, 1999.
6. National Association of Emergency Medical Technicians: *PHTLS: basic and advanced prehospital trauma life support,* ed 5, St Louis, 2003, Mosby.
7. Haynes B et al: Catheter introducers for rapid fluid resuscitation, *Ann Emerg Med* 12(10):606, 1983.

CHAPTER

22

Soft Tissue Trauma

OBJECTIVES

Upon completion of this chapter, the paramedic student will be able to:

1. Describe the normal structure and function of the skin.
2. Describe the pathophysiological responses to soft tissue injury.
3. Discuss pathophysiology as a basis for key signs and symptoms, and describe the mechanism of injury and signs and symptoms of specific soft tissue injuries.
4. Outline management principles for prehospital care of soft tissue injuries.
5. Describe, in the correct sequence, patient management techniques for control of hemorrhage.
6. Identify the characteristics of general categories of dressings and bandages.
7. Describe prehospital management of specific soft tissue injuries not requiring closure.
8. Discuss factors that increase the potential for wound infection.
9. Describe the prehospital management of selected soft tissue injuries.

KEY TERMS

abrasion: A partial-thickness injury caused by scraping or rubbing away of a layer or layers of skin.

amputation: A complete or partial loss of a limb caused by mechanical force.

avulsion: A full-thickness skin loss in which the wound edges cannot be approximated.

compartment syndrome: The result of a crush injury, usually caused by compressive forces or blunt trauma to muscle groups confined in tight fibrous sheaths with minimal ability to stretch.

crush injury: Injury from exposure of tissue to a compressive force sufficient to interfere with the normal structure and metabolic function of the involved cells and tissues.

crush syndrome: A life-threatening and sometimes preventable complication of prolonged immobilization; a pathological process that causes destruction, alteration, or both of muscle tissue.

hematoma: A closed injury characterized by blood vessel disruption and swelling beneath the epidermis.

puncture wound: An open injury that results from contact with a penetrating object.

rhabdomyolysis: An acute, sometimes fatal, disease characterized by destruction of skeletal muscle.

The skin and its accessory organs are the primary cosmetic structures of the body. These structures perform many functions that are critical to survival. The paramedic must understand soft tissue trauma fully. This understanding will help the paramedic to assess life-threatening injury quickly. This understanding also will help the paramedic to intervene to promote normal healing and function.

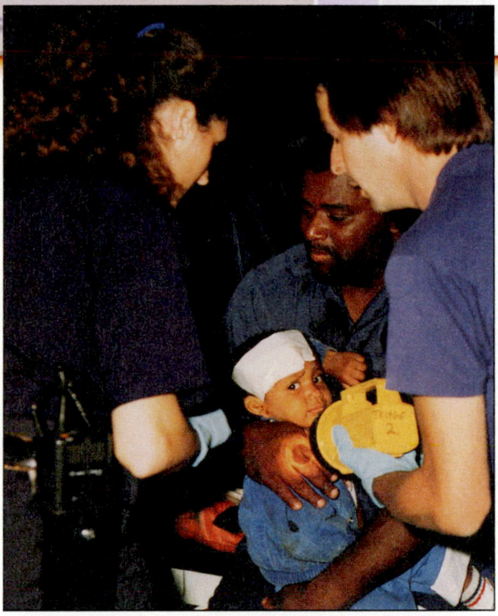

NOTE Each year about 40 million persons in the United States seek care in emergency departments for soft tissue injuries that result from falls, motor vehicle crashes, blunt and penetrating trauma, and burns. Although most soft tissue injuries are not life threatening, more than 73,000 persons died as a result of these injuries in 2001.[1]

ANATOMY AND PHYSIOLOGY

The skin is a tough, supple membrane that covers the entire body. The skin constitutes the largest and most dynamic organ of the body, covering more than 20 sq ft and making up 16% of total body weight. The skin comprises two distinct layers of tissue: the outer layer (epidermis) and the inner layer (dermis) (Fig. 22-1).

Epidermis

The epidermis is a thin, nonvascular epithelial tissue that derives its nourishment from the capillaries of the dermis. Although the epidermis is only as thick as a page of this text, the epidermis is composed of five layers: stratum basale, the innermost layer; stratum spinosum; stratum granulosum; stratum lucidum; and stratum corneum, the most superficial layer of the epidermis. The stratum corneum is composed of about 20 layers of dead skin cells that are filled with the waterproofing protein keratin.

Dermis

The dermis lies beneath the epidermis. The dermis contains connective tissue, elastic fibers, blood vessels, lymph vessels, and motor and sensory fibers. The dermis also houses other structures of the integumentary system. These other structures include hair, nails, and sebaceous and sweat glands. This layer of skin offers protection against bacterial invasion. The dermis helps maintain fluid balance as well.

Connective tissue and elastic fibers in the dermis give skin its strength and elasticity. Blood vessels in the dermis nourish all skin cells. They also aid in body temperature regulation through vasoconstriction or vasodilation. Nerves in the dermis generate impulses to dermal muscles and glands. These nerves also are responsible for carrying impulses away from sensory receptors in the skin in response to pain, touch, heat, and cold.

CRITICAL THINKING

Predict the effects of destruction of a large segment of skin, which includes the dermis, based on your knowledge of its functions.

The dermis has a reservoir of defensive and regenerative elements. These elements combat infection and repair deep

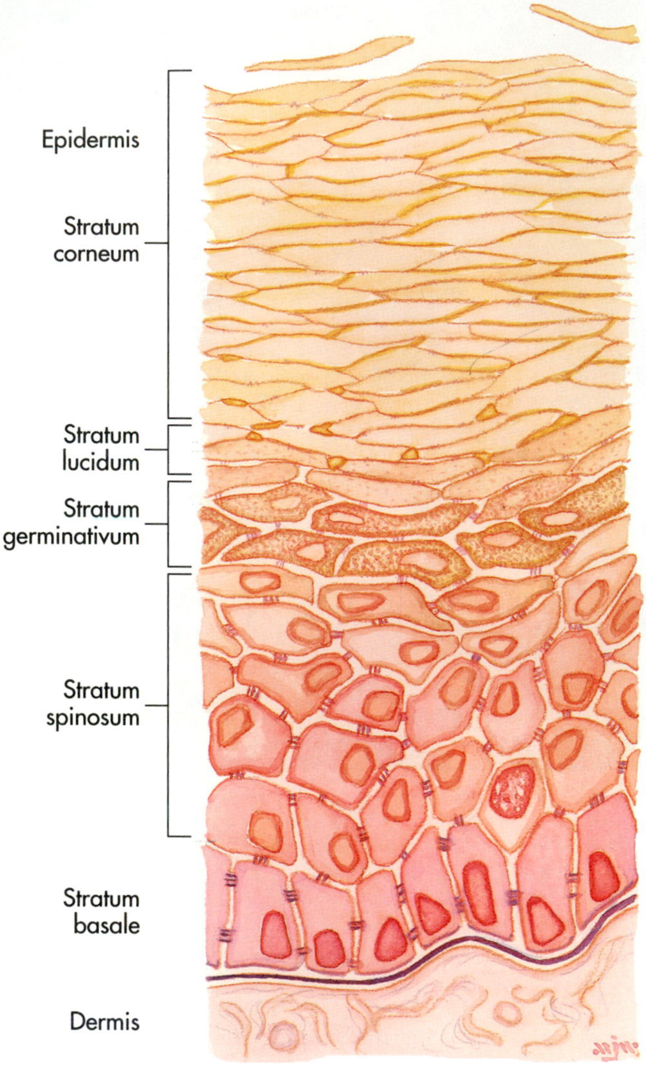

FIGURE 22-1 ■ Tissue layers of the skin.

wounds. They do this by use of specialized white blood cells, lymphatics, and other cellular components.

The dense layer of fibrous tissue beneath the dermis is the deep fascia. This layer provides for insulation, cushioning, caloric reserve, and body substance and shape. The primary function of this tissue is to support and protect underlying structures.

PATHOPHYSIOLOGY

Surface trauma can disrupt the normal distribution of body fluids and electrolytes. Surface trauma also can interfere with the maintenance of body temperature. The two physiological responses to surface trauma are vascular and inflammatory reactions. These reactions can lead to healing, scar formation, or both. The extent and success of these responses are influenced by the amount of tissue that has been disrupted.

Hemostasis of Wound Healing

As described in Chapter 21, hemostasis is the initial physiological response to wounding. This vascular reaction involves vasoconstriction, formation of a platelet plug, coagulation, and the growth of fibrous tissue into the blood clot that permanently closes and seals the injured vessel.

Vasoconstriction resulting from injury is rapid but temporary. In response to injury, severed blood vessels constrict and retract with the aid of the surrounding subcutaneous tissues. This vessel spasm slows blood loss immediately. Vasoconstriction may close the ends of the injured vessels completely. The vasoconstriction response usually is sustained for as long as 10 minutes. During this time, blood coagulation mechanisms are activated to produce a blood clot.

Platelets adhere to injured blood vessels and to collagen in the connective tissue that surrounds the injured vessel. As platelets contact collagen, they swell, become sticky, and secrete chemicals that activate other surrounding platelets.

FIGURE 22-2 ■ The complex clotting mechanism can be distilled into three basic steps: release of platelet factors at the injury site, formation of thrombin, and trapping of red blood cells in fibrin to form a clot.

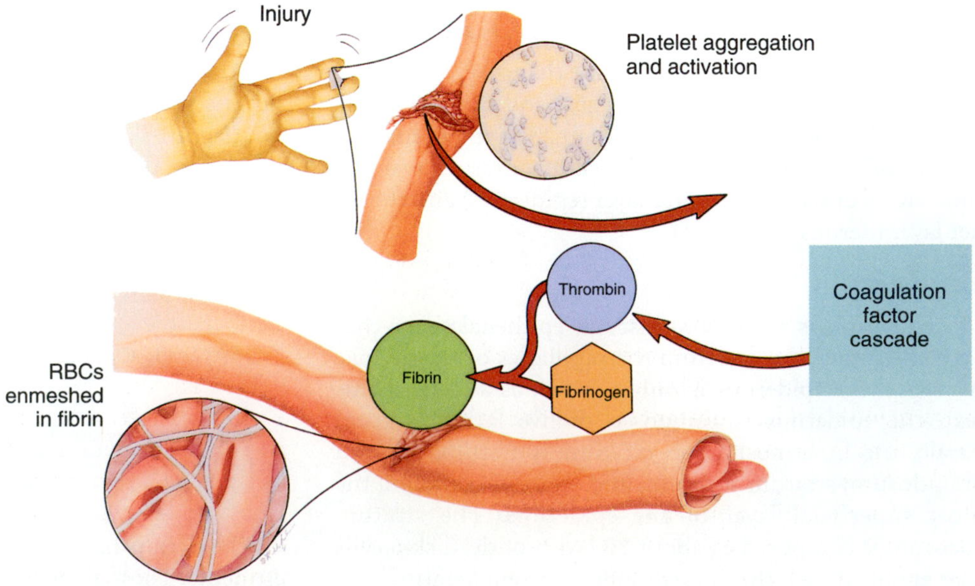

This process causes the platelets to adhere to one another. The process creates a platelet plug in the injured vessel. If the opening in the vessel wall is small, the plug may be sufficient to stop blood loss completely. For larger wounds, however, a blood clot is necessary to arrest the flow of blood (Fig. 22-2).

Blood coagulation occurs as a result of a chemical process that begins within seconds of a severe vessel injury and within 1 to 2 minutes of a minor wound. Coagulation progresses rapidly; within 3 to 6 minutes after the rupture of a vessel, the entire end of the vessel is filled with a clot. Within 30 minutes the clot retracts and the vessel is sealed further. The blood-clotting mechanism is a complex process and includes the following three mechanisms:

1. Prothrombin activator is formed in response to rupture or damage of the blood vessel.
2. Prothrombin activator stimulates the conversion of prothrombin to thrombin.
3. Thrombin acts as an enzyme to convert fibrinogen into fibrin threads. These threads entrap platelets, blood cells, and plasma to form the clot.

The process of hemostasis usually is protective. Hemostasis is required for survival. In some instances, though, hemostasis can result in responses that threaten life and function. For example, blood clots that form in atherosclerotic vessels can lead to myocardial infarction or stroke. (See Chapter 29.)

Certain diseases or genetic factors that interrupt the clotting process (also referred to as the clotting cascade) can impair hemostasis. Thus they retard the process of clot formation. Examples include hemophilia, thrombocytopenia (low platelet count), and liver disease, which affects the production of clotting factors. Various drugs also can impair coagulation. ***Aspirin*** decreases platelet activity. Warfarin suppresses the ability of the liver to make certain clotting factors. In any patient with impaired hemostasis, even minor trauma can result in uncontrollable and life-threatening hemorrhage.

CRITICAL THINKING

List some drugs that may impair the normal clotting functions.

Inflammatory Response

The release of chemicals from the injured vessel and various blood components (platelets, white blood cells) causes localized vasodilation of arterioles, precapillary sphincters, and venules, increasing the permeability of the affected capillaries and vessels. Plasma, plasma proteins, electrolytes, and chemical substances from the leaking venules accumulate in the extracellular space for about 72 hours after the injury. Blood flow increases to the area of injury. This increase supplies the metabolic demands of the tissues during healing and results in the redness, swelling, and pain associated with inflammation.

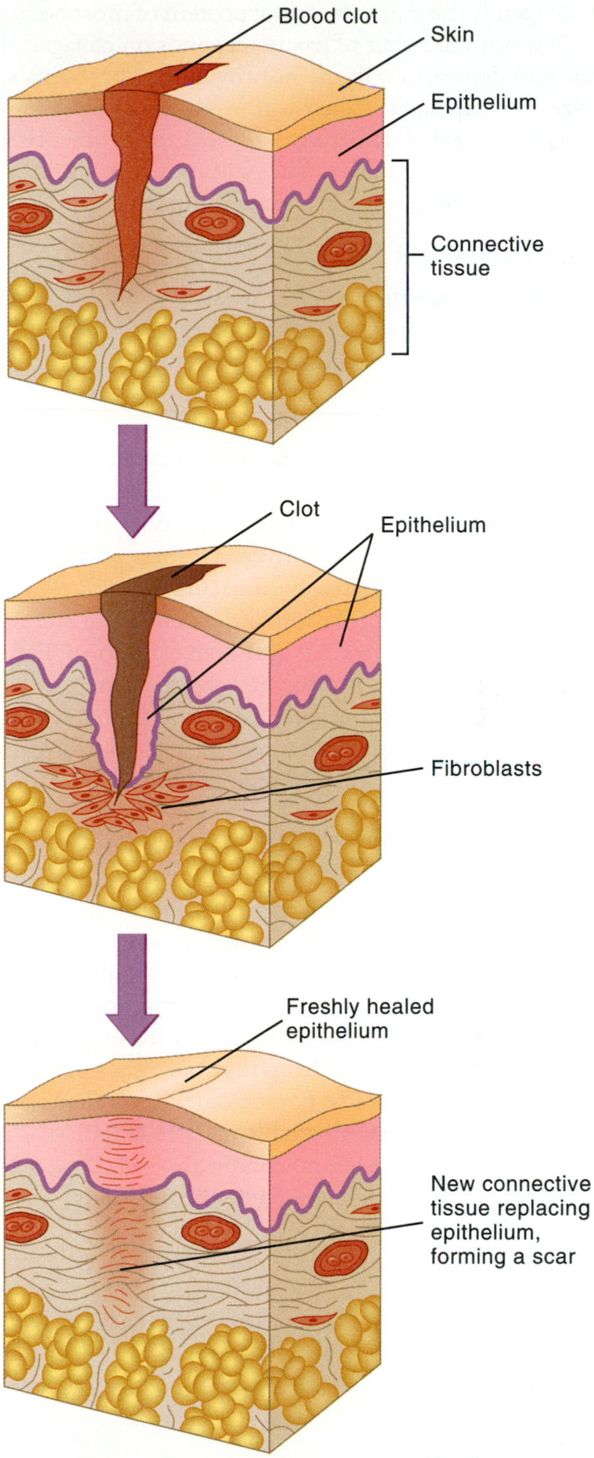

FIGURE 22-3 ■ Healing of a minor wound.

The transportation of granulocytes, lymphocytes, and macrophages to the injured area also increases local blood flow. These specialized cells prepare the wound for healing. They clear foreign bodies and dead tissue. They trigger neovascularization (new vessel formation) as well. Within 12 hours of the injury, new epithelial cells are regenerated. (This is the epithelialization phase.) These cells begin the process of healing through the reestablishment of skin layers (Fig. 22-3).

Collagen is the main structural protein of most body tissues. The normal repair of tissues depends on collagen synthesis and deposition. In the healthy body, fibroblasts synthesize and deposit collagen within 48 hours after injury. Collagen increases the tensile strength of the tissue. However, most injured tissue will not regain its full strength and function until at least 4 months later.[2]

Alterations of Wound Healing

Many factors can affect or alter wound healing. These include anatomic factors, concurrent drug use, medical condition and disease, and wounds that are high-risk.

ANATOMIC FACTORS

Some tissues of the body heal better and faster than others because of the body region and the amount of tension on the tissues (lines of tension). The elasticity of the skin and lines of tension vary in different areas of the body. Moreover, they are affected by muscular contraction and the body movements of flexion and extension. Thus these factors affect wound healing and scar formation. For example, a soft tissue injury to the forearm generally heals better and faster than one over a joint. Other anatomical factors that may affect wound healing and scar formation adversely include oily skin and pigmentation.

CONCURRENT DRUG USE, EXISTING MEDICAL CONDITIONS, AND DISEASE

Certain factors can delay or interfere with the normal wound-healing process through various mechanisms. For instance, a patient's concurrent drug use can interfere with or delay this process. Existing medical conditions also may have this effect. In addition, disease can delay or interfere with the process. Common drugs that can alter wound healing include corticosteroids, nonsteroidal antiinflammatory drugs (***aspirin***), penicillin, colchicine, anticoagulants, and antineoplastic agents. Medical conditions and diseases that can result in delayed healing include the following:

- Advanced age
- Severe alcoholism
- Acute uremia
- Diabetes
- Hypoxia
- Peripheral vascular disease
- Malnutrition
- Advanced cancer
- Hepatic failure
- Cardiovascular disease

HIGH-RISK WOUNDS

High-risk wounds have an increased potential for infection because of the location of the wound or the nature of the wounding force. Examples of high-risk wounds include those located on or near the hands, feet, and perineal areas. Wound forces that are associated with a high risk for infection include those produced by human and animal bites, foreign bodies, and injection (e.g., high-pressure grease guns). Other high-risk wounds are those contaminated with organic material or that have a significant amount of dead (devitalized) tissue; crush wounds; and any wounds in patients who are immunocompromised or who have poor peripheral circulation.

ABNORMAL SCAR FORMATION

Abnormal scar formation can result in a keloid or hypertrophic scar. A keloid is the excessive accumulation of scar tissue that extends beyond the original wound borders. This abnormal scar is more common in darkly pigmented patients. The scar also is more common in those who have injuries to the ears, upper extremities, lower abdomen, or sternum. A hypertrophic scar has an excess accumulation of scar tissue within the original wound borders. This scar is more common in areas of high tissue stress such as the flexion creases across joints.

WOUNDS REQUIRING CLOSURE

Although all serious wounds should be evaluated by a physician, the paramedic should expect the following types of wounds to require closure:

- Wounds to cosmetic regions (e.g., face, lips, and eyebrows)
- Gaping wounds
- Wounds over tension areas (e.g., joints)
- Degloving injuries (described later in this chapter)
- Ring finger injuries
- Skin tearing

Many techniques are used to close a wound, including suture, tape, staples, and tissue adhesives.

PATHOPHYSIOLOGY AND ASSESSMENT OF SOFT TISSUE INJURIES

Soft tissue injuries are classified as closed or open. This classification depends on the absence or presence of a break in the continuity of the epidermis. Soft tissue wounds often are the most evident injury. However, they generally are considered low-priority injuries, unless life-threatening hemorrhage or associated airway compromise is present.

Closed Wounds

Closed soft tissue injuries usually are associated with little blood loss. However, some of these injuries can cause significant hemorrhage in the cavities of the thorax, abdomen, pelvis, or soft tissues of the legs. This text classifies closed wounds as contusion, **hematoma,** and **crush injury.**

CONTUSIONS AND HEMATOMATA

Blunt trauma causes contusions and hematomata. A contusion is characterized by blood vessel disruption beneath the epidermis. A contusion results in swelling, pain, and ecchymosis (bruising) that can occur 24 to 48 hours after the

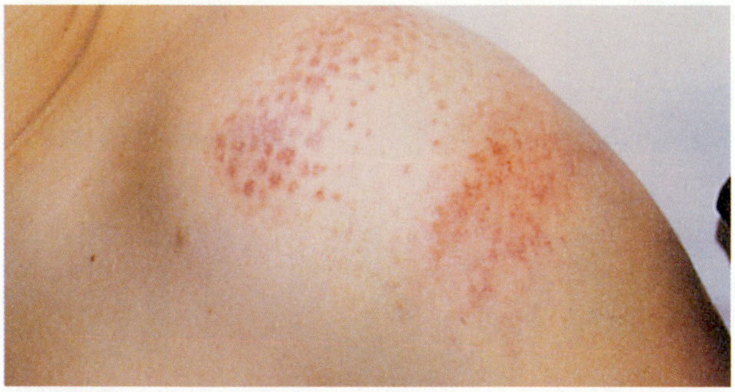

FIGURE 22-4 ■ Spotty bruising on a well-padded part of the shoulder.

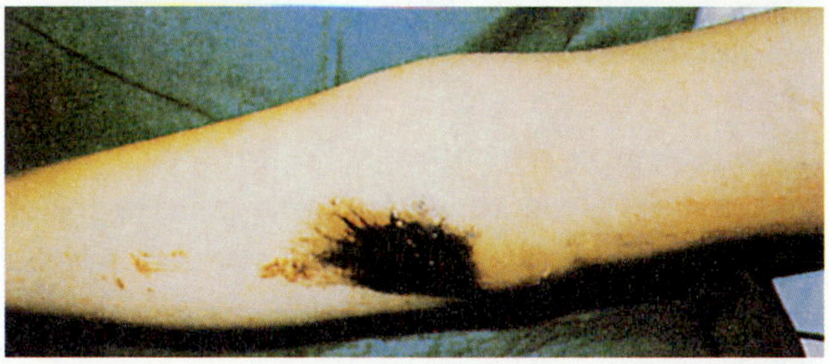

FIGURE 22-6 ■ Deep abrasion caused by a fall from a bicycle.

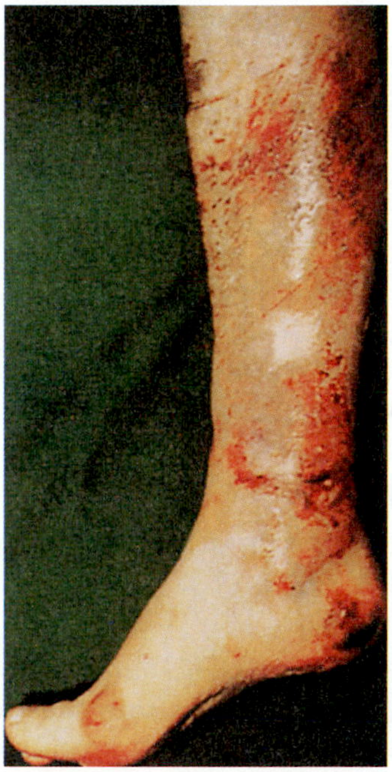

FIGURE 22-5 ■ Appearance of a woman's leg after it had been run over by the wheel of a milk van.

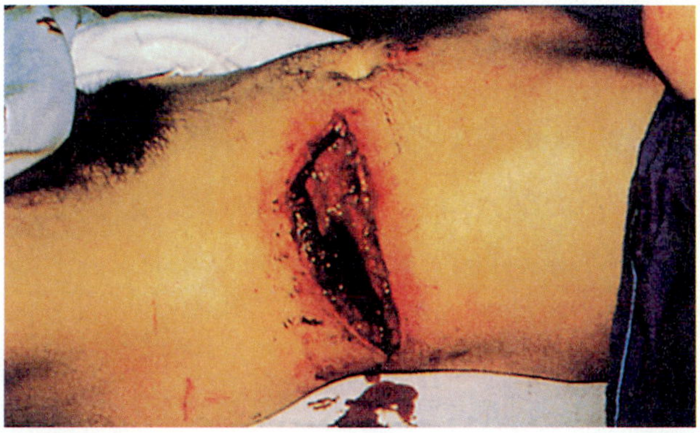

FIGURE 22-7 ■ Large wound caused by a broken power saw.

injury. A hematoma is a collection of blood beneath the skin. A hematoma may occur with a contusion. However, the hematoma represents a larger amount of tissue damage and the disruption of larger vessels (Fig. 22-4). These wounds usually are superficial. Sometimes, though, they are associated with underlying fractures, vascular involvement, and significant hemorrhage.

CRUSH INJURY

Crush injury can occur when a crushing force is applied to a body area (Fig. 22-5). These injuries can be severe. Sometimes they are associated with internal organ rupture, major fractures, and hemorrhagic shock. Overlying skin may remain intact with crush injury, even in the presence of severe injury and shock. Crush injuries are described further later in this chapter.

> **CRITICAL THINKING**
> What are some mechanisms of crush injury?

Open Wounds

Open soft tissue injuries are classified as **abrasion,** laceration, puncture, **avulsion, amputation,** and bites. (Note: Burns that include open and closed injury are addressed in Chapter 23.)

ABRASION

An abrasion is a partial-thickness skin injury. Abrasion is caused by the scraping or rubbing away of a layer or layers of skin (Fig. 22-6). The wound usually results from friction with a hard object or surface. (For example, abrasions occur in sports injuries and motorcycle crashes.) Although these wounds often are superficial, they are painful and are at high risk for infection from contamination.

LACERATION

A laceration results from a tear, a split, or an incision of the skin (Fig. 22-7). Lacerations most often are caused by a knife or other sharp object, resulting in a linear wound or incision. The sizes and depths of lacerations vary

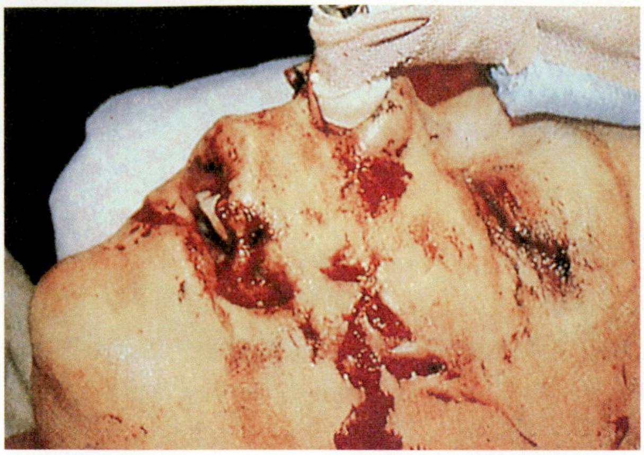

FIGURE 22-8 ■ Puncture wounds caused by broken glass from a shattered windshield.

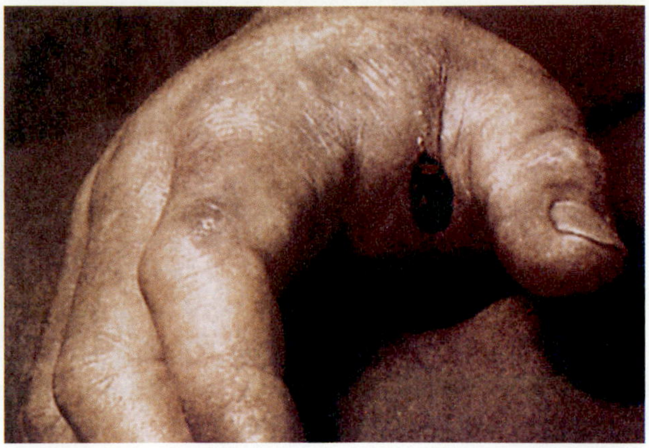

FIGURE 22-10 ■ Injection of paraffin into the hand resulted in amputation of the index finger.

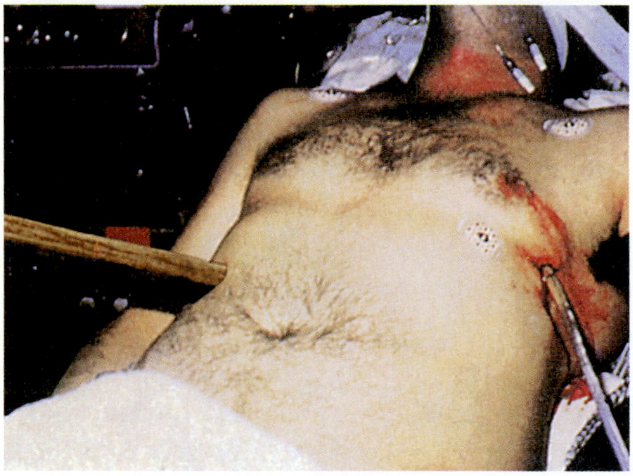

FIGURE 22-9 ■ Piece of wood impaled in the right side of the chest, piercing the diaphragm and lacerating the spleen, stomach, and liver.

greatly depending on the injury sites and wounding mechanism. Lacerations can be sources of significant bleeding.

PUNCTURE

Contact with a sharp, pointed object commonly causes a **puncture wound** (Fig. 22-8). (Examples of such objects include a wooden splinter, needle, staple, glass, or nail.) The entrance wound generally is small. Yet these injuries often may be associated with deep penetration and injury to underlying tissues. Punctures can be hard to assess in the prehospital setting. Even an injury that appears to be minor can conceal a considerable amount of internal damage.

In some penetrating injuries, the object remains embedded or impaled in the wound (Fig. 22-9). If this occurs to the chest or abdomen, severe bleeding can occur. In addition, major underlying damage to internal organs can occur. Examples include the following:

- Chest injury
- Pneumothorax (simple, open, tension)
- Hemothorax
- Pericardial tamponade
- Penetrating heart wound
- Rupture of the esophagus, aorta, diaphragm, main stem bronchus
- Abdominal injury
- Hollow and solid organ damage
- Peritonitis (bacterial, chemical)
- Evisceration

CRITICAL THINKING

Why should a person always seek medical care to have a penetrating object removed?

The injection of a substance into the body under high pressure also can cause a puncture wound (Fig. 22-10). (Examples include grease, paint, turpentine, dry-cleaning fluids, and molten plastics.) These injuries often have life- or limb-threatening potential. They often require rapid surgical decompression and débridement. These injuries usually are associated with minimal bleeding. In addition, they may not appear serious. Numbness and blanching of the involved area often occur because of increased tissue pressure of the injected substance. Most patients with injection injuries are surgical emergencies. Moreover, most of these patients are at high risk for developing **compartment syndrome.** Definitive care for injection injuries usually requires surgery and hospitalization to prevent infection. Amputation may be needed if treatment is delayed.

AVULSION

An avulsion is a full-thickness skin loss (Fig. 22-11) in which the wound edges cannot be approximated. Frequently involved body areas are the ear lobes, nose tip, and fingertips. A common cause of avulsion injury is industrial equipment, such as meat slicers or sawing devices. Another common cause is domestic violence, such as human bites.

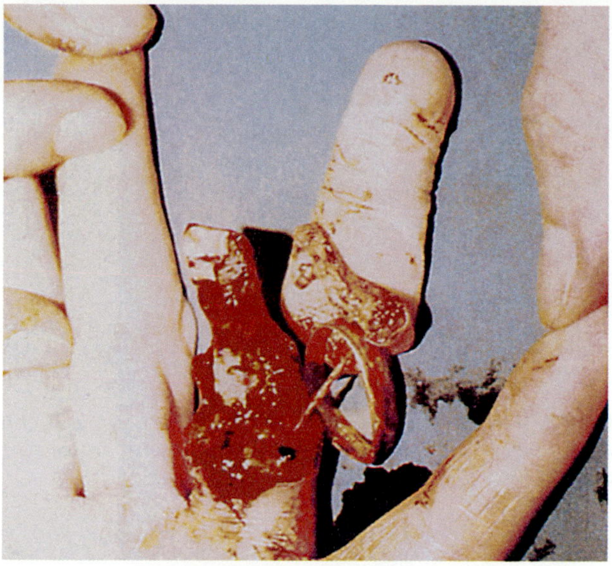

FIGURE 22-11 ■ Ring avulsion injury.

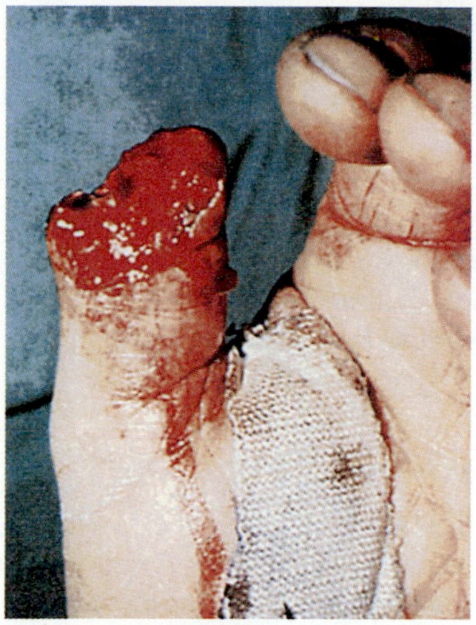

FIGURE 22-13 ■ Amputation of the fingertip.

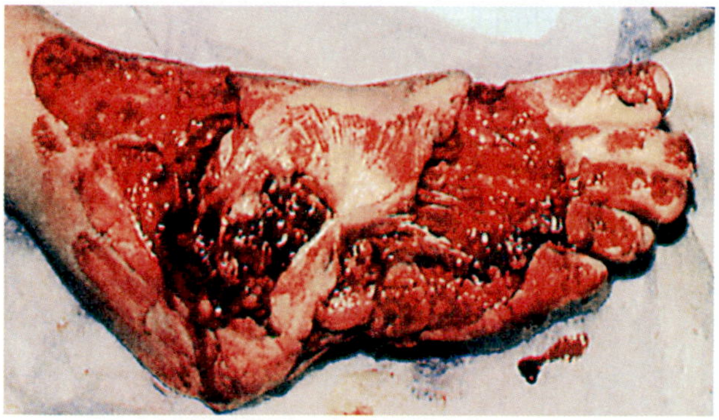

FIGURE 22-12 ■ Degloving injury of the foot.

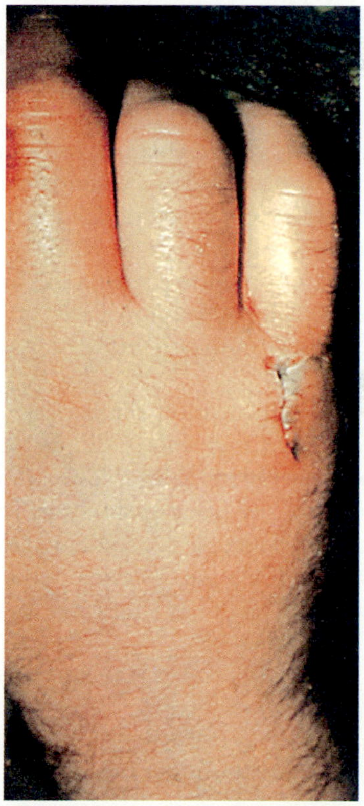

FIGURE 22-14 ■ Human bite to the hand.

A degloving injury is a type of avulsion. In this injury, shearing forces separate the skin from the underlying tissues (Fig. 22-12). A common cause of such an injury is industrial machinery. This machinery may entangle an extremity, producing circumferential tearing. Another common cause is finger jewelry that gets caught on a stationary object. This can produce a shearing of the soft tissue and possibly of the bone of the digit. Another common cause is machinery that entraps hair. This results in scalp avulsion. Degloving injuries sometimes are associated with underlying skeletal damage. They also sometimes are associated with massive loss of tissue in the affected area. Bleeding can be significant.

AMPUTATION

Traumatic amputation involves a complete or partial loss of a limb by a mechanical force (Fig. 22-13). The digits, lower leg, hand and forearm, and the distal part of the foot most often are injured in this way. Bleeding is a possible fatal complication of an amputation injury. In cases in which a complete amputation has occurred, injured arteries often retract. Hemorrhage may be less severe than in partial amputation injuries.

BITES

An animal or human bite wound frequently is a combination of puncture, laceration, avulsion, and crush injury (Fig. 22-14). The pressure from a bite can be as great as 400 psi. The bite can involve deep structures such as tendons, muscles, and bones. Complications from bite wounds, particularly human bites, include abscesses, lymphangitis, cellulitis, osteomyelitis, tenosynovitis, tuberculosis, hepatitis B, and tetanus. Although it is theoretically possible for a human bite to transmit human immunodeficiency virus, the Centers for Disease Control and Prevention suggest that the potential for salivary transmission of the virus is remote.[3] Other less common complications of mammalian bites include the transmission of diseases such as actinomycosis, syphilis, and rarely, rabies. All patients who have been bitten should seek physician evaluation.

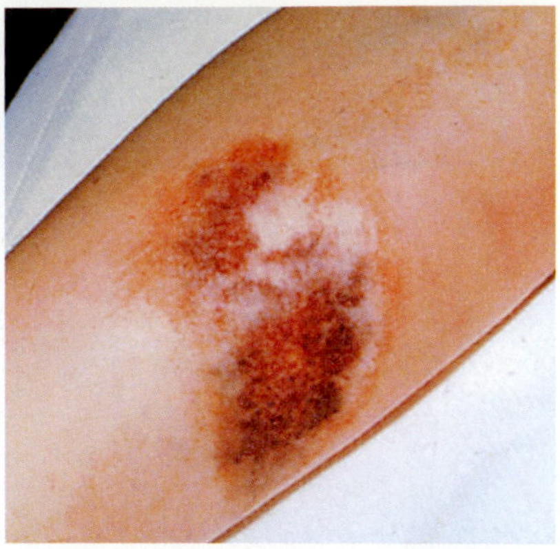

FIGURE 22-15 ■ Appearance that can follow prolonged crushing, as when an unconscious person lies on a body part for several hours.

CRITICAL THINKING

Consider that you are caring for a person who has sustained an animal bite. Aside from caring for the patient's wounds and documenting that care, what other concerns and responsibilities do you have?

Crush Injury

Crush injury is one of the three injuries that occurs when tissue is exposed to a compressive force. This force can be sufficient to interfere with the normal structure and metabolic function of the involved cells and tissues. The degree of injury produced by the crushing force depends on three things: the amount of pressure applied to the body, the amount of time the pressure remains in contact with the body, and the specific body region in which the injury occurs. A massive crush injury to vital organs can cause immediate death.

Crush injury usually involves the upper or lower extremities, torso, or pelvis. Crush injury can result from entrapment under a heavy object, as in a foundation collapse, or from some other massive compressive force. Examples of situations that can cause crush injury include the following:

- Collapse of masonry or steel structures
- Collapse of earth (e.g., mud slides and earthquakes)
- Motor vehicle crashes
- Warfare injuries
- Industrial incidents
- Prolonged application of a pneumatic antishock garment and improperly applied casts

COMPARTMENT SYNDROME

Compartment syndrome is a result of crush injury and is a surgical emergency (Fig. 22-15). Compartment syndrome usually results from compressive forces or blunt trauma to muscle groups confined in tight fibrous sheaths with minimal ability to stretch (below the knee, above the elbow). Other less common causes of compartment syndrome include the following:

- Extreme exertional exercise
- Low-level repetitive injury
- Electrical injury
- Hemorrhage into a compartment (e.g., coagulopathy among hemophiliacs)
- Circumferential deep burns and electrical burns
- Vascular occlusion
- High-pressure injection injuries
- Immobility with the development of pressure necrosis (e.g., among alcoholics, drug addicts, and victims of stroke)

CRITICAL THINKING

Why would alcoholics, drug addicts, and stroke victims be at risk for compartment syndrome?

Compartment syndrome develops as associated hemorrhage and edema increase pressure in the closed fascial space (compartment). This results in ischemia to the muscle. This ischemia causes further muscle cell swelling. The intracompartmental pressure continues to rise. As this occurs, circulation is compromised. Irreversible tissue damage from lack of oxygen develops within several hours to several days after injury. In addition to muscular damage, any nerves that travel through the compartment can undergo necrosis if the condition remains untreated. Signs and symptoms of compartment syndrome in an extremity include those of vascular insufficiency (the five *P*'s; Box 22-1). Other signs and symptoms that can indicate the presence of compartment syndrome include the following:

- Pain seemingly out of proportion to injury
- Swelling (tautness of the compartment)
- Tenderness to palpation
- Weakness of the involved muscle groups
- Pain on passive stretch (earliest finding)

The recognition of compartment syndrome calls for a high degree of suspicion based on patient history and mechanism of injury. Compartment syndrome most often is associated with tibial fracture of the lower leg. Yet compartment syndrome also can occur with crush injury or fracture of the femur, forearm, or upper arm. Delayed treat-

BOX 22-1 Five P's of Vascular Insufficiency

1. **P**ain
2. **P**aresis (late finding)
3. **P**aresthesia
4. **P**allor (variable)
5. **P**ulselessness (late finding)

ment can result in nerve death, muscle necrosis, and **crush syndrome.**

CRUSH SYNDROME

Crush syndrome is a life-threatening and sometimes preventable complication of prolonged immobilization or compression. The syndrome is a pathological process that causes destruction or alteration of muscle tissue. Crush syndrome is rare and is most likely to occur in catastrophic events in which patient rescue and extrication are delayed beyond 4 to 6 hours. (Examples of such events are earthquake or building collapse.) The prehospital management of crush syndrome often determines patient outcome.

The exact mechanism of crush syndrome is unknown. The compressive forces of entrapment are believed to produce a pathological process. This process disrupts vascular integrity and causes loss of structure of the cell and the cell membranes. Patients with crush syndrome may appear stable for hours or days, as long as the compressive forces remain in place. But when the patient is released from the entrapment, three harmful processes occur at the same time that can lead to death:

1. Oxygen-rich blood returns to the ischemic extremity. This produces a pooling of intravascular volume into crushed tissue. This reperfusion reduces total circulating volume, which in turn often leads to shock.
2. With the return of oxygen-rich blood, various toxic substances and waste products of anaerobic metabolism are released into the systemic circulation. This causes metabolic acidosis. High levels of intracellular solutes and water are released from damaged cells. This results in hyperkalemia, hyperuricemia, hypocalcemia, and hyperphosphatemia.
3. Myoglobin is released from the damaged muscle cells of the injured extremity. Myoglobin is filtered through the kidneys **(rhabdomyolysis)** and results in acute renal failure.

Blast Injuries

As described in Chapter 20, severe injuries can result from an initial air blast, from flying debris, and from secondary contact with another object as the victim is thrown by the blast. Examples of situations that can result in blast injury include natural gas or gasoline explosions, fireworks explosions, explosions in grain elevators, and terrorist bombs. Scene and personal safety is of the highest importance. Paramedics should not enter the scene where a blast injury occurred until the scene has been made safe by the authorities. (The appropriate authorities include, for example, law enforcement, fire service, specialized rescue teams, hazardous materials teams, and other public service agencies.)

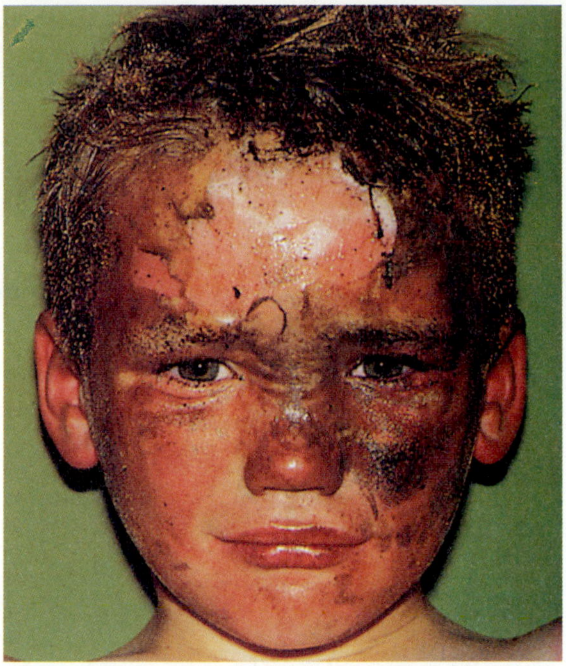

FIGURE 22-16 ■ Blast injury to the face. His eardrums were normal. He was admitted because of the risk of swelling to his face and airway with potential airway obstruction.

Injuries from blasts can be superficial or deep (Fig. 22-16). The deep injuries can injure internal organs. Patients who suffer blast injury require rapid stabilization (airway and ventilatory support with spinal precautions; circulatory support) and rapid transportation for physician evaluation. Blast injuries and associated trauma can be hard to identify in the prehospital setting. These patients will need extensive evaluation in a trauma center. Compression injuries that occur to air-filled organs include rupture of the eardrum, sinuses, lungs, stomach, and intestines.

CRITICAL THINKING

What injury do you suspect if a patient who has suffered a blast injury has a sudden onset of hearing loss?

MANAGEMENT PRINCIPLES FOR SOFT TISSUE INJURIES

Personal and scene safety is always the priority in any emergency response. If indicated, law enforcement and rescue personnel should assure the paramedic that the scene is safe for entry and that any perpetrators have been apprehended. Help from other public service agencies also may be needed if other types of dangers exist. Examples of such dangers may include hazardous materials or bombs.

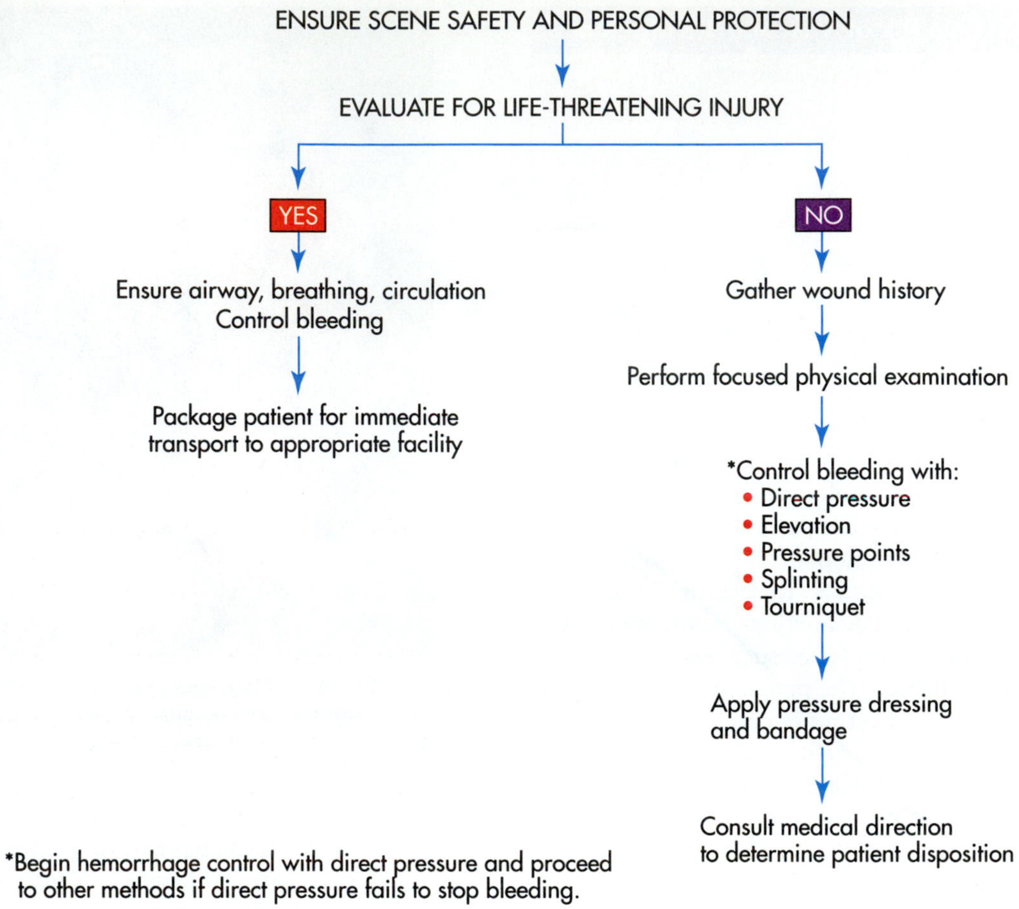
ENSURE SCENE SAFETY AND PERSONAL PROTECTION
EVALUATE FOR LIFE-THREATENING INJURY
YES
NO
Ensure airway, breathing, circulation
Control bleeding
Package patient for immediate transport to appropriate facility
Gather wound history
Perform focused physical examination
*Control bleeding with:
• Direct pressure
• Elevation
• Pressure points
• Splinting
• Tourniquet
Apply pressure dressing and bandage
Consult medical direction to determine patient disposition
*Begin hemorrhage control with direct pressure and proceed to other methods if direct pressure fails to stop bleeding.

FIGURE 22-17 ■ Treatment plan for a patient with soft tissue injury.

Treatment Priorities

The assessment of life-threatening injuries and resuscitation precedes evaluation and intervention of non–life-threatening soft tissue injuries. The paramedic should evaluate wounds that do not pose a threat to life later in the physical exam. General wound assessment should include a history of the wounding event and a careful examination of the injury. Fig. 22-17 shows a treatment plan based on assessment findings for a patient with soft tissue injury.

Wound History

A wound history should include the following:

- Time of injury
- Environment where the injury occurred (risk of infection is greater in unclean environments)
- Mechanism of injury and likelihood of concurrent or associated injuries
- Volume of blood loss
- Severity of pain
- Medical history, including use of medications that may impair hemostasis
- Tetanus immunization

Physical Examination

Physical examination of a wound should include the following:

- Inspection of the wound for bleeding, size, depth, presence of foreign bodies, amount of tissue lost, edema, and deformity
- Inspection of the area surrounding the wound for damage to underlying structures, arteries, nerves, tendons, or muscle

CRITICAL THINKING

Will you perform this physical examination on every wound in the prehospital setting?

- Assessment of sensory or motor function of the extremity
- Evaluation of the perfusion status of the wound and tissue distal to the wound
- Palpation of the injury and associated structures to evaluate capillary refill, distal pulses, tenderness, temperature, edema, and crepitus (if underlying bony injury is suspected)

A

B

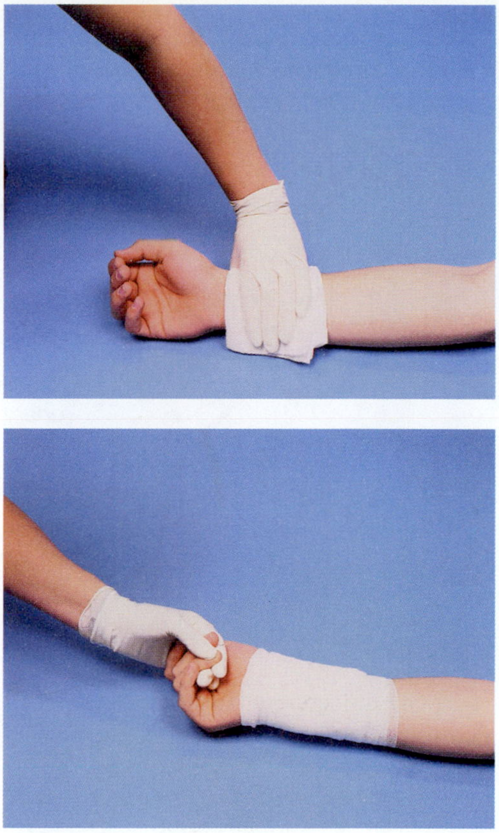

FIGURE 22-18 ■ A, Application of direct pressure to control hemorrhage. B, Pressure dressing.

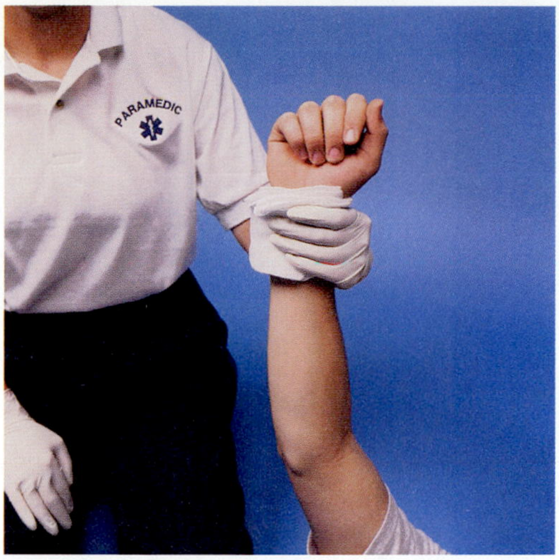

FIGURE 22-19 ■ Elevation to control hemorrhage.

HEMORRHAGE AND CONTROL OF BLEEDING

Blood loss often is associated with soft tissue injury. The blood loss may result from damage to arteries, veins, capillaries, or a combination of these. Generally, arterial bleeding is characterized as bright red and spurting. Venous bleeding is dark reddish-blue and flowing. Capillary bleeding is bright red and oozing. But differentiation among the types of vessel hemorrhage often is difficult. In the prehospital setting the main concern in hemorrhage, regardless of origin, is to control bleeding.

Methods of hemorrhage control include direct pressure, elevation, pressure point, immobilization by splinting, pneumatic pressure devices (air splints, pneumatic antishock garment), and rarely the use of tourniquets. As in any patient encounter in which contact with body fluids is likely, the paramedic must take personal protective measures.

Direct Pressure

The paramedic can control external hemorrhage by applying direct pressure over the injury site (Fig. 22-18). Direct pressure controls most types of hemorrhage within 4 to 6 minutes. To maintain control, a pressure dressing can be applied over the site and held in place with a self-adherent roller bandage. The paramedic must continue direct pressure, even with a pressure dressing. Once the dressing has been applied, the paramedic should not remove it because removal can disrupt the fresh blood clot. If bleeding resumes and the dressing becomes soaked with blood, a second dressing should be applied on top of the first one and held in place with direct pressure until the bleeding is controlled.

Elevation

The paramedic can control or reduce venous bleeding in an extremity by elevating the extremity above the level of the heart (Fig. 22-19). Elevation alone usually does not control hemorrhage. Elevation should be considered a supplement to direct pressure.

Pressure Point

Pressure-point control may become necessary if direct pressure and elevation have not controlled hemorrhage. The chosen artery must be proximal to the injury site. In addition, the artery must overlie a bony structure against which it can be compressed. Examples of pressure-point sites include the temporal artery to control bleeding from the scalp, the brachial artery to control bleeding from the forearm, and the femoral artery to control bleeding from the leg (Fig. 22-20). Pressure-point control (Fig. 22-21) should be maintained for at least 10 minutes. Continued compression of the pressure point may be needed during patient transport. The paramedic may need to complement combinations of direct pressure, elevation, and proximal pressure-point compression to control vigorous hemorrhage.

CRITICAL THINKING

Why should the pressure point chosen to control hemorrhage be proximal to the injury?

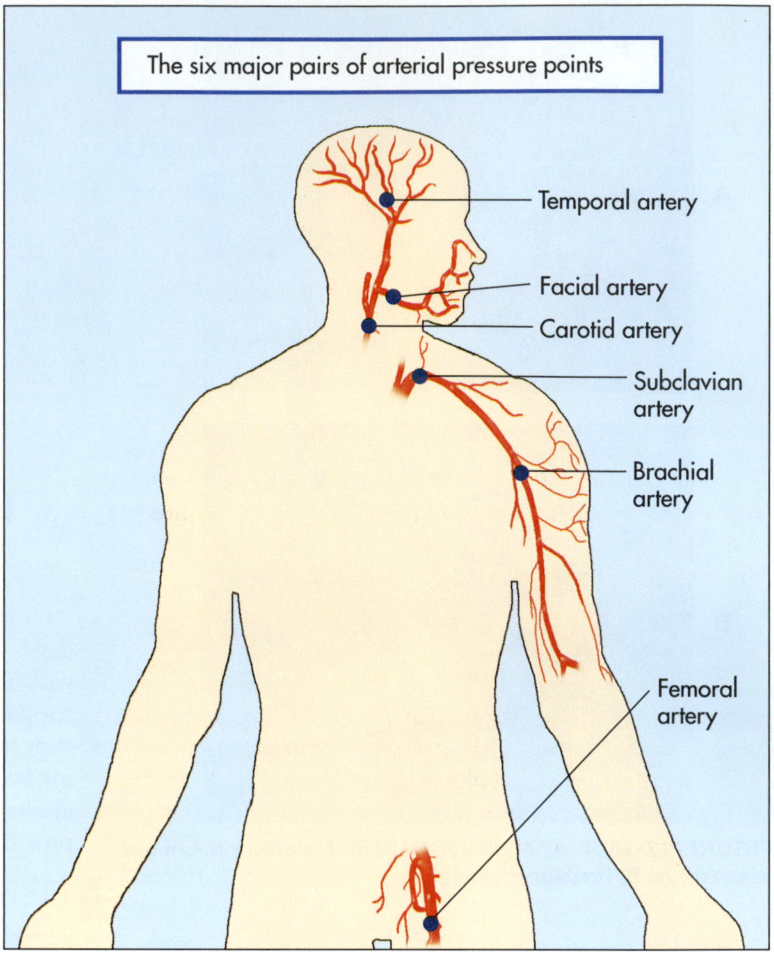

FIGURE 22-20 ■ Arterial pressure points.

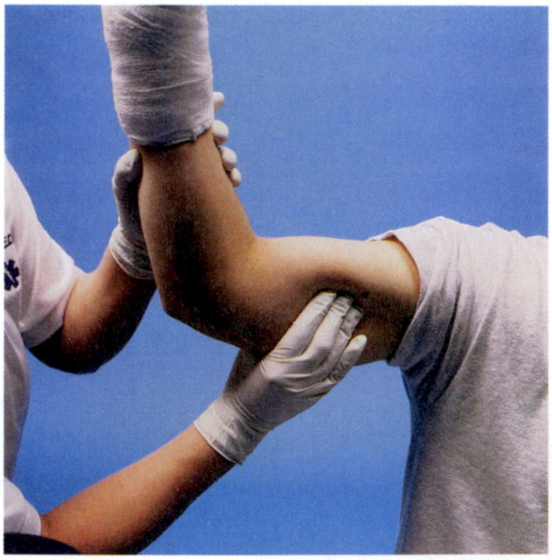

FIGURE 22-21 ■ Pressure-point control.

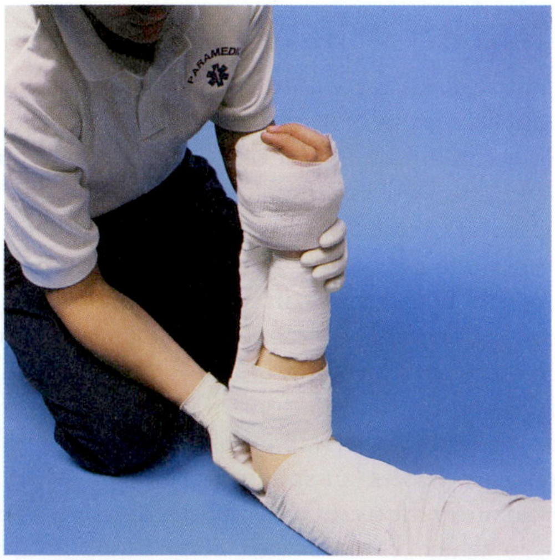

FIGURE 22-22 ■ Immobilization by splinting to control hemorrhage.

Immobilization by Splinting

Patient movement promotes the flow of blood. This movement can disrupt the clot or increase vascular injury. Thus patients should be immobilized whenever possible (Fig. 22-22). The paramedic can immobilize extremity injuries with appropriate splinting devices. The patient can be immobilized fully with a long spine board. Immobilization is not effective alone as a method to control bleeding. Immobilization should be used as an adjunct.

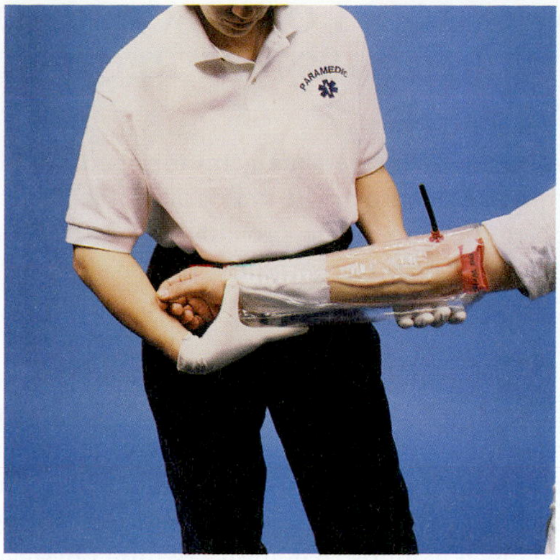

FIGURE 22-23 ■ Application of pneumatic pressure device to control hemorrhage.

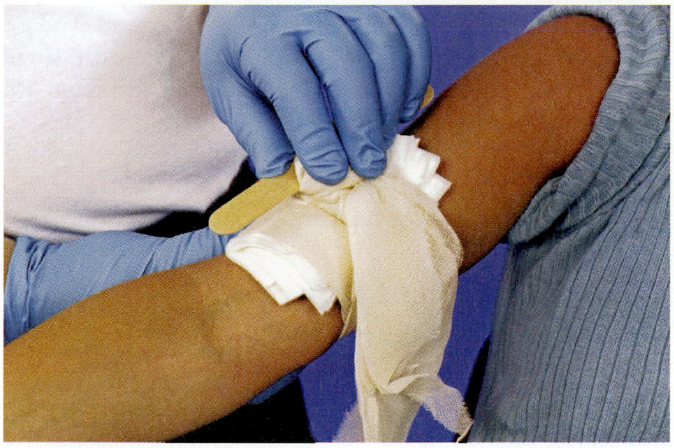

FIGURE 22-24 ■ Application of a tourniquet to control hemorrhage.

Pneumatic Pressure Devices

Pneumatic pressure devices can provide uniform direct pressure to an immobilized injury site. (Examples of such devices are inflatable air splints applied to an extremity or the use of the pneumatic antishock garment.) These devices should be applied over a dressed wound only after other methods have controlled the bleeding (Fig. 22-23).

Tourniquet

The use of a tourniquet has little or no indication in the emergency management of hemorrhage (Fig. 22-24). Use of a tourniquet is associated with damage to nerves and blood vessels and with the eventual loss of the extremity. A poorly applied tourniquet can produce venous occlusion, only restricting the outflow but not the inflow of blood and producing an increase in blood loss. Thus the use of a tourniquet should be a last resort only. Use of a tourniquet should be considered only when all other methods have failed and when its use is essential to save the patient's life. An example of such an extreme circumstance is a partial or complete traumatic amputation of a limb. Even in these cases, other methods of hemorrhage control often are effective. Guidelines for application of a tourniquet are as follows:

1. Consult with medical direction.
2. Select a site for the tourniquet. The site should be about 2 inches proximal to the wound and over the supplying brachial or femoral artery. A blood pressure cuff applied over the brachial artery also can act as a tourniquet. If a blood pressure cuff is used, note the time of application on the cuff itself.
3. Place the tourniquet (commercially prepared or wide, flat material) within 2 inches of the wound and over the artery to be compressed. Never use thin material such as rope or twine because it may damage underlying tissue. If a blood pressure cuff is used as a tourniquet, inflate the cuff until the cuff pressure exceeds the arterial pressure or to the point at which the hemorrhage stops.
4. Place the pad (a roll of gauze or thick folded dressings) over the artery to be compressed.
5. Encircle the tourniquet twice around the extremity and pad, and tie it in a half knot over the pad.
6. Place a windlass (stick, pen, or similar object) on the half knot, and secure it in place with a square knot.
7. Tighten the windlass by twisting *only* until hemorrhage stops. Secure the windlass in that position. Never loosen the tourniquet once it is tightened.
8. Note the time of tourniquet application and secure it to the patient, or clearly mark "TK" on the patient's forehead. Document the tourniquet procedure on the patient care report.

DRESSING MATERIALS USED WITH SOFT TISSUE TRAUMA

A variety of bandages and dressings are used in trauma care. The six general categories of dressings are as follows:

1. *Sterile dressings* are processed to eliminate bacteria. They should be used whenever infection of the wound is a concern.
2. *Nonsterile dressings* are not sterilized. They can be used when infection is not a prime concern.
3. *Occlusive dressings* do not allow the passage of air through the material. These dressings are useful in treating wounds of the thorax and major vessels where negative pressure can cause air to enter the body, resulting in a pneumothorax or air embolism, respectively (see Chapter 26).
4. *Nonocclusive dressings* allow air to pass through the material and are indicated for managing most soft tissue injuries.
5. *Adherent dressings* attach to the wound surface by incorporating wound exudate into the dressing mesh. Use of

these dressings sometimes can assist in controlling acute bleeding.

6. *Nonadherent dressings* allow the passage of wound exudate and do not adhere to the wound surface. These dressings do not damage the wound when removed and often are used after wound closure.

Bandages hold dressings in place. Bandages are classified as absorbent, nonabsorbent, adherent, and nonadherent. Like dressings, bandages are sterile or nonsterile.

Complications of Improperly Applied Dressings and Bandages

Improperly applied dressings and bandages can harm the patient and can cause discomfort. For example, dressings that are applied too loosely often do not stop bleeding. Bandages that are applied too tightly can cause tissue ischemia and structural damage to vessels, nerves, tendons, muscles, and skin.

Basic Concepts of Open Wound Dressing

The basic concepts of open wound dressing include the following steps:

1. Assess the wound for size, depth, location, and contamination.
2. Properly prepare the wound for dressing. Prehospital care usually is limited to cleaning the injured surface of gross contaminants by irrigation of the wound with sterile water or normal saline. Do not attempt extensive débridement in the prehospital setting. Apply antibacterial ointment if the patient is not allergic (per protocol).
3. Apply the appropriate dressing.
4. Secure the dressing in place with bandages or gauze wrappings.
5. Tape the loose ends of the bandage.

MANAGEMENT OF SPECIFIC SOFT TISSUE INJURIES NOT REQUIRING CLOSURE

The paramedic encounters many minor open wounds that do not require closure or the evaluation of a physician. In these cases the paramedic provides basic first aid. The paramedic also provides instructions for self-care to the patient.

Dressings and Bandages

Depending on the nature and location of the patient's injury, dressings, bandages, and immobilization may be indicated to care for the wound properly. (Fig. 22-25 illustrates basic dressing and bandaging procedures for various wounds.) Open wounds that always require physician evaluation include those with the following:

- Neural, muscular, or vascular compromise
- Tendon or ligament compromise
- Heavy contamination
- Cosmetic complications (e.g., facial trauma)
- Foreign bodies

Patients with soft tissue injuries that pose a threat to life or limb require rapid assessment, stabilization, and rapid transportation for physician evaluation.

Evaluation

Local protocol may permit the paramedic to manage and release the patient with minor soft tissue injury to the patient's own care. Local protocol also may allow the paramedic to manage and refer the patient to the patient's private physician for follow-up care. Some emergency medical services systems allow paramedics to provide tetanus vaccine. Paramedics also may be permitted to give written and verbal instructions regarding care to patients who will not be transported by ambulance for physician evaluation.

A

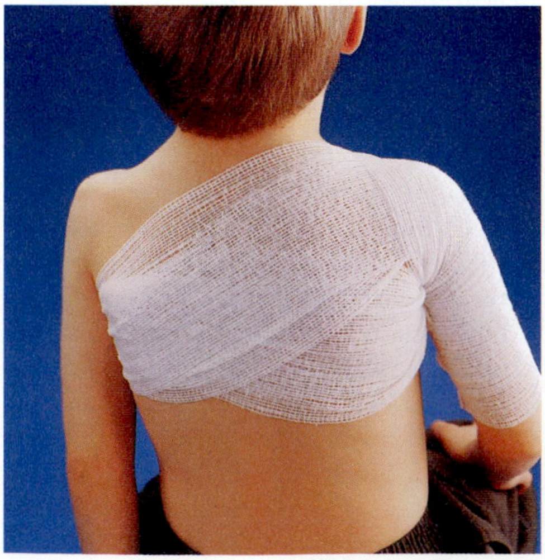

B

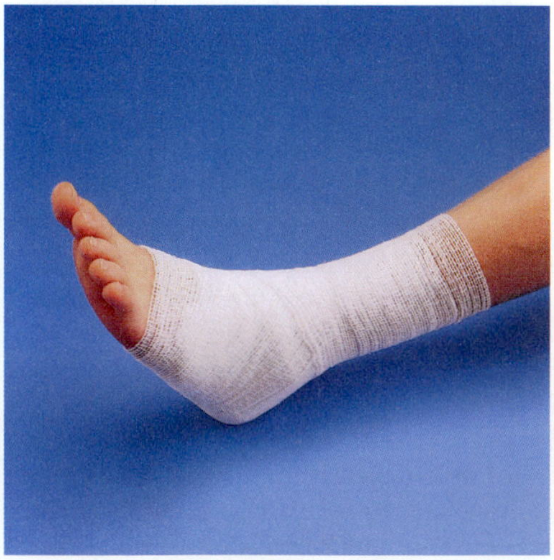

FIGURE 22-25 ■ Types of dressings. **A,** Shoulder dressing. **B,** Ankle dressing.

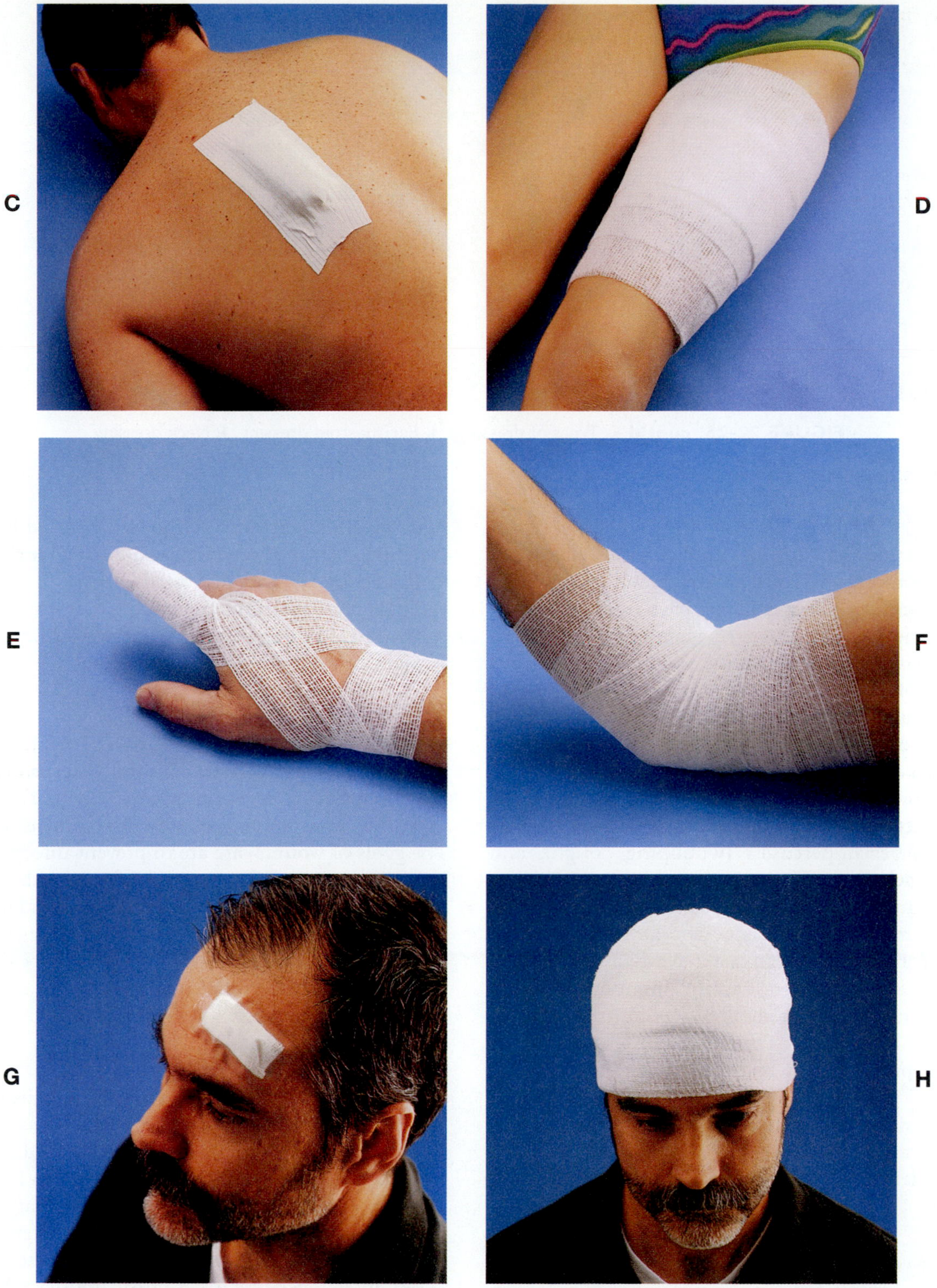

FIGURE 22-25, cont'd ■ Types of dressings. **C,** Torso dressing. **D,** Thigh dressing. **E,** Finger dressing. **F,** Elbow dressing. **G,** Forehead dressing. **H,** Scalp dressing. *Continued*

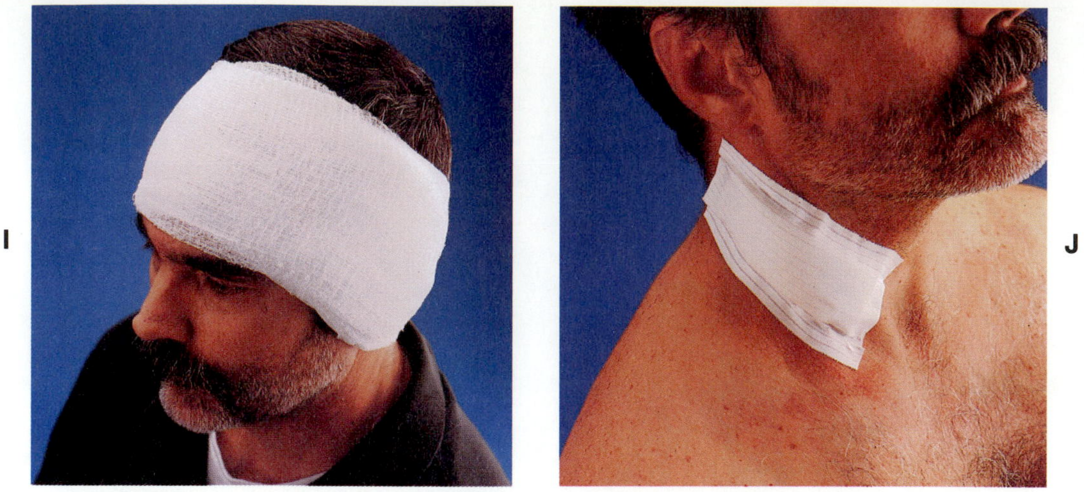

FIGURE 22-25, cont'd ■ Types of dressings. **I,** Ear/mastoid dressing. **J,** Neck dressing.

TETANUS VACCINE

Tetanus is a serious and at times fatal disease. Tetanus is a disease of the central nervous system caused by the infection of a wound with spores of the bacterium *Clostridium tetani.* The patient can be protected against tetanus by periodic immunization with a tetanus vaccine. About half a million cases of tetanus occur across the world each year. In the United States only about 100 cases are reported each year. All cases occur in nonimmunized persons. Tetanus infection occurs mostly in those over 50 years of age.

Adults receive a combined immunization against diphtheria and tetanus, and children receive vaccinations against diphtheria, pertussis (whooping cough), and tetanus routinely in the United States. After initial immunization during childhood, children receive booster vaccines every 5 to 10 years. Patients who have not been immunized before against tetanus receive tetanus immune globulin because it confers instant immunity. During wound care, the paramedic should ascertain the patient's last tetanus immunization. The paramedic also should determine any prior allergic reactions to tetanus preparations. Normal side effects from the vaccine include slight fever, sore injection site, or minor rash. The tetanus vaccine is contraindicated in infants less than 6 weeks of age, in pregnant patients, and in those who are hypersensitive to the vaccine.

CRITICAL THINKING

Why is it crucial for you to be knowledgeable about and to ask the patient about tetanus vaccination if the vaccine is not carried on your ambulance?

PATIENT INSTRUCTIONS

Verbal and written instructions sometimes are referred to as a "patient instruction sheet." These instructions relate to wound care (Fig. 22-26). Paramedics should give instructions to all patients who are not transported for physician evaluation. These instructions should include the following:

- Protection and care of wounded area
- Dressing change and follow-up
- Wound cleansing recommendations
- Signs of wound infection

Wound Infection

Infection is a common complication of soft tissue injury. It results from a break in the continuity of the skin and subsequent exposure to the nonsterile external environment. Most infections are minor. However, some can be serious. The goals of wound care are to prevent infection and protect from infection. Factors that influence the likelihood of infection include unclean wounds and wound mechanisms (e.g., wounds contaminated by soil, dirt, or grease) and a patient's poor state of health. These factors can have both local and systemic complications and can affect the patient's general recovery.

Causes of Wound Infection

Many factors can cause wound infection. Nine of the most common factors are as follows[4]:

1. *Time.* The risk of infection can be reduced greatly if the wound is cleaned and repaired within 8 to 12 hours after injury. Bacterial proliferation to a level that can result in infection can occur as early as 3 hours after injury.
2. *Mechanism.* Lacerations caused by fine cutting forces resist infection better than crush injuries. High-velocity missile injuries can produce internal damage that may not be apparent for several days.
3. *Location.* Injuries of the foot, lower extremity, hand, and perineum have a higher-than-normal risk for infection.
4. *Severity.* The more tissue damage produced by the injury, the higher the risk for infection.
5. *Contamination.* The presence of foreign matter in a wound decreases resistance to infection. Of particular concern are wounds contaminated by soil, saliva, and feces.

WOUND CARE INSTRUCTION SHEET

Patient name: ______________________________

1. Call your physician. He/she may have further instructions to offer for your care.
2. Keep the wound and dressing as dry as reasonably possible, since water aids bacterial growth.
3. Remove the dressing applied after 2 days.
4. Check for signs of infection:
   a. Swelling
   b. Excessive redness
   c. Pain
   d. Heat—either locally or systemically as reflected by a fever
   e. Excessive drainage from wounds
5. Reapply a sterile gauze dressing, taping it down at the edges. Repeat this every 2 days until the wound heals.
6. Wounds in areas of high mobility, such as around joints, are subject to excessive tension. Appropriate precautions should be taken to decrease the motion of the affected joint to assist in healing.

Other instructions: ______________________________

____

____

Treatment rendered: ______________________________

Tetanus: Yes / No Type: ______________________________

I hereby acknowledge that I have read the instructions above, that they have been explained to me, that I understand them, and that I have received a copy of them.

I understand that I have had emergency treatment only and that I may be released before all of my medical problems are known and treated. I will arrange for the follow-up care as instructed.

______________________________ ______________________________
Responsible Party's Signature Relationship

______________________________ ______________________________
Witness Title

Original to Patient Care Report
Copy to Patient

____
Date/Time

FIGURE 22-26 ■ Sample instruction sheet for wound care.

6. *Preparation.* Body, facial, and head hair removed by clipping versus shaving is less likely to result in wound infection. Shaving can cause additional injury by abrading the skin and potentially moving skin flora into the larger wound.
7. *Cleansing.* Wound cleansing should be performed with normal saline and a high-pressure syringe.
8. *Technique of repair.* Wounds at high risk for infection (e.g., animal bites) may need to be cleaned, débrided, left open for 4 to 5 days, and then closed through traditional techniques.
9. *General patient condition.* Elderly patients and patients with concurrent illness or preexisting disease (e.g., diabetes) often are less able to ward off infection.

Assessment of Wound Healing

A paramedic can assess a wound for proper healing by doing the following:

- Examine dressings for excess drainage. Change saturated dressings to prevent contamination of the wound.
- Examine wounds for early signs of infection or delayed healing. Inflammation, edema, and bloody drainage are normal during the first 3 days but should subside gradually as the wound heals.

Signs of wound infection include increasing inflammation or edema, purulent drainage, foul odor, persistent pain, delayed healing, and fever. If any of these is present, the paramedic should consult with medical direction. Medical direction may advise patient transport to the emergency department or may direct patient referral to a private physician for follow-up care.

SPECIAL CONSIDERATIONS FOR SOFT TISSUE INJURIES

As stated before, assessment of life-threatening injuries and resuscitation precede evaluation of and intervention for non–life-threatening soft tissue injuries. After ensuring adequate airway, breathing, and circulatory status (with spinal precautions if indicated); controlling severe hemorrhage; and maintaining normal body temperature, the paramedic can proceed with wound care. Special considerations for specific wounds are described in the following sections.

Penetrating Chest or Abdominal Injury

Open wounds to the chest or abdomen must be covered properly with sterile and occlusive dressings. Open chest wounds can involve severe pulmonary injuries. These injuries can include pneumothorax and tension pneumothorax (described in Chapter 26). Major complications of penetrating abdominal injury include hemorrhage from a major vessel or solid organ and perforation of a segment of bowel (see Chapter 27). The paramedic should observe the following guidelines in managing a penetrating wound to the chest or abdomen in which an impaled object is present:

1. Do not remove the impaled object; severe hemorrhage or damage to underlying structures can occur.
2. Do not manipulate the impaled object unless it is necessary to shorten the object for extrication or for patient transportation.
3. Control bleeding with direct pressure applied around the impaled object.
4. Stabilize the object in place with bulky dressings; immobilize the patient to prevent movement.

Avulsion

Prehospital management of avulsed tissue varies by protocol, but two guidelines generally apply:

1. If the tissue is still attached to the body, do the following:
   a. Clean the wound surface of gross contaminants with sterile saline.
   b. Gently fold the skin back to its normal position.
   c. Control bleeding, dress the wound with bulky pressure dressings, and maintain direct pressure.
2. If the tissue is completely separated from the body, do the following:
   a. Control the bleeding with application of direct pressure.
   b. Retrieve the avulsed tissue if possible, but do not delay transport to locate amputated body parts.
   c. Wrap the tissue in gauze, either dry or moistened with lactated Ringer's or saline solution (per protocol).
   d. Seal the tissue in a plastic bag.
   e. Place the sealed bag on crushed ice; never place tissue directly on ice.

CRITICAL THINKING

Why should you use normal saline or lactated Ringer's solution instead of sterile water to wrap or clean avulsed tissue?

Amputations

As with other open wounds, hemorrhage control for amputation should be managed initially with direct pressure and elevation. The wound may require use of a tourniquet. However, use of a tourniquet should be avoided if possible. The resultant damage can interfere with reimplantation attempts. An amputated limb should be retrieved and managed in the same manner as avulsed tissue.

Crush Syndrome

Crush syndrome is complex and is difficult to diagnose and treat because of the many variables involved. These variables include the extent of tissue damage, duration and force of compression, patient's general health, and associated injuries. The management of crush syndrome is controversial. A medical direction physician who is familiar with this pathological process must supervise the prehospital care.

Paramedics should consider possible crush syndrome when prolonged immobilization or compression occurs. The emergency care must be coordinated with rescue efforts. That way, the timing of the release from entrapment follows medical treatment. This will help to prevent hypovolemic shock and crush syndrome. The steps in patient care management are as follows[4]:

1. Provide airway and ventilatory support. This includes high-concentration oxygen administration.
2. Maintain body temperature.
3. Aggressively hydrate the patient with D5$^1/_2$NS (5% dextrose in water with 0.45% normal saline) to manage hypovolemia and to maintain urine output.
4. Alkalinize the urine with sodium bicarbonate to control hyperkalemia and acidosis that can prevent acute myoglobinuric renal failure and sudden cardiac dysrhythmias. Manage severe hyperkalemia with ***insulin*** and ***dex-***

trose (per medical direction). ***Calcium chloride*** generally is not indicated unless a danger of hyperkalemia dysrhythmia exists.

5. Consider ***mannitol*** per medical direction to hydrate the kidneys and to maintain urine output. Do not administer loop diuretics such as ***furosemide,*** which may acidify the urine.
6. Use of arterial tourniquets before the release of a crushed limb can be beneficial. If intracompartmental pressure is greater than 40 mm Hg, fasciotomy may be indicated to preserve the limb and cutaneous sensation. Performing a field fasciotomy carries an increased risk for infection and sepsis and requires special training and authorization from medical direction.
7. A physician may need to perform surgical amputation when extrication is impossible.
8. After extrication, care may include transporting the patient for hyperbaric oxygen treatment to restore tissue perfusion and to decrease tissue necrosis and muscle edema. (Hyperbaric therapy is described further in Chapter 38.)

SUMMARY

- The skin and its accessory organs are the main cosmetic structures of the body. These structures perform many functions that are critical to survival. The skin is composed of two distinct layers of tissue: the outer layer (epidermis) and the inner layer (dermis).
- Surface trauma can disrupt the normal distribution of body fluids and electrolytes. Surface trauma also can interfere with the maintenance of body temperature. The two physiological responses to surface trauma are vascular and inflammatory reactions. These can lead to healing, scar formation, or both. Many factors can affect or alter wound healing.
- Soft tissue injuries are classified as closed or open. Classification is determined by the absence or presence of a break in the continuity of the epidermis. Closed wounds include contusions, hematomata, and crush injury. Open wounds are classified as abrasion, laceration, puncture, avulsion, amputation, and bite.
- Assessment of life-threatening injuries and resuscitation precedes evaluation and intervention of non-life-threatening soft tissue injuries. General wound assessment should include a history of the event that caused the wound and a careful examination of the injury.
- Methods of hemorrhage control include direct pressure, elevation, pressure point, immobilization by splinting, and pneumatic pressure devices.
- The general categories of dressings used in trauma care are sterile, nonsterile, occlusive, nonocclusive, adherent, and nonadherent. The general categories of bandages are absorbent, nonabsorbent, adherent, and nonadherent.
- Depending on the nature and location of the patient's injury, dressings, bandages, and immobilization may be indicated to care for a wound properly.
- The goals of wound care are to prevent infection and protect from infection. Factors that influence the likelihood of infection include unclean wounds and wound mechanisms and a patient's poor state of health.
- Special considerations for specific wounds include penetrating chest or abdominal injury, avulsion, amputations, and crush syndrome.

REFERENCES

1. National Safety Council: *Injury facts,* Itasca, Ill, 2002, The Council.
2. Rosen P, Barkin R: *Emergency medicine: concepts and clinical practice,* ed 5, St Louis, 2003, Mosby.
3. Centers for Disease Control and Prevention, US Department of Health and Human Services, Public Health Service: *Guidelines for prevention and transmission of human immunodeficiency virus and hepatitis B virus to health-care and public safety workers,* Atlanta, 1989, The Department.
4. US Department of Transportation, National Highway Traffic Safety Administration: *EMT-Paramedic national standard curriculum,* Washington, DC, 1998, US Government Printing Office.

CHAPTER

23

Burns

OBJECTIVES

Upon completion of this chapter, the paramedic student will be able to:

1. Describe the incidence, patterns, and sources of burn injury.
2. Describe the pathophysiology of local and systemic responses to burn injury.
3. Classify burn injury according to depth, extent, and severity based on established standards.
4. Discuss the pathophysiology of burn shock as a basis for key signs and symptoms.
5. Outline the physical examination of the burned patient.
6. Describe the prehospital management of the patient who has sustained a burn injury.
7. Discuss pathophysiology as a basis for key signs, symptoms, and management of the patient with an inhalation injury.
8. Outline the general assessment and management of the patient who has a chemical injury.
9. Describe specific complications and management techniques for selected chemical injuries.
10. Describe the physiological effects of electrical injuries as they relate to each body system based on an understanding of key principles of electricity.
11. Outline assessment and management of the patient with electrical injury.
12. Describe the distinguishing features of radiation injury and considerations in the prehospital management of these patients.

KEY TERMS

eschar: A scab or dry crust resulting from a thermal or chemical burn.

full-thickness burn: A burn injury in which the entire thickness of the epidermis and dermis is destroyed; also known as a third-degree burn.

inhalation injury: An upper and/or lower airway injury that results from thermal and/or chemical exposure.

Lund and Browder chart: A method to estimate burn injury that assigns specific numbers to each body part and that accounts for developmental changes in percentages of body surface area.

partial-thickness burn: A burn injury that extends through the epidermis to the dermis; considered a deep partial-thickness injury if it extends to the basal layers of the skin; also known as a second-degree burn.

rule of nines: A method to estimate burn injury that divides the total body surface area into segments that are multiples of 9%.

superficial burn: A burn injury in which only a superficial layer of epidermal cells is destroyed; also known as a first-degree burn.

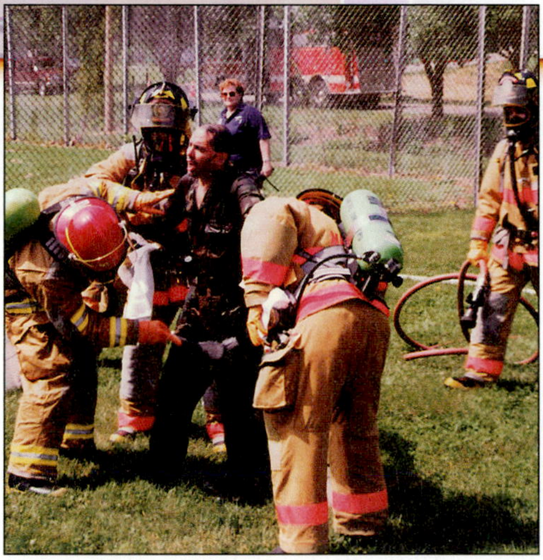

The management of burns often poses a challenge for the paramedic. Understanding the long-term results of a serious burn injury is important. Appropriate prehospital management can reduce morbidity and mortality for burn patients.

INCIDENCE AND PATTERNS OF BURN INJURY

Burns are a devastating form of trauma. They are associated with high mortality rates, lengthy rehabilitation, cosmetic disfigurement, and permanent physical disabilities. Each year, more than 2 million Americans seek medical attention for burns. Of these, 70,000 persons are hospitalized and up to 10,000 die as a result of thermal injury or burn-related infection.[1] Box 23-1 lists common complications that contribute to thermal injury deaths.

Morbidity and mortality rates from burn injury follow significant patterns regarding gender, age, and socioeconomic status. For example, two thirds of all fire fatalities are men; the death rate from thermal injury is highest among children and older adults; and three fourths of all fire deaths occur in the home, with the highest incidence in lower-income households.[2] A key part of the professional role of the paramedic is community education. This education should stress prevention as the most effective management of these injuries. (See Chapter 3.)

BOX 23-1 Physiological and Systemic Complications of Thermal Injuries

Depending on the severity of thermal injury, physiological and systemic complications may include the following:

- Acidosis
- Anoxia
- Dysrhythmias
- Electrolyte loss
- Fluid loss
- Heart failure
- Hypothermia
- Hypovolemia
- Hypoxia
- Infection
- Liver failure
- Renal failure

Major Sources of Burns

A burn injury is caused by contact between energy and living cells. The source of this energy may be thermal, chemical, electrical, or radiation.

THERMAL BURNS

The majority of burns are thermal. These burns commonly result from flames, scalds, or contact with hot substances. (*Frostbite* is also a thermal injury. Frostbite is addressed in Chapter 38.) Studies have shown that surface temperatures of 44° C (111° F) do not produce burns unless exposure time exceeds 6 hours.[3] At temperatures between 44° C and 51° C (111° F and 124° F), the rate of epidermal necrosis approximately doubles with each degree of temperature rise. At 70° C (185° F) or greater, the exposure time required to cause transepidermal necrosis is less than 1 second. The degree of tissue destruction depends on the temperature and on the duration of exposure. Factors that influence the ability of the body to resist burn injury include the water content of the skin tissue;

thickness and pigmentation of the skin; presence or absence of insulating substances such as skin oils or hair; and peripheral circulation of the skin, which affects dissipation of heat. Anatomy and physiology of the skin is presented in Chapters 6 and 22. The reader should refer to those chapters for review.

> **CRITICAL THINKING**
>
> Based on these facts and your knowledge of life span development, who would you predict would have a deeper burn from the same energy source: an 18-year-old or a 75-year-old? Why?

CHEMICAL BURNS

Chemical burns are caused by substances that are capable of producing chemical changes in the skin, with or without the production of heat. Heat may be generated during the burning process. Yet the chemical changes in the skin, not the heat, produce the greatest injury. Chemical burns differ from thermal burns. With chemical burns, the topical agent usually adheres to the skin for prolonged periods, producing continuous tissue destruction. The severity of the chemical injury is related to the type of agent, its concentration and volume, and the duration of contact. Chemical agents that often cause burn injury include acids and alkalis. These agents are found in many household cleaning products and organic compounds. Chemical burns are associated with high morbidity. This is especially the case when they involve the eyes. **Inhalation injury** (described later in this chapter) may also result from thermal and/or chemical exposure.

ELECTRICAL BURNS

Electrical injuries (including lightning injuries) result from direct contact with an electrical current. Electrical injuries can also result from arcing of electricity between two contact points near the skin. In a direct contact injury the current itself is not considered to have any thermal properties. The potential energy of the current, however, is changed into thermal energy. This transformation occurs when electricity meets the electrical resistance of biological tissue interposed between the entrance and exit sites. Arc injuries are localized at the termination of current flow. They are caused by the intense heat or flash that occurs when the current "jumps," making contact with the skin. Flame burn also may occur as a result of arcing if the heat generated ignites clothing or other fuel source near the patient.

> **CRITICAL THINKING**
>
> Electrical energy is transformed to heat, causing tissue damage in a human being. Then why does an electrical cord not feel hot when you touch it?

RADIATION BURNS

Radiation injury is caused by *ionizing* and *nonionizing* radiation (described later in this chapter). Burns may result from a high level of radiation exposure to a specific body area. However, radiation injuries make up a small percentage of burn injuries.

Local Response to Burn Injury

Burn injury immediately destroys cells or so fully disrupts their metabolic functions that cellular death ensues. Cellular damage is distributed over a spectrum of injury. Some cells are destroyed instantly. Others are irreversibly injured. Some injured cells, though, may survive if rapid and appropriate intervention is provided in the prehospital setting and in-hospital care.

Major thermal burns have three distinct zones of injury (*Jackson's thermal wound theory*). These zones usually appear in a bull's-eye pattern (Fig. 23-1). The central area of the burn wound, which has sustained the most intense contact with the thermal source, is the *zone of coagulation.* In this area, coagulation necrosis of the cells has occurred, and the tissue is nonviable. The *zone of stasis* surrounds the critically injured area. It consists of potentially viable tissue despite the serious thermal injury. In this zone, cells are ischemic because of clotting and vasoconstriction. The cells die within 24 to 48 hours after injury if no supportive measures are undertaken. At the periphery of the zone of stasis is the *zone of hyperemia.* This zone has increased blood flow as a result of the normal inflammatory response. The tissues in this area recover in 7 to 10 days if infection or profound shock does not develop.

Tissue damage from burns depends on the degree of heat and on the duration of exposure to the thermal source. As a rule, the burn wound swells rapidly because of the release of chemical mediators. These mediators cause an increase in capillary permeability and a fluid shift from the intravascular space into the injured tissues. The increased permeability is accentuated by injury to the sodium pump in the cell walls. As sodium moves into the injured cells, it causes an increase in osmotic pressure. This increase in osmotic pressure increases the inflow of vascular fluid into the wound. Finally, the normal process of evaporative loss of water to the environment is accelerated (5 to 15 times that of normal skin) through the burned tissue. In a small wound, these physiological alterations produce a classic local inflammatory response (pain, redness, swelling) without major systemic effects. If the wound covers a large area, however, these local tissue responses can produce effects throughout the body and life-threatening hypovolemia.

Systemic Response to Burn Injury

As local events occur at the injury site, other organ systems become involved in a general response to the stress caused by the burn. One of the earliest manifestations of the systemic effects of a large thermal injury is hypovolemic shock. This hypovolemic shock is known as *burn shock* (described later in this chapter). Burn shock is associated with a decrease in ve-

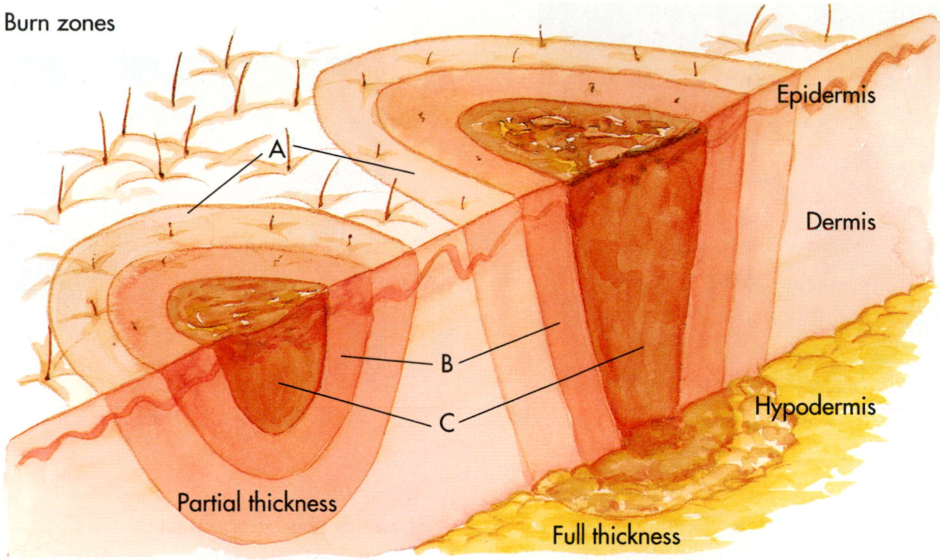

FIGURE 23-1 ■ Three zones of intensity: (A) zone of hyperemia (peripheral); (B) zone of stasis (intermediate); and (C) zone of coagulation (central).

BOX 23-2 Systemic Responses to Major Burn Injury

- Pulmonary response
  Hyperventilation to meet increased metabolic needs
- Gastrointestinal response
  Decrease in splanchnic perfusion that may lead to mucosal hemorrhage and transient adynamic ileus
  Vomiting and aspiration
  Stress ulcers
- Musculoskeletal response
  Decreased range of motion from immobility and edema
  Possible osteoporosis and demineralization (late)
- Neuroendocrine response
  Increased amounts of circulating epinephrine and norepinephrine and transient elevation of aldosterone levels
- Metabolic response
  Elevated metabolic rate, particularly with infection or surgical stress
- Immune response
  Altered immunity, resulting in increased susceptibility to infection
  Depressed inflammatory response
- Emotional response
  Physical pain
  Isolation from loved ones and familiar surroundings
  Fear of disfigurement, deformities, and disability
  Altered self-image
  Depression

nous return, decreased cardiac output, and increased vascular resistance. Burn shock can lead to renal failure. Box 23-2 lists other systemic responses to major burn injury.

CLASSIFICATIONS OF BURN INJURY

Burns must be assessed and classified (body surface area involvement and depth) as correctly as possible in the field. This will help to ensure the proper treatment and transport to a proper facility. It also will help to monitor the progression of tissue damage. However, this usually is not possible in the prehospital setting because of the progressive nature of the injury. The amount of tissue damage may not be evident for hours or even days after a burn injury.

Depth of Burn Injury

Burns are classified in terms of depth as superficial, partial-thickness, and full-thickness. Superficial and **partial-thickness burns** usually heal without surgery. This is the case, at least, if the burns are uncomplicated by infection or shock. **Full-thickness burns** usually require skin grafts. Other depth classifications may be preferred by medical direction.

SUPERFICIAL BURNS

Superficial burns are also known as *first-degree burns.* These burns characteristically are painful, red, and dry and blanch with pressure (Fig. 23-2). Superficial burns usually occur after prolonged exposure to low-intensity heat or a short-duration flash exposure to a heat source. In these burns, only a superficial layer of epidermal cells is destroyed. The

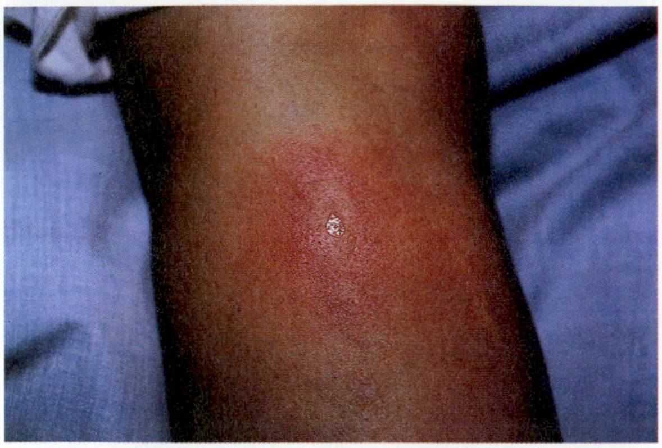

FIGURE 23-2 ■ Superficial burn.

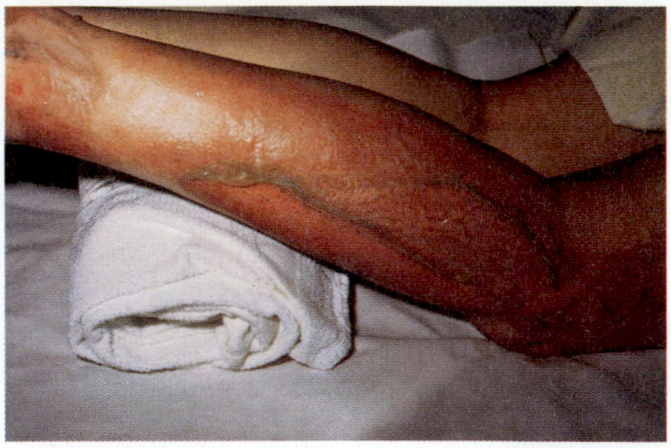

FIGURE 23-4 ■ Deep partial-thickness burn.

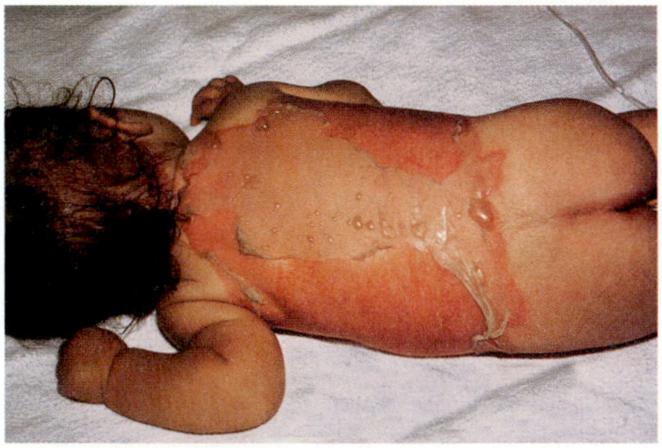

FIGURE 23-3 ■ Superficial partial-thickness second-degree burn.

cells slough (peel away from healthy tissue underneath the wound) without residual scarring. Superficial burn injuries usually heal within 2 to 3 days. An example of a superficial burn is *sunburn.*

PARTIAL-THICKNESS BURNS

Partial-thickness burns are also known as *second-degree burns.* These burns may be divided into two groups: superficial partial-thickness and deep partial-thickness wounds. The superficial partial-thickness injury is characterized by blisters. It often is caused by skin contact with hot but not boiling water or other hot liquids, explosions producing flash burns, hot grease, and flame.

In superficial partial-thickness and deep partial-thickness burns (Fig. 23-3), injury extends through the epidermis to the dermis. However, the basal layers of the skin are not destroyed, and the skin regenerates within a few days to a week. Edematous fluid infiltrates the dermal-epidermal junction, creating the blisters characteristic of this depth of wound. Intact blisters provide a seal. This seal protects the wound from infection and excessive fluid loss. (For this reason, blisters should not be broken in the prehospital setting.) The injured area usually is red, wet, and painful and may blanch when the tissue around the injury is compressed. In the absence of infection, these wounds heal without scarring, usually within 14 days.

If the depth of the partial-thickness burn involves the basal layer of the dermis, the burn is considered a deep partial-thickness burn (Fig. 23-4). As in superficial partial-thickness burns, edema forms at the epidermal-dermal junction. Sensation in and around the wound may be diminished because of the destruction of basal-layer nerve endings. The injury may appear red and wet or white and dry. The appearance depends on the degree of vascular injury. Wound infection and subsequent sepsis and fluid loss are major complications of these injuries. If uncomplicated, deep partial-thickness burns generally heal within 3 to 4 weeks. Skin grafting may be needed to promote timely healing and minimize thick scar tissue formation. The formation of thick scar tissue may restrict joint movements severely and may cause persistent pain and disfigurement.

FULL-THICKNESS BURNS

In full-thickness burns (also known as *third-degree burns*), the entire thickness of the epidermis and dermis is destroyed; thus skin grafts are necessary for timely and proper healing (Fig. 23-5). The wound is characterized by coagulation necrosis of the cells. The wound appears pearly white, charred, or leathery. A definitive sign of a full-thickness burn is a translucent surface in the depths of which thrombosed veins are visible. **Eschar,** a tough, nonelastic coagulated collagen of the dermis, is present in these injuries.

Sensation and capillary refill are absent in full-thickness burns because small blood vessels and nerve endings are destroyed. This often results in large plasma volume loss, infection, and sepsis. Natural wound healing may produce contracture deformity and severe scarring. Therefore surgical intervention with skin grafting is necessary to close full-thickness wounds, minimize complications, and allow restoration of maximal function.

Some burn classifications also describe a full-thickness injury (sometimes called a *fourth-degree burn*) that penetrates the subcutaneous tissue, muscle, fascia, periosteum, or bone. These burns often result from incineration-type exposure and electrical burns in which the heat is great enough to destroy tissues below the skin.

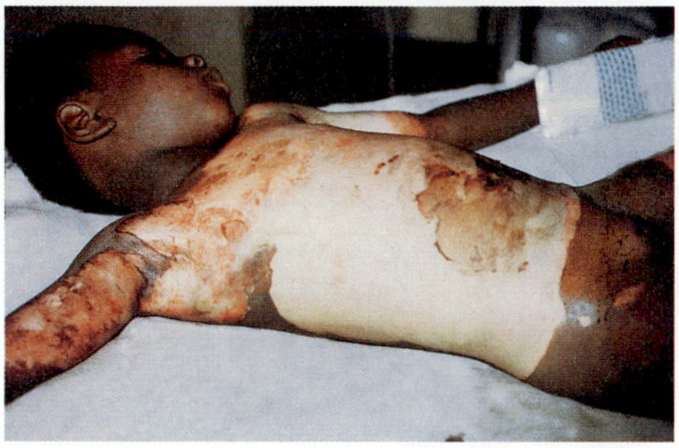

FIGURE 23-5 ■ Full-thickness burn.

Extent and Severity of Burn Injury

There are several methods to evaluate the extent of burn injury. Two common methods include the **rule of nines** and the **Lund and Browder chart.** The paramedic should use a method for determining the extent of burn injury approved by medical direction. Use of any method to evaluate a burn injury should never delay patient care or transport.

RULE OF NINES

The rule of nines commonly is used in the prehospital setting. The measurement divides the total body surface area (TBSA) into segments that are multiples of 9%. This method provides a rough estimate of burn injury size and is most accurate for adults and children older than 10 years of age. Fig. 23-6 explains the rule of nines.

CRITICAL THINKING

Why is the calculation of body surface area different for children less than 10 years of age?

If the burn is irregularly shaped or has a scattered distribution throughout the body, the rule of nines is hard to apply. In these cases, burn size can be estimated by visualizing the patient's palm as an indicator of percentage. (This is the rule of palms.) The surface of the patient's palm equals about 1% of the TBSA.

NOTE Only partial- and full-thickness burns are included when calculating total body surface area. For large burns, total body surface area may be calculated more easily by subtracting the percentage of unburned area from 100.

LUND AND BROWDER CHART

The Lund and Browder chart (Fig. 23-7) is a more accurate method of determining the area of burn injury because it assigns specific numbers to each body part. The chart is used to measure burns in infants and young children. It allows for developmental changes in percentages of body surface area. For example, the adult head is 9% of TBSA, but the newborn head is 18% of TBSA.

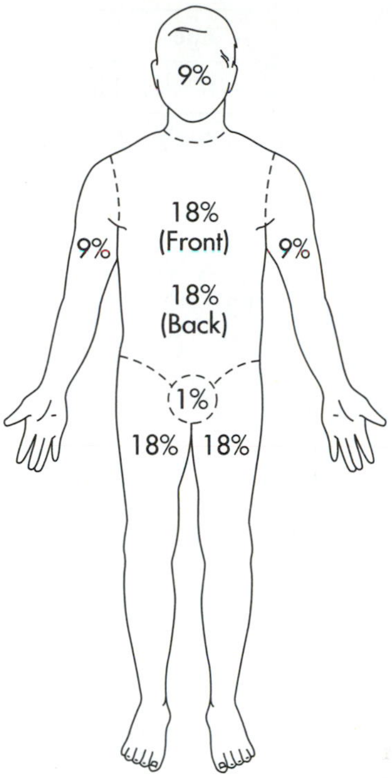

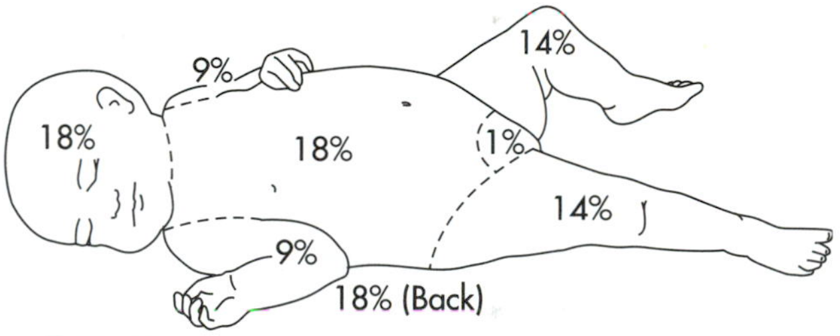

FIGURE 23-6 ■ The rule of nines. **A,** Adult. **B,** Infant.

AMERICAN BURN ASSOCIATION CATEGORIZATION

The American Burn Association has devised a method of categorizing burns to determine severity. The method is based on extent, depth, and location of burn injury; age of the patient; etiological agents involved; presence of inhalation injury; and coexisting injuries or preexisting illness. Using these criteria, burn injuries are categorized as *major, moderate,* and *minor* (Box 23-3).

In determining severity, the paramedic also must consider factors such as the patient's age, the presence of concurrent medical or surgical problems, and the complications that accompany certain types of burns, such as those of the face and neck, hands and feet, and genitalia. For example, burns of the face and neck may cause respiratory compromise. They also may interfere with the ability to eat or drink. Burns of the hands and feet may interfere with ambulation and activities of daily living. Perineal burns present a high risk of infection because of the contaminants in this region. These burns may disrupt the normal patterns of elimination.

Age	0-1	1-4	5-9	10-14	15
A—1/2 of head	9 1/2%	8 1/2%	6 1/2%	5 1/2%	4 1/2%
B—1/2 of one thigh	2 3/4%	3 1/4%	4%	4 1/4%	4 1/2%
C—1/2 of one leg	2 1/2%	2 1/2%	2 3/4%	3%	3 1/4%

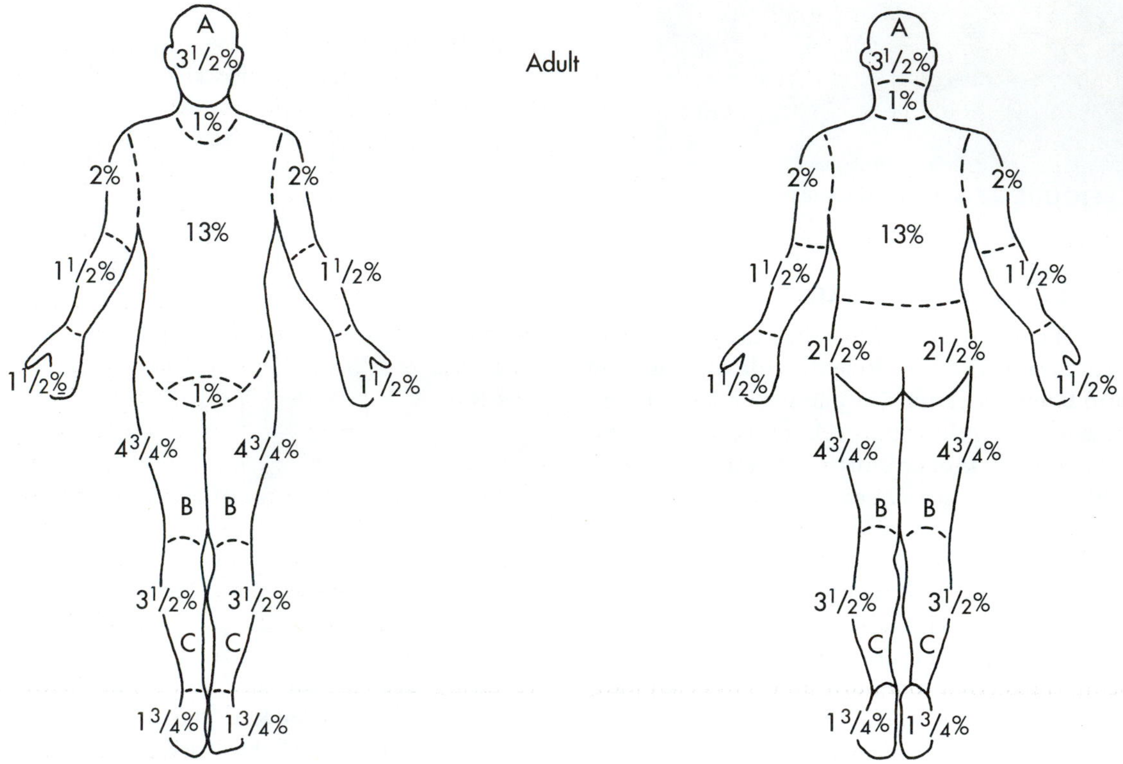

FIGURE 23-7 ■ Lund and Browder chart.

BOX 23-3 Classification of Burn Severity

Major Burns

1. Partial-thickness burns greater than 25% of body surface area (BSA) in adults or greater than 20% of BSA in children or the elderly
2. Full-thickness burns greater than 10% of BSA
3. All burns involving the face, eyes, ears, hands, feet, or perineum that may result in functional or cosmetic impairment
4. Burns caused by caustic chemical agents
5. High-voltage electrical injury
6. Burns complicated by inhalation injury, major trauma, or poor-risk patients

Moderate Burns

1. Partial-thickness burns 15% to 25% of BSA in adults and 10% to 20% of BSA in children or the elderly
2. Less than 10% of BSA full-thickness burns
3. Not involving risk to areas to specialized function such as the face, eyes, ears, hands, feet, or perineum

Minor Burns

1. Burns less than 15% of BSA in adults or 10% of BSA in children or the elderly
2. Less than 2% full-thickness burns
3. No functional or cosmetic risk to areas or specialized function

Adapted from the American Burn Association Injury Severity Grading System.

Burn Center Referral Criteria

Many emergency medical services (EMS) use the categories or other criteria determined by medical direction as the basis for determining which patients need transport to specialized burn centers. According to the Committee on Trauma of the American College of Surgeons and the American Burn Association, burn injuries usually requiring referral to a burn center include the following 10 guidelines.*

A burn unit may treat adults or children or both.

Burn injuries that should be referred to a burn unit include the following[4]:

1. Partial-thickness burns greater than 10% total body surface area.
2. Burns that involve the face, hands, feet, genitalia, perineum, or major joints.
3. Third-degree burns in any age group.
4. Electrical burns, including lightning injury.
5. Chemical burns.
6. Inhalation injury.
7. Burn injury in patients with preexisting medical disorders that could complicate management, prolong recovery, or affect mortality.
8. Any patients with burns and concomitant trauma (such as fractures) in which the burn injury poses the greatest risk of morbidity or mortality. In such cases, if the trauma poses the greater immediate risk, the patient may be initially stabilized in a trauma center before being transferred to a burn unit. Physician judgment will be necessary in such situations and should be in concert with the regional medical control plan and triage protocols.
9. Burned children in hospitals without qualified personnel or equipment for the care of children.
10. Burn injury in patients who will require special social, emotional, or long-term rehabilitative intervention.

PATHOPHYSIOLOGY OF BURN SHOCK

As stated previously, shock can occur from large body surface area burns. Burn shock results from local and systemic responses to thermal trauma that lead to edema and accumulation of vascular fluid in the tissues in the area of injury. Locally, a brief initial decrease in blood flow to the area occurs (this is the *emergent phase*). This is followed by a considerable increase in arteriolar vasodilation. A concurrent release of vasoactive substances from the burned tissue causes increased capillary permeability. This in turn produces intravascular fluid loss and wound edema (the *fluid shift phase*). The fluid shifts cause cardiovascular changes such as a compromised cardiac output, increased systemic vascular resistance, and reduced peripheral blood flow.

*Reprinted from Committee on Trauma, American College of Surgeons: *Resources for optimal care of the injured patient,* Chicago, 1999, American College of Surgeons. Chapter 14.

> **NOTE** Hypovolemia caused by burn trauma usually is not seen in the prehospital setting. This is because burn edema develops over the first several hours after the burn. A hypovolemic patient with burns should be evaluated at the scene for other injuries. These other injuries may be responsible for the volume loss.

Hypovolemia results from fluid loss in the injured tissues and fluid that evaporates from the body because of the loss of the skin. Despite the compensatory effort of the body to retain sodium and water, sodium is lost and potassium is released into the extracellular fluid. The blood becomes concentrated. In severe burns, red blood cells may burst (hemolyze). When combined with hemolysis, rhabdomyolysis, and subsequent hemoglobinuria and myoglobinuria seen with major burns and electrical injury, this hypovolemic state can lead to renal failure. (See Chapter 7.) Impaired peripheral blood flow can damage tissue further and can result in metabolic acidosis.

The greatest loss of intravascular fluid occurs in the first 8 to 12 hours. This loss is followed by a continued, moderate loss over the next 12 to 16 hours. At some point within 24 hours, the leaking of fluid from the cells greatly diminishes (this is the *resolution phase*). At this point, a balance between the intravascular space and the interstitial space is reached. Peripheral vascular resistance will increase in response to hypovolemia and the resulting decrease in cardiac output. With volume replacement, cardiac output can increase to levels above normal (this is the *hypermetabolic phase* of thermal injury) (Fig. 23-8).

Fluid Replacement

Within minutes of a major burn injury, all capillaries in the circulatory system (not just those in the area of the burn) lose the ability to retain fluid. This increase in capillary permeability prevents the creation of an osmotic gradient between the intravascular and extravascular space. This change allows colloid solutions to equilibrate quickly across the capillaries and into the surrounding tissue. The process of burn shock continues for about 24 hours, at which time the normal capillary permeability is restored.[5] Therefore therapy for burn shock is aimed at supporting the patient's vital organ function through the period of hypovolemic shock. Crystalloid solution (e.g., lactated Ringer's solution or normal saline) usually is considered the fluid of choice in initial resuscitation.

Several fluid resuscitation formulae consider body size and extent of burned body surface area. These formulae

> **NOTE** Fluid resuscitation in burn-injured persons is controversial. Medical direction may recommend that fluid resuscitation not be initiated in the prehospital setting if transport to a hospital can be accomplished within 30 minutes.[6] Transport should not be delayed to initiate intravenous therapy.

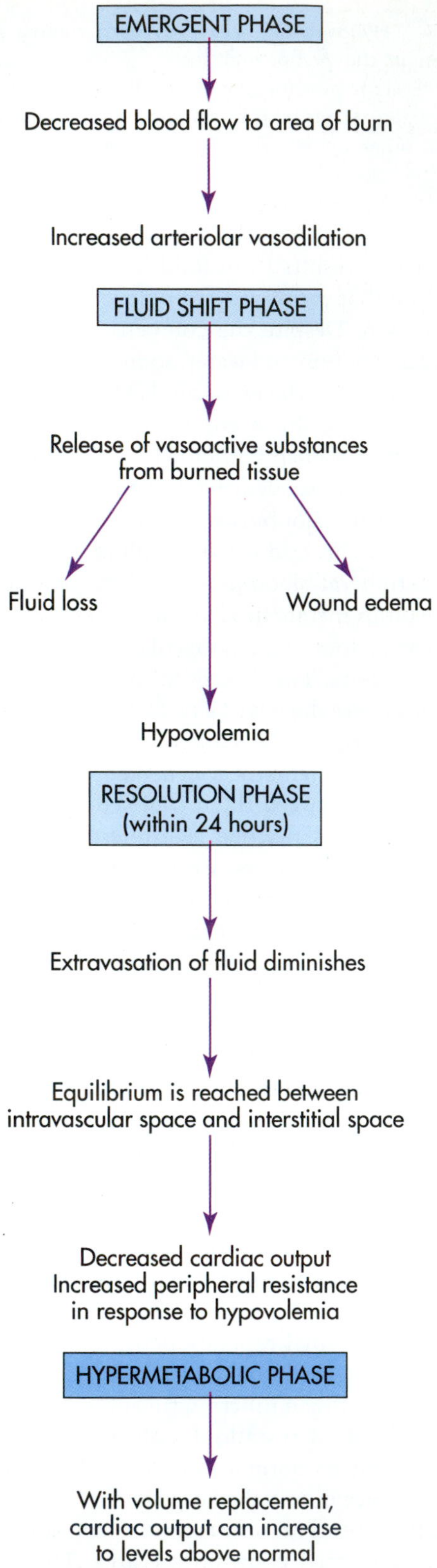
EMERGENT PHASE
Decreased blood flow to area of burn
Increased arteriolar vasodilation
FLUID SHIFT PHASE
Release of vasoactive substances from burned tissue
Fluid loss
Wound edema
Hypovolemia
RESOLUTION PHASE (within 24 hours)
Extravasation of fluid diminishes
Equilibrium is reached between intravascular space and interstitial space
Decreased cardiac output
Increased peripheral resistance in response to hypovolemia
HYPERMETABOLIC PHASE
With volume replacement, cardiac output can increase to levels above normal

FIGURE 23-8 ■ Phases of burn shock.

have proved clinically useful in replacing fluids. The two most common formulae for estimating fluid replacement are the Parkland formula and the modified Brooke formula. These formulae have been combined into the consensus formula. All three formulae call for half of the total calculated amount of fluid to be infused over the first 8 hours from the time of the injury. The second half is to be infused over the following 16 hours. Fluid resuscitation must be guided by regular monitoring of measures of hemodynamic function, including the patient's vital signs, respiratory rate, lung sounds, capillary refill, and in some cases, urinary output. *When determining the percentage of burn for fluid resuscitation, the paramedic should calculate only partial- and full-thickness burns.*

CONSENSUS FORMULA

The consensus formula is applied as follows:

1. The first 24 hours: 4 mL/kg lactated Ringer's solution or normal saline multiplied by percent of TBSA burned
   a. 50% of the calculated amount infused in the first 8 hours
   b. 25% of the calculated amount infused in the second 8 hours
   c. 25% of the calculated amount infused in the third 8 hours

   Example:

   A patient who weighs 100 kg has 30% body surface area (BSA) burns. Total fluid to be infused in the first 24 hours at 4 mL/kg is calculated as follows: 4 mL × 30% BSA × 100 kg = 12,000 mL. Of the 12,000 mL, 6000 mL should be infused in the first 8 hours at a rate of 750 mL/hr. Note that the volume of fluid actually infused may be adjusted according to patient needs as prescribed by medical direction.

The amount and type of fluids required after the first 24 hours are vastly different from those administered during the first 24 hours. Fluid replacement is dictated by the patient's response to the burn and the treatment regimen.

ASSESSMENT OF THE BURN PATIENT

As with any other trauma patient, emergency care for a burn patient begins with making sure the scene is safe and with an initial assessment. In this assessment the paramedic should recognize and treat injuries that pose a threat to life. In burn patients, however, the dramatic appearance of burns, the patient's intense pain, and the characteristic odor of burnt flesh may distract the paramedic from life-threatening problems. A confident assessment by the EMS provider and direction of efforts away from the burn wound and toward the patient as a whole are crucial.

Initial Assessment

The evaluation of the patient's airway is a major concern in the initial assessment. The evaluation is a big concern for the patient with an inhalation injury (described later in this chapter). The paramedic should observe for stridor

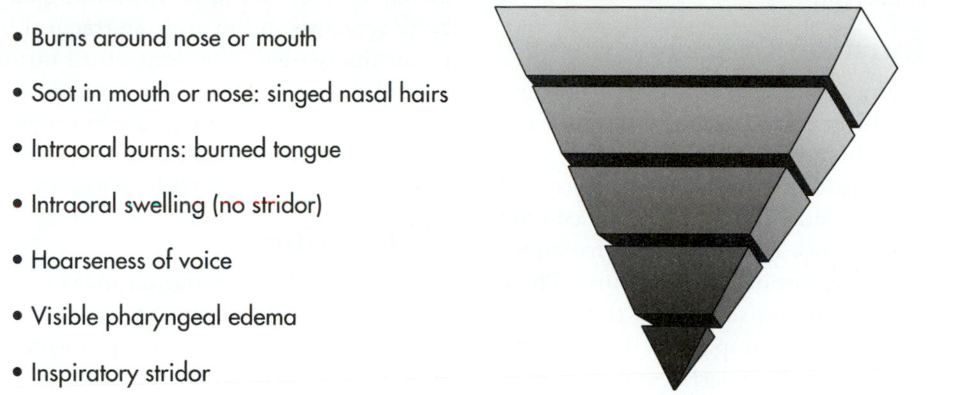

• Burns around nose or mouth
• Soot in mouth or nose: singed nasal hairs
• Intraoral burns: burned tongue
• Intraoral swelling (no stridor)
• Hoarseness of voice
• Visible pharyngeal edema
• Inspiratory stridor

FIGURE 23-9 ■ Probability of upper airway obstruction.

(an ominous sign that indicates the patient's upper airway is at least 80% narrowed), facial burns, soot in the nose or mouth, singed facial or nasal hair, edema of lips and the oral cavity, coughing, inability to swallow secretions in the pharynx, hoarse voice, and circumferential neck burns. Airway management should be aggressive with these patients (Fig. 23-9).

> **CRITICAL THINKING**
>
> Consider a patient who has a large burn. Your initial assessment reveals that the airway is patent. Why should you perform frequent reassessment of the airway?

The paramedic should evaluate breathing for rate, depth, and the presence of wheezes, crackles, or rhonchi. The paramedic should evaluate the patient's circulatory status by assessing the presence, rate, character, and rhythm of pulses; capillary refill; skin color and temperature; pulse oximetry, which may be inaccurate in the presence of carbon monoxide; and obvious arterial bleeding.

The paramedic should determine the patient's neurological status by using the AVPU (alert, verbal, painful, unresponsive) scale. (A similar method can be used as well.) The paramedic should evaluate carefully any deviations from normal for underlying cause. Abnormalities include hypoxia, decreased cerebral perfusion from hypovolemia, and cerebral injury resulting from head trauma. After the initial assessment the paramedic should obtain a history of the event while performing the physical examination.

An accurate history from the patient or bystanders can help the paramedic to determine the potential for inhalation injury, concomitant trauma, or preexisting conditions that may influence the physical examination or patient outcome. When obtaining the patient history, the paramedic should ascertain the following information:

1. What is the patient's chief complaint (e.g., pain or dyspnea)?
2. What were the circumstances of the injury?
   - Did the injury occur in an enclosed space?
   - Were explosive forces involved?
   - Were hazardous chemicals involved?
   - Is there related trauma?
3. What was the source of the burning agent (e.g., flame, metal, liquid, or chemical)?
4. Does the patient have any significant medical history?
5. What medications does the patient take (including recent ingestion of illegal drugs or alcohol)?
6. Did the patient lose consciousness at any time? (Suspect inhalation injury.)
7. What is the status of tetanus immunization?

Physical Examination

At the start of the physical exam, the paramedic should obtain a full set of vital signs. The paramedic should obtain blood pressure in an unburned extremity, if available. If all extremities are burned, the paramedic may place sterile gauze under the blood pressure cuff and attempt to auscultate a blood pressure. Patients with severe burns or preexisting cardiac or medical illness should be monitored by electrocardiogram. Lead placement may need to be modified to avoid placing electrodes over burned areas (see Chapter 29). Field care and hospital destination are determined by the depth, size, location, and extent of burned tissue and the presence of associated illness or injury.

GENERAL PRINCIPLES IN BURN MANAGEMENT

Goals for prehospital management of the severely burned patient include preventing further tissue injury, maintaining the airway, administering oxygen and ventilatory support, providing fluid resuscitation (per protocol), providing rapid transport to an appropriate medical facility, using clean technique to minimize the patient's exposure to infectious agents, and providing psychological and emotional support. Patients with burns also should be evaluated for other types of trauma that pose a threat to life. Some will have additional injuries associated with the burn event. Examples include blunt or penetrating trauma sustained in automobile crashes, blast injury, and skeletal or spinal injury from attempts to escape the thermal source or contact with electrical current.

Stopping the Burning Process

The first step in managing any burn is to stop the burning process. This step must be achieved with the safety of the emergency crew in mind because it often occurs in proximity to the source that caused the burn. With superficial burns the burning process can be terminated by cooling the local area with cold (but not ice-cold) water. Ice, snow, or ointments should not be applied to the burn. These agents may increase the depth and severity of thermal injury. In addition, ointments may impair or delay assessment of the injury when the patient arrives in the emergency department.

In cases of severe burns the paramedic should move the patient rapidly and safely from the burning source to an area of safety if possible. A person whose clothing is in flames or smoldering should be placed on the floor or ground and rolled in a blanket to smother the flames or should be doused with large quantities of the cleanest available water. (Cold water to decrease skin temperature rapidly is preferred.) Contaminated water sources, such as lakes or rivers, should be avoided. These patients should never be allowed to run or remain standing. Running may fan the flame, and an upright position may increase the likelihood of the patient's hair being ignited.

NOTE The National Fire Protection Association developed a training program called *Stop, Drop, and Roll.* The program was designed to teach children and adults that in the event their clothing catches fire, they should: *stop* (do not run); *drop* (cover your face with your hands and drop to the ground in a prone position); and *roll* (to smother the fire until the flames are extinguished).

The paramedic should remove the patient's clothing completely while cooling the burn so that heat is not trapped under the smoldering cloth. If pieces of smoldering cloth have adhered to the skin, the paramedic should cut, not pull, them away. Melted synthetic fabrics that cannot be removed should be soaked in cold water to stop the burning process. After the burn is cooled, the paramedic should cover the patient who has a large body surface area injury with a clean, preferably sterile sheet, over which blankets can be placed when ambient temperatures are low. The duration of cooling is controversial; cooling should continue at least until pain is relieved and probably for a total duration of 15 to 30 minutes.[7]

Airway, Oxygen, and Ventilation

The paramedic should evaluate the adequacy of airway and breathing in all burn patients.The paramedic should give humdified high-concentration oxygen, if it is available, to any patient with severe burns and should assist breathing as needed. If inhalation injury is suspected, the paramedic should observe the patient closely for signs of impending airway obstruction. Life-threatening laryngeal edema may be progressive and may make tracheal intubation difficult if not impossible. The decision to intubate these patients should not be delayed. The paramedic should make every attempt to intubate the patient's lungs with a normal (not smaller) size endotracheal tube. These patients often are hard to ventilate, even with an appropriately sized tube.

Circulation

The need for fluid resuscitation is based on three things: the severity of the injury, the patient's vital signs, and on transport time to the receiving hospital. Some authorities contend that prompt intervention of intravenous therapy in the critically burned patient is essential to prevent long-term complications such as burn shock and renal failure. (The paramedic should consult with medical direction and follow local protocol regarding fluid replacement.)

If intravenous therapy is to be performed, the paramedic should initiate it with a large-bore catheter in a peripheral vein in an unburned extremity. (The arm is the preferred site.) If an unburned site is not available, the paramedic may insert the catheter through burned tissue, although the risk of subsequent infection is greater. The paramedic should take care to secure the catheter with a dressing; tape may not adhere to the injured area as the tissue begins to leak fluid.

The administration of pain medication is an early intervention. Medical direction may recommend that patients with large burns be given ***morphine, meperidine,*** or other analgesic agents (e.g., ***nitrous oxide*** or ***fentanyl***) intravenously. Some of these medications can cause vasodilation and respiratory depression. Thus fluid resuscitation and ventilation support must be adequate. Other pharmacological therapy that may be given after arrival in the emergency department includes topical applications (e.g., silver sulfadiazine or special synthetic dressings), oral analgesics, and tetanus immunization.

CRITICAL THINKING
How should you administer pain medicine to a patient with a large burn? Why did you choose this route?

At times, transport of the burn patient is delayed. A lengthy interfacility transport may be anticipated as well. In either case, other patient care procedures may be required. One such procedure includes the placement of a nasogastric tube. This will prevent gastric distention or vomiting. Another procedure is the placement of an indwelling urinary catheter. This will measure urine output and maintain patency of the urethra in patients with burns to the genitalia. (See Chapter 48.)

Special Considerations

All burn injuries warrant good patient assessment and care. However, burns of specific body regions require special consideration. These include burns to the face and extremities and circumferential burns.

Burns of the face swell rapidly. These burns may be associated with airway problems. The head of the ambulance stretcher should be elevated at least 30 degrees, if not contraindicated by spinal trauma, to minimize the edema. If the patient's ears are burned, the paramedic should aviod use of a pillow to minimize additional injury to the area.

If burns involve the extremities or large areas of the body, the paramedic should remove all rings, watches, and other jewelry as soon as possible. This will help to prevent vascular compromise with increased wound edema. The paramedic should assess peripheral pulses frequently and should elevate the burned limb above the patient's heart if possible.

CRITICAL THINKING

What life- or limb-threatening problems can develop from this swelling?

Burn injuries that encircle a body region can pose a threat to the patient's life or limbs. Circumferential burns that occur to an extremity may produce a tourniquet-like effect that may quickly compromise circulation. The effect can cause irreversible damage to the limb. Circumferential burns of the chest can severely restrict movement of the thorax. These burns may impair chest wall compliance significantly. If this occurs, the depth of respirations is reduced; tidal volume is decreased; and the patient's lungs may become difficult to ventilate, even by mechanical means. Definitive treatment for circumferential burns involves an in-hospital surgical procedure known as *escharotomy.* In this procedure, incisions are made through deep burns to reduce compartment pressure and allow adequate blood volume to flow to and from the affected limb or thorax.

INHALATION BURN INJURY

Smoke inhalation injury is present in about 20% to 35% of all patients admitted to burn centers[8]; more than 50% of the 12,000 fire deaths each year are related directly to smoke inhalation or inhalation injury.[1] Prehospital considerations in caring for patients with inhalation injury include recognition of the dangers inherent in the fire environment, pathophysiology of inhalation injury, and early detection and treatment of impending airway or respiratory problems.

Smoke inhalation most often occurs in a closed environment such as a building, a vehicle, or an airplane. Such injury is caused by the accumulation of toxic by-products of combustion. Inhalation injury also can occur in an open space. Therefore all burn victims should be evaluated for this injury. Dangers that contribute to inhalation injury in a fire environment are as follows:

- Heat
- Consumption of oxygen by the fire
- Production of carbon monoxide
- Production of other toxic gases

Inhalation injury also may occur in the absence of significant thermal injury from exposure to toxic gases (e.g., carbon monoxide).

Pathophysiology

Smoke inhalation and inhalation injury can produce a large number of complications. For this text, these complications are classified as carbon monoxide poisoning, inhalation injury above the glottis *(supraglottic)*, and inhalation injury below the glottis *(infraglottic)*.

Carbon Monoxide Poisoning

Carbon monoxide is a colorless, odorless, tasteless gas produced by incomplete burning of carbon-containing fuels. Carbon monoxide does not harm lung tissue physically. However, it displaces oxygen off the hemoglobin molecule, forming carboxyhemoglobin. The result is low circulating volumes of oxygen despite normal partial pressures. In addition, the presence of carboxyhemoglobin requires that tissues be hypoxic before oxygen is released from the hemoglobin to fuel the cells. This condition is reversible.

Carbon monoxide has about 250 times the attraction to hemoglobin that oxygen has. Therefore small concentrations of carbon monoxide in inspired air can result in severe physiological impairments, including tissue hypoxia, inadequate cellular oxygenation, inadequate cellular and organ function, and eventually death. The physical effects of carbon monoxide poisoning are related to the level of carboxyhemoglobin in the blood (Box 23-4).

NOTE As discussed in Chapter 19, the pulse oximeter is unreliable in determining effective oxygenation in a patient with carbon monoxide poisoning.

Treatment of the patient with carbon monoxide poisoning includes ensuring a patent airway, providing adequate

BOX 23-4 Physical Effects of Carbon Monoxide Blood Levels

Carbon monoxide levels less than 10% usually do not cause symptoms; they are common in smokers, traffic police, truck drivers, and others who are exposed to carbon monoxide chronically. At carbon monoxide levels of 20% a healthy patient may complain of headache, nausea, vomiting, and loss of manual dexterity. At 30% the patient may become confused and lethargic, and electrocardiogram abnormalities may be present. At levels between 40% and 60%, coma may develop. Levels above 60% often are fatal. Tachypnea and cyanosis usually are not present in these patients because arterial oxygen tension is normal. Patients with high carboxyhemoglobin levels may have a skin appearance that is bright red. More commonly, though, the patient has normal or pale skin and lip coloration.

ventilation, administering high-concentration oxygen, and possible pharmacological therapy (sodium thiosulfate) for severely poisoned patients. The half-life of carbon monoxide at room air is about 4 hours. This half-life can be reduced to 30 to 40 minutes if 100% oxygen and adequate ventilation are provided. The use of hyperbaric oxygen therapy may be recommended in treating carbon monoxide poisoning. The therapy promotes increased oxygen uptake by hemoglobin molecules that have not yet been bound to carbon monoxide. The paramedic should follow local protocol.

In addition to carbon monoxide, other gases (e.g., cyanide and hydrogen sulfide) may be released when some materials are burned. The inhalation of these toxic gases can result in inhalation poisoning (e.g., *thiocyanate intoxication*). This may require pharmacological therapy (e.g., cyanide antidote kit), further described in Chapter 36.

CRITICAL THINKING

Can carbon monoxide poisoning be ruled out if the patient does not have these signs or symptoms?

Inhalation Injury above the Glottis

The structure and function of the airway superior to the glottis makes it susceptible to injury if exposed to high temperatures. The upper airway is vascular and has a large surface area. This allows the upper airway to normalize temperatures of inspired air. Because of this design, actual thermal injury to the lower airway is rare. The upper airway sustains the impact of injury when environmental air is superheated.

Thermal injury to the airway can result in immediate edema of the pharynx and larynx (above the level of the true vocal cords). This can progress rapidly to complete airway obstruction. Signs and symptoms of upper airway inhalation injury include the following (Fig. 23-10):

- Facial burns
- Singed nasal or facial hairs
- Carbonaceous sputum
- Edema of the face, oropharyngeal cavity, or both
- Signs of hypoxemia
- Hoarse voice
- Stridor
- Brassy cough
- Grunting respirations

Prompt assessment of the airway is critical in these patients. The paramedic must establish and protect the airway. If impending airway obstruction is suspected, early nasotracheal or orotracheal intubation may be warranted because progressive edema can make intubation hazardous if not impossible.

Inhalation Injury below the Glottis

The two main mechanisms of direct injury to the lung tissue (parenchyma) are heat and toxic material inhalation. Thermal injury to the lower airway is rare. One cause of such injury is the inhalation of superheated steam. This steam has 4000 times the heat-carrying capacity of dry air. Another cause is the aspiration of scalding liquids. Explosions are another cause. These occur as the patient is breathing high concentrations of oxygen under pressure.

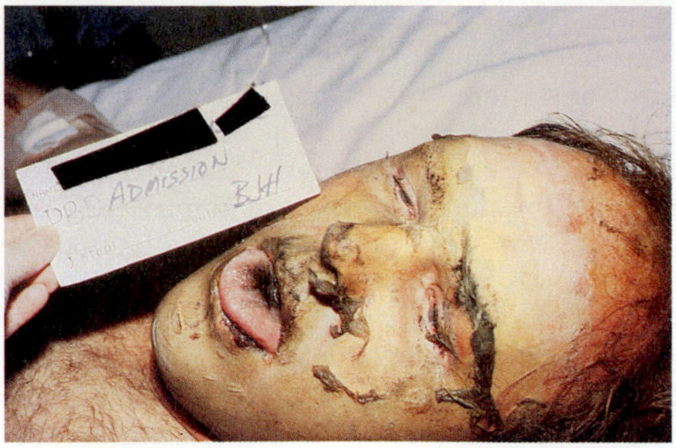

FIGURE 23-10 ■ Inhalation injury.

Most lower airway injuries in fires result from the inhalation of toxic chemicals. Such chemicals include the gaseous by-products of burning materials. Signs and symptoms of lower airway injury may be immediate, but more often they are delayed. Signs and symptoms may begin several hours after the exposure and include the following:

- Wheezes
- Crackles or rhonchi
- Productive cough
- Signs of hypoxemia
- Spasm of bronchi and bronchioles

Prehospital care should be directed at maintaining a patent airway providing high-concentration oxygen and ventilatory support. Specific airway and ventilatory management should be guided by online/direct medical control. This may include nasal or oral tracheal intubation and drug therapy with bronchodilators.

CHEMICAL BURN INJURY

Caustic chemicals often are present in the home and workplace. Unintentional exposure is common. Three types of caustic agents often are associated with burn injuries. These are alkalis, acids, and organic compounds. Alkalis are strong bases with a high pH. Alkalis include hydroxides and carbonates of sodium, potassium, ammonium, lithium, barium, and calcium. These compounds commonly are found in oven cleaners, household drain cleaners, fertilizers, heavy industrial cleaners, and the structural bonds of cement and concrete. Strong acids are in many household cleaners, such as rust removers, bathroom cleaners, and swimming pool acidifiers (Fig. 23-11).

Organic compounds are chemicals that contain carbon. Most organic compounds, such as wood and coal, are harmless chemicals. However, several organic compounds produce caustic injury to human tissue. These compounds include phenols and creosote and petroleum products such as gasoline. In addition to their role in producing chemical burns, or-

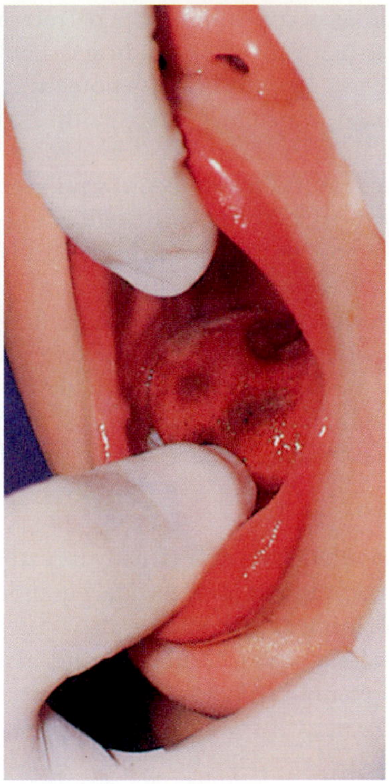

FIGURE 23-11 ■ Intraoral chemical burns sustained by a boy who had ingested bleach.

ganic compounds may be absorbed by the skin. Absorption in turn may cause serious systemic effects. The severity of chemical injury is related to the chemical agent, concentration and volume of the chemical, and duration of contact.

Assessment

While obtaining the patient history, the paramedic should collect facts regarding the exposure factors. When dealing with a chemical exposure, the paramedic should determine the following:

- Type of chemical substance. If the container is available and can be transported safely, it should be taken to the medical facility.
- Concentration of chemical substance
- Volume of chemical substance
- Mechanism of injury (local immersion of a body part, injection, splash)
- Time of contamination
- First aid administered before EMS arrival
- Appearance (chemical burns vary in color)
- Pain

Management

As with all burn injuries, the safety of the rescuers must be the first priority in managing the victim of chemical injury. (Law enforcement, fire service, and special rescue personnel may be needed to secure the scene before entry.) The paramedic must consider the use of protective gear before entering the scene. Depending on the scene and the chemical agent(s), decontamination may be required. Personal protection may include gloves, eye shields, protective garments, and appropriate breathing apparatus. A response to a hazardous materials incident requires special safety considerations and trained rescue personnel (see Chapter 53). The treatment of chemical injuries does not vary much from that of thermal burns during the initial assessment. Treatment is directed at stopping the burning process. This can best be achieved by the following:

1. Remove all clothing, including shoes. These can trap concentrated chemicals.
2. Brush off powdered chemicals.
3. Irrigate the affected area with vast amounts of water.
   a. In otherwise stable patients, irrigation takes priority over transport. That is the case unless irrigation can be continued en route to the emergency department.
   b. If a large body surface area is involved, a shower should be used for irrigation, if available.

CHEMICAL BURN INJURY TO THE EYES

Chemical exposure to the eyes (e.g., from mace, pepper spray, or other irritants) may cause damage ranging from superficial inflammation *(chemical conjunctivitis)* to severe burns. Patients with these conditions have local pain, visual disturbance, lacrimation (tearing), edema, and redness of surrounding tissues. Management guidelines include flushing the eyes with water. This can be done by using a mild flow from a hose, intravenous tubing, or water from a container. (The affected eye should be irrigated from the medial to the lateral aspect. This will help to avoid flushing the chemical into the unaffected eye.) Irrigation should be continued during transport. If contact lenses are present, they should be removed. When retracting the lids to irrigate the eyes, the paramedic should take care to apply pressure only to the bony structures surrounding the eye. The paramedic should avoid applying pressure on the globe.

Some EMS services use nasal cannulas to irrigate both eyes at the same time. The cannula is placed over the bridge of the nose; the nasal prongs are pointing down toward the eyes. The cannula is attached to an intravenous administration set using normal saline or lactated Ringer's solution, and the fluid is run continually into both eyes (Fig. 23-12). Irrigation lenses (e.g., *Morgan therapeutic lens*) may be useful for prolonged eye irrigation in adults, provided that edema is absent and there are no lacerations or penetrating wounds of the globe or eyelids. The use of these devices in the prehospital setting is controversial. Their use requires special training and authorization from medical direction. A chemical burn to the eye can be frightening for the patient. The patient may fear loss of sight from the injury. The paramedic should attempt to calm the patient. The paramedic also should explain the importance of thorough eye irrigation, which may be uncomfortable. This often improves the patient's cooperation.

USE OF ANTIDOTES OR NEUTRALIZING AGENTS

According to the American Burn Association, no agent has been found to be superior to water for treating most chemical burns.[9] Thus the use of antidotes or neutralizing agents

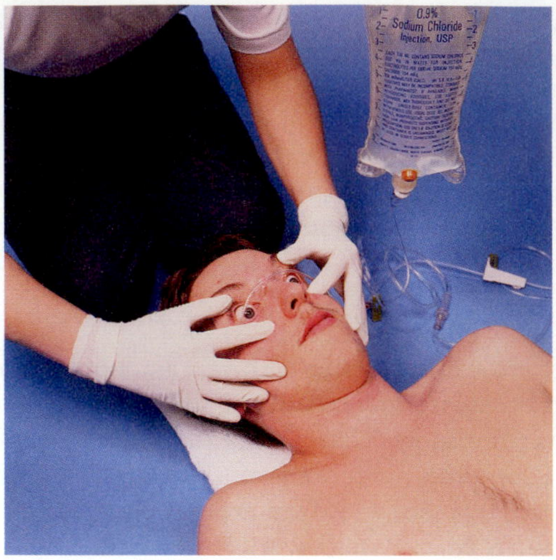

FIGURE 23-12 ■ Use of nasal cannula for eye irrigation.

should be avoided in initial prehospital management of most burn injuries. Many neutralizing agents produce heat. They may increase injury when applied to the wound.

In special circumstances, such as when an industrial complex within a response area is known to use a chemical agent with a specific antidote, medical direction may elect to have the EMS stock the neutralizer. In this case, paramedics should receive special training on the indications, contraindications, use, and side effects of these agents.

Specific Chemical Injuries

The main treatment for most chemical burns is copious irrigation with water. However, a number of chemical injuries call for further discussion and include those from petroleum, hydrofluoric acid, phenols, ammonia, and alkali metals. Personal safety is a priority when working around any of these chemicals.

PETROLEUM

In the absence of flame, products such as gasoline and diesel fuel can cause significant chemical burns if prolonged contact occurs. (This may occur, for example, with entrapment in a vehicle that is surrounded by spilled gasoline.) At first, the injury may appear to be only a superficial or partial-thickness burn. In fact, though, it may be a full-thickness injury. Systemic effects such as central nervous system depression, organ failure, and death may result from the absorption of various hydrocarbons. In addition, lead toxicity can occur if the exposure was from gasoline that contained tetraethyl lead.

HYDROFLUORIC ACID

Hydrofluoric acid is one of the most corrosive materials known. The acid is used in industry for cleaning fabrics and metals, for glass etching, and in the manufacture of silicone chips for electronic equipment. The hydrogen ion and fluoride ion are damaging to tissue. Fluoride hinders several chemical reactions that are required for cell survival. Fluoride also continues to penetrate and kill cells even when it is neutralized by binding to calcium or magnesium. Thus endogenous or exogenous hydrofluoric acid has the potential to produce deep, painful, and severe injuries. If large body surface areas are involved, the patient may experience severe hypocalcemia and even death. This is true with exposure to high concentrations of the acid also. Even the most minor-appearing wounds that involve hydrofluoric acid should be evaluated at a proper medical facility.

Irrigation of the exposed area with large amounts of water should be started immediately. On arrival in the emergency department, treatment may include subcutaneous injection of 10% ***calcium gluconate*** directly into the burn site.

PHENOL

Phenol *(carbolic acid)* is an aromatic hydrocarbon. Phenol is derived from coal tar and is used widely in industry as a disinfectant in cleaning agents. Phenol also is used in the manufacture of plastics, dyes, fertilizers, and explosives. Skin contact with phenol can result in local tissue coagulation and systemic toxicity if the agent is absorbed. A soft tissue injury from phenol exposure may be painless because of the anesthetic properties of the agent. Minor exposures may cause central nervous system depression and dysrhythmias. Patients with significant exposures (10% to 15% TBSA) may require systemic support. These patients should be observed carefully for signs of respiratory failure.

Wounds should be irrigated with large volumes of water. After irrigation, medical direction may advise that the wound be swabbed with a suitable solvent such as glycerol, vegetable oil, or soap and water to bind phenol and prevent its systemic absorption.

AMMONIA

Ammonia is a noxious, irritating gas. Ammonia also is a strong alkali that is very soluble in water. Ammonia is hazardous if introduced into the eye and may result in tissue necrosis and blindness. The patient with an ammonia burn to the eye probably will have swelling or spasm of the eyelids. These injuries must be irrigated with water or a balanced salt solution for up to 24 hours.

Respiratory injury from ammonia vapors depends on two things; the concentration and duration of exposure. For example, short-term, high-concentration exposure usually results in upper airway edema. However, long-term, low-concentration exposure may damage the lower respiratory tract. The initial care for patients with respiratory injury includes high-concentration oxygen administration, ventilatory support as needed, and rapid transport to an appropriate medical facility.

ALKALI METALS

Sodium and potassium are highly reactive metals. They can ignite spontaneously. Water generally is contraindicated when these metals are imbedded in the skin because they react with water and produce large amounts of heat.

BOX 23-5 Principles of Electricity

Tissue damage produced by electric current is a function of six factors: amperage, voltage, resistance, type of current, current pathway, and duration of current flow.

1. *Amperage.* Amperage is a measure of the current flow (intensity) per unit of time. One ampere is a passage of 1 coulomb of charge per second past any point in the circuit. Thus a 10-amp flow means that 10 coulombs of electricity are passing a point per second.
2. *Voltage.* Voltage is a continuous force (tension) applied to any electric circuit that produces a flow of electricity. Volts are the driving force for electrical current. One volt is the force needed to drive 1 amp of current in a circuit with 1 ohm of resistance. High-voltage electrical injuries result from contact with a source of 1000 volts or greater. High-tension accidents usually range from 7200 to 19,000 volts. Yet they may involve current with as high as 100,000 to 1 million volts.
3. *Ohm.* An ohm is a measure of the *resistance* of an electrical conductor. Electrical resistance is composed of four factors: (1) resistivity, the capacity of a material to resist current flow; (2) the size of the object pathway; (3) the length of the object pathway; and (4) temperature. Resistance to the flow of electricity varies greatly within the body because various tissues have different resistance to current flow. Tissue resistance to electrical flow in the body is highest in bone and decreases progressively through the fat, skin, muscle, blood, and nerve tissue.
4. *Type of current.* Two basic forms of electric current are in common usage: direct current (DC) and alternating current (AC). The type of current can influence patterns and severity of injury. Direct current flows in one direction only. Direct current often is used in industry; it is the type of current produced by batteries. Direct current commonly is used in electrosurgical devices and defibrillators and is characterized by high amperage and low voltage.

   Alternating current reverses the direction of flow at regular intervals (60-cycle current has 60 reversals per second). These alterations in current direction can cause tetanic muscle contractions. These contractions may "freeze" the victim to the source until the current is terminated. Household current in the United States generally is alternating current and either 120 or 220 volts. Alternating current is a more common cause of electrical injury.
5. *Current pathway.* Electricity normally flows along a continuous pathway. This pathway is known as an electric circuit. The current pathway can be unpredictable. However, as a rule, low-voltage current (less than 1000 volts) follows the path of least resistance. High-voltage current follows the shortest path. In either case, the greater the current flow, the greater the heat generated.

   The pathway of the current through the body is important because it gives a clue as to what anatomical structures are damaged. For example, if the current travels from one hand to the other, it may flow across the heart and provoke ventricular fibrillation or other dysrhythmias.
6. *Duration of flow.* Tissue injury results from the conversion of electrical energy into heat. The amount of heat produced is directly proportional to the square of the current strength multiplied by the resistance of the tissue multiplied by the duration of the current flow (Joule's law). Therefore injury is directly proportional to the duration of contact with the electrical source.

Physically removing the metal or covering it with oil minimizes the thermal injury.

ELECTRICAL BURN INJURIES

Electrical injuries account for 4% to 6.5% of admissions to burn centers and are responsible for about 500 deaths each year.[2] Good patient care and personal safety at the scene of an electrocution depends on understanding how electricity flows (current) through the body (Box 23-5).

Types of Electrical Injury

Three basic types of injury may occur as a result of contact with electric current. These are *direct contact burns, arc injuries,* and *flash burns.* Direct contact burns occur when electric current directly penetrates the resistance of the skin and underlying tissues. The hand and wrist are common entrance sites. The foot is a common exit site (Fig. 23-13). Although the skin may initially resist current flow, continued contact with the source lessens resistance and permits increased current flow. The greatest tissue damage occurs directly under and adjacent to the contact points and may include fat, fascia, muscle, and bone. Tissue destruction may be massive at the entrance and exit sites; however, injury to the area between these wounds is what poses the greatest threat to the patient's life.

Arc injuries occur when a person is close enough to a high-voltage source that the current between two contact points near the skin overcomes the resistance in the air, passing the current flow through the air to the bystander. Temperatures generated by these sources can be as high as 2000° C to 4000° C (3632° F to 7232° F). The arc may jump as far as 10 feet.

Flame and flash burn injuries can occur when the heat of electrical current ignites a nearby combustible source. Common injury sites include the face and eyes *(welder's flash).* Flash burns also may ignite a person's clothing or cause fire in the surrounding environment. No electrical current passes through the body in this type of burn.

Effects of Electrical Injury

Electrical injuries often are unpredictable. They vary according to the parameters that have been described. Yet certain physiological effects should be expected by the paramedic crew.

The skin is almost always the first point of contact with electrical current. Direct contact and passage of the current through tissue may cause wide areas of coagulation necrosis. The entrance site is often a bull's-eye wound. The site may appear dry, leathery, charred, or depressed. The exit wound may be ulcerated and may appear exploded. Areas of tissue may be missing.

A

B

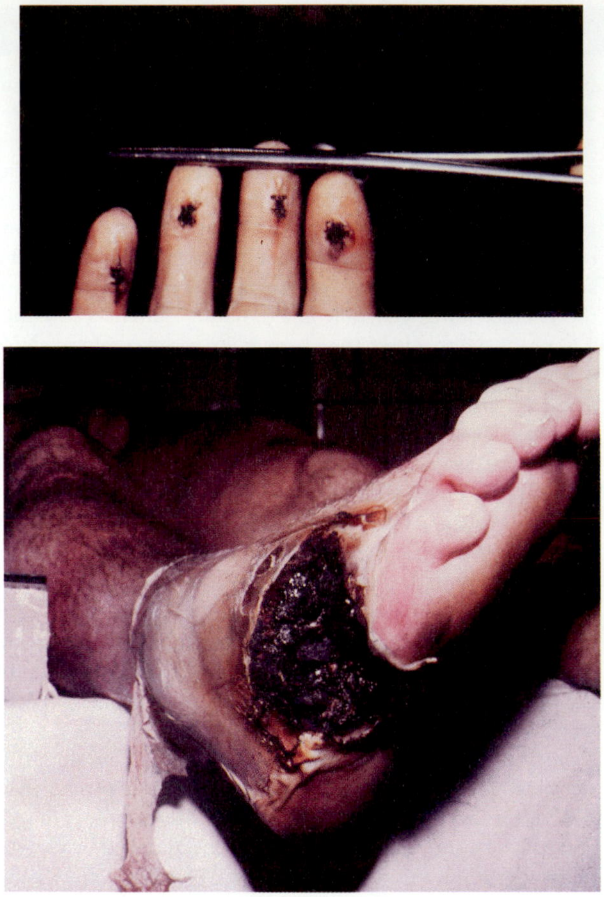

FIGURE 23-13 ■ Direct contact burn. **A,** Entry wound (hand). **B,** Exit wound (foot).

Oral burns often are seen in children younger than 2 years of age. These wounds usually are caused by chewing or sucking on a low-tension electrical cord. Oral burns may be associated with injury to the tongue, palate, and face.

Hypertension and tachycardia associated with a large release of catecholamines is a common finding in electrical injury. Electrical current also may cause significant dysrhythmias (including ventricular fibrillation and asystole) and damage to the myocardium as it passes through the body. The patient may have suffered cardiac arrest. If early rescue and resuscitation can be initiated, success rates are high.

Nerve tissue is a good conductor of electrical current. Thus nerve tissue often may be affected in electrical injuries. Central nervous system damage may result in seizures or coma with or without focal neurological findings. Peripheral nerve injury may lead to motor or sensory deficits. These deficits may be permanent. If the current passes through the brainstem, respiratory arrest or depression, cerebral edema, or hemorrhage may rapidly lead to death.

Electrical injury can cause extensive necrosis of blood vessels. This may not be evident upon the arrival of EMS. However, such injuries can cause immediate or delayed internal hemorrhage or arterial or venous thrombosis and embolism with subsequent complications.

Damage within the extremities after an electrical burn is similar to crush injury (described in Chapter 22). Severe muscle necrosis releases myoglobin. Bursting of the red blood cells (hemolysis) releases hemoglobin. Both of these large molecules can precipitate in the renal tubules, producing acute renal failure. Some patients may require amputation of the affected extremity. This results from decreased circulation and compartment syndrome. In the electrocuted patient, severe muscle spasms can produce bony fractures. These spasms also may produce dislocations, even of major joints. A patient may fall after the electrical shock as well. In such a fall, the patient may sustain skeletal trauma. This trauma may include damage to the cervical spine.

Acute renal failure is a serious complication that affects about 10% of significant direct-contact electrical injuries. Acute renal failure may result from a combination of myoglobin or hemoglobin precipitating out of solution in the renal tubules, disseminated intravascular coagulation caused by tissue damage, hypovolemic shock, and direct current damage. Acute renal failure is not of immediate consequence in the prehospital setting. Yet prompt fluid resuscitation and management of shock may have a positive impact on a number of these patients.

Ventilation may be impaired when electrical burns produce central nervous system injury or chest wall dysfunction. If the respiratory center is disrupted, hypoventilation can lead to instant patient death. Contact with any alternating current sources also has been known to produce respiratory arrest and death from tetany of the muscles of respiration.

Conjunctival and corneal burns and ruptured tympanic membranes are common in some electrical injuries. Cataracts and hearing loss also may appear as late as 1 year after the event.

A number of other internal structures may be damaged from electrical injury. These structures include the abdominal organs and urinary bladder. Submucosal hemorrhage may occur in the bowel; various forms of ulceration are possible. Each patient requires a thorough physical assessment and a high degree of suspicion for associated trauma.

Assessment and Management

Patient assessment should begin by ensuring that no hazards exist for the rescuers or bystanders. If the patient is still in contact with the electrical source, the paramedic should summon the electric company, fire department, or other specially trained personnel before approaching the patient. Once the scene is safe, the patient intervention may begin.

CRITICAL THINKING

What will you do if you respond to a scene and there is a child still in contact with electrical current and who is having tetanic movements? A large crowd has gathered around and is screaming at you to help. The fire department is 3 minutes away. How will you feel?

INITIAL ASSESSMENT

The initial assessment should proceed as it does for all other trauma patients. The paramedic should take care to immobilize the cervical spine. If the patient is not breathing, assisted ventilation should proceed immediately. The paramedic should perform intubation as soon as possible because apnea may persist for lengthy periods. A patient who is breathing should have a patent airway maintained. Respirations should be supported with supplemental high-concentration oxygen as well. If the patient is in cardiac arrest, the paramedic should initiate resuscitation efforts according to protocol. If possible, the paramedic should obtain a history that includes the following:

- Patient's chief complaint (e.g., injury or disorientation)
- Source, voltage, and amperage of the electrical injury
- Duration of contact
- Level of consciousness before and after the injury
- Significant medical history

> **NOTE** The source, voltage, and type of current (alternating current versus direct current) is essential information for the attending physician to estimate internal damage from external wounds.

PHYSICAL EXAMINATION

The physical exam should be thorough. The paramedic should search for entrance and exit wounds or any associated trauma caused by tetany or a fall. The paramedic should recall that there may have been multiple pathways of current. This would mean multiple wounds. The paramedic should remove all of the patient's clothing and jewelry. The paramedic should examine the areas between the patient's fingers and toes for sites of entry or exit. The paramedic carefully should assess distal pulses, motor function, and sensation in all extremities and document the finding to monitor for possible development of compartment syndrome. The paramedic should cover entrance and exit wounds with sterile dressings and should manage any associated trauma appropriately.

Internal damage from electrical current may be much more significant than external wounds. Frequent reassessment is necessary because of the progressive nature of electrical injury. In addition, electrocardiogram monitoring should be implemented at the scene and continued during patient transport. As previously discussed, electrical injury may cause a variety of dysrhythmias, some of which can be lethal.

MANAGEMENT

Early administration of fluids is critical for patients with severe electrical injury. Fluid administration helps to prevent hypovolemia and subsequent renal failure. If possible, the paramedic should establish two large-bore intravenous lines. These should be in an extremity without entry or exit wounds. The fluid of choice generally is lactated Ringer's solution or normal saline without glucose. The flow rate should be determined by the patient's clinical status.

In the emergency department or during interhospital transfer, the patient's intravenous fluid rates will be regulated to maintain a urine output of 75 to 100 mL/hr. This rate decreases the potential for renal damage caused by myoglobin. Emergency department management may include the administration of ***sodium bicarbonate*** to help maintain an alkaline urine. Alkalinity in turn increases the solubility of hemoglobin and myoglobin and decreases the risk of renal failure.

Lightning Injury

Lightning strikes the earth about 7.4 million times each year and accounts for about 70 deaths each year.[2] Lightning can deliver direct current of up to 200,000 amps at a potential of 100 million or more volts, with temperatures that vary between 16,000° F and 60,000° F (8871° C and 33,315° C). Lightning injuries can occur from a direct strike or by a side flash (splash) between a victim and a nearby object that has been struck by lightning. About 30% of those struck by lightning die. Lightning strikes are most common in Florida, Texas, and North Carolina.

Lightning strikes produce tissue injuries that differ from other types of electrical injury because the pathway of tissue damage often is *over* rather than *through* the skin (Fig. 23-14). The duration of the lightning is short ($^1/_{100}$ to $^1/_{1000}$ second). Thus skin burns are less severe than those seen with other high-voltage current. In fact, full-thickness burns are rare. Common lightning burns are linear, feathery, and punctate (pinpoint). In addition, depending on the severity of the strike, the patient may suffer cardiac and respiratory arrest. These are the most common causes of death in lightning injuries.

Lightning injuries may be classified as minor, moderate, or severe. The patients with minor lightning injuries usually are conscious. These patients often are confused and amnesic. Burns or other signs of injury are rare. The vital signs of these patients usually are stable.

The patients with moderate injury may be combative or comatose. These patients may have associated injuries from the impact of the lightning strike. Superficial and partial-thickness burns are common, as is tympanic membrane rupture. These patients may have serious internal organ damage. They should be observed carefully for signs and symptoms of cardiorespiratory dysfunction.

Severe lightning injuries include those that cause immediate brain damage, seizures, respiratory paralysis, and cardiac arrest. The prehospital care is directed at basic and advanced life support measures and rapid transport to a proper facility.

ASSESSMENT AND MANAGEMENT

Like all other emergency responses, scene safety is the first priority. If the electrical storm is still in progress, all patient care should take place in a sheltered area. To prevent injury from subsequent lightning strikes, the paramedic crew

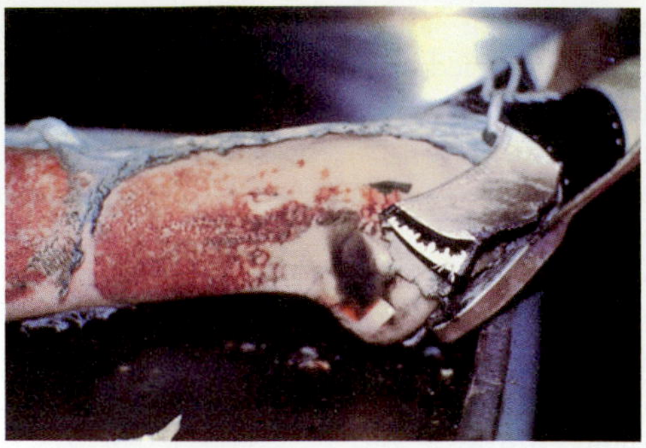

FIGURE 23-14 ■ Lightning injury.

should stay away from objects that project from the ground. Such objects include trees, fences, and high buildings. The crew also should avoid areas of open water. If rescue attempts in an open area are necessary, the paramedic should stay low to the ground.

The prehospital management of lightning injuries is the same as for other severe electrical injuries. Initial patient care is directed at airway and ventilatory support; basic and advanced life support; patient immobilization; fluid resuscitation to prevent hypovolemia and renal failure; pharmacological therapy (per protocol) to manage seizures (if present) and promote excretion of myoglobin and to treat dysrhythmias; wound care; and rapid transport to a proper facility.

> **NOTE** Cardiopulmonary resuscitation should be initiated immediately for patients who appear dead because resuscitation is possible after lightning injury.

RADIATION EXPOSURE

The most common radiation incidents involve sealed radioactive sources used in industrial radiography and nondestructive testing. The victims of these types of incidents rarely require emergency care. However, EMS may be called to building fires and crashes that may involve radioactive materials. Thus an understanding of the hazards of radiation exposure is important. As with all incidents involving hazardous materials, the paramedic crew should never enter the scene until it has been made safe by the proper authorities.

Safety issues regarding radiation have been excellent overall throughout the world. However, hazards associated with radiation became well known as a result of two incidents. First, the serious potential for disaster occurred at Three Mile Island in Pennsylvania in 1979. Second, a disastrous incident occurred at the Chernobyl Nuclear Power Station in the Soviet Union in 1986.

> **CRITICAL THINKING**
> What industries in your area use radioactive materials? Is there a preplan for accidents at that site?

Characteristics of Radioactive Particles

Radioactive particles generally are classified into three types: *alpha, beta,* and *gamma.* Alpha particles are large. They travel only a few millimeters. They have little penetrating ability. In fact, alpha particles may be stopped by paper, clothing, or skin. These particles are considered the least dangerous external radiation source. However, if alpha particles enter the body through inhalation, ingestion, or absorption, they can damage internal organs and interfere with the chemical functions of the body. Alpha radiation is considered the most dangerous form of internal radiation exposure.

Beta particles are one seven thousandth the size of alpha particles. Yet beta particles have much more energy and penetrating power. Beta particles can penetrate subcutaneous tissue. They usually enter the body through damaged skin, ingestion, or inhalation. Protection from alpha and beta radiation requires full protective clothing, including a positive-pressure self-contained breathing apparatus.

Gamma rays and x-rays are the most dangerous forms of penetrating radiation. They require lead shields for protection. Gamma rays have 10,000 times the penetrating power of alpha particles. They have 100 times the penetrating power of beta particles. Protective clothing does not stop gamma rays. Gamma rays pose internal and external hazards. They may produce localized skin burns and extensive internal damage.

Harmful Effects from Radiation Exposure

Nonionizing radiation includes radio waves and microwaves. Nonionizing radiation usually is not thought to be dangerous. Ionizing radiation is produced by nuclear weapons, reactors, radioactive material, and x-ray machines. Although rare, the exposure to ionizing radiation poses a threat to victims and rescue workers.

The amount of emitted radiation is expressed in *roentgens* and indicates the ionization produced in the air by gamma or x-ray radiation. Other units used to measure radiation are the *rad* (radiation absorbed dose), and the *rem* (roentgen equivalent man). A rad is a measure of the amount of ionized radiation being emitted and the amount that has been absorbed and is active within the body tissues. A rem is used to assess the biological effects of the various types of radiation. For emergency purposes, rescue workers should assume that 1 roentgen equals 1 rad equals 1 rem.

Doses of less than 100 rem usually do not cause significant acute problems. Doses from 100 to 200 rem may cause symptoms. Yet the doses are not life threatening. When an exposure of 200 rem is neared, nausea, vomiting, and diarrhea begin within 2 to 4 hours. After an exposure of 450 rems, 50% mortality can be expected within 30 days if no

BOX 23-6 Types of Radiation Injury

The harmful effects from radiation may be classified as external irradiation, contamination by radioactive materials, incorporation of radioactive materials, and combined radiation injury.

External irradiation occurs when all or part of the body is exposed to penetrating radiation from an external source. An example of external irradiation is a medical x-ray. The degree of radiation injury depends on the intensity of radiation, which in turn depends on the duration of exposure. Degree of injury also depends on the distance from the source. A patient who has been exposed to large amounts of radiation may have nausea, vomiting, and diarrhea. In severe cases, additional symptoms may include weight loss, hair loss, fever, bleeding, mouth and throat sores, skin burns, lowered body resistance, vesiculation, and ulceration. The effects from this type of radiation are not contagious; there are no risks to the rescuer in providing care.

Contamination occurs when radioactive materials in the form of gases, liquids, or solids are released into the environment. These materials contaminate persons internally, externally, or both. When radioactive material remains on the patient's clothing or skin or in open wounds, a potential hazard is present for the rescuer and the patient. Patients who have been contaminated should be considered medical emergencies. They may pose significant risk to emergency providers.

Incorporation refers to the uptake of radioactive materials by body cells, tissues, and target organs such as bone, liver, thyroid, or kidney. Incorporation is impossible unless contamination has occurred.

A combination radiation injury involves external irradiation, contamination, incorporation, or some combination of these. This type of exposure usually is the result of a major incident. Exposure may be complicated by a patient's physical injury.

After exposure to radiation, a person may be at risk for delayed complications. Such complications include cell and chromosomal changes, subsequent reproductive genetic aberrations, cell death, and sterility. Diseases such as anemia and forms of cancer may develop as well.

medical care is given. Victims of radiation rarely show immediate signs or symptoms of exposure. Thus all victims of possible exposure should be presumed to have a radiation injury until proved otherwise (Box 23-6.)

NOTE An object or a person who has been exposed to radiation is not radioactive. Only the presence of the radioactive residue poses a threat to rescuers.

Emergency Response to Radiation Accidents

If the EMS crew has been advised that radioactive materials are present at an emergency scene, they should approach the site with caution. They should not enter the scene until it has been secured by proper authorities (see Chapter 53). Rescue personnel, emergency vehicles, and the command post should be positioned 200 to 300 feet upwind of the site. Emergency workers should not eat, drink, or smoke at the site or in any rescue vehicle. The proper local authorities should be contacted (state radiological health office, local specialists). Medical direction should be notified as well. Protective clothing suitable for other hazardous material releases should be worn by all emergency workers. In addition, dose meters should be available for all rescue personnel. Self-contained breathing apparatus should be used if fire, smoke, or gas is present.

Personal Protection from Radiation

The Federal Emergency Management Agency recommends that basic radiation protection for the rescuer and the patient include the following four factors[10]:

1. *Time:* The less time spent in a radiation field, the less radiation exposure. If adequate personnel are available, a rotating team approach can be used to keep individual radiation exposure to a minimum.
2. *Distance:* The farther a person is from the source of radiation, the lower the radiation dose. Even moving several feet away from a radioactive source greatly reduces the level of exposure.
3. *Shielding:* The general principle of shielding is that the denser the material, the greater its ability to stop the passage of radiation. Lead shields provide the best protection from exposure. However, vehicles, mounds of dirt, and pieces of heavy equipment placed between the radiation source and the rescuer and victim also can diminish exposure levels. Protective clothing and self-contained breathing apparatus may provide adequate protection from all alpha and some beta radiation, but protective clothing does not prevent penetration of gamma rays. If adequate shielding is not readily available, rescuers should use the time and distance factors to reduce radiation exposure.
4. *Quantity:* Limiting the amount of radioactive material in a specific area lessens the radiation exposure. Examples include removing contaminated clothing, bagging all contaminated items, and moving containers of radioactive material from the area.

Emergency Care for Victims of Radiation Exposure

A patient who has been irradiated is not radioactive. But when external contamination occurs and radioactive material remains on the patient's clothing and skin or in open wounds, the rescuer should consult with medical direction. The rescuer also should follow agency protocol. The effects of radiation exposure may be instant (e.g., burns) or delayed.

With the exception of dealing with contaminants and containing their spread, there are no emergency care procedures specific to radiation injury. All external bleeding should be controlled, the spine immobilized, open wounds covered, and fractures stabilized in normal fashion. The EMS crew should move the patient away from the source of radiation as soon as possible. Lifesaving care should not be delayed for patient transfer or decontamination procedures. Intravenous fluid replacement should be initiated if indicated. (Strict aseptic technique should be used.) If an intravenous line is not needed for specific therapy, its use should be avoided to prevent introducing contaminants into the body.

Radiation Decontamination Procedures

Radiation emergencies involving patients may be defined in two ways: clean and dirty. *Clean* means that the patient was exposed but not contaminated. *Dirty* means that the patient was contaminated. Only properly trained personnel (e.g., hazardous materials teams and qualified county, state, or federal health department personnel) should attempt to decontaminate radiation victims at the scene. A patient who is to be transported to a hospital for decontamination should be isolated from the environment (described in Chapter 53). Also, all patient effects should be transported with the patient.

SUMMARY

- Each year more than 2 million Americans seek medical attention for burns. Morbidity and mortality rates from burn injury follow significant patterns regarding gender, age, and socioeconomic status. A burn injury is caused by an interaction between thermal, chemical, electrical, or radiation energy and biological matter.
- Tissue damage from burns depends on the degree of the heat and on the duration of exposure to the thermal source. As local events occur at the injury site, other organ systems become involved in a general response to the stress caused by the burn.
- Burns are classified in terms of depth as superficial, partial-thickness, and full-thickness. The rule of nines provides a rough estimate of burn injury size (extent) and is most accurate for adults and for children older than age 10. The Lund and Browder chart is a more accurate method of determining the area of burn injury. Severity of burn injury and burn center referral guidelines are based on standards that take into account the depth, extent, and severity of the burn wound; the source of injury; patient age; presence of concurrent medical or surgical problems; and the body region that is burned.
- Shock after thermal injury results from edema and accumulation of vascular fluid. These tissue changes occur in the area of injury and can produce systemic hypovolemia if the burn area is large.
- Emergency care for a burn patient begins with the initial assessment. The goal is to recognize and treat life-threatening injuries.
- Goals for prehospital management of the severely burned patient include preventing further tissue injury, maintaining the airway, administering oxygen and ventilatory support, providing fluid resuscitation, providing rapid transport to an appropriate medical facility, using aseptic (clean) technique to minimize the patient's exposure to infectious agents, managing pain, and providing psychological and emotional support.
- Prehospital considerations in caring for patients with inhalation injury include recognition of the dangers inherent in the fire environment, pathophysiology of inhalation injury, and early detection and treatment of impending airway or respiratory problems.
- The severity of chemical injury is related to three things: the chemical agent, the concentration and volume of the chemical, and the duration of contact. Treatment is directed at stopping the burning process by using copious irrigation.
- Three types of injury may occur as a result of contact with electrical current: direct contact burns, arc injuries, and flash burns. Once the scene is safe, patient intervention may begin. Internal damage from electrical current may be much more significant than external wounds.
- Persons who are injured by radiation rarely require emergency care. Radioactive particles are classified into three types: alpha, beta, and gamma. The Federal Emergency Management Agency recommends that basic radiation protection for the rescuer and the patient include four factors: minimize time in the radiation field; maintain a safe distance from the source; place shielding between the rescuers and the source; and limit the amount of radioactive material in a specific area.

REFERENCES

1. National Institute of General Medical Sciences, National Institutes of Health: *Trauma, burn, shock and injury: facts and figures,* Bethesda, Md, 1999, The Institute.
2. National Safety Council: *Injury facts,* Itasca, Ill, 2001, The Council.
3. Achauer B: *Management of the burned patient,* Norwalk, Conn, 1987, Appleton & Lange.
4. Committee on Trauma American College of Surgeons: *Resources for optimal care of the injured patient,* Chicago, 1999, The Committee.
5. Faldmo L et al: Management of acute burns and shock resuscitation, *AACN Clin Issues Crit Care Nurs* 4(2):351, 1993.
6. Rosen P, Barkin R: *Emergency medicine: concepts and clinical practice,* ed 5, St Louis, 2003, Mosby.
7. American Heart Association: Guidelines 2000 for cardiopulmonary resuscitation and emergency cardiovascular care, International Consensus on Science, *Circulation* 102(8):79, 2000.
8. US Department of Transportation, National Highway Traffic Safety Administration: *EMT-Paramedic national standard curriculum,* Washington, DC, 1998, The Department.
9. *Advanced burn life support provider manual,* Chicago, IL, 2001, American Burn Association.
10. Federal Emergency Management Agency: Radiological emergency management. http://www.fema.gov. Accessed January 14, 2005.

CHAPTER

24

Head and Facial Trauma

OBJECTIVES

Upon completion of this chapter, the paramedic student will be able to:

1. Describe the mechanisms of injury, assessment, and management of maxillofacial injuries.
2. Describe the mechanisms of injury, assessment, and management of ear, eye, and dental injuries.
3. Describe the mechanisms of injury, assessment, and management of anterior neck trauma.
4. Describe the mechanisms of injury, assessment, and management of injuries to the scalp, cranial vault, or cranial nerves.
5. Distinguish between types of traumatic brain injury based on an understanding of pathophysiology and assessment findings.
6. Outline the prehospital management of the patient with cerebral injury.
7. Calculate a Glasgow Coma Scale, trauma score, Revised Trauma Score, and pediatric trauma score when given appropriate patient information.

KEY TERMS

antegrade amnesia: The loss of memory for events that occurred immediately after recovery of consciousness.

Battle's sign: Ecchymosis over the mastoid process caused by a fracture of the temporal bone.

cerebral perfusion pressure: A measure of the amount of blood flow to the brain calculated by subtracting the intracranial pressure from the mean systemic arterial blood pressure.

Cushing's triad: Increased systolic pressure, widened pulse pressure, and decrease in the pulse and respiratory rate, which result from increased intracranial pressure.

decerebrate posturing: A position in which a comatose patient's arms are extended and internally rotated and the legs are extended with the feet in forced plantar flexion; usually observed in patients who have compression of the brainstem.

decorticate posturing: A position in which the comatose patient's upper extremities are rigidly flexed at the elbows and at the wrists; usually observed in patients who have a lesion in the mesencephalic region of the brain.

intracerebral hematoma: An accumulation of blood or fluid within the tissue of the brain.

Le Fort fracture: A fracture pattern that can be produced in the midface region.

mean arterial pressure: The arithmetic mean of the blood pressure in the arterial portion of the circulation.

raccoon's eyes: Ecchymosis of one or both orbits caused by fracture of the base of the sphenoid sinus.

retrograde amnesia: The loss of memory for events that occurred before the event that precipitated the amnesia.

subarachnoid hematoma: A collection of blood or fluid in the subarachnoid space.

Head injuries affect nearly 4 million persons each year in the United States, and about 50,000 patients with severe head trauma die each year before reaching the emergency department.[1] The categories of head trauma discussed in this chapter include maxillofacial trauma; ear, eye, and dental trauma; anterior neck trauma; and trauma to the skull and brain.

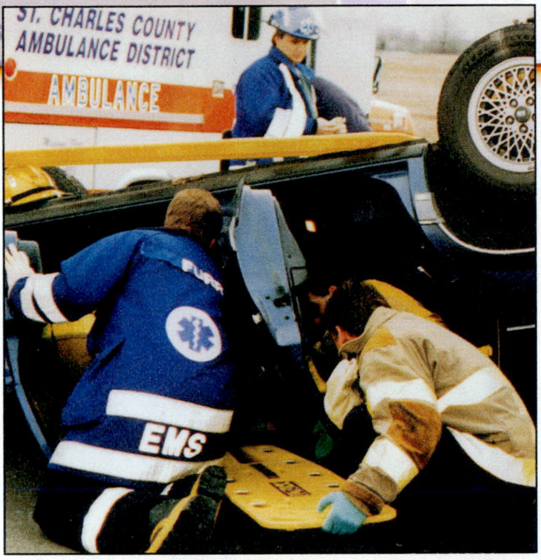

MAXILLOFACIAL INJURY

In descending order of frequency, major causes of maxillofacial trauma are motor vehicle crashes, home injuries, athletic injuries, animal bites, intentional violent acts, and industrial injuries. Maxillofacial trauma may include soft tissue injuries and facial fractures.

Soft Tissue Injuries

The face receives its blood supply from the branches of the internal and external carotid arteries. These branches provide a rich vascular supply. As a result, soft tissue injuries to the face often appear to be serious (Fig. 24-1). With the exception of a compromised upper airway and the potential for heavy bleeding, however, damage to the tissues of the maxillofacial area is seldom life threatening. Depending on the mechanism of injury, facial trauma may range from minor cuts and abrasions to more serious injuries. The more serious injuries may involve extensive soft tissue lacerations and avulsions. If possible, the paramedic should obtain a thorough history from the patient. The history should include mechanism of injury; events leading up to the injury; time of injury; associated medical problems; and allergies, medications, and last oral intake.

CRITICAL THINKING

Why might it be difficult to obtain a history from a patient with this type of injury?

MANAGEMENT

The management of soft tissue injuries was described in Chapter 22. The key principles of wound management include the control of bleeding with direct pressure and pressure bandages. The paramedic also should use spinal precautions if indicated by mechanism of injury (described in Chapter 25). The paramedic also should pay close attention to airway management. Soft tissue injuries to the nose and mouth are common with facial injuries. The paramedic should assess the patient's airway for obstruction caused by blood, vomitus, bone fragments, broken teeth, dentures, and damage to the anterior neck. Suction may be needed to clear the patient's airway. Also, oral or nasal adjuncts, tracheal intubation, or cricothyrotomy may be required to ensure adequate ventilation and oxygenation.

Facial Fractures

Facial bones can withstand tremendous forces from the impact of energy. However, facial fractures are common after blunt trauma. The anatomical structure of the facial bones allows stepwise fracture to absorb the impact of blunt trauma. Blunt trauma injuries may be classified anatomically as fractures to the mandible, midface, zygoma, orbit, and nose. Signs and symptoms of facial fractures include the following:

- Asymmetry of cheek bone prominences
- Crepitus
- Dental malocclusion
- Discontinuity of the orbital rim
- Displacement of the nasal septum
- Ecchymosis

A

B

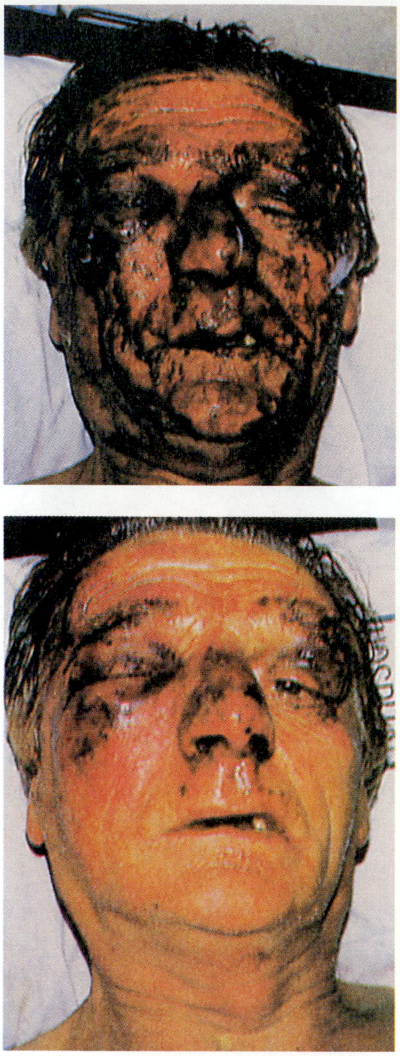

FIGURE 24-1 ■ **A,** Appearance of a patient after being attacked. **B,** Appearance of same man after cleansing.

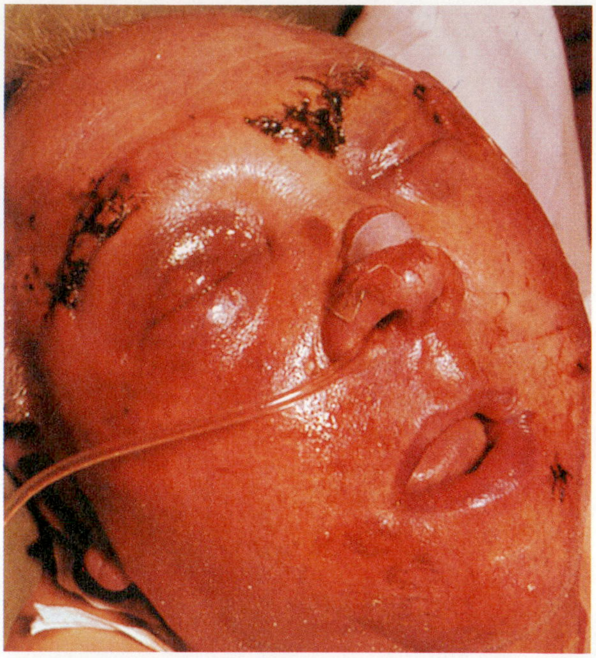

FIGURE 24-2 ■ Fracture of the middle third of the face.

- Lacerations and bleeding
- Limitation of forward movement of the mandible
- Limited ocular movements
- Numbness
- Pain
- Swelling
- Visual disturbances

FRACTURES OF THE MANDIBLE

The mandible is the single facial bone in the lower third of the face. (See Chapter 6.) Because of its prominence, fractures to this bone rank second in frequency after nasal fractures. The mandible is a hemicircle of bone. It may break in multiple locations, often distant from the point of impact. Signs and symptoms specific to mandibular fractures include malocclusion (patients may complain that their teeth do not "feel right" when their mouths are closed), numbness in the chin, and inability to open the mouth. The patient also may have difficulty swallowing and may have excessive salivation. Most patients with mandibular fractures require hospitalization.

Anterior dislocation of the mandible in the absence of fracture also may occur as a result of blunt trauma to the face (rare), an abnormally wide yawn, and dental treatment requiring that the jaws remain open for long periods. In these cases, the condylar head advances forward beyond the articular surface of the temporal bone. The jaw-closing muscles spasm. As a result, the mouth becomes locked in a wide-open position. The patient usually feels severe pain from the spasm. The patient also experiences anxiety and discomfort that perpetuate the spasm. Mandibular dislocations are reduced manually in the emergency department with the aid of a muscle relaxant or sedative or in the operating room with a general anesthetic.

CRITICAL THINKING

What will be your patient care priority with these patients?

FRACTURES OF THE MIDFACE

The middle third of the face includes the maxilla, zygoma, floor of the orbit, and nose. Fractures to this region result from direct or transmitted force. (For example, fractures may result from blunt trauma to the mandible with the energy transmitted to produce fractures to the maxilla.) These injuries often are associated with central nervous system injury and spinal trauma (Fig. 24-2).

In 1901 a cadaver study done by Le Fort described three patterns of injuries **(Le Fort fractures).** These injuries occur in the midface region (Fig. 24-3). The Le Fort I fracture involves the maxilla up to the level of the nasal fossa.

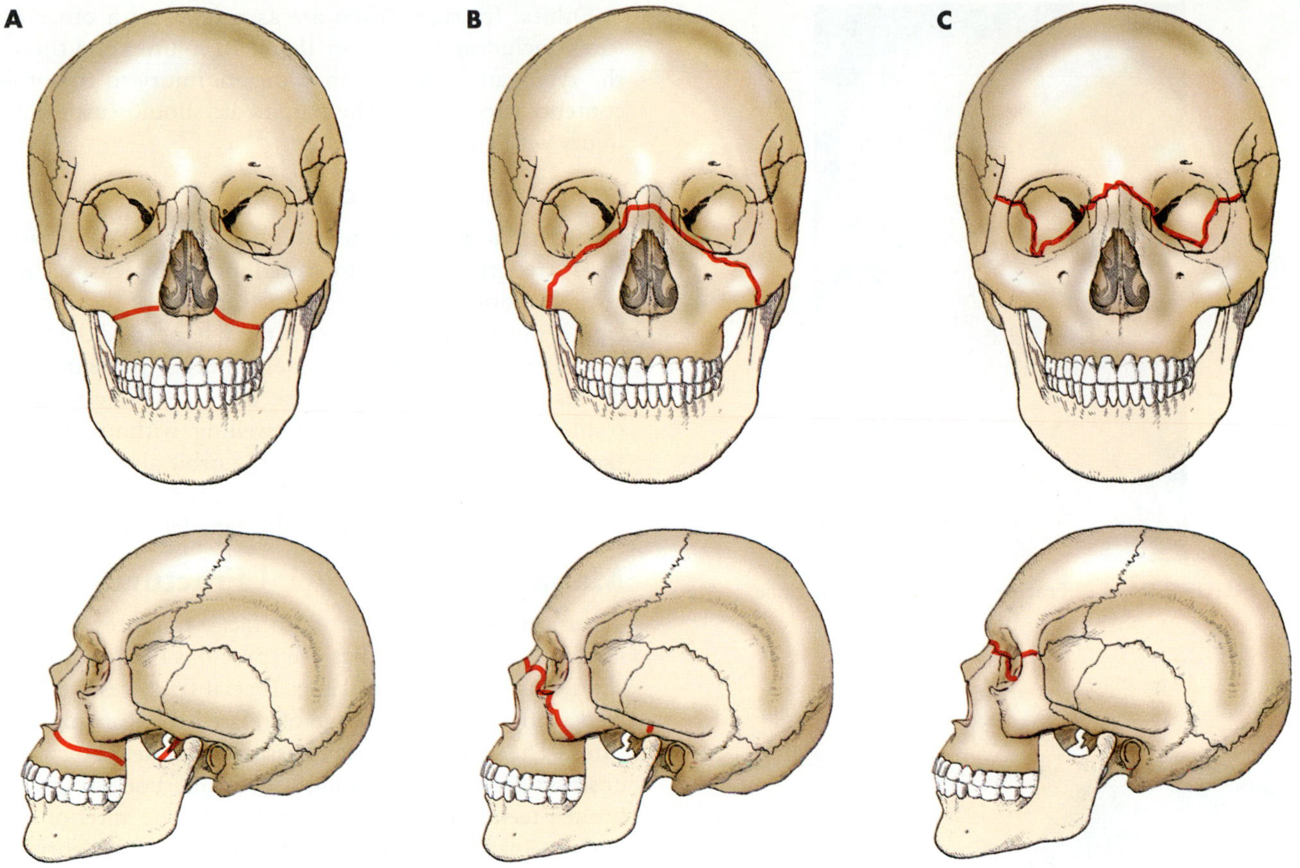

FIGURE 24-3 ■ **A,** Le Fort I facial fractures (lateral and frontal views). **B,** Le Fort II fractures (lateral and frontal views). **C,** Le Fort III fractures (lateral and frontal views).

The Le Fort II involves the nasal bones and medial orbits. The fracture line generally is shaped like a pyramid. The Le Fort III results in craniofacial dislocation and involves all of the bones of the face. Depending on the severity of injury, different combinations of Le Fort fractures may be present.

Signs and symptoms specific to midface fractures include midfacial edema, unstable maxilla, lengthening of the face (donkey face), epistaxis, numb upper teeth, nasal flattening, and cerebrospinal fluid rhinorrhea (cerebrospinal fluid leakage caused by ethmoid cribriform plate fracture). Patients with midface fractures require hospitalization. These patients (particularly those with Le Fort II and III fractures) are at risk of having serious airway problems. Because of the extent of the fractures, a risk exists of placing the nasogastric or even nasotracheal tubes into the brain tissue.

▶**NOTE** As described in Chapter 19, nasal airways, nasogastric tubes, and nasotracheal intubation are contraindicated in patients who have fractures of the basal skull or facial bones. Cerebrospinal fluid leakage from the ear or nose should be allowed to drain freely. The paramedic should make no attempts to control cerebrospinal fluid leakage with direct pressure.

FRACTURES OF THE ZYGOMA

The zygoma (malar eminence) articulates with the frontal, maxillary, and temporal bones. The zygoma commonly is called the *cheek bone.* Rarely does it get fractured because of its sturdy construction. When fractures occur, they usually are a result of physical assaults and vehicle crashes. Zygomatic fractures often are associated with orbital fractures and manifest similar clinical signs (Fig. 24-4). The two are distinguished by x-ray exam. Signs and symptoms specific to zygomatic fractures include flatness of a usually rounded cheek area; numbness of the cheek, nose, and upper lip (particularly if an orbital fracture is involved); epistaxis; and altered vision.

FRACTURES OF THE ORBIT

The orbital contents are protected by a bony ring. The ring resembles a pyramid, with the apex pointed toward the back of the head. The bones of the walls, floor, and roof of the orbit are thin and are fractured easily by direct blows and transmitted forces. In addition, many orbital fractures are associated with other facial injuries, such as Le Fort II and III fractures.

A blowout fracture to the orbit can occur when an object of greater diameter than that of the bony orbital rim strikes the globe of the eye and surrounding soft tissue (Fig. 24-5). This impact pushes the globe into the orbit and in turn com-

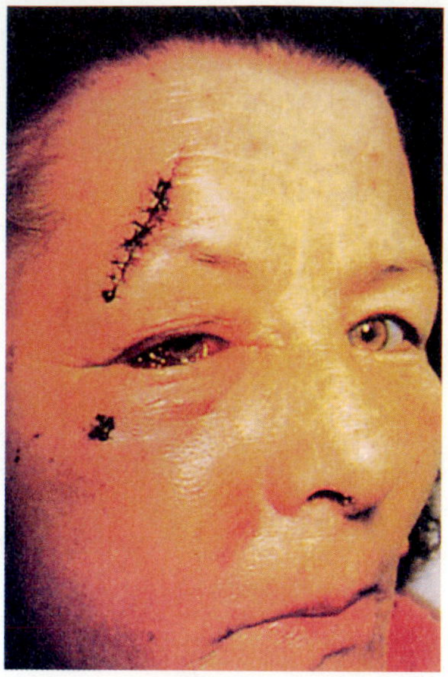

FIGURE 24-4 ■ Fracture of the zygomatic bone.

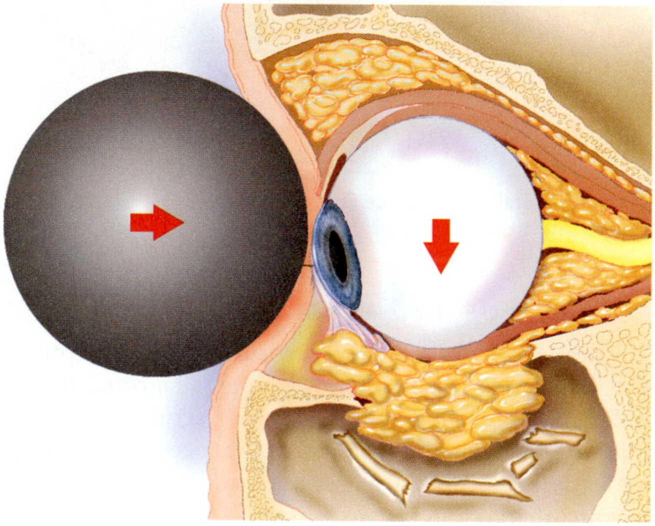

FIGURE 24-5 ■ Artist's impression of a blowout fracture caused by the impact of a ball.

presses the orbital contents. The sudden increase in intraocular pressure is transmitted to the orbital floor. The orbital floor is the weakest part of the orbital structure. If the orbital floor fractures, the orbital contents may be forced into the maxillary sinus, where soft tissue and extraocular muscles may be trapped in the defect. Signs and symptoms of blowout fractures include periorbital edema, subconjunctival ecchymosis, diplopia (double vision), enophthalmos (recessed globe), epistaxis, anesthesia in the region of the infraorbital nerve (anterior cheek), and impaired extraocular movements.

CRITICAL THINKING

How do you assess a patient's eye movement?

Orbital fractures often are associated with other fractures, including the LeFort II and III injuries and those of the zygomatic complex. In addition, injury to the orbital contents is common. The paramedic should suspect such injury with any facial fracture.

FRACTURES OF THE NOSE

Of all the facial bones the nasal bones have the least structural strength. They are fractured most frequently. The external portion of the nose, formed mostly of hyaline cartilage, is supported mainly by the nasal bones and the frontal processes of the maxillary bones. Injuries to the nose may depress the dorsum of the nose, displace it to one side, or result only in epistaxis and swelling without apparent skeletal deformity. Fractures to the orbit also may be present. In children, minimal displacement of nasal bones can result in growth changes and ultimate deformity.

Management of Facial Fractures

When caring for a patient with facial fractures, the paramedic should assume that the spine has been injured and should use spinal precautions. (Facial fractures are associated with a high percentage of related cervical spine fractures.) The paramedic should assess the patient's airway for obstruction caused by blood, vomitus, bone fragments, broken teeth, dentures, and damage to the anterior neck. Suction may be needed to clear the airway of debris and fluid. The paramedic may need to maintain the airway with an oral or nasal adjunct (in the absence of suspected midface or basal skull fracture), tracheal intubation, or cricothyrotomy if indicated.

Bleeding usually can be controlled by direct pressure and pressure bandages. Epistaxis may be severe and should be controlled by applying external pressure to the anterior nares. To prevent blood from draining down the throat, mild epistaxis is best controlled in the conscious patient by instructing the patient to sit upright or to lean forward (in the absence of spinal injury) while compressing the nares. An unconscious patient should be positioned on the side (if not contraindicated by injury). If bleeding is severe, the paramedic should evaluate the patient for hemorrhagic shock.

CRITICAL THINKING

Why would you not want the blood to drain posteriorly?

Nasal and Ear Foreign Bodies

The insertion of foreign bodies (e.g., beans and crayons) in the nose or ear is common in children. Foreign bodies may cause infection if they are not detected and removed. These patients may need to be transported for physician evaluation. The paramedic should remove a foreign body from the ear if it can be retrieved easily. As a rule, a foreign body in the nose should not be removed in the prehospital setting unless it is contributing to airway compromise or unless it can be removed easily without equipment.

EAR, EYE, AND DENTAL TRAUMA

The ears, eyes, or teeth may be injured separately or along with other forms of head trauma. Injury to these regions may be minor. Yet such injuries may result in permanent sensory function loss and disfigurement. Regardless of the severity, the paramedic should evaluate ear, eye, and dental trauma and treat it only after identifying and managing life-threatening problems.

Ear Trauma

Trauma to the ear may include lacerations and contusions, thermal injuries, chemical injuries, traumatic perforations, and barotitis.

LACERATIONS AND CONTUSIONS

Lacerations and contusions usually result from blunt trauma. They are particularly common in victims of domestic violence (Fig. 24-6). These injuries are treated by direct pressure to control bleeding. In addition, the application of ice or cold compresses decreases soft tissue swelling. If a portion of the outer ear (pinna) has been avulsed, the paramedic should retrieve the avulsed tissue if possible. The paramedic should wrap the tissue in moist gauze, seal it in plastic, place it on ice, and transport it with the patient for surgical repair. Cartilage tears often heal poorly and are easily infected.

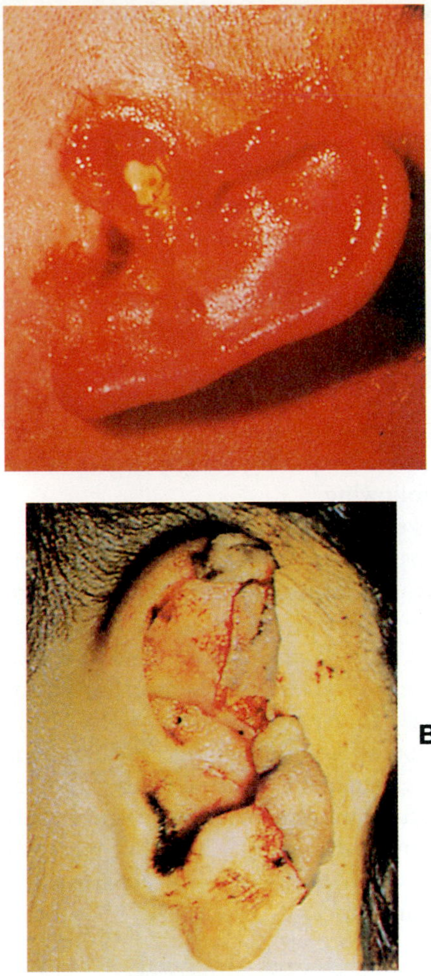

A

B

FIGURE 24-6 ■ **A,** Partially detached pinna. **B,** Loss of rim.

THERMAL INJURIES

Thermal injuries may occur from prolonged exposure to extreme cold. They also may occur from exposure of lesser duration to extreme heat. Contact with hot liquids or electrical currents also can lead to thermal injury. Prehospital treatment usually is limited to dressings to prevent contamination and transportation for evaluation by a physician.

CHEMICAL INJURIES

Strong acids or alkalis produce burns on contact. Emergency care consists of copious irrigation. After irrigation, the paramedic should bathe the ear and ear canal with saline or sterile water, allowing the irrigation liquid to remain in the ear canal for 2 to 3 minutes. The paramedic should repeat this procedure 3 or 4 times and afterward dry the ear and cover it to prevent contamination. The patient should be transported for evaluation by a physician.

TRAUMATIC PERFORATIONS

The tympanic membrane can be perforated. Perforation can occur by objects such as a cotton-tipped applicator and by changes in pressure. Pressure injuries may result from explosions (blast injuries) or scuba diving (barotrauma). These injuries usually heal spontaneously without treatment. Still, evaluation by a physician is advised.

If the injury is caused by a penetrating object, the paramedic should stabilize the object in place. The paramedic should cover the ear to prevent further contamination. The inner or middle ear canal may have been contaminated (e.g., by swimming water or a foreign object). In that case, antibiotic therapy usually is prescribed. Serious complications that may result from perforations include facial nerve palsy frequently accompanied by temporal bone fractures, hearing loss, and vertigo.

BAROTITIS

Barotitis occurs when a person is exposed to changes in barometric pressure great enough to produce inflammation and injury to the middle ear. Barotitis can result, for example, from flying at high altitudes and from scuba diving.

Gas pressure in the air-filled spaces of the middle ear normally equals that of the environment. Boyle's law (further described in Chapter 38) states that at constant temperature, the volume of gas is inversely proportional to the pressure. On ascent, gas expands. On descent, it contracts. Therefore when gases become trapped or partially trapped, they expand in direct proportion to the decrease in pressure. When trapped gas cannot reach equilibrium with environmental pressure, pain and the sensation of a blocked ear may develop. To equalize the pressure in the middle ear, the patient can be directed to bear down (Valsalva's maneuver), yawn, swallow, and move the lower jaw. These methods may cause the eustachian tube to open, which will equalize the pressure in the middle ear cavity.

Eye Trauma

More than 2000 eye and orbital injuries are estimated to occur each day in the United States.[2] Common causes of eye injury are blunt and penetrating trauma from motor vehicle crashes, sport and recreational activities, and violent altercations; chemical exposure from household and industrial accidents; foreign bodies; and animal bites and scratches.

EVALUATION

Acute eye injuries may be difficult to identify because a patient with normal vision may have a serious underlying injury. Symptoms requiring a high degree of suspicion include the following:

- Obvious trauma with eye injury
- Visual loss or blurred vision that does not improve with blinking, indicating possible damage to the globe, ocular contents, or optic nerve
- Loss of a portion of the visual field, indicating possible detachment of the retina, hemorrhage into the eye, or optic nerve injury

Evaluation of eye injury should include a thorough history and measurement of visual acuity, pupillary reaction, and extraocular movements. Assessing the patient's vision will be a rough estimation at best. The patient's vision will be reevaluated in the emergency department under controlled circumstances.

CRITICAL THINKING

Aside from trauma, what are some other causes of visual disturbances?

History. A thorough history should include the following information:

- Exact mode of injury
- Previous ocular, medical, and drug history, including cataracts, glaucoma, and presence of hepatitis or human immunodeficiency virus
- Use of eye medications
- Use of corrective glasses or contact lenses
- Presence of ocular prostheses
- Duration of symptoms and treatment interventions that may have been attempted before emergency medical services arrival

Visual Acuity. The measurement of visual acuity is usually the first step in any examination of the patient's eyes. (The exception is a chemical burn to the eye. In this case, irrigation should come before measurement of visual acuity.) To measure visual acuity, the paramedic should use a handheld visual acuity chart (e.g., Snellen chart). The paramedic also may use any printed material with small, medium, and large point sizes (e.g., an intravenous fluid bag). The paramedic should record the distance that the printed item was held from the patient's face.

The paramedic should assess the vision of each eye separately while covering the other eye. (No pressure should be applied.) The paramedic should test the injured eye first for acuity comparison to the uninjured eye. If the patient wears corrective lenses, the paramedic should measure acuity with lenses first and then without lenses. Illiterate or non-English-speaking patients require an alternative method of evaluation. Such methods may include finger counting, hand motion, and presence or absence of light perception. Abnormal responses to any of these methods indicate significant loss of vision.

CRITICAL THINKING

The assessment of visual acuity may be difficult on some calls. What factors in the prehospital setting may make it difficult?

▶NOTE The two types of vision are central and peripheral. Central vision results from images falling on the macula of the retina. Peripheral vision is the ability to see objects that reflect light waves on areas of the retina other than the macula.

PUPILLARY REACTION

Pupils should be black, round, and equal in size. The pupils also should react to light in the same way and at the same time. Both eyes should constrict in response to light and dilate in response to dark. Abnormal pupillary responses after blunt trauma to the eye are common. Abnormal responses may be caused by tearing. More commonly, though, they are caused by direct trauma to the pupillary sphincter muscle. Abnormal responses also may suggest a more serious injury involving the optic nerve or globe. Causes of pupil abnormalities in the absence of recent injury include drug use, cataracts, previous surgical procedures, ocular prosthesis, anisocoria (normal or congenital unequal pupil size), central nervous system disease, strokes, and previous injury. The paramedic should document all of the patient's pupil abnormalities.

EXTRAOCULAR MOVEMENTS

Extraocular muscles are responsible for movements of the globe, or eyeball. Voluntary muscles are innervated by cranial nerves III, IV, and VI. The muscles are attached to the outside of the eyeball and bones of the orbit and move the globe in any desired direction. Involuntary eye muscles are innervated by sympathetic nerves. These muscles are located within the eye. Examples of involuntary eye muscles are the iris and the ciliary muscle. These muscles dilate and constrict the pupil and change the shape of the lens, respectively.

To evaluate the extraocular movement of the eyes (described in Chapter 11), the paramedic should instruct the patient to visually track the movement of an object. (For example, the object may be a finger, pencil, or penlight.) The paramedic should ask the patient to track the object up, down, to the right, and to the left. Abnormalities in move-

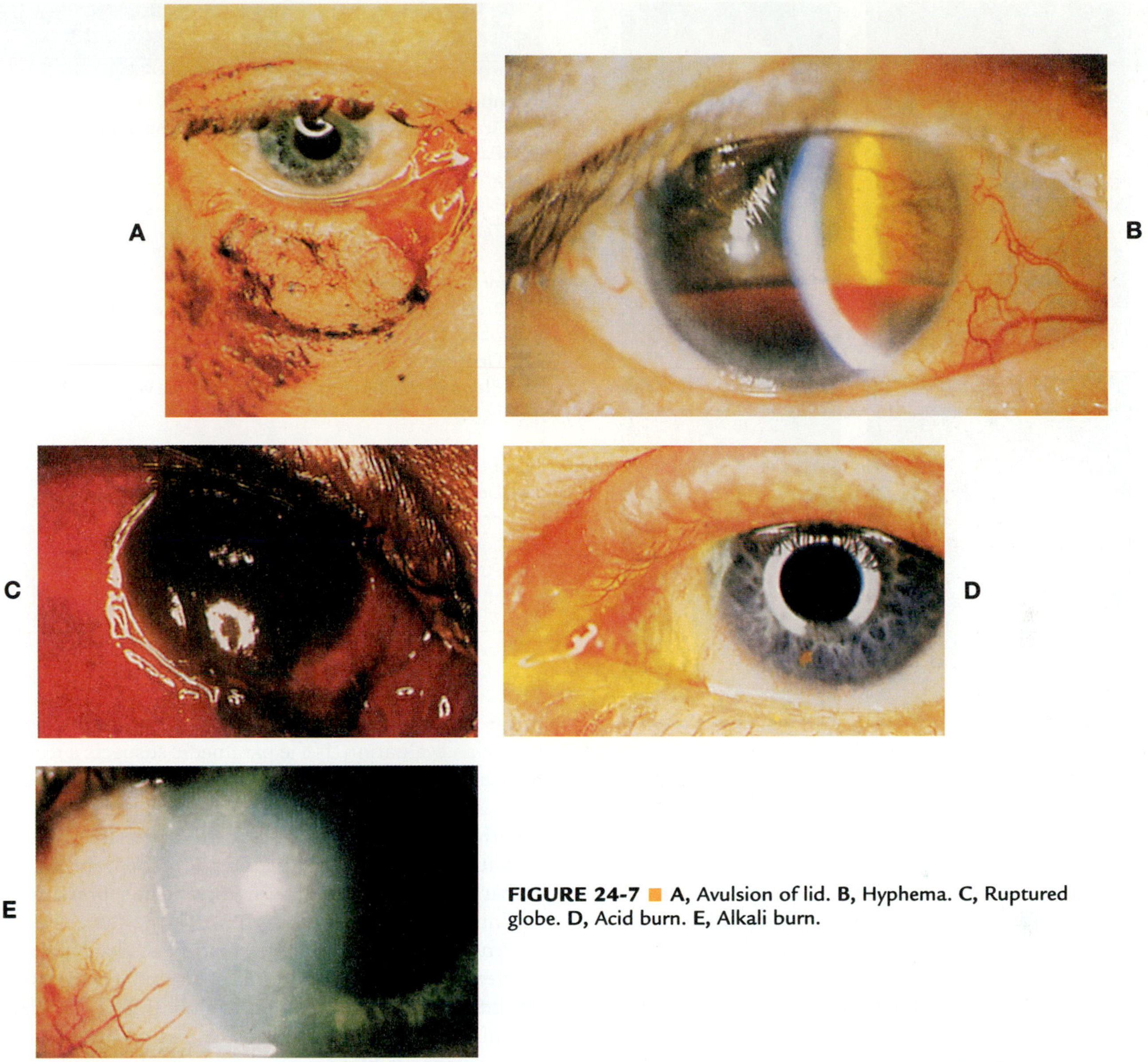

FIGURE 24-7 ■ **A,** Avulsion of lid. **B,** Hyphema. **C,** Ruptured globe. **D,** Acid burn. **E,** Alkali burn.

ment may indicate orbital content edema, cranial nerve injury, contusions or lacerations of extraocular muscles, or muscle entrapment in a fracture. Patients with limited or abnormal extraocular movements often complain of double vision in one or more directions of gaze. The paramedic should document all findings.

EVALUATION AND MANAGEMENT OF SPECIFIC EYE INJURIES

Few eye injuries are truly urgent. However, all victims of ocular trauma should be evaluated by a physician. Some patients need specialized care by an ophthalmologist. If the paramedic suspects a serious injury that may call for specialized care, the paramedic should advise medical direction as soon as possible. That way, services will be ready when the patient arrives in the emergency department (Fig. 24-7).

Foreign bodies in the cornea, conjunctiva, or eyelid usually cause the patient to complain of the sensation of something in the eye (especially when opening and closing the eyelids) and profuse tearing. If a foreign body is suspected, the paramedic should inspect the inner surface of the upper and lower lid and conjunctiva. The paramedic should remove the foreign body by gentle, copious irrigation with clear fluid. (For example, tap water, normal saline, or sterile water would work.) Medical direction may recommend that an ophthalmic anesthetic such as ***tetracaine*** be applied for patient comfort. The paramedic should advise and remind the patient not to touch or rub the eye after the administration of ***tetracaine***. Serious eye injury can result.

Corneal abrasion occurs when the outer layers of the cornea are rubbed away. The injury often results from a foreign body scratching the cornea and is common in those who wear contact lenses. Patients with a corneal abrasion

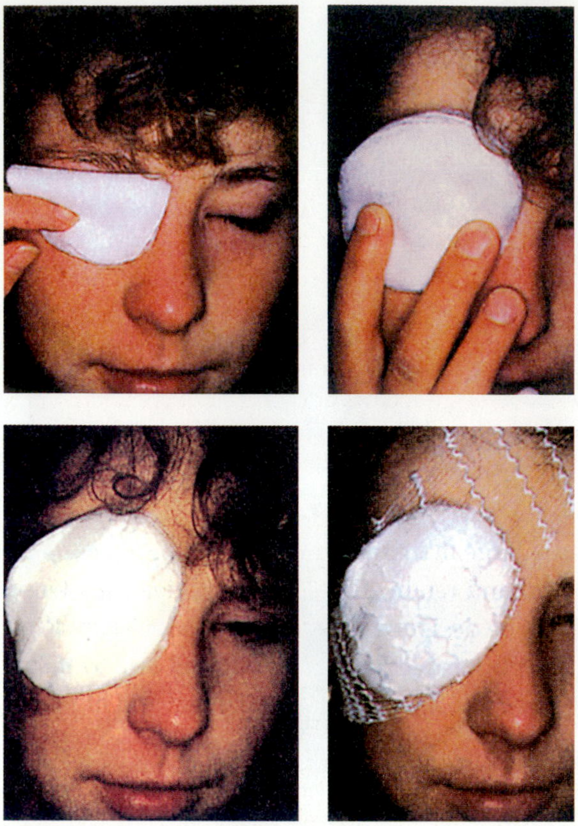

A B C D

FIGURE 24-8 ■ **A,** A folded pad is placed over the closed eye. **B,** A second unfolded pad is placed over the top of the first pad. **C,** Tape is applied along the length of the pad. **D,** The pads are secured firmly in place.

usually complain of pain and foreign body sensation under the upper eyelid, photophobia (abnormal light sensitivity), excessive tearing, and sometimes a decrease in visual acuity. Often these signs and symptoms are delayed. The prehospital management of corneal abrasion is gentle irrigation with clear fluid. Management also involves the application of a double patch to eyes to prevent the injured eye from moving when the uninjured eye moves, causing aggravation (Fig. 24-8). Corneal abrasions generally heal within 24 to 48 hours.

CRITICAL THINKING

Will the patient with a suspected corneal abrasion need to be evaluated by a physician?

Blunt trauma to the eye or its adjacent structures may result in a contusion injury, traumatic hyphema (bleeding into the anterior chamber), or globe or scleral rupture. Box 24-1 lists the signs and symptoms of these injuries.

Blunt injury to the eye may be associated with other serious injuries. Such injuries include orbital fracture, vitreous hemorrhage, and dislocation of the lens. The prehospital care should be limited to the control of any bleeding with gentle, direct pressure; protection of the eye with a metal shield or cardboard cup; and rapid transport for physician evaluation. If the paramedic suspects a traumatic hyphema or globe or scleral rupture, the patient's head and spine should be immobilized. The paramedic should elevate the head of the spine board 40 degrees to decrease intraocular pressure and instruct the patient to avoid any activity that might increase intraocular pressure (e.g., straining and coughing).

BOX 24-1 Signs and Symptoms of Eye Injuries

Contusion Injury

- Traumatic dilation or constriction of the pupil
- Pain
- Photophobia
- Blurred vision
- Tears of the iris (tear-shaped pupil)

Traumatic Hyphema

- Traumatic dilation or, less commonly, constriction of the pupil
- Decrease in visual acuity
- Blood in the anterior chamber (may be visible with penlight)

Globe or Scleral Rupture

- Decrease in visual acuity to hand movements or light perception
- Lowered intraocular pressure (soft eye)
- Pupil irregularity
- Hyphema

Penetrating injury to the eye may be associated with embedded foreign bodies, lid avulsions, and lacerations to the lids, sclera, or cornea. Penetrating globe injuries can damage retinal structures and can cause a loss of vitreous humor and subsequent blindness. The paramedic should control any bleeding by gentle, direct pressure. The globe should be protected from dehydration or contamination from foreign material. One way is to cover the orbital area with plastic or damp, sterile dressings and an eye shield.

The paramedic should stabilize foreign bodies protruding from the eye and should cover these with a cardboard cup and secure the cup with tape. The unaffected eye should also be covered to prevent consensual movement. The paramedic should not attempt to remove the object. If needed, the penetrating object may be shortened for transport (*after* consulting with medical direction.) Oxygen and intravenous fluids also may be recommended in these cases.

Chemical injury to the eye (described in Chapter 23) may be associated with loss of corneal epithelial tissue, globe perforation, and scarring and deformation of eyelids and conjunctiva. These injuries are true emergencies. They require immediate intervention. A chemical exposure generally mandates extensive, continuous irrigation of both eyes

BOX 24-2 Removal of Contact Lenses

Removal of Hard and Rigid Gas-Permeable Lenses

1. With gloved hands, separate the eyelids so that the margins of the lids are beyond the top and bottom edges of the lens.
2. Gently pass the eyelids down and forward to the edges of the lens.
3. Move the eyelids toward each other, forcing the lens to slide out between them.
4. Store the lens in a container with water or saline, and label the container with the patient's name. If a contact lens container is not available, store each lens in a separate container and label as left or right.
5. If lens removal is difficult, gently move the lens downward from the cornea to the conjunctiva overlying the sclera until arrival in the emergency department.

Note: Special suction cups are also available for the removal of hard and rigid contact lenses. This device should be moistened with saline or sterile water before contacting the lens.

Removal of Soft Lenses

1. With gloved hands, pull down the lower eyelid.
2. Gently slide the soft lens down onto the conjunctiva.
3. Using a pinching motion, compress the lens between the thumb and index finger.
4. Remove the lens from the eye.
5. Store the lens in a container (marked right or left) with water or saline, and label the container with the patient's name.

with a neutral fluid for 20 minutes before patient transport (if effective irrigation can be performed) and while en route to the emergency department.

CRITICAL THINKING

Should you wait until contacting medical direction before you begin irrigation of the eye?

CONTACT LENSES

Contact lenses are of three general types: hard, soft hydrophilic, and rigid gas-permeable. Hard lenses are microlenses that sometimes are prescribed for astigmatism (these lenses rarely are used today). Soft (hydrophilic) lenses usually are large in diameter (extending onto the conjunctiva). Soft lenses may be designed for daily or extended wear. Rigid gas-permeable lenses are similar in size to microlenses. These lenses have a low water content and high oxygen permeability.

As a rule, paramedics should not attempt to remove contact lenses in patients with eye injuries. To do so may cause more damage and may aggravate the injury. If management of an eye injury is complicated by the presence of contact lenses (e.g., chemical burns to the eyes), medical direction may recommend that the lenses be removed. If the patient is unable to remove the lenses, the paramedic may be instructed to do so (Box 24-2).

Dental Trauma

The adult normally has 32 teeth. Each tooth consists of two sections: the crown, which projects above the gingiva (the portion of the oral mucosa surrounding the tooth), and the root, which fits into the bony socket (alveolus) of the maxilla or mandible. Three layers make up the hard tissues of the teeth: the enamel, the dentin (ivory), and the cementum. The soft tissues of the teeth include the pulp and the periodontal membrane (Fig. 24-9).

The teeth and associated alveolar process may be injured alone or along with fractures of the jaw or facial bones. The two most common types of dental trauma involve fractures and avulsions of the anterior teeth. If a tooth is fractured, the paramedic should search the oral cavity carefully for tooth fragments. Removal of fragments reduces the risk of aspiration and obstruction of the airway. Lacerations and avulsions to the tongue and surrounding mucous membranes often occur with dental trauma. These injuries often are painful and may bleed profusely. They may compromise the patient's airway as well.

Tooth avulsions are common, and many teeth can be saved with proper emergency treatment.[3] Permanent teeth that have been avulsed have a good survival rate if reimplanted and stabilized within 1 hour. (Deciduous teeth, or milk teeth, generally are not reimplanted. They may become fused to the bone, delaying formation and eruption of the permanent tooth.) If the avulsed tooth has been out of the patient's mouth for less than 15 minutes, medical direction may recommend reimplanting the tooth into the original socket. The paramedic should take care not to reimplant the tooth backward and also should be alert for possible aspiration. If reimplantation is impossible, the paramedic should follow the guidelines established by the American Dental Association and the American Association of Endodontists:

1. Never place an avulsed tooth in anything that can dry or crush the outside of the tooth.
2. Do not handle the tooth roughly. Do not rinse it off or rub, scrape, or disinfect the outside of the tooth in any way. (Any adherent membrane or fibrous tissue should be left in place to avoid stripping off the periodontal membrane and ligament, which are critical to the survival of a reimplanted tooth.)
3. Place the tooth in a nurturing, break-resistant storage device (e.g., Emergency Tooth Preserving System). This device should have a tightly fitted top and soft inner walls.
4. Store the tooth in a pH-balanced, isotonic, glucose-, calcium-, and magnesium-enriched cell-preserving fluid (e.g., Hank's solution). Use refrigerated fresh whole milk as the best alternative storage medium. (Powdered milk is not suitable.) For short periods (1 hour or less), use sterile saline. Do not use tap water because it damages the periodontal ligament.
5. Advise medical direction of avulsed teeth so that appropriate services will be available when the patient arrives in the emergency department.

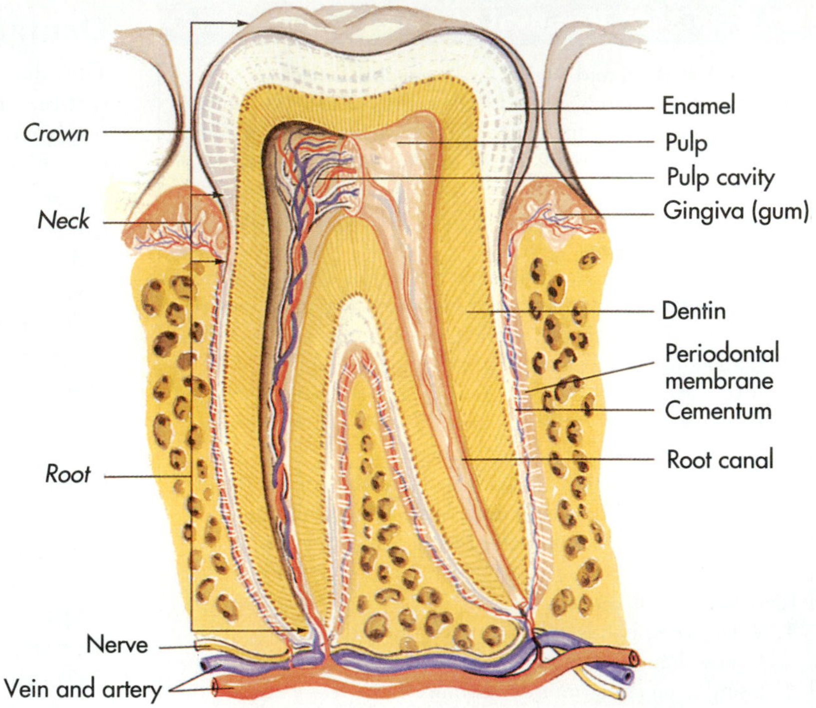

FIGURE 24-9 ■ Longitudinal section of a tooth.

ANTERIOR NECK TRAUMA

Anterior neck injuries are caused by blunt and penetrating trauma (Fig. 24-10). These injuries may result in damage to the skeletal structures, vascular structures, nerves, muscles, and glands of the neck. Common mechanisms of injury to the anterior neck are as follows:

- Strangulation injuries from clothing, jewelry, or personal equipment getting caught in machinery
- All-terrain vehicles and other small motor vehicles (clothesline injuries to the neck from running into wires, ropes, or fences)
- Blows to the neck
- Contact sports (boxing, karate, basketball, football, hockey)
- Hangings
- Horseback riding
- Hyperextension and hyperflexion injuries
- Industrial injuries
- Missile injury from firearms
- Motor vehicle crashes
- Neck striking dashboard or steering column
- Snow skiing
- Sport and recreational activities
- Stab wounds (knives, screwdrivers, ice picks)
- Violent altercations
- Water sports (jet skiing, water skiing)

With blunt and penetrating neck injuries, the paramedic should assume the patient has a cervical spine injury also. The paramedic must assume such injury until ruled out by clinical examination and x-ray films (radiography) of the cervical region of the neck. X-ray examination alone does not rule out cervical spine injury (see Chapter 25).

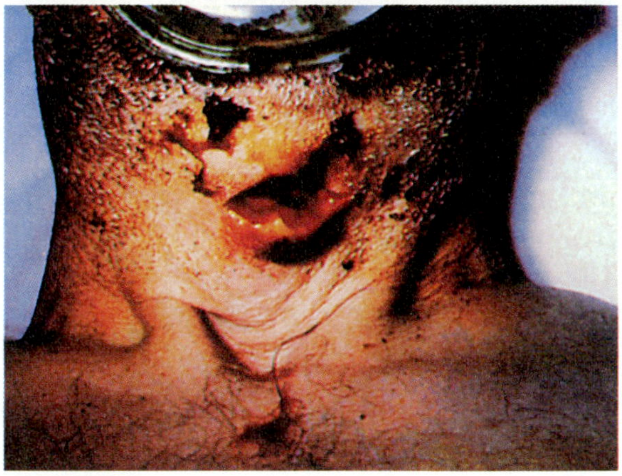

FIGURE 24-10 ■ A self-inflicted stab wound that had entered the pharynx.

Evaluation

For purposes of evaluating the trauma patient, the neck can be divided into three zones defined by horizontal planes (Fig. 24-11).[1] Zone I represents the base of the neck. This zone extends from the sternal notch to the top of the clavicles or the cricoid cartilage. Injuries to this zone have the highest mortality rate because of the risk of injury to major vascular and thoracic structures (subclavian vessels and jugular veins, lungs, esophagus, trachea, cervical spine, cervical nerve roots).

Zone II extends from the clavicles or cricoid cartilage cephalad to the angle of the mandible. The carotid artery, jugular vein, trachea, larynx, esophagus, and cervical spine are the vital structures in this zone. Because of the

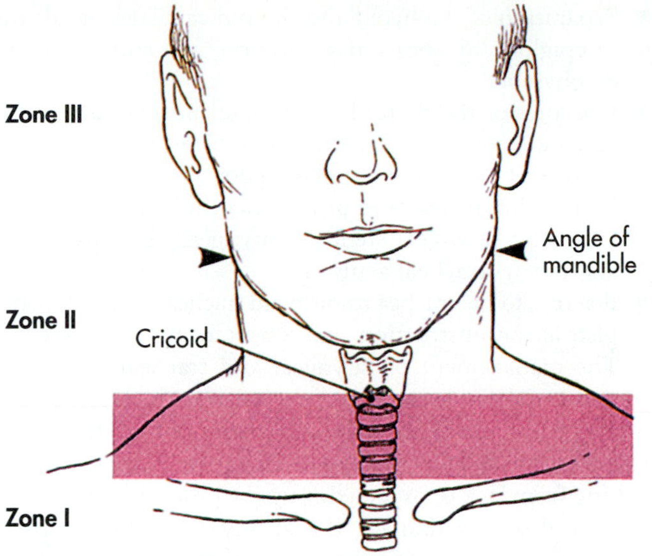

FIGURE 24-11 ■ Zones of the neck. The junction of zone I and zone II is described variously as the cricoid cartilage or top of the clavicles.

relative size of zone II, injuries to this zone are the most common. However, they have a lower mortality rate than zone I injuries.

Zone III is the part of the neck above the angle of the mandible. The risk of injury to the distal carotid artery, salivary glands, and pharynx is greatest in this zone.

Soft Tissue Injuries

Soft tissue injuries to the neck from blunt trauma often produce hematomata and associated edema or direct laryngeal or tracheal injury. Both of these can result in airway compromise. Penetrating trauma may produce lacerations and puncture wounds with resultant vascular, laryngotracheal, or esophageal injury. Blunt trauma may cause vascular injuries as well. However, this is uncommon. As with all trauma victims, initial evaluation and resuscitation must begin with rapid assessment, control of the airway, and consideration for spinal injury.

> **CRITICAL THINKING**
> Is prehospital airway control always possible in patients with anterior neck injuries?

HEMATOMATA AND EDEMA

Edema of the pharynx, larynx, trachea, epiglottis, and vocal cords may produce enough pressure in the neck tissues to obstruct the airway completely. If the airway is compromised (evidenced by dyspnea, inspiratory stridor, cyanosis, or changes in voice quality), the paramedic should consider oral or nasal intubation with spinal precautions. Intubation stabilizes damaged areas of the neck, protects the airway, and provides a means for ventilatory support. (A slightly smaller endotracheal tube may be needed to ensure passage through the airway.)

> **NOTE** Crushed or severed airways can be blocked totally or partially by attempts at oral or nasal intubation. In these cases (if the patient is moving air), rapid transport with high-concentration oxygen is perhaps the most prudent course.

When direct intubation is impossible because of blood, vomitus (that cannot be removed by suction), or progressive edema, a cricothyrotomy or translaryngeal cannula ventilation (described in Chapter 19) may be indicated. Another measure that may help in treating edematous airways includes the administration of cool, humidified oxygen. Yet another measure is the slight elevation of the patient's head. (This can be done if it is not contraindicated by the injury.)

LACERATIONS AND PUNCTURE WOUNDS

Lacerations and puncture wounds may be superficial or deep. Superficial wounds usually can be managed by covering the wound. The covering helps to prevent further contamination. Deep wounds are associated with more serious injuries to underlying structures. These injuries may require aggressive airway therapy and ventilatory support, suction, hemorrhage control by direct pressure, and fluid replacement. Signs and symptoms of significant penetrating neck trauma include the following:

- Active bleeding
- Dysphagia
- Dyspnea
- Hematemesis
- Hemoptysis
- Hoarseness
- Large or expanding hematoma
- Mobility and crepitus
- Neurological deficit (stroke, brachial plexus injury, spinal cord injury)
- Pulse deficit
- Shock
- Stridor
- Subcutaneous emphysema
- Tenderness to palpation

> **CRITICAL THINKING**
> Why is rapid transport crucial when caring for a patient who has anterior neck injuries?

VASCULAR INJURY

Blood vessels are the most commonly injured structures in the neck; they may be injured by blunt or penetrating trauma. Vessels at risk of injury include the carotid, vertebral, subclavian, innominate, and internal mammary arteries and the jugular and subclavian veins. Laceration of these major vessels can result in rapid exsanguination (death from extensive blood loss) if bleeding is not controlled.

Securing the airway (with spinal precautions) and providing adequate ventilatory support is the first priority. The next priority is to control hemorrhage. This can be achieved with constant, direct pressure. The paramedic should apply pressure only to the affected vessels. Thus blood flow to the brain will not be obstructed completely. If bleeding cannot be controlled in this manner, medical direction may advise applying direct pressure with a gloved finger to the vessel.

> **NOTE** Under no circumstances should cervical vessels be clamped with hemostats in the prehospital setting. Doing so may traumatize critical vascular structures and may produce permanent nerve injury.

If the paramedic suspects a venous injury, the patient should be kept supine or in a slight Trendelenburg position. This will help to prevent air embolism (a rare but lethal complication). If the paramedic suspects an air embolism (described in Chapter 18), the paramedic should turn the immobilized patient on the left side. The patient's head should be lower than the feet in an attempt to trap the air embolus in the right ventricle.

Fluid replacement for hypovolemia should be guided by medical direction. Fluid replacement may include using large-bore catheters and isotonic crystalloid (lactated Ringer's solution or normal saline). If penetrating injury to the base of the neck (zone I) has occurred, upper extremity venous drainage may be compromised by the laceration. In this event, placement of at least one intravenous line in a lower extremity should be considered. Medical direction may advise that a second intravenous line be placed in the upper extremity on the side opposite the injury.

> **CRITICAL THINKING**
> Why might application of pneumatic antishock garment be harmful with this type of injury?

LARYNGEAL OR TRACHEAL INJURY

Injury from blunt or penetrating trauma to the anterior neck may cause fracture or dislocation of the laryngeal and tracheal cartilages, hemorrhage, or swelling of the air passages. All of these injuries can compromise the airway and cause respiratory distress. Airway injury can lead to death in head and neck trauma patients. Thus rapid and judicious control of the airway and prevention of aspiration are crucial. In addition, a high degree of suspicion for associated vascular disruption and esophageal, chest, and intraabdominal injury is a critical aspect of preventing death. Injuries that may be associated with laryngeal and tracheal trauma include the following:

- Fracture of the hyoid bone resulting in laceration and distortion of the epiglottis
- Separation of the hyoid and thyroid cartilages resulting in epiglottis dislocation, aspiration, and subcutaneous emphysema
- Fractures of the thyroid cartilage resulting in epiglottis and vocal cord avulsion, arytenoid dislocation, and aspiration of blood and bone fragments
- Dislocation or fracture of the cricothyroid resulting in long-term laryngeal stenosis, laryngeal nerve paralysis, and laryngotracheal avulsion
- Fracture to the trachea resulting in tracheal avulsion, complete airway obstruction, and subcutaneous emphysema

The management of laryngeal and tracheal trauma is controversial. Some medical direction agencies recommend oral or nasal intubation. Other agencies hold that intubation attempts may contribute to the potential for injury resulting from lack of oxygen during the procedure. These attempts also may damage the airway structures further. Alternative methods of airway management include use of bag-valve-mask ventilation, cricothyrotomy, and translaryngeal cannula ventilation.

> **NOTE** Airway procedures that involve entry through the neck generally are avoided in the field because of the associated risks. As a rule, these patients should be well ventilated with a bag-valve-mask device. They should be transported rapidly to the receiving facility for surgical tracheotomy as well. As described in Chapter 19, translaryngeal cannula ventilation is hazardous in the presence of complete airway obstruction. Incorrectly used, this technique does not provide adequate exhalation of gases and air. The technique may result in carbon dioxide retention and significant injury from high pressure developing in the chest and airways (barotrauma).

If penetrating trauma causes complete disruption of the laryngotracheal structure, medical direction may recommend dissection through the wound. That way, the exposed distal trachea can be cannulated directly with a cuffed endotracheal tube. Regardless of the method chosen, emergency care is directed at securing the airway with spinal precautions, providing adequate ventilatory support, controlling hemorrhage, treating for shock, and providing rapid transport to an appropriate medical facility for definitive surgical care.

ESOPHAGEAL INJURY

Esophageal injuries should be suspected in patients with trauma to the neck or chest. Specific injuries that require a high degree of suspicion for associated esophageal injury include tracheal fractures, penetrating trauma from stab or gunshot wounds, and ingestion of caustic substances.

Esophageal injury is difficult to diagnose. It may be overlooked as the paramedic focuses on more obvious injuries that pose a threat to life. Signs and symptoms may include subcutaneous emphysema, neck hematoma, and bleeding from the mouth and nose.

Esophageal perforation is associated with a high mortality rate. Death results from mediastinitis caused by the release of gastric contents into the thoracic cavity. If not contraindicated by mechanism of injury, the paramedic should place the patient with a suspected esophageal tear in a semi-Fowler position. (This is an inclined position. The upper half of the body is raised by elevating the head or stretcher about 30 degrees.) This position will help to prevent reflux of gastric contents.

CRITICAL THINKING

Are these signs and symptoms so unique that you will be able to distinguish esophageal injury as the cause, versus other kinds of traumatic conditions?

HEAD TRAUMA

The anatomical components of the skull are the scalp, followed by the cranial vault, under which are the dural membrane, the arachnoid membrane, the pia, and the brain substance. Injuries to the skull may be classified as soft tissue injuries to the scalp and skull fractures.

NOTE All patients with head or neck trauma must be assumed to have a spinal injury. This must be the case until injury is ruled out by clinical examination and x-ray films in the emergency department. (Spinal precautions [including helmet removal] are presented in Chapter 25.) This text assumes that spinal precautions will be used for all patients with a significant mechanism of injury.

Soft Tissue Injuries to the Scalp

The most common scalp injury is an irregular linear laceration. Like the face, the scalp is very vascular. Thus scalp lacerations may bleed heavily (Fig. 24-12). They also may result in hypovolemia, particularly in infants and children. Other, less frequent scalp injuries include stellate wounds, avulsions, and subgaleal hematomata.

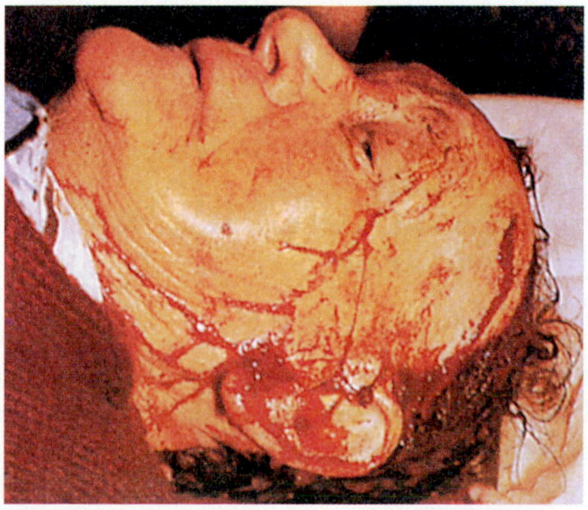

FIGURE 24-12 ■ Even small wounds from the scalp can bleed profusely.

Management of soft tissue injuries to the scalp includes efforts to prevent contamination of open wounds, use of direct pressure or pressure dressings to decrease blood loss, and fluid replacement if needed. The potential for underlying skull fracture and brain and spinal trauma also exists with these injuries. Scalp lacerations that are the only injury rarely produce life-threatening complications. However, such lacerations can result in excessive blood loss. If not contraindicated by injury, the paramedic should position all patients with head or facial trauma on a stretcher or spine board with the head elevated 30 degrees (semi-Fowler position).

Skull Fractures

Skull fractures may be classified as *linear fractures, basilar fractures, depressed fractures,* and *open vault fractures* (Fig. 24-13). Complications associated with these injuries are cranial nerve injury, vascular involvement (e.g., meningeal artery and dural sinuses), infection, underlying brain injury, and dural defects caused by depressed bone fragments. As with all injuries to the head, the paramedic should consider the possibility of a spinal injury. Proper spinal precautions should be maintained.

LINEAR FRACTURES

Linear fractures (seen as straight lines on x-ray film) account for 80% of all fractures to the skull.[4] Such fractures usually are not depressed. Often linear fractures occur without an overlying scalp laceration. As an isolated injury, these fractures usually have a low rate of complication. But if the fracture is associated with scalp laceration, infection is possible. Linear fractures that cross the meningeal groove in the temporal-parietal area, midline, or occipital area may lead to epidural bleeding from the middle cerebral artery.

CRITICAL THINKING

Will you be able to detect linear skull fractures during a physical examination in the prehospital setting?

BASILAR SKULL FRACTURES

Basilar skull fractures usually are associated with major impact trauma. These injuries may occur when the mandibular condyles perforate into the base of the skull. More commonly, though, they result from an extension of a linear fracture into the floor of the anterior and middle fossae. Basilar skull fractures can be difficult to see on x-ray films. They usually are diagnosed clinically by the following signs and symptoms:

- Ecchymosis over the mastoid process resulting from fracture to the temporal bone **(Battle's sign)** (Fig. 24-14, *A*)
- Ecchymosis of one or both orbits caused by fracture of the base of the sphenoid sinus **(raccoon's eyes)** (Fig. 24-14, *B*)
- Blood behind the tympanic membrane caused by fractures of the temporal bone (hemotympanum)
- Cerebrospinal fluid leakage, which can result in bacterial meningitis

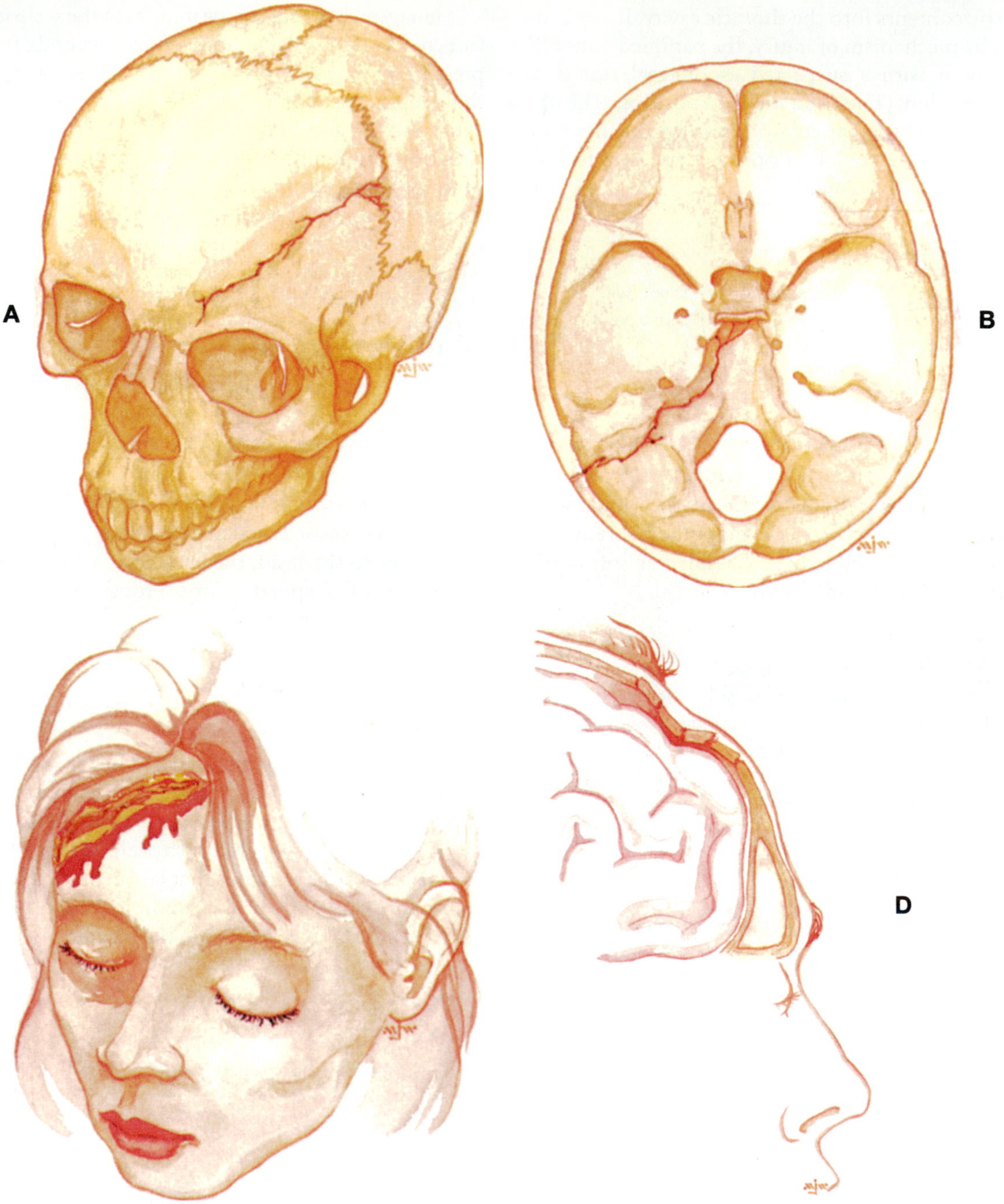

FIGURE 24-13 ■ Skull fractures. **A,** Linear skull fracture. **B,** Basilar skull fracture. **C,** Open vault fracture. **D,** Depressed skull fracture.

> **NOTE** Battle's sign and raccoon's eyes usually do not occur until some time after the injury. If they are present on the arrival of emergency medical services, the bruising is most likely the result of a prior injury.

Other complications associated with basilar skull fractures include cranial nerve injuries and massive hemorrhage from vascular involvement of the carotid artery. Treatment for basilar skull fractures includes bed rest, in-hospital observation, and evaluation for hearing loss caused by acoustic nerve injury.

DEPRESSED SKULL FRACTURES

Depressed skull fractures usually result from a relatively small object striking the head at high speed. Thus they commonly are associated with scalp lacerations (Fig. 24-15). The frontal and parietal bones most often are affected by these fractures. Thirty percent of patients with depressed skull fractures are estimated to have associated hematomata and

A

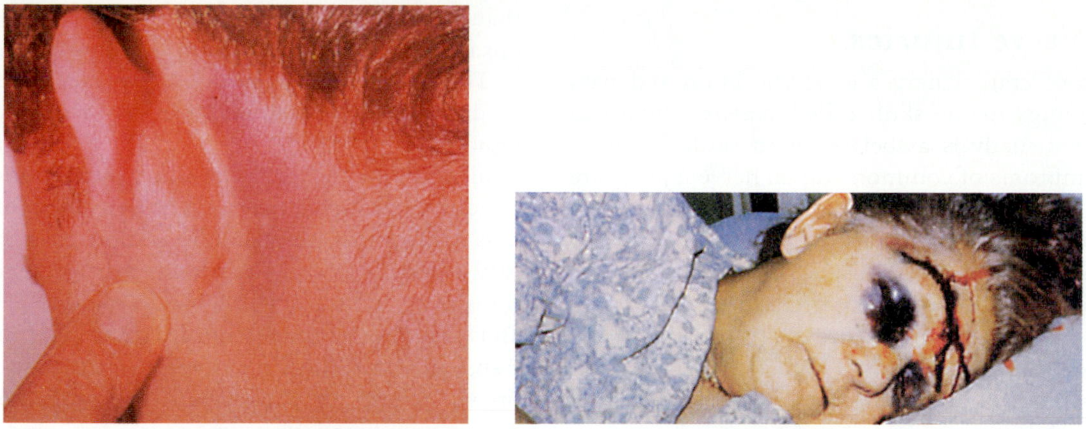

B

FIGURE 24-14 ■ A, Battle's sign. B, Raccoon's eyes.

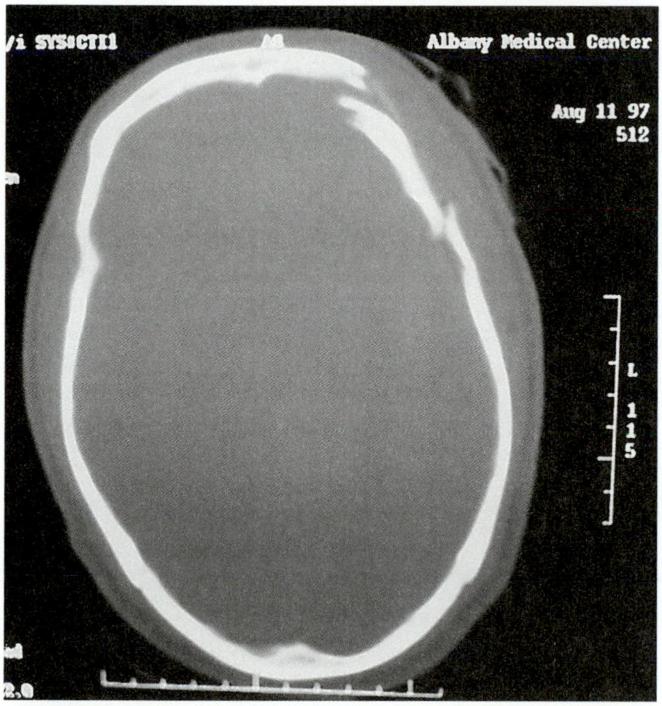

FIGURE 24-15 ■ Head computed tomography scan showing a depressed skull fracture.

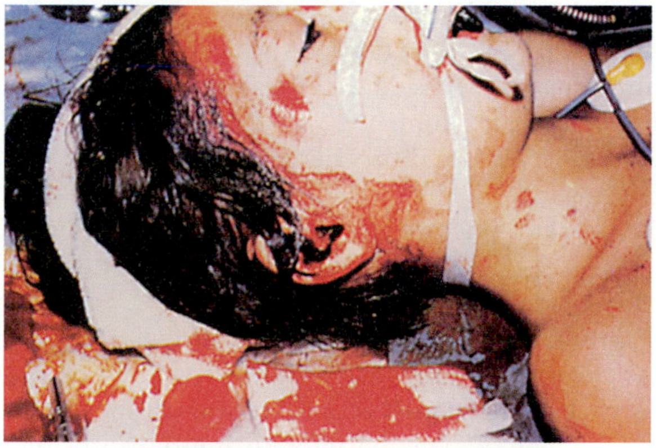

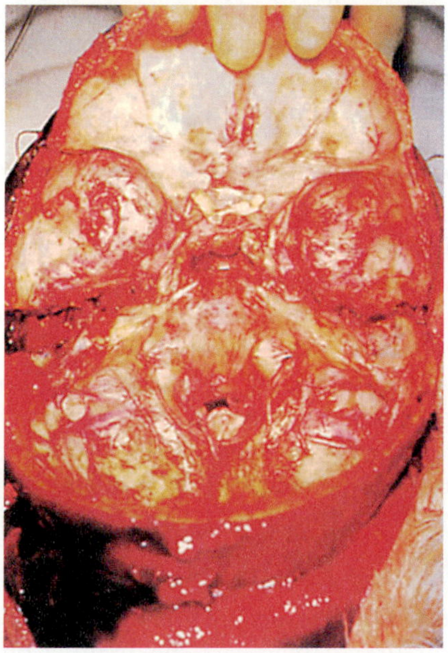

FIGURE 24-16 ■ Severe fracture of the base of the skull.

cerebral contusions.[4] If the depression is greater than the thickness of the skull, dural laceration also is likely. Patients with depressed skull fractures often require surgical removal of the bone fragments (craniectomy).

OPEN VAULT FRACTURES

Open vault fractures result when an opening exists between a scalp laceration and brain tissue (Fig. 24-16). Because of the nature of these injuries and the force required to produce them, they often are associated with multiple trauma to other systems. They have a high mortality rate. Exposure of brain tissue to the external environment may lead to infection (meningitis). Open vault fractures require surgical repair. Prehospital management usually is limited to spinal immobilization, ventilatory support, efforts to prevent contamination, and rapid transportation to an appropriate medical facility.

Cranial Nerve Injuries

Twelve pairs of cranial nerves leave the brain and pass through openings in the skull called *foramina.* Injury to cranial nerves usually is associated with skull fractures. Signs and symptoms of common cranial nerve injuries are as follows:

Cranial nerve I (olfactory nerve)
- Loss of smell
- Impairment of taste (dependent on food aroma)
- Hallmark of basilar skull fracture

Cranial nerve II (optic nerve)
- Blindness in one or both eyes
- Visual field defects

Cranial nerve III (oculomotor nerve)
- Ipsilateral (same side), dilated, fixed pupil
- Especially compression by the temporal lobe
- Mimicking of direct ocular trauma

Cranial nerve VII (facial nerve)
- Immediate or delayed facial paralysis
- Basilar skull fracture

Cranial nerve VIII (auditory nerve)
- Deafness
- Basilar skull fracture

BRAIN TRAUMA

A *brain injury* is defined by the National Head Injury Foundation as "a traumatic insult to the brain capable of producing physical, intellectual, emotional, social, and vocational change."[4] Traumatic brain injury can be divided into two categories. The first is *primary brain injury.* The second is *secondary brain injury.* Primary brain injury refers to direct trauma to the brain and to the associated vascular injuries that occurred from the initial injury. Secondary brain injury results from intracellular and extracellular derangements that probably were initiated at the time of the injury. These derangements may include hypoxia, hypocapnia, and hypercapnia from airway compromise, aspiration of gastric contents, and thoracic injury; anemia and hypotension from external and internal hemorrhage; and hyperglycemia or hypoglycemia that can injure ischemic brain tissue further. The adverse effects of secondary brain injury can be minimized. They perhaps can be reversed, if they are recognized and properly managed in the prehospital setting. Brain injuries can be classified as mild and moderate diffuse injury, diffuse axonal injury, and focal injury.[5]

Mild Diffuse Injury (Concussion)

Concussion is a fully reversible brain injury. It does not result in structural damage to the brain. Concussion is caused by a mild to moderate impact to the skull, movement of the brain within the cranial vault, or both. Concussion occurs when the function of the brainstem (particularly the reticular activating system) or both cerebral cortices is disturbed temporarily. This results in a brief altered level of consciousness. (This is usually less than 5 minutes.) If the patient has been unconscious for more than 5 minutes, the paramedic should suspect a more serious injury caused by contusion or hemorrhage.

The loss of consciousness usually is followed by periods of drowsiness, restlessness, and confusion, with a fairly rapid return to normal behavior. The patient may have no recall of the events before the injury **(retrograde amnesia).** In addition, amnesia may exist after recovery of consciousness **(antegrade amnesia).** This short-term memory loss may produce anxiety. The patient may ask repetitive questions (e.g., "Where am I? What happened?"). Other signs and symptoms of concussion are vomiting; combativeness; transient visual disturbances (e.g., light flashes and wavy lines); defects in equilibrium and coordination; and changes in blood pressure, pulse rate, and respiration (rare). After physician evaluation, treatment usually consists of in-hospital or home observation by a reliable observer for 24 to 48 hours.

CRITICAL THINKING

Consider the patient with a new onset of retrograde or antegrade amnesia. Why should the patient not be considered a reliable historian?

A concussion injury affects the patient most severely at the time of impact but is followed by improvement. Concussion is the most common type of brain injury. It also is the least serious. *Any patient whose condition worsens over time or whose level of consciousness deteriorates rather than improves must be suspected of having a more serious injury.* Therefore documentation of baseline measurements of level of consciousness, memory status, and neurological function (e.g., Glasgow Coma Scale or AVPU [alert, verbal, painful, unresponsive] scale) in any victim of head injury is important.

Moderate Diffuse Injury

Moderate injuries are those that result in minute petechial bruising of brain tissue. The involvement of the brainstem and reticular activating system leads to unconsciousness. These injuries account for 20% of all severe head injuries and 45% of all cases of diffuse injury.[4] Often these patients will have basilar skull fracture. Most patients will survive the injury. Yet permanent neurological impairment is common.

A patient with moderate diffuse injury initially will be unconscious, followed by persistent confusion, disorientation, and amnesia of the event. During recovery, these patients often experience an inability to concentrate, frequent periods of anxiety, uncharacteristic mood swings, and sensorimotor deficits (e.g., an altered sense of smell). Patients with moderate diffuse injury are managed as are those with concussion; frequent reassessments of the level of consciousness and assurance of an adequate airway and tidal volume are necessary. If possible, patients with head injury should be moved to a quiet, calm area. Exposure to bright lights should be avoided. (Patients often are photophobic.) Also, constant reorientation of the patient may be necessary.

Diffuse Axonal Injury

Diffuse axonal injury (DAI) is the severest form of brain injury. It results from brain movement within the skull from acceleration or deceleration forces. These forces cause shearing, stretching, or tearing of nerve fibers with subsequent axonal (nerve cell) damage. Diffuse axonal injury may be classified as mild, moderate, or severe. Mild DAI is associated with coma of 6 to 24 hours and has a mortality rate of 16%.[4] Moderate DAI is more common and is distinguished by coma lasting more than 24 hours and abnormal posturing (described later). The associated mortality rate of moderate DAI approaches 24%.[6]

CRITICAL THINKING

Can a patient with a diffuse axonal injury die as a result of that injury?

Severe DAI was once known as a *brainstem injury*. Severe DAI involves severe mechanical shearing of many axons in both cerebral hemispheres extending to the brainstem. Severe DAI occurs in 16% of all severe head injuries and in 36% of all cases of DAI.[4] These patients often are unconscious for prolonged periods. They may exhibit abnormal posturing and other signs of increased intracranial pressure (ICP). The prehospital care for these patients is focused on ensuring an adequate airway and tidal volume. Hypoxia must be prevented in all patients with head injury. (This helps to avoid secondary injury to brain tissue.)

Focal Injury

Focal injuries are specific, grossly observable brain lesions. Included in this category are lesions that result from skull fracture (previously described), contusion, edema with associated increased ICP, ischemia, and hemorrhage.

The brain occupies 80% of the intracranial space. The brain is divided into four areas: the brainstem (consisting of the medulla, pons, and midbrain), the diencephalon (including the thalamus and hypothalamus), the cerebrum, and the cerebellum. The intracranial contents consist of brain water (58%), brain solids (25%), cerebrospinal fluid (7%), and intracranial blood (10%).

CEREBRAL CONTUSION

A cerebral contusion is bruising of the brain in the area of the cortex or deeper within the frontal (most common), temporal, or occipital lobes (Fig. 24-17). This bruising produces a structural change in the brain tissue. Bruising results in greater neurological deficits and abnormalities than are seen with concussions. These abnormalities may include seizures, hemiparesis, aphasia, and personality changes. If the brainstem also is contused, the patient may lose consciousness. In some cases, the comatose state may be prolonged. It may last hours to days or longer. Of the patients who die from head injury, 75% have cerebral contusions at autopsy.[4]

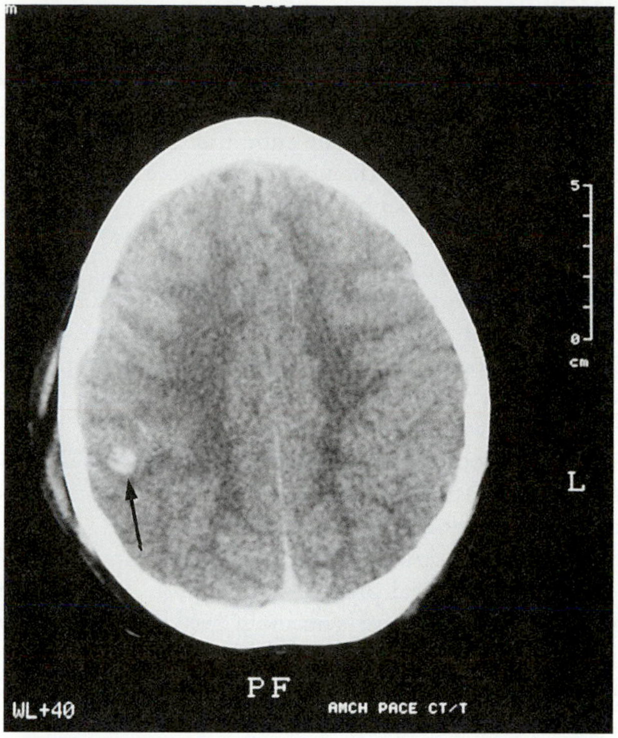

FIGURE 24-17 ■ Head CT scan demonstrating a cerebral contusion.

If applied force is enough to cause the brain to be displaced against the irregular surfaces of the skull, tiny blood vessels in the pia mater may rupture. The brain substance may be damaged locally at the site of impact *(coup)*. Or the brain may be damaged on the opposite, or contralateral, side *(contrecoup)*. Contrecoup injuries often are caused by deceleration of the head. This may occur, for example, in a fall or motor vehicle crash.

As a rule, cerebral contusions usually heal without intervention. As with patients with concussion, these patients usually improve. However, the time to heal and level of improvement differ in these two conditions. The most important complication associated with cerebral contusion is increased ICP manifested by headache, nausea, vomiting, seizures, and a declining level of consciousness. These signs usually are delayed responses to the injury. Therefore they usually are not seen in the prehospital emergency setting.

EDEMA

Major injuries to the brain often result in swelling of the brain tissue with or without associated hemorrhage. The swelling results from humoral and metabolic responses to injury. Swelling leads to considerable increases in ICP. This in turn can lead to decreased cerebral perfusion (described later) or herniation.

ISCHEMIA

Ischemia can result from vascular injuries, secondary vascular spasm, or increased ICP. In any case, focal or more global infarcts can result.

HEMORRHAGE

The same forces that result in concussion and contusion also may cause serious vascular damage. This damage may result in hemorrhage into or around brain tissue. These injuries may cause epidural or subdural hematomata. The hematomata compress the underlying brain tissue, or produce intraparenchymal hemorrhage (bleeding directly into the brain tissue). This bleeding often results from cerebral contusions and skull fractures.

Cerebral Blood Flow. Although the brain accounts for only 2% of adult weight, 20% of total body oxygen use and 25% of total body glucose use are devoted to brain metabolism.[4] Oxygen and glucose delivery are controlled by cerebral blood flow.

Cerebral blood flow is a function of **cerebral perfusion pressure** (CPP) and resistance of the cerebral vascular bed. Cerebral blood flow is the difference between the **mean arterial pressure** (MAP) and the ICP (CPP = MAP − ICP). Normal mean arterial pressure ranges from 85 to 95 mm Hg. Intracranial pressure is normally less than 70 to 80 mm Hg. Thus normal CPP is between 70 and 80 mm Hg. (Cerebral perfusion pressure of 60 mm Hg is the critical minimum threshold.) As ICP approaches mean arterial pressure, the gradient for flow decreases and cerebral blood flow decreases. That is, when ICP increases, CPP decreases. As CPP decreases, vessels in the brain dilate (cerebral vasodilation). This results in increased cerebral blood volume (increasing ICP) and further cerebral vasodilation. In most emergency medical services systems, CPP is not calculated because mean arterial pressure and ICP are not measured in the prehospital setting. However, maintaining a systolic blood pressure of at least 90 mm Hg also may help maintain adequate mean arterial pressure.[7]

> **CRITICAL THINKING**
> What happens to the flow of oxygen to the brain, and carbon dioxide from the brain to the capillaries, when intracranial pressure is increasing and cerebral perfusion pressure is decreasing?

Vascular tone in the normal brain is regulated by carbon dioxide pressure (P_{CO_2}), oxygen pressure (P_{O_2}), and autonomic and neurohumoral control; P_{CO_2} has the greatest effect on intracerebral vascular diameter and subsequent resistance. For example, if P_{CO_2} is increased from 40 to 80 mm Hg, cerebral blood flow is doubled. This results in increased brain blood volume and ICP.

Intracranial Pressure. The normal range of ICP is 0 to 15 mm Hg. When ICP rises above this level, the body has difficulty maintaining adequate CPP, usually because of an expanding mass or diffuse swelling. Cerebral blood flow is diminished when the CPP is not adequate. As the cranial vault continues to fill (because of brain edema or expanding hematoma), the body tries to compensate for the decline in CPP by a rise in mean arterial pressure (Cushing reflex). Yet this increase in cerebral blood flow further elevates the ICP. As pressure continues to increase, cerebrospinal fluid is displaced to make up for the expansion. If unresolved, the brain substance may herniate over the edge of the tentorium. (This is one of three extensions of the dura mater that separates the cerebellum from the occipital lobe of the cerebrum.) Or it may herniate through the foramen magnum (Fig. 24-18).

Early signs and symptoms of increased ICP include headache, nausea and vomiting, and altered level of consciousness (Box 24-3). These signs and symptoms eventually are followed by increased systolic pressure, widened pulse pressure, and a decrease in the pulse and irregular respiratory pattern **(Cushing's triad).** As the volume continues to expand in the cranial vault, herniation of the temporal lobe of the brain through the tentorium may occur. The herniation causes compression of cranial nerve III. This produces a dilated pupil and loss of the light reflex on the side of compression. The patient rapidly becomes unresponsive to verbal and painful stimuli. The patient may exhibit the ominous signs of **decorticate posturing.** (This is characterized by extension of the legs and flexion of the arms at the elbows.) Or the patient may exhibit **decerebrate posturing.** (This is characterized by extension of all four extremities [Fig. 24-19].)

> **CRITICAL THINKING**
> Why is cranial nerve III affected by this shift in brain tissue?

Respiratory Patterns. As ICP continues to rise, abnormal respiratory patterns (described in Chapter 19) may develop. Respiratory abnormalities associated with increased ICP and significant brainstem injury include hypoventilation, Cheyne-Stokes breathing (which may accompany decorticate posturing), central neurogenic hyperventilation (which may accompany decerebrate posturing), and ataxic breathing. The clinical significance of decorticate (flexion) and decerebrate (extension) posturing and respiratory patterns are not of major clinical importance other than to identify the need for intervention and treatment (intubation and consideration of immediate neurosurgical intervention).

> **▶NOTE** Some motion of the limbs, albeit abnormal, is better than no motion of the limbs. (No motion indicates a worse level of neurological function.)

TYPES OF BRAIN HEMORRHAGE

Traditionally, brain hemorrhages are classified according to their location as epidural, subdural, subarachnoid, or cerebral (intraparenchymal) (Fig. 24-20).

Epidural Hematoma. An epidural hematoma (accounting for 0.5% to 1% of all head injuries[4]) is a collection of blood between the cranium and the dura in the epidural space (Fig. 24-21). The hematoma usually is a rapidly de-

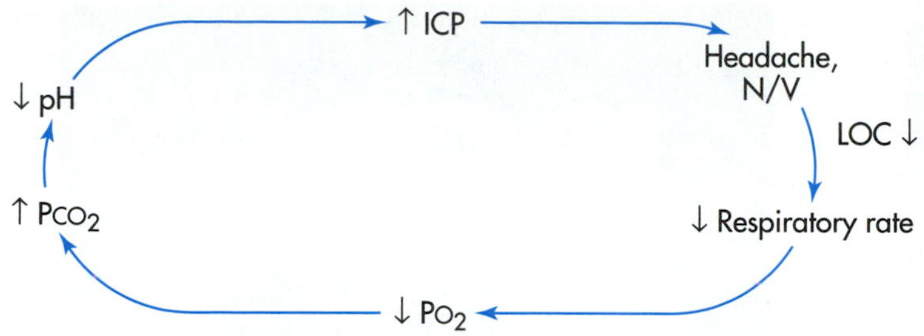

FIGURE 24-18 ■ Effects of increased intracranial pressure.

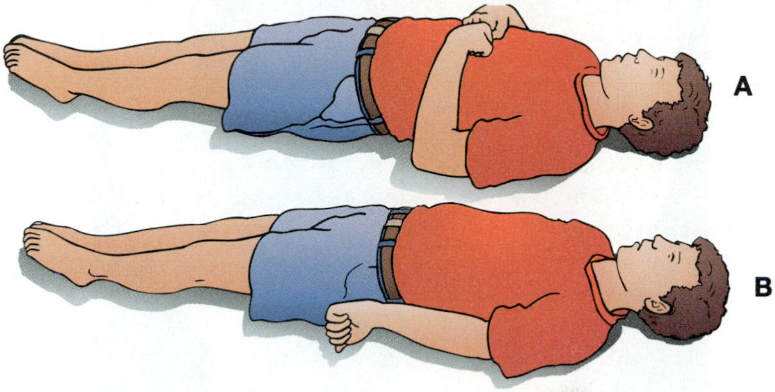

FIGURE 24-19 ■ **A,** Abnormal flexion (decorticate posturing). **B,** Abnormal extension (decerebrate posturing).

BOX 24-3 Levels of Increasing Intracranial Pressure

Cerebral Cortex and Upper Brainstem

Blood pressure rises; pulse rate slows.
Pupils remain reactive.
Cheyne-Stokes respirations may be present.
Patient initially will try to localize and remove painful stimuli (eventually withdraws and flexion occurs).
All effects are reversible at this stage.

Middle Brainstem

Wide pulse pressure and bradycardia are present.
Pupils become nonreactive or sluggish.
Central neurogenic hyperventilation develops.
Abnormal posturing (extension) occurs.
Few patients function normally with injury at this level.

Lower Portion of Brainstem/Medulla

Pupil is "blown" (fixed and dilated) on same side of injury.
Respirations become ataxic.
Patient will be flaccid.
Pulse rate is irregular.
QRS, S-T, and T wave changes will be present.
Blood pressure will fluctuate.
These patients generally do not survive.

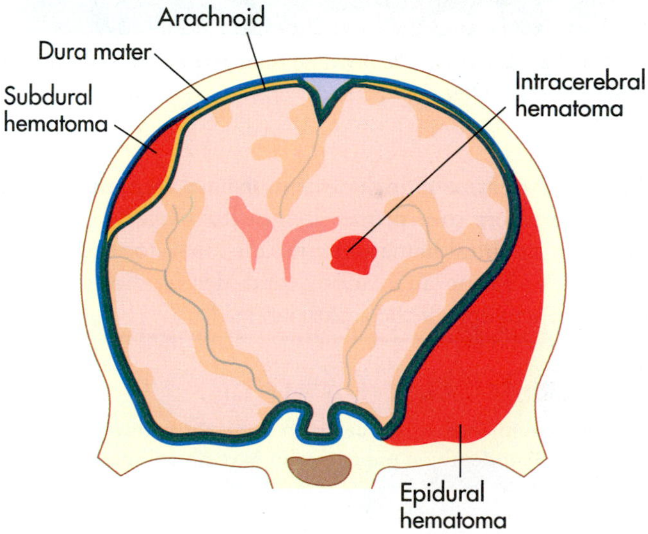

FIGURE 24-20 ■ Varieties of intracranial hemorrhage.

veloping lesion. Usually the hematoma is associated with a laceration or tear of the middle meningeal artery. This hemorrhage often occurs as a result of a linear or depressed skull fracture in the temporal bone. Yet bleeding from other sites can produce epidural hemorrhage as well. If the source of hemorrhage is mostly venous, deterioration usually is not as rapid because low-pressure vessels bleed more slowly.

Fifty percent of patients with epidural hematoma have a transient loss of consciousness, followed by a lucid interval in which neurological status returns to normal. (The remaining 50% of patients with acute epidural hematoma never recover consciousness.) The lucid interval usually lasts between 6 and 18 hours. During this time the hematoma enlarges. As ICP rises, the patient develops a headache with lethargy, decreasing level of consciousness, and contralateral hemiparesis. In the early stages of an epidural hematoma, the patient may complain only of headache and drowsiness.

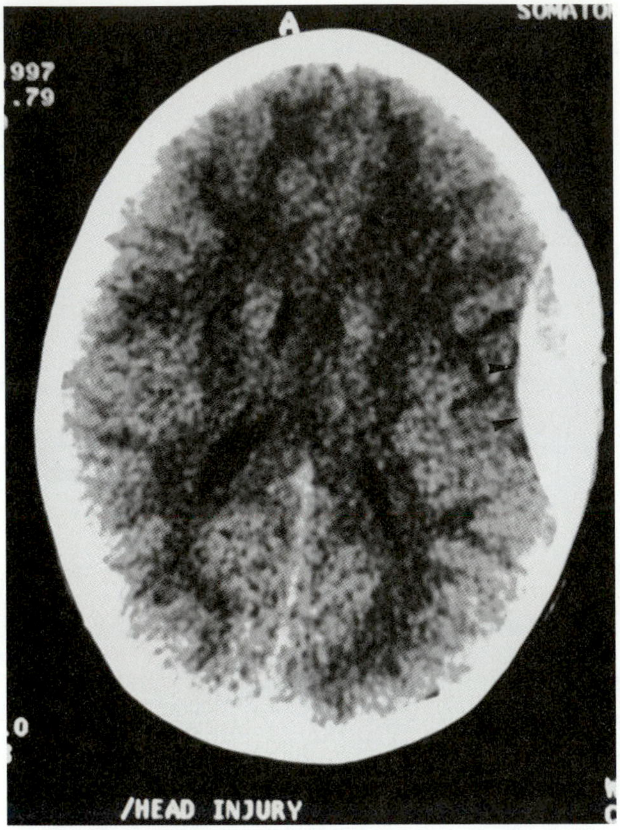

FIGURE 24-21 ■ Head computed tomography scan showing an epidural hematoma.

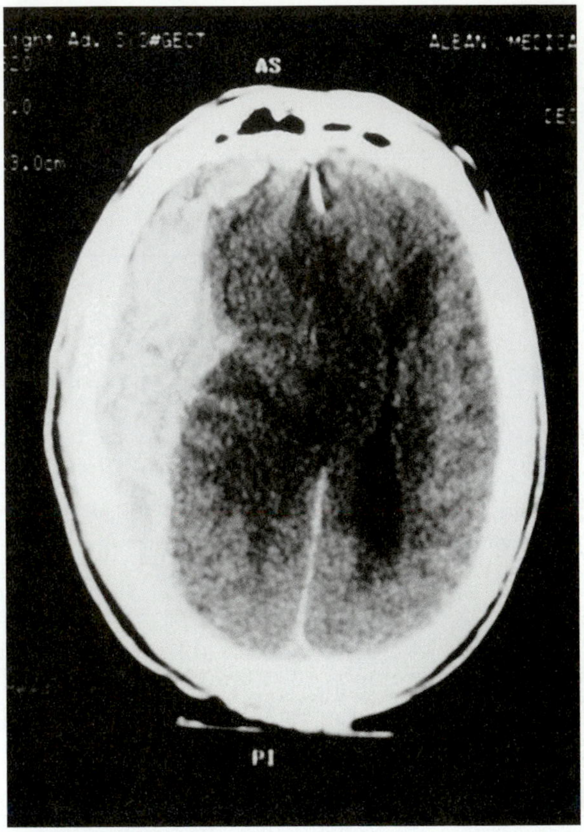

FIGURE 24-22 ■ Head computed tomography scan showing an acute subdural hematoma.

Definitive treatment includes immediate recognition and rapid transport to a proper facility for surgery. Common causes of epidural hematoma include low-velocity blows to the head, violent altercations, and deceleration injuries. About 15% to 20% of these patients die.[4]

CRITICAL THINKING

What could account for delays in surgical treatment, causing subsequent death, in patients who have an epidural hematoma?

Subdural Hematoma. A subdural hematoma is a collection of blood between the dura and the surface of the brain in the subdural space (Fig. 24-22). This injury usually results from bleeding of the veins that bridge the subdural space. Associated contusion or laceration of the brain often is present. The hematoma often results from blunt head trauma. Commonly the hematoma is associated with skull fracture. Subdural hematomata are classified as *acute* (50% to 80% mortality rate), *subacute* (25% mortality rate), and *chronic* (20% mortality rate).[4] Classification depends on the time lapse between the injury and development of symptoms. As a general rule, if symptoms occur within 24 hours, the hematoma is considered acute; between 2 and 10 days, subacute; and after 2 weeks, chronic. Subdural hematomata are more common than epidural hematomata.

Signs and symptoms of subdural hematoma are similar to those of epidural hematoma and include headache, nausea and vomiting, decreasing level of consciousness, coma, abnormal posturing, paralysis, and in infants, bulging fontanelles. These findings may be subtle because of the slow development of the hematoma in the subacute and chronic phases. Definitive care consists of surgery to remove the blood from the hematoma. Individuals at increased risk of developing subdural hematoma include older adults and patients with clotting deficiencies (e.g., alcoholics, hemophiliacs, and persons who take anticoagulants) and patients with cortical atrophy (older adults, alcoholics).

Subarachnoid Hematoma. A **subarachnoid hematoma** refers to intracranial bleeding into the cerebrospinal fluid. This results in bloody cerebrospinal fluid and meningeal irritation (Fig. 24-23). Bleeding that results from trauma, rupture of an aneurysm, or arteriovenous anomaly may extend into the brain if the force of the bleeding from the broken vessel is sudden and severe. Patients with this injury often complain of a sudden and severe headache. The headache initially may be localized. Then the headache spreads (from meningeal irritation) and becomes dull and throbbing. Other characteristics of a subarachnoid hemorrhage include dizziness, neck stiffness, unequal pupils, vomiting, seizures, and loss of consciousness. Severe hemorrhage may result in coma and death. Permanent brain damage is common in those who survive.

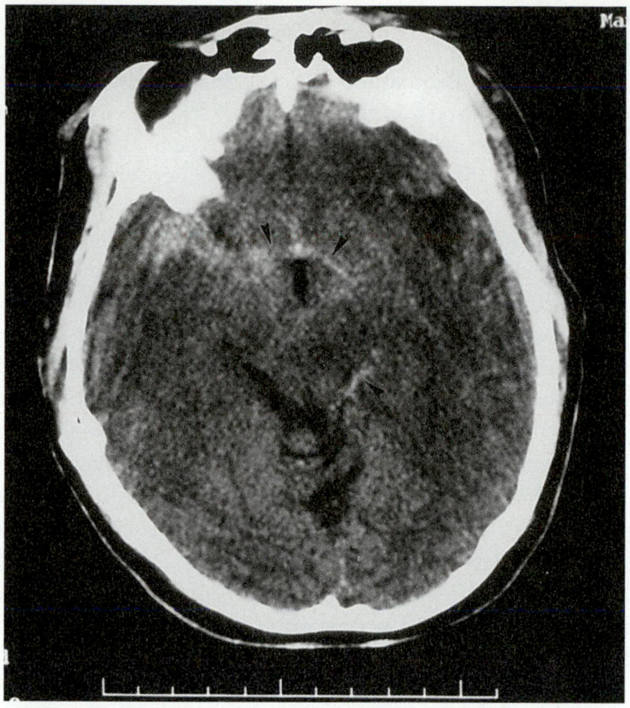

FIGURE 24-23 ■ Head computed tomography scan showing a traumatic subarachnoid hemorrhage.

> **CRITICAL THINKING**
> What causes the vomiting, seizures, and loss of consciousness in a patient with subarachnoid hemorrhage?

Cerebral Hematoma. An **intracerebral hematoma** may be defined as a collection of more than 5 mL of blood somewhere within the substance of the brain, most commonly in the frontal or temporal lobe.[4] This injury can result from multiple lacerations produced by penetrating head trauma (gunshot wound). The injury also may result from a high-velocity deceleration injury (automobile crash) in which vessels are torn as the brain moves across rough surfaces of the skull. Increased ICP can produce an intracerebral hematoma as the result of the brain being compressed.

Cerebral hematoma often is associated with subdural hemorrhage and skull fracture. Signs and symptoms may be immediate or delayed. This depends on the size and location of the hemorrhage. Once symptoms appear, the patient usually deteriorates rapidly. The mortality rate after surgical evacuation of the hematoma (if possible) is more than 40%.[4]

PENETRATING INJURY

Penetrating injuries to the brain usually are caused by missiles fired from handguns and stab wounds caused by sharp objects. Such objects include knives, scissors, screwdrivers, and nails. Less often, penetrating trauma may result from falls and high-velocity vehicle crashes. Associated injuries include skull fracture; damage to cerebral arteries, veins, or venous sinuses; and intracranial hemorrhage. Complications include infection and posttraumatic epilepsy. Definitive care for these injuries requires neurosurgical intervention.

ASSESSMENT AND NEUROLOGICAL EVALUATION

Prehospital management of the patient with a head injury is determined by a number of factors, including the mechanism and severity of injury and the patient's level of consciousness. Associated injuries affect the priorities of emergency care.

Airway and Ventilation. The initial step in treating all patients with head trauma is to ensure an open airway with spinal precautions. The next step is to provide adequate ventilation with high-concentration oxygen. Airway management may include oral or nasal adjuncts, multilumen devices, or nasal or tracheal intubation to maintain and protect the airway. Tracheal intubation and ventilatory support usually are recommended in all patients with head injuries who have a Glasgow Coma Scale (GCS) score of 8 or less[4] (described later in the chapter).

> **CRITICAL THINKING**
> Imagine what a patient with a Glasgow Coma Scale score of 8 or lower would look like. Why should these patients be intubated? What if the Glasgow Coma Scale score improves rapidly?

Patients with head injuries are likely to vomit. If the patient has a decreased level of consciousness after the airway is secured, a nasogastric tube should be inserted to empty the stomach. In the presence of facial fractures, rhinorrhea (cerebrospinal fluid discharge from the nose), or otorrhea (cerebrospinal fluid discharge from the ear), an orogastric tube rather than a nasogastric tube should be inserted. Use of this tube helps to avoid possible intubation of the cranial cavity through the fracture site. In addition, the patient should be well stabilized on a long spine board for safe repositioning. Suction equipment with large-bore suction catheters should be available as well.

Ventilatory support should be focused on maintaining adequate oxygenation and optimizing cerebral perfusion. Capnography and pulse oximetry should be used to maintain oxygen saturation at a level of 95% or greater. Aggressive hyperventilation reduces carbon dioxide; it can lead to secondary brain injury through cerebral vasoconstriction and a decrease in cerebral blood flow. (Routine prophylactic hyperventilation should be avoided.) Thus in the absence of capnography to guide ventilatory support, normal ventilations should be provided at 10 breaths/min for adults; 20 breaths/min for children; and 25 breaths/min for infants. With evidence of herniation (Box 24-4), the patient should be hyperventilated at the following rates: 20 breaths/min for adults; 30 breaths/min for children; and 35 breaths/min for infants. These rates should yield a Pco_2 of about 35 mm Hg.[7]

Circulation. After the airway has been secured (maintaining spinal protection), support of the patient's cardiovascular function becomes the next priority. The paramedic

BOX 24-4 Indicators of Herniation for Hyperventilation

An unresponsive patient with the following:

Bilateral, dilated, unresponsive pupils *or* asymmetric pupils (>1 mm)

and

Abnormal extension (decerebrate) posturing *or* no motor response to painful stimuli

BOX 24-5 Systolic Blood Pressure Thresholds Defining Hypotension in Head-Injured Patients

<65 mm Hg in patients from birth to 1 year of age
<75 mm Hg in patients 2 to 5 years of age
<80 mm Hg in patients 6 to 12 years
<90 mm Hg in patients 13 years or older

Source: Brain Trauma Foundation.

should control major external bleeding and should assess the patient's vital signs. Assessment establishes a baseline for future evaluations. A cardiac monitor will detect changes in rhythm (particularly bradycardia and tachycardia) that can occur with increasing ICP and brainstem injury. The blood pressure of every patient should be maintained at normal levels with fluid replacement (per medical direction). A single episode of hypotension doubles mortality and increases morbidity in the patient with traumatic brain injury.[7] Therefore the paramedic should administer intravenous fluids to support oxygen delivery and to avoid hypertension or limit hypotension to the shortest duration possible. Systolic blood pressure thresholds that can be used to define hypotension in head-injured patients are listed in Box 24-5.

Persistent hypotension from an isolated head injury is a rare and terminal event. The exception is head injury in infants and small children. *Closed head injury in the adult does not produce hypovolemic shock.* Thus a patient with head injuries who also is hypotensive should be evaluated for other injuries that could cause hemorrhage. The paramedic also should evaluate the patient for the possibility of neurogenic shock from spinal cord trauma. Infusion of isotonic fluids (lactated Ringer's solution or normal saline) may be indicated for hemorrhagic shock. However, these fluids probably should be used cautiously in patients with hypotension caused by neurogenic shock. In the latter patient group, vasopressors also may be helpful in maintaining blood pressure. Neurogenic shock may be distinguished from hemorrhagic shock by the following:

- A relatively bradycardic response (e.g., a pulse of 80 with a blood pressure of 80 mm Hg)
- Skin that often is warm and dry (not cool and clammy)
- No evidence of significant blood loss or hypovolemia
- Paralysis and loss of spinal reflexes

Neurological Examination. Conscious patients should be interviewed to determine their memory status before and after the injury and to learn of significant medical history (e.g., heart disease, hypertension, diabetes, epilepsy, medication use, alcohol or other drug use, and allergies). The history also should include the mechanism of injury and the events that led up to the injury. (For example, the history may detail a loss of consciousness before or after the injury incident.)

The paramedic should evaluate the motor skills of conscious patients. Evaluation determines the patient's ability to follow commands and helps the paramedic to note any paralysis. (Hemiparesis or hemiplegia, especially with a sensory deficit on the same side, indicates brain damage rather than spinal trauma.) If the patient is unconscious on emergency medical services arrival, the paramedic should interview bystanders about the history of the event. The paramedic also should ask bystanders about the length of time the patient has been unconscious. The most important indicator of increasing ICP is deterioration in the patient's sensorium. Thus the paramedic should evaluate the level of consciousness using the GCS every 5 minutes. A decrease of 2 points with a GCS score of 9 or lower is significant; it indicates significant injury.[7]

CRITICAL THINKING

How reliable will the patient be regarding the duration of his or her loss of consciousness?

After the patient has been resuscitated and stabilized, the paramedic should assess the patient's pupils for symmetry, size, and reactivity to light. Abnormal pupillary responses may indicate an increase in ICP and cranial nerve involvement. *Asymmetric pupils* differ more than 1 mm in size. *Dilated pupils* are greater than or equal to 4 mm in adults. A *fixed pupil* shows less than 1 mm change in response to bright light. (The paramedic should evalute pupil size every 5 minutes.) Alcohol and some other drugs can cause abnormal pupillary reactions, but the reactions commonly are bilateral (except for certain eye drops, if placed in one eye). If the patient is conscious, the paramedic also should evaluate extraocular movement. (See Chapter 11.)

NOTE The initial pupil evaluation and the Glasgow Coma Scale establish the baseline against which all subsequent neurological evaluations are compared.[7]

Fluid Therapy. In the absence of hypotension, fluid therapy normally should be restricted in a patient with head injury to minimize cerebral edema. If the patient is hemodynamically stable, the paramedic should establish an intravenous line of crystalloid fluid to keep the vein open. If significant hypovolemia is present from another injury, the paramedic should give the patient an isotonic fluid bolus. (This should be guided by medical direction.) The patient also should be transported rapidly to a proper facility. In this case, the injury causing hypovolemia usually is more immediately life threatening than the head injury. As a rule, hypotension in the presence of head injury initially should be managed with fluid boluses to maintain a systolic blood pressure of 90 to 100 mm Hg in the adult male less than 40 years of age.[4]

Drug Therapy. Prehospital use of drugs for the treatment of head injuries is controversial. Drugs that may be prescribed by medical direction to decrease cerebral edema or circulating blood volume may include ***mannitol*** and hypertonic saline. (Both are controversial.) Medical direction may require the insertion of an indwelling urinary catheter for careful monitoring of urine output before starting diuretic therapy. Hypotension leading to hypoperfusion may occur as a complication of diuretic use in patients with head injuries.

▶NOTE The administration of glucose (dextrose 50%) is contraindicated in patients with head injuries unless hypoglycemia is confirmed. Intravenously administered dextrose 50% may worsen cerebral damage.

Anticonvulsant agents such as ***lorazepam*** and ***diazepam*** are used to control seizure activity in head-injured patients. As a rule, these drugs are not used in the initial management of head injuries because of their sedating effects. Some medical direction agencies may prescribe these agents to protect against seizures. Prevention of seizures avoids the rise in ICP that often accompanies sudden seizure activity. Intravenously administered ***lidocaine*** has been shown to control increases in ICP that normally occur during endotracheal intubation.[4]

In addition, the use of sedatives and paralytics for some patients with head injuries may be indicated for airway management. These drugs also may be used to aid in the transport of combative patients (especially in aeromedical transport). The paramedic should follow local protocol. The paramedic also should consult with medical direction regarding the use of these drugs.

INJURY RATING SYSTEMS

Several injury rating systems are used to triage, guide patient care, predict patient outcome, identify changes in patient status, and evaluate trauma care in epidemiological studies and quality assurance reviews. (These also are known as *indexes* or *scales*.) These indexes are important to prehospital personnel. They aid in determining patient care needs with reference to hospital resources. Rating systems commonly used in emergency care include the Glasgow Coma Scale, trauma score, Revised Trauma Score, and pediatric trauma score.

Glasgow Coma Scale

The GCS evaluates eye opening, verbal and motor responses, and brainstem reflex function. The scale is considered one of the best indicators of eventual clinical outcome[4] and should be part of any neurological examination for patients with head injury (Table 24-1). A GCS score of 9 to 13 indicates moderate traumatic brain injury; a GCS score of 8 or less indicates a severe traumatic brain injury. (Note: The lowest possible score is 3; the highest possible score is 15.) Hypoxemia and hypotension have been shown to affect GCS scoring negatively. Thus GCS should be measured after the initial assessment. The score should be measured after a clear airway is established. Also, the GCS should be measured after necessary ventilation and circulatory resuscitation have been performed. Unresponsive patients with a GCS score of 3 to 8 should be transported to a trauma center with traumatic brain injury capabilities.[7]

TABLE 24-1 Glasgow Coma Scale

CRITERIA	POINTS ASSIGNED TO SCORE
Eye Opening	
Spontaneous eye opening	4
Eye opening on command	3
Eye opening to painful stimulus	2
No eye opening	1
Best Verbal Response	
Answers appropriately (oriented)	5*
Gives confused answers	4
Inappropriate response	3
Makes unintelligible noises	2
Makes no verbal response	1
Best Motor Response	
Follows commands	6
Localizes painful stimuli	5
Withdraws from pain	4
Responds with abnormal flexion to painful stimuli (decorticate)	3
Responds with abnormal extension to painful stimuli (decerebrate)	2
Gives no motor response	1
Total	—

From National Association of Emergency Medical Technicians: *PHTLS basic and advanced prehospital trauma life support,* St Louis, 2003, Mosby.
*It generally is agreed that a full verbal score of 5 should be assigned to a child less than 2 years of age who cries after stimulation.
Example: A head-injured patient with an eye opening response to pain would be assigned a 2 (E2); with no verbal response would be assigned a 1 (V1); with decerebrate posturing would be assigned a 2 (M2). The Glasgow Coma Scale score for this patient would be 5.

Trauma Score/Revised Trauma Score

The trauma score was developed in 1980 to predict outcome for patients with blunt or penetrating injuries. This score has limited use in the prehospital setting. The trauma score does not predict adequately the mortality for isolated, severe head injury.

The Revised Trauma Score was published in 1989. The Revised Trauma Score uses the GCS with measurements for systolic blood pressure and respiratory rate that are divided into five intervals. A range of values for these physiological measurements is assigned a number between 0 and 4. These numbers then are added to give a total between 0

TABLE 24-2 Revised Trauma Score

VARIABLE	SCORE (POINTS)	START OF TRANSPORT	END OF TRANSPORT
A. Ventilatory Rate			
10-29/min	4		
>29/min	3		
6-9/min	2		
1-5/min	1		
0	0		
B. Systolic Blood Pressure			
>89 mm Hg	4		
76-89 mm Hg	3		
50-75 mm Hg	2		
1-49 mm Hg	1		
No pulse	0		
C. Glasgow Coma Scale Score			
13-15	4		
9-12	3		
6-8	2		
4-5	1		
<4	0		
Trauma score total + A + B + C			

Adapted from Champion HR et al: A revision of the trauma score, *J Trauma* 29(5):624, 1989.
Example: At the start of transport, a head-injured patient has spontaneous ventilations at 30 breaths/min (score of 3); a systolic pressure of 80 mm Hg (score of 3); and a Glasgow Coma Scale score of 12 (score of 3); providing a Revised Trauma Score of 9. At end of transport, the patient has spontaneous ventilations of 18 breaths/min (score of 4); a systolic pressure of 62 (score of 2); and a Glasgow Coma Scale score of 7 (score of 2), providing a Revised Trauma Score of 8.

TABLE 24-3 Pediatric Trauma Score

COMPONENT	+2	+1	+1
Size	Child/adolescent >20 kg	Toddler 11-20 kg	Infant <10 kg
Airway	Normal	Assisted: O_2 mask, cannula	Intubated: endotracheal tube, cricothyroidotomy
Consciousness	Awake	Obtunded, lost consciousness	Coma, unresponsive
Systolic blood pressure	90 mm Hg	51-90 mm Hg	<50 mm Hg
	Good peripheral pulses, perfusion	Carotid, femoral pulse palpable	Weak or no pulse
Fracture	None seen or suspected	Single closed fracture anywhere	Open or multiple fractures
Cutaneous	No visible injury	Confusion, abrasion, laceration <7 cm through fascia	Tissue loss, any gunshot wound or stab through fascia

From National Association of Emergency Medical Technicians: *PHTLS basic and advanced prehospital trauma life support,* St Louis, 2003, Mosby.

and 12. (A score of 0 indicates the most critical. A score of 12 indicates the least critical; Table 24-2) Calculating the Revised Trauma Score en route to the receiving hospital provides baseline measurements. This can be helpful to the physician in managing the patient's care. In some emergency medical services systems, this score is calculated after arrival at the emergency department using data from radio reports and the prehospital care report.

Pediatric Trauma Score

The pediatric trauma score grades six characteristics commonly seen in pediatric trauma patients. These are size (weight), airway, consciousness, systolic blood pressure, fracture, and cutaneous injury (Table 24-3). The pediatric trauma score has a significant inverse linear relationship with patient mortality. A child with a pediatric trauma score less than 8 should be cared for in an appropriate pediatric trauma center.[7]

Patient size (weight) is one of the first parameters to assess. The smaller the child, the greater the risk for severe injury because of an increased ratio of body surface to volume. The risk also is greater because of the potential for limited physiological reserve.

The child's airway is scored by potential difficulty in management. Scoring also is by the type of care required to ensure adequate ventilation and oxygenation. Respiratory failure is the main cause of death in most pediatric patients. Aggressive management to control the airway should be started without delay.

As with adult patients, the most critical factor in assessing the central nervous system of a child is a change in the level of consciousness. Any change in the level of consciousness will reduce this score—no matter how brief the time.

The assessment of systolic blood pressure in the pediatric patient is critical because the circulating volume is notably less than the adult. Because of a normal child's healthy heart and excellent reserve capacity, children often do not show classic signs of shock until they have lost about 25% of their circulating volume. Any child who has a systolic blood pressure less than 50 mm Hg is in obvious jeopardy.[8]

A child's skeleton is more pliable than that of the adult. It allows traumatic forces to be sent through the body and to the organs. Thus a fracture in the pediatric patient is a sign that serious injury likely has occurred.

Like fractures, cutaneous injury in the pediatric patient is a potential contributor to mortality and disability. These injuries include open and visible wounds and penetrating trauma.

For example, a head-injured child who is 8 years of age weighs 34 kg (+2); has spontaneous respirations (+1); is unresponsive (+1); has a systolic pressure of 86 mm Hg with palpable femoral pulses (+1); no visible fractures (+2); and an abrasion on the head with minimal bleeding (+1). The pediatric trauma score for this patient is 8.

SUMMARY

- Major causes of maxillofacial trauma are motor vehicle crashes, home accidents, athletic injuries, animal bites, intentional violent acts, and industrial injuries.
- With the exception of compromised airway and the potential for significant bleeding, damage to the tissues of the maxillofacial area is seldom life threatening. Blunt trauma injuries may be classified as fractures to the mandible, midface, zygoma, orbit, and nose.
- Injury to the ears, eyes, or teeth may be minor or may result in permanent sensory function loss and disfigurement. Trauma to the ear may include lacerations and contusions, thermal injuries, chemical injuries, traumatic perforation, and barotitis. Evaluation of the eye should include a thorough history. Evaluation also should include measurement of visual acuity, pupillary reaction, and extraocular movements.
- Anterior neck injuries may result in damage to the skeletal structures, vascular structures, nerves, muscles, and glands of the neck.
- Injuries to the skull may be classified as soft tissue injuries to the scalp and skull fractures. Skull fractures may be classified as linear fractures, basilar fractures, depressed fractures, and open vault fractures.
- The categories of brain injury include DAI and focal injury. Diffuse axonal injury may be mild (concussion), moderate, or severe. Focal injuries are specific, grossly observable brain lesions. Included in this category are lesions that result from skull fracture, contusion, edema with associated increased ICP, ischemia, and hemorrhage.
- The prehospital management of a patient with head injuries is determined by a number of factors. One factor is the mechanism of injury. A second factor is the severity of injury. A third factor is the patient's level of consciousness. Associated injuries affect the priorities of care.
- Several injury rating systems are used to triage, guide patient care, predict patient outcome, identify changes in patient status, and evaluate trauma care. Rating systems commonly used in emergency care include the Glasgow Coma Scale, trauma score/Revised Trauma Score, and pediatric trauma score.

REFERENCES

1. Rosen P, Barkin R: *Emergency medicine: concepts and clinical practice,* ed 5, St Louis, 2003, Mosby.
2. National Safety Council: *Injury facts,* Itasca, Ill, 1999, The Council.
3. American Association of Endodontists: *Treating the avulsed permanent tooth,* Chicago, 1998, The Association.
4. US Department of Transportation, National Highway Traffic Safety Administration: *EMT-Paramedic national standard curriculum,* Washington, DC, 1998, The Department.
5. Hickey J: *The clinical practice of neurological and neurosurgical nursing,* ed 4, Philadelphia, 1997, Lippincott.
6. Cardona V et al, editors: *Trauma nursing: from resuscitation through rehabilitation,* ed 2, Philadelphia, 1994, WB Saunders.
7. Gabriel E et al: Guidelines for prehospital management of traumatic brain injury, brain trauma foundation, *J Neurotrauma* 19:111-174, 2002.
8. National Association of Emergency Medical Technicians: *PHTLS: basic and advanced prehospital trauma life support,* ed 5, St Louis, 2003, Mosby.

CHAPTER 25

Spinal Trauma

OBJECTIVES

Upon completion of this chapter, the paramedic student will be able to:

1. Describe the incidence, morbidity, and mortality related to spinal injury.
2. Predict mechanisms of injury that are likely to cause spinal injury.
3. Describe the anatomy and physiology of the spine and spinal cord.
4. Outline the general assessment of a patient with suspected spinal injury.
5. Distinguish between types of spinal injury.
6. Describe prehospital evaluation and assessment of spinal cord injury.
7. Identify prehospital management of the patient with spinal injuries.
8. Distinguish between spinal shock, neurogenic shock, and autonomic hyperreflexia syndrome.
9. Describe selected nontraumatic spinal conditions and the prehospital assessment and treatment of them.

KEY TERMS

anterior cord syndrome: A spinal cord injury usually seen in flexion injuries; caused by pressure on the anterior aspect of the spinal cord by a ruptured intervertebral disk or fragments of the vertebral body extruded posteriorly into the spinal canal.

axial loading: Vertical compression of the spine that results when direct forces are transmitted along the length of the spinal column.

Brown-Séquard syndrome: A hemitransection of the spinal cord. In the classic presentation, pressure on half of the spinal cord results in weakness of the upper and lower extremities on the ipsilateral (same) side and loss of pain and temperature sensation on the contralateral (opposite) side.

central cord syndrome: A spinal cord injury commonly seen with hyperextension or flexion cervical injuries; characterized by greater motor impairment of the upper than lower extremities.

distraction: A spinal injury that occurs if the cervical spine is stopped suddenly while the weight and momentum of the body pull away from it.

neurogenic hypotension: Hypotension following spinal shock; caused by a loss of sympathetic tone to the vessels.

spinal shock: A temporary loss of all types of spinal cord function distal to a cord injury.

subluxation: A partial dislocation.

transection: A complete or incomplete lesion to the spinal cord.

More than 200,000 victims of spinal injury currently are living in the United States, and more than 10,000 new spinal cord injuries will occur this year.[1] Of these, an estimated 4200 persons will die before they are admitted to a hospital. Education in injury prevention, prehospital assessment, and proper handling and transportation of these patients can decrease morbidity and mortality.

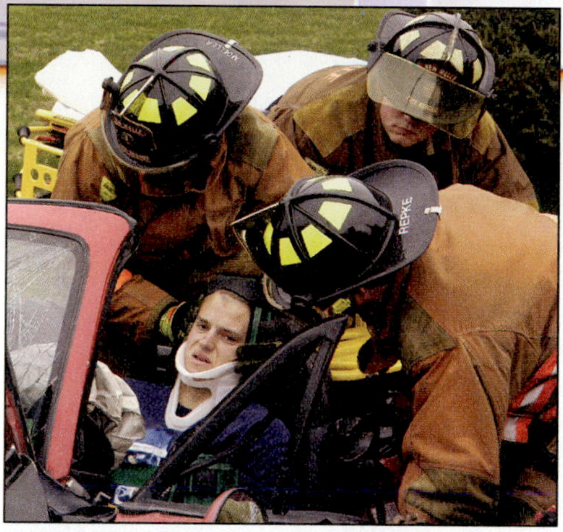

SPINAL TRAUMA: INCIDENCE, MORBIDITY, AND MORTALITY

Most spinal cord injuries (SCIs) result from motor vehicle crashes (48%). The next largest cause is falls (21%). Penetrating injuries from acts of violence (15%) and injuries from sports (14%) follow. The median age of spinal injury victims is 25 years, with men outnumbering women four to one.[1] The incidence of SCI is highest in men between ages 16 and 30 years.

> **CRITICAL THINKING**
> Why do you think this group is at increased risk for spinal injuries?

Forty percent of trauma patients with neurological deficit will have a temporary or permanent SCI. In addition to the devastating emotional and psychological impact on victims and their families, the annual cost to society exceeds $5 billion. The cost of lifelong care for a 25-year-old victim with a permanent SCI is estimated at $1.7 million.[2] Injury prevention strategies can have a positive effect on incidence, morbidity, and mortality associated with spinal trauma (see Chapter 3).

TRADITIONAL SPINAL ASSESSMENT CRITERIA

Assessment of suspected SCIs traditionally has focused on mechanism of injury (MOI). Spinal immobilization was required for two specific patient groups: (1) unconscious injury victims and (2) any patient with a motion injury. This MOI standard covers all patients with a potential for spinal injury, yet the standard is not always practical in the prehospital setting. The accuracy of prehospital assessment can be strengthened by applying clear, clinical guidelines (clinical criteria) for evaluating SCI, which includes the following signs and symptoms

- Altered level of consciousness (Glasgow Coma Scale score less than 15)
- Spinal pain or tenderness
- Neurological deficit or complaint
- Anatomical deformity of spine
- Evidence of alcohol or other drugs
- Distracting injury
- Inability to communicate

Mechanism of Injury/ Nature of Injury

When determining MOI in a patient who may have spinal trauma, the paramedic can classify the MOI as *positive, negative,* or *uncertain.*[3] This method, combined with the clinical criteria for spinal injury listed previously, can help the paramedic identify situations in which spinal immobilization is appropriate. When in doubt, the paramedic should use full spinal precautions (Fig. 25-1).

> **CRITICAL THINKING**
> What are the disadvantages of immobilizing a patient on a long spine board?

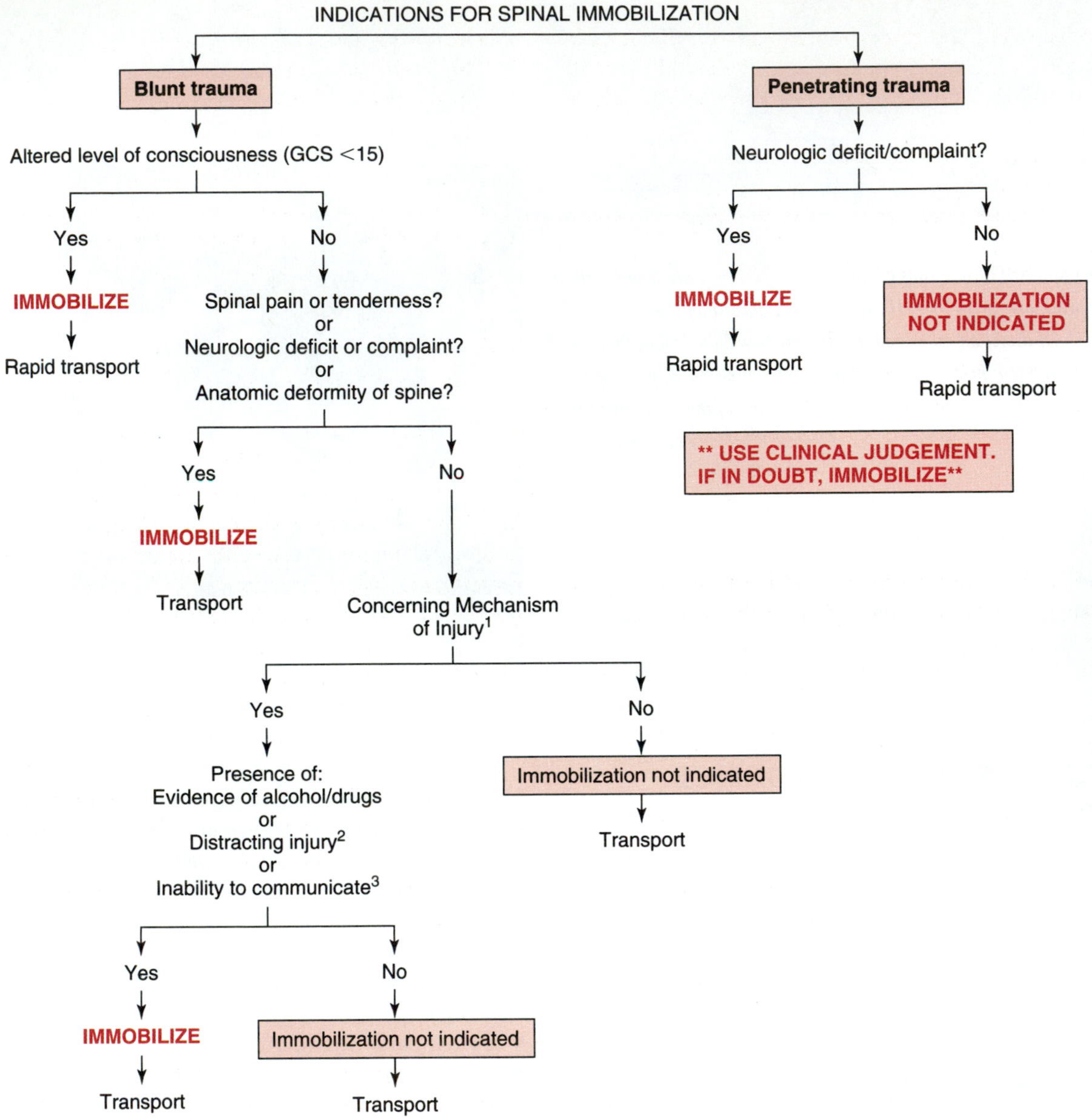

Notes:

[1]Concerning Mechanisms of Injury

- Any mechanism that produced a violent impact to the head, neck, torso, or pelvis (e.g., assault, entrapment in structural collapse, etc.)
- Incidents producing sudden acceleration, deceleration, or lateral bending forces to the neck or torso (e.g., moderate- to high-speed MVC, pedestrian struck, involvement in an explosion, etc.)
- Any fall, especially in the elderly
- Ejection or fall from any motorized or human-powered transportation device (e.g., scooters, skateboards, bicycles, motor vehicles, motorcycles or recreational vehicles)
- Victim of shallow-water diving incident

[2]Distracting Injury

Any injury that may have the potential to impair the patient's ability to appreciate other injuries. Examples of distracting injuries include a) long bone fracture; b) a visceral injury requiring surgical consultation; c) a large laceration, degloving injury, or crush injury; d) large burns, or e) any other injury producing acute functional impairment.

(Adapted from Hoffman JR, Wolfson AB, Todd K. Mower WR: Selective cervical spine radiography in blunt trauma: methodology of the National Emergency X-Radiography Utilization Study [NEXUS], *Ann Emerg Med* 461, 1998.)

[3]Inability to communicate. Any patient who, for reasons not specified above, cannot clearly communicate so as to actively participate in their assessment. Examples: speech or hearing impaired, those who only speak a foreign language, and small children.

FIGURE 25-1 ■ Indications for spinal immobilization.

POSITIVE MECHANISM OF INJURY

In a positive MOI, the forces exerted on the patient are highly suggestive of SCI. A positive MOI always calls for full spinal immobilization. Examples of positive MOIs include the following:

- High-speed motor vehicle crashes
- Falls from greater than 3 times the patient's height
- Violent situations occurring near the patient's spine (e.g., blunt and penetrating injuries)
- Sports injuries
- Other high-impact situations

In the absence of signs and symptoms of SCI, some medical direction agencies may recommend that a patient with a positive MOI *not* be immobilized.[3] Medical direction bases this action on the paramedic's assessment, a reliable patient history, and the absence of distracting injuries (described later in this chapter).

NEGATIVE MECHANISM OF INJURY

A negative MOI includes events in which force or impact does not suggest a likely spinal injury. In the absence of SCI signs and symptoms, negative MOI injuries do not require spinal immobilization. Examples of negative MOIs include the following:

- Dropping an object on the foot
- Twisting an ankle while running
- Isolated soft tissue injury

UNCERTAIN MECHANISM OF INJURY

At times, the impact or force involved in the injury is unknown or uncertain. Thus clinical criteria must be the basis used to determine the need for spinal immobilization (Box 25-1). Examples of uncertain MOIs include the following:

- Tripping or falling to the ground and hitting the head
- Falls from 2 to 4 feet
- Low-speed motor vehicle crashes (fender benders)

Assessment of Uncertain Mechanism of Injury. When evaluating the need for spinal immobilization in which the MOI is uncertain, the paramedic must ensure that the patient is reliable. A reliable patient is one who is calm, cooperative, sober, alert, and oriented. The following are examples of patients who would be considered unreliable:

- Those who have acute stress reactions from sudden stress of any type
- Those who have brain injury
- Those who are intoxicated
- Those who have abnormal mental status
- Those who have distracting injuries
- Those who have problems communicating

BOX 25-1 Clinical Criteria versus Mechanism of Injury

- Initial management is based solely on mechanism of injury.
- *Positive* mechanism of injury requires spinal immobilization.
- *Negative* mechanism of injury (without signs and symptoms) requires no spinal immobilization.
- *Uncertain* mechanism of injury requires further clinical assessment and evaluation to determine need for spinal immobilization.

CRITICAL THINKING

The reliability of a patient is not always easy to assess quickly in the prehospital setting. Why is this?

REVIEW OF SPINAL ANATOMY AND PHYSIOLOGY

As described in Chapter 6, the spinal column is composed of 33 bones (vertebrae). These bones are divided into five sections. The sections include 7 cervical, 12 thoracic, 5 lumbar, 5 sacral (fused), and 4 coccygeal (fused) vertebrae. The anterior elements of the spine include vertebral bodies, intervertebral disks, and anterior and posterior longitudinal ligaments that connect the vertebral bodies anteriorly and inside the canal (Fig. 25-2).

Each vertebra consists of a solid body (bearing most of the weight of the vertebral column), a posterior and anterior arch, a posterior spinous process, and in some vertebrae, a transverse process. Ligaments between the spinous processes provide support for the movements of flexion and extension. Those between the laminae provide support during lateral flexion. The spinal cord lies in the spinal canal. The spinal nerve roots pass out through the vertebral foramen.

GENERAL ASSESSMENT OF SPINAL INJURY

Spinal injury most often results from the spine being forced beyond its normal range and limits of motion (Fig. 25-3). The adult skull weighs 16 to 22 lb. The skull sits on top of the first cervical vertebra (C1), or the atlas. The second cervical vertebra (C2), or the axis and its odontoid process, allow the head to move with about a 180-degree range of motion. Because of the weight and position of the head in relation to the thin neck and cervical vertebrae, the cervical spine is particularly susceptible to injury (27% to 33% of all SCIs occur in the C1 to C2 region).[3] Other spinal components that affect physiological limits of motion are the posterior neck muscles and the sacrum. The posterior neck muscles allow up to 60 degrees of flexion and 70 degrees of extension without stretching of the spinal cord. The sacrum is joined to the pelvis by immovable joints.

The specific MOIs that often cause spinal trauma are axial loading; extremes of flexion, hyperextension, or hyperrotation; excessive lateral bending; and **distraction.** These mechanisms may result in stable and unstable injuries. This is based on the extent of damage to spinal structures and the relative strength of the structures remaining intact.

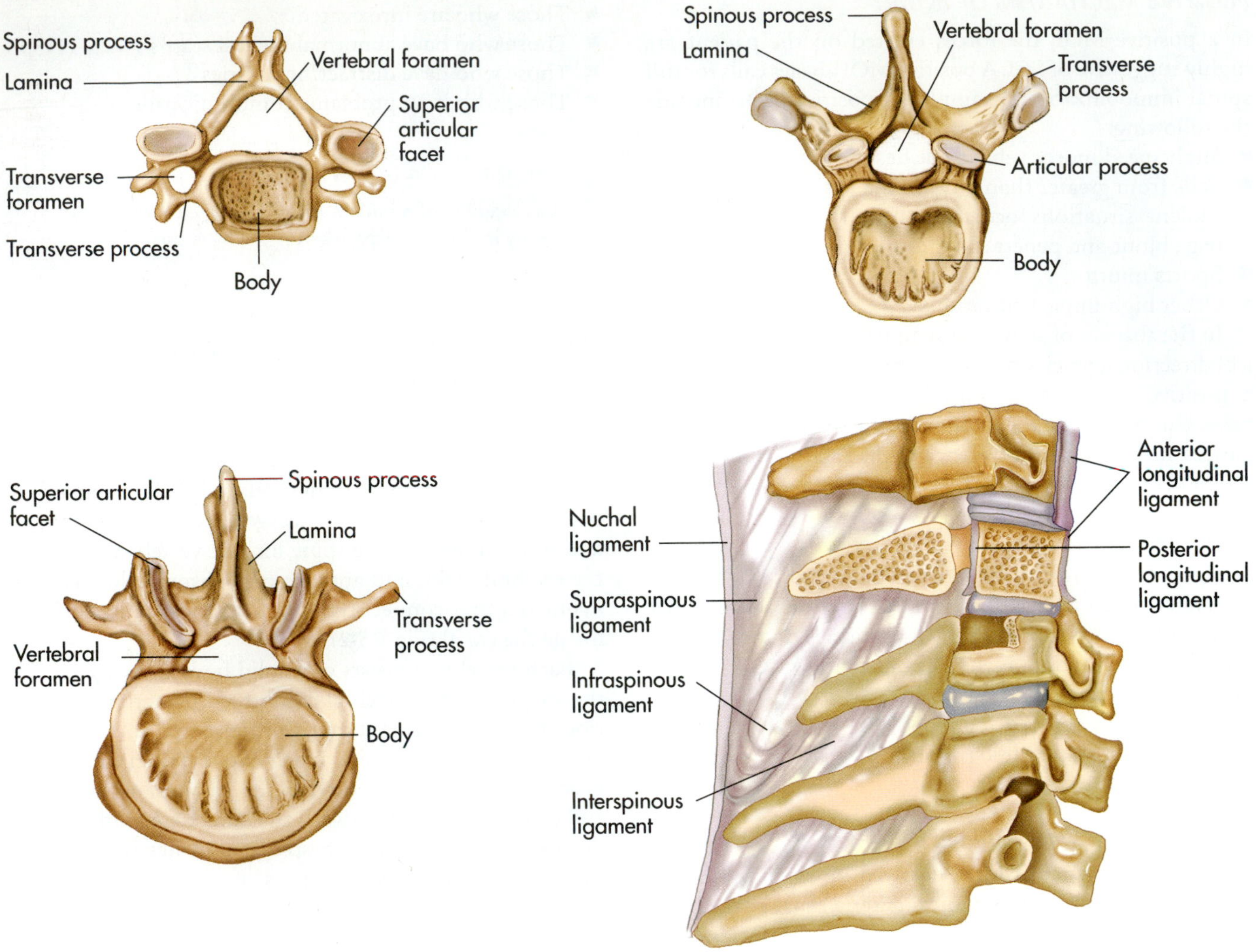

FIGURE 25-2 ■ Vertebral bodies and elements of the spine.

Axial Loading

Axial loading (vertical compression) of the spine results when direct forces are sent down the length of the spinal column. Examples include striking the head against the windshield of a car, shallow diving injuries, vertical falls, and being struck on the head or a helmet with a heavy object. These forces may produce compression fracture or a crushed vertebral body without SCI and most commonly occur from T12 to L2.[3]

Flexion, Hyperextension, and Hyperrotation

Extremes in flexion, hyperextension, or hyperrotation may result in fracture, ligament injury, or muscle injury. Spinal cord injury is caused when one or more of the cervical vertebrae dislocate **(subluxation)** and are forced into the spinal canal. This injures the spinal cord. Examples of these motion extremes include rapid acceleration or deceleration forces from motor vehicle crashes, hangings, and midfacial skeletal or soft tissue trauma. Serious injuries often are the result of a combination of loading *and* rotational forces. These forces produce displacement or fracture of one or more vertebrae.

Lateral Bending

Excessive lateral bending may result in dislocations and bony fractures to the cervical and thoracic spine. The injury occurs as a sudden lateral impact moves the torso sideways. Initially, the head tends to remain in place. Then the head is pulled along by the cervical attachments. Examples of lateral bending include side or angular collisions from motor vehicle crashes and injuries from contact sports. The mechanism of this lateral force requires less movement to produce an injury than flexion or extension forces in frontal or rear impacts.

Distraction

Distraction may occur if the cervical spine is stopped suddenly while the weight and momentum of the body pull away from it. This force or stretching may result in tearing and laceration of the spinal cord. Examples of distraction

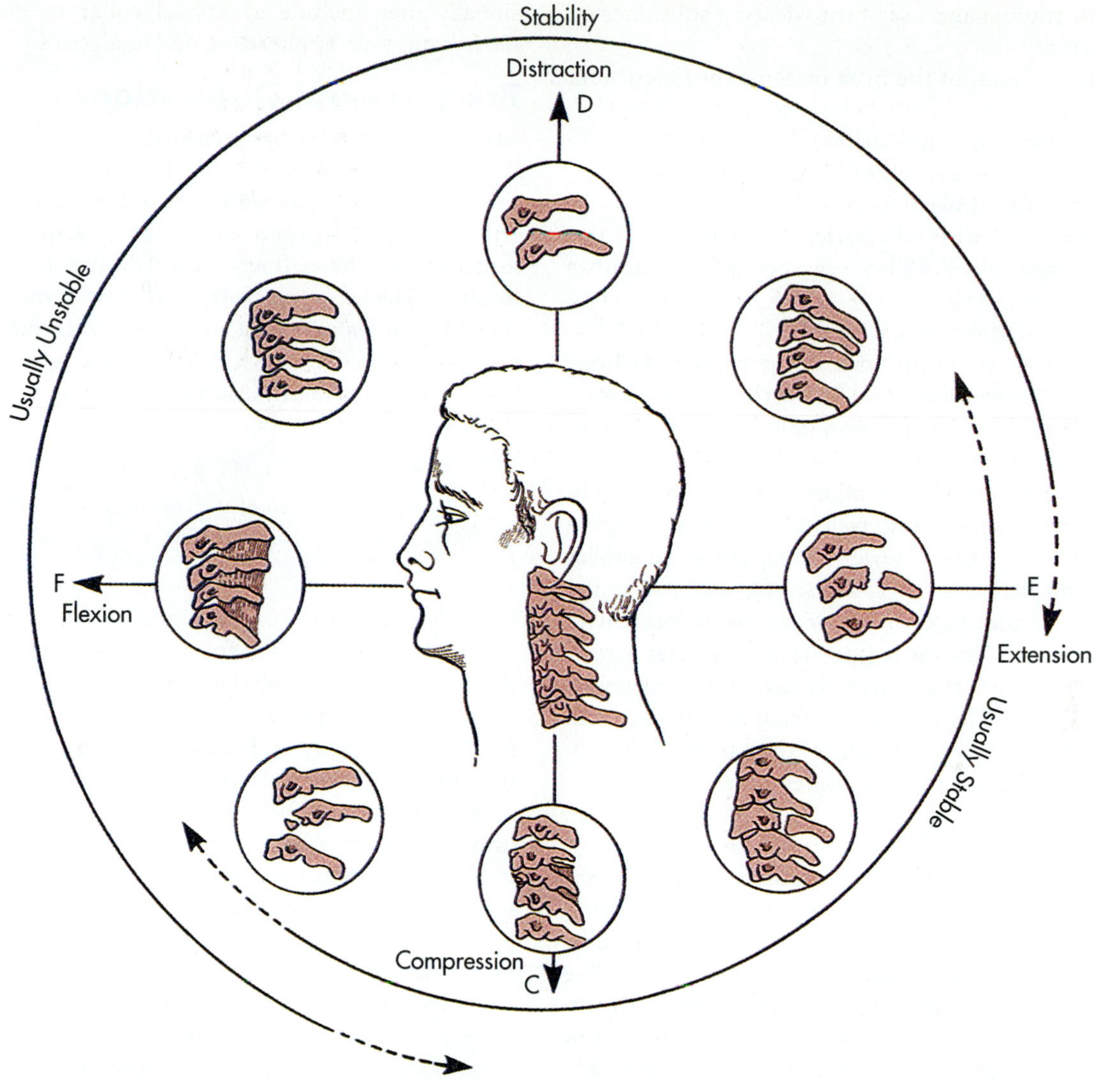

FIGURE 25-3 ■ Mechanisms of cervical spine injury and fracture or dislocation. The mechanism of cervical injury (flexion versus extension) determines the type of cervical spine fracture or dislocation.

include intentional or unintentional hangings (e.g., suicide or school yard or playground injuries).

Other Mechanisms

Other less common mechanisms of spinal injury include blunt and penetrating trauma and electrical injury. The spinal cord, like the brain, may suffer concussions, contusions, and lacerations. The spinal cord may develop hematomata and edema in response to blunt trauma. Examples include spinal injuries that result from direct blows such as from falling tree limbs or other heavy objects.

Penetrating trauma to the spine may be caused by missile-type injuries or stab wounds to the neck, chest, or abdomen. These forces may result in laceration of the spinal cord or nerve roots over a wide area. At times penetrating trauma may produce a complete **transection** (lesion). In addition, areas of edema or contusion adjacent to the laceration may disrupt cord tissue.

Spinal trauma may occur from direct electrical injury. Trauma also may occur from the violent muscle spasms that accompany electrical shock (described in Chapter 23).

CLASSIFICATIONS OF SPINAL INJURY

Spinal injuries may be classified as sprains and strains, fractures and dislocations, sacral and coccygeal fractures, and cord injuries. Regardless of the specific injury, all patients with suspected spinal trauma and signs and symptoms of SCI should be immobilized. Unnecessary movement should be avoided until injury to the spine or spinal cord can be excluded by clinical examination and radiography. An unstable spine can be ruled out only by radiography or lack of any potential mechanism for the injury. As a guideline, the paramedic should assume the presence of spine injury and an unstable spine with the following[3]:

- Significant trauma and use of intoxicating substances
- Seizure activity
- Complaints of pain in the neck or arms (or paresthesia in the arms)
- Neck tenderness on examination
- Unconsciousness as a result of head injury
- Significant injury above the clavicle
- A fall more than 3 times the patient's height
- A fall and fracture of both heels (associated with lumbar fractures)
- Injury from a high-speed motor vehicle crash

Spinal injury (bony injury) can occur with or without SCI. Likewise, a patient may have SCI without bony injury. *Spinal cord injury without radiological abnormality* is a more common finding in children.

The damage produced by the injury forces can be complicated further by the patient's age (calcification from the aging process), preexisting bone diseases (osteoporosis, spondylosis, rheumatoid arthritis, Paget's disease), and congenital spinal cord anomalies (e.g., fusion or narrow spinal canal). Spinal cord neurons do not regenerate to any great extent. Thus any injury to the central nervous system that causes destruction of tissue often results in irreparable damage and permanent loss of function. The role of the paramedic in protecting this critical area cannot be overemphasized.

Sprains and Strains

Sprains and strains usually result from hyperflexion and hyperextension forces. A hyperflexion sprain occurs when the posterior ligamentous complex tears at least partially. This sprain also can result in tears of the joint capsules. The sprain may allow partial dislocation (subluxation) of the intervertebral joints. Hyperextension strains are common in low-speed, rear-end car crashes. They are known commonly as *whiplash*. Injury occurs as the person is thrown backward against the posterior thorax during impact. This action damages anterior soft tissues of the neck.

CRITICAL THINKING

How can the paramedic distinguish between cervical sprain/strain and spinal fracture in the prehospital setting?

With sprains and strains, local pain may be produced by spasms of the neck muscles and injury to the vertebrae, intervertebral disks, and ligamentous structures. The pain usually is described as a nonradiating, aching soreness of the neck or back muscles. The discomfort often varies in intensity and with changes in posture.

On examination, a deformity of the spine may be palpable if dislocation (subluxation) has occurred. The patient may complain of associated point tenderness and swelling. Until the SCI is ruled out by x-ray exam, the paramedic should treat these patients as having unstable cervical spine injuries with a potential for damage to the spinal cord. After the diagnosis is confirmed, treatment of cervical sprain or strain usually is symptomatic. Treatment occasionally may include a cervical collar to decrease neck movement, heat application, and analgesics.

Fractures and Dislocations

The most frequently injured spinal regions in descending order are C5 to C7, C1 to C2, and T12 to L2.[3] Of these injuries, the most common are wedge-shaped compression fractures and teardrop fractures or dislocations. Neurological deficits associated with these fractures and dislocations vary with the location. They also vary with the extent of injury. Although the spine and spinal cord are close to each other, the spine can be fractured without SCI and vice versa. In addition, spinal injuries at multiple levels are common.

CRITICAL THINKING

Look at an illustration of the spinal column. Why do you think these areas are susceptible to fractures?

Wedge-shaped fractures (Fig. 25-4) are hyperflexion injuries. They usually result from compressive force applied to the anterior portion of the vertebral body. This results in stretching of the posterior ligaments. (These injuries often result from injuries and falls in industrial settings.) These fractures usually occur in the mid or lower cervical segments or at T12 and L1. They generally are considered stable because the posterior ligaments rarely are disrupted totally.

Teardrop fractures and dislocations (Fig. 25-5) are unstable injuries. They result from a combination of severe hyperflexion and compression forces and often are seen in motor vehicle crashes. During impact, the vertebral body is fractured. The anterior-inferior corner of the vertebral body is pushed forward. Unlike simple wedge fractures, these fractures may be associated with neurological damage. These are among the most unstable injuries of the spine. A number of other spinal injuries are associated with the mechanisms of flexion, extension, rotation, and axial loading. Most of these are unstable and require careful immobilization.

Sacral and Coccygeal Fractures

The majority of serious spinal injuries occur in the cervical, thoracic, and lumbar regions. One reason for this is the location of the spinal cord and its termination in the adult spine at about L2. Another reason is the protection provided by the ring structure of the pelvis and the musculature of the buttocks and lower back. However, fractures through the foramina of S1 and S2 are fairly common. They may compromise several sacral nerve elements. Such fractures may result in loss of perianal sensory motor function. They also may result in damage to the bladder and bladder sphincters.

The sacrococcygeal joint also may be injured as a result of direct blows and falls. Patients often complain that they have "broken their tailbone." They often experience moderate pain from the mobile coccyx. Diagnosis usually is confirmed by a physician through a rectal examination.

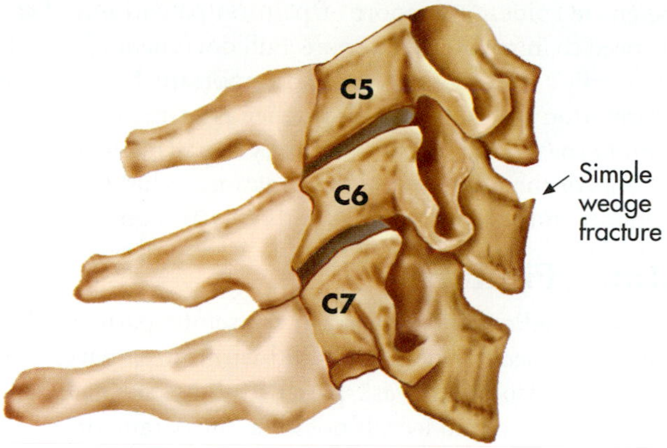

FIGURE 25-4 ■ Lateral view of simple wedge fracture.

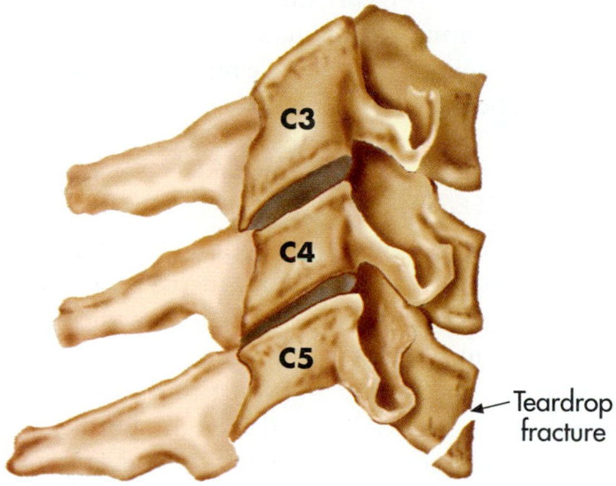

FIGURE 25-5 ■ Lateral view of teardrop fracture.

Cord Injuries

Spinal cord injuries may be classified further as *primary* and *secondary* injuries. Primary injuries occur at the time of impact. Secondary injuries occur after the initial injury. This type of injury can include swelling, ischemia, and movement of bony fragments. Like other tissues, the spinal cord can be concussed, contused, compressed, and lacerated. All of these mechanisms can cause temporary or permanent loss of cord-mediated functions distal to the injury from compression or ischemia. Bleeding from damaged blood vessels also can occur in the tissue of the spinal cord. Bleeding can cause an obstruction to spinal blood supply. The severity of these injuries depends on the amount and type of force that produced them and the duration of the injury.

CORD LESIONS

Lesions (transections) to the spinal cord are classified as *complete* or *incomplete*. Complete lesions usually are associated with spinal fracture or dislocation. Patients have total absence of pain, pressure, and joint sensation. They also have complete motor paralysis below the level of injury. Autonomic nervous system dysfunction may be associated with complete cord lesions. This depends on the level of cord involvement. Manifestations of autonomic dysfunction include the following:

- Bradycardia caused by loss of sympathetic autonomic activity
- Hypotension caused by loss of vasomotor control and peripheral vascular resistance
- Priapism
- Loss of sweating and shivering
- Poikilothermy (body temperature varying with ambient temperature)
- Loss of bowel and bladder control

CRITICAL THINKING

Why should you immobilize a patient who already is showing signs and symptoms of a complete cord lesion?

The paramedic should be familiar with signs and symptoms of several incomplete spinal cord syndromes. Knowledge of these rare syndromes helps the emergency medical services provider understand the MOI. Such knowledge also helps the paramedic to understand the potential for further injury. The three syndromes indicating incomplete lesions of the spinal cord are as follows:

1. **Central cord syndrome:** Central cord syndrome commonly occurs with hyperextension or flexion cervical injuries. The syndrome is characterized by greater motor impairment of the upper than lower extremities. Signs and symptoms of central cord syndrome are as follows:
   - Paralysis of the arms
   - *Sacral sparing* (the preservation of sensory or voluntary motor function of the perineum, buttocks, scrotum, or anus)
2. **Anterior cord syndrome:** Anterior cord syndrome usually is seen in flexion injuries. The syndrome is caused by pressure on the anterior aspect of the spinal cord by a ruptured intervertebral disk or fragments of the vertebral body forced posteriorly into the spinal canal. Signs and symptoms include the following:
   - Decreased sensation of pain and temperature below the level of the lesion (including lesions of the sacral region)
   - Intact light touch and position sensation
   - Paralysis
3. **Brown-Séquard syndrome:** Brown-Séquard syndrome is a hemitransection of the spinal cord. This syndrome may result from a ruptured intervertebral disk or the pushing of a fragment of vertebral body on the spinal cord. This often occurs after knife or missile injuries. In the classic presentation, pressure on half of the spinal cord results in weakness of the upper and lower extremities on the ipsilateral (same) side. Pressure also results in loss of pain and temperature sensation on the contralateral (opposite) side.

CRITICAL THINKING

How will the prehospital care differ for a patient who has signs or symptoms of one of these syndromes?

PHARMACOLOGICAL THERAPY FOR INCOMPLETE CORD INJURY

The benefits of pharmacological agents (glucocorticoids, ***naloxone,*** calcium channel blockers, GM-1 ganglioside, and others) in the management of incomplete cord injury are controversial. These drugs are thought to provide some type of damage control following some SCIs. Some of the drugs are thought to work by reducing the toxicity of excitatory amino acids that cause cells to die; others, by encouraging the growth of new neurons or by reducing inflammation of the injured spinal cord and the bursting open of damaged cells.[2] Of these, only ***methylprednisolone*** currently is used routinely for human victims of SCI.[1]

Methylprednisolone is a synthetic steroid that reduces posttraumatic spinal cord edema and inflammation. ***Methylprednisolone*** routinely is used in victims of SCI. Studies have found that patients treated with this drug within 8 hours of injury show significant neurological improvement at 6 weeks compared with patients who were treated with a placebo.[4] Paramedics should consult with medical direction and follow local protocol regarding the use of these drugs in the prehospital setting.

EVALUATION AND ASSESSMENT OF SPINAL CORD INJURY

Spinal cord trauma should be evaluated only after all injuries that pose a threat to life have been assessed and treated. As with any scenario of serious illness or injury, the paramedic's first priority must be scene survey (including ensuring personal safety) and assessment of the patient's airway, breathing, and circulation. The second priority is to preserve spinal cord function and avoid secondary injury to the spinal cord.

The primary injury to the spine occurs at impact. Thus the critical role of paramedics is to prevent secondary injury. A secondary injury could result from unnecessary movement of an unstable spinal column, hypoxemia, edema, or shock (which may reduce perfusion of the injured cord). These goals are best met by maintaining a high degree of suspicion for the presence of spinal trauma (based on scene survey, kinematics, and history of the event), providing early spinal immobilization, and rapidly correcting any volume deficit through fluid replacement, pneumatic antishock garment application (per protocol), and oxygen administration.

After any life-threatening problems found in the initial assessment are treated, the paramedic should perform a neurological examination. This examination may be done in the field. The exam also may be done en route to the receiving hospital if the patient's condition requires rapid transport. Any movement of the patient for performing a general or neurological examination must be accompanied by continuous, manual protection and in-line stabilization of the spine. Once the spine is stabilized, the paramedic should palpate the entire spine. Any report of pain on palpation indicates the need to immobilize the spine. Full documentation of the paramedic's findings provides an important baseline. This information will be useful for further assessment and evaluation of the patient in the emergency department. The components of the neurological examination include evaluation of motor and sensory findings and reflex responses.

Motor Findings

The paramedic should question conscious patients about pain in the neck or back with and without palpation. The paramedic also should ask patients about their ability to move their arms and legs. If possible, the paramedic should test the strength and motion of all four extremities. The paramedic can do this by asking the patient to flex the elbows (biceps, C6), extend the elbows (triceps, C7), and abduct/adduct the fingers (C8, T1). In unconscious patients, painful stimuli in the hands and lower extremities may initiate an involuntary muscle reflex unless the patient is in profound coma.

UPPER EXTREMITY NEUROLOGICAL FUNCTION ASSESSMENT

To test interosseous muscle function (controlled by T1 nerve roots), the paramedic should instruct the patient to spread the fingers of both hands. The paramedic should instruct the patient to keep the fingers apart while the paramedic squeezes the second and fourth fingers. Normal resistance should be springlike and equal on both sides.

To test the extensors of the hands and fingers (controlled by C7 nerve roots), the paramedic should instruct the patient to hold his or her wrists or fingers straight out and to keep them out while the paramedic presses down on the fingers. (The arm should be supported at the wrist to avoid testing arm function and other nerve roots.) The paramedic should feel moderate resistance with moderate pressure. Both sides of the patient should be evaluated if not contraindicated by injury.

LOWER EXTREMITY NEUROLOGICAL FUNCTION ASSESSMENT

To test plantar flexors of the foot (controlled by S1 and S2 nerve roots), the paramedic should place his or her hands at the sole of each foot and instruct the patient to push against the hands. Both sides should feel equal and strong.

To test dorsal flexors of the foot and great toe (controlled by L5 nerve roots), the paramedic should hold the patient's foot (with fingers on toes) and instruct the patient to pull the feet back or toward the nose. Both sides should feel equal and strong.

Sensory Findings

In conscious patients, sensory examination should be performed with light touch on each hand and each foot (while the patient's eyes are closed) to evaluate the ability to feel this type of stimuli. (Light touch is carried by more than one nerve tract.) Sensation should be equal on both sides. The paramedic also should question the patient about weakness, numbness, paresthesia, or radicular pain (shooting pain that travels along a nerve).

If the patient cannot feel light touch or is unconscious, the paramedic may evaluate sensation by gently pricking the hands and soles of the feet. A sharp object that will not penetrate the skin is useful. (For example, the end of a pen or broken cotton-tipped applicator can be used.) One method of evaluation moves from head to toe; recording the level at which sensation stops or the unconscious patient ceases to respond to a painful stimulus by marking that location on the patient's skin with ink or a marker. Another method is to begin the sensory assessment by moving from an area of no sensation to an area where sensation begins. The paramedic would note the area where sensation begins with ink or marker. (These marks make it possible to compare sensory level accurately after repeated examinations.) Lack of response to stimulation in the upper extremities indicates cord damage in the cervical region; failure of only the lower extremities to respond indicates cord injury in the thoracic region, lumbar regions, or both.

CRITICAL THINKING

How will you respond to the patient who fearfully asks you, "Why can't I move or feel my arms or legs?"

Dermatomes (described in Chapter 6) correspond to spinal nerves (Table 25-1), so the following four landmarks may be useful for a quick sensory evaluation in the prehospital setting[3]:

1. C2 to C4 dermatomes provide a collar of sensation around the neck and over the anterior chest to below the clavicles.
2. T4 dermatome provides sensation to the nipple line.
3. T10 dermatome provides sensation to the umbilicus.
4. S1 dermatome provides sensation to the soles of the feet.

Reflex Responses

Reflex responses seldom are evaluated in the prehospital setting. However, some abnormal responses are observed easily. These responses may indicate autonomic nerve injury. These responses include loss of temperature control, hypotension, bradycardia, and priapism. Another pathological reflex includes the presence of Babinski's sign (the plantar reflex). This is a reflex movement in which the great toe bends upward when the outer edge of the sole of the foot is scratched (Fig. 25-6). Babinski's sign (which may indicate a spinal cord lesion in the older child or adult) is a normal and expected response in children under 2 years of age.

Other Methods of Evaluation

A visual inspection of the spine may reveal the presence of injury and its level. For example, transection of the cord above C3 often results in respiratory arrest. Lesions that occur at C4 may result in paralysis of the diaphragm. However, transections that occur at C5 to C6 usually spare the diaphragm, allowing diaphragmatic breathing. This occurs because the intercostal muscles are innervated sequentially between C4 to C5 and T12. As a result, intercostal muscle groups may be paralyzed with cervical or thoracic spinal cord lesions below the level where diaphragmatic nerves are located. (The higher the lesion, the greater the loss of intercostal muscle function.)

The patient's body position also may offer clues about neurological injury. For example, a patient with a SCI at C6 may lie with the arms flexed at the elbows and wrists (the "holdup" position).

TABLE 25-1 Common Nerve Root and Motor/Sensory Correlation

NERVE ROOT	MOTOR	SENSORY
C3, C4	Trapezius (shoulder shrug)	Top of shoulder
C3 to C5	Diaphragm	Top of shoulder
C5, C6	Biceps (elbow flexion)	Thumb
C7	Triceps (elbow extension) Wrist/finger extension	Middle finger
C8, T1	Finger abduction/adduction	Little finger
T4	Nipple	
T10	Umbilicus	
L1, L2	Hip flexion	Inguinal crease
L3, L4	Quadriceps	Medial thigh/calf
L5	Great toe/foot dorsiflexion	Lateral calf
S1	Knee flexion	Lateral foot
S1, S2	Foot plantar flexion	
S2 to S4	Anal sphincter tone	Perianal

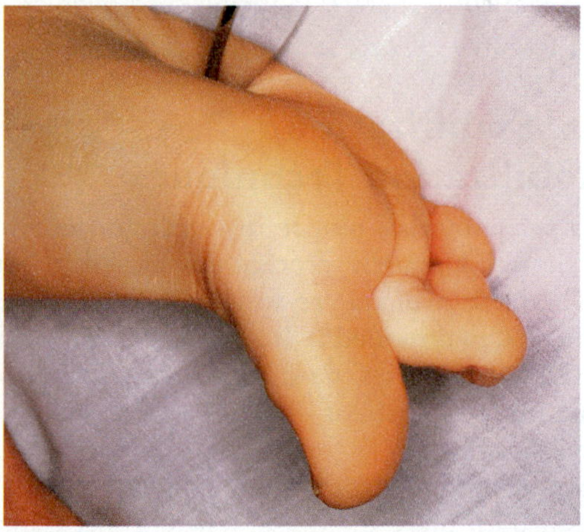

FIGURE 25-6 ■ Babinski's sign: dorsiflexion of the great toe with or without fanning of the toes.

GENERAL MANAGEMENT OF SPINAL INJURIES

A significant spinal injury still may be present, even though the patient may not show signs of spinal injury. More than 50% of patients with cervical spinal injuries have normal responses to motor, sensory, and reflex examinations.[1] Thus if the paramedic suspects a spinal injury for any reason, the paramedic must protect the patient's spine. An estimated 15% of secondary SCIs are preventable with proper immobilization.[3] In addition, the patient's ability to walk does not rule out the need for spinal precautions. As previously stated, an unstable spine can be ruled out only by clinical examination, radiography, and the lack of any potential mechanism for spinal injury. General principles of spinal immobilization include the following:

1. The primary goal is to prevent further injury.
2. The spine should be treated as a long bone with a joint at either end (the head and pelvis).
3. The paramedic should always use complete spinal immobilization. (Splinting and isolation of a specific injury site is impossible. Having spine fractures in more than one location also is common.)
4. Spinal immobilization begins in the initial assessment and must be maintained until the spine is immobilized completely on a long spine board.
5. The patient's head and neck must be placed in a neutral, in-line position unless contraindicated by condition or MOI. (Neutral positioning allows for the most space for the spinal cord, thereby reducing cord hypoxia and excess pressure.)

Spinal Stabilization/ Immobilization Techniques

As soon as a potential spine injury is recognized, the paramedic should manually protect the patient's head and neck. The basic principle to follow is that the head and neck must be maintained in line with the long axis of the body. If other injuries need treatment, the paramedic must maintain the patient's head and neck position without interruption.

A number of devices for immobilizing the spinal column are designed for prehospital use. When properly applied to patients who are sitting, standing, or lying, these devices can provide adequate spinal protection. However, no device should be considered for use until the head and neck have been stabilized with manual in-line immobilization.

> **NOTE** All spinal immobilization techniques discussed in this text follow the guidelines recommended by the Prehospital Trauma Life Support Committee of the National Association of Emergency Medical Technicians in cooperation with the Committee on Trauma of the American College of Surgeons.[4]

MANUAL IN-LINE IMMOBILIZATION

Manual in-line immobilization can be done from almost any patient position. It should be applied without traction on the head. Only enough tension should be applied to relieve the weight of the head from the cervical spine. After manual immobilization has been initiated, it must be continued without stopping until the head and spine are immobilized to a proper device (short spine board or vest, long spine board).

Contraindications for moving the patient's head to an in-line position follow. If any of these contraindications exist, all manual movement of the patient's head should stop. At that point, the head and neck should be stabilized in the position found. Contraindications include the following:

- Resistance to movement
- Neck muscle spasm
- Increased pain
- The presence or increase in neurological deficits during movement (e.g., numbness, tingling, and loss of motor function)
- Compromise of the airway or ventilation
- Severe misalignment of the head away from the midline of the shoulders and body axis (rare)

Manual Immobilization From the Sitting or Standing Patient's Side

1. Stand alongside the patient, holding the back of the head with one hand. Place the thumb and first finger of the other hand on each cheek, just below the zygomatic arch (Fig. 25-7).
2. Tighten the position of both hands without moving the head or neck.
3. Move the head to an in-line position if needed. Maintain this position by bracing the elbows against your torso for support.

Manual In-line Immobilization From the Front of the Sitting or Standing Patient

1. Stand in front of the patient and place the thumb of each hand on the patient's cheeks, just below the zygomatic arch.
2. Place the little fingers of each hand on the posterior aspect of the patient's skull.
3. Spread the remaining fingers of each hand on the lateral planes of the head and increase the strength of the grip (Fig. 25-8).
4. Move the head to an in-line position if needed. Maintain this position by bracing the elbows against your torso for support.

Manual In-Line Immobilization With a Supine Patient

1. Kneel or lie at the patient's head and place the thumbs of each hand just below the zygomatic arch of each cheek (Fig. 25-9).
2. Place the little fingers of each hand on the posterior aspect of the patient's skull.
3. Spread the remaining fingers of each hand on the lateral planes of the head and increase the strength of the grip.
4. Move the head to an in-line position if needed. Maintain this position by bracing the elbows against your torso or ground surface for support.

Logroll With Spinal Precautions. Logrolling methods are used to move patients with a possible spinal injury. Examples include moving patients onto a mechanical immobilization device and turning patients from a prone to a supine position. Logrolling maneuvers require at least four rescuers. With four, the rescuers can provide for adequate

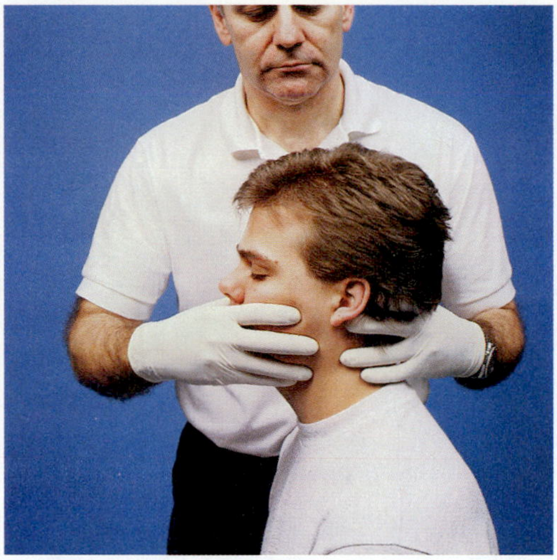

FIGURE 25-7 ■ Manual in-line immobilization from the side.

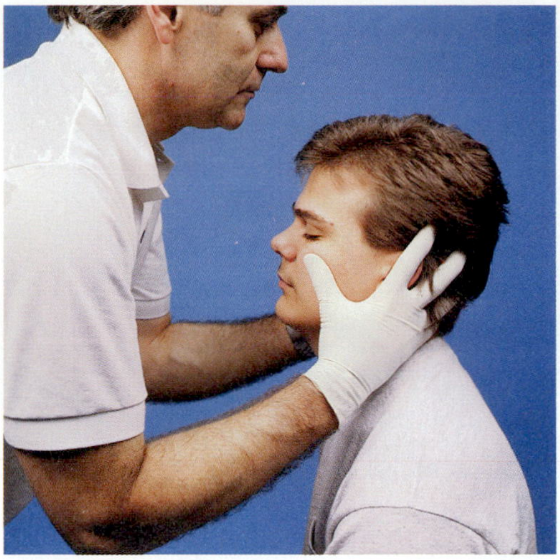

FIGURE 25-8 ■ Manual in-line immobilization from the front.

spinal protection. The position of the patient's arms during a logrolling maneuver may affect thoracic-lumbar motion and further compromise the stability of the spine. One method that may minimize lateral motion and help to maintain neutral alignment of the pelvis and legs is to position the patient with arms extended at the side. The patient's palms should be on the lateral thighs.

Logroll of the Supine Patient. The following steps should be used for logrolling of patients in the supine position (Fig. 25-10).

1. Rescuer 1 should be positioned at the patient's head. Rescuer 1 should provide in-line manual stabilization. Another rescuer should apply a rigid cervical collar and place a long spine board at the patient's side. (If a spinal injury with paralysis is obvious or if shock is suspected, the pneumatic antishock garment should be prepared on the spine board per protocol.)
2. Rescuers 2 and 3 should be positioned at the patient's midthorax and knees. The patient's arms should be extended at the sides, palms on lateral thighs. The legs should be brought together for neutral alignment.
3. Rescuer 2 grasps the far side of the patient at the shoulder and wrist. Rescuer 3 grasps the hips (just distal of the wrists) and both lower extremities at the ankles.
4. In one organized move, the rescuers slowly logroll the patient onto his or her side. At the same time, they slide the spine board under the patient. In-line support of the patient's head must be maintained. This is done by rotating the head exactly with the torso to avoid flexion or hyperextension. In addition, the ankles must be elevated slightly to maintain lateral and anterior-posterior alignment.
5. Rescuer 4 positions the long spine board by placing the device flat on the ground or at a 30- to 40-degree angle against the patient's back.
6. In one organized move, the rescuers slowly logroll and center the patient on the long spine board.

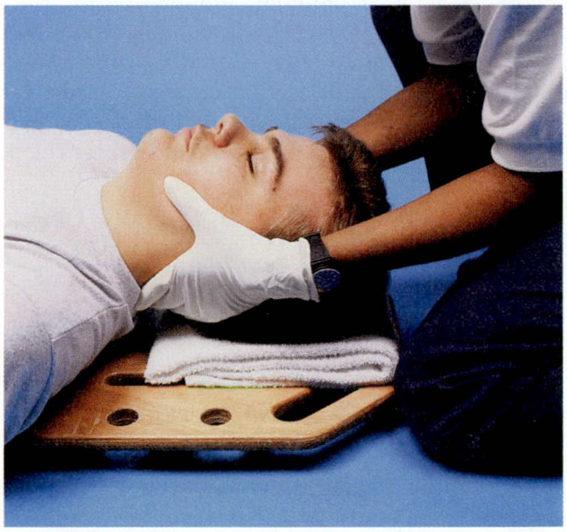

FIGURE 25-9 ■ Manual in-line immobilization with a supine patient.

Logroll of the Prone Patient. The basic principles used in logrolling supine patients can be applied to a patient who is in a prone or semiprone position. The procedure uses the same initial alignment of the patient's arms and legs. The rescuers have the same responsibilities for maintaining alignment. There are two major differences in this logroll maneuver. These are Rescuer 1's hand position during the logroll and the application of the rigid cervical collar, which can be applied only after the patient is in a supine position (Fig. 25-11).

1. Rescuer 1 places his or her hands in a position that provides in-line stabilization and that accommodates rotation of the patient with the torso.
2. In one organized move, the rescuers rotate the patient away from the direction of the initial prone position.
3. A rescuer places the long spine board on a flat surface or positions it between the patient's back and the rescuers at the patient's side.

A

B

C

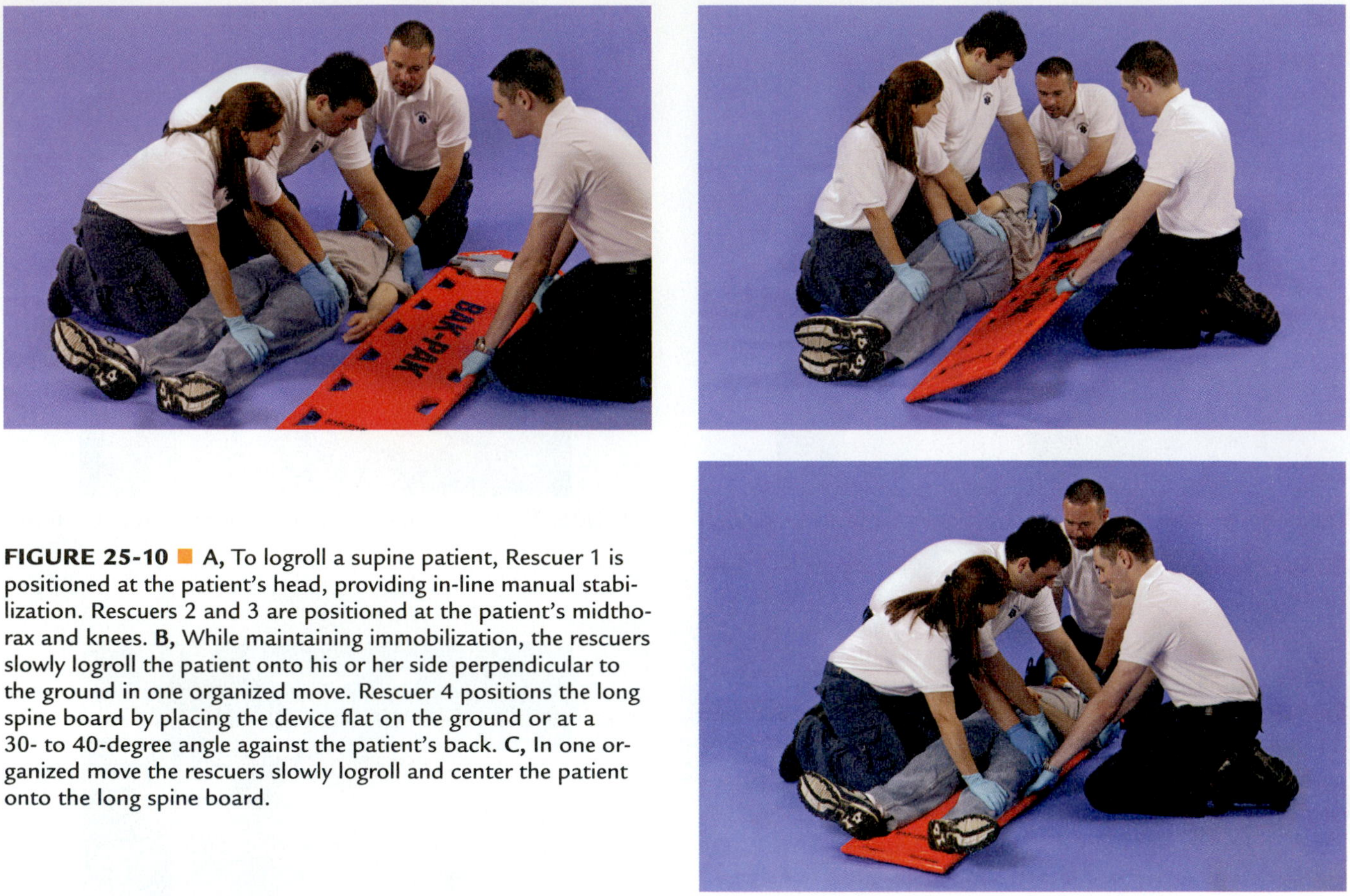

FIGURE 25-10 ■ **A,** To logroll a supine patient, Rescuer 1 is positioned at the patient's head, providing in-line manual stabilization. Rescuers 2 and 3 are positioned at the patient's midthorax and knees. **B,** While maintaining immobilization, the rescuers slowly logroll the patient onto his or her side perpendicular to the ground in one organized move. Rescuer 4 positions the long spine board by placing the device flat on the ground or at a 30- to 40-degree angle against the patient's back. **C,** In one organized move the rescuers slowly logroll and center the patient onto the long spine board.

4. In one organized move, the rescuers slowly logroll and center the patient on the long spine board.
5. A rescuer applies a rigid cervical collar.

MECHANICAL DEVICES

Spinal immobilization equipment covered includes rigid cervical collars, short spine boards, and long spine boards. This text presents only *general* principles of spinal immobilization by mechanical devices. The specific methods of application vary by device. Paramedics should become familiar with the equipment used in their locale. They also should follow the application guidelines of the manufacturer.

Rigid Cervical Collars. Rigid cervical collars are designed to protect the cervical spine from compression. These devices may reduce movement and some range of motion of the head. However, they do not by themselves provide adequate immobilization of the spine. These devices must always be used along with manual in-line stabilization or immobilization by a suitable device (e.g., vest, short spine board, or long spine board). To apply a rigid cervical collar, the paramedic should follow these general steps, which demonstrate the application of the Stifneck Collar (Fig. 25-12):

1. Rescuer 1 applies manual in-line immobilization from behind the patient and maintains this position throughout the procedure.
2. Rescuer 2 properly angles the collar for placement.
3. Rescuer 2 positions the collar bottom.
4. Rescuer 2 sets the collar in place around the patient's neck.
5. Rescuer 2 secures the collar with the Velcro straps.
6. Rescuer 1 spreads his or her fingers and maintains support until the patient is secured to a short or long spine board.

Rigid cervical collars come in a number of sizes (or they are adjustable). They can accommodate the range of physical characteristics of patients. Choosing the proper size reduces flexion or hyperextension of the neck. These movements may occur during patient extrication and packaging. These movements also may result from acceleration and deceleration forces that normally occur during patient transport. The following guidelines apply to the use of rigid cervical collars:

- Rigid cervical collars must not inhibit the patient's ability to open the mouth. They also must not inhibit the patient's ability to clear his or her airway in case vomiting occurs.
- Rigid cervical collars must not obstruct airway passages or hinder ventilation.
- Rigid cervical collars should be applied only after the head has been brought into a neutral in-line position.

Short Spine Boards. Short spine boards or other short spine extrication devices are used to splint the cervical and

A B C D

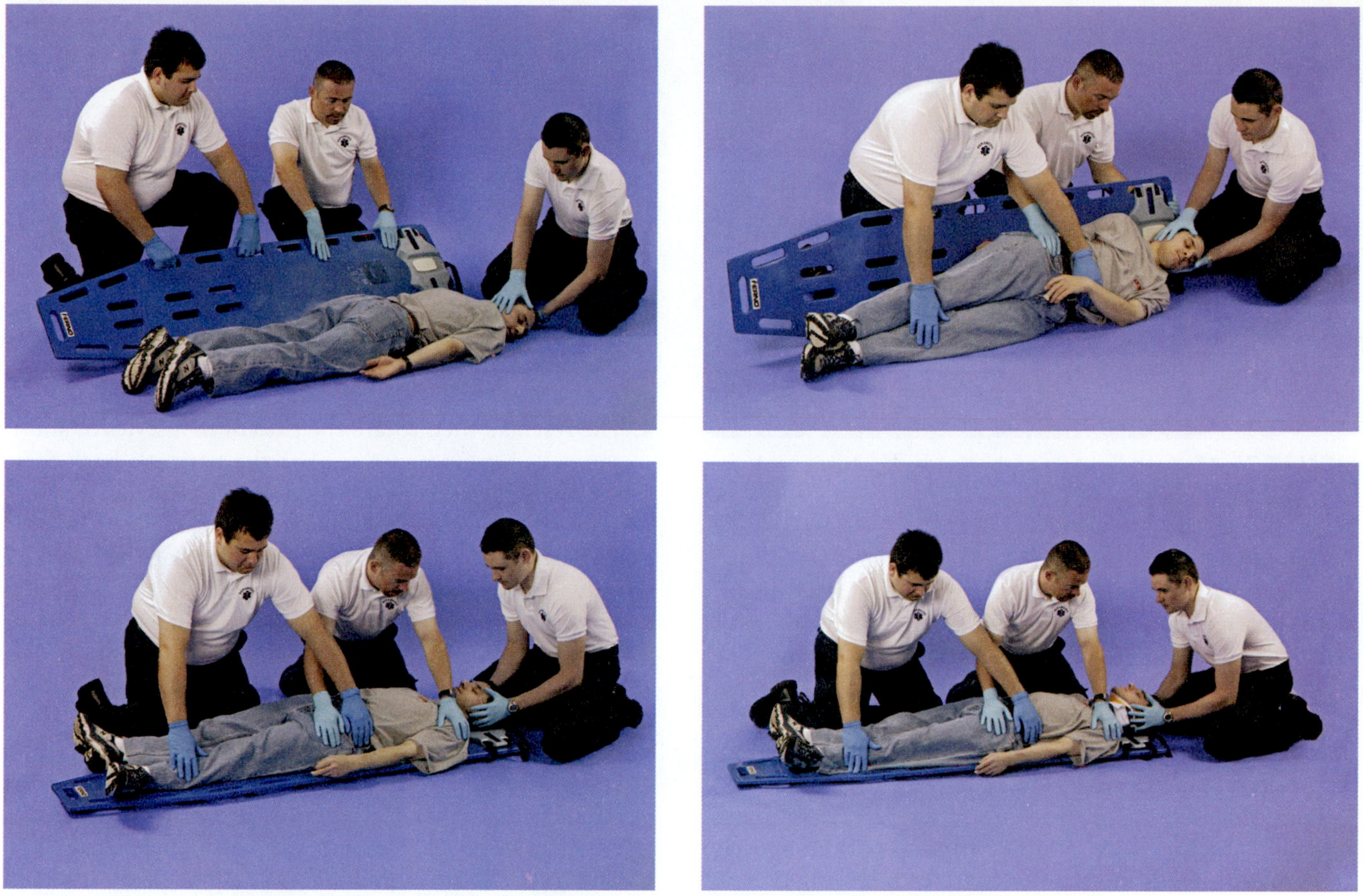

FIGURE 25-11 ■ **A,** Rescuer 1 places his or her hands in a position that provides in-line stabilization and that accommodates the rotation of the patient with the torso. Rescuer 2 positions the long spine board. **B,** In one organized move the rescuers rotate the patient away from the direction of his or her initial prone position. **C,** In one organized move the rescuers slowly logroll and center the patient onto the long spine board. **D,** Another rescuer then applies a rigid cervical collar.

thoracic spine. These devices vary in design. They are available from a number of manufacturers. In general, short spine boards are used to provide spinal immobilization when the patient is sitting or is in a confined space. After short spine board immobilization, the patient is moved to a long spine board device for complete spinal immobilization. Examples of short spine boards include the plastic or synthetic half backboard, the Kendrick extrication device, the Oregon Spine Splint II, and the Hare extrication device. General principles of short spine board application, demonstrated with the Kendrick extrication device, are as follows (Fig. 25-13):

CRITICAL THINKING

When would the use of the short board *not* be indicated for spinal column immobilization?

1. After manual in-line immobilization and the application of a rigid cervical collar, place the short spine board device behind the patient. The board should be posi-

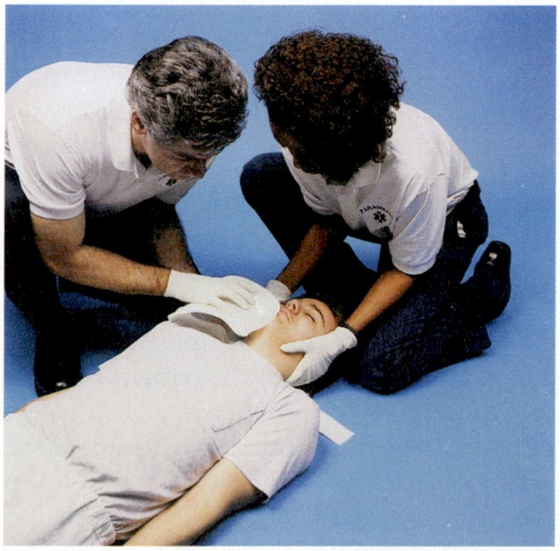

FIGURE 25-12 ■ Rescuer 2 positions the collar and secures it with Velcro straps.

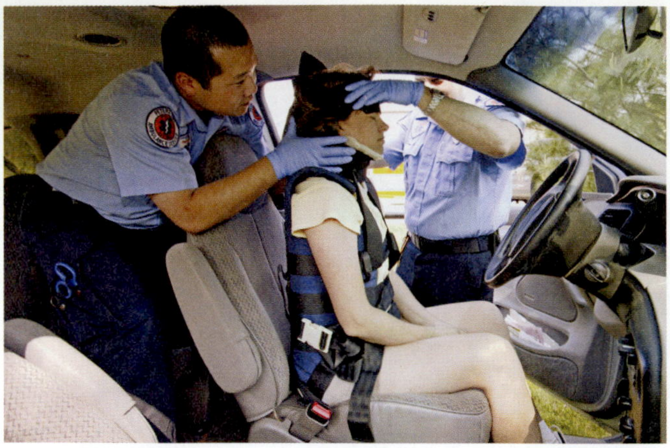

FIGURE 25-13 ■ Application of the Kendrick extrication device.

tioned snugly beneath the patient's axillae; this will prevent it from moving up the torso.

2. Immobilize the upper and middle torso by fastening the upper, middle, and lower chest straps. The upper strap can be relatively tight without impairing chest excursion. The middle and lower straps should be snug so that fingers cannot be slipped beneath the straps. Readjust as needed.
3. Position and fasten each groin strap separately, forming a loop. These straps prevent the Kendrick extrication device from moving up and the lower end from moving laterally.
4. Pad the device as needed and secure the head to the short spine board.
5. Carefully move the patient as a unit to a long spine board by rotating the patient and Kendrick extrication device onto the board. Hold the legs proximal to the knees and lift them during the transition.

> **NOTE** The use of a short spine board should be considered only if the patient's condition allows. If the patient is unstable because of life-threatening injury, the need for immediate resuscitation, or if the time required to apply the device would jeopardize the patient's life (e.g., a patient with a carotid pulse, but absent radial pulse), the patient's head and neck should be stabilized with manual, in-line support, and the patient should be moved as a unit to a long spine board.

6. Center the patient on the long spine board, release the leg straps, and slowly lower the patient's legs to an in-line position.
7. Secure the patient and Kendrick extrication device to the long spine board, maintaining a neutral in-line position with the long axis of the body. Then slightly loosen the Kendrick extrication device chest straps.

RAPID EXTRICATION

The steps required for rapid extrication may vary depending on the size and make of the vehicle. They also may vary based on the patient's location inside the vehicle. A general description of the steps required for rapid extrication are listed:

Three or More Rescuers (Fig. 25-14)

1. Rescuer 1 supports the patient's head and neck. Rescuer 1 uses manual in-line stabilization from behind the patient or from the patient's side. Rescuer 1 maintains this stabilization throughout the extrication process.
2. After a rapid initial assessment, Rescuer 2 applies a rigid cervical collar and positions a long spine board near the vehicle.
3. Rescuer 3 manually stabilizes and controls movement of the patient's upper and lower torso and legs during extrication.
4. The rescuers then rotate the patient in a series of short, controlled movements so that the patient's back faces the open doorway. Rescuer 2 exits the vehicle. Rescuer 2 assumes control of manual stabilization from outside the vehicle. Rescuer 1 assumes control of the patient's lower torso and legs. Each movement during the rotation of the patient should be coordinated, stopping so that the rescuers and the patient can be repositioned as needed to limit unwanted patient movement.
5. A rescuer should insert the foot end of the long spine board on the car seat at the patient's buttocks and should position the head end on the ambulance stretcher. Rotation of the patient continues until the patient can be positioned onto the long spine board.
6. The rescuers center and secure the patient on the long spine board as described later.

Two Rescuers (Fig. 25-15)

1. Rescuer 1 supports the patient's head and neck. Rescuer 1 uses manual in-line stabilization from behind the patient or from the patient's side. Rescuer 1 maintains this stabilization throughout the extrication process.
2. After a rapid initial assessment, Rescuer 2 applies a rigid cervical collar and places a prerolled blanket around the patient. Rescuer 2 places the center of the blanket roll at the patient's midline on the rigid cervical collar. Rescuer 2 then wraps the ends of the blanket roll around the cervical collar and places them under the patient's arms. Rescuer 2 positions a long spine board near the vehicle.
3. Using the ends of the blanket roll, the rescuers rotate the patient in a series of short, controlled movements so that the patient's back faces the open doorway. Each movement during the rotation of the patient should be coordinated, stopping so that the rescuers and the patient can be repositioned as needed to limit unwanted patient movement.
4. Rescuer 1 takes control of the blanket ends, moving them under the patient's shoulders, and moves the patient by the blanket while Rescuer 2 controls the patient's lower torso, pelvis, and legs.
5. The rescuers center and secure the patient on the long spine board as described next.

Long Spine Board with Supine Patient. Like short spine boards, long spine boards are available in a variety of configurations. These include plastic and synthetic spine

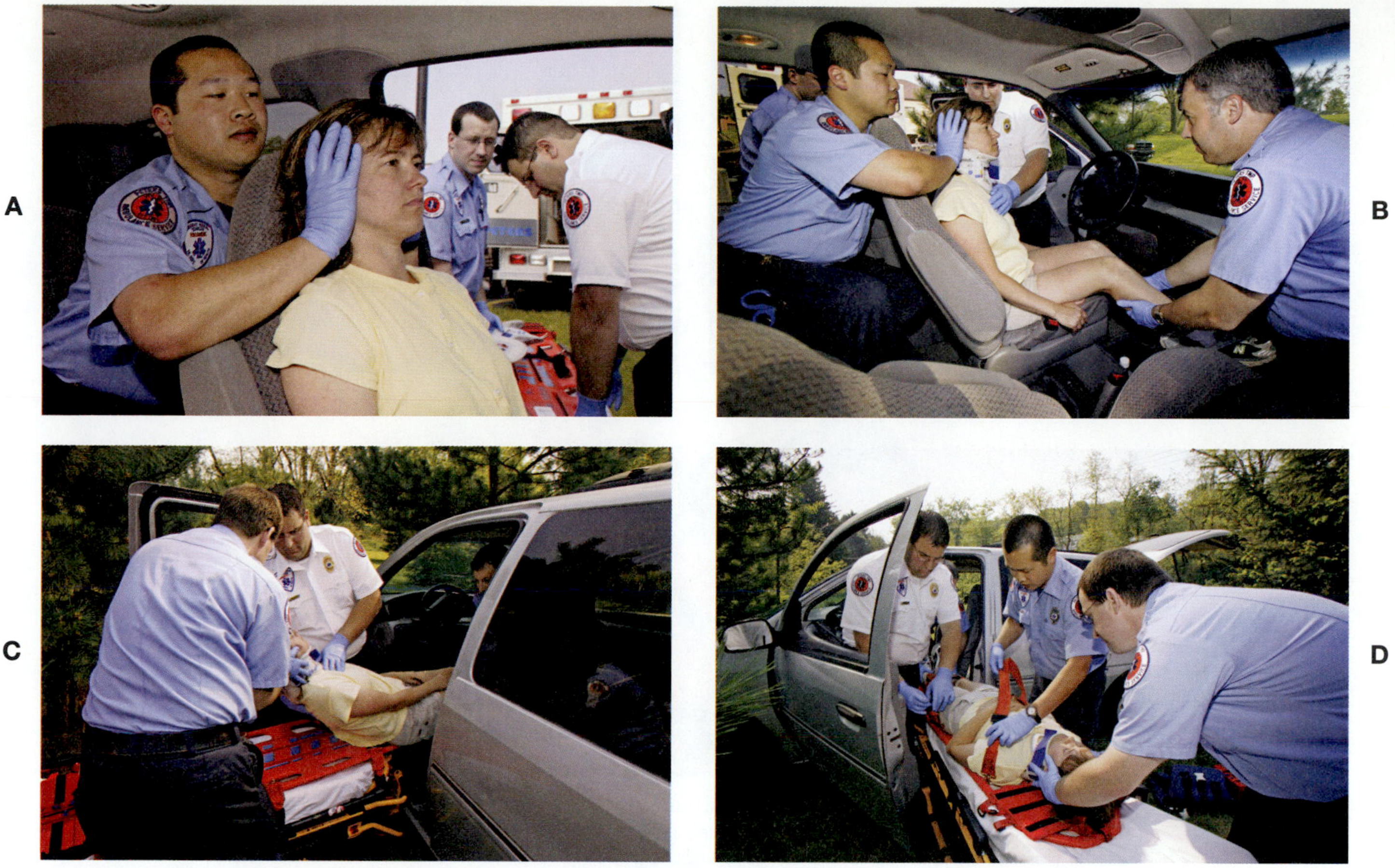

FIGURE 25-14 ■ **A,** Rescuer 1 supports the patient's head and neck and uses manual in-line stabilization throughout the procedure. **B,** After a rapid primary assessment, Rescuer 2 helps support the patient's midthorax as Rescuer 3 frees the patient's lower extremities for extrication. **C,** The rescuers carefully lower the patient onto the long spine board. **D,** The rescuers center and secure the patient on the long spine board.

boards, metal alloy spine boards, vacuum mattress splints, and split litters (scoop stretchers) that must be used along with a long spine board. The following description of securing patients on a long spine board may be applied to any long spinal immobilization device.

Immobilization of the torso to a long spine board must be done before immobilization of the head. This will prevent angulation of the cervical spine. The torso must not be allowed to move up, down, or to either side. Straps should be placed at the shoulders or chest to avoid compression and lateral movement of the thorax, around the midtorso, and across the iliac crest to prevent movement of the lower torso. The paramedic should take care not to tighten the straps to the point of reducing chest wall movement.

After immobilization of the torso, the head and neck should be immobilized in a neutral, in-line position. When most adults are placed on a long or short spinal device, a large space is produced between the back of the head and the spine board. Therefore noncompressible padding (e.g., commercial padding or folded towels) should be added (body shims). This can be done before securing the head (Fig. 25-16, *A*). The amount of padding required for in-line immobilization varies by patient and must be evaluated on an individual basis. Too little padding may cause hyperextension of the head, and too much padding may cause flexion; both may increase spinal cord damage. Children have proportionally larger heads than adults and may require padding under the torso to allow the head to lie in a neutral position on the board (Fig. 25-16, *B*). The padding (if needed) should be firm and should extend the full length and width of the torso from the buttocks to the top of the shoulders to prevent movement and misalignment of the spine.

The head is secured to the spinal device by placing commercial pads or rolled blankets on both sides of the head and securing them with the included straps, 2- to 3-inch tape strips, or a self-adhering firm wrap (e.g., Colban, Medi-Rip, or Elastoplast). (Elastic or gauze bandages do not prevent movement.) The upper forehead should be secured across the supraorbital ridge. The lower portion of the head should be secured across the anterior portion of the rigid cervical collar. Chin straps, sandbags, and intravenous bags are considered less optimal in immobilizing the head to a spinal device.

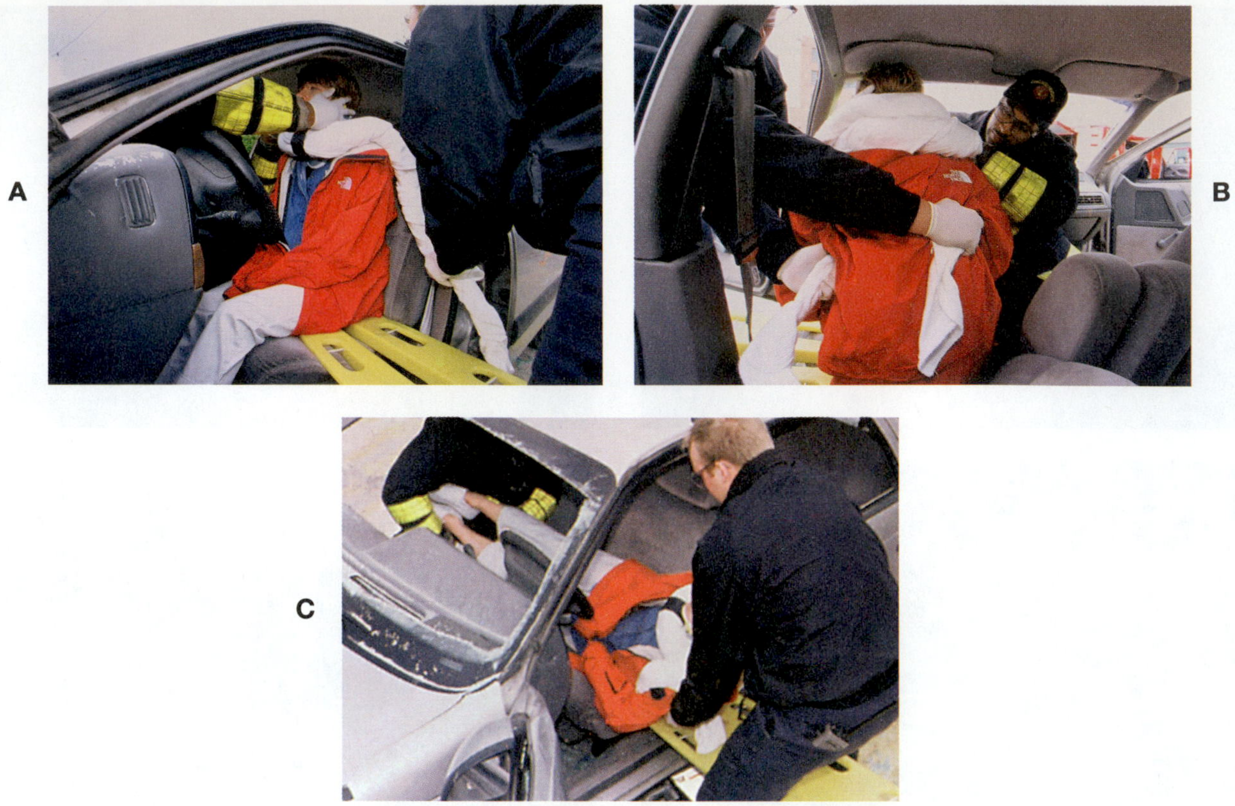

FIGURE 25-15 ■ **A,** Rescuer 1 suppports the patient's head and neck and uses manual in-line stabilization throughout the procedure. **B,** After assessment and application of a cervical collar, a rescuer positions the center of a blanket roll at the patient's midline on the cervical collar. The rescuer wraps the ends of the blanket roll around the cervical collar and places them under the patient's arms. **C,** The rescuers rotate the patient using the ends of the blanket roll until the patient's back faces the open doorway.

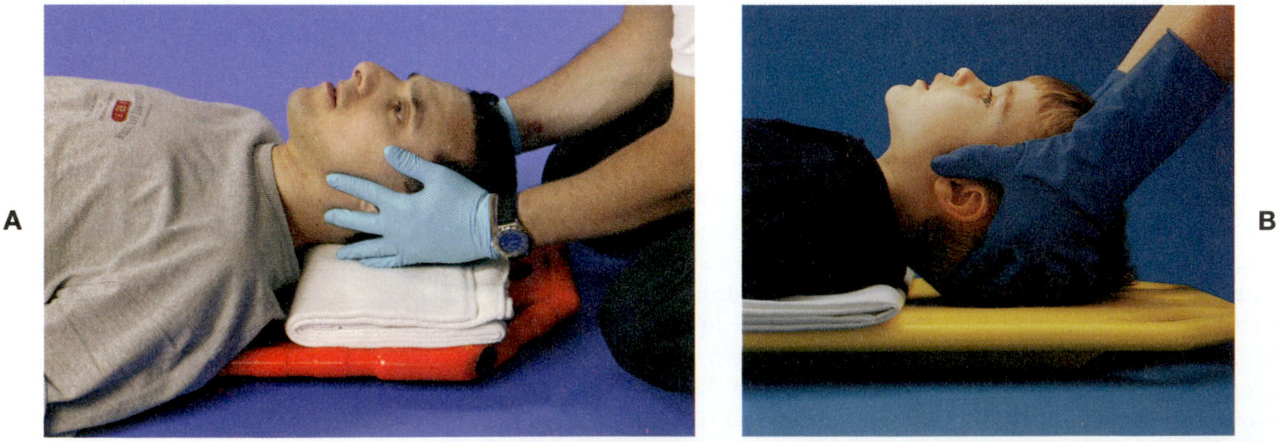

FIGURE 25-16 ■ Padding requirements for adult (**A**) and pediatric (**B**) patients.

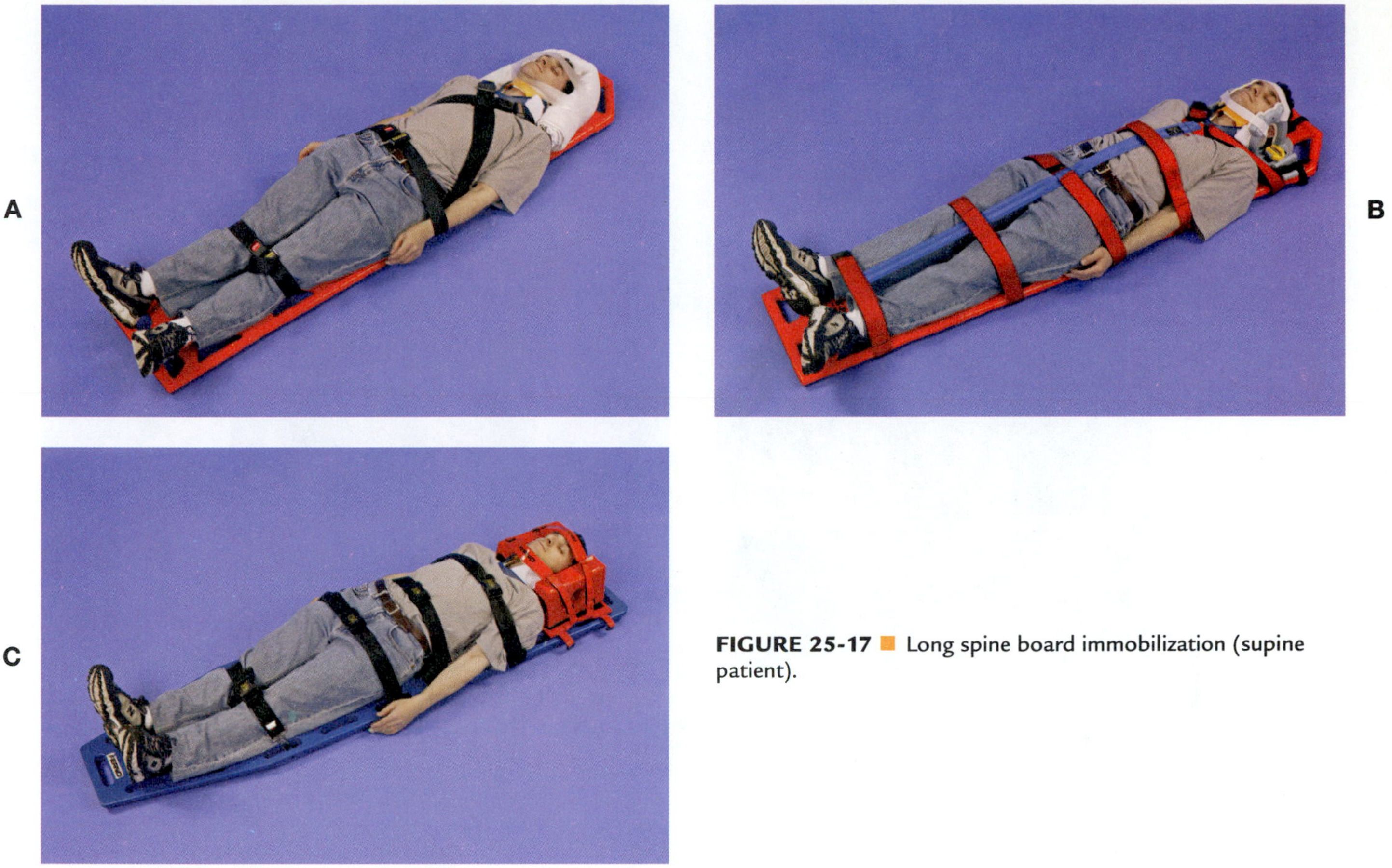

FIGURE 25-17 ■ Long spine board immobilization (supine patient).

The patient's legs should be secured to the long spine board. Two or more straps can be applied above and below the knees. Towels, blankets, or suitable padding may be placed on both sides of the patient's lower legs. This will minimize movement and will help to maintain the patient's central position on the spinal device (Fig. 25-17).

Before moving the patient, the patient's arms should be secured to the spinal device for safety. This is best achieved by placing the patient's arms at his or her side. (The patient's palms should be facing the body.) The arms should be secured with a separate strap placed across the forearms and torso.

Long Spine Board with Standing Patient. Patients who are standing also may be secured to a long spine board using the following technique (Fig. 25-18):

1. Rescuer 1 applies manual in-line immobilization from behind the patient or in front of the patient. Rescuer 1 maintains this position throughout the procedure. Rescuer 2 applies a rigid cervical collar
2. Rescuer 2 slides the long spine board behind the patient from the side and presses it against the patient.
3. Rescuers 2 and 3 stand on either side of the patient and insert the hand that is closest to the patient under the patient's armpit and grasp the nearest handhold of the backboard without moving the patient's shoulders. The rescuers grab the higher handhold on the board with their other hands and lower the patient and backboard to the ground while maintaining manual in-line immobilization.
4. Once on the ground, the rescuers secure the patient to the long backboard as described.

IMMOBILIZING PEDIATRIC PATIENTS

As with adult patients, prehospital care of a pediatric patient with suspected spine trauma should be managed with manual in-line immobilization, a rigid cervical collar, and a long spinal immobilization device. Many different pediatric immobilization devices are available from manufacturers (Fig. 25-19). If pediatric immobilization devices are not available, children may be secured on an adult long spine board. (A great deal of padding, however, is needed to fill voids. The padding also helps to prevent movement.)

Helmet Issues

The purpose of helmets is to protect the head and brain. Helmets are not intended to protect the neck. (This leaves the cervical spine open to injury.) The various types of helmets include full-face or open-face designs (used in motorcycling, bicycling, in-line skating, and other activities), and helmets designed for sports such as football and motocross. Factors that the paramedic should consider when determining the need to remove a helmet from an injured

A

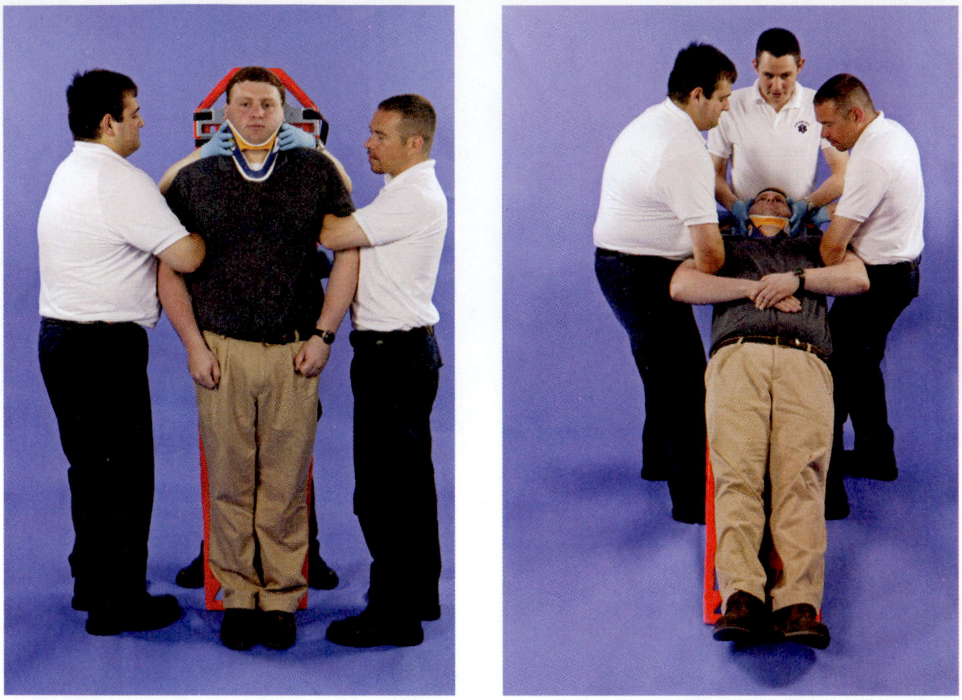

B

FIGURE 25-18 ■ **A,** While Rescuer 1 maintains manual in-line stabilization, Rescuers 2 and 3 support the patient. **B,** In one organized move the rescuers lower the patient to the ground onto the long spine board for further immobilization.

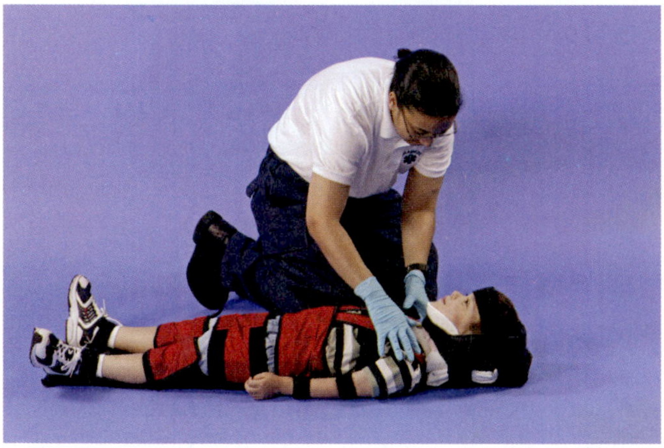

FIGURE 25-19 ■ Infant and pediatric immobilization board.

patient who requires airway management and spinal immobilization include the following:

- Athletic trainers may have special equipment (and training) to remove face pieces from sports helmets, allowing easier access to the patient's airway.
- Sports garb (e.g., shoulder pads) could compromise the cervical spine further if only the helmet were removed.
- The firm fit of a helmet may provide firm support for the patient's head.

Helmet Removal

Patients who are wearing full-face helmets must have the helmet removed early in the assessment process. Removing the helmet allows the rescuers to assess and manage a patient's airway and ventilatory status completely. In addition, rescuers can look for bleeding. The bleeding may be hidden by the helmet. They also can move the patient's head (from the flexed position cause by large helmets) into neutral alignment. The paramedic should consult with medical direction if the patient complains of increased pain during removal of the helmet or if the helmet is hard to remove in the field. The following steps in full-face helmet removal are recommended by the American College of Surgeons Committee on Trauma[4]:

1. Rescuer 1 immobilizes the helmet and head in an in-line position (Fig. 25-20). Rescuer presses his or her palms on each side of the helmet with the fingertips curled over the lower margin of the helmet.
2. Rescuer 2 removes the face shield and chin strap. Rescuer 2 assesses the patient's airway and ventilatory status.
3. Rescuer 2 grasps the patient's mandible by placing the thumb at the angle of the mandible on one side and two fingers at the angle on the other side. Rescuer 2 places his or her other hand under the neck at the base of the skull, taking over in-line immobilization of the patient's head.
4. Rescuer 1 carefully spreads the sides of the helmet away from the patient's head and ears. Rescuer 1 then rotates the helmet rotated toward the rescuer to clear the patient's nose. Rescuer 1 then removes the helmet from the patient's head in a straight line. Just before removing the helmet from under the patient's head, Rescuer 1 assumes in-line immobilization by squeezing the sides of the helmet against the patient's head.
5. Rescuer 2 repositions his or her hands to support the head and to prevent it from dropping as the helmet is re-

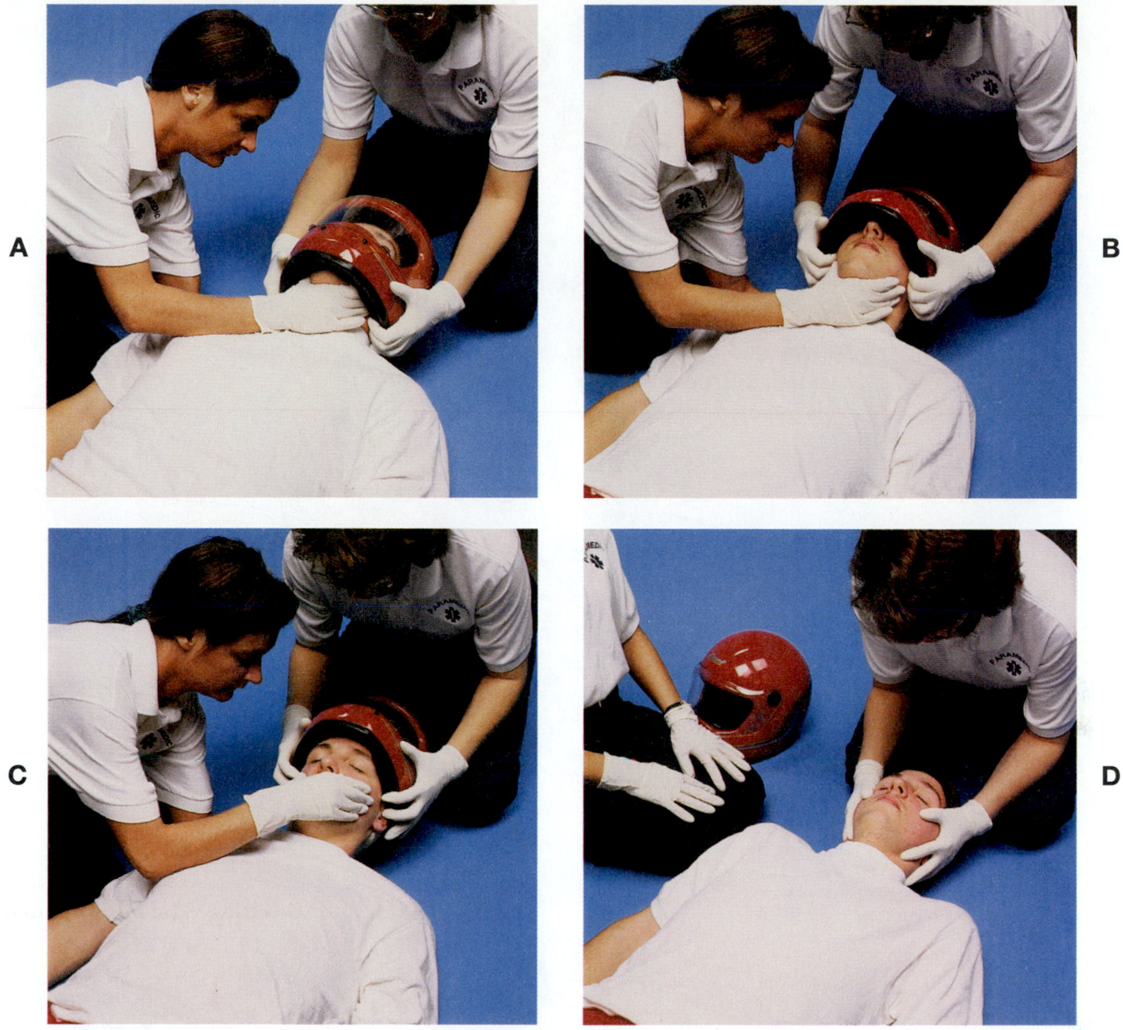

FIGURE 25-20 ■ **A,** Rescuer 1 immobilizes the helmet and head in an in-line position. Rescuer 2 grasps the patient's mandible by placing the thumb at the angle of the mandible on one side and two fingers at the angle on the other side. Rescuer 2 places the other hand under the patient's neck at the base of the skull, producing in-line immobilization of the patient's head. **B,** Rescuer 1 carefully spreads the sides of the helmet away from the patient's head and ears. **C,** Rescuer 1 then rotates the helmet toward the rescuer to clear the nose and remove it from the patient's head in a straight line. **D,** After the removal of the helmet, Rescuer 1 applies in-line immobilization. Another rescuer applies a rigid cervical collar.

moved completely. This is accomplished by the rescuer placing a hand farther up on the occipital area of the head and by grasping the maxilla with the thumb and first fingers of the other hand on each side of the nose. After securing this position, Rescuer 2 takes over in-line immobilization.

6. Rescuer 1 rotates the helmet about 30 degrees, following the curvature of the patient's head. Rescuer 1 completely removes the helmet by carefully pulling it in a straight line.
7. After removal of the helmet, Rescuer 1 applies in-line immobilization, and Rescuer 2 applies a rigid cervical collar.

> **NOTE** A key point to remember during helmet removal is that in-line immobilization must be maintained throughout the procedure. Thus the rescuers should never remove their hands from the patient at the same time. In addition, the helmet must be rotated in one direction to clear the nose. The helmet must be rotated in the opposite direction to clear the back of the patient's head.

Spinal Immobilization in Diving Incidents

Most diving incidents involve injury to the patient's head, neck, and spine. If the patient is still in the water when emergency medical services arrives, the patient should be managed as follows:

1. Ensure scene and personal safety. Only rescuers trained in water rescue should enter the water (Fig. 25-21).

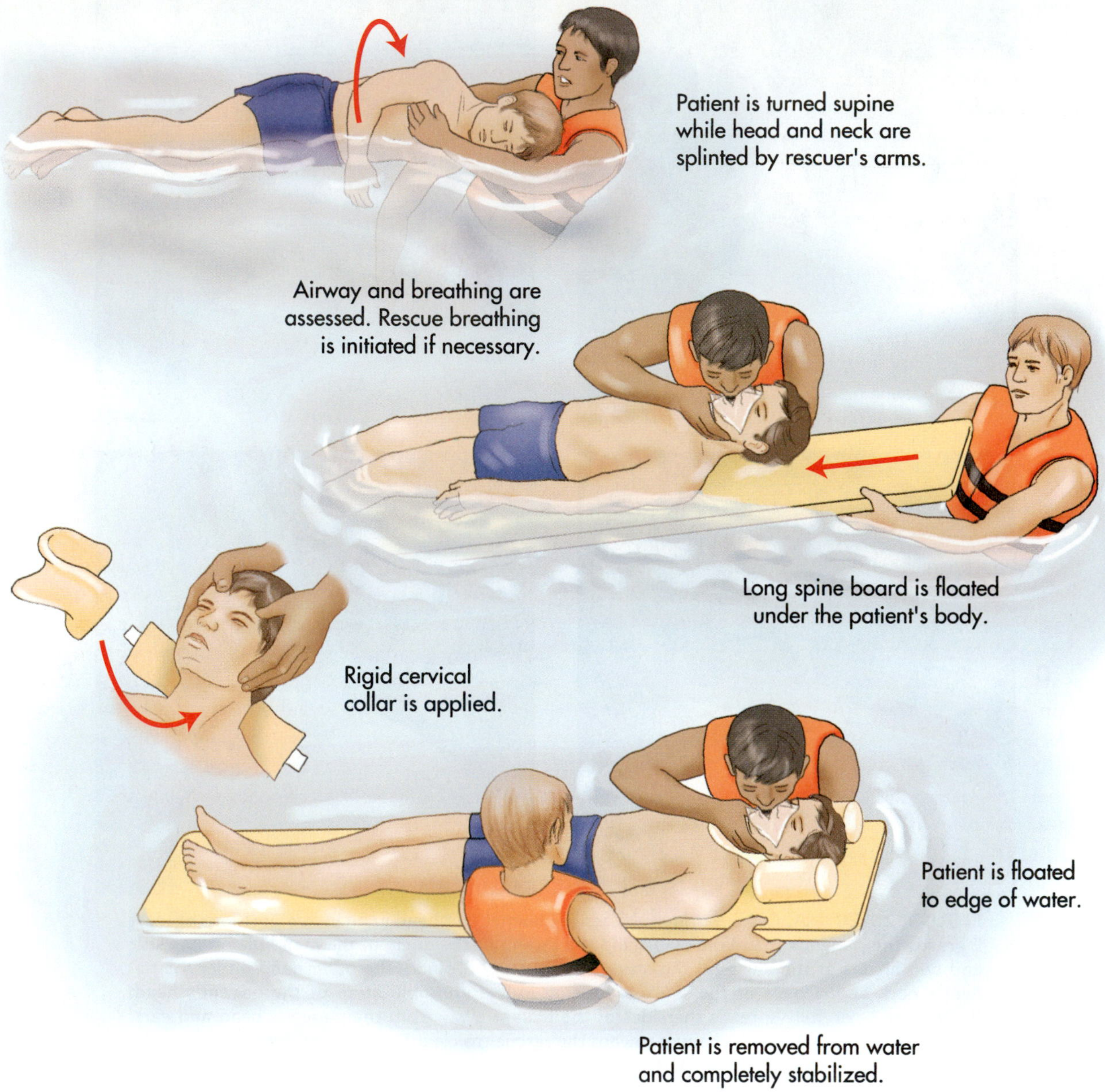

Patient is turned supine while head and neck are splinted by rescuer's arms.
Airway and breathing are assessed. Rescue breathing is initiated if necessary.
Long spine board is floated under the patient's body.
Rigid cervical collar is applied.
Patient is floated to edge of water.
Patient is removed from water and completely stabilized.

FIGURE 25-21 ■ Extrication of a diving accident victim. Rescue breathing with barrier protection can begin in the water.

2. Float a supine patient to a shallow area without unnecessary movement of the spine.
3. Approach a prone patient from the top of the head. Position one arm under the patient to support the head, neck, and torso. Place the other arm across the patient's head and back, splinting the head and neck between the rescuer's arms. Carefully turn the patient to a supine position and quickly assess airway and breathing. (The paramedic may initiate rescue breathing while in the water.)
4. A second rescuer slides a long spine board or other rigid device under the patient's body while the first rescuer continues to support the patient's head and neck without flexion or extension. Apply a rigid cervical collar. Maintain manual in-line immobilization throughout the rescue.
5. Float the spinal immobilization device to the edge of the water and lift it out.
6. The patient should be immobilized completely on the long spine board as previously described.

CORD INJURY PRESENTATIONS

Three cord injury presentations deserve special mention. These include spinal shock, **neurogenic hypotension,** and autonomic hyperreflexia syndrome.

Spinal Shock

Spinal shock refers to a temporary loss of all types of spinal cord function distal to the injury. Signs and symptoms of spinal shock include flaccid paralysis distal to the injury site and loss of autonomic function, which may be demonstrated by hypotension, vasodilation, loss of bowel and bladder control, priapism, and loss of thermoregulation. Spinal shock does not always involve permanent, primary injury. The autonomic dysfunction usually resolves within 24 hours. Rarely, though, spinal shock may last a few days to a few weeks. Careful handling of these patients to avoid secondary injury is crucial. Initial management includes full spinal immobilization, high-concentration oxygen administration, positioning the secured patient in a Trendelenburg position (elevating the foot end of the long spine board) providing it does not impair ventilation, and administering crystalloids intravenously (per protocol).

Neurogenic Hypotension

Neurogenic hypotension (neurogenic shock) following spinal shock results from the blockade of vasoregulatory fibers, motor fibers, and sensory fibers. This block produces a loss of sympathetic tone to the vessels or vasodilation. Patients with neurogenic hypotension often have relative hypotension (a systolic blood pressure of 80 to 100 mm Hg); warm, dry, and pink skin (from cutaneous vasodilation); and relative bradycardia.

Neurogenic hypotension is rare. Initially, it should not be considered as a cause of hypovolemia in the patient with a spine injury. The paramedic should consider other causes of hypotension, including internal hemorrhage, cardiac tamponade, and tension pneumothorax. If hypotension is severe, the paramedic should initate shock management (per protocol).

Autonomic Hyperreflexia Syndrome

Autonomic hyperreflexia syndrome may occur after resolution of spinal shock and is associated with chronic SCI in patients who have injuries at T6 or above.[3] (The syndrome often is caused by a distended bladder or rectum.) The effects of this syndrome result from a massive, uncompensated cardiovascular response that stimulates the sympathetic nervous system. The stimulation of sensory receptors below the level of cord injury causes the intact autonomic nervous system to respond with spasms of the arterioles. These spasms in turn increase blood pressure. The baroreceptors sense the rise in blood pressure. They stimulate the parasympathetic nervous system. This decreases heart rate and sends the message to the peripheral and visceral vessels to dilate. Because of the cord injury, however, vasodilation is not possible. Thus blood pressure continues to rise and could pose a threat to life. The characteristics of this syndrome include the following:

- Paroxysmal hypertension (up to 300 mm Hg)
- Pounding headache
- Blurred vision
- Sweating (above the level of injury) with flushing of the skin
- Increased nasal congestion
- Nausea
- Bradycardia (30 to 40 beats/min)
- Distended bladder or rectum

Emptying of the bladder or bowel often relieves the syndrome. Blood pressure may need to be controlled with antihypertensive agents. These patients are best managed in the hospital setting under close physician supervision.

NONTRAUMATIC SPINAL CONDITIONS

The nontraumatic spinal conditions to be discussed in this chapter include low back pain, degenerative disk disease, spondylosis, herniated intervertebral disk, and spinal cord tumors.

Low Back Pain

Between 60% and 90% of the U.S. population is estimated to experience some form of low back pain.[5] Low back pain usually affects the area between the lower rib cage and the gluteal muscles. The pain often radiates into the thighs. About 1% of those with low back pain have sciatica. (This is pain in the lumbar nerve root accompanied by neurosensory and motor deficits in the thigh and leg.) Most low back pain is idiopathic. That makes a precise diagnosis difficult. Causes of this condition include the following:

- Tension from tumors
- Disk prolapse
- Bursitis
- Synovitis
- Degenerative joint disease
- Abnormal bone pressure
- Inflammation caused by infection (e.g., osteomyelitis)
- Fractures
- Ligament strains

CRITICAL THINKING

What are some other medical conditions that may cause the patient to have a chief complaint of low back pain?

Risk factors associated with low back pain include occupations that require repetitive lifting, exposure to vibrations from vehicles or industrial machinery, and osteoporosis (elderly women report more symptoms than men).

Low back pain must come from innervated structures. However, deep pain and the way it is referred to other parts of the body vary by individual. Although the disk has no specific innervation, irritation of surrounding membranes that have pain receptors often occurs. (This occurs especially in the presence of disk prolapse.) The source of most low back pain occurs at L3, L4, L5, and S1. Other areas of abundant pain receptors are found in anterior and posterior longitudinal ligaments that are vulnerable to strains and sprains.

Degenerative Disk Disease

Degenerative disk disease is a common finding in persons older than 50 years of age. The causes of this condition include deterioration of the tissue of the intervertebral disk that occur with aging. The associated narrowing of the disk results in instability of the spine and can cause occasional low back pain.

Spondylosis

Spondylosis is a structural defect of the spine. It involves the lamina or vertebral arch. Spondylosis usually occurs in the lumbar spine between superior and inferior articulating surfaces. (Rotational stress fractures are common at the affected site.) Heredity appears to be a key factor for this condition.

Herniated Intervertebral Disk

Herniated intervertebral disk (herniated nucleus pulposus) refers to a tear in the posterior rim of the capsule that encloses the gelatinous center of the disk. Rupture of the disk usually is caused by trauma, degenerative disk disease, and improper lifting (most common). Men between the ages of 30 and 50 are more prone to develop this condition. Disks that most commonly are affected are L5-S1 and L4-L5. (Herniated intervertebral disk also at times occurs in the cervical area at C5-C6 and C6-C7.) These injuries may have an immediate onset. They also may develop over months to years.

Spinal Cord Tumors

Tumors in the spinal cord may develop from cord compression, degenerative changes in bones and joints, or from an interruption in the blood supply to the cord. These tumors are classified by cell type, growth rate, and structure of origin. Clinical manifestations depend on tumor type and location. The manifestations may include bilateral or asymmetrical motor dysfunction, paresis, spasticity, pain, temperature dysfunction, sensory changes, and other abnormalities.

ASSESSMENT AND MANAGEMENT OF NONTRAUMATIC SPINAL CONDITIONS

As stated before, nontraumatic spinal conditions such as low back pain are difficult to diagnose. The assessment and management are based on the patient's chief complaint, the physical examination, and through the evaluation of associated risk factors. Signs and symptoms that commonly are seen with nontraumatic spinal conditions include the following:

- Discomfort
- Difficulty in standing erect
- Pain with straining (e.g., coughing, sneezing)
- Limited range of motion
- Alterations in sensation, pain, and temperature
- Upper extremity pain or paresthesia that increases with motion
- Motor weakness

The management of patients with back pain in the prehospital setting mainly is supportive. Management focuses on decreasing the patient's pain and discomfort. Some patients are best managed with immobilization on a full spine board or vacuum-type stretcher. These devices prevent movement. Full spinal immobilization is not required unless the condition is a result of trauma. The in-hospital evaluation may include various testing such as computed tomography, electromyelography, and magnetic resonance imaging.

SUMMARY

- Most SCIs are the result of motor vehicle crashes. Other causes are falls, penetrating injuries from acts of human violence, and sport injuries.
- The paramedic can classify the MOI as positive, negative, or uncertain. This classification is combined with the clinical guidelines for evaluating SCI, which include the following signs and symptoms: pain, tenderness, painful movement, deformity, cuts/bruises over spinal area, paralysis, paresthesias, and weakness. This system can help to identify cases in which spinal immobilization is appropriate.
- The spinal column is composed of 33 vertebrae. These are divided into five sections. The sections are 7 cervical, 12 thoracic, 5 lumbar, 5 sacral (fused), and 4 coccygeal (fused).
- The specific mechanisms of injury that frequently cause spinal trauma are axial loading; extremes of flexion, hyperextension, or hyperrotation; excessive lateral bending; and distraction.
- Spinal injuries may be classified as sprains and strains, fractures and dislocations, sacral and coccygeal fractures, and cord injuries. The spinal cord may sustain a primary or a secondary injury. Lesions (transections) of the spinal cord are classified as complete or incomplete.

- With spinal injuries, the first priority is to evaluate and manage any threats to life. The second priority is to preserve spinal cord function. This includes avoiding secondary injury to the spinal cord. These goals are best met by maintaining a high degree of suspicion for the presence of spinal trauma, by providing early spinal immobilization, by rapidly correcting any volume deficit, and by administering oxygen.
- General principles of spinal immobilization include prevention of further injury; treating the spine as a long bone with a joint at either end (the head and pelvis); always using complete spinal immobilization; beginning spinal immobilization in the initial assessment and maintaining it until the spine is immobilized completely on the long spine board; and, placing the patient's head in a neutral, in-line position, unless contraindicated.
- Spinal shock refers to a temporary loss of all types of spinal cord function distal to the injury.
- Neurogenic shock produces a loss of sympathetic tone to the vessels. This causes relative hypotension; warm, dry, and pink skin; and relative bradycardia.
- Autonomic hyperreflexia syndrome results from a massive, uncompensated cardiovascular response that stimulates the sympathetic nervous system. This response in turn causes an increase in blood pressure and other symptoms.
- Some nontraumatic spinal conditions include low back pain, degenerative disk disease, spondylolysis, herniated intervertebral disk, and spinal cord tumors. The management of patients with nontraumatic back pain in the prehospital setting is mainly supportive. The goal is to help patients decrease their pain and discomfort.

REFERENCES

1. Rosen P, Barkin R: *Emergency medicine: concepts and clinical practice,* ed 5, St Louis, 2003, Mosby.
2. Foundation for Spinal Cord Injury Prevention: *Spinal cord injury facts,* Detroit, 1999, National Spinal Cord Injury Statistical Center. www.fscip.org/facts.
3. US Department of Transportation, National Highway Traffic Safety Administration: *EMT-Paramedic national standard curriculum,* Washington, DC, 1998, The Department.
4. National Association of Emergency Medical Technicians: *PHTLS: basic and advanced prehospital life support,* ed 5, St Louis, 2003, Mosby.
5. McCance K, Huether S: *Pathophysiology: the biological basis for disease in adults and children,* ed 2, St Louis, 1994, Mosby.

CHAPTER 26

Thoracic Trauma

OBJECTIVES

Upon completion of this chapter, the paramedic student will be able to:

1. Discuss the factor and mechanism of injury associated with thoracic trauma.
2. Describe the mechanism of injury, signs and symptoms, and management of skeletal injuries to the chest.
3. Describe the mechanism of injury, signs and symptoms, and prehospital management of pulmonary trauma.
4. Describe the mechanism of injury, signs and symptoms, and prehospital management of injuries to the heart and great vessels.
5. Outline the mechanism of injury, signs and symptoms, and prehospital care of the patient with esophageal and tracheobronchial injury and diaphragmatic rupture.

KEY TERMS

Beck triad: A combination of three symptoms that characterize cardiac tamponade: elevated central venous pressure, muffled heart sounds, and hypotension.

closed pneumothorax: A collection of air or gas in the pleural space that causes the lung to collapse without exposing the pleural space to atmospheric pressure.

flail chest: A chest wall injury in which three or more adjacent ribs are fractured in two or more places.

hemothorax: The accumulation of blood and other fluid in the pleural space caused by bleeding from the lung parenchyma or damaged vessels.

open pneumothorax: A chest wall injury that exposes the pleural space to atmospheric pressure.

pulmonary contusion: Bruising of the lung tissue that results in rupture of the alveoli and interstitial edema.

tension pneumothorax: An accumulation of air or gas in the pleural cavity that can lead to collapse of the lung.

traumatic asphyxia: A severe crushing injury to the chest and abdomen that causes an increase in the intrathoracic pressure. The increased pressure forces blood from the right side of the heart into the veins of the upper thorax, neck, and face.

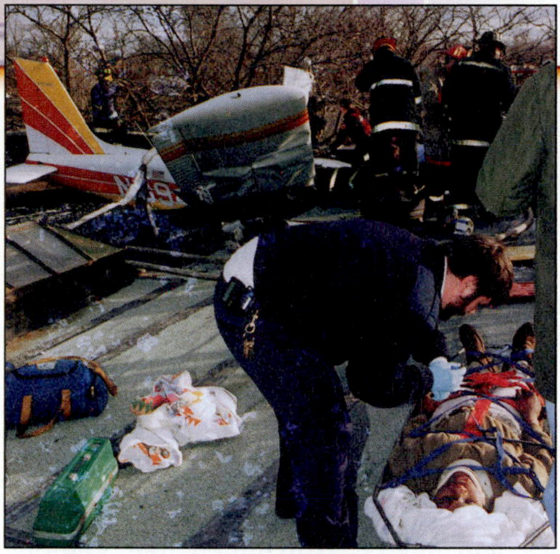

Chest injuries are directly responsible for more than 20% of all traumatic deaths (regardless of mechanism) and account for about 16,000 deaths per year in the United States.[1] Chest injuries are caused by blunt trauma, penetrating trauma, or both. They often are the result of motor vehicle crashes, falls from heights, blast injuries, blows to the chest, chest compression, gunshot wounds, and stab wounds. Thoracic trauma may be classified as skeletal injury, pulmonary injury, heart and great vessel injury, and diaphragmatic injury. (Anterior neck trauma is discussed in Chapter 24.)

SKELETAL INJURY

Skeletal injuries may be caused by blunt or penetrating trauma. The injuries discussed in this chapter include clavicular fractures, rib fractures, flail chest, and sternal fractures (see Chapter 6 for a review of the structures that make up the thoracic cavity).

Clavicular Fractures

The clavicle is the most commonly fractured bone. An isolated clavicular fracture is seldom a significant injury (Fig. 26-1). It is common in children who fall on their shoulders or outstretched arms. It also is common in athletes involved in contact sports. Treatment usually involves applying a clavicle strap or a sling and swathe that immobilizes the affected shoulder and arm (see Chapter 28). These injuries usually heal well within 4 to 6 weeks.

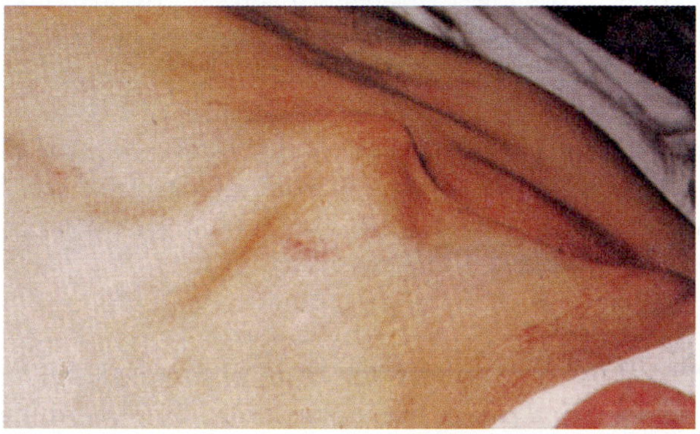

FIGURE 26-1 ■ Fracture of the left clavicle seen from above the left shoulder. (From London PS: *A colour atlas of diagnosis after recent injury.* Ipswich, England, 1990, Wolfe Medical Publications.)

Signs and symptoms of clavicular fractures include pain, point tenderness, and evident deformity. The subclavian vein or artery may be injured when the clavicle is broken. Bony fragments from the fracture may puncture a vessel, resulting in a hematoma or venous thrombosis. However, this is rare.

Rib Fractures

Rib fractures most often occur on the lateral aspect of the third through eighth ribs, where the ribs are least protected by musculature (Fig. 26-2). Fractures are more likely to occur in adults than in children. This is because younger patients have more resilient cartilage. Morbidity or mortality from rib fractures depends on the patient's age and the number and location of the fractures.

> **CRITICAL THINKING**
> Why would you expect greater underlying pulmonary injury in a child versus an adult with rib fractures?

Simple rib fractures usually are very painful. However, they rarely are life-threatening. Most patients can localize the fracture by pointing to the area. (This is confirmed by palpation.) Sometimes movement or grating of the bone ends *(crepitus)* can be felt. One complication of rib fracture is splinting, which leads to atelectasis. Another complication is ventilation-perfusion mismatch (ventilated alveoli that are not perfused or perfused alveoli that are not ventilated). The goal of treatment is to relieve the pain. The paramedic should en-

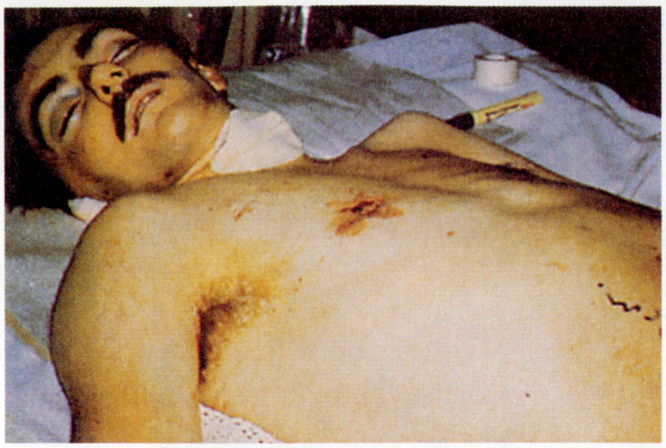

FIGURE 26-2 ■ Chest wall asymmetry caused by rib fractures. (From London PS: *A colour atlas of diagnosis after recent injury.* Ipswich, England, 1990, Wolfe Medical Publications.)

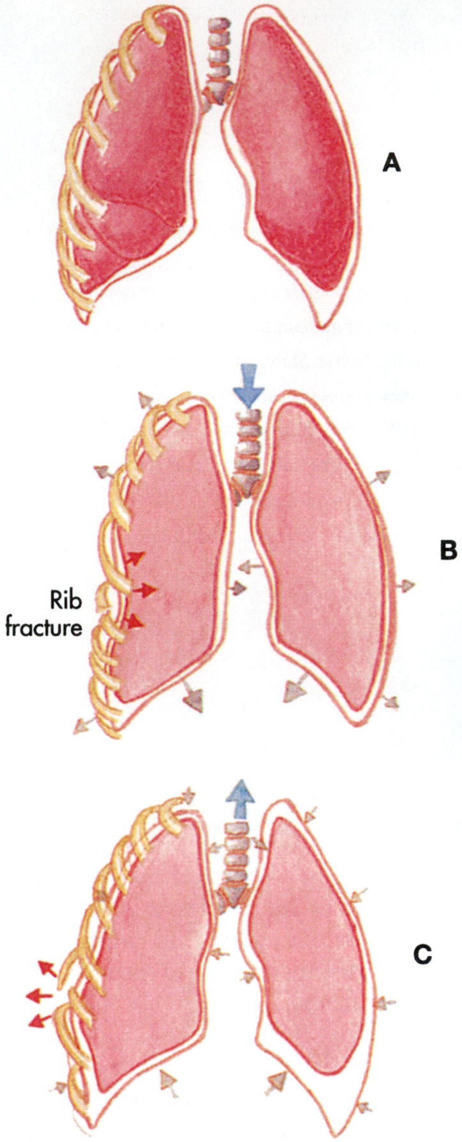

FIGURE 26-3 ■ Flail chest. **A,** Normal lungs. **B,** Flail chest during inspiration. **C,** Flail chest during expiration.

courage the patient to cough and to breathe deeply. Pain may be relieved by splinting the patient's arm against the chest wall with a sling and swathe. (Circumferential splinting should not be used.) Administration of analgesics per protocol also may help. Based on the mechanism of injury, the paramedic should consider the possibility of more serious trauma, such as closed pneumothorax and internal bleeding. Fractures to the lower ribs (eighth through twelfth) may be associated with injuries to the spleen, kidneys, or liver.

Great force is required to fracture the first and second ribs. This is due to their shape. It also is due to the protected location of these ribs provided by the scapulae, clavicles, and upper chest musculature. Fractures of the first and second ribs may be associated with myocardial contusion, bronchial tears, and vascular injury.

Flail Chest

A **flail chest** may occur when three or more adjacent ribs are fractured in two or more places (Fig. 26-3). This injury usually is not detected in the prehospital setting. This is because of the muscle spasm that accompanies the injury. Within 2 hours after the injury, however, the muscle spasm subsides. At that point, the injured segment of the chest wall may begin to move in a paradoxical (contrary) fashion with inspiration and expiration.

> **NOTE** In paradoxical breathing, part of the lung deflates during inspiration and inflates during expiration. This condition commonly is associated with chest trauma. An open chest wound or a rib cage injury is an example of this type of trauma.

Causes of flail chest include vehicle crashes, falls, industrial accidents, assault, and birth trauma. The mortality rate is 20% to 40% because of associated injuries.[2] The mortality rate increases with advanced age, seven or more rib fractures, three or more associated injuries, shock, and head injury.

During inspiration the diaphragm descends. This lowers the intrapleural pressure. The unstable chest wall is pushed ("sucked") inward by the negative intrathoracic pressure as the rest of the chest wall expands. During expiration, the diaphragm rises, and the intrapleural pressure exceeds atmospheric pressure. This causes the unstable chest wall to move outward. Patients with flail chest often develop hypoxia. This is because of the lung contusions usually related to this injury. Bleeding from the alveoli and the lung tissue causes the contusion. It is associated with decreased vital capacity and vascular shunting of deoxygenated blood. Signs and symptoms of flail chest include tenderness and bony crepitus on palpation and paradoxical motion (a late sign).

Prehospital management of patients with flail chest includes assisting ventilation with positive pressure by means of a bag-valve-mask, use of high-concentration supplemental oxygen, and fluid replacement as needed. Field stabilization of the flail segment is controversial. In one method, the paramedic tries to splint the flail segment in the inward position with simple hand pressure, bulky dressings, or towels taped to the chest wall. This splinting can reduce vital capacity. However, it may increase the efficiency of ventilation. Many authorities recommend intubation and positive-pressure ventilation (internal splinting) in patients with respiratory distress and a flail chest. Intubation also may be indicated if the chest injury is associated with shock, other severe injuries, head injury, or pulmonary disease, or if it occurs in a patient over 65 years of age. A large percentage of patients with significant chest injury progress to respiratory failure. This requires long-term ventilatory support and hospitalization. Prehospital use of positive end-expiratory pressure (PEEP) to keep alveoli open at the end of exhalation may be recommended by some medical direction agencies. This procedure requires special equipment and training (see Chapter 30).

CRITICAL THINKING

Why is positive-pressure ventilation the treatment of choice for this injury?

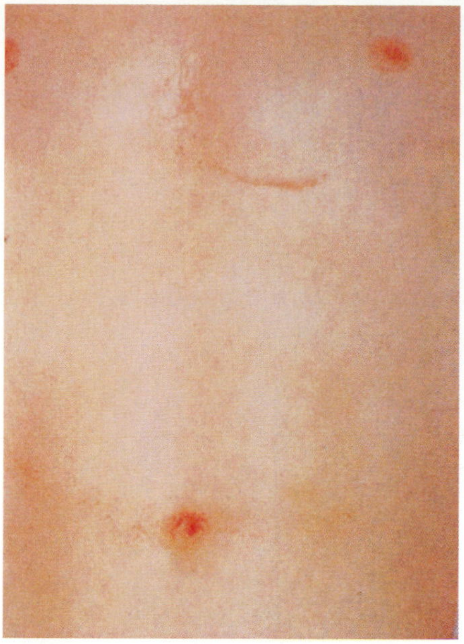

FIGURE 26-4 ■ Well-marked band of spotty bruising caused by a steering wheel impact. (From London PS: *A colour atlas of diagnosis after recent injury.* Ipswich, England, 1990, Wolfe Medical Publications.)

Sternal Fractures

Sternal fractures are uncommon but serious. They usually result from a direct blow to the chest (e.g., striking a steering column or dashboard) or from a massive crush injury (Fig. 26-4). Sternal fractures usually are very painful. They may be associated with an unstable chest wall, myocardial injury, or cardiac tamponade. They occur in only 5% to 8% of patients with blunt chest trauma. However, the mortality rate is 25% to 45%.[2] Signs and symptoms include a history of significant anterior chest trauma, tenderness, and abnormal motion or crepitation over the sternum. Prehospital management includes maintaining a high degree of suspicion for associated injuries, airway maintenance, ventilatory support, electrocardiographic (ECG) monitoring, and rapid transport to an appropriate medical facility. Associated injuries that often contribute to serious disability or death include the following:

- Pulmonary and myocardial contusion
- Flail chest
- Vascular disruption of thoracic vessels (rare)
- Intraabdominal injuries
- Head injury

Pulmonary Injury

Pulmonary injuries may be classified as closed pneumothorax, tension pneumothorax, open pneumothorax, hemothorax, pulmonary contusion, and traumatic asphyxia. Any of these injuries can result in difficulty in breathing (respiratory insufficiency). Prehospital treatment must be directed at ensuring an open airway, providing ventilatory support, correcting immediately life-threatening ventilatory problems (e.g., tension pneumothorax), and rapid transport for definitive care.

CLOSED PNEUMOTHORAX

A **closed pneumothorax** (simple pneumothorax) is caused by the presence of air in the pleural space. This air causes the lung to partly or totally collapse (Fig. 26-5). A common cause of pneumothorax is a fractured rib that penetrates the underlying lung. Pneumothoraces also may occur without rib fractures. They may be caused by excessive pressure on the chest wall against a closed glottis (paper bag effect; see Chapter 20). They also may be caused by rupture or tearing of the lung parenchyma and visceral pleura from no demonstrable cause (spontaneous pneumothorax). Closed pneumothorax occurs in 10% to 30% of patients with blunt chest trauma and in almost 100% of patients with penetrating chest trauma.[2]

CRITICAL THINKING

How does high-flow oxygen promote faster resolution of a closed pneumothorax?

The signs and symptoms of a closed pneumothorax include chest pain, dyspnea, and tachypnea. Breath sounds may be diminished or absent on the affected side. Treatment includes ventilatory support with high-concentration oxygen. The patient should be watched carefully for signs of a tension pneumothorax. The person should be transported in a semisitting position of comfort unless this position is contraindicated by the mechanism of injury. If

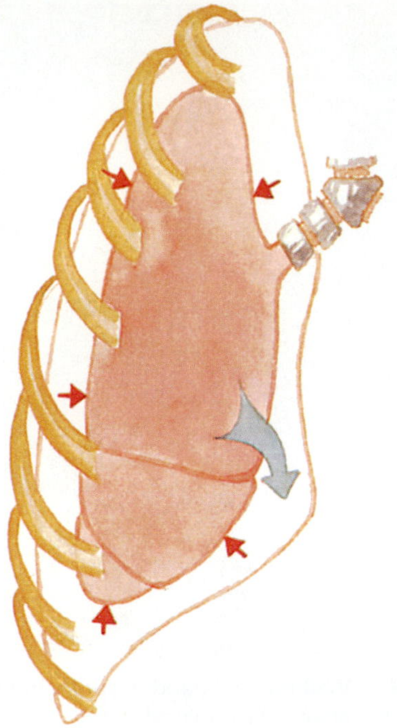

FIGURE 26-5 ■ Closed (simple) pneumothorax.

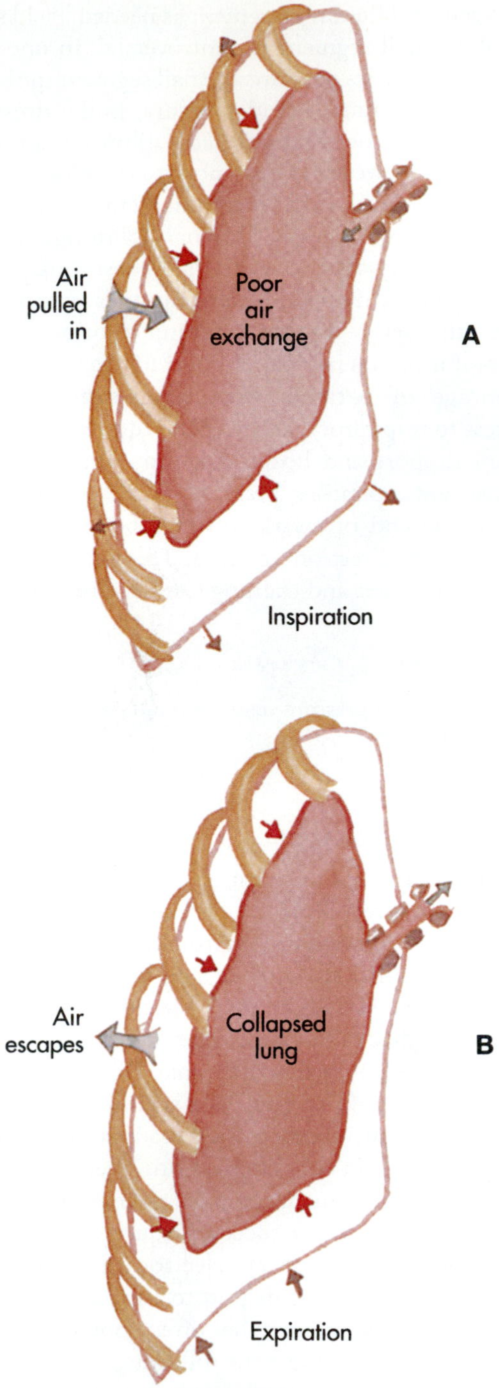

FIGURE 26-6 ■ Open pneumothorax. **A,** Air enters the pleural cavity during inspiration. **B,** Air exits the pleural cavity during expiration.

the patient's respiratory rate is below 12 or above 28 breaths per minute, ventilatory assistance with a bag-valve-mask may be indicated.

Most healthy patients have large circulatory and ventilatory reserve capacities. Therefore closed pneumothoraces usually do not pose a threat to life. However, life-threatening consequences may develop if the pneumothorax is a tension pneumothorax, if it occupies more than 40% of the hemithorax, or if it occurs in a patient with shock or preexisting pulmonary or cardiovascular diseases.

Open Pneumothorax

An **open pneumothorax** develops when a chest injury exposes the pleural space to atmospheric pressure (Fig. 26-6). The severity of the injury is directly proportional to the size of the wound. When a chest wound is larger than the normal pathway for air through the nose and mouth, atmospheric pressure forces the air through the open wound and into the thoracic cavity during inspiration. As the air builds up in the pleural space, the lung on the injured side collapses. The lung begins to shift toward the uninjured side. Very little air enters the tracheobronchial tree to be exchanged with intrapulmonary air on the affected side. This results in decreased alveolar ventilation and decreased perfusion. The normal side also is adversely affected. That is because expired air may enter the lung on the collapsed side. It then is rebreathed into the functioning lung with the next ventilation. This may result in severe ventilatory dysfunction, hypoxemia, and death unless the situation is quickly recognized and corrected.

> **NOTE** A small open chest wound may function like a ball-valve mechanism. That is, it may allow air in but not out. The accumulation of air may result in a shift in the patient's mediastinum, reducing the preload.

Signs and symptoms of open pneumothorax include shortness of breath, pain, and a sucking or gurgling sound as air moves in and out of the pleural space through the open chest wound (thus the term *sucking chest wound*). Prehospital

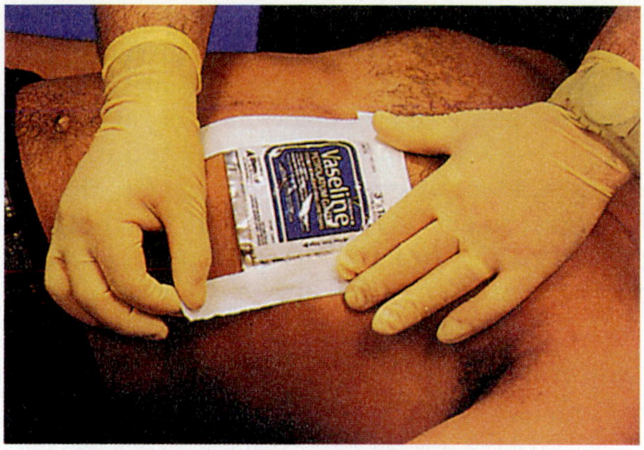

FIGURE 26-7 ■ Sealing a chest wound.

treatment of an open pneumothorax proceeds as follows (Fig. 26-7):

1. Close the chest wound. This can be done by applying a sterile plastic dressing and securing it with tape. Medical direction may advise that only three sides of the dressing be taped. This provides a venting mechanism (or one-way valve). It also allows spontaneous decompression of a developing tension pneumothorax. The paramedic should closely monitor for the development of a tension pneumothorax if the patient's dressing does not provide a venting mechanism.
2. Provide ventilatory support with high-concentration oxygen. Airway management includes assisting ventilations with a bag-valve device and intubation.
3. Treat the patient for shock by administering crystalloid per protocol.
4. Rapidly transport the patient to an appropriate medical facility.

Tension Pneumothorax

When air in the thoracic cavity cannot exit the pleural space, a **tension pneumothorax** may develop (Fig. 26-8). This is a true emergency. It results in profound hypoventilation. Tension pneumothorax may result in death if it is not immediately recognized and managed.

When air is allowed to leak into the pleural space during inspiration and becomes trapped during expiration, the pleural pressure increases. This increase in pressure produces a shift in the mediastinum. It further compresses the lung on the uninjured side. In addition, compression of the vena cava reduces venous return to the heart. This results in a decrease in cardiac output. The signs and symptoms of a tension pneumothorax include the following:

- Anxiety
- Cyanosis
- Increasing dyspnea
- Tracheal deviation (a late sign)
- Tachycardia
- Hypotension or unexplained signs of shock
- Diminished or absent breath sounds on the injured side
- Distended neck veins (unless the patient is hypovolemic)

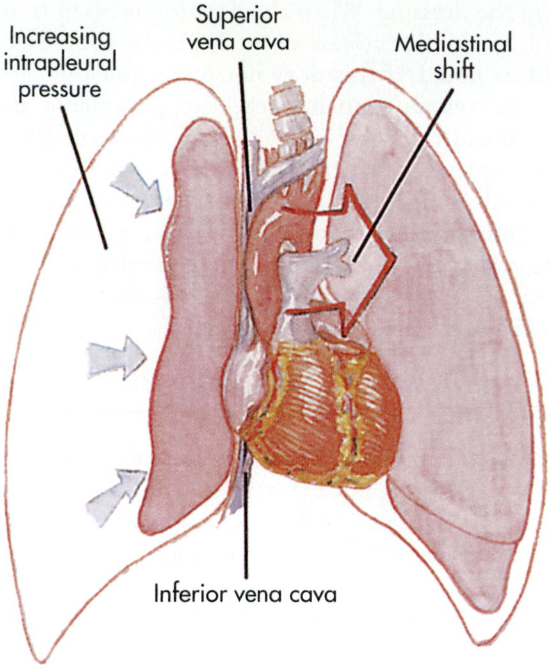

FIGURE 26-8 ■ Tension pneumothorax.

- Unequal expansion of the chest (tension does not fall with respiration)
- Subcutaneous emphysema

CRITICAL THINKING
Why might the neck veins be distended in a patient with a tension pneumothorax?

Tension pneumothorax may be confirmed by x-ray films in the hospital setting. However, waiting for x-ray confirmation is less than optimal management. In the prehospital setting, a suspected tension pneumothorax should be managed aggressively. It is evidenced by increasing dyspnea, compromised ventilation, tachycardia, tachypnea, unilateral decreased or absent breath sounds, and hyperresonance on percussion. Emergency care is directed at reducing the pressure in the pleural space; that is, returning the intrapleural pressure to atmospheric or subatmospheric levels.

NOTE The value of chest percussion in the prehospital setting is questionable. In the field, it should not be the only method used to identify a tension pneumothorax or hemothorax.[3] As a rule, hyperresonance on percussion points to the presence of air *(pneumothorax)*; dullness on percussion points to the presence of blood and other fluid *(hemothorax)*.

TENSION PNEUMOTHORAX ASSOCIATED WITH PENETRATING TRAUMA

Sealing an open pneumothorax with an occlusive dressing may produce a tension pneumothorax. In such cases the increased pleural pressure can be relieved by momentarily removing the dressing. When the dressing is lifted from the wound, an audible release of air from the thoracic cavity should be noted. If this does not occur and the patient's condition remains unchanged, the paramedic should gently spread the chest wound open. This will allow the trapped air to escape. After the pressure has been released, the wound should again be sealed. The dressing may need to be removed more than once to relieve pleural pressure during transport. If the tension is not relieved with this procedure, thoracic decompression (needle thoracentesis) should be performed.

TENSION PNEUMOTHORAX ASSOCIATED WITH CLOSED TRAUMA

A tension pneumothorax that develops in a patient with closed chest trauma must be relieved through thoracic decompression. This can be done with a large-bore needle. It also can be done with a commercially available thoracic decompression kit.

For needle decompression, a 2-inch, 12- or 14-gauge hollow needle or catheter is inserted into the affected pleural space, usually in the second intercostal space in the midclavicular line (Fig. 26-9). The needle should be inserted just above the third rib. This point is used to avoid the nerve, artery, and vein that lie just beneath each rib. After insertion of the needle, an audible rush of air should be noted. This is pressure escaping from the pleural space (confirming the tension pneumothorax). At this point, the patient should show signs of improvement (i.e., the patient will be easier to ventilate, or the person's breathing will be less labored). The needle or catheter should be secured in place with tape.

> **CRITICAL THINKING**
>
> Put your finger on the point on your chest where a needle would be inserted for decompression of a tension pneumothorax.

If time and circumstances allow, a one-way valve can be constructed to close off the hub of the needle during inspiration, preventing reentry of air into the pleural space. This can be done by cutting a finger from a sterile glove (rinsed with sterile water) and making a small hole at the fingertip. The finger is slipped over the hub of the needle and secured with a rubber band. An alternative method is to attach spe-

A

B

C

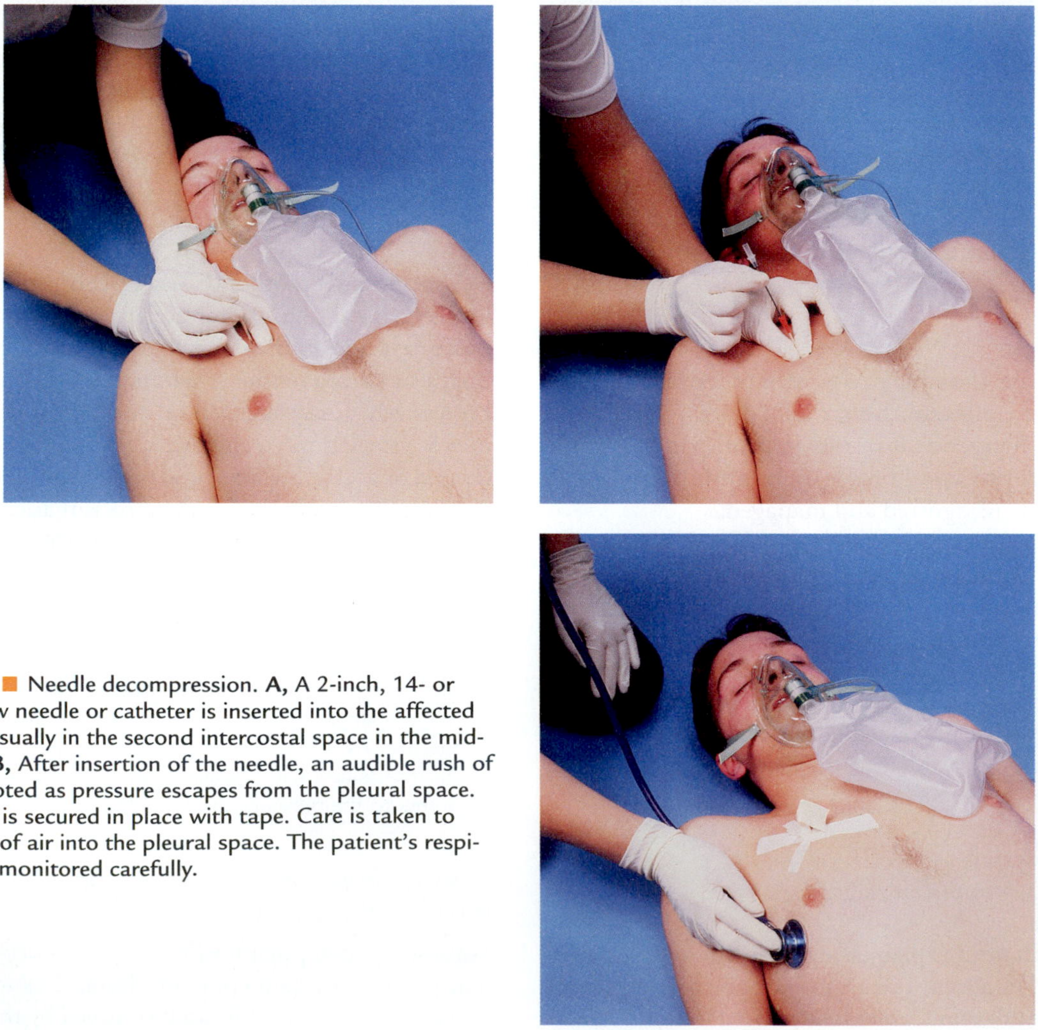

FIGURE 26-9 ■ Needle decompression. **A,** A 2-inch, 14- or 16-gauge hollow needle or catheter is inserted into the affected pleural space, usually in the second intercostal space in the midclavicular line. **B,** After insertion of the needle, an audible rush of air should be noted as pressure escapes from the pleural space. **C,** The catheter is secured in place with tape. Care is taken to prevent reentry of air into the pleural space. The patient's respiratory status is monitored carefully.

cial tubing and a flutter valve (per protocol) to the hub of the needle. Both methods allow air to escape from but not enter the pleural space. If the tension is not relieved with initial decompression, a second or third needle may need to be inserted.[2]

HEMOTHORAX

A **hemothorax** is the accumulation of blood in the pleural space. It is caused by bleeding from the lung parenchyma or damaged vessels (Fig. 26-10). If this condition is associated with a pneumothorax, it is called a *hemopneumothorax.* Blood loss may be massive in these patients; each side of the thorax can hold 30% to 40% (2000 to 3000 mL) of the patient's blood volume.[2] (A severed intercostal artery can easily bleed 50 mL per minute.) Thus patients with a hemothorax often have hypovolemia and hypoxemia.

As blood continues to fill the pleural space, the lung on the affected side may collapse. In rare cases the mediastinum may even shift away from the hemothorax. This would compress the unaffected lung. The resultant effects of respiratory and circulatory compromise are responsible for the following signs and symptoms:

- Tachypnea
- Dyspnea
- Cyanosis (often not evident in hemorrhagic shock)
- Diminished or decreased breath sounds (dullness on percussion)
- Hypovolemic shock
- Narrow pulse pressure
- Tracheal deviation to the unaffected side (rare)

Prehospital care for patients with a hemothorax is directed at correcting ventilatory and circulatory problems. This involves administration of high-concentration oxygen; ventilatory support with bag-valve-mask, intubation, or both; administration of volume-expanding fluids to correct the hypovolemia; and rapid transport to an appropriate medical facility. Hemothorax associated with great vessel or cardiac injury has a high mortality rate: 50% of these patients die immediately; 25% live for 5 to 10 minutes; and 25% may live longer than 30 minutes.[2]

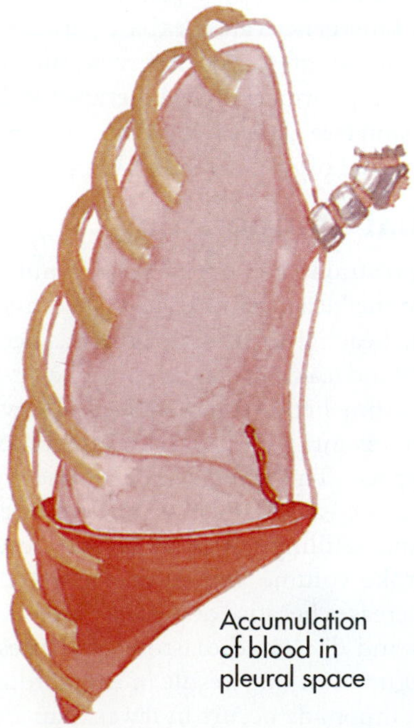

FIGURE 26-10 ■ Hemothorax.

CRITICAL THINKING

Hemothorax is associated with a higher mortality rate than a simple (closed) pneumothorax. Why is that the case?

Pulmonary Contusion

Pulmonary contusion most often is caused by rapid deceleration forces. (Such forces may be created by motor vehicle crashes and by injuries that result in a flail chest.) These forces push the lung against the chest wall. This results in rupture of the alveoli, with hemorrhage and swelling of the lung tissue. More than 50% of patients with blunt chest trauma have pulmonary contusion.[2]

During sudden inertial deceleration and direct impact, fixed and mobile parts of the lung move at varying speeds. The result is stretching and shearing of alveoli and intravascular structures. (This is the *inertial effect.*) This kinetic wave of energy is partly reflected at the alveolar membrane surface. The remainder causes a localized release of energy. (This is the *spalding effect.*) Overexpansion of air in the lungs occurs after the primary energy wave has passed *(implosion effect)*. Then low-pressure rebound shock waves cause overstretching and damage to lung tissue. The combination of these events results in alveolar and capillary damage with bleeding into the lung tissue and alveoli. The contused area of the lung is unable to function properly after injury. Therefore profound hypoxemia may develop. The degree of respiratory complication is directly related to the size of the contused area.

The signs and symptoms of pulmonary contusion are subtle at first. They should be suspected based on the kinematics of the event and the presence of associated injuries. Common signs and symptoms include the following:

- Tachypnea
- Tachycardia
- Cough
- Hemoptysis
- Apprehension
- Respiratory distress
- Dyspnea
- Evidence of blunt chest trauma
- Cyanosis

CRITICAL THINKING

Will you always be able to distinguish between simple pneumothorax and pulmonary contusion in the prehospital setting? Why or why not?

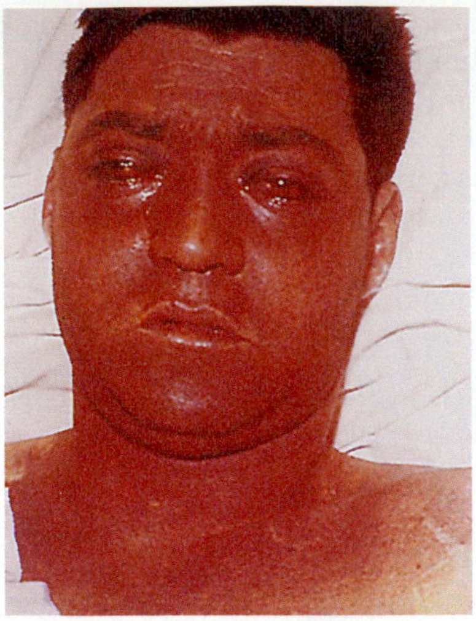

FIGURE 26-11 ■ Discoloration of traumatic asphyxia, which results from forcible compression of the chest. (From London PS: *A colour atlas of diagnosis after recent injury*. Ipswich, England, 1990, Wolfe Medical Publications.)

Emergency care for pulmonary contusion includes ventilatory support and administration of high-concentration oxygen. Patients with associated injuries or preexisting pulmonary or cardiovascular disease should be closely monitored in case ventilations need to be assisted with a bag-valve device, intubation, or both. Pulmonary contusions may be associated with a major chest injury. However, they generally heal spontaneously over several weeks.

Traumatic Asphyxia

The term **traumatic asphyxia** is used to describe a severe crushing injury to the chest and abdomen (Fig. 26-11). It results from an increase in intrathoracic pressure. This pressure increase forces blood from the right side of the heart into the veins of the upper thorax, neck, and face. The forces involved in this phenomenon may cause lethal injury, but traumatic asphyxia alone is not life-threatening[1] (although brain hemorrhages, seizures, coma, and death have been documented to occasionally occur).

Signs and symptoms of traumatic asphyxia include reddish purple discoloration of the face and neck (the skin below the area remains pink), jugular vein distention, and swelling or hemorrhage of the conjunctiva (subconjunctival petechiae may appear). Emergency care is directed at ensuring an open airway, providing adequate ventilation, and caring for associated injuries. The paramedic should be ready to manage hypovolemia and shock when the compressive force is released.

HEART AND GREAT VESSEL INJURY

Trauma to the heart and to the great vessels (i.e., the aorta, pulmonary arteries and veins, and superior and inferior venae cavae) may be caused by the force of blunt or penetrating injuries. The injuries discussed in this section are myocardial contusion, pericardial tamponade, myocardial rupture, and traumatic aortic rupture.

Myocardial Contusion

The clinical findings in **myocardial contusion** are often subtle and frequently overlooked for several reasons: (1) multiple injuries direct attention elsewhere; (2) often little evidence of thoracic injury is present; and (3) signs of cardiac injury may not be present on initial examination. Contusions to the myocardium usually are caused by a vehicle collision. In these cases the chest wall strikes the dashboard or steering column. (Sternal and multiple rib fractures are common.) Therefore a deformed dashboard or steering column should alert the paramedic to the possibility of a cardiac injury. Blunt myocardial injury occurs in 16% to 76% of patients who suffer blunt trauma to the chest.[2]

CRITICAL THINKING

How would you manage a cardiac rhythm disturbance resulting from a myocardial contusion?

The extent of injury may vary. The injury may be only a localized bruise. It also may be a full-thickness injury to the wall of the heart with hemorrhage and edema. Blood may accumulate in the pericardium *(hemopericardium)* as a result of a tear in the epicardium or endocardium. This, in turn, may result in cardiac rupture or a traumatic myocardial infarction. The fibrinous reaction at the contusion site may lead to delayed rupture or ventricular aneurysm.

Patients with a myocardial contusion may have no symptoms, or they may complain of chest pain similar to that seen with a myocardial infarction. Other signs and symptoms include ECG abnormalities, a new cardiac murmur, pericardial friction rub (late), persistent tachycardia, and palpitations. Emergency care for these patients is similar to that for myocardial infarction: oxygen administration, ECG monitoring, and pharmacological therapy for dysrhythmias and hypotension (see Chapter 29). Any intervention that increases myocardial oxygen consumption should be avoided.

Pericardial Tamponade

Penetrating trauma (and, in rare cases, blunt trauma) may cause tears in the heart chamber walls. This allows blood to leak from the heart. If the pericardium has been torn sufficiently, this blood leaks into the thoracic cavity. The patient rapidly dies from hemorrhage. Often, however, the pericardium remains intact. In such cases the blood enters the pericardial space. This causes an increase in pericardial pressure. The increased pressure prevents the heart from expanding and refilling with blood. This results in a decrease in stroke volume and cardiac output. Myocardial perfusion decreases because of pressure effects on the walls of the heart and decreased diastolic pressures. Associated ischemic dysfunction may result in myocardial infarction. Pericardial tamponade occurs in fewer than 2% of patients who suffer chest trauma.[2]

NOTE Penetrating injuries, such as those caused by some knife and gunshot wounds, may result in death from hemorrhage rather than tamponade. This happens when the wound is large enough that the pericardium cannot contain the blood in the pericardial space. Gunshot wounds have a higher mortality rate than stab wounds.[2]

At first, most patients with pericardial tamponade have peripheral vasoconstriction. (The diastolic blood pressure rises more than the systolic blood pressure. This causes a decrease in pulse pressure.) These patients are also tachycardic. The increase in heart rate compensates for the decrease in cardiac output. Up to this point, pericardial tamponade and hemorrhagic shock have similar signs. Yet a key clinical finding often allows differentiation of the two forms of shock. This clinical finding was first described by Beck in 1935. It and two other clinical clues make up the **Beck triad.** The Beck triad is seen in only 30% of patients with pericardial tamponade.[2]

The Beck triad consists of elevated central venous pressure (evidenced by jugular vein distention), muffled heart sounds, and hypotension. The first element of the Beck triad, elevated central venous pressure, is the single best way to distinguish pericardial tamponade from hemorrhagic shock.[1] Other signs and symptoms of pericardial tamponade include the following:

- Tachycardia
- Respiratory distress
- Narrow pulse pressure
- Cyanosis of the head, neck, and upper extremities

NOTE Paramedics must keep in mind that problems other than pericardial tamponade can cause hypotension and elevated central venous pressure. The most common alternative causes are tension pneumothorax in trauma victims and cardiogenic shock. Patients with tamponade and hemorrhage may not have an elevated venous pressure at first.

Two other findings in pericardial tamponade may include *pulsus paradoxus* and *electrical alternans*. Pulsus paradoxus is a systolic blood pressure that drops more than 10 to 15 mm Hg during inspiration compared with expiration. (Normally this drop is minimal.) The excessive decline in systolic pressure occurs in cardiac tamponade when pleural pressure is reduced during inspiration. The reduction of pleural pressure provides some relief from the tamponade and causes the inspiratory fall in arterial flow and systolic pressure. (Pulsus paradoxus is difficult to measure in the prehospital setting.) Electrical alternans refers to a change in the amplitude of a patient's ECG waveforms that decrease with every other cardiac cycle. It is a rare finding in cardiac tamponade.

Pericardial tamponade is a true emergency. Pericardial blood must be removed in these patients. Also, the bleeding must be stopped if the patient is to survive the injury. Prehospital management includes careful monitoring, oxygen administration, fluid replacement, and rapid transport to an appropriate medical facility. Treatment at the medical facility involves needle pericardiocentesis to remove blood from the pericardial sac. Removal of as little as 20 mL may drastically improve cardiac output.[2]

Myocardial Rupture

Myocardial rupture occurs when blood-filled chambers of the ventricles are compressed with enough force to rupture the chamber wall, septum, or valve. The injury is nearly always immediately fatal, but death may be delayed for 2 to 3 weeks (after blunt trauma).[2] Motor vehicle crashes are responsible for most cases of myocardial rupture, accounting for 15% of fatal thoracic injuries.[1] Other proposed mechanisms include the following:

- Deceleration or shearing forces that disrupt the inferior and superior venae cavae
- Upward displacement of blood (causing an increase in intracardiac pressure) after abdominal trauma
- Direct compression of the heart between the sternum and vertebrae
- Laceration from a rib or sternal fracture
- Complications of myocardial contusion

A significant mechanism of injury often is a factor in these cases. Also, signs and symptoms of congestive heart failure and cardiac tamponade are present. Prehospital care for these patients is mainly supportive. It includes airway and ventilatory support and rapid transport for definitive care. It is crucial that paramedics consider the possibility of a tension pneumothorax in these patients. The signs and symptoms of tension pneumothorax mimic those of myocardial rupture with tamponade.

Traumatic Aortic Rupture

Traumatic aortic rupture is thought to be a result of shearing forces. These forces develop between tissues that decelerate at different rates. Common mechanisms of injury include rapid deceleration in high-speed motor vehicle crashes, falls from great heights, and crushing injuries. It has been estimated that one in six people who die in motor vehicle crashes has a rupture of the aorta.[1] Of these patients, 80% to 90% die at the scene as a result of massive hemorrhage. About 10% to 20% survive the first hour. This is because the bleeding is tamponaded by the surrounding adventitia of the aorta and intact visceral pleura. Of these individuals, 30% have ruptures within 6 hours. For these reasons, rapid and pertinent evaluation and transport to an appropriate medical facility are critical. Aortic rupture is responsible for 15% of all deaths from blunt trauma.[2]

The usual site of damage to the aorta is in the distal arch. This is just beyond the takeoff of the left subclavian artery and proximal to the ligamentum arteriosum (Fig. 26-12). The ligamentum arteriosum and descending thoracic arch are somewhat fixed. On the other hand, the transverse portion of the arch is somewhat mobile. If shearing forces exceed the tensile strength of the arch, the junction of the mobile and fixed points of attachment may be partly torn. If the outer layer of tissue around the aorta remains intact, the patient may survive long enough for surgical repair.

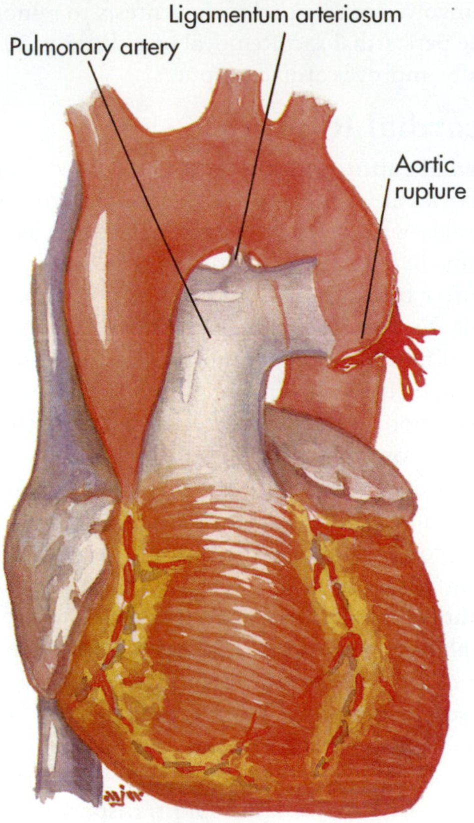

FIGURE 26-12 ■ Aortic rupture.

Aortic rupture is a severe injury. (The fatality rate is 80% to 90% within the first hour.) Any trauma patient who has unexplained shock and an appropriate mechanism of injury (rapid deceleration) should be suspected of having a ruptured aorta. Blood pressure may be normal or elevated, with a significant difference between the two arms. In addition, upper extremity hypertension with absent or weak femoral pulses can occur in these patients. (This is thought to result from compression of the aorta by the expanding hematoma.) Other patients have hypertension because of increased activity of the sympathetic nervous system. About 25% of these patients have a harsh systolic murmur that can be heard over the pericardium or between the scapulae. In rare cases these patients may have paraplegia without a cervical or thoracic spine injury. This occurs as a consequence of decreased blood flow through the anterior spinal artery. The anterior spinal artery is in the thoracic region. It is composed of branches from the posterior intercostal arteries. These in turn are branches of the thoracic aorta.

▶NOTE A difference in pulse quality between the arms and lower torso or between the left and right arms is sometimes detected with aortic rupture. Therefore checking both radial and femoral pulses is important.[3]

Prehospital management of these patients includes advising medical direction of the suspected rupture, administration of high-concentration oxygen, ventilatory support with spinal precautions, judicious fluid replacement (avoiding overhydration), and rapid transport for surgical repair.

▶NOTE Fluid replacement should be limited in patients who have a stable blood pressure. This helps to prevent an increase in pressure in the remaining aortic wall tissue.

Penetrating Wounds of the Great Vessels

Penetrating wounds of the great vessels usually involve injury to the chest, abdomen, or neck. These wounds often are accompanied by massive hemothorax, hypovolemic shock, cardiac tamponade, and enlarging hematomas that may cause compression of the vena cava, trachea, esophagus, great vessels, and heart. Prehospital care for patients with penetrating injury to the great vessels is directed at providing airway and ventilatory support, managing hypovolemia with judicious fluid therapy (guided by medical direction), and rapid transport for definitive care.

OTHER THORACIC INJURIES

Other injuries that may be associated with blunt or penetrating trauma to the thorax include esophageal and tracheobronchial injuries (see Chapter 24) and diaphragmatic rupture.

Esophageal and Tracheobronchial Injuries

Esophageal injuries most often are caused by penetrating trauma. (For example, these may be caused by projectile or knife wounds.) They also can result from spontaneous perforation caused by cancer and from anatomic distortions caused by diverticulas or gastric reflux, both of which can lead to violent vomiting.[2] Assessment findings may include pain, fever, hoarseness, dysphagia, respiratory distress, and shock. If esophageal perforation occurs in the cervical region, local tenderness, subcutaneous emphysema, and resistance to neck movement may be noted. Esophageal perforation that occurs lower in the thoracic region may result in mediastinal and subcutaneous emphysema, inflammation of the mediastinum, and splinting of the chest wall.

Tracheobronchial injuries are rare. They occur in fewer than 3% of victims of blunt or penetrating chest trauma. However, the mortality rate for these injuries is over 30%.[2] Most injuries occur within 3 cm (about 1½ inches) of the carina. However, they can occur anywhere along the tracheobronchial tree. Signs and symptoms of tracheobronchial injury include the following:

- Severe hypoxia
- Tachypnea
- Tachycardia

- Massive subcutaneous emphysema
- Dyspnea
- Respiratory distress
- Hemoptysis

Emergency care for patients with an esophageal or a tracheobronchial injury is directed at providing airway, ventilatory, and circulatory support and rapid transport for definitive care at an appropriate medical facility.

NOTE A tension pneumothorax that does not improve after needle decompression or the absence of a continuous flow of air from the needle after decompression should alert the paramedic to the possibility of a tracheobronchial injury.

Diaphragmatic Rupture

As described in Chapter 6, the diaphragm is a sheet of voluntary muscle. This sheet of muscle separates the abdominal cavity from the thoracic cavity. Sudden compression of the abdomen (such as with blunt trauma to the trunk) results in a sharp increase in intraabdominal pressure. When this occurs, the pressure differences may cause abdominal contents to rupture through the thin diaphragmatic wall and enter the chest cavity (Fig. 26-13). Diaphragmatic rupture is detected more often on the left side than on the right side. However, rupture on either side may allow intraabdominal organs to enter the thoracic cavity. There they may cause compression of the lung, resulting in reduced ventilation, decreased venous return, decreased cardiac output, and shock. Because of the mechanical forces involved, patients with diaphragmatic rupture often have multiple injuries.

Signs and symptoms of a ruptured diaphragm include abdominal pain, shortness of breath, and decreased breath sounds. If most of the abdominal contents are forced into the chest, the abdomen may have a hollow or empty appearance. Also, bowel sounds may be heard in the chest. Prehospital management includes oxygen administration, ventilatory support as needed (positive pressure may worsen the injury), volume-expanding fluids, and rapid transport with the patient in a supine position to an appropriate medical facility for surgical repair. Some medical direction agencies also may recommend that a nasogastric tube be placed to empty the stomach and reduce abdominal pressure.

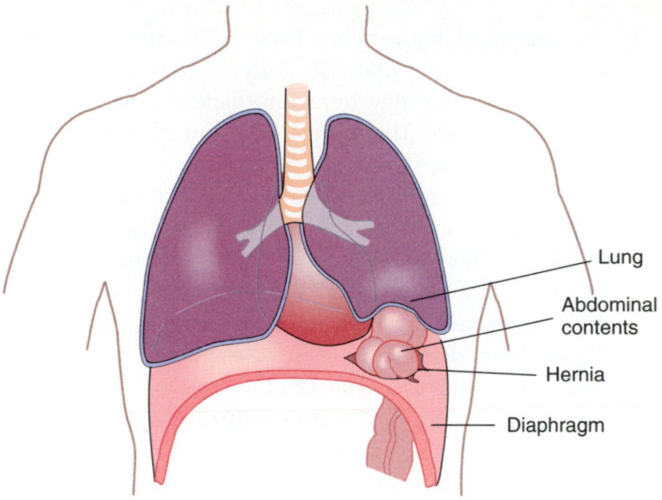

FIGURE 26-13 ■ Diaphragmatic rupture. Sudden compression of the abdomen may increase intraabdominal pressure, causing the abdominal contents to rupture through the thin diaphragmatic wall and enter the chest cavity.

SUMMARY

- Thoracic injuries are caused by blunt or penetrating trauma. Such trauma often is caused by motor vehicle crashes, falls from heights, blast injuries, blows to the chest, chest compression, gunshot wounds, and stab wounds.
- Fractures of the clavicle, ribs, or sternum, as well as flail chest, may be caused by blunt or penetrating trauma. Complications of skeletal trauma of the chest may include cardiac, vascular, or pulmonary injuries.
- Closed pneumothorax may be life-threatening if (1) it is a tension pneumothorax, (2) it occupies more than 40% of the hemithorax, or (3) it occurs in a patient in shock or a preexisting pulmonary or cardiovascular disease. Open pneumothorax may result in severe ventilatory dysfunction, hypoxemia, and death unless it is quickly recognized and corrected. Tension pneumothorax is a true emergency. It results in profound hypoventilation. It may result in death if it is not quickly recognized and managed. Hemothorax may result in massive blood loss. These patients often have hypovolemia and hypoxemia. Pulmonary contusion results when trauma to the lung causes alveolar and capillary damage. Severe hypoxemia may develop. The degree of hypoxemia is directly related to the size of the contused area. Traumatic asphyxia results from forces that cause an increase in intrathoracic pressure. When it occurs alone, it often is not lethal. However, brain hemorrhages, seizures, coma, and death have been reported after these injuries.

Continued

- The extent of injury from myocardial contusion may vary. The injury may be only a localized bruise. However, it also may be a full-thickness injury to the wall of the heart. The full-thickness injury may result in cardiac rupture, ventricular aneurysm, or a traumatic myocardial infarction. Pericardial tamponade occurs if 150 to 200 mL of blood enters the pericardial space suddenly. This results in a decrease in stroke volume and cardiac output. *Myocardial rupture* is an acute traumatic perforation of the ventricles or atria. It is nearly always immediately fatal. However, death may be delayed for several weeks after blunt trauma. Aortic rupture is a severe injury. The mortality rate in the first hour is 80% to 90%. The paramedic should consider the possibility of aortic rupture in any trauma patient who has unexplained shock after a rapid deceleration injury.
- Esophageal injuries most often are caused by penetrating trauma (e.g., projectile and knife wounds). Tracheobronchial injuries are rare (occurring in fewer than 3% of victims of blunt or penetrating chest trauma), but the mortality rate is over 30%. A tension pneumothorax that does not improve after needle decompression or the absence of a continuous flow of air from the needle after decompression should alert the paramedic to the possibility of a tracheobronchial injury.
- Diaphragmatic ruptures may allow abdominal organs to enter the thoracic cavity. There they may cause compression of the lung, resulting in reduced ventilation, decreased venous return, decreased cardiac output, and shock.

REFERENCES

1. Rosen P, Barkin R: *Emergency medicine: concepts and clinical practice,* ed 5, St Louis, 2003, Mosby.
2. US Department of Transportation, National Highway Traffic Safety Administration: *EMT-paramedic national standard curriculum,* Washington, DC, 1998, The Department.
3. National Association of Emergency Medical Technicians: *PHTLS: basic and advanced prehospital life support,* ed 5, St Louis, 2003, Mosby.

SUGGESTED READINGS

Emergency Nurses Association: *Sheehy's emergency nursing: principles and practice,* ed 5, St Louis, 2003, Mosby.

Ferrera P et al: *Trauma management,* St Louis, 2001, Mosby.

Roberts J, Hedges J: *Clinical procedures in emergency medicine,* ed 3, Philadelphia, 1998, WB Saunders.

CHAPTER 27

Abdominal Trauma

OBJECTIVES

Upon completion of this chapter, the paramedic student will be able to:

1. Identify mechanisms of injury associated with abdominal trauma.
2. Describe mechanisms of injury, signs and symptoms, and complications associated with abdominal solid organ, hollow organ, retroperitoneal organ, and pelvic organ injuries.
3. Outline the significance of injury to intraabdominal vascular structures.
4. Describe the prehospital assessment priorities for a patient suspected of having an abdominal injury.
5. Outline the prehospital care of a patient with abdominal trauma.

KEY TERMS

hematuria: The abnormal presence of blood in the urine.

hemoperitoneum: The presence of extravasated blood in the peritoneal cavity.

Kehr sign: Pain in the left shoulder thought to be caused by referred pain secondary to irritation of the adjacent diaphragm.

peritonitis: Inflammation of the serous membrane that covers the abdominal wall.

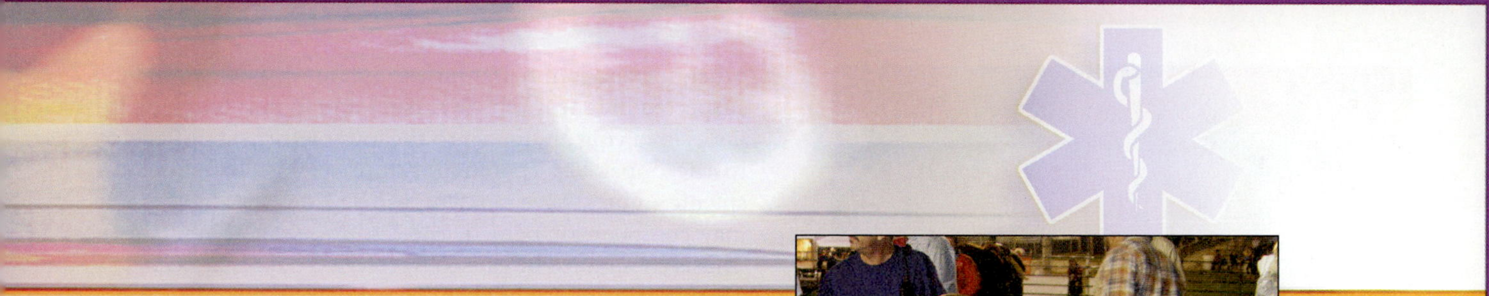

Abdominal trauma may not be easy to evaluate in the prehospital setting. It can cause many injuries to multiple organs. Physical findings may be absent, minimal, or exaggerated. Also, patients may have different perceptions of pain. Pain perception varies as a result of preexisting conditions, shock, alcohol or other drug use, head injury, or other factors. Therefore the paramedic must have a high degree of suspicion based on the mechanism of injury and kinematics. Death from abdominal trauma usually is a result of ongoing hemorrhage and the delay of surgical repair.

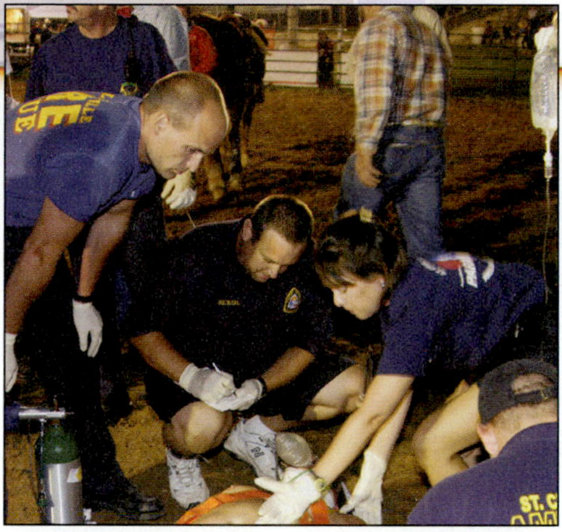

NOTE Like most other types of trauma, many abdominal injuries can be prevented. An important prevention strategy is taking part in community programs that promote safety. (For example, one could work to promote gun safety legislation.) Another crucial approach is stressing the importance of using personal restraints (see Chapter 3).

BOX 27-1 Prehospital Care for Abdominal Injury

1. Secure the airway with spinal precautions.
2. Provide ventilatory support.
3. Provide wound management.
4. Manage shock with fluid replacement and pneumatic antishock garment (per protocol).
5. Rapidly transport the patient for definitive care.

MECHANISMS OF ABDOMINAL INJURY

Abdominal injury may result from blunt or penetrating trauma. Regardless of the organ injured, management usually is limited to securing the airway with spinal precautions, providing ventilatory support, providing wound management, managing shock with fluid replacement and application of a pneumatic antishock garment (PASG) (per protocol), and rapidly transporting the patient for definitive care (Box 27-1).

Blunt Trauma

Blunt trauma to abdominal organs usually is caused by compression or shearing forces (see Chapter 20). Compression forces may cause the abdominal organs to be crushed between solid objects (e.g., between the steering column and the spinal vertebrae). Shearing forces may cause a tear or rupture of the solid organs or blood vessels. This occurs when the tissues are stretched at their points of attachment (stabilizing ligaments or blood vessels). The severity of injury usually is related to the degree and duration of force applied. It also is related to the type of abdominal structure injured (fluid filled, gas filled, solid, or hollow). Blunt abdominal trauma may be caused by motor vehicle and motorcycle collisions (including injuries that result from the use of personal restraints), pedestrian injuries, falls, assaults, and blast injuries. The car is the major cause of blunt abdominal trauma (Fig. 27-1). Automobile-automobile and automobile-pedestrian crashes have been cited as causes in 50% to 75% of cases, blows to the abdomen in about 15% of cases, and falls in 6% to 9% of cases.[1]

CRITICAL THINKING
Young children are more susceptible to abdominal injuries than adults. Why?

Penetrating Trauma

Penetrating injury may result from stab wounds, gunshot wounds, or impalement. A major complication of this type of trauma is hemorrhage from a major vessel or solid organ.

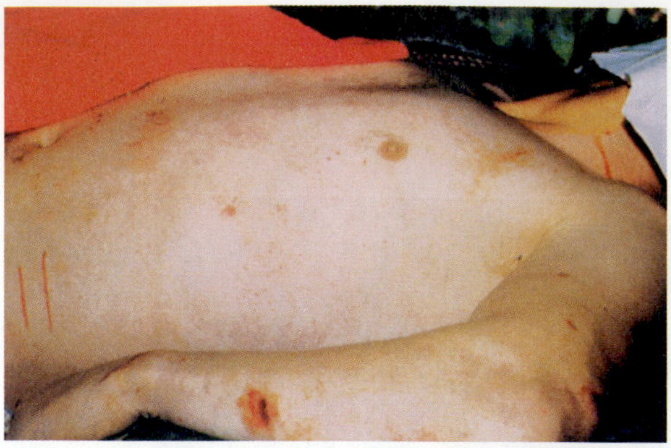

FIGURE 27-1 ■ Marks of impact on the front-seat passenger in a car crash. The victim suffered rupture of the diaphragm and spleen.

Another is perforation of a segment of bowel. As a rule, injuries caused by penetrating trauma do not have as high a mortality rate as those caused by blunt trauma.[2]

SPECIFIC ABDOMINAL INJURIES

An abdominal injury may be classified as a solid organ, hollow organ, retroperitoneal organ, pelvic organ, or vascular injury (Fig. 27-2). (See Chapter 6 for a review of the abdominal anatomy.)

Solid Organ Injury

Injury to solid organs usually results in rapid and significant blood loss. The two solid organs most often injured are the liver and spleen. Both of these organs are primary sources of life-threatening hemorrhage.

> **CRITICAL THINKING**
>
> When does shock associated with injury to the liver or spleen develop?

LIVER

The liver is the largest organ in the abdominal cavity. Because of its location, it often is injured by trauma to the eighth through twelfth ribs on the right side of the body (Fig. 27-3). It also is often injured by trauma to the upper central part of the abdomen. Injury to the liver should be suspected in any patient with a steering wheel injury, lap belt injury, or history of epigastric trauma. After an injury to the liver, blood and bile escape into the peritoneal cavity. This results in the signs and symptoms of shock and peritoneal irritation (abdominal pain, tenderness, rigidity), respectively. The liver is damaged in about 19% of cases of blunt abdominal trauma and in about 37% of cases of penetrating trauma.[1]

SPLEEN

The spleen lies in the upper left quadrant of the abdomen. It is slightly protected by the organs that surround it medially and anteriorly. It also is protected by the lower portion of the rib cage. Injury to the spleen often is associated with other intraabdominal injuries. Splenic injury should be suspected in motor vehicle crashes and in falls or sports injuries involving an impact to the lower left chest or flank or to the upper left abdomen. About 40% of patients with splenic injures have no symptoms. However, the patient may complain of pain in the left shoulder **(Kehr sign).** This is thought to be caused by referred pain that occurs as a result of irritation of the adjacent diaphragm by a splenic hematoma or **hemoperitoneum.** The spleen is damaged in about 41% of cases of blunt abdominal trauma and in about 7% of cases of penetrating trauma.[1]

Hollow Organ Injury

Injuries to the hollow abdominal organs may result in sepsis, wound infection, and abscess formation, particularly if trauma to the intestine remains undiagnosed for an extended period. With injuries to solid organs, hemorrhage is the major cause of symptoms. In contrast, injury to the hollow organs results in symptoms from spillage of their contents (this spillage results in **peritonitis**) (Box 27-2).

STOMACH

Because of its protected location in the abdomen, the stomach is not often injured by blunt trauma. However, penetrating trauma may cause gastric transection or laceration. Patients with either of these injuries may show signs of peritonitis rather quickly as a result of leakage of acidic gastric contents. The diagnosis of injury to the stomach usually is confirmed during surgery or when nasogastric drainage returns blood. The stomach is damaged in about 1% of cases of blunt abdominal trauma and in about 19% of cases of penetrating trauma.[1]

COLON AND SMALL INTESTINE

The colon and small intestine, like the stomach and duodenum, are more likely to be injured as a result of penetrating trauma than blunt trauma. (For example, the injury may be caused by a gunshot wound to the abdomen or buttocks.) However, the large and small bowel also may be injured by compression forces in high-speed motor vehicle crashes. They also may sustain deceleration injuries associated with the wearing of personal restraints. Considerable force is required to cause an injury to the colon or small intestine. Therefore other injuries usually are present. Peritoneal contamination with bacteria is a common problem. With blunt abdominal trauma, the colon is damaged in about 6% of cases and the small intestine in about 7% of cases. With penetrating abdominal trauma, the colon is damaged in about 16% of cases and the small intestine in about 26% of cases.[1]

Retroperitoneal Organ Injury

Injury to the retroperitoneal organs (kidneys, ureters, pancreas, duodenum) may occur as a result of blunt or penetrating trauma to the anterior abdomen, posterior abdomen (particularly the flank area), or thoracic spine. Hemorrhage within the retroperitoneal area may be mas-

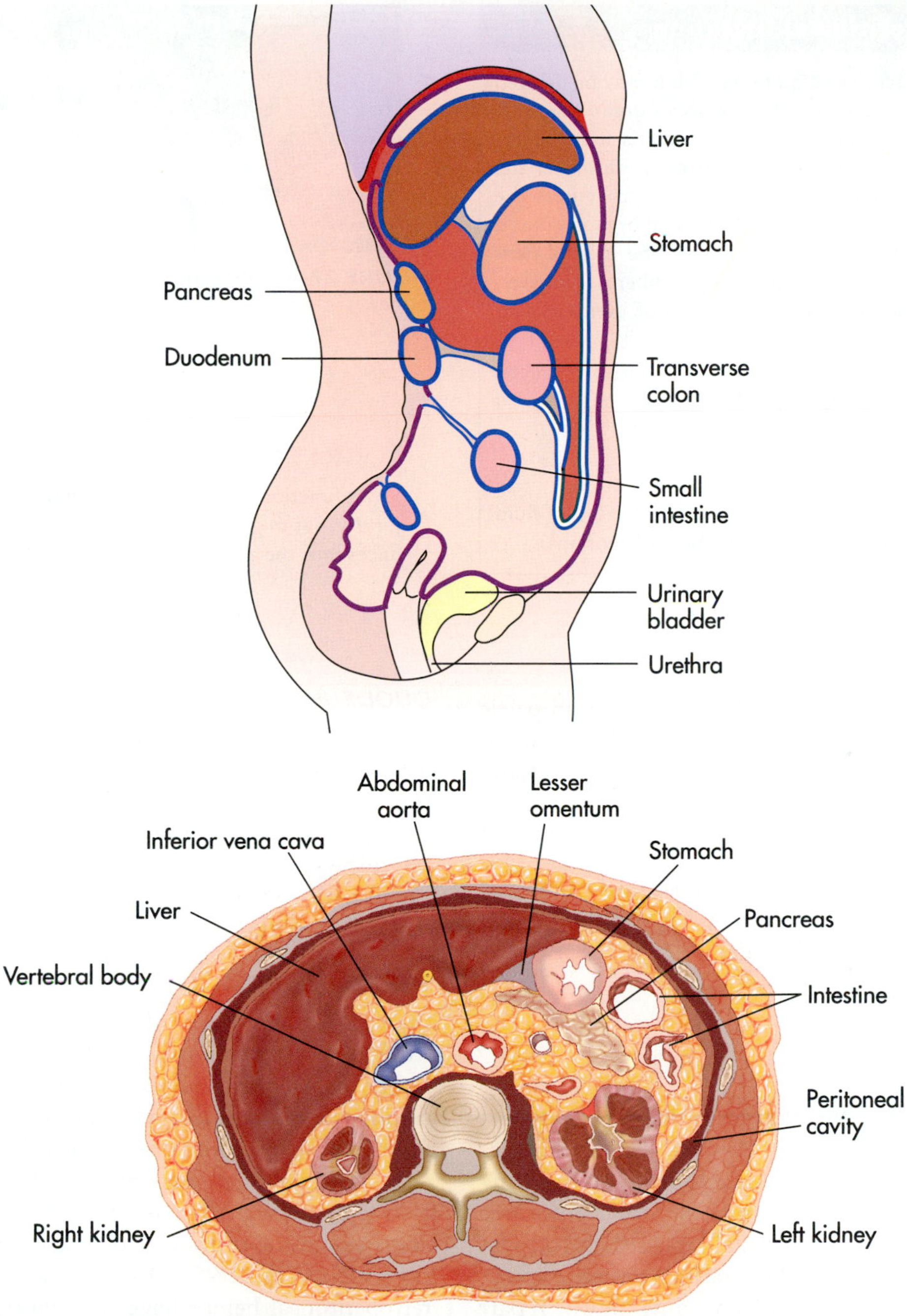

FIGURE 27-2 ■ Hollow, solid, retroperitoneal, and pelvic organs.

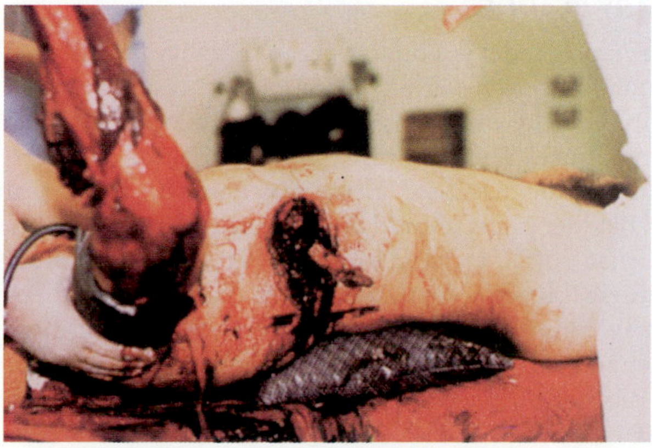

FIGURE 27-3 ■ Liver injury visible beneath broken rib caused by high-speed vehicle crash.

BOX 27-2 Peritoneal Irritation

Peritonitis usually is acute and quite painful. It may be delayed for hours or days after injury to a hollow viscus organ. It results from the spillage of enzymes, acids, and bacteria into the abdominal cavity. The spillage causes chemical irritation of the peritoneum. The peritoneum is the membrane that lines the wall of the abdomen and covers the abdominal organs. (Blood is not a chemical irritant to the abdomen.) The pain of peritonitis usually is localized (via somatic nerve fibers). However, it also may be diffuse. Signs and symptoms of peritonitis include the following:

- Pain
- Tenderness on percussion or palpation
- Guarding, rigidity
- Fever (if untreated)
- Distention (a late finding)

Note: The adult abdomen can accommodate 1.5 L of fluid without the belly looking bloated (abdominal distention).

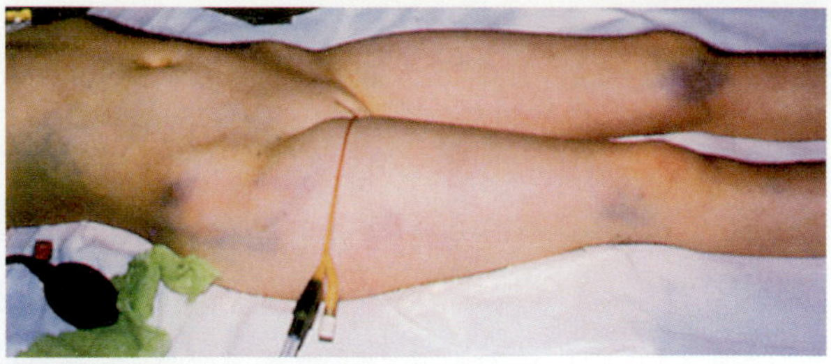

FIGURE 27-4 ■ Bruising caused by rupture of the liver and right kidney.

CRITICAL THINKING

What functions of the pancreas may be disrupted after injury? What might be the effects of spillage of pancreatic juices into the abdominal cavity?

sive. Most retroperitoneal hemorrhages result from pelvic or lumbar fractures. Retroperitoneal structures are damaged in about 9% of cases of blunt abdominal injuries and in about 11% of cases of penetrating trauma.[1]

NOTE Bruising of the flanks (Turner sign) or around the umbilicus (Cullen sign) indicates retroperitoneal hemorrhage (Fig. 27-4). However, these signs usually are delayed 12 hours to several days.

KIDNEYS

The kidneys are solid organs that lie in the retroperitoneal space. They may be injured by abdominal trauma. Injuries may involve contusion, fractures, and lacerations, resulting in hemorrhage, extravasation of urine, or both. Contusions usually are self-limiting. They usually heal with bed rest and forced fluids. Fractures and lacerations are more severe. They may require surgical repair, depending on which part of the kidney is damaged.

URETERS

The ureters are hollow organs that are rarely injured by blunt trauma. This is because of their flexible structure. When injury occurs, it usually is the result of penetrating abdominal or flank wounds (e.g., stab wounds, firearm injuries).

PANCREAS

The pancreas is a solid organ that lies within the retroperitoneal space. Injury to the pancreas is rare. When it occurs, it usually is caused by compressive or penetrating forces on the upper left quadrant, as in steering wheel and bicycle handlebar impalement. The pancreas more often is injured by penetrating trauma (particularly firearms) than by blunt trauma.

DUODENUM

The duodenum, which lies across the lumbar spine, is seldom injured. This is due to its location in the retroperitoneal area, near the pancreas. When great force from blunt trauma or a penetrating injury occurs, the duodenum may be crushed or lacerated. Injury to this organ usually is associated with concurrent pancreatic trauma; it is confirmed through surgery.

Pelvic Organ Injury

Injury to pelvic organs (bladder, urethra) usually results from motor vehicle crashes that cause pelvic fractures. Other, less frequent causes of pelvic organ injury are penetrating trauma, straddle-type injuries from falls, pedestrian injuries, and some sexual acts. The pelvis supports and protects multiple organ systems. Therefore the risk of associated injury is high. The most common associated injuries are those to the urinary bladder and urethra. Fractures of the pelvis (Fig. 27-5) often are associated with severe retroperitoneal hemorrhage. The mortality rate for pelvic fractures ranges from 6.4% to 19%.[1] (Pelvic fractures are further described in Chapter 28.)

URINARY BLADDER

The urinary bladder is a hollow organ that may be ruptured by blunt trauma, penetrating trauma, or pelvic fracture. Rupture is more likely if the bladder is distended at the time of injury. With rupture, the integrity of the peritoneum may be disrupted. Urine may enter the peritoneal cavity. Bladder injury should be suspected in inebriated patients that suffer trauma to the lower abdomen. Gross **hematuria** (blood in the urine) may be present. The patient also may complain of being unable to void. The urinary bladder and surrounding structures are damaged in about 6% of cases of abdominal trauma.[1]

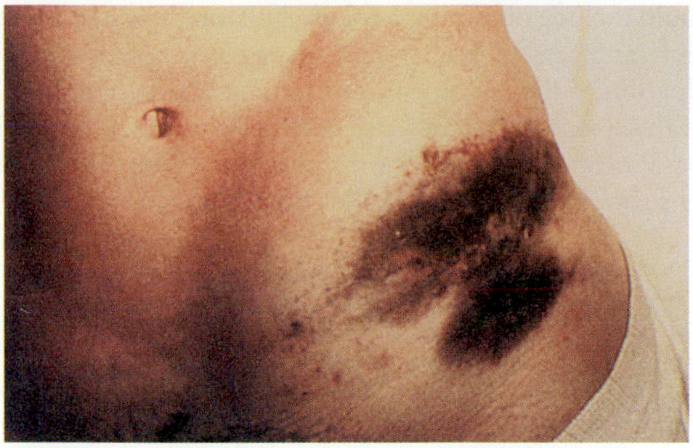

FIGURE 27-5 ■ Massive swelling and bruising from a pelvic fracture.

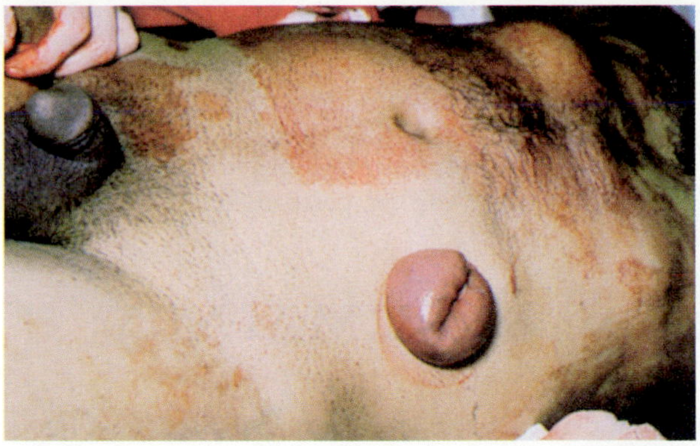

FIGURE 27-6 ■ A loop of gut that emerged through a stab wound to the abdomen.

URETHRA

A tear in the urethra occurs more often in men than in women. It usually occurs as a result of blunt trauma associated with pelvic fracture. The patient may complain of abdominal pain and of being unable to urinate. Blood at the meatus indicates urethral injury. An indwelling urinary catheter should not be used in these patients.

VASCULAR STRUCTURE INJURIES

Injuries to arterial and venous vessels in the abdomen can be life-threatening because of their potential for massive hemorrhage. These injuries usually are caused by penetrating trauma. However, they may also be the result of compression or deceleration forces on the abdomen. As in solid organ injury, vascular injury usually is marked by hypovolemia. In some cases vascular injuries are associated with a palpable abdominal mass. The major vessels most often injured are the aorta, the inferior vena cava, and the renal, mesenteric, and iliac arteries and veins (see Chapter 6). Injury to major vessels in the abdomen has a high mortality rate. Immediate surgical repair is often required.

CRITICAL THINKING

How can you attempt to manage shock when major vessels have been injured as a result of a severe pelvic fracture?

ASSESSMENT OF ABDOMINAL TRAUMA

The most significant sign of severe abdominal trauma is unexplained shock. The mechanism of injury and the classic presentation of hypovolemia are important indicators. Other signs and symptoms that should alert the paramedic to the possibility of severe abdominal trauma are abdominal wall injuries (e.g., bruising and discoloration of the abdomen, abrasions) and the following:

- Obvious bleeding
- Pain and abdominal tenderness or guarding
- Abdominal rigidity and distention
- Evisceration (Box 27-3)
- Rib fractures
- Pelvic fractures

However, the absence of these signs and symptoms does not rule out an abdominal injury. The paramedic must maintain a high degree of suspicion based on the nature of the injury.

BOX 27-3 Evisceration

Evisceration is the protrusion of an internal organ or the peritoneal contents through a wound or surgical incision, especially in the abdominal wall (Fig. 27-6). The presence of an evisceration from abdominal trauma generally is associated with major abdominal injury. In the prehospital setting the wound is managed by covering the eviscerated contents with moist, sterile gauze or a dressing. This helps to prevent further contamination and drying. No attempt should be made to replace eviscerated organs into the peritoneal cavity; this would increase the risk of infection. It also would complicate surgical evaluation of the injury.

MANAGEMENT OF ABDOMINAL TRAUMA

Emergency care of patients with abdominal trauma usually is limited to two courses of action: (1) stabilizing the patient's condition and (2) rapidly transporting the patient to a hospital for surgical repair of the injury.

The following are the most important components of on-scene care:

- A thorough scene survey to identify forces involved in abdominal trauma
- Rapid evaluation of the patient and the mechanism of injury
- Airway maintenance with spinal precautions
- Administration of high-concentration oxygen
- Ventilatory support as needed

- Reduction of hemorrhage by application of pressure
- Fluid replacement with volume expanders
- Use of a PASG (per protocol)
- Cardiac monitoring

En route to the hospital, a full physical examination and ongoing assessment can be performed. These procedures should include obtaining a focused history, vital sign assessment (and reassessment), and inspection, percussion, and palpation of the abdomen (see Chapter 11). Auscultation of the abdomen for the presence of bowel sounds can establish a baseline measurement for hospital personnel. This assessment should never delay patient transport.

SUMMARY

- Blunt trauma to abdominal organs usually results from compression or shearing forces.
- Penetrating injury may result from stab wounds, gunshot wounds, or impalement.
- The two solid organs most often injured are the liver and the spleen. Both of these organs are primary sources of death from hemorrhage. Injuries to the hollow abdominal organs may result in sepsis, wound infection, and abscess formation.
- Injury to the retroperitoneal organs (kidneys, ureters, pancreas, duodenum) may cause massive hemorrhage.
- Injury to the pelvic organs (bladder, urethra) usually results from motor vehicle crashes that cause pelvic fractures.
- Injuries to abdominal vascular structures may be life-threatening. This is due to their potential for massive hemorrhage.
- The most significant sign of severe abdominal trauma is unexplained shock.
- Emergency care of patients with abdominal trauma usually is limited to two courses of action: (1) stabilizing the patient's condition and (2) rapidly transporting the patient to a hospital for surgical repair of the injury.

REFERENCES

1. Rosen P, Barkin R: *Emergency medicine: concepts and clinical practice,* ed 4, St Louis, 1998, Mosby.
2. US Department of Transportation, National Highway Traffic Safety Administration: *EMT-paramedic national standard curriculum,* 1998, Washington, DC, The Department.

SUGGESTED READINGS

Emergency Nurses Association: *Sheehy's emergency nursing: principles and practice,* ed 5, St Louis, 2003, Mosby.

Ferrera P et al: *Trauma management,* St Louis, 2001, Mosby.

National Association of Emergency Medical Technicians: *PHTLS: basic and advanced prehospital life support,* ed 5, St Louis, 2003, Mosby.

Roberts J, Hedges J: *Clinical procedures in emergency medicine,* ed 3, Philadelphia, 1998, WB Saunders.

CHAPTER

28

Musculoskeletal Trauma

OBJECTIVES

Upon completion of this chapter, the paramedic student will be able to:

1. Describe the features of each class of musculoskeletal injury.
2. Describe the features of bursitis, tendonitis, and arthritis.
3. Given a specific patient scenario, outline the prehospital assessment of the musculoskeletal system.
4. Outline general principles of splinting.
5. Describe the significance and prehospital management principles for selected upper extremity injuries.
6. Describe the significance and prehospital management principles for selected lower extremity injuries.
7. Identify prehospital management priorities for open fractures.
8. Describe the principles of realignment of angular fractures and dislocations.
9. Outline the process for referral of patients with a minor musculoskeletal injury.

KEY TERMS

DCAP-BTLS: An acronym for wound assessment: deformity, contusions, abrasions, penetrations or punctures, burns, tenderness, lacerations, and swelling.

false movement: An unnatural movement of an extremity, usually associated with fracture.

fracture: A break in the continuity of bone or cartilage.

joint dislocation: An injury that occurs when the normal articulating ends of two or more bones are displaced.

sprain: A partial tearing of a ligament caused by a sudden twisting or stretching of a joint beyond its normal range of motion.

strain: An injury to the muscle or its tendon from overexertion or overextension.

Musculoskeletal trauma occurs in 70% to 80% of patients who suffer a traumatic injury (occurring as an isolated injury or with other injuries).[1] Trauma to an extremity is seldom life-threatening. However, early recognition and management may prevent long-term disability.

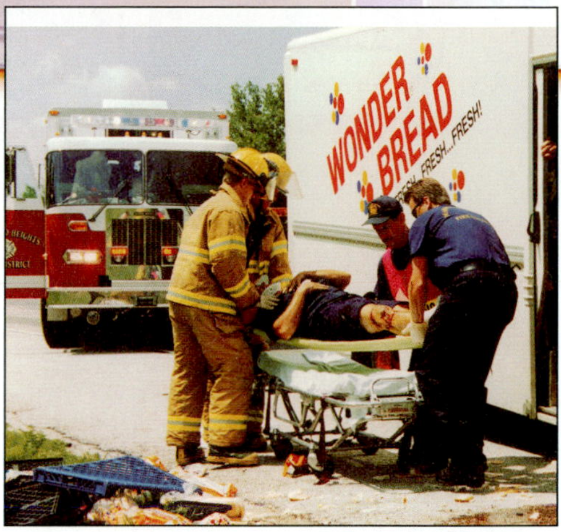

NOTE Extremity trauma usually results from motor vehicle crashes, falls, acts of violence, and contact sports.[2] Prevention strategies include proper sports training (working with athletic trainers on the use of protective equipment), use of personal restraints, gun safety education, and fall prevention (e.g., high-rise window guards) (see Chapter 3).

CLASSIFICATIONS OF MUSCULOSKELETAL INJURIES

The musculoskeletal system and associated neurovascular structures are made up of bones, nerves, vessels, muscles, tendons, ligaments, and joints (see Chapter 6). Injuries that result from traumatic forces to these tissues include fractures, sprains, strains, and joint dislocations. The paramedic should not attempt to differentiate these injuries in the prehospital setting. Patients suspected of having trauma to an extremity should be managed as though a fracture exists. Problems associated with musculoskeletal injuries include the following:

- Hemorrhage
- Instability
- Loss of tissue
- Simple laceration and contamination
- Interruption of blood supply
- Nerve damage
- Long-term disability

CRITICAL THINKING

How could long-term disability result from a musculoskeletal injury?

Musculoskeletal injuries can result from direct trauma (e.g., blunt force applied to an extremity), indirect trauma (e.g., a vertical fall that produces a spinal fracture distant from the site of impact), or pathological conditions (e.g., some forms of arthritis; malignancy). Paramedics should consider kinematics when caring for a patient with a musculoskeletal injury. They also should carefully evaluate the scene (see Chapter 20).

Fractures

A **fracture** is any break in the continuity of bone or cartilage (Fig. 28-1). It may be complete or incomplete, depending on the line of fracture through the bone. Fractures also are classified as *open* or *closed,* depending on the integrity of the skin near the fracture site (Box 28-1). Fractures of long bones may result in moderate to severe hemorrhage within the first 2 hours. As much as 550 mL of blood may be released in the lower leg from a tibial or fibular fracture, 1000 mL of blood in the thigh from a femoral fracture, and 2000 mL of blood from a pelvic fracture.[1]

As described in Chapter 6, the head of long bones in children is separated from the shaft of the bone by the epiphyseal plate until the bone stops growing. Fractures that involve the epiphyseal plate are called *epiphyseal fractures.* These are serious injuries. They may result in separation or fragmentation of the growth plate. They also may result in permanent bending or deformity of an extremity (Fig. 28-2).

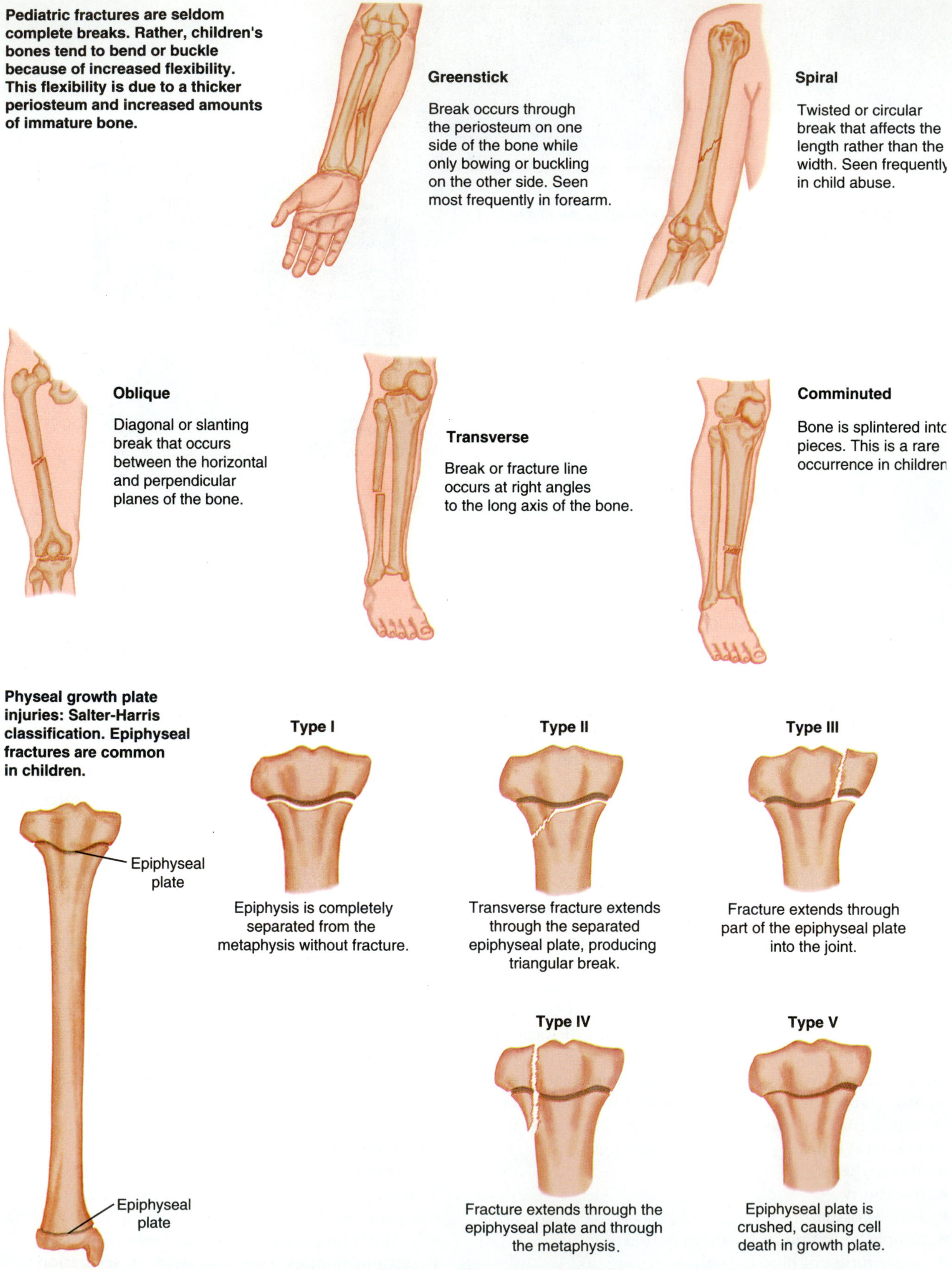
Pediatric fractures are seldom complete breaks. Rather, children's bones tend to bend or buckle because of increased flexibility. This flexibility is due to a thicker periosteum and increased amounts of immature bone.
Greenstick
Break occurs through the periosteum on one side of the bone while only bowing or buckling on the other side. Seen most frequently in forearm.
Spiral
Twisted or circular break that affects the length rather than the width. Seen frequentl
in child abuse.
Oblique
Diagonal or slanting break that occurs between the horizontal and perpendicular planes of the bone.
Transverse
Break or fracture line occurs at right angles to the long axis of the bone.
Comminuted
Bone is splintered intc pieces. This is a rare occurrence in children
Physeal growth plate injuries: Salter-Harris classification. Epiphyseal fractures are common in children.
Epiphyseal plate
Epiphyseal plate
Type I
Epiphysis is completely separated from the metaphysis without fracture.
Type II
Transverse fracture extends through the separated epiphyseal plate, producing triangular break.
Type III
Fracture extends through part of the epiphyseal plate into the joint.
Type IV
Fracture extends through the epiphyseal plate and through the metaphysis.
Type V
Epiphyseal plate is crushed, causing cell death in growth plate.

FIGURE 28-1 ■ Bone fractures. **A**, Complete and incomplete. **B**, Comminuted and transverse. **C**, Impacted. **D**, Oblique and spiral. (Courtesy David J. Mascaro and Associates.)

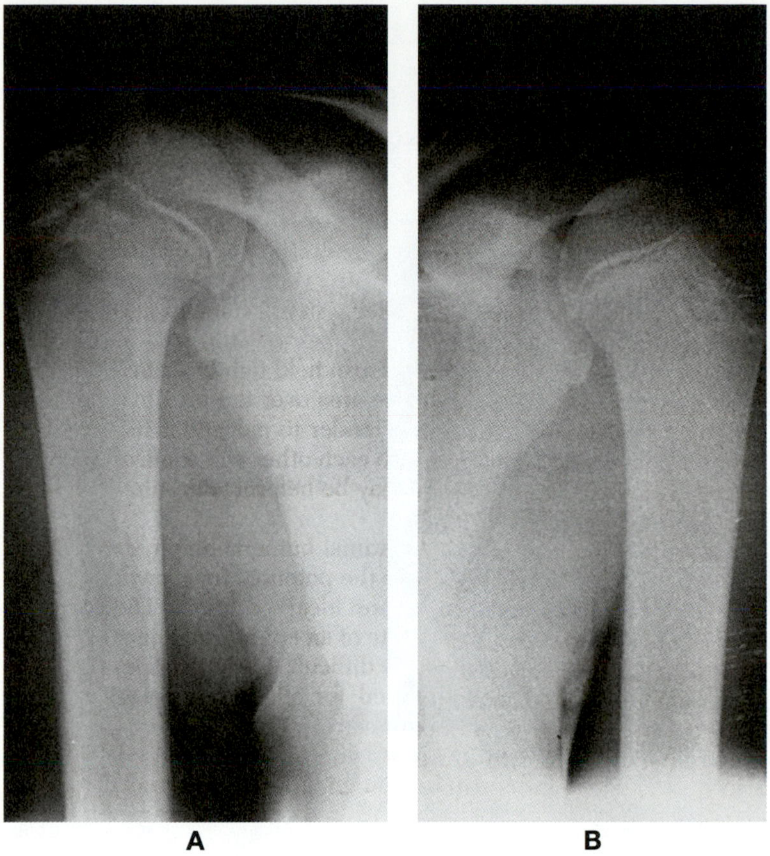

FIGURE 28-2 ■ **A,** Fracture of the proximal humeral epiphysis. Normal left side **(B)** is included for comparison.

BOX 28-1 Classification of Fractures

Open: A break in which a protruding bone or penetrating object causes a soft tissue injury
Closed: A break in the bone that has not yet penetrated the soft tissue or skin
Comminuted: A fracture that involves several breaks in the bone, resulting in multiple bone fragments
Greenstick: A break in which the bone is bent but only broken on the outside of the bend (common in children)
Spiral: A break caused by a twisting motion
Oblique: A break at a slanting angle across a bone
Transverse: A break that occurs at right angles to the long axis of the bone
Stress: A break (especially in one or more of the foot bones) caused by repeated, long-term, or abnormal stress
Pathological: A break resulting from weakness in bone tissue caused by neoplasm or malignant growth
Epiphyseal: A break that involves the epiphyseal growth plate of a child's long bone; may result in permanent angulation or deformity and may cause premature arthritis

Sprains

A **sprain** is a partial tearing of a ligament. It is caused by sudden twisting or stretching of a joint beyond its normal range of motion (Fig. 28-3). Two common areas for sprains are the knee and the ankle. Sprains are graded by severity (Box 28-2). A first-degree sprain has no joint instability. This is because only a few fibers of the ligament are torn. Swelling and hemorrhage are minimal. (Repeated first-degree sprains can result in stretching of the ligaments.) A second-degree sprain causes more disruption than a first-degree injury. The joint usually is still intact, but swelling and bruising are increased. In third-degree sprains the ligaments are completely torn. If third-degree sprains are accompanied by a dislocation, nerve or blood vessel compromise to the extremity is possible. Some second-degree sprains and most third-degree sprains have the same presentation as a fracture.

The application of ice to an injury during the first 24 hours generally reduces pain and swelling. After that time, heat (e.g., warm soaks) often is prescribed to increase circulation.

Strains

A **strain** is an injury to the muscle or its tendon from overexertion or overextension. Strains commonly occur in the back and arms and may be accompanied by a significant

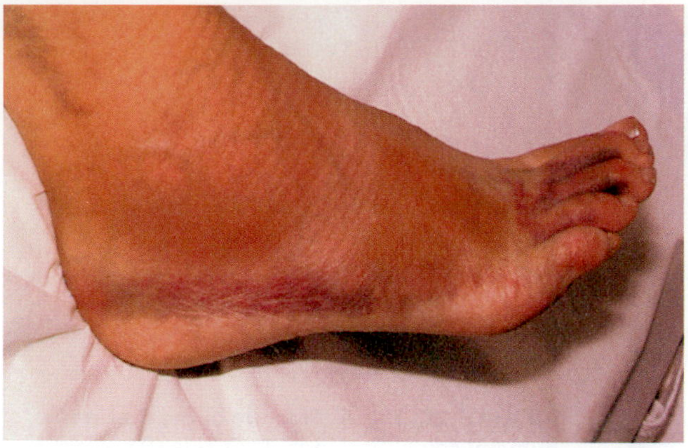

FIGURE 28-3 ■ Swelling and bruising from a sprain of a lateral ligament.

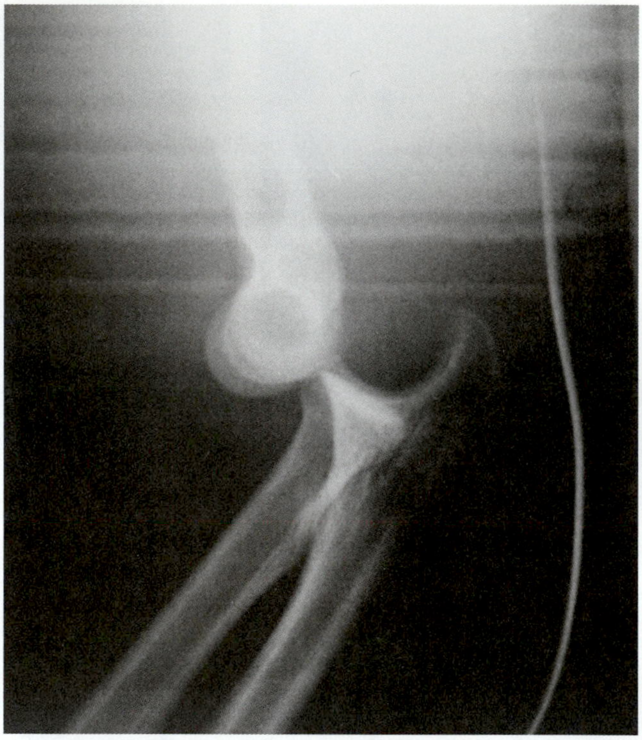

FIGURE 28-4 ■ Posterior elbow dislocation.

BOX 28-2 Grading of Sprains by Severity

First-Degree Sprain
No joint instability
Minimal swelling/hemorrhage

Second-Degree Sprain
Joint usually intact
Increased swelling/ecchymosis

Third-Degree Sprain
Total disruption of ligaments
Possible nerve or vascular compromise

loss of function. Severe strains may cause an avulsion of bone from the tendon attachment site.

Joint Dislocations

A **joint dislocation** occurs when the normal articulating ends of two or more bones are displaced (Fig. 28-4). Joints that often are dislocated are those of the shoulders, elbows, fingers, hips, knees, and ankles. Dislocation should be suspected when a joint is deformed or does not move with normal range of motion. A complete dislocation is called a *luxation;* an incomplete dislocation is called a *subluxation.* All dislocations can result in great damage and instability.

CRITICAL THINKING

Why do dislocations have a high rate of vascular or nerve damage?

INFLAMMATORY AND DEGENERATIVE CONDITIONS

Several inflammatory and degenerative conditions (Box 28-3) may manifest as or may be complicated by an extremity injury. These include bursitis, tendonitis, and arthritis.

BOX 28-3 Age-Associated Changes in Bones

As a person ages, morphological changes occur in the bones. Some of the changes may increase the chance of injury or complicate the healing process. These morphological changes include the following:

- A decrease in the water content of the intervertebral disks (increasing the risk of herniation)
- Loss of about 1 to 2 cm (½ to ¾ inch) in height, resulting in a shortened trunk and the formation of an arc-shaped vertebral column that is prone to injury
- Thoracic rigidity caused by ossification of costal cartilage (may lead to shallow breathing)
- Porous and brittle bones that are prone to fracture
- Bone disorders (e.g., osteoporosis) that increase the risk of fracture

Bursitis

Bursitis is inflammation of a bursa (a small, fluid-filled sac that acts as a cushion at a pressure point near joints). The most important bursae are around the knee, elbow, and shoulder (Fig. 28-5). The condition usually is a result of pressure (e.g., prolonged kneeling on a hard surface), friction, or slight injury to the membranes surrounding the joint. Management generally consists of rest, ice, and analgesics. The condition usually subsides after this treatment. In rare cases, bursectomy (surgical excision of a bursa) may be performed.

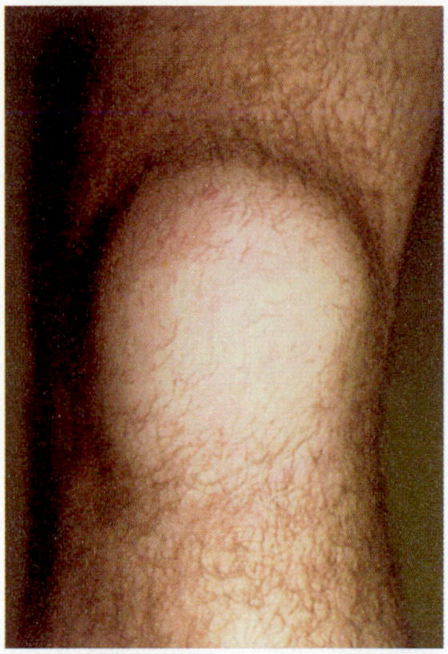

FIGURE 28-5 ■ Prepatellar bursa (housemaid's knee).

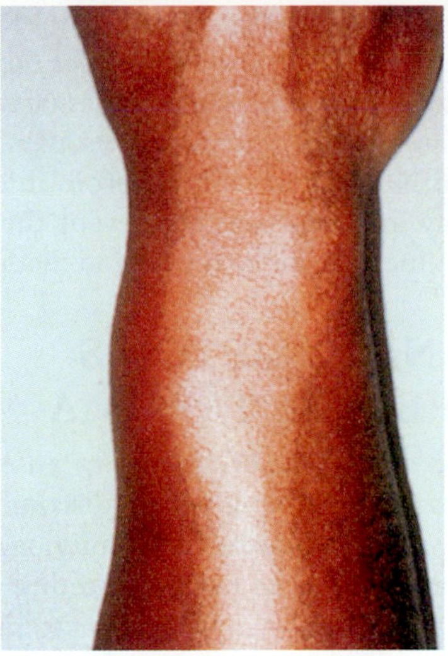

FIGURE 28-6 ■ Swelling of the tendons over the radial side of the wrist.

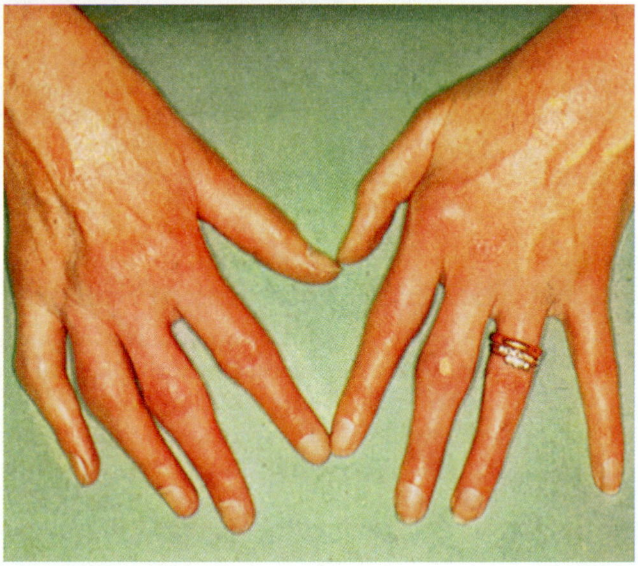

FIGURE 28-7 ■ Rheumatoid arthritis.

Tendonitis

Tendonitis is inflammation of a tendon. It often is caused by injury (Fig. 28-6). Symptoms include pain, tenderness, and sometimes restricted movement of the muscle attached to the affected tendon (e.g., pain in the shoulder when the arm is raised above a certain angle). Management usually includes nonsteroidal antiinflammatory drugs (NSAIDs) and sometimes corticosteroid drugs that are injected around the tendon.

Arthritis

Arthritis is inflammation of a joint. It is characterized by pain, swelling, stiffness, and redness (see Chapter 45). The condition is not a single disease. Rather, the term refers to joint disease (involving one or many joints) that can occur from a number of causes. Arthritis varies in severity from a mild ache and stiffness to severe pain and, later, joint deformity.

Osteoarthritis (degenerative arthritis) is the most common form of arthritis. It results from wear and tear on the joints. Osteoarthritis begins in middle age. The pain from this condition generally is managed with antiinflammatory agents.

Rheumatoid arthritis is the most severe type of inflammatory joint disease. It is an autoimmune disorder. The body's immune system acts against and damages joints and surrounding soft tissues. Many joints, most often those in the hands, feet, and arms, become extremely painful, stiff, and deformed (Fig. 28-7). Drugs used to treat this condition include NSAIDs to reduce pain and antirheumatic drugs and immunosuppressive agents to arrest or slow the progress of the disease.

Gouty arthritis is a form of joint disease in which uric acid builds up in joints in the form of crystals, causing inflammation. The first attack of this form of arthritis usually involves only one joint (e.g., the base of the big toe).

This first attack usually lasts a few days. Subsequent attacks may be more severe and may affect more joints (e.g., knee, ankle, wrist, foot, and small joints of the hand). Pain and inflammation from gouty arthritis are controlled with large doses of NSAIDs or corticosteroid injections. Other treatment may include drugs to prevent the formation of uric acid or to increase its excretion and diet modifications.

SIGNS AND SYMPTOMS OF EXTREMITY TRAUMA

The signs and symptoms of trauma to an extremity vary. They may be subtle complaints of discomfort. However, they also may include obvious deformity or open fracture. Field evaluation should be rapid, assuming significant injury. Common signs and symptoms of extremity trauma include the following:

- Pain on palpation or movement
- Swelling, deformity
- Crepitus
- Decreased range of motion
- **False movement** (unnatural movement of an extremity)
- Decreased or absent sensory perception or circulation distal to the injury (evidenced by alterations in skin color and temperature, distal pulses, and capillary refill)

CRITICAL THINKING

How can a paramedic tell a serious sprain from a fracture in the prehospital setting?

ASSESSMENT OF MUSCULOSKELETAL INJURIES

For the purposes of musculoskeletal assessment, patients can be divided into four classes:

- Those with life- or limb-threatening injuries or conditions, including life- or limb-threatening musculoskeletal trauma
- Those with other life- or limb-threatening injuries and only simple musculoskeletal trauma
- Those with no other life- or limb-threatening injuries but with life- or limb-threatening musculoskeletal trauma
- Those with only isolated injuries that are not life or limb threatening

The paramedic should perform an initial assessment to determine whether the patient has any conditions that pose a threat to life. Such conditions must be dealt with first. Paramedics must never overlook musculoskeletal trauma. They also must never allow a frightful, but noncritical, musculoskeletal injury to distract from the priorities of care.

Evaluation of an injured extremity should always include checking the "six *Ps*": *p*ain, *p*allor, *p*aresthesia, *p*ulses, *p*aralysis, and *p*ressure (Box 28-4). The paramedic also should evaluate an extremity's neurovascular status by assessing the distal pulse, motor function, and sensation (before and after movement or splinting). In addition, the paramedic should inspect and palpate the injured area for **DCAP-BTLS:**

*D*eformity
*C*ontusions
*A*brasions
*P*enetrations or punctures
*B*urns
*T*enderness
*L*acerations
*S*welling

If possible, the assessment should include comparison with the opposite, uninjured extremity. If trauma to an extremity is suspected, the extremity should be splinted.

NOTE This text presents methods to immobilize fractures and dislocations for isolated extremity injuries. Again, seldom does trauma to an extremity pose a threat to life. Therefore patients with multiple-system traumatic injury should first be managed for conditions that compromise the airway, breathing, and circulation (including internal and external hemorrhage in the extremities) and spinal stability. Rapid transport may be indicated by the patient's condition or mechanism of injury. If this is the case, injured extremities can be stabilized by fully immobilizing the patient on a long spine board (Fig. 28-8).

General Principles of Splinting

The goal of splinting is immobilization of the injured body part. Immobilization by splinting helps alleviate pain; decreases tissue injury, bleeding, and contamination of an open wound; and simplifies and facilitates transport of the patient. The general principles of splinting are listed in Box 28-5.

TYPES OF SPLINTS

A wide variety of splints and splinting materials are available. Splints can be broadly categorized as rigid splints, soft or formable splints, and traction splints.

The shape of a rigid splint cannot be changed. The body part must be positioned to fit the splint's design. Examples of rigid splints include board splints, contoured metal and plastic splints, and some cardboard splints (Fig. 28-9). Rigid splints should be padded before use to accommodate for shape and patient comfort.

Soft or formable splints can be molded into a variety of shapes and configurations to accommodate the injured body part. Examples of soft or formable splints include pillows, blankets, slings and swathes, vacuum splints, some cardboard splints, wire ladder splints, and padded, flexible aluminum splints (Fig. 28-10). Inflatable air splints also are considered soft or formable splints. However, they are not designed to be used for injuries to the knee or elbow.

Traction splints are specifically designed for midshaft femoral fractures. These splints do not apply or maintain enough traction to reduce a femoral fracture. However,

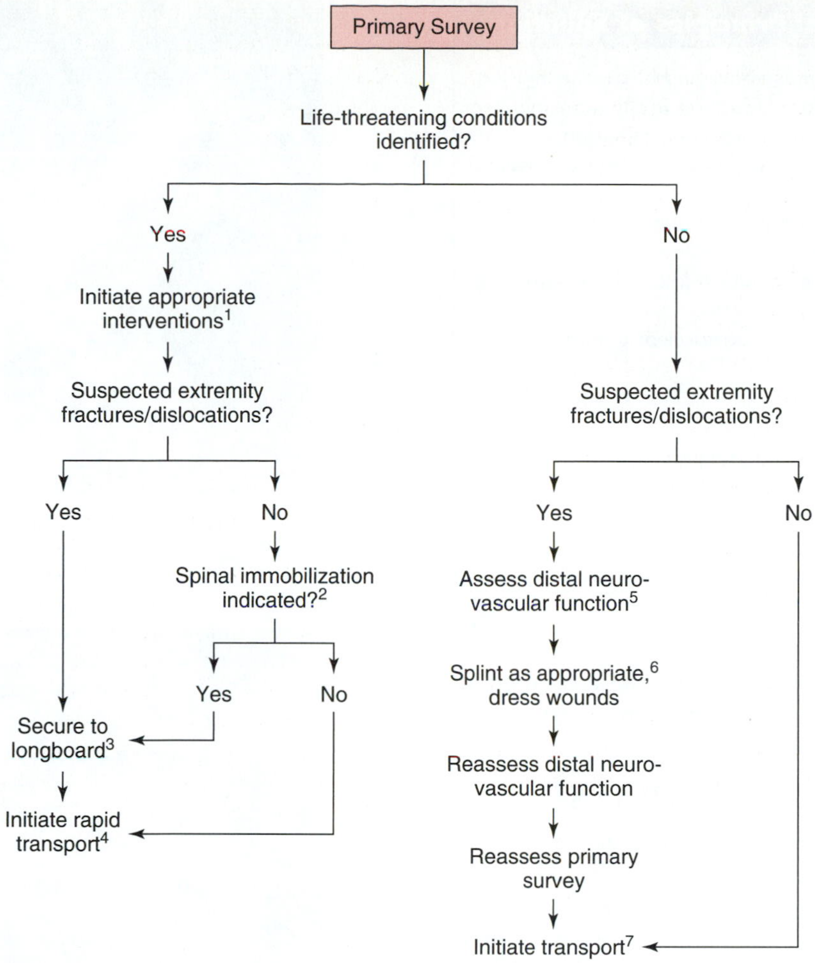

[1]Airway management, ventilatory support, shock therapy.

[2]See Indications for Spinal Immobilization algorithm.

[3]Injured extremities are immobilized in anatomic position by securing to longboard.

[4]Transport to closest appropriate facility (trauma center, if available); assess distal neurovascular function and apply traction splint (if suspected femur fracture) as time permits.

[5]Assess perfusion (pulses and capillary refilling) and neurologic function (motor and sensory) distal to the suspected fracture or dislocation.

[6]Use appropriate splinting technique to immobilize suspected fracture or dislocation; if suspected midshaft femur fracture, apply traction splint.

[7]Transport to closest appropriate facility.

FIGURE 28-8 ■ Evaluating extremity trauma.

BOX 28-4 Six *P*s of Musculoskeletal Assessment

Pain or tenderness	Pulses (diminished or absent)
Pallor (pale skin or poor capillary refill)	Paralysis (inability to move)
Paresthesia (pins-and-needles sensation)	Pressure

BOX 28-5 General Principles of Splinting

1. Splint joints and bone ends above and below the injury.
2. Immobilize open and closed fractures in the same manner.
3. Cover open fractures to minimize contamination.
4. Check pulses, sensation, and motor function before and after splinting.
5. Stabilize the extremity with gentle in-line traction to a position of normal alignment.
6. Immobilize a long bone extremity in a straight position that can be splinted easily.
7. Immobilize dislocations in a position of comfort; ensure good vascular supply.
8. Immobilize joints as found; joint injuries are aligned only if no distal pulse is felt.
9. Apply cold to reduce swelling and pain.
10. Apply compression to reduce swelling.
11. Elevate the extremity if possible.

Note: Immobilization requires a minimum of two rescuers.

they provide enough traction to stabilize and align it. Examples include Thomas half-ring, Hare traction, and Sager traction splints (Fig. 28-11).

UPPER EXTREMITY INJURIES

Upper extremity injuries can be classified as fractures or dislocations to the shoulder, humerus, elbow, radius and ulna, wrist, hand, and finger (Fig. 28-12). Clavicular injury is discussed in Chapter 26. Most upper extremity injuries can be adequately immobilized with a sling and swathe.

Shoulder Injury

Shoulder injuries are common in older adults. This is due to a weaker bone structure. Shoulder injuries often result from a fall on an outstretched arm. Patients with an anterior fracture or dislocation (accounting for 90% of cases) often have the affected arm and shoulder close to the chest (with the lateral aspect of the shoulder appearing flat instead of rounded). In addition a deep depression between the head of the humerus and the acromion laterally ("hollow shoulder") may be visible. Patients with posterior fracture or dislocation may be found with the arm above the head. Management of shoulder injuries includes the following:

1. Assessment of neurovascular status
2. Application of a sling and swathe (Fig. 28-13)
3. Application of ice

NOTE Ice should be placed in a plastic bag and applied for 20-minute periods to the injury site. Refreezable packs of gelled solution are inefficient and should not be used.

Based on the position of the affected arm and shoulder, a makeshift splint may need to be devised to hold the injury in place. For example, with some fractures or dislocations,

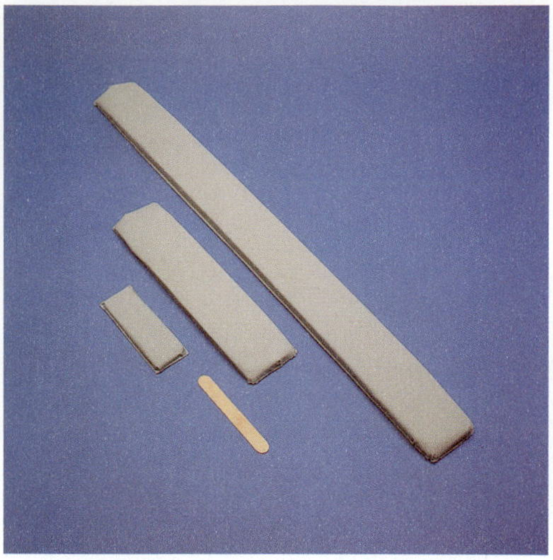

FIGURE 28-9 ■ Rigid splints.

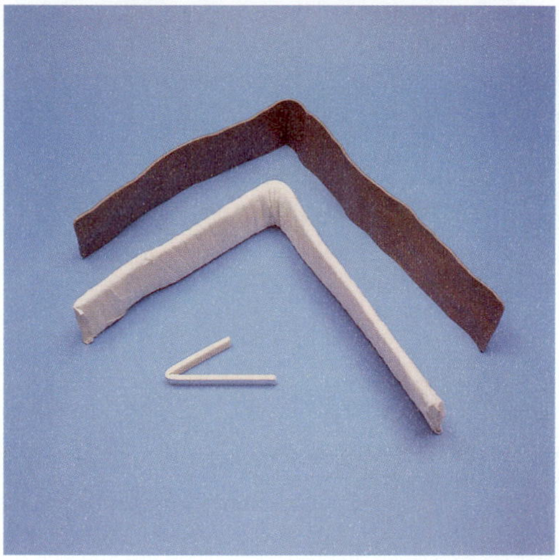

FIGURE 28-10 ■ Formable splints.

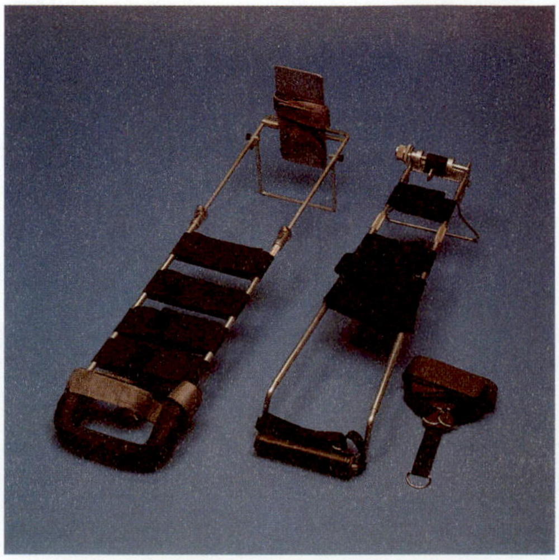

FIGURE 28-11 ■ Traction splints.

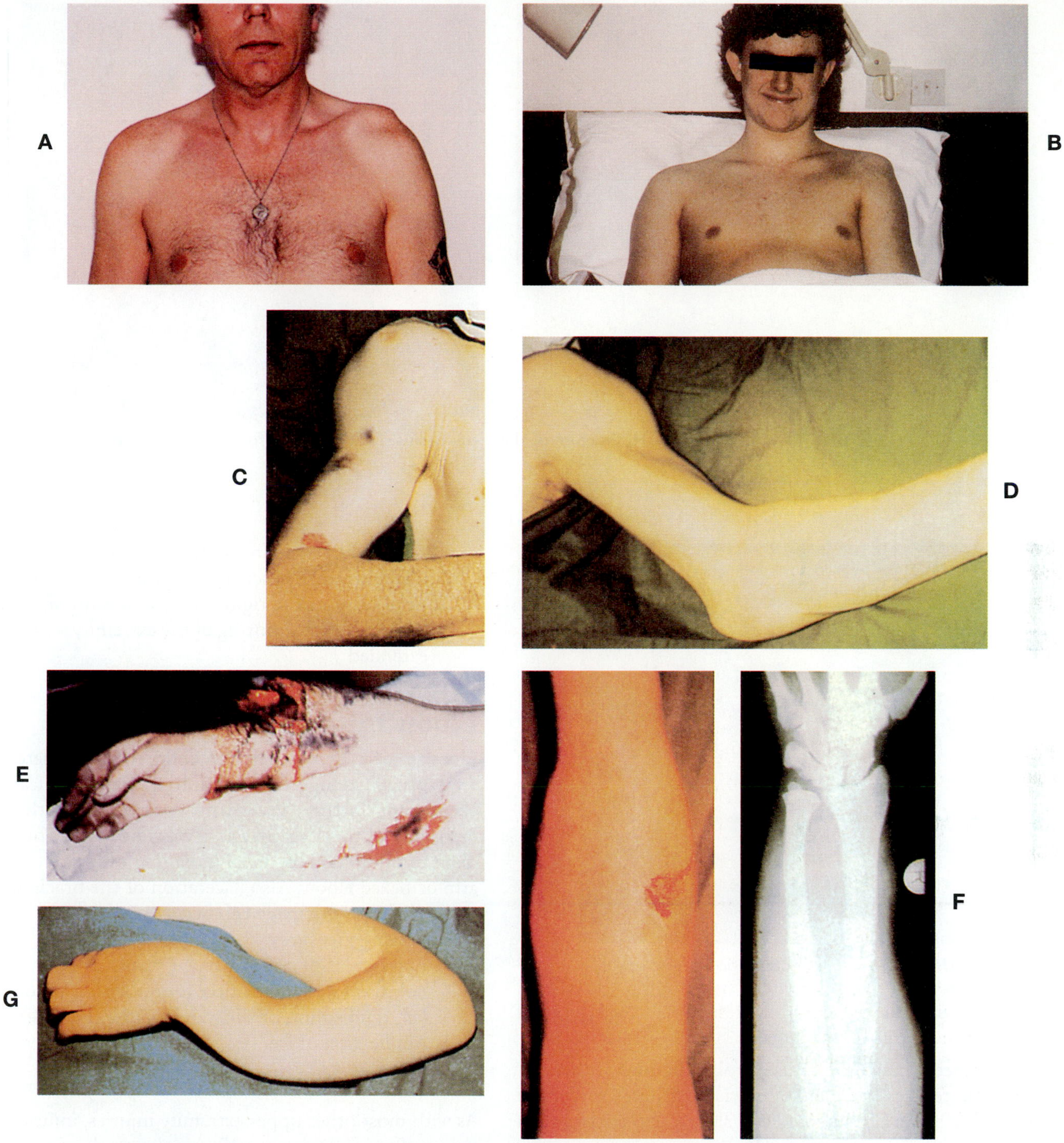

FIGURE 28-12 ■ **A,** Complete separation of the left acromioclavicular joint. **B,** Anterior dislocation of the left shoulder. **C,** Fracture of the proximal humerus. **D,** Posterior dislocation of the elbow joint with marked deformity. **E,** Severe open fracture of the forearm. **F,** Penetration of the forearm caused by a nail gun. **G,** Greenstick fracture with marked deformity. *Continued*

H

I

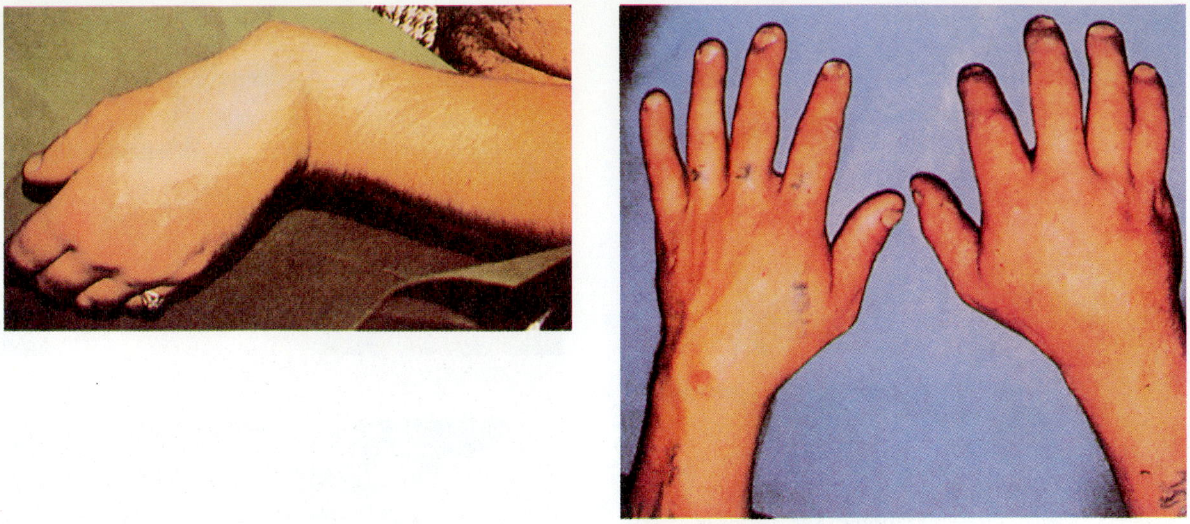

FIGURE 28-12, cont'd ■ **H,** Fracture of the distal radius. **I,** Hand injury from a motorcycle crash.

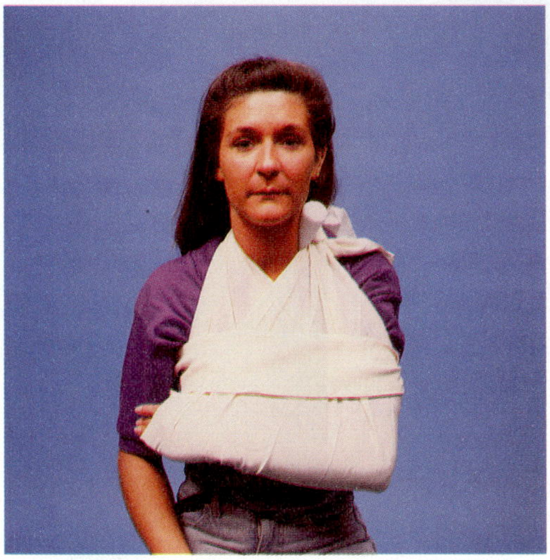

FIGURE 28-13 ■ Immobilization of the shoulder.

the paramedic may need to use a rolled blanket with a cravat at the center. The blanket roll is positioned under the elevated arm and secured like a sling. The arm is then swathed to prevent movement. If the patient's arm is positioned above the head, it should be splinted in position. Alternatively, traction can be applied on the long axis of the arm to obtain a better position for immobilization.

Humeral Injury

Upper arm fractures are common in older adults and children. They often are difficult to stabilize. Radial nerve damage may be present if a fracture occurs in the middle or distal portion of the humeral shaft. A fracture of the humeral neck may cause axillary nerve damage. Internal hemorrhage into the joint also may be a complication. Management includes the following measures:

1. Assessment of neurovascular status
2. Realignment if vascular compromise is present
3. Application of a rigid splint and sling and swathe (Fig. 28-14) or splinting of the extremity with the arm extended
4. Application of ice

Elbow Injury

Elbow injuries are common in children and athletes. They are especially dangerous in children. They may lead to ischemic contracture (Volkmann contracture) with serious deformity of the forearm and a clawlike hand. The mechanism of injury usually involves falling on an outstretched arm or flexed elbow. Also, laceration of the brachial artery and radial nerve damage can occur. Management includes the following measures:

1. Assessment of neurovascular status
2. Splinting in the position found with a pillow, blanket, rigid splint, or sling and swathe (Fig. 28-15)
3. Application of ice

Radial, Ulnar, or Wrist Injury

As with most other upper extremity injuries, injuries to the radius, ulna, and wrist usually are the result of a fall on an outstretched arm. Wrist injuries may involve the distal radius, the ulna, or any of the eight carpal bones. The most common wrist injury is a fracture with a "silver fork" deformity of the distal radius with dorsal angulation (Colles fracture) (Fig. 28-16). Forearm injury is common in both children and adults. Management includes the following measures:

1. Assessment of neurovascular status
2. Splinting in the position found with rigid or formable splints or a sling and swathe (Fig. 28-17)
3. Application of ice and elevation

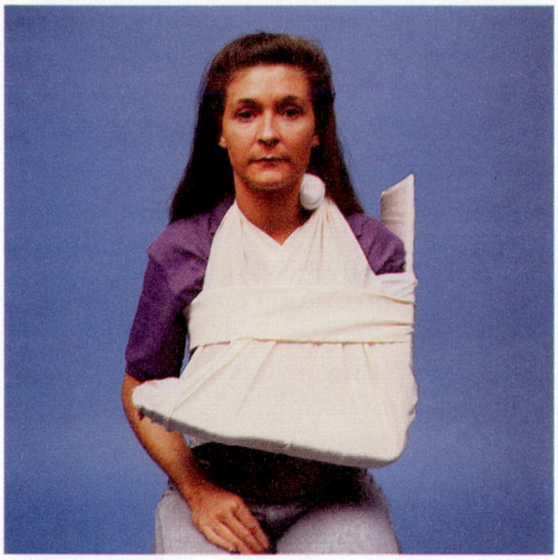

FIGURE 28-14 ■ Immobilization of the humerus.

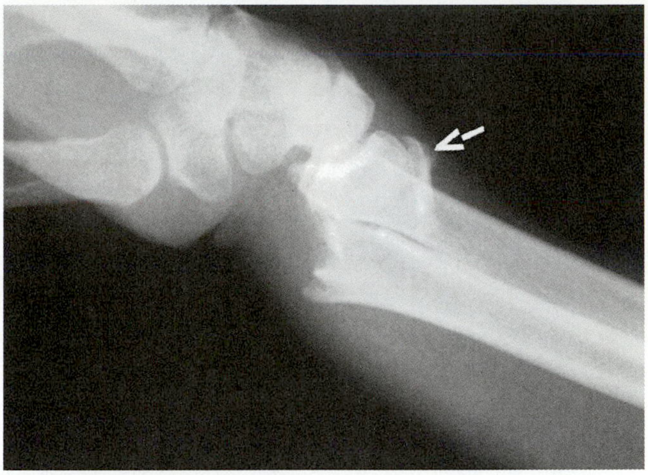

FIGURE 28-16 ■ Colles fracture (arrow shows dorsal angulation of distal radius fragment).

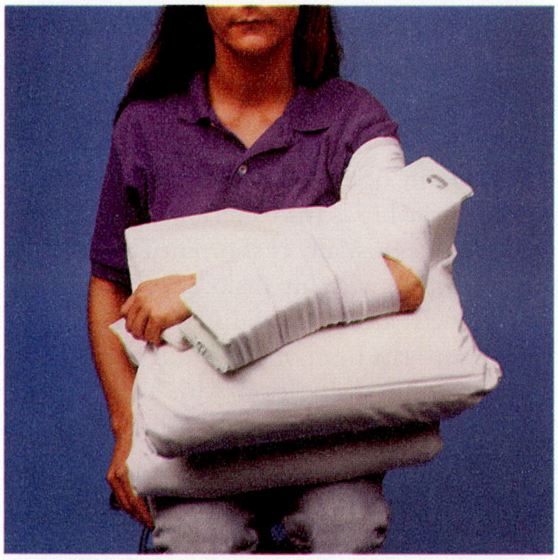

FIGURE 28-15 ■ Immobilization of the elbow.

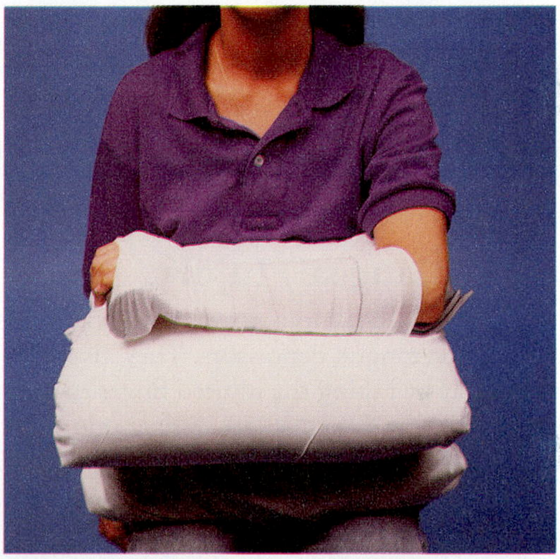

FIGURE 28-17 ■ Immobilization of the forearm.

CRITICAL THINKING

What effect does a cold pack have on musculoskeletal injuries?

Hand (Metacarpal) Injury

Injury to the hand often results from contact sports, violence (fighting), and work-related crushing injuries. A common metacarpal injury is boxer's fracture. This results from direct trauma to a closed fist, resulting in fracture of the fifth metacarpal bone (Fig. 28-18). These injuries also may be associated with hematomas and open wounds. Boxer's fracture is the most common metacarpal fracture, but any of the metacarpals can be fractured, depending on the mechanism of injury. Hand injuries should be splinted in the position of function (as with a hand grasping a football). Rigid or formable splints (previously described for a

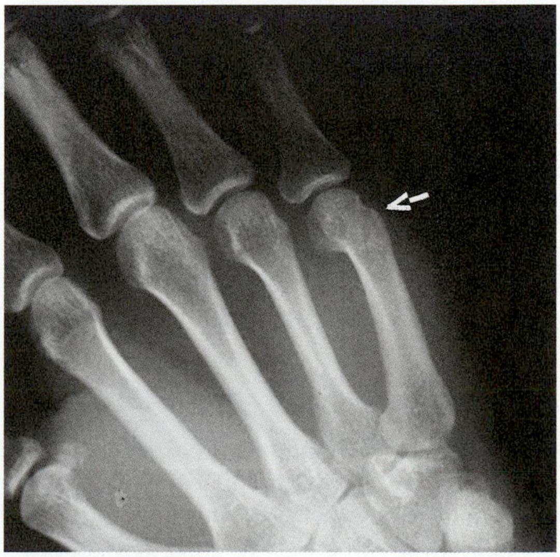

FIGURE 28-18 ■ Boxer's fracture (*arrow*).

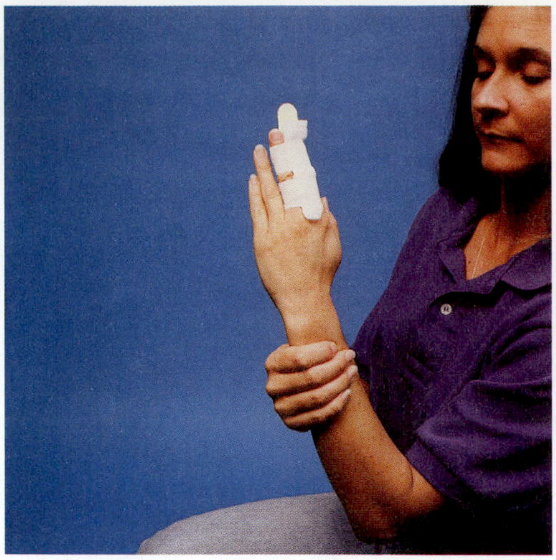

FIGURE 28-19 ■ Immobilization of the finger.

radial, ulnar, or wrist injury) may be used. Management includes the following measures:

1. Assessment of neurovascular status
2. Splinting with a rigid or formable splint (pillow, blanket) in the position of function
3. Application of ice and elevation

Finger (Phalangeal) Injury

Injured fingers may be immobilized with foam-filled aluminum splints or tongue depressors. They also may be immobilized simply by taping the injured finger to an adjacent one ("buddy splinting") (Fig. 28-19). Finger injuries are common. However, they should not be considered trivial. Serious injuries include fractures of the thumb. Also, any open or markedly comminuted fractures of the hand or fingers are serious. Management includes the following measures:

1. Assessment of neurovascular status
2. Splinting as previously described
3. Application of ice and elevation

LOWER EXTREMITY INJURIES

Lower extremity injuries include fractures of the pelvis and fractures or dislocations of the hip, femur, knee and patella, tibia and fibula, ankle and foot, and phalanx (Fig. 28-20). Compared with upper extremity injuries, lower extremity injuries are associated with greater forces. They also are associated with more significant blood loss. They are more difficult to manage in patients with multiple injuries, and they may be life-threatening (e.g., femoral and pelvic fractures).

Pelvic Fracture

As described in Chapter 27, blunt or penetrating injury to the pelvis may result in fracture, severe hemorrhage, and associated injury to the urinary bladder and urethra. The pelvis is surrounded by heavy muscles and other soft tissues. Therefore deformity may be difficult to see (Fig. 28-21). Injury to the pelvis should be suspected based on the mechanism of injury or tenderness on palpation of the iliac crests (see Chapter 12). Trauma to the abdomen and pelvic area may be complicated by pregnancy (see Chapter 42). Management includes the following measures:

1. Administration of high-concentration oxygen
2. Management for shock (pneumatic antishock garment [PASG] per protocol)
3. Full-body immobilization on a long spine board (adequately padded for comfort)
4. Regular monitoring of vital signs
5. Rapid transport (essential)

> **NOTE** The pneumatic antishock garment (PASG) may help to arrest hemorrhage by tamponading bleeding vessels in the pelvis or lower extremities (see Chapter 21). It also may be used to stabilize pelvic and lower extremity fractures. Decisions on the use of the PASG are made per local protocol and according to medical direction.

Hip Injury

Hip injuries commonly occur in older adults as a result of a fall. They commonly occur in younger patients as a result of major trauma. If the hip is fractured at the femoral head and neck, the affected leg usually is shortened and externally rotated. By comparison, with hip dislocation the affected leg is usually shortened and internally rotated (Fig. 28-22). (Fractures closer to the head of the femur may manifest similar to an anterior hip dislocation, with a shortened and internally rotated leg.) Management includes the following measures:

1. Assessment of neurovascular status
2. Splinting with a long spine board (Fig. 28-23) and generously padding the patient for comfort during transport (slight flexion of the knee or padding beneath the knee may improve comfort)
3. Frequent monitoring of vital signs

Femoral Injury

Injury to the femur usually results from major trauma, such as may occur with motor vehicle crashes and pedestrian injuries. It also is a fairly common result of child abuse.

Fractures of the femur result in powerful thigh muscle contractions. These contractions cause the bone fragments to ride back and forth over each other. The patient generally has a shortened leg that is externally rotated and midthigh swelling from hemorrhage, which can be life-threatening (Fig. 28-24). These fractures should be immobilized in the field with a traction splint. Management includes the following measures:

1. Administration of high-concentration oxygen
2. Management for shock
3. Assessment of neurovascular status
4. Application of a traction splint (Fig. 28-25)
5. Regular monitoring of vital signs

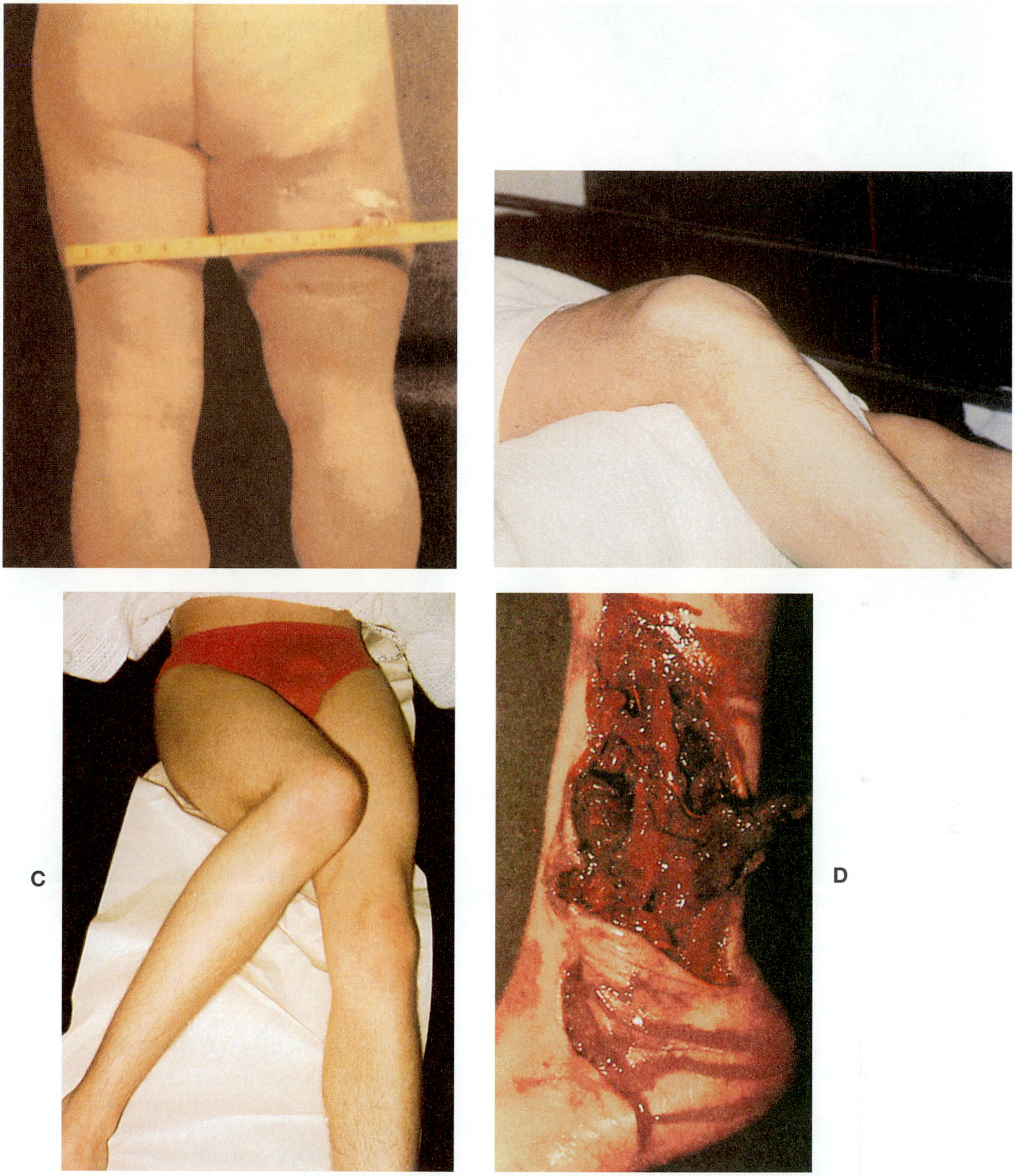

A B C D

FIGURE 28-20 ■ A, The diameter of the right thigh represents an increase in volume of 2 to 3 L of blood. B, Lateral dislocation of the right patella. C, Posterior dislocation of the right hip. D, Open fracture of the lower leg.

Continued

E

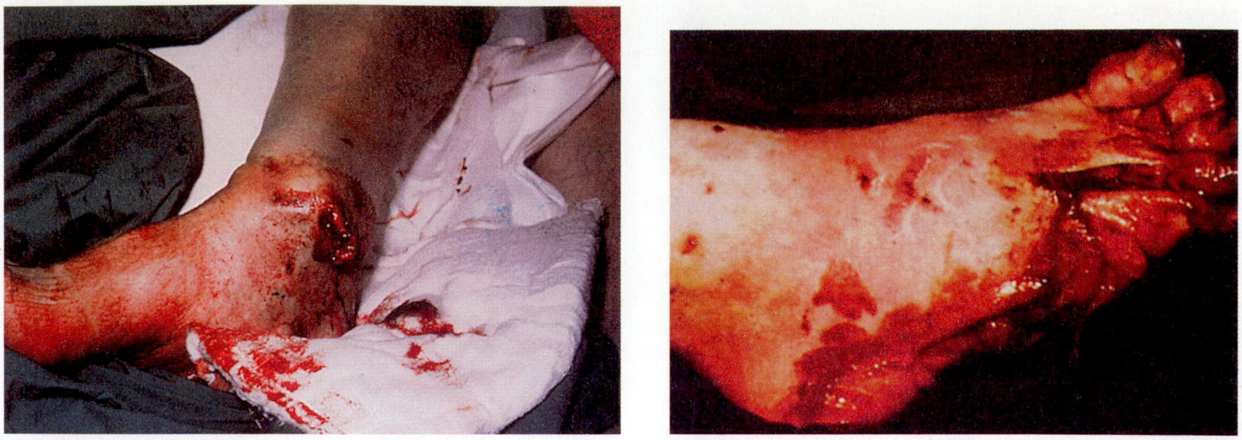

F

FIGURE 28-20, cont'd ■ **E,** Subtalar dislocation. **F,** Foot that was run over by the wheel of a railway coach.

A

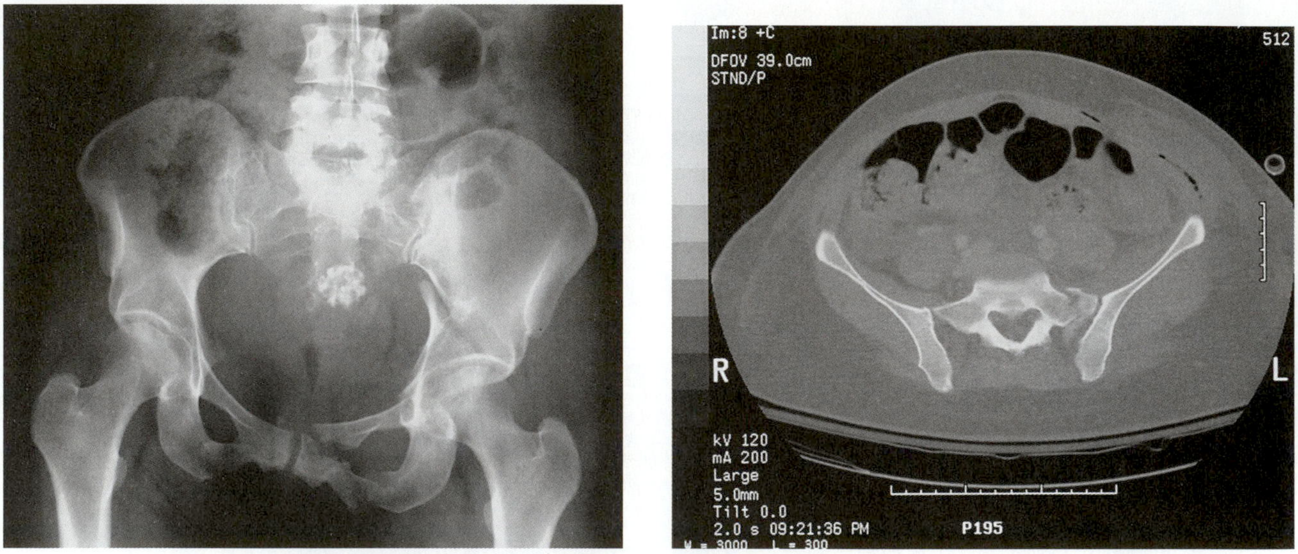

B

FIGURE 28-21 ■ Lateral compression injury. **A,** Anteroposterior projection demonstrating the characteristic horizontal anterior ring fracture and ipsilateral sacral crush fracture. **B,** The sacral fracture is well visualized on the pelvic CT.

▶**NOTE** Traction splints should be used only to immobilize midshaft femoral fractures. They should not be used with fractures of the lower third of the leg, pelvic fractures, hip injury, knee injury, or avulsion or amputation of the ankle and foot. The patient should be placed on a long spine board before the traction splint is applied.

When more than one injury contributes to the development of shock, the PASG and traction splint may be used together (per local protocol for the use of the PASG). The traction splint should be applied *over* the PASG only after it has been inflated. Any traction device placed under the PASG may promote continued hemorrhage, tissue damage, and compromised circulation to the injured extremity.

Knee and Patellar Injury

Fractures of the knee (supracondylar fracture of the femur, intraarticular fracture of the femur or tibia) and fractures and dislocations of the patella commonly result from motor vehicle crashes, pedestrian injuries, contact sports, and falls on a flexed knee (Fig. 28-26). The popliteal artery is close to the knee joint. Injury to the knee can also injure the popliteal artery, particularly with posterior dislocations. Management includes the following measures:

1. Assessment of neurovascular status
2. Splinting in the position found with a rigid or formable splint (Fig. 28-27) that effectively immobilizes the hip and ankle (traction splints should not be used to immobilize a knee or patellar injury)
3. Application of ice and elevation, if possible

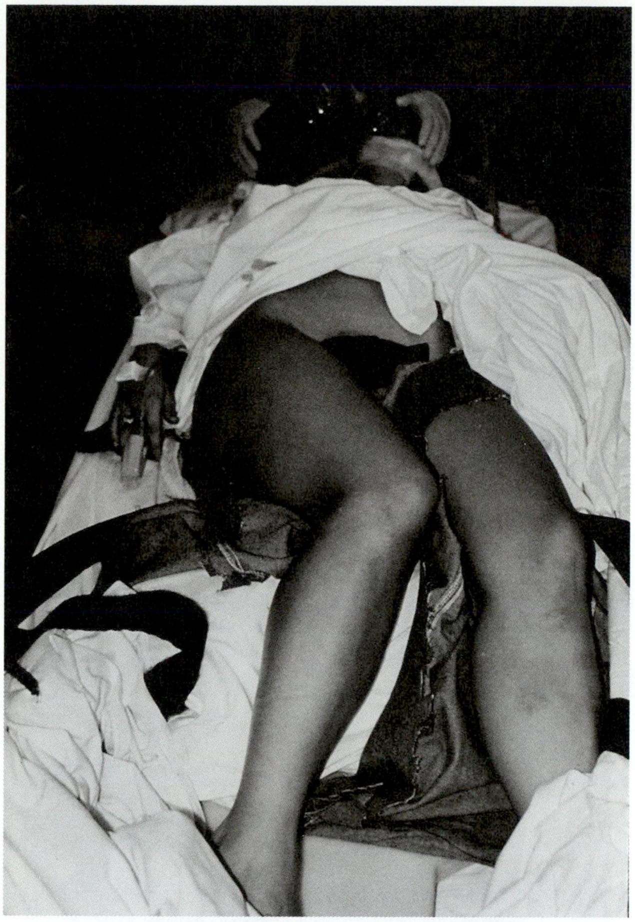

FIGURE 28-22 ■ Young woman with internal rotation, adduction, and shortening of right femur, consistent with her right posterior hip dislocation.

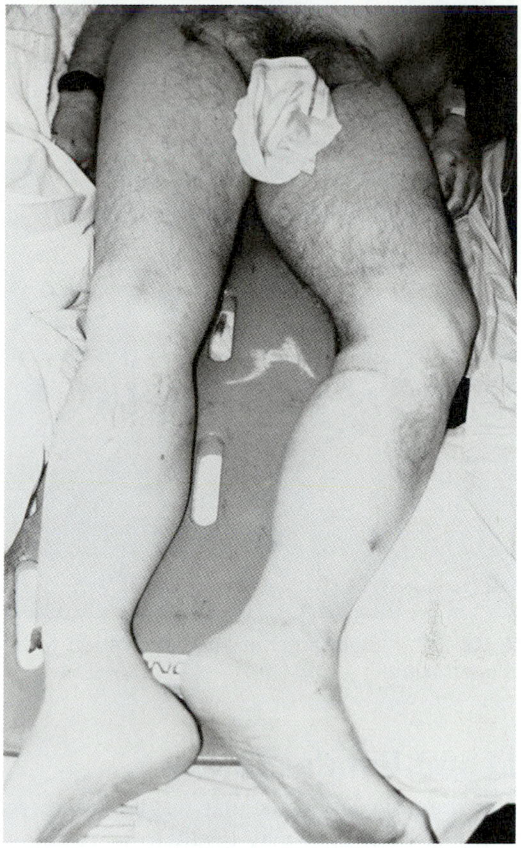

FIGURE 28-24 ■ Young man with external rotation, abduction, and shortening of the left femur, consistent with his midshaft fracture. Also note right tibia fracture.

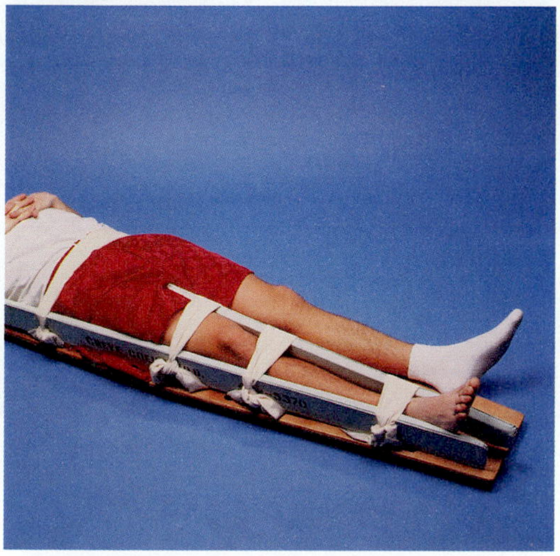

FIGURE 28-23 ■ Immobilization of the hip.

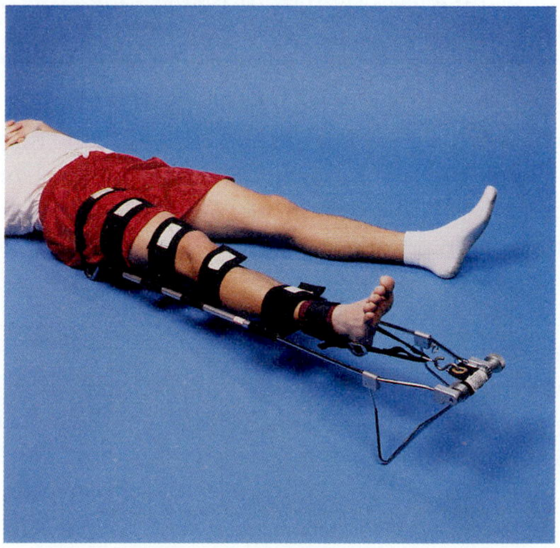

FIGURE 28-25 ■ Application of a traction splint.

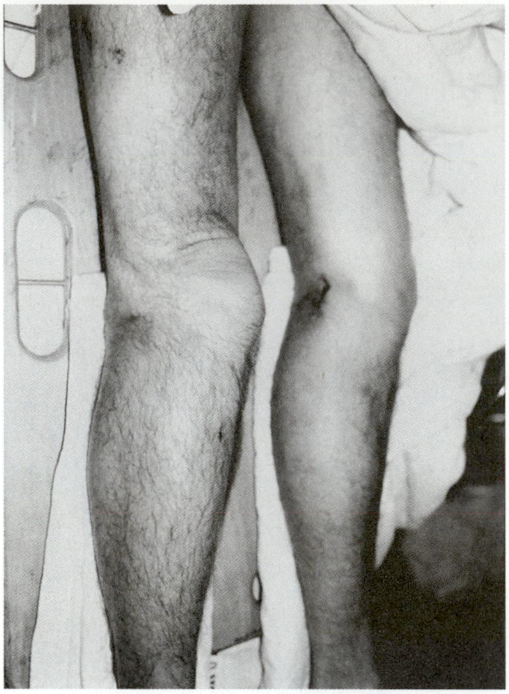

FIGURE 28-26 ■ Right anterior knee dislocation with overriding of tibia on femur.

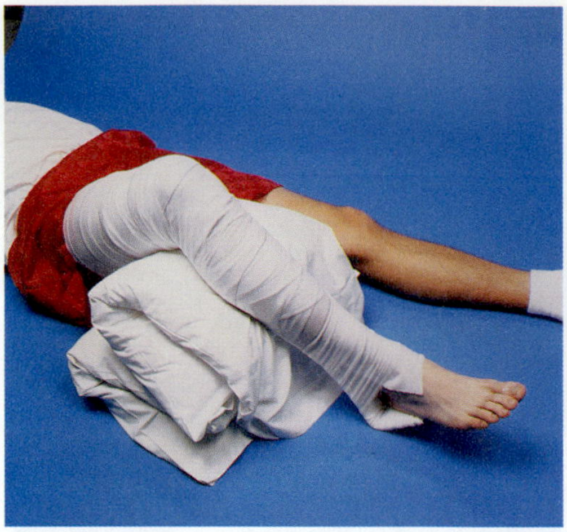

FIGURE 28-27 ■ Immobilization of the knee.

Tibial and Fibular Injury

Injuries to the tibia and fibula may result from direct or indirect trauma. They also may result from twisting injury (Fig. 28-28). If the injury is associated with the knee, popliteal vascular injury should be suspected. Management includes the following measures:

1. Assessment of neurovascular status
2. Splinting with a rigid or formable splint (Fig. 28-29)
3. Application of ice and elevation

Foot and Ankle Injury

Fractures and dislocations of the foot and ankle may result from a crush injury, a fall from a height, or a violent rotating or twisting force (Fig. 28-30). The patient usually complains of point tenderness. The person also often is hesitant to bear weight on the extremity. Management includes the following measures:

1. Assessment of neurovascular status
2. Application of a formable splint, such as a pillow, blanket, or air splint (Fig. 28-31)
3. Application of ice and elevation

Phalangeal Injury

Toe injuries often are caused by "stubbing" the toe on an immovable object. These injuries usually are managed by buddy taping the toe to an adjacent toe. This helps to support and immobilize the injury. Management includes the following measures:

1. Assessment of neurovascular status
2. Buddy splinting
3. Application of ice and elevation

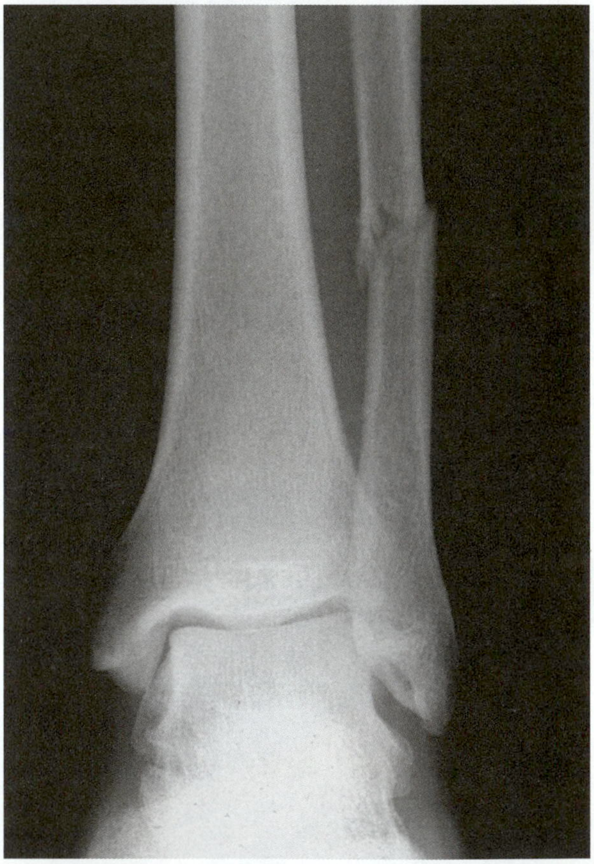

FIGURE 28-28 ■ Isolated fibular shaft fracture. This patient sustained a direct blow to the lateral leg to produce this transverse fracture. A fracture in this location should arouse suspicion of associated injury to knee ligaments or ankle injury.

OPEN FRACTURES

Patients with open fractures require special care and evaluation by the paramedic. Fractures may be opened in two ways. They may be opened *from within,* as when a bone fragment pierces the skin, or they may be opened *from without* (e.g., after

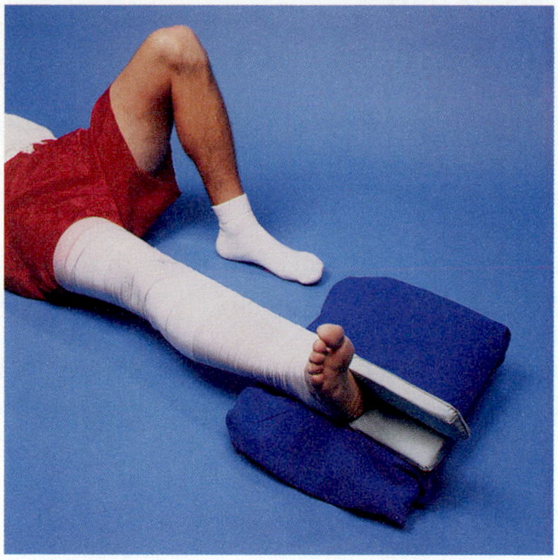

FIGURE 28-29 ■ Immobilization of the lower leg.

a gunshot wound). An open fracture also may have made contact with the skin some distance from the fracture site. Although most open fractures are obvious because of associated hemorrhage, a small puncture wound may not be immediately apparent, and bleeding may be minimal. Therefore the paramedic must consider any soft tissue wound in the area of a suspected fracture to be evidence of an open fracture.

Open fractures are considered a true surgical emergency because of the potential for infection. Most authorities agree that open wounds associated with fractures should be covered with sterile, dry dressings. They should not be irrigated in the field or soaked with any type of antiseptic solution. Hemorrhage should be controlled with direct pressure and pressure dressings.

If a bone end or bone fragment is visible, it should be covered with a dry, sterile dressing and splinted. Bone ends that slip back into the wound during immobilization should be noted and reported to the receiving hospital so that the bone can be cleaned in surgery.

STRAIGHTENING ANGULAR FRACTURES AND REDUCING DISLOCATIONS

Angular fractures and dislocations may make it difficult to apply a splint. In some cases they also may make it difficult to extricate and transport a patient. Paramedics may need to attempt manipulation of a fracture or dislocation. They may need to do this to aid transport or to improve circulation to the injured extremity. If this is the case, medical direction should be consulted.

> **NOTE** Limb-threatening injuries include knee dislocation, fracture or dislocation of the ankle, and subcondylar fractures of the elbow.[1] These serious injuries require rapid transport for evaluation by a physician.

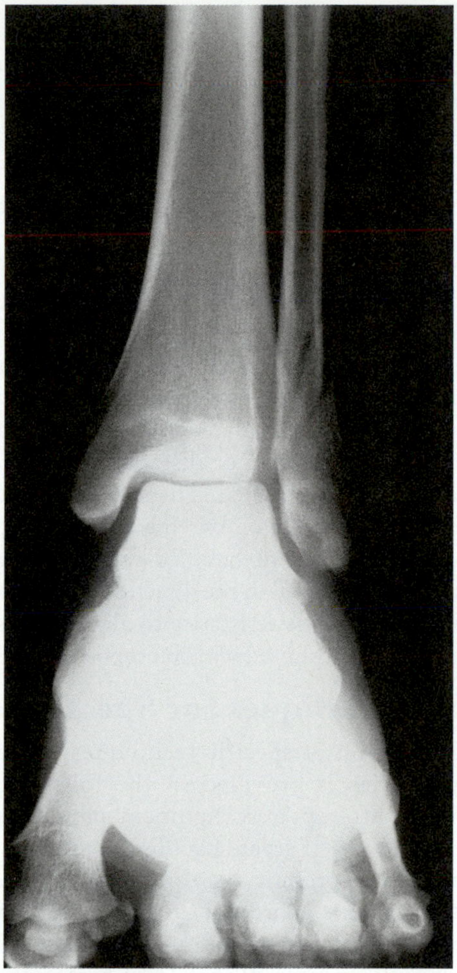

FIGURE 28-30 ■ Weber B ankle fracture. The fracture lines extend obliquely from the mortise. The medial joint line (between medial malleolus and talus) is somewhat widened. This patient had deltoid ligament rupture and was later treated with surgery.

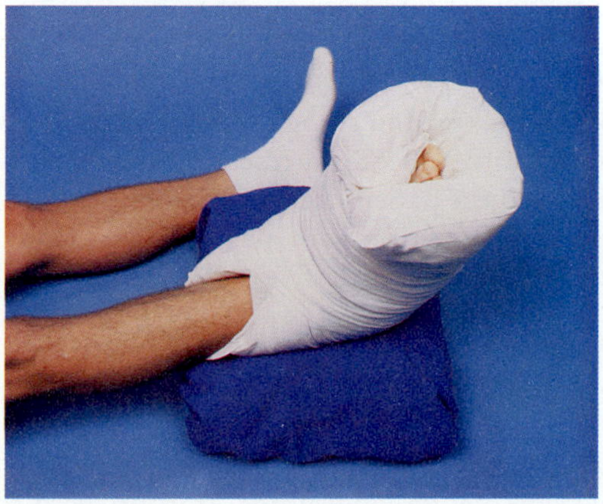

FIGURE 28-31 ■ Immobilization of the foot and ankle.

> **CRITICAL THINKING**
> Aside from narcotic analgesics, what other drugs may be indicated to relieve muscle spasm, provide anesthesia, and relax the patient while a dislocation or fracture is reduced?

As a rule, fractures and dislocated joints should be immobilized in the position of injury, and the patient should be transported as quickly as possible to the emergency department for realignment (reduction). However, if transport is delayed or prolonged, and if circulation is impaired, an attempt should be made to reposition a grossly deformed fracture or dislocated joint. The exception is the elbow. The elbow should never be manipulated in the prehospital setting. A grossly deformed fracture or dislocation elsewhere often can be realigned if required. This usually can be done without causing more damage or extreme discomfort to the patient. The injury should be handled carefully. Gentle, firm traction should be applied in the direction of the long axis of the extremity. If obvious resistance to alignment is felt, the extremity should be splinted without repositioning.

Specific Techniques for Specific Joints

A brief description of specific techniques for realigning extremity injuries is provided in the following discussion.[1] Only *one* attempt at realignment should be made. It should be done *only* if severe problems with nerve or vascular function are present (e.g., an extremely weak or absent distal pulses). Moreover, the attempt should be made *only* after consultation with medical direction. Manipulation (if indicated) should be performed as soon as possible after the injury. It should not be performed if the patient has other severe injuries. If not contraindicated by other injuries, the use of analgesics (e.g., ***midazolam***) for the realignment procedure should be considered. The paramedic should always assess and document pulse, sensation, and motor function before and after manipulating any injured extremity or joint.

FINGER REALIGNMENT

1. Apply in-line traction along the shaft of the finger.
2. Continue with slow, steady traction until the finger is realigned and the patient feels relief from pain.
3. Immobilize the finger with a splint device or by buddy splinting.

SHOULDER REALIGNMENT

1. Attempt realignment only in the absence of severe back injury.
2. Check circulatory and sensory status.
3. Apply slow, gentle longitudinal traction, with countertraction exerted on the axilla.
4. Slowly bring the extremity to the midline. (Do not apply force.) Realign in the anatomical position while maintaining traction.
5. Immobilize with a sling and swathe.

HIP REALIGNMENT

1. Apply in-line traction along the shaft of the femur with the hip and knee flexed at 90 degrees.
2. Continue with slow, steady traction to relax the muscle spasm. Successful realignment is indicated by a "pop" into the joint, a sudden relief of pain, and easy manipulation of the leg to full extension.
3. Immobilize the leg in full extension with the patient positioned on a long spine board. Reevaluate pulses and neurovascular status.
4. If full extension is not achieved, immobilize the leg at a flexion not to exceed 90 degrees with pillows or blankets. Place the patient supine.

KNEE REALIGNMENT

1. Apply gentle, steady traction while moving the injured joint into normal position.
2. Successful realignment is indicated by a "pop" into the joint, resolution of deformity, relief of pain, and increased mobility.
3. Immobilize the leg in full extension (or slight flexion for comfort). Position the patient supine on a long spine board.

A knee dislocation should not be confused with a patellar dislocation. (Patellar dislocation is not a limb-threatening injury.) An attempt should be made to reposition a dislocation of the knee into anatomical position if transport time is delayed or prolonged more than 2 hours. This should be done even if distal circulation is normal. Realignment should not be attempted if the dislocation is associated with other severe injuries.[1]

ANKLE REALIGNMENT

1. Apply in-line traction on the talus while stabilizing the tibia.
2. Successful realignment is noted by a sudden rotation to a normal position.
3. Immobilize the ankle in the same manner as for a fracture.

REFERRAL OF PATIENTS WITH MINOR MUSCULOSKELETAL INJURY

Some patients with a minor musculoskeletal injury (e.g., a minor sprain) do not require transport by emergency medical services. To make this determination, the paramedic should follow these guidelines:

- Evaluate the need for immobilization.
- Evaluate the need for radiography. This is based on the patient's condition and the mechanism of injury.

> **CRITICAL THINKING**
> What should be documented for calls involving minor musculoskeletal injuries?

- Evaluate the need for emergency department assessment versus the patient going to his or her private physician. This is based on the patient's condition and the mechanism of injury.
- Consult with medical direction.

Patients who are not transported to the hospital should be given advice on how to care for the injury. (An instruction sheet should explain techniques for immobilization, elevation, cold, heat, rest, use of analgesics, and indications for physician follow-up.) If any doubt exists about the seriousness of the patient's injury, the person should be transported to the emergency department for evaluation by a physician.

SUMMARY

- Injuries that can result from traumatic force on the musculoskeletal system include fractures, sprains, strains, and joint dislocations. Problems associated with musculoskeletal injuries include hemorrhage, instability, loss of tissue, simple laceration and contamination, interruption of blood supply, and long-term disability.
- Several inflammatory and degenerative conditions may manifest as or may be complicated by extremity injury. These include bursitis, tendonitis, and arthritis.
- Common signs and symptoms of extremity trauma include pain on palpation or movement, swelling or deformity, crepitus, decreased range of motion, false movement, and decreased or absent sensory perception or circulation distal to the injury.
- Once the paramedic has assessed for life-threatening conditions, the extremity injury should be examined for pain, pallor, paresthesia, pulses, paralysis, and pressure. In addition, DCAP-BTLS should be evaluated for the injured extremity.
- Immobilization by splinting helps alleviate pain; reduces tissue injury, bleeding, and contamination of an open wound; and simplifies and facilitates transport of the patient. Splints can be categorized as rigid, soft or formable, and traction splints.
- Upper extremity injuries can be classified as fractures or dislocations of the shoulder, humerus, elbow, radius and ulna, wrist, hand, and finger. Most upper extremity injuries can be adequately immobilized by application of a sling and swathe.
- Lower extremity injuries include fractures of the pelvis and fractures or dislocations of the hip, femur, knee and patella, tibia and fibula, ankle and foot, and toes.
- Most open fractures are obvious because of associated hemorrhage. However, a small puncture wound may not be initially apparent. In addition, bleeding may be minimal. Therefore the paramedic must consider any soft tissue wound in the area of a suspected fracture to be evidence of an open fracture. Open fractures are considered a true surgical emergency. This is due to the potential for infection.
- Only *one* attempt at realignment should be made. This should be done *only* if severe neurovascular compromise is present (e.g., extremely weak or absent distal pulses). Moreover, it should be done *only* after consultation with medical direction.
- The paramedic should evaluate the need for emergency department assessment versus having the patient see his or her private physician. This need is determined by the patient's condition and the mechanism of injury.

REFERENCES

1. US Department of Transportation, National Highway Traffic Safety Administration: *EMT-paramedic national standard curriculum,* Washington, DC, 1998, The Department.
2. Rosen P, Barkin R: *Emergency medicine: concepts and clinical practice,* ed 5, St Louis, 2003, Mosby.

SUGGESTED READINGS

Emergency Nurses Association: *Sheehy's emergency nursing: principles and practice,* ed 5, St Louis, 2003, Mosby.

Ferrera PC et al: *Trauma management: an emergency medicine approach,* St Louis, 2001, Mosby.

National Association of Emergency Medical Technicians: *PHTLS: basic and advanced prehospital life support,* ed 5, St Louis, 2003, Mosby.

Roberts J, Hedges J: *Clinical procedures in emergency medicine,* ed 3, Philadelphia, 1998, WB Saunders.

PART SEVEN

IN THIS PART

CHAPTER 29 Cardiology

CHAPTER

29

Cardiology

OBJECTIVES

Upon completion of this chapter, the paramedic student will be able to:

1. Identify risk factors and prevention strategies associated with cardiovascular disease.
2. Describe the normal physiology of the heart.
3. Discuss electrophysiology as it relates to the normal electrical and mechanical events in the cardiac cycle.
4. Outline the activity of each component of the electrical conduction system of the heart.
5. Outline the appropriate assessment of a patient who may be experiencing a cardiovascular disorder.
6. Describe basic monitoring techniques that permit electrocardiogram interpretation.
7. Explain the relationship of the electrocardiogram tracing to the electrical activity of the heart.
8. Describe in sequence the steps in electrocardiogram interpretation.
9. Identify the characteristics of normal sinus rhythm.
10. When shown an electrocardiogram tracing, identify the rhythm, site of origin, possible causes, clinical significance, and prehospital management that is indicated.
11. Describe prehospital assessment and management of patients with selected cardiovascular disorders based on knowledge of the pathophysiology of the illness.
12. List indications, contraindications, and prehospital considerations when using selected cardiac interventions, including basic life support, monitor-defibrillators, defibrillation, implantable cardioverter defibrillators, synchronized cardioversion, and transcutaneous cardiac pacing.
13. List indications, contraindications, dose, and mechanism of action for pharmacological agents used to manage cardiovascular disorders.
14. Identify appropriate actions to take in the prehospital setting to terminate resuscitation.

KEY TERMS

atrioventricular dissociation: A conduction disturbance in which atrial and ventricular contractions occur rhythmically but are unrelated to each other.

automaticity: A property of specialized excitable tissue that allows self-activation through spontaneous development of an action potential.

bundle of Kent: An accessory pathway between the atria and ventricles outside of the conduction system; a congenital anomaly that causes Wolff-Parkinson-White syndrome.

cardiac ejection fraction: The percentage of ventricular blood volume released during a contraction.

hypertensive encephalopathy: A set of symptoms—including headache, convulsions, and coma—that results solely from elevated blood pressure.

P wave: The first complex of the electrocardiogram, representing depolarization of the atria.

paroxysmal nocturnal dyspnea: An abnormal condition of the respiratory system characterized by sudden attacks of shortness of breath, profuse sweating, tachycardia, and wheezing that awaken a person from sleep; often associated with left ventricular failure and pulmonary edema.

Cardiovascular disease accounts for more than 930,000 deaths in the United States each year. About two thirds of sudden death from coronary disease takes place outside the hospital and usually occurs within 2 hours after onset of symptoms.[1] A large number of these deaths can be prevented. They can be prevented by rapid entry into the emergency medical services system, prompt provision of cardiopulmonary resuscitation, and early defibrillation.

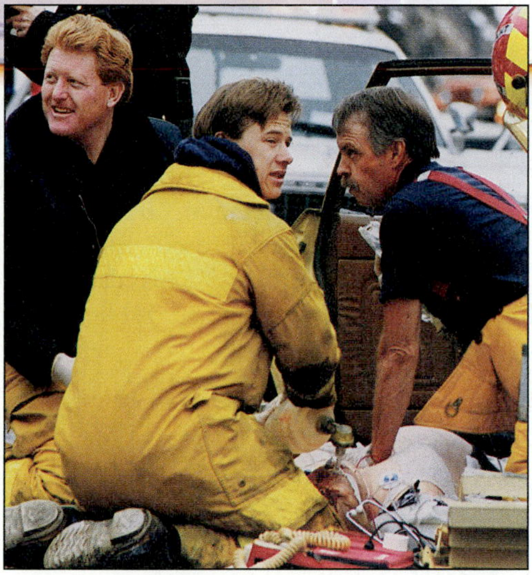

paroxysmal supraventricular tachycardia: An ectopic rhythm in excess of 100 beats per minute and usually faster than 170 beats per minute that begins abruptly with a premature atrial or junctional beat and is supported by an atrioventricular nodal reentry mechanism or by an atrioventricular reentry involving an accessory pathway.

P-R interval: The time elapsing between the beginning of the P wave and the beginning of the QRS complex in the electrocardiogram.

premature atrial complex: A cardiac dysrhythmia characterized by an atrial beat occurring before the expected excitation and indicated on the electrocardiogram as an early P wave.

premature junctional contraction: A cardiac dysrhythmia that occurs during sinus rhythm earlier than the next expected sinus beat and is caused by premature discharge of an ectopic focus in the atrioventricular junctional tissue.

premature ventricular complex: A cardiac dysrhythmia characterized by a ventricular beat preceding the expected electrical impulse and indicated on the electrocardiogram as an early, wide QRS complex without a preceding related P wave.

proarrhythmia: A new or worsened rhythm disturbance seemingly generated by antidysrhythmic therapy.

QRS complex: The principal deflection in the electrocardiogram, representing ventricular depolarization.

Q-T interval: The time elapsing from the beginning of the QRS complex to the end of the T wave, representing the total duration of electrical activity of the ventricles.

R-on-T phenomenon: The occurrence of a ventricular depolarization during a vulnerable period of relative refractoriness.

refractory period: The period after effective stimulation during which excitable tissue fails to respond to a stimulus of threshold intensity.

resting membrane potential: The electrical charge difference inside a cell membrane measured relative to just outside the cell membrane.

ST segment: The early part of repolarization in the electrocardiogram of the right and left ventricles.

Starling's law of the heart: A rule that the force of the heartbeat is determined by the length of the fibers making up the myocardial walls.

T wave: A deflection in the electrocardiogram after the QRS complex, representing ventricular repolarization.

threshold potential: The value of the membrane potential at which an action potential is produced as a result of depolarization in response to a stimulus.

torsades de pointes: An unusual bidirectional ventricular tachycardia.

U wave: The gradual deviation from the T wave in the electrocardiogram, thought to represent the final stage of repolarization of the ventricles.

ventricular bigeminy: A cardiac rhythm disturbance characterized by two ventricular beats in rapid succession followed by a longer interval.

ventricular tachycardia: A tachycardia that usually originates in the Purkinje fibers.

ventricular trigeminy: A cardiac dysrhythmia characterized by three ventricular beats in rapid succession followed by a longer interval.

CRITICAL THINKING

How many of your friends or family have had a heart attack or stroke? How has that illness affected their lives?

RISK FACTORS AND PREVENTION STRATEGIES

Although death rates from myocardial infarction have declined over the past several decades, coronary artery disease and resultant sudden death is still a major cause of morbidity and mortality and is the most prominent medical emergency in the United States today.[1] This decline in death rates is due in large part to heightened public awareness, increased availability of automated external defibrillators, improved cardiovascular diagnosis and therapy, use of cardiovascular drugs by persons at high risk, improved revascularization techniques, and improved and more aggressive risk factor modification.

Risk Factors and Risk Factor Modifications

Persons at high risk for cardiovascular disease include those with diabetes, hypertension, hypercholesterolemia, hyperlipidemia, a family history of premature cardiovascular disease, and known coronary artery disease. Their risk can be increased considerably if they have additional risk factors. Some of these factors include obesity, cigarette smoking, and a sedentary lifestyle (Box 29-1). Clearly, some risk factors cannot be changed. Other risk factors, however, can be changed or modified through the following:

- Cessation of smoking
- Medical management and control of blood pressure, diabetes, cholesterol, and lipid disorders
- Exercise
- Weight loss
- Diet
- Stress reduction

Modifying cardiovascular risk factors can slow the rate of development of arterial disease. It also can reduce the incidence of acute myocardial infarction, sudden death, renal failure, and stroke.

Prevention Strategies

Paramedics and other health care professionals can support and practice prevention activities against the development of cardiovascular disease. These strategies include educational programs about nutrition in their communities, cessation of smoking (smoking prevention for children), early recognition and management of hypertension and cardiac symptoms, and prompt intervention (including cardiopulmonary resuscitation and early use of an automated external defibrillator). These and other prevention strategies may help reduce risk factors at a young age. They also may have the greatest impact on risk factor modification. (See Chapter 3.)

BOX 29-1 Risk Factors for Cardiovascular Disease

Risk Factors	Possible Contributing Risk Factors
Age	Obesity
Carbohydrate intolerance	Oral contraceptive use
Cigarette smoking	Personality type
Cocaine use	Poor diet
Diabetes	Psychosocial tensions
Family history	Sedentary lifestyle
Hypercholesterolemia	Stress
Hyperlipidemia	
Hypertension	
Prior myocardial infarction	

SECTION ONE
ANATOMY AND PHYSIOLOGY OF THE HEART

ANATOMY

The anatomy of the heart is described and illustrated in Chapter 6. Readers are encouraged to refer to that chapter for a review.

The coronary arteries are the sole suppliers of arterial blood to the heart. They deliver 200 to 250 mL of blood to the myocardium each minute during rest (Fig. 29-1). The left coronary artery carries about 85% of the blood supply to the myocardium. The right coronary artery carries the rest. The coronary arteries begin just above the aortic valve where the aorta exits the heart. These arteries run along the epicardial surface. They divide into smaller vessels as they penetrate the myocardium and the endocardial (inner) surface.

The left main coronary artery supplies the left ventricle, interventricular septum, and part of the right ventricle. Its two main branches are the left anterior descending and the circumflex arteries. The right coronary artery supplies the right atrium and ventricle, part of the left ventricle, and the conduction system. Its two major branches are the right anterior descending and the marginal branch. In addition to the blood supply provided by these arteries, many connections (anastomoses) exist between arterioles to provide backup (collateral) circulation. These anastomoses play a key role in providing alternative routes of blood flow in the event of blockage in one or more of the coronary vessels.

CRITICAL THINKING

Why is collateral circulation important?

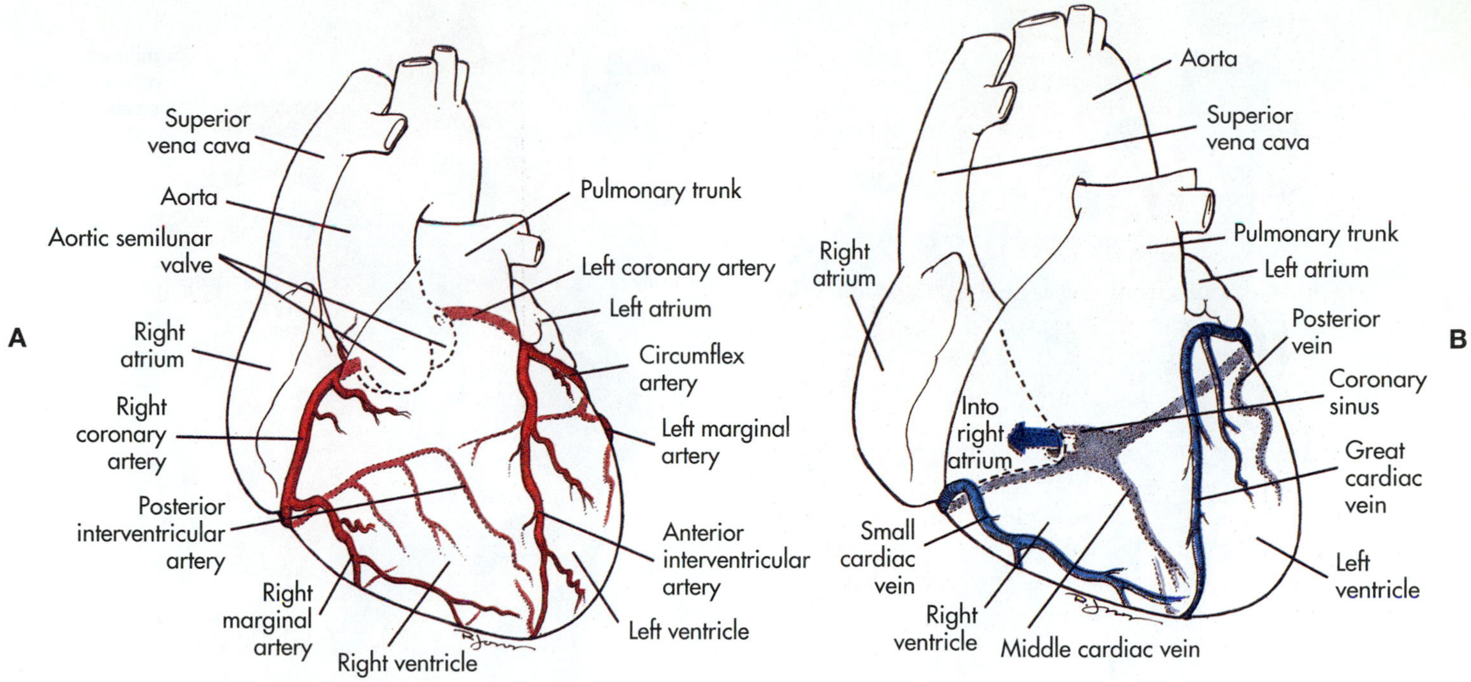

FIGURE 29-1 ■ Blood vessels providing circulation of the heart. **A,** Arteries. **B,** Veins. The anterior surface of the heart is represented. The vessels of the anterior surface are seen directly and have a darker color, whereas the vessels of the posterior surface are seen through the heart and have a lighter color.

Coronary capillaries allow for the exchange of nutrients and metabolic wastes. The capillaries merge to form coronary veins. These veins deliver most of the blood to the coronary sinus. The coronary sinus empties directly into the right atrium. The coronary sinus is the major vein draining the myocardium.

PHYSIOLOGY

The heart can be thought of as two pumps in one. One is a low-pressure pump (right atrium and right ventricle). This pump supplies blood to the lungs. The second is a high-pressure pump (left atrium and left ventricle). This pump supplies blood to the body. The right atrium receives venous blood from the systemic circulation and from the coronary veins. Most of this deoxygenated blood in the right atrium then passes to the right ventricle as the ventricle relaxes from the previous contraction. Once the right ventricle receives about 70% of its volume, the right atrium contracts. The blood remaining in the atrium is pushed into the ventricle. Contraction of the right ventricle pushes blood against the tricuspid valve (forcing it closed) and through the pulmonic valve (forcing it open). This allows the blood to enter the lungs via the pulmonary arteries. From the pulmonary arteries, the deoxygenated blood enters the capillaries in the lungs where gas exchange takes place.

From the lungs the blood travels through four pulmonary veins back to the left atrium. The mitral valve opens, and blood flows to the left ventricle. Once the left ventricle receives about 70% of its volume, the left atrium contracts. The remaining blood is pushed into the ventricle. The blood passing from the left atrium to the left ventricle opens the bicuspid valve when the ventricle relaxes to complete left ventricular filling. As the left ventricle contracts, blood is pushed against the bicuspid valve (closing it) and against the aortic valve (opening it). This allows blood to enter the aorta. From the aorta, blood is distributed first to the heart itself and then throughout the systemic arterial circulation.

NOTE The atria work mainly as "primer pumps." Under most conditions, the ventricles can pump enough blood to maintain adequate blood flow to the body without the help of the atria. However, under stress, the heart may pump 300% to 400% more blood than during rest. In such conditions, the priming action of the atria becomes key in maintaining pumping efficiency.

Cardiac Cycle

The pumping action of the heart is a product of rhythmic, alternate contraction (systole) and relaxation (diastole) of the atria and ventricles. (When *systole* and *diastole* are used without reference to specific chambers, they mean *ventricular systole* or *diastole.*) These heartbeats occur about 70 times per minute in resting adults. These rhythmic contractions of the heart chambers are responsible for blood movement (Fig. 29-2).

VENTRICULAR SYSTOLE AND DIASTOLE

As the ventricles begin to contract, ventricular pressure exceeds atrial pressure. This causes the atrioventricular valves to close. As the contraction proceeds, ventricular pressure

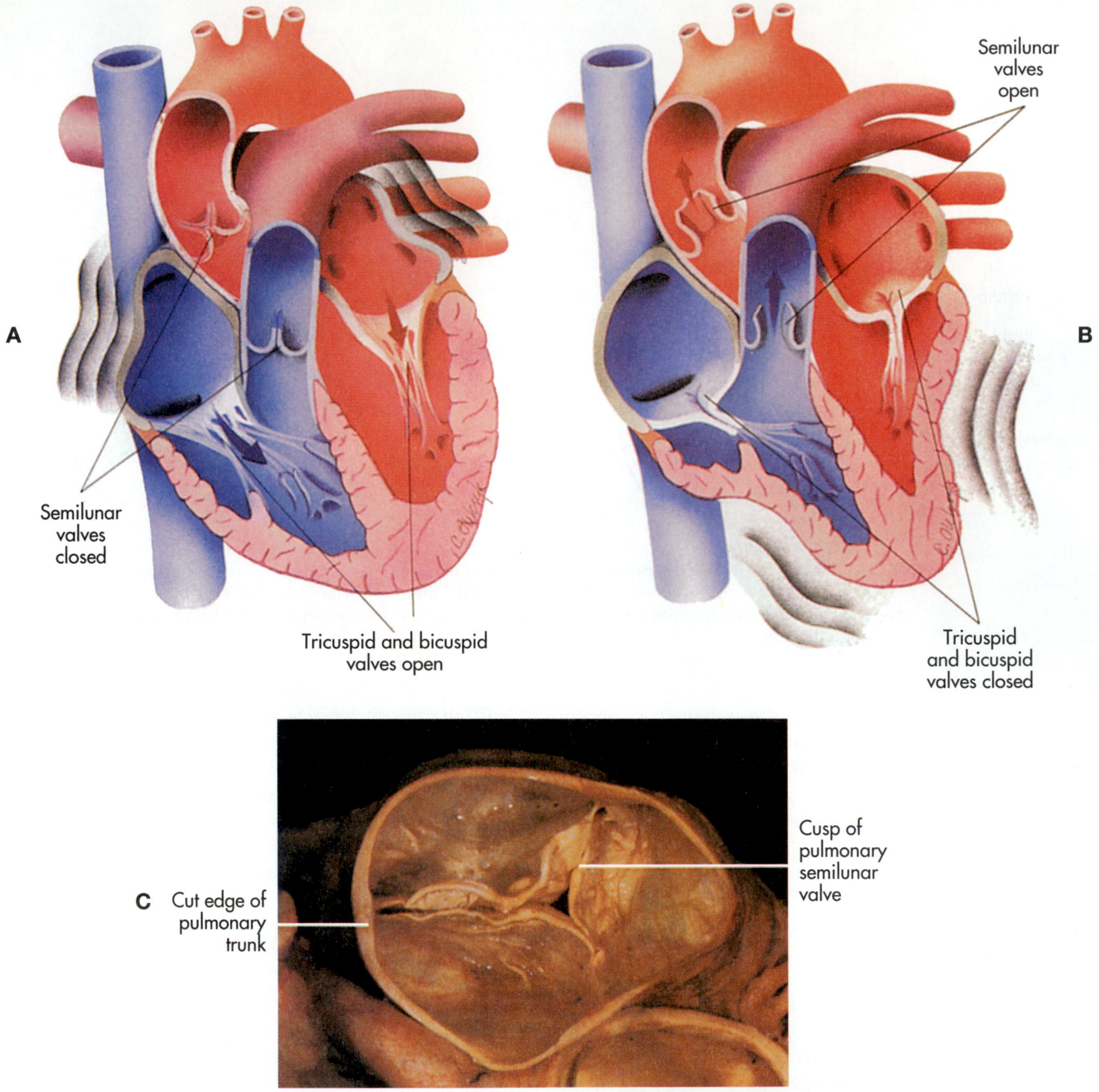

FIGURE 29-2 ■ Heart action. **A,** During atrial systole (contraction), cardiac muscle in the atrial wall contracts, forcing blood through the atrioventricular valves and into the ventricles. **B,** During the ventricular systole that follows, the atrioventricular valves close, and blood is forced out of the ventricles through the semilunar valves into the arteries. **C,** The pulmonary semilunar valves as seen from above (superior).

continues to rise. Pressure rises until it exceeds that in the pulmonary artery on the right side of the heart and in the aorta on the left side. At that time, the pulmonary and aortic valves open. Then blood flows from the ventricles into those arteries (ejection).

After ventricular contraction, ventricular relaxation begins. Ventricular pressure falls rapidly. When the pressure falls below the pressure in the aorta or the pulmonary trunk, blood is forced back toward the ventricles. This closes the pulmonic and aortic valves. As ventricular pressure drops below atrial pressure, the tricuspid and mitral valves open. Then blood flows from the atria into the ventricles. Atrial systole occurs during ventricular diastole.

CRITICAL THINKING

What would happen if the valves were scarred and became stiff?

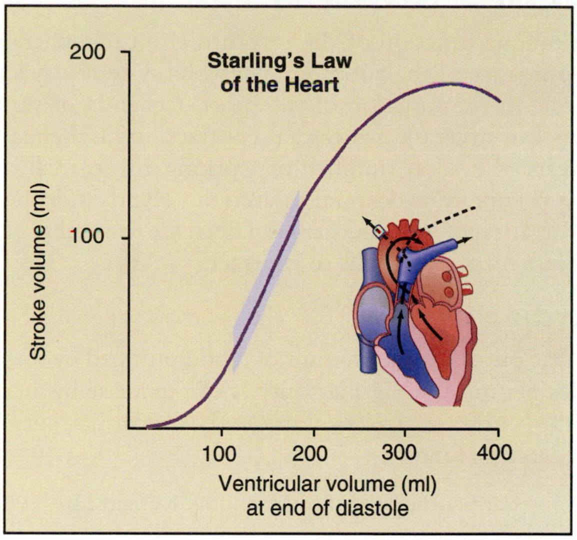

FIGURE 29-3 ■ Starling's law of the heart.

Stroke Volume

The stroke volume is the amount of blood ejected from the heart with each ventricular contraction. Stroke volume depends on three factors: preload (the volume of blood returning to the heart), afterload (the resistance against the heart muscle must pump), and myocardial contractility.

PRELOAD

During diastole, blood flows from the atria into the ventricles. The volume of blood returning to each ventricle is the end-diastolic volume. This volume normally reaches 120 to 130 mL. As the ventricles empty during systole, their volume decreases to 50 to 60 mL (end-systolic volume). Therefore the amount of blood ejected during each cardiac cycle (stroke volume) is about 70 mL.

In a patient with a healthy heart the capacity to increase stroke volume is great. The strong contraction of a heart during exercise, for example, can reduce the volume returning to each ventricle to as little as 10 to 30 mL. If large amounts of blood flow into the ventricles during diastole, their end-diastolic volume can be as much as 200 to 250 mL. In this way, stroke volume can increase to more than double that of normal. The ability of the heart to pump more strongly when it has a larger preload is explained by **Starling's law of the heart.**

CRITICAL THINKING

When you blow up a balloon, why does the balloon act like the heart muscle?

According to Starling's law (Fig. 29-3), myocardial fibers contract more forcefully when they are stretched. (This ability of stretched muscle to contract with increased force is a quality of all striated muscle; it is not just a quality of cardiac muscle.) When the ventricles are filled with larger-than-normal volumes of blood (increased preload), they contract with greater-than-normal force to deliver all of the blood to the systemic circulation.

The most important feature of the ability of the heart to handle changes in venous blood return is that changes in arterial pressure have minimal effect on cardiac output. In other words, the heart can pump a small amount of blood or a large amount. The amount depends on the amount of venous return. The heart just adapts as long as the total quantity of blood does not exceed the limit that the heart can pump. Venous return is the most important factor in stroke volume, with arterial pressure causing a lesser effect in the form of afterload. Starling's law and its effect on stroke volume can be applied only up to a certain limit of muscle fiber stretching. Beyond that limit, muscle fiber stretch actually diminishes the strength of contraction. At that point the heart begins to fail.

NOTE Preload is more important in determining cardiac output than afterload.

AFTERLOAD

Afterload is a result of peripheral vascular resistance. An increase in peripheral vascular resistance decreases stroke volume. The decrease is due to the increased pressure in the aorta that the ventricular muscle must overcome to open the aortic valve and push blood through. However, a decrease in peripheral vascular resistance increases stroke volume if there is enough volume of fluid in the system.

CRITICAL THINKING

What condition will increase the afterload?

MYOCARDIAL CONTRACTILITY

The unique function of the myocardial muscle fibers and the influence of the autonomic nervous system play a major role in the function of the heart. Ischemia or various drugs can decrease myocardial contractility. Ischemia can decrease the total number of working myocardial cells. (This occurs in myocardial infarction.) Hypoxia or the administration of beta-blockers can decrease the ability of the separate myocardial cells to contract.

Cardiac Output

Cardiac output is the amount of blood pumped by the ventricles per minute. Cardiac output can increase by increasing the heart rate, stroke volume, or both. Cardiac output is calculated as follows:

$$\text{Cardiac output} = \text{Stroke volume} \times \text{Heart rate}$$

Peripheral vascular resistance changes cardiac output by affecting the stroke volume. Vasodilation of the arteries, for example, decreases afterload. This produces an increase in cardiac output. In contrast, vasoconstriction increases afterload. In turn, this tends to decrease cardiac output. However, the body responds to the decrease by constricting the venous circulation. This increases the amount of blood returning to the heart and causes the heart to contract more forcefully (Starling's law). These actions help to maintain or increase cardiac output.

Nervous System Control of the Heart

In addition to the heart regulating its behavior, the autonomic nervous system also controls the behavior of the heart. The autonomic nervous system greatly influences the heart rate, conductivity, and contractility. The autonomic nervous system innervates the atria and ventricles. The atria are well supplied with large numbers of sympathetic and parasympathetic nerve fibers. Yet the ventricles mainly are supplied by sympathetic nerves.

The parasympathetic nervous system mainly is concerned with vegetative functions. In contrast, the sympathetic nervous system helps prepare the body to respond to stress. These sympathetic and parasympathetic control systems work in a check-and-balance manner. They stimulate the heart to increase or decrease cardiac output according to the metabolic demands of the body.

CRITICAL THINKING

Consider how you regulate the hot and cold taps in a shower. How is the behavior of the autonomic nervous system similar?

PARASYMPATHETIC CONTROL

Parasympathetic control of the heart is through the vagus nerve. Control by these nerve fibers has a continuous restraining influence on the heart, primarily by decreasing the heart rate and, to a lesser extent, contractility. The vagus nerve may be stimulated in several ways. Examples include the Valsalva maneuver, carotid sinus massage (described later in this chapter), pain, and distention of the urinary bladder. Acetylcholine is the chemical mediator of the parasympathetic nervous system.

Strong parasympathetic stimulation can decrease the heart rate to 20 or 30 beats per minute. Yet such stimulation generally has little effect on stroke volume. In fact, stroke volume may increase with a decreased heart rate. This occurs because the longer time interval between heartbeats allows the heart to fill with a larger amount of blood and thus contract more forcefully (Starling's law).

SYMPATHETIC CONTROL

Sympathetic nerve fibers originate in the thoracic region of the spinal cord. They form groups of nerve fibers called ganglia. Their postganglionic fibers release the chemical norepinephrine. This chemical stimulates an increase in the heart rate (positive chronotropic effect). Norepinephrine also stimulates an increase in the force of muscle contraction (positive inotropic effect). Sympathetic stimulation of the heart causes coronary arteries to dilate. It also causes constriction of peripheral vessels. These two effects, dilation and constriction, help to increase blood and oxygen supply to the heart. The cardiac effects of norepinephrine result from stimulation of alpha- and beta-adrenergic receptors.

NOTE As described in Chapter 17, *inotropic* refers to the force of energy of muscular contractions; *chronotropic* refers to the regularity and rate of the heartbeat; and *dromotropic* refers to conduction velocity. The effects are classified as positive or negative. For example, a positive inotropic effect would increase the strength of contraction. However, a negative dromotropic effect would decrease the speed of conduction.

Strong sympathetic stimulation of the heart may increase the heart rate notably. When rates are significantly high (greater than 150 beats per minute), the time available for the heart to fill is decreased. This produces a decrease in stroke volume.

Hormonal Regulation of the Heart

Impulses from the sympathetic nerves are sent to the adrenal medulla at the same time that they are sent to all blood vessels. In response, the adrenal medulla secretes the hormones epinephrine and norepinephrine into the circulating blood in response to increased physical activity, emotional excitement, or stress.

Epinephrine has basically the same effect on cardiac muscles as norepinephrine. Epinephrine increases the rate and force of contraction. In addition, epinephrine causes blood vessels to constrict in the skin, kidneys, gastrointestinal tract, and other organs (viscera). Epinephrine also causes dilation of skeletal and coronary blood vessels. Epinephrine from the adrenal glands takes longer to act on the heart than direct sympathetic innervation does. Yet the effect lasts longer. Norepinephrine causes constriction of peripheral blood vessels in most areas of the body and stimulates cardiac muscle as well.

Role of Electrolytes

Myocardial cells, like all other cells of the human body, are bathed in an electrolyte solution. The major electrolytes that affect cardiac function (described in the next section) are calcium, potassium, and sodium. Magnesium is a major intracellular cation. It plays an important role as well.

CRITICAL THINKING

What drugs can alter the normal balance of electrolytes in the body?

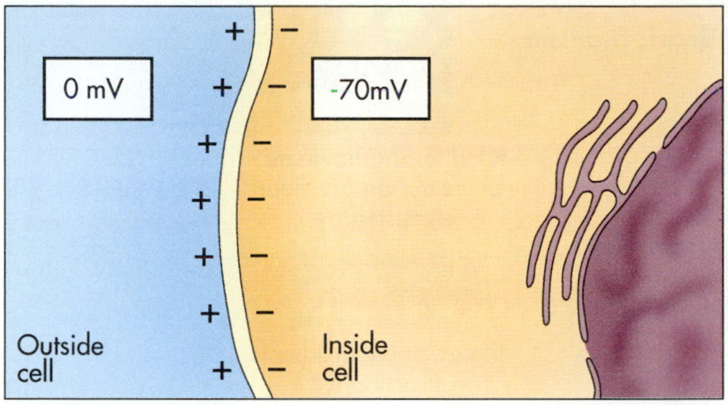

FIGURE 29-4 ■ Electrical activity of cardiac cells and membrane potentials.

SECTION TWO
ELECTROPHYSIOLOGY OF THE HEART

Caring for patients with cardiac disease is based on understanding how the heart works, including the mechanical and electrical functions. Understanding why and how the electrical conduction system can malfunction is crucial for the paramedic. The paramedic also must understand the effect that lack of oxygen to the cells (myocardial ischemia) has on cardiac rhythms. Two basic groups of cells within the myocardium are vital for cardiac function. One group is the specialized cells of the electrical conduction system. These cells are responsible for the formation and conduction of electrical current. The second group is the working myocardial cells. These cells possess the property of contractility. They do the actual pumping of the blood.

ELECTRICAL ACTIVITY OF CARDIAC CELLS AND MEMBRANE POTENTIALS

As described in Chapter 7, ions are charged particles. These particles are positive or negative. The charge depends on the ability of the ion to accept or to donate electrons. In solutions containing electrolytes, particles with unlike (opposite) charges attract each other, and the particles with like charges push away from each other. This results in a tendency to produce ion pairs. These ion pairs help to keep the solution neutral.

Electrically charged particles may be thought of as small magnets. They require energy to pull them apart if they have opposite charges. They also require energy to push them together if they have like electrical charges. Thus separated particles with opposite charges have an electrical magnetic-like force of attraction. This gives them potential energy (Fig. 29-4). The electrical charge creates a membrane potential between the inside and the outside of the cell. The electrical charge (potential difference) between the inside and outside of cells is expressed in millivolts (1 mV equals 0.001 volt). This potential energy is released when the cell membrane separating the ions becomes permeable.

Resting Membrane Potential

When the cell is in its resting state, the electrical charge difference is the **resting membrane potential.** The term *potential* is used in the electrical sense as a synonym for *voltage.* The inside of the cell is negative compared with the outside of the cell membrane. Also, the resting membrane potential is recorded from the inside of the cell. Thus resting membrane potential is reported as a negative number (about −70 to −90 mV).

The resting membrane potential is a result of the balance between two opposing forces. One of these forces is the concentration gradient of ions (mainly potassium) across a permeable cell membrane. The other is the electrical forces produced by the separation of positively charged ions from their negative ion pair. The resting membrane potential mainly is established by the difference between the intracellular potassium ion level and the extracellular potassium ion level. The ratio of 148:5 produces a large chemical gradient for potassium ions to leave the cell. Yet the negative intracellular charge relative to the extracellular charge tends to keep potassium ions in the cell (Fig. 29-5).

Sodium ions are positively charged ions on the outside of the cell. These ions have a chemical and electrical gradient. This gradient tends to cause them to move intracellularly. Depolarization (electrical conduction) takes place when sodium ions rush into the cell. This rush into the cell makes the cell more positive on the inside compared with the outside.

Diffusion through Ion Channels

The cell membrane is relatively permeable to potassium. The cell membrane is less permeable to calcium chloride. Moreover, the membrane is minimally permeable to

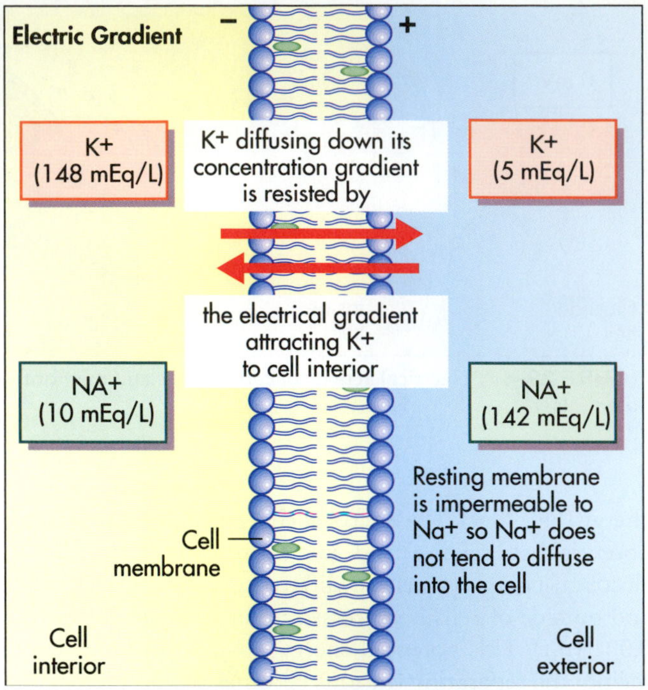

FIGURE 29-5 ■ At equilibrium (resting conditions), the tendency for potassium ions to diffuse out of the cell is opposed by the potential difference (electrical gradient) across the cell membrane. Because the resting membrane is not permeable to sodium ions, sodium ions do not tend to diffuse into the cell. (Sims/illustrator Rusty Jones.)

sodium. The cell membrane appears to have individual protein-lined channels. These channels allow passage of a specific ion or group of ions. Permeability is influenced by electrical charge, size, and the proteins that open and close the channels (gating proteins).

The potassium ion channels are smaller than the sodium ion channels. Thus they prevent sodium from passing into the cell. Potassium ions are small enough to pass through sodium ion channels, but the cell favors sodium entering the cell during rapid depolarization (the rapid entry of sodium ions into cells). Rapid depolarization creates a local area of current known as the *action potential.* After one patch of membrane is depolarized, the electrical charge spreads along the cell surface. This opens more channels (Fig. 29-6).

NOTE *Depolarization* occurs when the resting membrane potential changes from being more negatively charged on the inside of the cell to being more positively charged on the inside of the cell. This is followed by muscle contraction. *Repolarization* occurs when charges inside the cell return to normal (become more negatively charged on the inside), allowing the cell to return to its normal resting state.

The contribution of unpaired ions to the resting membrane potential depends on two factors. The first factor is the diffusion of ions through the membrane by way of the ion channels. This creates an imbalance of charges. The second factor is the active transport of ions through the membrane by way of the sodium-potassium exchange pump. This also creates an imbalance of charges.

CRITICAL THINKING

Which of these processes of electrolyte transfer requires energy for it to occur?

Sodium-Potassium Exchange Pump

The specialized sodium-potassium exchange pump actively pumps sodium ions out of the cell and potassium ions into the cell. Thus this pump separates the ions across the membrane against their concentration gradients. Potassium ions are transported into the cell. This increases their concentration in the cell. Sodium ions are transported out of the cell. This increases their concentration outside the cell (Fig. 29-7).

The sodium-potassium exchange pump normally transports three sodium ions out for every two potassium ions taken in. Thus more positively charged ions are transferred outward than inward. This returns the cell to its resting state. In the resting state of the cell, the number of negative charges inside the cell is equal to the number of positive charges outside the cell.

Pharmacological Actions

In cardiac muscle, sodium and calcium ions can enter the cell through two separate channel systems in the cell membrane. These are the fast channels and slow channels. Fast channels are sensitive to small changes in membrane potential. As the cell drifts toward threshold level (the point at which a cell depolarizes), fast sodium channels open. This results in a rush of sodium ions into the cell and in rapid depolarization. The slow channel has selective permeability to calcium and to a lesser extent to sodium. Calcium plays an electrical role. Calcium contributes to the number of positive charges in the cell. Calcium also plays a contractile role. Calcium is the ion required for cardiac muscle contraction to occur.

An understanding of ion channels helps the paramedic understand how the heart rate and contractility responds to drugs. For example, calcium channel blockers selectively block the slow channel. Examples of such drugs are ***verapamil*** and ***diltiazem.*** These drugs limit the movement of calcium ions into the cell without altering its voltage. Other examples, such as ***procainamide*** (a type I antidysrhythmic) owe much of their antidysrhythmic effects to their ability to block the fast inward sodium channel.

CELL EXCITABILITY

Nerve and muscle cells are capable of producing action potentials. This is known as *excitability.* When these cells are stimulated, a series of changes in the resting membrane potential normally causes depolarization of a small region of the cell membrane. The stimulus may be strong enough to depolarize a cell membrane to a level called the **threshold potential.** If this is the case, an explosive series of permeability changes takes place. This causes an action potential to spread over the entire cell membrane.

Propagation of Action Potential

An action potential at any point on the cell membrane acts as a stimulus to adjacent regions of the cell membrane.

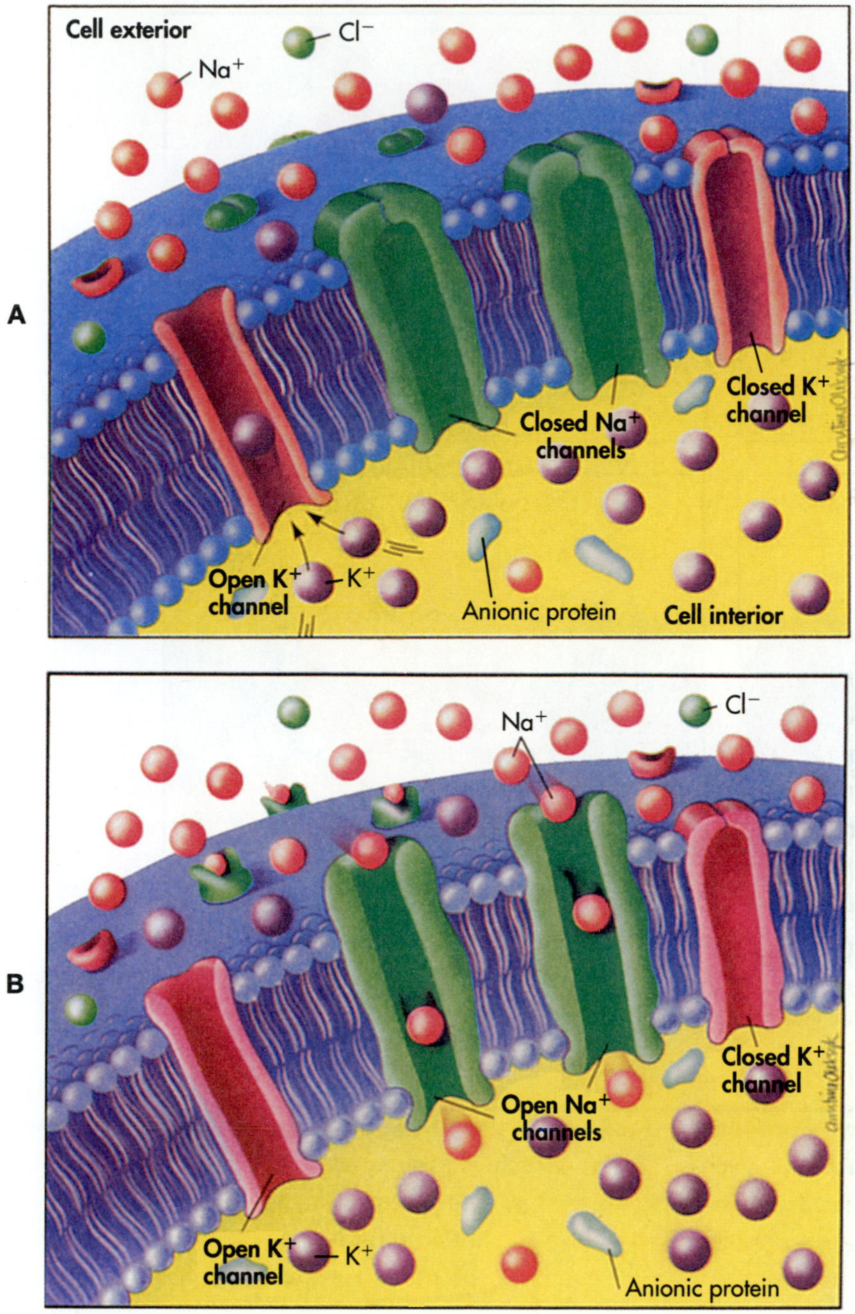

FIGURE 29-6 ■ Effect of a stimulus that causes a voltage change across the cell membrane on the permeability of the cell membrane. **A,** Sodium channels remain closed in a resting or unstimulated cell membrane. **B,** Depolarization of the cell membrane causes sodium channels to open. Sodium ions then diffuse down their concentration gradient into the cell, causing depolarization of the cell membrane.

Thus the excitation process, once started, is spread along the length of the cell and onto the next cell and so on. A stimulus that is strong enough to cause a cell to reach threshold and depolarize (action potential) spreads quickly from one cell to another. (This is the *all-or-none principle.*) The cardiac action potential can be divided into five phases (phases 0 to 4) (Fig. 29-8).

PHASE 0

Phase 0 is the rapid depolarization phase. This phase represents the rapid upstroke of the action potential. This occurs when the cell membrane reaches threshold potential. During this phase, the fast sodium channels open momentarily. In this moment, the sodium channels permit rapid entry of sodium into the cell. As the positively charged ions flow into the cell, the inside of the cell becomes positively charged compared with the outside, leading to muscular contraction.

PHASE 1

Phase 1 is the early rapid repolarization phase. During this phase, the fast sodium channels close, the flow of sodium into the cell stops, and potassium continues to be lost from the cell. This results in a decrease in the number of positive electrical charges inside the cell and a drop in the membrane potential. This returns the cell membrane to its resting permeability state.

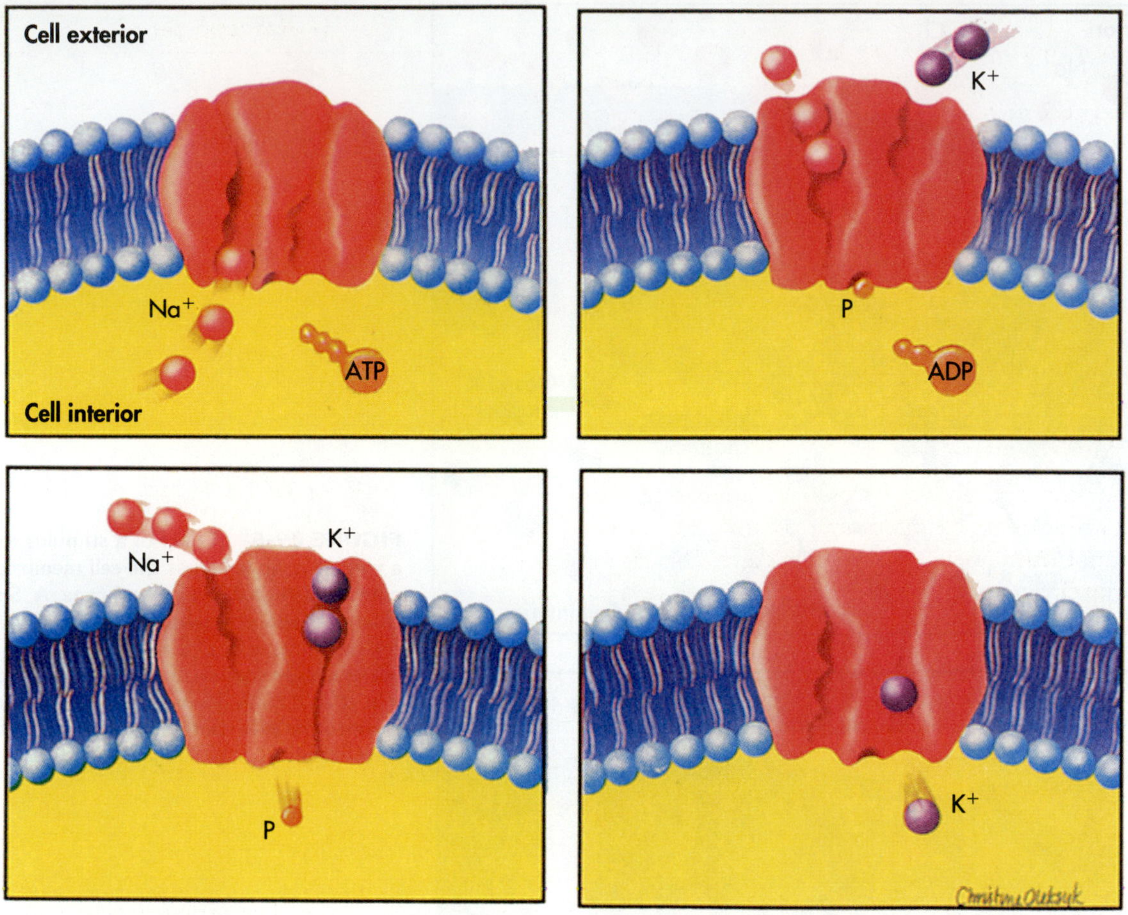

FIGURE 29-7 ■ The sodium-potassium exchange pump actively transports sodium ions out of the cell across the cell membrane and potassium ions into the cell across the cell membrane. Adenosine triphosphate is used as the energy source, and the pump can transport up to three sodium ions for every two potassium ions transported.

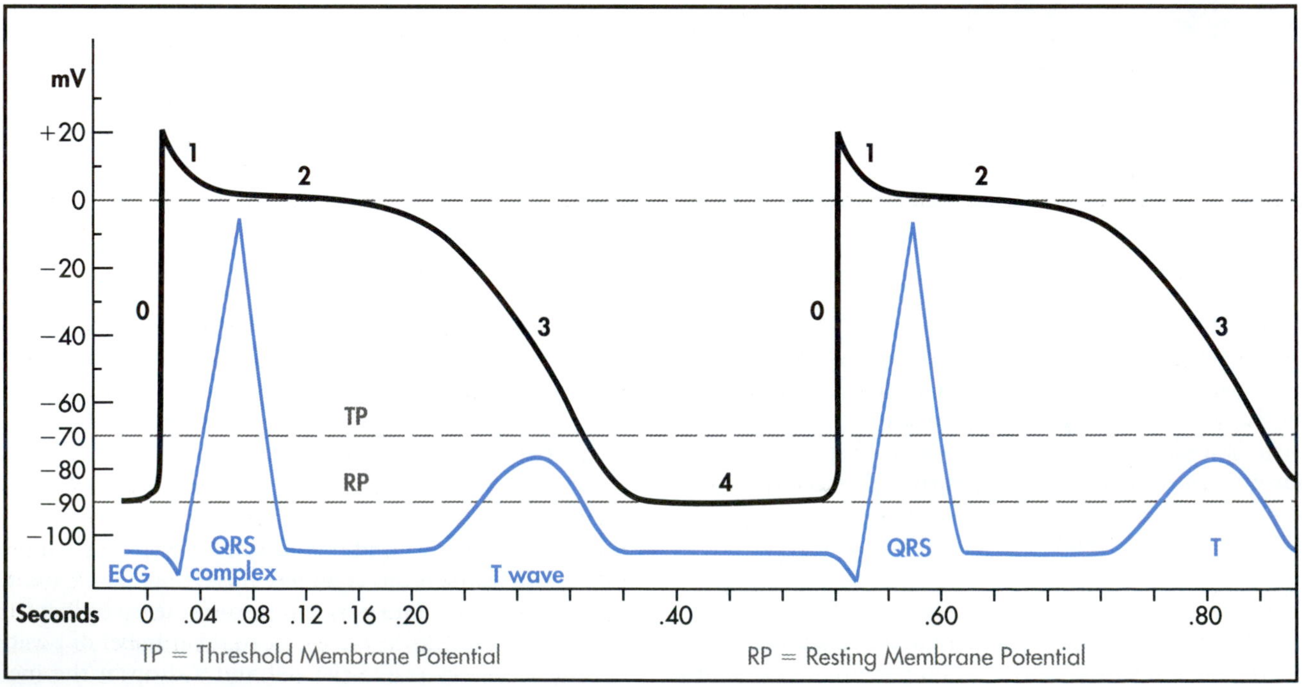

FIGURE 29-8 ■ Cardiac action potential of myocardial cells.

PHASE 2

Phase 2 is the plateau phase. Phase 2 is the prolonged phase of repolarization of the action potential. During this phase, calcium enters the myocardial cells. This triggers a large secondary release of calcium from intracellular storage sites and initiating contraction. Calcium slowly enters the cell through the slow calcium channels. At the same time, potassium continues to leave the cell. The inward calcium current maintains the cell in a prolonged depolarization state. This allows time for completion of one muscle contraction before another depolarization begins. This phase also stimulates the release of intracellular stores of calcium and aids in the contraction process.

PHASE 3

Phase 3 is the terminal phase of rapid repolarization. It results in the inside of the cell becoming negative. The membrane potential also returns to its resting state. This phase is initiated by closing of the slow calcium channels and by an increase in permeability with an outflow of potassium. Repolarization is completed by the end of this phase.

PHASE 4

Phase 4 represents the period between action potentials, when the membrane has returned to its resting membrane potential. During this phase, the inside of the cell is negatively charged with respect to the outside. However,the cell still has an excess of sodium inside and of potassium outside. This activates the sodium-potassium exchange pump. The excess sodium is transported out of the cell and the potassium is transported back into the cell. During phase 4, pacemaker cells have a slow depolarization from their most negative membrane potential to a level at which threshold is reached, and phase 0 begins all over again.

Refractory Period of Cardiac Muscle

Cardiac muscle, like all excitable tissue, has a **refractory period** or resting period. During the *absolute refractory period,* the cardiac muscle cell cannot respond to any stimulation. If the depolarization phase of cardiac muscle is prolonged, the refractory period also is prolonged (Fig. 29-9).

The refractory period ensures that the cardiac muscle is fully relaxed before another contraction begins. The refractory period of the ventricles is of about the same duration as that of the action potential. The refractory period of the atrial muscle is much shorter than that of the ventricles. This allows the rate of atrial contraction to be much faster than that of the ventricles. There also is a *relative refractory period.* During this time, the muscle cell is harder than normal to excite. Still, the cell can be stimulated.

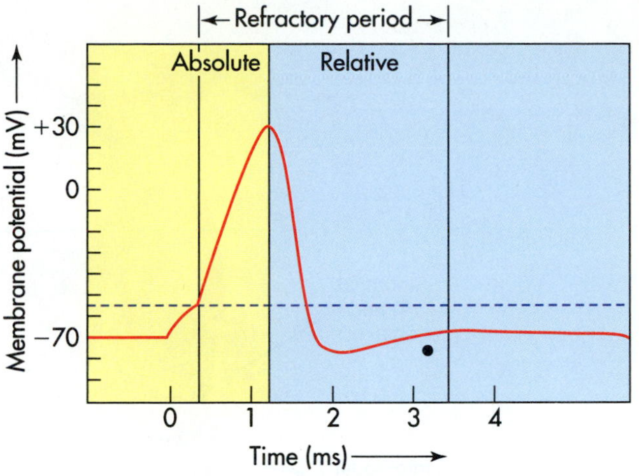

FIGURE 29-9 ■ Refractory period.

> **CRITICAL THINKING**
> How are the relative and absolute refractory periods of the heart similar to the flushing mechanism of your toilet?

ELECTRICAL CONDUCTION SYSTEM OF THE HEART

The conduction system of the heart has two nodes and a bundle branch (Fig. 29-10). The two nodes are in the right atrium. They are named according to their location. The sinoatrial node is located by the opening of the superior vena cava. The atrioventricular node is located by the right atrioventricular valve. The atrioventricular node and the bundle of His form the atrioventricular junction. This junction serves as the only electrical link between the atria and ventricles in a normal heart. The bundle of His reaches into the interventricular septum. There the bundle of His divides into right and left bundle branches. The left bundle branch then subdivides into the anterior and posterior branches, which provide pathways for impulse conduction. A third branch of the left bundle branch also innervates the interventricular septum and the base of the heart.

The right and left bundle branches are on either side of the septum and reach to the apical portions of the right and left ventricles. The bundle branches subdivide into smaller branches. The smallest branches are called Purkinje fibers. The Purkinje fibers spread electrical impulses through the myocardial fibers. This results in contraction of the heart muscle. The rapid conduction along these fibers causes all ventricular cells to contract at more or less the same time.

Pacemaker Activity

In skeletal and most smooth muscle, the individual cells contract only in response to hormones or nerve impulses from the central nervous system. But unlike most other muscle cells, cardiac fibers have specialized cells that are known as pacemaker cells. These cells can generate electrical impulses spontaneously. (This is known as **automaticity.**) Pacemaker cells depolarize in a repetitive manner. This rhythmic activity occurs because the pacemaker cells can depolarize without

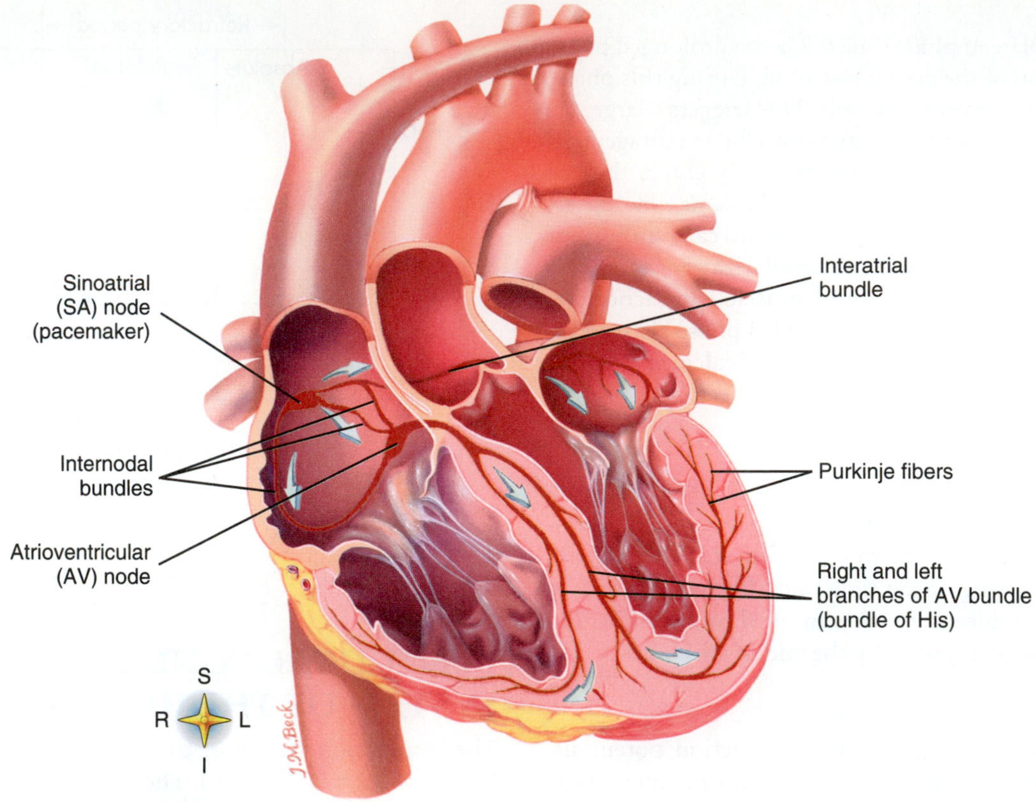

FIGURE 29-10 ■ Conduction system of the heart. Impulses *(arrows)* travel across the wall of the right atrium from the sinoatrial node to the atrioventricular node. The atrioventricular bundle extends from the atrioventricular node through the fibrous skeleton and into the interventricular septum, where it divides into right and left bundle branches. The bundle branches descend to the apex of the ventricle and then branch repeatedly for distribution throughout the ventricular walls.

an outside stimulus. Sometimes the sinoatrial node may fail to generate an electrical impulse. If this occurs, other pacemaker cells take over. These pacemaker cells are capable of spontaneous depolarization and subsequent spread of an action potential. However, their rate is slower.

Sequence of Excitation in Cardiac Muscle

Under normal conditions the chief pacemaker of the heart is the sinoatrial node. This is because the sinoatrial node reaches its threshold for depolarization at a faster rate than do other pacemakers. The rapid rate of the sinoatrial node normally prevents the slower pacemakers from taking over. If impulses from the sinoatrial node do not develop normally, however, the next pacemaker to reach its threshold level would take over the pacemaker duties.

Because of automaticity, cardiac cells can act as a fail-safe means for initiating electrical impulses. The backup cells (intrinsic pacemakers) are arranged in cascade fashion: the farther from the sinoatrial node, the slower the intrinsic firing rate. In order, the location of cells with pacemaker capabilities and rates of spontaneous discharge are the sinoatrial node (60 to 100 discharges per minute); atrioventricular junctional tissue (40 to 60 discharges per minute); and the ventricles, including the bundle branches and Purkinje fibers (20 to 40 discharges per minute) (Fig. 29-11).

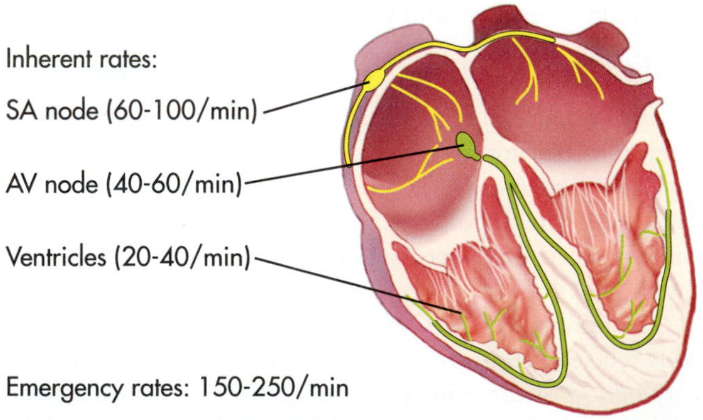

FIGURE 29-11 ■ Intrinsic pacemakers in the atria, atrioventricular node, and ventricles can discharge at their own inherent rate when normal pacemaking fails.

From the sinoatrial node the excitation spreads throughout the right atrium. Through internodal tracts, impulses travel directly from the right to the left atrium and to the base of the right atrium. This results in virtually simultaneous contraction of both atria. About 0.04 second is required for the impulse of the sinoatrial node to spread to the atrioventricular node. From there, propagation of the action potentials within the atrioventricular node is slow compared with the rate in the rest of the conducting system. As a result, a delay of 0.11 second occurs from the time the action potentials reach the atrioventricular node until they pass to the atrioventricular bundle. The total delay of 0.15 second allows atrial contraction to be completed before ventricular contraction begins.

After leaving the atrioventricular node, the impulse picks up speed. The impulse travels rapidly through the bundle of His and the left and right bundle branches. The action potential passes quickly through the individual Purkinje fibers. The impulse ends in near simultaneous stimulation and contraction of the left and right ventricles. Ventricular contraction begins at the apex. Once stimulated, the special arrangement of muscle layers in the wall of the heart produce a wringing action that proceeds toward the base of the heart.

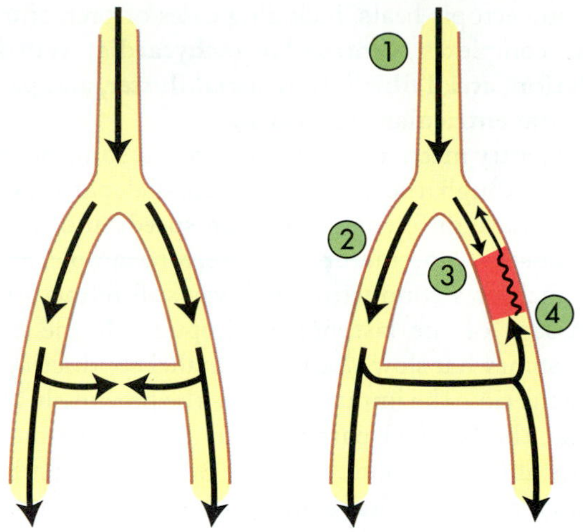

FIGURE 29-12 ■ Reentry within terminal Purkinje fibers. **A,** Conduction through normal Purkinje fibers. The conduction velocity is uniform. **B,** Conduction through a severely depressed segment of terminal Purkinje fibers. The impulse *(1)* travels normally through normal tissue *(2)* and is blocked at the severely depressed tissue *(3)* but returns, with delay, through this tissue from the opposite direction.

Autonomic Nervous System Effects on Pacemaker Cells

The effects of autonomic nervous system stimulation on the heart rate are mediated by acetylcholine and norepinephrine. Acetylcholine causes the cell membrane of the sinoatrial node to take more time to reach its threshold. Thus acetylcholine decreases the heart rate. Parasympathetic effects also may result from stimulation of the vagus nerve. This occurs in vigorous carotid sinus massage. Excessive vagal stimulation may result in asystole. (This is the absence of electrical and mechanical activity in the heart.) This is why asystole at times is referred to as the ultimate bradycardia.

CRITICAL THINKING
What else can cause vagal stimulation?

Norepinephrine increases the heart rate by increasing the rate of depolarization. The result is an increase in pacemaker discharge rate in the sinoatrial node. As a result, sympathetic stimulation leads to an increase in the heart rate. The force of cardiac contractions also increases.

Mechanisms of Ectopic Electrical Impulse Formation

An ectopic beat results when cells other than those in the sinoatrial node cause the heart to contract. These beats are called *premature beats* because they occur early in the cycle before the sinoatrial node normally would discharge. The new pacemaker is called an *ectopic focus.* Depending on the location of the ectopic focus, the premature beats may be of atrial origin **(premature atrial complexes)**, junctional origin **(premature junctional contractions)**, or ventricular origin **(premature ventricular complexes)**. The ectopic focus may be intermittent or may be sustained and may assume the pacemaker duties of the heart (i.e., the pacemaker site that fires the fastest controls the heart).

The two basic ways ectopic impulses are generated are by enhanced automaticity and reentry.

ENHANCED AUTOMATICITY

Enhanced automaticity is caused by an acceleration in depolarization. The cells reach threshold prematurely. As a result, the rate of electrical impulse formation in potential pacemakers increases.

Enhanced automaticity is responsible for dysrhythmias in Purkinje fibers and other myocardial cells. This condition may occur following release of excess catecholamines (i.e., norepinephrine and epinephrine), digitalis toxicity, hypoxia, hypercapnia, myocardial ischemia or infarction, increased venous return (preload), hypokalemia or other electrolyte abnormalities, or ***atropine*** administration.

REENTRY

Reentry is the reactivation of myocardial tissue for the second or subsequent time by the same impulse (Fig. 29-12). Reentry occurs when the progression of an electrical impulse is delayed, blocked, or both in one or more segments of the electrical conduction system of the heart. A delayed or blocked impulse can enter cardiac cells that have just become repolarized. This reentry may produce single or repetitive ectopic beats. Reentry dysrhythmias can occur in the sinoatrial node, atria, atrioventricular junction, bundle branches, or Purkinje fibers. Reentry is the most common mechanism in producing ectopic beats, including cases of premature ventricular complexes, **ventricular tachycardia, ventricular fibrillation, atrial fibrillation, atrial flutter,** and **paroxysmal supraventricular tachycardia.**

The reentry mechanism requires that at some point conduction through the heart takes parallel pathways. The pathways have different conduction speeds and refractory characteristics. A premature impulse, for example, may find one branch of a conducting pathway still refractory from the passage of the last normal impulse. If the impulse passes (somewhat slowly) along a parallel conducting pathway, by the time the impulse reaches the previously blocked pathway, the blocked pathway may have had time to recover its ability to conduct. If the two parallel paths connect at an area of excitable myocardial tissue, the depolarization process from the slower path may enter the now repolarized tissue and give rise to a new impulse spawned from the original impulse. Common causes of delayed or blocked electrical impulses include myocardial ischemia, certain drugs, and hyperkalemia.

SECTION THREE ASSESSMENT OF THE PATIENT WITH CARDIAC DISEASE

ASSESSMENT

A focused evaluation of any patient should include three things. First, it should identify a chief complaint. It also should cover the history of the event and significant medical history. It should include a physical examination as well. These elements are crucial in determining the cause of the emergency. They also aid in directing initial patient care. In addition, they help in anticipating issues during transport to a medical facility. The following discussion of patient assessment explains the approach to the patient with a cardiovascular problem.

> **CRITICAL THINKING**
>
> What emotions might the patient who has called you for a cardiovascular complaint be feeling?

Chief Complaint

Cardiovascular disease may cause a variety of symptoms. The paramedic should obtain an appropriate history of each symptom. The paramedic should apply this to form a diagnostic impression of any patient with a possible coronary event. Common chief complaints include chest pain or discomfort, including shoulder, arm, neck, or jaw pain or discomfort; dyspnea; syncope; and abnormal heartbeat or palpitations.

In some patients (e.g., some women, older adults, and patients with diabetes), cardiovascular problems commonly have atypical symptoms. Such symptoms include mental status changes, abdominal or gastrointestinal symptoms (including persistent heartburn), and vague complaints of being ill.

CHEST PAIN OR DISCOMFORT

Chest pain or discomfort is the most common chief complaint of patients with myocardial infarction. Yet many causes of chest pain are not related to cardiac disease. (Examples include pulmonary embolus, pleurisy, and reflux esophagitis.) Thus a history of chest pain is key. The OPQRST method (or a similar method) should be used to obtain the following information when possible:

Onset/Origin: Ask the patient to describe the pain or discomfort. What does it feel like? What were you doing when the pain began? Have you ever had this type of pain before? Is it the same or different than last time?

Provokes: Try to determine the events surrounding the patient's symptoms. What do you think might have caused this pain? Does anything you do make the pain better or worse? Does the pain go away when you rest? Have you taken ***nitroglycerin*** for the pain, and if so, did it help? Does the pain get worse when you exercise, walk, or when you eat certain foods?

Quality: Ask the patient to describe the pain or discomfort using his or her own words. Common descriptions for the quality of chest pain associated with a coronary event include sharp, tearing, burning, heavy, and squeezing.

Region: Ask the patient to localize the pain. With one finger, point to where the pain hurts most. Does the pain move (radiate) to another area of the body or does it stay in one place? If the pain moves, where does it move to? (Cardiac chest pain often radiates to the arms, neck, jaw, and back.)

Severity: Ask the patient to rate the pain or discomfort to establish a baseline. On a scale of 1 to 10, with 10 being the worst pain you have ever had, what number would you use to describe this pain? If you had pain like this before, is it worse than the last time, or not as bad as the last time?

Time: Try to determine the length of the pain episode and document it. How long have you had this pain? Is the pain better or worse than it was when you called emergency medical services? Is the pain constant, or does it come and go?

> **CRITICAL THINKING**
>
> What factors may influence a person's perception and description of pain?

NOTE Chest pain is one of the most common complaints of cocaine users. The use of cocaine can cause serious cardiac toxicity because of the effect of the drug on the heart. Cocaine also stimulates the central nervous system and that also stimulates the cardiovascular system. Although rare, acute myocardial infarction can occur in these patients, even in the absence of risk factors for ischemic heart disease.[1]

DYSPNEA

Dyspnea often is associated with myocardial infarction. Dyspnea is a main symptom of pulmonary congestion that is caused by heart failure. Other common causes of dyspnea that may be unrelated to heart disease include chronic obstructive pulmonary disease, respiratory infection, pulmonary embolus, and asthma. Historical factors important in differentiating breathing difficulties include the following:

- Duration and circumstances of onset of dyspnea
- Anything that aggravates or relieves the dyspnea, including medications
- Previous episodes
- Associated symptoms
- Orthopnea
- Prior cardiac problems

SYNCOPE

Syncope is caused by a sudden decrease in oxygenated blood to the brain. Cardiac causes of syncope result from events that decrease cardiac output. The most common cardiac disorders associated with syncope are dysrhythmias. Other causes of syncope in the patient include stroke, drug or alcohol intoxication, aortic stenosis, pulmonary embolism, and hypoglycemia. In the older patient, syncope may be the only symptom of a cardiac problem. Young persons who are healthy may have a syncopal episode. This episode may result from stimulation of the vagus nerve (vasovagal syncope). Stimulation of the vagus nerve can produce hypotension and bradycardia. The history of a syncopal event should include the following:

- Presyncope aura (nausea, weakness, light-headedness)
- Circumstances of occurrence (e.g., patient's position before the event, severe pain, or emotional stress)
- Duration of syncopal episode
- Symptoms before syncopal episode (palpitation, seizure, incontinence)
- Other associated symptoms
- Previous episodes of syncope

CRITICAL THINKING

Syncopal events often occur in public places, such as a church. How can you decrease the feelings of embarrassment that the patient may have during this situation?

ABNORMAL HEARTBEAT AND PALPITATIONS

Many patients are aware of their own heartbeat. They may be even more aware if it is irregular (skipping beats) or rapid (fluttering). Palpitations sometimes are a normal occurrence. However, they also may indicate a serious dysrhythmia. Important information to obtain from these patients includes the following:

- Pulse rate
- Regular versus irregular rhythm
- Circumstances of occurrence
- Duration
- Associated symptoms (chest pain, diaphoresis, syncope, confusion, dyspnea)
- Previous episodes and frequency
- Medication (drug stimulant) or alcohol use

Significant Medical History

Medical history is a vital part of any patient assessment. If possible, the paramedic should determine the following:

1. *Is the patient taking prescription medications, particularly cardiac medications?* Common medications that should alert the paramedic to a possible coronary event include ***nitroglycerin, propranolol*** and other beta-blockers, ***digoxin***, ***furosemide*** and other diuretics, antihypertensives, and antihyperlipidemic agents. The paramedic should ask the patient about his or her compliance with medications as well. The paramedic also should ask about the use of any nonprescription drugs such as over-the-counter medications, ***aspirin,*** and herbal supplements. Alcohol use or illicit drug use may be a contributing factor in the patient's chief complaint. (This may include, for example, the use of cocaine or methamphetamines.)
2. *Is the patient being treated for any other illness?* A medical history that includes angina pectoris, previous myocardial infarction, coronary artery bypass, or angioplasty procedures increases the likelihood of a significant coronary event. Chronic illness such as heart failure, hypertension, diabetes, and lung disease are also indicators that heart disease may be present.
3. *Does the patient have any allergies?* Few emergency drugs given in the prehospital setting have the potential to cause an allergic reaction. However, medication allergies (e.g., an allergy to radiographic dye) may be important in the course of the patient's care. The paramedic should document these allergies and report them to medical direction.
4. *Does the patient have risk factors for a heart attack?* Examples of risk factors include older age, tobacco use, diabetes, family history of heart disease, obesity, an increased serum cholesterol level (hypercholesterolemia), and illicit drug use.
5. *Does the patient have an implanted pacemaker or implantable cardioverter defibrillator?* The presence of these devices (described later in this chapter) indicates a significant coronary history.

Physical Examination

The classic presentation of myocardial infarction is pain or discomfort beneath the sternum. The pain often lasts more than 30 minutes. (The pain often is described as *crushing, pressure, squeezing,* or *burning.*) Associated signs and symptoms may include apprehension, diaphoresis, dyspnea, nausea and vomiting, and a sense of impending doom (e.g., patients feel that they are going to die). Yet at times the presentation is atypical. The paramedic's skill in gathering a relevant medical history and performing a focused physical examination will direct the patient care. For example, patients with myocardial ischemia may deny that they have chest pain. They may need to be asked specifically about a tightness or squeezing in the chest.

CRITICAL THINKING

Think of a way to ask a patient a question about chest pain that cannot be answered with a simple yes or no.

When caring for a patient who has chest pain caused by heart problems, the paramedic should understand that the patient is frightened. Chest pain is associated with life-threatening consequences. These patients should be calmed and reassured to decrease their anxiety.

INITIAL ASSESSMENT

In most medical emergencies involving conscious patients, the main elements of the initial assessment (airway, breathing, and circulation) can be evaluated during the initial paramedic-patient encounter. For example, an appropriate verbal exchange between the paramedic and the conscious patient will establish that the patient is alert, oriented, and has adequate cardiorespiratory function. However, the initial assessment for a patient with a possible coronary event should include a more in-depth evaluation of the patient's level of consciousness, respirations, pulse, and blood pressure.

A change in the patient's level of consciousness (e.g., light-headedness or confusion) may indicate decreased cerebral perfusion caused by poor cardiac output. If possible, the paramedic should determine the normal level of functioning for the patient. The paramedic can do this by interviewing the patient, family members, or others who are familiar with the patient (e.g., neighbors and nursing staff). In addition, the paramedic should evaluate the patient's vital signs and include a respiratory assessment, an assessment of the patient's pulse for rate and regularity, and an initial measurement of the patient's blood pressure. These findings will give the paramedic a baseline from which to guide patient care.

PHYSICAL EXAMINATION

The physical examination of the patient with cardiac disease should be organized and complete. The paramedic should use a look-listen-feel approach (see Chapter 11).

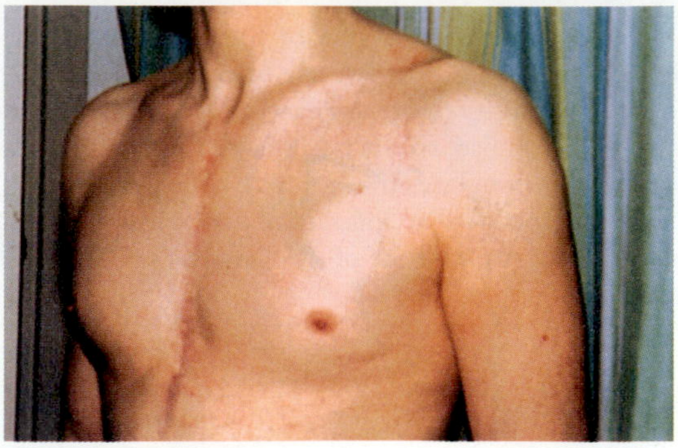

FIGURE 29-13 ■ Midsternal scar and implanted cardiac device.

Look

- Skin: Pale and diaphoretic skin may indicate peripheral vasoconstriction and sympathetic stimulation. Cyanosis is an indicator of poor oxygenation. The paramedic should consider using pulse oximetry to measure hemoglobin oxygenation.
- Jugular veins: An increase in central venous pressure from heart failure and cardiac tamponade can produce distention of internal jugular veins. Jugular vein distention is best evaluated with the patient's head elevated at 45 degrees. Distention may be hard to assess in obese patients.
- Peripheral and presacral edema: Edema can result from chronic back pressure in the systemic venous circulation. Edema is most obvious in dependent areas. (For example, these areas may include the ankles and the sacral region of patients who are bedridden.) Edema can be classified as *nonpitting.* (Minimal or no depression of tissue occurs after removal of finger pressure.) Or edema can be *pitting.* (Depression of tissue remains after removal of finger pressure.)
- Additional indicators of cardiac disease: More subtle signs of cardiac disease that may be found on a visual inspection include a midsternal scar from coronary surgery, a ***nitroglycerin*** patch on the skin, an implanted pacemaker or implantable cardioverter defibrillator in the left upper chest (Fig. 29-13) or abdominal wall, and medical alert identification necklaces or bracelets.

Listen

- Lung sounds: The paramedic should assess the patient's chest visually for accessory muscle use in breathing before listening to lung sounds. Lung sounds should be clear and equal bilaterally. Adventitious breath sounds may indicate pulmonary congestion or edema.

CRITICAL THINKING

What breath sounds might you hear if the patient has congestive heart failure or pulmonary edema?

- Heart sounds: Abnormal heart sounds may indicate congestive heart failure in adult patients. (Box 29-2).

BOX 29-2 Heart Sounds

Heart sounds typically can be auscultated with a stethoscope during ventricular systole and diastole. When the ventricles contract, both atrioventricular valves close at nearly the same time. This closure causes a vibration of the valves and surrounding fluid. Vibration results in a low-pitched sound (often described as a "lubb"). Closing of the aortic and pulmonary semilunar valves at the end of ventricular systole produces a higher-pitched sound (described as "dubb"). These normal heart sounds are referred to as S_1 and S_2, respectively.

Rarely, a third heart sound can be heard near the end of the first third of diastole (S_3). The third heart sound (caused by turbulent flow of blood into the ventricles) may be normal but may be an indicator of congestive heart failure. A fourth heart sound (S_4) may be heard during the end of diastole. This sound is thought to result from turbulence and chamber stretching from the atrial contraction during this part of the cardiac cycle and is often a sign of congestive heart failure in adults. The S_3 and S_4 contribute to "gallop" rhythms, which are useful clinical indicators of congestive heart failure. Heart sounds are difficult to distinguish in the field. The evaluation of heart sounds should never delay emergency care or transport; they do not alter prehospital patient management.

S_1: First heart sound occurs with closure of atrioventricular valves during ventricular systole.

S_2: Second heart sound occurs with closure of aortic and pulmonic valves and signifies the beginning of ventricular diastole.

S_3: Extra heart sound is heard after S_2 and is compatible with heart failure but not always present. It also may be a normal finding in some patients.

S_4: Extra heart sound is heard in late diastole (just before S_1); it is associated with atrial contractions and often is heard in patients with congestive heart failure.

Heart sounds are best heard at the **point of maximum impulse**. The point of maximum impulse is the location at which the apical impulse is most readily visible or palpable. This is often in the fifth intercostal space, just medial to the left midclavicular line. Heart sounds are difficult to distinguish in the prehospital setting. They also do not alter prehospital care. The evaluation of heart sounds should never delay other patient care measures or transportation

- Carotid artery bruit: Bruits are murmurs that indicate turbulent blood flow through a vessel. (This is most commonly from atherosclerosis.) The presence of a bruit in a patient with cardiac disease is evaluated at the carotid artery with a stethoscope and should always be assessed before performing carotid sinus massage (described later in this chapter). If a carotid artery bruit is present, carotid sinus massage is contraindicated. The procedure may dislodge plaque in the artery and cause a stroke.

Feel

- Skin: The paramedic should assess the patient's skin with the back of the hand for diaphoresis or fever.
- Pulse: The paramedic should assess the pulse for rate, regularity, and equality. A pulse deficit in peripheral and apical pulse sites may indicate a rhythm disturbance or vascular disease. The paramedic should note any pulse deficit and report it to medical direction.
- Thorax and abdomen: The paramedic should check the thorax and abdomen of a patient with cardiac disease for chest wall tenderness and pulsating masses. Chest wall tenderness is not uncommon in patients with acute myocardial infarction. A pulsating mass or distention in the abdomen or epigastric area may indicate an abdominal aneurysm.

SECTION FOUR
ELECTROCARDIOGRAM MONITORING

The electrocardiogram is a graphic representation of the electrical activity of the heart. The electrocardiogram is produced by the electrical events in the atria and ventricles and is an important diagnostic tool. The electrocardiogram helps to identify a number of cardiac abnormalities. These include abnormal heart rates and rhythms, abnormal conduction pathways, hypertrophy or atrophy of portions of the heart, and the approximate location of ischemic or infarcted cardiac muscle.

An evaluation of the electrocardiogram requires a systematic approach. The paramedic analyzes the electrocardiogram and then relates it to the clinical assessment of the patient. The electrocardiogram tracing is a picture of the electrical activity of the heart. It does not offer details on mechanical events such as force of contraction or blood pressure.

CRITICAL THINKING

Aside from blood pressure, how will you evaluate the mechanical activity of the heart?

BASIC CONCEPTS OF ELECTROCARDIOGRAM MONITORING

The summation of all the action potentials transmitted through the heart during the cardiac cycle can be measured on the surface of the body. This measurement is obtained by applying electrodes on the surface of the body. These electrodes are connected to an electrocardiogram machine. The voltage changes are fed to the machine, amplified, and displayed visually on the oscilloscope, graphically on electrocardiogram paper, or both. Voltage may be positive (seen

TABLE 29-1 Comparison of Various Leads

LEADS	TYPE OF LEAD	POLARITY
I, II, III	Limb lead	Bipolar
aV_R, aV_L, aV_F	Limb lead	Unipolar
V_1-V_6	Chest lead	Unipolar

From Phalen T: *The 12-lead ECG in acute myocardial infarction*, St Louis, 1996, Mosby.

as an upward deflection on the electrocardiogram tracing); negative (seen as a downward deflection on the electrocardiogram tracing); or isoelectric, when no electrical current is detected (seen as a straight baseline on the electrocardiogram tracing).

Electrocardiogram Leads

Electrocardiogram machines can offer many views of the electrical activity of the heart. They monitor voltage changes using electrodes applied to the body. Each pair of electrodes is referred to as a *lead.* A standard electrocardiogram views the electrical activity of the heart from 12 leads.

An electrocardiogram lead can consist of two surface electrodes, one positive and the other negative. Or the lead consists of one positive surface electrode and one reference point. A lead composed of two electrodes is called a *bipolar lead.* A lead composed of a single positive electrode and a reference point is a unipolar lead. Bipolar leads constitute the standard limb leads (I to III). Unipolar leads make up the augmented limb leads (aV_R, aV_L, and aV_F) and the precordial leads (V_1 to V_6) (Table 29-1).

Each lead assesses the electrical activity of the heart from a slightly different view. The various leads produce different electrocardiogram tracings. If the electricity moves toward a positive electrode, the electrocardiogram tracing for that lead shows an upward deflection. If the wave moves away from a positive electrode, a negative deflection appears on the electrocardiogram tracing (Fig. 29-14).

STANDARD LIMB LEADS

Standard limb leads record the difference in electrical potential between the left arm, the right arm, and the left leg electrodes, which represent the axes (the average direction of the electrical activity of the heart) of the standard limb leads. If these axes are moved so that they cross a common midpoint without altering their orientation, they form a triaxial reference system. (This is three intersecting lines of reference.) Lead I is a lateral (leftward) lead. It assesses the electrical activity of the heart from a vantage point that is defined as 0 degrees on a circle. This circle is divided into an upper negative 180 degrees and a lower positive 180 degrees. Leads II and III are inferior leads. They assess the electrical activity of the heart from vantage points of +60 degrees and +120 degrees, respectively (Fig. 29-15). The electrodes of the three bipolar leads are placed on the following areas of the body:

Lead	Positive electrode	Negative electrode
I	Left arm	Right arm
II	Left leg	Right arm
III	Left leg	Left arm

AUGMENTED LIMB LEADS

Augmented limb leads record the difference in electrical potential between the respective extremity lead sites and a reference point with zero electrical potential at the center of the electrical field of the heart. As a result, the axis of each lead is formed by the line from the electrode site (on the right arm, left arm, or left leg) to the center of the heart. The aV_R, aV_L, and aV_F leads intersect at different angles than the standard limb leads and produce three other intersecting lines of reference, which together with the standard limb leads make up the hexaxial reference system. Augmented limb leads use the same set of electrodes as the standard limb leads. They measure an axis between the two bipolar leads by electronically combining the negative electrodes. Augmented limb leads augment the voltage of the positive lead to increase the size of the electrocardiogram complexes.

Lead aV_L acts as a lateral (leftward) lead. It records the electrical activity of the heart from a vantage point that looks down from the left shoulder (−30 degrees). Lead aV_F acts as an inferior lead. It records the electrical activity of the heart from a vantage point that looks up from the left lower extremity (+90 degrees). Lead aV_R is a distant recording electrode. It looks down at the heart from the right shoulder. Based on these lead descriptions, the lateral, or left-sided, leads are I and aV_L. The inferior leads are II, III, and aV_F (Fig. 29-16).

CRITICAL THINKING

Why is aV_R seldom used in electrocardiogram analysis? What "view" of the heart does it provide?

MODIFIED LEAD RECORDING

Placement of the limb leads can be altered to mimic the precordial leads (V_1 to V_6). This can help to evaluate conduction in specific areas of the heart. These leads are referred to as *modified chest leads* and become MCL_1 to MCL_6. Modified chest leads that are useful for monitoring cardiac activity in the prehospital setting are MCL_1 and MCL_6. These leads may help to distinguish between supraventricular tachycardia and ventricular tachycardia. They also can help diagnose conduction blocks in the bundle branches (described later in this chapter).

When MCL_1 is viewed, the positive electrode is placed in the V_1 position. (This is the fourth intercostal space, just to the right of the patient's sternum.) The negative electrode is placed anteriorly, just below the lateral end of the left clavicle. Electrical activity in MCL_6 is observed by placing the positive electrode on the left midaxillary line at the level of the fifth intercostal space (as for lead V_6). The negative electrode is placed anteriorly, just below the left shoulder (Fig. 29-17).

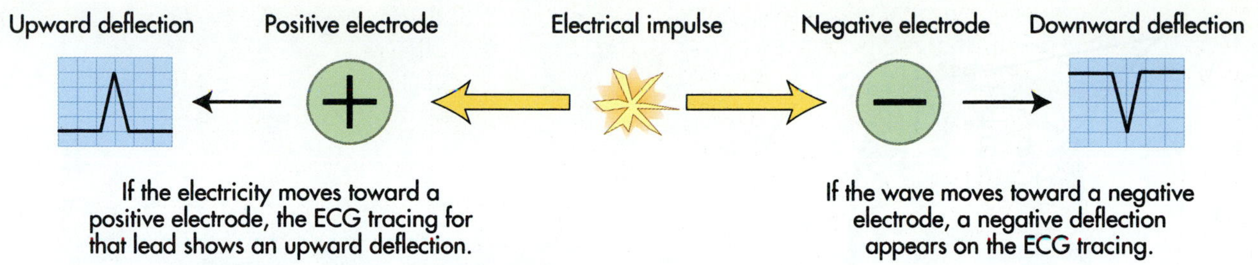

FIGURE 29-14 ■ Rule of electrical flow.

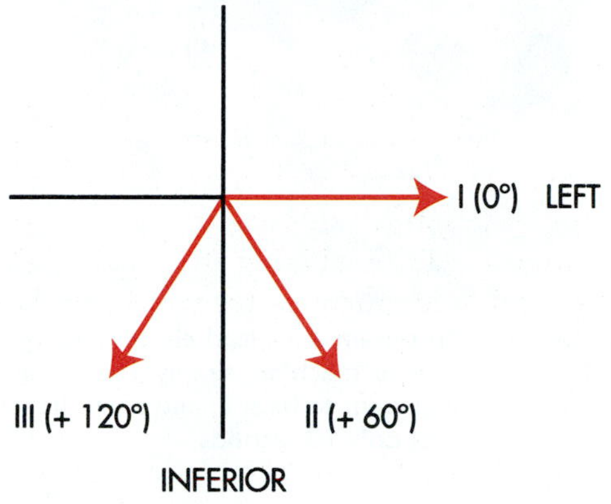

FIGURE 29-15 ■ Electrical vantage points of the three standard limb leads.

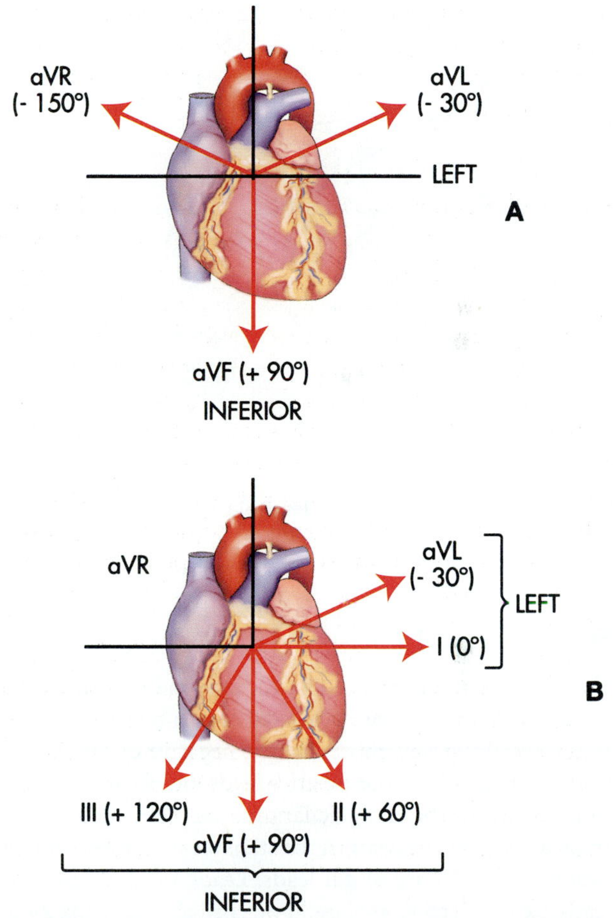

FIGURE 29-16 ■ **A,** Electrical vantage points of the three augmented limb leads. **B,** Combined electrical vantage points. Leads II, III, and aV_F are considered inferior leads; leads I and aV_L are considered lateral leads.

Routine Electrocardiogram Monitoring

Routine monitoring of cardiac rhythm in the prehospital setting, emergency department, or coronary care unit usually is obtained in lead II or MCL_1. These are the best leads to monitor for dysrhythmias because of their ability to display waves on the ECG that represent atrial depolarization (P waves). A good deal of information can be gathered from a single monitoring lead. In many cases, cardiac monitoring by a single lead is sufficient. For example, a paramedic can determine how fast the heart is beating and how regular. The paramedic also can determine how long conduction lasts in various parts of the heart.

Single-lead monitoring has its limitations. It may fail to reveal various abnormalities (particularly ST segment changes that signal myocardial injury or infarction) in the electrocardiogram tracing.

12-Lead Electrocardiogram Monitoring

A 12-lead electrocardiogram is obtained through 10 electrodes: 4 limb leads (right arm, right leg, left arm, left leg) and 6 chest leads (V_1 to V_6) (Fig. 29-18). The 4 limb leads provide readings of leads I, II, and III and aV_F, aV_L, and aV_R. Each lead of the 12-lead electrocardiogram views the left ventricle from the position of its positive electrode. Monitoring 12 leads is performed with a 12-lead monitor. This obtains the leads at the same time and provides a readout in conventional three- or four-column format. As described later in this chapter, 12-lead electrocardiogram monitoring can be used to do the following:

- Identify ST segment and T wave changes relative to myocardial ischemia, injury, and infarction.
- Identify ventricular tachycardia in wide-complex tachycardia.
- Determine the electrical axis and the presence of fascicular blocks.
- Determine the presence and location of bundle branch blocks.

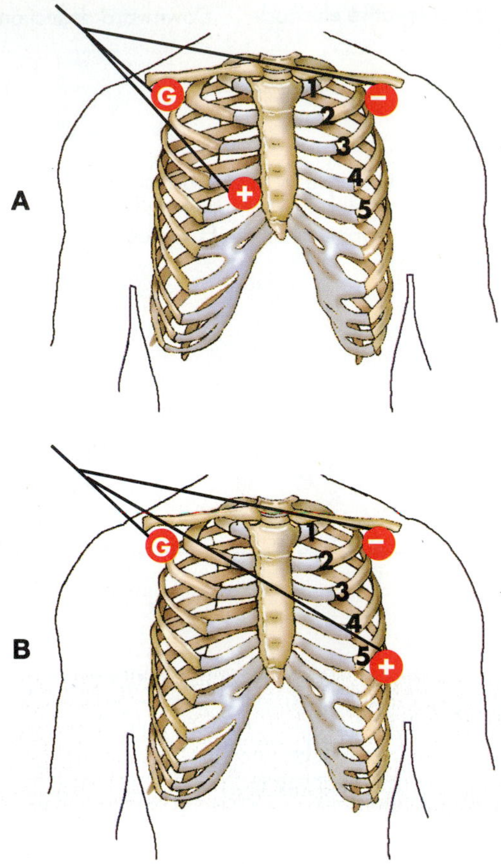

FIGURE 29-17 ■ Monitor lead placement for MCL_1 **(A)** and MCL_6 **(B)**.

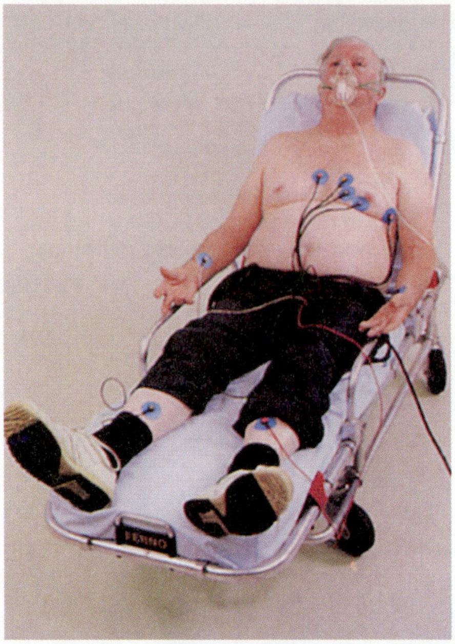

FIGURE 29-18 ■ To obtain a 12-lead electrocardiogram when using a 12-lead monitor or machine, simply attach the cables to the electrodes, ask the patient to be still, and push the record button. Acquisition requires only 10 seconds.

Precordial Leads

The 6 precordial leads used in 12-lead (and 9-lead) electrocardiogram monitoring are projected through the anterior chest wall toward the patient's back (the negative end of each chest lead) (Fig. 29-19). These positive leads are placed on the chest in reference to the thoracic landmarks. They record the electrical activity of the heart in the transverse or horizontal plane. Leads V_1 and V_2 are septal leads. Leads V_2 to V_4 are anterior leads. Leads V_4 to V_6 are lateral precordial leads (Box 29-3).

BOX 29-3 15-Lead Electrocardiogram

The wall of the right ventricle and the posterior wall of the left ventricle are areas of the heart that are hard to evaluate with the six precordial leads. Electrocardiogram monitoring that includes 12 leads plus V_{4R}, V_8, and V_9 leads (15-lead electrocardiogram) increases sensitivity for myocardial infarctions that occur in these areas (e.g., isolated posterior myocardial infarction). For 15-lead electrocardiogram monitoring, the V_{4R} lead is placed at the fifth intercostal space in the right anterior midclavicular line. The V_8 lead is placed at the posterior fifth intercostal space in the right midscapular line. The V_9 lead is placed between the V_8 lead and the spinal column at the posterior fifth intercostal space.

Note: Fifteen-lead electrocardiograms are not performed routinely in the prehospital setting.

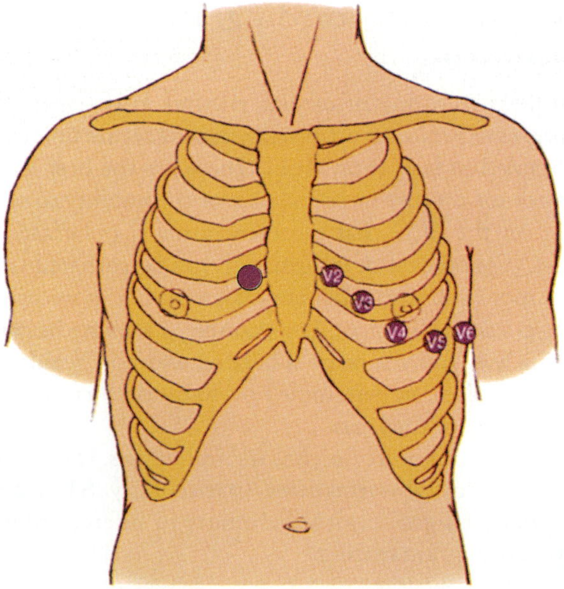

FIGURE 29-19 ■ Proper chest lead placement.

Proper placement of the chest leads at specific intercostal spaces is essential for an accurate reading. One method to locate the appropriate intercostal spaces is as follows[2] (Fig. 29-20):

STEP-BY-STEP SKILL

FIGURE 29-20 ■

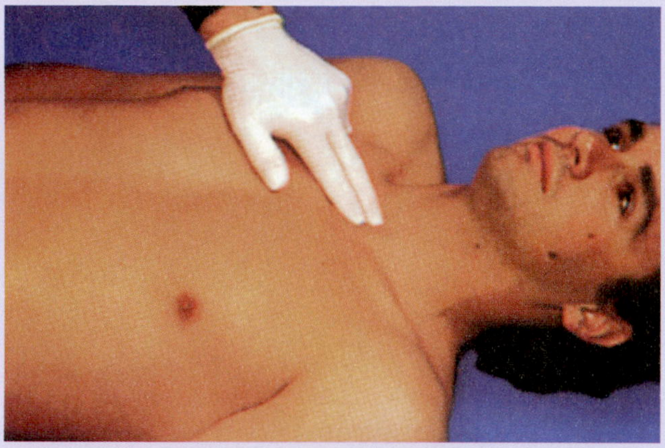

A ■ Locate the jugular notch.

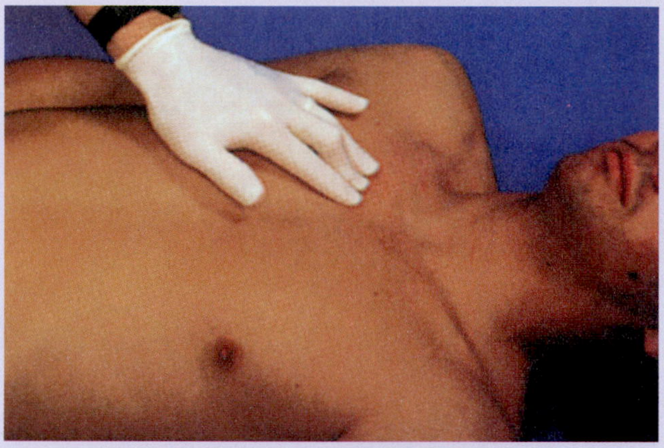

B ■ Palpate for the angle of Louis.

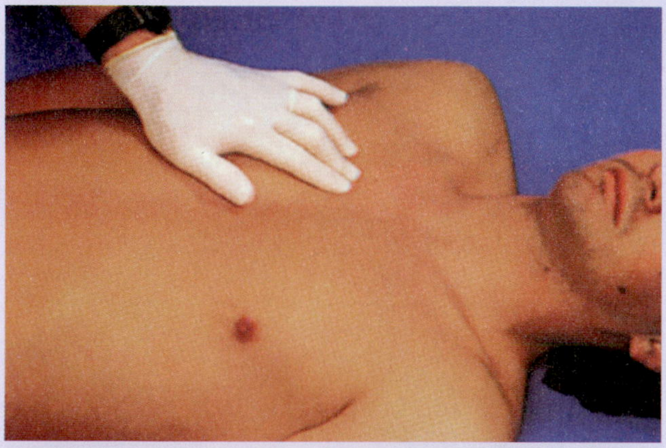

C ■ Follow the angle of Louis to the patient's right until it articulates with the second rib.

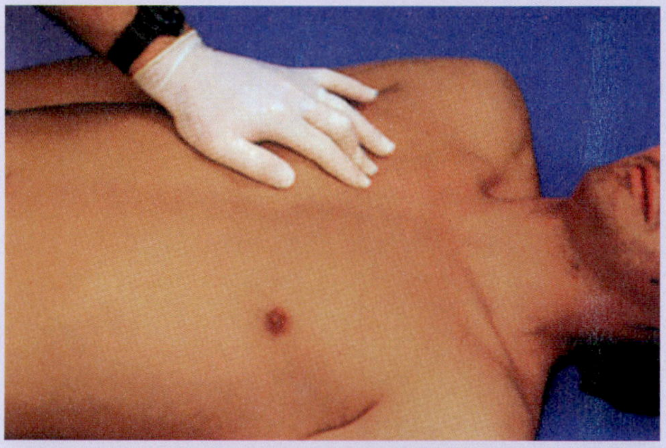

D ■ Locate the second intercostal space (immediately below the second rib).

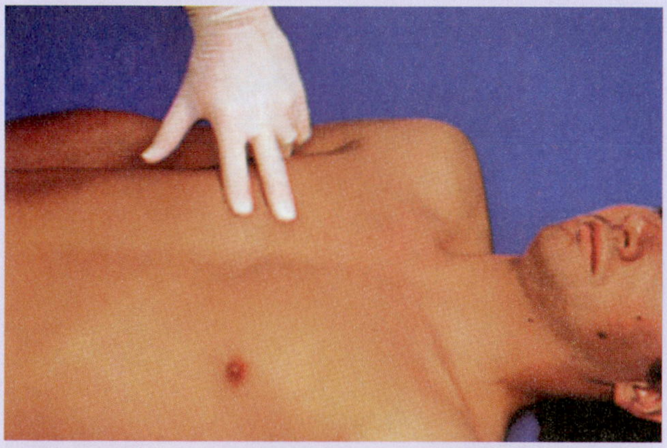

E ■ From the second intercostal space the third and fourth intercostal spaces can be found.

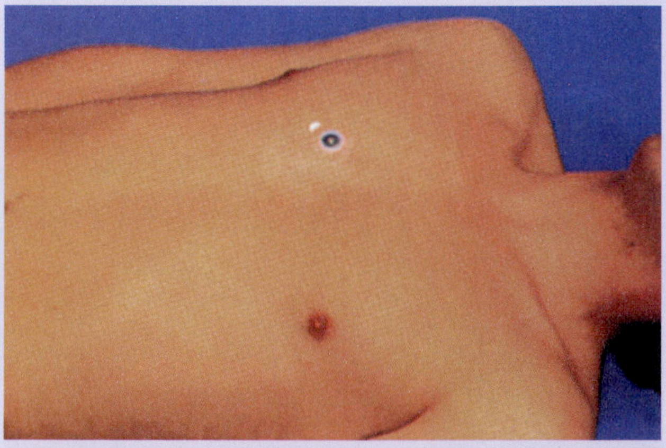

F ■ Lead V_1 is positioned in the fourth intercostal space just to the right of the sternum.

Continued

STEP-BY-STEP SKILL

FIGURE 29-20, cont'd ■

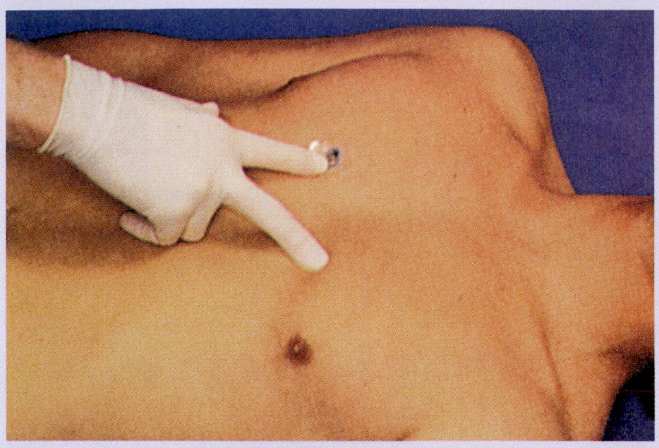

G ■ From the V_1 position, find the corresponding intercostal space on the left side of the sternum.

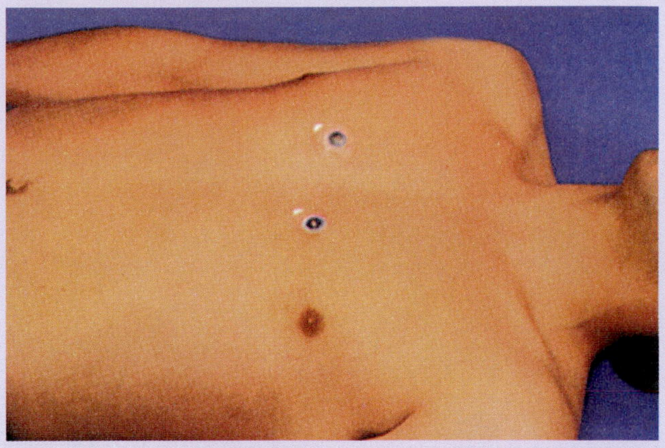

H ■ Place the V_2 electrode in the fourth intercostal space just to the left of the sternum.

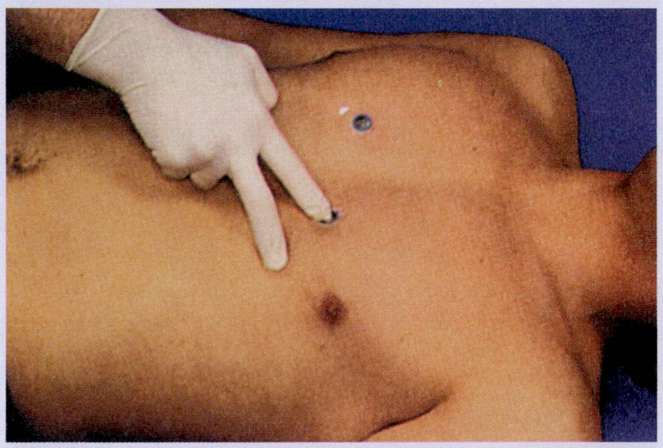

I ■ From the V_2 position, locate the fifth intercostal space and follow it to the midclavicular line.

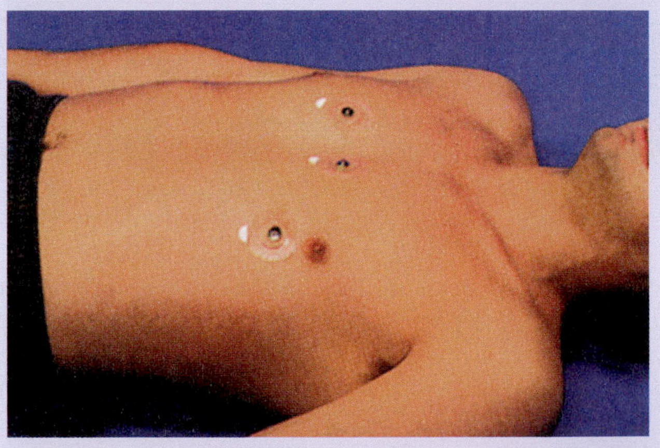

J ■ Position the V_4 electrode in the fifth intercostal space in the midclavicular line.

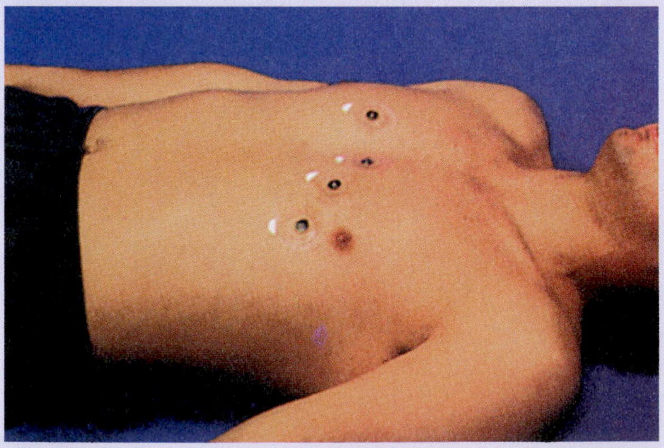

K ■ Lead V_3 is positioned halfway between V_2 and V_4.

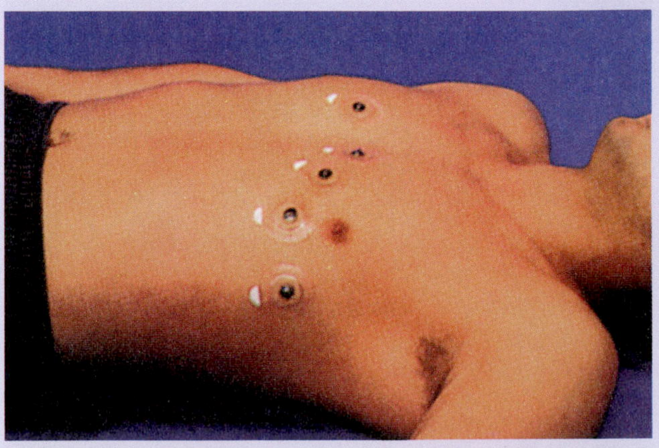

L ■ Lead V_5 is positioned in the anterior axillary line, level with V_4.

Continued

STEP-BY-STEP SKILL

FIGURE 29-20, cont'd ■

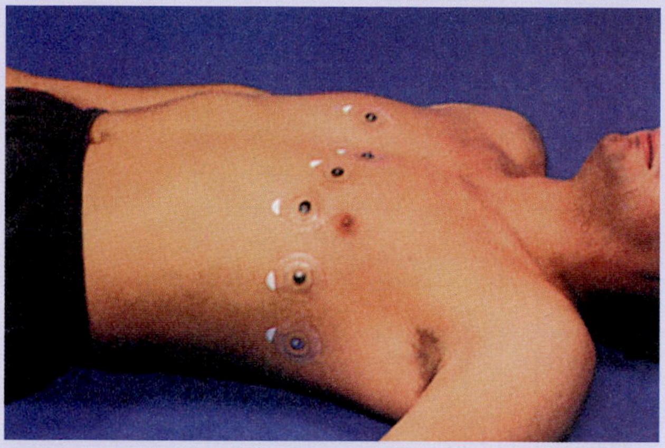

M ■ Lead V_6 is positioned in the midaxillary line, level with V_4.

1. Locate the jugular notch and move downward until the sternal angle is found.
2. Follow the articulation to the right sternal border to locate the second rib. Just below the second rib is the second intercostal space.
3. Move down two intercostal spaces and position the V_1 electrode in the fourth intercostal space, just to the right of the patient's sternum.
4. Move across the sternum to the corresponding intercostal space and position V_2 to the left of the patient's sternum.
5. From V_2, palpate down one intercostal space and follow the fifth intercostal space to the midclavicular line to place the V_4 electrode.
6. Place lead V_3 midway between V_2 and V_4.
7. Place V_5 in the anterior axillary line in a straight line with V_4 (where the arm joins the chest).
8. Place V_6 in the midaxillary line, level with V_4 and V_5. (It may be more convenient to place V_6 first, and then V_5.) In women, place the V_4 to V_6 electrodes under the left breast to avoid any errors in the electrocardiogram tracing that may occur from breast tissue.

CRITICAL THINKING

Consider that your patient is female. You are performing 12-lead electrocardiogram tracing. What measures can you take to decrease her potential discomfort or embarrassment?

Another method to obtain the six precordial leads in select patient groups is to use a single electrode (e.g., UNI-LEAD Electrode System). This system uses a single cable (based on the adult patient's size as small, medium, or large) and a connector. This eliminates individual precordial lead wires. It also reduces electrode placement error.

9-Lead Electrocardiogram Monitoring

In the absence of a 12-lead machine, a standard 3-lead monitor can be used to obtain a multilead (9-lead) electrocardiogram reading. (The 9-lead electrocardiogram does not include aV_R, aV_L, or aV_F but still provides valuable information about the lateral, anterior, and inferior wall.) To obtain a 9-lead reading from a standard 3-lead monitor, the paramedic should enable the diagnostic setting of the machine (if available) and follow these steps:

1. Run leads I, II, and III first. Obtain a representative sample of each lead and label it.
2. Leave the monitor in lead III (the negative electrode at the left shoulder) and move the left leg cable (the red lead wire) to each of the modified chest lead positions (from V_1 to V_6) to obtain a readout. Label each sample.
3. Arrange the readouts in a standard 9-lead order: I, II, and III in the first column; MCL_1, MCL_2, and MCL_3 in the middle column; and MCL_4, MCL_5, and MCL_6 in the last column (Fig. 29-21).

CRITICAL THINKING

What effect will improper lead placement have on the "view" of the heart and the analysis of the electrocardiogram tracing?

Application of Monitoring Electrodes

The most commonly used electrodes for continuous electrocardiogram monitoring are pregelled, stick-on disks. These disks can be applied easily to the chest wall. The paramedic should observe the following guidelines to minimize artifacts in the signal and to make effective contact between the electrode and the skin:

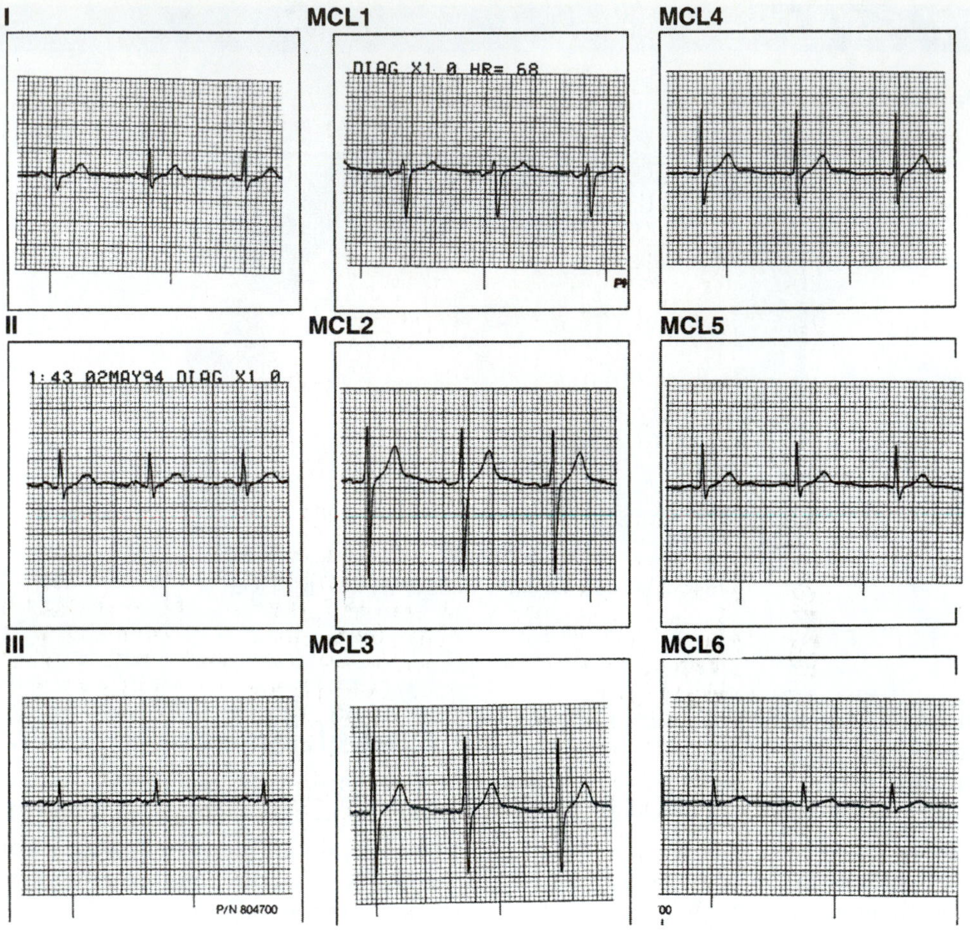

FIGURE 29-21 ■ Nine-lead electrocardiogram readout.

> **CRITICAL THINKING**
> Why should alcohol or benzoin not be used under defibrillator pads?

1. Choose an appropriate area of skin, avoiding large muscle masses and large quantities of hair, which may prevent the electrode from lying flat against the skin.
2. Cleanse the area with alcohol to remove dirt and body oil. When attaching electrodes to the extremities, use the inner surfaces of the arms and legs. If necessary, trim excess body hair before placing the electrodes. If the patient is extremely diaphoretic, use tincture of benzoin to aid in securing application or use diaphoretic electrodes.
3. Attach the electrodes to the prepared site.
4. Attach the electrocardiogram cables to electrodes. Most electrocardiogram cables are marked for right arm, left arm, and left leg application.
5. Turn on the electrocardiogram monitor and obtain a baseline tracing.

If the signal is poor, the paramedic should recheck the cable connections. The paramedic also should check the effectiveness of the patient's skin contact with the electrodes. Other common causes of a poor signal include body hair, dried conductive gel, poor electrode placement, and diaphoresis.

Electrocardiogram Graph Paper

The paper used in recording electrocardiograms is standardized to allow comparative analysis of an electrocardiogram wave. The graph paper is divided into squares 1 mm in height and width. The paper is divided further by darker lines every fifth square vertically and horizontally. Each large square is 5 mm high and 5 mm wide (Fig. 29-22).

As the graph paper moves past the stylus of the electrocardiogram machine, it measures time and amplitude. Time is measured on the horizontal plane (side to side). When the electrocardiogram is recorded at the standard paper speed of 25 mm per second, each small square is equal to 1 mm (0.04 second) and each large square (the dark vertical lines) is equal to 5 mm (0.20 second). These squares measure the length of time it takes an electrical impulse to pass through a specific part of the heart.

Amplitude is measured on the vertical axis (top to bottom) of the graph paper. Each small square of the graph pa-

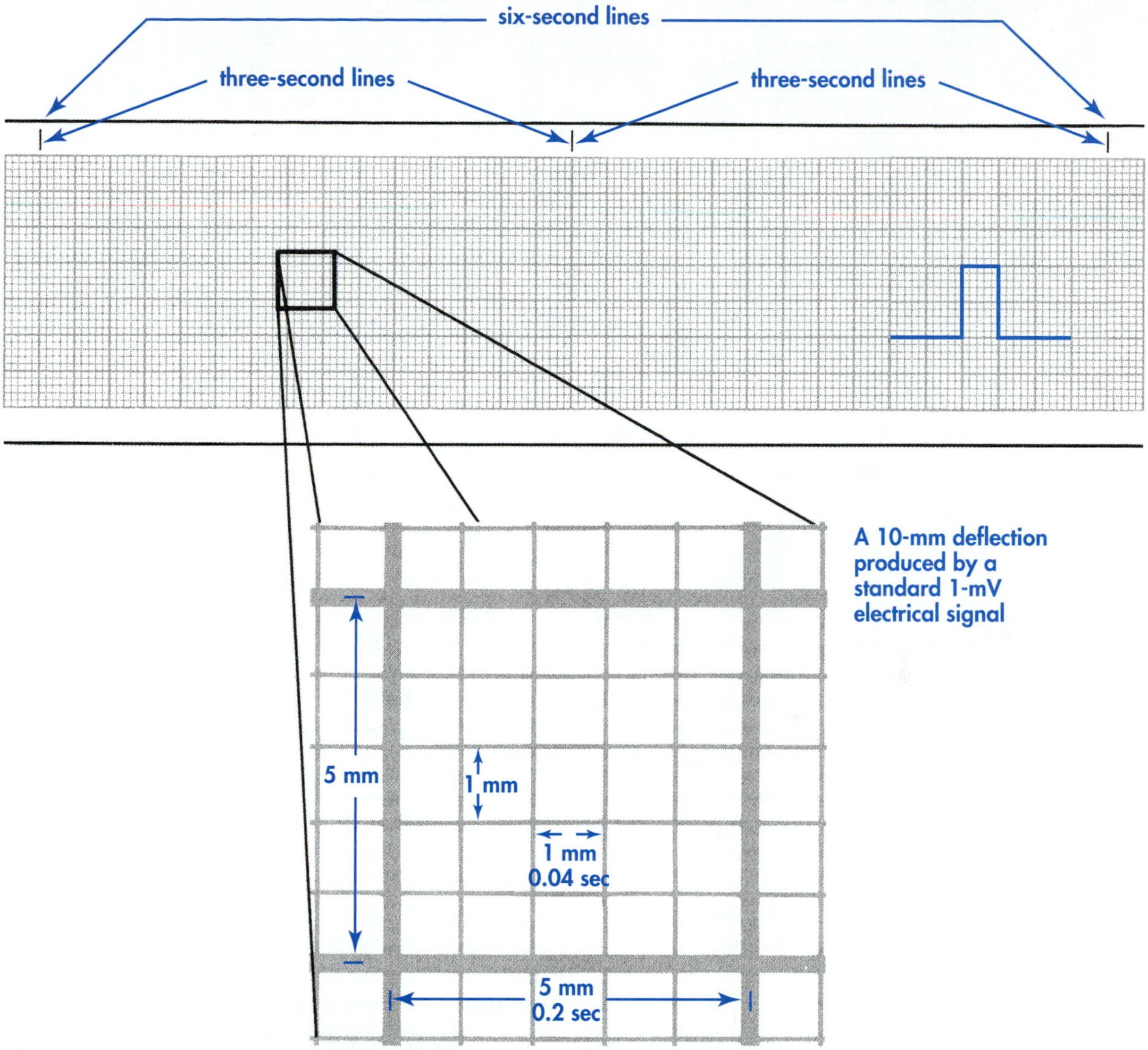

FIGURE 29-22 ■ Electrocardiogram graph paper.

per is equal to 0.1 mV. Each large square (five small squares) is equal to 0.5 mV. The sensitivity of the 12-lead electrocardiogram machine is standardized. When properly calibrated, a 1-mV electrical signal produces a 10-mm deflection (two large squares) on the electrocardiogram tracing. Electrocardiogram machines equipped with calibration buttons should have a calibration curve placed at the beginning of the first electrocardiogram tracing (generally a 1-mV burst, represented by a 10-mm "block" wave).

Time-interval markings are denoted by short vertical lines and usually are located on the top of the electrocardiogram graph paper. When the electrocardiogram is recorded at the standard paper speed, the distance between each short vertical line is 75 mm (3 seconds). Each 3-second interval contains 15 large squares (0.2 second multiplied by 15 squares equals 3 seconds). These markings are used as a method of heart rate calculation (i.e., counting the number of QRS complexes in 6 seconds and multiplying by 10).

RELATIONSHIP OF THE ELECTROCARDIOGRAM TO ELECTRICAL ACTIVITY

Each waveform seen on the oscilloscope or recorded on the electrocardiogram graph paper represents the conduction of an electrical impulse through a certain part of the heart. All waveforms begin and end at the isoelectric line. This line represents the absence of electrical activity in cardiac tissue. A deflection above the baseline is positive. It indicates an electrical flow toward the positive electrode. A deflection below the baseline is negative. It indicates an electrical flow away from the positive electrode.

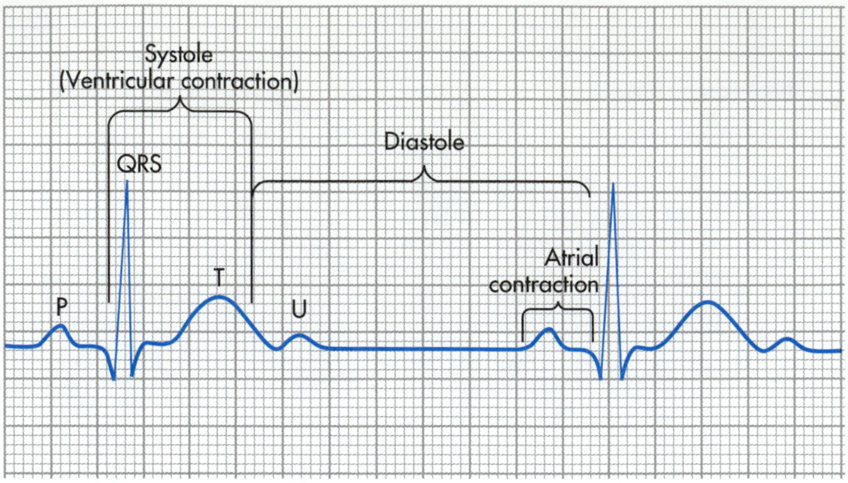

FIGURE 29-23 ■ Summary of the electrical basis of the electrocardiogram.

The normal electrocardiogram consists of a **P wave, QRS complex,** and **T wave.** At times, a **U wave** also can be seen after the T wave. If present, the U wave usually is a positive deflection. The U wave may be associated with electrolyte abnormalities. Other key parts of the electrocardiogram that should be evaluated include the **P-R interval, ST segment,** and **Q-T interval.** The combination of these waves represents a single heartbeat, or one complete cardiac cycle (Fig. 29-23). The electrical events of the cardiac cycle are followed by their mechanical counterparts. The descriptions of electrocardiogram waveform components refer to those that would be seen in lead II monitoring.

P Wave

The P wave is the first positive (upward) deflection on the electrocardiogram, representing atrial depolarization. It usually is rounded and precedes the QRS complex. The P wave begins with the first positive deflection from the baseline and ends at the point where the wave returns to the baseline. The duration of the P wave normally is 0.10 second or less, and its amplitude is 0.5 to 2.5 mm. The P wave usually is followed by a QRS complex. However, if conduction disturbances are present, a QRS complex does not always follow each P wave.

P-R Interval

The P-R interval is the time it takes for an electrical impulse to be conducted through the atria and the atrioventricular node up to the instant of ventricular depolarization. The P-R interval is measured from the beginning of the P wave to the beginning of the next deflection on the baseline (the onset of the QRS complex). The normal P-R interval is 0.12 to 0.20 second (three to five small squares on the graph paper). The P-R interval depends on the heart rate and the conduction characteristics of the atrioventricular node. When the heart rate is fast, the P-R interval normally is of shorter duration than when the heart rate is slow. A normal P-R interval indicates that the electrical impulse has been conducted through the atria, atrioventricular node, and bundle of His normally and without delay.

QRS Complex

The QRS complex generally is composed of three individual waves: the Q, R, and S waves. The QRS complex begins at the point where the first wave of the complex deviates from the baseline. It ends where the last wave of the complex begins to flatten at, above, or below the baseline. The direction of the QRS complex may be predominantly positive (upright), predominantly negative (inverted), or biphasic (partly positive, partly negative). The shape of the normal QRS complex is narrow and sharply pointed (when conduction is normal). Its duration generally is 0.08 to 0.10 second (two to two and a half small squares on the graph paper) or less, and its amplitude normally varies from less than 5 mm to more than 15 mm.

The Q wave is the first negative (downward) deflection of the QRS complex on the electrocardiogram. However, it may not be present in all leads. The Q wave represents depolarization of the interventricular septum or a pathological change. The R wave is the first positive deflection after the P wave. Subsequent positive deflections in the QRS complex that extend above the baseline and that are taller than the first R wave are called *R prime (R′)*, *R double prime (R″)*, and so on. The S wave is the negative deflection that follows the R wave. Subsequent negative deflections are called *S prime (S′)*, *S double prime (S″)*, and so on. Although there may be only one Q wave, there can be more than one R wave and one S wave in the QRS complex. The R and S waves represent the sum of electrical forces resulting from depolarization of the right and left ventricles (Fig. 29-24).

CRITICAL THINKING

What is the import of a QRS complex duration of 0.10 second?

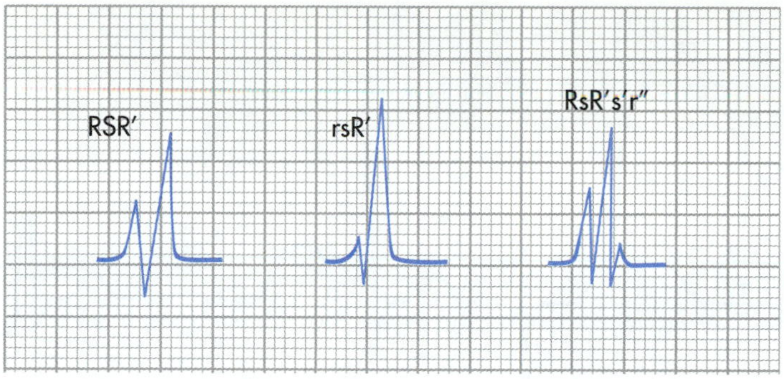

FIGURE 29-24 ■ QRS complexes with more than one positive or negative deflection.

The QRS complex follows the P wave. The QRS complex marks the approximate beginning of mechanical systole of the ventricles, which continues through the onset of the T wave. The QRS complex represents ventricular depolarization. This includes the conduction of an electrical impulse from the atrioventricular node through the bundle of His, Purkinje fibers, and the right and left bundle branches. This impulse results in ventricular depolarization.

ST Segment

The ST segment represents the early phase of repolarization of the right and left ventricles. It immediately follows the QRS complex and ends with the onset of the T wave. The point at which it takes off from the QRS complex is called the *J point*. In a normal electrocardiogram, the ST segment begins at baseline and has a slight upward slope.

The position of the ST segment commonly is judged as normal or abnormal using the baseline of the P-R or T-P interval as a reference. Deviations above this baseline are referred to as *ST segment elevation*. Deviations below baseline are referred to as *ST segment depression* (Fig. 29-25). Certain conditions can cause depression or elevation of the P-R interval, thus affecting the reference for ST segment abnormalities. Usually the baseline from the end of the T wave to the beginning of the P wave maintains its isoelectric position and can be used as a reference. Abnormal ST segments may be seen in infarction, ischemia, and pericarditis; after digitalis administration; and in other disease states.

T Wave

The T wave represents repolarization of the ventricular myocardial cells. The wave occurs during the last part of ventricular contraction. The T wave is identified as the first deviation from the ST segment and ends where the T wave returns to the baseline. This wave may be above or below the isoelectric line. The T wave usually is slightly rounded and slightly asymmetrical. Deep and symmetrically inverted T waves may indicate cardiac ischemia. A T wave elevated more than half the height of the QRS complex (peaked T wave) may indicate new onset of ischemia of the myocardium or hyperkalemia.

Q-T Interval

The Q-T interval is measured from the beginning of the QRS complex to the end of the T wave (Fig. 29-26). It represents the time from the beginning of ventricular depolarization until the end of ventricular repolarization. During the start of the Q-T interval, the heart is completely unable to respond to electrical stimuli. (This is the absolute refractory period.) During the latter portion of this interval (from the peak of the T wave onward), the heart may be able to respond to premature stimuli. This is called the relative refractory period. During this period, premature impulses may depolarize the heart. Commonly prescribed medications that may prolong the Q-T interval include quinidine, ***procainamide***, and disopyramide. These antidysrhythmics, by virtue of their effect on the Q-T interval, may lead to potentially lethal dysrhythmias, including ventricular tachycardia, ventricular fibrillation, and an unusual bidirectional ventricular dysrhythmia called **torsades de pointes** (described later in this chapter).

▶**NOTE** If the heart rate is fewer than 100 beats per minute, the Q-T interval probably is prolonged if it is greater than half of the R-R interval.[3]

Artifacts

Artifacts are marks on the electrocardiogram display or tracing caused by activities other than the electrical activity of the heart (Fig. 29-27). Common causes of artifacts are improper grounding of the electrocardiogram machine, patient movement, loss of electrode contact with the patient's skin, patient shivering or tremors, and external chest compression. Two types of artifacts deserve special mention. One is alternating current interference (60-cycle interference). The other one is biotelemetry-related interference.

Alternating current interference may occur in a poorly grounded electrocardiogram machine. Or interference may occur when an electrocardiogram is obtained near high-tension wires, transformers, and some household appliances. This

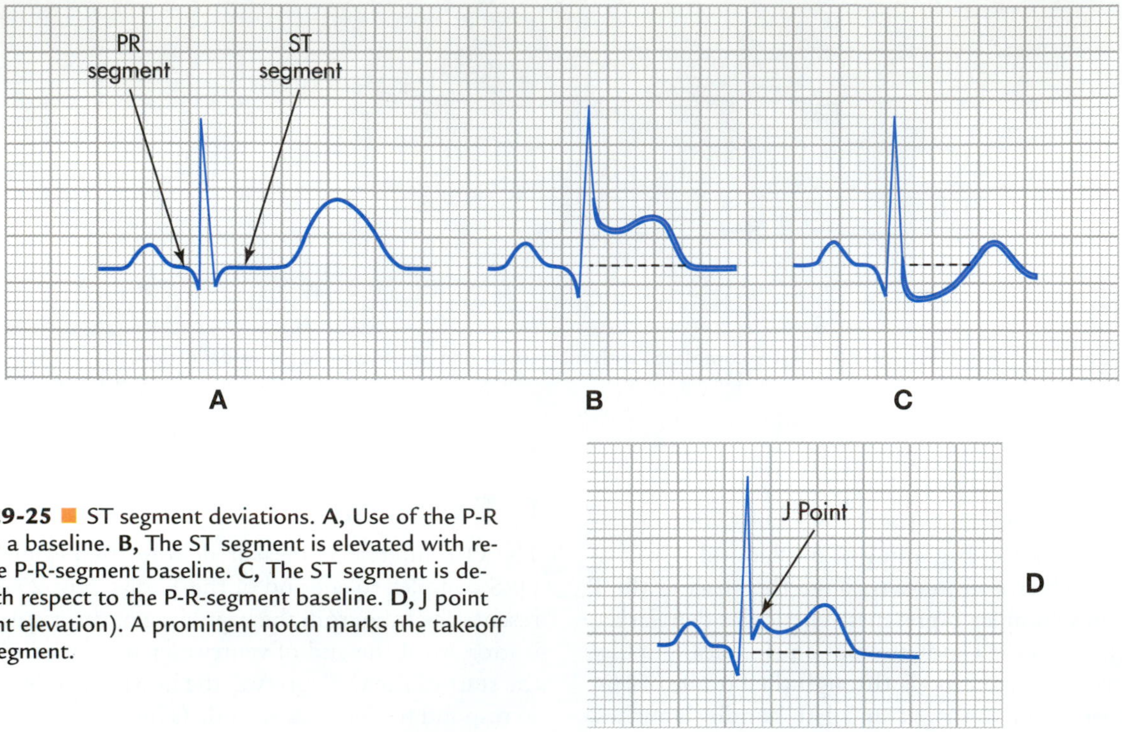

FIGURE 29-25 ■ ST segment deviations. **A,** Use of the P-R segment as a baseline. **B,** The ST segment is elevated with respect to the P-R-segment baseline. **C,** The ST segment is depressed with respect to the P-R-segment baseline. **D,** J point (ST segment elevation). A prominent notch marks the takeoff of the ST segment.

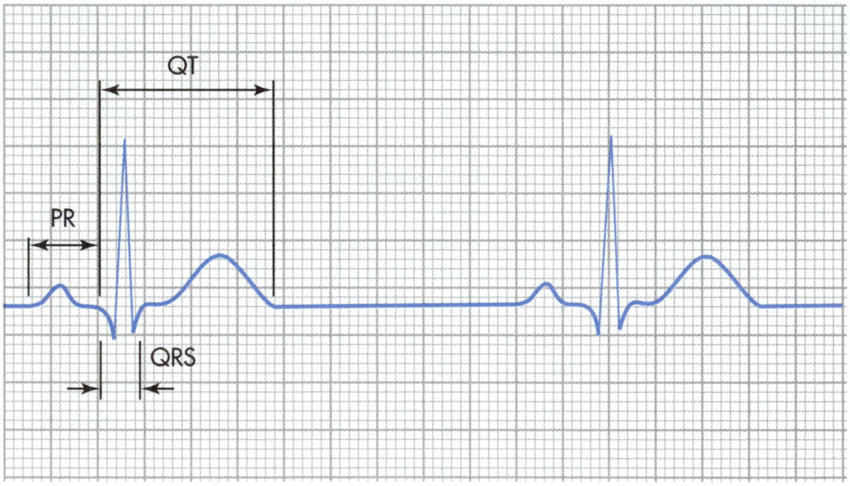

FIGURE 29-26 ■ P-R, Q-T, and QRS intervals.

results in a thick baseline made up of 60-cycle waves. The P waves may not be discernible because of the interference. Yet the QRS complex usually is visible. Alternating current interference also may be caused by the patient or the lead cable touching a metal object such as a bed rail. Placing a blanket between the metal object and the patient may correct the interference.

Biotelemetry-related interference may occur when biotelemetry electrocardiogram signals are received poorly. This may result from weak batteries or from electrocardiogram transmission in areas with poor signaling conditions. Interference also may result if the transmitter is located a distance away from a base station receiver. Biotelemetry-related interference may produce sharp spikes and waves that have a jagged appearance.

SECTION FIVE
ELECTROCARDIOGRAM INTERPRETATION

STEPS IN RHYTHM ANALYSIS

Evaluation of an electrocardiogram requires a systematic approach to analyzing a given rhythm. Numerous methods can be used for rhythm interpretation. This text uses a method that first looks at the QRS complex (the most im-

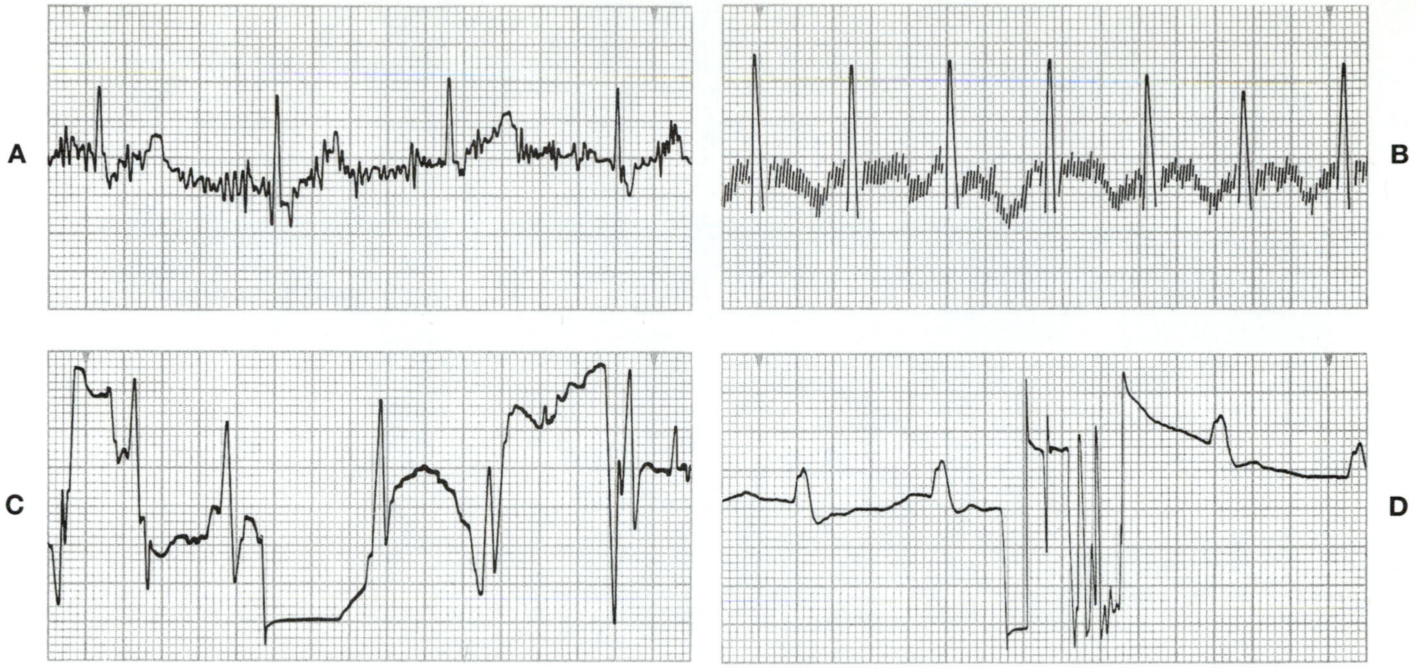

FIGURE 29-27 ■ Artifacts. **A,** Muscle tremors. **B,** Alternating current (60-cycle) interference. **C,** Loose electrodes. **D,** Biotelemetry.

portant observation in life-threatening dysrhythmias); followed by P waves and the relationship between the P waves and the QRS; rate; rhythm; and finally the P-R interval. Regardless of the method chosen to analyze a given rhythm, the paramedic should use a consistent format. This section of the text discusses rhythm interpretation as it pertains to standard 3-lead electrocardiogram monitoring. Evaluation of 12-lead electrocardiogram monitoring is presented later in this chapter.

Five questions the paramedic must ask in any rhythm analysis to determine the presence or potential for life-threatening rhythm disturbances are as follows:

1. Is the patient sick?
2. What is the heart rate?
3. Are there normal-looking QRS complexes?
4. Are there normal-looking P waves?
5. What is the relationship between the P waves and the QRS complexes?

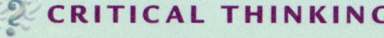

CRITICAL THINKING

What does the electrocardiogram tell you about perfusion?

Step 1: Analyze the QRS Complex

The paramedic should analyze the QRS complex for regularity and width. QRS complexes less than or equal to 0.10 second wide (less than three small squares) are supraventricular in origin. These complexes are normal. Complexes that are equal to or greater than 0.12 second wide may indicate a conduction abnormality in the ventricles. Or they may indicate that the focus originates in the ventricles and is abnormal (Fig. 29-28). When evaluating an abnormal QRS width, the paramedic should identify the lead with the widest QRS complex because a portion of the QRS complex may be hidden or hard to see in some leads.

Step 2: Analyze the P Waves

The normal P wave in lead II is positive and smoothly rounded and usually precedes each QRS complex, indicating that the pacemaker originates in the sinoatrial node (Fig. 29-29). Therefore the paramedic should observe the following five components when evaluating P waves:

1. Are P waves present?
2. Are the P waves regular (can they be mapped out similar to R-R intervals [described later])?
3. Is there one P wave for each QRS complex, and is there a QRS complex following each P wave?
4. Are the P waves upright or inverted?
5. Do they all look alike? (P waves that look alike and are regular are likely from the same pacemaker.)

Step 3: Analyze the Rate

Analysis of the heart rate may be done in a number of ways. The methods for calculating the heart rate presented in this text are heart rate calculator rulers, the triplicate method, the R-R method, and the 6-second count method.

The heart rate is determined by analyzing the ventricular rate (QRS complex). An adequate rate of ventricular contraction is responsible for cardiac output. However, if the atrial and ventricular rates differ (as may occur in certain dysrhythmias), they should be calculated separately. The

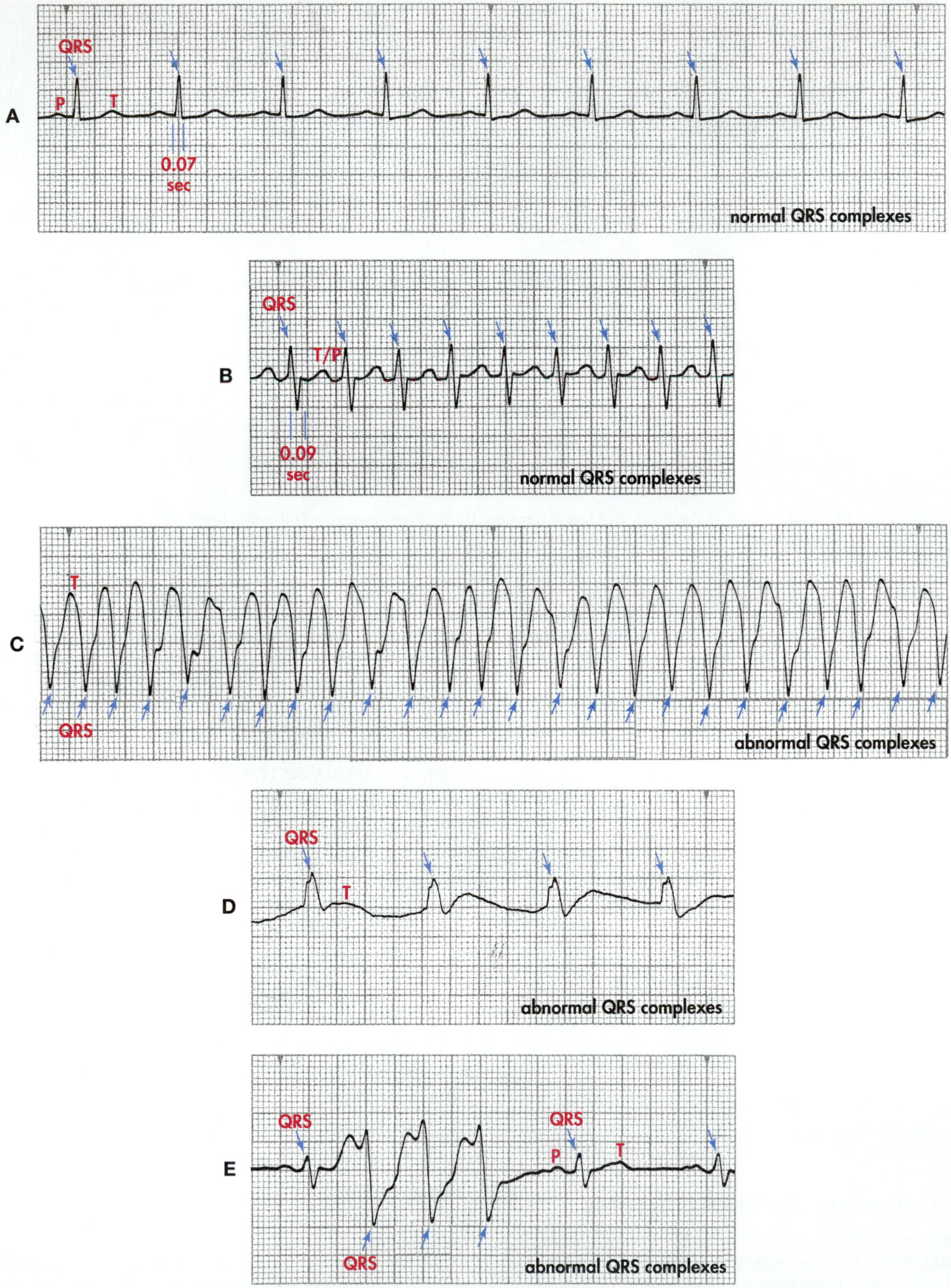

FIGURE 29-28 ■ A and B, Normal QRS complexes. C to E, Abnormal QRS complexes.

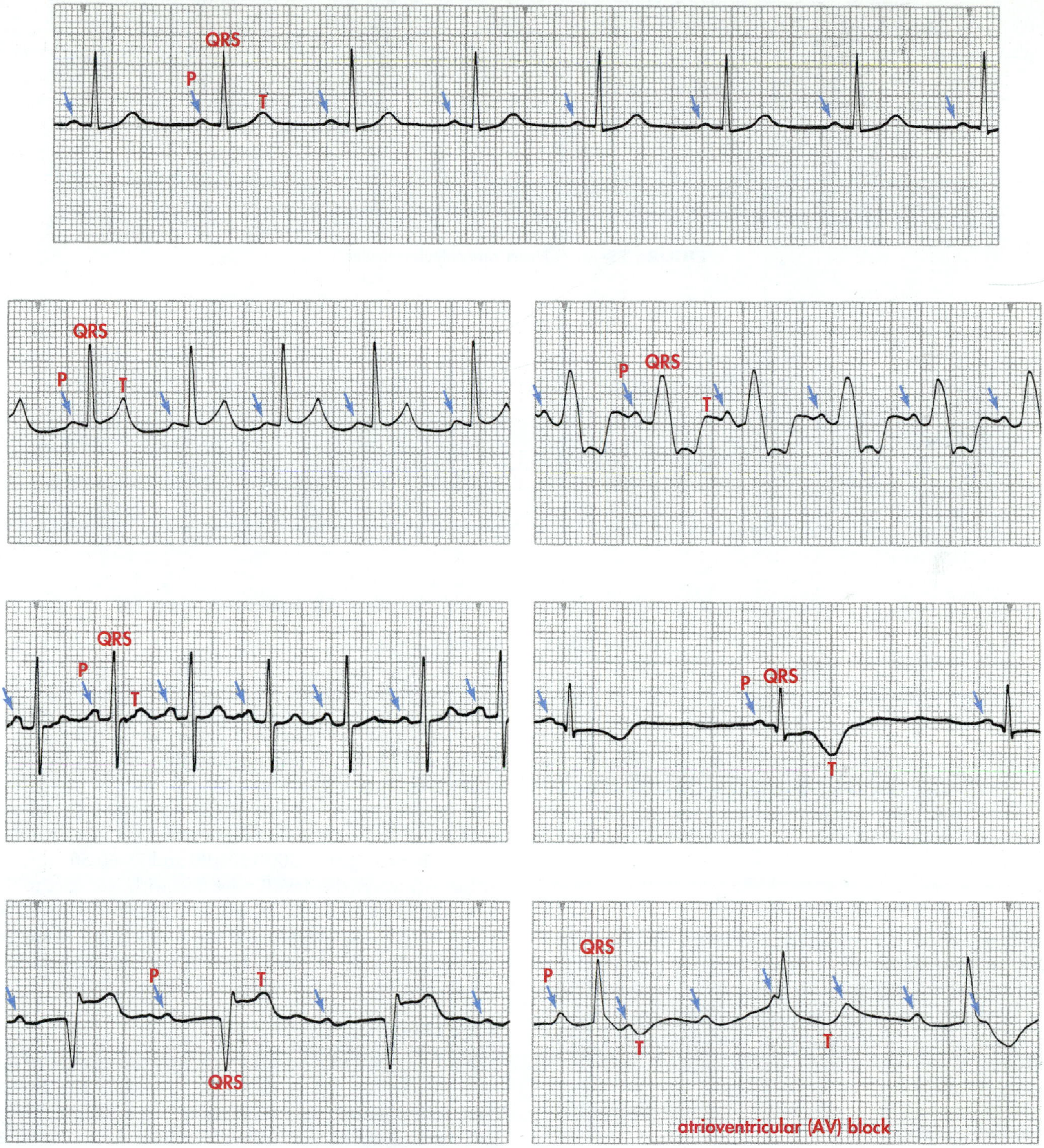

FIGURE 29-29 ■ Normal P waves.

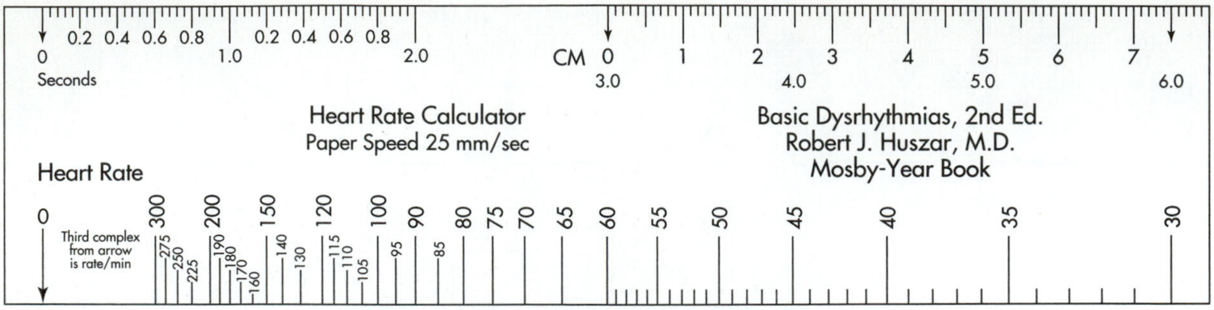

FIGURE 29-30 ■ Heart rate calculator ruler.

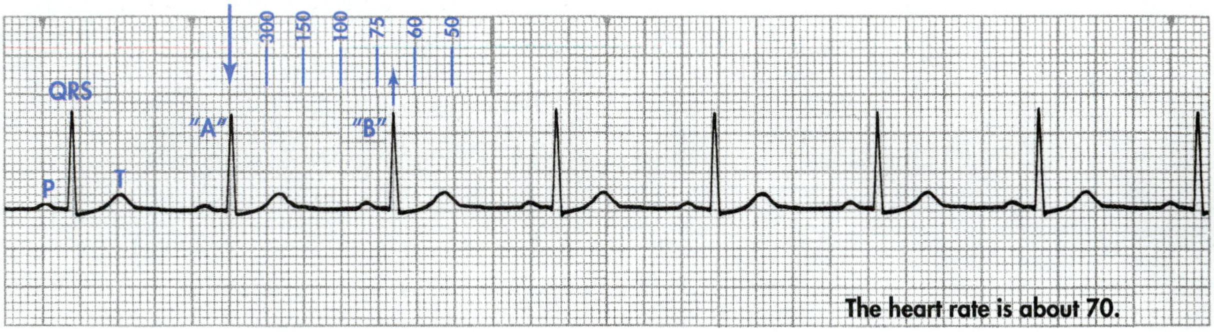

FIGURE 29-31 ■ Triplicate method.

normal adult heart rate is between 60 and 99 beats per minute. If the ventricular rate is less than 60 beats per minute, it is considered a bradycardia; if the rate is equal to or greater than 100 beats per minute, it is considered a tachycardia.

HEART RATE CALCULATOR RULERS

Heart rate calculator rulers (Fig. 29-30) are available from a number of manufacturers. The paramedic should follow the directions that come with the rulers. Heart rate calculator rulers are reasonably accurate if the rhythm is regular. Still, a mechanical device or tool should not be relied on solely to determine the heart rate because one may not be readily available.

TRIPLICATE METHOD

The triplicate method of determining the heart rate (Fig. 29-31) is accurate only under two circumstances. One, the rhythm is regular. Two, the heart rate is greater than 50 beats per minute. The method requires memorizing two sets of numbers. These are 300-150-100 and 75-60-50. These numbers are derived from the distance between the heavy black lines (each representing $^1/_{300}$ minute). Thus two $^1/_{300}$-minute units are equal to $^2/_{300}$ minute, which is equal to $^1/_{150}$ minute, or a heart rate of 150 beats per minute; three $^1/_{300}$-minute units are equal to $^3/_{300}$ minute, which is equal to $^1/_{100}$ minute, or a heart rate of 100 beats per minute. Using these triplicates, the paramedic can calculate heart rate as follows:

1. Select an R wave that lines up with a dark vertical line.
2. Number the next six dark vertical lines consecutively from left to right as 300-150-100 and 75-60-50.
3. Identify where the next R wave falls with reference to the six dark vertical lines. If the R wave falls on 75, the heart rate is 75 beats per minute. If the R wave falls halfway between 100 and 150, the heart rate is about 125 beats per minute.

R-R METHOD

The R-R method may be used several different ways to calculate the heart rate. Like the triplicate method, the rhythm must be regular to obtain an accurate reading. However, the R-R method works equally well for slow rates. The three methods are as follows:

Method 1. Measure the distance in seconds between the peaks of two consecutive R waves. Then divide this number into 60 to obtain the heart rate (Fig. 29-32).

Method 2. Count the large squares between the peaks of two consecutive R waves. Divide this number into 300 to obtain the heart rate (Fig. 29-33).

Method 3. Count the small squares between the peaks of two consecutive R waves. Divide this number into 1500 to obtain the heart rate (Fig. 29-34).

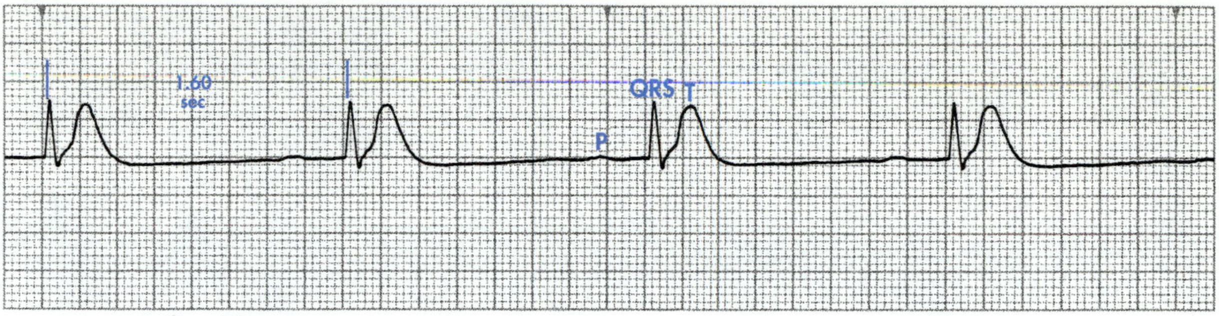

The heart rate $= \dfrac{60}{1.60 \text{ sec}} = 37.5$ or, rounded off, 38.

FIGURE 29-32 ■ R-R interval method 1.

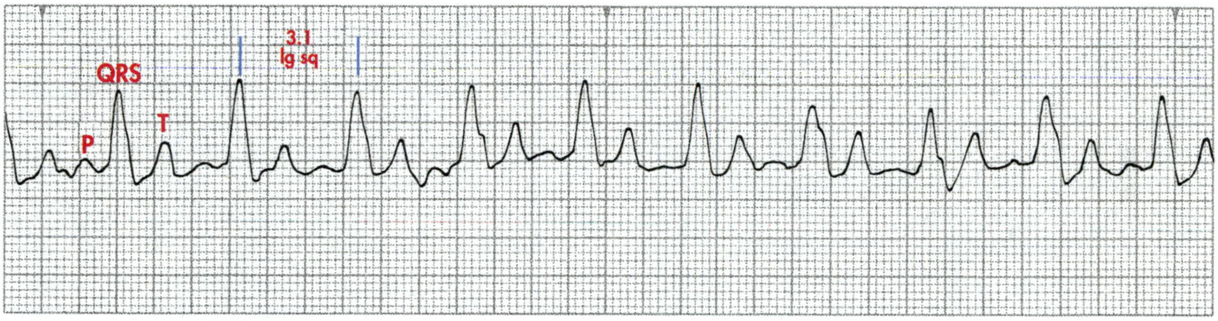

The heart rate $= \dfrac{300}{3.1 \text{ lg sq}} = 97.$

FIGURE 29-33 ■ R-R interval method 2.

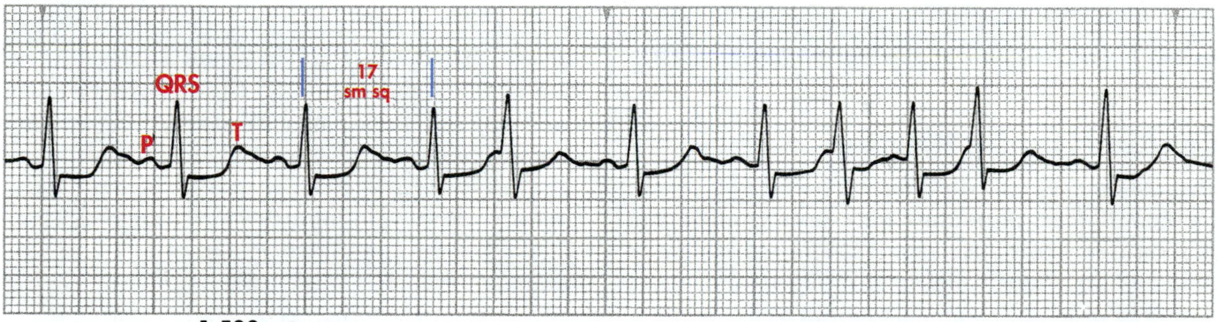

The heart rate $= \dfrac{1{,}500}{17 \text{ sm sq}} = 88.$

FIGURE 29-34 ■ R-R interval method 3.

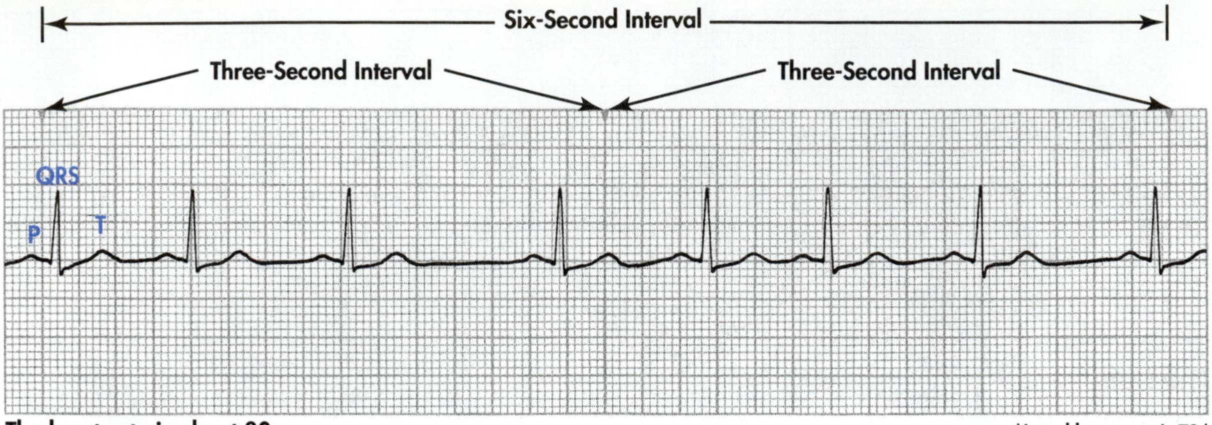

FIGURE 29-35 ■ Six-second count method.

6-SECOND COUNT METHOD

The 6-second count method (Fig. 29-35) is the least accurate method of determining the heart rate. The method is useful, however, for quickly obtaining an approximate rate in regular and irregular rhythms.

As previously stated, the short vertical lines at the top of most electrocardiogram graph papers are divided into 3-second intervals when run at a standard speed of 25 mm per second. Two of these intervals are equal to 6 seconds. The heart rate is calculated by counting the number of QRS complexes in a 6-second interval. This number is multiplied by 10.

> **CRITICAL THINKING**
>
> Which of these rate calculation methods is fastest? Which is most accurate?

Step 4: Analyze the Rhythm

To analyze the ventricular rhythm, the paramedic should compare the R-R intervals on the electrocardiogram tracing in a systematic way from left to right. This measurement may be taken using electrocardiogram calipers or pen and paper. Using calipers, the paramedic should place one tip of the caliper on the peak of one R wave and adjust the other tip so that it rests on the peak of the adjacent R wave. The paramedic then uses the caliper to map the distance of the R-R interval to evaluate evenness and regularity.

In the absence of calipers, the paramedic may use a similar method of evaluating the R-R interval using pen and paper. The paramedic places the straight edge of the paper near the peaks of the R waves and marks off the distance between the two other consecutive R waves. The paramedic then compares this R-R interval with the other R-R intervals in the electrocardiogram tracing (Fig. 29-36).

If the distances between the R waves are equal or vary by less than 0.16 second (four small squares), the rhythm is regular. If the shortest and longest R-R intervals vary by more than 0.16 second, the rhythm is irregular. Irregular rhythms may be classified further. They may be classified as *regularly irregular.* In this case, the irregularity has a pattern; it is also called "group beating." Irregular rhythms also may be *occasionally irregular.* In this case, only one or two R-R intervals are unequal. Finally, irregular rhythms may be *irregularly irregular.* In this case, the rhythm is totally irregular. No relationship is seen between the R-R intervals (Fig. 29-37).

Step 5: Analyze the P-R Interval

The P-R interval indicates the time it takes for an electrical impulse to be conducted through the atria and atrioventricular node. The interval should be constant across the electrocardiogram tracing. A prolonged P-R interval (greater than 0.20 second) indicates a delay in the conduction of the impulse through the atrioventricular node or bundle of His. The delay is called an *atrioventricular block.* A short P-R interval (less than 0.12 second) indicates that the impulse progressed from the atria to the ventricles through pathways other than the atrioventricular node (Fig. 29-38). This is known as an *accessory pathway syndrome,* the most common of which is Wolff-Parkinson-White syndrome (described later in this chapter).

Analyzing a Rhythm Using the Five Steps

To review, the normal sequence of atrial and ventricular activation as it relates to the electrocardiogram tracing is as follows: Each P wave (atrial depolarization) is followed by a normal QRS complex (ventricular depolarization) and T wave (ventricular repolarization). All QRS complexes are preceded by P waves; the P-R interval is within normal limits, and the R-R interval is regular. The five steps in electrocardiogram rhythm interpretation can be applied to the rhythm in Fig. 29-39.

Text continued on p. 713

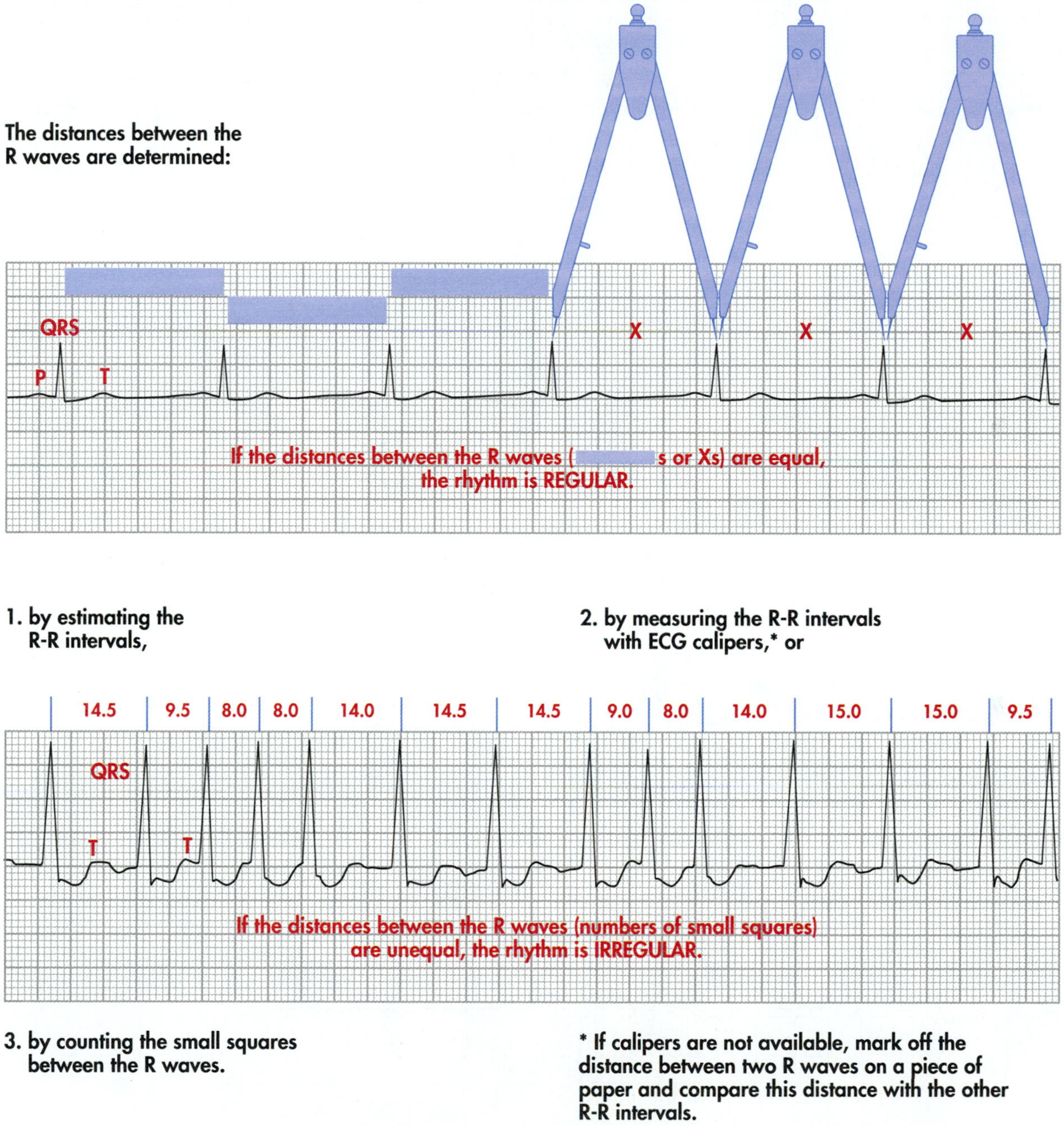
The distances between the R waves are determined:
QRS
P
T
X
X
X
If the distances between the R waves (s or Xs) are equal, the rhythm is REGULAR.
1. by estimating the R-R intervals,
2. by measuring the R-R intervals with ECG calipers,* or
14.5
9.5
8.0
8.0
14.0
14.5
14.5
9.0
8.0
14.0
15.0
15.0
9.5
QRS
T
T
If the distances between the R waves (numbers of small squares) are unequal, the rhythm is IRREGULAR.
3. by counting the small squares between the R waves.
* If calipers are not available, mark off the distance between two R waves on a piece of paper and compare this distance with the other R-R intervals.

FIGURE 29-36 ■ Determining the rhythm.

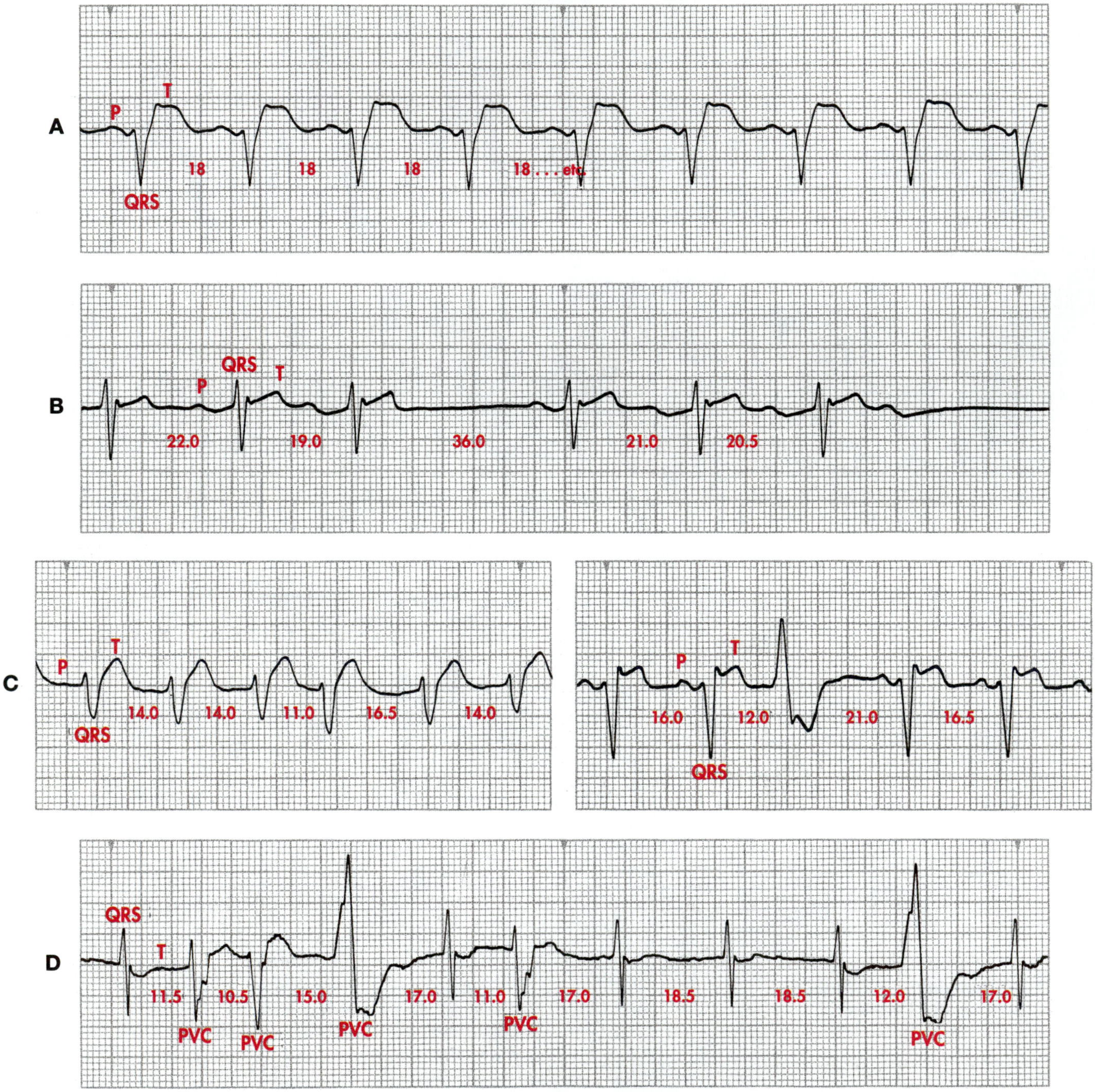

FIGURE 29-37 ■ **A,** Regular rhythm. **B,** Regularly irregular rhythm. **C,** Occasionally irregular rhythm. **D,** Irregularly irregular rhythm.

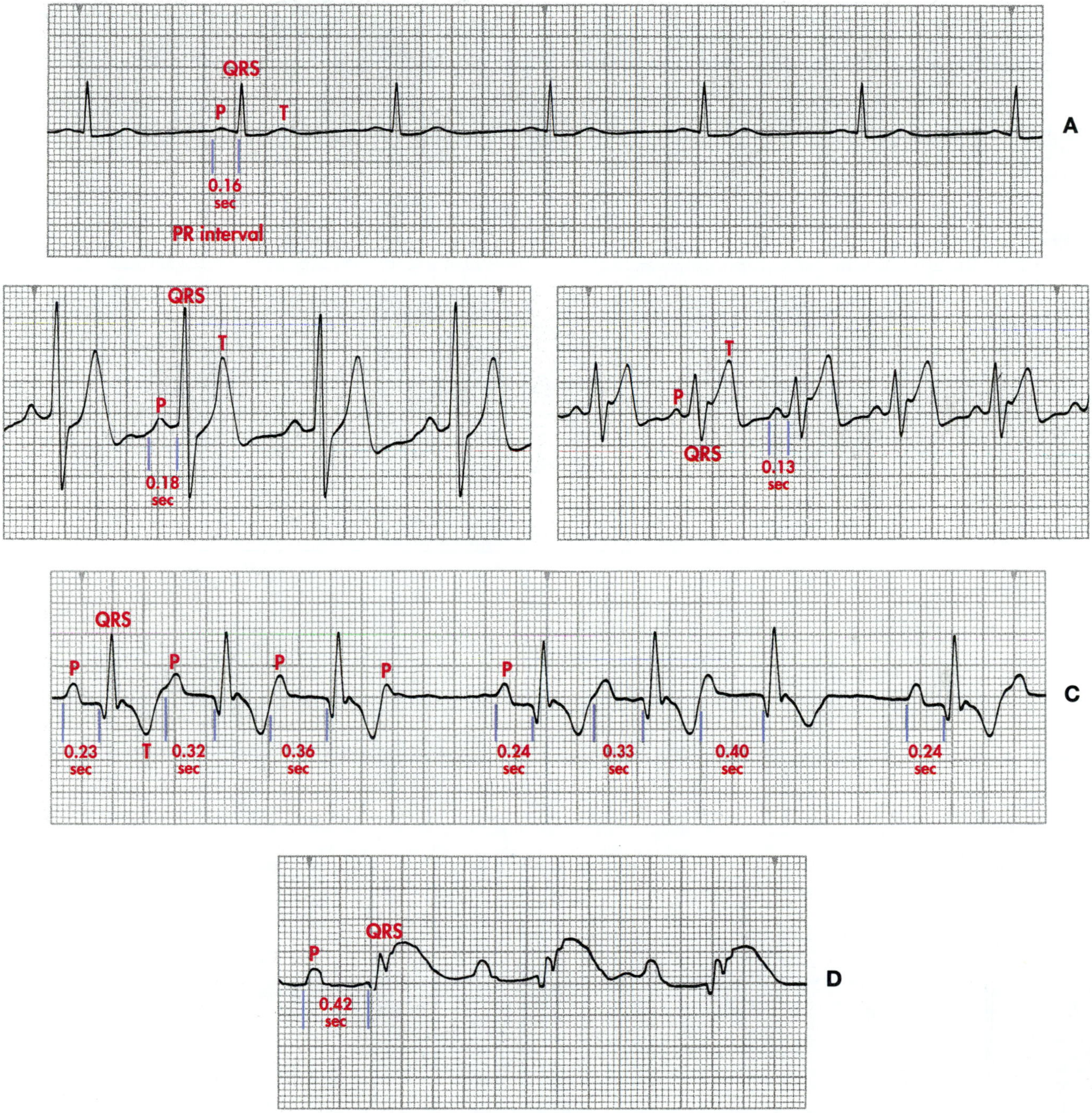

FIGURE 29-38 ■ A and B, Normal P-R intervals. C and D, Abnormal P-R intervals.

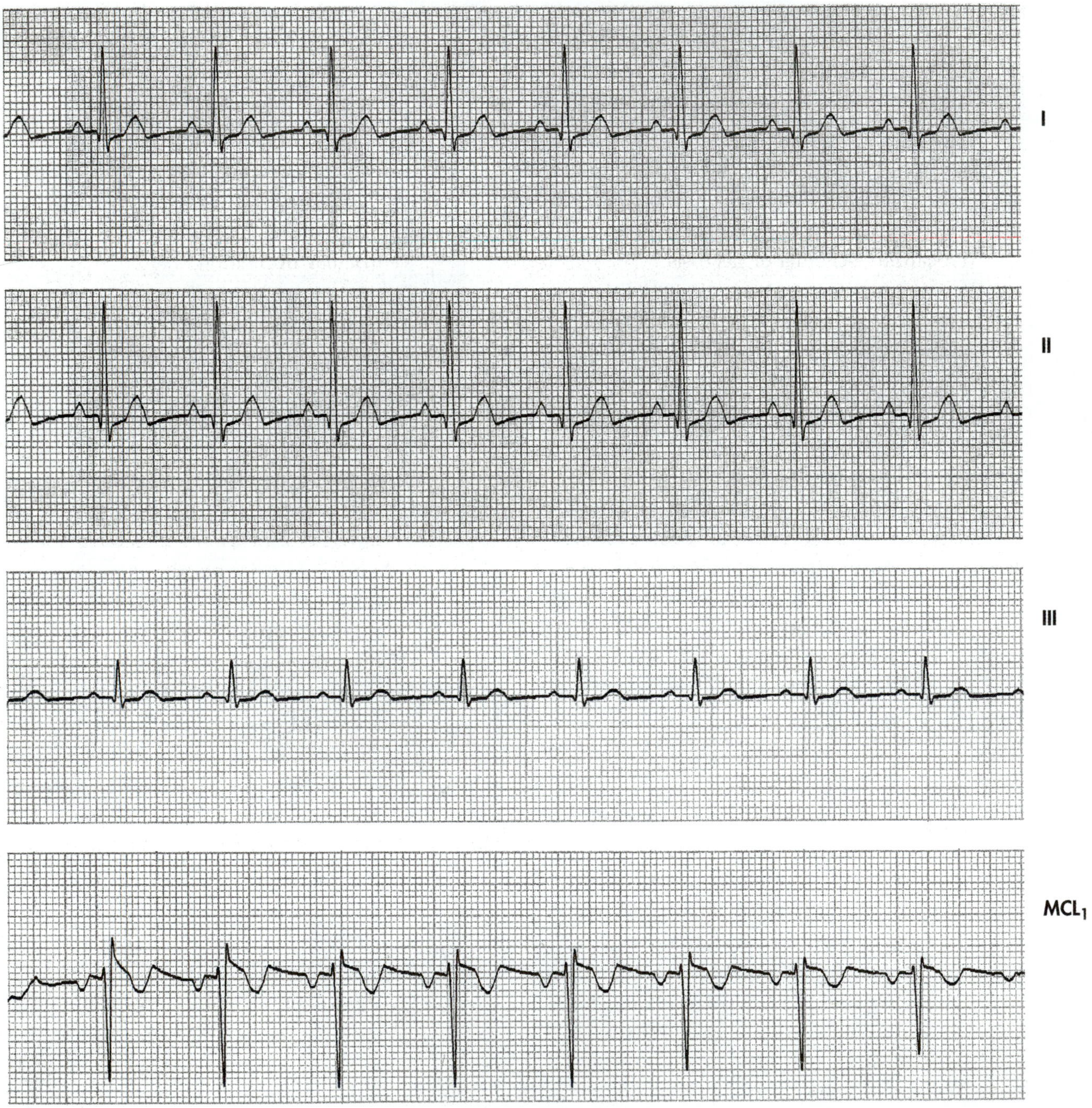

FIGURE 29-39 ■ Normal sinus rhythm.

SECTION SIX
INTRODUCTION TO DYSRHYTHMIAS

Cardiac dysrhythmias can result from a number of physiological, pharmacological, and disease processes, including the following:

- Myocardial ischemia or necrosis
- Autonomic nervous system imbalance
- Distention of heart chambers
- Acid-base abnormalities
- Hypoxemia
- Electrolyte imbalance
- Drug effects or toxicity
- Electrical injury
- Hypothermia
- Central nervous system injury

In addition to these potential causes of dysrhythmias, some cardiac rhythm disturbances are normal. They may be seen even in patients who have healthy hearts. (For example, a patient may have sinus tachycardia from stress or anxiety.) *Regardless of the cause or type of dysrhythmia, management should focus on the patient and the underlying cause. Management should not focus merely on the dysrhythmia.*

> **NOTE** Special considerations regarding cardiac rhythm disturbances and resuscitation for infant and pediatric patients are addressed in Chapters 43 and 44.

CLASSIFICATION OF DYSRHYTHMIAS

Classification by Rate and Pacemaker Site

The classification of dysrhythmias can be based on a number of factors, including changes in automaticity versus disturbances in conduction, cardiac arrest (lethal) rhythms and noncardiac arrest (nonlethal) rhythms, and site of origin. For learning purposes, this text classifies rhythms by rate and pacemaker site (e.g., ventricular tachycardia and sinus bradycardia) and includes the following five groups:

1. Dysrhythmias originating in the sinoatrial node
   a. Sinus bradycardia
   b. Sinus tachycardia
   c. Sinus dysrhythmia
   d. Sinus arrest
2. Dysrhythmias originating in the atria
   a. Wandering pacemaker
   b. Premature atrial complex
   c. Paroxysmal supraventricular tachycardia
   d. Atrial flutter
   e. Atrial fibrillation
3. Dysrhythmias originating in the atrioventricular node and surrounding tissues
   a. Premature junctional contraction
   b. Junctional escape complexes or rhythms
   c. Accelerated junctional rhythm
4. Dysrhythmias originating in the ventricles
   a. Ventricular escape complexes or rhythms
   b. Premature ventricular complex
   c. Ventricular tachycardia
   d. Ventricular fibrillation
   e. Asystole
   f. Artificial pacemaker rhythms
5. Dysrhythmias that are disorders of conduction
   a. Atrioventricular blocks
      (1) First-degree atrioventricular block
      (2) Second-degree atrioventricular block type I (or Wenckebach)
      (3) Second-degree atrioventricular block type II
      (4) Third-degree atrioventricular block
   b. Disturbances of ventricular conduction
   c. Pulseless electrical activity
   d. Preexcitation syndrome: Wolff-Parkinson-White syndrome

> **NOTE** Broadly speaking, there are only four cardiac arrest rhythms. These are ventricular fibrillation, pulseless ventricular tachycardia, asystole, and assorted pulseless electrical activity rhythms. The two noncardiac arrest rhythms (precollapse or precardiac arrest rhythms) that are important to consider in prehospital care are those that are too slow (fewer than 60 beats per minute) and those that are too fast (more than 120 beats per minute).[1]

The text presents each dysrhythmia in lead II. For comparison, the same dysrhythmia also is shown as it would appear in leads I, III, and MCL_1. The text discusses how to recognize the dysrhythmia and the emergency treatment for patients with each dysrhythmia. All treatments in this chapter follow the recommendations of the American Heart Association. All treatments are referenced to the American Heart Association algorithms.

Use of Algorithms for Classification

Algorithms are lists used to summarize information. Some algorithms contain prehospital and in-hospital management recommendations. The following nine guidelines apply to the use of all algorithms[1]:

BOX 29-4 Classes of Recommendations 2000

Class I
Definitely recommended
Interventions always acceptable, safe, and effective
Considered standard of care
Interventions supported by excellent research-based evidence

Class IIa
Acceptable and useful
Interventions acceptable, safe, and useful
Considered intervention of choice
Interventions supported by good research-based evidence

Class IIb
Acceptable and useful
Interventions acceptable, safe, and useful
Considered as an optional or alternative intervention
Interventions supported by fair research-based evidence
Indeterminate
Interventions in early stages of research and documentation or lack sufficient quantity or quality of research
No recommendation until further research is available

Class III
Unacceptable, not useful; may be harmful
Intervention with no evidence of benefit; may be harmful to patient
Evidence of benefit is completely lacking, or research suggests or confirms harm

From American Heart Association: *Guidelines 2000 for cardiopulmonary and emergency cardiovascular care,* International Consensus on Science, Dallas, 2000, The Association.

1. First, manage the patient, not the monitor.
2. Algorithms for cardiac arrest presume that the condition under discussion continually persists, that the patient remains in cardiac arrest, and that cardiopulmonary resuscitation is always performed.
3. Apply different interventions when appropriate indications exist.
4. The algorithms are designed to outline the most common assessments and actions performed for the majority of patients, but they are not designed to be all-inclusive or restrictive.[4] The flow diagrams present treatments mostly in sequential order of priority. Next to a treatment or pharmacological agent may be a class recommendation (Box 29-4). The footnotes to the algorithm contain additional important information related to assessment, treatment, and evaluation.
5. Adequate airway, ventilation, oxygenation, chest compression, and defibrillation are more important than administration of medications. These measures take precedence over initiating an intravenous line or injecting pharmacological agents.
6. Several medications (***epinephrine, lidocaine,*** and ***atropine***) can be administered via an endotracheal tube. The endotracheal dose is 2 to 2½ times the intravenous dose for adults.
7. With a few exceptions, intravenous medications should always be administered rapidly in bolus method.
8. After each intravenous medication, give a 20- to 30-mL bolus of intravenous fluid. Also, immediately elevate the extremity. This enhances delivery of drugs to the central circulation. This delivery may take 1 to 2 minutes.
9. Last, manage the patient, not the monitor.

DYSRHYTHMIAS ORIGINATING IN THE SINOATRIAL NODE

Most sinus dysrhythmias result from increases or decreases in vagal tone (parasympathetic nervous system). The sinoatrial node generally receives sufficient inhibitory parasympathetic impulses from the vagus nerve to keep the sinoatrial node within the normal rate of 60 to 100. However, if vagal nerve activity increases, the heart rate becomes bradycardic. If the vagus nerve is slowed or blocked, the heart rate increases and results in sinus tachycardia. Dysrhythmias that originate in the sinoatrial node include sinus bradycardia, sinus tachycardia, sinus dysrhythmia, and sinus arrest. Electrocardiogram features common to all sinoatrial node dysrhythmias include the following:

- Normal duration of QRS complex (in the absence of bundle branch block)
- Upright P waves in lead II
- Similar appearance of all P waves
- Normal duration of P-R interval (in the absence of atrioventricular block)

Sinus Bradycardia

DESCRIPTION

Sinus bradycardia results from slowing of the pacemaker rate of the sinoatrial node (Fig. 29-40).

ETIOLOGY

The following are possible causes of sinus bradycardia:

- Intrinsic sinus node disease
- Increased parasympathetic vagal tone
- Hypothermia
- Hypoxia
- Drug effects (e.g., digitalis, beta-blockers, and calcium channel blockers)
- Myocardial infarction

RULES FOR INTERPRETATION (LEAD II MONITORING)

Sinus bradycardia has the following characteristics on the electrocardiogram:

QRS complex: Less than 0.12 second, provided there is no ventricular conduction disturbance
P waves: Normal and upright; one P wave before each QRS complex
Rate: Less than 60 beats per minute

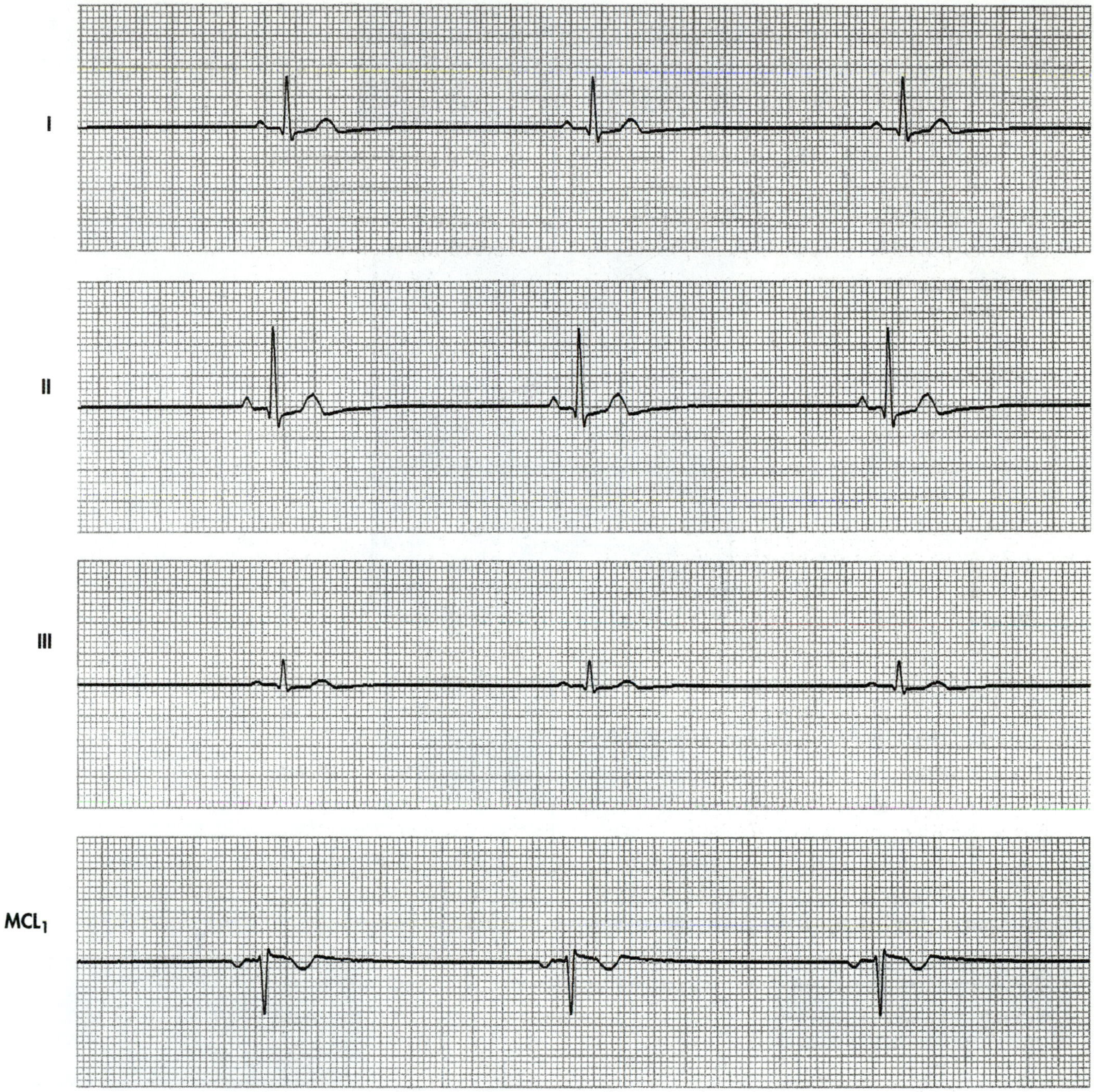

FIGURE 29-40 ■ Sinus bradycardia.

Rhythm: Regular

P-R interval: 0.12 to 0.20 second and constant (normal), provided no atrioventricular block is present

CLINICAL SIGNIFICANCE

Decreased rate may compromise cardiac output. It may result in hypotension, angina pectoris, or central nervous system symptoms (e.g., light-headedness, vertigo, and syncope). Sinus bradycardia can result from nausea and vomiting. Sinus bradycardia is associated with overstimulation of the vagus nerve that can result in fainting (vasovagal syncope). However, sinus bradycardia may be beneficial. It may reduce myocardial oxygen consumption when the patient is having a heart attack. Sinus bradycardia also may follow the use of carotid sinus pressure (carotid sinus massage). This dysrhythmia is common during sleep and in well-conditioned athletes.

CRITICAL THINKING

Take a poll of your classmates. How many have a resting heart rate 60 beats per minute?

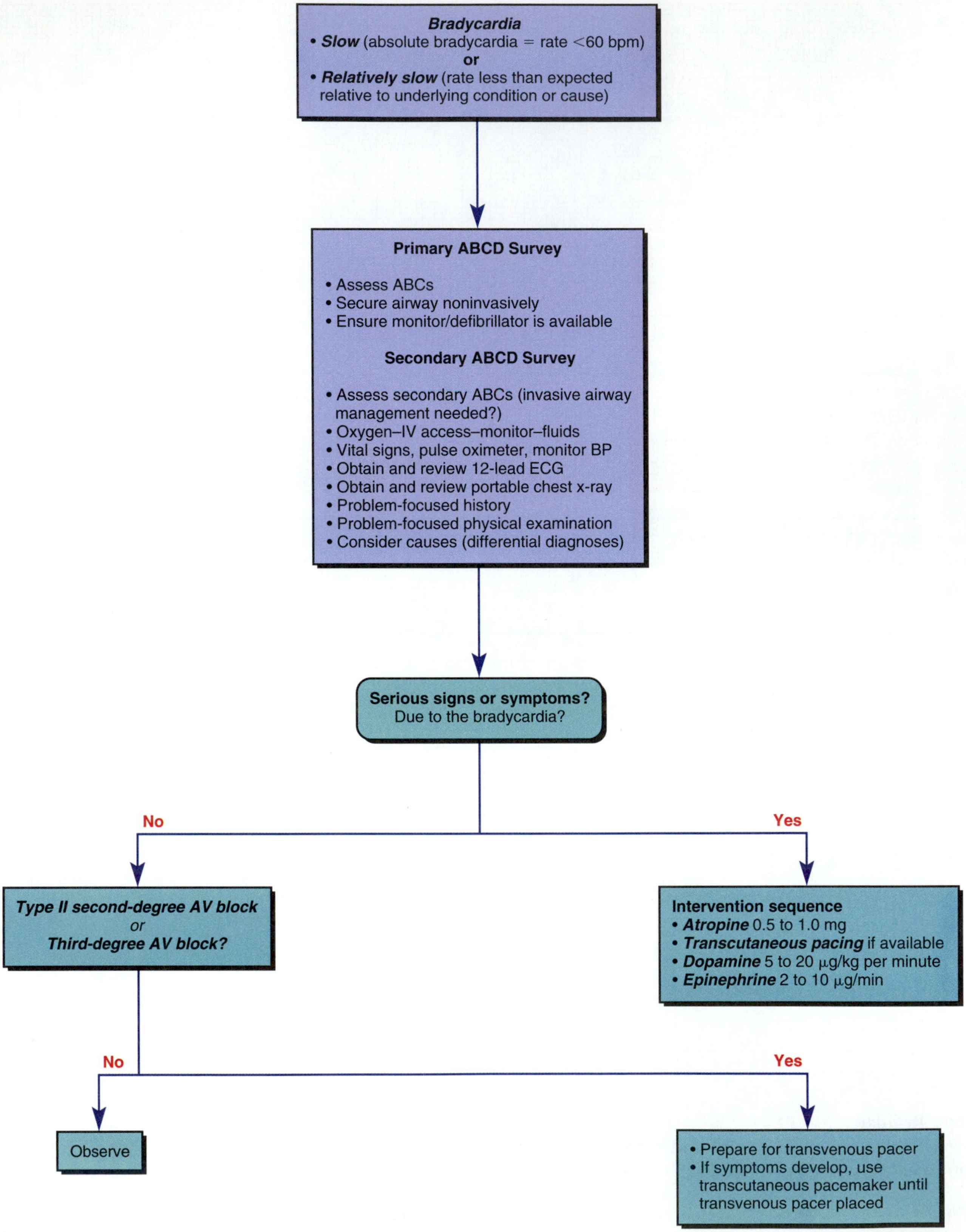

FIGURE 29-41 ■ Bradycardia algorithm.

MANAGEMENT

Prehospital intervention usually is unnecessary unless hypotension, altered mental status caused by inadequate perfusion, or ventricular irritability is present. (These are more common with rates of less than 50 beats per minute.) Management for symptomatic bradycardia is aimed at increasing the heart rate to improve cardiac output. Inotropic support also may be required (Fig. 28-41). Treatment options for symptomatic bradycardia include oxygen, transcutaneous pacing (described later in this chapter), ***atropine,*** a ***dopamine*** infusion, an ***epinephrine*** infusion, and an ***isoproterenol*** infusion. Transcutaneous pacing is considered a Class I intervention for all symptomatic bradycardias. If the patient fails to respond to ***atropine*** or is critically unstable, the paramedic should begin pacing immediately. Pacing is indicated for symptomatic bradycardias that are related to a conduction delay or block at or below the His-Purkinje level (infranodal). The paramedic should consider sedation for the patient to decrease discomfort caused by the electrical pacer stimuli.

For mild symptoms related to the bradycardia, ***atropine*** may be administered intravenously. Administration may be repeated every 3 to 5 minutes as needed. The frequency of ***atropine*** administration is based on the patient's condition. ***Atropine*** should be administered at shorter intervals, every 3 minutes, for severely unstable patients.

Atropine should be used with caution in the patient with an acute myocardial infarction. ***Atropine*** can increase the heart rate, increasing myocardial oxygen demand. This in turn can worsen ischemia or increase the size of the infarction. ***Atropine*** may be beneficial for the treatment of nodal blocks and asystole. However, ***atropine*** is contraindicated for infranodal blocks such as second-degree type II and complete heart block with a wide QRS complex. ***Atropine*** rarely increases the heart rate in infranodal atrioventricular blocks. In fact, it may actually worsen the rhythm. (***Atropine*** can increase the sinus rate and speed conduction through the atrioventricular node. This increase in impulses gives the diseased His-Purkinje system less time to recover. This can cause a second-degree block to progress to a third-degree or complete block.)

If hypotension persists after ***atropine*** administration, the paramedic should add a ***dopamine*** infusion (Box 29-5). Also, if the patient remains hypotensive and severely distressed with adequate transcutaneous pacing, the paramedic may start a ***dopamine*** infusion.

An ***epinephrine*** infusion can be used for symptomatic bradycardia (Box 29-6). Generally, this occurs after ***atropine*** administration and transcutaneous pacing fail to improve the patient's condition. However, an ***epinephrine*** infusion may be administered earlier if the patient displays severe symptoms and is deteriorating quickly.

In the treatment of symptomatic bradycardia, ***isoproterenol*** should be used only as an immediate and temporary measure to improve the unstable patient (Box 29-7). ***Isoproterenol*** is a pure beta-agonist producing an increase in rate and force of contractions (positive chronotropic and inotropic properties). The potent effects of ***isoproterenol*** may increase myocardial oxygen consumption, exacerbate ischemia, and induce dysrhythmias. ***Isoproterenol*** is not the treatment of choice for symptomatic bradycardia (Box 29-8). If ***isoproterenol*** is used, it should be administered only in low doses.

BOX 29-5 Dopamine Infusion

- Low-dose dopamine: 1 to 5 μg/kg per minute. A low dose of dopamine produces a dopaminergic effect that increases renal, mesenteric, and cerebrovascular vessel dilation.
- Moderate-dose dopamine: 5 to 10 μg/kg per minute. At moderate doses, dopamine improves contractility, cardiac output, and blood pressure through $alpha_1$- and $beta_1$-receptor stimulation.
- High-dose dopamine: 10 to 20 μg/kg per minute. Higher doses of dopamine have an alpha-adrenergic effect producing peripheral arterial and venous vasoconstriction. See Chapter 17 for calculating dopamine infusions.

BOX 29-6 Epinephrine Infusion

Epinephrine infusions generally are used for critically unstable patients with bradycardia close to a pulseless state or asystole. An epinephrine infusion may be prepared by mixing 1 mg of epinephrine 1:1000 into 500 mL of 5% dextrose in water or 0.9% normal saline. The concentration is 2 μg/mL. The recommended rate of infusion is 2 to 10 μg/min.

BOX 29-7 Isoproterenol Infusion

Mix 1 mg of isoproterenol in 250 mL of normal saline, lactated Ringer's solution, or 5% dextrose in water. Infuse at 2 to 10 μg/min, titrated to adequate heart rate.

BOX 29-8 Sequence of Care for Symptomatic Bradycardia

Atropine
Transcutaneous cardiac pacing (if available)
Dopamine
Epinephrine infusion
Isoproterenol infusion

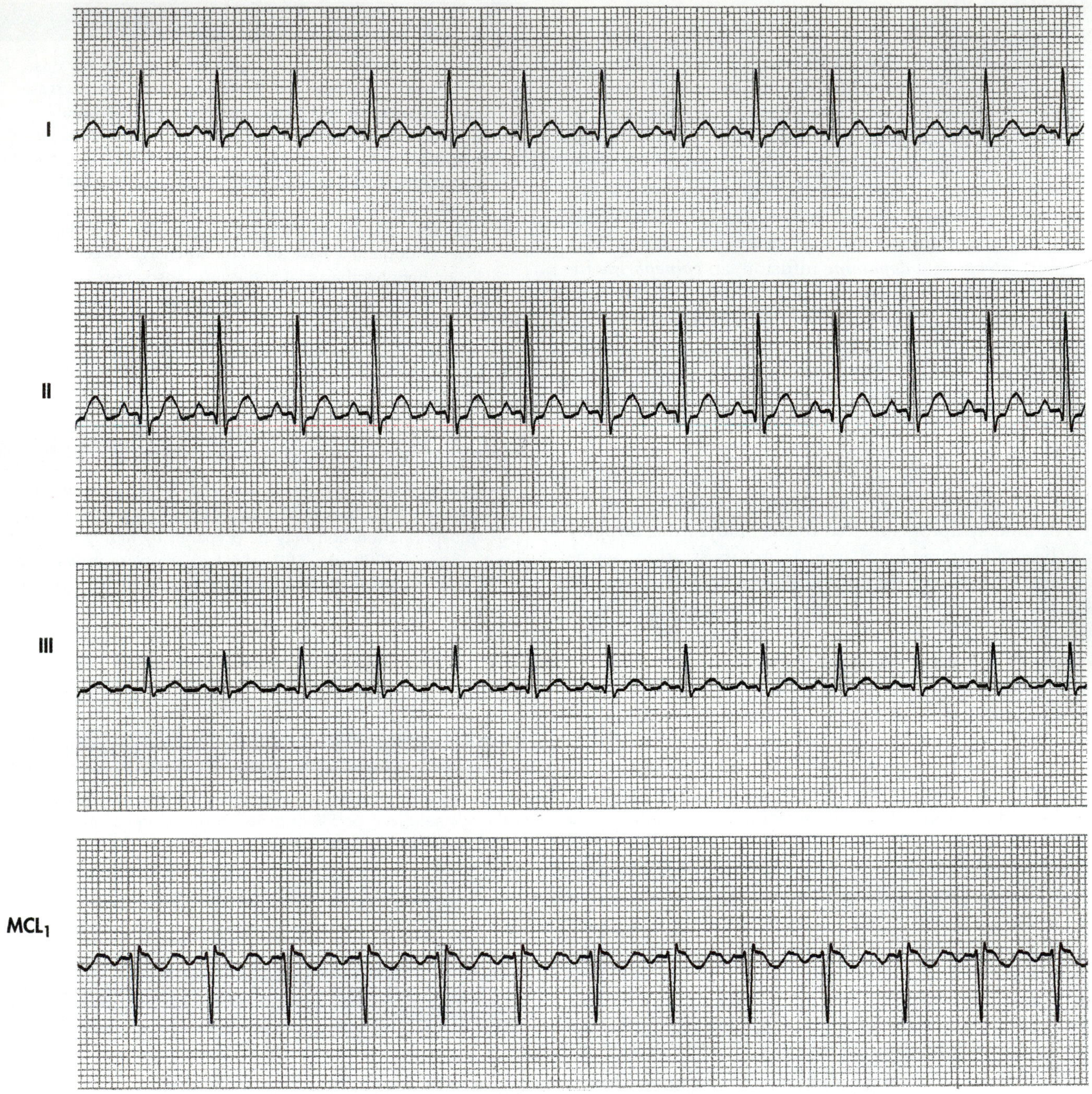

FIGURE 29-42 ■ Sinus tachycardia.

Sinus Tachycardia

DESCRIPTION

Sinus tachycardia results from an increase in the rate of sinus node discharge (Fig. 29-42).

> **CRITICAL THINKING**
> What effect will the excitement and commotion of the arrival of your ambulance likely have on the heart rate and blood pressure of a conscious, alert patient?

ETIOLOGY

Sinus tachycardia is common and may result from multiple factors, including the following:

- Exercise
- Fever
- Anxiety
- Ingestion of caffeine or alcohol
- Smoking
- Hypovolemia
- Hyperthyroidism

- Anemia
- Congestive heart failure
- Administration of ***atropine*** or any vagolytic or sympathomimetic drug (e.g., cocaine, phencyclidine, ***epinephrine,*** and ***isoproterenol***)

RULES FOR INTERPRETATION (LEAD II MONITORING)

Sinus tachycardia has the following characteristics on the electrocardiogram:

QRS complex: Less than 0.12 second, provided there is no ventricular conduction disturbance
P waves: Normal and upright; one before each QRS complex
Rate: Equal to or greater than 100 beats per minute
Rhythm: Regular
P-R interval: 0.12 to 0.20 second (normal), provided no atrioventricular conduction block is present

CLINICAL SIGNIFICANCE

Sinus tachycardia in healthy individuals generally is not significant. If tachycardia is associated with myocardial infarction, however, it may increase the oxygen requirements of the heart, increase myocardial ischemia, and predispose the patient to more serious rhythm disturbances.

MANAGEMENT

Sinus tachycardia usually does not require treatment. When the underlying cause is removed, the tachycardia usually resolves gradually and spontaneously.

Sinus Dysrhythmia

DESCRIPTION

Sinus dysrhythmia is present when the difference between the longest and shortest R-R intervals is greater than 0.16 second (Fig. 29-43).

ETIOLOGY

Sinus dysrhythmia usually is normal. It often is related to the respiratory cycle and to changes in intrathoracic pressure. These changes cause the heart rate to increase during inspiration and to decrease during expiration. Although sinus dysrhythmia sometimes occurs normally in healthy persons, it is more common in patients with heart disease or myocardial infarction. It also is more common in patients receiving certain drugs such as ***digoxin*** and ***morphine***.

RULES FOR INTERPRETATION (LEAD II MONITORING)

Sinus dysrhythmia has the following characteristics on the electrocardiogram:

QRS complex: Less than 0.12 second, provided no ventricular conduction disturbance is present
P waves: Normal and upright; one P wave before each QRS complex
Rate: Usually 60 to 99 beats per minute (varies with respiration)
Rhythm: Irregular (changes occur in cycles and usually follow the patient's respiratory pattern)
P-R interval: 0.12 to 0.20 second and constant (normal)

CLINICAL SIGNIFICANCE

Sinus dysrhythmia is common in children, young adults, and older adults. It may be associated with palpitations, dizziness, and syncope (rare).

MANAGEMENT

Sinus dysrhythmia usually is not significant. It seldom requires treatment.

Sinus Arrest

DESCRIPTION

Sinus arrest results from a problem with the ability of the sinoatrial node to fire automatically (Fig. 29-44). The failure of the sinus node causes short periods of cardiac standstill. This occurs until lower-level pacemakers discharge (escape beats) or the sinus node resumes its normal function.

ETIOLOGY

Sinus arrest may be precipitated by an increase in parasympathetic tone on the sinoatrial node, hypoxia or ischemia, excessive administration of digitalis or ***propranolol,*** hyperkalemia, or damage to the sinoatrial node (acute myocardial infarction, degenerative fibrotic disease).

RULES FOR INTERPRETATION (LEAD II MONITORING)

Sinus arrest has the following characteristics on the electrocardiogram:

QRS complex: Less than 0.12 second, provided there is no bundle branch conduction disturbance
P waves: Normal and upright. If the electrical impulse is not generated by the sinoatrial node or blocked from entering the atria, atrial depolarization does not occur and the P wave is dropped.
Rate: Normal to slow, depending on the frequency and duration of sinus arrest
Rhythm: Irregular when sinus arrest is present
P-R interval: P-R intervals (when the P wave is present) of the underlying rhythm are normal (0.12 to 0.20 second) in the absence of atrioventricular block. Junctional escape beats may occur with no P waves.

CLINICAL SIGNIFICANCE

Frequent or prolonged episodes of sinus arrest may decrease cardiac output. The overall heart rate slows and the atria do not contract, so ventricular filling is reduced. If an escape pacemaker does not take over, ventricular asystole may result. This would cause light-headedness followed by syncope. With this dysrhythmia, there is danger that sinus node activity will cease completely. Also, there is danger that an escape pacemaker may not take over pacing. (This would result in asystole.)

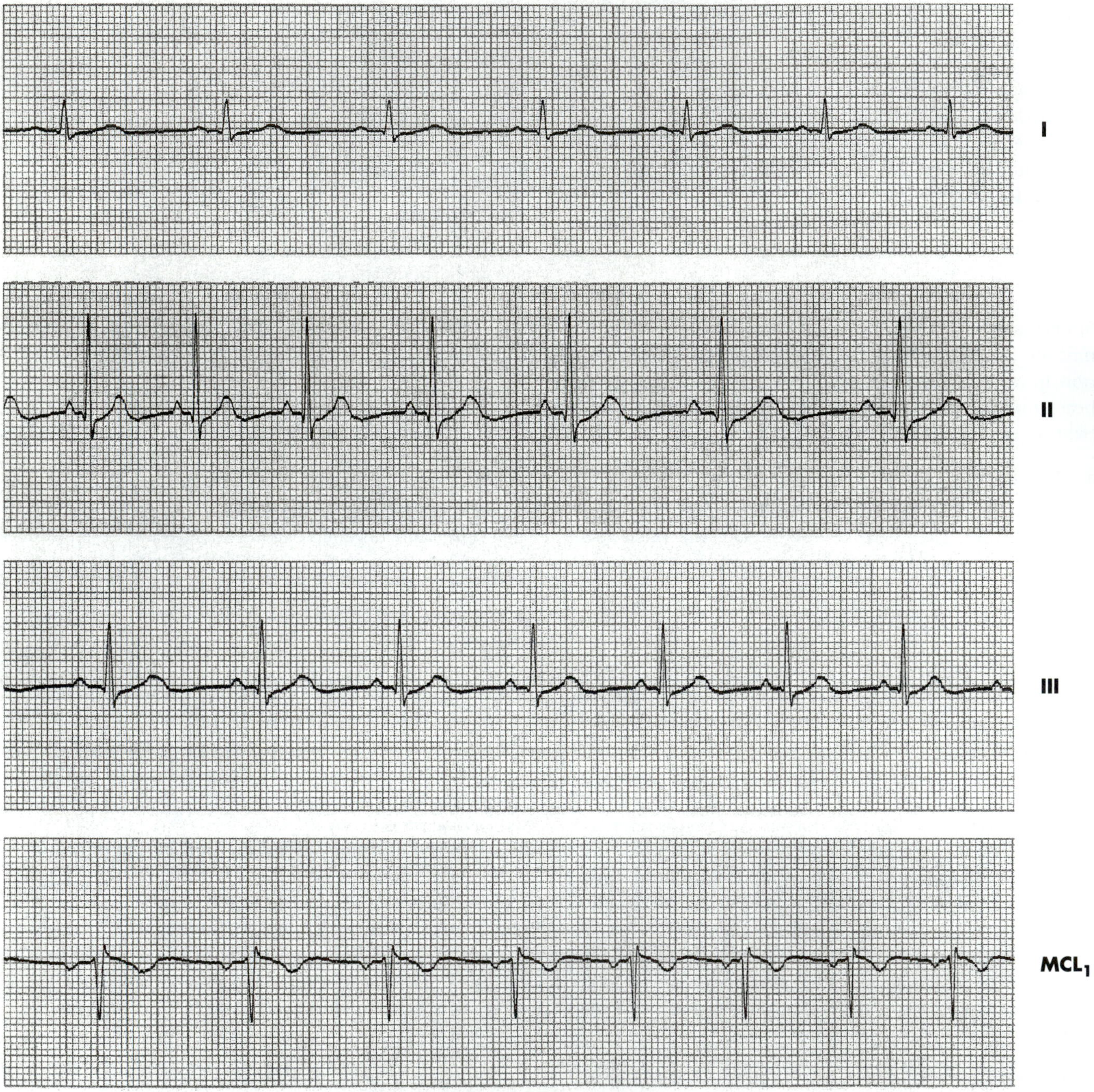

FIGURE 29-43 ■ Sinus dysrhythmia.

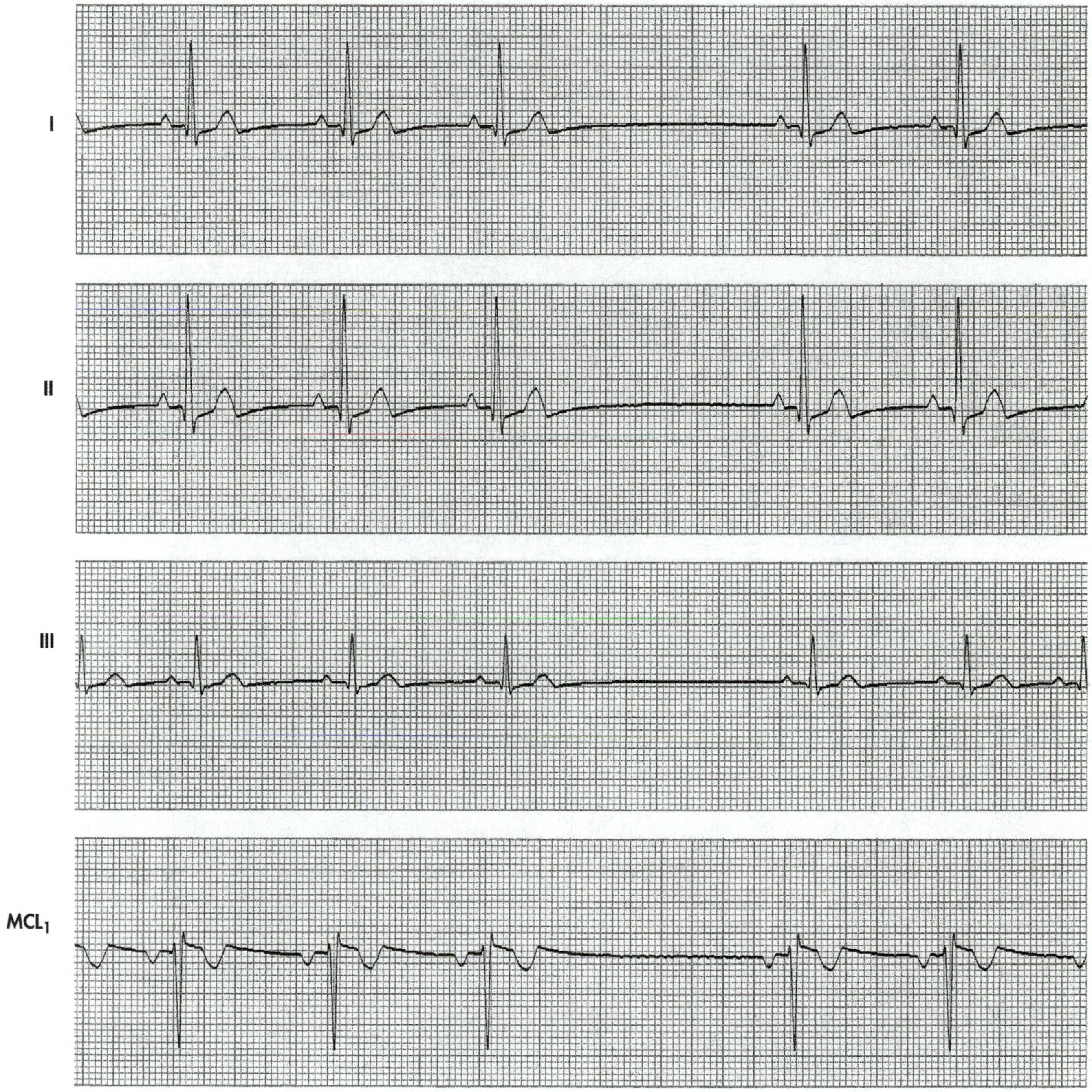

FIGURE 29-44 ■ Sinus arrest.

MANAGEMENT

If the patient is asymptomatic, close observation is all that is required. In patients with bradycardia that produces symptoms, management may include the administration of ***atropine*** or transcutaneous cardiac pacing (Fig. 29-40).

DYSRHYTHMIAS ORIGINATING IN THE ATRIA

Atrial dysrhythmias may begin in the tissues of the atria or in the atrioventricular junction. Common causes of atrial dysrhythmias are ischemia, hypoxia, and atrial dilation caused by congestive heart failure, mitral valve abnormalities, or increased pulmonary artery pressures. Atrial dysrhythmias include wandering pacemaker, premature atrial complexes, paroxysmal supraventricular tachycardia, atrial flutter, and atrial fibrillation. Electrocardiogram features common to all atrial dysrhythmias (provided there is no ventricular conduction disturbance) include the following:

- Normal QRS complexes
- P waves (if present) that differ in appearance from sinus P waves
- Abnormal, shortened, or prolonged P-R intervals

Wandering Pacemaker

DESCRIPTION

Wandering pacemaker (or wandering atrial pacemaker) occurs when the pacemaker shifts from the sinus node to another pacemaker site in the atria or the atrioventricular junction (Fig. 29-45). The shift in the site usually is transient, back and forth along the sinoatrial node, atria, and atrioventricular junction.

ETIOLOGY

Wandering pacemaker is a type of sinus dysrhythmia. It may be normal in the very young, older adults, and well-conditioned athletes. The dysrhythmia generally is caused by pressure on the vagus nerve related to respiration. This stimulation or pressure on the vagus nerve causes the sinoatrial node and atrioventricular junction pacemaker rates to slow. Other causes include associated underlying heart disease and the administration of digitalis. Another type of wandering atrial pacemaker is multifocal atrial tachycardia. This rhythm disturbance looks like a wandering pacemaker. However, multifocal atrial tachycardia is associated with rates often in the 120- to 150-per-minute range. Moreover, it is always considered pathological. Multifocal atrial tachycardia most often is found in patients with severe chronic obstructive pulmonary disease. Treatment of the lung disease may help to stop this rhythm. Multifocal atrial tachycardia often is mistaken for atrial fibrillation with rapid ventricular response.

RULES FOR INTERPRETATION (LEAD II MONITORING)

Wandering pacemaker has the following characteristics on the electrocardiogram:

QRS complex: Usually less than 0.12 second, provided no conduction block occurs in the bundle branches

P waves: Change in P wave morphology from beat to beat. In lead II the P waves may be upright, rounded, notched, inverted, biphasic, or buried in the QRS complex.

Rate: Usually 60 to 99 beats per minute. The rate may slow gradually when the pacemaker site shifts from the sinoatrial node to the atria or atrioventricular junction and may increase when the pacemaker site shifts back to the sinoatrial node.

Rhythm: Irregular

P-R interval: Varies

CLINICAL SIGNIFICANCE

A wandering pacemaker usually does not produce serious signs and symptoms. Other atrial dysrhythmias (such as atrial fibrillation) sometimes result from this dysrhythmia.

MANAGEMENT

Sometimes a wandering pacemaker is a benign rhythm. In those instances, no management is required. Multifocal atrial tachycardia, however, may be precipitated by acute exacerbation of emphysema, congestive heart failure, or acute mitral valve regurgitation. Management is aimed at the underlying cause. Oxygen administration is usually the initial treatment of choice for multifocal atrial tachycardia.

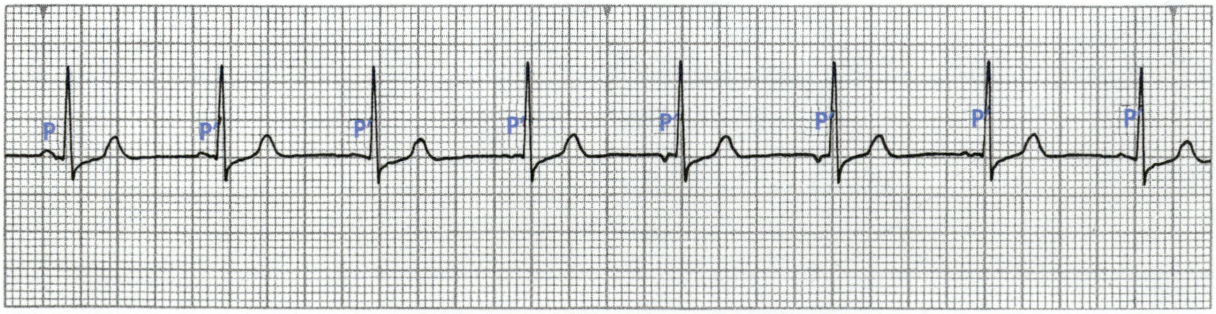

FIGURE 29-45 ■ Wandering atrial pacemaker.

Premature Atrial Complex

DESCRIPTION

A premature atrial complex is a single electrical impulse originating in the atria, outside the sinus node (Fig. 29-46). The impulse creates a premature atrial complex (P wave). If conducted through the atrioventricular node, the impulse also causes a QRS complex before the next expected sinus beat. Because the premature atrial complex usually depolarizes the sinoatrial node prematurely, the timing of the sinoatrial node is reset. The next expected P wave of the underlying rhythm appears earlier than it would have if the sinoatrial node had not been disturbed (noncompensatory pause). Premature atrial complexes may originate from a single ectopic pacemaker site. Or they may originate from multiple sites in the atria. Premature atrial complexes probably result from enhanced automaticity or a reentry mechanism.

CRITICAL THINKING

What will you feel when you palpate the pulse of a patient with premature atrial complexes?

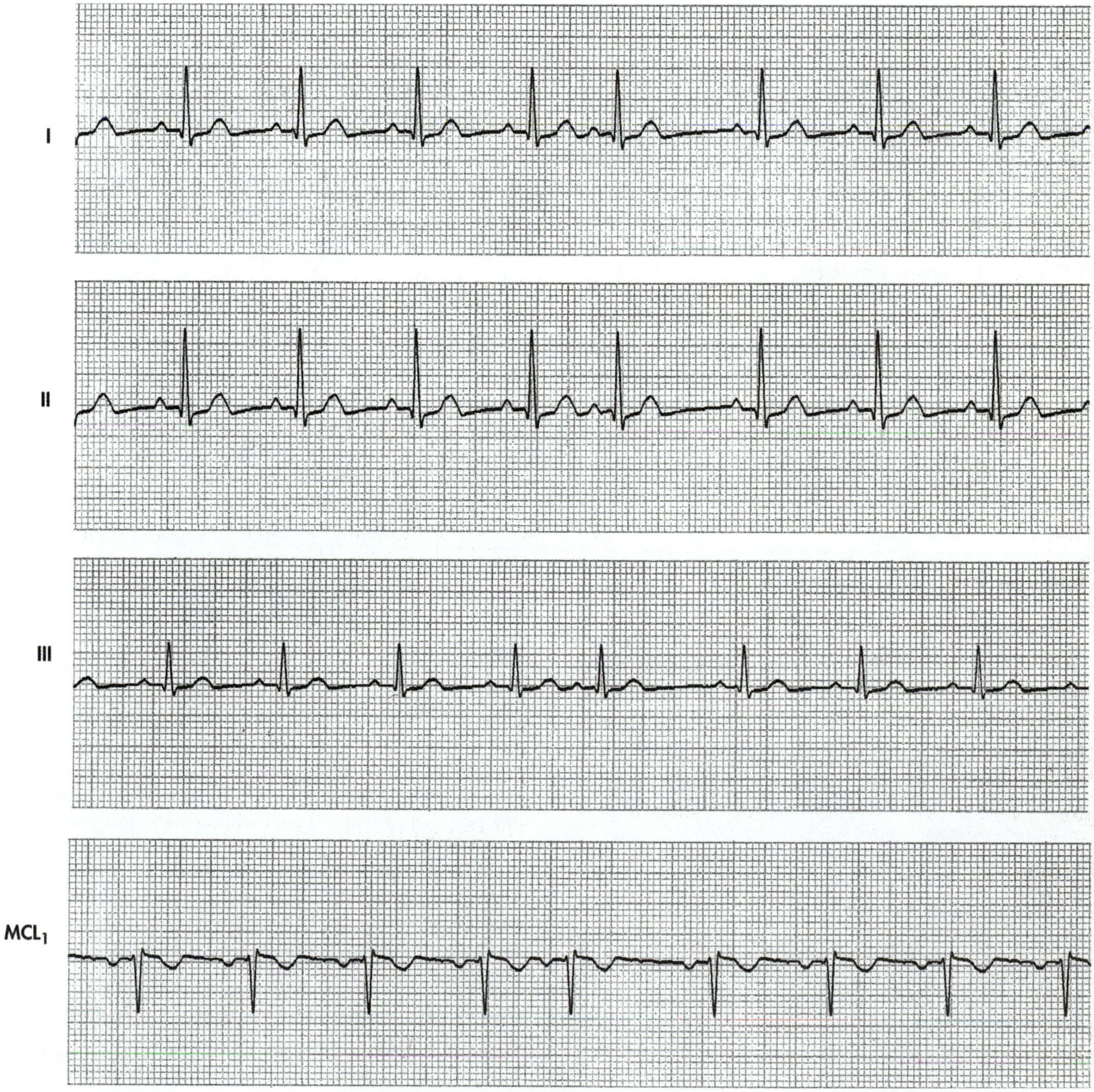

FIGURE 29-46 ■ Premature atrial complex.

ETIOLOGY

Premature atrial complexes may result from the following:

- Increase in catecholamines and sympathetic tone
- Use of caffeine, tobacco, or alcohol
- Use of sympathomimetic drugs ***(epinephrine, isoproterenol, norepinephrine)***
- Electrolyte imbalance
- Hypoxia
- Digitalis toxicity
- Cardiovascular disease
- In some cases, no apparent cause

RULES FOR INTERPRETATION (LEAD II MONITORING)

Premature atrial complexes have the following characteristics on the electrocardiogram:

QRS complex: Usually less than 0.12 second. The QRS complex may be greater than 0.12 second and appear bizarre if the premature atrial complex is conducted abnormally. The QRS complex may be absent as a result of a temporary complete atrioventricular block (nonconducted premature atrial complex) that occurs during the refractory period of the atrioventricular node or ventricles.

P waves: The P wave of a premature atrial complex differs in shape from a sinus P wave. It occurs earlier than the next expected sinus P wave and may be so early that it is superimposed or hidden in the preceding T wave. The paramedic should evaluate the preceding T wave to see whether its morphology is altered by the presence of a P wave.

Rate: Depends on the underlying rhythm

Rhythm: Usually the underlying rhythm is sinus and regular with irregular premature beats when the premature atrial complexes occur.

P-R interval: Usually in the normal range but differs from those of the underlying rhythm. The P-R interval of a premature atrial complex varies from 0.20 second when the pacemaker site is near the sinoatrial node to 0.12 second when the pacemaker site is near the atrioventricular junction.

> **NOTE** Premature atrial complexes with aberrancy may resemble premature ventricular complexes. Distinguishing between these two types of dysrhythmias is important so as to manage the patient properly.

CLINICAL SIGNIFICANCE

Isolated premature atrial complexes in healthy patients are not significant. Frequent premature atrial complexes that occur in patients with heart disease may lead to serious supraventricular dysrhythmias such as multifocal atrial tachycardia, atrial tachycardia, atrial flutter, atrial fibrillation, or paroxysmal supraventricular tachycardia.

MANAGEMENT

Prehospital care usually only requires observation. If nonconducted premature atrial complexes are frequent and the patient becomes symptomatic from bradycardia, transcutaneous cardiac pacing or ***atropine*** may be indicated (Fig. 29-40).

Supraventricular Tachycardia and Paroxysmal Supraventricular Tachycardia

DESCRIPTION

Supraventricular tachycardias include paroxysmal reentrant supraventricular tachycardia, nonparoxysmal atrial tachycardia, multifocal atrial tachycardia, junctional tachycardia, atrial flutter, and atrial fibrillation (Fig. 29-47). This section presents paroxysmal supraventricular tachycardia, a supraventricular tachycardia that begins abruptly.

> **NOTE** Junctional tachycardia, ectopic atrial tachycardia, and multifocal atrial tachycardia are known as *automatic supraventricular tachycardia*.

Paroxysmal supraventricular tachycardia can originate in the atria or atrioventricular junction (Fig. 29-48). Paroxysmal atrial tachycardia starts in the atria, whereas paroxysmal junctional tachycardia starts in the junction. The dysrhythmia results from rapid atrial or junctional impulse firing that overrides the rate of the sinoatrial node. The impulse reenters the atrioventricular node at the same time that it is conducted to the ventricles (to produce the QRS complex). The cycle and the tachycardia continue until the reentry pathway is interrupted. Paroxysmal supraventricular tachycardia is characterized by repeated episodes (paroxysms) of atrial tachycardia. These episodes often have a sudden onset (lasting minutes to hours). They often have an abrupt termination as well.

ETIOLOGY

In most cases, paroxysmal supraventricular tachycardia is a reentry tachycardia. The electrical impulses are caught in a cycle that continuously circulates around the atrioventricular node. Paroxysmal supraventricular tachycardia may occur at any age. This tachycardia is not commonly associated with underlying heart disease. This tachycardia is rare in patients with myocardial infarction. Precipitating factors include stress, overexertion, tobacco use, and caffeine consumption. Paroxysmal supraventricular tachycardia also is common in patients who have Wolff-Parkinson-White syndrome.

RULES FOR INTERPRETATION (LEAD II MONITORING)

Paroxysmal supraventricular tachycardia has the following characteristics on the electrocardiogram:

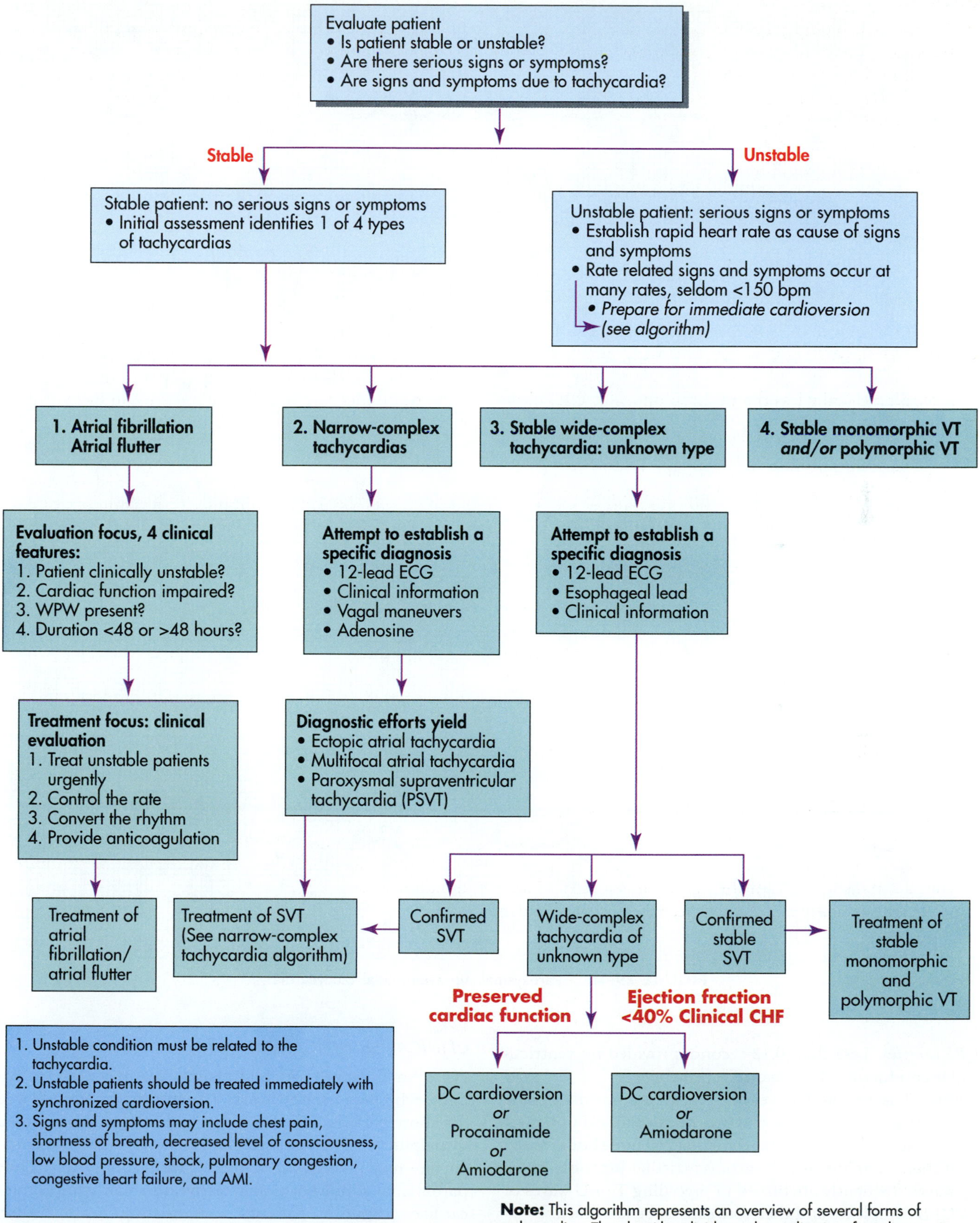
Evaluate patient
• Is patient stable or unstable?
• Are there serious signs or symptoms?
• Are signs and symptoms due to tachycardia?
Stable
Unstable
Stable patient: no serious signs or symptoms
• Initial assessment identifies 1 of 4 types of tachycardias
Unstable patient: serious signs or symptoms
• Establish rapid heart rate as cause of signs and symptoms
• Rate related signs and symptoms occur at many rates, seldom <150 bpm
• Prepare for immediate cardioversion (see algorithm)
1. Atrial fibrillation Atrial flutter
2. Narrow-complex tachycardias
3. Stable wide-complex tachycardia: unknown type
4. Stable monomorphic VT and/or polymorphic VT
Evaluation focus, 4 clinical features:
1. Patient clinically unstable?
2. Cardiac function impaired?
3. WPW present?
4. Duration <48 or >48 hours?
Attempt to establish a specific diagnosis
• 12-lead ECG
• Clinical information
• Vagal maneuvers
• Adenosine
Attempt to establish a specific diagnosis
• 12-lead ECG
• Esophageal lead
• Clinical information
Treatment focus: clinical evaluation
1. Treat unstable patients urgently
2. Control the rate
3. Convert the rhythm
4. Provide anticoagulation
Diagnostic efforts yield
• Ectopic atrial tachycardia
• Multifocal atrial tachycardia
• Paroxysmal supraventricular tachycardia (PSVT)
Treatment of atrial fibrillation/ atrial flutter
Treatment of SVT (See narrow-complex tachycardia algorithm)
Confirmed SVT
Wide-complex tachycardia of unknown type
Confirmed stable SVT
Treatment of stable monomorphic and polymorphic VT
Preserved cardiac function
Ejection fraction <40% Clinical CHF
DC cardioversion or Procainamide or Amiodarone
DC cardioversion or Amiodarone
1. Unstable condition must be related to the tachycardia.
2. Unstable patients should be treated immediately with synchronized cardioversion.
3. Signs and symptoms may include chest pain, shortness of breath, decreased level of consciousness, low blood pressure, shock, pulmonary congestion, congestive heart failure, and AMI.

Note: This algorithm represents an overview of several forms of tachycardias. The algorithm divides tachycardias into four diagnostic categories that will be discussed in the following pages.

FIGURE 29-47 ■ The tachycardia overview algorithm.

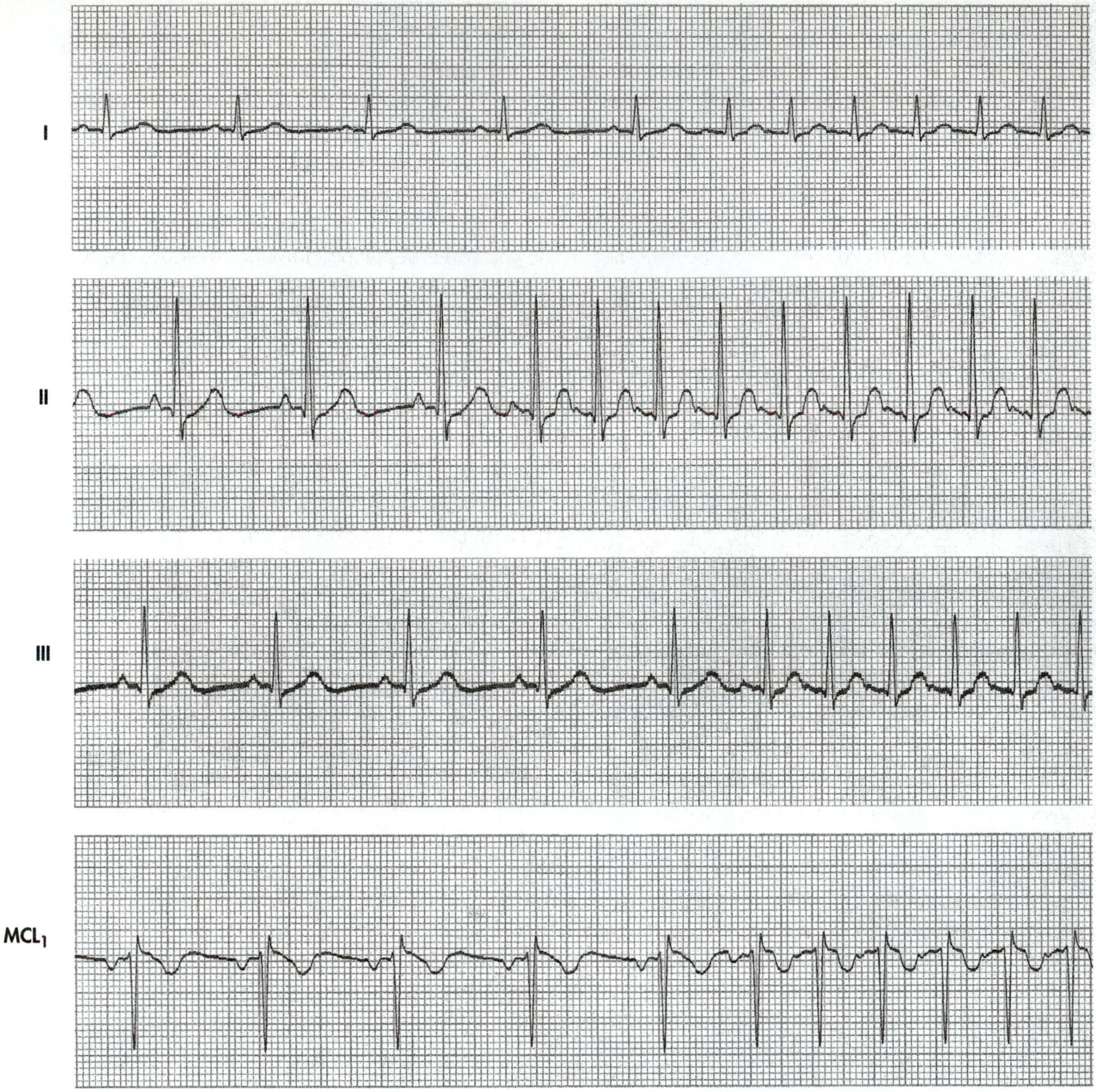

FIGURE 29-48 ■ Paroxysmal supraventricular tachycardia.

QRS complex: Less than 0.12 second, provided no ventricular conduction disturbance is present

P waves: The ectopic P waves differ from the normal sinus P waves. In lead II the P waves may be normal and upright if the pacemaker site is near the sinoatrial node but inverted if they originate near the atrioventricular junction. The P waves frequently are buried in preceding T or U waves or QRS complexes and therefore cannot be identified.

Rate: 150 to 250 beats per minute

Rhythm: Regular except at onset and termination

P-R interval: If P waves are discernible, the P-R interval often is shortened but may be normal or, rarely, prolonged.

CLINICAL SIGNIFICANCE

Paroxysmal supraventricular tachycardia may occur in patients who have healthy hearts. Patients may tolerate it well for short periods. Often the dysrhythmia is accompanied by palpitations, nervousness, and anxiety. A rapid ventricular rate may prevent the ventricles from filling fully. Thus paroxysmal supraventricular tachycardia can compromise cardiac output in patients with existing heart disease. Decreased perfusion may cause confusion, vertigo, lightheadedness, and syncope and may precipitate angina pectoris, hypotension, or congestive heart failure. In addition, paroxysmal supraventricular tachycardia increases the oxygen requirement of the heart. This may increase myocardial ischemia and may increase the frequency and severity of the patient's chest pain.

> **▶NOTE** The distinctions among ventricular tachycardia, nonparoxysmal supraventricular tachycardia, and paroxysmal supraventricular tachycardia may be difficult to make. However, they are crucial. Two critical points to remember are these. First, if the patient displays serious signs and symptoms, particularly if the ventricular rate is greater than 150 beats per minute, the paramedic should prepare for immediate cardioversion. Second, if the tachycardia complex appears wide, the paramedic should manage the rhythm as ventricular tachycardia. These two clinical rules should help manage the most difficult tachydysrhythmias. Use of modified chest leads may help identify these rhythms.

MANAGEMENT

The paramedic should manage symptomatic paroxysmal supraventricular tachycardia promptly (Fig. 29-49). This will help to reverse the consequences of the reduced cardiac output and increased workload on the heart. If the patient is stable (conscious with normal blood pressure and without chest pain, congestive heart failure, or pulmonary edema), the paramedic should attempt the following techniques to terminate paroxysmal supraventricular tachycardia.

Vagal Maneuvers. Vagal maneuvers slow the heart and decrease the force of atrial contraction by stimulating the vagus nerve. Vagal maneuvers may be used to interrupt and end paroxysmal supraventricular tachycardia. The patient should be stable. Vagal maneuvers should be used only under medical direction. Continuous electrocardiogram monitoring and an intravenous line must be in place before beginning these procedures. In addition, ***atropine, lidocaine,*** and airway equipment should be readily available.

Valsalva Maneuver. The paramedic should place the patient in a sitting or semisitting position with the head tilted down. The paramedic then instructs the patient to take in a deep breath and to bear down as if to have a bowel movement. The forced expiration against a closed glottis stimulates the vagus nerve and may terminate the tachycardia. The procedure may be repeated if unsuccessful.

Ice Pack Maneuver. Placing an ice pack on the patient's anterior neck may stimulate the vagus nerve because of the mammalian diving reflex (see Chapter 38). (In the pediatric patient, this technique is performed with a washcloth soaked in ice water. The washcloth is placed across the patient's face, about to nostril level.) The paramedic should not attempt the ice pack maneuver if ischemic heart disease is present or suspected. The procedure may be repeated (per medical direction) if unsuccessful.

Unilateral Carotid Sinus Pressure. Carotid sinus pressure stimulates the carotid bodies located in the carotid arteries. The body interprets this localized pressure as an increase in blood pressure. This activates the autonomic nervous system and stimulates the vagus nerve. The heart rate slows in an attempt to lower blood pressure. The paramedic should auscultate the carotid arteries for the presence of a bruit (described in Chapter 11) before applying carotid sinus pressure. The paramedic should not apply carotid sinus pressure if bruits are present, if the patient is an older adult, or if the patient is known to have carotid artery disease or cerebral vascular disease. Possible complications from the procedure include cerebral emboli, stroke, syncope, sinus arrest, asystole, and increased degree of atrioventricular block.[1] The procedure for carotid sinus massage is as follows:

1. Position yourself behind the patient, who is lying supine with the neck extended and the head turned away from the side of the applied pressure.
2. Gently palpate each carotid artery to confirm the presence of equal pulses. If pulses are unequal, or if one is absent, do not apply carotid sinus pressure.
3. Auscultate (while the patient holds his or her breath for 4 to 5 seconds) for the presence of bruits.
4. To apply carotid sinus pressure, place the index and middle fingers over the artery on the neck just below the angle of the jaw. Compress the artery firmly against the vertebral column while massaging the area. (Inform the patient that he or she may experience some pain or discomfort.) Maintain pressure no longer than 5 to 10 seconds. Discontinue the massage immediately if bradycardia or signs of heart block develop or if the tachycardia breaks. *Apply pressure to only one carotid sinus at a time. Applying bilateral carotid sinus pressure may interfere with cerebral circulation.*
5. Observe the electrocardiogram monitor and run a strip during the procedure and obtain a tracing. Repeat the procedure in 2 to 3 minutes if it is ineffective.

> **CRITICAL THINKING**
> You perform carotid sinus massage on a patient with bruits or known carotid artery disease. What might occur?

Pharmacological Therapy. If vagal maneuvers fail or are contraindicated and the patient remains stable, administration of ***adenosine*** (the initial drug of choice), ***verapamil, diltiazem,*** or other antidysrhythmics may end paroxysmal supraventricular tachycardia.

> **CRITICAL THINKING**
> What are some of the side effects of verapamil?

> **▶NOTE** The administration of ***verapamil*** to a patient with ventricular tachycardia can be lethal. The paramedic must use the patient's signs and symptoms rather than just electrocardiogram criteria when distinguishing between paroxysmal supraventricular tachycardia with aberrant conduction and ventricular tachycardia. If the complexes are wide and ventricular tachycardia is suspected, the paramedic should manage the rhythm like ventricular tachycardia.

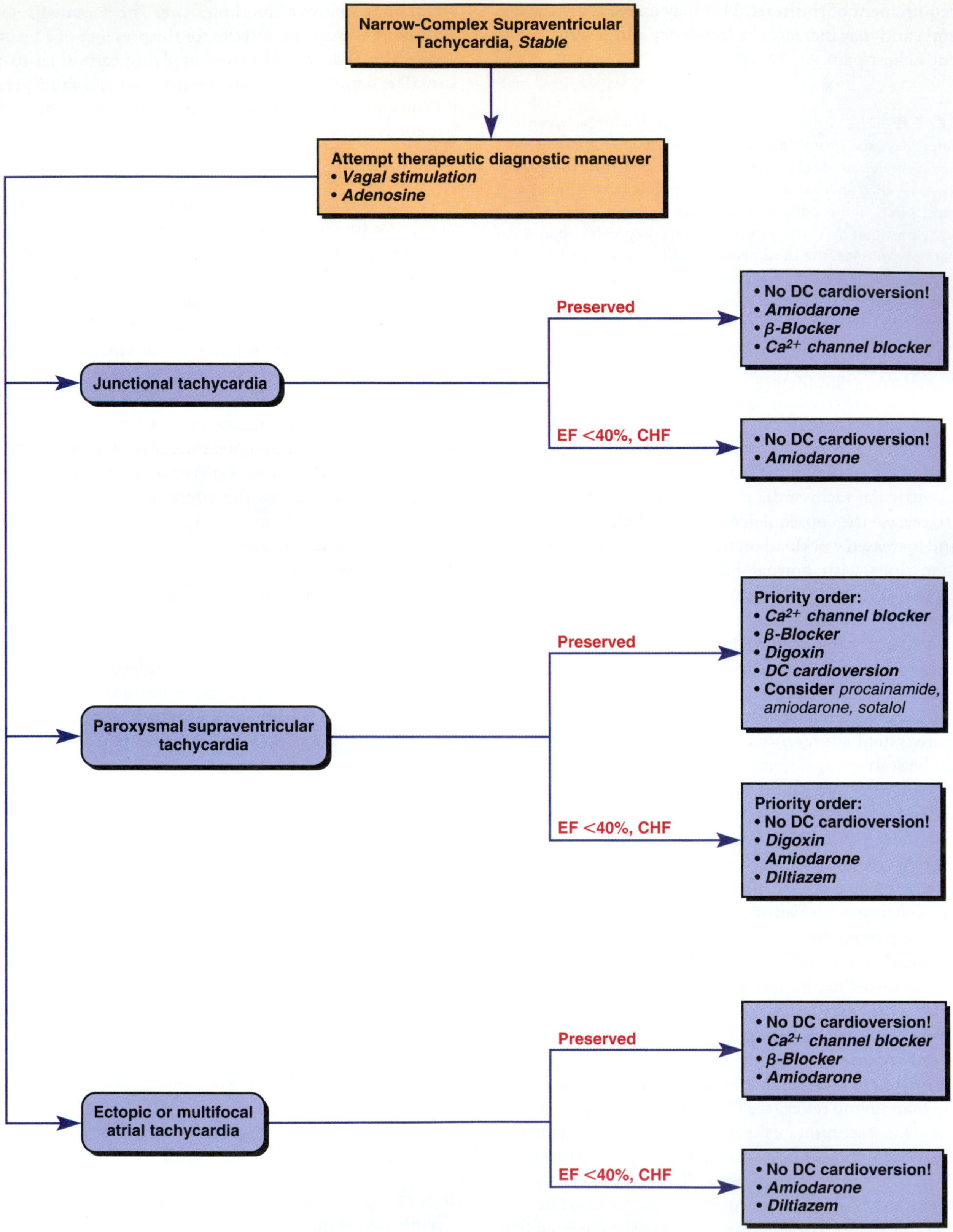

FIGURE 29-49 ■ Narrow-complex supraventricular tachycardia.

BOX 29-9 Sequence of Care for Narrow-Complex Supraventricular Tachycardias

1. Vagal maneuvers
2. ***Adenosine***
3. Consider antidysrhythmics
   a. Calcium channel blockers (Class I)
      - ***Diltiazen***
      - ***Verapamil***
   b. Beta-blockers (Class II)
      - Esmolol
      - ***Metoprolol***
   c. ***Digoxin*** (Class IIb)
   d. ***Amiodarone*** (Class IIa)
   e. ***Procainamide*** (Class IIa)
   f. ***Flecainide*** (Class IIa)
   g. Propafenone (Class IIa)
   h. Sotalol (Class IIa)

Drug treatment recommended by the American Heart Association for stable narrow-complex supraventricular tachycardias is based on rhythm interpretation and the stability of the patient (Box 29-9). Technically, treatment is based on the percentage of blood pumped by the left ventricle with each contraction or **cardiac ejection fraction.** (A cardiac ejection fraction between 55% and 75% is considered normal; Fig. 29-49.) Persons with heart disease possibly may experience a rapid heart rate and yet remain clinically stable. These patients are often chronically ill with heart disease and have adjusted to a reduced level of cardiac function. Based on patient history and physical examination, the paramedic should be able to distinguish between acute and chronic or stable congestive heart failure. A *sudden* onset of signs and symptoms of congestive heart failure with impaired cardiac function (e.g., jugular vein distention, dyspnea, tachycardia, chest pain, or decreased level of consciousness) indicates that the patient is unstable.

Junctional tachycardia in adults is rare; it is not paroxysmal. Ectopic atrial tachycardia is also not paroxysmal. It often will continue after drug treatment to block conduction through the atrioventricular node. Unlike reentry dysrhythmias, ectopic atrial tachycardia, multifocal atrial tachycardia, and sinus tachycardia are not responsive to electrical cardioversion.

For simplicity, in paroxysmal supraventricular tachycardia, vagal maneuvers and ***adenosine*** should be used first to end the tachydysrhythmia. With preserved ejection fraction (a hemodynamically stable patient condition without evidence of congestive heart failure), the primary pharmacological treatment options include calcium channel blockers (Class I), beta-blockers (Class I), ***amiodarone*** (Class IIa), or digitalis (Class IIb).

Persistent or recurrent paroxysmal supraventricular tachycardia may be treated with antidysrhythmic agents such as ***procainamide, amiodarone,*** flecainide, propafenone, and sotalol (all are Class IIa). These agents most likely will be used after diagnosis and evaluation by a physician. As of yet, intravenously administered flecainide, propafenone, and sotalol are not approved for use in the United States.

The consecutive use of calcium channel blockers, beta-blockers, and primary antidysrhythmics is discouraged. The general rule is to use only one antidysrhythmic agent; using several can result in more dysrhythmias and a drop in blood pressure. Furthermore, the paramedic should avoid negative inotropic drugs (***verapamil,*** beta-blockers, flecainide, ***procainamide,*** propafenone, and sotalol) in hemodynamically unstable patients with impaired cardiac function.

Many drug treatments are available for narrow- and wide-complex tachycardias (ventricular rate 150) (Box 29-9). However, when serious signs and symptoms point to poor perfusion and instability in either type of tachycardia, synchronized electrical cardioversion is the treatment of choice. Cardioversion should commence with a synchronized shock of 50 J. If this fails, the energy may be increased to 100, 200, 300 and then 360 J. Sedation should be considered before the cardioversion (if time permits) (see Fig. 29-71).

NOTE Cardioversion encompasses vagal, pharmacological, and electrical therapy. The term, however, commonly is used to describe electrical cardioversion.

CRITICAL THINKING

Why is the drug ***midazolam*** an ideal sedative before cardioversion?

Atrial Flutter

DESCRIPTION

Atrial flutter is almost always a result of a rapid atrial reentry focus (Fig. 29-50). Atrial flutter not slowed by preexisting atrioventricular block usually manifests a 2:1 atrioventricular conduction ratio. (That is, 50% of the atrial impulses are conducted through the ventricles and may look like supraventricular tachycardia.) Yet 3:1, 4:1, and greater conduction ratios are not uncommon. These ratios produce a discrepancy between atrial and ventricular rates. The conduction ratios may be constant or variable. Atrial flutter may be seen with atrial fibrillation (atrial fib-flutter). Rarely, atrial flutter may conduct 1:1. This results in rapid ventricular rates that cause the patient to become unstable quickly.

ETIOLOGY

Atrial flutter usually is seen in middle-aged and older patients who have heart disease. At times, atrial flutter also occurs in patients who have healthy hearts. The dysrhythmia commonly is associated with the following:

- Cardiomyopathy
- Cardiac hypertrophy
- Digitalis toxicity (rare)

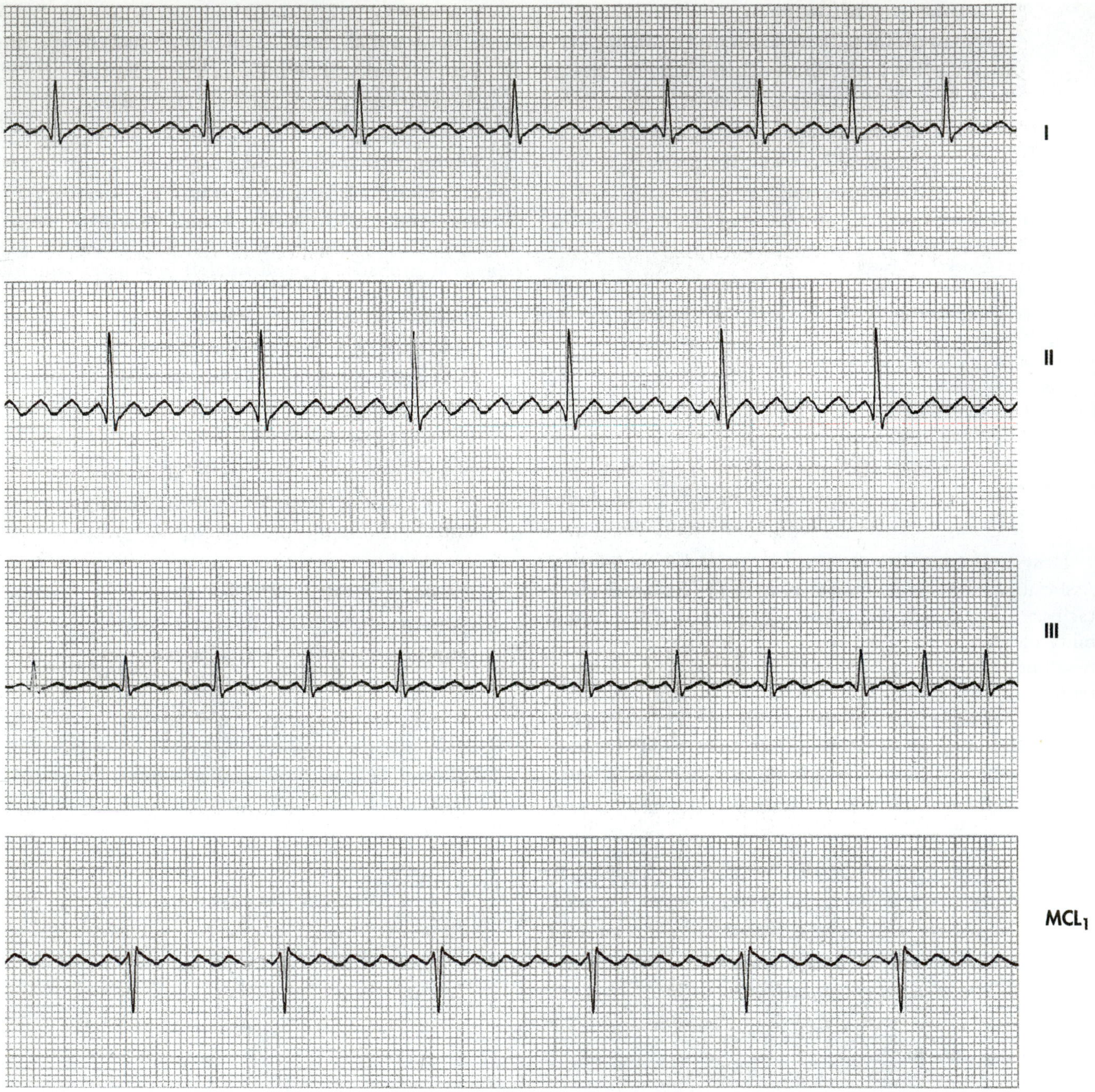

FIGURE 29-50 ■ Atrial flutter.

- Hypoxia
- Congestive heart failure
- Pericarditis
- Myocarditis

RULES FOR INTERPRETATION (LEAD II MONITORING)

Atrial flutter has the following characteristics on the electrocardiogram:

QRS complex: Less than 0.12 second, unless ventricular conduction disturbance (aberrancy) is present

P waves: Normal P waves are absent. The flutter waves (F waves) usually resemble a sawtooth or picket fence pattern. The flutter waves represent atrial depolarization in an abnormal direction that is followed by atrial repolarization.

▶ **NOTE** Flutter waves may be hard to identify when there is a 2:1 ratio of atrial to ventricular complexes. The paramedic should suspect 2:1 flutter when the rhythm is regular and the ventricular rate is 150 beats per minute.

Rate: The atrial rate is 250 to 300 beats per minute; the ventricular rate is regular but often is less than the atrial rate.

Rhythm: The atrial rhythm is regular; the ventricular rate is usually regular. However, the ventricular rate may be irregular if the atrioventricular conduction ratio varies.

P-R interval: Usually is constant but may vary

CLINICAL SIGNIFICANCE

With a normal ventricular rate, atrial flutter usually is well tolerated by the patient. A rapid ventricular rate produces the same signs and symptoms of decreased cardiac output as seen in patients with atrial tachycardia. In addition, in some flutter rhythms (particularly a 2:1 atrial flutter), the atria do not contract regularly and empty before each ventricular contraction. The loss of the "atrial kick" results in incomplete filling of the ventricles. This may decrease cardiac output further.

▶**NOTE** The pulse rate of a patient with this dysrhythmia (and other tachycardias) might not be the same as the heart rate. This is because not all heart contractions produce enough output of blood to create a palpable pulse.

Atrial Fibrillation

DESCRIPTION

Atrial fibrillation results from multiple areas of reentry within the atria (Fig. 29-51). It also can result from ectopic atrial pacemakers. (The activity of the sinoatrial node is suppressed completely by atrial fibrillation.) Atrial fibrillation produces chaotic impulses too numerous for all to be conducted by the atrioventricular node through the ventricles. Atrioventricular conduction is random. This results in an irregular ventricular response. Usually the response is rapid unless the patient is taking medication (e.g., ***digoxin***) to slow the ventricular rate.

ETIOLOGY

Sudden onset (paroxysmal) atrial fibrillation may occur in young adults after heavy alcohol ingestion. (This fibrillation is known as the "holiday heart" syndrome.) Atrial fibrillation also may occur as a result of acute stress. It usually does not require treatment. Chronic atrial fibrillation may be intermittent. It often is associated with rheumatic heart disease, congestive heart failure, and atherosclerotic heart disease. Chronic atrial fibrillation usually requires drug therapy with digitalis (or calcium channel blocker or beta-blocker) therapy. This slows the ventricular rate to 80 to 100 beats per minute. Atrial fibrillation may be a stable rhythm that does not require management. Less commonly, atrial fibrillation may occur in cardiomyopathy, acute myocarditis and pericarditis, and chest trauma. It rarely is caused by digitalis toxicity. However, a slow, regular ventricular response with atrial fibrillation could be the result of digitalis toxicity.

RULES FOR INTERPRETATION (LEAD II MONITORING)

Atrial fibrillation has the following characteristics on the electrocardiogram:

QRS complex: Less than 0.12 second, provided there is no ventricular conduction disturbance

P waves: P waves and organized atrial contractions are absent. Fibrillation waves (F waves) may be fine (less than 1 mm) or coarse (greater than 1 mm). Fine F waves may be so small that they appear as a wavy or flat (isoelectric) line or absent. The F waves are irregularly shaped, rounded (or pointed), and dissimilar.

Rate: The atrial rate is 350 to 700 beats per minute (cannot be counted); the ventricular rate varies greatly, depending on conduction through the atrioventricular node (average 150 to 180 beats per minute, if uncontrolled).

Rhythm: Irregularly irregular

P-R interval: None

▶**NOTE** Irregularly irregular rhythms are most likely to be atrial fibrillation.

CLINICAL SIGNIFICANCE

The atrial kick is lost in atrial fibrillation. This loss reduces cardiac output by as much as 15%. This loss, coupled with a rapid ventricular response, may cause cardiovascular decompensation (angina pectoris, myocardial infarction, congestive heart failure, or cardiogenic shock).

MANAGEMENT OF ATRIAL FIBRILLATION/ ATRIAL FLUTTER

The American Heart Association algorithm "Tachycardia: Atrial Fibrillation and Atrial Flutter" has three categories: atrial fibrillation or atrial flutter with normal heart function, impaired heart function, and Wolff-Parkinson-White syndrome (described later in this chapter). Each condition is managed by controlling rate or converting rhythm (Fig. 29-52).

A risk of emboli formation exists when atrial fibrillation or atrial flutter has been present for more than 48 hours. This formation of emboli in the heart increases the risk of "throwing a clot" or systemic embolization. This most often occurs when the atrial fibrillation is converted suddenly to a sinus rhythm. The algorithm cautions against converting atrial fibrillation or atrial flutter without first giving the patient drugs that prevent blood from clotting. Electrical cardioversion and the use of antidysrhythmic agents that may convert the rhythm should be avoided unless the patient is unstable or hemodynamically compromised.[4]

Using drugs to control heart rate is the recommended initial treatment for stable, rapid atrial fibrillation or atrial flutter regardless of how long the patient has had it. Specific drug treatment depends on the patient's condition and how stable the patient is. Using several different drugs can cause a dysrhythmia to develop (a **proarrhythmia**). The paramedic should use only one drug from the list of suggested drug treatments.

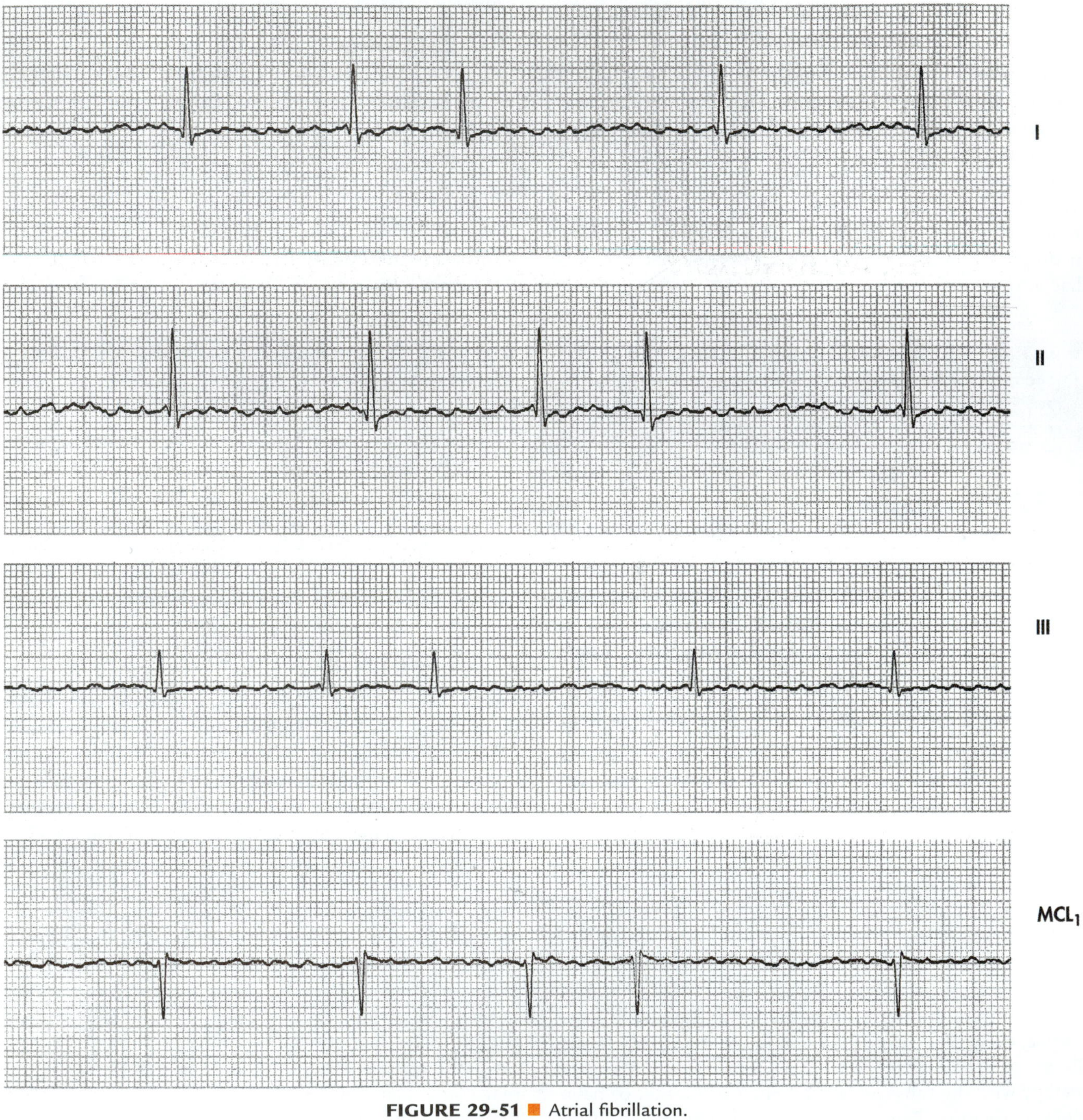

FIGURE 29-51 ■ Atrial fibrillation.

Atrial Fibrillation/Atrial Flutter Algorithm

Perform Primary ABCD Survey (Basic Life Support)

(Correct critical problems IMMEDIATELY as they are identified)

- Assess responsiveness, **A**irway, **B**reathing, **C**irculation, ensure availability of monitor/**D**efibrillator

Perform Secondary ABCD Survey (Advanced Life Support)

- Administer oxygen, establish IV access, attach cardiac monitor, administer fluids as needed (O_2, IV, monitor, fluids)
- Assess vital signs, attach pulse oximeter, and monitor blood pressure
- Obtain and review 12-lead ECG, portable chest x-ray, perform a focused history and physical exam

Is the patient stable or unstable?
Is the patient experiencing serious signs and symptoms due to the tachycardia?
Is the patient's cardiac function normal or impaired?
Attempt to identify patient's cardiac rhythm using 12-lead ECG, clinical information.
Is Wolff-Parkinson-White syndrome (WPW) present? If yes, see WPW algorithm
Has atrial fibrillation/atrial flutter been present for more or less than 48 hours?

STABLE PATIENT			
Normal Cardiac Function		**Impaired Cardiac Function**	
Onset < 48 hours **Control Rate**	**Onset > 48 hours** **Control Rate**	**Onset < 48 hours** **Control Rate**	**Onset > 48 hours** **Control Rate**
Calcium channel blocker (Class I) **OR** Beta-blockers (Class I) **OR** Digoxin (IIb)	Calcium channel blocker (Class I) **OR** Beta-blocker (Class I) **OR** Digoxin (IIb)	Diltiazem (IIb) **OR** Amiodarone (IIb) **OR** Digoxin (IIb) Note: Impaired cardiac function = ejection fraction <40% or CHF	Diltiazem (IIb) **OR** Amiodarone (IIb) **OR** Digoxin (IIb)
Convert Rhythm	**Convert Rhythm**	**Convert Rhythm**	**Convert Rhythm**
Cardioversion **OR** Amiodarone (IIa) **OR** Procainamide (IIa) **OR** Ibutilide (IIa) **OR** Flecainide (IIa) **OR** Propafenone (IIa)	Delayed cardioversion **OR** Early cardioversion	Cardioversion **OR** amiodarone (IIb)	Delayed cardioversion **OR** Early cardioversion

Delayed cardioversion:

Anticoagulation therapy for 3 weeks before cardioversion, for at least 48 hours in conjunction with cardioversion, and for at least 4 weeks after successful cardioversion. Early cardioversion: IV heparin immediately, transesophageal echocardiography (TEE) to r/o atrial thrombus, cardioversion within 24 h, anticoagulation x 4 wks

FIGURE 29-52 ■ Atrial fibrillation/atrial flutter algorithm.

Continued

UNSTABLE PATIENT

If hemodynamically unstable, perform synchronized cardioversion: **Atrial fibrillation:** 100 J, 200 J, 300 J, 360 J, or equivalent biphasic energy. Atrial flutter: 50 J, 100 J, 200 J, 300 J, 360 J, or equivalent biphasic energy.

MEDICATION DOSING

Amiodarone*,† 150 mg IV bolus over 10 minutes followed by an infusion of 1 mg/min for 6 hours and then a maintenance infusion of 0.5 mg/min. Repeat supplementary infusions of 150 mg as necessary for recurrent or resistant dysrhythmias. Maximum total daily dose 2 g.

Beta-blockers *Esmolol:* 0.5 mg/kg over 1 minute followed by a maintenance infusion at 50 mcg/kg/min for 4 minutes. If inadequate response, administer a second bolus of 0.5 mg/kg over 1 minute and increase maintenance infusion to 100 mcg/kg/min. The bolus dose (0.5 mg/kg) and titration of the maintenance infusion (addition of 50 mcg/kg/min) can be repeated every 4 minutes to a maximum infusion of 300 mcg/kg/min. *Metoprolol:* 5 mg slow IV push over 5 minutes x 3 as needed to a total dose of 15 mg over 15 minutes. *Propranolol:* 0.1-mg/kg slow IV push divided in 3 equal doses at 2-3 minute intervals. Do not exceed 1 mg/min. Repeat after 2 minutes if necessary. *Atenolol:* 5 mg slow IV (over 5 min). Wait 10 min then give second dose of 5 mg slow IV (over 5 min).

Calcium channel blockers‡,§ *Diltiazem* 0.25 mg/kg over 2 min (e.g., 15 to 20 mg). If ineffective, 0.35 mg/kg over 2 min (e.g., 20-25 mg) in 15 min. Maintenance infusion 5 to 15 mg/h, titrated to heart rate if chemical conversion successful. Calcium chloride (2 to 4 mg/kg) may be given slow IV push if borderline hypotension exists before diltiazem administration. *Verapamil*–2.5 to 5.0 mg slow IV push over 2 min. May repeat with 5 to 10 mg in 15 to 30 min. Maximum dose 20 mg.

Ibutilide Adults 60 kg: 1 mg (10-mL) over 10 min. May repeat x 1 in 10 min. Adults < 60 kg: 0.01 mg/kg IV over 10 min.

Procainamide|| 100 mg over 5 minutes (20 mg/min). Maximum total dose 17 mg/kg. Maintenance infusion 1 to 4 mg/min.

Flecainide, propafenone IV form not currently approved for use in the United States

Sotaolol 1 to 1.5 mg/kg IV slowly at a rate of 10 mg/min

*Cotter G et al: Conversion of recent onset paroxysmal atrial fibrillation to normal sinus rhythm: the effect of no treatment and high-dose amiodarone: a randomized, placebo-controlled study [see comments], *Eur Heart J* 20:1833, 1999.
†Clemo HF et al: Intravenous amiodarone for acute heart rate control in the critically ill patient with atrial tachyarrhythmias, *Am J Cardiol* 81:594, 1998.
‡Ellenbogen KA et al: A placebo-controlled trial of continuous intravenous diltiazem infusion for 24-hour heart rate control during atrial fibrillation and atrial flutter: a multicenter study, *J Am Coll Cardiol* 18:891, 1991.
§Salerno DM et al: Efficacy and safety of intravenous diltiazem for treatment of atrial fibrillation and atrial flutter, *Am J Cardiol* 63:1046, 1989.
||Chapman MJ et al: Management of atrial tachyarrhythmias in the critically ill: a comparison of intravenous procainamide and amiodarone, *Intensive Care Med* 19:48, 1993.

FIGURE 29-52, cont'd ■ Atrial fibrillation/atrial flutter algorithm.

In patients with a rapid atrial fibrillation or flutter and normal left ventricular function, calcium channel blockers, beta-blockers, and digitalis are recommended. For patients who are exhibiting signs of *impaired* heart function such as pulmonary congestion, diminished peripheral perfusion, or poor ejection fraction (less than 40%), digitalis, ***diltiazem,*** and ***amiodarone*** are recommended. ***Amiodarone*** has a potential for rhythm conversion. Thus ***amiodarone*** should be reserved for use within the first 48 hours of dysrhythmia onset when other medications for rate control have failed. The use of calcium channel blocking agents and beta-blocking agents warrants caution in the presence of congestive heart failure because of their negative inotropic properties. Beta-blocking agents also should be used with caution in patients with asthma and chronic obstructive pulmonary disease.

Patients with a known history of Wolff-Parkinson-White syndrome and who have experienced rapid atrial fibrillation or atrial flutter for less than 48 hours may be treated with ***amiodarone,*** flecainide, ***procainamide,*** or propafenone.

BOX 29-10 Atrial Fibrillation/Flutter

(with/without congestive heart failure)

Rate control	Diltiazem
Rhythm conversion	Nonemergent chemical or direct current cardioversion should be avoided and, when indicated, should be performed only by an experienced health care provider after careful evaluation and initiation of thromboembolic precautions.

If the patient has had the dysrhythmia for longer than 48 hours, the paramedic should avoid elective cardioversion unless anticoagulation drugs have been given. However, when serious signs or symptoms such as chest pain, shortness of breath, pulmonary congestion, decreased level of consciousness, or hypotension occur, the paramedic should cardiovert the patient immediately. The initial attempt at cardioversion for atrial flutter should consist of a synchronized shock of 50 J. If needed, the energy may be increased to 100, 200, 300, and 360 J. Because atrial fibrillation is a more difficult rhythm to convert and lower joule settings have been known to cause asystole, recommendations are initially to use a synchronized shock of 100 J, followed by 200, 300, and 360 J if necessary (Box 29-10).[4]

CRITICAL THINKING

What signs or symptoms would make you think these patients are unstable?

DYSRHYTHMIAS SUSTAINED OR ORIGINATING IN THE ATRIOVENTRICULAR JUNCTION

When the sinoatrial node and the atria cannot generate the electrical impulses needed to begin depolarization because of factors such as hypoxia, ischemia, myocardial infarction, and drug toxicity, the atrioventricular node or the area surrounding the atrioventricular node may assume the role of the secondary pacemaker. Rhythms that start in the atrioventricular node or atrioventricular junctional area are junctional rhythms. This type of rhythm usually is a benign dysrhythmia. Yet the paramedic must assess the rhythm to determine the patient's tolerance of the rhythm disturbance. Dysrhythmias that originate in the atrioventricular junction include premature junctional contractions, junctional escape complexes or junctional escape rhythms, and accelerated junctional rhythm.

In junctional rhythms, electrical impulses travel in a normal pathway from the atrioventricular junction through the bundle of His and bundle branches to the Purkinje fibers. The pathway ends in the ventricular muscle. Conduction through the ventricles proceeds normally. Thus the QRS complex usually is within normal limits of 0.04 to 0.10 second. However, the impulse that depolarizes the atria travels in a backward or retrograde motion. The retrograde depolarization of the atria results in one of the following three P wave characteristics: (1) inverted P waves in lead II with a short P-R interval, (2) absent P waves, or (3) retrograde P waves.

Premature Junctional Contraction

DESCRIPTION

A premature junctional contraction results from a single electrical impulse from the atrioventricular junction (Fig. 29-53). The impulse occurs before the next expected sinus impulse.

ETIOLOGY

Isolated premature junctional contractions may occur in a healthy person without apparent cause. Yet they more often are a result of heart disease or drug toxicity. Usually premature junctional contractions result from enhanced automaticity or a reentry mechanism. Premature junctional contractions have several causes:

- Digitalis toxicity
- Other cardiac medications (quinidine, ***procainamide***)
- Increased vagal tone on the sinoatrial node
- Sympathomimetic drugs (e.g., cocaine and methamphetamines)
- Hypoxia
- Congestive heart failure
- Damage to the atrioventricular junction

CRITICAL THINKING

Will the P wave be visible if it occurs during the QRS wave? Why?

RULES FOR INTERPRETATION (LEAD II MONITORING)

Premature junctional contractions have the following characteristics on the electrocardiogram:

QRS complex: Usually less than 0.12 second, provided there is no ventricular conduction disturbance

P waves: May be associated with premature junctional contractions. P waves can occur before, during, or after the QRS complex or can be absent. If present, P waves are abnormal, differing in size, shape, and direction from normal P waves.

Rate: The heart rate is that of the underlying rhythm

Rhythm: Usually regular, except when premature junctional contractions are present

P-R interval: Usually less than 0.12 second if the P wave precedes the QRS complex

CLINICAL SIGNIFICANCE

Occasional premature junctional contractions usually are not significant.

MANAGEMENT

No management is required.

Junctional Escape Complexes or Rhythms

DESCRIPTION

A junctional escape beat or rhythm (series of beats) occurs when the rate of the sinoatrial node falls below that of the atrioventricular junction (Fig. 29-54). The dysrhythmia also may occur when the electrical impulses from the sinoatrial node or atria fail to reach the atrioventricular junction because of sinoatrial or atrioventricular block. The escape complex or rhythm provided by the atrioventricular junction serves as a safety mechanism. This mechanism prevents cardiac standstill. The atrioventricular junction begins firing at an inherent rate of 40 to 60 beats per minute within about 1.0 to 1.5 seconds of not receiving an impulse from the sinoatrial node.

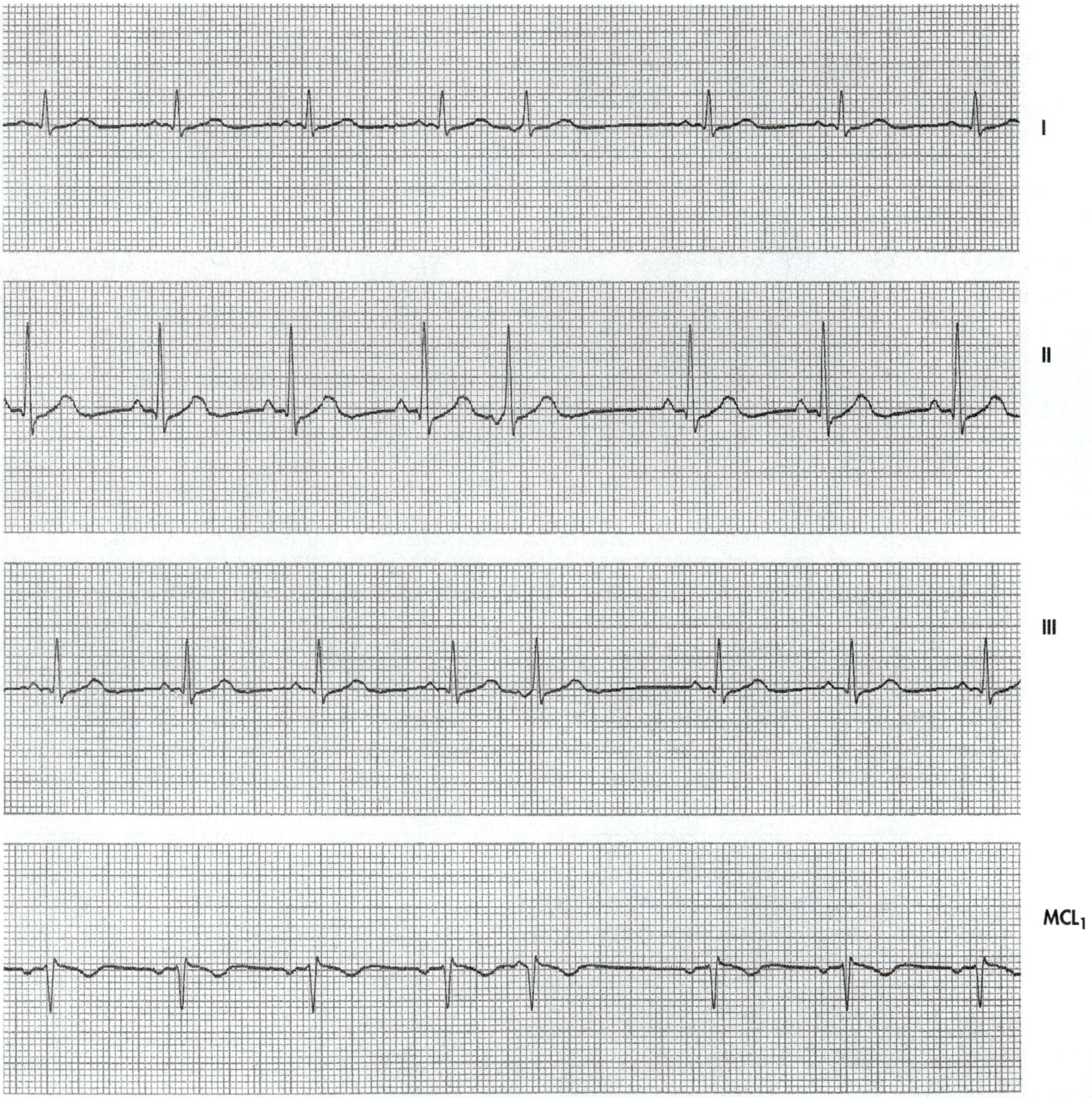

FIGURE 29-53 ■ Premature junctional contractions.

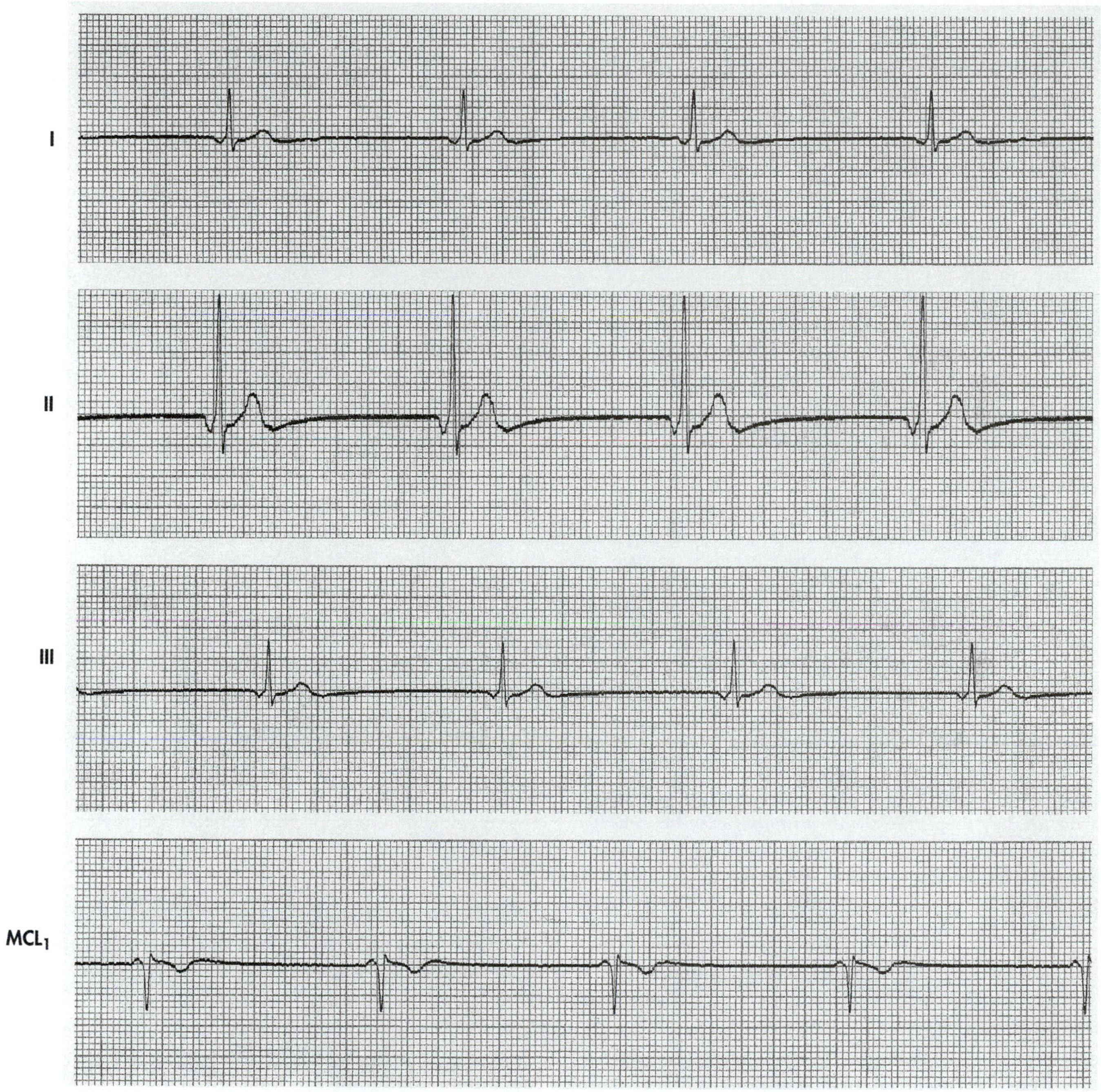

FIGURE 29-54 ■ Junctional escape complex or rhythm.

ETIOLOGY

A junctional escape complex or a junctional escape rhythm is a normal response. It may result from an increased vagal tone on the sinoatrial node, a pathological slowing of the sinoatrial discharge, or a complete atrioventricular block.

RULES FOR INTERPRETATION (LEAD II MONITORING)

Junctional escape complexes or rhythms have the following characteristics on the electrocardiogram:

QRS complex: Usually less than 0.12 second, provided no preexisting bundle branch block is present

P waves: May be present (with or without relationship to QRS complex) or absent. If P waves are present, they may occur before, after, or during the QRS complex. Depending on the pacemaker site, P waves may differ from normal P waves in size, shape, and direction and may be upright or inverted.

Rate: Usually 40 to 60 beats per minute but may be less

Rhythm: The ventricular rhythm usually is regular in junctional rhythm; it may be irregular if an isolated junctional escape complex is present.

P-R interval: If P waves precede the QRS complex, the P-R interval commonly is shortened (less than 0.12 second) and constant.

CLINICAL SIGNIFICANCE

Junctional bradycardias can cause decreased cardiac output. Thus patients can show signs and symptoms that are similar to those of other bradycardias. (For example, the signs may include light-headedness, hypotension, and syncope.) As a rule, patients tolerate junctional rhythms of 50 beats per minute or greater.

MANAGEMENT

Patients who are stable do not need to be treated. If the patient is symptomatic or if ventricular irritability is present, drug therapy (beginning with ***atropine***) may be indicated. In severe cases and in patients unresponsive to ***atropine***, external pacing may be necessary. If the sinoatrial node is diseased or damaged, the patient may need a permanent pacemaker (see Fig. 29-40).

Accelerated Junctional Rhythm

DESCRIPTION

Accelerated junctional rhythm results from increased automaticity of the atrioventricular junction (Fig. 29-55). This increase causes it to discharge faster than its intrinsic rate. (The intrinsic rate is 40 to 60 beats per minute.) This rate in turn overrides the main (sinoatrial node) pacemaker. The rate of this dysrhythmia (usually 60 to 99 beats per minute) does not truly constitute a tachycardia. Thus the dysrhythmia is termed *accelerated junctional rhythm.* In this text, rapid junctional rhythms equal to or greater than 100 beats per minute (paroxysmal junctional tachycardia or nonparoxysmal junctional tachycardia) and caused by a reentry mechanism are discussed with other supraventricular tachycardias.

ETIOLOGY

An accelerated junctional rhythm commonly is a result of digitalis toxicity. Other causes of this problem include excessive catecholamine administration, damage to the atrioventricular junction, inferior wall myocardial infarction (described later in this chapter), and rheumatic fever.

RULES FOR INTERPRETATION (LEAD II MONITORING)

Accelerated junctional rhythm has the following characteristics on the electrocardiogram:

QRS complex: Usually is less than 0.12 second, provided there is no preexisting bundle branch block

P waves: May be present (with or without relationship to the QRS complex), absent (retrograde atrioventricular block), or buried in the QRS complex. If present, P waves usually are inverted and appear before or after the QRS complex.

Rate: Usually 60 to 99 beats per minute

Rhythm: Regular

P-R interval: If the P wave occurs before the QRS complex, the P-R interval will be less than 0.12 second. If the P wave follows the QRS complex, it technically is an R-P interval and usually is less than 0.20 second.

CLINICAL SIGNIFICANCE

Accelerated junctional rhythm usually is well tolerated by the patient. However, the presence of heart disease and lack of oxygen to the heart muscle may cause more serious dysrhythmias.

MANAGEMENT

Accelerated junctional rhythm generally requires no immediate treatment.

> **CRITICAL THINKING**
>
> Do you need to start an intravenous line on these patients, since no drug therapy is indicated?

DYSRHYTHMIAS ORIGINATING IN THE VENTRICLES

Ventricular dysrhythmias usually are considered a threat to life. Ventricular rhythm disturbances generally result from failure of the atria, atrioventricular junction, or both to initiate an electrical impulse. Such disturbances also can result from enhanced automaticity or reentry pathways in the ventricles. Enhanced automaticity and

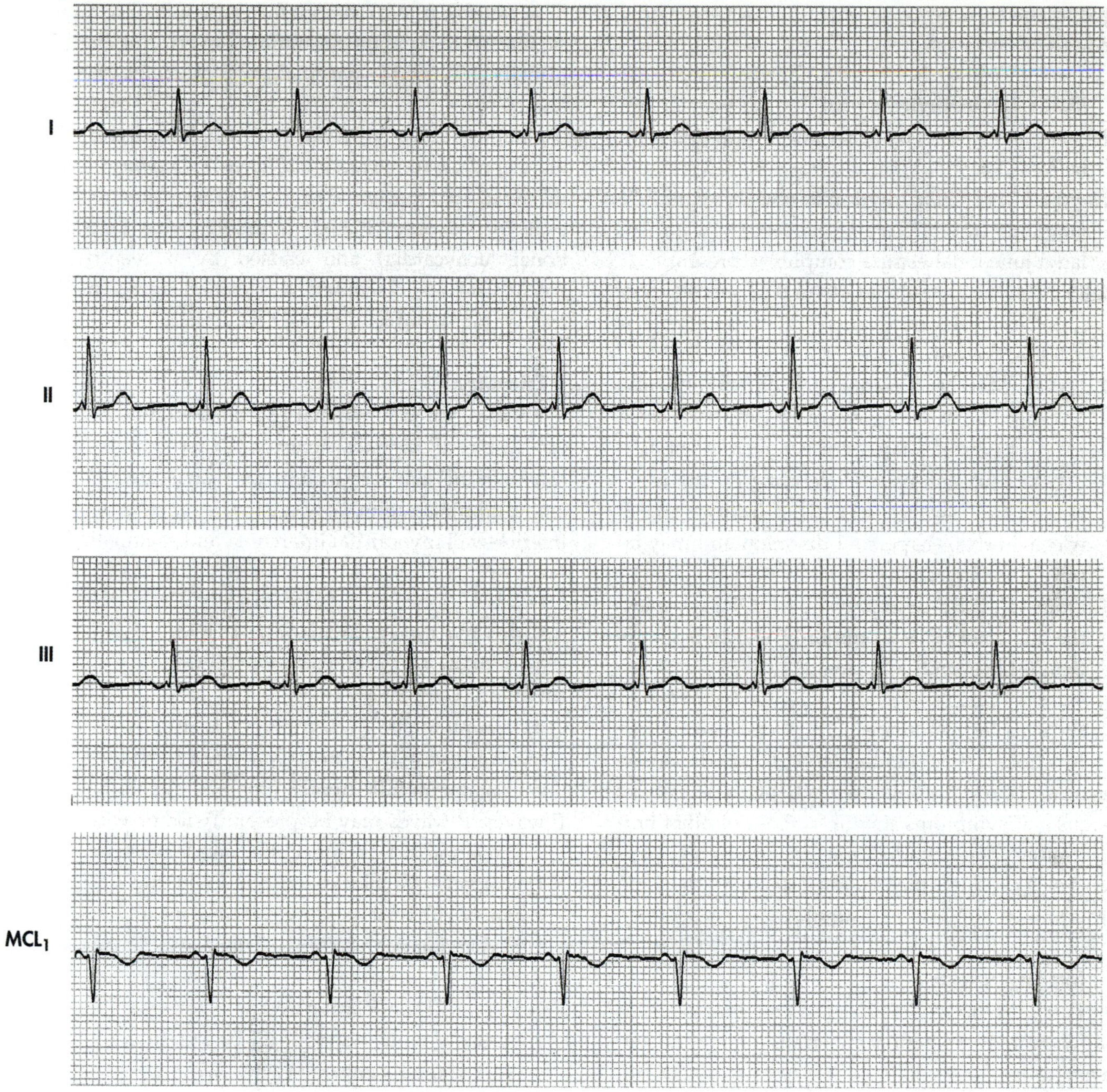

FIGURE 29-55 ■ Accelerated junctional rhythm.

rentry can lead to premature ventricular complexes, ventricular tachycardia, and even ventricular fibrillation. Ventricular dysrhymias often are associated with myocardial ischemia or infarction. The ventricle is the least efficient pacemaker of the heart. It usually generates only 20 to 40 impulses per minute. But the ventricle may discharge at rates up to 99 impulses per minute (accelerated idioventricular rhythm) or even faster (ventricular tachycardia) because of increased automaticity. Dysrhythmias originating in the ventricles include ventricular escape complexes or rhythms, premature ventricular complexes, ventricular tachycardia, ventricular fibrillation, asystole, and artificial pacemaker rhythm.

Because electrical impulses of ventricular origin start in the lower portion of the heart (the ventricular muscle, bundle branches, or Purkinje fibers), the electrical impulse must travel in a retrograde conduction pathway to depolarize the atria. The impulse may travel in an antegrade direction to depolarize the ventricles. This depends on the site of initiation of the impulse. Regardless of the direction of depolarization, the normal, rapid conducting pathways are bypassed, producing the following three electrocardiogram features:

1. QRS complexes are wide and bizarre in appearance. They are 0.12 second or greater in duration.
2. P waves may be hidden in the QRS complex. (This is because the atria are depolarized at about the same time as the ventricles.) Or they may be superimposed on every second or third QRS complex when ventricular tachycardia with **atrioventricular dissociation** (P waves that have no set relation to the QRS complexes) is present.
3. ST segments usually deviate from baseline. T waves frequently are sloped off in the opposite direction of the QRS complex.

Ventricular Escape Complexes or Rhythms

DESCRIPTION

A ventricular escape complex (isolated impulse) or rhythm (series of complexes) is also known as *idioventricular rhythm* (Figs. 29-56 and 29-57). The dysrhythmia results when impulses from higher pacemakers fail to fire or to reach the ventricles. It also results when the rate of discharge of higher pacemaker sites falls to less than that of the ventricles. Like the junctional escape complex or rhythm, this

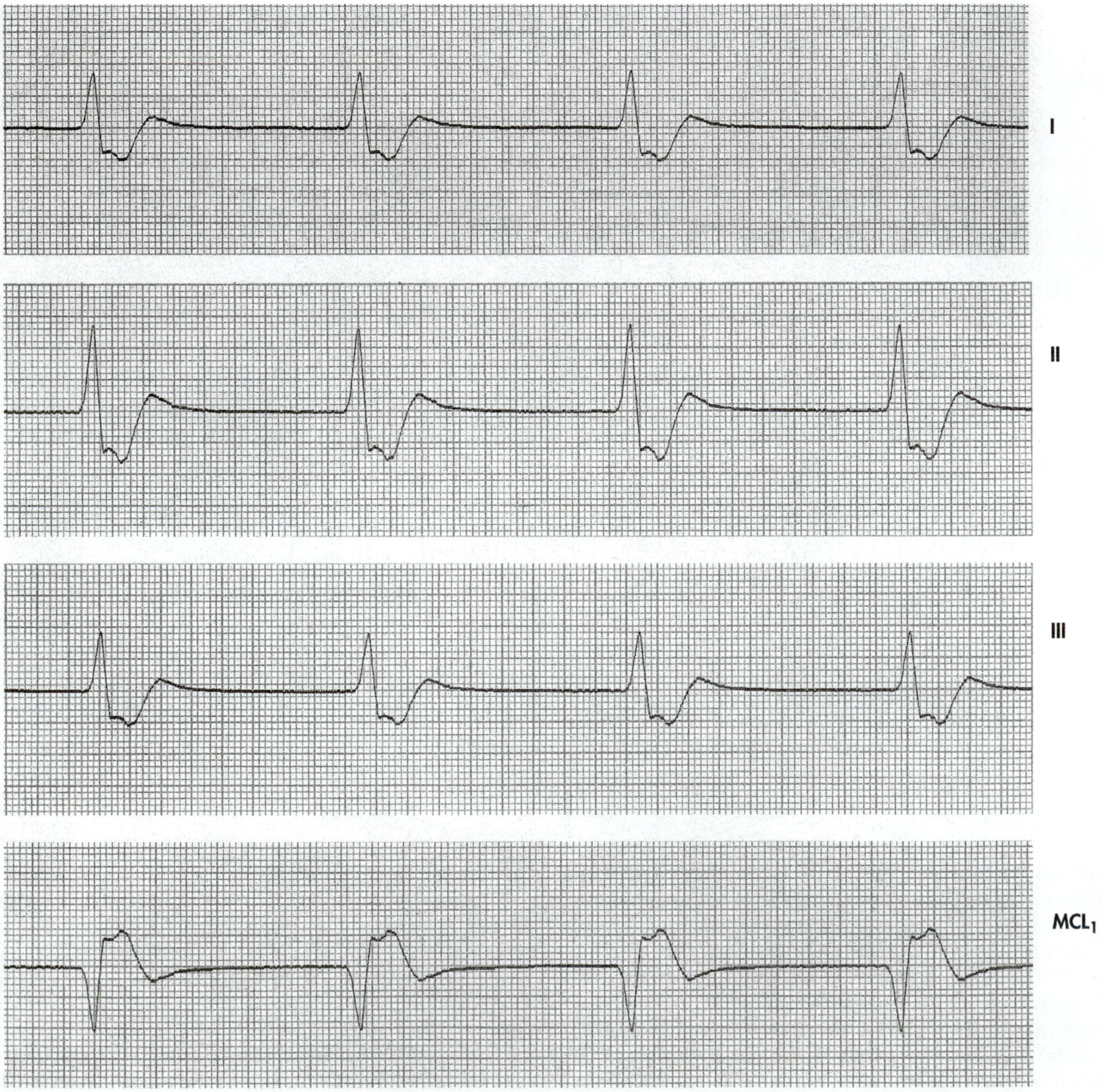

FIGURE 29-56 ■ Ventricular escape rhythm.

dysrhythmia serves as a compensatory mechanism to prevent cardiac standstill.

ETIOLOGY

Ventricular escape rhythms occur in two ways. First, the rate of impulse formation of the dominant pacemaker (usually the sinoatrial node) can fall below that of the ventricles. Second, the escape pacemaker in the atrioventricular junction can fail or fall below that of the pacemaker in the ventricles. This dysrhythmia often is seen as the first rhythm after defibrillation.

RULES FOR INTERPRETATION (LEAD II MONITORING)

Ventricular escape complexes or rhythms have the following characteristics on the electrocardiogram:

QRS complex: Generally exceed 0.12 second and are bizarre in appearance. The shape of the QRS complex may vary in any given lead.

P waves: May be absent. If they are present and have no set relationship to the QRS complex, then a third-degree atrioventricular block should be suspected.

Rate: Usually 20 to 40 beats per minute; may be lower

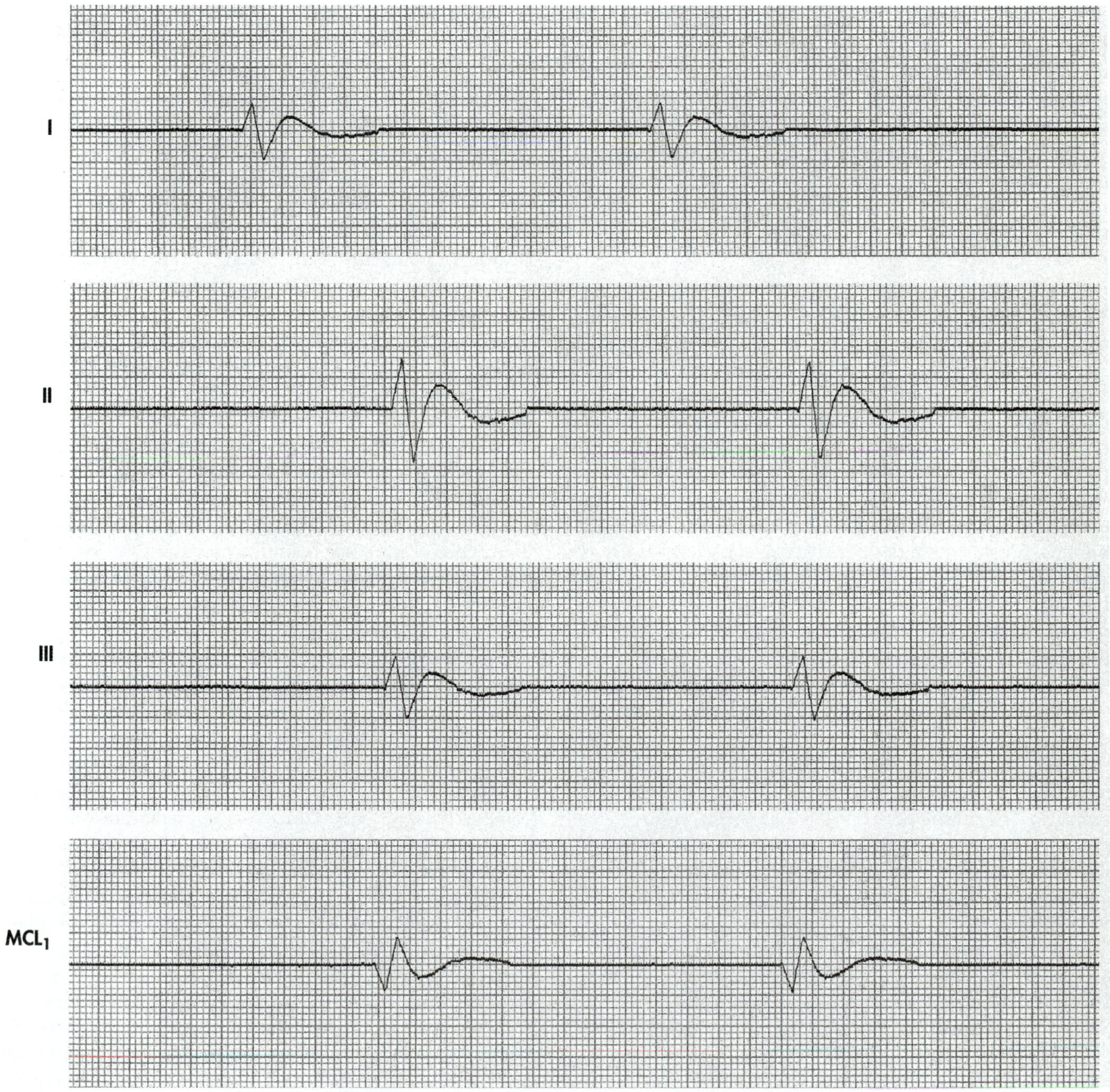

FIGURE 29-57 ■ "Dying heart" or agonal rhythm.

Rhythm: The ventricular rhythm usually is regular but may be irregular.

P-R interval: If P waves are present, the P-R interval is variable and irregular.

CLINICAL SIGNIFICANCE

A ventricular escape rhythm generally produces symptoms. This dysrhythmia is manifested by hypotension, decreased cardiac output, and decreased perfusion of the brain and other vital organs, often resulting in syncope and shock. Patient assessment is essential because the escape rhythm may be perfusing or nonperfusing (pulseless electrical activity).

MANAGEMENT

If the rhythm is perfusing, management must be directed at increasing the heart rate by administering oxygen, transcutaneous cardiac pacing, and/or ***dopamine.*** Managing the escape rhythm with ***lidocaine*** likely would be lethal, and so is contraindicated. If the rhythm is nonperfusing, the paramedic should initiate basic life support measures. The paramedic also should follow the treatment guidelines for pulseless electrical activity (Fig. 29-58).

> **CRITICAL THINKING**
> Why might ***lidocaine*** be harmful in this situation?

Premature Ventricular Complex

DESCRIPTION

A premature ventricular complex is a single ectopic impulse arising from an irritable focus in either ventricle (bundle branches, Purkinje fibers, or ventricular muscle) that occurs earlier than the next expected sinus beat (Fig. 29-59). This dysrhythmia is common and can occur with any underlying cardiac rhythm. The dysrhythmia results from enhanced automaticity or a reentry mechanism.

When the ventricles initiate a premature ventricular complex, the atria may or may not respond and depolarize. If atrial depolarization does not occur, a P wave is seen on the electrocardiogram. If atrial depolarization does occur, the P wave occurs but often is hidden in the QRS complex. The reason for this is the timing and large electrical force of ventricular depolarization blocking out the electrical activity from the atrial depolarization. The altered sequence of ventricular depolarization results in a wide, bizarre QRS complex. Depolarization may be deflected in the opposite direction from the QRS complex in the underlying rhythm. Or it may be deflected in the same direction. (This depends on the location of the focus and the lead selected.) The T wave that immediately follows the premature ventricular complex usually is deflected in the opposite direction from the QRS complex of the premature ventricular complex because of the altered sequence of repolarization.

> **CRITICAL THINKING**
> Why is the QRS deflection opposite the underlying rhythm?

A premature ventricular complex usually does not depolarize the sinoatrial node or interrupt its rhythm. (For instance, the P wave of the underlying rhythm that follows the premature ventricular complex occurs at its expected time but is obstructed by the premature ventricular complex and finds the ventricles refractory.) Thus the ectopic impulse usually is followed by a full compensatory pause. Compensatory pauses are confirmed by measuring the interval between the R wave before the premature ventricular complex and the R wave after it. If the pause is compensatory, the distance is at least 2 times the R-R interval of the underlying rhythm. At times, a premature ventricular complex falls between two sinus beats without interrupting the rhythm. (This is called an *interpolated premature ventricular complex;* Fig. 29-60).

Premature ventricular complexes may originate from a single ectopic pacemaker site (unifocal premature ventricular complexes) or from multiple sites in the ventricles (multifocal premature ventricular complexes) (Fig. 29-61). Unifocal premature ventricular complexes look alike. Multifocal premature ventricular complexes have varying shapes and sizes.

Multifocal premature ventricular complexes are thought of as more dangerous than unifocal premature ventricular complexes. In general, this is because they result from increased myocardial irritability. A premature ventricular complex that occurs at about the same time as ventricular activation by a normal impulse can cause ventricular depolarization to occur at the same time. This *fusion beat* results in a QRS complex that has the characteristics of a premature ventricular complex and the QRS complex of the underlying rhythm (Fig. 29-62). Fusion beats confirm that the ectopic impulse is located in the ventricle rather than the atria.

Frequently, premature ventricular complexes occur in patterns of grouped beating. **Ventricular bigeminy** occurs when every other complex is a premature ventricular complex. **Ventricular trigeminy** occurs when every third complex is a premature ventricular complex. Quadrigeminy occurs when every fourth complex is a premature ventricular complex (Fig. 29-63). Consecutive premature ventricular complexes that are not separated by a complex of the underlying rhythm also can occur on the electrocardiogram: couplets, or salvos, are two premature ventricular complexes in a row, and triplets are three premature ventricular complexes in a row (a definition for ventricular tachycardia). These terms also may be used to describe patterns of premature atrial complexes and premature junctional contractions.

Like multifocal premature ventricular complexes, frequently occurring premature ventricular complexes usually indicate that the ventricles are highly irritable. These types of premature ventricular complexes can trigger life-threatening dysrhythmias such as ventricular tachycardia and ventricular

Pulseless Electrical Activity
(**PEA** = rhythm on monitor, without detectable pulse)

↓

Primary ABCD Survey

Focus: *basic CPR and defibrillation*

- **Check** responsiveness
- **Activate** emergency response system
- **Call** for defibrillation

A Airway: open the airway
B Breathing: provide positive-pressure ventilations
C Circulation: give chest compressions
D Defibrillation: assess for and shock VF/pulseless VT

↓

Secondary ABCD Survey

Focus: *more advanced assessments and treatments*

A Airway: place airway device as soon as possible
B Breathing: confirm airway device placement by exam plus confirmation device
B Breathing: secure airway device; purpose-made tube holders preferred
B Breathing: confirm effective oxygenation and ventilation
C Circulation: establish IV access
C Circulation: identify rhythm → monitor
C Circulation: administer drugs appropriate for rhythm and condition
C Circulation: assess for occult blood flow ("pseudo-EMT")
D Differential Diagnosis: search for and treat identified reversible causes

↓

Review for most frequent causes

- Hypovolemia
- Hypoxia
- Hydrogen ion — acidosis
- Hyper-/hypokalemia
- Hypothermia
- "Tablets" (drug OD, accidents)
- Tamponade, cardiac
- Tension pneumothorax
- Thrombosis, coronary (ACS)
- Thrombosis, pulmonary (embolism)

↓

Epinephrine 1 mg IV push, repeat every 3 to 5 minutes

↓

Atropine 1 mg IV (if PEA rate is ***slow***), repeat every 3 to 5 minutes as needed, to a total dose of 0.04 mg/kg

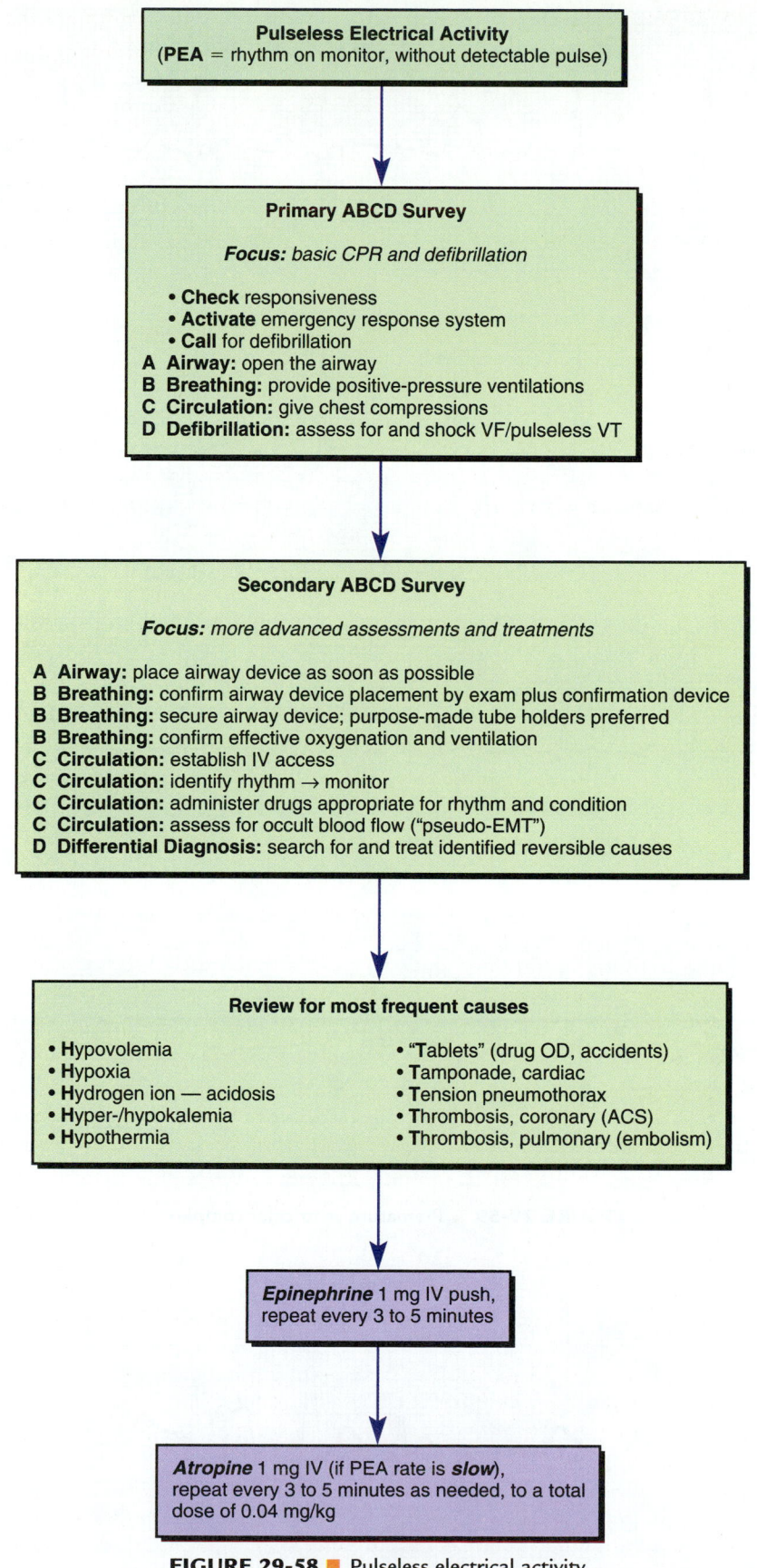

FIGURE 29-58 ■ Pulseless electrical activity.

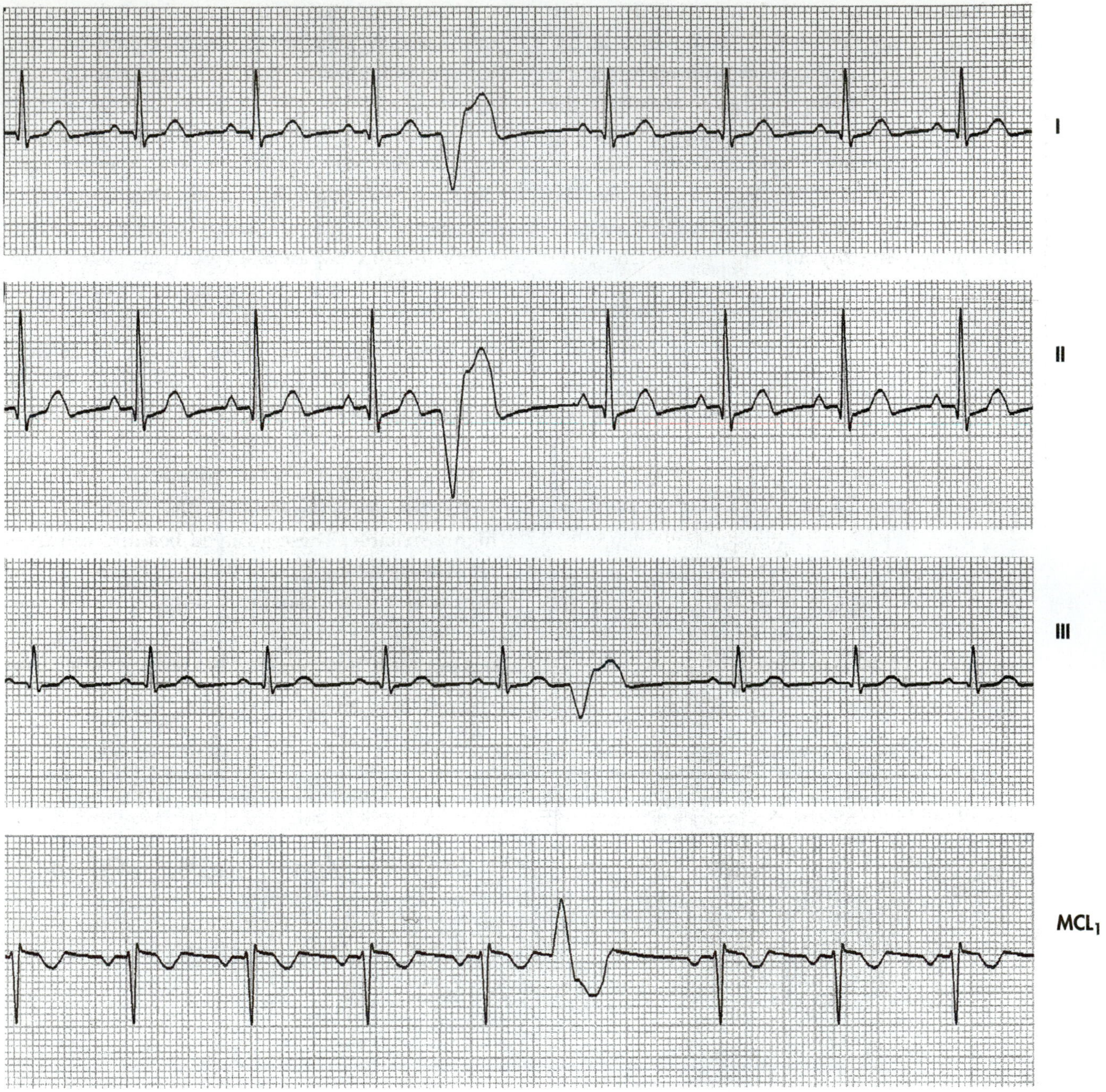

FIGURE 29-59 ■ Premature ventricular complexes.

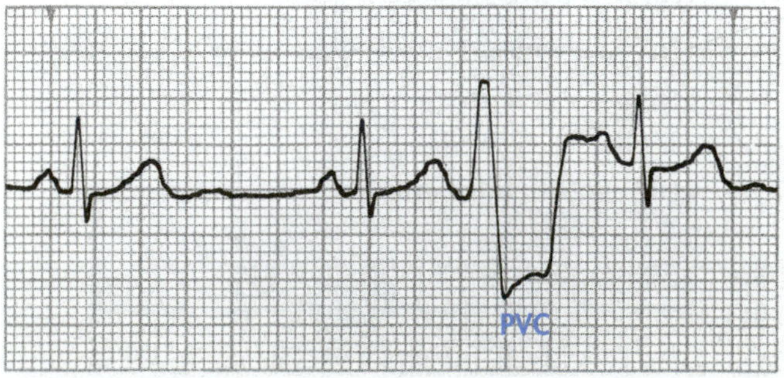

FIGURE 29-60 ■ Interpolated premature ventricular complex.

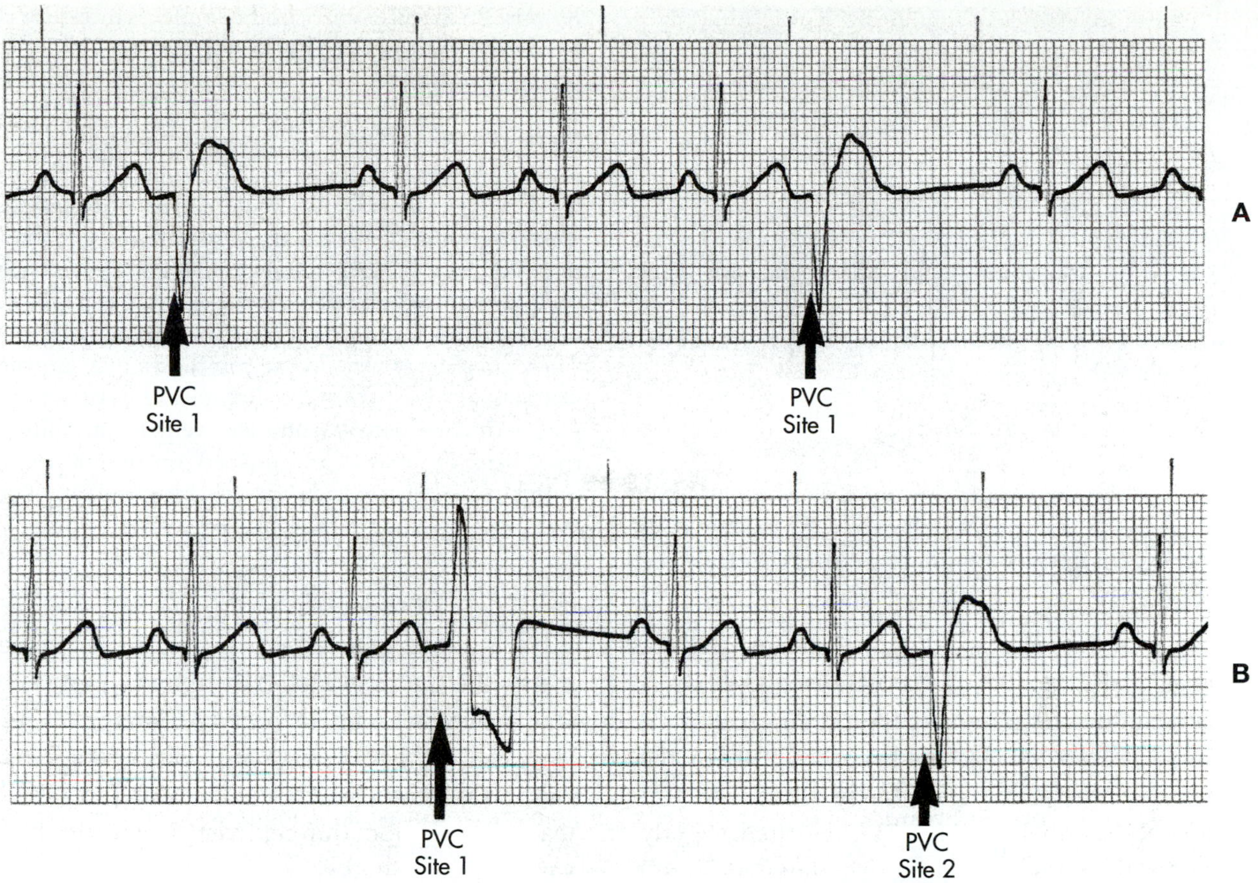

FIGURE 29-61 ■ **A,** Unifocal premature ventricular complexes. **B,** Multifocal premature ventricular complexes.

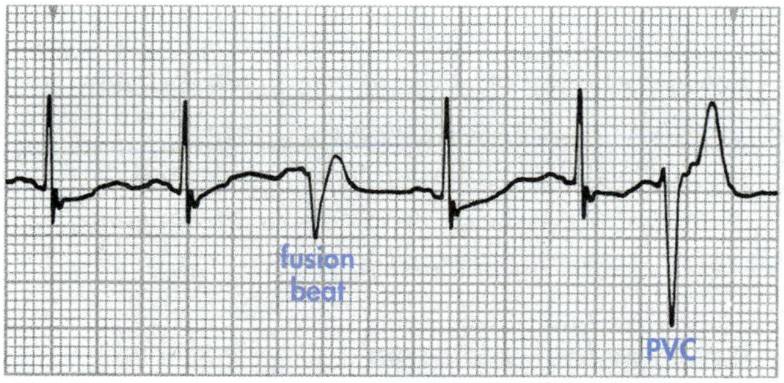

FIGURE 29-62 ■ Fusion beat with premature ventricular complex.

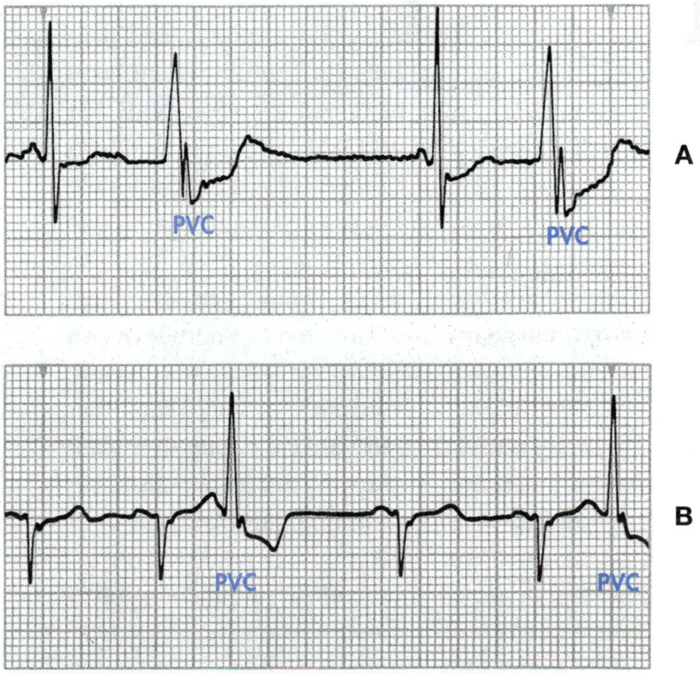

FIGURE 29-63 ■ **A,** Bigeminy (unifocal premature ventricular complexes). **B,** Trigeminy (unifocal premature ventricular complexes).

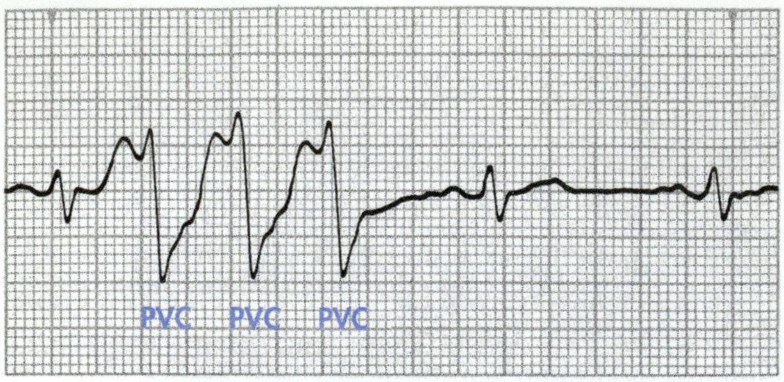

FIGURE 29-64 ■ R-on-T phenomenon (unifocal premature ventricular complexes).

fibrillation. This is especially the case if they occur during the T wave (relative refractory phase) of the cardiac cycle. During this period, the heart muscle is at its greatest electrical instability.

During this period, some of the ventricular muscle fibers may be repolarized partially. Others may be repolarized completely. Still others may be completely refractory. Stimulation of the ventricles in the vulnerable period by an electrical impulse such as a premature ventricular complex, cardiac pacemaker, or cardioversion may cause ventricular fibrillation or ventricular tachycardia. The occurrence of a ventricular depolarization during the relative refractory period is known as the **R-on-T phenomenon** (Fig. 29-64).

ETIOLOGY

Isolated premature ventricular complexes do occur in healthy persons without apparent cause. They usually are of no significance. Pathological premature ventricular complexes usually are a result of one or more of the following:

- Myocardial ischemia
- Hypoxia
- Acid-base and electrolyte imbalance
- Hypokalemia
- Congestive heart failure
- Increased catecholamine and sympathetic tone (as in emotional stress)
- Ingestion of stimulants (alcohol, caffeine, tobacco)
- Drug toxicity
- Sympathomimetic drugs (cocaine; stimulants such as phencyclidine, ***epinephrine,*** and ***isoproterenol***)

RULES FOR INTERPRETATION (LEAD II MONITORING)

Premature ventricular complexes have the following characteristics on the electrocardiogram:

QRS complex: Equal to or greater than 0.12 second; frequently distorted and bizarre

P waves: May be present or absent. If they are present, they usually are of the underlying rhythm and have no relationship to the premature ventricular complex.

Rate: Depends on the underlying rhythm and the number of premature ventricular complexes

Rhythm: Premature ventricular complexes interrupt the regularity of the underlying rhythm.

P-R interval: None

CLINICAL SIGNIFICANCE

Premature ventricular complexes that occur in patients without heart disease usually do not produce serious signs and symptoms, although these patients may complain of skipped beats. Premature ventricular complexes that occur with heart disease (myocardial ischemia) may result from enhanced automaticity, a reentry mechanism, or both. These premature ventricular complexes may trigger lethal ventricular dysrhythmias. Premature ventricular complexes do not permit complete ventricular filling. Also, they may produce a diminished or nonpalpable pulse (nonperfusing premature ventricular complex). If the premature ventricular complexes occur often enough and occur early enough in the cardiac cycle, cardiac output drops.

Warning signs of serious ventricular dysrhythmias in patients with myocardial ischemia include frequent premature ventricular complexes, the presence of multifocal premature ventricular complexes, early premature ventricular complexes (R-on-T phenomenon), and patterns of grouped beating.

MANAGEMENT

Premature ventricular complexes that occur in patients without symptoms and without known heart disease seldom require treatment. In patients with myocardial ischemia, frequent premature ventricular complexes must be treated promptly with oxygen and drugs (e.g., ***lidocaine*** and ***procainamide***).

CRITICAL THINKING

Consider this situation. A ***lidocaine*** drip is not regulated properly and infuses too rapidly. What signs and symptoms might the patient develop?

Ventricular Tachycardia

DESCRIPTION

Ventricular tachycardia is a dysrhythmia defined by three or more consecutive ventricular complexes occurring at a rate of more than 100 beats per minute (Fig. 29-65). This dysrhythmia overrides the primary pacemaker. This dysrhythmia starts suddenly and is triggered by a premature ventricular complex. During ventricular tachycardia, the atria and ventricles are not beating in step with each other. If ventricular tachycardia continues, the patient's condition may become unstable. Ventricular tachycardia can produce unconsciousness. Occasionally, it can even lead to loss of a perfusing pulse. Yet some patients in ventricular tachycardia may be able to walk and talk. The misconception that ventricular tachycardia cannot be associated with reasonable blood pressure may result in a patient being inappropriately managed. The origin of ventricular tachycardia is enhanced automaticity or reentry.

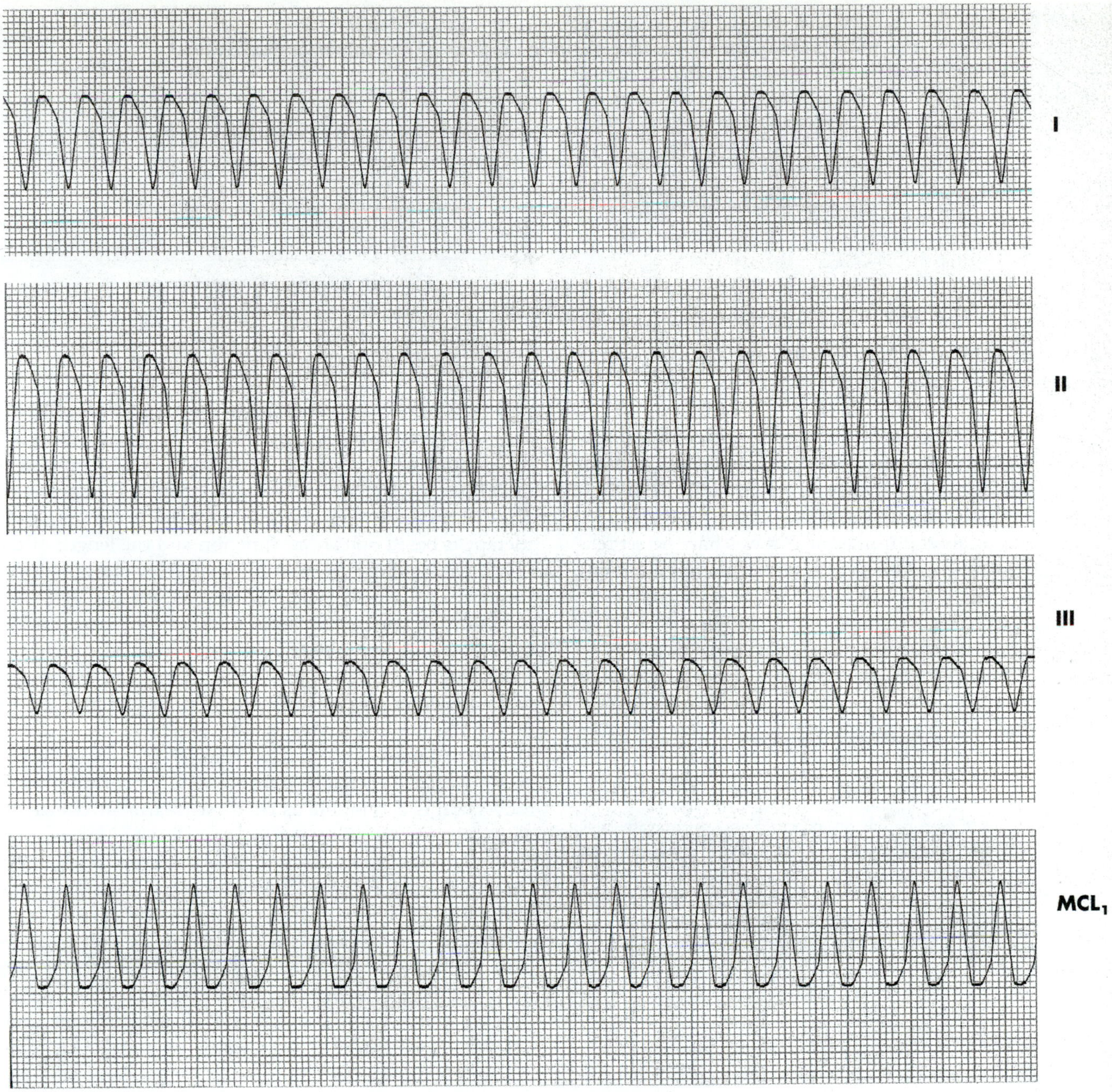

FIGURE 29-65 ■ Ventricular tachycardia.

ETIOLOGY

Like premature ventricular complexes, ventricular tachycardia usually occurs in the presence of myocardial ischemia or significant cardiac disease. Other causes of ventricular tachycardia include the following:

- Acid-base and electrolyte imbalance
- Hypokalemia
- Congestive heart failure
- Increased catecholamine and sympathetic tone (as in emotional stress)
- Ingestion of stimulants (alcohol, caffeine, tobacco)
- Drug toxicity (digitalis, tricyclic antidepressants)
- Sympathomimetic drugs (cocaine, methamphetamines)
- Prolonged Q-T interval (may be caused by drugs, metabolic problems, or be congenital)

> **▶NOTE** Patients with a history of heart attacks with subsequent tachycardias and who are now experiencing a wide-complex tachycardia very likely are in ventricular tachycardia.

▶NOTE Torsades de pointes means "twisting around a point." The condition is a form of ventricular tachycardia characterized by QRS complexes that gradually change back and forth from one shape and direction to another over a series of beats (Fig. 29-66). Torsades de pointes usually is caused by one of a number of conditions that prolong the Q-T interval. These include hypokalemia or hyperkalemia, hypomagnesemia, certain antidysrhythmic medications (quinidine or ***procainamide***), and tricyclic antidepressant overdose.

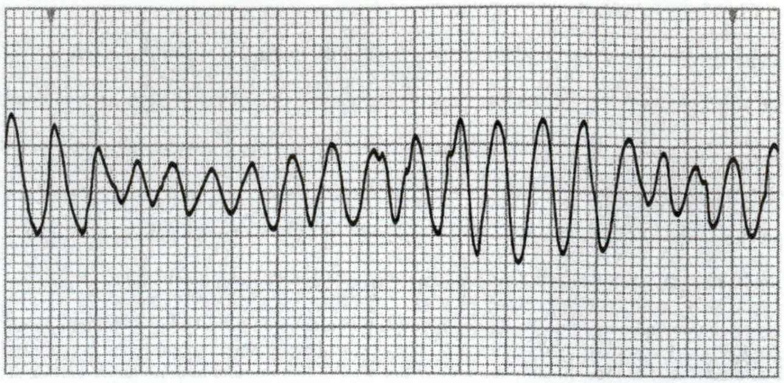

FIGURE 29-66 ■ Torsades de pointes.

RULES FOR INTERPRETATION (LEAD II MONITORING)

Ventricular tachycardia has the following characteristics on the electrocardiogram:

QRS complex: Equal to or greater than 0.12 second and usually distorted and bizarre. The QRS complexes generally are identical, but if fusion beats are present, one or more QRS complexes may differ in size, shape, and direction.

P waves: May be absent. If present, P waves have no set relation to the QRS complex (atrioventricular dissociation). P waves occur at a slower rate than the ventricular focus and are superimposed on the QRS complexes.

Rate: Usually between 100 and 250 beats per minute

Rhythm: Usually regular (unless drug induced) but may be slightly irregular

P-R interval: If P waves are present, the P-R interval varies widely.

▶NOTE Atrioventricular dissociation may precipitate cannon A waves. (These are waves of pulse pressure that are visible in the jugular veins of a patient in ventricular tachycardia.) The cannon A waves result from the right atrium pumping against a closed tricuspid valve that in turn directs the waves of pressure into the jugular veins. Atrioventricular dissociation is diagnostic of ventricular tachycardia.

CLINICAL SIGNIFICANCE

Ventricular tachycardia usually indicates significant heart disease. The rapid rate and the loss of atrial kick cause a drop in cardiac output and decreased coronary artery and cerebral perfusion. The severity of symptoms varies with the rate of the ventricular tachycardia and how much heart disease is present. Ventricular tachycardia may be perfusing or nonperfusing; that is, it may produce a pulse or it may not. Ventricular tachycardia also may lead to ventricular fibrillation.

MANAGEMENT

Treatment for patients with ventricular tachycardia is based on their signs and symptoms and the presence or absence of torsades de pointes (Fig. 29-66). As with supraventricular tachycardias, the paramedic should obtain a history and identify the rhythm (see Fig. 29-47). Management of wide-complex tachycardias of unknown type includes synchronized cardioversion and administration of ***amiodarone*** or ***procainamide*** (Fig. 29-67). Ventricular tachycardia treatment depends on whether the QRS complex is monomorphic (having the same morphology) or polymorphic (having varying morphology). Furthermore, drug therapy is based on cardiac function and the length of the Q-T intervals (Figs. 29-68 and 29-69). However, any wide-complex tachycardia that occurs with serious signs and symptoms—such as chest pain, dyspnea, decreased level of consciousness, or hypotension—may require immediate synchronized cardioversion. Patients that have ventricular tachycardia without a pulse should be treated as if it were ventricular fibrillation (Fig. 29-70).

Synchronized cardioversion (Fig. 29-71) is an effective treatment for ventricular tachycardia. Synchronized cardioversion is acceptable as the first treatment choice for all wide-complex tachycardias, regardless of cardiac function. If synchronized cardioversion is not preferred as the first intervention, several drug therapy treatments are available.

Monomorphic ventricular tachycardia treatment guidelines are based on heart function (ejection fraction) (Box 29-11). Signs and symptoms of failing heart function are pulmonary congestion and decreased level of consciousness. Management of monomorphic ventricular tachycardia with preserved heart function is drug therapy with ***procainamide,*** sotalol, ***amiodarone,*** or ***lidocaine.*** Failing heart function with monomorphic ventricular tachycardia requires administration of ***amiodarone*** or ***lidocaine*** and then, if necessary, synchronized cardioversion.

The patient with polymorphic ventricular tachycardia is usually unstable. This type of ventricular tachycardia can degenerate into ventricular fibrillation quickly. With polymorphic ventricular tachycardia, the paramedic should check to see whether the patient is suffering from torsades de pointes. This type of ventricular tachycardia is usually a product of a prolonged Q-T interval. If torsades de pointes is suspected, treatment needs to be quick. The first action is to discontinue any medications that may prolong the Q-T interval. The second step is to correct any electrolyte imbalances present. Other interventions include ***magnesium sulfate*** intravenously and temporary overdrive pacing. ***Isoproterenol*** may

Wide-Complex Tachycardia of Unknown Origin*

Perform Primary ABCD Survey (Basic Life Support)

(Correct critical problems IMMEDIATELY as they are identified)

- Assess responsiveness, **A**irway, **B**reathing, **C**irculation, ensure availability of monitor/**D**efibrillator

Perform Secondary ABCD Survey (Advanced Life Support)

- Administer oxygen, establish IV access, attach cardiac monitor
- Administer fluids as needed (O_2, IV, monitor, fluids)
- Assess vital signs, attach pulse oximeter, and monitor blood pressure
- Obtain and review 12-lead ECG, portable chest x-ray, perform a focused history and physical exam

Is the patient stable or unstable?
Is the patient experiencing serious signs and symptoms due to the tachycardia?

Use 12-lead ECG/clinical information to help clarify rhythm diagnosis

Rhythm confirmed as SVT Go to narrow-QRS tachycardia algorithm	Wide-Complex Tachycardia of Unknown Origin Stable Patient	Rhythm confirmed as VT Go to VT algorithm

	Normal Cardiac Function	Impaired Cardiac Function
	Sync cardioversion **OR** Procainamide (IIb) **OR** Amiodarone (IIb)	Sync cardioversion **OR** Amiodarone (IIb) Note: Impaired cardiac function = ejection fraction <40% or CHF

If medication therapy ineffective, perform synchronized cardioversion

UNSTABLE PATIENT

If hemodynamically unstable, sync 100 J, 200 J, 300 J, and 360 J or equivalent biphasic energy. If hypotensive (systolic BP < 90), unresponsive, or if severe pulmonary edema exists, defibrillate with same energy.

MEDICATION DOSING:

Amiodarone 150 mg IV bolus over 10 min. if chemical conversion successful, follow with IV infusion of 1 mg/min for 6 hours and then a maintenance infusion of 0.5 mg/min. Repeat supplementary infusions of 150 mg as necessary for recurrent or resistant dysrhythmias. Maximum total daily dose 2 g.

Procainamide† 100 mg over 5 min (20 mg/min). Maximum total dose 17 mg/kg. If chemical conversion successful, maintenance infusion 1 to 4 mg/min.

*The American Heart Association in Collaboration with the International Liaison Committee on Resuscitation (ILCOR). Part 7: Era of Reperfusion Section
†Ryan TJ et al: ACC/AHA guidelines for the management of patients with acute myocardial infarction: 1999 update: a report of the American College of Cardiology/American Heart Association Task Force on Practice Guidelines (Committee on Management of Acute Myocardial Infarction).

FIGURE 29-67 ■ Wide-complex tachycardia of unknown origin.

be administered as a temporary measure while pacing therapy is begun. Other medications include ***phenytoin*** and ***lidocaine.***

Polymorphic ventricular tachycardia with a *prolonged* baseline Q-T interval suggestive of torsades de pointes usually is treated with intravenously administered ***magnesium sulfate.*** This dysrhythmia also is treated with synchronized cardioversion beginning at 200 J (Box 29-12). Polymorphic ventricular tachycardia with a *normal* baseline Q-T interval also can be treated with synchronized cardioversion. In addition, pharmacological agents for treatment of polymorphic ventricular tachycardia (with a normal baseline Q-T interval) consist of ***amiodarone, lidocaine, procainamide,*** sotalol, beta-blockers, and ***phenytoin.***

Drugs given to treat dysrhythmias can cause dysrhythmias; this is called proarrhythmic. Sequential use of two or more antidysrhythmic drugs increases the incidence of bradycardias, hypotension, and torsades de pointes. Avoiding use of more than one antidysrhythmic agent in treating narrow or wide QRS complex tachydysrhythmias is strongly recommended. In most cases, after an adequate dose of a single drug is unsuccessful in ending the dysrhythmia, synchronized cardioversion is the next treatment (Fig. 29-71).

Text continued on p. 755

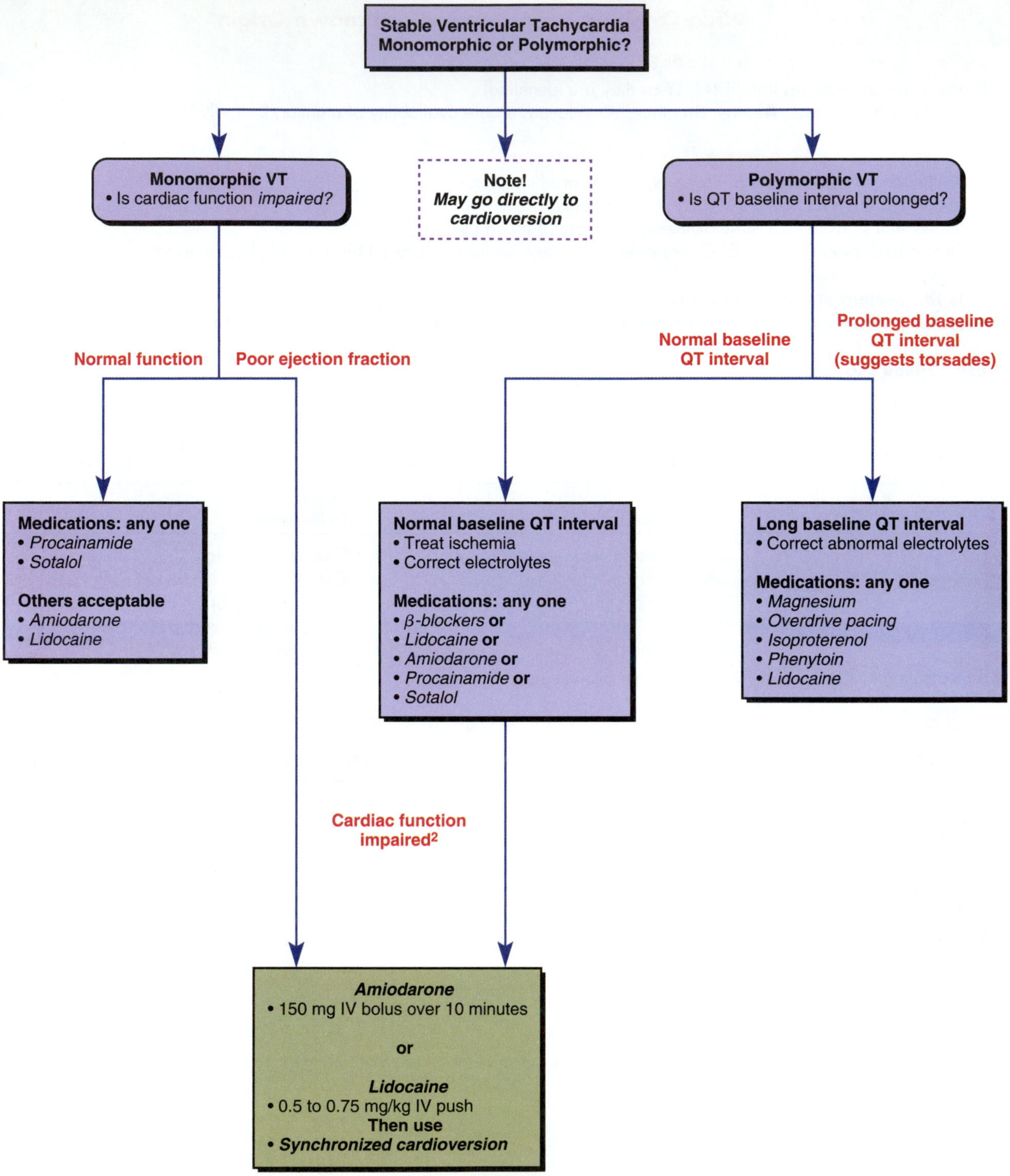

FIGURE 29-68 ■ Stable ventricular tachycardia (monomorphic or polymorphic).

Polymorphic Ventricular Tachycardia*, †

Perform Primary ABCD Survey (Basic Life Support)

(Correct critical problems IMMEDIATELY as they are identified)

- Assess responsiveness, **A**irway, **B**reathing, **C**irculation, ensure availability of monitor/**D**efibrillator

Perform Secondary ABCD Survey (Advanced Life Support)

- Administer oxygen, establish IV access, attach cardiac monitor, administer fluids as needed (O_2, IV, monitor, fluids)
- Assess vital signs, attach pulse oximeter, and monitor blood pressure
- Obtain and review 12-lead ECG, portable chest x-ray, perform a focused history and physical exam

Is the patient stable or unstable?
Is the patient experiencing serious signs and symptoms due to the tachycardia?

Determine if the rhythm is monomorphic or polymorphic VT and determine patient's QT interval.

Polymorphic VT Normal QT interval STABLE PATIENT		Polymorphic VT Prolonged QT interval (Suggests Torsades de Pointes) STABLE PATIENT	
Normal Cardiac Function	**Impaired Cardiac Function**	**Normal Cardiac Function**	**Impaired Cardiac Function**
Treat ischemia if present Correct electrolyte abnormalities May proceed directly to electrical therapy or use **one** of the following: Amiodarone (IIb) Lidocaine (IIb) Procainamide (IIb) Sotalol (IIb) Beta-blockers (Indeterminate). (Indeterminate)	May proceed directly to electrical therapy or **use** one of the following: Amiodarone (IIb) Lidocaine (indeterminate).	DC meds that prolong QT Correct electrolyte abnormalities May proceed directly to electrical therapy or use **one** of the following: Magnesium (Indeterminate) Overdrive pacing with or without beta-blocker (Indeterminate) Phenytoin (Indeterminate) Lidocaine (Indeterminate)	May proceed directly to electrical therapy or use the following: Amiodarone (IIb) Lidocaine (Indeterminate) Isoproterenol Note: Impaired cardiac function = ejection fraction <40% or CHF

If medication therapy ineffective, use electrical therapy.

FIGURE 29-69 ■ Polymorphic ventricular tachycardia.

Continued

UNSTABLE PATIENT

Sustained (>30 seconds or causing hemodynamic collapse) polymorphic VT should be treated with an unsynchronized shock using an initial energy of 200 J; if unsuccessful, a second shock of 200 to 300 J should be given, and, if necessary, a third shock of 360 J.*

MEDICATION DOSING

Amiodarone 150 mg IV bolus over 10 min. If chemical conversion successful, follow with IV infusion of 1 mg/min for 6 hours and then a maintenance infusion of 0.5 mg/min. Repeat supplementary infusions of 150 mg as necessary for recurrent or resistant dysrhythmias. Maximum total daily dose 2 g.

Beta-blockers *Esmolol:* 0.5 mg/kg over 1 minute followed by a maintenance infusion at 50 mcg/kg/min for 4 minutes. If inadequate response, administer a second bolus of 0.5 mg/kg over 1 minute and increase maintenance infusion to 100 mcg/kg/min. The bolus dose (0.5 mg/kg) and titration of the maintenance infusion (addition of 50 mcg/kg/min) can be repeated every 4 minutes to a maximum infusion of 300 mcg/kg/min.
Metoprolol: 5 mg slow IV push over 5 minutes x 3 as needed to a total dose of 15 mg over 15 minutes.
Atenolol: 5 mg slow IV (over 5 min). Wait 10 min then give second dose of 5 mg slow IV (over 5 min).

Isoproterenol Can be used as a temporizing measure until overdrive pacing can be instituted if no evidence of coronary artery disease, ischemic syndromes, or other contraindications. 2 to 10 mcg/min. Mix 1 mg in 500-mL NS or D5W.

Lidocaine 1 to 1.5 mg/kg initial dose. Repeat dose 1/2 the initial dose every 5 to 10 min. Maximum total dose 3 mg/kg. If chemical conversion successful, maintenance infusion 1 to 4 mg/min. If impaired cardiac function, dose = 0.5-0.75 mg/kg IV push. May repeat every 5 to 10 min. Maximum total dose 3 mg/kg. If chemical conversion successful, maintenance infusion 1 to 4 mg/min.

Magnesium‡ Loading dose of 1 to 2 g mixed in 50 to 100-mL over 5 to 60 min IV. If chemical conversion successful, follow with 0.5 to 1.0 g/h IV infusion.

Phenytoin 250 mg IV at a rate of 25-50 mg/min in NS using a central vein.

Procainamide 100 mg over 5 min (20 mg/min). Maximum total dose 17 mg/kg. If chemical conversion successful, maintenance infusion 1 to 4 mg/min.

Sotalol 1 to 1.5 mg/kg IV slowly at a rate of 10 mg/min

*Ryan TJ et al: ACC/AHA guidelines for the management of patients with acute myocardial infarction: 1999 update: a report of the American College of Cardiology/American Heart Association Task Force on Practice Guidelines (Committee on Management of Acute Myocardial Infarction).

†The American Heart Association in Collaboration with the International Liaison Committee on Resuscitation (ILCOR). Part 7: Era of Reperfusion Section 1: Acute Coronary Syndromes (Acute Myocardial Infarction): A Consensus on Science. *Circulation* 2000; 102 (suppl I):I-163.

‡Tzivoni D et al: Treatment of torsade de pointes with magnesium sulfate, *Circulation* 77:392, 1988.

FIGURE 29-69, cont'd ■ Polymorphic ventricular tachycardia.

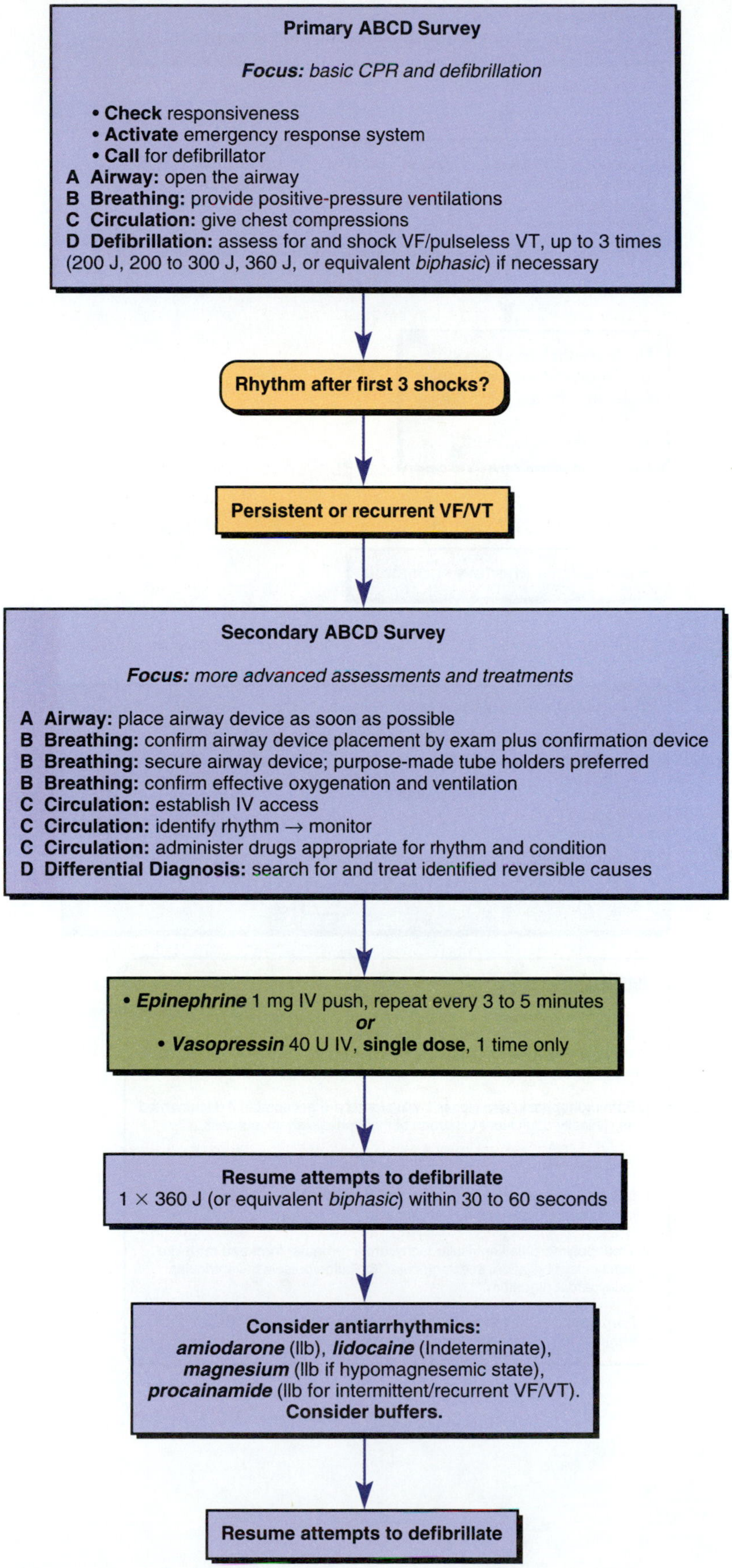
Primary ABCD Survey
Focus: basic CPR and defibrillation
• Check responsiveness
• Activate emergency response system
• Call for defibrillator
A Airway: open the airway
B Breathing: provide positive-pressure ventilations
C Circulation: give chest compressions
D Defibrillation: assess for and shock VF/pulseless VT, up to 3 times (200 J, 200 to 300 J, 360 J, or equivalent biphasic) if necessary
Rhythm after first 3 shocks?
Persistent or recurrent VF/VT
Secondary ABCD Survey
Focus: more advanced assessments and treatments
A Airway: place airway device as soon as possible
B Breathing: confirm airway device placement by exam plus confirmation device
B Breathing: secure airway device; purpose-made tube holders preferred
B Breathing: confirm effective oxygenation and ventilation
C Circulation: establish IV access
C Circulation: identify rhythm → monitor
C Circulation: administer drugs appropriate for rhythm and condition
D Differential Diagnosis: search for and treat identified reversible causes
• Epinephrine 1 mg IV push, repeat every 3 to 5 minutes
or
• Vasopressin 40 U IV, single dose, 1 time only
Resume attempts to defibrillate
1 × 360 J (or equivalent biphasic) within 30 to 60 seconds
Consider antiarrhythmics:
amiodarone (IIb), lidocaine (Indeterminate),
magnesium (IIb if hypomagnesemic state),
procainamide (IIb for intermittent/recurrent VF/VT).
Consider buffers.
Resume attempts to defibrillate

FIGURE 29-70 ■ Ventricular fibrillation/pulseless ventricular tachycardia.

Tachycardia
With serious signs and symptoms related to the tachycardia

↓

If ventricular rate is >150 bpm, prepare for **immediate *cardioversion.*** May give brief trial of medications based on specific arrhythmias. Immediate cardioversion is generally not needed if heart rate is ≤150 bpm.

↓

Have available at bedside
- Oxygen saturation monitor
- Suction device
- IV line
- Intubation equipment

↓

Premedicate whenever possible

↓

Synchronized cardioversion

- Ventricular tachycardia
- Paroxysmal supraventricular tachycardia
- Atrial fibrillation
- Atrial flutter

→ 100 J, 200 J, 300 J, 360 J monophasic energy dose (or clinically equivalent biphasic energy dose)

Notes:

1. Effective regimens have included a sedative (eg, ***diazepam, midazolam, barbiturates, etomidate, ketamine, methohexital***) with or without an analgesic agent (eg, ***fentanyl, morphine, meperidine***). Many experts recommend anesthesia if service is readily available.
2. Both monophasic and biphasic waveforms are acceptable if documented as clinically equivalent to reports of monophasic shock success.
3. Note possible need to resynchronize after each cardioversion.
4. If delays in synchronization occur and clinical condition is critical, go immediately to unsynchronized shocks.
5. Treat polymorphic ventricular tachycardia (irregular form and rate) like ventricular fibrillation: see ventricular fibrillation/pulseless ventricular tachycardia algorithm.
6. Paroxysmal supraventricular tachycardia and atrial flutter often respond to lower energy levels (start with 50 J).

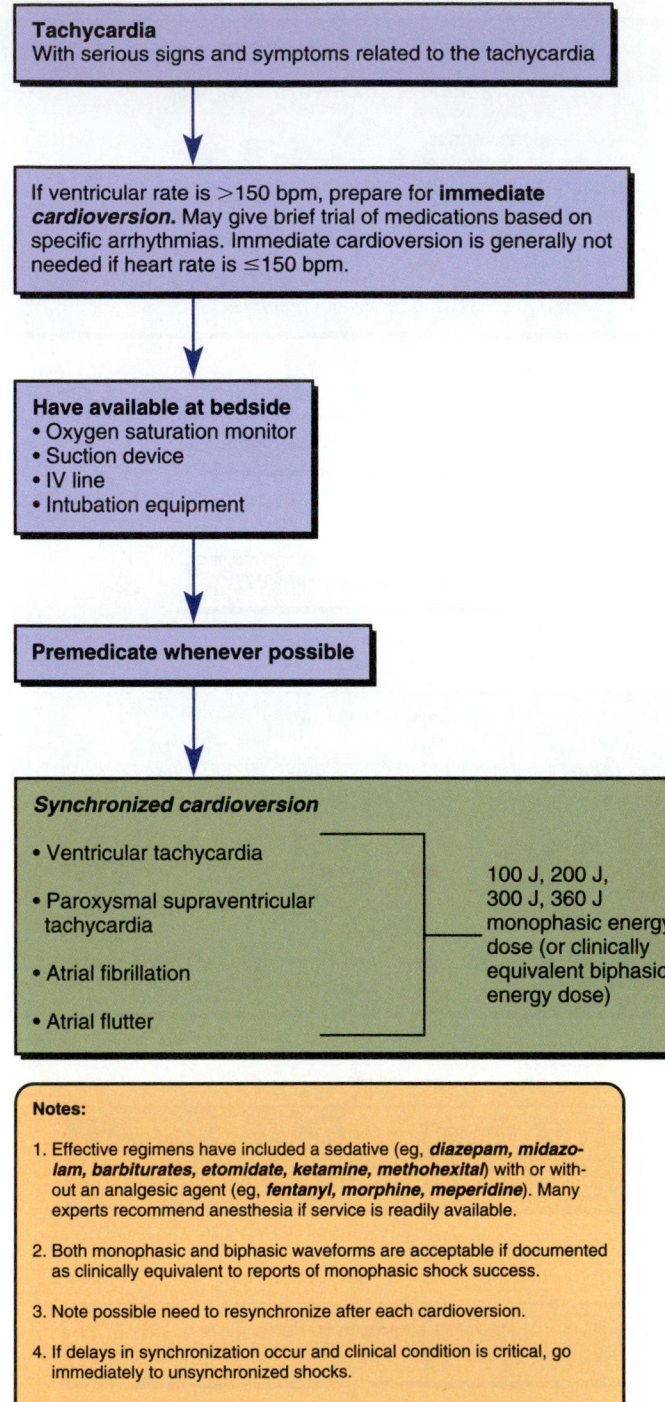

FIGURE 29-71 ■ Synchronized cardioversion.

BOX 29-11 Sequence of Care for Perfusing Monomorphic Ventricular Tachycardia

1. Consider synchronized cardioversion
2. Consider antidysrhythmics:
   a. Normal heart function
      - Procainamide (Class IIa)
      - Sotalol (Class IIa)
      - Amiodarone
      - Lidocaine
   b. Impaired heart function
      - Amiodarone
      - Lidocaine
3. Synchronized cardioversion

BOX 29-12 Sequence of Care for Perfusing Polymorphic Ventricular Tachycardia

- Consider synchronized cardioversion
- Treat ischemia and electrolyte imbalances
- Consider antidysrhythmics
  - ***Amiodarone*** (Class IIb)
  - ***Lidocaine*** (Class IIb)
  - ***Procainamide*** (Class IIb)
  - Sotalol (Class IIa)
  - Beta-Blockers (Class Indeterminate)
  - ***Phenytoin*** (Class Indeterminate)

If rhythm is suggestive of torsades de pointes:

- Discontinue any medications known to prolong the QT interval
- Correct electrolyte imbalances
- Consider antidysrhythmics
  - ***Magnesium Sulfate*** (Class Indeterminate)
  - Overdrive pacing
    - Beta-Blockers (as an adjunct to pacing)
  - ***Isoproterenol*** (temporary measure while overdrive pacing initiated)
  - ***Phenytoin*** (Class Indeterminate)
  - ***Lidocaine*** (Class Indeterminate)
- Severe hemodynamically unstable polymorphic VT should be treated as pulseless VT using the VF/Pulseless VT algorithm.

American Heart Association. Guidelines 2000 for Cardiopulmonary Resuscitation and Emergency Cardiovascular Care, International Consensus on Science. *Supplement to Circulation.* 2000;102(8): 115–116, 159, 163–165.

NOTE Torsades de pointes is a special form of ventricular tachycardia. It may not respond to the recommended antidysrhythmics ***lidocaine*** and ***magnesium sulfate***. The first step is to stop medications that are known to prolong the Q-T interval. This step also includes correcting any electrolyte or metabolic disorders. Overdrive pacing may be used to try to control ventricular rate. At times, ***isoproterenol*** is useful in abolishing torsades de pointes. It decreases repolarization rates and causes a sinus tachycardia overdrive. ***Magnesium sulfate*** also has been shown to suppress runs of torsades de pointes. It therefore is crucial to search for an underlying cause of this rhythm and to institute corrective measures if possible.

Pulseless ventricular tachycardia is treated like ventricular fibrillation.

Monitored adult patients who become pulseless may be managed with a solitary precordial thump when a defibrillator is not readily available.[1] A precordial thump may terminate a dysrhythmia by causing ventricular depolarization and allowing a normal, organized rhythm to return. To deliver a precordial thump, the arm and wrist should be parallel to the long axis of the sternum. This will help to avoid rib fractures and other injury. The paramedic delivers the thump to the midsternum with the heel of the fist from 10 to 12 inches above the patient's chest.

12-LEAD STRATEGIES FOR WIDE-COMPLEX TACHYCARDIAS

If an unstable patient's QRS complex is wide (greater than 0.12 second) and fast (greater than 150 beats), immediate cardioversion may be indicated. If the patient is stable, however, the following steps in multilead assessments may help distinguish between ventricular tachycardia and other wide-complex tachycardias[5]:

1. Assess leads I, II, III, MCL_1 (V_1), and MCL_6 (V_6). If the QRS complex is negative in leads I, II, and III and positive in MCL_1 (V_1), the rhythm indicates ventricular tachycardia (Fig. 29-72). If these criteria are not met, proceed to step 2.
2. Assess the QRS deflection in MCL_1 (V_1) and MCL_6 (V_6). Regardless of the QRS deflection in leads I, II, and III, positive QRS deflections with a single peak, a taller left "rabbit ear," or an RS complex with a fat R wave or slurred S wave in MCL_1 (V_1) indicates ventricular tachycardia. A negative QS complex, a negative RS complex, or any wide Q wave in MCL_6 (V_6) also indicates ventricular tachycardia (Fig. 29-73).
3. A negative QRS complex in lead I, positive QRS complex in leads II and III, and a negative QRS complex in MCL_1 (V_1) indicates ventricular tachycardia (Fig. 29-74).
4. If all precordial leads (V leads) are positive or negative (precordial concordance), the rhythm indicates ventricular tachycardia (Fig. 29-75).
5. If the RS interval is greater than 0.10 second in any V lead (increased ventricular activation time), the rhythm indicates ventricular tachycardia (Fig. 29-76).

NOTE These steps involve identifying the predominant direction of flow of impulses in the heart (axis), further described later in this chapter.

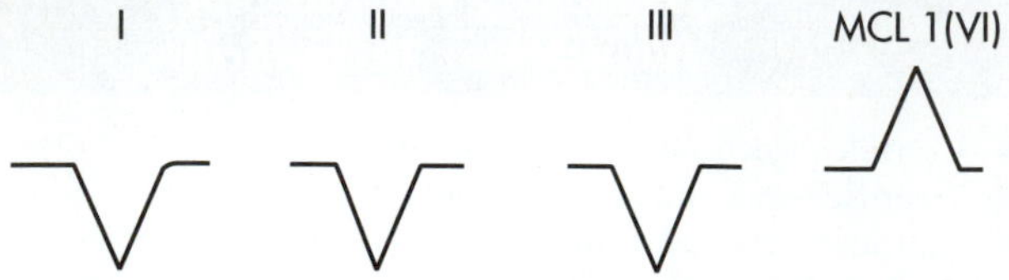

FIGURE 29-72 ■ Criteria for ventricular tachycardia.

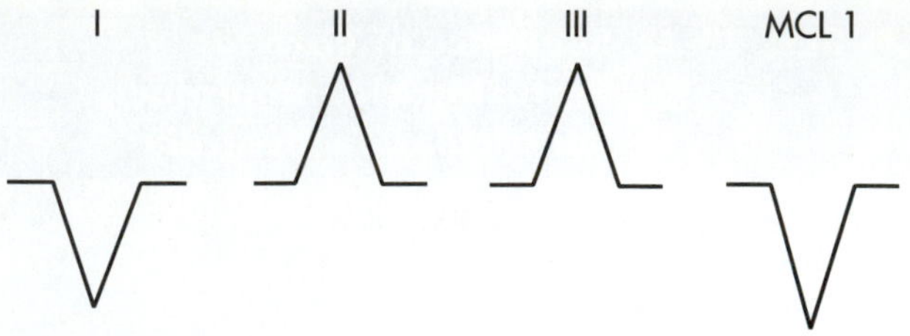

FIGURE 29-74 ■ Right axis deviation and a downward MCL_1 indicates ventricular tachycardia.

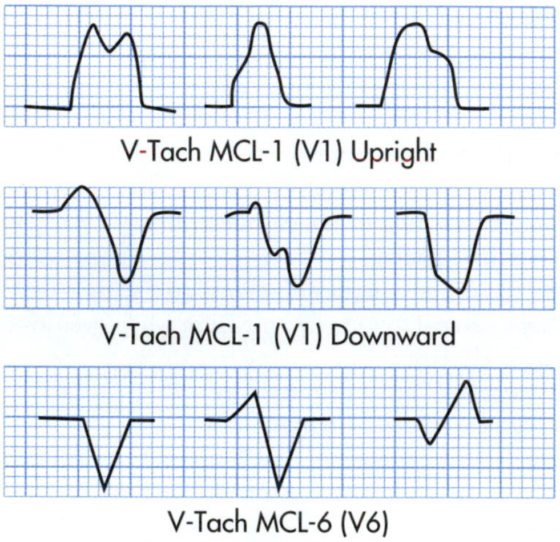

FIGURE 29-73 ■ Step 1: A QRS complex that is negative in leads I, II, III, and positive in MCL_1 (V_1) indicates ventricular tachycardia. Step 2: Assess the QRS complex in MCL_1 (V_1) and MCL_6 (V_6). Step 3: Assess the QRS complex in leads I, II, III and MCL_1 (V_1).

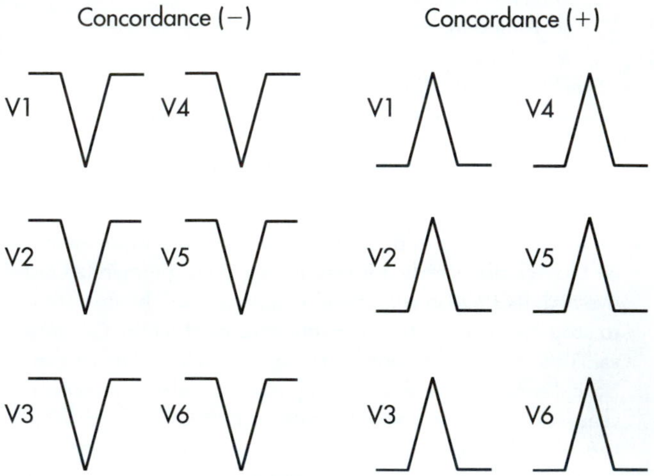

FIGURE 29-75 ■ Ventricular tachycardia-concordance.

▶NOTE Non-ventricular tachycardia precordial concordance may occur in patients who have Wolff-Parkinson-White syndrome and associated left bundle branch block.

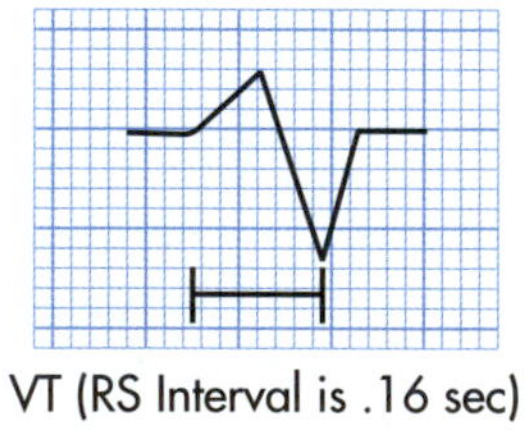

FIGURE 29-76 ■ RS interval.

CRITICAL THINKING

Why is it crucial to distinguish between ventricular tachycardia and wide-complex tachycardias in stable patients?

CRITICAL THINKING

How will you manage a patient with ventricular tachycardia, chest pain, or difficulty breathing if you cannot establish an intravenous line?

Ventricular Fibrillation

DESCRIPTION

Ventricular fibrillation is a quivering of the ventricles and results in pulselessness (Fig. 29-77). Organized ventricular contraction does not occur. Ventricular fibrillation is the most common initial rhythm disturbance in sudden cardiac arrest. It results from multifocal reentry foci in the ventricles.

ETIOLOGY

Ventricular fibrillation most commonly is associated with significant heart disease. The dysrhythmias also may be precipitated by premature ventricular complexes, the R-on-T phenomenon (rarely), or a sustained ventricular tachycardia. Other causes include the following:

- Myocardial ischemia
- Acute myocardial infarction
- Third-degree atrioventricular block with a slow ventricular escape rhythm
- Cardiomyopathy
- Digitalis toxicity
- Hypoxia
- Acidosis

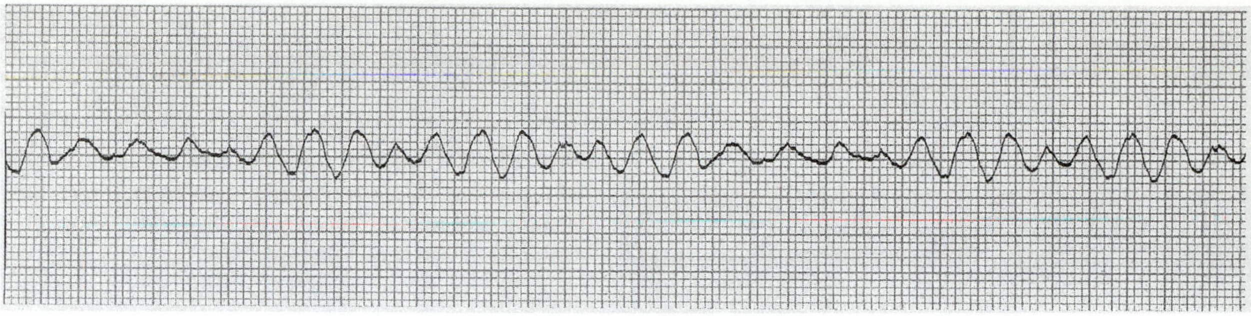

FIGURE 29-77 ■ Ventricular fibrillation.

- Electrolyte imbalance (hypokalemia, hyperkalemia, submersion)
- Electrical injury
- Drug overdose or toxicity (cocaine, tricyclic antidepressants)

RULES FOR INTERPRETATION (ALL LEADS)

Ventricular fibrillation has the following characteristics on the electrocardiogram:

QRS complex: Absent
P waves: Absent
Rate: No coordinated ventricular contractions are present. The unsynchronized ventricular impulses occur at rates from 300 to 500 beats per minute.
Rhythm: Irregularly irregular
P-R interval: Absent

Because organized depolarizations of the atria and ventricles are absent, P waves, QRS complexes, ST segments, and T waves are absent. Ventricular fibrillatory waves are seen on the oscilloscope as bizarre, rounded or pointed. They also appear considerably different in shape. They vary at random from positive to negative as well. These waves represent twitching of small individual groups of muscle fibers. Fibrillatory waves less than 3 mm in amplitude are called *fine* ventricular fibrillation. Those greater than 3 mm are called *coarse* ventricular fibrillation (Fig. 29-78). The fibrillatory waves may be so fine that they appear as a flat line, resembling ventricular asystole.

> ▶**NOTE** Coarse ventricular fibrillation usually indicates the recent onset of ventricular fibrillation. It readily can be converted by prompt defibrillation. The presence of fine ventricular fibrillation that approaches asystole often means that a considerable delay has occurred since collapse and that successful defibrillation is more difficult.[2]

CLINICAL SIGNIFICANCE

Ventricular fibrillation causes all life functions to cease because of the lack of circulating blood flow. The dysrhythmia initially may result in light-headedness. Ventricular fibrillation usually is followed within seconds by loss of consciousness, apnea, and if untreated, death.

MANAGEMENT

For adult resuscitation, management of ventricular fibrillation and pulseless ventricular tachycardia is the most important sequence because most adult cardiac arrests result from these two rhythm disturbances and the vast majority of successful resuscitations result from the appropriate management of these two dysrhythmias (see Fig. 29-70).[1] Ventricular fibrillation and nonperfusing ventricular tachycardia are managed alike: basic life support (if a defibrillator is not immediately available), defibrillation, endotracheal intubation, and pharmacological therapy (***epinephrine, lidocaine, amiodarone,*** and in some cases ***magnesium*** and ***procainamide***) (Box 29-13).

Ventricular Asystole

DESCRIPTION

Ventricular asystole (cardiac standstill) refers to the absence of all ventricular activity (Fig. 29-79).

ETIOLOGY

Ventricular asystole may be the cause of cardiac arrest. It also may occur in complete heart block when there is no escape pacemaker. The dysrhythmia usually is associated with extensive heart disease. It often follows ventricular tachycardia, ventricular fibrillation, pulseless electrical activity, or an agonal escape rhythm in the dying heart. When faced with an isoelectric line on the monitor, the paramedic should confirm asystole as the rhythm. The paramedic can do this by changing placement of the leads by 90 degrees or switching to a second lead on the monitor.

> ▶**NOTE** If the monitor appears to show asystole, fine ventricular fibrillation still may be the underlying rhythm. Asystole should be confirmed in two leads (90 degrees apart) to rule out fine ventricular fibrillation so that the patient may be identified as "shockable."

RULES FOR INTERPRETATION (ALL LEADS)

Ventricular asystole has the following characteristics on the electrocardiogram:

QRS complexes: Absent
P waves: Absent or present

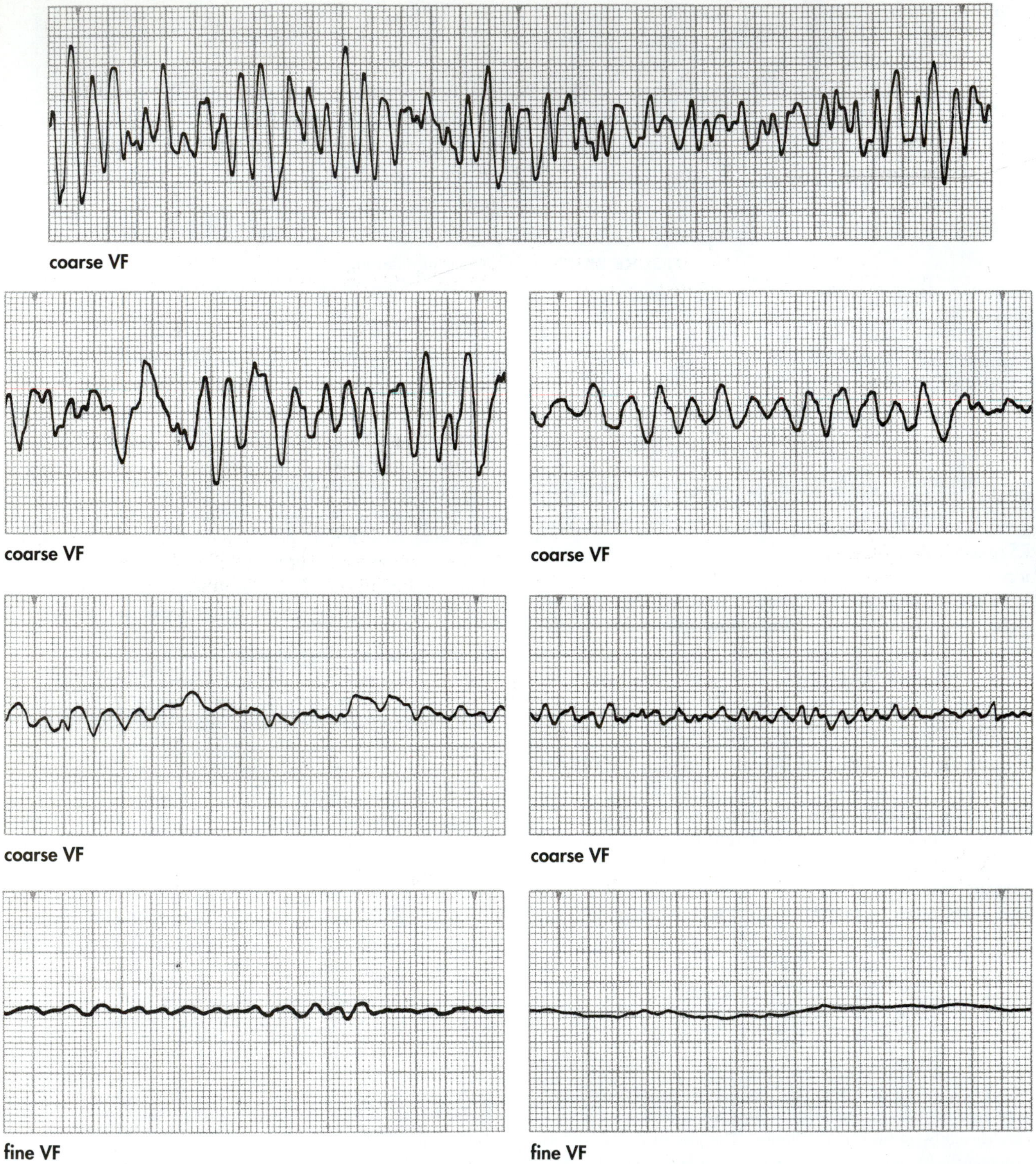

FIGURE 29-78 ■ Coarse and fine ventricular fibrillation.

BOX 29-13 Sequence of Care for Ventricular Fibrillation and Pulseless Ventricular Tachycardia

Basic life support measures
Defibrillation
Endotracheal intubation/IV access
Epinephrine
Vasopressin
Antidysrhythmics
- ***Amiodarone***
- ***Lidocaine***
- ***Magnesium sulfate***
- ***Procainamide***

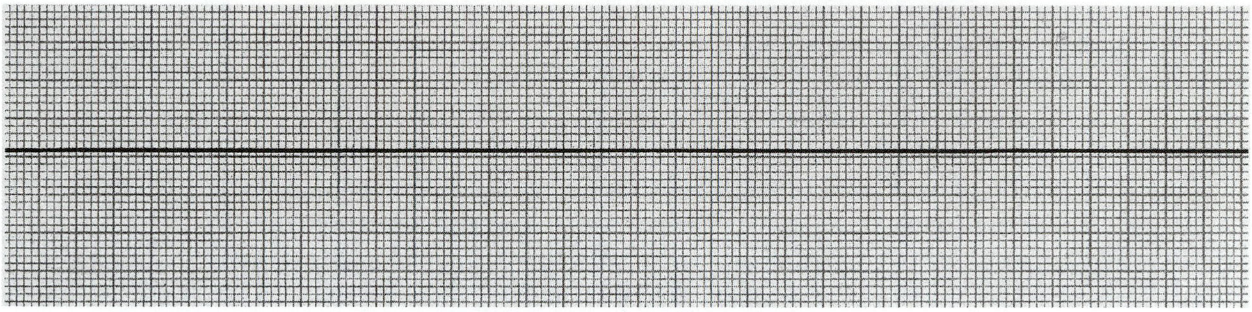

FIGURE 29-79 ■ Ventricular asystole.

Rate: Absent
Rhythm: Absent
P-R Interval: Absent

CLINICAL SIGNIFICANCE

Ventricular asystole produces no cardiac output and is an ominous dysrhythmia. Asystole often confirms death. The chance for resuscitation is small.

MANAGEMENT

The management for ventricular asystole is basic life support, endotracheal intubation, and pharmacological therapy (***epinephrine, atropine,*** and possibly ***sodium bicarbonate***) (Fig. 29-80). If fine ventricular fibrillation is suspected, defibrillation is indicated. However, defibrillating asystole "just in case" is not recommended.[1] The stopping of resuscitation efforts in the prehospital setting after meeting medical protocol is indicated for this patient situation. Potential causes of asystole that the paramedic should consider before cessation of resuscitative efforts include hypoxia, hyperkalemia, hypothermia, drug overdose, and acidosis (Box 29-14).

CRITICAL THINKING

What benefit is there to the community and to the patient's family when resuscitation is halted in the field after following all appropriate guidelines?

Artificial Pacemaker Rhythms

DESCRIPTION

Artificial pacemakers generate a rhythm (Fig. 29-81). They generate this rhythm by regular electrical stimulation of the heart through an electrode implanted in the heart. The electrode is connected to a power source (a battery cell implanted subcutaneously, typically the right or left side of the chest). The tip of the pacemaker wire is at the apex of the right ventricle (ventricular pacemaker), in the right atrium (atrial pacemaker), or in both locations (dual-chamber pacemaker). These devices are placed in patients with complete heart block. They also are used by patients who have episodes of severe symptomatic bradycardia.

Some pacemakers fire continuously at a preset rate regardless of the patient's own electrical activity. These are known as *fixed-rate* or *asynchronous pacemakers.* They rarely are used today. Other pacemakers fire only if the patient's own rate drops below the preset rate of the pacemaker. (Thus they act as an escape rhythm.) These are known as *demand pacemakers.* Atrial and ventricular demand pacemakers pace the atria and ventricles when the intrinsic rate of the paced chamber drops dangerously low. *Atrial synchronous ventricular pacemakers* are in step with the patient's atrial rhythm. This type of pacemaker paces the ventricle after the patient's atria contract. This pacemaker is useful in patients with normal sinus node activity but various degrees of atrioventricular block. *Atrioventricular sequential pacemakers* pace the atria first and then the ventricles when normal impulses are absent or slowed in either or both chambers. If regular atrial activity is too slow, for example, then both chambers are paced sequentially to maintain the atrial kick. If the atrial rate is adequate, the atrial pacer does not fire. The ventricular pacemaker still fires if the ventricular rate is below a preset rate. This pacemaker is ideal for sick sinus syndrome and sinus arrest.

A class of newer pacemakers are rate-responsive pacemakers. These pacemakers can adjust their pacing rates to a patient's needs. They do this by sensing when cardiac output should be increased. Several methods of sensing metabolic

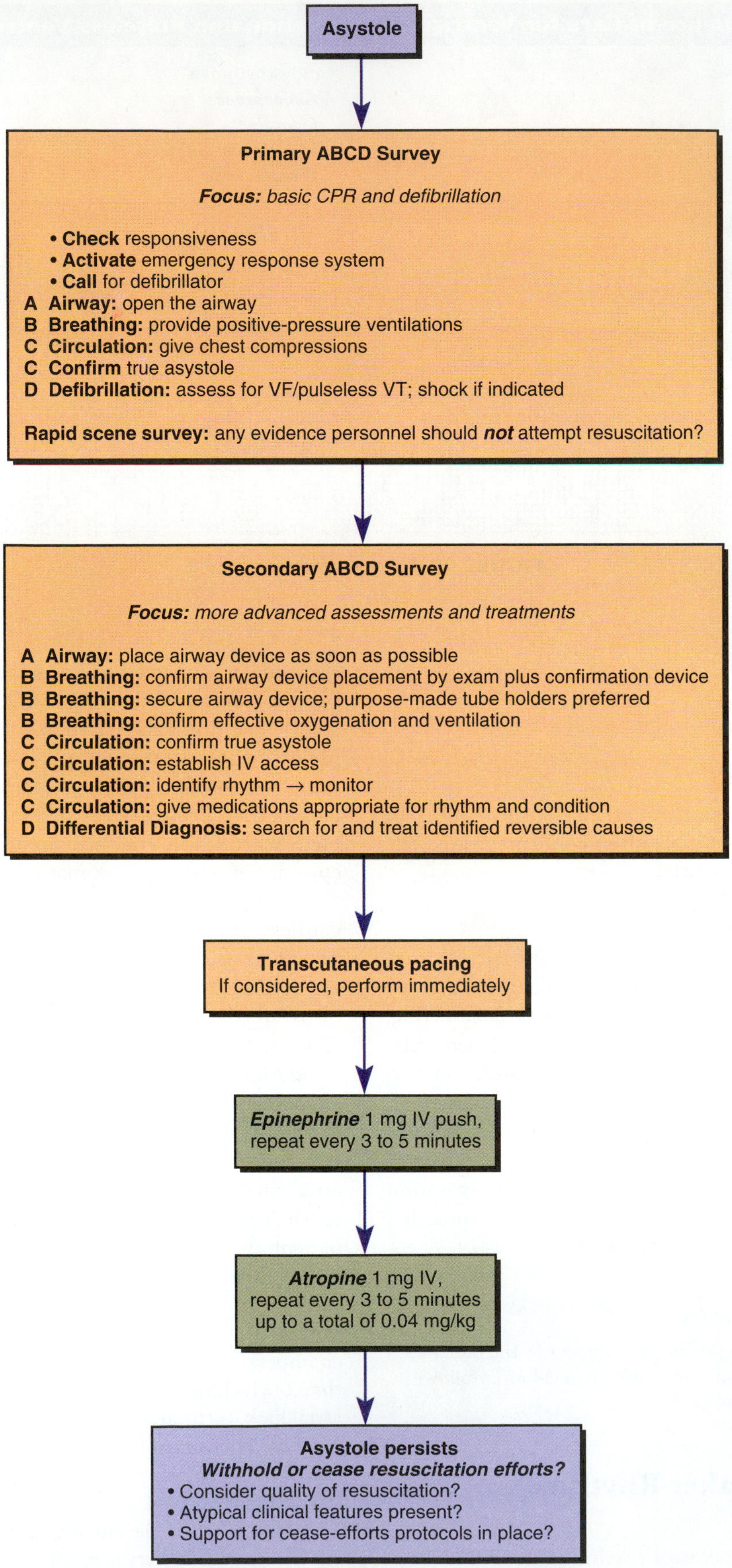
Asystole
Primary ABCD Survey
Focus: basic CPR and defibrillation
• Check responsiveness
• Activate emergency response system
• Call for defibrillator
A Airway: open the airway
B Breathing: provide positive-pressure ventilations
C Circulation: give chest compressions
C Confirm true asystole
D Defibrillation: assess for VF/pulseless VT; shock if indicated
Rapid scene survey: any evidence personnel should not attempt resuscitation?
Secondary ABCD Survey
Focus: more advanced assessments and treatments
A Airway: place airway device as soon as possible
B Breathing: confirm airway device placement by exam plus confirmation device
B Breathing: secure airway device; purpose-made tube holders preferred
B Breathing: confirm effective oxygenation and ventilation
C Circulation: confirm true asystole
C Circulation: establish IV access
C Circulation: identify rhythm → monitor
C Circulation: give medications appropriate for rhythm and condition
D Differential Diagnosis: search for and treat identified reversible causes
Transcutaneous pacing
If considered, perform immediately
Epinephrine 1 mg IV push, repeat every 3 to 5 minutes
Atropine 1 mg IV, repeat every 3 to 5 minutes up to a total of 0.04 mg/kg
Asystole persists
Withhold or cease resuscitation efforts?
• Consider quality of resuscitation?
• Atypical clinical features present?
• Support for cease-efforts protocols in place?

FIGURE 29-80 ■ Asystole: the silent heart algorithm.

BOX 29-14 Sequence of Care for Asystole

Basic life suport
Endotracheal intubation/IV access
TCP
Epinephrine
Atropine
Sodium bicarbonate (possibly)

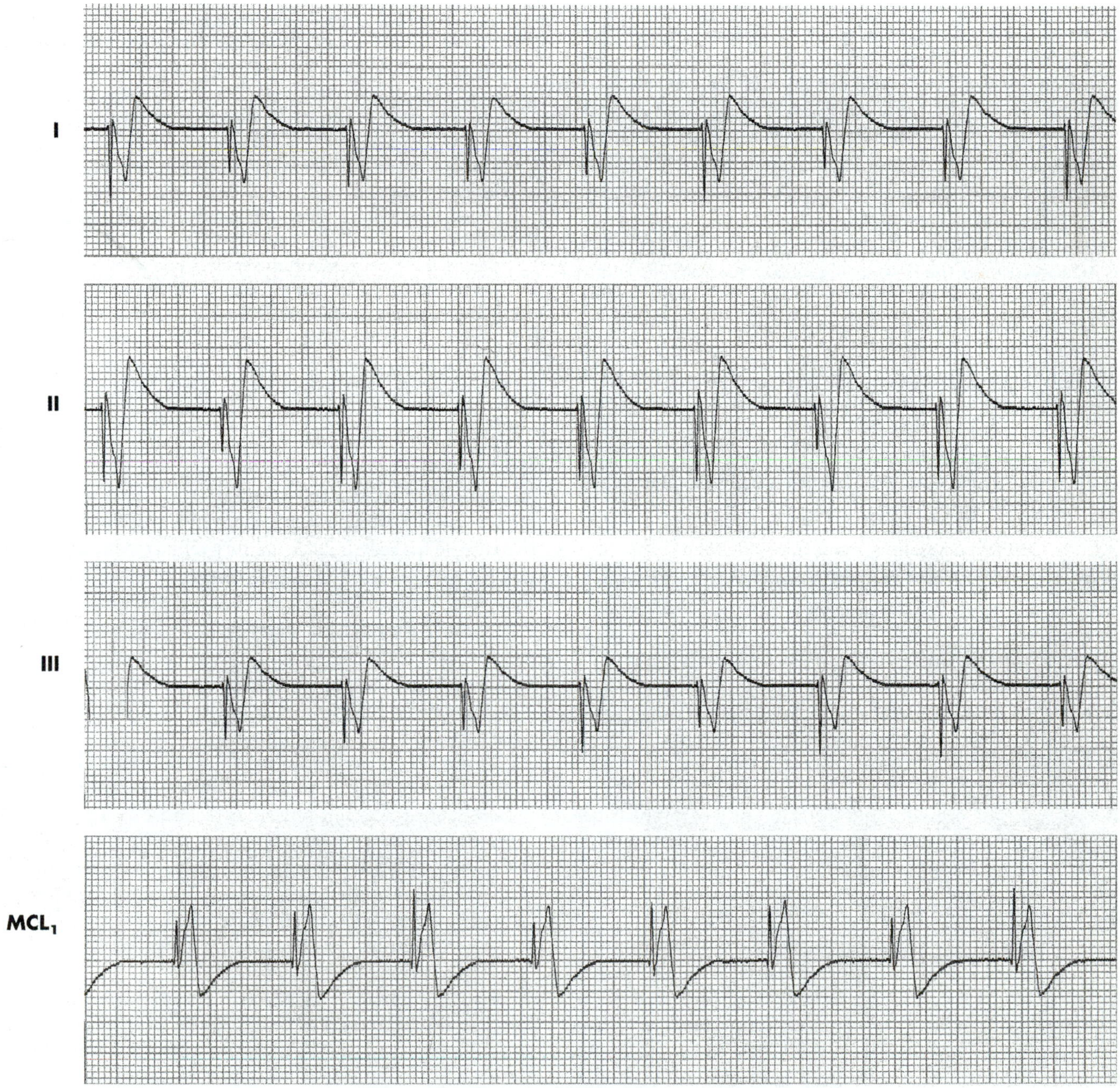

FIGURE 29-81 ■ Artificial pacemaker rhythms.

activity are used. However, the most popular rate-responsive pacers detect patient movement to determine the best firing rate. These devices are popular. They can increase cardiac output and increase tolerance of physical activity. At times these pacemakers may increase the patient's pacing rate inappropriately. They may do this if they sense muscle movement that is not caused by increased patient activity.

RULES FOR INTERPRETATION (LEAD II MONITORING)

Artificial pacemaker rhythms have the following characteristics on the electrocardiogram:

QRS complex: If pacemaker induced, QRS complexes are 0.12 second or greater. Their appearance usually is bizarre, resembling a premature ventricular complex. The pacemaker is said to be "capturing" if each pacemaker spike elicits a QRS complex. If only the atria are being paced, the QRS complexes usually are normal, provided no bundle branch block is present. With demand pacemakers, some of the patient's own QRS complexes may be present. These normal QRS complexes occur without pacemaker spikes.

P waves: May be present or absent, normal or abnormal. The relationship of the P waves to the pacemaker (QRS) complex varies by type of artificial pacemaker. Pacemaker spikes precede QRS complexes induced by ventricular pacemakers, whereas dual-chambered pacemakers also produce an atrial spike followed by a P wave. The pacemaker spike is a narrow deflection on the oscilloscope and represents the electrical discharge of the pacemaker. Pacemaker spikes indicate only that a pacemaker is discharging. They provide no information about ventricular contraction or perfusion.

CRITICAL THINKING

If the pacemaker fails, what rhythms might you see on the monitor?

Rate: Varies according to the preset rate of the pacemaker. Typically the rate is 60 to 80 beats per minute.

Rhythm: Regular if pacing is constant; irregular if pacing occurs only on demand

P-R interval: The presence and duration of P-R intervals depend on the underlying rhythm and vary by the type of artificial pacemaker.

CLINICAL SIGNIFICANCE

Pacemaker spikes indicate that the patient's heart rate is being regulated by an artificial pacemaker. Pacemaker spikes followed by QRS complexes indicate electrical capture. If spikes do not elicit a QRS complex, the pacemaker is not capturing the ventricle electrically. Thus there will be no ventricular contraction. A large percentage of pacemaker failures occur within the first month after implantation (Box 29-15).

BOX 29-15 Four Potential Causes of Pacemaker Malfunction

1. Battery failure: Most implanted pacemakers today use a lithium-iodine cell power source. This source provides stable voltage output for about 80% to 90% of the life of the battery. (The battery life is 5 to 10 years or more.) Battery failure usually slows the pacemaker rate. It also usually decreases the spike amplitude. If the battery fails, the patient may have bradycardia or asystole.
2. Runaway pacemakers: Runaway pacemakers are ones that develop rapid discharge rates that may reach 300 beats per minute. This occurs as the batteries decrease their voltage output. This type of failure rarely is seen in pacemakers used today because the newer power sources provide a gradual increase in rate as their batteries run low.
3. Failure of the sensing device in demand pacemakers: Demand pacemakers may fail to shut off when patients have an adequate rate of their own. When this occurs, there is a competition between the natural and artificial pacemakers of the heart. The pacemaker may discharge during the vulnerable period of the cardiac cycle. This may result in dysrhythmias.
4. Failure to capture: A failure of the pacemaker to capture may result from a variety of causes. These may include battery failure, loose or broken catheter electrode wires, inoperable electrodes, and a shift in the location of the catheter tip. In such cases, pacemaker spikes usually are present. However, they are not followed by P waves or QRS complexes.

MANAGEMENT

Pacemaker failure is a true emergency. It requires immediate recognition. It also requires rapid transport for definitive care. (This may include battery replacement or temporary pacemaker insertion.) The paramedic should not delay transport while attempting to stabilize these patients. The following five principles apply to treating patients with pacemakers:

1. When examining an unconscious patient, be alert for battery packs implanted under the skin. Also be alert for any medical alert information.
2. Manage all dysrhythmias per the appropriate algorithm.
3. Manage ventricular irritability with ***lidocaine*** without fear of suppressing ventricular response to a pacemaker rhythm.
4. Defibrillate patients with artificial pacemakers in the usual manner. However, do not discharge paddles directly over the implanted battery pack.
5. Transcutaneous cardiac pacing, if indicated, may be used in the usual manner.

Besides pacemakers, implantable cardioverter defibrillators also are common. The battery packs of these devices are located in the subcutaneous tissues of the abdominal wall. Emergency cardiac care can be given as usual. These devices present no danger to rescuers. However, paramedics should wear gloves to help avoid unpleasant sensations when the device discharges. (Implantable cardioverter defibrillators are described further later in this chapter.)

DYSRHYTHMIAS THAT ARE DISORDERS OF CONDUCTION

Delay or blockage of the electrical impulse conduction in the heart is called a *heart block.* Heart blocks can occur anywhere in the atria between the sinoatrial node and the atrioventricular node or in the ventricles between the atrioventricular node and the Purkinje fibers. These conduction problems can be caused by diseased tissue in the conduction system. Or they may be caused by a physiological block, as occurs in atrial fibrillation or atrial flutter. Causes of heart blocks include atrioventricular junctional ischemia, atrioventricular junctional necrosis, degenerative disease of the conduction system, electrolyte imbalances (e.g., hyperkalemia), and drug toxicity, especially with digitalis.

Classifications

Conduction blocks may be classified based on several characteristics: site of block (e.g., left bundle branch block), degree of block (e.g., second-degree atrioventricular block), or category of atrioventricular conduction disturbances (e.g., type I). This text presents the dysrhythmias by degree and location. One should note, however, that the term *degree* does not reflect directly the gradients of severity when applied to the classification of heart blocks. Any evaluation of heart block must consider the specific rates of the atria and ventricles, the patient's clinical presentation, and the findings of a complete history and physical examination before one determines the clinical severity of atrioventricular conduction disturbances. The dysrhythmias discussed in this section include first-degree atrioventricular block; second-degree atrioventricular block type I (or *Wenckebach*); second-degree atrioventricular block type II; third-degree atrioventricular block (complete heart block); and ventricular conduction disturbances, including bundle branch blocks and hemiblocks.

Atrioventricular Blocks

The discussion of conduction disturbances of the heart begins with the atrioventricular blocks.

FIRST-DEGREE ATRIOVENTRICULAR BLOCK

Description. First-degree atrioventricular block is not a true block (Fig. 29-82). Rather, the disturbance is a delay in conduction, usually at the level of the atrioventricular node. First-degree atrioventricular block is not considered a rhythm in itself because it usually is superimposed on another rhythm. Thus the paramedic also must identify the underlying rhythm (e.g., sinus bradycardia with first-degree atrioventricular block).

Etiology. First-degree atrioventricular block may occur for no apparent reason. The dysrhythmia sometimes is associated with myocardial ischemia, acute myocardial infarction, increased vagal (parasympathetic) tone, or digitalis toxicity.

Rules for Interpretation (Lead II Monitoring). First-degree atrioventricular block has the following characteristics on the electrocardiogram:

QRS complex: Typically normal (less than 0.12 second), with an atrioventricular conduction ratio of 1:1 (a QRS complex follows each P wave)
P waves: Present, identical waves that precede each QRS complex
Rate: The rate is that of the underlying sinus or atrial rhythm.
Rhythm: The rhythm is that of the underlying rhythm.
P-R interval: A prolonged (greater than 0.20 second), constant P-R interval is the hallmark of first-degree atrioventricular block and often is the only alteration in the electrocardiogram.

Clinical Significance. As a general rule, first-degree atrioventricular block has little or no clinical significance because all of the impulses are conducted to the ventricles. Rarely, though, a newly developed first-degree atrioventricular block progresses to a more serious atrioventricular block.

Management. This dysrhythmia usually does not require treatment.

SECOND-DEGREE ATRIOVENTRICULAR BLOCK TYPE I (WENCKEBACH)

Description. Type I second-degree atrioventricular block is an intermittent block (Fig. 29-83). It usually occurs at the level of the atrioventricular node. The conduction delay progressively increases from beat to beat until conduction to the ventricle is blocked. This dysrhythmia produces a characteristic cyclical pattern in which the P-R intervals get progressively longer until a P wave occurs that is not followed by a QRS complex. By the time the sinoatrial node fires again, atrioventricular conduction has had time to recover. Then the sequence starts over.

Etiology. Type I second-degree atrioventricular block often occurs in acute myocardial infarction or acute myocarditis. Other causes include increased vagal tone, ischemia, drug toxicity (digitalis, ***propranolol, verapamil***), head injury, and electrolyte imbalance.

Rules for Interpretation (Lead II Monitoring). Second-degree atrioventricular block type I has the following characteristics on the electrocardiogram:

QRS complex: Usually less than 0.12 second. Commonly, the atrioventricular conduction ratio (P waves to QRS complexes) is 5:4, 4:3, 3:2, or 2:1; the pattern may be constant or variable. A constant 2:1 block makes it difficult to distinguish between type I and type II blocks.
P waves: Upright and uniform and preceding the QRS complex when the QRS complex occurs
Rate: The atrial rate is that of the underlying sinus or atrial rhythm. The ventricular rate may be normal or slow but always is slightly less than the atrial rate.

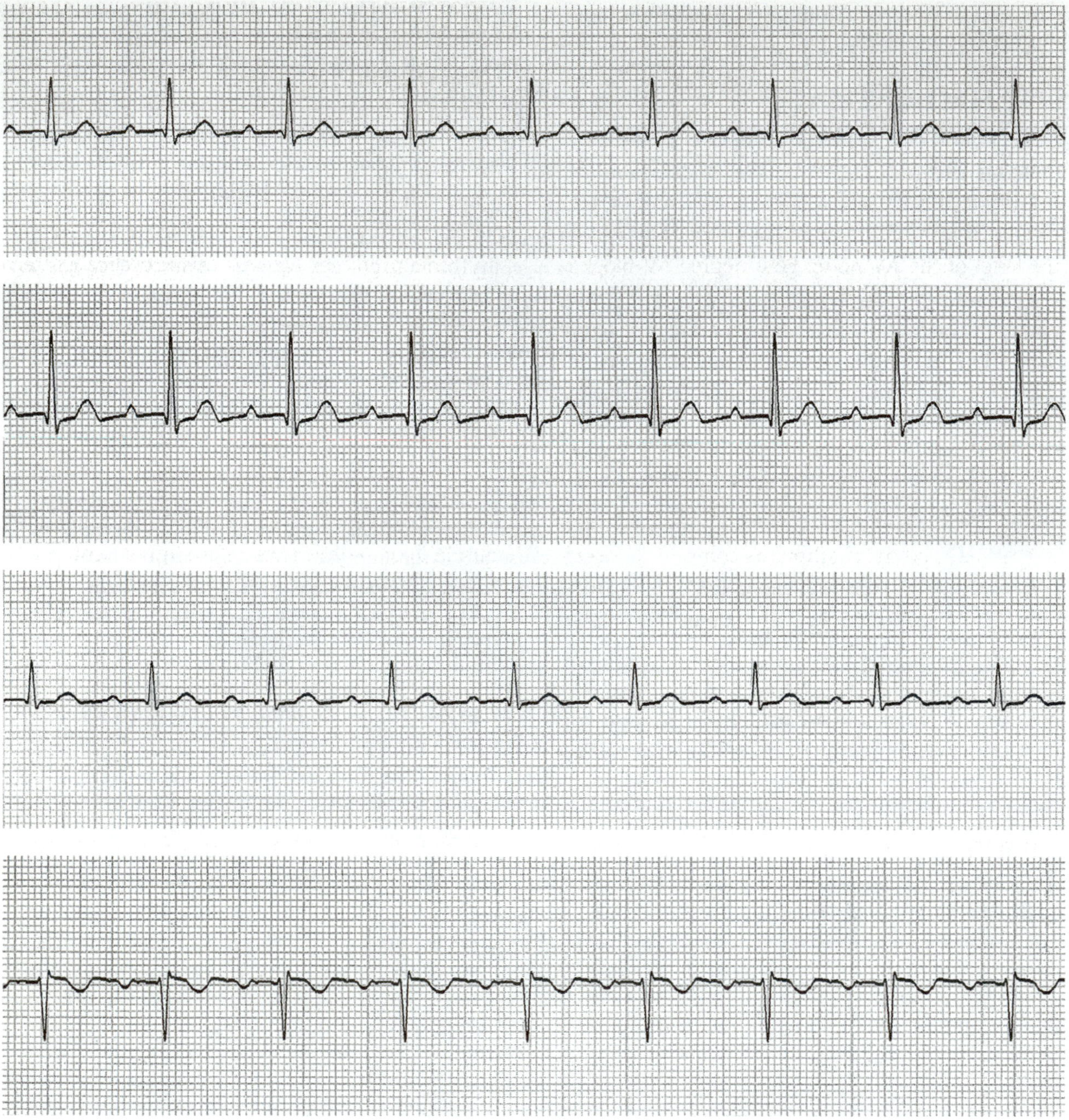

FIGURE 29-82 ■ First-degree atrioventricular block.

Rhythm: The atrial rhythm is regular; the ventricular rhythm is irregular (characteristic group beating).

P-R interval: Progressively lengthens before the nonconducted P wave. The P-P interval is constant, but the R-R interval decreases until the dropped beat (producing grouping of QRS complexes).

Clinical Significance. Type I second-degree atrioventricular block usually is a transient and reversible phenomenon. However, it can progress to a more serious atrioventricular block. If dropped beats occur often, the patient may show signs and symptoms of decreased cardiac output.

NOTE Atrioventricular block, in which the P-R interval before a dropped beat is prolonged and the P-R interval after the dropped beat is shortened by comparison, is the most common form of second-degree block.

Management. No management is required if the patient is asymptomatic. If the dropped beats compromise the heart rate and cardiac output, administration of ***atropine,*** transcutaneous cardiac pacing, or both may be indicated (see Fig. 29-40).

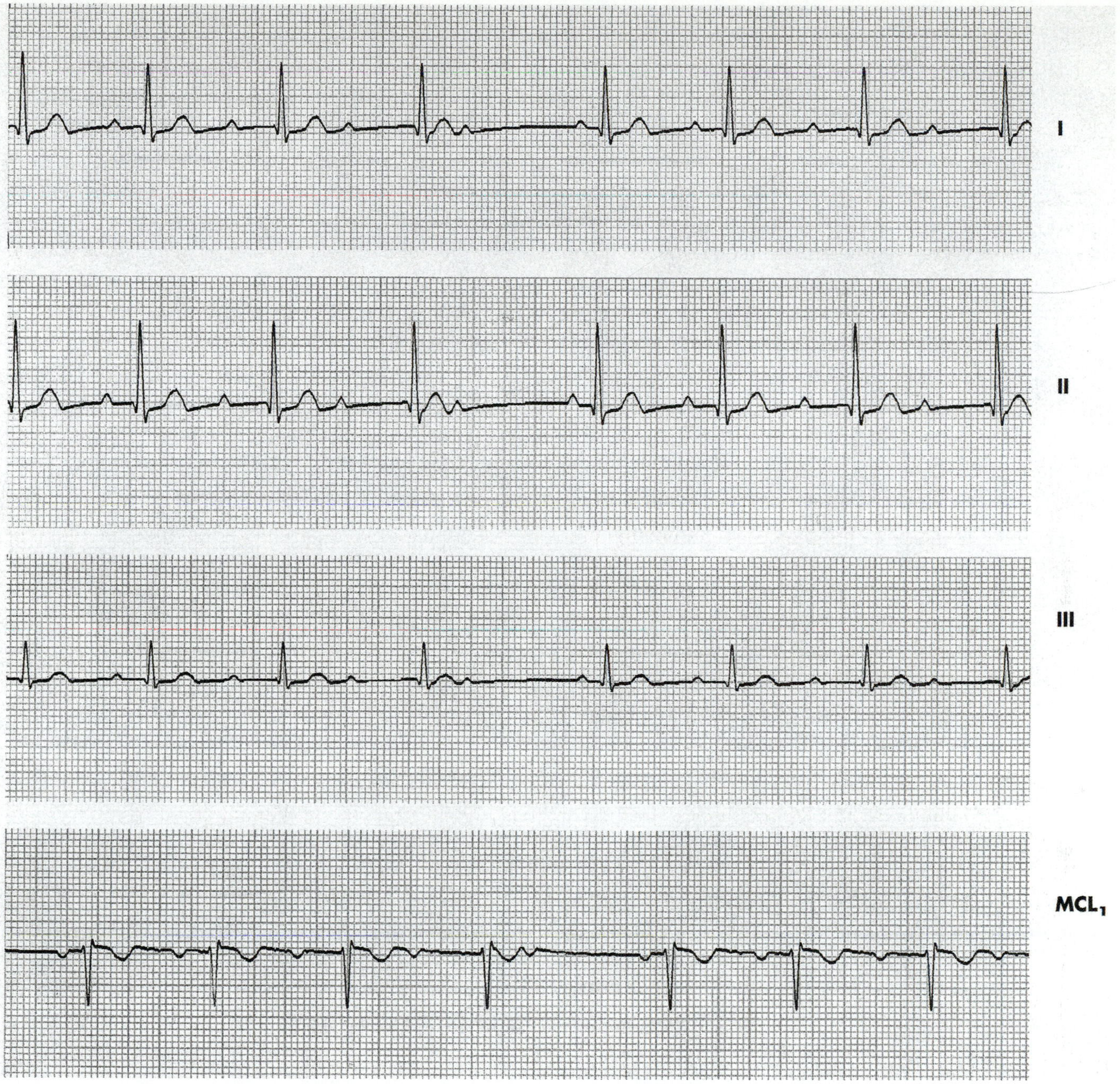

FIGURE 29-83 ■ Second-degree atrioventricular block, type I.

SECOND-DEGREE ATRIOVENTRICULAR BLOCK TYPE II

Description. Type II second-degree atrioventricular block is an intermittent block (Fig. 29-84). This dysrhythmia occurs when atrial impulses are not conducted to the ventricles. Unlike type I, this block is characterized by consecutive P waves being conducted with a constant P-R interval before a dropped beat. This variation of atrioventricular block usually occurs in a regular sequence with the conduction ratios (P waves to QRS complexes), such as 2:1, 3:2, and 4:3 (Fig. 29-85). Type II second-degree atrioventricular block usually occurs below the bundle of His.

When at least two consecutive P waves fail to be conducted to the ventricles, the atrioventricular block is referred to as a *high-grade atrioventricular block* (Fig. 29-86). Clinically, serious high-grade atrioventricular blocks and those that are less serious are distinguished by the atrial and ventricular rates. A 2:1 block might be considered high grade (and certainly is clinically significant) when the patient's underlying atrial rate is 60 beats per minute. However, such a block is of much less concern if the patient's atrial rate is 120 beats per minute.

A type II 2:1 atrioventricular block sometimes may be difficult to distinguish from a type I 2:1 atrioventricular

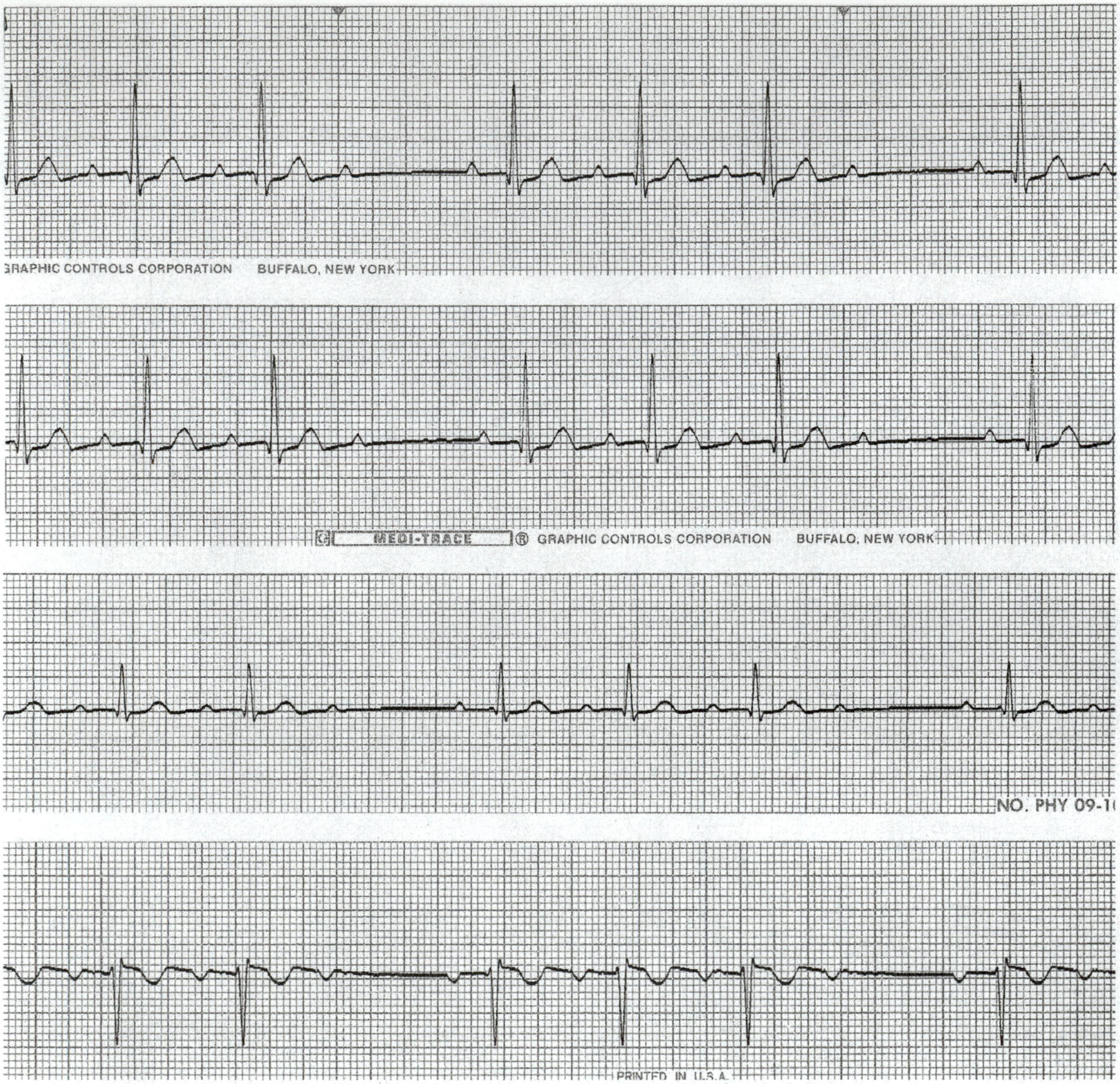

FIGURE 29-84 ■ Second-degree atrioventricular block, type II.

block. When assessing a patient who has two atrial complexes for each QRS complex, the paramedic should evaluate the normal cycle. If the normally conducted cycle has a prolonged P-R interval (greater than 0.20 second), a narrow QRS complex (less than 0.12 second, indicating the absence of bundle branch block), and an adequate escape rate, the patient probably has a type I 2:1 atrioventricular block. If the conducted QRS complex has a normal P-R interval, a wide QRS complex (greater than 0.12 second, which indicates the presence of a bundle branch block), and an adequate escape rate, a type II 2:1 atrioventricular block is most likely (Fig. 29-87).

Etiology. Type II second-degree atrioventricular block usually is associated with acute myocardial infarction that occurs in the septum. Unlike type I second-degree atrioventricular block, type II normally does not result solely from increased parasympathetic tone or drug toxicity.

Rules for Interpretation (Lead II Monitoring). Second-degree atrioventricular block type II has the following characteristics on the electrocardiogram:

QRS complex: May be abnormal (equal to or greater than 0.12 second) because of bundle branch block

P waves: Upright and uniform. Some P waves will not be followed by QRS complexes.

Rate: The atrial rate is unaffected and is that of the underlying sinus, atrial, or junctional rhythm. The ventricular rate is less than that of the atrial rate and is often bradycardic.

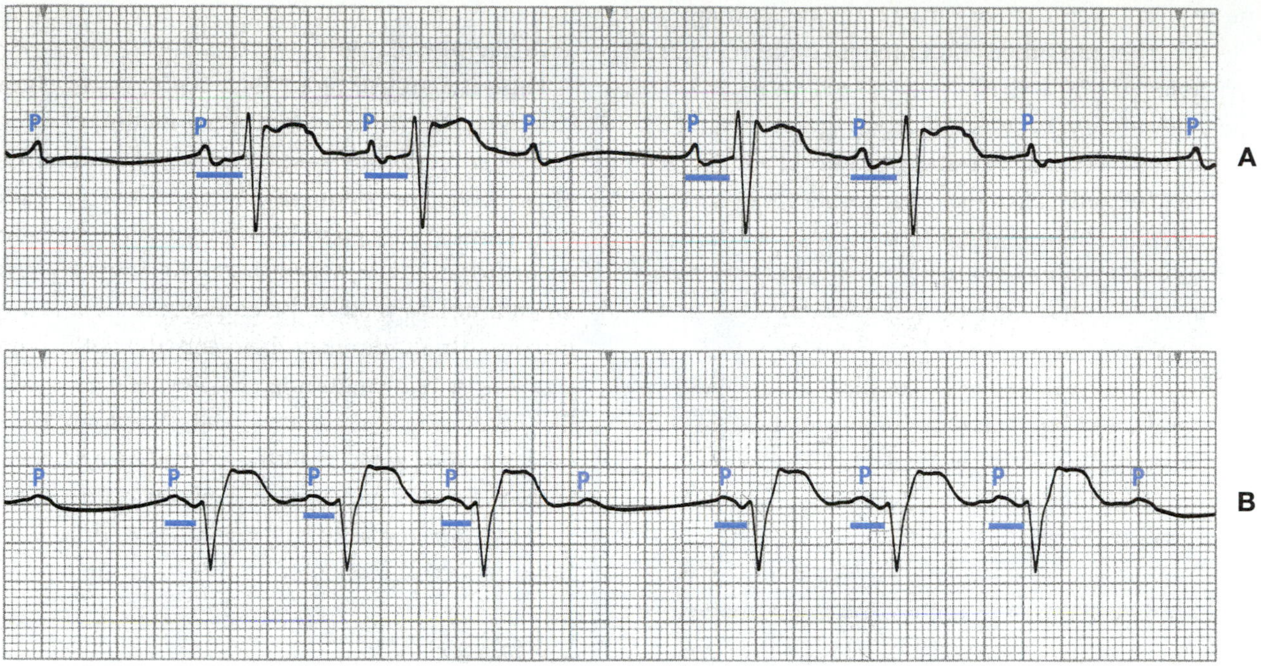

FIGURE 29-85 ■ **A,** A 3:2 atrioventricular block. **B,** A 4:3 atrioventricular block.

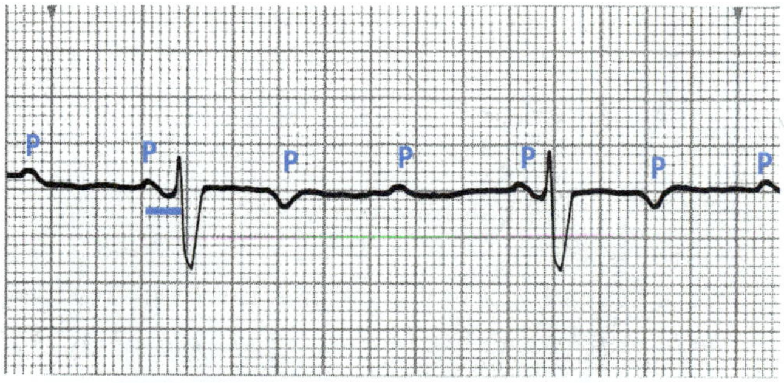

FIGURE 29-86 ■ A 3:1 high-grade atrioventricular block.

Rhythm: Regular or irregular, depending on whether the conduction ratio is constant or variable

P-R interval: Usually is constant for conducted beats and may be greater than 0.20 second

Clinical Significance. Type II second-degree atrioventricular block is a serious dysrhythmia. The dysrhythmia is usually thought of as malignant in the emergency setting (unlike type I atrioventricular blocks, which usually are considered benign). Slow ventricular rates may result in signs and symptoms of hypoperfusion. This dysrhythmia may progress to a more severe heart block. It may even progress to ventricular asystole.

Management. Regardless of the patient's initial condition, pacemaker insertion is the treatment for the patient. Prehospital care for symptomatic patients may consist of transcutaneous cardiac pacing and possibly the administration of ***atropine*** (see Fig. 29-41).

THIRD-DEGREE HEART BLOCK

Description. Third-degree atrioventricular block results from complete electrical block at or below the atrioventricular node (infranodal) (Fig. 29-88). The dysrhythmia is said to be present when the opportunity for conduction between the atria and the ventricles is present but conduction does not occur. In this condition the sinoatrial node serves as the pacemaker for the atria. An ectopic focus serves as a pacemaker in the ventricles. The result is that P waves and QRS complexes occur rhythmically. Yet the rhythms are unrelated to each other (atrioventricular dissociation). The only electrical link between the atria and the ventricles is the atrioventricular node and bundle of His.

> **NOTE** ***Atropine*** should be used with caution in patients with complete heart block and wide-complex ventricular escape beats and also for patients with type II second-degree heart block.[1] (Atropine may increase the degree of block or cause third-degree atrioventricular block.) Many patients with heart block cannot be managed effectively in the prehospital setting with only medication. Immediate transport to an emergency department is indicated.

Etiology. Common causes of third-degree atrioventricular block include increased vagal tone (which may produce a transient atrioventricular dissociation), septal necrosis, acute myocarditis, digitalis, beta-blocker or calcium

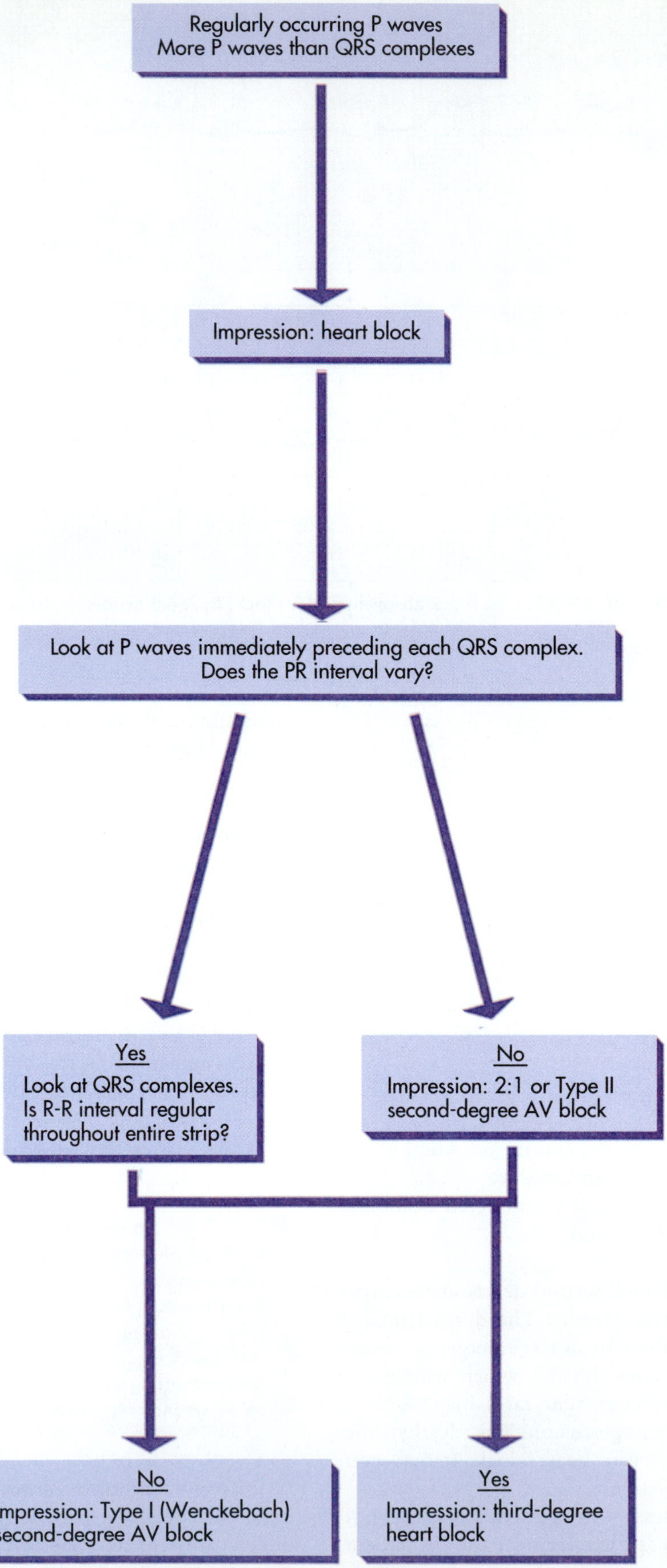

FIGURE 29-87 ■ Identifying heart blocks.

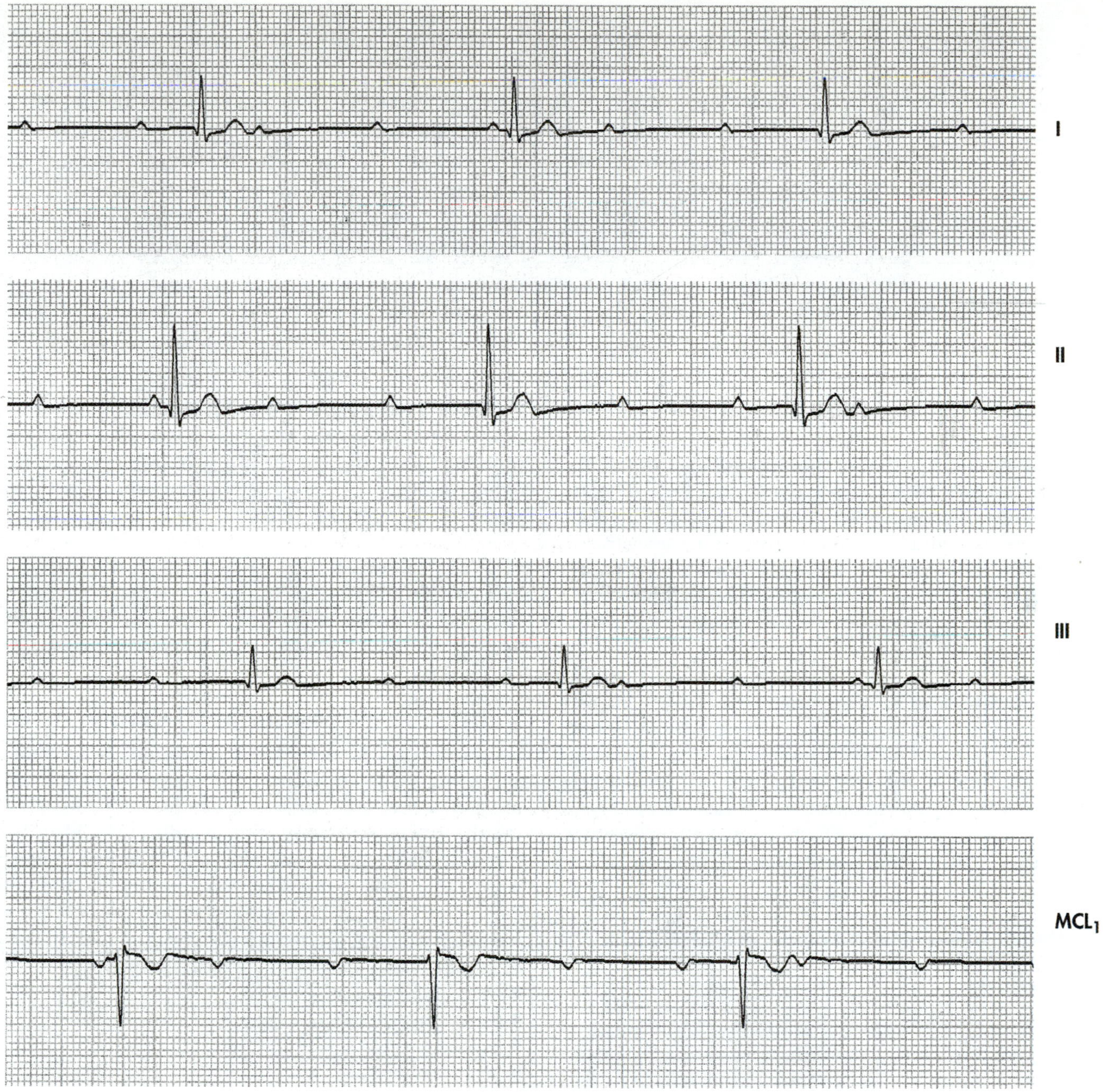

FIGURE 29-88 ■ Third-degree atrioventricular block.

channel blocker toxicity, and electrolyte imbalance. The dysrhythmia also may occur in older adults from chronic degenerative changes in the conduction system.

> **CRITICAL THINKING**
>
> When P waves and QRS complexes do not appear to be related to each other on the electrocardiogram, the paramedic should look at the shape of QRS-T waves. QRS-T waves altered by superimposed P waves suggests atrioventricular dissociation. Atrioventricular dissociation suggests third-degree atrioventricular block.

Rules for Interpretation (Lead II Monitoring). Third-degree heart block has the following characteristics on the electrocardiogram:

QRS complex: May be less than 0.12 second if the escape focus is below the atrioventricular node and above the bifurcation of the bundle branches or 0.12 second or greater if the escape focus is ventricular. A narrow QRS complex in third-degree heart block is less common than a wide QRS complex.

P waves: Present but with no relationship to the QRS complexes. In cases of atrial flutter or fibrillation, complete

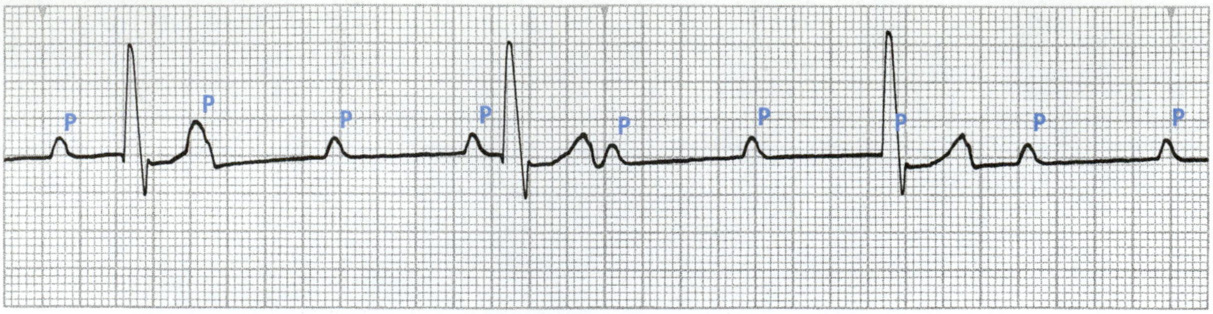

FIGURE 29-89 ■ Third-degree block demonstrating P waves superimposed on the QRS complex and T waves.

heart block is manifested by a slow, regular ventricular response.

Rate: The atrial rate is that of the underlying sinus or atrial rhythm. The ventricular rate typically is 40 to 60 beats per minute if the escape focus is junctional and less than 40 beats per minute if the escape focus is in the ventricles.

Rhythm: The atrial and ventricular rhythms usually are regular. The rhythms are independent of each other.

P-R interval: No relation exists between atrial and ventricular activity (Fig. 29-89).

Clinical Significance. The patient may have signs and symptoms of severe bradycardia and decreased cardiac output. These are the result of slow ventricular rate and asynchronous action of the atria and ventricles. Third-degree atrioventricular block associated with wide QRS complexes is an ominous sign. The dysrhythmia potentially is lethal. Patients with this rhythm often present as unstable.

> **NOTE** Complete atrioventricular block in the presence of atrial fibrillation often is caused by drug toxicity (usually digitalis). Almost always some atrioventricular block occurs with atrial fibrillation or flutter. Yet complete atrioventricular block is recognized by a slow, regular ventricular response. (Response is usually less than 60 beats per minute.) The QRS complex may be normal if the escape focus is from above the bifurcation of the bundle branches.

Management. Pacemaker insertion is the definitive treatment for symptomatic third-degree atrioventricular block. Pacemaker insertion is also the treatment for asymptomatic third-degree heart block with bundle branch block. Initial prehospital care includes transcutaneous cardiac pacing or administration of ***dopamine*** to increase the ventricular rate if needed and administration of ***epinephrine, isoproterenol,*** and possibly ***atropine*** to stimulate atrioventricular conduction or to increase the rate of a junctional escape rhythm if sanctioned by medical direction.

Transcutaneous cardiac pacing is a class I intervention for all symptomatic bradycardias. Pacing should be applied as soon as possible if the patient's condition is unstable (see Fig. 29-41). ***Atropine*** (a parasympatholytic) is unlikely to help patients with complete heart block. The vagus nerve innervates the atria, and the focus controlling the heart in a third-degree block is most often in the ventricles. Thus ***atropine*** will likely have no effect on the ventricular rate.

> **CRITICAL THINKING**
> What should you tell the patient before initiating transcutaneous cardiac pacing?

Ventricular Conduction Disturbances

Ventricular conduction disturbances (bundle branch blocks and hemiblocks) are delays or interruptions in the transmission of electrical impulses. These disturbances occur below the level of bifurcation of the bundle of His. Identifying these blocks is important. It helps to identify the patient who is at an increased risk of severe bradycardia and third-degree heart block. This is especially true when the patient has other forms of atrioventricular block. Common causes of bundle branch block include the following:

- Acute heart failure
- Acute myocardial infarction
- Aortic stenosis
- Cardiomyopathy
- Hyperkalemia
- Infection (e.g., carditis)
- Ischemic heart disease
- Trauma

BUNDLE BRANCH ANATOMY

To review, the bundle of His begins at the atrioventricular node and divides to form the left and right bundle branches (Fig. 29-90). The right bundle branch continues toward the apex and spreads throughout the right ventricle. The left bundle branch subdivides into the anterior and posterior fascicles and spreads throughout the left ventricle. Conduction of electrical impulses through the Purkinje fibers stimulates the ventricles to contract.

With normal conduction, the first part of the ventricle to be stimulated is the left side of the septum. The electrical im-

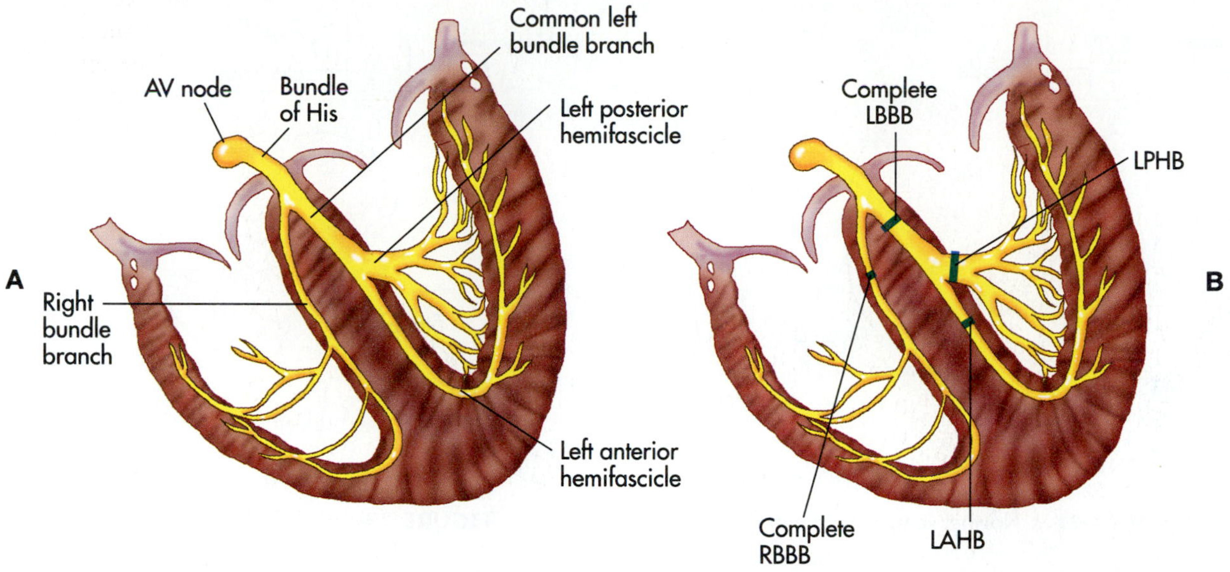

FIGURE 29-90 ■ **A,** Simplified illustration showing the major divisions of the ventricular conduction system. After passing through the atrioventricular node and the bundle of His, the electrical impulse is carried to the right and common left bundle branches. The latter structure divides into the left anterior and posterior hemifascicles. **B,** Possible sites of block and the conduction deficits that may be produced.

pulse then traverses the septum to stimulate the other side. Shortly thereafter, the left and right ventricles at the same time are stimulated. The left ventricle is normally much larger and thicker than the right ventricle. Thus its electrical activity predominates over that of the right ventricle.

COMMON ELECTROCARDIOGRAM FINDINGS

When an electrical impulse is blocked from passing through the right or left bundle branch, one ventricle depolarizes and contracts before the other. Ventricular activation no longer occurs at the same time. Thus the QRS complex widens (often with a slurred or notched appearance known as *rabbit ears*). The hallmark of bundle branch block is a QRS complex that is equal to or greater than 0.12 second. The two criteria for bundle branch block recognition are as follows:

- A QRS complex equal to or greater than 0.12 second
- QRS complexes produced by supraventricular activity

> **NOTE** *Bundle branch block* and *hemiblock (fascicular block)* are terms used to describe abnormal conduction of impulses from above the bundle branches to the ventricles. These patterns of abnormal or aberrant conduction must be recognized as different from beats of ventricular origin. Beats of ventricular origin can have similar QRS complex shapes.

Ventricular conduction disturbances are identified best by monitoring leads MCL_1 and MCL_6 (or by monitoring V_1 and V_6 with a 12-lead machine). These leads permit the easiest differentiation of the right and left bundle branch blocks. For electrocardiogram evaluation the paramedic should ensure that the electrodes are placed properly for leads I, II, and III. Lead MCL_1 looks at right and left bundle branches and should be monitored during transport of these patients.[6] For the purpose of this discussion, the reader should assume that all MCL_1 descriptions can be applied to V_1 when using 12-lead monitoring.

Normal Conduction. In normal ventricular stimulation the electrical impulse reaches the septum first. Then the impulse travels from the left endocardium to the right endocardium of the septum (Fig. 29-91). This impulse generates a small R wave in MCL_1. The rest of the impulses mainly are conducted away from the MCL_1 electrode. This yields a negative deflection. Thus during normal conduction, MCL_1 mainly is negative. The QRS complex also usually is 0.08 to 0.10 second wide (the same as any other narrow QRS complex).

Right Bundle Branch Block. In right bundle branch block the left bundle branch performs normally. Thus the left branch activates the left side of the heart before the right (Fig. 29-92). When the left ventricle is activated initially, the impulse travels away from the MCL_1 electrode. This yields a negative deflection (S wave). The electrical impulse then travels across the interventricular septum and activates the right ventricle. Because the impulse is coming back toward the MCL_1 electrode, a large positive deflection (R wave) occurs. This results in the RSR′ pattern seen in MCL_1 in patients with right bundle branch block. The QRS (or in this case, RSR) complex is at least 0.12 second. Whenever the two criteria for bundle branch block are met and MCL_1 displays an RSR′ pattern, right bundle branch block should be suspected.

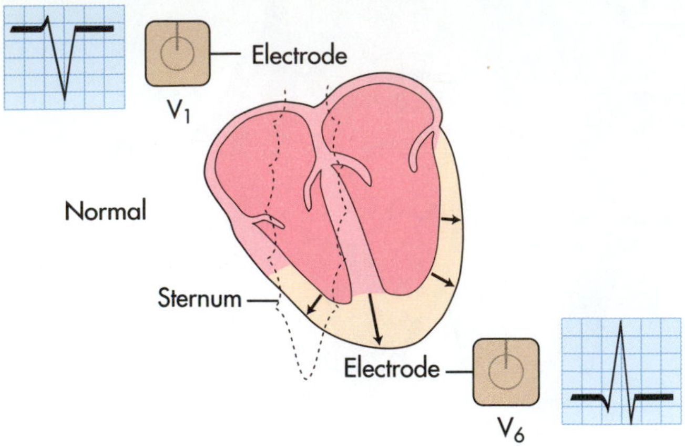

FIGURE 29-91 ■ Normal ventricular conduction.

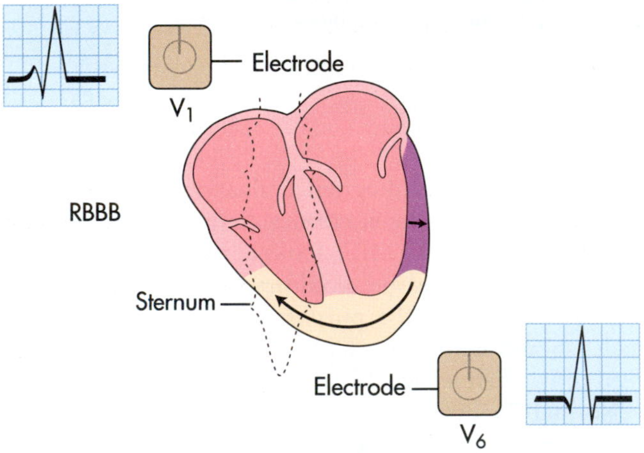

FIGURE 29-92 ■ Right bundle branch block.

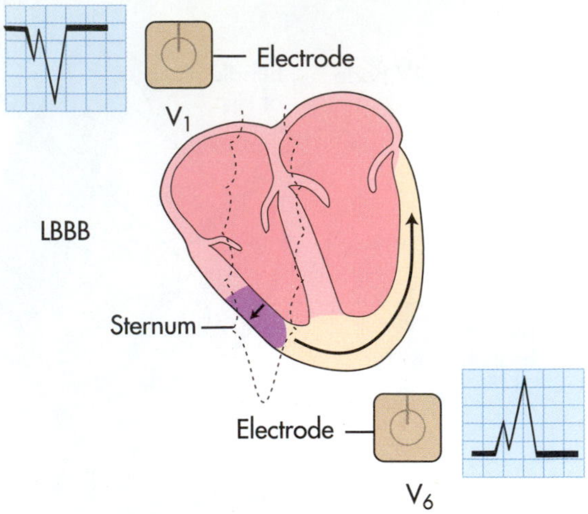

FIGURE 29-93 ■ Left bundle branch block.

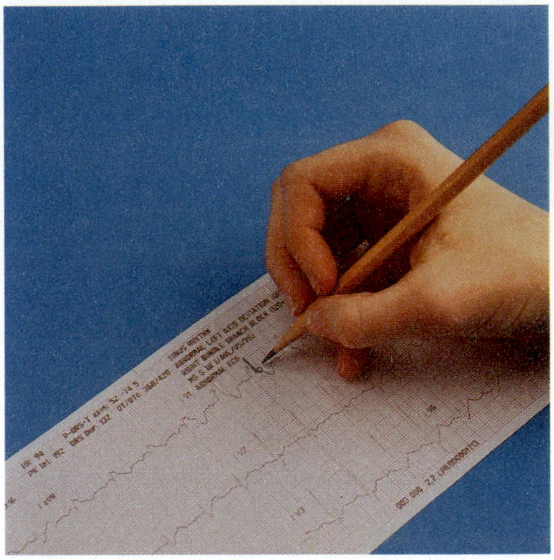

FIGURE 29-94 ■ To distinguish left from right bundle branch blocks, find the J point of the QRS complex, draw a line backward into the QRS complex, and fill in the triangle created by this line and the last portion of the QRS complex. The direction the triangle points distinguishes the two types of blocks.

BOX 29-16 Determining Right or Left Bundle Branch Block

When lead MCL_1 is monitored, the bundle branch block may be determined by the following procedure (see also Fig. 29-94).

1. Find a QRS complex that is at least 0.12 second wide.
2. Count backward three small boxes from the beginning of the QRS and move straight up to see the J point.
3. Draw a line backward from the J point into the QRS complex.
4. Fill in the triangle that is created by this line and the last portion of the QRS complex.
5. If the triangle points up, it is a right bundle branch block.
6. If the triangle points down, it is a left bundle branch block.

Left Bundle Branch Block. In the more serious left bundle branch block, the fibers that usually stimulate the interventricular septum are blocked. This blockage alters normal septal activation and sends it in the opposite direction (Fig. 29-93). This yields an initial Q wave in MCL_1 instead of the normal small R wave. The right ventricle then is activated, producing a positive deflection R wave in MCL_1; this impulse travels across the interventricular septum to the left ventricle. Because the impulse is leading away from MCL_1, the lead shows a deep, wide S wave (QS pattern) (Fig. 29-94). As with right bundle branch block, the activation takes at least 0.12 second. Whenever the two criteria for bundle branch block are met and a QS pattern is seen in MCL_1, a left bundle branch block should be suspected (Box 29-16). Patients with new left bundle branch

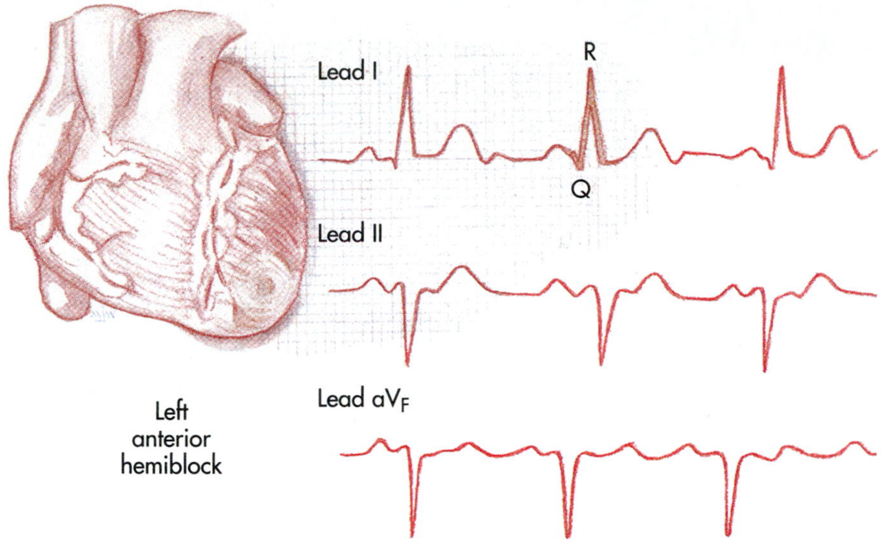

FIGURE 29-95 ■ Anterior hemiblock.

block have lost a lot of myocardium; left ventricular failure may develop and may lead to death.

Anterior Hemiblock. Anterior hemiblocks (anterior hemifascicular blocks) occur more often than posterior hemiblocks (posterior hemifascicular blocks). The anterior fascicle of the left bundle branch is a longer and thinner structure. Its blood supply comes mainly from the left anterior descending coronary artery. Anterior hemiblock is characterized by left axis deviation in a patient who has a supraventricular rhythm (Fig. 29-95). Other electrocardiogram findings associated with an anterior hemiblock include a normal QRS complex (less than 0.12 second) or a right bundle branch block, a small Q wave followed by a tall R wave in lead I, and a small R wave followed by a deep S wave in lead III. In a patient who has an anterior hemiblock with a right bundle branch block, impulses can be conducted only through the ventricles by way of the posterior fascicle of the left bundle branch. These patients are at high risk of developing complete heart block.

CRITICAL THINKING

What rhythms are produced by supraventricular activity?

Posterior Hemiblock. The posterior fascicle of the left bundle branch is not blocked as easily as the anterior fascicle. As a result, posterior hemiblock occurs less often. Posterior hemiblock is identified by right axis deviation with a normal QRS complex or a right bundle branch block (Fig. 29-96). A diagnosis of posterior hemiblock requires excluding right ventricular hypertrophy. This is difficult to do in the prehospital setting, if not impossible. For practical purposes, posterior hemiblock can be assumed in patients with right axis deviation and a QRS complex of normal width or with a right bundle branch block. (Other electrocardiogram findings that indicate the presence of a posterior hemiblock include a small R wave followed by a deep S wave in lead I and a small Q wave followed by a tall R wave in lead III.)

Bifascicular Block. *Bifascicular block* refers to the blockage of two of three pathways for ventricular conduction. This condition occurs with right bundle branch block with anterior or posterior hemiblock and in left bundle branch block. Bifascicular block decreases myocardial contractility and cardiac output. Patients with this condition may develop complete heart block suddenly and without warning. As a rule, the more branches that have impaired conduction, the greater the chance a patient will develop complete atrioventricular block (especially in patients with acute myocardial infarction).

MULTILEAD DETERMINATION OF THE AXIS AND HEMIBLOCKS

The axis is the direction of impulse flow in the heart that stimulates contraction. Identifying the axis can be useful in determining the presence of hemiblocks. Hemiblocks are evaluated best by looking at the QRS complexes in leads I, II, and III. The axis is considered *normal* when the QRS deflection is positive (upright) in all bipolar leads; *physiological left* (which may be normal in some patients) when the QRS deflection is positive in leads I and II but negative (inverted) in lead III; *pathological left* when the QRS deflection is positive in lead I and negative in leads II and III (indicating an anterior hemiblock); *right axis* when the QRS deflection is negative in lead I, negative or positive in lead II, and positive in lead III (pathological in any adult and indicative of a posterior hemiblock); and *extreme right* ("no man's land") when the QRS deflection is negative in all three leads (indicating that the rhythm is ventricular in origin) (Table 29-2).

MANAGEMENT OF BUNDLE BRANCH BLOCKS AND HEMIBLOCKS

No specific treatment is necessary for bundle branch blocks or hemiblocks. However, if other conditions (e.g., hypoxia, ischemia, electrolyte imbalance, or drug toxicity) are causing a block, these conditions should be treated. Some emergency medications administered to patients with cardiac

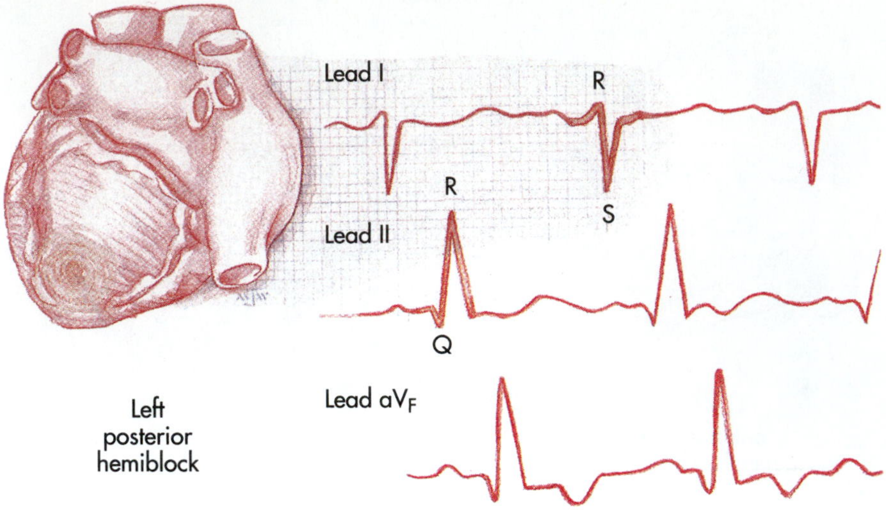

FIGURE 29-96 ■ Posterior hemiblock.

TABLE 29-2 Identifying Axis by QRS Complex

AXIS	LEAD I	LEAD II	LEAD III	INDICATIONS
	QRS COMPLEX			
Normal	Upright	Upright	Upright	May be normal
Physiological left	Upright	Upright	Inverted	May be normal
Pathological left	Upright	Inverted	Inverted	Anterior hemiblock
Right axis	Inverted	Inverted or upright	Upright	Posterior hemiblock
Extreme right	Inverted	Inverted	Inverted	Ventricular in origin

disease (e.g., ***procainamide, digoxin,*** and ***verapamil*** or ***diltiazem***) can slow electrical impulse conduction through the atrioventricular node. To administer these medicines safely, the paramedic must ensure that the patient is not at a high risk of developing full heart block. Those at such risk include the following:

- Any patient with type II atrioventricular block
- Any patient with evidence of disease in both bundle branches
- Any patient with two or more blocks of any kind (e.g., prolonged P-R interval and anterior hemiblock, right bundle branch block and anterior hemiblock, type I atrioventricular block, and left bundle branch block)

Prehospital care for these patients should include management of any accompanying signs and symptoms, transport, constant electrocardiogram monitoring, and anticipation of the possible need for external pacing. Emergency pacing has been recommended for the following four indications[1]:

1. Hemodynamically compromising bradycardias
2. Bradycardias with malignant escape rhythms unresponsive to pharmacological therapy
3. Overdrive pacing of refractory supraventricular or ventricular tachycardia unresponsive to pharmacological therapy or cardioversion
4. Bradyasystolic cardiac arrest (in rare situations)

The American Heart Association also recommends pacing readiness in the setting of acute myocardial infarction for patients with symptomatic sinus node dysfunction; type II second-degree atrioventricular block; third-degree heart block; or newly acquired left, right, or alternating bundle branch block or bifascicular block.[1]

Pulseless Electrical Activity

The term *pulseless electrical activity* (also known as *electromechanical dissociation*) (Fig. 29-97) is defined as the absence of a detectable pulse and the presence of some type of electrical activity other than ventricular tachycardia or ventricular fibrillation.[1] The outcome of pulseless electrical activity almost always is poor; that is, unless an underlying cause can be identified and corrected. The paramedic must maintain circulation for the patient with basic and advanced life support techniques while searching for a correctable cause.

CRITICAL THINKING

What rhythms might you see on the monitor when a patient is in pulseless electrical activity?

Correctable causes of pulseless electrical activity are cardiac tamponade, tension pneumothorax, hypoxemia, acido-

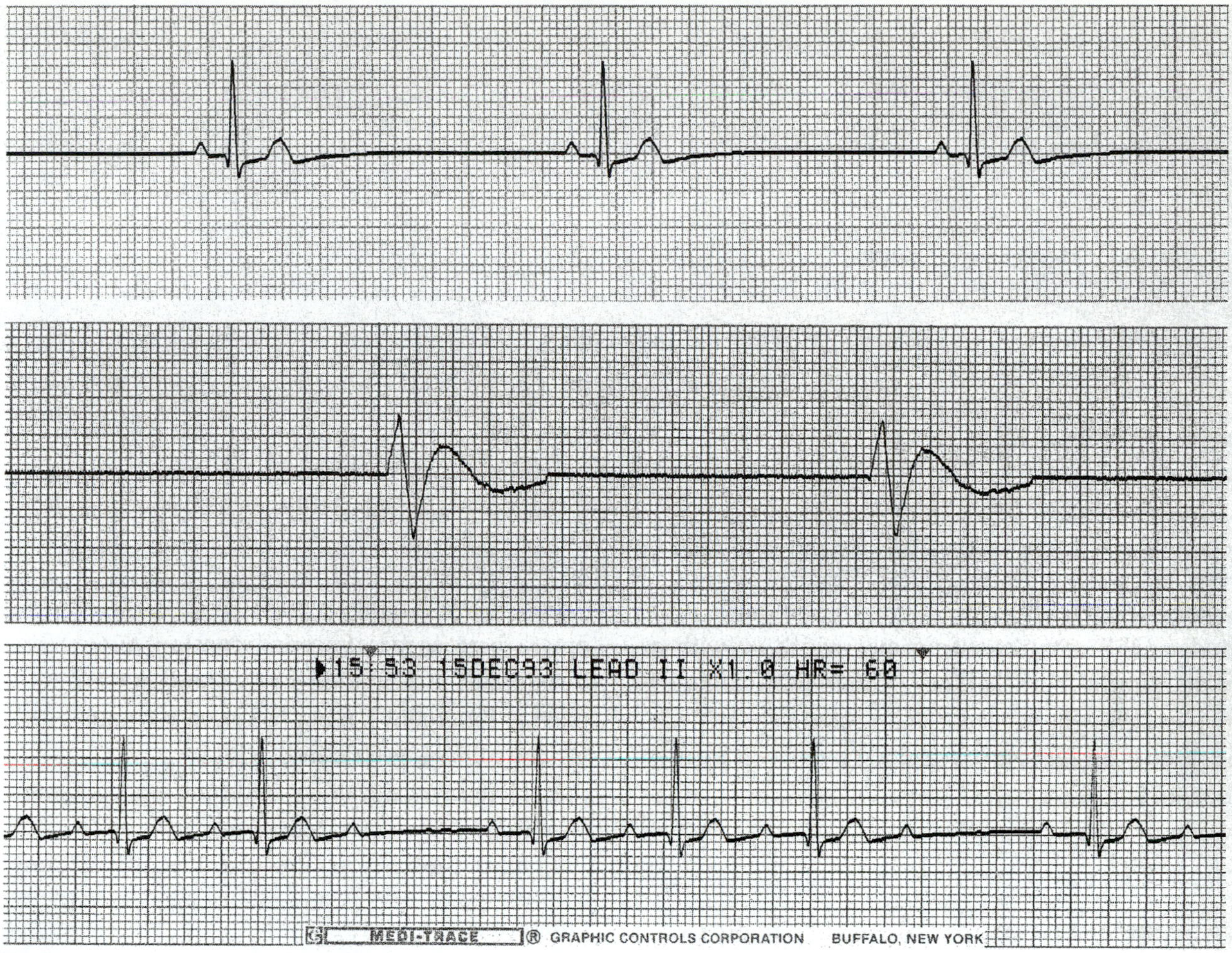

FIGURE 29-97 ■ Various pulseless electrical activity rhythms as seen in lead II.

sis, hyperkalemia, hypothermia, and overdoses of, for example, tricyclic antidepressants, beta-blockers, and digitalis. Other less correctable causes include massive myocardial damage from infarction, prolonged ischemia during resuscitation, profound hypovolemia, and massive pulmonary embolism. Patients in profound shock of any type (including anaphylactic, septic, neurogenic, and hypovolemic) may have pulseless electrical activity. The paramedic should manage tension pneumothorax with needle decompression. If the patient is hypoxic, the paramedic should manage the patient by improving oxygenation and ventilation. If acute hypovolemia is present (because of hemorrhage), the paramedic should begin fluid resuscitation with volume expanders. The paramedic should manage acidosis by ensuring adequate cardiopulmonary resuscitation and hyperventilation. If preexisting acidosis (e.g., diabetic ketoacidosis) or hyperkalemia is suspected (e.g., a patient on home dialysis), the use of ***sodium bicarbonate*** may be indicated. ***Calcium*** is a specific therapy for hyperkalemia and calcium channel blocker toxicity. Both of these conditions can produce pulseless electrical activity. Besides calcium channel blockers, other drugs when taken in toxic amounts can produce wide-complex pulseless electrical activity. These overdoses can be managed with specific therapy. The therapy may be effective in reestablishing a perfusing rhythm (see Fig. 29-58).

CRITICAL THINKING

What patient care measures should you take in this case?

Preexcitation Syndromes

Preexcitation syndrome (anomalous or accelerated atrioventricular conduction) is associated with an abnormal conduction pathway between the atria and ventricles. This pathway bypasses the atrioventricular node, bundle of His, or both. This allows the electrical impulses to initiate depolarization of the ventricles earlier than usual. The most common preexcitation syndrome is Wolff-Parkinson-White syndrome.

WOLFF-PARKINSON-WHITE SYNDROME

Description. In some hearts, an accessory muscle bundle (known as the **bundle of Kent** or the *Kent fibers*) connects the lateral wall of the atrium and the ventricle, bypassing the atrioventricular node. This produces an early activation of the ventricle (Wolff-Parkinson-White syndrome).[6] Wolff-

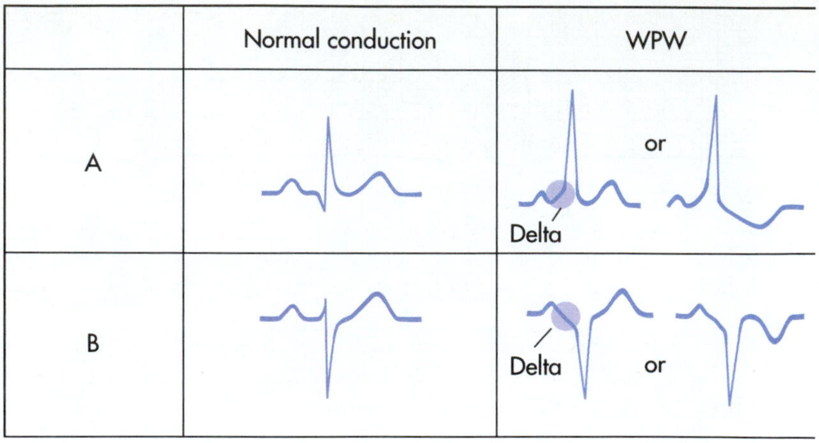

FIGURE 29-98 ■ Characteristic findings in Wolff-Parkinson-White syndrome (short P-R interval, QRS widening, and delta wave) compared with normal conduction. **A,** Usual appearance of Wolff-Parkinson-White syndrome in leads where the QRS complex is predominantly upright. **B,** Appearance of Wolff-Parkinson-White syndrome; the QRS complex is predominantly negative.

Parkinson-White syndrome is thought to be of minor clinical significance; that is, unless a tachycardia is present. In that case, the syndrome can become life threatening.

Etiology. Wolff-Parkinson-White syndrome may occur in young, healthy persons (mainly men) without apparent cause. The syndrome also may occur in multiple members of a family. It may be present in successive generations.

Rules for Interpretation (Lead II Monitoring). Wolff-Parkinson-White syndrome has the following characteristics on the electrocardiogram:

QRS complex: May be normal or wide (depending on whether conduction is retrograde or anterograde along the bundle of Kent). Conduction that occurs normally down the atrioventricular node and simultaneously in an anterograde fashion along the accessory pathway results in a meeting of the two waves or depolarization that forms a fusion (delta wave). A delta wave is evidenced by slurring or notching of the onset of the QRS complex and is a diagnostic finding in Wolff-Parkinson-White syndrome. (Not all leads show the delta wave.) One should note that QRS widening may simulate right or left bundle branch block.

P waves: Normal

Rate: Normal unless associated with rapid supraventricular tachycardia

Rhythm: Regular

P-R interval: Usually less than 0.12 second because the normal delay at the atrioventricular node does not occur

The three characteristic electrocardiogram findings in Wolff-Parkinson-White syndrome are a short P-R interval, a delta wave, and QRS widening (Fig. 29-98).

Clinical Significance. Patients with Wolff-Parkinson-White syndrome are highly susceptible to bouts of paroxysmal supraventricular tachycardias. The reason is that the accessory pathway provides a ready-made reentry circuit. This allows continued transmission of the impulse from the atria to the ventricles. The majority of tachydysrhythmias seen in Wolff-Parkinson-White syndrome occur with the wave of depolarization progressing from the atrioventricular node to the bundle of His to the accessory pathway. In the accessory pathway the impulse is conducted in a retrograde direction to the atria. Therefore the majority of tachydysrhythmias seen in Wolff-Parkinson-White syndrome are narrow complexes. Patients with Wolff-Parkinson-White syndrome may have attacks of paroxysmal tachydysrhythmias for many years. However, these attacks are not always benign. The atrioventricular node may be bypassed. Conduction rates also can greatly exceed those in patients whose atrioventricular node is part of the reentry circuit. This leads to rapid tachycardias. These can precipitate congestive heart failure and even death from ventricular fibrillation.

Management. Recognition of Wolff-Parkinson-White syndrome is crucial (Fig. 29-99). Differentiating the syndrome from ventricular tachycardia and uncomplicated supraventricular tachycardia also is key. Many emergency drugs used to manage other reentry tachycardias (e.g., ***adenosine***) are contraindicated in Wolff-Parkinson-White syndrome because they can ease conduction over the abnormal pathway. Management must be based on the patient's signs and symptoms. If the patient's heart rate is normal, no emergency care is required. If the patient has a rapid tachycardia, emergency treatment to restore a normal rhythm is needed. The treatment is aimed at blocking conduction through the accessory pathways from the atria to the ventricles.

Prehospital care may include pharmacological therapy for specific dysrhythmias, vagal maneuvers and administration of ***adenosine*** for paroxysmal supraventricular tachycardia, or cardioversion for severe clinical deterioration. ***Verapamil*** is contraindicated in wide-QRS complex tachycardia because the drug can speed conduction down the accessory pathway (greater than 280 beats per minute). This increase in conduction may lead to ventricular fibrillation and sudden death. Thus in patients with wide-QRS complex tachycardia, the drug treatment depends on signs and symptoms and their severity. ***Amiodarone*** or ***lidocaine*** are the first drugs of choice for presumed ventricular tachycardia. ***Adenosine*** and ***procainamide*** are the first choices for presumed supraventricular tachycardia and supraventricular tachycardia with aberrant conduction. The paramedic should perform cardioversion without delay in patients with rapid ventricular rates (greater than 150 beats per minute) who are unstable.

Wolff-Parkinson-White (WPW) Syndrome

Perform Primary ABCD Survey (Basic Life Support)

(Correct critical problems IMMEDIATELY as they are identified)

- Assess responsiveness, **A**irway, **B**reathing, **C**irculation, ensure availability of monitor/**D**efibrillator

Perform Secondary ABCD Survey (Advanced Life Support)

- Administer oxygen, establish IV access, attach cardiac monitor, administer fluids as needed (O_2, IV, monitor, fluids)
- Assess vital signs, attach pulse oximeter, and monitor blood pressure
- Obtain and review 12-lead ECG, portable chest x-ray, perform a focused history and physical exam

Is the patient stable or unstable?
Is the patient experiencing serious signs and symptoms due to the tachycardia?
Is the patient's cardiac function normal or impaired?

Attempt to identify patient's cardiac rhythm using 12-lead ECG, clinical information.

Is Wolff-Parkinson-White syndrome (WPW) present? (e.g., young patient, HR > 300, ECG: short PR interval, wide QRS, delta wave)
Has WPW been present for more or less than 48 hours?

NORMAL CARDIAC FUNCTION		IMPAIRED CARDIAC FUNCTION	
Onset < 48 hours	Onset > 48 hours	Onset < 48 hours	Onset > 48 hours
Control Rate	**Control Rate**	**Control Rate**	**Control Rate**
Cardioversion **OR** Amiodarone (IIb) **OR** Procainamide (IIb) **OR** Flecainide (IIb) **OR** Propafenone (IIb) **OR** Sotalol (IIb)	Use antiarrhythmics with extreme caution because of embolic risk	Cardioversion **OR** amiodarone (IIb) Note: Impaired cardiac function = ejection fraction <40% or CHF	Use antiarrhythmics with extreme caution because of embolic risk
Convert Rhythm	**Convert Rhythm**	**Convert Rhythm**	**Convert Rhythm**
Cardioversion **OR** Amiodarone (IIb) **OR** Procainamide (IIb) **OR** Flecainide (IIb) **OR** Propafenone (IIb) **OR** Sotalol (IIb)	Delayed cardioversion **OR** Early cardioversion	Cardioversion	Delayed cardioversion **OR** Early cardioversion

Delayed cardioversion:
Anticoagulation therapy for 3 weeks before cardioversion, for at least 48 hours in conjunction with cardioversion, and for at least 4 weeks after successful cardioversion. **Early cardioversion:** IV heparin immediately, transesophageal echocardiography (TEE) to r/o atrial thrombus, cardioversion within 24 h, anticoagulation x 4 wks

MEDICATION DOSING

Amiodarone* 150 mg IV bolus over 10 minutes followed by an infusion of 1 mg/min for 6 hours and then a maintenance infusion of 0.5 mg/min. Repeat supplementary infusions of 150 mg as necessary for recurrent or resistant dysrhythmias. Maximum total daily dose 2 g.

Procainamide 100 mg over 5 minutes (20 mg/min). Maximum total dose 17 mg/kg. Maintenance infusion 1–4 mg/min.

Flecainide, propafenone IV form not currently approved for use in the United States

Sotalol 1 to 1.5 mg/kg IV slowly at a rate of 10 mg/min

*Chapman MJ et al: Management of atrial tachyarrhythmias in the critically ill: a comparison of intravenous procainamide and amiodarone, *Intensive Care Med* 19:48, 1993.

FIGURE 29-99 ■ Wolff-Parkinson-White syndrome algorithm.

SECTION SEVEN
SPECIFIC CARDIOVASCULAR DISEASES

PATHOPHYSIOLOGY AND MANAGEMENT OF CARDIOVASCULAR DISEASE

Many true medical emergencies are cardiovascular in nature. Cardiovascular emergencies often result from atherosclerosis of the coronary arteries or peripheral arteries. The following specific medical conditions are discussed in this section:

- Atherosclerosis
- Angina pectoris
- Myocardial infarction
- Left ventricular failure and pulmonary edema
- Right ventricular failure
- Cardiogenic shock
- Cardiac tamponade
- Thoracic and abdominal aneurysm
- Acute arterial occlusion
- Noncritical peripheral vascular disorders
- Hypertension

Pathophysiology of Atherosclerosis

Atherosclerosis is a disease process characterized by progressive narrowing of the lumen of medium and large arteries (e.g., the aorta and its branches, cerebral arteries, and coronary arteries). The process results in the development of thick, hard atherosclerotic plaque. This plaque is referred to as atheromata or *atheromatous lesions.* These lesions most often are found in areas of turbulent blood flow. Such areas include vessel bifurcations or in vessels with decreased lumen diameter.

Atherosclerosis is thought to result from damage to the endothelial cell from mechanical or chemical injury and perhaps excess inflammation (Box 29-17). This response includes platelet adhesion and clotting. Smooth muscle cells may move from the middle muscle layer into the lining of the artery. In the lining the muscle cells form an atheroma. Over time, the atheromata become fibrous and hardened. In time, they partially or fully obstruct the opening of the arteries. In most cases, some collateral circulation develops to make up for the narrowed vessels.

BOX 29-17 Role of Inflammation in Heart Attacks

Studies have suggested that painless inflammation deep within the body plays an important role in the trigger of heart attacks.[7] The inflammation may arise from sources such as chronic gum disease, lingering urinary tract infections, and others. Inflammation may weaken the walls of the blood vessels, allowing fatty buildups to burst. Inflammation can be measured in those at risk for heart disease by testing the blood for elevated white blood cell count and for C-reactive protein. This is a chemical in the blood that is necessary for fighting injury and infection. C-reactive protein can be lowered with cholesterol-lowering drugs, aspirin, and other medications and through diet and exercise.

MAJOR RISK FACTORS

Atherosclerosis occurs to some extent in all middle-aged and older persons. The disease occurs in some young persons as well. Atherosclerosis is thought to be inherited. It usually is seen at a younger age in men than in women. Associated risk factors include age, family history of heart disease, and diabetes. Some other risk factors can be reduced or eliminated. These include cigarette smoking, obesity, hypertension, and hypercholesterolemia. Some research has shown that plaque formation is not only preventable but also reversible.[1]

EFFECTS

Atherosclerosis has two major effects on blood vessels. First, the disease disrupts the innermost lining of the vessels. This causes a loss of vessel elasticity and an increase in the formation of clots. Second, the atheroma reduces the diameter of the vessel lumen. This decreases the blood supply to tissues. Both effects result in an insufficient supply of nutrients to the tissue. This is especially true under conditions of increased tissue demand for nutrients and oxygen.

The severity of this insufficiency is related to the extent of narrowing (stenosis) of the blocked artery. Severity also depends on how long the atheroma took to develop, and the patient's ability to develop collateral circulation around the obstruction. For example, a patient who gradually develops an atherosclerotic occlusion in an artery of a lower extremity may compensate well through collateral circulation. The patient may experience only mild, intermittent pain during periods of exercise. In contrast, sudden-onset occlusion in a coronary artery (following an acute thrombus) almost always results in ischemia, injury, and necrosis to the area of the myocardium supplied by the affected artery.

Angina Pectoris

Angina pectoris is a symptom of myocardial ischemia; the term literally means "choking pain in the chest." Angina is caused by an imbalance between myocardial oxygen supply and demand. The result is a buildup of lactic acid and carbon dioxide in ischemic tissues of the myocardium. These metabolites irritate nerve endings that produce anginal pain. The most common cause of angina pectoris is atherosclerotic disease of the coronary arteries (Box 29-18). A temporary occlusion caused by spasm of a coronary artery with or without atherosclerosis (Prinzmetal's angina) also

BOX 29-18 Other Conditions That May Mimic Angina Pectoris

Acromioclavicular disease	Herpes zoster
Chest wall syndrome	Hiatal hernia
Chest wall trauma	Pancreatitis
Chest wall tumors	Peptic ulcer disease
Cholecystitis	Pleural irritation
Costochondritis	Pneumothorax
Dyspepsia	Pulmonary embolism
Esophageal disease	Respiratory infection
Gastric reflux	Thoracic aortic dissection

can cause angina pectoris. Emotional stress and any activity that increases myocardial oxygen demand may cause anginal pain, particularly in patients with atherosclerosis. Myocardial ischemia in turn may put the patient at risk for cardiac dysrhythmias.

NOTE Several conditions can mimic signs and symptoms of heart disease and angina pectoris. These include cholecystitis, peptic ulcer disease, aneurysm, hiatal hernia, pulmonary embolism, pancreatitis, pleural irritation, and respiratory infection (Box 29-18).

STABLE ANGINA

Angina pectoris generally is classified as *stable* or *unstable.* Stable angina usually is precipitated by physical exertion or emotional stress. The pain usually lasts 1 to 5 minutes. Yet pain may last as long as 15 minutes. Angina is relieved by rest, ***nitroglycerin,*** or oxygen. Stable angina attacks usually are similar and are always relieved by the same mode of therapy.

UNSTABLE ANGINA

Unstable angina (preinfarction angina) denotes an anginal pattern that has changed in its ease of onset, frequency, intensity, duration, or quality. (This includes any new-onset anginal chest pain.) Unstable angina may occur during periods of light exercise or at rest. The pain usually lasts 10 minutes or more. The pain is relieved less promptly with cessation of activity or ***nitroglycerin*** than with stable angina. Unstable angina mimics acute myocardial infarction. The two are sometimes difficult to differentiate in the prehospital setting. Patients with unstable angina are at increased risk of acute myocardial infarction and sudden death.

The pain of angina usually is described by the patient as a pressure, squeezing, heaviness, or tightness in the chest. Although 30% of patients with angina feel pain only in the chest, others describe the pain as radiating to the shoulders, arms, neck, and jaw and through the chest to the back. Associated signs and symptoms include anxiety, shortness of breath, nausea or vomiting, and diaphoresis. The patient history often reveals previous attacks of angina. Many times the patient will have taken ***nitroglycerin*** before arrival of emergency medical services. If so, the paramedic should determine the age of the ***nitroglycerin*** prescription (***nitroglycerin*** is unstable and quickly loses its strength), the amount of ***nitroglycerin*** taken, and its effect. If the pain is not relieved by rest and medication, the paramedic should suspect a myocardial infarction.

MANAGEMENT

All patients with chest pain and signs and symptoms of myocardial ischemia should be managed as though an acute myocardial infarction were evolving. The goal of management is to increase the coronary blood supply, decrease the myocardial oxygen demand, or both. Management guidelines include the following:

1. Place the patient at rest physically and emotionally.
2. Administer oxygen.
3. Administer ***aspirin*** (per protocol).
4. Initiate intravenous therapy for any drugs that may be needed.
5. If pain is present on arrival of emergency medical services, use pharmacological therapy. This may include sublingual or topical ***nitroglycerin*** followed by ***morphine.***
6. Monitor the electrocardiogram for dysrhythmias. Whenever possible (and if scene time is not delayed), record a 3-lead or 12-lead electrocardiogram, or both, during pain. (The electrocardiogram may be normal during a pain-free period.) Also measure, record, and communicate any ST segment changes.
7. Transport the patient for physician evaluation.

Myocardial Infarction

Acute myocardial infarction occurs with a sudden and total blockage or near blockage of blood flowing through an affected coronary artery to an area of heart muscle. This blockage results in ischemia, injury, and necrosis to the area of the myocardium distal to the occlusion. Acute myocardial infarction most often is associated with atherosclerotic heart disease.

PRECIPITATING EVENTS

The process of myocardial infarction is complex. It generally begins with the formation of an atherosclerotic plaque involving the intimal layer of a coronary artery. The plaque disrupts the smooth arterial lining and results in an uneven surface. This creates turbulent blood flow. The plaque may rupture. If rupture occurs, the injured tissue is exposed to circulating platelets. This results in the formation of a thrombus that occludes the artery. As the thrombus enlarges, it further reduces blood flow in the coronary vessel.

Acute thrombotic occlusion generally is accepted as the cause of most myocardial infarctions. Other factors that may lead to acute myocardial infarction include coronary spasm, coronary embolism, severe hypoxia, hemorrhage into a diseased arterial wall, and reduced blood flow after any form of shock. All of these may result in an inadequate amount of blood reaching the myocardium.

TYPES AND LOCATIONS OF INFARCTS

The myocardial cells beyond the occluded artery die (infarct) from lack of oxygen. The size of the infarct is determined by the needs of the tissue supplied by the occluded vessel, by the presence of collateral circulation, and by the time it takes to reestablish blood flow. Therefore emergency care is directed at the following:

- Increasing oxygen supply by administering supplemental oxygen
- Decreasing the metabolic needs and providing collateral circulation
- Reestablishing perfusion to the ischemic myocardium as quickly as possible after the onset of symptoms

The majority of acute myocardial infarctions involve the left ventricle or interventricular septum. These areas are supplied by either of the two major coronary arteries. (However, some patients sustain damage to the right ventricle.) If the occlusion is in the left coronary artery, the result is an anterior, lateral, or septal wall infarction. Inferior wall infarction (of the inferior-posterior wall of the left ventricle) usually is a result of right coronary artery occlusion.

Infarction also can be classified into one of three ischemic syndromes based on the rupture of an unstable plaque in an epicardial artery: unstable angina, non–Q wave myocardial infarction, and Q wave myocardial infarction.[1] All three of these acute coronary syndromes share common risk factors. The management of each overlaps a good deal. Sudden cardiac death may occur with any of these syndromes:

1. Unstable angina. In unstable angina the early thrombus has not obstructed coronary blood flow completely. This partial occlusion produces symptoms of ischemia. The blockage eventually may result in complete occlusion and produce a non–Q wave myocardial infarction. Fibrinolytic therapy (described later in this chapter) is not effective in unstable angina. In fact, such therapy may accelerate the occlusion. Therapy with antiplatelet agents, however, is most effective at this time because the thrombus is rich in platelets.
2. Non–Q wave myocardial infarction. Non–Q wave myocardial infarction occurs as microemboli from the thrombus become lodged in the coronary arteries. This produces minimal damage to the myocardium. Yet these patients are at highest risk for progression to myocardial infarction. Non–Q wave infarcts are evident only with ST segment depression or T wave abnormalities.
3. Q wave myocardial infarction. A Q wave myocardial infarction occurs when the thrombus occludes the coronary vessel for a prolonged period. The infarct is diagnosed by the development of abnormal Q waves in two or more contiguous (adjacent) leads. (Abnormal Q waves are greater than 5 mm in depth or greater than 0.04 second in duration) (Fig. 29-100). The clot is rich in thrombin. Thus early management with fibrinolytics may help to limit the size of the infarct.

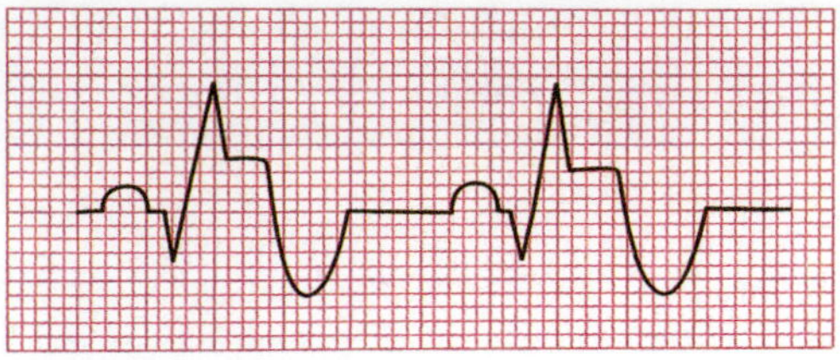

FIGURE 29-100 ■ Pathological Q waves.

DEATH OF MYOCARDIUM

When blood flow to the myocardium ceases, a series of events begins. Cells switch from aerobic to anaerobic metabolism. This results in the release of lactic acid and an increase in tissue carbon dioxide levels. These changes contribute to ischemic pain (angina). As cells lose their ability to maintain their electrochemical gradients, they begin to swell and depolarize. These initial changes are reversible. But within a few hours, if collateral flow and reperfusion are inadequate, much of the muscle distal to the occlusion dies. The area surrounding the necrotic tissue may survive because of collateral circulation. However, surviving tissue may become the origin of dysrhythmias (Fig. 29-101).

Scar tissue replaces the infarcted area in a process that takes about 8 weeks. The process starts with deposits of connective tissue on about the twelfth day. Scar tissue is durable. Yet it lacks elasticity, does not contract, and conducts electrical impulses poorly in the damaged area of the myocardium. The left ventricle, however, can lose as much as 25% of its muscle and still function as an effective pump. Areas with poor perfusion after a large myocardial infarction may not develop strong scar tissue. This may result in an aneurysm. Such an aneurysm can greatly decrease the effective ventricular contractility. An aneurysm also may lead to the development of serious dysrhythmias.

The damaged myocardium is most susceptible to rupture during the first 1 to 2 weeks after a myocardial infarction because the scar tissue has not reached adequate strength. For this reason, patient activity is limited. Prevention of hypertension and excitement during this period also is usually necessary. Even so, the length of hospitalization of patients with uncomplicated myocardial infarctions has decreased. Today, most patients resume activity within 2 to 3 days. Most leave the hospital within 7 to 10 days. Many patients get a stress test before they are discharged. This test determines the patient's exercise tolerance level and whether ischemia or dysrhythmias are present during exercise. The result of this test helps determine what activities the patient may resume after discharge.

DEATHS FOLLOWING MYOCARDIAL INFARCTION

Deaths following myocardial infarction usually result from lethal dysrhythmias (ventricular tachycardia, ventricular fibrillation, and cardiac standstill), pump failure (cardiogenic shock and congestive heart failure), or myocardial tis-

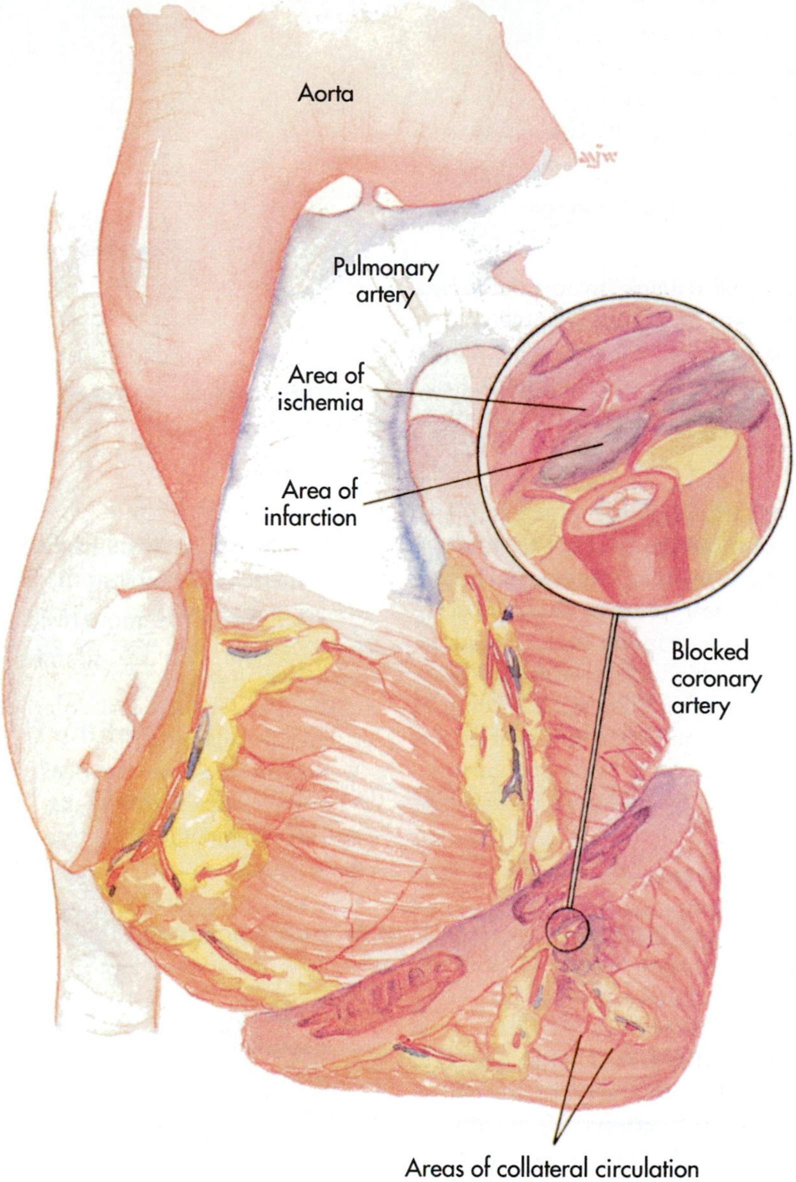

FIGURE 29-101 ■ Area of infarct.

sue rupture (rupture of the ventricle, septum, or papillary muscle). Fatal dysrhythmias are the most common cause of death from myocardial infarction. Deaths that occur within the first 2 hours after the onset of illness or injury are *sudden deaths*. The majority of patients who suffer sudden death have no immediate warning symptoms.

▶**NOTE** *Sudden death* is defined as a sudden dysrhythmic death that occurs within the first 2 hours of cardiac ischemic symptoms.[1] More than 50% of cardiac deaths occur with no evidence of infarction on autopsy when resuscitation attempts fail. Sudden death without infarction is a main reason for the widespread availability of automated external defibrillators. (Another reason is the fact that the most common death-producing dysrhythmia is ventricular fibrillation.)

SIGNS AND SYMPTOMS

Some patients with acute myocardial infarction—particularly diabetic patients, some women, and those in the older age groups—may have only symptoms of dyspnea, syncope, or confusion. However, substernal chest pain is present in 70% to 90% of patients with acute myocardial infarction. The pain generally has the same characteristics and locations as anginal pain. The pain also may radiate to the arms, neck, jaw, or back. The following signs and symptoms may accompany the pain and occasionally are present even in the absence of pain (silent myocardial infarction):

- Agitation
- Anxiety
- Cyanosis
- Diaphoresis
- Dyspnea

- Nausea and vomiting
- Palpitations
- Sense of impending doom

CRITICAL THINKING

How can the prehospital recognition of acute myocardial infarction affect the care of the patient at the hospital?

The chest pain associated with acute myocardial infarction often is constant. The pain also often is not altered or alleviated by ***nitroglycerin*** or other cardiac medications, rest, changes in body position, or breathing patterns. With angina pectoris, the onset often occurs during periods of activity. In contrast, the onset of pain in more than half of all patients with acute myocardial infarction occurs during rest. Most patients have had warning anginal pains (preinfarction angina) hours or days before the attack. Many patients deny the possibility of an evolving myocardial infarction. They may blame the chest pain or discomfort to unrelated causes such as fatigue or indigestion. Denial delays the request for emergency medical services assistance during the most critical phase of the illness. According to the American Heart Association, more than 50% of deaths from ischemic heart disease occur outside the hospital within the first 2 hours after the onset of pain.[1]

CRITICAL THINKING

Why do you think patients deny that their signs and symptoms may be due to a heart attack?

Vital signs vary. They depend on the extent of damage to the heart muscle and conduction system. They also depend on the degree and type of autonomic nervous system response. (Inferior myocardial infarctions often show a mainly parasympathetic response. In contrast, anterior myocardial infarctions commonly show a mainly sympathetic response.) For example, the patient's blood pressure may be normal, elevated (sympathetic discharge), or low (parasympathetic discharge or pump failure). The pulse rate depends on the presence or absence of dysrhythmias. The pulse rate may be normal, tachycardic, bradycardic, regular, or irregular. Respirations may be normal or increased.

COMMON ELECTROCARDIOGRAM FINDINGS

When the heart muscle is damaged, the damaged area is unable to contract effectively. This area remains in a constant depolarized state. The flow of current between the pathologically depolarized and normally repolarized areas produces abnormal ST segment elevation on the electrocardiogram tracing (Fig. 29-102). The most accurate way to measure ST segment elevation is to draw a baseline from the end of the T wave to the start of the P wave. ST segment elevation greater than or equal to 0.5 mV in at least two contiguous electrocardiogram leads indicates acute myocardial infarction. However, the initial electrocardiogram may not show ST segment elevation in patients who are experiencing infarction. Even if infarction is present, ST segment elevation is a poor indicator of whether the infarction will be Q wave or non-Q wave infarction. ST segment elevation also may be caused by conditions other than acute myocardial infarction. These conditions include the following:

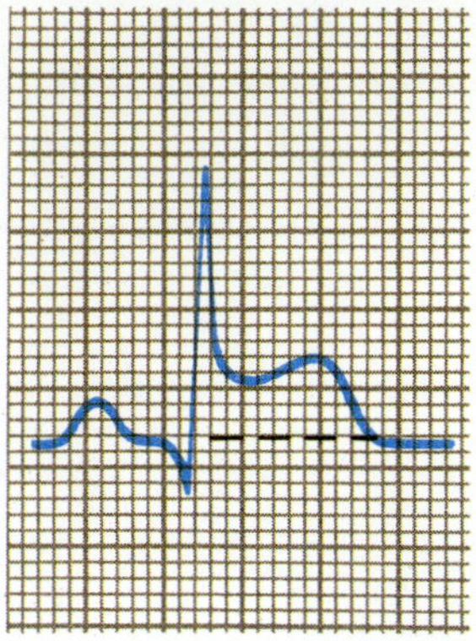

FIGURE 29-102 ■ ST segment elevation likely to present with acute injury.

- Left bundle branch block
- Some ventricular rhythms
- Left ventricular hypertrophy
- Pericarditis
- Ventricular aneurysm
- Early repolarization

NOTE When ST segment elevation is present in a patient suspected of having an acute myocardial infarction, the paramedic should notify the physician. The paramedic also should transmit an electrocardiogram for evaluation (per protocol).

USE OF A 12-LEAD ELECTROCARDIOGRAM TO ASSESS INFARCTS

Early recognition and management of acute myocardial infarction sometimes can salvage a damaged myocardium ("time is muscle"). Paramedics can play an important role in identifying these patients by using the five-step analysis for infarct recognition[2]:

Step 1: Identify the rate and rhythm. The recognition and management of life-threatening rhythms is more important than obtaining a 12-lead electrocardiogram monitoring for infarct location.

Step 2: Identify the area of infarct. ST segment elevation is the most reliable indicator during the first hours of infarction. ST segment elevation can be present before serious tissue damage has occurred. If ST segment elevation is present in a patient with chest pain, the paramedic should identify the degree of elevation and visualize cardiac anatomy to predict which coronary artery is oc-

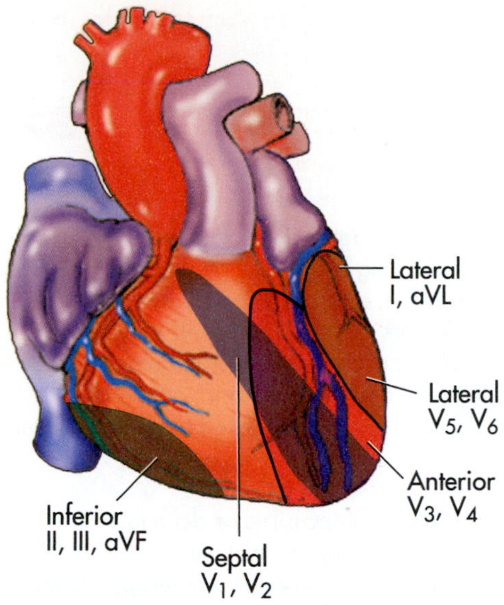

FIGURE 29-103 ■ Multilead assessment of the heart.

TABLE 29-3 ST Segment Elevation and Location of Infarct

LEAD	LOCATION OF INFARCT	CORONARY ARTERY INVOLVED
II, III, aV_F	Inferior wall (most common)	Right
V_1, V_2	Septal wall	Left
V_3, V_4	Anterior wall (most lethal)	Left
I, aV_L, V_5, V_6	Lateral wall	Left
V_4-V_6	Right ventricle	Right

cluded. The paramedic should use a systematic approach for multilead assessment. One method is to begin by monitoring the inferior leads (II, III, aV_F), followed by septal leads (V_1, V_2), anterior leads (V_3, V_4), and lateral leads (V_5, V_6, I, aV_L). The paramedic then evaluates each lead for ST segment elevation (the most important sign of injury), deep symmetrically inverted T waves (a sign of ischemia), ST segment depression (a reciprocal change to ST elevation), and pathological Q waves (Table 29-3 and Fig. 29-103).

▶**NOTE** Sulfonylurea drugs (diabetes drugs), such as glyburide or glipizide, may lessen the magnitude of ST segment elevation in the presence of an infarct.* Thus a careful check of all patients with a cardiac event for a diabetic history is crucial.

*Diabetes drugs can mask severity of heart attack, *Reuters Health* Sep 29, 2003.

At times, the extent of the infarction can be gauged by the number of leads showing ST segment elevation. The degree of ST segment elevation is also important. For example, large infarcts often show an ST elevation of 7 mm or more in inferior leads and an ST elevation of 12 mm or more in anterior leads. ST segment elevation or new or presumably new left bundle branch block is suspicious for injury.

Step 3: When evaluating the electrocardiogram, the paramedic must consider other conditions that could be responsible for ST segment changes (as described before). These "infarct impostors" also may be present in a patient who *is* experiencing acute myocardial infarction. With the exception of left bundle branch block (which makes the interpretation of myocardial infarction difficult), left ventricular hypertrophy looks less like an infarction. Ventricular rhythms often produce Q waves *and* ST segment elevation. Ventricular rhythms also will not have reciprocal ST depression. Electrocardiogram changes with pericarditis are subtle. In addition, early repolarization produces no clinical symptoms.

Step 4: Assess the patient's clinical presentation. An assessment of the clinical condition is just as crucial as the electrocardiogram findings. Thus obtaining a thorough patient history and performing a physical examination should be incorporated into the electrocardiogram interpretation. Not all patients with acute myocardial infarction have classic signs and symptoms. So the paramedic should maintain a high degree of suspicion in the absence of pain. (This should be the case especially with diabetic patients, older adults, and postmenopausal women.) A significant number of patients with acute myocardial infarction have no early electrocardiogram changes. The clinical picture is therefore important.

Step 5: Recognize the infarction and initiate care. When all indications point to acute myocardial infarction, the paramedic will need to take steps to speed the process of data collection, physician evaluation, and thrombolysis (when appropriate). This will help to reduce the time from infarct to treatment. Clinical presentation and electrocardiogram findings that suggest an acute myocardial infarction must be confirmed by medical direction to determine whether fibrinolytic therapy is appropriate.

MANAGEMENT OF AN UNCOMPLICATED ACUTE MYOCARDIAL INFARCTION

All patients with anginal chest pain are assumed to have an acute myocardial infarction until proved otherwise (Fig. 29-104). Any patient with chest pain should be transported to a medical facility for physician evaluation. This is regardless of the apparent severity on emergency medical services arrival, the patient's age, or associated complaints. The primary goals of prehospital care are to relieve pain and apprehension, to prevent the development of serious dysrhythmias, and to limit the size of the infarct.

The paramedic should obtain a full patient history while conducting the physical examination and during initial

Initial Assessment and General Treatment of the Patient with an Acute Coronary Syndrome.

PREHOSPITAL	EMERGENCY DEPARTMENT

Initial Assessment (Goal: targeted clinical exam and 12-lead ECG within 10 minutes)

PREHOSPITAL

- Obtain a brief, targeted history/physical exam (determine age, gender; S/S, pain presentation including location of pain, duration, quality, relation to effort, time of symptom onset; history CAD, CAD risk factors present?) History of Viagra use?
  Assess vital signs, determine oxygen saturation

If above consistent with possible or definite ACS:

- Use checklist (yes-no); focus on eligibility for reperfusion therapy; evaluate contraindications to aspirin and heparin
- Establish IV access, ECG monitoring
- Administer aspirin 162 to 325 mg (chewed) if no reason for exclusion
- Obtain 12-lead ECG (machine interpretation or transmission of ECG to physician)
- Draw blood for initial serum cardiac marker levels (to lab on arrival in emergency department)

Consider triage to facility capable of angiography and revascularization if any of the following are present:
- Signs of shock
- Pulmonary edema (rales > halfway up)
- Heart rate 100 beats/min and SBP 100 mm Hg

EMERGENCY DEPARTMENT

RN triage for rapid care
- Targeted history - determine age, gender, S/S, pain presentation including location of pain, duration, quality, relation to effort, time of symptom onset; history CAD, CAD risk factors present? History of Viagra use?
- Assess vital signs, determine oxygen saturation
- Establish IV access, ECG monitoring
- Obtain 12-lead ECG (present to physician for review)

Physician evaluation

If above consistent with possible or definite ACS:
- Brief, targeted history/physical exam
- Evaluate eligibility for reperfusion therapy + contraindications to aspirin and heparin
- Administer aspirin 162 to 325 mg (chewed) if no reason for exclusion
- Administer nitroglycerin as indicated
- Evaluate 12-lead ECG—categorize patient into one of three groups: ST-elevation or new or presumably new LBBB; ST-depression/transient ST-segment/T wave changes; normal or nondiagnostic ECG
- Obtain serial ECGs in patients with history suggesting MI and nondiagnostic ECG
- Obtain baseline serum cardiac marker levels (CK-MB, Troponin T or I, myoglobin)
- Obtain lab specimens (CBC, lipid profile, electrolytes, coagulation studies)
- Obtain portable chest x-ray
- Evaluate results

Routine Measures

- Oxygen 4 L/min by nasal cannula for first 2 to 3 hours (Class IIa)
- Oxygen 4 L/min by cannula, titrate if pulmonary congestion, $SaO_2 < 90\%$ (Class I)
- Aspirin 162 to 325 mg–chewed (if hypersensitivity exists, ticlopidine); may administer via rectal suppository (325 mg) if nausea, vomiting, upper GI disorder present
- NTG SL or spray (ensure IV access, SBP > 90 mm Hg, HR > 50 beats/min, no RV infarction)
- Morphine 2 to 4 mg IV if pain not relieved with NTG; may repeat every 5 min (ensure SBP > 90 mm Hg)

FIGURE 29-104 ■ Acute myocardial infarction algorithm.

patient care. Time is of the essence. Thus the following aspects of patient care are a high priority:

1. Place the patient at rest or in a comfortable position. This will help to decrease anxiety and the heart rate. Thus it will decrease oxygen demand.
2. Administer low-concentration oxygen (3 to 4 L/min) via the nasal cannula. Patients with respiratory compromise need a higher oxygen concentration.
3. Initiate transport quickly. (Do this without audible or visual warning devices if the patient is stable.) This will help decrease patient anxiety.
4. Administer ***aspirin*** (per protocol).
5. Consider the use of pulse oximetry.
6. Establish an intravenous line with normal saline or lactated Ringer's solution to keep the vein open.
7. Obtain baseline vital signs. Repeat the assessment often. Vital sign assessment should include auscultation of the lungs for heart failure indicators (presence of crackles).
8. Attach electrocardiogram electrodes, document initial rhythm, and monitor for dysrhythmias.
9. Administer medications (per protocol) for the relief of pain and the management of dysrhythmias:
   a. Medications that may be used for analgesia and to decrease preload and afterload include ***nitroglycerin*** and ***morphine.***

Management of ST-Segment Elevation MI.

ST-segment elevation 1 mm in two or more anatomically contiguous leads or new, or presumably new, LBBB

Confirm diagnosis by signs/symptoms, ECG, serum cardiac markers

All patients with ST-segment elevation MI should receive (if no contraindications):

- Antiplatelet therapy - aspirin 162–325 mg (chewed)
- Anti-ischemia therapy (beta-blockers, NTG IV if ongoing ischemia or uncorrected hypertension)
- Antithrombin therapy - heparin (if using fibrin-specific lytics)
- ACE inhibitors (after 6 hours or when stable)–especially with large or anterior MI, heart failure without hypotension (SBP > 100 mm Hg), previous MI

Symptom onset 12 hours?

Patient Eligible for Reperfusion?

Goals–
- Fibrinolytics: Door-to-drug time < 30 min
- Primary PCI: Door-to-dilation time 90 ± 30 min

- Yes → Signs of cardiogenic shock or contraindications in fibrinolytics?
  - Yes → PCI; Medical management
  - No → Can cath lab be mobilized within 60 min?
    - Yes → PCI
    - No → Fibrinolysis (alteplase, reteplase, streptokinase, anisteplase, or tenecteplase)
- No → Persistent or stuttering symptoms of EG changes?
  - Yes → Cardiac cath, medical management
  - No → Medical management

Symptom onset > 12 hours?

Persistent Symptoms	Resolution of Symptoms
Consider reperfusion	Medical management
Medical management	

Note: PCI = percutaneous coronary intervention (angioplasty ± stent).

FIGURE 29-104, cont'd ■ Acute myocardial infarction algorithm.

Continued

b. Medications that may be used to manage the various dysrhythmias include ***lidocaine, procainamide, atropine, verapamil, adenosine, magnesium, propranolol,*** and ***amiodarone.***

FIBRINOLYTIC THERAPY

Studies have shown that an acute intracoronary thrombus can be dissolved (thereby restoring blood flow to the ischemic area) with salvage of ischemic myocardium if a fibrinolytic agent is administered within 6 hours after the onset of symptoms.[1] Some emergency medical services are authorized by medical direction to administer these agents in the prehospital setting. However, the American Heart Association recommends that prehospital systems focus on early diagnosis; field administration of fibrinolytics should occur in special circumstances when a physician is present or if transport time exceeds 90 minutes.[1]

Common fibrinolytic agents include ***streptokinase, tissue plasminogen activator,*** and ***reteplase.*** All of these agents work through activation of the plasma protein plasminogen to dissolve the coronary thrombus. Plasminogen is converted to plasmin (the active form). The plasmin degrades fibrin, the basic component of a clot (thrombus). ***Aspirin*** and ***heparin*** are part of the "fibrinolytic package."

Management of Unstable Angina/Non-ST-Segment Elevation MI

ECG changes in 2 or more anatomically contiguous leads:
ST-segment depression > 1 mm or T wave inversion > 1 mm or
Transient (<30 min) ST-segment/T wave changes > 1 mm with discomfort

Confirm diagnosis by signs/symptoms, ECG, serum cardiac markers

- Aspirin 162–325 mg (chewed) if not already administered (and no contraindications) (antiplatelet therapy)
- Heparin IV (antithrombin therapy)

If high-risk patient give:
- Aspirin + glycoprotein IIb/IIa inhibitors (i.e., Integrilin, Aggrastat, ReoPro) + IV heparin OR.
- Aspirin + glycoprotein IIb/IIa inhibitors + SC low molecular weight heparin

High-risk criteria
- Persistent ("stuttering") symptoms/recurrent ischemia; left ventricular (LV) dysfunction, CHF; widespread EG changes; prior MI, positive troponin or CK-MB

Anti-ischemic therapy
- Beta-blockers–if patient not previously on beta-blockers or inadequately treated on current dose of beta-blocker (if no contraindications)
- NTG sublingual tablet or spray, followed by IV NTG if symptoms persist despite sublingual NTG therapy and initiation of beta-blocker therapy (and SBP > 90 mm Hg)
- Morphine 2 to 4 mg IV (if discomfort is not relieved or symptoms recur despite antiischemic therapy)–may repeat every 5 min (ensure SBP > 90 mm Hg)

Assess clinical status–is patient clinically stable?

YES
- Continue in-hospital observation
- Consider stress testing

NO
Cardiac cath
- If anatomy suitable for revascularization–PCI, CABG
- If anatomy unsuitable–medical management

Management of Patient with a Suspected Acute Coronary Syndrome and Nondiagnostic/Normal ECG

Nondiagnostic or Normal ECG
Evaluate signs/symptoms, serial ECGs, serum cardiac markers

Aspirin + other therapy as appropriate

- Assess patient's clinical risk of death/nonfatal MI
- History and physical exam
- Obtain follow-up serum cardiac marker levels, serial ECG monitoring
- Continue evaluation and treatment in emergency department chest pain unit or monitored bed
- Consider radionuclide, echocardiography

FIGURE 29-104, cont'd ■ Acute myocardial infarction algorithm.

A fibrinolytic agent can dissolve beneficial and pathological thrombi. Thus the drug is administered selectively. Most emergency medical services systems using fibrinolytic agents establish inclusion-exclusion criteria similar to the following[4]:

1. Patient inclusion criteria
   - Chest pain suggesting acute myocardial infarction for at least 20 minutes
   - Onset of symptoms less than 12 hours
   - Oriented and able to give informed consent
   - ST segment elevation equal to or greater than 0.5 mm (0.5 mV) in two or more contiguous leads
   - Under 75 years of age
2. Patient exclusion criteria

   Absolute Contraindications
   - History of intracranial bleeding or stroke
   - Other stroke or cerebrovascular accident in less than 1 year

- Internal bleeding (menses excluded)
- Suspected aortic dissection

Relative Contraindications

- Pregnancy or postpartum state
- Uncontrolled hypertension
- Major surgery within 3 weeks
- Intracranial tumor
- Thoracic aortic aneurysm
- Cardiopulmonary resuscitation in the nontrauma patient that has been in progress less than 10 minutes
- Trauma (within 2 to 4 weeks)
- Known bleeding disorder or current use of anticoagulants
- Terminal illness

Congestive Heart Failure

Congestive heart failure is a condition in which the heart is unable to pump blood at a rate to meet the metabolic needs of the tissues. The condition affects about 5 million Americans and is responsible for 7000 to 10,000 hospital admissions each year.[8] Congestive heart failure most often is caused by volume overload, pressure overload, loss of myocardial tissue, and impaired contractility. All of these can impair left ventricular function. This text discusses congestive heart failure in terms of left ventricular failure and pulmonary edema and of right ventricular failure.

LEFT VENTRICULAR FAILURE AND PULMONARY EDEMA

Left ventricular failure occurs when the left ventricle fails to work as an effective forward pump. This causes a back-pressure of blood into the pulmonary circulation. This condition may be caused by a number of forms of heart disease. These forms may include ischemic, valvular, and hypertensive heart disease. If left unmanaged, significant left ventricular failure results in pulmonary edema.

In left ventricular failure, blood is delivered to the left ventricle. Yet the blood is not fully ejected from the ventricle. The increase in end-diastolic blood volume increases left ventricular end-diastolic pressure. This pressure is transmitted to the left atrium. Pressure then is transmitted to the pulmonary veins and capillaries. As pulmonary capillary hydrostatic pressure increases, the plasma portion of blood is forced into the alveoli. There plasma mixes with air. This results in the typical finding in pulmonary edema: foamy, blood-tinged sputum. If left unmanaged, the progressive fluid buildup can result in death from hypoxia. Myocardial infarction is a common cause of left ventricular failure. Thus all patients with pulmonary edema (particularly those with an abrupt onset) also should be suspected of having an acute myocardial infarction.

NOTE **Paroxysmal nocturnal dyspnea** is an abnormal condition of the respiratory system. This dyspnea is characterized by sudden attacks of shortness of breath, profuse sweating, tachycardia, and wheezing that awaken a person from sleep. This dyspnea often is associated with left ventricular failure and pulmonary edema.

BOX 29-19 Signs and Symptoms of Left Ventricular Failure

- Severe respiratory distress
  - Orthopnea
  - Spasmodic cough that may produce foamy, blood-tinged sputum
  - History of paroxysmal nocturnal dyspnea (a sudden episode of dyspnea that occurs after lying down)
- Severe apprehension, agitation, confusion
- Cyanosis (if severe)
- Diaphoresis
- Adventitious lung sounds
  - Bilateral crackles that do not clear with coughing (usually present at the base of the lungs and up to the level of the scapulae)
  - Rhonchi (fluid in upper airways)
  - Wheezes (reflex airway spasm, sometimes referred to as cardiac asthma)
- Jugular vein distention (indicative of back-pressure through the right heart and into the venous system)
- Abnormal vital signs
  - Blood pressure: possibly elevated
  - Pulse rate: rapid to compensate for low stroke volume; possibly irregular if dysrhythmias are present
- Regular alterations of weak and strong beats without changes in the length of cycle (pulsus alternans)
  - Respirations: rapid, labored
- Level of consciousness (Patient may be anxious, agitated, uncooperative, or obtunded because of poor cerebral perfusion or hypoxia.)
- Chest pain
  - Presence or absence of pain
  - Possible masking by respiratory distress

Left ventricular failure results in a reduction of stroke volume. This in turn initiates several compensatory mechanisms that restore cardiac output and organ perfusion (tachycardia, vasoconstriction, and activation of the renin-angiotensin-aldosterone system). However, these mechanisms often increase myocardial oxygen demand. Thus they further decrease the ability of the myocardium to contract. Box 29-19 lists the signs and symptoms of left ventricular failure and pulmonary edema.

Management. Pulmonary edema is an acute and critical emergency (Fig. 29-105). It may lead to death unless it is treated rapidly. Emergency management is directed at decreasing the venous return to the heart, improving myocardial contractility, decreasing myocardial oxygen demand, improving ventilation and oxygenation, and rapidly transporting the patient to a medical facility.

Emergency care entails patient positioning, oxygenation, ventilatory support as needed, and pharmacological therapy. As in any other true emergency, the paramedic should perform a full but focused patient history and examination while initiating treatment. No characteristic electrocardiogram changes are associated with pulmonary

Management of Acute Pulmonary Edema

Perform Primary ABCD Survey (Basic Life Support)

(Correct critical problems IMMEDIATELY as they are identified)
- Assess responsiveness, **A**irway, **B**reathing, **C**irculation, ensure availability of monitor/**D**efibrillator

Perform Secondary ABCD Survey (Advanced Life Support)

(Obtain arterial blood gas before oxygen administration if possible)
- Administer oxygen, establish IV access, attach cardiac monitor (O_2, IV, monitor)
- Assess vital signs, attach pulse oximeter, & monitor blood pressure
- Obtain & review 12-lead ECG, portable chest x-ray
- Perform a focused history and physical exam

If feasible and BP permits, place patient in sitting position with feet dependent
- Increases lung volume and vital capacity
- Decreases work of respiration
- Decreases venous return, decreases preload

If systolic BP > 100 mm Hg:
- Sublingual nitroglycerin–1 tablet or 2 sprays every 5 minutes (max 3 tablets) until IV nitroglycerin or nitroprusside can take effect
- Furosemide IV 0.5 to 1.0 mg/kg (typically 20 to 80 mg) can repeat in 30 minutes if symptoms persist and BP stable
- Consider morphine IV 2-4 mg

Consider additional preload/afterload reduction–nitroglycerin or nitroprusside IV, ACE inhibitors
- Nitroglycerin IV–start at 5 mcg/min and increase gradually until mean systolic pressure falls by 10% to 15%, avoid hypotension (SBP <90 mm hg)" **OR**
- Nitroprusside IV (If SBP > 100 mm Hg)–0.1 to 5 mcg/kg/min

Evaluate early for:
- Readily reversible cause and institute appropriate intervention (e.g., cardiac dysrhythmias, tamponade)
- Myocardial ischemia/infarction (Institute appropriate intervention–candidate for fibrinolytic therapy? PTCA?

If patient is refractory to above therapies, hypotensive, or in cardiogenic shock:
- Consider fluid or IV inotropic and/or vasopressor agents (e.g., dobutamine, dopamine, norepinephrine)
- Consider pulmonary and systemic arterial catheterization
- Obtain echocardiogram to assist in diagnosis, evaluation, and reparability of culprit lesion or condition
- Consider need for mechanical circulatory assistance (balloon pump)

FIGURE 29-105 ■ Acute pulmonary edema/hypotension/shock algorithm.

edema. However, the paramedic should obtain an initial tracing. The paramedic also should monitor the patient's rhythm continuously for evidence of myocardial irritability and dysrhythmias.

The paramedic should place the patient in a sitting position with the legs dependent. This position increases lung volume and vital capacity. It also diminishes the work of respiration. It decreases venous return to the heart as well.

The paramedic should administer high-concentration oxygen using a well-fitted face mask. Preferably the mask should be a non-rebreathing mask to optimize the amount of inspired oxygen. Some patients may require (and will tolerate) positive-pressure assistance (including continuos positive airway pressure or biphasic positive airway pressure). Positive pressure assistance helps reduce pulmonary edema. This also reduces the need for high levels of inspired oxygen. If possible, the paramedic should use a pulse oximeter to ensure arterial oxygen saturation of at least 90%. If this cannot be achieved with 100% oxygen or if there are signs of cerebral hypoxia or progressive hypercapnia, endotracheal intubation and assisted ventilations may be indicated.

The following three medications may be used to decrease venous return, enhance contractile function of the myocardium, and reduce dyspnea:

1. ***Nitroglycerin***
   a. Induction of peripheral vasodilation
   b. Possible reduction of preload and afterload, thereby reducing the myocardial workload and improving cardiac function
2. ***Furosemide***
   a. Direct relaxant (dilating) effect on the venous system within 5 minutes

Management of Hypotension/Shock-Suspected Pump Problem

Perform Primary ABCD Survey (Basic Life Support)

(Correct critical problems IMMEDIATELY as they are identified)

- Assess responsiveness, **A**irway, **B**reathing, **C**irculation, ensure availability of monitor/**D**efibrillator

Perform Secondary ABCD Survey (Advanced Life Support)

- Administer oxygen, establish IV access, attach cardiac monitor, administer fluids as needed (O_2, IV, monitor, fluids)
- Assess vital signs, attach pulse oximeter, and monitor blood pressure
- Obtain and review 12-lead ECG, portable chest x-ray,
- Perform a focused history and physical exam

Hypotension–suspected pump problem

If breath sounds are clear, consider fluid challenge of 250 to 500 -mL NS to ensure adequate ventricular filling pressure before vasopressor administration

Marked hypotension (systolic BP < 70 mm Hg)/cardiogenic shock

Pharmacologic management:[i]

- Norepinephrine infusion (0.5 to 30 mcg/min) until SBP 80 mm Hg
- Then attempt to change to dopamine 5 to 15 mcg/kg/min until SBP 90 mm Hg
- IV dobutamine (2 to 20 mcg/kg/min) can be given simultaneously in an attempt to reduce magnitude of dopamine infusion

Consider balloon pump or patient transfer to a cardiac interventional facility

Moderate hypotension (systolic BP 70 to 90 mm Hg)ii

- Dopamine 5 to 15 mcg/kg/min
- If BP remains low despite dopamine doses > 20 mcg/kg/min, may substitute norepinephrine in doses of 0.5 to 30 mcg/min
- Once SBP ≥ 90 with dopamine, add dobutamine 2 to 20 mcg/kg/min and attempt to taper off dopamine

Systolic BP 90 mm Hg[iii iv]

- Dobutamine 2 to 20 mcg/kg/min

Dosing:

Norepinephrine IV	0.5 to 30 mcg/min
Dopamine IV	5 to 15 mcg/kg/min
Dobutamine IV	2 to 20 mcg/kg/min

FIGURE 29-105, cont'd ■ Acute pulmonary edema/hypotension/shock algorithm.

Continued

b. Diuretic effect that reduces intravascular volume
c. May lead to electrolyte imbalance

3. ***Morphine***
   a. Decrease of venous return by dilation of the capacitance vessels of the peripheral venous bed (reduces preload)
   b. Reduction of myocardial work
   c. Reduction of anxiety

All of these medications can lower blood pressure. Thus one must take care in patients with pulmonary edema and hypotension (blood pressure less than 100 mm Hg systolic).

> **CRITICAL THINKING**
> What happens to the diffusion of oxygen and carbon dioxide in the lungs during this process?

RIGHT VENTRICULAR FAILURE

Right ventricular failure most often results from left ventricular failure that produces elevated pressure in the pulmonary vascular system. This pressure causes resistance to pulmonary blood flow. It also increases the workload of the right side of the heart to overcome the resistance. Over time, the right ventricle fails as an effective forward pump. This causes back-pressure of blood into the systemic venous circulation. When the pressure in the systemic venous circulation becomes too high, the plasma portion of the blood is forced out into the interstitial tissues of the body. This results in edema, particularly in the dependent areas of the body. (For example, edema occurs in the lower extremities and the sacrum of patients who are bedridden.) Right ventricular failure can result from several diseases. These include chronic hypertension (in which left ventricular failure

Management of Hypotension/Shock–Suspected Volume Problem

Perform Primary ABCD Survey (Basic Life Support)

(Correct critical problems IMMEDIATELY as they are identified)
- Assess responsiveness, **A**irway, **B**reathing, **C**irculation, ensure availability of monitor/**D**efibrillator

Perform Secondary ABCD Survey (Advanced Life Support)
- Administer oxygen, establish IV access, attach cardiac monitor, administer fluids as needed (O_2, IV, monitor, fluids)
- Assess vital signs, attach pulse oximeter, and monitor blood pressure
- Obtain and review 12-lead ECG, portable chest x-ray,
- Perform a focused history and physical exam

Hypotension–suspected volume (or vascular resistance) problem

Volume replacement
- Fluid challenge (250 to 500-mL IV boluses–reassess)
- Blood transfusion (if appropriate)
- If cause known, institute appropriate intervention (e.g., septic shock, anaphylaxis)
- Consider vasopressors, if indicated, to improve vascular tone if no response to fluid challenge(s)

Management of Hypotension/Shock–Suspected Rate Problem

Perform Primary ABCD Survey (Basic Life Support)

(Correct critical problems IMMEDIATELY as they are identified)
- Assess responsiveness, **A**irway, **B**reathing, **C**irculation, ensure availability of monitor/**D**efibrillator

Perform Secondary ABCD Survey (Advanced Life Support)
- Administer oxygen, establish IV access, attach cardiac monitor, administer fluids as needed (O_2, IV, monitor, fluids)
- Assess vital signs, attach pulse oximeter, and monitor blood pressure
- Obtain and review 12-lead ECG, portable chest x-ray,
- Perform a focused history and physical exam

Hypotension - suspected rate problem

If rate too slow–bradycardia algorithm

If rate too fast–determine width of QRS, then use appropriate tachycardia algorithm

FIGURE 29-105, cont'd ■ Acute pulmonary edema/hypotension/shock algorithm.

usually precedes right ventricular failure), chronic obstructive pulmonary disease, pulmonary embolism, valvular heart disease, and infarction of the right ventricle.

Box 29-20 lists the signs and symptoms of right ventricular failure. When left and right ventricular failure occur at the same time, signs and symptoms of each may be present. Table 29-4 can help the paramedic differentiate between the two.

Management. Right ventricular failure is often a chronic condition. It usually is not a medical emergency in itself. Yet if right ventricular failure is associated with pulmonary edema or hypotension, it may be a medical emergency. The paramedic should be prepared to manage the patient for either of these situations. Patient management for right ventricular failure includes the following:

1. Placing the patient at rest in a sitting or semi-Fowler position (head elevated)
2. Administering high-concentration oxygen
3. Obtaining baseline vital signs and an electrocardiogram tracing
4. Initiating an intravenous line to keep the vein open or to manage hypotension
5. Monitoring the electrocardiogram
6. Managing symptoms of left ventricular failure, if present

BOX 29-20 Signs and Symptoms of Right Ventricular Failure

- Tachycardia
- Venous congestion
  - Engorged liver, spleen, or both
  - Venous distention: distention and pulsation of the neck veins
- Peripheral edema
  - Lower extremities or entire body (anasarca)
  - Sacral region in bedridden patients
  - Pitting edema
- Fluid accumulation in serous cavities
  - Abdominal cavity (ascites)
  - Pericardium (pericardial effusion)
  - *Note:* Patients often can tolerate large quantities of effusion without compromise when the effusion develops over an extended period.
- History
  - Often previous myocardial infarction in patients with chronic congestive failure
  - Frequent medication history of digitalis and diuretics to control heart failure

TABLE 29-4 Symptoms and Signs of Chronic Heart Failure

RIGHT VENTRICULAR DYSFUNCTION		LEFT VENTRICULAR DYSFUNCTION		NONSPECIFIC FINDINGS	
SYMPTOMS	**SIGNS**	**SYMPTOMS**	**SIGNS**	**SYMPTOMS**	**SIGNS**
Abdominal pain	Peripheral edema	Dyspnea on exertion	Bibasilar crackles	Exercise intolerance	Tachycardia
Anorexia	Jugular venous distention	Paroxysmal nocturnal dyspnea	Pulmonary edema	Fatigue	Pallor
Nausea	Engorged liver	Orthopnea	S_3 gallop	Weakness	Cyanosis of digits
Bloating	Engorged spleen	Tachypnea	Pleural effusion	Nocturia	Cardiomegaly
Constipation	—	Cough	Chest pain	Central nervous system symptoms	Agitation
Ascites	—	Hemoptysis	Diaphoresis		

NOTE Hypotension caused by right ventricular failure (often seen in right ventricular infarction) can mimic cardiogenic shock. In this case, fluid administration helps normalize left ventricular filling. Administration of fluids is crucial and helps the hypotensive patient regain a normal blood pressure. (This is just the opposite of the hypotension associated with cardiogenic shock, where administration of fluids worsens the condition.) Management may include 250-mL intravenous boluses of normal saline over 5 to 10 minutes. This will help to increase myocardial strength (Starling's law). Fluid administration also improves contractility. Close observation of the patient and vital signs is crucial.

Cardiogenic Shock

Cardiogenic shock is the most extreme form of pump failure. It occurs when left ventricular function is so compromised that the heart cannot meet the metabolic needs of the body. The result is a significant decrease in stroke volume (resulting from ineffective myocardial contraction), cardiac output, and blood pressure. All of these result in an inadequate supply of blood to the organs. Cardiogenic shock occurs in 5% to 10% of patients with acute myocardial infarction. It may be the result of acute left- or right-sided heart failure.

By definition, cardiogenic shock is present when shock persists after correction of existing dysrhythmias, volume deficit, or decreased vascular tone. Cardiogenic shock usually is caused by extensive myocardial infarction (often involving more than 40% of the left ventricle) or by diffuse ischemia. Even with aggressive therapy, cardiogenic shock has a mortality rate of 70% or higher.[9]

In addition to the signs and symptoms of myocardial infarction, patients in cardiogenic shock show clinical evidence of hypoperfusion to vital organs and significant systemic hypotension similar to that found in other forms of shock. (This makes it difficult to differentiate the exact cause of shock.) This evidence includes the following:

- Acidosis
- Altered level of consciousness
- Cool, clammy, cyanotic, or ashen skin
- Hypoxemia
- Profound hypotension (systolic blood pressure usually less than 80 mm Hg)
- Pulmonary congestion (crackles)
- Sinus tachycardia or other dysrhythmias
- Tachypnea

In the early stages of cardiogenic shock, the patient's heart tries to compensate. The heart rate increases. If possible, the heart also increases contractility and cardiac output. If the condition is managed inadequately, the heart progresses toward hypodynamic failure with depressed contractility, reduced stroke volume, and subsequent hypoperfusion (see Chapter 21).

MANAGEMENT

Patients in cardiogenic shock are ill. (See Fig. 29-105.) These patients need rapid transport to a medical facility. Transport should not be delayed attempting field treatment. Prehospital care should include airway management and ventilatory support with high-concentration oxygen, placement of the patient in a supine position (or semi-Fowler position, if the patient is dyspneic), insertion of an intravenous line with normal saline or lactated Ringer's solution to keep the vein open, electrocardiogram monitoring, correction of dysrhythmias, and frequent evaluation of vital signs (including auscultation of the lungs and observation for jugular venous distention). A patient in respiratory failure may require intubation and ventilatory support.

> **CRITICAL THINKING**
> Consider unstable patients with signs and symptoms indicating cardiogenic shock. How should you respond when they ask you, "Am I going to die?"

Drug therapy may include drugs that strengthen the force of contraction (inotropic agents) to improve cardiac output. Such agents include ***dopamine*** or ***dobutamine.*** The use of vasodilator drugs to reduce afterload generally is reserved for in-hospital coronary care settings. In such settings, blood pressure can be evaluated more accurately. If left-sided heart failure and pulmonary edema also are present, they should be treated at the same time.

> **CRITICAL THINKING**
> What dose of each of these drugs should be given for this condition?

Cardiac Tamponade

Cardiac tamponade (described in Chapter 26) is defined as impaired diastolic filling of the heart caused by increased intrapericardial pressure and volume.[9] As the pressure of the buildup in pericardial fluid compresses the atria and ventricles, they are unable to fill adequately. This results in a decrease in ventricular filling, and stroke volume is decreased. The condition may have a gradual onset. This may result from a cancerous growth or infection. Or the condition may be acute, resulting from trauma to the chest, including cardiopulmonary resuscitation. Cardiac tamponade also may result from renal disease or hypothyroidism. Signs and symptoms of cardiac tamponade include the following:

- Chest pain
- Decreased systolic pressure (a late sign)
- Ectopy
- Electrocardiogram changes (usually inconclusive)
- Elevated venous pressure (an early sign) with associated jugular vein distention
- Faint or muffled heart sounds
- Low-voltage QRS complexes and T waves
- Pulsus paradoxus
- ST segment elevation or nonspecific T wave changes
- Tachycardia

As described in Chapter 26, the most important reliable signs of cardiac tamponade are elevated venous pressure associated with hypotension and tachycardia (Beck's triad).

> **CRITICAL THINKING**
> Why would fluid resuscitation with large amounts of fluid not be indicated in this situation?

MANAGEMENT

First, the paramedic must obtain a thorough history to attempt to identify the cause of cardiac tamponade. Then the paramedic performs a physical examination. Prehospital care is directed at ensuring an adequate airway and ventilatory support and providing rapid transport for physician evaluation and possible drainage of the pericardial sac (pericardiocentesis). A fluid bolus may help support the circulatory system temporarily if the patient becomes hypotensive. However, definitive management requires drainage of the pericardial sac. Cardiac tamponade may result in death if the condition is not relieved.

> **CRITICAL THINKING**
> Why is drainage of the pericardial sac not done routinely in the prehospital setting?

Thoracic and Abdominal Aortic Aneurysms

Aneurysm is a nonspecific term that means "dilation of a vessel." Aneurysm may result from atherosclerotic disease (most common), infectious disease (primarily syphilis), traumatic injury, or certain genetic disorders (e.g., Marfan syndrome). Fig. 29-106 illustrates the branches of the aorta. Abdominal aortic aneurysm and dissecting aneurysm of the aorta are presented here.

Most aneurysms develop at a weak point in the wall of an artery. This weak point results from degenerative changes in the medial layer. Weakening of the supportive elements of the vessel wall allows dilation. This causes turbulence and increasing lateral pressure. The aneurysm tends to enlarge over time as the lateral pressure increases in the dilated segment. Eventually the aneurysm may rupture. This in turn may produce life-threatening hemorrhage.

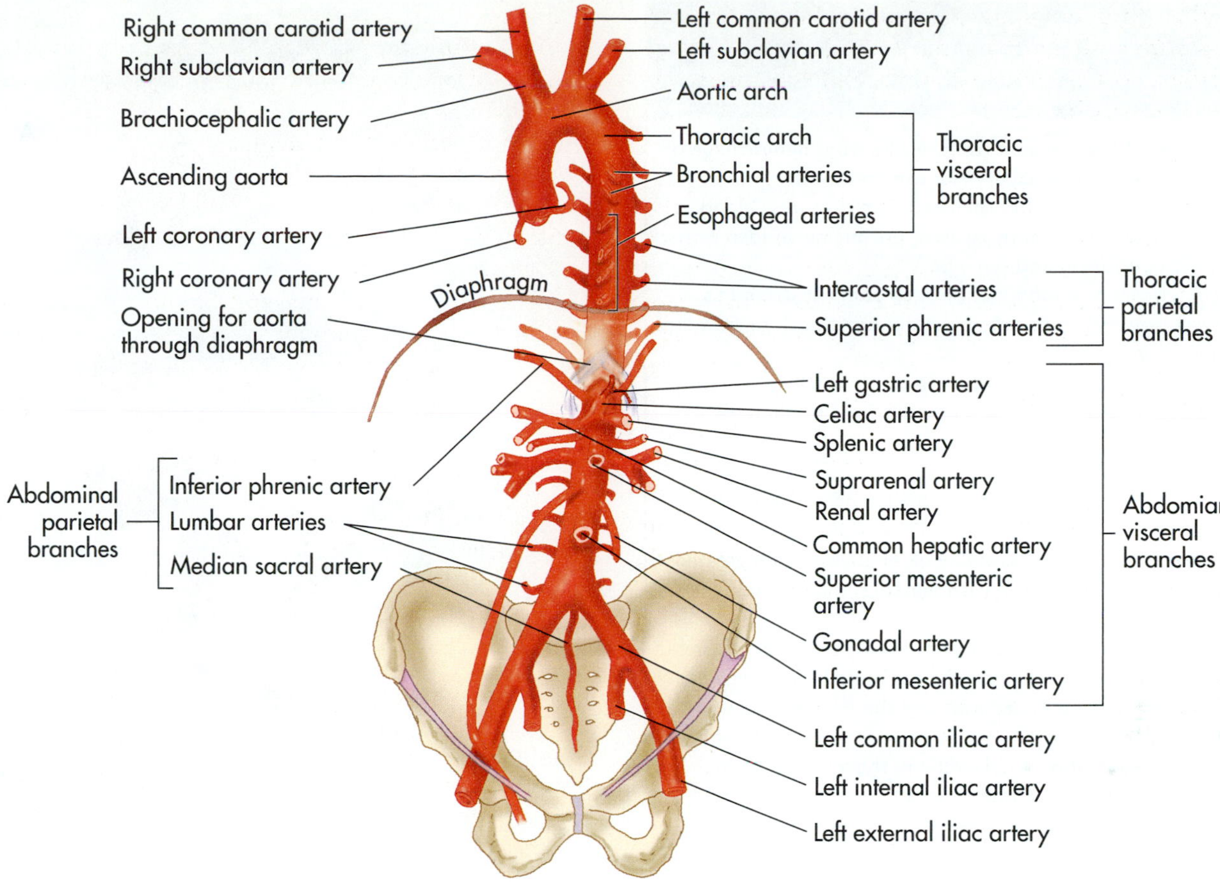

FIGURE 29-106 ■ Branches of the aorta: aortic arch, thoracic aorta, abdominal aorta, and their branches.

ABDOMINAL AORTIC ANEURYSM

Abdominal aortic aneurysms affect about 2% of the population.[9] The most common site for an abdominal aortic aneurysm is below the renal arteries and above the branching of the common iliac arteries. Abdominal aortic aneurysm is 10 times more common in men. Moreover, this aneurysm is most prevalent between the ages of 60 and 70. An abdominal aneurysm usually is asymptomatic as long as it is stable. However, if the aneurysm begins to expand or leak, symptoms will indicate impending rupture (Box 29-21).

Rupture of an abdominal aortic aneurysm may begin with a small tear in the intima. This small tear allows blood to leak into the wall of the aorta. As the process continues with increasing pressure, the tear may extend through the outer layer of the vessel. Then the tear may cause bleeding into the retroperitoneal space. If bleeding is tamponaded by the retroperitoneal tissues, the patient may be normotensive on the arrival of emergency medical services. If the rupture opens into the peritoneal cavity, however, massive fatal hemorrhage may follow. In either case, major blood loss results, and hypovolemic shock ensues.

Often a patient with a rupturing aneurysm will have syncope followed by hypotension with bradycardia despite a large amount of blood loss. The reason for bradycardia is stimulation of the vagus nerve. The aorta has fibers of the vagus nerve wrapped around it. When the aorta tears, the tear stretches these fibers, which in turn produces bradycardia. The bradycardia is present despite the hemorrhagic shock condition, which usually produces hypotension and tachycardia in the patient.

Management. Patients with a leaking or a ruptured abdominal aneurysm appear ill. They usually need immediate surgery to repair the vessel. Twenty percent of patients with an abdominal aortic aneurysm rupture their aneurysm before reaching the hospital, and 80% of these patients die.[10] Thus early recognition and rapid transport can prevent the death of these patients.

In most cases, prehospital care should be limited to gentle handling, oxygen administration, cardiac monitoring (myocardial infarctions may be associated with advanced aneurysms), initiation of volume-expanding intravenous fluids while en route to the receiving hospital, and alerting the receiving facility to prepare for imminent surgery.

Pulsatile masses (if present) are fragile and in most cases are membrane thin. The paramedic should avoid aggressive examination or deep palpation of the mass. Palpation may cause the mass to rupture. Examination, if needed, can be

BOX 29-21 Signs and Symptoms of a Leaking or Ruptured Abdominal Aortic Aneurysm

- Unexplained hypotension (that results from hemorrhage or a compensatory vasovagal response mechanism)
- Unexplained syncope (As the aneurysm ruptures, blood pressure drops transiently to zero, producing sudden cerebral hypoperfusion and syncope.)
- Sudden onset of abdominal or back pain (described as *tearing* or *ripping*) from the physical trauma itself or from inflammation
- Low back or flank pain (radiating to the thigh, groin, testicle, or perineum) that is unrelieved by rest or changes in position
- Signs of peritoneal irritation
- Urge to defecate (caused by retroperitoneal leakage of blood)
- Pulsatile, tender mass that may be palpated when greater than 5 cm and that usually is located above the umbilicus, left of the midline
- Distal pulses (femoral artery and below) that may be present or absent, depending on the patient's blood pressure, the occurrence of a dissection, and the degree of peripheral vascular disease
- Possible presentation as bleeding in the gastrointestinal tract if the aneurysm erodes into it

made by auscultation. This may reveal a sound similar to that of a systolic murmur or bruit.

The management of hypotension varies and depends on whether the aneurysm is leaking or ruptured. A patient with a suspected leaking aneurysm can be maintained with mildly hypotensive blood pressure to try to prevent rupture during the transport. (The hypotension associated with small leaks is thought to result from a compensatory vasovagal mechanism.) In these patients, fluid resuscitation should be minimal and less aggressive than in patients who have a ruptured aneurysm.

If rupture has occurred, hypotension, tachycardia, and loss of the pulsating mass may develop suddenly. The patient also may become unresponsive. This often is followed by full cardiac and respiratory arrest. These patients require rapid and aggressive resuscitation (intubation, ventilation, fluid replacement, and rapid transport for surgery).

ACUTE DISSECTING AORTIC ANEURYSM

Acute dissection (separation of the arterial wall) is the most common aortic catastrophe, affecting 5 to 10 persons per million population each year (3 times as many as ruptured abdominal aortic aneurysm).[11] Factors that can lead to the development of dissecting aneurysm are systemic hypertension, atherosclerosis, congenital abnormalities, degenerative changes in the connective tissue of the aortic media (cystic medial necrosis), trauma, and pregnancy. The syndrome affects men twice as often as women. The syndrome also is more common in African Americans.

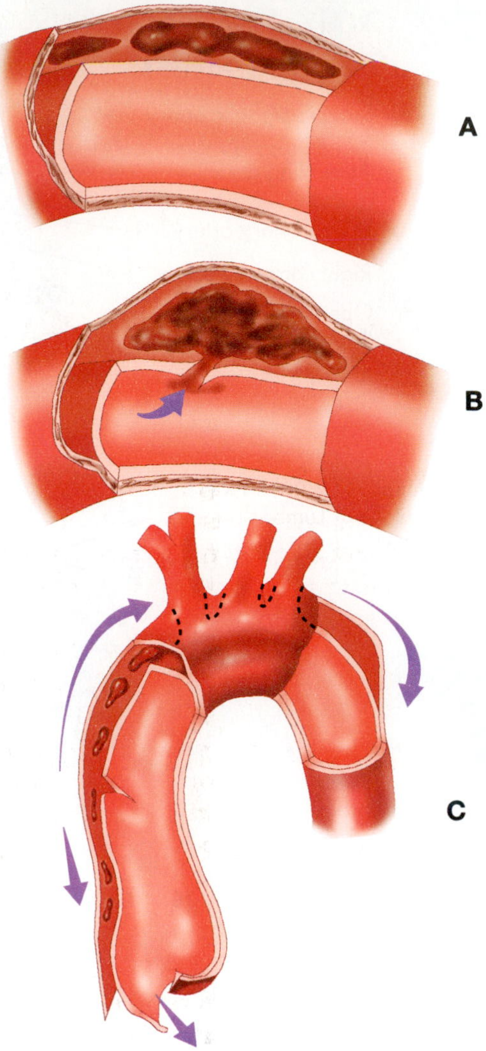

FIGURE 29-107 ■ Pathogenesis of dissecting aneurysms. **A,** Medial and intimal degeneration in aortic wall set stage. **B,** Hemodynamic forces acting on aortic wall produce intimal tear, directing bloodstream into diseased media. **C,** Resulting dissecting hematoma is propagated in both directions by pulse wave produced with each myocardial contraction.

A dissecting aneurysm of the aorta results from a small tear in the intimal layer of the vessel wall (Fig. 29-107). After the tear, the process of dissection begins. The tear in the inner wall allows blood to move between the inner and outer layers. This creates a false passage between the layers of the vessel wall. Blood that enters the false passage results in the formation of a hematoma. As a result, this can rupture through the outer wall (adventitia) at any time, usually into the pericardial or pleural cavity.

Any area of the aorta may be involved. But in the majority of cases the site of a dissecting aneurysm is in the ascending aorta. Once begun, the aneurysm may extend distally or proximally to involve all of the thoracic and abdominal aorta and tributaries, the coronary arteries, the aortic valve, and the carotid and subclavian vessels. Any vessels (including the carotid and other aortic arch vessels) bypassed by the dissection have their blood flow decreased. As a result, aortic dissection may cause the following:

- Syncope
- Stroke
- Absent or reduced pulses
- Heart failure resulting from sudden aortic valve regurgitation
- Pericardial tamponade
- Acute myocardial infarction

Signs and Symptoms. The signs and symptoms of a dissecting aortic aneurysm depend on the site of the intimal tear (ascending or descending aorta). They also depend on the extent of dissection. More than 70% of patients with acute dissecting aneurysm of the aorta complain of severe pain in the back, epigastrium, abdomen, or extremities. They often describe this pain as the most intense pain they have ever experienced. The pain usually is sudden in onset. Pain may be characterized by the patient as "ripping," "tearing," or "sharp and cutting, like a knife." Pain often originates in the back (between the scapulae). The pain possibly extends down into the legs. The patient with acute dissection may appear "shocky," with pallor, sweating, and peripheral cyanosis (from impaired perfusion), even when blood pressure is normal or elevated. If the patient is hypotensive, the paramedic should suspect cardiac tamponade or aortic rupture.

CRITICAL THINKING

What other condition has signs and symptoms similar to abdominal aortic aneurysm?

It may be difficult to distinguish the pain of aortic dissection from that of myocardial infarction or pulmonary embolism in the prehospital setting. The following distinctive features may help:

1. Severity of pain is maximal from the onset (compared with crescendo pain characteristic of acute myocardial infarction).
2. Pain may migrate from the anterior portion of the chest or interscapular area downward as dissection progresses.
3. Significant differences in blood pressure occur between the left and right arm or between the arms and the legs.
4. Peripheral pulses are unequal.
5. Neurological deficits result from occlusion of a cerebral vessel.

NOTE Blood pressure may differ significantly in the two arms if the dissection occludes either subclavian artery, leading to loss of blood pressure in the affected upper extremity.

Management. The goals of managing suspected aortic dissection in the prehospital setting are the relief of pain and rapid transport to a medical facility. (The transport should not be delayed; analgesics should be administered en route to the hospital.) The emergency medical services crew should be ready to initiate intubation. They also should be ready to assist ventilation in case the patient begins to decompensate. Other prehospital care measures include the following:

- Gently handling the patient
- Decreasing anxiety
- Administering high-concentration oxygen
- Beginning a large-bore intravenous line of crystalloid solution (Fluids should be kept to a minimum unless severe hypotension is present.)
- Giving analgesia (e.g., ***morphine*** or ***fentanyl***) per medical direction if the diagnosis is strongly suspected

Definitive in-hospital care generally includes reducing the myocardial contractile force to stop progressive dissection (with antihypertensives and beta-blockers), monitoring of intraarterial pressure, and possibly surgical repair.

Acute Arterial Occlusion

Sudden occlusion of an artery can occur. Occlusion most commonly is caused by trauma, embolus, or thrombosis. The severity of the ischemic episode depends on the site of occlusion. Severity also depends on how much collateral circulation is around the blockage. Vascular occlusion caused by thrombosis is a complication of atherosclerosis. Occlusions caused by emboli may indicate an abnormal cardiac rhythm, particularly atrial fibrillation.

CRITICAL THINKING

Why does atrial fibrillation put the patient at increased risk for emboli?

Arterial occlusion may follow blunt or penetrating trauma; it often is associated with long bone fractures. These injuries vary from injuries to the lining of a vessel to a vessel being severed completely. The occlusion usually is evident because there are no signs of circulation in the tissue or limb.

An embolism occurs when a blood clot breaks away and enters the arterial system. The clot travels until it reaches a narrow point in a vessel. This is often at a branching site of an artery. Ninety percent of peripheral emboli originate in the heart. Thus a history of cardiac disease (e.g., dysrhythmia, myocardial infarction, or valvular heart disease) favors a diagnosis of embolic occlusion, particularly when the patient has an asymptomatic opposite extremity with normal pulses. The most common sites of embolic occlusion are the abdominal aorta, common femoral artery, popliteal artery, carotid artery, brachial artery, and mesenteric artery (Fig. 29-108).

Thrombosis usually results from atherosclerotic disease. It usually occurs at a site of severe narrowing of a vessel. Unlike an embolus, thrombosis usually develops over time. As the thrombosis gets larger, collateral blood supply also can become occluded, causing progressive ischemia. The location of the ischemic pain often is related to the site of occlusion:

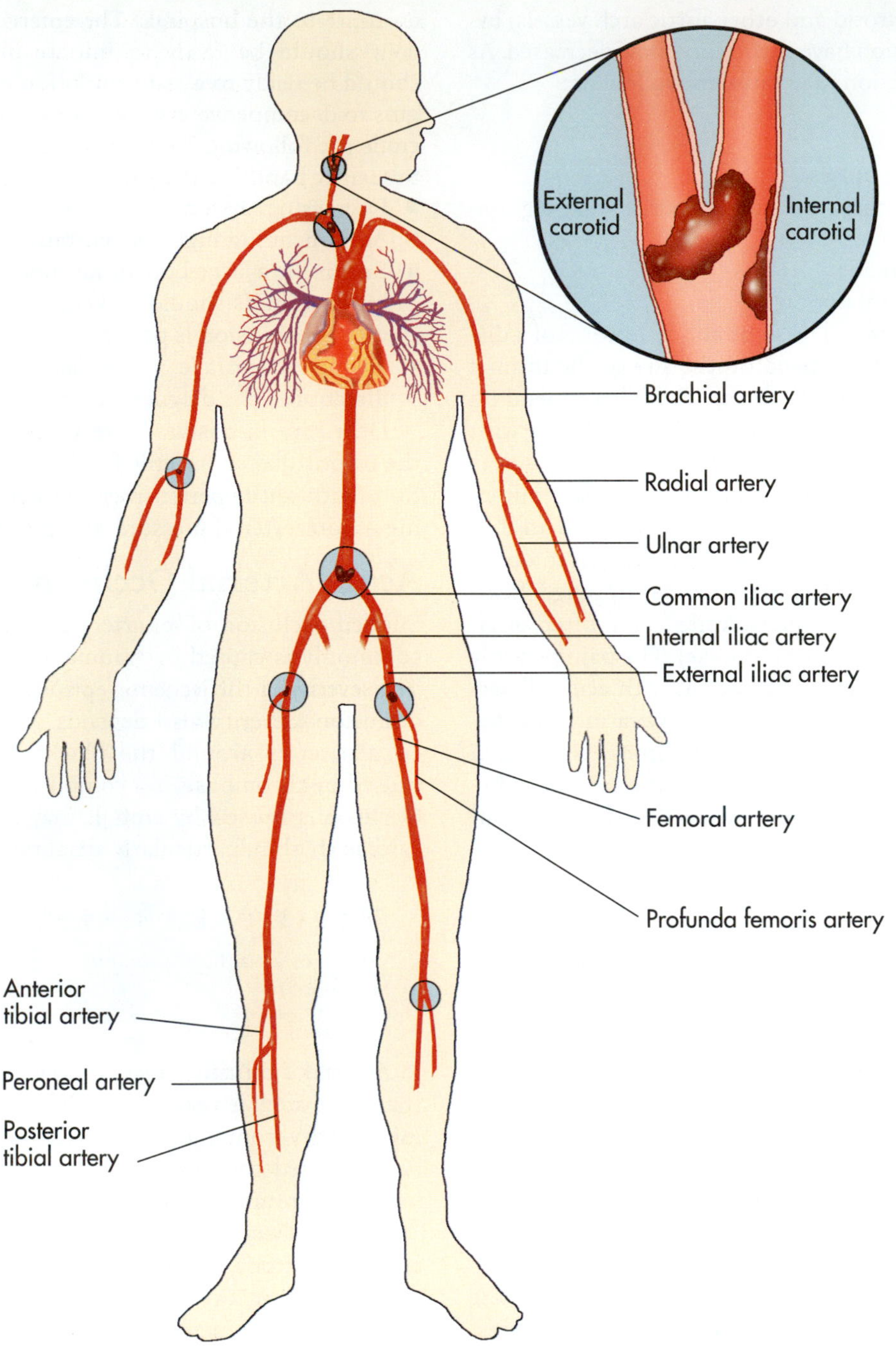

FIGURE 29-108 ■ Common sites of embolic arterial occlusion.

- Terminal portion of the abdominal aorta: pain in both hips or lower limbs
- Iliac artery: pain in the buttocks or hip on the involved side
- Femoral artery: claudication (cramplike pain) in the calf of the involved leg
- Mesenteric artery: severe abdominal pain

If severe ischemia persists, muscle necrosis occurs. Thrombotic occlusion is seen most often in men, smokers, and those over 60 years of age. Common sites of atherosclerotic (thrombotic) occlusions are depicted in Figure 29-109.

SIGNS AND SYMPTOMS

Regardless of the origin of the occlusion, the signs and symptoms of ischemia are the same and include the following:

- Pain in the extremity that may be severe and sudden in onset or absent as a result of paresthesia
- Pallor (skin also may be mottled or cyanotic)
- Lowered skin temperature distal to the occlusion
- Changes in sensory and motor function
- Diminished or absent pulse distal to the injury
- Bruit over the affected vessel
- Slow capillary filling
- Sometimes shock (particularly in mesenteric occlusion)

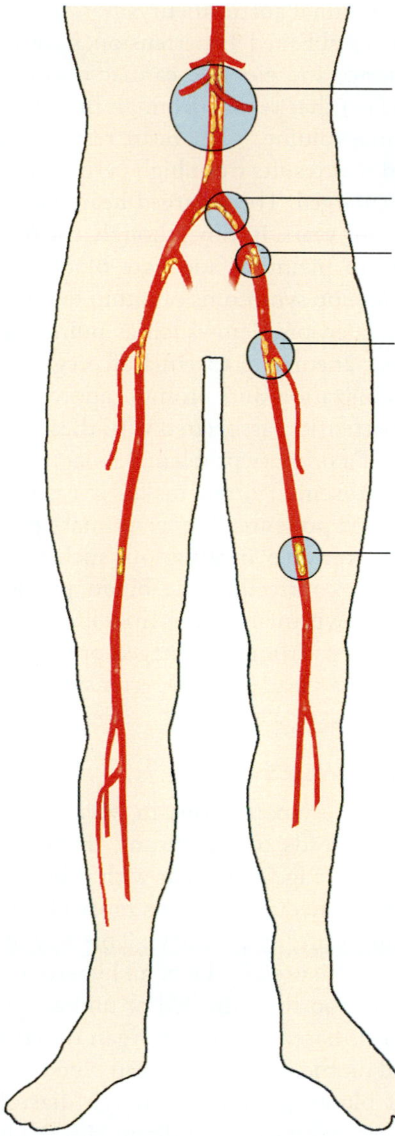

FIGURE 29-109 ■ Common sites of atherosclerotic occlusive disease.

> **NOTE** Some patients with vascular occlusion will have unequal blood pressure readings in the arms. Systolic readings in the arms that differ by 15 mm Hg or more suggest vascular disease. (A normal difference of 5 to 10 mm Hg exists between arms.)

MANAGEMENT

Acute arterial occlusion in an extremity is serious and painful. Occlusion may be limb threatening if blood flow is not reestablished within 4 to 8 hours. The affected limb should be immobilized and protected. In addition, the patient should be transported for physician evaluation. Patients with mesenteric occlusion should be managed for shock with oxygen and intravenous fluids. Analgesics also may be prescribed by medical direction to relieve pain. In-hospital, definitive care may include anticoagulant or fibrinolytic therapy, transluminal arterial dilation using a balloon catheter, embolectomy, or vascular reconstruction.

Noncritical Peripheral Vascular Conditions

Noncritical peripheral vascular conditions include varicose veins, superficial thrombophlebitis (described in Chapter 7), and acute deep vein thrombosis. Of these conditions, deep vein thrombosis is the only one that can cause life-threatening pulmonary embolus. Predisposing factors to venous thrombosis include the following:

- Birth control pills
- Coagulopathies
- History of trauma
- Malignancy
- Pregnancy
- Recent immobilization (e.g., leg fracture)
- Sepsis
- Smoking
- Stasis or inactivity (e.g., bedridden patients or long air flights)
- Varicose veins (usually a benign condition)

ACUTE DEEP VEIN THROMBOSIS

Occlusion of the deep veins is a serious, common problem. Occlusion may involve any portion of the deep venous system. However, occlusion is much more common in the lower extremities. Risk factors for deep vein thrombosis include recent lower extremity trauma, recent surgery, advanced age, recent myocardial infarction, inactivity, confinement to bed, congestive heart failure, cancer, previous thrombosis, oral contraceptive therapy, and obesity. Signs and symptoms of acute deep vein thrombosis include the following:

- Pain
- Edema
- Warmth
- Erythema or bluish discoloration
- Tenderness

MANAGEMENT

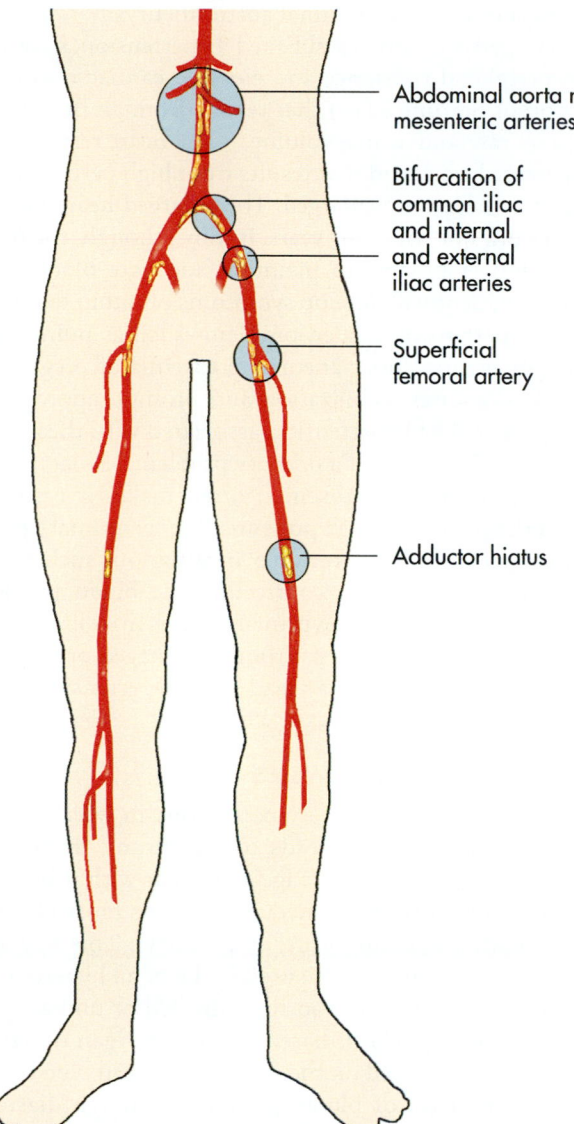

Patients with acute deep vein thrombosis require hospitalization. Prehospital care usually is limited to immobilization and elevation of the extremity and transport for physician evaluation. Deep vein thrombosis in the calf of the leg usually is much less serious than deep vein thrombosis of the thigh. The latter has a higher incidence of associated pulmonary embolus. Definitive care includes bed rest,

TABLE 29-5 Categories for Blood Pressure Levels in Adults (Age 18 Years and Older)*

	BLOOD PRESSURE LEVEL (MM HG)		
CATEGORY	SYSTOLIC		DIASTOLIC
Normal	<120	and	<80
Prehypertension	120-139	or	80-89
High blood pressure			
Stage 1	140-159	or	90-99
Stage 2	160-179		100-109
Stage 3	≥160	or	≥100

*For those not taking medicine for high blood pressure and not having a short-term serious illness. These categories are from the National High Blood Pressure Education Program.

BOX 29-22 Signs and Symptoms of Hypertensive Emergencies

- Altered mental status
- Changes in visual acuity
- Electrocardiogram changes
- Epistaxis
- Headache
- Nausea and vomiting
- Paroxysmal nocturnal dyspnea
- Seizures
- Shortness of breath
- Tinnitus
- Vertigo

administration of anticoagulants or occasionally fibrinolytic agents, and rarely thrombectomy.

Hypertension

Hypertension is a common disorder, afflicting about 23% of the U.S. population, and is directly responsible for about 23,000 deaths per year.[12] Hypertension often is defined by a resting blood pressure consistently greater than 140/90 mm Hg (hypertension, Stage 1).[13] The several categories of hypertension are based on the level of blood pressure, symptomatology, and urgency of need for intervention (Table 29-5 and Box 29-22). For the purpose of this textbook, two general categories are presented. One is chronic hypertension. The other group is hypertensive emergencies. (These emergencies include **hypertensive encephalopathy.**) A common cause of hypertension is the patient who has stopped taking the medication or other therapy prescribed by the physician.

CHRONIC HYPERTENSION

Chronic hypertension has an adverse effect on the function of the heart and blood vessels. It requires the heart to perform more work than normal. This leads to hypertrophy of the cardiac muscle and left ventricular failure. Chronic hypertension increases the rate at which atherosclerosis develops. This in turn increases the probability of cardiovascular, cerebrovascular, and peripheral vascular disease and the risk of aneurysm formation. Conditions commonly associated with chronic, uncontrolled hypertension are cerebral hemorrhage and stroke, myocardial infarction, renal failure (caused by vascular changes in the kidney), and development of thoracic or abdominal aortic aneurysm.

Many persons with established hypertension have elevated peripheral resistance and elevated cardiac output (a function of Starling's law) that results from an increase in the heart rate and stroke volume.[11] The heart responds to the increased workload that results from high peripheral resistance by becoming enlarged. The enlarged heart may be able to work fine for many years. In time, though, the heart will no longer be able to maintain adequate blood flow. Then the patient will develop symptoms of pump failure.

Any hypertension-related problem—such as pulmonary edema, dissecting aortic aneurysm, toxemia of pregnancy, or stroke—requires stabilization and prompt, appropriate management. The hypertension associated with these situations often is a result of a primary problem. Managing the primary problem (e.g., toxemia) often makes it easier to control the patient's blood pressure. But the primary problem may not easily be correctable. In situations such as dissecting aortic aneurysm, controlling the blood pressure also is key to managing the primary problem. A life-threatening problem that develops from unmanaged or partially managed hypertension may lead to a hypertensive emergency.

HYPERTENSIVE EMERGENCIES

Hypertensive emergencies are conditions in which an increase in blood pressure leads to significant, irreversible damage to organs. This damage can occur within hours if the hypertension is not treated. The organs most likely to be at risk are the brain, heart, and kidneys. This now uncommon condition is experienced by 1% of all hypertensive patients whose illness is poorly controlled or unmanaged. As a rule, the diagnosis is based on loss of organ function. Diagnosis also is based on the rate of the rise in blood pressure, not the level of blood pressure (although diastolic blood pressure usually is greater than 100 mm Hg). All hypertensive emergencies (except hypertension in ischemic stroke) require a 5% to 20% reduction in blood pressure within a few hours of discovery to avoid permanent organ damage. For blood pressure readings to range from 220/120 mm Hg to 240/140 mm Hg in hypertensive emergencies is not uncommon.

Hypertensive emergencies include the following clinical conditions: (1) myocardial ischemia with hypertension, (2) aortic dissection with hypertension, (3) pulmonary edema with hypertension, (4) hypertensive intracranial hemorrhage, (5) toxemia, and (6) hypertensive encephalopathy. Hypertension per se may not be the cause of the first five conditions. However, they all can be made worse by untreated hypertension. The sixth condition, hypertensive encephalopathy, results solely from elevated blood pressure and concurrently raised intracranial pressure.

Persistent hypertension produces brain damage (hypertensive encephalopathy). It results in a decrease in blood and oxygen to the brain (cerebral hypoperfusion). It also damages the tissues that make up the blood-brain barrier. This results in *fluid exudation* into the brain tissue. Hypertensive encephalopathy may progress over several hours from initial symptoms of severe headache, nausea, vomiting, aphasia, hemiparesis, and transient blindness to seizures, stupor, coma, and death. The condition is a true emergency. It requires immediate transport to a medical facility for definitive care. The goal of therapy is controlled but rapid lowering of blood pressure to normalize cerebral blood flow. If blood pressure is lowered too fast, infarction of end organs (heart, kidney, brain) may occur.

CRITICAL THINKING

Why do patients fail to take medicines that are prescribed for hypertension?

Prehospital management of these patients includes the following:

- Supportive care
- Calming the patient
- Oxygen therapy
- Intravenous line to keep the vein open
- Electrocardiogram monitoring
- Rapid transport

In most cases, drug therapy for hypertensive emergencies is not initiated in the prehospital setting. However, in severe cases of hypertensive encephalopathy or if transport is delayed, medical direction may recommend the administration of antihypertensives such as ***nitroglycerin*** or ***labetalol.*** These drugs induce arteriolar vasodilatation and may cause the blood pressure to decrease.

CRITICAL THINKING

How will fluid leak into the brain affect intracranial pressure and cerebral perfusion pressure?

SECTION EIGHT
TECHNIQUES OF MANAGING CARDIAC EMERGENCIES

This section addresses various procedures, techniques, and equipment used in managing cardiac emergencies. These include basic life support, mechanical cardiopulmonary resuscitation devices, monitor-defibrillators (manual, fully automated, and semiautomated), defibrillation, automatic implantable cardioverter defibrillators, synchronized cardioversion, and transcutaneous cardiac pacing. This section also offers an overview of managing a cardiac arrest as it applies to working within an advanced cardiac life support system. The reader is encouraged to review the dysrhythmias and drug therapy presented previously in this text.

BASIC CARDIAC LIFE SUPPORT

Basic cardiac life support provides circulation and respiration of a victim of cardiac arrest until advanced cardiac life support (ACLS) is available. According to the American Heart Association, "the highest hospital discharge rate—a measure of resuscitation success—is achieved in patients for whom CPR [cardiopulmonary resuscitation] is initiated within 4 minutes of the time of the arrest and who, in addition, are provided with ACLS management within 8 minutes of their arrest. The victim whose heart and breathing have stopped for less than 4 minutes has an excellent chance for recovery if CPR is administered immediately. After 4 to 6 minutes without circulation, brain damage may occur; after 6 minutes brain damage will almost always occur."[14] Cardiac arrest most often is associated with cardiovascular disease and is precipitated by ventricular fibrillation or ventricular asystole. Cardiac arrest also may result from noncardiac causes such as poisonings, drug overdose, toxic inhalation, trauma, and foreign body airway obstruction.

Physiology of Circulation via External Chest Compression

Two mechanisms are thought to be responsible for blood flow during cardiopulmonary resuscitation. The first is direct compression of the heart between the sternum and the spine. This increases pressure within the ventricles enough to provide blood flow to the lungs and body organs. The second mechanism to provide blood flow is the increased pressure in the chest cavity that gets transmitted to the vessels in the chest. This causes forward blood flow through the heart. Which mechanism contributes more to blood flow is unknown. Other mechanisms not currently known may be involved as well. Artificial circulation generates only about 20% to 30% of the normal output of the heart.[14]

Research has been conducted for many years on ways to improve cardiopulmonary resuscitation. These methods include simultaneous chest compressions and ventilation, abdominal compression with synchronized ventilation, cardiopulmonary resuscitation augmented by pneumatic antishock garments, interposed abdominal compression, continuous abdominal binding, and plunger mechanisms for chest compression that cause active compression and active expansion. However, no alternative method has been shown to improve survival or circulation unequivocally. Table 29-6 presents the standards of cardiopulmonary resuscitation as recommended by the American Heart Association and the American Red Cross.

TABLE 29-6 Basic Life Support for Healthcare Providers

	SUMMARY OF ABCD MANEUVERS			
CARDIOPULMONARY RESUSCITATION/ RESCUE BREATHING	**MANEUVER**	**ADULT (8 YEARS OF AGE AND OLDER)**	**CHILD (1 TO 8 YEARS OF AGE)**	**INFANT (LESS THAN 1 YEAR OF AGE)**
Establish unresponsiveness. Activate emergency medical services system or appropriate resuscitation team.				
A—Airway (head tilt–chin lift or jaw thrust)	Head tilt–chin lift (If trauma is present, use jaw thrust.)	Head tilt–chin lift (If trauma is present, use jaw thrust.)	Head tilt–chin lift (If trauma is present, use jaw thrust.)	Head tilt–chin lift (If trauma is present, use jaw thrust.)
B—Breathing (look, listen, and feel for no more than 10 seconds.)	Initial	Two breaths at 2 seconds/breath	Two breaths at 1 to 1½ seconds/breath	Two breaths at 1 to 1½ seconds/breath
• *If victim is breathing or resumes effective breathing,* place in the recovery position.	Subsequent	10 to 12 breaths/min (approximate)	20 breaths/min (approximate)	20 breaths/min (approximate)
• *If victim is not breathing,* give two slow breaths using pocket mask or bag-mask. Allow for exhalation between breaths.	Foreign-body airway obstruction	Heimlich maneuver	Heimlich maneuver	Back blows and chest thrusts
C—Circulation (breathing, coughing, movement, including pulse for no more than 10 seconds from carotid artery in child and adult, brachial or femoral artery in infant)	Pulse check*	Carotid artery	Carotid artery	Brachial or femoral artery
• *If signs of circulation/pulse are present but breathing is absent,* provide rescue breathing (one breath every 4 to 5 seconds for adult, one breath every 3 seconds for infant or child).	Compression landmarks	Lower half of sternum	Lower half of sternum	One finger's width below intermammary line
• *If signs of circulation/pulse are absent,* begin chest compressions interposed with breaths.	Compression method	Heel of one hand, other hand on top	Heel of one hand	Two or three fingers or two thumb-encircled hands
• *If signs of circulation/pulse are present but 60 beats/min in infant or child with poor perfusion,* begin chest compressions.	Compression depth	1½ to 2 inches	1 to 1½ inches or about one third to one half the depth of chest	½ to 1 inch or about one half the depth of chest
Continue basic life support.	Compression rate	About 100/minute	About 100/minute	At least 100/min (newborn: 120/minute)

From American Heart Association: *Guidelines 2000 for cardiopulmonary resuscitation and emergency cardiovascular care,* International Consensus on Science, Dallas, 2000, The Association.

*Note: Pulse check is performed by health care providers but is not expected of lay rescuers. Lay rescuers are taught to check for signs of circulation (e.g., normal breathing, coughing, and movement) in response to two rescue breaths given to the unresponsive, nonbreathing victim.

Continued

TABLE 29-6 Basic Life Support for Healthcare Providers, cont'd

SUMMARY OF ABCD MANEUVERS				
CARDIOPULMONARY RESUSCITATION/ RESCUE BREATHING	MANEUVER	ADULT (8 YEARS OF AGE AND OLDER)	CHILD (1 TO 8 YEARS OF AGE)	INFANT (LESS THAN 1 YEAR OF AGE)
C—Circulation, cont'd				
Integrate procedures appropriate for newborn resuscitation, pediatric advanced life support, or advanced cardiovascular life support at earliest opportunity.	Compression/ ventilation ratio	15:2 (single rescuer or two rescuers. Pause for ventilation with unprotected airway.) 12-15 breaths/min (1 breath every 4-5 seconds) with asynchronous chest compressions with protected airway	5:1 (Pause for ventilation until trachea is intubated.)	5:1 (Pause for ventilation until trachea is intubated.) 3:1 for intubated newborn (two rescuers)
D—Defibrillation				
Defibrillation using automatic external defibrillators is now considered an integral part of adult basic life support by health care providers.	Automatic external defibrillator	Per local emergency medical services protocol	Not yet recommended for use in infants and children	

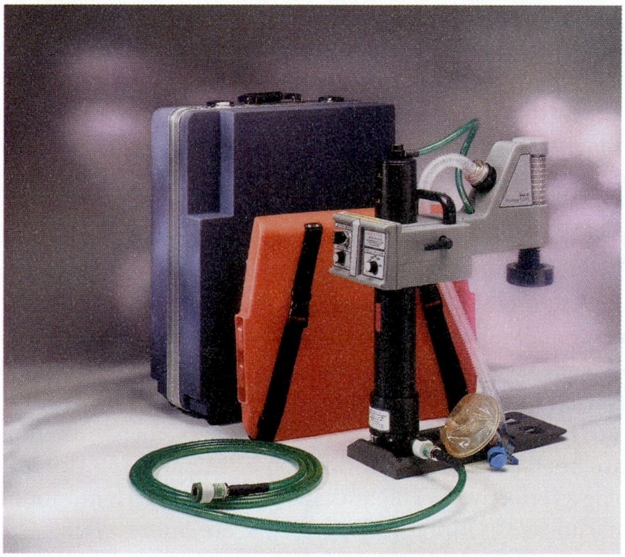

FIGURE 29-110 ■ Mechanical cardiopulmonary resuscitation device.

Mechanical Cardiopulmonary Resuscitation Devices

A number of mechanical devices can be used to produce external chest compression. Some devices provide chest compression and synchronized ventilation in the patient with cardiac arrest (Fig. 29-110). These devices are designed to standardize cardiopulmonary resuscitation technique, eliminate rescuer fatigue, free other rescuers to participate in advanced cardiac life support procedures, and ensure adequate compression during patient transport. In addition, these devices permit acceptable electrocardiogram recordings during compressions and defibrillation without interruption of cardiopulmonary resuscitation. The American Heart Association recommends that the use of mechanical cardiopulmonary resuscitation devices be limited to adult patients. The use of mechanical cardiopulmonary resuscitation devices requires special training. It also requires authorization from medical direction. Emergency medical services providers should follow the directions supplied with the equipment.

Monitor-Defibrillators

Cardiac monitor-defibrillators are classified as manual or automated external defibrillators. The latter may be semiautomated or fully automated. The paramedic should be familiar with the monitor-defibrillators used in the local emergency medical services system or community settings.

MANUAL MONITOR-DEFIBRILLATORS

Monitor-defibrillators are available from a number of equipment manufacturers in a variety of designs and capabilities. All consist of the following:

- Paddle or patch electrodes (with "quick look" capability)
- Defibrillator controls
- Synchronizer switch
- Oscilloscope
- Patient cable and lead wires
- Controls for monitoring

In addition, some manual monitor-defibrillators contain special features such as data recorders, transcutaneous cardiac pacing capabilities, and 12-lead monitoring.

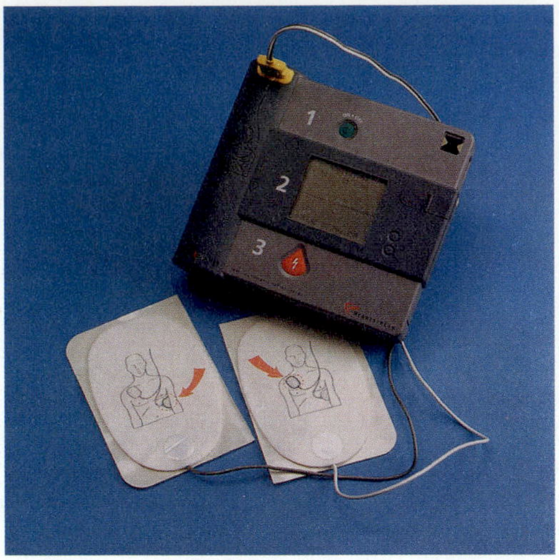

FIGURE 29-111 ■ R2 automated defibrillator.

AUTOMATED EXTERNAL DEFIBRILLATORS

Automated external defibrillators (Fig. 29-111) analyze the electrocardiogram signal. They evaluate the frequency, amplitude, and shape of the electrocardiogram waves. They are designed to be used by persons with little training. They increase the number of persons who are able to use a defibrillator in a cardiac arrest emergency. Automated external defibrillators are available for adult and pediatric patients. (See Chapter 44.)

> **NOTE** An increasing number of states have laws that allow community-based first-responder defibrillation programs using automated external defibrillators. These programs and others (e.g., automated external defibrillators located in airports and on public airlines) are supported by the American Heart Association and other groups. Recently, the Food and Drug Administration approved nonprescription sales of some automated external defibrillators for home use.

All automated external defibrillators are attached to the patient by two adhesive monitor-defibrillator pads (electrodes) and connecting cables. Automated external defibrillators are available from a number of manufacturers. They have a variety of features and controls as well. Most units provide programmable modules, data recorders, and voice messages to the operator. All users should become familiar with the automated external defibrillator device used in their system. Moreover, they should follow the recommendations of the manufacturer.

A fully automated defibrillator requires only that the operator attach the defibrillation pads and turn on the device. The rhythm is analyzed in the internal circuitry of the automated external defibrillator. If a shockable rhythm is detected, the automated external defibrillator charges capacitors and delivers a shock.

A semiautomated defibrillator requires the operator to press an "analyze" button to interpret the rhythm and a "shock" button to deliver the shock. The operator presses the shock control only when the automated external defibrillator identifies a shockable rhythm and "advises" the operator to press the shock button.

> **CRITICAL THINKING**
> What safety measure is still the duty of the automated external defibrillator operator?

Automated external defibrillators have four safety features:

1. They can analyze electrocardiogram waves.
2. They have built-in filters that check for QRS-like signals, radio transmission waves, 60-cycle interference, and loose or poor electrode contact.
3. Most are programmed to detect spontaneous patient movements, continued heartbeat and blood flow, and movement of the patient by others.
4. They make multiple evaluations of the rhythm before making a shock advisory or delivering a shock.

BIPHASIC TECHNOLOGY

In the past, defibrillation has used monophasic waveforms, in which the current travels in only one direction. Current travels from positive pad to negative pad. These defibrillators require high energy to defibrillate a patient effectively. In fact, they may deliver more energy than is needed for some patients. These machines also require large batteries, energy storage capacitors, inductors, and large, high-voltage mechanical devices.

Most newer automated external defibrillators and implantable defibrillators use biphasic waveform technology. This technology predicts a patient's energy requirements and chest wall impedance. The shock then is delivered by a current that travels in one direction, is stopped, and then is reversed to travel in the opposite direction, allowing for effective defibrillation to occur with lower energy for most patients.[15] (Biphasic defibrillation of 115 and 130 J appears to be as effective as 200 and 360 J delivered with monophasic shocks.[16]) Biphasic waveforms are more effective at lower energy than monophasic waveforms. Thus automated external defibrillators (using smaller batteries) have become smaller, lighter, more durable. They also have become less expensive to manufacture.

DEFIBRILLATION

Defibrillation is the delivery of electrical current through the chest wall. The purpose is to terminate ventricular fibrillation and pulseless ventricular tachycardia. The shock depolarizes a large mass of myocardial cells at once. If about 75% of these cells are in the resting state (depolarized) after the shock is delivered, a normal pacemaker may resume discharging. Early defibrillation is supported by the following rationale[1]:

- The most frequent initial rhythm in sudden cardiac arrest is ventricular fibrillation.

- The most effective management for ventricular fibrillation is electrical defibrillation.
- The probability of successful defibrillation decreases rapidly over time.
- Ventricular fibrillation tends to convert to asystole within a few minutes.

The modern defibrillator is designed to deliver an electrical shock via paddle, patches, or pads to the patient's chest. The defibrillator accepts the electrical charge from the battery source. It stores the charge in the capacitor. Then it releases the current into the patient in a short, controlled burst (within 5 to 30 milliseconds).

Paddle Electrodes

Paddle electrodes are designated by location of use as "apex" or "sternum." This allows the operator to view an approximation of lead II though the "quick look" function. (If the paddles are reversed in polarity or location, a negative QRS complex is noted.) With reference to defibrillation, however, the position of the paddles is unimportant.

The position of the paddles on the chest wall is important during shock delivery (Fig. 29-112). The paddles should be placed so that the heart (mainly the ventricles) is in the path of the current and the distance between the electrodes and the heart is minimized. This helps ensure adequate delivery of current through the heart. Bone is not a good conductor. For that reason, the paddles should not be placed over the sternum. As recommended by the American Heart Association, one paddle should be placed to the right of the upper sternum below the right clavicle, and the other to the left of the nipple in the midaxillary line.[1] (The anterior-posterior position also is acceptable.) Most manufacturers have adult and pediatric paddles available. Adult paddles are usually 10 to 13 cm in diameter. Pediatric paddles are used for children less than 1 year of age. They are 4.5 cm in diameter.

The resistance to current by the chest wall is called *impedance.* Impedance is determined by body size, bone structure, skin properties, underlying health conditions, and other variables. The greater the resistance, the less current delivered. Dry, unprepared skin has high impedance. To reduce resistance, the paramedic should place electrode gel, gel pads, or electrode paste between the paddles and the skin. The paramedic should hold the paddles firmly in place with about 20 to 25 pounds of pressure. (Prepackaged self-adhesive monitor-defibrillator pads also may be used.) Whichever method is chosen to decrease impedance, the paramedic should take care to prevent contact (bridging) between the two conductive areas on the chest wall. If contact between the two areas is made, superficial burns of the skin may result. The effective current also may bypass the heart (arcing). Even when gels or pads and proper techniques are used, minor skin damage may occur.

Stored and Delivered Energy

Electrical energy is commonly measured in *joules* (watt seconds). One joule of electrical energy is the product of 1 V (potential) multiplied by 1 A (current) multiplied by 1 second. Delivered energy is about 80% of stored energy because of losses within the circuitry of the defibrillator and resistance to the flow of current across the chest wall. As a rule, 80% of stored energy approximates the number of joules delivered to the patient. The American Heart Association currently recommends that initial defibrillation be attempted 3 times (200, 200 to 300, and 360 J) and delivered in succession (Box 29-23).[1] The pediatric initial defibrillation generally is 2 J/kg. This is followed by 4 J/kg if needed.

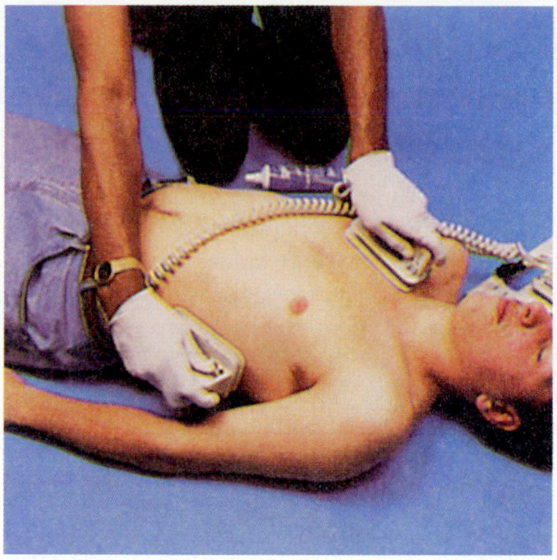

FIGURE 29-112 ■ Correct paddle placement for defibrillation.

Procedure

The following is the procedure for defibrillation as recommended by the American Heart Association:

1. Turn on defibrillator.
2. Select energy level at 200 J for monophasic defibrillators (or clinically equivalent biphasic energy).
3. Set "lead select" switch on "paddles" (or lead I, II, or III if monitor leads are used).
4. Apply gel to paddles, or position conductor pads on patient's chest.
5. Position paddles or remote defibrillation pads on patient (sternum-apex).
6. Visually check the monitor display and assess the rhythm. (Subsequent steps assume ventricular tachycardia/ventricular fibrillation is present.)
7. Announce to the team members, *"Charging the defibrillator. Stand clear!"*
8. Press "charge" button on the apex paddle (right hand) or defibrillator controls.
9. When defibrillator is fully charged, state firmly in a forceful voice the following chant (or some suitable equivalent) before each shock.
   - *"I am going to shock on three. One, I'm clear."* (Check to make sure you are clear of contact with the patient, the stretcher, and the equipment.)
   - *"Two, you're clear."* (Make visual check to ensure that no one continues to touch the patient or stretcher. In particular, do not forget about the person providing

> **BOX 29-23 Current-Based Defibrillation**
>
> *Current-based defibrillation* has been studied as an alternative to traditional defibrillation. With current-based defibrillation, the defibrillator operator selects electrical current (amperes) versus energy (joules). This method avoids the problem of low-energy selection in the presence of high impedance (resulting in current flow that is too low and failure to defibrillate). It also avoids the problem of high-energy selection in the presence of low impedance (resulting in excessive current flow, myocardial damage, and failure to defibrillate). The optimal current for ventricular defibrillation[2] appears to be 30 to 40 A.

ventilations. That person's hands should not be touching the ventilatory adjuncts, including the tracheal tube. Turn oxygen off or direct flow away from the patient's chest.)

- *"Three, everybody's clear."* (Check yourself one more time before pressing the "shock" buttons.)

10. Apply 25 psi of pressure on both paddles.
11. Press the two paddle "discharge" buttons simultaneously.
12. Check the monitor. If ventricular fibrillation/ventricular tachycardia remains, recharge the defibrillator at once. Check a pulse if there is any question about the rhythm display (e.g., a lead has been dislodged or the paddles are not displaying the correct signal).
13. Shock at 200 to 300 J for monophasic defibrillators (or clinically equivalent biphasic energy level), repeating the same verbal statements noted in step 9.

Operator and Personnel Safety

The following 10 guidelines are designed to ensure safe defibrillator use[17]:

1. Make certain that all personnel are clear of the patient, bed, and defibrillator before making a defibrillation attempt.
2. Do not make contact with the patient except through the defibrillator paddle handles.
3. Do not use excessive gel or coupling material, which can become a contact between the patient's chest and the paddle handles. Do not discharge paddles over a pacemaker or implantable cardioverter defibrillator generator or ***nitroglycerin*** paste. Remove ***nitroglycerin*** patches before defibrillation.
4. To prevent gel from the patient's chest from being transferred to the paddle handles, do not have one person perform cardiopulmonary resuscitation and defibrillation alternately.
5. Apply gel or paste before turning on the defibrillator.
6. Do not "open air" discharge the defibrillator to get rid of an unwanted charge. Turn the defibrillator off to "dump" the charge.
7. Do not fire the defibrillator with the paddles placed together. This can cause pits on the paddles that can increase the risk of burns to the patient.
8. Treat equipment with respect. It is safe when used properly. Do not touch the metal electrodes or hold the paddles to your body when the defibrillator is on.
9. Clean the paddles after use. Even dry gel presents a conductive pathway that could endanger the operator during a subsequent defibrillation attempt or equipment checkout procedure.
10. Routinely check the defibrillator (including batteries) to make sure the equipment is functioning properly. Follow the recommendations of the manufacturer.

Defibrillator Use in Special Environments

On occasion a patient requires defibrillation in a special environment (e.g., in inclement weather). The guidelines in operator and personnel safety always apply. However, additional precautions are taken in special situations.

A patient can be defibrillated in wet conditions, such as near water, in rain, or in snowy weather. The patient's chest should be kept dry between the defibrillator electrode sites. The operator's hands and the paddle handles should be kept as dry as possible. In a rainstorm, it would be safest to find shelter.

Depending on the defibrillator and its equipment specifications, the device may not be guaranteed to work properly in nonpressurized aircraft. In addition, some electrical interference may occur between the radio equipment in the aircraft and the monitor-defibrillator or vice versa. This is affected by the distance and angle between the defibrillator and the radio equipment. Studies have demonstrated that defibrillation with current equipment would be expected to be safe in all types of rotary aircraft used for emergency medical transport.[18] Still the medical crew should always inform the pilot(s) when electrical therapy is being used. In addition, the paramedic should consult with the pilot(s) to make sure the flight instruments are well shielded from electromagnetic interference.

IMPLANTABLE CARDIOVERTER DEFIBRILLATORS

Implantable cardioverter defibrillators commonly are implanted through an incision in the sternum. This incision is similar to that used for coronary artery bypass surgery. However, left lateral thoracotomy, subcostal, and subxiphoid approaches also are used (Fig. 29-113). During implantation, the two defibrillation patches of the implantable cardioverter defibrillator are placed on the epicardium. The patches are usually opposite each ventricle to increase the effectiveness of the device. The device is tested in the operating room. A pair of sensors is attached to the surface of the left ventricle to monitor cardiac rhythm. The leads are connected to the biphasic defibrillator device. The device is placed surgically in the left upper quadrant of the abdomen. (An outline of the generator usually can be felt or seen under the patient's skin.)

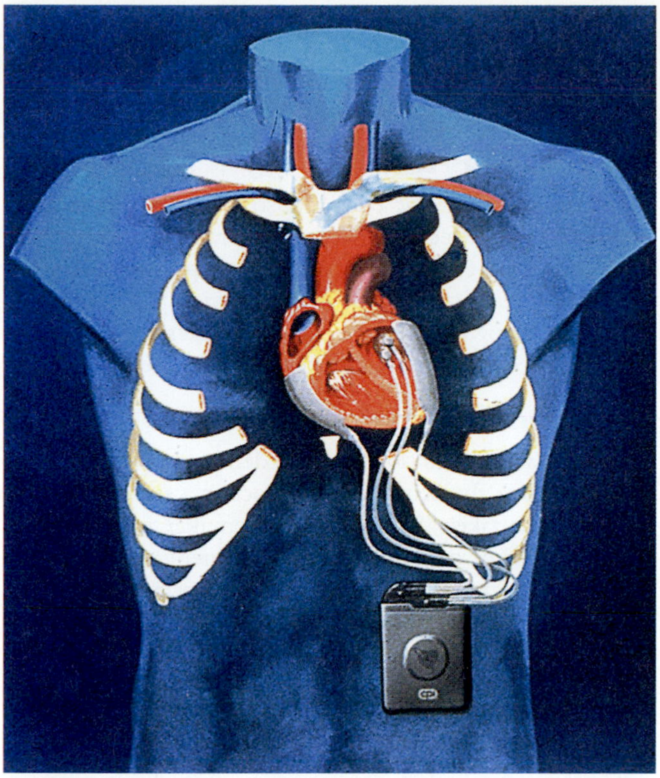

FIGURE 29-113 ■ Automatic implantable cardioverter defibrillator.

CRITICAL THINKING

What type of patients will have these devices?

The implantable cardioverter defibrillator works by monitoring the patient's cardiac rhythm, rate, and QRS complex morphology. When a monitored ventricular rate exceeds the preprogrammed rate, the implantable cardioverter defibrillator delivers a shock of about 6 to 30 J through the patches to restore a normal sinus rhythm. The device requires 10 to 30 seconds to sense ventricular tachycardia or ventricular fibrillation and to charge the capacitor before delivering the shock. If defibrillation does not restore a normal sinus rhythm, the implantable cardioverter defibrillator will charge again. Then it will deliver up to four shocks. A complete sequence of five shocks, if required, may take up to 2 minutes. If the tachycardia or fibrillation persists after five shocks, no further shocks are delivered. Once a slower rhythm is restored (i.e., sinus or idioventricular) for at least 35 seconds, the device can deliver another series of up to five shocks if ventricular tachycardia or ventricular fibrillation recurs.

CRITICAL THINKING

Consider a conscious patient whose device is firing repeatedly in response to the presence of a ventricular rhythm. How can you lessen the patient's discomfort and anxiety?

The paramedic must manage patients with implantable cardioverter defibrillators as if they did not have a device. The paramedic should follow standard advanced cardiac life support protocols if the patient is in cardiac arrest or in any other way medically unstable. The American Heart Association recommends the following four guidelines when caring for a patient with an implantable cardioverter defibrillator[1]:

1. If the implantable cardioverter defibrillator discharges while the rescuer is touching the victim, the rescuer may feel the shock. However, the shock will not be dangerous. Personnel shocked by implantable cardioverter defibrillators report sensations similar to contact with an electrical current.
2. Implantable cardioverter defibrillators are protected against damage from traditional transchest defibrillation shocks. However, they require an implantable cardioverter defibrillator readiness check after external defibrillation occurs.
3. If ventricular fibrillation or ventricular tachycardia is present despite an implantable cardioverter defibrillator, an external shock should be given immediately, because the implantable cardioverter defibrillator likely has failed to defibrillate the heart. After an initial series of shocks, the implantable cardioverter defibrillator will become operative again only if a period of nonfibrillatory rhythm occurs to reset the unit.
4. Implantable cardioverter defibrillator units generally use patch electrodes. These electrodes cover a portion of the epicardial surface. They may reduce the amount of current delivered to the heart from transthoracic shocks. Thus if transthoracic shocks of up to 360 J fail to defibrillate a patient with an implantable cardioverter defibrillator, the chest electrode positions should be changed immediately (e.g., anterior-apex to anteroposterior). The transthoracic shocks should be repeated. The different electrode positions could increase transthoracic current flow. This in turn may facilitate defibrillation.

Because the implantable cardioverter defibrillator can be deactivated and activated with a magnet, patients with implantable cardioverter defibrillators should be kept away from strong magnets. This will prevent accidental deactivation or reactivation of the device. The ability to use a magnet to deactivate and reactivate many of these devices can be useful when the unit is not working properly. However, use of a handheld magnet to turn the unit off or back on should be considered only with the advice and under the direction of a physician.

SYNCHRONIZED CARDIOVERSION

Synchronized cardioversion (or countershock) is used to terminate dysrhythmias other than ventricular fibrillation and pulseless ventricular tachycardia. Defibrillation (unsynchronized cardioversion) delivers the shock on the operator's command and with no regard as to where the shock occurs in the cardiac cycle. In contrast, synchronized cardioversion is designed to deliver the shock about 10 milliseconds after the peak of the R wave of the cardiac cycle. This avoids the vulnerable relative refractory period of the ventricles. Synchronization may reduce the energy required to end the dysrhythmia. It also may decrease the chance of causing another dysrhythmia.

When the defibrillator is placed in the synchronized mode, the electrocardiogram displayed on the oscilloscope shows a marker denoting where in the cardiac cycle the energy will be discharged. This marker should appear on the R wave; if it does not, the paramedic should select another lead. Adjustment of the electrocardiogram size may be needed if the marker does not appear. The procedure for synchronized cardioversion is as follows:

1. Consider sedation.
2. Turn on defibrillator (monophasic or biphasic).
3. Attach monitor leads to the patient ("white to right, red to ribs, what's left over to the left shoulder") and ensure proper display of the patient's rhythm.
4. Enlarge the synchronization mode by pressing the "sync" control button.
5. Look for markers on R waves indicating sync mode.
6. If necessary, adjust monitor gain until sync markers occur with each R wave.
7. Select appropriate energy level.
8. Position conductor pads on patient (or apply gel to paddles).
9. Position paddles on patient (sternum-apex).
10. Announce to team members: *"Charging defibrillator. Stand clear!"*
11. Press "charge" button on apex paddle (right hand).
12. When the defibrillator is charged, begin the final clearing chant. State firmly in a forceful voice the following chant before each shock:
    - *"I am going to shock on three. One, I'm clear."* (Check to make sure you are clear of contact with the patient, the stretcher, and the equipment.)
    - *"Two, you're clear."* (Make visual check to ensure that no one continues to touch the patient or stretcher. In particular, do not forget about the person providing ventilations. That person's hands should not be touching the ventilatory adjuncts, including the tracheal tube. Turn oxygen off or direct flow away from the patient's chest.)
    - *"Three, everybody's clear."* (Check yourself one more time before pressing the "shock" buttons.)
13. Apply 25 psi pressure on both paddles.
14. Press the "discharge" buttons simultaneously.
15. Check the monitor. If tachycardia persists, increase the joules according to the electrical cardioversion algorithm.
16. Reset the sync mode after each synchronized cardioversion because most defibrillators default back to the unsynchronized mode. This default allows an immediate shock if the cardioversion produces ventricular fibrillation.

TRANSCUTANEOUS CARDIAC PACING

Transcutaneous cardiac pacing (also known as *external cardiac pacing*) is an effective emergency therapy for bradycardia, complete heart block, asystole, and suppression of some malignant ventricular tachydysrhythmias. These devices have been recognized by the American Heart Association. They are used to treat bradycardia and asystole.

Artificial Pacemakers

Artificial pacemakers (Fig. 29-114) deliver repetitive electrical currents to the heart. They can act as a substitute for a natural pacemaker. The natural pacemaker may have become blocked or dysfunctional. The patient with severe sinus bradycardia, heart block, or idioventricular rhythm who is capable of generating a pulse with cardiac contractions may respond to an external pacing device and produce a perfusing pulse. Sinus bradycardia also may be paced. Generally, though, sinus bradycardia responds well to ***atropine.*** Most patients in cardiac arrest do not respond to pacing because the heart does not receive adequate perfusion. Thus the heart cannot achieve effective contractions.

The two modes of transcutaneous cardiac pacing are nondemand (asynchronous) pacing and demand pacing. Most devices provide both modes. An asynchronous pacemaker delivers timed electrical stimuli at a selected rate. This occurs regardless of the patient's own cardiac activity. These pacing devices are used less often than demand pacers. That is because they may discharge during the vulnerable period of the cardiac cycle (producing the R-on-T phenomenon). The asynchronous mode generally is used only as a last resort, usually in asystole. This mode also can be used when artifact on the electrocardiogram interferes with

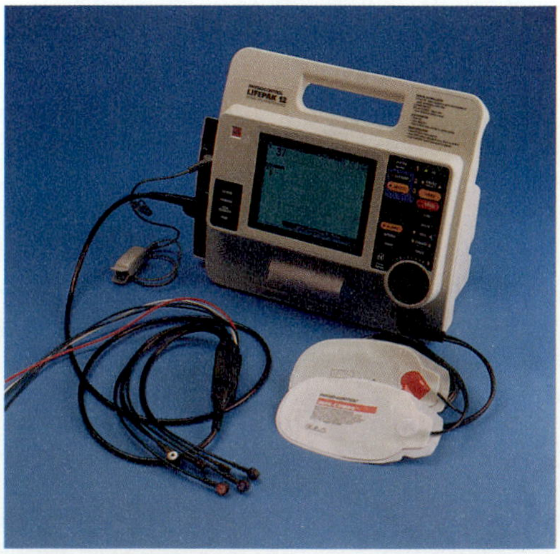

FIGURE 29-114 ■ Life Pack 12 3D Biphasic defibrillator/monitor.

the ability of the machine to sense the patient's own heart beat. Another use for asynchronous pacing is in overriding the high heart rates in tachydysrhythmias (e.g., torsades de pointes). This should be attempted only if other means of controlling the dysrhythmia have failed.

Demand pacing senses the patient's QRS complex. The pacemaker delivers electrical stimuli only when needed. Demand pacing is much safer to apply than the nondemand mode. When the pacemaker senses an intrinsic beat, the pacemaker is inhibited. If no beats are sensed, the pacemaker delivers pacing stimuli at a selected rate. The device usually is set to discharge at a rate between 70 and 80 beats per minute beginning with 50 mA. The charge then is increased in increments of 5 to 10 mA of electricity, and mechanical capture is achieved. Generally, the patient's clinical condition (blood pressure, level of consciousness, skin color, and temperature) improves at this point.

The paramedic should ensure that each pacemaker spike on the oscilloscope is followed by a QRS complex. If not, the current should be increased gradually until there is consistent capture. Unfortunately, motion artifact often makes electrocardiogram confirmation of electrical capture difficult. The only accurate method of monitoring mechanical function of the heart produced by the pacing device is the presence of a pulse with each QRS complex. Thus the paramedic must monitor the patient's pulse constantly. The paramedic should assess the patient's pulse rate and blood pressure on the patient's right side. This will help to minimize interference from muscle artifact.

Procedure

The procedure for transcutaneous pacing is as follows:

1. Gather the required equipment.
2. Explain the procedure to the patient.
3. Connect the patient to a cardiac monitor and obtain a rhythm strip.
4. Obtain baseline vital signs.
5. Apply pacing electrodes (avoid large muscle masses) and attach the pacing cable and pacing device. (The electrodes should be placed in the anterior-posterior position, avoiding the diaphragm.)
6. Select the pacing mode.
7. Select the pacing rate (usually 80 beats per minute); set the current (begin with 50 mA and then increase the current until ventricular capture is obtained).
8. Activate the pacemaker, observing the patient and the electrocardiogram.
9. Obtain rhythm strips as appropriate.
10. Continue monitoring the patient and anticipate further therapy.

NOTE As with synchronized cardioversion, selecting the "pacing mode" should result in the appearance of light markers on intrinsic beats. Paramedics should ensure that this occurs. That way, they will know the demand mode is activated and working properly.

Indications and Contraindications

The primary indications for transcutaneous cardiac pacing in the prehospital setting are symptomatic bradycardia, heart block associated with reduced cardiac output that is unresponsive to ***atropine,*** pacemaker failure, and asystole. As stated before, cardiac pacing rarely is effective in cardiac arrest. It also is ineffective in pulseless electrical activity unless the underlying cause of pulseless electrical activity is corrected. Use of cardiac pacing is not advised in patients with open wounds or burns to the chest or for patients in a wet environment.

CRITICAL THINKING

Why should patient movement be minimized during transcutaneous cardiac pacing?

Electrode Placement

Proper electrode placement is key in providing effective external pacing (Fig. 29-115). The paramedic should apply the negative (anterior) electrode to the left of the sternum. The electrode should be centered as close as possible to the point of maximal cardiac impulse. The paramedic should place the positive (posterior) electrode directly behind the anterior electrode. The electrode should be to the left of the thoracic spinal column. In rare cases the posterior placement cannot be used. Then the positive electrode can be placed in line with the patient's left nipple at the midaxillary line. (Anterior-anterior placement may produce pronounced chest muscle twitching.) The electrodes should be applied to clean, dry skin without localized trauma or infection.

The conscious patient most likely will experience some pain and discomfort during transcutaneous cardiac pacing. This is related directly to the intensity of muscle contractions and the amount of applied current. Ideally, analgesia or sedation of the patient should be provided.

CARDIAC ARREST AND SUDDEN DEATH

It is becoming increasingly evident that patients who cannot be resuscitated in the prehospital setting rarely survive. This is the case even if they are resuscitated temporarily in the emergency department (Box 29-24). The patient's best chance for survival is to have rapid and appropriate treatment in the field. However, endotracheal intubation and intravenous access take time to complete. Thus maintaining ventilation and compressions and rapidly transporting the patient to the nearest medical facility should be considered. Initial defibrillation should always be attempted as soon as possible. However, prolonged field resuscitation in the face of difficulties with intravenous access and intubation almost always is destined to fail.

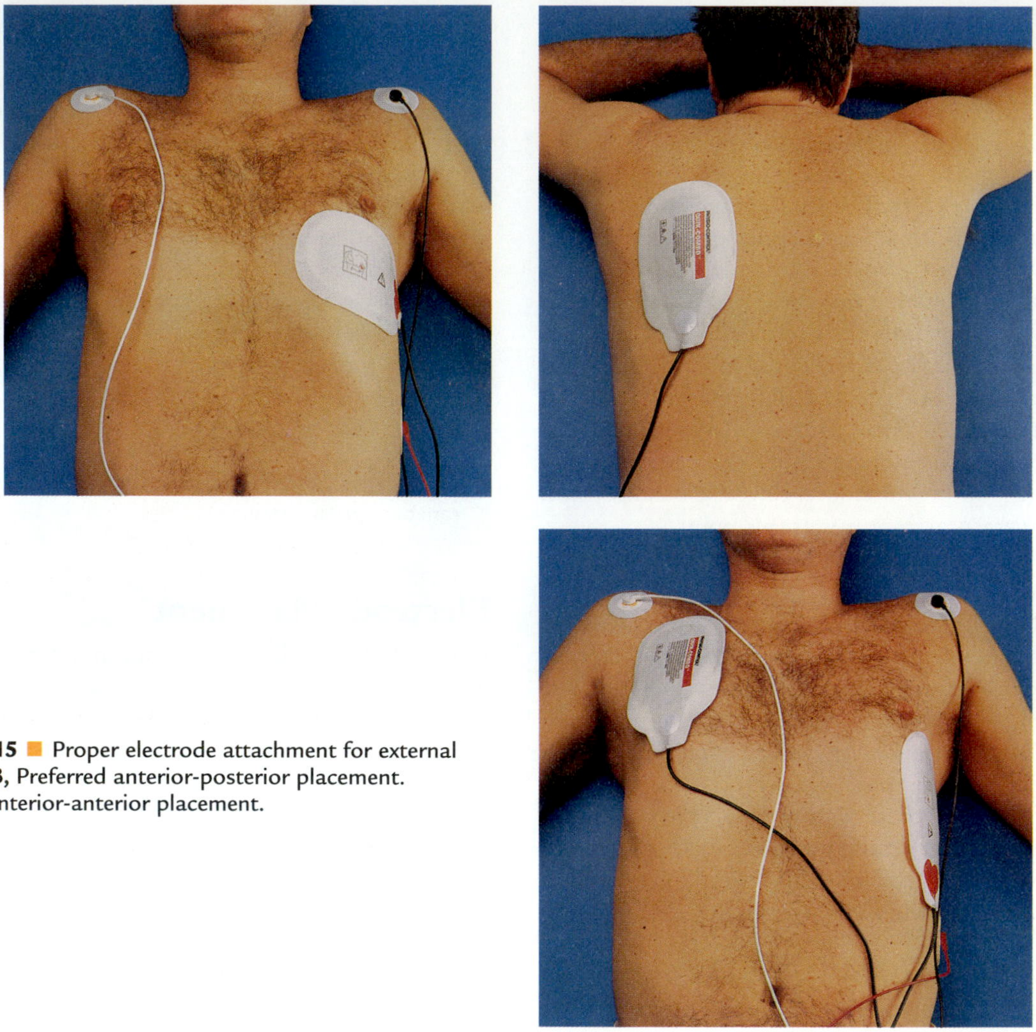

FIGURE 29-115 ■ Proper electrode attachment for external pacing. A and B, Preferred anterior-posterior placement. C, Alternative anterior-anterior placement.

BOX 29-24 Related Terminology

Resuscitation: To provide efforts to return spontaneous pulse and breathing to the patient in full cardiac arrest
Survival: Resuscitation of a patient who survives to hospital discharge
Return of spontaneous circulation: Resuscitation of a patient to the point of having a pulse without cardiopulmonary resuscitation; may or may not have return of spontaneous respirations; the patient may or may not survive

Much research is under way in the area of emergency cardiac care. Some of the research deals with various drugs to improve cardiac and neurological outcomes after resuscitation. A fairly large number of patients regain cardiac function but never regain consciousness. Thus a good deal of interest has arisen in how to improve cerebral perfusion after cardiac arrest. This research may lead to a variety of new drugs to be used by paramedics during resuscitation in the future.

TERMINATION OF RESUSCITATION

According to the American Heart Association, health care professionals are expected to provide basic life support and advanced cardiac life support as part of their professional duty to respond, with the following exceptions[4]:

- When a person lies dead, with obvious clinical signs of irreversible death
- When attempts to perform cardiopulmonary resuscitation would place the rescuer at risk of physical injury
- When the patient or surrogate has indicated that resuscitation is not desired

The association has advised further that termination of resuscitative efforts in the prehospital setting follow rules established by the local emergency medical services system. These rules are established by medical direction. The rules should include consideration for advance directives and no cardiopulmonary resuscitation orders (described in Chapter 4). If at any time paramedics are presented with an advance directive (e.g., a written directive, living will, or durable power of attorney) that indicates a patient should not be resuscitated, they should follow established protocol or immediately consult with medical direction.

Criteria for Terminating Resuscitation

Resuscitation (in some cases) may be stopped appropriately if asystole persists. The termination of resuscitative efforts should occur only after reviewing the quality of the resuscitation attempt. Termination of efforts also should occur only after one considers the presence of unusual clinical features. Questions about the resuscitation attempt to be considered include the following[4]:

- Has there been an adequate trial of basic life support and advanced cardiac life support?
- Has the patient's trachea been intubated?
- Has effective ventilation been provided?
- If ventricular fibrillation was present, was the patient defibrillated?
- Was intravenous access obtained?
- Were ***epinephrine*** and ***atropine*** administered?
- Have reversible causes been ruled out?
- Has the asystole been documented continuously for more than 5 to 10 minutes after all of the foregoing have been accomplished?

Finally, the presence of unusual clinical features such as drowning or profound hypothermia, young age, toxins or electrolyte abnormalities, and drug overdose may be indicators that continued resuscitation is appropriate. Termination of resuscitation in the prehospital setting should be guided by medical direction.

Procedure for Termination of Resuscitation

The process for terminating resuscitation in the field varies by protocol. The paramedic must follow the guidelines set by medical direction. When termination is considered to be appropriate, the paramedic should contact medical direction to convey the following information:

- Medical condition of the patient
- Known causes of the arrest
- Any treatment provided
- Family's appraisal of the situation and any resistance or uncertainty

While gathering and giving this information to medical direction, the paramedic should maintain ongoing documentation of the event. (This should include continuous electrocardiogram monitoring.) Documentation will help in the review of the call. The review usually is performed for quality assurance in most emergency medical services systems.

CRITICAL THINKING

Consider that you have just terminated resuscitation in the home. What resources can you contact to help the family?

Special Considerations

In addition to the needs of the patient, grief support for the family must be considered. Support services vary by agency. Often a paramedic (or other emergency medical services personnel) will be assigned to stay with the family for a period of time. At times, a community agency referral will be arranged.

Law enforcement officers may have more duties at the scene as part of their professional role. These duties may include an on-scene determination that the patient be assigned to a medical examiner. This may occur when the death or event is suspicious, or when a patient's private physician refuses or hesitates to sign the death certificate.

SUMMARY

- Persons at high risk for cardiovascular disease include those with diabetes, a family history of premature cardiovascular disease, and prior myocardial infarction. Prevention strategies include community educational programs in nutrition, cessation of smoking (smoking prevention for children), and screening for hypertension and high cholesterol.
- The left coronary artery carries about 85% of the blood supply to the myocardium. The right coronary artery carries the rest. The pumping action of the heart is a product of rhythmic, alternate contraction and relaxation of the atria and ventricles. The stoke volume is the amount of blood ejected from each ventricle with one contraction. Stroke volume depends on preload, afterload, and myocardial contractility. Cardiac output is the amount of blood pumped by each ventricle per minute.
- In addition to the intrinsic control of the body in regulating the heart, extrinsic control by the parasympathetic and sympathetic nerves of the autonomic nervous system is a major factor influencing the heart rate, conductivity, and contractility. Sympathetic impulses cause the adrenal medulla to secrete epinephrine and norepinephrine into the blood.

- The major electrolytes that influence cardiac function are calcium, potassium, sodium, and magnesium. The electrical charge (potential difference) between the inside and outside of cells is expressed in millivolts. When the cell is in a resting state, the electrical charge difference is referred to as a resting membrane potential. The specialized sodium-potassium exchange pump actively pumps sodium ions out of the cell. It also pumps potassium ions into the cell. The cell membrane appears to have individual protein-lined channels. These channels allow for passage of a specific ion or group of ions.
- Nerve and muscle cells are capable of producing action potentials. This property is known as *excitability.* An action potential at any point on the cell membrane stimulates an excitation process. This process is spread down the length of the cell and is conducted across synapses from cell to cell.
- The contraction of cardiac and skeletal muscle is believed to be activated by calcium ions. This results in a binding between myosin and actin myofilaments.
- The conduction system of the heart is composed of two nodes and a conducting bundle. One of the nodes is the sinoatrial node. The other is the atrioventricular node.
- Common chief complaints of the patient with cardiovascular disease include chest pain or discomfort, including shoulder, arm, neck, or jaw pain or discomfort; dyspnea; syncope; and abnormal heartbeat or palpitations. Paramedics should ask patients suspected of having a cardiovascular disorder whether they take prescription medications, especially cardiac drugs. Paramedics should ask whether patients are being treated for any serious illness as well. They also should ask whether patients have a history of myocardial infarction, angina, heart failure, hypertension, diabetes, or chronic lung disease. In addition, paramedics should ask whether patients have any allergies or have other risk factors for heart disease.
- After performing the initial assessment of the patient with cardiovascular disease, the paramedic should look for skin color, jugular venous distention, and the presence of edema or other signs of heart disease. The paramedic should listen for lung sounds, heart sounds, and carotid artery bruit. The paramedic should feel for edema, pulses, skin temperature, and moisture.
- The electrocardiogram represents the electrical activity of the heart. The electrocardiogram is generated by depolarization and repolarization of the atria and ventricles.
- Routine monitoring of cardiac rhythm in the prehospital setting usually is obtained in lead II or MCL_1. These are the best leads to monitor for dysrhythmias because they allow visualization of P waves. A 12-lead electrocardiogram can be used to help identify changes relative to myocardial ischemia, injury, and infarction; distinguish ventricular tachycardia from supraventricular tachycardia; determine the electrical axis and the presence of fascicular blocks; and determine the presence of bundle branch blocks.
- The paper used to record electrocardiograms is standardized. This allows comparative analysis of an electrocardiogram wave.
- The normal electrocardiogram consists of a P wave, QRS complex, and T wave. The P wave is the first positive deflection on the electrocardiogram. The P wave represents atrial depolarization. The P-R interval is the time it takes for an electrical impulse to be conducted through the atria and the atrioventricular node up to the instant of ventricular depolarization. The QRS complex represents ventricular depolarization. The ST segment represents the early part of repolarization of the right and left ventricles. The T wave represents repolarization of the ventricular myocardial cells. Repolarization occurs during the last part of ventricular systole. The Q-T interval is the period from the beginning of ventricular depolarization (onset of the QRS complex) until the end of ventricular repolarization or the end of the T wave.
- The steps in electrocardiogram analysis include analyzing the QRS complex, P waves, rate, rhythm, and P-R interval.
- Dysrhythmias originating in the sinoatrial node include sinus bradycardia, sinus tachycardia, sinus dysrhythmia, and sinus arrest. Most sinus dysrhythmias are the result of increases or decreases in vagal tone.
- Dysrhythmias originating in the atria include wandering pacemaker, premature atrial complexes, paroxysmal supraventricular tachycardia, atrial flutter, and atrial fibrillation. Common causes of atrial dysrhythmias are ischemia, hypoxia, and atrial dilation caused by congestive heart failure or mitral valve abnormalities.
- When the sinoatrial node and the atria cannot generate the electrical impulses needed to begin depolarization because of factors such as hypoxia, ischemia, myocardial infarction, and drug toxicity, the atrioventricular node or the area surrounding the atrioventricular node may assume the role of the secondary pacemaker. Dysrhythmias originating in the atrioventricular junction include premature junctional contractions, junctional escape complexes or rhythms, and accelerated junctional rhythm.
- Ventricular dysrhythmias pose a threat to life. Ventricular rhythm disturbances generally result from failure of the atria, atrioventricular junction, or both to initiate an electrical impulse. They also may result from enhanced automaticity or reentry phenomena in the ventricles. Dysrhythmias originating in the ventricles include ventricular escape complexes or rhythms, premature ventricular complexes, ventricular tachycardia, ventricular fibrillation, asystole, and artificial pacemaker rhythm.

- Partial delays or full interruptions in cardiac electrical conduction are called *heart blocks*. Causes of heart blocks include atrioventricular junctional ischemia, atrioventricular junctional necrosis, degenerative disease of the conduction system, and drug toxicity. Dysrhythmias that are disorders of conduction are first-degree atrioventricular block, type I second-degree atrioventricular block (Wenckebach), type II second-degree atrioventricular block, third-degree atrioventricular block, disturbances of ventricular conduction, pulseless electrical activity, and preexcitation (Wolff-Parkinson-White) syndrome.
- Atherosclerosis is a disease process characterized by progressive narrowing of the lumen of medium and large arteries. Atherosclerosis has two major effects on blood vessels. First, the disease disrupts the intimal surface. This causes a loss of vessel elasticity and an increase in thrombogenesis. Second, the atheroma reduces the diameter of the vessel lumen. Thus this decreases the blood supply to tissues.
- Angina pectoris is a symptom of myocardial ischemia. Angina is caused by an imbalance between myocardial oxygen supply and demand. Prehospital management includes placing the patient at rest, administering oxygen, initiating intravenous therapy, administering nitroglycerin and possibly morphine, monitoring the patient for dysrhythmias, and transporting the patient for physician evaluation.
- Acute myocardial infarction occurs when a coronary artery is blocked and blood does not reach an area of heart muscle. This results in ischemia, injury, and necrosis to the area of myocardium supplied by the affected artery. Death caused by myocardial infarction usually results from lethal dysrhythmias (ventricular tachycardia, ventricular fibrillation, and cardiac standstill), pump failure (cardiogenic shock and congestive heart failure), or myocardial tissue rupture (rupture of the ventricle, septum, or papillary muscle). Some patients with acute myocardial infarction, particularly those in the older age groups, have only symptoms of dyspnea, syncope, or confusion. However, substernal chest pain is usually present in patients with acute myocardial infarction (70% to 90% of patients). ST segment elevation greater than or equal to 0.5 mV in at least two side-by-side electrocardiogram leads indicates an acute myocardial infarction. However, some patients infarct without ST segment elevation changes. Other conditions also can produce ST segment elevation. Prehospital management of the patient with a suspected myocardial infarction should include placing the patient at rest; administering oxygen at 3 to 4 L per minute via nasal cannula; frequently assessing vital signs and breath sounds; initiating an intravenous line with normal saline or lactated Ringer's solution to keep the vein open; monitoring for dysrhythmias; administering medications such as nitroglycerin, morphine, and aspirin; and screening for risk factors for fibrinolytic therapy.
- Left ventricular failure occurs when the left ventricle fails to function as an effective forward pump. This causes a back-pressure of blood into the pulmonary circulation. This in turn may lead to pulmonary edema. Emergency management is directed at decreasing the venous return to the heart, improving myocardial contractility, decreasing myocardial oxygen demand, improving ventilation and oxygenation, and rapidly transporting the patient to a medical facility.
- Right ventricular failure occurs when the right ventricle fails as a pump. This causes back-pressure of blood into the systemic venous circulation. Right ventricular failure is not usually a medical emergency in itself; that is, unless it is associated with pulmonary edema or hypotension.
- Cardiogenic shock is the most extreme form of pump failure. It usually is caused by extensive myocardial infarction. Even with aggressive therapy, cardiogenic shock has a mortality rate of 70% or higher. Patients in cardiogenic shock need rapid transport to a medical facility.
- *Cardiac tamponade* is defined as impaired filling of the heart caused by increased pressure in the pericardial sac.
- Abdominal aortic aneurysms are usually asymptomatic. However, signs and symptoms will signal impending or active rupture. If the vessel tears, bleeding initially may be stopped by the retroperitoneal tissues. The patient may be normotensive on the arrival of emergency medical services. If the rupture opens into the peritoneal cavity, however, massive fatal hemorrhage may follow.
- Acute dissection is the most common aortic catastrophe. Any area of the aorta may be involved. However, in 60% to 70% of cases the site of a dissecting aneurysm is in the ascending aorta, just beyond the takeoff of the left subclavian artery. The signs and symptoms depend on the site of the intimal tear. They also depend on the extent of dissection. The goals of managing suspected aortic dissection in the prehospital setting are relief of pain and immediate transport to a medical facility.
- Acute arterial occlusion is a sudden blockage of arterial flow. Occlusion most commonly is caused by trauma, an embolus, or thrombosis. The most common sites of embolic occlusion are the abdominal aorta, common femoral artery, popliteal artery, carotid artery, brachial artery, and mesenteric artery. The location of ischemic pain is related to the site of occlusion.
- Noncritical peripheral vascular conditions include varicose veins, superficial thrombophlebitis, and acute deep vein thrombosis. Of these conditions, deep vein thrombosis is the only one that can cause a life-threatening problem. This problem is pulmonary embolus.

- Hypertension often is defined by a resting blood pressure that is consistently greater than 140/90 mm Hg. Chronic hypertension has an adverse effect on the heart and blood vessels. It requires the heart to perform more work than normal. This leads to hypertrophy of the cardiac muscle and left ventricular failure. Conditions associated with chronic, uncontrolled hypertension are cerebral hemorrhage and stroke, myocardial infarction, and renal failure.
- Hypertensive emergencies are conditions in which a blood pressure increase leads to significant, irreversible end-organ damage within hours if not treated. The organs most likely to be at risk are the brain, heart, and kidneys. As a rule, the diagnosis is based on altered end-organ function and the rate of the rise in blood pressure, not on the level of blood pressure.
- Basic cardiac life support helps to maintain the circulation and respiration of a victim of cardiac arrest. Basic life support is continued until advanced cardiac life support is available. Two mechanisms are thought to be responsible for blood flow during cardiopulmonary resuscitation. One is direct compression of the heart between the sternum and the spine. This increases pressure within the ventricles to provide blood flow to the lungs and body organs. The second one is increased intrathoracic pressure transmitted to all intrathoracic vascular structures. This creates an intrathoracic-to-extrathoracic pressure gradient. This gradient causes blood to flow out of the thorax. A number of mechanical devices provide external chest compression. Others provide chest compression with ventilation in the cardiac arrest patient.
- Cardiac monitor-defibrillators are classified as manual or automated external defibrillators. Defibrillation is the delivery of electrical current through the chest wall. Its purpose is to terminate ventricular fibrillation and certain other nonperfusing rhythms.
- Implantable cardioverter defibrillators work by monitoring the patient's cardiac rhythm. When a monitored ventricular rate exceeds the preprogrammed rate, the implantable cardioverter defibrillator delivers a shock of about 6 to 30 J through the patches. This is an attempt to restore a normal sinus rhythm.
- Synchronized cardioversion is designed to deliver a shock about 10 milliseconds after the peak of the R wave of the cardiac cycle. (Thus the device avoids the relative refractory period.) Synchronization may reduce the amount of energy needed to end the dysrhythmia. It also may decrease the chances of causing another dysrhythmia.
- Transcutaneous cardiac pacing is an effective emergency therapy for bradycardia, complete heart block, asystole, and suppression of some malignant ventricular dysrhythmias. Proper electrode placement is important for effective external pacing.
- What is becoming more and more evident is that patients who cannot be resuscitated in the prehospital setting rarely survive. This is the case even if they are resuscitated temporarily in the emergency department. Cessation of resuscitative efforts in the prehospital setting should follow system-specific criteria established by medical direction.

REFERENCES

1. American Heart Association: *Advanced cardiac life support,* Dallas, 1997, The Association.
2. Phalen T: *The 12-lead ECG in acute myocardial infarction,* St Louis, 1996, Mosby.
3. Marriott H, Conover M: *Advanced concepts in arrhythmias,* ed 2, St Louis, 1989, Mosby.
4. American Heart Association: *Guidelines 2000 for cardiopulmonary resuscitation and emergency cardiovascular care,* International Consensus on Science, Dallas, 2000, The Association.
5. Page B: *12-lead ECG interpretation workshop,* St Louis, 1998, Multi-lead Medics.
6. Taigman M, Cannon S: Reading bundle branch blocks, *J Emerg Med Serv JEMS* 15(5):41, 1990.
7. American Heart Association/Centers for Disease Control and Prevention Scientific Statement: Markers of inflammation and cardiovascular disease: application to clinical and public health practice, *Circulation* 107:499-511, 2003.
8. ACC/AHA guidelines for the evaluation and management of chronic heart failure in the adult: executive summary, *Circulation* 104:2926-3007, 2001.
9. Rosen P, Barkin R: *Emergency medicine: concepts and clinical practice,* ed 4, St Louis, 1998, Mosby.
9. US Department of Transportation, National Highway Traffic Safety Administration: *Paramedic national standard curriculum,* p. 114, Washington, DC, 1998, The Department.
10. Grubbs T: The ultimate emergency: managing aortic aneurysms, *J Emerg Med Serv JEMS* 16(10):56, 1991.
11. Little R, Little W: *Physiology of the heart,* ed 4, St Louis, 1989, Mosby.
12. National Vital Statistics Reports, vol 50, No 15, 2000.
13. National Joint Committee on Hypertension: *The sixth report of the Joint National Committee on Prevention, Detection, Evaluation, and Treatment of High Blood Pressure,* Washington, DC, 1998, National Institutes of Health, National Heart Lung and Blood Institute.
14. American Heart Association: *Basic life support for healthcare providers,* Dallas, 1997, The Association.
15. *The forerunner biphasic waveform technical note,* Seattle, 1997, Heartstream.
16. Brady G et al: Multicenter comparison of trunicated biphasic shocks and standard damped sine wave monophasic shocks for transthoracic ventricular defibrillation, *Pacing Clin Electrophysiol* 19:678, 1996.
17. Higgins S: *Defibrillation: what you should know,* Redmond, Texas, 1978, Physio-Control.
18. Dedrick D et al: Defibrillation safety in emergency helicopter transport, *Ann Emerg Med* 18(1):69, 1989.

PART EIGHT

IN THIS PART

CHAPTER 30 Pulmonary Emergencies

CHAPTER 31 Neurology

CHAPTER 32 Endocrinology

CHAPTER 33 Allergies and Anaphylaxis

CHAPTER 34 Gastroenterology

CHAPTER 35 Urology

CHAPTER 36 Toxicology

CHAPTER 37 Hematology

CHAPTER 38 Environmental Conditions

CHAPTER 39 Infectious and Communicable Diseases

CHAPTER 40 Behavioral and Psychiatric Disorders

CHAPTER 41 Gynecology

CHAPTER 42 Obstetrics

CHAPTER

30

Pulmonary Emergencies

OBJECTIVES

Upon completion of this chapter, the paramedic student will be able to:

1. Distinguish the pathophysiology of respiratory emergencies related to ventilation, diffusion, and perfusion.
2. Describe the causes, complications, signs and symptoms, and prehospital management of patients diagnosed with obstructive airway disease, pneumonia, adult respiratory distress syndrome, pulmonary thromboembolism, upper respiratory infection, spontaneous pneumothorax, hyperventilation syndrome, and lung cancer.

KEY TERMS

bronchiectasis: An abnormal dilation of the bronchi caused by a pus-producing infection of the bronchial wall.

hyperventilation syndrome: Abnormally deep or rapid breathing that leads to excessive loss of carbon dioxide, resulting in respiratory alkalosis.

spontaneous pneumothorax: A condition that results when a subpleural bleb ruptures, allowing air to enter the pleural space from within the lung.

status asthmaticus: A severe, prolonged asthma exacerbation that has not been broken with repeated doses of bronchodilators.

Respiratory emergencies are common in the prehospital setting. They account for 28% of the chief complaints in all EMS calls.[1] Each year more than 300,000 people die as a result of respiratory emergencies in the United States.[2] Therefore patients with respiratory emergencies require the highest priority of care. The paramedic must be able to assess a patient with respiratory distress quickly, identify the cause, initiate management, and provide appropriate care en route to the hospital.

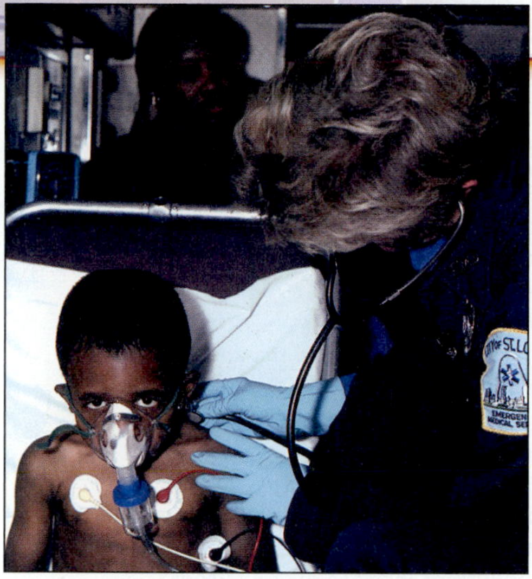

PATHOPHYSIOLOGY

A variety of problems can affect the pulmonary system's ability to achieve gas exchange. Gas exchange must occur to provide for cellular needs and the excretion of wastes (see Chapters 6 and 19). Specific disorders responsible for respiratory emergencies include those related to ventilation, diffusion, and perfusion. Risk factors associated with the development of respiratory disease are listed in Box 30-1. Smoking prevention and cessation programs are a key prevention strategy for avoiding respiratory illness. Controlling air pollution is another. A third important factor is smoke-free workplaces and public locations (see Chapter 3). The following discussion of physiology serves as a review.

▶**NOTE** There are many pulmonary diseases. These diseases act in different ways on a number of body systems. However, all respiratory problems (acute or chronic) can be categorized as affecting ventilation, diffusion, or perfusion. Treatment can be started rapidly and effectively once the problem has been identified as a ventilation, diffusion, or perfusion problem (or a combination of defects) (Table 30-1).

Ventilation

Ventilation is the process of air movement into and out of the lungs. For ventilation to occur, the following must be intact:

- Neurological control (to initiate ventilation)
- Nerves between the brain stem and the muscles of respiration
- Functional diaphragm and intercostal muscles
- Patent upper airway
- Functional lower airway
- Alveoli that are functional and have not collapsed

Specific pathophysiologies associated with ventilation include upper and lower airway obstruction, chest wall impairment, and problems in neurological control. Emergency treatments for ventilation problems include making sure the upper and lower airways are open and clear and providing assisted ventilations.

Diffusion

Diffusion is the process of gas exchange. This gas exchange occurs between the air-filled alveoli and the pulmonary capillary bed. Gas exchange is driven by simple diffusion. In simple diffusion, gases move from areas of high concentration to areas of low concentration. (This occurs until the concentrations are equal.) For diffusion to occur, the following must be intact:

- Alveolar and capillary walls that are not thickened
- Interstitial space between the alveoli and capillary wall that is not enlarged or filled with fluid

Specific pathophysiologies associated with diffusion include inadequate oxygen concentration in ambient air, alveolar disorders, interstitial space disorders, and capillary bed disorders. Emergency treatment for diffusion problems includes providing high-concentration oxygen. Treatment is

BOX 30-1 Risk Factors Associated with the Development of Respiratory Disease

Intrinsic Factors

Genetic predisposition may influence the development of these conditions:

- Asthma
- Obstructive lung disease
- Cancer

Cardiac or circulatory disorders may influence the development of these conditions:

- Pulmonary edema
- Pulmonary emboli

Stress may increase the following:

- Severity of respiratory complaints
- Frequency of exacerbations of asthma and chronic obstructive pulmonary disease (COPD)

Extrinsic Factors

Smoking increases the following:

- Prevalence of COPD and cancer
- Severity of virtually all respiratory disorders

Environmental pollutants increase the following:

- Prevalence of COPD
- Severity of all obstructive airway disorders

TABLE 30-1 Ventilation, Diffusion, and Perfusion Problems

PROBLEM	EXAMPLE
Ventilation	
Upper airway obstruction	Foreign body, epiglottitis
Lower airway obstruction	Asthma, airway edema
Chest wall impairment	Trauma, muscular dystrophy
Neurogenic dysfunction	Central nervous system (CNS)–depressant drugs, stroke
Diffusion	
Inadequate oxygen in ambient air	Fire environment, carbon monoxide (CO) poisoning
Alveolar disorder	Lung disease, inhalation injury
Interstitial space disorder	Pulmonary edema, near-drowning
Capillary bed disorder	Severe atherosclerosis
Perfusion	
Inadequate blood volume or hemoglobin levels	Shock, anemia
Impaired circulatory blood flow	Pulmonary embolus
Capillary wall disorder	Trauma

also directed at reducing inflammation in the interstitial space.

Perfusion

Perfusion is the process of circulation of the blood through the lung tissues (capillary bed). For perfusion to occur, the following must be intact:

- Adequate blood volume
- Adequate hemoglobin in the blood
- Pulmonary capillaries that are not blocked
- Efficient pumping by the heart that provides a smooth flow of blood through the pulmonary capillary bed

Specific pathophysiologies associated with perfusion include inadequate blood volume, impaired circulatory blood flow, and capillary wall disorders. Emergency treatment for perfusion problems includes providing an adequate circulating blood volume. In addition, the blood must have enough hemoglobin to carry adequate oxygen supplies. Treatment also may be needed to increase the heart's ability to pump effectively.

SCENE SIZE-UP AND RESCUER SAFETY

Sometimes the air a patient is breathing may not have enough oxygen or may have poisonous or toxic gases. This can lead to breathing difficulties. During the scene size-up, it is critical to ensure a safe environment for all emergency medical services (EMS) workers. This should be done before treatment efforts are started. Rescue personnel with special training and equipment should be used as needed to ensure scene safety.

Patient Care

INITIAL ASSESSMENT

A primary focus of the initial assessment is to detect any life-threatening conditions. This and starting resuscitation take priority over detailed assessment. Signs of life-threatening respiratory distress in adults include the following:

- Alterations in mental status
- Severe cyanosis
- Absent breath sounds
- Audible stridor
- Inability to speak one or two words without dyspnea
- Tachycardia
- Pallor and diaphoresis
- Retractions and/or the use of accessory muscles to assist breathing

FOCUSED HISTORY AND PHYSICAL EXAMINATION

The paramedic should find out the patient's chief complaints. These may include dyspnea, chest pain, productive or nonproductive cough, hemoptysis (coughing up blood from the respiratory tract), wheezing, and signs of respiratory infection (e.g., fever, increased sputum production). The history should focus on the patient's previous experiences with similar or the same symptoms. The patient's objective description of severity often is an accurate indicator of the severity of the current episode if the condition is chronic.

Asking the patient, "What happened the last time you had an attack this bad?" is very useful for predicting what will happen with this episode. The following is a sample of questions that might be asked in order to obtain a focused history for a patient with respiratory distress. This format uses the acronym OPQRST (onset, provocation, quality, severity, and time):

Onset: "What were you doing when the breathing difficulty began? Do you think anything might have triggered it? Did your breathing difficulty begin gradually or was it sudden in onset? Did you experience any pain when the breathing difficulty began?"

Provocation: "Does lying down or sitting up make your breathing better or worse? Do you have any pain when you breathe? If so, does the pain increase when you take a deep breath or does it stay the same?"

Quality: "Is it more difficult to breathe when you inhale or exhale? If you have pain when you breathe, would you describe it as sharp or dull?"

Severity: "On a scale of 1 to 10 (with 10 being the worst), how would you rate the difficulty of your breathing?"

Time: "What time did the breathing difficulty start? Has it been constant since it began? If you've had this type of difficulty before, how long did it last?"

Unknown Pulmonary Diagnosis

If paramedics do not know a patient's diagnosed condition, they should try to determine whether it is related mainly to ventilation, diffusion, or perfusion or to a combination of defects. They may be able to determine this from the patient's medication history. After obtaining a history of the current illness, paramedics should obtain a medication history that includes current medications, medication allergies, cardiac medications, and pulmonary medications (e.g., oxygen therapy; inhaled, oral, or parenteral sympathomimetics; inhaled or oral corticosteroids; cromolyn sodium; methylxanthines; antibiotics).

> **NOTE** It is important to ask patients whether they have been intubated before because of breathing difficulty. A history of previous intubation indicates severe pulmonary disease. It also suggests that intubation may be required again.

PHYSICAL EXAMINATION

The physical examination begins with a general impression of the patient. The paramedic should note the patient's position, mental status, ability to speak, respiratory effort, and skin color (see Chapter 12). Vital signs should be assessed, with the following considerations kept in mind[1]:

- *Pulse rate:* Tachycardia is a sign of hypoxemia. It may result from the use of sympathomimetic medications. Bradycardia caused by respiratory problems is a warning sign of severe hypoxemia and imminent cardiac arrest.
- *Blood pressure:* Hypertension may result from the use of sympathomimetic medications.
- *Respiratory rate:* The respiratory rate is not an accurate sign of respiratory status unless it is very slow. Trends are essential in evaluating a patient with chronic respiratory disease. A slowing rate in a patient who is not improving suggests exhaustion and impending respiratory insufficiency. Abnormal patterns (see Chapter 19) that may be seen in patients with respiratory disease include eupnea, tachypnea, Cheyne-Stokes respirations, central neurogenic hyperventilation, Kussmaul respirations, ataxic respirations, apneustic respirations, and apnea.

The patient's face and neck should be assessed for pursed-lip breathing and use of accessory muscles. Pursed-lip breathing helps maintain pressure in the airways (even during exhalation). This pressure helps to support bronchial walls that have lost their support as a result of disease. The use of accessory muscles can quickly result in respiratory fatigue. The patient should be questioned about sputum production. An increasing amount of sputum suggests infection. Thick, green, or brown sputum may indicate pneumonia; yellow or pale gray sputum may be related to allergic or inflammatory causes; pink, frothy sputum is associated with severe and late stages of pulmonary edema. The patient's neck should be evaluated for jugular vein distention. It may be a sign of right-sided heart failure resulting from severe pulmonary congestion.

The patient's chest should be inspected for injury. It also should be inspected for any indicators of chronic disease. (An example is a barrel chest from long-standing chronic obstructive pulmonary disease.) Other components of the chest examination include noting accessory muscle use or retractions to facilitate breathing, evaluating chest wall symmetry, and auscultating the patient's lungs for normal and abnormal breath sounds.

The patient's extremities should be assessed for peripheral cyanosis, clubbing of the fingers, and carpopedal spasm. Peripheral cyanosis is caused when a large amount of the hemoglobin in the blood is not carrying oxygen. Clubbing is an abnormal enlargement of the ends of the fingers. It indicates long-standing chronic hypoxemia. Carpopedal spasms are spasms of the hands, thumbs, feet, or toes. They often are associated with hypocapnia. They result from long periods of rapid, deep respiration. All of these are crucial findings in a patient with respiratory disease. They should be documented on the patient care report. They also should be communicated to medical direction.

DIAGNOSTIC TESTING

Diagnostic testing that may be appropriate for some patients with respiratory disease includes pulse oximetry, the use of peak flow meters, and capnometry. Pulse oximeters measure oxygen saturation. Peak flow meters (described later in this chapter) provide a baseline assessment of airflow for patients with obstructive lung disease. Capnometry can help determine proper placement of the endotracheal tube in intubated patients. Pulse oximetry and capnometry are described in Chapter 19.

OBSTRUCTIVE AIRWAY DISEASE

Obstructive airway disease is a major health problem in the United States. It affects some 17 million Americans.[2] Predisposing factors that contribute to obstructive pulmonary disease include smoking, environmental pollution, industrial exposures, and various pulmonary infectious processes. Obstructive airway disease is a triad of distinct diseases that often coexist. They are chronic bronchitis and emphysema (together referred to as chronic obstructive pulmonary disease [COPD]) and asthma. These diseases are presented separately in this chapter. However, the paramedic must remember that patients often have all three in different degrees.

> **CRITICAL THINKING**
>
> Will patients with chronic obstructive pulmonary disease (COPD) always be able to "name" their disease when you ask about their history?

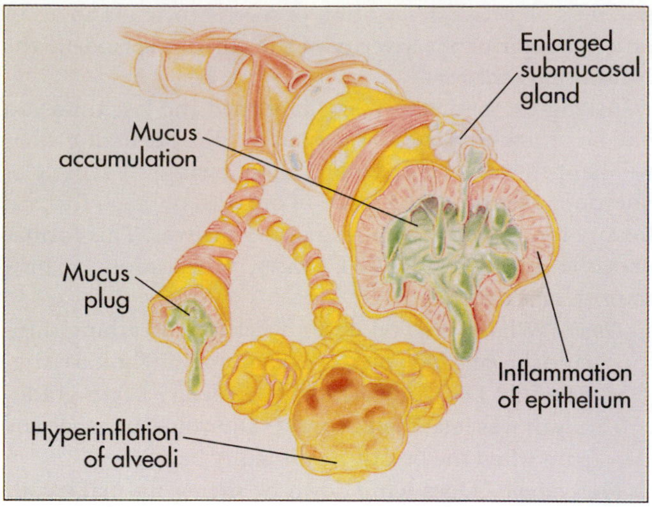

FIGURE 30-1 ■ Chronic bronchitis. Bronchi are filled with excess mucus.

Chronic Bronchitis

Chronic bronchitis is a condition involving inflammatory changes and excessive mucus production in the bronchial tree (Fig. 30-1). It affects about 20% of men in the United States. The disease is characterized by an increase in the number and size of mucus-producing glands. This results from prolonged exposure to irritants. (Most often the irritant is cigarette smoke.) The condition is diagnosed clinically by the presence of cough with sputum production on most days for at least 3 months of the year and for at least 2 consecutive years.[1] The alveoli are not seriously affected. Also, diffusion remains relatively normal.

Patients with severe chronic bronchitis have a low oxygen pressure (Po_2). (These patients sometimes are called "blue bloaters" when they appear cyanotic.) They have a low Po_2 because of changes in the ventilation-perfusion relationships in the lung and hypoventilation. The hypoventilation leads to hypercapnia (high levels of carbon dioxide [CO_2]), hypoxemia (low levels of oxygen [O_2]), and increases in arterial carbon dioxide pressure (Pco_2). Patients with chronic bronchitis have frequent respiratory infections. These eventually cause scarring of lung tissue. In time, irreversible changes occur in the lung. These changes may lead to emphysema or bronchiectasis. **Bronchiectasis** is an abnormal dilation of the bronchi. It is caused by a pus-producing infection of the bronchial wall.

Emphysema

Emphysema results from pathological changes in the lung. It is the end stage of a process that progresses slowly for many years. The disease is characterized by permanent abnormal enlargement of the air spaces beyond the terminal bronchioles, destruction of the alveoli, and collapse of the alveoli (Fig. 30-2). The disease reduces the number of alveoli available for gas exchange. It also reduces the elasticity of the remaining alveoli. This loss of elasticity leads to trapping of air in the alveoli. Thus residual volume increases, whereas vital capacity remains somewhat normal.

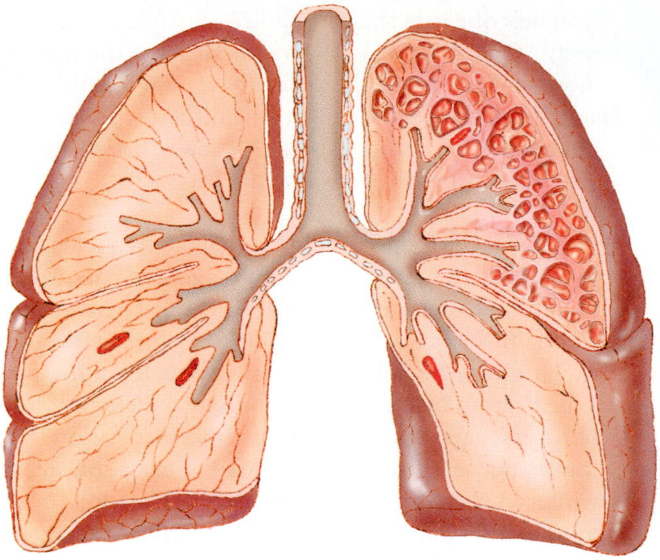

FIGURE 30-2 ■ Cystic changes of lobar emphysema resulting from destruction of alveoli.

The reduction in arterial Po_2 leads to increased production of red blood cells. This is called *polycythemia* (i.e., an elevated hematocrit value.) This elevation in hematocrit is much more common in the "blue bloater" than in the "pink puffer." (That is, it is more common in a patient with chronic bronchitis than in one with mainly emphysema.) This is because the patient with chronic bronchitis is more

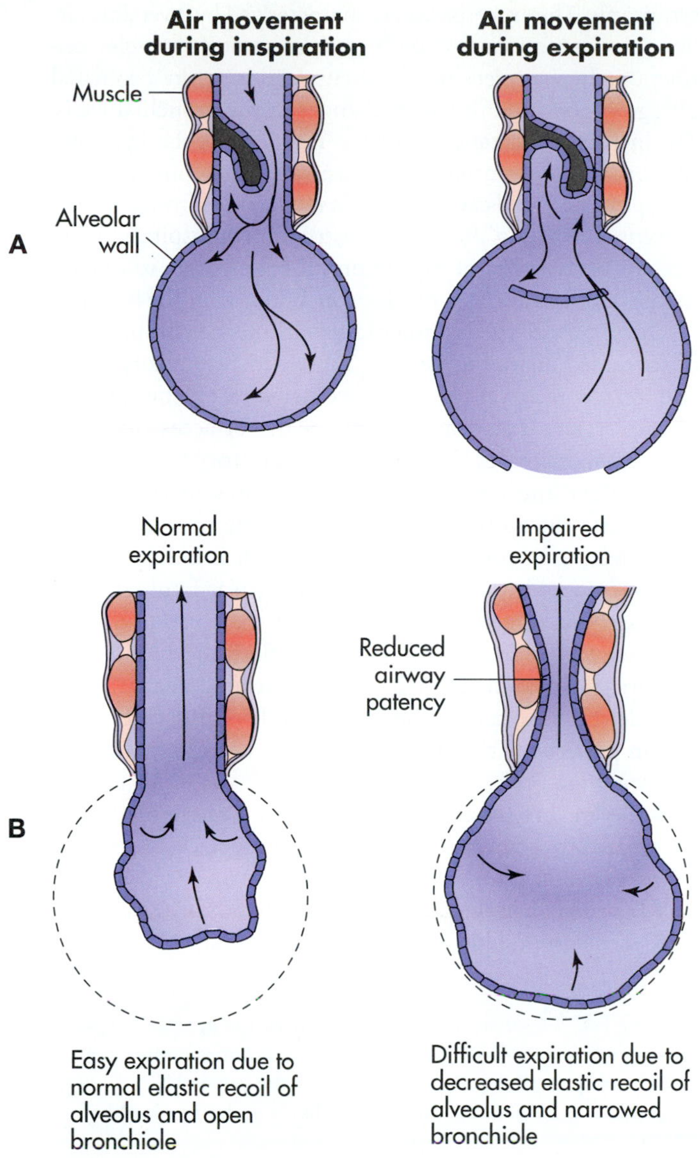

FIGURE 30-3 ■ **A,** Mechanisms of air trapping in chronic obstructive pulmonary disease (COPD): Mucus plugs and narrowed airways cause air trapping and hyperinflation on expiration. During inspiration, the airways enlarge, allowing gas to flow past the obstruction. This mechanism of air trapping occurs in asthma and chronic bronchitis. **B,** Mechanism of air trapping in emphysema: Damaged or destroyed alveolar walls no longer support and hold open the airways, and alveoli lost their property of elastic recoil. Both these factors contribute to airway collapse during expiration.

often chronically hypoxemic. Decreases in alveolar membrane surface area and in the number of pulmonary capillaries in the lung reduce the area for gas exchange and increase resistance to pulmonary blood flow.

Patients with emphysema have some resistance to airflow into and out of the lungs. Yet most of the hyperexpansion is caused by air trapped in the alveoli as a result of the loss of elasticity (Fig. 30-3). Patients with chronic bronchitis have increased airway resistance during inspiration and expiration. In contrast, patients with emphysema have increased airway resistance only on expiration. Normally a passive, involuntary act, expiration becomes a muscular act in patients with COPD. Over time, the chest becomes rigid (barrel shaped). Then, the patient must use accessory muscles of the neck, chest, and abdomen to move air into and out of the lungs. Full deflation of the lungs becomes more and more difficult. Finally, it becomes impossible. Often the patient with emphysema is thin. This is due to poor dietary intake. It also is due to the increased caloric consumption required by the work of breathing (Table 30-2). Patients with emphysema often develop *bullae* (thin-walled cystic lesions in the lung) from the destruction of alveolar walls. When bullae collapse, they increase the problems with air exchange seen in these patients. They also can lead to pneumothorax.

TABLE 30-2 Comparison of Signs and Symptoms of Emphysema and Chronic Bronchitis

EMPHYSEMA	CHRONIC BRONCHITIS
Thin, barrel-chest appearance	Typically overweight
Nonproductive cough	Productive cough with sputum
Wheezing and rhonchi	Coarse rhonchi
Pink complexion	Chronic cyanosis
Extreme dyspnea on exertion	Mild, chronic dyspnea
Prolonged inspiration (pursed-lip breathing)	Resistance on inspiration and expiration

CRITICAL THINKING

What effect might application of a cervical collar, use of a short spine board or vest, and immobilization supine on a long backboard have on a patient with chronic obstructive pulmonary disease (COPD) who has sustained trauma?

ASSESSMENT OF COPD

Patients with COPD usually are aware of and have adapted to their illness. A request for emergency care indicates that a significant change has occurred in the patient's condition. The patient with COPD usually has an acute episode of worsening dyspnea that is manifested even at rest, an increase or change in sputum production, or an increase in the malaise that accompanies the disease. Other common complaints include inability to sleep and recurrent headaches.

Paramedics responding to the call are likely to find the patient with COPD in respiratory distress. Often the patient is sitting upright. The person may be leaning forward to aid breathing. The individual frequently is using pursed-lip breathing to maintain positive airway pressures, in addition to using accessory muscles. Increased hypoxemia and hypercarbia may be indicated by tachypnea, diaphoresis, cyanosis, confusion, irritability, and drowsiness.

Other physical findings include wheezes, rhonchi, and crackles (see Chapter 11). Breath sounds and heart sounds also may be diminished. This is due to reduced air exchange and the increased diameter of the thoracic cavity. In late stages of decompensation, the patient may have peripheral cyanosis, clubbing of the fingers, and signs of right-sided heart failure. The patient's electrocardiogram (ECG) may reveal cardiac dysrhythmias or signs of right atrial enlargement; these include tall, peaked P waves in leads II, III, and AVF (see Chapter 29).

MANAGEMENT

The main goal of prehospital care for these patients is the correction of hypoxemia through improved airflow. This can be achieved through administration of oxygen and drug therapy. However, drug therapy can cause serious side effects and complications. This particularly may be the case if the patient has used medication before the paramedics arrive. Therefore it is crucial for paramedics to obtain a thorough medical history regarding medication use, home oxygen use, and drug allergies.

An intravenous (IV) line should be established in all patients in respiratory distress. A cardiac monitor also should be applied. If the patient has a productive cough, coughing should be encouraged. Any sputum should be collected. This should be delivered with the patient for laboratory analysis.

Some patients with COPD rely on a hypoxic drive for ventilatory effort. However, the paramedic should never withhold oxygen because of fear of decreasing hypoxic drive while providing emergency care in the prehospital setting. High-concentration oxygen should be administered with a nonrebreather mask if indicated. Pulse oximetry to measure oxygen saturation should be considered. Some of these patients require ventilatory assistance.

The medications used in the prehospital setting to relieve bronchospasm and reduce constricted airways are the beta agonists (e.g., ***metaproterenol*** and ***albuterol***). Other drugs that may be given after evaluation by a physician include steroids ***(methylprednisolone),*** nebulized anticholinergics (e.g., ***atropine***), and occasionally methylxanthines (e.g., ***aminophylline***) for bronchodilation and stimulation of the respiratory drive.[3] (See the Emergency Drug Index for specific drug therapy.)

Asthma

Asthma, or reactive airway disease, is a common disorder that affects 10 to 15 million Americans (4% to 5% of the U.S. population). It is responsible for 4000 to 5000 deaths each year.[3] Asthma is most common in children and young adults. Yet it can occur in any decade of life. Aggravating factors tend to be extrinsic (external) in children. In contrast, they tend to be intrinsic (internal) in adults (Fig. 30-4). Childhood asthma often improves or resolves with age. Adult asthma usually persists.

PATHOPHYSIOLOGY OF AN ASTHMA EXACERBATION

Asthma generally occurs in acute episodes of variable duration. Between these episodes, the patient is somewhat free of symptoms. The exacerbation is characterized by reversible airflow obstruction caused by bronchial smooth muscle contraction; hypersecretion of mucus, resulting in bronchial plugging; and inflammatory changes in the bronchial walls. The increased resistance to airflow leads to alveolar hypoventilation, marked ventilation-perfusion mismatching (leading to hypoxemia), and carbon dioxide retention (stimulating hyperventilation) (Fig. 30-5). The obstruction of inspiration and marked obstruction of expiration causes pressure to remain high in the airways, as a result of air trapping in the lungs.

During an acute asthma exacerbation, the combination of increased airway resistance, increased respiratory drive, and air trapping creates excessive demand on the muscles of respiration. This leads to greater use of accessory muscles. It also increases the chance of respiratory fatigue. If labored breathing continues, high pressures in the thorax can reduce the amount of blood returning to the left ventricle (left ventricular preload). The result is a drop in cardiac output and systolic blood pressure (near-fatal asthma). Pulsus paradoxus also may be seen. If the episode continues, hypoxemia and changes in blood flow and blood pressure may lead to death. Most asthma-related deaths occur outside the hospital. In the prehospital setting, cardiac arrest in patients with severe asthma has been linked to the following factors[4]:

- Severe bronchospasm and mucous plugging, which leads to asphyxia (the most common cause of asthma-related deaths)
- Cardiac dysrhythmias caused by hypoxia
- Tension pneumothorax (often bilateral)

> **NOTE** *Caution:* Thoracic decompression in a patient with severe refractory asthma without pneumothorax might result in puncture of the visceral pleura of the hyperinflated lung, producing a pneumothorax (most likely under tension).[5]

Other conditions that may be present in patients with near-fatal asthma include cardiac disease, pulmonary disease, acute allergic bronchospasm or anaphylaxis, drug use or misuse (beta blockers, cocaine, and opiates), and recent discontinuation of long-term corticosteroid therapy (associated with adrenal insufficiency).

ASSESSMENT

When paramedics arrive, the asthmatic patient usually is sitting upright. The person may be leaning forward with hands on knees (tripod position). Also, the patient may be using accessory muscles to aid breathing. The typical asthmatic patient is in obvious respiratory distress. Respirations are rapid and loud, and audible wheezing may be present. The patient's mental status should be noted and monitored carefully. Lethargy, exhaustion, agitation, and confusion are serious signs of impending respiratory failure. An initial history must be obtained quickly. Questions about the onset of the current problem, its relative severity, the precipitating cause, medication use, and allergies should be specific and to the point.

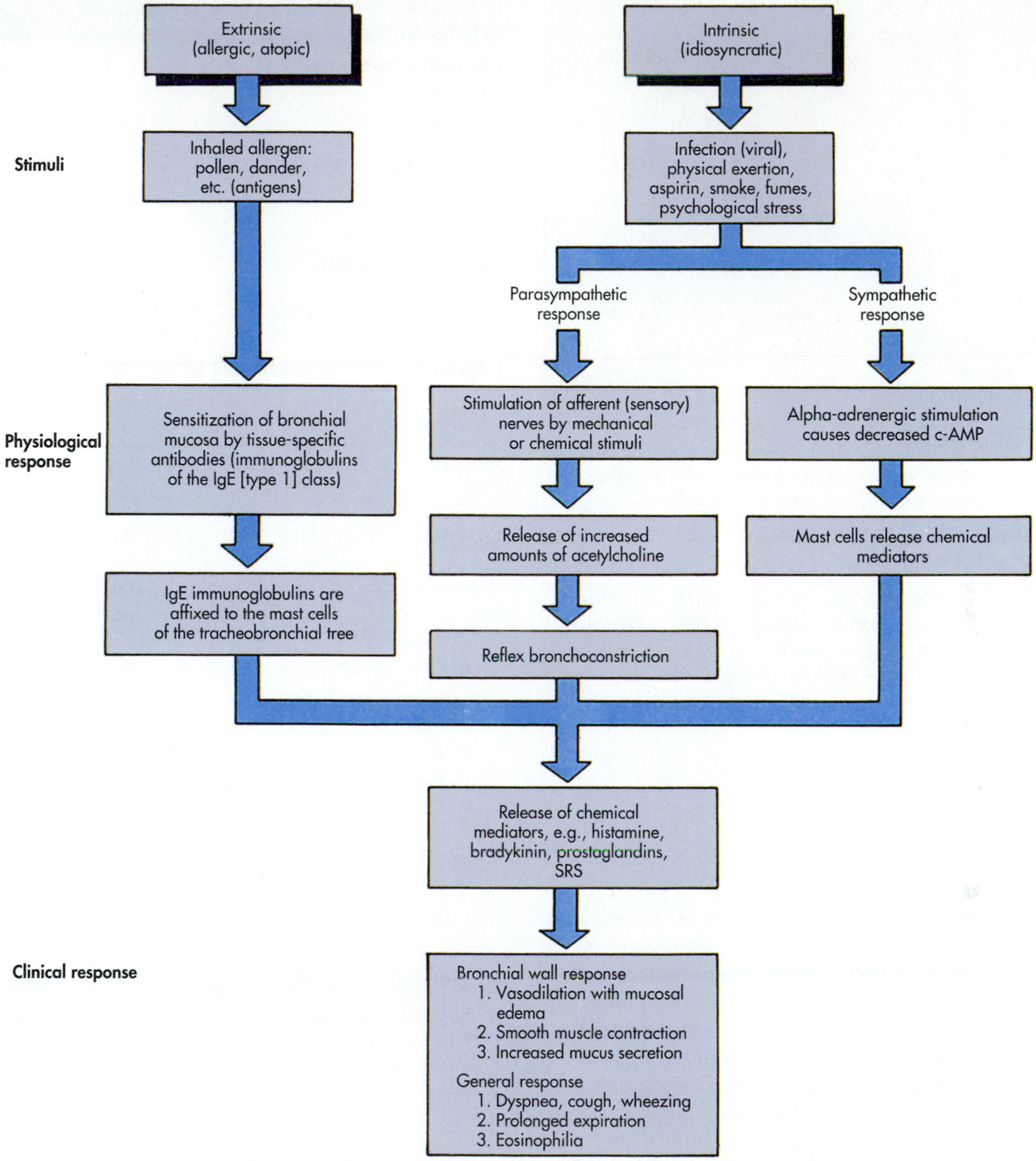

FIGURE 30-4 ■ Extrinsic and intrinsic bronchial asthma.

It is crucial to find out whether the patient has needed intubation to manage previous asthma attacks.

On auscultation, a prolonged expiratory phase may be noted. Usually wheezing is heard from the movement of air through the narrowed airways. Inspiratory wheezing (unlike inspiratory stridor) does not indicate upper airway occlusion. It suggests that the large and midsize muscular airways are obstructed. This indicates more obstruction than if only expiratory wheezes are heard. Inspiratory wheezes also may suggest that the large airways are filled with secretions. A silent chest (i.e., no audible wheezing or air movement) may indicate such severe obstruction that the flow of air is too low to generate breath sounds. Other signs of severe asthma include the following:

- Reduced level of consciousness
- Diaphoresis and pallor
- Retractions
- Inability to speak after only one or two words
- Poor, floppy muscle tone
- Pulse rate greater than 130 beats per minute
- Respirations greater than 30 breaths per minute
- Pulsus paradoxus greater than 20 mm Hg
- Altered mental status or severe agitation

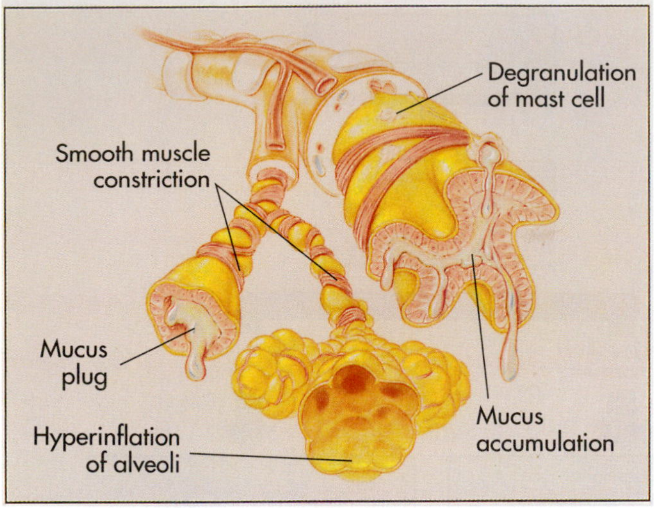

FIGURE 30-5 ■ With bronchial asthma, thick mucus, mucosal edema, and smooth muscle spasm obstruct the small airways. Breathing becomes labored, and expiration is difficult.

BOX 30-2 Asthma Medications

Nebulized Beta$_2$ Agonists
Albuterol
Metaproterenol

Corticosteroids (IV)
Methylprednisone
Hydrocortisone

Aminophylline (IV)

Magnesium Sulfate (IV)

Epinephrine or Terbutaline (SQ or IM)

Heliox (helium/oxygen)

IV, Intravenous; *SQ,* subcutaneous; *IM,* intramuscular.

NOTE Asthma attacks are true medical emergencies. Paramedics should manage these episodes aggressively. Deterioration of the patient's condition can be expected and also rapid. It also can be fatal. Therefore the paramedic must monitor the patient carefully and continuously. Initial patient management should be directed at ensuring an adequate airway, providing supplemental oxygen, and reversing the bronchospasm.

MANAGEMENT

After administration of high-concentration oxygen, drug therapy is provided (Box 30-2). Drug therapy is based on the patient's age. It also is based on the patient's use of medications before the arrival of paramedics. The initial drugs prescribed by medical direction probably will be fast-acting agents (e.g., ***albuterol***). ***Albuterol*** is the current cornerstone of asthma treatment in the United States. It stimulates beta-adrenergic receptors. It therefore acts as a rapid bronchodilator. Side effects include brief tachycardia and tremors.

Medical direction also may prescribe rehydration. This can be accomplished through the administration of IV fluids. All patients with acute asthma should be transported in a position of comfort. This helps to maximize the use of respiratory muscles. These patients should also be monitored for cardiac rhythm disturbances.

CRITICAL THINKING

Consider that the patient is unable to hold the nebulizer mouthpiece or needs to be ventilated using a bag-valve device. What can you do to promote bronchodilation?

In some cases endotracheal (ET) intubation is required for a patient having a severe asthma attack. If a conscious patient requires ET intubation, the paramedic should consult with medical direction and consider the following critical actions[4]:

- Provide adequate sedation with ***ketamine***, a benzodiazepine, or barbiturate
- Paralyze the patient with ***succinylcholine*** or ***vecuronium***
- Immediately after intubation, administer 2.5 to 5 mg ***albuterol*** directly into the ET tube
- Confirm ET tube placement with primary and secondary confirmation methods (see Chapter 19).
- Ventilate at 8 to 10 breaths per minute to allow for the escape of air and to avoid sudden hypotension (especially in elderly patients with emphysema)

NOTE Even after intubation, ventilating the patient may be difficult. The absence of any significant obstruction to airflow immediately after tracheal intubation suggests that the diagnosis of acute asthma may have been incorrect, and the problem may be in the upper airway.[4]

Pulmonary Function Tests. Pulmonary function tests measure the peak expiratory flow rate (PEFR). These tests can help to determine the severity of an asthma attack. They also can help the paramedic assess the effectiveness of treatment of the airway obstruction. Peak flow meters (Fig. 30-6) can be used in the prehospital setting for this purpose. Their use requires a cooperative patient. (One who can make a maximal respiratory effort.) It also requires coaching by the paramedic.

To determine a baseline airflow (before drug administration), the paramedic should instruct the patient to inflate the lungs fully and forcefully exhale as quickly as possible into the flow meter. (Children should be reminded to breathe out as if they were blowing out candles or blowing up a balloon.) The reading is recorded in liters per minute.

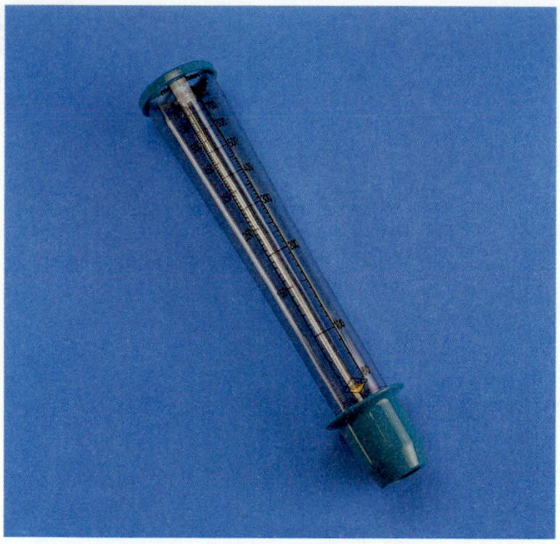

FIGURE 30-6 ■ Peak flow meter.

This measurement should be taken two more times. The highest of the three readings is chosen as the peak value flow. This measurement is then compared with standard tables based on height, gender, and race (Table 30-3). A PEFR measurement with variabilityless than 20% is considered mild; 20% to 30% is moderate; and more than 30% is severe. Peak flow measurements should be repeated throughout the course of management to evaluate the patient's response to drug therapy.

▶**NOTE** Most children under 5 years of age cannot adequately perform peak expiratory flow rate (PEFR) tests. Also, this test should not be used with a patient in severe respiratory distress. Drug therapy to reverse the bronchospasm is the priority.

STATUS ASTHMATICUS

Status asthmaticus is a severe, prolonged asthma attack that has not been broken with repeated doses of bronchodilators. It may be of sudden onset. (For example, it may result from spasm of the airways.) It can also be subtle in onset, resulting from a viral respiratory infection or prolonged exposure to one or more allergens. Status asthmaticus is a true emergency. It calls for early recognition and immediate transport of the patient. These patients are in danger of respiratory failure.

The treatment of patients for status asthmaticus is the same as that for acute asthma attacks. Yet the urgency of rapid transport is more important. In addition, these patients usually are dehydrated. They typically require IV fluid administration. The patient's respiratory status should be monitored closely. Also, high-concentration oxygen should be administered. The need for intubation and aggressive ventilatory support should be anticipated. Continuous bronchodilator therapy may be ordered by medical direction.

CRITICAL THINKING

When a patient treated for status asthmaticus is reassessed, would decreasing respiratory and heart rates indicate a good outcome or a bad one? Why?

Differential Considerations

Wheezing commonly is associated with asthma. However, it may be present in *all* types of obstructive lung disease. Also, it may be present with other conditions that cause dyspnea (Table 30-4). For example, tachypnea, wheezing, and respiratory distress may indicate heart failure, pneumonia, pulmonary edema, pulmonary embolism, pneumothorax, toxic inhalation, foreign body aspiration, and various other pathological states. Appropriate emergency care is based on the patient assessment and an accurate history.

PNEUMONIA

Pneumonia is a group of specific infections (not a single disease) that cause an acute inflammatory process of the respiratory bronchioles and the alveoli. It is the fifth most common cause of death from infectious disease in the United States[1] (Fig. 30-7). Pneumonia can be caused by bacterial, viral, or fungal infection; associated risk factors include cigarette smoking, alcoholism, exposure to cold, and extremes of age (the very young and very old). These diseases may be spread by respiratory droplets. They may be spread by contact with infected individuals. They also may be spread by breathing in bacteria from one's own nose and mouth.

Pneumonia may be classified as the viral, bacterial, mycoplasmal, or aspiration type. Pneumonia generally manifests with classic signs and symptoms (*typical pneumonia*). These include a productive cough, pleuritic chest pain, and fever that produces "shaking chills." It also may cause nonspecific complaints. (This particularly may be the case in older adults and debilitated patients.) Nonspecific complaints may include a nonproductive cough, headache, fatigue, and sore throat (*atypical pneumonia*).

▶**NOTE** Community-acquired pneumonia is an infection that is acquired from the environment. This category includes infections acquired indirectly as a result of the use of medications that change the body's ability to fight off disease. The occurrence of these infections has risen in recent years. This is due to the increased percentage of the population over age 65. It also is due to the increasing number of patients taking immunosuppressive drugs for malignancy, transplantation, or autoimmune disease.

Viral Pneumonia

Influenza A is the most common type of viral pneumonia (Box 30-3). It often occurs as epidemics in populations of small groups such as schoolchildren, army recruits, and nursing

TABLE 30-3 Predicted Average Peak Expiratory Flow

Note: These charts are for informational purposes only. Spirometry should be used for diagnosis and staging. "Personal best" measures should be used for the asthma treatment plan.

PREDICTED AVERAGE PEAK EXPIRATORY FLOW FOR NORMAL CHILDREN AND ADOLESCENTS (L/MIN)

HEIGHT (INCHES)	MALES AND FEMALES	HEIGHT (INCHES)	MALES AND FEMALES
43	147	56	320
44	160	57	334
45	173	58	347
46	187	59	360
47	200	60	373
48	214	61	387
49	227	62	400
50	240	63	413
51	254	64	427
52	267	65	440
53	280	66	454
54	293	67	467
55	307		

Modified from Polger G, Promedhat V: *Pulmonary function testing in children: techniques and standards*, Philadelphia, 1971, WB Saunders.

PREDICTED AVERAGE PEAK EXPIRATORY FLOW FOR NORMAL MALES (L/MIN)

	HEIGHT (INCHES)				
AGE	60	65	70	75	80
20	554	602	649	693	740
25	543	590	636	679	725
30	532	577	622	664	710
35	521	565	609	651	695
40	509	552	596	636	680
45	498	540	583	622	665
50	486	527	569	607	649
55	475	515	556	593	634
60	463	502	542	578	618
65	452	490	529	564	603
70	440	447	515	550	587

Modified from Leiner GC et al: Expiratory peak flow rate: standard values for normal subjects_use as a clinical test of ventilatory function, *Am Resp Dis* 88:644, 1963.

PREDICTED AVERAGE PEAK EXPIRATORY FLOW FOR NORMAL FEMALES (L/MIN)

	HEIGHT (INCHES)				
AGE	55	60	65	70	75
20	390	423	460	496	529
25	385	418	454	490	523
30	380	413	448	483	516
35	375	408	442	476	509
40	370	402	436	470	502
45	365	397	430	464	495
50	360	391	424	457	488
55	355	386	418	451	482
60	350	380	412	445	475
65	345	375	406	439	468
70	340	369	400	432	461

Modified from Leiner GC et al: Expiratory peak flow rate: standard values for normal subjects use as a clinical test of ventilatory function, *Am Resp Dis* 88:644, 1963.

TABLE 30-4 Disease and Symptoms Associated with Wheezing

DISEASE	SYMPTOMS
Asthma	Productive cough, tightness in chest
Bacterial pneumonia	Productive cough, pleuritic pain
Chronic bronchitis	Chronic, productive cough
Emphysema	Cough
Foreign body aspiration	Cough
Heart failure	Cough, orthopnea, nocturnal dyspnea
Pneumothorax	Sudden, sharp pleuritic pain
Pulmonary disease	Tachypnea, cough, congestion
Pulmonary embolism	Sudden, sharp pleuritic pain
Toxic inhalation	Cough, pain

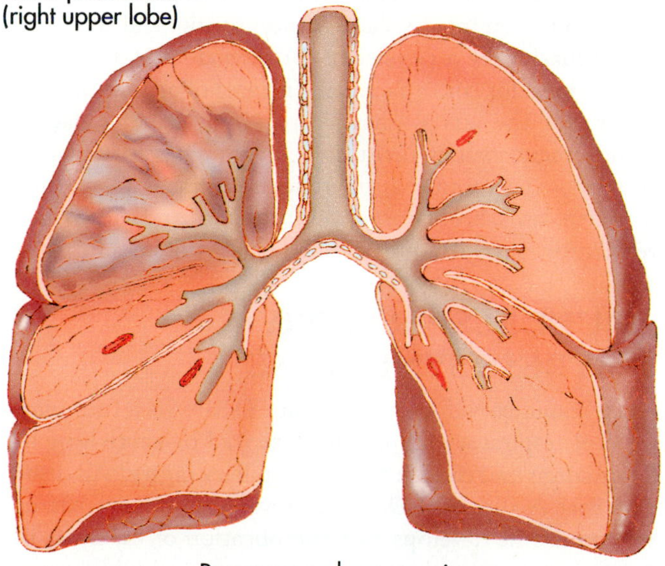

FIGURE 30-7 ■ *Pneumonia* is an inflammatory process of the respiratory bronchioles and alveoli. It is caused by infection.

home residents. The interstitial infection caused by the virus predisposes the patient to secondary bacterial pneumonia.

Bacterial Pneumonia

The pneumococcus bacillus *(Streptococcus pneumoniae)* accounts for 90% of bacterial pneumonias. It affects 1 in 500 people each year. The peak incidence is in winter and early spring. A vaccine that is now available is 80% to 90% effective against this type of pneumonia in adults. Bacterial pneumonia can result from the aspiration of mucus and saliva. Therefore patients in a coma or with seizures, suppressed cough reflex, and increased secretions are predisposed to developing the disease. Other predisposing risk factors that may contribute to the development of bacterial pneumonia include the following:

BOX 30-3 Influenza

Influenza is an acute, febrile disease that affects the entire body. It is associated with viral infection of the upper and lower respiratory tracts. It usually is characterized by the abrupt onset of a severe, protracted cough, fever, headache, muscle ache, and mild sore throat. Of all the viruses, the influenza and parainfluenza viruses are the most common causes of serious respiratory infections. Moreover, they have high morbidity and mortality rates.

Influenza viruses A, B, and C (and their many strains) are known for their potential to quickly cause respiratory infections after exposure. (It usually occurs within 24 to 48 hours.) The virus is inhaled in respiratory droplets from infected individuals (such as when an infected person sneezes). The droplets penetrate the surface of upper respiratory tract mucosal cells. The virus eventually spreads to the lower respiratory tract. There it causes cell inflammation and destruction of the cilia. Without the cilia, clearing the airways of infected mucus is more difficult. Consequently, a secondary bacterial infection often develops. This may result in pneumonia or acute respiratory failure. (This is particularly the case in patients with chronic lung disease.)

Influenza has the potential for widespread epidemics in high-risk populations. (These include adults and children with chronic cardiorespiratory or metabolic disorders, residents of nursing homes and other institutions, and health care workers.) Current vaccines are effective against some strains of the virus. These vaccines have minimal side effects. If uncomplicated, influenza is self-limiting. Acute symptoms last 2 to 7 days. These are followed by a convalescent period of about 1 week.

- Infection
  - Upper respiratory infection (influenza)
  - Postoperative infection
- Foreign body aspiration
- Alcohol or other drug addiction
- Cardiac failure
- Stroke
- Syncope
- Pulmonary embolism
- Chronic illness
  - Chronic respiratory disease
  - Diabetes mellitus
  - Congestive heart failure
- Prolonged immobilization
- Compromised immune status

Mycoplasmal Pneumonia

Mycoplasmal pneumonia is caused by infection with *Mycoplasma pneumoniae.* It causes mild upper respiratory infection in school-age children and young adults. Transmission is believed to occur by means of infected respiratory secretions.

NOTE All EMS workers should consider getting vaccinated against pneumonia.

Therefore the condition spreads quickly among family members. This form of pneumonia can be treated effectively with antibiotics.

Aspiration Pneumonia

Aspiration pneumonia is an inflammation of the lung tissue (parenchyma). It results when foreign material enters the tracheobronchial tree. The syndrome is common in patients who have an altered level of consciousness (e.g., from head injury, seizure activity, use of alcohol or other drugs, anesthesia, infection, shock) and in intubated patients and those who have aspirated foreign bodies. Factors common to victims of aspiration include depression of the cough or gag reflex, inability of the patient to handle secretions or gastric contents, and inability to protect the airway.

Aspiration pneumonia may be nonbacterial. (For example, it may develop after aspiration of stomach contents, toxic materials, or inert substances) It typically is called *pneumonitis*. This distinguishes it from infectious pneumonia or bacterial pneumonia (as a secondary complication). Bacterial aspiration pneumonia has a poor prognosis, even with antibiotic therapy.

Management

The type and degree of damage done by pneumonia depend on the cause of the disease. In viral and mycoplasmal pneumonias, the inflammatory response in the bronchi damages the cilia and the epithelium. This causes congestion. In some cases it causes hemorrhage. Signs and symptoms include chest pain, cough, fever, dyspnea, and occasionally hemoptysis. Patients usually complain of general malaise. They also complain of upper respiratory and gastrointestinal symptoms. Auscultation of the chest may reveal wheezing and fine crackles. In uncomplicated cases the symptoms usually resolve in 7 to 10 days.

Bacterial pneumonia begins with infection in the alveoli. In time, this infection fills the alveoli with fluid and purulent sputum. The infection spreads from alveolus to alveolus. As this occurs, large areas of the lung, even entire lobes, may become consolidated. (That is, they may become filled with fluid and cellular debris.) Consolidation reduces the available surface area of respiratory membranes. It also decreases the ventilation-perfusion ratio. Both of these effects may lead to hypoxemia. Patients with bacterial pneumonia usually have acute shaking chills, tachypnea, tachycardia, cough, and sputum production. The sputum may be rust colored (classic for pneumococcus). More often, though, it is yellow, green, or gray. Additional symptoms include malaise, anorexia, flank or back pain, and vomiting. If the disease is uncomplicated and treated with antibiotics, the patient begins to recover within 3 to 5 days. Antibiotics usually are continued for a total of 7 to 10 days.

The physiological effects of aspiration pneumonia are based on the volume and pH of the aspirated substances. If the pH is below 2.5 (as may occur in the aspiration of stomach contents), atelectasis, pulmonary edema, hemorrhage, and cell necrosis may occur. The alveolar-capillary membrane may be damaged as well. This, in turn, may lead to fluid buildup in the alveoli. In severe cases, it may lead to adult respiratory distress syndrome (described in the next section). The patient's signs and symptoms vary with the scenario and the severity of the insult (e.g., near-drowning, foreign body aspiration, aspiration of gastric contents). Clinical features may include dyspnea, cough, bronchospasm, wheezes, rhonchi, crackles, cyanosis, and pulmonary and cardiac insufficiency. Of these patients, 25% to 45% develop pulmonary infection.

CRITICAL THINKING

What measures can the paramedic take to reduce a patient's risk of aspiration?

Prehospital care for patients with pneumonia includes airway support, oxygen administration, ventilatory assistance as needed, IV fluids to support blood pressure and to thin and loosen mucus, cardiac monitoring, and transport for evaluation by a physician. (Bronchodilator drugs may also be used for some patients.) In cases of aspiration, suctioning of the airway may be required. General patient management usually includes bed rest, analgesics, decongestants, expectorants, antipyretics, and antibiotic therapy. In severe cases, bronchoscopy, intubation, and mechanical ventilation may be required for some patients.

ADULT RESPIRATORY DISTRESS SYNDROME

Adult respiratory distress syndrome (ARDS) is a fulminant form of respiratory failure characterized by acute lung inflammation and diffuse alveolar-capillary injury.[6] All disorders that result in ARDS cause severe pulmonary edema. The syndrome develops as a complication of injury or illness such as trauma, gastric aspiration, cardiopulmonary bypass surgery, gram-negative sepsis, multiple blood transfusions, oxygen toxicity, toxic inhalation, drug overdose, pneumonia, and infections. Regardless of the specific cause, increased capillary permeability (high-permeability noncardiogenic pulmonary edema) results in a clinical condition in which the lungs are wet and heavy, congested, hemorrhagic, and stiff, with decreased perfusion capacity across alveolar membranes. The lungs become noncompliant. This requires the patient to increase the pressure in the airways to breathe.

The pulmonary edema associated with ARDS leads to severe hypoxemia, intrapulmonary shunting, reduced lung compliance and, in some cases, irreversible parenchymal lung damage. Unique to this syndrome is the fact that most patients who develop this condition have healthy lungs before the event that caused the disease. ARDS is more common in men than in women. The mortality rate is over 65%. Complications include respiratory failure, cardiac dysrhythmias, disseminated intravascular coagulation, barotrauma, congestive heart failure, and renal failure (Box 30-4).

BOX 30-4 Severe Acute Respiratory Syndrome (SARS)

Severe acute respiratory syndrome, a viral disease, emerged in China in November 2003. To date SARS has affected about 8000 people in 29 countries. More than 770 SARS-related deaths have been reported worldwide. (None of these have been in the United States.)* SARS is thought to be caused by a new member of the coronavirus family. It is spread by direct contact with the respiratory secretions or body fluids of an infected person. Signs and symptoms of the disease include cough, shortness of breath, difficulty breathing, hypoxia, chills, and body ache (clinical findings of respiratory illness), as well as fever over 100.4° F (38° C).

The exact etiology of the illness has not yet been determined. Also, no specific treatment recommendations have been made. However, the Centers for Disease Control and Prevention recommend empiric therapy. This includes coverage for organisms associated with any community-acquired pneumonia of unclear etiology. It also includes administration of drugs with activity against both typical and atypical respiratory pathogens.† Until transmission of the disease is better understood, clinicians evaluating a person suspected of having SARS should use standard precautions (including hand hygiene, gowns, and gloves) together with respiratory protection (e.g., N-95 respirator), and eye protection.

From *Frequently asked questions about SARS.*
*Centers for Disease Control and Prevention. http://www.cdc.gov/mmwr/preview/mmwrhtml/mm5249a2.htm. Accessed September 21, 2004.
†Centers for Disease Control and Prevention. http://www.cdc.gov.ncidod/sars. Accessed April 23, 2003.

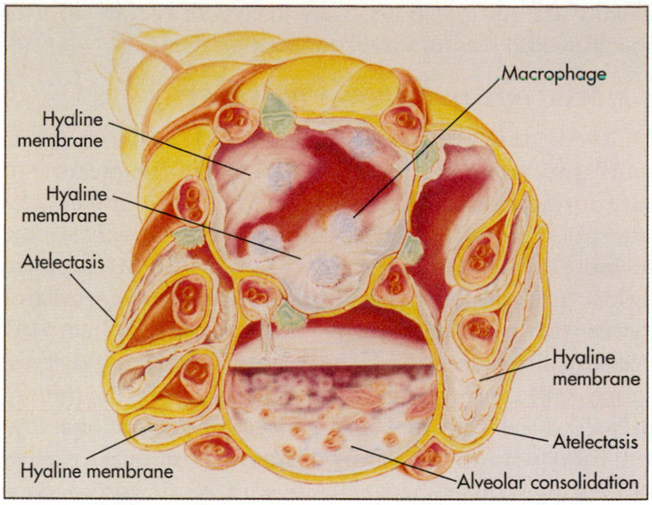

FIGURE 30-8 ■ Cross-sectional view of alveoli in adult respiratory distress syndrome.

Management

All patients with ARDS should be given high-concentration oxygen and ventilatory support. Depending on the underlying cause of ARDS, prehospital management may include fluid replacement to maintain cardiac output and peripheral perfusion; drug therapy to support mechanical ventilation; the use of pharmacological agents (e.g., corticosteroids) to stabilize pulmonary, capillary, and alveolar walls; and diuretics (all of these treatments are controversial).

Patients with ARDS usually have tachypnea, labored breathing, and impaired gas exchange 12 to 72 hours after the initial injury or medical crisis. The syndrome often results from another illness or injury. Therefore paramedics should consider the cause of the underlying problem. They also should provide supplemental oxygen and ventilatory support to improve arterial oxygenation (assessed by pulse oximetry). Most patients with moderate to severe respiratory distress require mechanical ventilation. This ventilation includes the use of positive end-expiratory pressure (PEEP) or continuous positive airway pressure (CPAP). Both of these provide positive-pressure ventilation. Both PEEP and CPAP increase Po_2 by reducing pressure in the lungs.

NOTE Positive end-expiratory pressure (PEEP) and continuous positive airway pressure (CPAP) may have unfavorable effects on the circulation. Such effects include decreased venous return, decreased cardiac output, and pulmonary barotrauma. This type of ventilatory support requires special training. It also requires authorization from medical direction.

POSITIVE END-EXPIRATORY PRESSURE

PEEP maintains a degree of positive pressure at the end of exhalation. This keeps the alveoli open and pushes fluid from the alveoli back into the interstitium or capillaries (Fig. 30-8). In the prehospital setting, ventilatory support with PEEP can be provided through intubation and the use of a Boehringer valve or other special PEEP delivery devices. The Boehringer valve is a cylinder in which a metal ball is suspended. It is connected to the expiratory port of a bag-valve device. The valve (available in pressures of 5, 10, and 15 cm H_2O) creates PEEP by forcing the patient to exhale against the weight of the metal ball.

CONTINUOUS POSITIVE AIRWAY PRESSURE

Continuous positive airway pressure (CPAP) transmits positive pressure into the airways of a spontaneously breathing patient throughout the respiratory cycle. The increase in airway pressure allows for better diffusion of gases and reexpansion of collapsed alveoli. This results in improvement of gas exchange and a reduction in the work of breathing. CPAP can be applied invasively (through an ET tube, creating PEEP). It also can be applied noninvasively through a face or nose mask. Mask CPAP is provided through a tight-fitting face mask. The face mask is connected to a battery-operated breathing circuit. This breathing circuit has an adjustable fraction of inspired oxygen (FIo_2) and a PEEP valve that delivers pressures of 5 to 10 cm H_2O. CPAP reduces the inspiratory work of breathing and lowers mean airway pressures. In addition to its use in patients with pulmonary congestion, CPAP also may benefit patients with acute blunt and penetrating pulmonary injury and those with obstructive airway disease.[3] Patients who receive CPAP usually are quite anxious. They likely will require a lot of coaching and reassurance from the paramedic.

BIPHASIC POSITIVE AIRWAY PRESSURE

Biphasic positive airway pressure (BiPAP) combines partial ventilatory support and CPAP. This allows the pressure to vary during each breath cycle. When the patient inhales, the pressure is similar to CPAP. When the patient exhales, the pressure drops, making it easier to breathe. BiPAP is applied by face mask or nose mask through a noninvasive ventilator device with two settings. The device provides a 5 cm H_2O pressure difference between inspiratory positive airway pressure (IPAP) and expiratory positive airway pressure (EPAP). BiPAP is a leak-tolerant system (CPAP is not). It allows IPAP and EPAP settings to be titrated (adjusted) to reach a desired PEEP range. In selected patients with respiratory distress caused by COPD, pulmonary edema, pneumonia, and asthma, BiPAP may eliminate the need for ET intubation.

PULMONARY THROMBOEMBOLISM

Pulmonary thromboembolism (pulmonary embolism [PE]) is a blockage of a pulmonary artery. The artery is blocked by a clot or other foreign material that has traveled there from another part of the body (Fig. 30-9). Usually pulmonary embolisms originate in the lower extremities. PE is a somewhat common disorder that affects about 650,000 people each year in the United States. Of this number about 50,000 (fewer than 10%) die, 10% within the first hour after blockage.[3] Pulmonary embolism is responsible for 5% of all sudden deaths.[1]

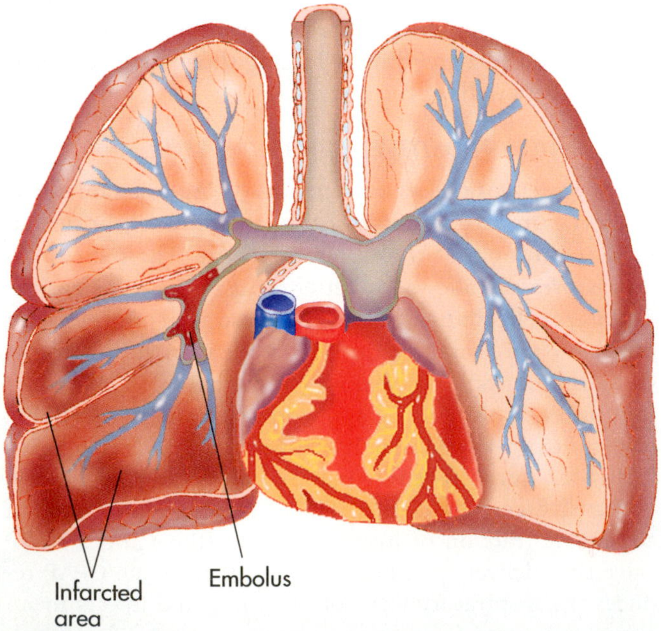

FIGURE 30-9 ■ *Pulmonary embolism (PE)* is the blockage of a pulmonary artery by foreign matter, such as a thrombus. The blockage usually arises from a peripheral vein, fat, air, or tumor tissue. The result is obstruction of the blood supply to the lung tissue.

PE usually begins as a venous disease. It most often is caused by migration of a thrombus from the large veins of the lower extremities, but it also can occur as a result of fat, air, sheared venous catheters, amniotic fluid, or tumor tissue. The clot or embolus dislodges and travels through the venous system to the right side of the heart. From there it migrates to the pulmonary arteries, obstructing the blood supply to a section of lung. The most common sites of thrombus formation are the deep veins of the legs and pelvis. Six factors that contribute to the development of venous thrombosis are listed in Box 30-5.

When one or more pulmonary arteries are blocked, an area does not receive blood flow; however, it continues to be ventilated. In response to the lack of blood flow, vasoconstriction occurs. If the vascular obstruction is severe (blockage of 60% or more of the pulmonary vascular supply), hypoxemia, acute pulmonary hypertension, systemic hypotension, and shock may rapidly occur, with subsequent death.

BOX 30-5 Contributing Factors in the Development of Venous Thrombosis

Venostasis
- Extended travel
- Prolonged bed rest
- Obesity
- Advanced age
- Burns
- Varicose veins

Venous Injury
- Surgery of the thorax, abdomen, pelvis, or legs
- Fractures of the pelvis or legs

Increased Blood Coagulability
- Malignancy
- Use of oral contraceptives
- Congenital or acquired coagulation disorders

Pregnancy

Disease
- Chronic lung disease
- Congestive heart failure
- Sickle cell anemia
- Cancer
- Atrial fibrillation
- Myocardial infarction
- Previous pulmonary embolism
- Previous deep vein thrombosis
- Infection
- Diabetes mellitus

Multiple Trauma
- Long bone fracture
- Pelvic fracture

Signs and Symptoms

An embolus may be small, moderate, or massive. Thus patients with PE may have very different presentations. A patient may have a wide variety of signs and symptoms. These depend on the location and size of the clot. They may include dyspnea, cough, hemoptysis (rare), pain, anxiety, syncope, hypotension, diaphoresis, tachypnea, tachycardia, fever, and distended neck veins. In addition, chest splinting, pleuritic pain, pleural friction rub, crackles, and localized wheezing may be present. The paramedic should consider a pulmonary embolism in any patient who has cardiorespiratory problems that cannot be otherwise explained, particularly when risk factors are present.

> **CRITICAL THINKING**
> Consider that you need to distinguish a pulmonary embolism (PE) from other conditions with similar signs and symptoms. What information in the patient assessment may help?

Management

Prehospital care mainly is supportive. Supplemental high-concentration oxygen should be administered, a cardiac monitor applied, pulse oximetry used, and an IV line of normal saline or lactated Ringer's solution established. The patient should be transported in a position of comfort. Definitive care requires hospitalization and in-hospital treatment with fibrinolytic or ***heparin*** therapy.

UPPER RESPIRATORY INFECTION

Upper respiratory infections (URIs) affect the nose, throat, sinuses, and larynx. They are among the most common of all illnesses, affecting nearly 80 million people each year.[1] These illnesses include the common cold, pharyngitis, tonsillitis, sinusitis, laryngitis, and croup. They rarely are life-threatening. However, they often exacerbate underlying pulmonary conditions. They also may lead to significant infections in patients with suppressed immune function. A key action for preventing the spread of respiratory infections is hand washing. Another crucial action is covering the mouth when sneezing or coughing.

A variety of bacteria and viruses can cause URIs. Group A streptococci are responsible for 20% to 30% of cases; 50% of cases have no demonstrated bacterial or viral cause.[1] Signs and symptoms of upper respiratory infection include the following:

- Sore throat
- Fever
- Chills
- Headache
- Facial pain (sinusitis)
- Purulent nasal drainage
- Halitosis (bad breath)
- Cervical adenopathy (enlarged cervical lymph nodes)
- Erythematous pharynx (pharyngeal inflammation/irritation)

> **CRITICAL THINKING**
> When might an upper respiratory infection (URI) become life-threatening? Think of two or three examples.

Management

Most URIs are self-limiting and require little or no prehospital treatment. Prehospital care is aimed at relieving the symptoms. This is especially true for patients who have underlying lung conditions. With such conditions, oxygen administration may be indicated. Other interventions that may be indicated for patients with underlying lung conditions include administration of bronchodilators or corticosteroids. If throat cultures are obtained at the scene, the family must be notified of the results. Follow-up by a physician is also required. The paramedic should follow local protocol.

SPONTANEOUS PNEUMOTHORAX

A primary **spontaneous pneumothorax** usually results when a bleb ruptures (a *bleb* is a cystic lesion on a lobe of the lung). This allows air to enter the pleural space from within the lung. This type of pneumothorax may occur in seemingly healthy individuals who are usually between 20 and 40 years of age. Often these patients are tall, thin men with long, narrow chests. (In contrast, a secondary spontaneous pneumothorax sometimes may develop from an underlying disease, such as COPD.) In recent years the number of spontaneous pneumothoraces has increased in some populations. These groups include individuals with acquired immunodeficiency syndrome (AIDS) who have pneumonia, and drug abusers who deeply inhale free-base cocaine, marijuana, or inhalants (e.g., glue or solvents).

Most primary spontaneous pneumothoraces that are well tolerated by the patient occupy less than 20% of a lung (partial pneumothorax). Signs and symptoms include shortness of breath and chest pain that often is sudden in onset, pallor, diaphoresis, and tachypnea. In severe cases in which the pneumothorax occupies more than 20% of the hemithorax, the following signs and symptoms may be present:

- Altered mental status
- Cyanosis
- Tachycardia
- Decreased breath sounds on the affected side
- Local hyperresonance to percussion
- Subcutaneous emphysema

> **NOTE** In severe cases a spontaneous pneumothorax may generate a tension pneumothorax. When this occurs, venous return to the heart is impaired. This can lead to total cardiovascular collapse.

Management

Prehospital care is based on the patient's symptoms. It also is based on the degree of respiratory distress. Administration of high-concentration oxygen is indicated to help resolve the pneumothorax, and airway, ventilatory, and circulatory support may be required in severe cases. These patients should be transported in a position of comfort for evaluation by a physician and possible decompression of the pleural space. Surgery may be indicated in some cases. This may be done to allow for lung reexpansion or to prevent recurrence.

HYPERVENTILATION SYNDROME

Hyperventilation syndrome is abnormally deep or rapid breathing. This type of breathing results in an excessive loss of carbon dioxide. (This, in turn, produces respiratory alkalosis.) As a result, the syndrome produces hypocarbia. The hypocarbia leads to cerebrovascular constriction, reduced cerebral perfusion, paresthesia, dizziness, or even feelings of euphoria. Several conditions can cause hyperventilation syndrome, including the following:

- Anxiety
- Hypoxia
- Pulmonary disease
- Cardiovascular disorders
- Metabolic disorders
- Neurological disorders
- Fever
- Infection
- Pain
- Pregnancy
- Drug use

> **CRITICAL THINKING**
> How can you distinguish between hyperventilation caused by anxiety and hyperventilation caused by a serious medical illness or toxic ingestion?

Signs and symptoms of hyperventilation syndrome include dyspnea with rapid breathing and a high minute volume, chest pain, facial tingling, and carpopedal spasm. Other assessment findings vary, based on the cause of the syndrome.

Management

If the syndrome clearly is caused by anxiety (psychogenic dyspnea, which is a diagnosis of exclusion), prehospital care is mainly supportive. It consists of calming measures and reassurance. Paramedics may suspect that the syndrome is a result of illness (e.g., diabetes, renal disease). They also may suspect drug ingestion. In either case care includes both oxygen administration and airway and ventilatory support. All patients who are hyperventilating should be calmed. Also, the paramedic should coach the patient's ventilations. If the hyperventilation is severe or complicated by illness or drug ingestion, transport for evaluation by a physician is indicated. The paramedic should consult with medical direction.

LUNG CANCER

Lung cancer is epidemic in the United States. An estimated 150,000 new cases are reported each year. Most cases of lung cancer develop in individuals between 55 and 65 years of age. Of the new cases reported, most patients die of the disease within 1 year; 20% have local lung involvement; 25% have spread to the lymph system, and 55% have distant metastatic cancer.[3] The most common cause of lung cancer is cigarette smoking. Heavy smokers (more than 20 cigarettes a day) have a 25 times greater chance of developing lung cancer than nonsmokers.[2] Other risk factors include passive smoking (exposure to someone else's cigarette smoke) and exposure to asbestos, radon gas, dust, coal products, ionizing radiation, and other toxins.

Pathophysiology

Like other cancers, lung cancer is the uncontrolled growth of abnormal cells. At least a dozen different cell types of tumors are associated with primary lung cancer (Fig. 30-10). The two major cell types of lung cancer are *small cell lung cancer* and *non–small cell lung cancer* (which is subcategorized as *squamous cell carcinoma, adenocarcinoma,* and *large cell carcinoma*). Each cell type has a different growth pattern. Each also has a different response to treatment. Most abnormal cell growth begins in the bronchi or bronchioles. The lung also is a fairly common site of metastasis for cancers from other primary sites (e.g., breast cancer).

Signs and Symptoms

The signs and symptoms of early-stage disease often are nonspecific. Smokers often attribute them to the effects of smoking. These include coughing, sputum production, lower airway obstruction (noted by wheezing), and respiratory illness (e.g., bronchitis). As the disease progresses, signs and symptoms may include the following:

- Cough
- Hemoptysis (which may be severe)
- Dyspnea
- Hoarseness or voice change
- Dysphagia
- Weight loss/anorexia
- Weakness

Patients with cancer may call paramedics because of complications resulting from chemotherapy or radiation therapy. Such therapy is toxic to both normal body cells and malignant cells. Associated complaints often include nausea and vomiting, fatigue, and dehydration. These patients should be offered emotional and psychological support.

> **CRITICAL THINKING**
> Should you assume that patients who have been diagnosed with lung cancer want "do not resuscitate" (DNR) status?

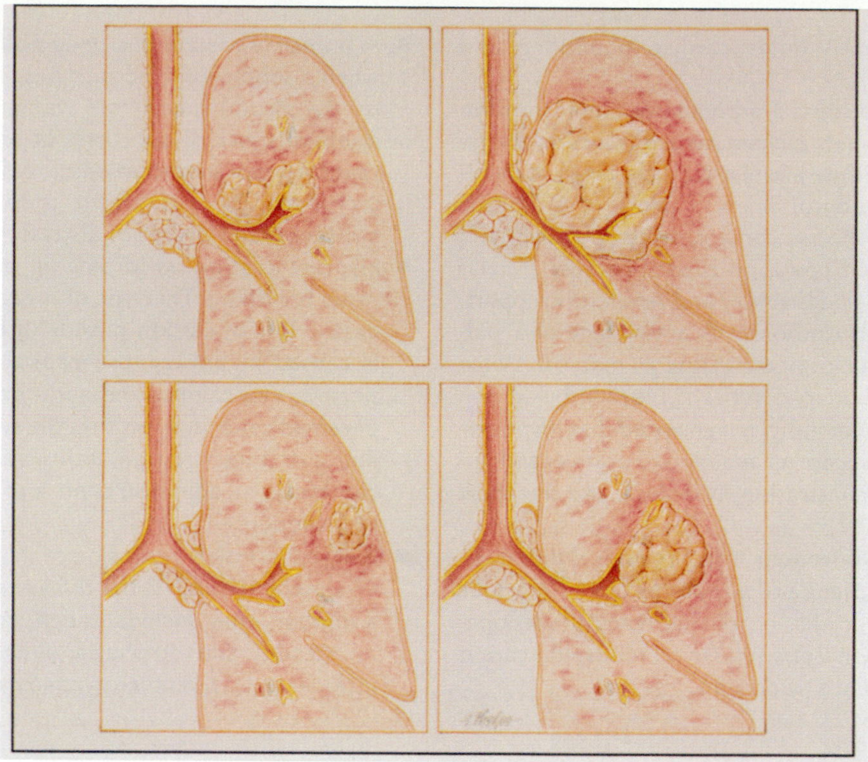

FIGURE 30-10 ■ Cancer of the lung. **A,** Squamous cell carcinoma. **B,** Small cell (oat cell) carcinoma. **C,** Adenocarcinoma. **D,** Large cell carcinoma.

Management

Most patients with lung cancer are aware of their disease. Prehospital management includes airway, ventilatory, and circulatory support; oxygen administration (based on symptoms and pulse oximetry); and transport for evaluation by a physician. Depending on the severity of the patient's condition, medical direction may recommend IV fluids to improve hydration and to thin sputum. They also may recommend drug therapy (e.g., bronchodilators and corticosteroids) to improve breathing. They may recommend analgesics to relieve pain as well. End-stage patients may have advance directives or "do not resuscitate" (DNR) orders. In these cases emotional support should also be offered to the family and loved ones.

SUMMARY

- Diseases responsible for respiratory emergencies include those related to ventilation, diffusion, and perfusion.
- Obstructive airway disease is a triad of distinct diseases that often coexist. These are chronic bronchitis, emphysema, and asthma. The patient with chronic obstructive pulmonary disease usually has an acute episode of worsening dyspnea that is manifested even at rest, an increase or change in sputum production, or an increase in the malaise that accompanies the disease. The main goal of prehospital care for these patients is the correction of hypoxemia through improved air flow.
- Asthma, or reactive airway disease, is characterized by reversible airflow obstruction caused by bronchial smooth muscle contraction; hypersecretion of mucus, resulting in bronchial plugging; and inflammatory changes in the bronchial walls. The typical patient with asthma is in obvious distress. Respirations are rapid and loud. Initial medications in the prehospital setting probably will have a short onset of action.
- Pneumonia is a group of specific infections (bacterial, viral, or fungal). These infections cause an acute inflammatory process of the respiratory bronchioles and the alveoli. Pneumonia usually manifests with classic signs and symptoms. These include a productive cough and associated fever that produces "shaking chills." Prehospital care of patients with pneumonia includes airway support, oxygen administration, ventilatory as-

Continued

sistance as needed, IV fluids, cardiac monitoring, and transport.

- Adult respiratory distress syndrome is a fulminant form of respiratory failure. It is characterized by acute lung inflammation and diffuse alveolar-capillary injury. It develops as a complication of illness or injury. In ARDS, the lungs are wet and heavy, congested, hemorrhagic, and stiff, with decreased perfusion capacity across alveolar membranes and includes airway and ventilatory support.
- Pulmonary thromboembolism is a blockage of a pulmonary artery by a clot or other foreign material. When one or more pulmonary arteries is blocked by an embolism, a section of lung is ventilated but hypoperfused. Prehospital care is mainly supportive and includes oxygen administration, IV access, and transport for definitive care.
- Upper respiratory infections affect the nose, throat, sinuses, and larynx. Signs and symptoms of a URI include sore throat, fever, chills, headache, cervical adenopathy, and an erythematous pharynx. Prehospital care is based on the patient's symptoms.
- A primary spontaneous pneumothorax usually results when a subpleural bleb ruptures. This allows air to enter the pleural space from within the lung. Signs and symptoms include shortness of breath and chest pain that often are sudden in onset, pallor, diaphoresis, and tachypnea. Prehospital care is based on the patient's symptoms and degree of distress.
- Hyperventilation syndrome is abnormally deep or rapid breathing. This type of breathing results in an excessive loss of carbon dioxide. If the syndrome clearly is caused by anxiety, prehospital care is mainly supportive (i.e., calming measures and reassurance). The paramedic may suspect that the syndrome is a result of illness or drug ingestion. If this is the case, care may include oxygen administration and airway and ventilatory support.
- Lung cancer is an expression of the uncontrolled growth of abnormal cells. As the disease progresses, signs and symptoms may include cough, hemoptysis, dyspnea, hoarseness, and dysphagia. Prehospital management includes airway, ventilatory, and circulatory support.

REFERENCES

1. US Department of Transportation, National Highway Traffic Safety Administration: *EMT-paramedic national standard curriculum,* Washington, DC, 1998, The Department.
2. American Lung Association: *Data and statistics,* http://www.lungusa.org/data/index.html. Accessed Feb. 18, 2005.
3. Rosen P, Barkin R: *Emergency medicine: concepts and clinical practice,* ed 4, St Louis, 1998, Mosby.
4. American Heart Association: Guidelines 2000 for cardiopulmonary resuscitation and emergency cardiovascular care, International Consensus on Science, *Circulation* 102*(8)*:237, 2000.
5. American Heart Association: Guidelines 2000 for cardiopulmonary resuscitation and emergency cardiovascular care, International Consensus on Science, *Circulation* 102*(8)*:240, 2000.
6. McCance L, Huether S: Pathophysiology: the biologic basis for disease in adults and children, ed 3, St Louis, 1998, Mosby.

CHAPTER 31

Neurology

OBJECTIVES

Upon completion of this chapter, the paramedic student will be able to:

1. Describe the anatomy and physiology of the nervous system.
2. Outline pathophysiological changes in the nervous system that may alter the cerebral perfusion pressure.
3. Describe the assessment of a patient with a nervous system disorder.
4. Describe the pathophysiology, signs and symptoms, and specific management techniques for each of the following neurological disorders: coma, stroke and intracranial hemorrhage, seizure disorders, headaches, brain neoplasm and brain abscess, and degenerative neurological diseases.

KEY TERMS

amyotrophic lateral sclerosis: One of a group of rare disorders in which the nerves that control muscular activity degenerate in the brain and spinal cord; also called Lou Gehrig disease.

Bell palsy: A condition in which paralysis of the facial muscles is caused by inflammation of the seventh cranial nerve; the condition usually is one sided and temporary and often develops suddenly.

central pain syndrome: Infection or disease of the trigeminal nerve (cranial nerve V).

cluster headache: A type of headache that occurs in bursts (clusters); also known as a *histamine headache.*

dystonia: A condition characterized by local or diffuse changes in muscle tone, resulting in painful muscle spasms, unusually fixed postures, and strange movement patterns.

epilepsy: A condition characterized by a tendency of the individual to have recurrent seizures (excluding those that arise from correctable or avoidable circumstances).

migraine: A severe, incapacitating headache that often is preceded by visual and/or gastrointestinal (GI) disturbances.

multiple sclerosis: A progressive disease of the central nervous system in which scattered patches of myelin in the brain and spinal cord are destroyed.

muscular dystrophy: An inherited muscle disorder of unknown cause marked by a slow but progressive degeneration of muscle fibers.

myoclonus: A condition characterized by rapid, uncontrollable contractions or spasms of muscles that occur at rest or during movement.

Parkinson disease: A disease caused by degeneration or damage (of unknown origin) to nerve cells in the basal ganglia in the brain.

peripheral neuropathy: Diseases and disorders that affect the peripheral nervous system, including the spinal nerve roots, cranial nerves, and peripheral nerves.

seizure: A temporary change in behavior or consciousness caused by abnormal electrical activity in one or more groups of neurons in the brain.

sinus headache: A headache characterized by pain in the forehead, nasal area, and eyes.

spina bifida: A congenital defect in which part of one or more vertebrae fails to develop completely, leaving a portion of the spinal cord exposed.

status epilepticus: Continuous seizure activity lasting 30 minutes or longer, or a recurrent seizure without an intervening period of consciousness.

tension headache: A headache caused by muscle contraction in the face, neck, and scalp.

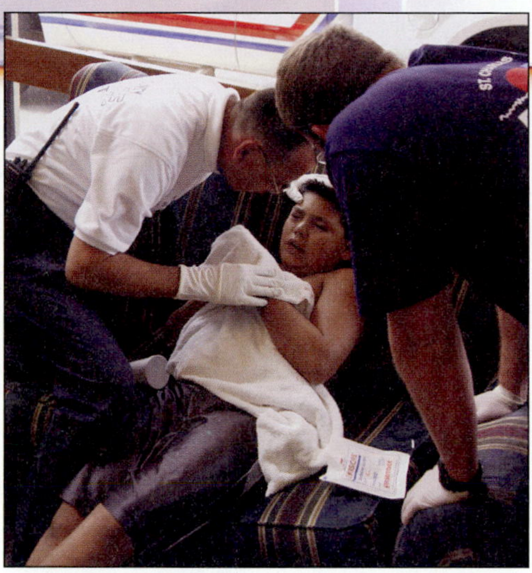

Acute disorders of the nervous system require rapid assessment and management. Paramedics must combine knowledge and skills with appropriate and aggressive intervention. These actions can help reduce mortality and morbidity. Proper recognition and treatment are the foundation for the greatest potential for rehabilitation and recovery.

ANATOMY AND PHYSIOLOGY OF THE NERVOUS SYSTEM

As described in Chapter 6, the nervous system is divided into two parts (Fig. 31-1). These two parts are the central nervous system (CNS) and the peripheral nervous system (PNS). The ability of the human body to maintain a state of balance *(homeostasis)* is chiefly the result of the nervous system's ability to coordinate and regulate the body's activities. To review, the CNS consists of the brain and spinal cord. Both of these are encased in and protected by bone. A total of 43 pairs of nerves originate from the CNS to form the PNS. Twelve pairs of cranial nerves originate from the brain. Thirty-one pairs of spinal nerves originate from the spinal cord.

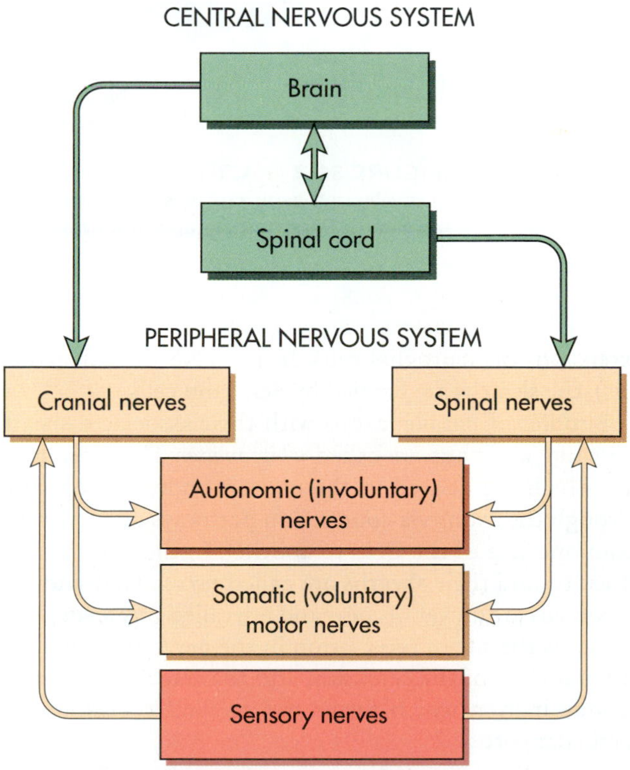

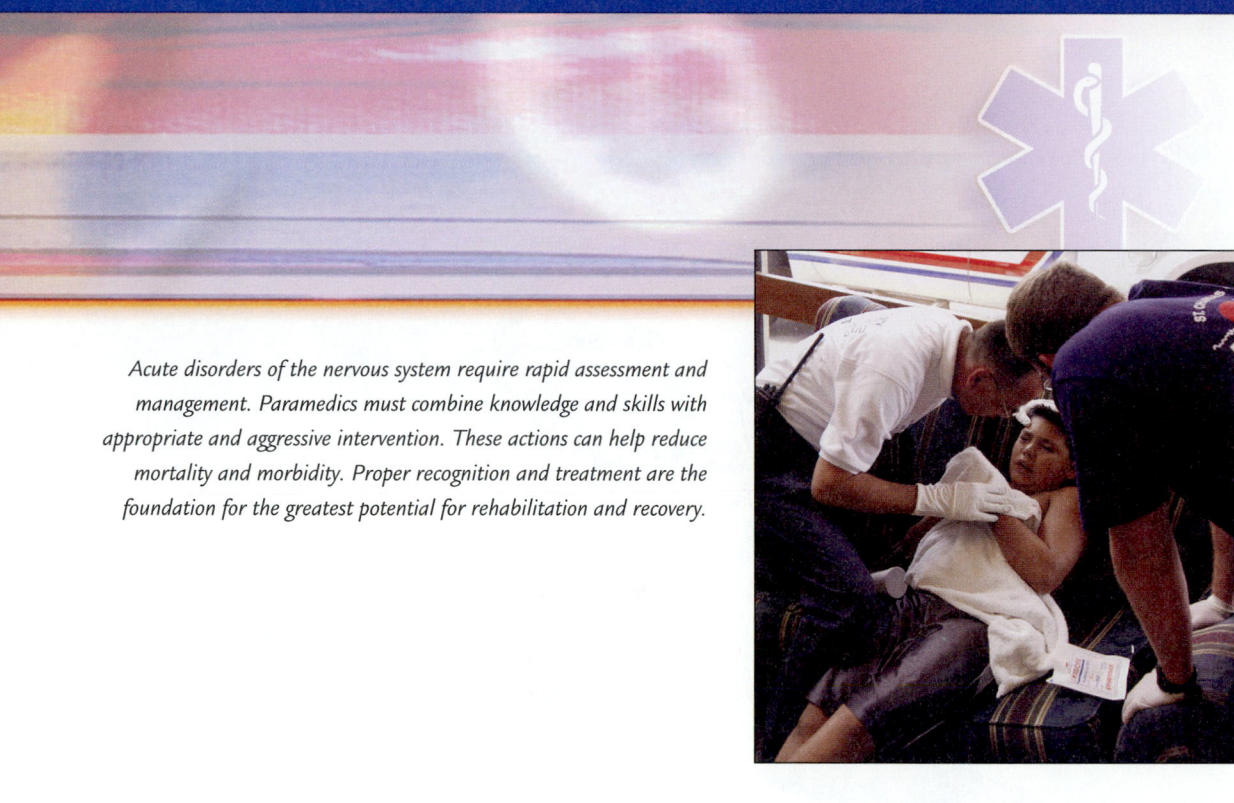

FIGURE 31-1 ■ Divisions of the nervous system.

Cells of the Nervous System

The cells of the nervous system include *neurons* (the basic units of the nervous system) and connective tissue cells known as *neuroglia* (specialized cells that protect and hold functioning neurons together). Each neuron has three main parts (Fig. 31-2): (1) the *cell body,* which has a single, relatively large nucleus with a prominent nucleolus; (2) one or more branching projections, called *dendrites;* and (3) a single, elongated projection, known as an *axon.* Dendrites transmit impulses to the cell bodies. Axons transmit impulses away from the cell bodies. Axons are surrounded by supportive and protective sheaths. In the CNS (unmyelinated axons), these sheaths are formed by the cytoplasmic

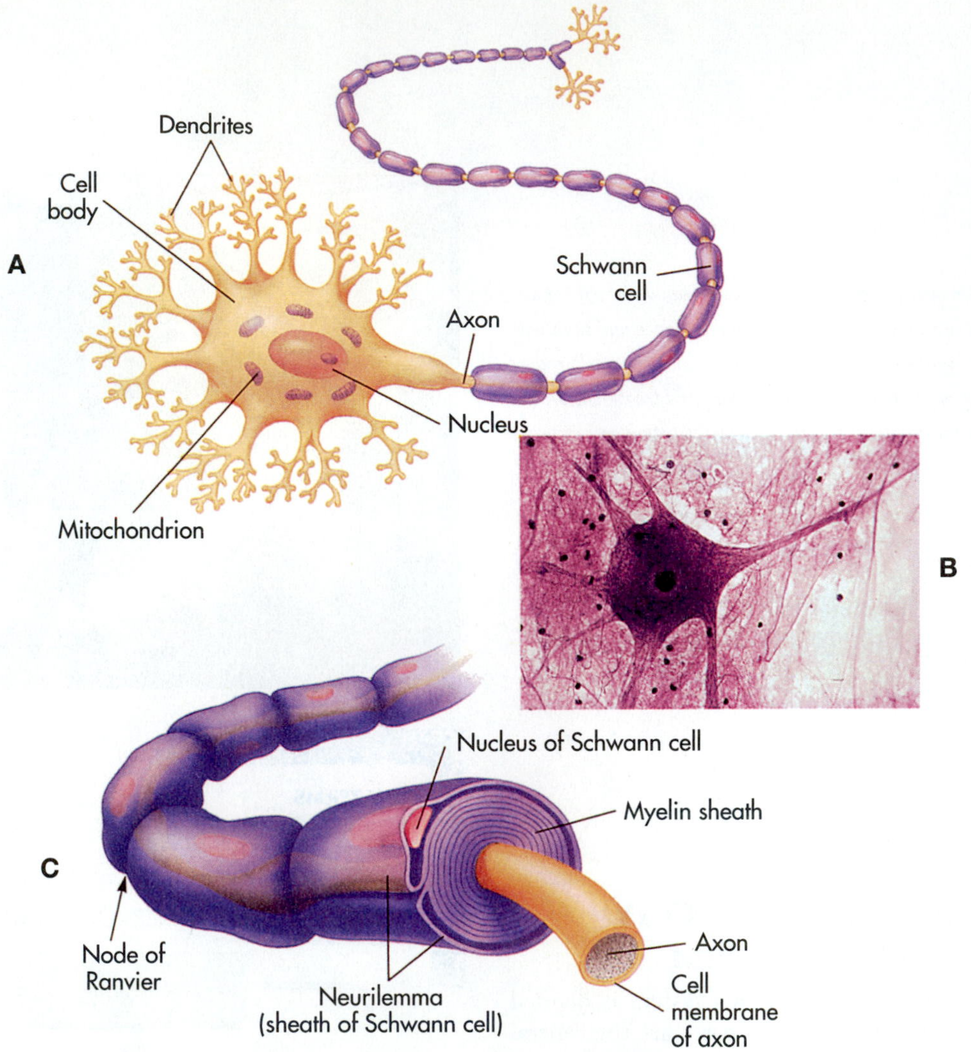

FIGURE 31-2 ■ **A,** Typical neuron showing dendrites, a cell body, and an axon. **B,** Segment of a myelinated axon cut to show detail of the concentric layers of the Schwann cell filled with myelin. **C,** Photomicrograph of a neuron.

extensions of neuroglial cells. In the PNS (myelinated axons), the sheaths are formed by Schwann cells.

Bundles of parallel axons with their associated sheaths are white and thus are called *white matter.* The *action potential,* which is initiated in the neuron body, is propagated through the axons via conduction pathways or nerve tracts from one area of the CNS to another. In the PNS, bundles of axons and their sheaths are called *nerves.* Collections of nerve cells are grayer in color and are called *gray matter.* Gray matter is the site of integration in the nervous system. The outer surface of the cerebrum and the cerebellum consists of gray matter, which forms the cerebral cortex and the cerebellar cortex.

Types of Neurons

Neurons are classified as sensory neurons, motor neurons, or interneurons. This is based on the direction in which they transmit impulses. *Sensory neurons* transmit impulses to the spinal cord and brain from all parts of the body. *Motor neurons* transmit impulses in the opposite direction, away from the brain and spinal cord. Also, they transmit impulses only to muscle and glandular epithelial tissue. *Interneurons* conduct impulses from sensory neurons to motor neurons. Sensory neurons also are called *afferent neurons.* Motor neurons are called *efferent neurons.* Interneurons are called *central* or *connecting neurons.*

Impulse Transmission

The transmission of nerve impulses in the nervous system is similar to the conduction of electrical impulses through the heart. In its resting state, the neuron is positively charged on the outside and negatively charged on the inside. When stimulated by pressure, temperature, or chemical changes, the permeability of the neuron's membrane to sodium ions increases. As a result, positively charged sodium ions rush into the interior of the neuron. This in-

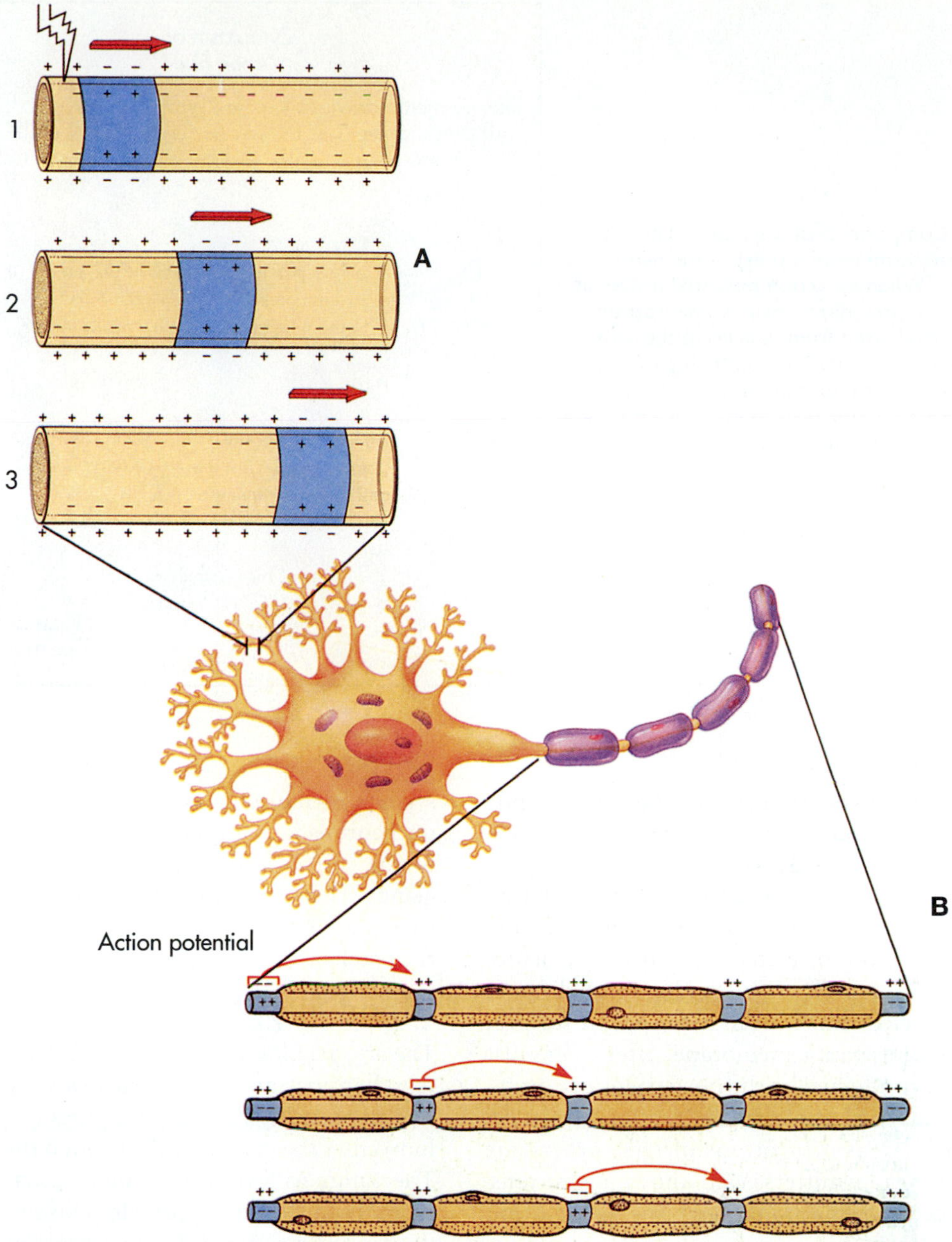

FIGURE 31-3 ■ Conduction of nerve impulses. **A,** In unmyelinated fiber, a nerve impulse (action potential) is a self-propagating wave of electrical disturbance. **B,** In myelinated fiber, the action potential "jumps" around the insulating myelin in a rapid type of conduction called *saltatory conduction.*

ward movement begins a wave of depolarization. The wave travels down the axon, resulting in the propagation of an action potential (Fig. 31-3).

CRITICAL THINKING

Think of examples of a pressure, a temperature, and a chemical stimulus to a nerve.

In unmyelinated axons, action potentials are spread along the entire axon membrane. Myelinated axons, however, have interruptions in the myelin sheaths. These are known as *nodes of Ranvier.* These nodes allow nerve impulses to "jump" from one node to the next without spreading along the entire length of the cell *(saltatory conduction).* Thus myelinated axons conduct action potentials faster than unmyelinated axons.

SYNAPSE

The membrane-to-membrane contact that separates the axon endings of one neuron *(presynaptic neuron)* from the dendrites of another neuron *(postsynaptic neuron)* is known as a *synapse.* The structures that compose a synapse are the presynaptic terminal, the synaptic cleft, and the plasma

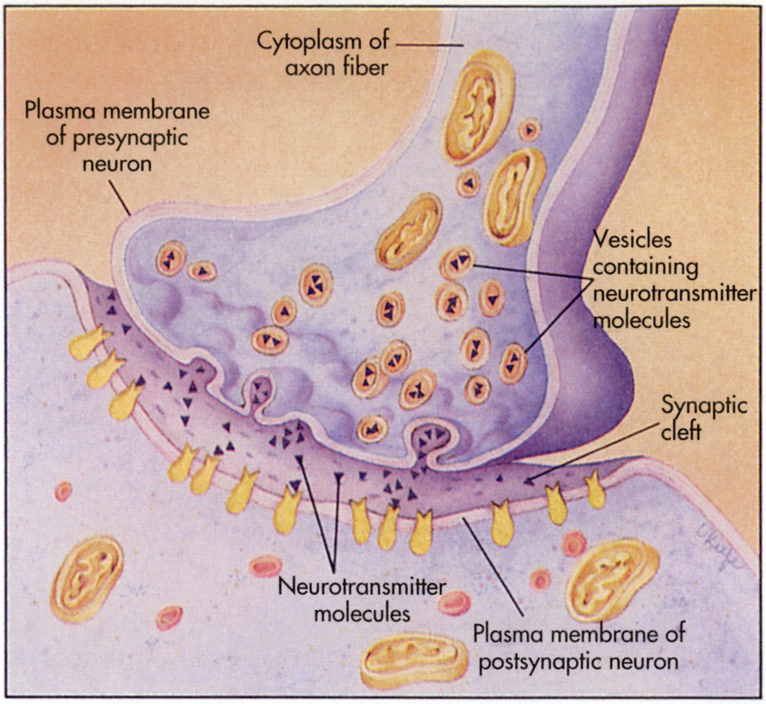

FIGURE 31-4 ■ Components of a synapse. The diagram shows an axon terminal of a presynaptic neuron and a synaptic cleft. When an action potential arrives at the axon terminal of a presynaptic neuron, neurotransmitter molecules are released from vesicles in the axon terminal into the synaptic cleft. The combining of neurotransmitter and receptor molecules in the plasma membrane of the postsynaptic neuron initiates impulse conduction in the postsynaptic neuron.

membrane of the postsynaptic neuron. Within each presynaptic terminal are synaptic vesicles. These contain neurotransmitter chemicals (Fig. 31-4).

Each action potential arriving at the presynaptic terminal initiates a series of specific events. These events result in the release of the neurotransmitter substance. The neurotransmitter chemical rapidly diffuses the short distance across the synaptic cleft. Then it binds to specific receptor molecules on the postsynaptic membrane. After an impulse is generated and is conducted by the postsynaptic neurons, neurotransmitter activity ends rapidly. Several substances have been identified as neurotransmitters; others are thought to be neurotransmitters. Well-known neurotransmitters include acetylcholine, norepinephrine, epinephrine, and dopamine.

Reflexes

One type of route traveled by nerve impulses is a *reflex* or *reflex arc*. A reflex is the basic unit of the nervous system that is capable of receiving a stimulus and generating a response. Reflexes allow conduction of impulses in one direction. They have several basic components: a sensory receptor, a sensory neuron, interneurons, a motor neuron, and an effector organ. Individual reflexes vary in complexity. Some function to remove the body from painful stimuli. Some prevent the body from suddenly falling or moving as a result of external forces. Others are responsible for maintaining a relatively constant blood pressure, body fluid pH, blood carbon dioxide level, and water intake. All reflexes are *homeostatic;* that is, they function to maintain healthy survival.

Action potentials initiated in sensory receptors spread along sensory axons in the PNS to the CNS. There they synapse with interneurons. Interneurons synapse with motor neurons in the spinal cord, which send their axons out of the spinal cord and through the PNS to muscles or glands. This causes the effector organ to respond. Fig. 31-5 shows the transmission of nerve impulses that results in the patellar (knee-jerk) reflex.

Blood Supply

The arterial blood supply to the brain comes from the vertebral arteries and the internal carotid arteries (Fig. 31-6). The right and left vertebral arteries (supplying the cerebellum) enter the cranial vault through the foramen magnum. They unite to form the midline basilar artery. The basilar artery branches to supply the pons and the cerebellum. It divides again to form the posterior cerebral arteries. These supply the posterior portion of the cerebrum.

The internal carotid arteries enter the cranial vault through the carotid canals. These vessels give rise to the anterior cerebral arteries. The anterior cerebral arteries supply blood to the frontal lobes of the brain. They end by forming the middle cerebral arteries. These supply a large portion of the lateral cerebral cortex. A posterior communicating artery branches off each internal carotid artery and connects with the ipsilateral posterior cerebral artery. The two posterior cerebral arteries are connected at their common origin from the basilar artery. The anterior cerebral arteries are connected by an anterior communicating artery. Thus they complete a circle around the pituitary gland and the brain. This is the *circle of Willis.* The circle of Willis provides an important safeguard. It helps to ensure the supply of blood to all parts of the brain in the event of a blockage in one of the vertebral or internal carotid arteries.

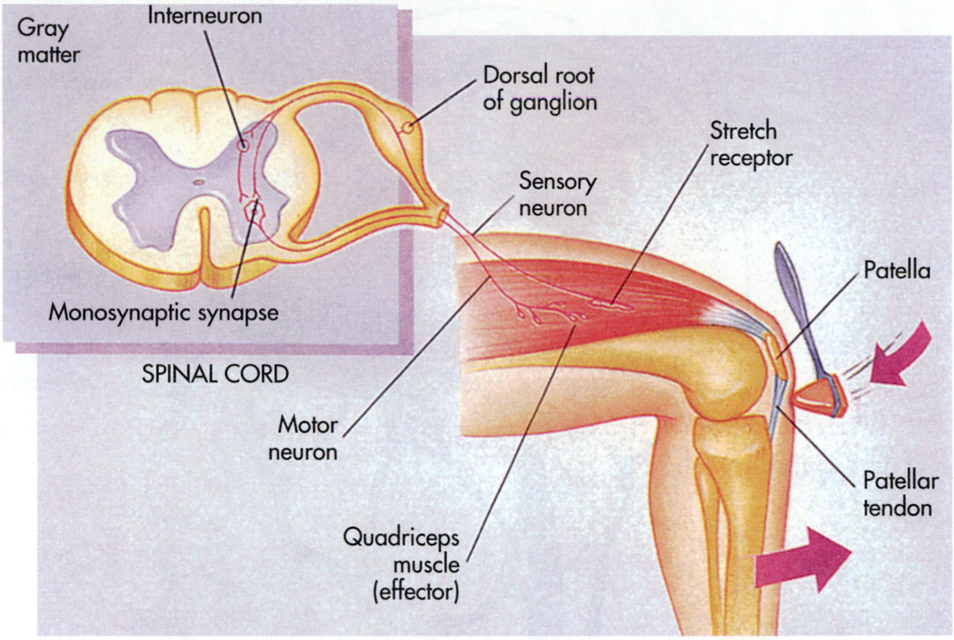

FIGURE 31-5 ■ Neural pathway involved in the patellar (knee-jerk) reflex.

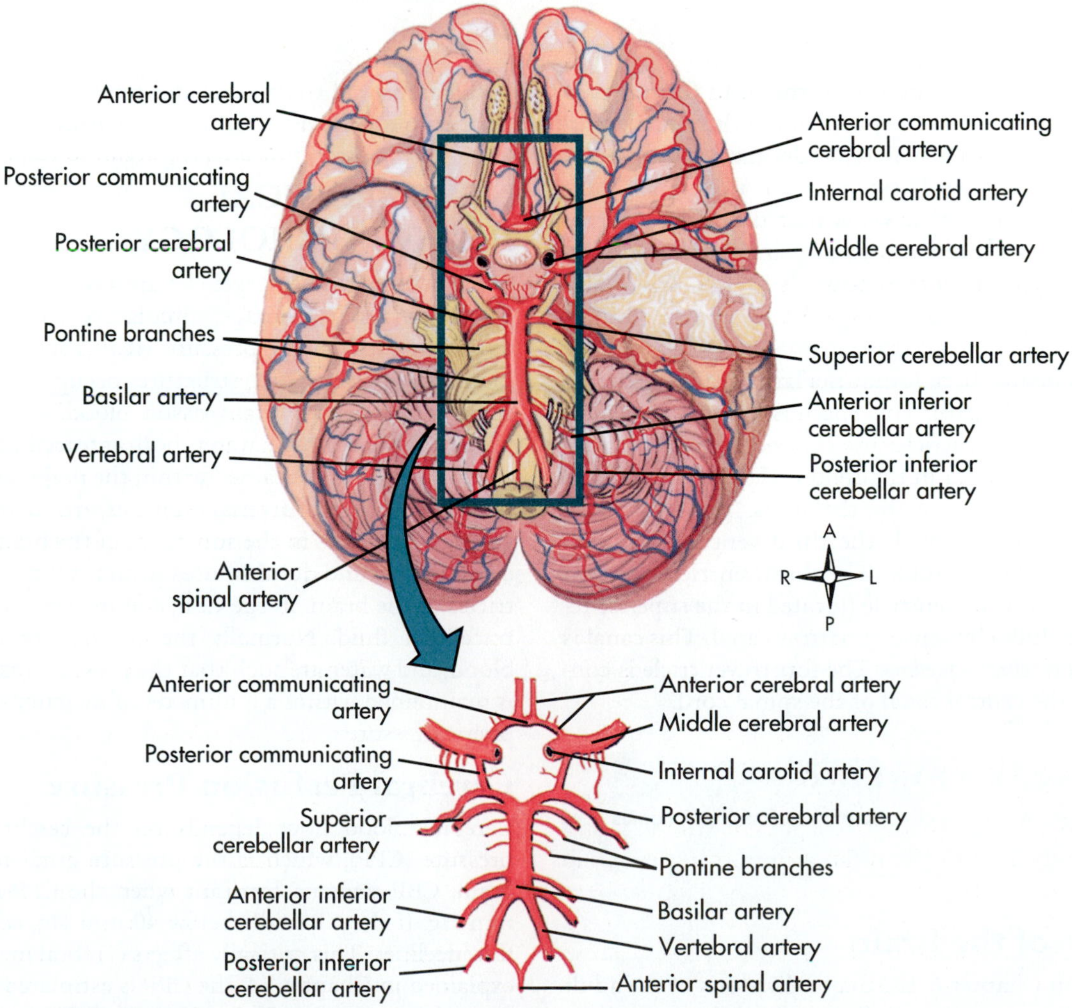

FIGURE 31-6 ■ Inferior view of the brain showing vertebral, basilar, and internal carotid arteries and their branches.

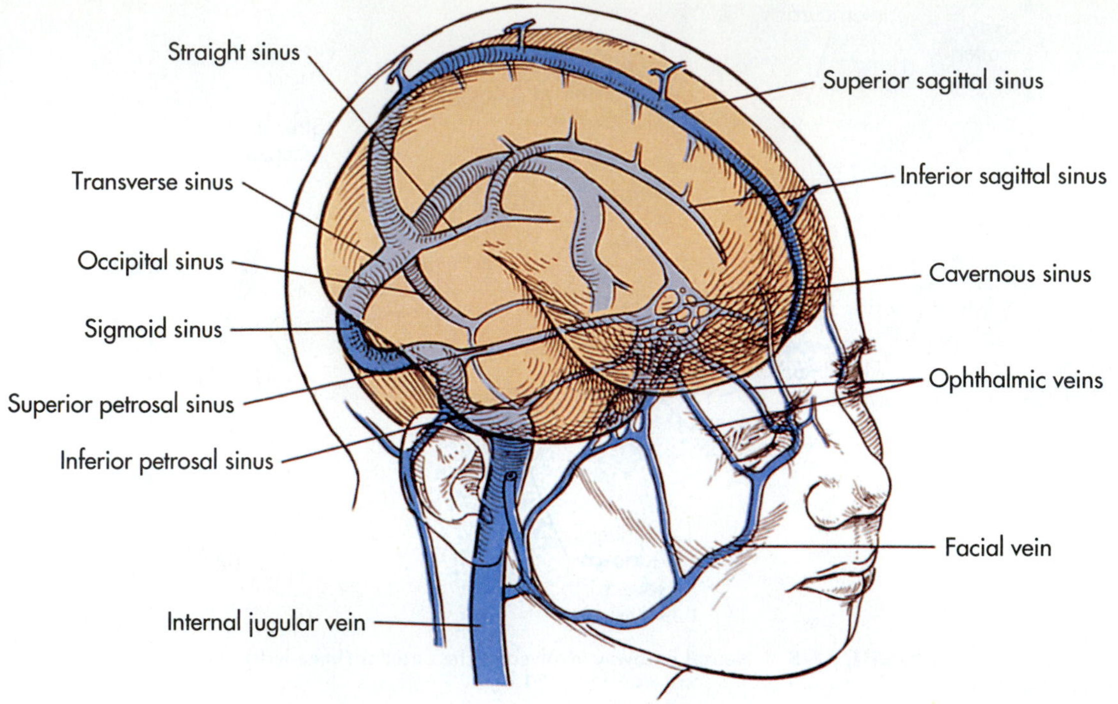

FIGURE 31-7 ■ Venous sinuses associated with the brain.

The veins that drain blood from the head form the venous sinuses. (These are the spaces in the dura mater surrounding the brain.) Eventually they drain into the internal jugular veins (Fig. 31-7). These veins exit the cranial vault and join with several other veins that drain the external head and face. The internal jugular veins join the subclavian veins on each side of the body.

Ventricles

Each cerebral hemisphere contains a large space filled with cerebrospinal fluid (CSF). This space is known as a *lateral ventricle.* The lateral ventricles are connected posteriorly. A third ventricle is located in the center of the diencephalon between the two halves of the thalamus. The two lateral ventricles communicate with the third ventricle through two interventricular foramina. The third ventricle communicates with the fourth ventricle (located in the superior region of the medulla) by way of a narrow canal. This canal is known as the *cerebral aqueduct.* The fourth ventricle is continuous with the central canal of the spinal cord.

CRITICAL THINKING

What happens if the flow in one of these canals becomes obstructed?

Divisions of the Brain

As described in Chapter 6, the major divisions of the adult brain are the brain stem (medulla, pons, midbrain, and site of the reticular formation), cerebellum, diencephalon (hypothalamus and thalamus), and cerebrum (Fig 31-8). (See Chapter 6 for a review of these structures.)

NEUROLOGICAL PATHOPHYSIOLOGY

Some neurological emergencies are a consequence of structural changes or damage, circulatory changes, or alterations in intracranial pressure (ICP) that affect cerebral blood flow (CBF). Three structures occupy the intracranial space. These are the brain tissue, blood, and water. Brain tissue contains mostly water, both intracellular and extracellular. Blood is contained within the major arteries in the base of the brain; in arterial branches, arterioles, capillaries, venules, and veins in the substance of the brain; and in the cortical veins and dural sinuses. Water is located in the ventricles of the brain, in the CSF, and in extracellular and intracellular fluid. Normally the volumes of brain tissue, blood, and water are such that the pressure inside the skull is maintained within a millimeter of mercury above atmospheric pressure.

Cerebral Perfusion Pressure

Cerebral blood flow depends on the cerebral perfusion pressure (CPP), which is the pressure gradient across the brain. CBF remains constant when the CPP is 50 to 160 mm Hg. If the CPP falls below 40 mm Hg, cerebral blood flow declines. This critically affects cerebral metabolism. As explained in Chapter 24, the CPP is estimated as the mean arterial pressure (MAP) minus the ICP. With mild to moderate elevation of the ICP, the MAP usually rises. The rise in

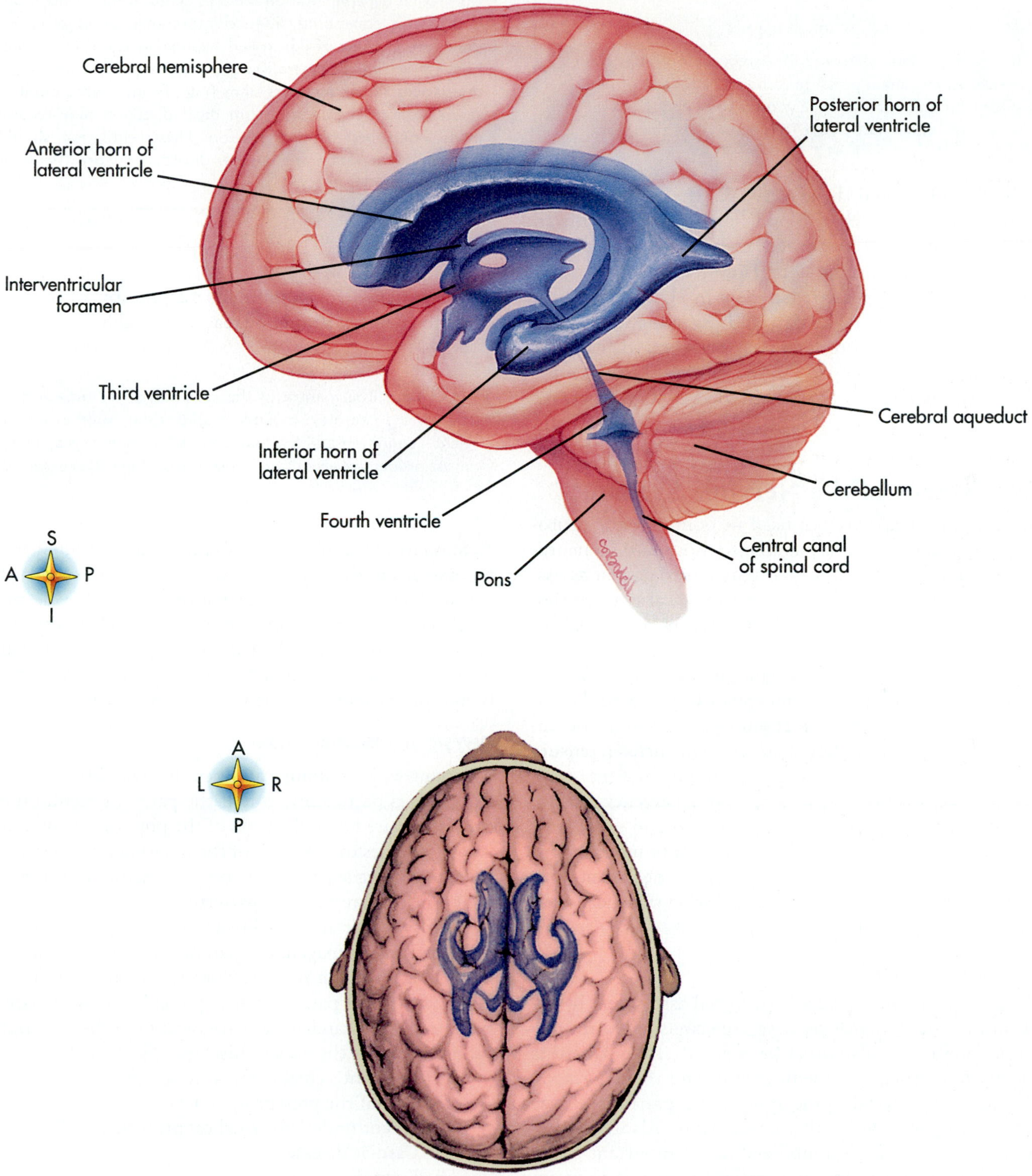

FIGURE 31-8 ■ Divisions of the brain.

the MAP causes cerebral blood vessels to constrict and prevents the increase in blood volume and CBF that normally would occur.

CRITICAL THINKING

Relate the difficulty created for cerebral blood flow by increased intracranial pressure to having a person push on a door from the outside while you try to open it from the inside. How much harder is it for you to open the door?

On the other hand, if the MAP falls, the cerebral arteries dilate, increasing cerebral blood flow. Therefore with an MAP of about 60 to 150 mm Hg, cerebral blood flow may be maintained in a constant state. However, when ICP elevations are marked (greater than 22 mm Hg), perfusion of brain tissue often decreases despite a rise in the systemic arterial pressure. Therefore, if a mass or cerebral edema develops, an immediate reduction in the volume of one or more of these components (brain tissue, blood, or water) must occur to prevent the ICP from rising and compressing brain tissue.

Assessment of the Nervous System

The assessment approaches used in nontraumatic neurological emergencies are very similar to those used for neurological trauma. The following discussion of patient assessment focuses on nontraumatic neurological emergencies. (Assessment of neurological trauma is addressed in Chapter 24.)

As with all patient encounters, care of a patient with a nontraumatic neurological emergency begins with the initial assessment. Paramedics should have a systematic approach for examining these patients. This helps to ensure that they do not miss signs and symptoms that may indicate an urgent condition. The goals of emergency care are (1) control of the airway, (2) stabilization and support of the cardiovascular system, (3) intervention to interrupt ongoing cerebral injury, and (4) protection of the patient from further harm while at the scene and during transport to an appropriate medical facility.

INITIAL ASSESSMENT

The paramedic should begin the initial assessment by determining the patient's level of consciousness. An open and patent airway also must be ensured. If the patient is unconscious when paramedics arrive and there is reason to suspect a cervical spine injury, the patient's airway should be opened with spinal precautions. Also, the cervical spine should be immobilized. It is important to remember that an unconscious patient is unable to maintain the airway. Therefore airway adjuncts may be indicated. (This includes tracheal intubation with appropriate spinal precautions.) The patient's airway also should be closely monitored for respiratory arrest. This may result from an increased ICP. The patient should be closely watched for vomiting or aspiration of stomach contents. Suction should be readily available.

BOX 31-1 Use of Controlled Hyperventilation

Controlled hyperventilation reduces cerebral blood flow, but it does not consistently reduce intracranial pressure (ICP). Therefore the use of controlled hyperventilation in the prehospital setting is generally not recommended. However, if the patient shows ominous signs (e.g., fixed, dilated pupil or severe abnormal posturing), medical direction may recommend controlled hyperventilation. Hyperventilation should attempt to maintain the carbon dioxide pressure (Pco_2) at about 30 mm Hg.

NOTE The mantra of the cardiologist is "time is muscle." Many neurologists agree. Rapid stabilization of the patient's condition and transport for definitive care may be the most prudent course of action in a neurological emergency.

Support of breathing and administration of supplemental oxygen should be provided for any patient experiencing a neurological emergency. Increased carbon dioxide pressure (Pco_2) or decreased oxygen pressure (Po_2) results in dilation of the blood vessels. This occurs presumably because of an increase in cerebral metabolic needs. As the Pco_2 drops, blood volume and blood flow to the brain are reduced.

PHYSICAL EXAMINATION

A patient with neurological illness may be difficult to assess. This is particularly true if the patient's mental function is impaired. Key elements of the physical examination may offer clues to the cause of the neurological emergency. These include the patient history, the history of the event, vital signs, and respiratory patterns.

History. After any life-threatening problems have been identified and managed, the paramedic should attempt to compile a thorough history. This information can be obtained from the patient (when possible) or from family members or bystanders. The following are the six important elements of the patient history:

1. The patient's chief complaint
2. Details of the presenting illness
3. Pertinent underlying medical problems
   a. Cardiac disease
   b. Lung disease
   c. Neurological disease (e.g., multiple sclerosis)
   d. Previous stroke
   e. Chronic seizures
   f. Diabetes
   g. Hypertension

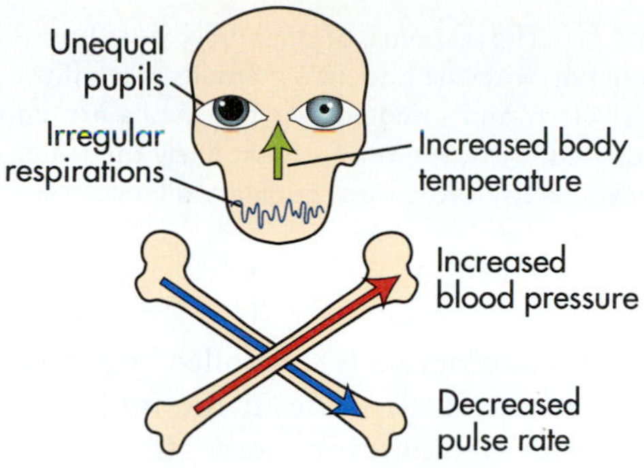

FIGURE 31-9 ■ Cushing triad.

4. Alcohol or other drug use
5. Previous history of similar symptoms
6. Recent injury (particularly head trauma)

If a loss of consciousness was involved, the paramedic should ascertain the events that led up to the unconscious state. This information may include the patient's position (sitting, standing, lying down), whether the person complained of a headache, and whether seizure activity or a fall occurred. At times no history is available. In such cases paramedics should assume that the onset of unconsciousness was acute. They also should assume that an intracranial hemorrhage is likely. In addition, they should be alert for any environmental clues. Examples include evidence of current prescribed medications, medical alert identification, recreational drugs, or alcohol or drug paraphernalia.

CRITICAL THINKING

How could having one of the conditions listed in the six important elements of the patient history result in a change in the patient's neurological status?

Vital Signs. The patient's vital signs should be checked and recorded often. This is important because the vital signs may change rapidly in patients with a neurological emergency. The patient's electrocardiogram (ECG) also should be monitored for dysrhythmias. These commonly occur with neurological problems.

The early stages of increased ICP are marked by an increase in systolic pressure, a widened pulse pressure, and a decrease in the pulse and respiratory rate (Cushing triad) (Fig. 31-9). In the terminal stages, the ICP continues to rise and brain tissue is compressed. As this occurs, body temperature usually remains elevated. However, the pulse rate generally drops. Also, the blood pressure falls, particularly after herniation occurs. Thus hypotension is a late and very serious sign.

Respiratory Patterns. The respiratory pattern of a patient with a neurological emergency may be normal or abnormal. Sometimes respiratory arrest is caused by damage to the lower respiratory centers in the medulla. Other times respiratory abnormalities of rate and rhythm occur. These abnormalities may provide clues to which area of the brain is involved. They also may indicate the severity of the neurological problem. Apnea can occur with loss of consciousness even with relatively minor head trauma. However, acute respiratory arrest usually results from involvement of the medullary respiratory center (brain stem compression or infarct). Damage to neural pathways (anywhere from the cortex down to the medulla) more often produces problems with the respiratory rhythm, rather than respiratory arrest. Abnormal respiratory patterns (see Chapter 19) include the following:

- Cheyne-Stokes respiration
- Central neurogenic hyperventilation
- Ataxic respiration
- Apneustic respiration
- Diaphragmatic breathing

CRITICAL THINKING

Consider a patient who has ataxic or apneustic respirations. Which respiratory control center is likely affected?

NEUROLOGICAL EVALUATION

Some neurological problems are obvious (e.g., paralysis). Others may be subtle (e.g., a decreasing level of awareness). A sudden or rapidly worsening level of consciousness is the single most suggestive sign of a serious neurological condition.[1]

Use of the mnemonic device AVPU (alert, verbal, painful, unresponsive) and the Glasgow Coma Scale (see Chapter 24) are quick, easy ways to determine the patient's baseline neurological status. These also allow comparisons for future management. Evaluation should be repeated and recorded often. In this way, changes in the patient's mental state can be detected as soon as possible.

When evaluating a patient's neurological status, the paramedic should report and record patient information with descriptive terms. These terms should be specific to responses to certain stimuli. (For example, "The patient has no recall of the event"; "The patient moves on command"; and "The patient does not open his eyes to painful stimuli.") Using clear descriptions of the patient's response allows others involved in the patient's care to follow the progression of the condition.

Posturing, Muscle Tone, and Paralysis. Significant neurological emergencies may be associated with abnormal or unusual posturing, paralysis of a limb or several limbs, or both. Generally, disturbances of posture result from flexor spasms, extensor spasms, or flaccidity. Abnormal flexor response of one or both arms with extension of the legs is called *decorticate rigidity*. This abnormal posturing is thought to result from damage to the cortex of the brain. Abnormal extensor response of the arms with extension of the legs is called *decerebrate rigidity*. Decerebrate rigidity has a worse prognosis than decorticate rigidity. It is thought to result from damage to the subcortical areas of the brain. Flaccidity usually is caused by brain stem or cord dysfunction. It has a dismal prognosis.

Abnormal reflexes are not uncommon with decorticate or decerebrate rigidity. Associated with this may be a positive Babinski sign (see Chapter 25). The patient with this type of brain damage may be incontinent of urine or feces or both.

Pupillary Reflexes. Examination of the pupils is very important in the unconscious patient. Often drug use can at least be suspected based on the appearance and reaction of the pupils (Fig. 31-10). If deviations from normal (in relative symmetry, size, and prompt reaction to light) are observed, it is crucial to note whether these deviations are unilateral or bilateral. If both pupils are dilated and do not react to light, the brain stem has probably been damaged. This may also occur when the brain has not received enough oxygen.

> **NOTE** The response of the pupils must be considered in conjunction with the patient's mental status. If the patient is awake, alert, and oriented, yet the pupils are unresponsive and dilated, this condition is most likely the result of topical medications used to induce pupillary dilation.

Pupillary constriction is controlled by parasympathetic fibers. These fibers originate in the midbrain. They accompany the oculomotor nerve (cranial nerve III). Pupillary dilation involves fibers that travel the entire brain stem and return in the cervical sympathetic nerves. Midbrain injury interrupts both pathways. Generally it results in fixed, midsize pupils. Compression of the third cranial nerve interrupts parasympathetic nerve actions. It is manifested by a unilateral, fixed, dilated pupil. Any unconscious patient who suddenly develops a fixed, dilated pupil probably has suffered a significant brain injury. This requires immediate transport to the proper medical facility.

Extraocular Movements. Conscious patients should be able to move their eyes in full directional ranges. As de-

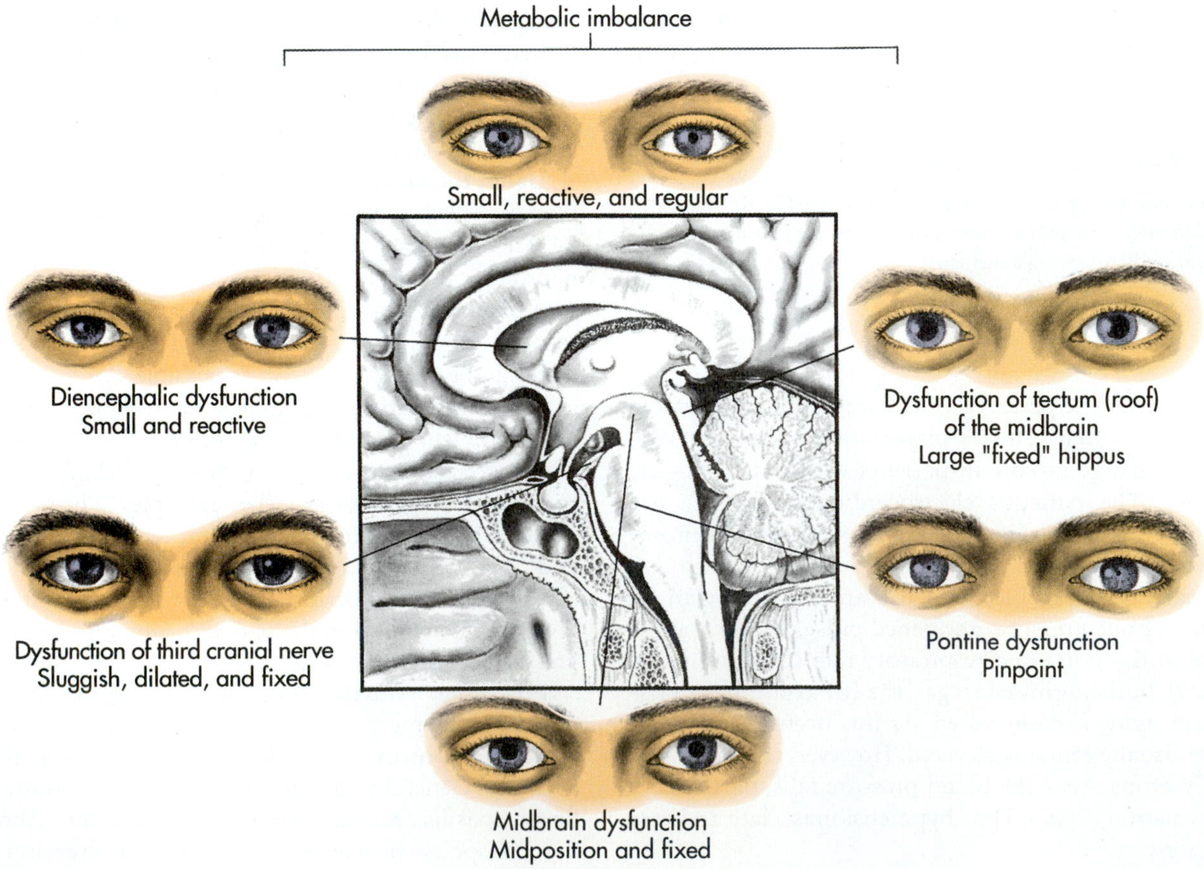

FIGURE 31-10 ■ Pupils at different levels of consciousness.

scribed in Chapter 12, paramedics can evaluate extraocular movements by asking the patient to follow their finger movements. For this test, the paramedic moves a finger to the extreme left and then up and down and to the extreme right and then up and down. Any deviations from normal should be recorded.

> **CRITICAL THINKING**
> Which cranial nerves control eye movements?

A deviation of both eyes to either side *(conjugate gaze)* at rest implies damage to brain tissue (a lesion). The lesion may have an *irritative focus.* In this focus, the eyes look away from the lesion. Alternatively, they may have a *destructive focus.* In this focus, the eyes look toward the lesion. A deviation of the eyes to opposite sides *(dysconjugate gaze)* at rest implies damage to the brain stem (Fig. 31-11).

PATHOPHYSIOLOGY AND MANAGEMENT OF SPECIFIC CENTRAL NERVOUS SYSTEM DISORDERS

Disorders of the nervous system have many causes. Specific causes discussed in this chapter include structural and metabolic coma, stroke and intracranial hemorrhage (including transient ischemic attack), seizure disorders, headaches, and brain neoplasm and brain abscess. Several degenerative neurological diseases also are discussed.

Coma

Coma is an abnormally deep state of unconsciousness. In such a state, the patient cannot be aroused by external stimuli. In general terms, only two mechanisms produce coma. Structural lesions (e.g., a tumor or abscess) are one mechanism. Structural lesions depress consciousness by destroying or pressing on the reticular activating system in the brain stem. The other mechanism is toxic-metabolic conditions. These involve the presence of toxins or the lack of oxygen or glucose. Either type of toxic-metabolic condition may result in depression of the cerebrum, with or without depression of the reticular activating system.

Within these two primary mechanisms there are six general causes of coma (Box 31-2). A mnemonic aid that may be useful for remembering the common causes of coma is AEIOU-TIPS (Box 31-3).

STRUCTURAL VERSUS TOXIC-METABOLIC COMA

Structural and toxic-metabolic causes of coma differ in two major ways. In patients with coma of structural origin, the neurological signs often are one sided, or asymmetrical. In toxic-metabolic coma, the neurological findings often are the same on both sides of the body. In addition, coma of toxic-metabolic origin often is slow to develop. In contrast, structural damage occurs instantly. Changes in pupil responses are the most important physical sign in distinguishing between structural and toxic-metabolic causes of

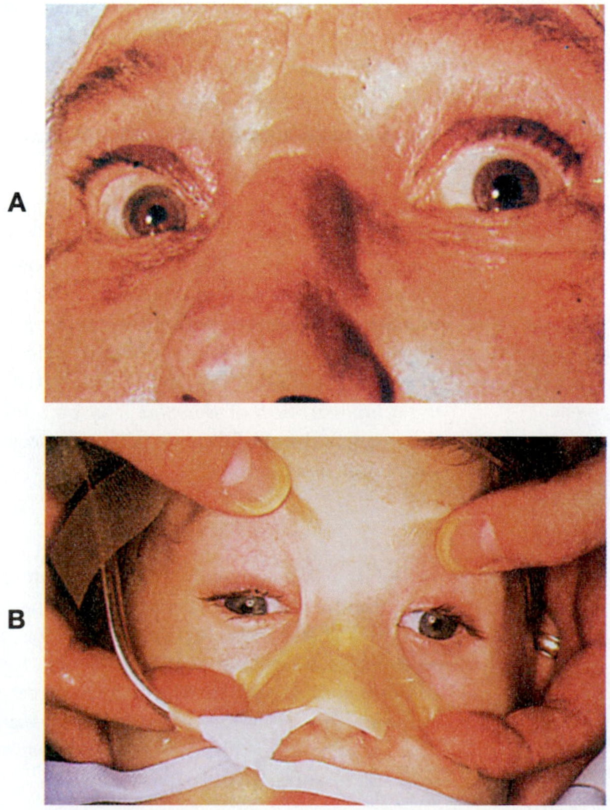

FIGURE 31-11 ■ **A,** Conjugate gaze. **B,** Dysconjugate gaze.

BOX 31-2 Six General Causes of Coma

Structural Origin
- Intracranial bleeding
- Head trauma
- Brain tumor or other space-occupying lesions

Metabolic System
- Anoxia
- Hypoglycemia
- Diabetic ketoacidosis
- Thiamine deficiency
- Kidney and liver failure
- Postictal phase of seizure

Drugs
- Barbiturates
- Narcotics
- Hallucinogenics
- Depressants
- Alcohol

Cardiovascular System
- Hypertensive encephalopathy
- Shock
- Dysrhythmias
- Stroke

Respiratory System
- Chronic obstructive pulmonary disease
- Toxic inhalation (e.g., carbon monoxide poisoning)

Infection
- Meningitis
- Sepsis

BOX 31-3 Common Causes of Coma: AEIOU-TIPS

A—Acidosis or alcohol
E—Epilepsy
I—Infection
O—Overdose
U—Uremia
T—Trauma
I—Insulin
P—Psychosis
S—Stroke

coma. Normal pupil responses suggest that the coma has a toxic-metabolic cause. Unresponsive or asymmetrical pupils suggest structural damage.

NOTE Comalike states can be mimicked by some psychiatric conditions. (A hysterical coma is one example.) In these conditions, the unconscious state has no physical cause. Patients who appear unconscious as a result of a psychiatric condition often vigorously blink and move the eyes. They also usually respond to annoying physical or verbal stimuli. In contrast, patients with organic sources of coma are unresponsive.

Unlike metabolic coma, structural coma follows a progressive pattern of deterioration. This pattern is caused by local pressure or compression in the brain. The syndrome often is sudden in onset. The patient's signs and symptoms are often one-sided, or asymmetrical (e.g., hemiparesis). As a rule, structural lesions damage the reticular activating system as a result of increased ICP and herniation of the brain. This type of injury requires rapid surgical correction.

A knowledge of the difference between toxic-metabolic coma and structural coma can help the paramedic to understand what is likely to occur next in the patient's condition.

ASSESSMENT AND MANAGEMENT

Regardless of the cause of coma, prehospital care is directed at support of vital functions, prevention of further deterioration of the patient's condition, and administration of medications, intravenous (IV) fluids, or both to manage potentially reversible causes of coma. As always, airway maintenance and ventilatory support with supplemental high-concentration oxygen are the first priorities in patient care. Rapid transport for definitive care may be indicated.

If respirations are abnormally slow or shallow, ventilations should be supported. If the patient is unconscious and has no gag reflex, the trachea should be intubated. After securing the airway, the paramedic should take the following steps to treat a patient in a coma of unknown origin:

1. Establish an IV line to keep the vein open or to manage hypotension (if present).
2. Monitor the patient's ECG.
3. Per protocol, draw a blood sample for laboratory analysis. If hypoglycemia is suspected, use a glucometer or other device to measure serum glucose levels (see Chapter 32). Administer ***50% dextrose*** if indicated (per protocol). If alcohol is suspected as the cause of the coma, administration of ***thiamine*** before glucose should be considered.
4. If no response is obtained with glucose administration, administer ***naloxone*** per protocol. This rules out or reverses narcotic depression.
5. If the patient remains in a comatose state, transport the person in a lateral recumbent position (if not con-

NOTE ***Thiamine*** is a B vitamin (B_1). It usually is found in adequate amounts in the normal diet. However, chronic alcoholism interferes with the intake, absorption, and utilization of ***thiamine.*** Serious neurological disease may result. The incidence of these alcohol-related neurological syndromes varies markedly in different regions of the United States. Therefore the administration of ***thiamine*** may be a local consideration. Paramedics should follow established protocols and consult with medical direction.

NOTE Patients who are dependent on narcotics may have frank withdrawal symptoms. The paramedic should be prepared to restrain a patient who may become violent as the ***naloxone*** reverses the narcotic effects. Repeated doses of ***naloxone*** may be needed. This is because the duration of some narcotics may be longer than that of ***naloxone.*** Doses should be titrated to keep the patient awake, responsive, and free of respiratory depression.

traindicated). This aids drainage of secretions. It also minimizes the chance of aspiration of stomach contents. Closely monitor the patient's airway. Have suction readily available. Protect the patient's eyes from corneal drying. This can be done by gently closing them and covering the lids with moist gauze pads.

Stroke and Intracranial Hemorrhage

Stroke is also known as cerebrovascular accident (CVA) or "brain attack." It is a sudden interruption in blood flow to the brain. It results in problems with a patient's neurological functioning. Stroke is a serious disease that affects more than 500,000 Americans each year.[2] It is associated with a 30-day mortality of about 10% to 15%. It also is the third leading cause of death in the United States. Frequently it leaves its survivors severely disabled. According to the American Heart Association (AHA), individuals who are more likely to suffer a stroke have prior risk factors that can be classified as modifiable and nonmodifiable. Modifiable risk factors include the following:

- High blood pressure
- Cigarette smoking
- Transient ischemic attacks
- Heart disease
- Diabetes mellitus
- Hypercoagulopathy
- High red blood cell count and sickle cell anemia
- Carotid bruit

Nonmodifiable risk factors include the following:

- Age
- Gender (men are at greater risk than women)
- Race (African-Americans are at greater risk than Caucasians)
- Prior stroke
- Heredity

The best way to prevent strokes is to identify individuals who are at risk. Then, as many risk factors as possible must be controlled. This can be achieved with modification of poor health habits and drug therapy.

PATHOPHYSIOLOGY

As described before, blood reaches the brain through four major vessels. These are the two carotid arteries and the two vertebral arteries. (The two carotid arteries provide about 80% of cerebral blood flow.) The two vertebral arteries combine to form the single basilar artery (supplying the remaining 20% of CBF). These two systems are interconnected at various levels. The principal level is the circle of Willis. In addition, collateral blood flow can be supplied to the brain through connections from blood vessels in the face to the dura and arachnoid coverings of the brain. The amount of collateral circulation varies from individual to individual. Beyond this, however, there is no collateral circulation in the depths of the brain. Therefore occlusion of any one of the more distal vessels may result in ischemia and infarction.

Normally, the CBF is maintained through autoregulation of cerebral vessels. These vessels constrict or dilate to preserve perfusion pressure even when the patient is hypotensive. Arterial cerebral perfusion is regulated by the level of oxygen and glucose supplied (ischemia and acidosis are profound vasodilators). Vessel occlusion or hemorrhage causes a sudden cessation of circulation to a portion of the brain. Autoregulatory mechanisms cannot readily correct this problem. The uncorrected ischemia that results within a short period of time leads to neuronal dysfunction and death. The onset and symptoms of the stroke depend on the area of the brain involved.

> **BOX 31-4 Classification of Strokes**
>
> **Ischemic Strokes**
> Ischemic strokes are caused by blood clots. This type of stroke accounts for 85% of all strokes. This is the only type of stroke for which fibrinolytics are administered. Ischemic strokes are divided into two classes, depending on the cause:
> 1. Cerebral thrombosis
> 2. Cerebral embolism
>
> **Hemorrhagic Strokes**
> Hemorrhagic strokes are caused by ruptured blood vessels. The two classes of hemorrhagic stroke are:
> 1. Intracerebral hemorrhage
> 2. Subarachnoid hemorrhage

> **CRITICAL THINKING**
> How much oxygen and glucose can the brain store for emergency situations?

TYPES OF STROKE

Stroke is a general term that refers to the neurological manifestations of a critical decrease in blood flow to a portion of the brain, regardless of the cause. The American Heart Association (AHA) has defined two primary categories of stroke: ischemic stroke (those caused by clots) and hemorrhagic stroke (those caused by bleeding). Each of these is subdivided into two classes. For ischemic stroke, these are cerebral thrombosis and cerebral embolism. For hemorrhagic stroke, they are intracerebral hemorrhage and subarachnoid hemorrhage (Box 31-4).

Determining the origin of a stroke frequently is difficult in the prehospital setting. Often it also is unnecessary. However, a paramedic who understands the various signs and symptoms of each type of stroke is better equipped to anticipate the course of patient care (Table 31-1). Documenting a thorough history and physical examination also helps others involved in the patient's care.

Ischemic Stroke. About 85% of strokes are the ischemic type. They are caused by a cerebral thrombosis. The thrombosis occurs as a result of atherosclerotic plaques or pressure from a mass in the brain itself. Stroke caused by cerebral thrombosis usually is associated with a long history of blood vessel disease. Therefore most of these patients are

TABLE 31-1 Differentiation of Ischemic and Hemorrhagic Strokes

ISCHEMIC STROKES	HEMORRHAGIC STROKES
Most common	Least common
Usually the result of atherosclerosis or tumor in the brain	Usually the result of cerebral aneurysms, AV malformations, hypertension
Develop slowly	Develop abruptly
Long history of vessel disease	Commonly occur during stress or exertion
May be associated with valvular heart disease and atrial fibrillation	May be associated with use of cocaine and other sympathomimetic amines
History of angina, previous strokes	May be asymptomatic before rupture

older. Most also have evidence of atherosclerotic disease in other areas of the body (angina pectoris, claudication, previous strokes). The signs and symptoms of thrombotic stroke usually are slower to develop than those of cerebral hemorrhage. These signs and symptoms include the following:

- Hemiparesis or hemiplegia on the side of the body opposite the lesion
- Numbness (decreased sensation) on the side of the body opposite the lesion
- Aphasia
- Confusion or coma
- Convulsions
- Incontinence
- Diplopia (double vision)
- Monocular blindness (painless visual loss in one eye)
- Numbness of the face
- Dysarthria (slurred speech)
- Headache
- Dizziness or vertigo
- Ataxia

Cerebral Embolus. A stroke caused by an embolus results when an intracranial vessel is blocked by a foreign substance. The vessel is occluded by a fragment of a foreign substance originating outside the CNS. Common sources of cerebral emboli include atherosclerotic plaques (originating from large vessels of the head, neck, or heart). Thrombi that develop on the valves or in the chambers of the heart are very common in patients with heart valve disease and atrial fibrillation. Other, rare causes include air embolism from a chest injury and fat embolism after long bone injury. Bacterial and fungal infections of the heart also can produce emboli. Women taking oral contraceptives and patients with sickle cell disease have an increased risk of developing a stroke (by both thrombotic and embolic origin). Signs and symptoms of cerebral embolus are similar to those of thrombotic stroke. However, embolic signs and symptoms develop more quickly. Also, they often are associated with an identifiable cause (e.g., atrial fibrillation).

Hemorrhagic Stroke. Cerebral hemorrhage accounts for about 15% of all strokes. A hemorrhage may occur anywhere in the brain and its structures. This includes the epidural, subdural, subarachnoid, intraparenchymal, and intraventricular spaces. The most common causes are cerebral aneurysms, arteriovenous (AV) malformations, and hypertension. Cerebral aneurysms and AV malformations are congenital anomalies. They can run in families. They often are asymptomatic until they rupture. Unlike thrombotic and embolic strokes, which have relatively high survival rates, cerebral hemorrhages are fatal in 50% to 80% of cases.[2]

Hemorrhagic strokes often occur during stress or exertion. Cocaine and other sympathetic-type drugs also may contribute to intracranial hemorrhage. (They do this through rapid elevation of blood pressure.) The onset of the stroke is sudden. It often begins with a headache. (This may be described as the worst headache of the patient's life.) The headache is accompanied by nausea, vomiting, and loss of consciousness. Often the patient loses consciousness or experiences a seizure at the time of the hemorrhage. The hemorrhage expands, and intracranial pressure (ICP) increases. As this occurs, the patient becomes comatose, with increasing hypertension and bradycardia (Cushing reflex).

CRITICAL THINKING

Why do you think mortality is higher for hemorrhagic stroke than for embolic stroke?

TRANSIENT ISCHEMIC ATTACKS

Transient ischemic attacks (TIAs) are often referred to as *little strokes*. They are episodes of cerebral dysfunction that affect a specific portion of the brain. They may last minutes to several hours. The patient returns to normal within 24 hours without permanent neurological deficit. A TIA is thought to be the most important indication of impending stroke; about 5% of patients who have a TIA go on to have a complete stroke within 1 month if untreated.[2] A TIA is the most important forecaster of a brain infarction.

The signs and symptoms of a TIA are the same as those that characterize stroke. They include weakness, paralysis, numbness of the face, and speech disturbances. All these correspond to vascular occlusion of a specific cerebral artery. Most patients who experience a TIA are hospitalized for close observation, evaluation, and treatment of vascular disease (e.g., endarterectomy, anticoagulant therapy).

BOX 31-5 Seven *Ds* of Stroke Management*

Detection: A patient, family member, or bystander recognizes the signs and symptoms of a stroke or transient ischemic attack (TIA) and calls EMS for help.
Dispatch: EMS dispatchers prioritize the call regarding a suspected stroke and dispatch the appropriate EMS team with high transport priority.
Delivery: EMS providers respond rapidly, confirm the signs and symptoms of stroke, and transport the patient (delivery) to an appropriate medical facility.
Door: An appropriate medical facility is a hospital that can provide fibrinolytic therapy within 1 hour of arrival at the emergency department (ED) door.
Data: A computed tomography (CT) scan is obtained.
Decision: Candidates for fibrinolytic therapy are identified.
Drug: Eligible patients are treated with fibrinolytic therapy.

*The first three *Ds* are the responsibility of the public and emergency medical services (EMS) providers. The fourth *D* is the responsibility of EMS, and the last three *Ds* are performed in the hospital.

BOX 31-6 Cincinnati Prehospital Stroke Scale

Facial Droop (have patient show teeth or smile)
- Normal—Both sides of face move equally well.
- Abnormal—One side of face does not move as well as the other side.

Arm Drift (patient closes eyes and holds both arms out)
- Normal—Both arms move the same *or* both arms do not move at all (other findings, such as pronator grip, may be helpful).
- Abnormal—One arm does not move *or* one arm drifts down compared with the other.

Speech (have the patient say, "You can't teach an old dog new tricks.")
- Normal—Patient uses correct words with no slurring.
- Abnormal—Patient slurs words, uses inappropriate words, *or* is unable to speak.

Note: If any one of these three signs is abnormal, the probability of a stroke is 72%.

Role of Paramedics in Stroke Care

In stroke care, the paramedic's role is to quickly identify a stroke event. Paramedics also should notify medical direction of the patient's condition. The patient then should be quickly transported to the proper facility for rapid, hospital-based evaluation and treatment. Key points in the management of stroke include the seven *Ds*: detection, dispatch, delivery, door, data, decision, and drug (Box 31-5). (The first three *Ds* are the responsibility of the public and emergency medical services [EMS] providers.)

NOTE About 85% of strokes occur at home. Public education programs focused on individuals at risk for stroke, their friends, and family members have been shown to reduce the time to arrival at the emergency department[3] (see Chapter 3). The "chain of survival" described by the American Heart Association (AHA) and the American Stroke Association (ASA) to improve stroke survival is made up of the following four links:

1. Rapid recognition and reaction to stroke warning signs
2. Rapid start of prehospital care
3. Rapid transport by emergency medical services (EMS) providers and hospital prenotification
4. Rapid diagnosis and treatment in the hospital

http://strokeassociation.org/presenter.jhtml?identifier=1018, accessed September 21, 2004.

ASSESSMENT

The initial examination of a patient who may have suffered a stroke (or TIA) follows the same sequence as for any other ill or injured patient in the emergency setting. The priorities are to maintain a patent airway and to provide adequate ventilatory support with supplemental high-concentration oxygen. If the patient is conscious and able to talk, a thorough history should be obtained. The following are important components of the patient history:

- Previous neurological symptoms (TIAs)
- Previous neurological deficits
- Initial symptoms and their progression
- Alterations in level of consciousness
- Precipitating factors
- Dizziness
- Palpitations
- Significant past medical history
  - Hypertension
  - Diabetes mellitus
  - Cigarette smoking
  - Oral contraceptive use
  - Cardiac disease
  - Sickle cell disease
  - Previous stroke

Cincinnati Prehospital Stroke Scale. In addition to the abnormal neurological signs and symptoms described previously, other methods can be used to diagnose stroke. One such method is the *Prehospital Stroke Scale*[4] developed in Cincinnati. This scale evaluates three major physical findings: facial droop, arm drift, and speech (Box 31-6). The paramedic can use this scale to help identify a stroke patient who needs rapid transport to a hospital. It also allows for prearrival notification of the receiving hospital.

Los Angeles Prehospital Stroke Screen. The Los Angeles Prehospital Stroke Screen (LAPSS) is another way to diagnose stroke. This screening tool requires the examiner to rule out other causes of altered level of consciousness (e.g., hypoglycemia or seizure). The examiner then must identify asymmetry (right versus left) in facial smile/grimace, grip, and arm strength (Box 31-7). Asymmetry in any category indicates a possible stroke. Like the Cincinnati stroke scale, the LAPSS can be used quickly in the prehospital setting.

BOX 31-7 Los Angeles Prehospital Stroke Screen (LAPSS)

For evaluation of acute, noncomatose, nontraumatic neurological complaint: If items 1 through 6 are **all checked "Yes"** (or "Unknown"), notify the receiving hospital before arrival of the potential stroke patient. If any are checked "No," follow the appropriate treatment protocol.

Interpretation: Ninety-three percent of patients with stroke have positive findings (all items checked "Yes" or "Unknown") (sensitivity = 93%). Of those with positive findings, 97% will have a stroke (specificity = 97%). The patient may still be having a stroke even if LAPSS criteria are not met.

Criteria	Yes	Unknown	No
1. Age >45	[ ]	[ ]	[ ]
2. History of seizures or epilepsy **absent**	[ ]	[ ]	[ ]
3. Symptom duration <24 hours	[ ]	[ ]	[ ]
4. At baseline, patient is **not** wheelchair bound or bedridden	[ ]	[ ]	[ ]
5. Blood glucose between 60 and 400 mg/dL	[ ]	[ ]	[ ]
6. **Obvious asymmetry** (right vs. left) in **any** of the following three categories **(must be unilateral):**	[ ]	[ ]	[ ]

	Equal	R Weak	L Weak
Facial smile/ grimace	[ ]	[ ] Droop	[ ] Droop
Grip	[ ]	[ ] Weak grip	[ ] Weak grip
	[ ]	[ ] No grip	[ ] No grip
Arm strength	[ ]	[ ] Drifts down	[ ] Drifts down
	[ ]	[ ] Falls rapidly	[ ] Falls rapidly

Modified from Kidwell CS et al: Design and retrospective analysis of the Los Angeles prehospital stroke screen (LAPSS), *Prehosp Emerg Care:* 2:267-273. 1998.

MANAGEMENT (FIG. 31-12)

Once the diagnosis of a stroke is suspected, *time in the field must be reduced.* This is because treatment must begin as soon as possible. (Less than 3 hours from onset is required for the use of fibrinolytics.[2]) Whenever possible, the paramedic should establish the time of onset of stroke signs and symptoms. This is important for determining whether fibrinolytics can be administered. Prehospital care is directed at managing the patient's airway, breathing, and circulation, and monitoring vital signs. Besides life support, the most important care a paramedic can provide a stroke victim is quick identification of the possible stroke and rapid transport of the patient for definitive care.

Airway. Paralysis of the muscles of the throat, tongue, and mouth can lead to partial or complete airway obstruction. (This is a major problem in acute stroke.) Frequent suctioning of the oropharynx and nasopharynx is required to prevent aspiration of saliva. If possible, the patient should be positioned to aid drainage of oral secretions.

CRITICAL THINKING

How can you detect paralysis of the muscles of the throat, tongue, and mouth on your physical exam?

Breathing. Inadequate ventilation should be managed with supplemental oxygen (in hypoxic patients) and positive-pressure ventilation. Hypoxia and hypercarbia can occur as a result of inadequate ventilation, contributing to cardiac and respiratory instability. Respiratory arrest should be managed with intubation and assisted ventilations. The paramedic should not routinely administer supplemental oxygen to victims of minor or moderate strokes who are not hypoxic (i.e., oxygen saturation is 90% or higher).[5]

Circulation. Cardiac arrest is uncommon. However, it may result from a respiratory arrest. Cardiac dysrhythmias occur frequently. Therefore the patient's ECG and blood pressure require constant monitoring. As described in Chapter 29, a difference in blood pressure readings in the upper extremities of 10 mm Hg or more may indicate aortic dissection and compromise of the brain's blood supply.

NOTE Many patients develop hypertension after a stroke. However, this usually does not require emergency treatment. Elevated blood pressure after a stroke is not a hypertensive emergency unless the patient has other medical indications, such as an acute myocardial infarction (AMI) or left ventricular failure. Management of hypertension in the prehospital setting is not recommended in cases of suspected stroke.[2]

Other Supportive Measures. If the airway is patent and the patient's condition permits, the individual should be kept supine. The head should be elevated 15 degrees. This aids venous drainage. Other patient care measures the paramedic can provide while en route to the receiving hospital include the following:

1. An IV line of lactated Ringer's solution or normal saline can be started (50 mL per hour).
2. A blood sample can be drawn for laboratory analysis per protocol.
3. Serum glucose analysis can be performed (***50% dextrose*** should be administered only if indicated).
4. Paralyzed extremities should be protected.
5. Normal body temperature should be maintained.
6. Any seizure activity should be controlled with benzodiazepines.
7. Comfort measures and reassurance should be provided.
8. Care should be taken to ensure gentle transport to the receiving hospital.

Paramedics must keep in mind that stroke patients have experienced a catastrophic event, one that may seriously affect their quality of life. They often are frightened, embar-

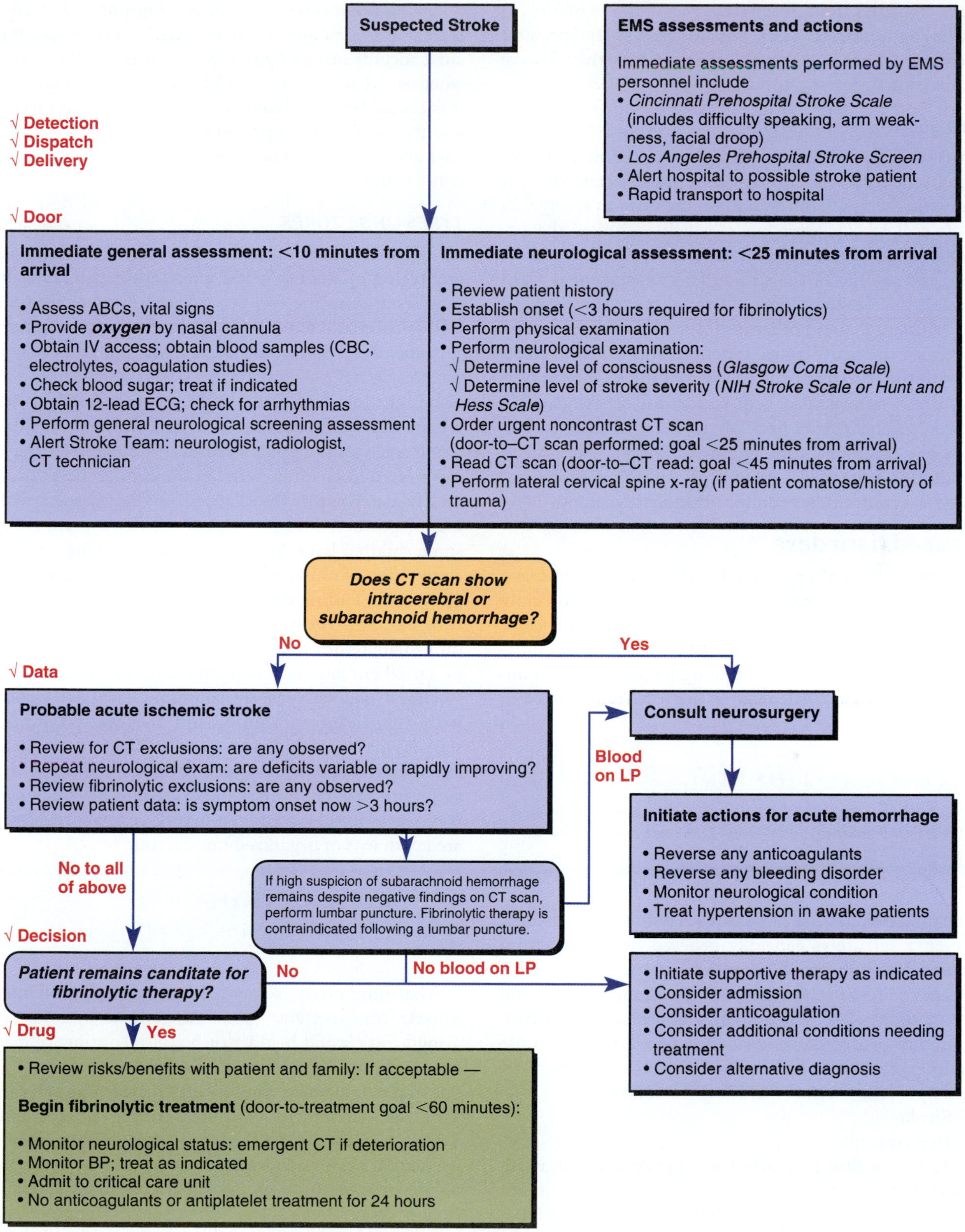
Suspected Stroke
EMS assessments and actions
Immediate assessments performed by EMS personnel include
• Cincinnati Prehospital Stroke Scale (includes difficulty speaking, arm weakness, facial droop)
• Los Angeles Prehospital Stroke Screen
• Alert hospital to possible stroke patient
• Rapid transport to hospital
√ Detection
√ Dispatch
√ Delivery
√ Door
Immediate general assessment: <10 minutes from arrival
• Assess ABCs, vital signs
• Provide oxygen by nasal cannula
• Obtain IV access; obtain blood samples (CBC, electrolytes, coagulation studies)
• Check blood sugar; treat if indicated
• Obtain 12-lead ECG; check for arrhythmias
• Perform general neurological screening assessment
• Alert Stroke Team: neurologist, radiologist, CT technician
Immediate neurological assessment: <25 minutes from arrival
• Review patient history
• Establish onset (<3 hours required for fibrinolytics)
• Perform physical examination
• Perform neurological examination:
√ Determine level of consciousness (Glasgow Coma Scale)
√ Determine level of stroke severity (NIH Stroke Scale or Hunt and Hess Scale)
• Order urgent noncontrast CT scan (door-to–CT scan performed: goal <25 minutes from arrival)
• Read CT scan (door-to–CT read: goal <45 minutes from arrival)
• Perform lateral cervical spine x-ray (if patient comatose/history of trauma)
Does CT scan show intracerebral or subarachnoid hemorrhage?
No
Yes
√ Data
Probable acute ischemic stroke
• Review for CT exclusions: are any observed?
• Repeat neurological exam: are deficits variable or rapidly improving?
• Review fibrinolytic exclusions: are any observed?
• Review patient data: is symptom onset now >3 hours?
Consult neurosurgery
Blood on LP
Initiate actions for acute hemorrhage
• Reverse any anticoagulants
• Reverse any bleeding disorder
• Monitor neurological condition
• Treat hypertension in awake patients
No to all of above
If high suspicion of subarachnoid hemorrhage remains despite negative findings on CT scan, perform lumbar puncture. Fibrinolytic therapy is contraindicated following a lumbar puncture.
√ Decision
Patient remains canditate for fibrinolytic therapy?
No
No blood on LP
• Initiate supportive therapy as indicated
• Consider admission
• Consider anticoagulation
• Consider additional conditions needing treatment
• Consider alternative diagnosis
√ Drug
Yes
• Review risks/benefits with patient and family: If acceptable —
Begin fibrinolytic treatment (door-to-treatment goal <60 minutes):
• Monitor neurological status: emergent CT if deterioration
• Monitor BP; treat as indicated
• Admit to critical care unit
• No anticoagulants or antiplatelet treatment for 24 hours

FIGURE 31-12 ■ Algorithm for suspected cases of stroke.

rassed, confused, and frustrated with their inability to move or communicate. These patients have special physical and emotional needs. As do all other patients, they deserve a compassionate, caring approach.

IN-HOSPITAL TREATMENT

On arrival at the emergency department, the non-hemorrhagic stroke patient is evaluated as a possible candidate for fibrinolytic therapy. This evaluation includes an emergency neurological stroke assessment, which identifies the patient's level of consciousness. It also identifies the type, location, and severity of the stroke. This assessment is aided by use of the Glasgow Coma Scale and other standardized scales. These scales and other in-hospital diagnostic studies help to measure neurological function. This function correlates with the severity of the stroke and the long-term outcome. These studies also help to identify stroke patients who would benefit from fibrinolytic therapy. Rapid evaluation of the computed tomography (CT) scan is critical to rule out an intracranial hemorrhage. An intracranial hemorrhage is a contraindication for fibrinolytic therapy.

Seizure Disorders

A **seizure** is a brief alteration in behavior or consciousness. It is caused by abnormal electrical activity of one or more groups of neurons in the brain. The annual incidence of seizure is estimated to be about 0.5% of the U.S. population. The highest incidence is among feverish children under 5 years of age. (Febrile seizures are further addressed in Chapter 44.)

> **CRITICAL THINKING**
>
> What feelings may parents experience after seeing their child have a febrile seizure? How should you respond to those feelings?

The underlying cause of seizures is not well understood. However, a seizure is generally believed to result from a structural lesion or problems with brain metabolism. This results in changes in the brain cell's permeability to sodium and potassium ions. When such changes occur, the neurons' ability to depolarize and emit an electrical impulse sometimes results in seizure activity. Seizures may be caused by several factors, including the following:

- Stroke
- Head trauma
- Toxins (including alcohol or other drug withdrawal)
- Hypoxia
- Hypoperfusion
- Hypoglycemia
- Infection
- Metabolic abnormalities
- Brain tumor or abscess
- Vascular disorders
- Eclampsia
- Drug overdose

In the prehospital setting, determining the cause of a seizure is not as important as other measures. Such measures include managing the complications and recognizing whether the seizure is reversible with therapy (e.g., whether it is caused by hypoglycemia). A tendency to have recurrent seizures is called **epilepsy.** (This does not include seizures that arise from correctable or avoidable causes, such as alcohol withdrawal.)

TYPES OF SEIZURES

All seizures are pathological. They may arise from almost any region of the brain and therefore have many clinical manifestations. The two most common types are generalized seizures and partial (focal) seizures.

Generalized Seizures. As the name implies, generalized seizures do not have a definable origin (focus) in the brain, although focal seizures may progress to generalized seizures. This class includes petit mal (absence seizures) and grand mal (tonic-clonic) seizures. Petit mal seizures occur most often in children between the ages of 4 and 12. They are characterized by brief lapses of consciousness without loss of posture. Often no motor activity is seen. However, some children have eye blinking, lip smacking, or isolated contraction of muscles. These seizures usually last less than 15 seconds. During this time, the patient is unaware of the surroundings. These seizures are followed by the patient's immediate return to normal. Most patients have remission by age 20 but later may develop grand mal seizures.

Grand mal seizures are common. They are associated with significant morbidity and mortality. Grand mal seizures may be preceded by an *aura.* (This is an olfactory or auditory sensation.) Often the patient recognizes the aura as a warning of the imminent convulsion. The seizure itself is characterized by a sudden loss of consciousness associated with loss of organized muscle tone.

> **CRITICAL THINKING**
>
> What could cause death after a grand mal seizure?

The tonic phase is marked by a sequence of extensor muscle tone activity (sometimes flexion) and apnea. Tongue biting and bladder or bowel incontinence may occur. The tonic phase lasts only seconds. It is followed by a bilateral clonic phase (rigidity alternating with relaxation). This usually lasts 1 to 3 minutes. During the clonic phase, a massive autonomic discharge occurs. This results in hyperventilation, salivation, and tachycardia.

After the seizure, the patient usually experiences a period of drowsiness or unconsciousness. This resolves over minutes to hours. On regaining consciousness, the patient often is confused and fatigued. The person also may show signs of a transient neurological deficit. This part of the seizure is known as the *postictal phase.* Grand mal seizures may be prolonged or may recur before the patient regains consciousness. When this occurs, the patient is said to be in **status epilepticus** (see discussion later in the chapter).

Partial Seizures. In generalized seizures, a specific seizure focus is unknown. In contrast, partial seizures arise from identifiable cortical lesions. Partial seizures may be classified as simple or complex. Simple partial seizures result mainly from seizure activity in the motor or sensory cortex. Simple motor seizures usually manifest as clonic activity that is limited to one body part. (For instance, this might be one hand, one arm or leg, or one side of the face.) Simple sensory seizures result in symptoms such as tingling or numbness of a body part or abnormal visual, auditory, olfactory, or taste symptoms. Patients with partial seizures generally do not lose consciousness. They usually maintain a somewhat normal mental status. However, the seizure focus may spread and lead to a generalized tonic-clonic seizure. Partial seizure activity that spreads in an orderly way to surrounding areas is known as a *jacksonian seizure.*

Complex partial seizures arise from focal seizures in the temporal lobe (psychomotor seizures). These manifest mainly as changes in behavior. The classic complex partial seizure is preceded by an aura. It is followed by abnormal repetitive motor behavior *(automatisms).* These may include lip smacking, chewing, or swallowing. During this time the patient will have no memory of the event. These seizures usually are brief, lasting less than 1 minute. The patient usually regains normal mental status quickly. Like simple partial seizures, complex partial seizures also may progress to a generalized tonic-clonic seizure.

> **NOTE** A hysterical seizure can mimic a true seizure. However, it stems from psychological causes. These seizures are not considered true seizures because they have no physical cause. Also, they do not respond to the usual treatments. Hysterical seizures, or *pseudoseizures,* usually can be ended by sharp commands or painful stimuli (e.g., a sternal rub). These maneuvers may help to distinguish between pathological and psychogenic seizure activity.

ASSESSMENT

The assessment process is determined by the patient's seizure state. In most cases the patient's seizure has ended before paramedics arrive. If possible, the assessment should include a thorough history and physical examination, including a neurological evaluation.

History. If the patient is in the postictal phase of the seizure, information can be gathered from family members or bystanders who saw the event. Important components of the patient history include the following:

1. History of seizures
   a. Frequency
   b. Compliance in taking prescribed medications (e.g., ***phenytoin,*** phenobarbital)
2. Description of seizure activity
   a. Duration of seizure
   b. Typical or atypical pattern of seizure for the patient
   c. Presence of aura
   d. Generalized or focal
   e. Incontinence
   f. Tongue biting
3. Recent or past history of head trauma
4. Recent history of fever, headache, nuchal rigidity (suggesting meningeal irritation)
5. Past significant medical history
   a. Diabetes
   b. Heart disease
   c. Stroke

Physical Examination. During the physical examination, maintaining a patent airway is always of prime importance. The paramedic also should be alert for signs of trauma (head and neck trauma, tongue injury, oral lacerations). These injuries may have occurred before or during the seizure. Also, the patient's mouth should be inspected for gingival hypertrophy (swelling of the gums). This is a sign of chronic ***phenytoin*** therapy. Other components of the physical examination include the following:

- Level of sensorium, including presence or absence of amnesia
- Cranial nerve evaluation, particularly pupillary findings
- Motor and sensory evaluation, including coordination (abnormalities may be caused by metabolic disturbances, meningitis, intracranial hemorrhage, and drug use)
- Evaluation for hypotension and hypoxia
- Presence of urine or feces (suggesting bladder or bowel incontinence)
- Automatisms
- Cardiac dysrhythmias

> **CRITICAL THINKING**
> What are signs and symptoms of ***phenytoin*** toxicity?

Syncope Versus Seizure. It may be difficult to determine whether the patient has experienced a syncopal episode (see Chapter 29) or a seizure. The main difference is in the symptoms the patient experiences before and after the event. The factors listed in Table 31-2 may aid differentiation of these two events.

MANAGEMENT

The first step in managing a patient with seizure activity is to protect the patient from injury. This is best achieved by removing obstacles in the patient's immediate area. If necessary, the patient can be moved to a safe environment such as a carpeted or soft, grassy area. *At no time should a patient with seizure activity be restrained, nor should objects be forced between the patient's teeth to maintain an airway.* Restraining activity may harm the patient or paramedic crew. Forcing objects into the oral cavity in an effort to secure an airway or prevent the patient from biting the tongue may evoke vomiting, aspiration, or spasm of the larynx.

Most patients with an isolated seizure can be properly managed in the postictal phase by being placed in a lateral recumbent position. This allows drainage of oral secretions

TABLE 31-2 Differentiation of Syncope and Seizure

CHARACTERISTIC	SYNCOPE	SEIZURE
Position	Syncope usually starts when patient is in a standing position.	Seizure may start with patient in any position.
Warning	Patient usually has a warning period of lightheadedness.	Patient has little or no warning.
Level of consciousness	Patient usually regains consciousness immediately on becoming supine; fatigue, confusion, and headache last less than 15 minutes.	Patient may remain unconscious for minutes to hours; fatigue, confusion, and headache last longer than 15 minutes.
Clonic-tonic activity	Clonic movements (if present) are of short duration.	Tonic-clonic movements occur during unconscious state.
Electrocardiographic (ECG) analysis	Bradycardia is caused by increased vagal tone associated with syncope.	Tachycardia is caused by muscular exertion associated with seizure activity.

and aids suctioning (if needed). Supplemental oxygen should be administered via a nonrebreather mask. The patient should be moved to a quiet place (away from onlookers). Patients often are embarrassed or self-conscious after a seizure. This is especially the case if incontinence has occurred. Paramedics should be sensitive to the physical and emotional needs of the patient.

Some patients should always be transported to the emergency department for care and evaluation by a physician. These include patients who have a history of seizures but who experienced a seizure that is different from the usual one, and patients with a seizure that is complicated by an unusual event (e.g., trauma). All patients who have experienced a seizure for the first time should be transported to the emergency department for evaluation by a physician. Depending on the patient's status and seizure history, an IV line may be necessary to administer drug therapy. However, few patients who experience an isolated seizure require drug therapy in the prehospital setting.

STATUS EPILEPTICUS

Status epilepticus is ongoing seizure activity that lasts 30 minutes or longer. The term also refers to recurrent seizures without a period of consciousness between them. Status epilepticus is a true emergency. Without immediate management, it can result in permanent neurological damage, respiratory failure, and death. Associated complications of status epilepticus include aspiration, brain damage, and fracture of long bones and the spine. The most common cause in adults is failure to take prescribed anticonvulsant medications.

Management. As in all patients with seizures, management priorities include securing the airway and providing ventilatory support, protecting the patient from injury, and, if indicated, transporting the patient to a medical facility for evaluation by a physician. In addition, management includes stopping the seizure activity with anticonvulsant medications (e.g., ***diazepam*** or ***lorazepam***).

After the airway has been secured with oral or nasal adjuncts (or with intubation of the trachea during the flaccid period between seizures), high-concentration oxygen should be administered. Also, ventilation should be supported with a bag-valve device. An IV line should be established to keep the vein open. It should be secured well with tape and roller bandage. A sample of the patient's blood should be drawn for laboratory analysis (per protocol). With authorization from medical direction, administration of the following medications may be considered:

- ***50% Dextrose*** by slow IV infusion (controversial unless hypoglycemia is suspected) to replace blood glucose lost during seizure activity or to correct hypoglycemia that caused the seizure
- ***Lorazepam*** (IV) or ***diazepam*** (IV) to stop the spread of the seizure focus.

Flumazenil should be available to reverse respiratory depression that may result from benzodiazepine sedation. ***Flumazenil*** also may cause seizures and must be used with caution in these patients.

While administering these drugs, paramedics should closely monitor the patient's blood pressure and respiratory status. They should be prepared for respiratory arrest. If the patient's blood pressure begins to fall or if the respiratory rate or effort decreases, paramedics should stop the drug therapy and consult with medical direction.

Headache

Headaches are painful and bothersome. However, most are minor health concerns. In addition, most are easily managed with analgesics. Headaches are categorized according to their underlying cause. The types of headaches are the **tension headache, migraine, cluster headache,** and **sinus headache.** Therapies that may be useful in managing these headaches include prescription and over-the-counter medications, herbal remedies, meditation, acupressure, aromatherapy, and others. Headache is an extremely common medical complaint; 40% of all Americans will have what they consider to be a serious headache at some time during their lives.[6] The pain associated with headaches arises from the meninges and from the scalp and its blood vessels and muscles.

Tension headaches are caused by muscle contractions of the face, neck, and scalp. They have a variety of causes.

Some of the causes include stress, persistent noise, eyestrain, and poor posture. The pain of tension headaches (usually described as dull, persistent, and nonthrobbing) may last for days or weeks. It can cause variable degrees of discomfort. These headaches can be short-lived and infrequent, or chronic in nature. Most tension headaches can be managed effectively with analgesics such as ***aspirin,*** acetaminophen, or ibuprofen.

Migraines are severe, incapacitating headaches. They often are preceded by visual and/or GI disturbances. These headaches usually begin with an intense, throbbing pain on one side of the head that may spread. They often are accompanied by nausea and vomiting. The symptoms of migraines are associated with constriction and dilation of blood vessels that may be brought on by an imbalance of serotonin or hormone fluctuations. Migraines also can be triggered by excessive caffeine use, various foods, changes in altitude, and extremes of emotions. A wide range of medications are prescribed for migraines. These include beta blockers, calcium channel blockers, antidepressants, and serotonin-inhibiting drugs.

Cluster headaches are headaches that occur in bursts (clusters). They often begin several hours after a person falls asleep. The pain may be severe. It usually is located in and around one eye. It generally is accompanied by nasal congestion and tearing. The painful episode often lasts 30 minutes to 2 hours. It then diminishes or disappears, recurring a day or so later. The headaches may occur every day for weeks or months before going into long periods of remission. Cluster headaches also are known as *histamine headaches.* This is because they are associated with the release of histamine from the body tissues. They are marked by symptoms of dilated carotid arteries, fluid accumulation under the eyes, tearing or lacrimation, and rhinorrhea. Cluster headaches generally are managed with antihistamines, corticosteroids, and calcium channel blockers. Cluster headaches seem to be more common in heavy smokers than in nonsmokers. Alcohol consumption and certain foods also may be implicated. The vast majority of sufferers are men.

Sinus headaches are characterized by pain in the forehead, nasal area, and eyes. They often produce a feeling of pressure behind the face. Allergies or inflammation or infection of the membranes lining the sinus cavities usually are responsible for the discomfort. Sinus headaches are managed with medications such as analgesics, antihistamines, and antibiotics to treat infection.

MANAGEMENT

Many causes of headaches can be avoided. For example, "triggers" can be identified, such as irregular meals, prolonged travel, noisy environments, and food additives (in susceptible individuals). Headaches such as those described in the preceding paragraphs seldom require prehospital emergency care. However, a full history of the headache should be obtained. This helps to identify a more serious cause of the headache, should one be present. For example, the headache may be a sign of an aneurysm or a stroke. Important assessment findings include the following:

- The patient's general health
- Previous medical conditions
- Medications used
- Previous experience with headaches
- The time of onset

After a patient history has been obtained and a neurological examination performed, prehospital care for patients with tension headaches, migraines, cluster headaches, and sinus headaches is mainly supportive. The paramedic should consult with medical direction to determine the appropriate follow-up care. Transport of the patient for evaluation by a physician may be indicated.

Brain Neoplasm and Brain Abscess

A brain tumor, or *neoplasm,* is a mass in the cranial cavity. This mass may be either malignant or benign. Heredity may play a role in the development of brain tumors. They also are associated with several risk factors, including exposure to radiation, tobacco use, dietary habits, some viruses, and the use of some medications.[1] The effects of the tumor depend on its size, location, and growth rate, and whether any evidence of hemorrhage or edema exists. Brain tumors may cause local and generalized manifestations. Local effects are caused by the destructive action of the tumor on a particular site in the brain and by compression, which reduces cerebral blood flow (Fig. 31-13). These effects are varied and may include the following[7]:

- Seizures
- Visual disturbances
- Unstable gait
- Cranial nerve dysfunction

> **NOTE** Central nervous system (CNS) tumors include both brain tumors and spinal cord tumors. The incidence of these tumors tends to increase up to age 70 and then decreases. CNS tumors are the second most common group of tumors in children.[7]

Lesions inside the cranial vault cause pain. They do this by distending or stretching the arteries and other pain-sensitive structures of the head and neck. Headache may be present but often is a late finding in the absence of hemorrhage, which may cause a sudden onset of pain.[6] The main treatment for a cerebral tumor is surgical or radiosurgical excision. Surgical decompression may be used if total excision is not possible. Chemotherapy and radiation also may be used.

A brain abscess is a buildup of purulent material (pus) surrounded by a capsule within the brain. It develops from a bacterial infection. The infection often begins in the nasal cavity, middle ear, or mastoid cells. The condition also may develop after surgery or penetrating cranial trauma, especially when bone fragments are retained in cranial tissue. Clinical manifestations of a brain abscess are associated with

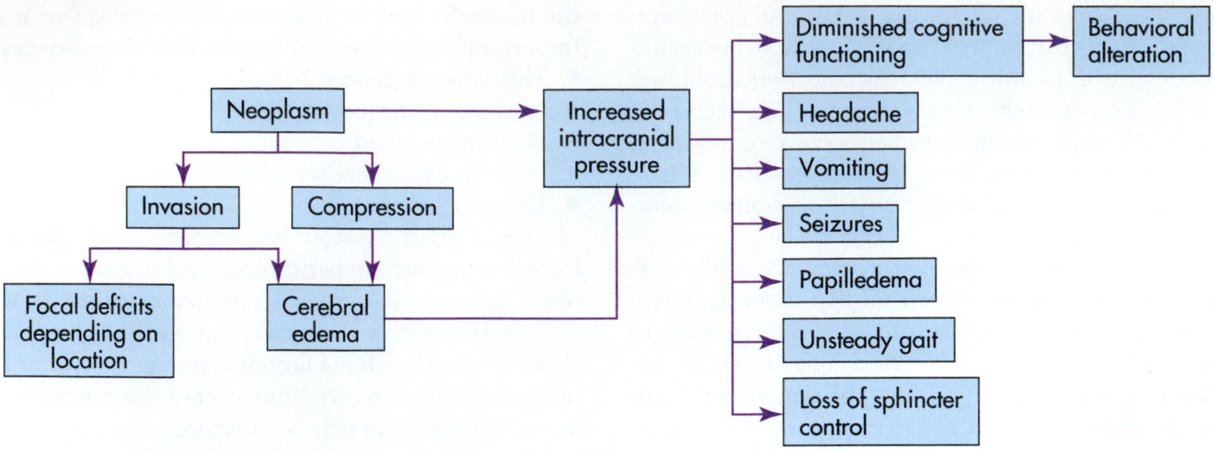

FIGURE 31-13 ■ Origin of signs and symptoms associated with an intracranial neoplasm.

intracranial infection (e.g., fever). They also are associated with an expanding intracranial mass (e.g., nausea, vomiting, seizures, and changes in mental status). Headache is the most common early symptom. The removal of fluid from the abscess or excision accompanied by antibiotic therapy generally is recommended to manage this disorder (controversial). The incidence of brain abscess is about 1 per 100,000 hospital admissions. The condition is twice as common in men as in women. The median age for abscess formation is 30 to 40 years of age.[7]

MANAGEMENT

Prehospital care of a patient with a brain neoplasm or abscess may range from providing comfort and emotional support during patient transport to managing seizure activity and providing airway, ventilatory, and circulatory resuscitation. If the patient's condition permits, a focused history should be obtained. Also, a neurological evaluation should be performed. Elements of the focused history for these patients should include the following:

- Past significant medical history (e.g., surgical removal of a tumor, radiation therapy)
- History and description of any headache
- Dizziness or loss of consciousness
- Seizure activity
- GI disturbances (vomiting, diarrhea)
- New onset of incoordination, difficulty walking, or maintaining balance
- Behavioral or cognitive changes
- Weakness or paralysis
- Vision disturbances

Degenerative Neurological Diseases

There are many degenerative neurological diseases. The pathophysiology of many of these disorders is not fully understood. Some diseases may involve Schwann cells, the CSF, or axons of the CNS. Others may result from circulatory and immunological disorders and exposure to bacterial toxins and chemicals. The following specific neurological diseases are discussed in this chapter:

- Muscular dystrophy
- Multiple sclerosis
- Dystonia
- Parkinson disease
- Central pain syndrome
- Bell palsy
- Amyotrophic lateral sclerosis
- Peripheral neuropathy
- Myoclonus
- Spina bifida
- Polio

MUSCULAR DYSTROPHY

Muscular dystrophy is an inherited muscle disorder. The cause is unknown. The disease is marked by a slow but progressive degeneration of muscle fibers. Different forms of the disease are classified by the age at which the symptoms appear, the rate at which the disease progresses, and the way in which it is inherited. Duchenne muscular dystrophy is the most common type. It affects 1 or 2 in 10,000 male children. It is inherited through a recessive sex-linked gene, therefore only males are affected and only females can pass on the disease.

Muscular dystrophy often is first diagnosed by the child's physician, who notices that the child is slow in learning to sit up and walk. The disease is confirmed through blood tests that reveal high levels of enzymes released from damaged muscle cells, through nerve conduction studies, and sometimes with muscle biopsy. Muscular dystrophy rarely is diagnosed before age 3. As the disease progresses, the child tends to walk with a waddle and has difficulty climbing stairs. Muscles (especially those in the calves) become bulky as wasted muscle is replaced by fat. By about age 12, affected children are no longer able to walk, and few survive their teenage years. Death usually results from pulmonary infections and heart failure.

CRITICAL THINKING

How can you determine a child's baseline level of functioning?

No effective treatment exists for muscular dystrophy. Parents or siblings of an affected child should receive genetic counseling. Some types of muscular dystrophy can be diagnosed before birth. This can be done through blood analysis and amniocentesis.

MULTIPLE SCLEROSIS

Multiple sclerosis (MS) is a progressive disease of the CNS. In this disease, scattered patches of myelin in the brain and spinal cord are destroyed. The cause of MS remains unknown. However, it is thought to be an autoimmune disease in which the body's defense system begins to treat the myelin in the CNS as foreign, gradually destroying it *(demyelination),* with subsequent scarring and nerve fiber damage.

MS is the most common acquired disease of the nervous system in young adults. It affects about 1 in every 1000 individuals. The ratio of women to men with the disease is 3 to 2. The symptoms, which may be active briefly in early adult life and resume years later, vary according to the parts of the brain and spinal cord affected. Symptoms range from numbness and tingling to paralysis and incontinence and may last several weeks to several months. Damage to the white matter in the brain may lead to fatigue, vertigo, clumsiness, unsteady gait, slurred speech, blurred or double vision, and facial numbness or pain. Some patients may have mild relapses and long symptom-free periods throughout life. Others may gradually become disabled from the first attack and are bedridden and incontinent in early middle life.

CRITICAL THINKING

Consider the patient who has been receiving long-term steroid therapy. This person is at risk for what conditions?

The disease is usually diagnosed by ruling out other diseases. Diagnostic tests that may help to identify MS include lumbar puncture, CT scanning, and magnetic resonance imaging (MRI) studies. Affected patients are managed with medications (e.g., corticosteroids, antidepressants, immune system medications). These help to control symptoms of an acute episode and to prevent it from getting worse. The disease also is managed with physical therapy to help maintain mobility and independence. Currently no cure exists for the disease.

DYSTONIA

The term **dystonia** refers to local or diffuse changes in muscle tone (usually abnormal muscle rigidity). These changes cause painful muscle spasms, unusually fixed postures, and strange movement patterns. Localized dystonia may result from *torticollis* (a painful neck spasm.) It also may result from *scoliosis* (an abnormal curvature of the spine). More generalized dystonia results from various neurological disorders. These include Parkinson disease and stroke. It also may be a feature of schizophrenia or a side effect of some antipsychotic drugs. Dystonia sometimes is managed with medications such as benztropine or ***diphenhydramine.*** These help to reverse the symptoms and to prevent their recurrence.

PARKINSON DISEASE

Parkinson disease is caused by degeneration of or damage to nerve cells in the basal ganglia in the brain. The cause is unknown. The degeneration causes a lack of dopamine. This prevents the basal ganglia from modifying nerve pathways that control muscle contraction. The result is muscles that are overly tense. This causes tremor, joint rigidity, and slow movement. Parkinson disease affects about 130 in 100,00 persons, and 50,000 new cases are diagnosed in the United States each year.[1] Left untreated, the disease progresses over 10 to 15 years to severe weakness and incapacity. Parkinson disease is the leading cause of neurological disability in people over 60 years of age. Currently about 500,000 people in the United States have the disease.[1]

Parkinson disease usually begins as a slight tremor in one hand, arm, or leg. In the early stages, the tremor is worse while the limb is at rest. In the later stages, the disease affects both sides of the body. It causes stiffness, weakness, and trembling of the muscles. Other symptoms include an unusual walking pattern (shuffling) that may break into uncontrollable, tiny running steps; constant trembling of the hands, sometimes accompanied by shaking of the head; a permanent rigid stoop; and an unblinking, fixed facial expression. Late in the disease, intellect may be affected. Speech becomes slow and hesitant as well. Depression is common.

At first Parkinson disease is managed with counseling, exercise, and special aids in the home. As the disease progresses, management may include various combinations of drugs to provide relief from specific symptoms. (For example, this may include levodopa. Levodopa is converted by the body into dopamine. It also may include anticholinergic agents.) Other management measures may include brain surgery to reduce tremor and rigidity and transplantation of dopamine-secreting adrenal tissue (experimental).

CENTRAL PAIN SYNDROME

Central pain syndrome refers to infection or disease of the trigeminal nerve (cranial nerve V). A common form of the syndrome is *tic douloureux* (trigeminal neuralgia). In this form, patients complain of paroxysmal episodes of excruciating pain (often described as recurrent bursts of an electric shock) that affect the cheek, lips, gums, or chin on one side of the face. The episode usually is very brief, lasting only a few seconds to minutes, but may be so intense that the person is unable to function during the attack. The pain often causes wincing; hence the name tic douloureux (literally, "painful twitch"). Central pain syndrome is unusual in individuals under age 50 but may be associated with MS in younger people. Attacks occur in bouts that may last weeks at a time.

The pain of trigeminal neuralgia usually begins from a trigger point on the face. It can be brought on by touching, washing, shaving, eating, drinking, or talking. The cause of the syndrome is unclear, therefore management is difficult. Treatment includes the use of drugs to inhibit nerve impulses (commonly carbamazepine) and sometimes surgery if the cause is a tumor or lesion.

BELL PALSY

Bell palsy (facial palsy) is a paralysis of the facial muscles. The paralysis is caused by inflammation of the seventh cranial nerve (Fig. 31-14). It usually is one sided and temporary. Also, it often develops suddenly. Bell palsy is the most common cause of facial paralysis, affecting 1 in 60 to 70 people in a lifetime.[1] The cause of the inflammation is unclear. However, it has been associated with many past or present infectious processes. These include Lyme disease, herpes viruses, mumps, and infection with the human immunodeficiency (HIV) virus.

> **CRITICAL THINKING**
> In the field, should you diagnose and release a patient who has Bell palsy?

Bell palsy usually causes the eyelid and corner of the mouth to droop on one side of the face. It sometimes is associated with numbness and pain. Depending on which branches of the nerve are affected, taste may be impaired, or sounds may seem oddly loud. Management involves the use of corticosteroids (controversial) to reduce inflammation of the nerve, along with analgesics. Recovery usually is complete within 2 weeks to 2 months. A key component of therapy is to protect the affected eye from corneal drying and injury. These may result because the paralysis prevents the eyelid from closing. Prevention of these conditions is best accomplished through the use of lubricating ointments and eye patches.

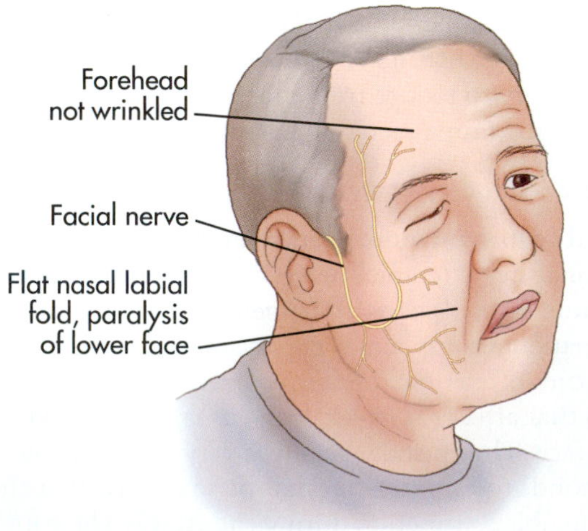

FIGURE 31-14 ■ Bell palsy.

AMYOTROPHIC LATERAL SCLEROSIS

Amyotrophic lateral sclerosis (ALS) is also called *Lou Gehrig disease*. It is one of a group of rare disorders (motor neuron disease). In these disorders, the nerves that control muscular activity degenerate in the brain and spinal cord. ALS usually affects people over the age of 50. It is more common in men than in women. One or two cases of ALS are diagnosed each year per 100,000 people in the United States.[7] About 10% of ALS cases are familial.

Motor neuron diseases may involve deterioration of both upper and lower neuron tracts. When only muscles of the tongue, jaw, face, and larynx are involved, the term *progressive bulbar palsy* is used. When only corticospinal processes are affected, the term *primary lateral sclerosis* is used. When only lower motor neurons are affected, the term *progressive spinal muscular atrophy* is used. *ALS* is used to describe neuron signs that predominate in the extremities and trunk.

Patients with ALS often first notice weakness in the hands and arms. This is accompanied by involuntary quivering *(fasciculations)*. The disease progresses to involve the muscles of all four extremities and those involved in respiration and swallowing. In the final stages of the disease, patients often are unable to speak, swallow, or move. However, awareness and intellect are maintained. Death usually occurs 2 to 4 years after the diagnosis. This is due to involvement of the respiratory muscles, aspiration pneumonia, and general inanition (starvation, failure to thrive). In some cases, life can be prolonged through the use of feeding tubes and ventilators. Care generally is aimed at providing emotional support and easing discomfort.

> **CRITICAL THINKING**
> Why is there a tendency to treat patients with amyotrophic lateral sclerosis (ALS) as if they have impaired intelligence?

PERIPHERAL NEUROPATHY

As the name implies, **peripheral neuropathy** refers to diseases and disorders that affect the peripheral nervous system. This includes the spinal nerve roots, cranial nerves, and peripheral nerves. Most neuropathies arise from damage to or irritation of either the axons or their myelin sheaths. This slows or fully blocks the passage of electrical signals. The various types of peripheral neuropathy are classified according to the site and distribution of damage. For example, damage to sensory nerve fibers may cause numbness and tingling, sensations of cold, or pain that often starts in the hands and feet and spreads toward the central body. Damage to motor nerve fibers may cause muscle weakness and muscle wasting. Damage that occurs to the nerves of the autonomic nervous system may result in blurred vision, impaired or absent sweating, fluctuations in blood pressure (and associated syncope), GI disorders, incontinence, and impotence.

Some peripheral neuropathies have no identifiable cause. Others may be related to specific causes, including the following:

- Diabetes
- Dietary deficiencies (especially of vitamin B)
- Alcoholism
- Uremia
- Leprosy
- Lead poisoning
- Drug intoxication
- Viral infection (e.g., Guillain-Barré syndrome)
- Rheumatoid arthritis
- Systemic lupus erythematosus
- Malignant tumors (e.g., lung cancer)
- Lymphomas
- Leukemias
- Inherited neuropathies (e.g., peroneal muscular atrophy)

When possible, management is aimed at the underlying cause. (For example, blood glucose control in a diabetic patient, and better nutrition.) If management is successful and the cell bodies of the damaged nerves have not been destroyed, full recovery from the neuropathy is possible.

MYOCLONUS

Myoclonus refers to rapid and uncontrollable muscular contractions (jerking) or spasms of one or more muscles. These occur at rest or during movement. The syndrome may be associated with disease of nerves and muscles. It also may be a symptom of a brain disorder (e.g., encephalitis) or seizure disorder. Myoclonus can occur in healthy individuals. An example is a limb "jump" that sometimes happens just before a person falls asleep. The condition is treated with medications to reduce the patient's symptoms. These may include barbiturates, clonazepam, and ***phenytoin***.

SPINA BIFIDA

Spina bifida is a congenital defect in which part of one or more vertebrae fails to develop completely. This leaves a portion of the spinal cord exposed. The condition can occur anywhere on the spine. However, it is most common in the lower back. Although the cause is unknown, spina bifida occurs in about 1 in every 1000 births. It is more likely to occur with extremes of maternal age. A woman who has given birth to one child with spina bifida is 10 times more likely than the average woman to give birth to another affected child (indicating the need for genetic counseling).

Types of Spina Bifida. The severity of spina bifida depends on how much nerve tissue is exposed after the neural tube has closed. The four types of spina bifida are spina bifida occulta, meningocele, myelomeningocele, and encephalocele. Currently the condition has no cure. Treatment includes surgery, medications, and physical therapy. Most patients with spina bifida live into adulthood.

Spina bifida occulta is the most common and least serious form. There is little external evidence of the defect. Meningocele (Fig. 31-15, *A*) is a type of spina bifida in which the nerve tissue of the spinal cord usually is intact and covered with a membranous sac of skin. Meningocele usually does not cause functional problems. However, it requires surgical repair early in life. Myelomeningocele (Fig. 31-15, *B*) is the severest form of spina bifida. The child often is severely handicapped. This type of spina bifida is marked by a raw swelling over the spine and a malformed spinal cord that may or may not be contained in a membranous sac. The legs of these children often are deformed. Also, the condition causes partial or complete paralysis and loss of sensation in all areas below the level of the defect. Associated abnormalities of myelomeningocele include hydrocephalus (excess CSF in the skull) with brain damage, cerebral palsy, epilepsy, and developmental delay. In the fourth and very rare type of spina bifida, encephalocele, the protrusion occurs through the skull. Severe brain damage is common with this condition.

POLIO

Polio (poliomyelitis) is caused by the poliovirus. The virus attacks with variable severity. It may range from not very apparent infection, to a febrile illness without neurological aftereffects, to aseptic meningitis, and finally to paralytic disease (including respiratory paralysis) and possibly death. The incidence of polio has declined in the United States, Canada, and Europe since the development of the Salk and Sabin vaccines in the 1950s. However, the disease may af-

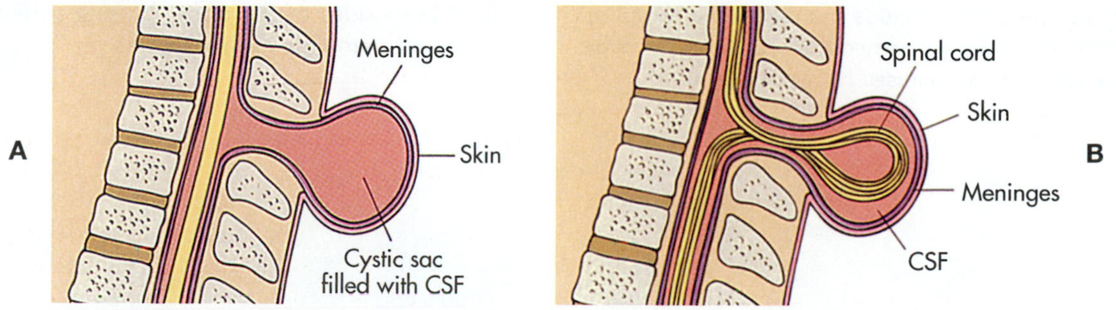

FIGURE 31-15 ■ **A,** Meningocele. **B,** Myelomeningocele.

fect nonimmune adults and indigent (particularly immigrant) children. It remains a serious risk for anyone not vaccinated and traveling in southern Europe, Africa, or Asia. Polio vaccinations are given during infancy. Usually they are given in doses at 2, 14, and 18 months of age in the United States. There is an optional extra dose at 6 months and a booster dose at 5 years.

CRITICAL THINKING

Ask your older friends or relatives about their memories of the polio epidemic. How did it affect their lives?

People infected with the poliovirus can pass large amounts of the virus in their feces. The virus then may be spread directly or indirectly to others by fingers-to-food transmission and by airborne transmission. Signs and symptoms of polio differ in the nonparalytic and paralytic forms. Fever, headache, sore throat, and malaise are common to both forms. However, the paralytic form of polio also is associated with generalized pain, weakness, muscle spasms, and paralysis of limbs and other muscles. If the infection spreads to the brain stem, the person may find it difficult or may be unable to swallow or breathe. A full recovery can be made from nonparalytic polio. Of those who become paralyzed, more than half eventually make a full recovery. (Some patients may develop "postpolio deterioration." They may have new weakness and pain from recovered muscles.) The disease is confirmed though CSF analysis, throat culture, or testing of fecal samples.

SUMMARY

- The human body's ability to maintain a state of balance, or *homeostasis,* results from the nervous system's regulatory and coordinating activities. The blood supply to the brain comes from the vertebral arteries and the internal carotid arteries.
- Some neurological emergencies are a consequence of structural changes or damage, circulatory changes, or alterations in intracranial pressure that affect cerebral blood flow.
- The initial survey should begin by determining the patient's level of consciousness and by ensuring an open and patent airway. Key elements of the physical examination that may provide clues to the nature of the neurological emergency include the patient history and the history of the event, vital signs, and respiratory patterns.
- *Coma* is an abnormally deep state of unconsciousness. The patient cannot be aroused from this state by external stimuli. In general, two mechanisms produce coma: structural lesions and toxic-metabolic states.
- *Stroke* is a sudden interruption in blood flow to the brain that results in a neurological deficit. Strokes can be classified as ischemic strokes or hemorrhagic strokes.
- A *seizure* is a brief alteration in behavior or consciousness. It is caused by abnormal electrical activity of one or more groups of neurons in the brain. In the prehospital setting, determining the cause of a seizure is not as important as other measures. These include managing the complications and recognizing whether the seizure is reversible with therapy (e.g., it is caused by hypoglycemia).
- The four fairly common types of headaches are tension headaches, migraines, cluster headaches, and sinus headaches.
- A brain tumor, or *neoplasm,* is a mass in the cranial cavity. This mass can be either malignant or benign. Heredity may play a role in the development of brain tumors. They also are associated with several risk factors. These include exposure to radiation, tobacco use, dietary habits, some viruses, and the use of some medications.
- A *brain abscess* is a buildup of purulent material (pus) surrounded by a capsule within the brain. It develops from a bacterial infection. The infection often starts in the nasal cavity, middle ear, or mastoid bone.
- Muscular dystrophy is an inherited muscle disorder. The cause is unknown. The disease is marked by a slow but progressive degeneration of muscle fibers.
- Damage to the white matter of the brain in multiple sclerosis may lead to fatigue, vertigo, clumsiness, unsteady gait, slurred speech, blurred or double vision, and facial numbness or pain.
- The term *dystonia* refers to local or diffuse changes in muscle tone. These may cause painful muscle spasms, unusually fixed postures, and strange movement patterns.
- Parkinson disease usually begins as a slight tremor in one hand, arm, or leg. In the later stages, the disease affects both sides of the body, causing stiffness, weakness, and trembling of the muscles.

- The term *central pain syndrome* refers to infection or disease of the trigeminal nerve.
- *Bell palsy* is paralysis of the facial muscles. It is caused by inflammation of the seventh cranial nerve. The condition is usually one sided and temporary. It often develops suddenly.
- Amyotrophic lateral sclerosis is also called *Lou Gehrig disease*. It is one of a group of rare nervous system disorders. In these disorders, the nerves that control muscular activity degenerate in the brain and spinal cord.
- Peripheral neuropathies usually arise from damage to or irritation of either the axons or their myelin sheaths. This slows or fully blocks the passage of electrical signals.
- The term *myoclonus* refers to rapid and uncontrollable muscle contractions or spasms. These occur at rest or during movement.
- *Spina bifida* is a congenital defect in which part of one or more vertebrae fails to develop completely. This leaves a portion of the spinal cord exposed.
- Polio is caused by a virus. The severity of the disease can range from unapparent infection, to a febrile illness without neurological aftereffects, to aseptic meningitis, and finally to paralytic disease and possibly death.

REFERENCES

1. US Department of Transportation, National Highway Traffic Safety Administration: *EMT-paramedic national standard curriculum,* 1998, Washington, DC, The Department.
2. American Heart Association: *Advanced cardiac life support,* Dallas, 1997, The Association.
3. American Heart Association: Guidelines 2000 for cardiopulmonary resuscitation and emergency cardiovascular care, International Consensus on Science, *Circulation* 102(8):204, 2000.
4. Kothari R et al: Early stroke recognition: developing an out-of-hospital stroke scale, *Acad Emerg Med* 4(10):986, 1997.
5. American Heart Association: Guidelines 2000 for cardiopulmonary resuscitation and emergency cardiovascular care, International Consensus on Science, *Circulation* 102(8):209, 2000.
6. Rosen P, Barkin R: *Emergency medicine: concepts and clinical practice,* ed 4, St Louis, 1998, Mosby.
7. McCance K, Huether S: Pathophysiology: the biologic basis for disease in adults and children, ed 2, St Louis, 1994, Mosby.

CHAPTER

32

Endocrinology

OBJECTIVES

Upon completion of this chapter, the paramedic student will be able to:

1. Describe how hormones secreted from endocrine glands help the body to maintain homeostasis.
2. Describe the anatomy and physiology of the pancreas and how its hormones work to maintain normal glucose metabolism.
3. Discuss pathophysiology as a basis for key signs and symptoms, patient assessment, and patient management for diabetes and diabetic emergencies of hypoglycemia, diabetic ketoacidosis, and hyperosmolar hyperglycemic nonketotic coma.
4. Discuss pathophysiology as a basis for key signs and symptoms, patient assessment, and patient management for disorders of the thyroid gland.
5. Discuss pathophysiology as a basis for key signs and symptoms, patient assessment, and patient management of Cushing syndrome and Addison disease.

KEY TERMS

Addison disease: A rare and potentially life-threatening disorder caused by a deficiency of the corticosteroid hormones normally produced by the adrenal cortex.

Cushing syndrome: A condition caused by an abnormally high circulating level of corticosteroid hormones produced naturally by the adrenal glands.

gluconeogenesis: The formation of glycogen from fatty acids and proteins rather than carbohydrates.

glycogenolysis: The breakdown of glycogen to glucose.

hyperosmolar hyperglycemic nonketotic (HHNK) coma: A diabetic coma in which the level of ketone bodies is normal. It is caused by hyperosmolarity of extracellular fluid and results in dehydration of intracellular fluid.

ketogenesis: The formation or production of ketone bodies.

myxedema: A condition that results from a deficiency in thyroid hormone.

thyrotoxicosis: A term that refers to any toxic condition that results from thyroid hyperfunction.

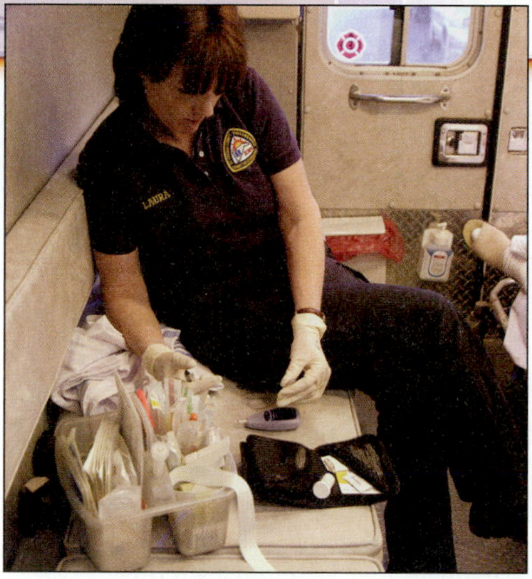

The endocrine system and the nervous system allow the body to regulate many functions. Some patients that paramedics treat will have endocrine system disorders. These disorders can range from minor changes in functioning to life-threatening conditions.

ANATOMY AND PHYSIOLOGY OF THE ENDOCRINE SYSTEM

As described in Chapter 6, the endocrine system is composed of ductless glands and tissues that produce and secrete hormones. The major endocrine glands are the pituitary, thyroid, and parathyroid glands; the adrenal cortex and medulla; the pancreatic islets; and the ovaries and testes (Fig. 32-1). Other specialized groups of cells that secrete hormones are found in the kidneys and the mucosa of the gastrointestinal (GI) tract.

Endocrine Gland Functions

Endocrine glands secrete hormones directly into the bloodstream. They regulate various metabolic functions. The products of endocrine glands travel via the blood (or tissue fluids). Thus they are able to exert their effects on the entire body. The endocrine hormones are released either in response to a change in the cellular environment or to maintain a normal level of certain hormones or substances. This integrated chemical and coordination system enables reproduction, growth and development, and the regulation of energy. Target organs and body tissues have hormone receptors and are able to respond to a certain hormone.

CRITICAL THINKING

How are hormones and their target organs like a lock and key?

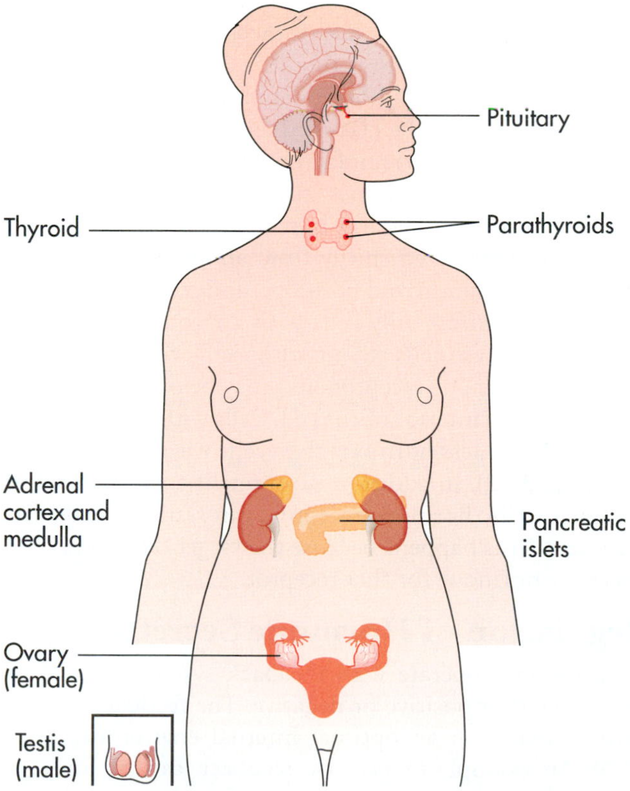

FIGURE 32-1 ■ Major endocrine glands.

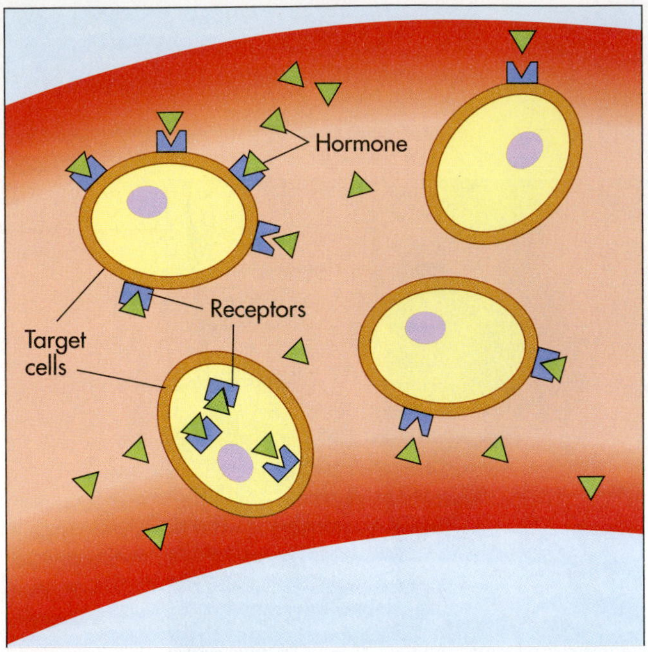

FIGURE 32-2 ■ Target cell concept. Cells with fewer receptor sites bind with less hormone than cells with many receptor sites.

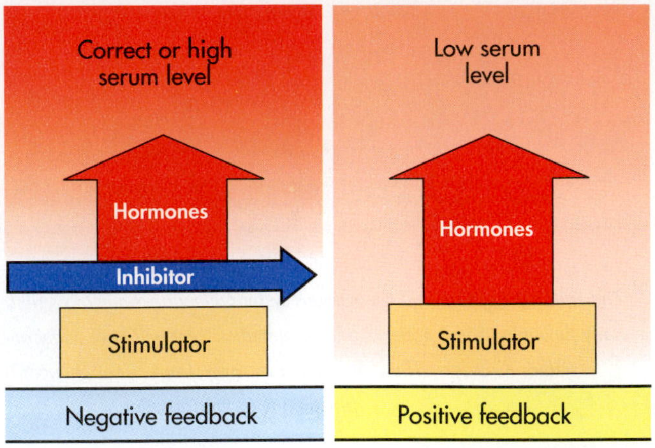

FIGURE 32-3 ■ Negative feedback.

HORMONE RECEPTORS

Most hormones can be categorized as proteins, polypeptides, derivatives of amino acids, or lipids. Each hormone may affect a specific organ or tissue, or each hormone may have a general effect on the entire body. (See Chapter 6 for a review of endocrine glands, hormones, and their functions.) Hormones also may be classified as steroid or nonsteroid. Steroid hormones are manufactured by endocrine cells from cholesterol. These hormones include cortisol, aldosterone, estrogen, progesterone, and testosterone. Nonsteroid hormones are synthesized chiefly from amino acids. These include insulin, parathyroid hormone, and others.

Hormones affect only cells with appropriate receptors. They act on these cells to initiate specific cell functions or activities. Hormone receptor sites may be on the cell membrane or in the interior of the cell. Cells with fewer receptor sites bind with less hormone than cells with many receptor sites (Fig. 32-2). In addition, abnormalities in or the presence of specific hormone receptors can result in endocrine disorders. This happens because the target cells completely reject the hormone for that receptor.

Regulation of Hormone Secretion

All hormones operate with feedback systems. These systems are either positive or negative. The feedback systems help to maintain an optimal internal environment (Fig. 32-3). An example of positive feedback can be found in childbirth. The hormone oxytocin stimulates and enhances labor contractions. As the baby moves toward the birth canal, pressure receptors in the cervix send messages to the brain to produce oxytocin. Oxytocin travels to the uterus through the bloodstream. It stimulates the muscles in the uterine wall to contract more strongly. The contractions intensify and increase until the baby is outside the birth canal. When the stimulus to the pressure receptors ends, oxytocin production stops. Labor contractions also stop.

Negative feedback is the mechanism most commonly used to maintain homeostasis. The term usually refers to an increase in the blood level of hormones or hormone-related substances. This increase suppresses further release of the hormone. For example, after a person eats a candy bar, the following occurs:

1. Glucose from the ingested lactose or sucrose is absorbed in the intestine. Consequently, the level of glucose in the blood rises.
2. The increase in the blood glucose concentration stimulates the pancreas to release insulin. Insulin facilitates the entry of glucose into the cells. As a result, the blood glucose level falls.
3. When the blood glucose level has dropped sufficiently, the endocrine cells in the pancreas stop producing and releasing insulin.

On the other hand, hormone production is stimulated when serum levels of the hormone fall. For example, the hypothalamus receptors monitor blood levels of thyroid hormones. Low blood levels of thyroid-stimulating hormone (TSH) cause the release of TSH-releasing hormone from the hypothalamus. This, in turn, causes the release of TSH from the anterior pituitary. TSH travels to the thyroid. There, it promotes the production of thyroid hormones. These, in turn, regulate the metabolic rate and body temperature.

SPECIFIC DISORDERS OF THE ENDOCRINE SYSTEM

Disorders of the endocrine system arise from the effects of an imbalance in the production of one or more hormones. They also arise from the effects of a change in the body's ability to use the hormones produced. The clinical effects of endocrine gland disorders are determined by the degree of dysfunction. They also are determined by the individ-

TABLE 32-1 Specific Disorders of the Endocrine System

GLAND	DISORDER
Pancreas	Diabetes mellitus (types 1 and 2)
	Hyperosmolar hyperglycemic nonketotic (HHNK) coma
Thyroid	Hyperthyroidism
	Hypothyroidism
	Myxedema
	Thyroid storm
	Thyrotoxicosis
Adrenal	Addison disease
	Cushing syndrome

ual's age and gender. Specific disorders of the endocrine system in this chapter include those found in Table 32-1.

DISORDERS OF THE PANCREAS: DIABETES MELLITUS

Diabetes mellitus is a systemic disease of the endocrine system. It usually results from a dysfunction of the pancreas. It is a complex disorder of fat, carbohydrate, and protein metabolism that affects more than 15.7 million Americans, both children and adults.[1] Diabetes mellitus is potentially lethal. It can put the patient at risk for several kinds of true medical emergencies.

Anatomy and Physiology of the Pancreas

The pancreas is important in the absorption and use of carbohydrates, fat, and protein. It is the chief regulator of glucose levels in the blood. The pancreas is located retroperitoneally adjacent to the duodenum on the right and extending to the spleen on the left. The healthy pancreas has exocrine and endocrine functions. To review, exocrine glands secrete substances through a duct onto the inner surface of an organ or the outer surface of the body. Endocrine glands are those that secrete chemicals directly (not through a duct) into the bloodstream. The exocrine portion consists of *acini* (glands that produce pancreatic juice) and a duct system. The duct system carries the pancreatic juice to the small intestine. The endocrine portion consists of pancreatic islets (islets of Langerhans) that produce hormones (Fig. 32-4).

ISLETS OF LANGERHANS AND PANCREATIC HORMONES

About 500,000 to 1 million pancreatic islets are dispersed among the ducts and the acini of the pancreas. Each islet is composed of beta cells, alpha cells, and other cells. The beta cells secrete insulin at a daily average of 0.6 units per kilogram of body weight. The alpha cells secrete glucagon. The other cells are of questionable function. Some of these are delta cells, which secrete the hormone somatostatin. This hormone inhibits the secretion of growth hormone. Nerves from both divisions of the autonomic nervous system innervate the pancreatic islets, and each islet is surrounded by a well-developed capillary network.

CRITICAL THINKING

Consider that part of a patient's pancreas must be removed as a result of traumatic injury. Will the patient still be able to produce insulin and glucagon?

INSULIN

Insulin is a small protein. It is released by the beta cells when blood glucose levels rise. The main functions of insulin are to increase glucose transport into cells, increase glucose metabolism by cells, increase liver glycogen levels, and decrease the blood glucose concentration toward normal (Box 32-1). Many of the functions of insulin antagonize the effects of glucagon.

GLUCAGON

Glucagon is a protein released by the alpha cells when blood glucose levels fall. Glucagon has two major effects. One effect is to increase blood glucose levels. It does this by stimulating the liver to release glucose stores from glycogen and other glucose storage sites. (This is called **glycogenolysis.**) The other effect is to stimulate **gluconeogenesis** (glucose formation) through the breakdown of fats and fatty acids, thereby maintaining a normal blood glucose level (Fig. 32-5).

GROWTH HORMONE

Growth hormone (GH) is a polypeptide hormone. It is produced and secreted by the anterior pituitary gland. GH secretion is triggered by many physiological stimuli. These include exercise, stress, sleep, and hypoglycemia. GH acts as an insulin antagonist. It decreases insulin actions on cell membranes. This reduces the capacity of muscles and adipose and liver cells to absorb glucose.

Regulation of Glucose Metabolism

Under normal conditions, the body maintains the serum glucose level in the blood at 60 to 120 mg/dL. An understanding of food intake and digestion is required to understand glucose metabolism.

DIETARY INTAKE

The three main organic components of food are carbohydrates, fats, and proteins. (Food also contains minerals and vitamins.) Carbohydrates are found in all sugary, starchy foods. They are a ready source of near-instant energy. They are the first food substances to enter the bloodstream after a meal is ingested. Carbohydrates yield the simple sugar glucose. If not "burned" for immediate energy, glucose is

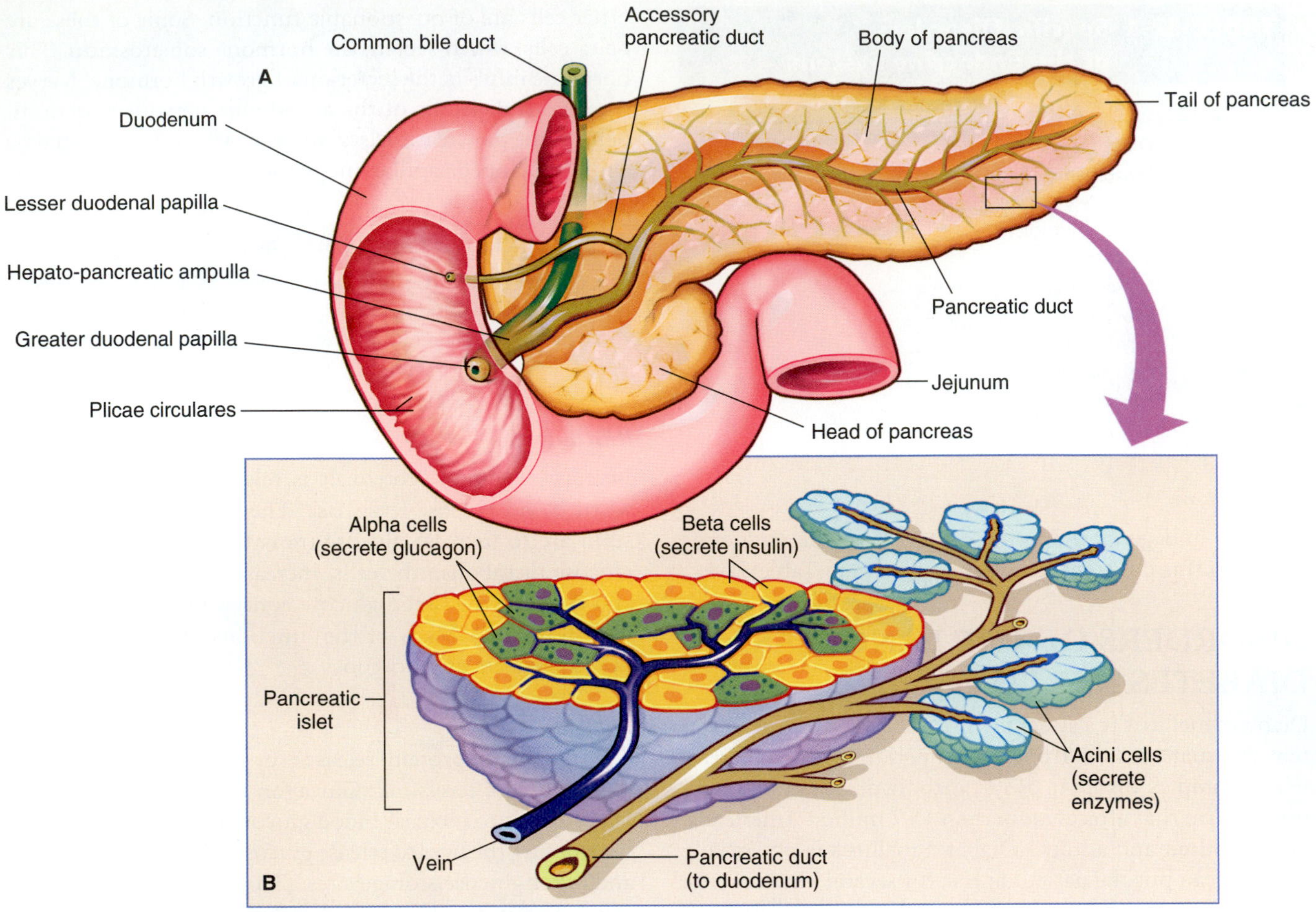

FIGURE 32-4 ■ Two pancreatic islets (islets of Langerhans), or hormone-producing areas, are evident among the pancreatic cells that produce the pancreatic digestive juice.

BOX 32-1 Primary Functions of Insulin

- To increase glucose transport into cells
- To increase glucose metabolism by cells
- To increase liver glycogen levels
- To decrease blood glucose concentration toward normal levels

stored in the liver and muscles as glycogen for short-term energy needs or converted into fat by adipose tissue and stored for intermediate and long-term needs.

PROCESS OF DIGESTION

Before food compounds can be used by body cells, they must be digested and absorbed into the bloodstream. Digestion begins in the mouth. It is accomplished by physical forces (chewing) and chemical (enzymatic) forces. This begins the process that reduces the food to soluble molecules and particles small enough to be absorbed. After food is swallowed, it enters the stomach. There, various nutrients are absorbed into the circulatory system. These nutrients include glucose, salts, water, and some other substances (alcohol and certain other drugs). The remaining material (chyme) is shunted from the stomach into the intestine for further digestion.

The duodenum signals the release of hormones that mobilize the pancreas to contribute its molecule-splitting enzymes and the gallbladder to release bile salts. These enzymes and salts neutralize acids. They also help emulsify fats. Carbohydrates are absorbed as simple sugars. Fats are absorbed as fatty acids and glycerol. Proteins are absorbed as amino acids. These nutrients are then carried from the intestine to the liver by way of the portal vein. Water and remaining salts are absorbed from food residues reaching the colon. The liver synthesizes glycogen from the absorbed glucose, lipoproteins from the absorbed fatty acids, and many proteins required for health from absorbed amino acids.

Carbohydrate Metabolism. The secretion of insulin is controlled by chemical, neural, and hormonal means. An increased concentration of blood glucose, parasympathetic stimulation, and gastrointestinal hormones involved with regulation of digestion cause beta cells of the pancreas to release insulin after dietary intake of carbohydrates. Insulin

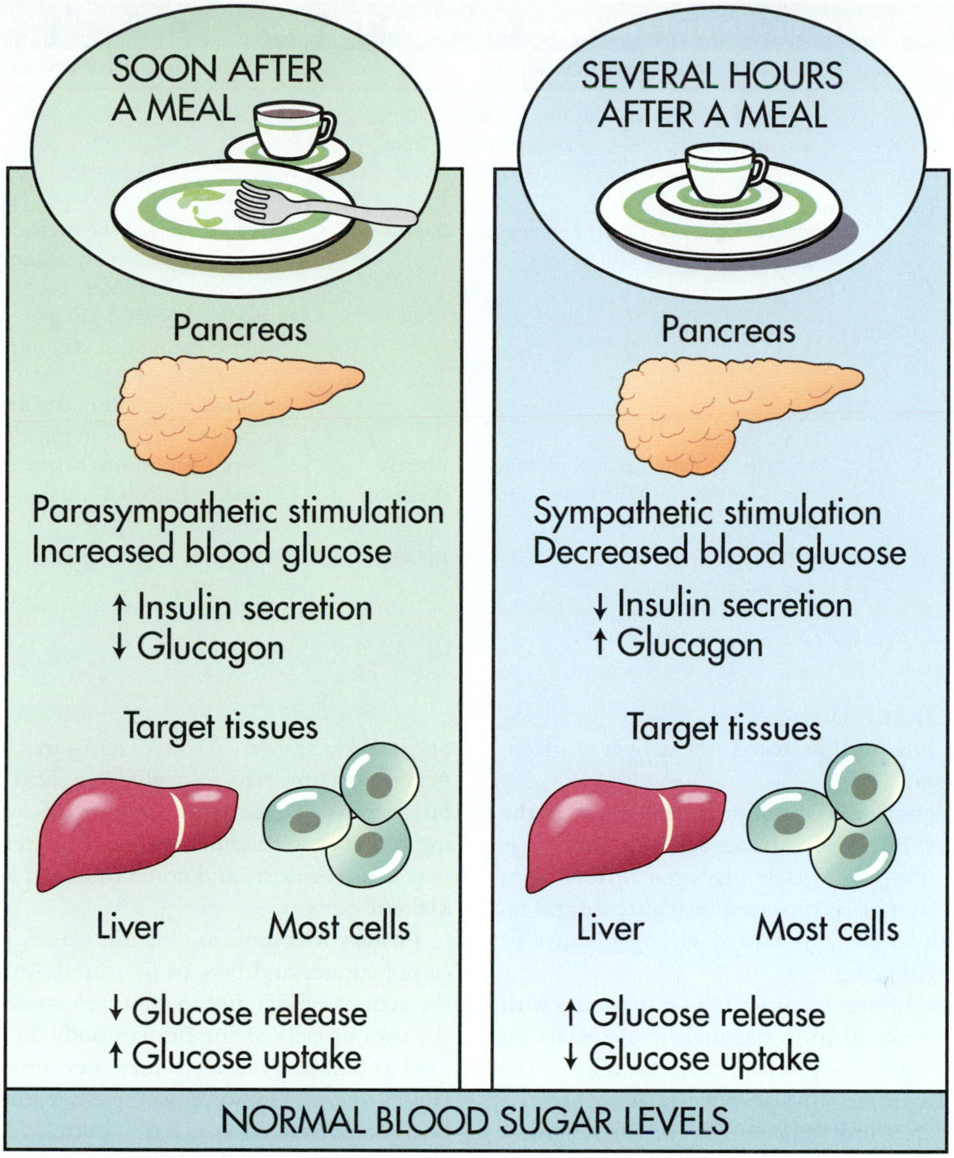

FIGURE 32-5 ■ Regulation of insulin and glucagon secretion. Sympathetic stimulation and decreasing concentrations of glucose increase the secretion of glucagon, which acts primarily on liver cells to increase the rate of glycogen breakdown and the secretion of glucose from the liver. The release of glucose from the liver helps maintain blood glucose levels. Increasing blood glucose levels has an inhibitory effect on glucagon secretion. Increasing concentrations of glucose and amino acids stimulate the beta cells of the islets to secrete insulin. In addition, parasympathetic stimulation causes insulin secretion. Insulin acts on most tissues to increase the uptake of glucose and amino acids. As the blood levels of glucose and amino acids decrease, the rate of insulin secretion also decreases.

travels through the blood to target tissues. There it combines with specific chemical receptors on the surface of the cell membrane to permit glucose to enter the cell (Table 32-2). This allows the cells to use glucose for energy. It also prevents the breakdown of alternative energy sources (proteins and fat cells). In addition, it promotes the uptake of glucose into the liver, where it is converted to glycogen for storage. This rapid uptake and storage of glucose normally prevents a large increase in blood glucose levels, even just after a normal meal.

CRITICAL THINKING

Why do diabetics eat carbohydrates instead of protein or fat when they sense that their glucose level is too low?

When the blood glucose level begins to fall, the liver releases glucose back into the circulating blood. Thus the liver removes glucose from the blood when it is in excess after dietary intake. Also, it returns it to the blood when it is needed between meals. Under normal circumstances, about

TABLE 32-2 Effects of Insulin and Glucagon on Target Tissues

TARGET TISSUE	RESPONSE TO INSULIN	RESPONSE TO GLUCAGON
Skeletal muscle, cardiac muscle, cartilage, bone, fibroblasts, leukocytes, and mammary glands	Increased glucose uptake and glycogen synthesis; increased uptake of certain amino acids	Little effect
Liver	Increased glycogen synthesis; increased use of glucose for energy (glycolysis)	Rapid increase in the breakdown of glycogen to glucose (glycogenolysis) and release of glucose into the blood Increased formation of glucose (gluconeogenesis) from amino acids and, to some degree, from fats Increased metabolism of fatty acids, resulting in increased ketones in the blood
Adipose cells	Increased glucose uptake, glycogen synthesis, fat synthesis, and fatty acid uptake; increased glycolysis	High concentrations cause breakdown of fats (lipolysis); probably unimportant under most conditions
Nervous system	Little effect except to increase glucose uptake in the satiety center	No effect

From Seeley R: *Anatomy and physiology*, ed 2, St Louis, 1992, Mosby.

60% of the glucose in a meal is stored in the liver as glycogen and released later.

If the muscles are not exercised after a meal, much of the glucose transported into the muscle cells by insulin is stored as muscle glycogen. Muscle glycogen differs from liver glycogen. It cannot be reconverted into glucose and released into the circulation. The stored glycogen must be used by the muscle for energy.

The brain is quite different from other body tissues with regard to glucose uptake. Insulin has little or no effect on the uptake or use of glucose by the brain; the cells of the brain do not have adequate storage capacity. Also, because the brain normally uses only glucose for energy, it cannot depend on stored supplies of glycogen. Thus it is essential that serum glucose be maintained at a level that provides adequate energy to these tissues. When the serum glucose level falls too low, signs and symptoms of hypoglycemia can develop quickly. These include progressive irritability, altered mental states, fainting, convulsions, and even coma.

Fat Metabolism. Only a limited amount of glycogen can be stored in the liver and skeletal muscles. Therefore one third of any glucose passing through the liver is converted to fatty acids. Under the influence of insulin, fatty acids are converted to triglycerides. (These are storable fats.) They are stored in adipose tissue. In the absence of insulin, the stored fat is broken down. The plasma concentration of free fatty acids rapidly increases. An inadequate level of insulin in the blood can result in high levels of triglycerides and cholesterol (in the form of lipoproteins) in the plasma. This is thought to contribute to the development of atherosclerosis in patients with serious diabetes.

If needed (as in the absence of insulin), fatty acids in the liver can be metabolized and used for energy. A byproduct of the breakdown of fatty acids in the liver is acetate. Acetate is converted to acetoacetic acid and beta hydroxybutyric acid. These products are released into the circulating blood as ketone bodies (see Chapter 7). Ketone bodies may cause acidosis and coma (diabetic ketoacidosis) in the diabetic patient.

Protein Metabolism. Insulin causes proteins, as well as carbohydrates and fats, to be stored. Amino acids (through the actions of GH and insulin) are actively transported into the various cells of the human body. Most amino acids are used as building blocks to form new proteins. (This is called *protein synthesis*.) However, some enter the metabolic cycle by being converted to glucose after initial breakdown in the liver.

In the absence of insulin, protein storage stops. Also, protein breakdown (particularly in muscle) begins. This releases large amounts of amino acids into the circulation. The excess amino acids are used directly for energy or as substrates for gluconeogenesis. The degradation of the amino acids leads to increased urea excretion in the urine. This "protein wasting" has serious effects in diabetes mellitus. It leads to extreme weakness and dysfunction of many organs.

GLUCAGON AND ITS FUNCTIONS

Glucagon has several functions that are the opposite of the functions of insulin. The most important is to increase the blood glucose concentration. Glucagon has two major effects on glucose metabolism. One is the breakdown of liver glycogen. The other is increased gluconeogenesis.

As the serum glucose level returns to normal (several hours after dietary intake), insulin secretion decreases with continued fasting. Then the blood sugar level begins to drop. As a result, glucagon, cortisol, GH, and epinephrine (from sympathetic stimulation) are secreted. This initiates

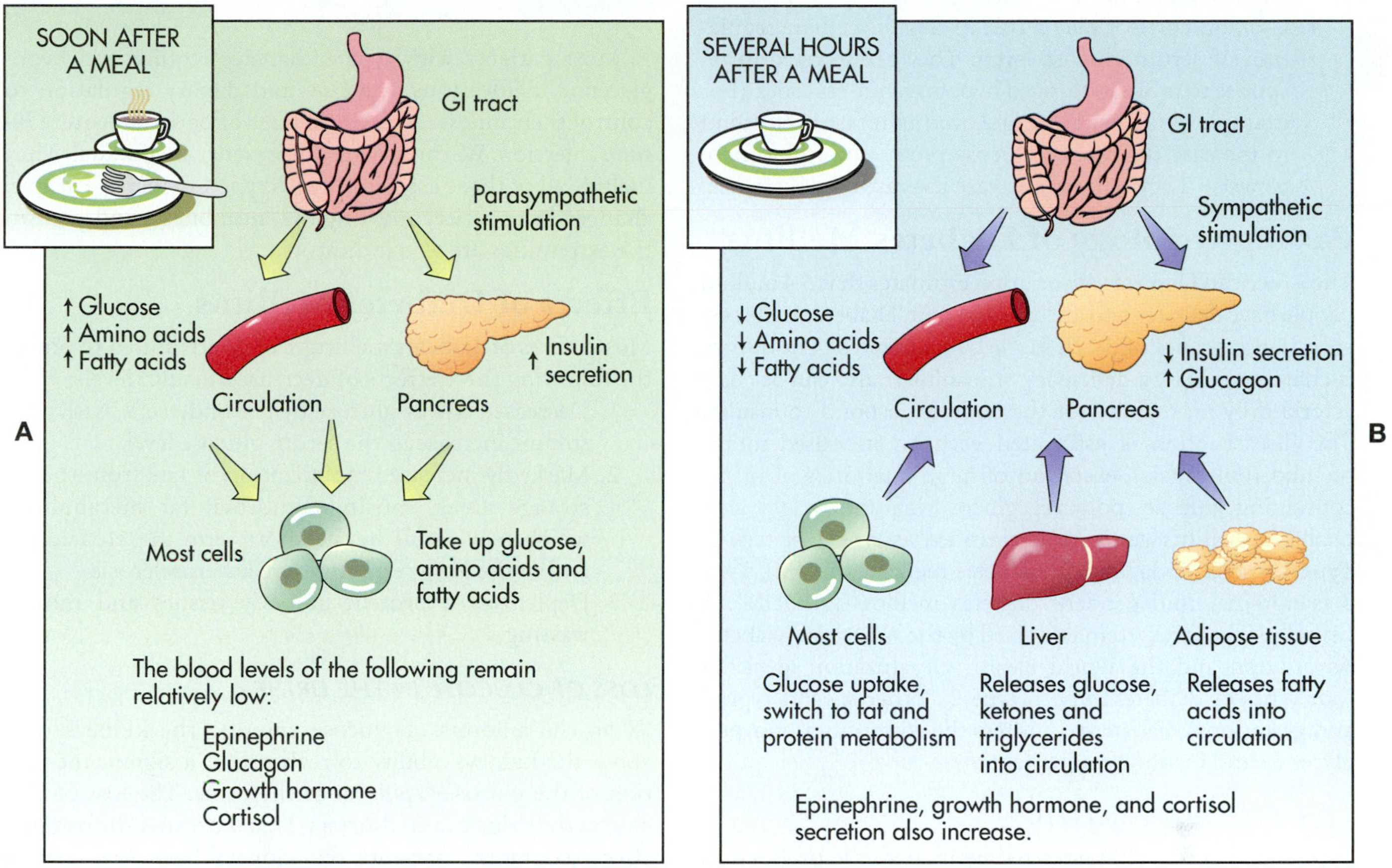

FIGURE 32-6 ■ A, Soon after a meal, glucose, amino acids, and fatty acids enter the bloodstream from the intestinal tract. Glucose and amino acids stimulate insulin secretion. Cells take up the glucose and amino acids and use them in their metabolism. **B**, Several hours after a meal, absorption from the intestinal tract decreases, and the blood levels of glucose, amino acids, and fatty acids decrease. As a result, insulin secretion decreases, and glucagon, epinephrine, and growth hormone (GH) secretion increases. Cell uptake of glucose decreases, and usage of fats and proteins increases.

the release of glucose from glycogen and other glucose-storage sites. Glycogen is converted back to glucose and released into the blood. Uptake of glucose by most tissues helps to maintain the blood glucose at levels necessary for normal function (Fig. 32-6).

CRITICAL THINKING

What signs and symptoms will the patient have in response to the release of epinephrine when blood glucose falls?

In summary, the four mechanisms for achieving adequate blood glucose regulation are as follows:

1. The liver functions as a blood glucose buffer system. It removes glucose from the blood when it is in excess (and stores it as glycogen). It also returns glucose to the blood when the glucose concentration and insulin secretion decline.
2. Insulin and glucagon function as a feedback control system. They work to maintain normal serum glucose concentrations. When serum glucose levels rise, insulin

is secreted to lower them toward normal. On the other hand, when serum glucose levels fall, glucagon is secreted to raise the serum glucose level toward normal.

3. Low serum glucose levels stimulate the sympathetic nervous system to secrete epinephrine. Epinephrine and, to a lesser degree, norepinephrine have a glucagon-like effect that promotes liver glycogenolysis.
4. GH and cortisol play a role in less immediate regulation of serum glucose levels. They are secreted in response to more prolonged hypoglycemic episodes. (For example, this might be a late overnight fast.) They tend to increase the rate of glucose production (gluconeogenesis). They tend to decrease the rate of glucose use.

Pathophysiology of Diabetes Mellitus

The American Diabetes Association estimates that 5.4 million people have diabetes and are unaware of it. Diabetes is the seventh leading cause of death in the United States.[1] The disease is characterized by a deficiency of insulin. It also can be characterized by an inability of the body to respond to insulin. The disease often is associated with an increased intake of fluid (polydipsia), excretion of large quantities of urine-containing glucose (polyuria, glucosuria), and weight loss. Diabetes mellitus generally is classified as type 1 or type 2. Type 1 is insulin-dependent diabetes mellitus (IDDM). Type 2 is non-insulin-dependent diabetes mellitus (NIDDM). A new classification system endorsed by the American Diabetes Association and the World Health Organization identifies four types of diabetes: type 1, type 2, "other specific types," and gestational diabetes to address the continuum of hyperglycemia and insulin requirements.[2]

TYPE 1 DIABETES MELLITUS

Type 1 diabetes is characterized by inadequate production of insulin by the pancreas. This form of diabetes affects 1 in every 10 diabetics. It may occur any time after birth. However, it usually occurs in teenagers and young adults. Heredity is a factor in type 1 diabetes. The disease appears to be an autoimmune phenomenon. It results from a genetic abnormality or susceptibility that causes the body to destroy its own insulin-producing cells. A person who has a parent or sibling with type 1 diabetes has a 10% chance of developing the disease by age 50.[1] Type 1 diabetes requires lifelong treatment with ***insulin*** injections, exercise, and diet regulation. The symptoms of type 1 diabetes usually appear suddenly. They include polyuria, polydipsia, dizziness, blurred vision, and rapid, unexplained weight loss.

TYPE 2 DIABETES MELLITUS

Type 2 diabetes usually is characterized by a decrease in the production of insulin by the pancreatic beta cells and diminished tissue sensitivity to insulin. The disease occurs most often in adults over 40 years of age and in those who are overweight. (Obesity predisposes a person to this form of diabetes. This is because larger amounts of insulin are needed for metabolic control in obese individuals than in those with normal weight.) Others at increased risk for type 2 diabetes are Native Americans, Hispanics, and African-Americans.

> **CRITICAL THINKING**
> Would patients with type 1 or type 2 diabetes have an increased risk of complications related to this disease?

Most patients with type 2 diabetes require oral hypoglycemic medications, exercise, and dietary regulation to control their illness. A small number of patients require ***insulin*** injection. Warning signs (if present) are gradual. They include all of those associated with type 1 diabetes. Fatigue, changes in appetite, and tingling, numbness, and pain in the extremities are also indicators.

Effects of Diabetes Mellitus

Most effects of diabetes mellitus can be attributed to one of the following three effects of decreased insulin levels:

1. Decreased use of glucose by the body cells, with a resultant increase in the serum glucose level
2. Markedly increased mobilization of fats from the fat storage areas, causing abnormal fat metabolism, which may result in the short term in ketoacidosis and in the long term in severe atherosclerosis
3. Depletion of protein in body tissues and muscle wasting

LOSS OF GLUCOSE IN THE URINE

When the amount of glucose entering the kidneys rises above the kidneys' ability to reabsorb it, a significant portion of the glucose "spills" into the urine. The loss of glucose in the urine causes diuresis. This is because the osmotic effect of glucose prevents the kidneys from reabsorbing fluid (osmotic diuresis). The effect is dehydration.

ACIDOSIS IN DIABETES

The shift from carbohydrate to fat metabolism results in the formation of ketone bodies. (These are called *ketoacids.*) Ketone bodies are strong acids. Continuous production of ketoacids leads to a metabolic acidosis. Often the respiratory system at least partly compensates for this acidosis (indicated by Kussmaul respirations). The kidneys' ability to clear the acid is overwhelmed by the continuous production of ketone bodies. Profound acidosis eventually occurs. This acidosis, along with the usually severe dehydration that occurs as a result of the osmotic diuresis, can lead to death. Treatment of this condition can be lifesaving.

Diabetes mellitus is a systemic disease with many long-term complications, including the following:

- Blindness (5000 diabetics lose their sight each year)
- Kidney disease (10% of all diabetics develop some form of kidney disease, including end-stage kidney failure, which requires dialysis or kidney transplant)
- Peripheral neuropathy, which results in nerve damage to the hands and feet and an increased incidence of foot infections

- Autonomic neuropathy, which damages the nerves controlling voluntary and involuntary functions and may affect sexual function, bladder and bowel control, and blood pressure
- Heart disease and stroke
  - High blood glucose and blood fat levels contribute to atherosclerosis.
  - Diabetics are two to four times as likely to develop heart disease as nondiabetics and are two to six times as likely to have a stroke.
- Peripheral vascular disease (also secondary to atherosclerosis), which results in the need for amputations

Management

The treatment of diabetes mellitus consists of drug therapy (***insulin*** or oral hypoglycemic agents), diet regulation, and exercise. These therapies allow patients to control their serum glucose levels. They also help restore normal metabolism. Pancreatic transplants remain an experimental treatment for diabetes mellitus.

INSULIN

Genetically engineered human ***insulin*** is available in rapid-, intermediate-, and long-acting preparations. (***Insulin*** is administered by injection; it is a protein that would be digested if it were consumed orally.) An insulin-dependent diabetic usually takes one or two doses of a long-acting ***insulin*** preparation each day. The person also takes additional amounts of a rapid-acting ***insulin*** (lasting only a few hours) at meal times.

Another way for the patient to self-administer ***insulin*** is with an insulin infusion pump. These devices allow for a continuous dose of ***insulin***. They are adjusted so that the blood glucose level is constantly controlled. The patient must regularly monitor the glucose level. This ensures adequate medication control. Medication balance is delicate. The same dosage of ***insulin*** that appears correct at one time may be too much or too little at another time. This depends on various factors. (Some of these include exercise and infection.)

ORAL HYPOGLYCEMIC AGENTS

Oral hypoglycemic agents stimulate the release of insulin from the pancreas. They are effective only in patients who have functioning beta cells (type 2 diabetes). Commonly prescribed oral hypoglycemic agents include chlorpropamide, tolazamide, tolbutamide, acetohexamide, glipizide, and glyburide. New drugs have been developed and approved by the U.S. Food and Drug Administration (FDA) to help treat type 2 diabetes. Pioglitazone increases a patient's sensitivity to insulin. Glyburide and metformin tablets lower blood sugar by causing more of the body's own insulin to be released, by decreasing the production and absorption of blood sugar, and by helping the body use its own insulin more effectively. These newer drugs have important side effects. They require careful patient monitoring (e.g., periodic tests for liver and kidney function).

Diabetic Emergencies

Three life-threatening conditions may result from diabetes mellitus: hypoglycemia (insulin shock), hyperglycemia (diabetic ketoacidosis), and **hyperosmolar hyperglycemic nonketotic (HHNK) coma.**

HYPOGLYCEMIA

Hypoglycemia is a syndrome related to blood glucose levels below 80 mg/dL. Symptoms usually occur at levels less than 60 mg/dL or at slightly higher blood glucose levels if the fall has been rapid. The condition also may occur in patients who are not diabetic. It usually is a result of excessive response to glucose absorption, physical exertion, alcohol or drug effects, pregnancy and lactation, or decreased dietary intake. In diabetics, hypoglycemic reactions usually are caused by the following:

- Too much ***insulin*** (or oral hypoglycemic medication)
- Decreased dietary intake (a delayed or missed meal)
- Unusual or vigorous physical activity

Less common causes and predisposing factors include the following:

- Chronic alcoholism (alcohol depletes liver glycogen stores)
- Adrenal gland dysfunction
- Liver disease (i.e., hepatic insufficiency or failure)
- Malnutrition
- Pancreatic tumor
- Cancer
- Hypothermia
- Sepsis
- Administration of beta blockers (e.g., ***propranolol***)
- Administration of salicylates in ill infants or children
- Intentional overdose with ***insulin***, oral hypoglycemic agents, or salicylates

Signs and Symptoms. The signs and symptoms of hypoglycemia usually appear quickly (often within minutes). They are related to the release of epinephrine as the body tries to compensate for a drop in blood sugar. In the early stages, the patient may complain of extreme hunger. He or she may demonstrate one or more of the following signs and symptoms because of decreased glucose availability to the brain:

- Nervousness, trembling
- Irritability
- Psychotic (combative) behavior
- Weakness and incoordination
- Confusion
- Appearance of intoxication
- Weak, rapid pulse
- Cold, clammy skin
- Drowsiness
- Seizures
- Coma (in severe cases)

Hypoglycemia should be suspected in any diabetic patient with behavioral changes, confusion, abnormal neurological signs, or unconsciousness. This condition is a true

BOX 32-2 Common Causes of Diabetic Ketoacidosis

- Inadequate insulin dose
- Failure to take insulin
- Infection
- Increased stress (trauma, surgery)
- Increased dietary intake
- Decreased metabolic rate
- Other, less common predisposing factors, including significant emotional stress, alcohol consumption (often associated with hypoglycemia), and pregnancy

emergency. It requires immediate administration of glucose to prevent permanent brain damage or death.

CRITICAL THINKING

Why might a call for a patient with diabetic ketoacidosis (DKA) be dispatched as a behavioral emergency?

DIABETIC KETOACIDOSIS

Diabetic ketoacidosis (DKA) results from an absence of or resistance to insulin (Box 32-2). The low insulin level prevents glucose from entering the cells. As a result, glucose accumulates in the blood. Consequently, the cells become starved for glucose and begin to use other sources of energy (principally fat). The metabolism of fat generates fatty acids and glycerol. The glycerol provides some energy to the cells, but the fatty acids are further metabolized to form ketoacids, resulting in acidosis.

Any acidosis increases the loss of potassium from the cells into the blood. This results in a high potassium concentration in the urine and a loss of total body potassium. In addition, the sodium concentration outside the cells usually decreases. It is replaced by increased amounts of hydrogen ions. This adds greatly to the acidosis. As blood sugar rises, the patient undergoes massive osmotic diuresis. This, combined with vomiting, causes dehydration and shock. The associated electrolyte imbalances may cause cardiac dysrhythmias and altered neuromuscular activity, including seizures.

Signs and Symptoms. The signs and symptoms of DKA usually are related to diuresis and acidosis. They usually are slow in onset (over 12 to 48 hours) and include the following:

- Diuresis
- Warm, dry skin
- Dry mucous membranes
- Tachycardia, thready pulse
- Postural hypotension
- Weight loss
- Polyuria
- Polydipsia
- Acidosis
- Abdominal pain (usually generalized)
- Anorexia, nausea, vomiting
- Acetone breath odor (fruity odor)
- Kussmaul respirations in an attempt to reduce carbon dioxide levels
- Decreased level of consciousness

DKA patients seldom are deeply comatose. Patients who are unresponsive should be assessed for another cause, such as head injury, stroke, or drug overdose.

CRITICAL THINKING

How can you distinguish Kussmaul respirations from hyperventilation?

HYPEROSMOLAR HYPERGLYCEMIC NONKETOTIC (HHNK) COMA

HHNK is a life-threatening emergency. It often occurs in older patients with type 2 diabetes or in patients with undiagnosed diabetes. The syndrome is easily mistaken for DKA. It differs from DKA in that enough insulin may be present to prevent metabolism of fats **(ketogenesis)** and the development of ketoacidosis. However, the amount of insulin may not be enough to prevent glucose use by peripheral tissues or to reduce gluconeogenesis by the liver. HHNK develops from sustained hyperglycemia that produces a hyperosmolar state. This is followed by an osmotic diuresis that results in marked dehydration and electrolyte losses. These patients usually have greater hyperglycemia (blood glucose levels of up to 1000 mg/dL) than those with DKA. This is because they are more dehydrated. They also have less ketone formation. This is because the presence of insulin in the liver directs free fatty acids into nonketogenic pathways. This results in less acidemia than in patients with DKA (Fig. 32-7).

HHNK tends to develop slowly, often over several days. It has a high mortality rate. Early signs and symptoms are mostly related to volume depletion. They include polyuria and polydipsia. Associated signs and symptoms may include orthostatic hypotension, dry mucous membranes, and tachycardia. CNS dysfunction may result in lethargy, confusion, and coma. Precipitating factors of HHNK coma include the following:

- Advanced age
- Preexisting cardiac or renal disease
- Inadequate insulin secretion or action (type 2 diabetes)
- Increased insulin requirements (stress, infection, trauma, burns, myocardial infarction)
- Medication use (thiazide and thiazide diuretics, glucocorticoids, ***phenytoin,*** sympathomimetics, ***propranolol,*** immunosuppressants)
- Supplemental parenteral and enteral feedings

ASSESSMENT OF THE DIABETIC PATIENT

A patient with a diabetic emergency may have a range of signs and symptoms. Many of these may mimic other, more commonly encountered conditions. Thus the paramedic must have a high degree of suspicion for illness related to diabetes.

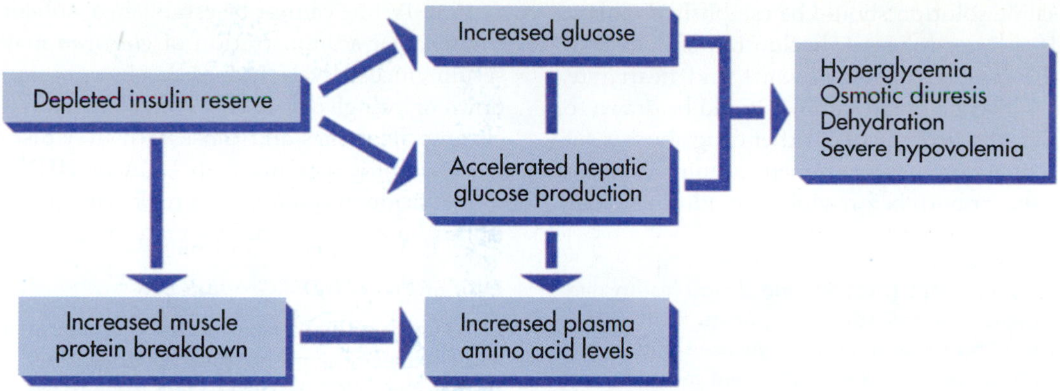

FIGURE 32-7 ■ Pathophysiology of hyperosmolar hyperglycemic nonketotic (HHNK) coma.

In addition to the patient assessment measures appropriate for any emergency patient encounter (initial assessment, physical examination, and treatment of life-threatening illness or injury), the paramedic should search for medical alert information, insulin syringes, and diabetic medications (***insulin*** is often kept in the refrigerator). Important components of the patient history in the assessment of diabetic patients include onset of symptoms, food intake, ***insulin*** or oral hypoglycemic use, alcohol or other drug consumption, predisposing factors (exercise, infection, illness, stress), and any associated symptoms.

MANAGEMENT OF THE CONSCIOUS DIABETIC PATIENT

If the diabetic patient is conscious and able to talk, a pertinent history should be obtained. The paramedic should do this while assessing the patient's airway, breathing, and circulation. If appropriate, the patient should be given glucose.

Protocols may include drawing a blood sample for laboratory testing before glucose is administered. Most EMS agencies use field glucose testing with Dextrostix, Chemstrips, or a glucometer (Fig. 32-8). Any patient who has a glucose reading below 80 mg/dL and who has signs and symptoms consistent with hypoglycemia should be given ***dextrose.*** Some patients who have experienced a diabetic reaction may be treated at the scene and released. Others may need to be transported for evaluation by a physician. The paramedic should consult with medical direction or follow the established protocol.

> **CRITICAL THINKING**
>
> What steps should you take before leaving the scene if the patient refuses transport after treatment with dextrose?

The methods of glucose administration vary. If the patient is alert, has a gag reflex, and is able to swallow, sugar may be administered orally. It may be given in the form of a candy bar, a glass of orange juice mixed with sugar, a nondiet soft drink, or by sublingual or buccal administration of a glucose gel preparation. An alternate method is to slowly administer ***50% dextrose*** through a stable peripheral vein (Box 32-3). (This dose may be repeated according to protocol.)

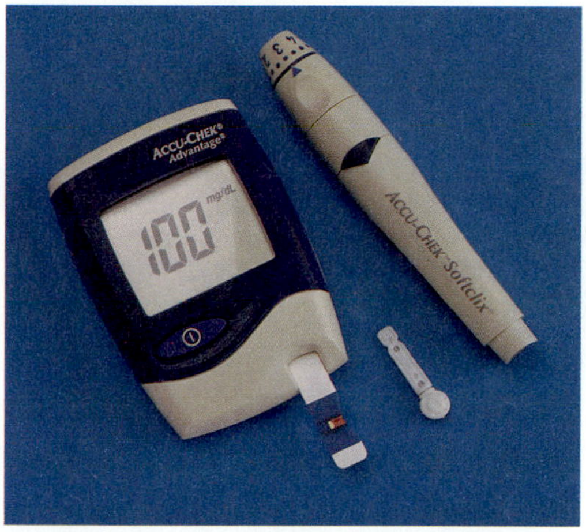

FIGURE 32-8 ■ Glucometer for measuring serum glucose levels.

> **BOX 32-3 Cautions for the Intravenous Administration of Glucose**
>
> - ***50% Dextrose*** should not be administered to infants or young children.
> - Administration of ***50% dextrose*** may lead to neurological complications in alcoholics and other patients with thiamine deficiency. Therefore administration of ***thiamine*** before or during the administration of ***dextrose*** should be considered for patients suspected of having a thiamine deficiency.

MANAGEMENT OF THE UNCONSCIOUS DIABETIC PATIENT

Prehospital management of any unconscious patient should be directed at airway management, administration of high-concentration oxygen, and ventilatory and circulatory support. Depending on protocol, an IV line of lactated Ringer's solution or a saline solution should be established. This replenishes fluids and electrolytes. (The flow rate should be determined by the patient's blood pressure and heart rate.) Before glucose is given, a blood sample should be drawn for laboratory analysis. If alcoholism or other drug abuse is suspected, medical direction may recommend administration of ***thiamine, naloxone,*** or both before glucose is administered.

▶ **NOTE** A patient's age (over 50) and clinical history may suggest a transient ischemic attack (TIA) or stroke. In such a case, administration of a concentrated glucose solution may worsen cerebral damage. (Consult with medical direction.) Otherwise, a patient in a coma of unknown origin should be given dextrose (if indicated by testing). (This is especially true if hypoglycemia cannot be ruled out.)

If an IV line cannot be established, subcutaneous or intramuscular administration of ***glucagon*** may help to raise serum glucose levels. It does this by stimulating the breakdown of liver glycogen. However, ***glucagon*** is not effective in chronic alcoholics and those with liver disease. Definitive treatment for patients with DKA or HHNK requires administration of ***insulin,*** fluid replacement, electrolyte monitoring, and in-hospital observation.

DIFFERENTIAL DIAGNOSIS

Determining the cause of a diabetic emergency sometimes is difficult in the prehospital setting. When the paramedic is not sure of the cause, all diabetic patients should receive glucose if indicated by testing. The difference in signs and symptoms in diabetic emergencies should help to identify the cause (Table 32-3).

TABLE 32-3 Differential Considerations in Diabetic Emergencies

FINDINGS	HYPOGLYCEMIA	HYPERGLYCEMIA	HHNK COMA
History			
Food intake	Insufficient	Excessive	Excessive
Insulin dosage	Excessive	Insufficient	Insufficient
Onset	Rapid	Gradual	Gradual
Infection	Uncommon	Common	Common
Gastrointestinal Tract			
Thirst	Absent	Intense	Intense
Hunger	Intense	Absent	Intense
Vomiting	Uncommon	Common	Uncommon
Respiratory System			
Breathing	Normal or rapid	Deep or rapid	Shallow/rapid
Breath odor	Normal	Acetone smell	Normal
Cardiovascular System			
Blood pressure	Normal	Low	Low
Pulse	Normal, rapid, or full	Rapid or weak	Rapid or weak
Skin	Pale or moist	Warm or dry	Warm or dry
Nervous System			
Headache	Present	Absent	Irritable
Consciousness	Irritability Seizure or coma	Restless Coma (rare)	Seizure or coma
Urine			
Sugar	Absent	Present	Present
Acetone	Usually absent	Usually present	Absent
Serum glucose levels	<60 mg/dL	>300 mg/dL	>600 mg/dL
Treatment response	Immediate (after glucose) (*Note:* if the hypoglycemic episode is prolonged or severe, response may be delayed and may require more than one dose.)	Gradual (within 6 to 12 hours after medication and fluid replacement)	Gradual (within 6 to 12 hours after medication and fluid replacement)

From Clark F et al: *Pharmacological basis of nursing,* ed 4, St Louis, 1993, Mosby.
HHNK, Hyperosmolar hyperglycemic nonketotic.

DISORDERS OF THE THYROID GLAND

Common disorders of the thyroid gland include hyperthyroidism and hypothyroidism. *Hyperthyroidism* is an excess of thyroid hormones in the blood, which may result in thyrotoxicosis. *Hypothyroidism* is an insufficiency of thyroid hormones in the blood, which may result in myxedema.

Thyrotoxicosis

The term **thyrotoxicosis** refers to any toxic condition that results from overproduction of the thyroid gland. *Hyperthyroidism* and *thyrotoxicosis* are names for common, milder forms of the disease. *Thyroid storm* is a life-threatening result of overactivity of the thyroid gland. It is a somewhat rare condition. The storm may occur spontaneously, or it may be brought on by infection, stress, or a thyroidectomy. Most cases of thyroid storm occur as a consequence of toxic diffuse goiter (Grave disease).[3] *Grave disease* is a type of excessive thyroid activity characterized by generalized enlargement of the gland (goiter), which leads to a swollen neck and, often, protruding eyes (exophthalmos) (Fig. 32-9). Grave disease most often occurs in young women. It may arise from an autoimmune process in which an antibody stimulates the thyroid cells.

Anatomy and Physiology of the Thyroid Gland

As described in Chapter 6, the thyroid gland is situated in the front of the neck just below the larynx. It consists of two lobes, one on each side of the trachea, joined by a narrower portion of tissue called the *isthmus* (Fig. 32-10).

Thyroid tissue is composed of two types of secretory cells. These are follicular cells and parafollicular cells (or C cells). Follicular cells make up most of the gland. They are arranged in the form of hollow, spherical follicles. They secrete the iodine-containing hormones thyroxine (T4) and triiodothyronine (T3). Parafollicular cells occur singly or in small groups in the spaces between the follicles. These cells secrete the hormone calcitonin, which helps regulate the level of calcium in the body.

Thyroid hormones play a key role in controlling body metabolism. They are essential in children for normal physical growth and mental development. The secretion of T3 and T4 is controlled by a feedback system. This system involves the pituitary gland and the hypothalamus. (The secretion of calcitonin is regulated directly by the level of calcium in the blood, independent of the pituitary gland or hypothalamus.)

Disorders of the thyroid gland may result from defects in the gland itself or from disruption of the hypothalamic-pituitary hormonal control system (Box 32-4). The disease advances in a slow fashion. (It may have nonspecific signs and symptoms over months to years.) It may culminate in an acute episode. Nonspecific signs and symptoms of thyroid hyperfunction include fatigue, anxiety, palpitations, sweating, weight loss, diarrhea, and heat intolerance.

In acute episodes of thyroid storm, signs and symptoms are those related to adrenergic hyperactivity. They may include the following:

- Severe tachycardia
- Heart failure
- Cardiac dysrhythmias

BOX 32-4 Causes of Thyroid Gland Disorders

- Congenital defects
- Genetic disorders
- Infection (thyroiditis)
- Tumors (benign or malignant)
- Autoimmune disorders
- Hormonal disorders during puberty or pregnancy
- Nutritional disorders

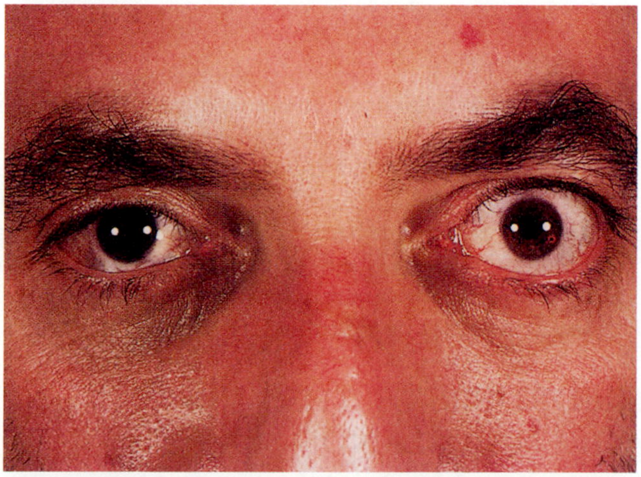

FIGURE 32-9 ■ Protrusion of the eyes in a patient with Grave disease. (From Epstein O et al: *Clinical examination,* ed 3, St Louis, 2003, Mosby.)

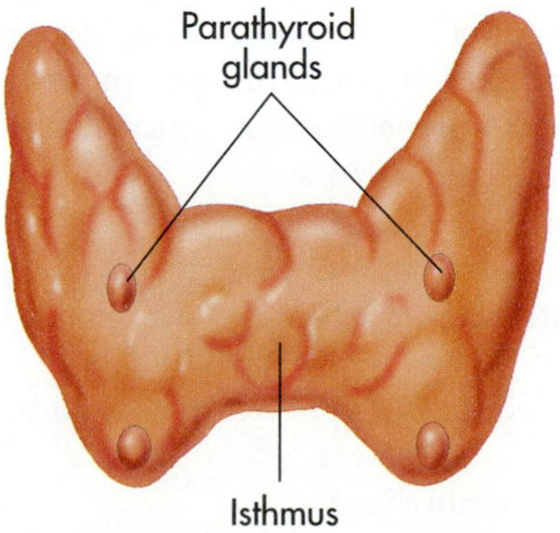

FIGURE 32-10 ■ Thyroid gland.

- Shock
- Hyperthermia
- Restlessness
- Agitation and paranoia
- Abdominal pain
- Delirium
- Coma

The paramedic should consider other causes of symptoms related to adrenergic hyperactivity—most notably the use of cocaine and amphetamines, hypoglycemia, and withdrawal from alcohol and other drugs.

CRITICAL THINKING

What medical emergencies could produce signs and symptoms similar to those of thyroid storm?

Management

Mild hyperthyroidism requires no emergency therapy. It is best managed with physician follow-up. By comparison, thyroid storm is a true emergency. It requires immediate treatment. Emergency care efforts are directed at providing airway, ventilatory, and circulatory support and rapid transport to an appropriate medical facility. In-hospital care focuses on inhibiting hormone synthesis, blocking hormone release and the peripheral effects of thyroid hormone with antithyroid drugs, and providing general support of the patient's vital functions.

Table 32-4 lists the signs and symptoms caused by hyperthyroidism and hypothyroidism.

Myxedema

Myxedema is a condition that results from a deficiency in thyroid hormone. It may be associated with inflammation of the thyroid gland (e.g., Hashimoto thyroiditis) or atrophy of the thyroid gland. It also may be a consequence of treatment for hyperthyroidism. Myxedema causes the buildup of mucinous material in the skin. This results in thickening and coarsening of the skin and other body tissues (most notably the lips and nose) (Fig. 32-11). The condition is most common in adults (especially women) over age 40.

Myxedema coma is a rare illness. In addition to myxedema, it is characterized by hypothermia and mental obtundation. Myxedema coma is a medical emergency that may be precipitated by the following factors:

- Exposure to cold
- Infection (usually pulmonary)
- Congestive heart failure
- Trauma
- Drugs (sedatives, hypnotics, anesthetics)
- Stroke
- Internal hemorrhage
- Hypoxia
- Hypercapnia
- Hyponatremia
- Hypoglycemia

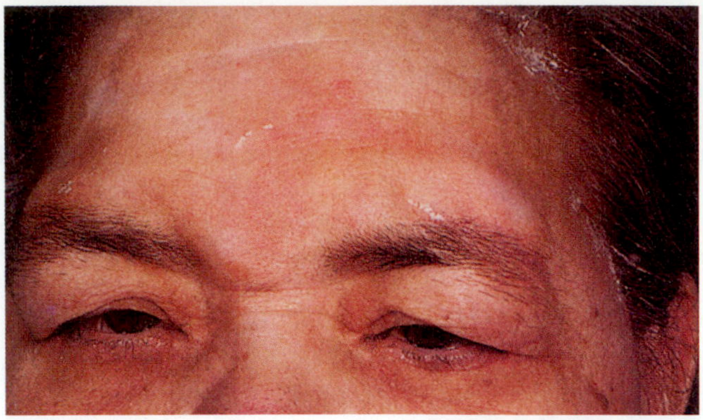

FIGURE 32-11 ■ Myxedema. (From Epstein O et al: *Clinical examination,* ed 3, St. Louis, 2003, Mosby.)

TABLE 32-4 Signs and Symptoms of Hyperthyroidism and Hypothyroidism

HYPERTHYROIDISM	HYPOTHYROIDISM
Exophthalmos	Facial edema
Goiter	Jugular venous distention (sometimes goiter)
Warm, flushed skin	Cool skin
Fever	Exposure to cold
Agitation/psychosis	Coma
Hyperactivity	Weakness
Weight loss	Weight gain
Common Medications	
Iodine	Levothyroxine (Synthroid)
Methimazole (Tapazole)	Liothyronine (Cytomel)
Propylthiouracil (Propacil)	Liotrix (Euthroid)

MANAGEMENT

Prehospital care is directed at managing life-threatening conditions (airway, ventilatory, and circulatory compromise) and providing rapid transport to an appropriate medical facility for evaluation by a physician. Once other causes of the coma have been ruled out and the patient's condition has been stabilized, treatment of myxedema can begin. Treatment involves oral administration of thyroxine. This treatment must be continued for life.

DISORDERS OF THE ADRENAL GLANDS

Two disorders of the adrenal gland are Cushing syndrome and Addison disease. Cushing syndrome is caused by excessive activity of the adrenal cortex. Addison disease is caused by inactivity of the adrenal cortex.

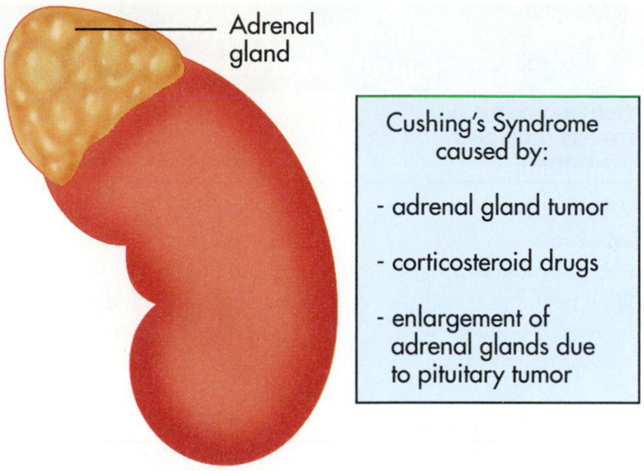

FIGURE 32-12 ■ Adrenal gland.

Cushing Syndrome

Cushing syndrome is caused by an abnormally high circulating level of corticosteroid hormones. These hormones are produced naturally by the adrenal glands (Fig. 32-12). This condition may be produced directly by an adrenal gland tumor. (The tumor causes excessive secretion of corticosteroids.) It also may be produced by administration of corticosteroid drugs. (These are used to treat conditions such as rheumatoid arthritis, inflammatory bowel disease, and asthma.) Finally, it may be produced by enlargement of both adrenal glands as a result of a pituitary tumor. The pituitary gland controls the activity of the adrenal gland by producing adrenocorticotropic hormone (ACTH). ACTH stimulates the cortex of the adrenal gland to grow. Cushing syndrome is rare. It mainly affects women 30 to 50 years of age.

People with Cushing syndrome have a characteristic appearance (Fig. 32-13). The face appears round ("moon face") and red (Fig. 32-14). Also, the trunk tends to become obese from disturbances in fat metabolism. The limbs become wasted from muscle atrophy. Acne develops, and purple stretch marks may appear on the abdomen, thighs, and breasts. The skin often thins and bruises easily. Weakened bones are at increased risk of fracture. Other features of the disease include the following:

- Increased body and facial hair
- Hump on the back of neck ("buffalo hump")
- Supraclavicular fat pads
- Weight gain
- Hypertension
- Psychiatric disturbances (depression, paranoia)
- Insomnia
- Diabetes mellitus

CRITICAL THINKING

How do you think patients who suffer from Cushing syndrome feel about their body image?

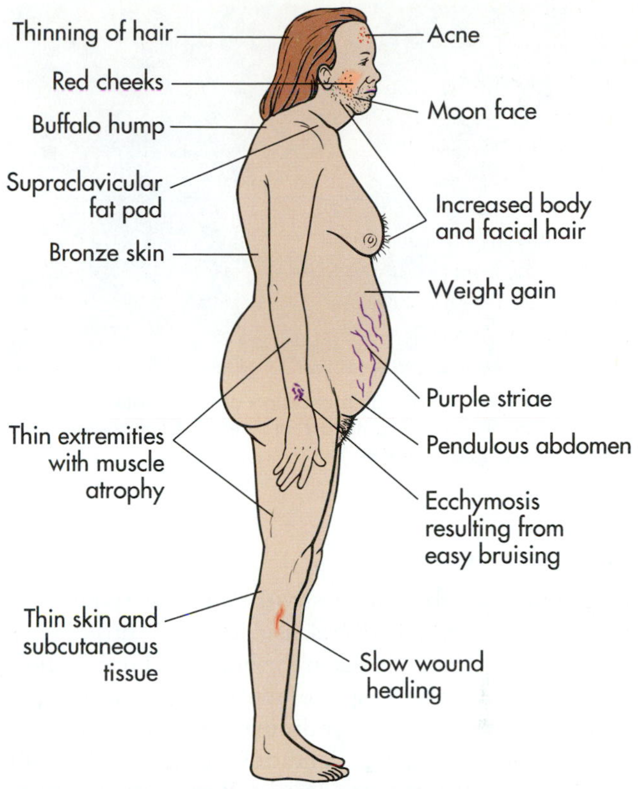

FIGURE 32-13 ■ Cushing syndrome. (From Lewis SM, Collier IC, Heitkemper MM: *Medical-surgical nursing: assessment and management of clinical problems*, ed 4, St Louis, 1996, Mosby.)

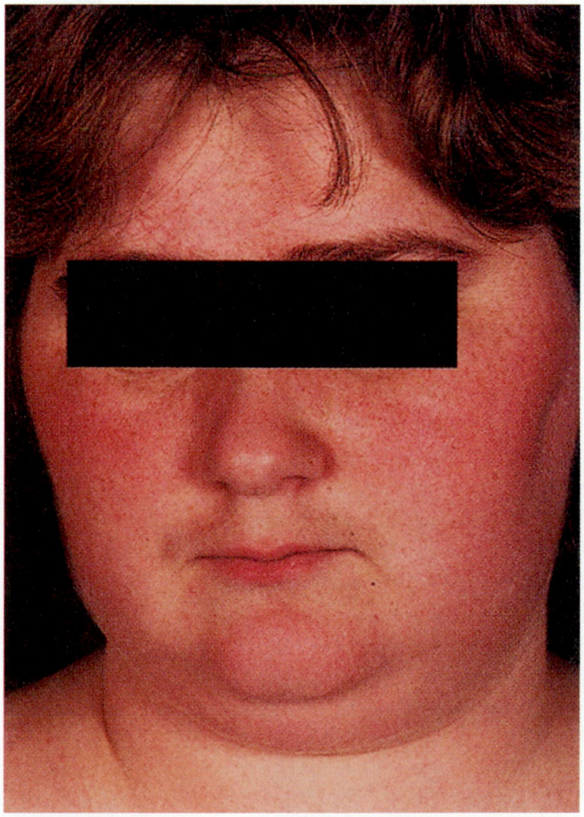

FIGURE 32-14 ■ Moon-faced appearance in a patient with Cushing syndrome. (From Epstein O et al: *Clinical examination*, ed 3, St. Louis, 2003, Mosby.)

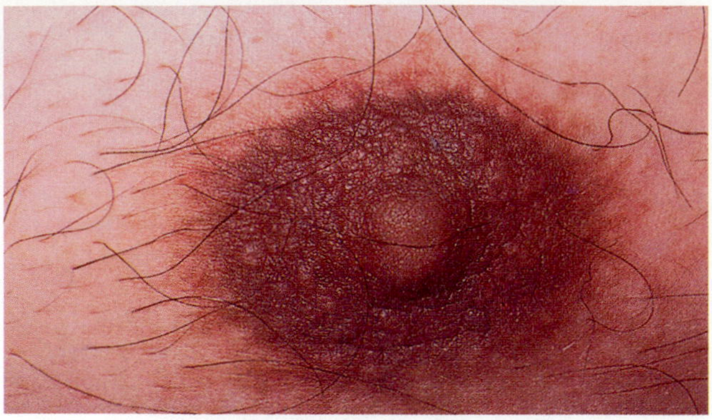

FIGURE 32-15 ■ Hyperpigmentation of the areola in a patient with Addison disease. (From Epstein O et al: *Clinical examination*, ed 3, St. Louis, 2003, Mosby.)

TABLE 32-5 Signs and Symptoms of Adrenal Gland Disorders

CORTICOSTEROID EXCESS (CUSHING SYNDROME)	ADRENAL INSUFFICIENCY (ADDISON DISEASE)
Weight gain	Weight loss
Weakness	Weakness
Hump on back of neck	Hypotension
Slow healing	Gastrointestinal disorders
Increased body and facial hair	Skin hyperpigmentation
Common Medications	
Aminoglutethimide (Cytadren)	Dexamethasone (Decadron)
Metyrapone (Metopirone)	Fludrocortisone (Florinef Acetate)

MANAGEMENT

Prehospital care for patients with Cushing syndrome is mainly supportive. The disease is diagnosed through measurement of hormone levels in the blood and urine, and by radiological imaging (e.g., computed tomography [CT] scan). If the cause of the syndrome is overtreatment with corticosteroid drugs, the condition usually is reversible when the drug dosages are adjusted. If the cause is a tumor or overgrowth of the adrenal gland, the gland may require surgical removal. If the tumor is in the pituitary gland, the usual treatment involves surgery, radiation, and medication. Treatment is usually successful. Lifelong hormone replacement therapy is required.

Addison Disease

Addison disease is a rare disorder. It can be life-threatening. The disease is caused by a deficiency of the corticosteroid hormones *cortisol* and *aldosterone*. These hormones are normally produced by the adrenal cortex. The disorder can be caused by any disease process that destroys the adrenal cortices. (Such disease processes may include adrenal hemorrhage or infarction, infections [tuberculosis, fungi, viruses], and autoimmune diseases.) However, the most common cause of Addison disease is shrinking of the adrenal tissue. When this occurs, production of corticosteroid hormones is inadequate to meet the body's metabolic requirements. Signs and symptoms associated with this disease include the following:

- Progressive weakness
- Progressive weight loss
- Progressive anorexia
- Skin hyperpigmentation (caused by increased hormone production by the pituitary gland, which stimulates melanin) (Fig. 32-15)
- Hypotension
- Hyponatremia
- Hyperkalemia
- GI disturbances (nausea, vomiting, diarrhea)

Addison disease usually has a slow onset. It also has a chronic course. The symptoms develop gradually over months to years. However, acute episodes *(addisonian crisis)* may be brought on by emotional and physiological stress. Examples of such stressors include surgery, alcohol intoxication, hypothermia, myocardial infarction, severe illness, trauma, hypoglycemia, and infection. During these events, the adrenal glands cannot increase the production of the corticosteroid hormones to help the body cope with stress. As a result, blood glucose levels drop; the body loses the ability to regulate the content of sodium, potassium, and water in body fluids (causing dehydration and extreme muscle weakness); blood volume and blood pressure fall; and the body may not be able to maintain circulation efficiently. In these situations, airway, ventilatory, and circulatory support are required in the prehospital setting.

MANAGEMENT

In-hospital treatment involves maintaining the patient's vital functions and correcting the sodium deficiency and dehydration. After the life-threatening episode has been managed, treatment consists of administration of corticosteroids. The patient often is advised to increase the dosage of these drugs during times of emotional and physiological stress. Table 32-5 presents a comparison of the signs and symptoms of Cushing syndrome and Addison disease.

SUMMARY

- The endocrine system consists of ductless glands and tissues. These glands and tissues produce and secrete hormones. Endocrine glands secrete their hormones directly into the bloodstream. They exert a regulatory effect on various metabolic functions. All hormones operate within feedback systems. (These are either positive or negative.) These systems work to maintain an optimal internal environment.
- The pancreatic islets are composed of beta cells, alpha cells, and other cells. The beta cells secrete insulin. The alpha cells secrete glucagon. The other cells are of questionable function. The chief functions of insulin are to increase glucose transport into cells, increase glucose metabolism by cells, increase the liver glycogen level, and decrease the blood glucose concentration toward normal. Glucagon has two major effects: (1) increase blood glucose levels by stimulating the liver to release glucose stores from glycogen and other glucose storage sites (glycogenolysis) and (2) stimulate gluconeogenesis through the breakdown of fats and fatty acids, thereby maintaining a normal blood glucose level.
- Diabetes mellitus is characterized by a deficiency of insulin or an inability of the body to respond to insulin. Diabetes generally is classified as type 1 or type 2. Type 1 is insulin dependent. Type 2 is non-insulin dependent. Type 1 diabetes requires lifelong treatment. This consists of insulin injections, exercise, and diet regulation. Most patients with type 2 diabetes require oral hypoglycemic medications, exercise, and dietary regulation to control the illness.
- Hypoglycemia is a syndrome related to blood glucose levels below 80 mg/dL. Any diabetic patient with behavioral changes or unconsciousness should be treated for hypoglycemia. This condition is a true emergency. It requires immediate administration of glucose to prevent permanent brain damage or death.
- Diabetic ketoacidosis results from an absence of or a resistance to insulin. The signs and symptoms of DKA are related to diuresis and acidosis. They usually are slow in onset.
- Hyperosmolar hyperglycemic nonketotic coma is a life-threatening emergency. It often occurs in older patients with type 2 diabetes. It also frequently occurs in undiagnosed diabetics. The hyperglycemia produces a hyperosmolar state. This is followed by an osmotic diuresis, dehydration, and electrolyte losses.
- Important components of the patient history in the assessment of diabetic patients include the onset of symptoms, food intake, insulin or oral hypoglycemic use, alcohol or other drug consumption, predisposing factors, and any associated symptoms.
- Any patient with a glucose reading below 80 mg/dL and signs and symptoms consistent with hypoglycemia should be given dextrose.
- Thyrotoxicosis is any toxic condition that results from overactivity of the thyroid gland.
- Thyroid storm is a life-threatening condition resulting from an overactive thyroid gland. Thyroid hormones play a key role in controlling body metabolism. They are essential in children for normal physical growth and development.
- Myxedema is a condition that results from a thyroid hormone deficiency. Myxedema coma is a rare illness. In addition to myxedema, it is characterized by hypothermia and mental obtundation. It is a medical emergency.
- Cushing syndrome is caused by an abnormally high circulating level of corticosteroid hormones. These are produced naturally by the adrenal glands.
- Addison disease is a rare but life-threatening disorder. It is caused by a deficiency of the corticosteroid hormones cortisol and aldosterone. These are normally produced by the adrenal cortex.

REFERENCES

1. American Diabetes Association: *Diabetes facts and figures.* www.diabetes.org/ada/facts.asp. Accessed Feb. 18, 2005.
2. American Diabetes Association: www.diabetes.org. Accessed Feb. 18, 2005.
3. Rosen P, Barkin R: *Emergency medicine: concepts and clinical practice*, ed 4, St Louis, 1998, Mosby.

SUGGESTED READINGS

Becker K et al: Principles and practice of endocrinology and metabolism, ed 3, Philadelphia, 2001, Lippincott Williams & Wilkins.
Kacsoh B: *Endocrine physiology*, McGraw-Hill/Appleton Lange, 2000.
William R et al: *Williams textbook of endocrinology*, ed 10, Philadelphia, 2002, WB Saunders.

CHAPTER

33

Allergies and Anaphylaxis

OBJECTIVES

Upon completion of this chapter, the paramedic student will be able to:

1. Describe the antigen-antibody response.
2. Differentiate between an allergic reaction and a normal immune response.
3. Describe signs and symptoms and management of local allergic reactions based on an understanding of the pathophysiology associated with this condition.
4. Identify allergens associated with anaphylaxis.
5. Describe the pathophysiology, signs and symptoms, and management of anaphylaxis.

KEY TERMS

eosinophil chemotactic factor of anaphylaxis: A group of active substances, including histamine and leukotrienes, that are released during an anaphylactic reaction.

leukotrienes: A class of biologically active compounds that occur naturally in leukocytes and that produce allergic and inflammatory reactions.

sensitization: An acquired reaction in which specific antibodies develop in response to an antigen.

thromboxanes: Antagonistic prostaglandin derivatives that are synthesized and released by degranulating platelets, causing vasoconstriction and promoting the degranulation of other platelets.

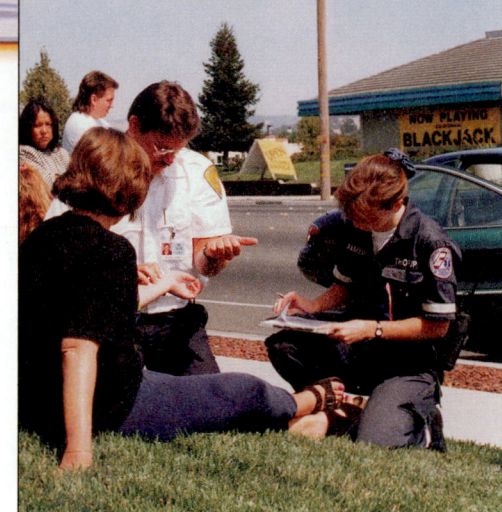

Anaphylaxis is an allergic reaction. Anaphylaxis is an immediate, systemic, life-threatening reaction. Anaphylaxis is associated with major changes in the cardiovascular, respiratory, and cutaneous systems. The prompt recognition and the proper drug therapy are vital to patient survival.

ANTIGEN-ANTIBODY REACTION

As described in Chapter 7, an antigen is a substance that induces the formation of antibodies. Antigens can enter the body by injection, ingestion, inhalation, or absorption. The antibodies bind to the antigen that produced them. Antibodies then aid in neutralizing the antigens and removing them from the body. This normal antigen-antibody reaction protects the body from disease by activating the immune response. Fig. 33-1 provides a brief summary of the immune response.

The immune responses normally are protective. However, they can become oversensitive. They can become directed toward harmless antigens to which human beings often are exposed. When this occurs, the response is termed *allergic*. The antigen or substance causing the allergic response is called an *allergen*. Common allergens include drugs, insects, foods, latex, animals, pollens and molds (Box 33-1). The healthy body responds to an antigen challenge through a collective defense system. This system is known as *immunity*. To review, immunity may be natural (present at birth). Immunity also may be acquired (resulting from exposure to a specific antigenic agent or pathogen). Finally, immunity may be induced artificially through immunization. (See Chapter 7.)

ALLERGIC REACTION

An allergic reaction is marked by an increased physiological response to an antigen after a previous exposure **(sensitization)** to the same antigen. The allergic reaction starts when a circulating antibody (immunoglobulin G [IgG] or IgM) combines with a specific foreign antigen, resulting in hypersensitivity reactions, or with antibodies bound to mast cells or basophils (IgE). As described in Chapters 7 and 17, hypersensitivity reactions are divided into four distinct types. These types are *type I* (IgE-mediated allergic reactions), *type II* (tissue-specific reactions), *type III* (immune-complex–mediated reactions), and *type IV* (cell-mediated reactions). A type I or immediate hypersensitivity reaction is the most dramatic. It may lead to life-threatening anaphylaxis. Box 33-2 gives examples of antigens that may cause hypersensitivity reactions (including anaphylaxis). Patients who have a known sensitivity to these or other agents should avoid exposure.

NOTE Anaphylactoid reactions are allergic reactions that are not mediated by an antigen-antibody reaction. These reactions present exactly like anaphylaxis. The distinction is not crucial in relation to treatment of an acute attack.[1]

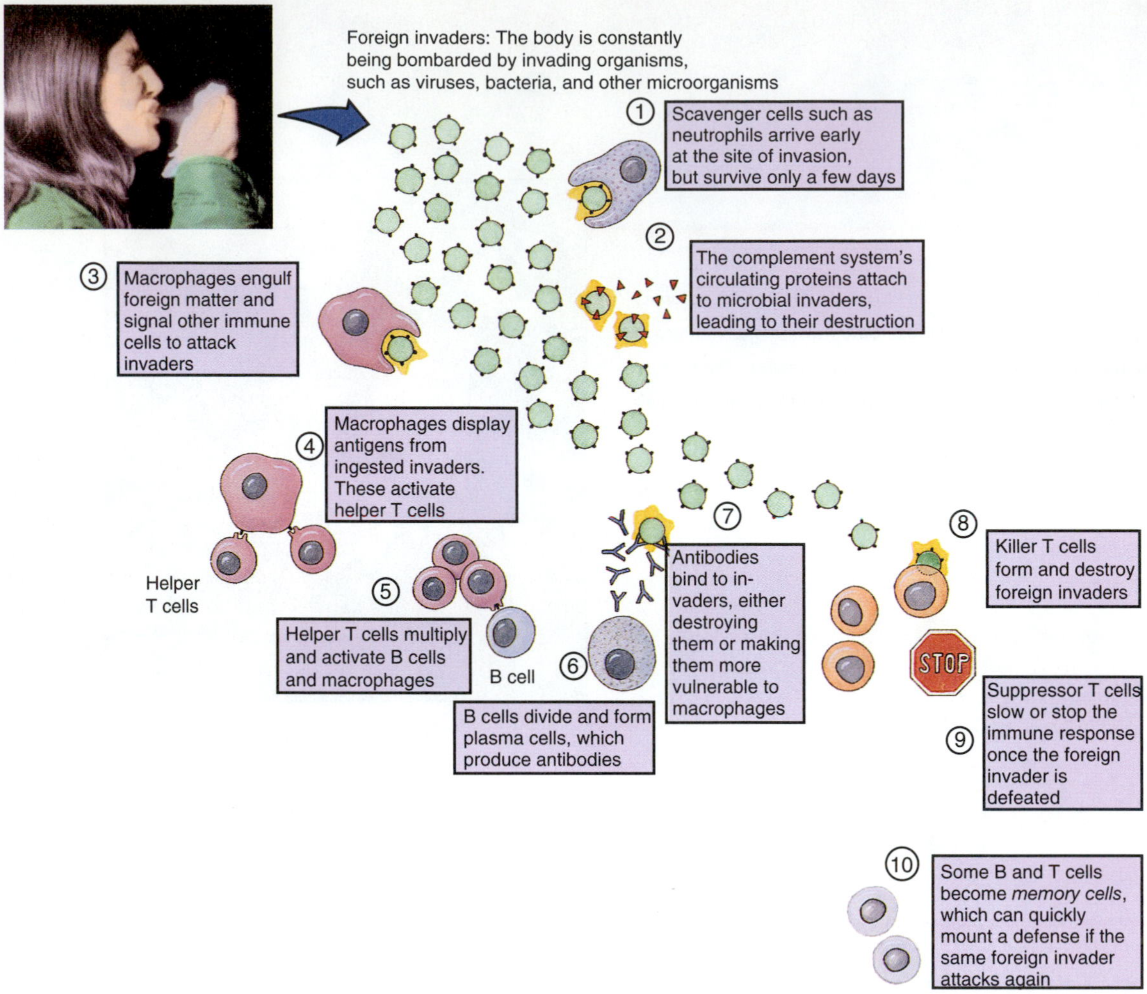
Foreign invaders: The body is constantly being bombarded by invading organisms, such as viruses, bacteria, and other microorganisms
1 Scavenger cells such as neutrophils arrive early at the site of invasion, but survive only a few days
2 The complement system's circulating proteins attach to microbial invaders, leading to their destruction
3 Macrophages engulf foreign matter and signal other immune cells to attack invaders
4 Macrophages display antigens from ingested invaders. These activate helper T cells
Helper T cells
5 Helper T cells multiply and activate B cells and macrophages
B cell
6 B cells divide and form plasma cells, which produce antibodies
7 Antibodies bind to invaders, either destroying them or making them more vulnerable to macrophages
8 Killer T cells form and destroy foreign invaders
STOP
9 Suppressor T cells slow or stop the immune response once the foreign invader is defeated
10 Some B and T cells become *memory cells*, which can quickly mount a defense if the same foreign invader attacks again

FIGURE 33-1 ■ A brief summary of the immune response.

LOCALIZED ALLERGIC REACTION

Localized allergic reactions (type IV) do not involve the entire body. In these cases, the sites of mast cell and basophil mediator release are limited. Common signs and symptoms of localized allergic reaction include the following:

- Conjunctivitis
- Rhinitis
- Angioedema
- Urticaria
- Contact dermatitis (Fig. 33-2)

Localized allergic reactions are best managed with drugs that compete for receptor sites with histamine. This competition prevents histamine from performing its physiological actions. Common antihistamines include over-the-counter oral and nasal decongestants and prescription and nonprescription ***diphenhydramine.*** Other medications that may be helpful for some local reactions include steroids and topical creams.

ANAPHYLAXIS

The term *anaphylaxis* comes from Greek. It means "against or opposite of protection." Anaphylaxis is the most extreme form of an allergic reaction, accounting for 400 to 800 deaths per year.[2] Anaphylaxis has a mortality rate of 3%. Thus rapid recognition and aggressive therapy are essential.

> **CRITICAL THINKING**
>
> Consider the list of allergens in Box 33-2. Based on this list, what are some likely locations to which you may be dispatched to care for a patient who is experiencing an anaphylactic reaction?

Causative Agents

Almost any substance can cause anaphylaxis. The antigenic agents most frequently associated with anaphylaxis are penicillin (by ingestion or injection), envenomation by

BOX 33-1 Latex Allergies

Today there is significant concern about latex allergy, especially among health care workers. The first published account of contact urticaria related to glove use was published in 1979; however, latex allergy was relatively unknown until after the acquired immunodeficiency syndrome epidemic in the mid-1980s and the resulting tremendous increase in glove usage. The prevalence of sensitization to latex has been reported to range from 2.9% to 4.7% among health care workers and from 7% to 10% among operating room staff. (In addition to latex gloves, health care workers and latex-sensitive patients can be exposed to latex on medical instruments, surgical equipment, and other appliances.) Those persons considered at high risk for latex allergy include the following:

- Individuals who have had significant and early exposure to latex (e.g., patients with spina bifida or genitourinary anomalies and others who have had multiple surgeries and catheterizations)
- Persons with a genetic propensity to develop allergies
- Asthmatics
- Health care workers and law enforcement and fire service personnel who regularly use latex gloves
- Workers in some occupations (e.g., rubber manufacturing employees, hairdressers, food handlers, auto mechanics, tollbooth operators)

Symptoms of latex allergy can range from mild discomfort to life-threatening anaphylaxis. Most often the first manifestation of a latex allergy is urticaria that typically is localized to the hands but may be widespread. A type I latex allergy can manifest itself in symptoms that include rash, lacrimation, rhinitis, wheezing, bronchospasm, laryngeal edema, hypotension, dysrhythmia, and, rarely, respiratory or cardiac arrest.

Many health care facilities, emergency medical services agencies, and other public service agencies have addressed this issue by developing "latex safe" environments and by using latex-free equipment for patients with latex allergy. For the health care provider the need for education, early recognition, prevention strategies, and the implementation of safe and effective practice is essential. The National Institute for Occupational Safety and Health and many professional organizations have recommended that health care workers wear low-protein, powder-free gloves when latex gloves are necessary and synthetic gloves when the risk of exposure to blood-borne pathogens is low. Individuals not exposed to blood or body fluids (e.g., food handlers and maintenance workers) should avoid latex gloves altogether. All patients should be questioned about latex allergy; persons with latex allergy should wear appropriate medical-alert identification. Sensitivity to latex should be documented on the patient care report, and this information should be conveyed to medical direction.

Source: Korniewicz D: Latex allergy: a current challenge, Asepsis on the Web 20(3), 1999. Retrieved Sept. 22, 2004 from www.jnjmedical.com/asepsis/latex_allg.asp.

BOX 33-2 Agents That May Cause Allergies and Anaphylaxis

Drugs and Biological Agents
Antibiotics
Anticancer agents
Aspirin
Cephalosporins
Chemotherapeutics
Insulin
Local anesthetics
Muscle relaxants
Nonsteroidal antiinflammatory agents
Opiates
Vaccines

Insect Bites and Stings
Bees
Fire ants
Wasps

Foods
Cod, halibut, shellfish (e.g., shrimp)
Cottonseed
Egg white
Food additives
Mango
Milk
Peanuts, soybeans
Sesame and sunflower seeds
Strawberries
Wheat and buckwheat

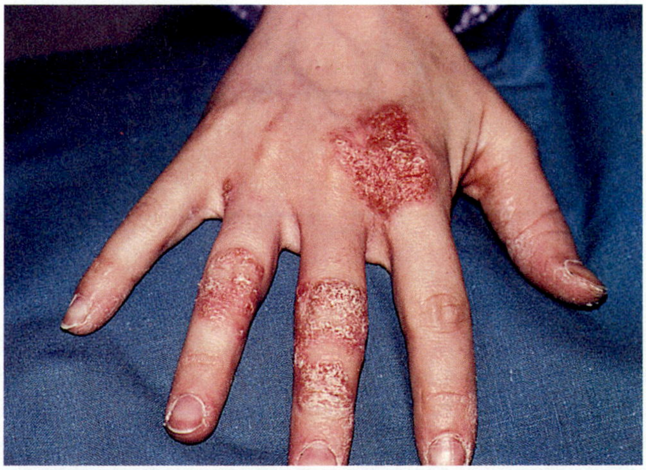

FIGURE 33-2 ■ Contact dermatitis caused by a delayed hypersensitivity leading to vesicles and scaling at the sites of contact.

stinging insects, and food (especially nuts and shellfish). Regardless of the offending antigen, the risk of anaphylaxis in sensitive persons increases with each exposure. To a lesser extent, the risk increases with the length of exposure or site of inoculation.

Pathophysiology

As described before, a person first must be exposed to a specific antigen to develop type I hypersensitivity. In the first exposure the antigen enters the body by injection, ingestion, inhalation, or absorption. Then the antigen activates the immune system. In susceptible persons, large amounts of IgE antibody are produced. Immunoglobulin E

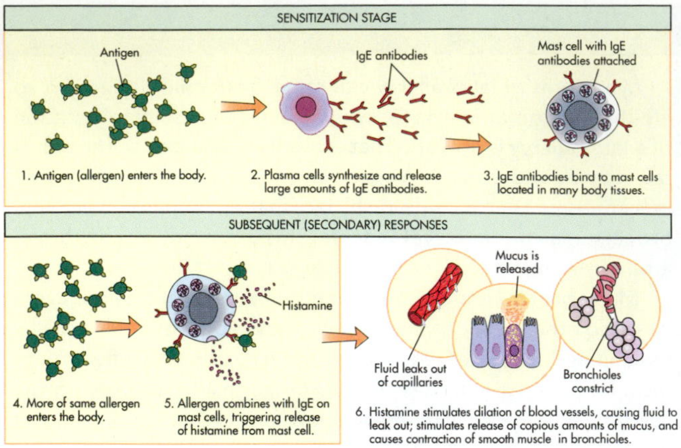

FIGURE 33-3 ■ Allergic reaction. Antigen stimulates the production of massive amounts of immunoglobulin E, a type of antibody produced by plasma cells. Immunoglobulin E attaches to mast cells. This is the sensitization stage. When the antigen enters again, it binds to the immunoglobulin E antibodies on the mast cells, triggering a massive release of histamine and other chemicals. Histamine in turn causes blood vessels to dilate and become leaky. This triggers the production of mucus in the respiratory tract. In some persons the chemicals released by the mast cells also cause the small air-carrying ducts in the lungs to constrict, making breathing difficult.

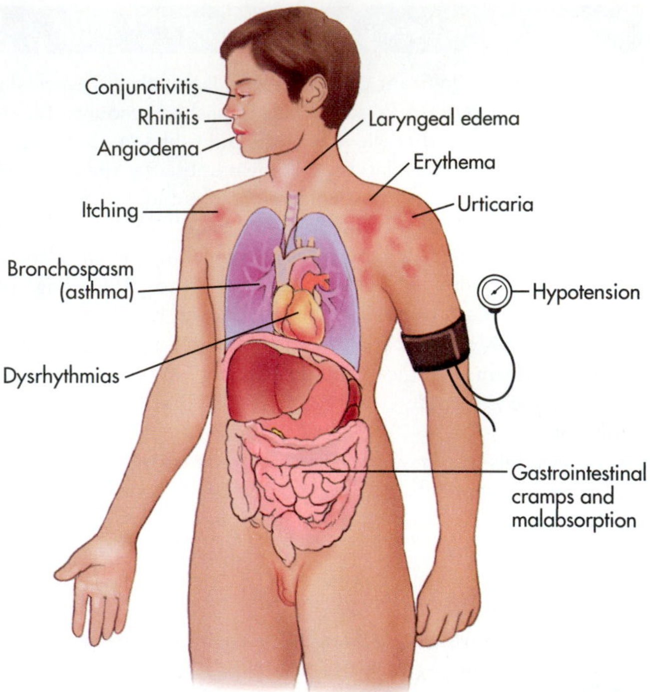

FIGURE 33-4 ■ Type I hypersensitivity reactions. Manifestation of allergic reactions as a result of type I hypersensitivity include itching, angioedema (swelling caused by exudation), edema of the larynx, urticaria (hives), bronchospasm (constriction of airways in the lungs), hypotension (low blood pressure), dysrhythmias (irregular heartbeat) because of anaphylactic shock, and gastrointestinal cramping caused by inflammation of the gastrointestinal mucosa.

BOX 33-3 Anaphylaxis

Three conditions must be met to sensitize an individual and generate an anaphylactic response:

1. An antigen-induced stimulation of the immune system with specific immunoglobulin E antibody formation
2. A latent period after the initial antigenic exposure for sensitization of mast cells and basophils to occur
3. Subsequent reexposure to the same specific antigen

antibodies leave the lymphatic system and bind to the cell membranes of basophils that are circulating in the blood and to mast cells that are in tissues surrounding the blood vessels. The antibodies remain on the cells. The antibodies are inactive until the same antigen is introduced into the body a second time (Fig. 33-3). With the next exposure to the specific antigen, the allergen cross-links at least two of the cell-bound IgE molecules. This results in degranulation (release of internal substances) of the mast cells and basophils and the onset of an anaphylactic reaction (Box 33-3).

The degranulation of the target cell is associated with the release of pharmacologically active chemical mediators from inside the affected basophils and mast cells (described in Chapter 6). These chemicals include histamine, **leukotrienes, eosinophil chemotactic factor of anaphylaxis,** heparin, kinins, prostaglandins, and **thromboxanes.** All of these chemicals mediate or trigger an internal systemic response.

Histamine increases the permeability of vessels. It also causes dilation of capillaries and venules. It also causes contraction of smooth muscle in the gastrointestinal tract and bronchial tree. An associated increase in gastric, nasal, and lacrimal secretions also occurs. This results in tearing and rhinorrhea. The increased capillary permeability allows plasma to leak into the interstitial space. This decreases the amount of fluid that is available for the heart to pump. The profound bodywide vasodilation further decreases cardiac preload. This in turn decreases stroke volume and cardiac output. These responses lead to flushing, urticaria, angioedema, and hypotension (Fig. 33-4). The onset of action of the histamine is rapid. Yet the effects of histamine are short lived because they are quickly broken down by enzymes. Fig. 33-5 illustrates the pathophysiology of anaphylactic shock.

Leukotrienes are the most potent bronchoconstrictors, which cause wheezing. These chemical mediators also cause coronary vasoconstriction and increased vascular permeability. Leukotrienes formerly were known as *slow-reacting substances of anaphylaxis* because their effects were delayed relative to histamine. The duration of action of these chemicals, however, is much longer than that of histamine.

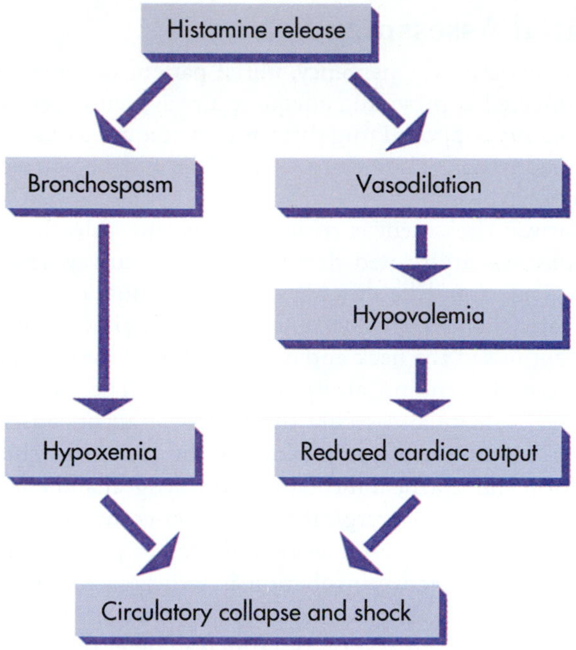

FIGURE 33-5 ■ Pathophysiology of anaphylactic shock.

TABLE 33-1 Conditions That May Mimic Anaphylaxis

SIGNS AND SYMPTOMS	POSSIBLE CAUSES
Stridor	Upper airway obstruction Foreign body aspiration Epiglottitis, angioedema, use of angiotensin-converting enzyme inhibitor, some panic disorders
Bronchospasm	Asthma, chronic obstructive pulmonary disease, bronchitis
Syncope	Vasovagal syncope Seizure Hypoglycemia Cardiac dysrhythmias

The process of anaphylaxis attracts eosinophils to the site of allergic inflammation. Eosinophils are thought to contain an enzyme that can deactivate leukotrienes. The remaining chemical mediators (heparin, neutrophil chemotactic factor, and kinins) exert varying effects that may include fever, chills, bronchospasm, and pulmonary vasoconstriction. These complex chemical processes can lead rapidly to upper airway obstruction and bronchospasm, dysrhythmias and cardiac ischemia, and circulatory collapse and shock.

Assessment Findings

An accurate history and physical assessment are required to tell the difference between severe allergic reactions and other conditions that may mimic anaphylaxis (Table 33-1). A flawed prehospital assessment in this group can threaten a patient's life. Disease entities that may present similar signs and symptoms of anaphylaxis include the following:

- Severe asthma with respiratory failure
- Upper airway obstruction
- Toxic or septic shock
- Pulmonary edema (with or without myocardial infarction)
- Drug overdose
- Hypovolemic shock

BOX 33-4 Signs and Symptoms of Anaphylaxis

Upper Airway
Hoarseness
Laryngeal or epiglottic edema
Rhinorrhea
Stridor

Lower Airway
Accessory muscle use
Bronchospasm
Decreased breath sounds
Increased mucous production
Wheezing

Cardiovascular System
Chest tightness
Dysrhythmias
Hypotension
Tachycardia

Gastrointestinal System
Abdominal cramps
Diarrhea
Nausea
Vomiting

Neurological System
Anxiety
Coma
Dizziness
Headache
Seizure
Syncope
Weakness

Cutaneous System
Angioedema
Edema
Erythema
Pruritus
Tearing of the eyes
Urticaria

RESPIRATORY EFFECTS

The initial signs of a breathing problem associated with anaphylaxis may vary. Signs may range from sneezing and coughing to complete airway obstruction (caused by laryngeal and epiglottic edema) (Box 33-4). The patient may complain of throat tightness and dyspnea. Stridor or voice changes also may be evident. Lower airway bronchospasm and associated hypersecretion of mucus caused by the actions of histamine, leukotrienes, and prostaglandins may produce wheezing and significant respiratory distress. Symptoms can develop with startling rapidity.

CARDIOVASCULAR EFFECTS

The cardiovascular manifestations of allergic reactions vary. They may range from mild hypotension to collapse and profound shock. Dysrhythmias are common. The dysrhythmias may be related to the severe hypoxia and loss of circulating fluid volume that occurs. The patient may complain of chest pain if myocardial ischemia is present.

CRITICAL THINKING
Which of these effects has the potential to cause death first?

GASTROINTESTINAL EFFECTS

Nausea, vomiting, diarrhea, and severe abdominal cramping may occur in a patient with an anaphylactic reaction. The increased gastrointestinal activity is related to smooth muscle contraction, increased mucous production, and outpouring of fluid from the gut wall into the intestinal lumen initiated by the chemical mediators.

NERVOUS SYSTEM EFFECTS

The nervous system responses are caused in large part by the impaired gas exchange and shock associated with anaphylaxis. At first the patient may be agitated and speak of a sense of impending doom. As hypoxia and shock worsen, brain functions deteriorate. This may result in confusion, weakness, headache, syncope, seizures, and coma.

CUTANEOUS EFFECTS

The most visible signs that distinguish anaphylaxis from other medical conditions relate to the skin. These signs are caused by the vasodilation induced by histamine release from the mast cells. Initially the patient may complain of warmth and itching. Physical examination often reveals diffuse redness and hives (urticaria). The hives are well-circumscribed wheals of 1 to 6 cm. Hives may be more reddened or pallid than the surrounding skin. Often they are accompanied by severe itching (Fig. 33-6). Significant swelling of the face and tongue and angioedema also may be present. This reflects involvement of deeper capillaries of the skin and mucous membranes. As hypoxia and shock continue, cyanosis appears.

NOTE Angioedema is a localized edematous reaction of the deep dermis or subcutaneous or submucosal tissues. It appears in the form of giant wheals. Patients with angioedema are at high risk for rapid deterioration.

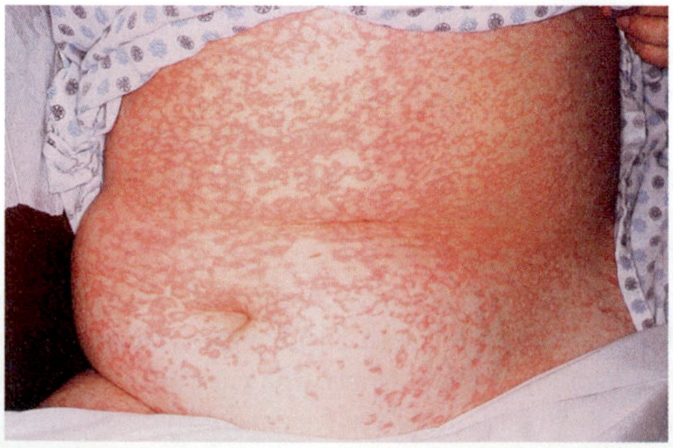

FIGURE 33-6 ■ Urticaria as a result of an allergic reaction. (Courtesy Gary Quick.)

Initial Assessment

As in any critical emergency, initial patient care measures are directed at providing adequate airway, ventilatory, and circulatory support. Drug therapy is the required treatment in anaphylaxis. Thus drug therapy should be started as quickly as possible.

Airway assessment is critical because most deaths from anaphylaxis are related directly to upper airway obstruction. The paramedic should evaluate the conscious patient for voice changes, stridor, or a barking cough. Complaints of tightness in the neck and dyspnea should alert the paramedic of impending airway obstruction. The paramedic should evaluate and secure the airway of an unconscious patient. If air movement is blocked, the paramedic should perform endotracheal intubation. If laryngeal and epiglottic edema is severe, surgical or needle cricothyrotomy (described in Chapter 19) may be indicated to provide airway access. Early, elective intubation is indicated for patients with hoarseness, lingual edema, and posterior or oropharyngeal swelling. If respiratory function deteriorates, medical direction may recommend tracheal intubation (with sedation) without paralytic agents.[1]

CRITICAL THINKING
How significant is stridor as a physical finding?

The paramedic should monitor the patient closely for signs of respiratory distress as indicated by pulse oximetry, skin color, accessory muscle use, wheezing, diminished breath sounds, and abnormal respiratory rates. The patient's circulatory status also may decline quickly. Thus the paramedic should assess pulse quality, rate, and location often.

History

A history may be hard to obtain. Yet it can be critical to rule out other medical emergencies that may mimic anaphylaxis. The paramedic should question the patient regarding the chief complaint and the rapidity of onset of symptoms. The signs and symptoms of anaphylaxis usually appear within 1 to 30 minutes of introduction of the antigen. The onset of a reaction can be delayed if the exposure is by the oral route.

Important medical history includes previous exposure and response to the suspected antigen. In addition, the paramedic should identify the method of exposure to the antigen. Injection of an antigen often produces the most rapid and severe response. Other significant history includes chronic or other illness and drugs that are used by the patient. Preexisting cardiac disease or bronchial asthma should cause the paramedic to anticipate severe complications as a result of the allergic reaction. Use of certain drugs, such as beta-blocking agents, may diminish the patient's response to ***epinephrine*** and may necessitate the administration of other medications. The paramedic also should determine whether the patient has an emergency ***epinephrine*** drug kit (e.g., EpiPen) and whether the medication was administered before the arrival of emergency medical services. Some patients with a history of allergic reaction may have taken an oral antihistamine (e.g., ***diphenhydramine***). Or they may have used aerosolized ***epinephrine*** (e.g., Primatene Mist or Medinhaler Epi). The patient's use of these drugs should be ascertained, if possible. Appropriate intervention, however, should not be delayed.

Physical Examination

The paramedic should assess vital signs often. In severe reactions, most patients initially are tachycardiac, tachypneic, and hypotensive if deterioration to cardiac arrest has not occurred. The paramedic should inspect the patient's face and neck for angioedema, hives, tearing, and rhinorrhea and should note the presence of erythema or urticaria on other body regions. Along with vital signs, the paramedic should assess airway and lung sounds often to evaluate the clinical progress of the patient. Such assessment also will help the paramedic to monitor the effectiveness of interventions. The paramedic should institute cardiac monitoring as soon as possible to aid in patient evaluation.

Key Interventions to Prevent Arrest

Organ involvement in anaphylaxis varies. This makes a standardized approach to patient management difficult. The following key interventions, however, commonly are used to manage anaphylaxis.[1]

1. Place the patient in position of comfort. Elevate the legs until replacement fluids improve blood pressure.
2. Administer high-concentration oxygen.
3. Give ***epinephrine*** to all patients with clinical signs of shock, airway swelling, or difficulty breathing. ***Epinephrine*** may be given by the IM, SQ, or IV route. (See the Emergency Drug Index.)
4. Initiate intravenous therapy with normal saline solution if hypotension is present and does not respond rapidly to ***epinephrine.*** A rapid infusion of 1 to 2 L (up to 4 L) may be needed initially.
5. Transport the patient for physician evaluation. Most patients will be observed carefully in the hospital for up to 24 hours. Many patients do not respond promptly to therapy, and symptoms may recur in some patients.

> **NOTE** Complications of intravenously administered ***epinephrine*** are significant. These include the development of uncontrolled systolic hypertension, vomiting, seizures, dysrhythmias, and myocardial ischemia. The intravenous route should be used only in patients with a critical life-threatening condition. Intravenous therapy is performed with extreme caution in rare circumstances and only with authorization from medical direction.

> **CRITICAL THINKING**
> How does ***epinephrine*** reverse the signs and symptoms of anaphylaxis?

OTHER DRUG THERAPY

Additional drug therapy may be helpful. However, ***epinephrine*** is the only drug that can reverse the life-threatening complications of anaphylaxis immediately. Pharmacological agents that may be used with ***epinephrine*** include antihistamine to antagonize the effects of histamine, beta-agonists to improve alveolar ventilation, corticosteroids to prevent a delayed reaction, ***glucagon*** (for patients unresponsive to ***epinephrine***, especially those taking antidysrhythmics [beta-blockers]), and perhaps vasopressors to manage protracted hypotension (Box 33-5).

> **NOTE** Beta-blockers may increase the incidence and severity of anaphylaxis and can produce a paradoxical response to ***epinephrine.***[1] In these cases, ***glucagon*** may be effective.

Key Interventions during Arrest

Cardiac arrest from anaphylaxis may be associated with profound vasodilation, intravascular collapse, tissue hypoxia, and asystole. Special considerations for resuscitation of these patients are described next.[1]

AIRWAY, OXYGENATION, AND VENTILATION

Swelling of the airway can make bag-mask ventilation and endotracheal intubation difficult or ineffective in patients with anaphylaxis. In addition, the landmarks for needle cricothyrotomy may not be visible because of severe

BOX 33-5 Additional Drug Therapy for Anaphylaxis

Antihistamines
Diphenhydramine
Hydroxyzine
Promethazine
Cimetidine
Ranitidine

Corticosteroids
Methylprednisolone
Hydrocortisone
Dexamethasone

Beta Agonists
Albuterol
Metaproterenol
Isoetharine

Antidysrhythmics
Amiodarone
Lidocaine and others

Vasopressors
Dopamine
Norepinephrine

Glucagon

swelling in the soft tissues of the neck. Fiberoptic intubation or digital intubation are alternative methods to consider in these situations (see Chapter 19).

SUPPORT OF CIRCULATION

Cardiac arrest from anaphylaxis requires rapid and aggressive volume replacement (2 to 4 L) to support circulation and the use of vasopressor drugs to support blood pressure. ***Epinephrine*** is the drug of choice for treatment of vasodilation and hypotension in cardiac arrest. The paramedic may need to administer ***epinephrine*** in high doses (see the EDI). In the presence of asystole or pulseless electrical activity (the most common arrest rhythms in anaphylaxis), the administration of ***atropine*** and transcutaneous pacing should be included (see Chapter 29). In addition, cardiac arrest from anaphylaxis may respond to prolonged periods of cardiopulmonary resuscitation. This may be the case especially when the patient is young and has a healthy heart and cardiovascular system.

SUMMARY

- Antibodies bind to the antigen that produced them. Antibodies aid in neutralizing the antigen and removing it from the body.
- Allergic reaction is an increased physiological response to an antigen after a previous exposure to the same antigen. Localized allergic reactions do not affect the entire body.
- Anaphylaxis is the most extreme form of allergic reaction. Rapid recognition and aggressive therapy are needed for patient survival.
- Almost any substance can cause anaphylaxis. The risk of anaphylaxis increases with the frequency of exposure.
- Symptoms of anaphylaxis may include sneezing and coughing; airway obstruction; wheezing; hypotension or vascular collapse; chest pain; nausea, vomiting, or diarrhea; and weakness, headache, syncope, seizures, or coma.

REFERENCES

1. American Heart Association: Guidelines 2000 for cardiopulmonary resuscitation and emergency cardiovascular care, International Consensus on Science, *Circulation* 102(8):241, 2000.
2. Rosen P, Barkin R: *Emergency medicine: concepts and clinical practice,* ed 4, St Louis, 1998, Mosby.

SUGGESTED READINGS

Altman L et al: *Allergy in primary care,* Philadelphia, 2000, WB Saunders.

Busse W, Gern J: *Contemporary diagnosis and management of allergic diseases and asthma,* ed 3, Newtown, Pa, 2003, Handbooks in Health Care.

Simmons F, Simons E: *Histamine and H-1 receptor antagonists in allergic disease,* New York, 1996, Marcel Dekker.

CHAPTER

34 Gastroenterology

OBJECTIVES

Upon completion of this chapter, the paramedic student will be able to:

1. Label a diagram of the abdominal organs.
2. Outline prehospital assessment of a patient who has abdominal pain.
3. Describe general prehospital management techniques for the patient with abdominal pain.
4. Describe signs and symptoms, complications, and prehospital management for the following gastrointestinal disorders: gastroenteritis, gastritis, colitis, diverticulosis, appendicitis, peptic ulcer disease, bowel obstruction, Crohn's disease, pancreatitis, esophagogastric varices, hemorrhoids, cholecystitis, and acute hepatitis.

KEY TERMS

acute gastroenteritis: Inflammation of the stomach and intestines with an associated sudden onset of vomiting, diarrhea, or both.

acute hepatitis: An inflammatory condition of the liver associated with the sudden onset of malaise, weakness, anorexia, intermittent nausea and vomiting, and dull right upper quadrant pain, usually followed within 1 week by the onset of jaundice, dark urine, or both, characterized by jaundice.

appendicitis: An acute inflammation of the appendix.

bowel obstruction: An occlusion of the intestinal lumen that results in blockage of normal flow of intestinal contents.

cholecystitis: Inflammation of the gallbladder, most often associated with the presence of gallstones.

chronic gastroenteritis: Inflammation of the stomach and intestines that accompanies numerous gastrointestinal disorders.

Crohn's disease: A chronic, inflammatory bowel disease of unknown origin, usually affecting the ileum, the colon, or both structures.

diverticulitis: Inflammation of one or more diverticula.

diverticulosis: The presence of pouchlike herniations through the muscular layer of the colon.

esophagogastric varices: A complex of longitudinal, tortuous veins at the lower end of the esophagus that become large and swollen as a result of portal hypertension.

hemorrhoids: Swollen, distended veins (internal, external, or both) in the rectoanal area.

involuntary guarding: An unconscious rigid contraction of the abdominal muscles; a sign of peritoneal inflammation.

pancreatitis: Inflammation of the pancreas, which causes severe epigastric pain.

peptic ulcer disease: Illness that results from a complex pathological interaction among the acidic gastric juice and proteolytic enzymes and the mucosal barrier.

rebound tenderness: A sign of peritoneal inflammation in which pain is caused by the sudden release of fingertip pressure on the abdomen.

referred pain: Visceral pain felt at a site distant from its origin.

somatic pain: Pain that arises from skeletal muscles, ligaments, vessels, or joints.

ulcerative colitis: An inflammatory condition of the large intestine characterized by severe diarrhea and ulceration of the mucosa of the intestine.

visceral pain: Deep pain that arises from smooth vasculature or organ systems.

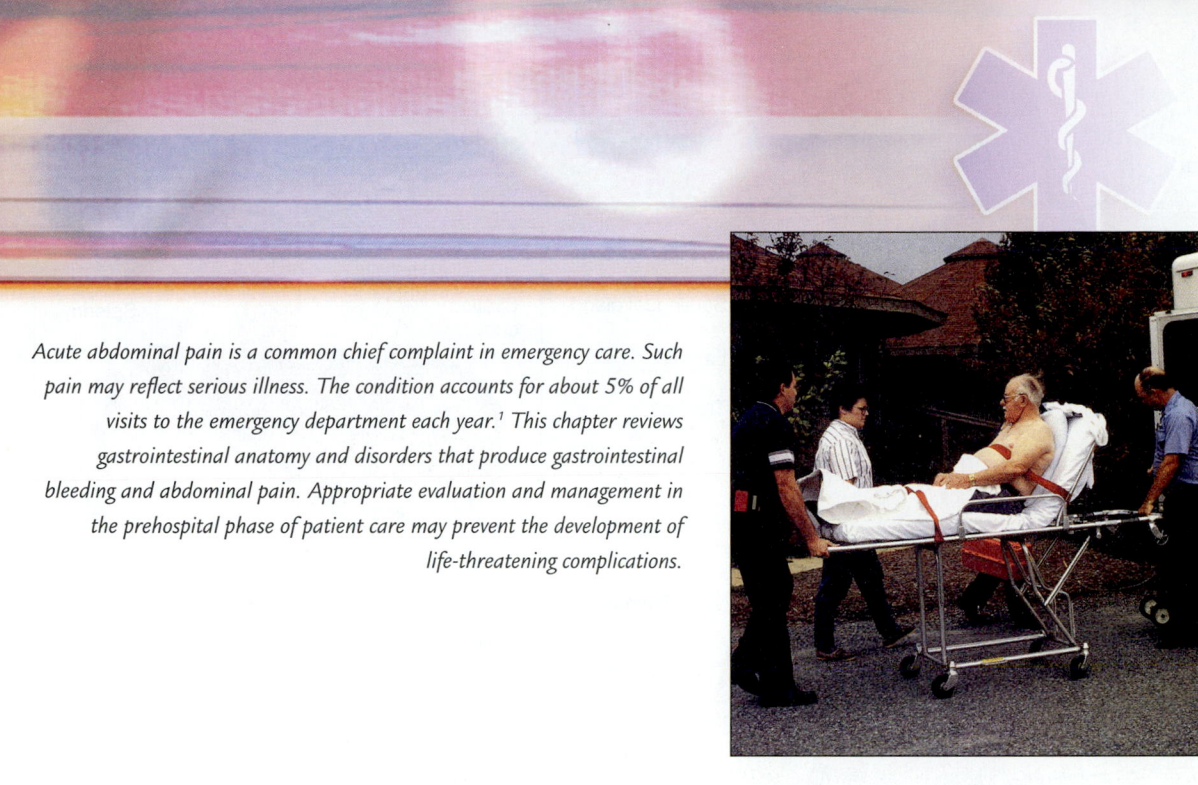

Acute abdominal pain is a common chief complaint in emergency care. Such pain may reflect serious illness. The condition accounts for about 5% of all visits to the emergency department each year.[1] This chapter reviews gastrointestinal anatomy and disorders that produce gastrointestinal bleeding and abdominal pain. Appropriate evaluation and management in the prehospital phase of patient care may prevent the development of life-threatening complications.

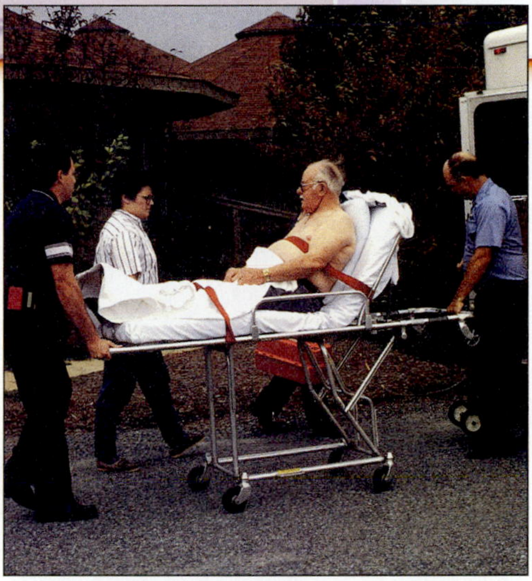

GASTROINTESTINAL ANATOMY

As described in Chapter 6, the gastrointestinal system provides the body with water, electrolytes, and other nutrients used by the cells. The major organs most often associated with the gastrointestinal system include the esophagus, stomach, small and large intestines, liver, gallbladder, and pancreas (Fig. 34-1). The genitourinary system also can produce abdominal pain and bleeding. This system is described in Chapters 35 and 41.

ASSESSMENT OF THE PATIENT WITH ACUTE ABDOMINAL PAIN

When caring for a patient with abdominal pain, the paramedic should begin the general assessment by ensuring that the scene is safe. This should include an initial scene size-up. The paramedic should determine whether the nature of the patient's abdominal pain is a result of trauma or a medical condition. This may be evident from the initial scene survey. The nature of the pain also may become evident by obtaining information from the patient, family, or bystanders. The paramedic should inspect the nearby area for medication bottles and signs of alcohol or other drug use. These signs may offer clues about the cause of the patient's condition. Any containers of emesis should be transported with the patient for laboratory analysis.

After the initial survey to ensure adequacy of airway, breathing, and circulation, assessment of the patient with acute abdominal pain begins with a thorough history focused on the chief complaint. The paramedic should assess and document the baseline vital signs. The paramedic should perform a systematic physical examination as well. This exam will help the paramedic to identify abdominal emergencies. These may indicate the development of shock or the need for immediate transport for surgical intervention.

History

When obtaining a history of abdominal pain, the paramedic should attempt to identify the location and type of pain and any associated signs and symptoms. Using the mnemonic OPQRST or a similar method can help the paramedic organize this information. Sample questions that might be included in the OPQRST evaluation include the following:

O (Onset): Was the onset of pain sudden? What were you doing when it started?

P (Provocative/palliative): What makes the pain better? What makes the pain worse? Does a sitting or lying position affect your discomfort?

Q (Quality): What does the pain feel like? Is it sharp, dull, burning, tearing?

R (Region): Where is the pain located? Does it travel (radiate) to another area of the body or does it stay in the same place?

S (Severity): Is the pain mild, moderate, or severe? What is the degree of discomfort on a scale of 1 to 10?

T (Time): When did the pain begin? Is it constant or intermittent? If intermittent, how long does the pain episode last?

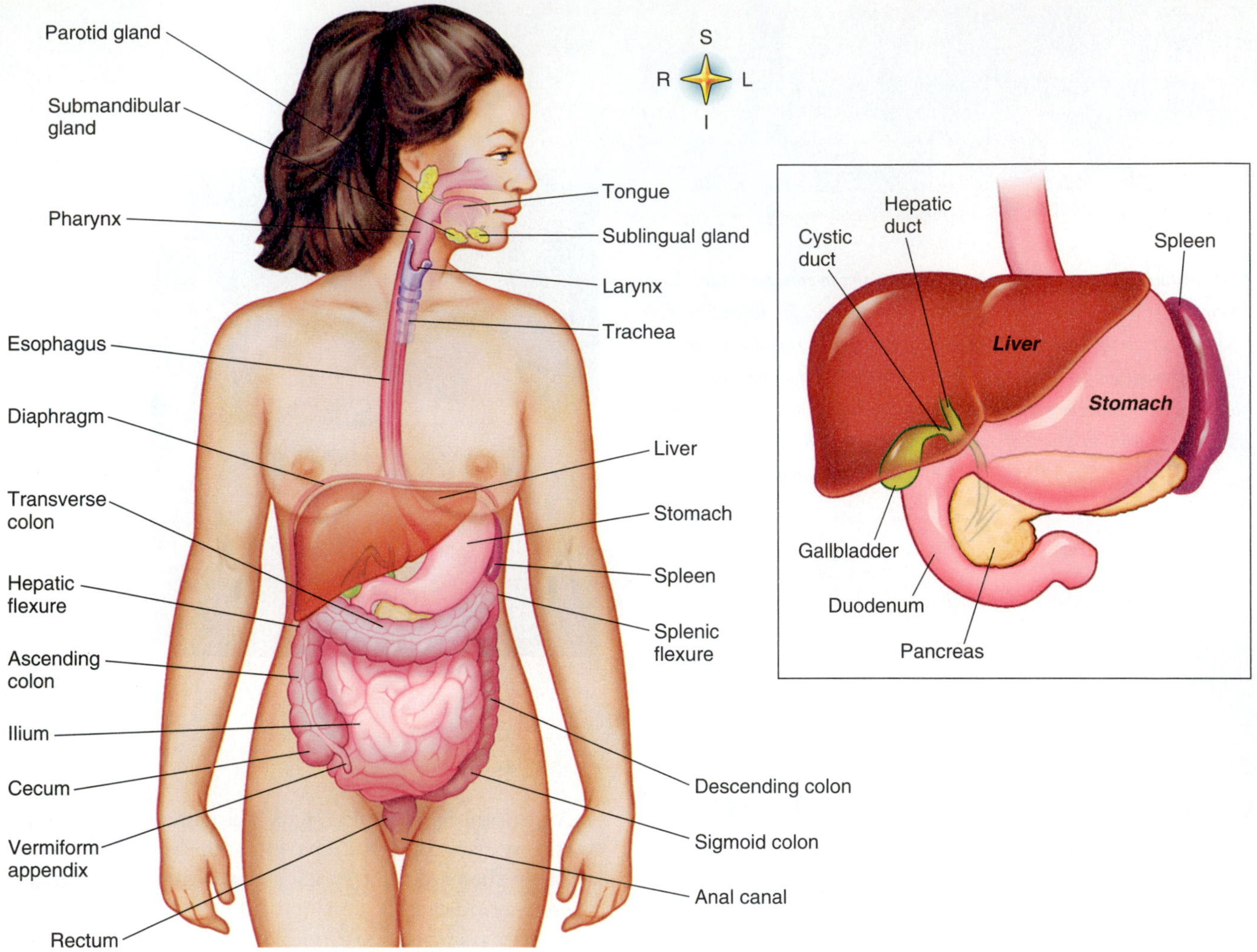

FIGURE 34-1 ■ Location of digestive organs.

Other key elements of a patient history can be obtained through a SAMPLE history (*S*igns and symptoms, *A*llergies, *M*edications, *P*ast medical history, *L*ast meal or oral intake, and *E*vents before the emergency). This will help to identify symptoms, allergies, medical history, last oral intake, and important events that preceded the patient's chief complaint. Of particular importance is significant medical history, such as hypertension or cardiac or respiratory disease that may manifest in abdominal pain; medication use; alcohol or other drug use; last bowel movement and any significant changes in the patient's bowel habits; and previous abdominal surgeries. Women of childbearing age also should be questioned about menstrual periods (including regularity and the date of the last menstrual period) and the possibility of pregnancy.

Persistent abdominal pain lasting 6 hours or longer warrants patient transport for physician evaluation. As a rule, patients with abdominal pain should not receive pain medication in the field. Analgesics can mask signs and symptoms that are critical for a physician to evaluate accurately the cause of a patient's pain. In addition, patients should not be permitted to eat or drink anything because surgery may be needed.

> **CRITICAL THINKING**
>
> What factors can influence a patient's perception and description of pain?

Location and Type of Abdominal Pain

To assess a specific disorder, the paramedic can use a method that relates anatomical location of gastrointestinal organs and structures to origin. Box 34-1 lists location of abdominal pain and possible causes of illness. The types of abdominal pain that may result from chronic or acute episodes may be classified as *visceral, somatic,* and *referred.*

VISCERAL PAIN

Visceral pain (or organ pain) is caused by the stimulation of autonomic nerve fibers that surround a hollow organ. Visceral pain also can be caused by the distention or

BOX 34-1 Location of Abdominal Pain and Possible Origins

Right Upper Quadrant
Cholecystitis
Hepatitis
Pancreatitis
Perforated ulcer
Renal pain (right)

Left Upper Quadrant
Gastritis
Pancreatitis
Renal pain (left)

Right Lower Quadrant
Abdominal aortic dissection or rupture
Appendicitis
Hernia
Ovarian cyst (right)
Ovarian or testicular torsion
Pelvic inflammatory disease
Ruptured ectopic pregnancy
Urinary calculus

Left Lower Quadrant
Abdominal aortic dissection or rupture

Left Lower Quadrant, cont'd
Diverticulitis
Hernia
Ovarian cyst (left)
Ovarian or testicular torsion
Pelvic inflammatory disease
Ruptured ectopic pregnancy
Urinary calculus

Epigastric Pain
Abdominal aortic aneurysm
Cholecystitis
Esophagitis
Gastritis
Myocardial ischemia
Pancreatitis

Diffuse Pain
Generalized peritonitis
Intestinal obstruction
Perforation

stretching of hollow organs or the ligaments. The patient usually describes the pain as cramping or gas-type pain. Patients usually say that the pain varies in intensity, increasing to a high degree of severity and then subsiding. Visceral pain generally is diffuse. Thus the pain is difficult to localize. Often the pain is centered at the umbilicus or lower in the midline. Visceral pain often is associated with other symptoms of autonomic nerve involvement such as tachycardia, diaphoresis, nausea, or vomiting. Common causes of visceral abdominal pain include early **appendicitis, pancreatitis, cholecystitis,** and intestinal obstruction.

SOMATIC PAIN

Somatic pain is produced by bacterial or chemical irritation of nerve fibers in the peritoneum (peritonitis). Unlike visceral pain, somatic pain usually is constant. Moreover, the pain is localized to a specific area. The patient often describes the pain as sharp or stabbing. Patients with somatic abdominal pain generally are hesitant to move about. They may lie on their back or side with legs flexed to prevent more pain from stimulation of the peritoneal area. These patients often exhibit **involuntary guarding** of the abdomen during the physical examination and **rebound tenderness** (signs of peritoneal inflammation). Common causes of somatic pain are appendicitis and an inflamed or perforated viscus (ulcer, gallbladder, or small or large intestine).

REFERRED PAIN

Referred pain is pain in a part of the body considerably removed from the tissues that cause the pain. This mechanism results from branches of visceral fibers that synapse in the spinal cord with the same second-order neurons that receive pain fibers from the skin. When these pain fibers are stimulated intensely, pain sensations spread. The patient experiences the pain in areas distant from the original source.

A knowledge of referred pain is important because many visceral ailments cause no other symptoms except referred pain. For example, cardiac pain may be referred to the neck and jaw, shoulders, pectoral muscles, and down the arms; biliary pain to the right subscapular area; renal colic to the genitalia and flank area; uterine and rectal pain to the low back; and a leaking aortic aneurysm to the lower back or buttocks. Fig. 34-2 illustrates surface areas of referred pain from visceral organs.

Signs and Symptoms

Although numerous signs and symptoms may be associated with acute abdominal pain, the following are the most common[2]:

1. Nausea, vomiting, anorexia
   Appendicitis
   Biliary tract disease
   Gastritis
   High intestinal obstruction
   Pancreatitis
2. Diarrhea
   Inflammatory process (gastroenteritis, **ulcerative colitis**)
3. Constipation
   Dehydration, obstruction, medication-induced decreased intestinal motility (codeine, ***morphine***)
4. Change in stool color
   Biliary tract obstruction (clay-colored stools)
   Lower intestinal bleeding (black, tarry stools)
5. Chills and fever
   Appendicitis
   Bacterial infection
   Cholecystitis
   Pyelonephritis

Vital Signs

Vital sign assessment should include evaluation and documentation of the patient's blood pressure; pulse rate (including electrocardiogram assessment); respiratory rate; and skin color, moisture, temperature, and turgor. If possible, the paramedic should check the patient for orthostatic pulse and blood pressure changes. As described in Chapter 21, a rise from a recumbent position to a sitting or standing position associated with a fall in systolic pressure (after 1 minute) of 10 to 15 mm Hg and/or a concurrent rise in pulse rate (after 1 minute) of 10 to 15 beats per minute indicates a significant volume depletion and a decrease in perfusion status. The paramedic also should perform an assessment of blood pressure, pulses, and capillary refill in each extremity as a consideration for aortic dissection (described in Chapter 29).

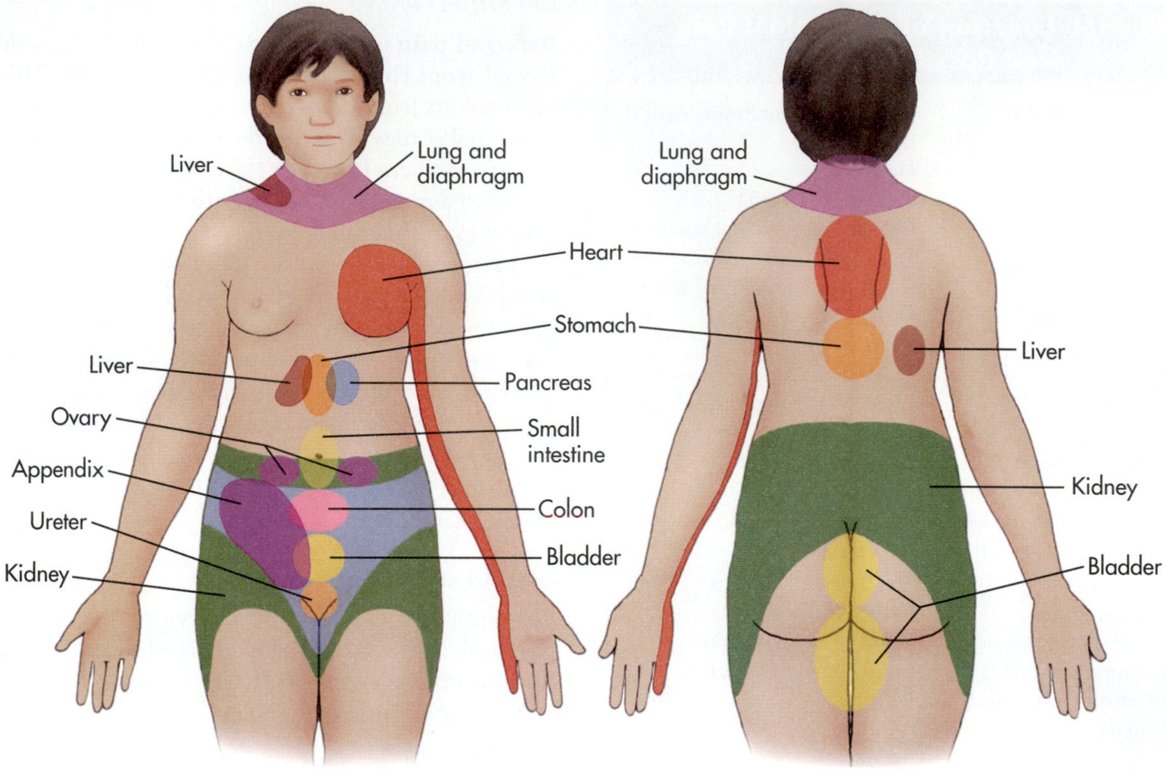

FIGURE 34-2 ■ Referred pain. **A**, Anterior view. **B**, Posterior view.

Physical Examination

The physical examination of a patient with acute abdominal pain includes the skills of inspection, auscultation, percussion, and palpation. If a life-threatening illness is suspected, rapid stabilization and transportation of the patient is the first priority. Further examination can be completed en route to the receiving hospital. Physical examination of the patient's abdomen is described in Chapter 11. However, the following discussion serves as a review. (Male and female physical examinations to evaluate genitourinary complaints are discussed in Chapter 35.)

INSPECTION

In the initial patient encounter, the paramedic should note the position in which the patient is lying. As stated before, many patients with abdominal peritoneal irritation lie on their sides. They often have their knees flexed and pulled in toward their chests. Other visual clues that may indicate abdominal pain are skin color, facial expressions such as grimacing, and the presence or absence of voluntary movement. The paramedic should remove the patient's clothing and inspect the abdominal wall for the presence of bruises, scars, ascites (Fig. 34-3) abdominal distention, or abdominal masses.

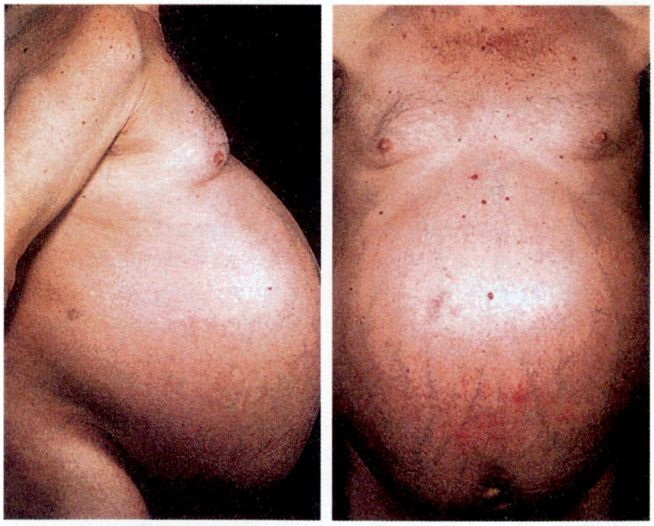

FIGURE 34-3 ■ Gross ascites in a male patient.

AUSCULTATION

Determining the presence or absence of bowel sounds by auscultation usually is done in the emergency department. But if auscultation is to be performed, it should be done for about 2 minutes in each quadrant before determining that bowel sounds are absent. (Auscultation should always precede palpation and percussion because these procedures may alter the intensity of bowel sounds.) Bowel sounds that are increased in number, duration, or intensity indicate the possibility of gastroenteritis or intestinal obstruction. Bowel sounds that are considerably decreased in number and intensity (or their absence) may indicate peritonitis or ileus (obstruction of the intestine).

PALPATION

The paramedic should begin palpation of the abdomen gently and avoid the painful area until after examining the rest of the abdomen. The paramedic should be alert to rigidity or spasm, tenderness or masses, and to the patient's facial expressions. These may provide clues about the severity of the pain. In addition, the paramedic should note whether the abdomen is soft or rigid.

PERCUSSION

If time permits, the paramedic may perform a general assessment of tympany and dullness by percussion to detect the presence of fluid, air, or solid masses in the abdomen. The paramedic should use a systematic approach and move from side to side or clockwise. Tenderness and abdominal skin temperature and color should be noted. To review, tympany is the major sound that should be noted during percussion because of the normal presence of air in the stomach and intestines. Dullness should be heard over organs and solid masses.

BOX 34-2 Emergency Care for Acute Abdominal Pain

1. High-concentration oxygen administration
2. Adequate intravenous access with a crystalloid solution (Application of the pneumatic antishock garment for the treatment of shock with acute abdominal pain is controversial and should be authorized by medical direction.)
3. Electrocardiogram monitoring
4. Rapid and gentle transport to an appropriate medical facility

BOX 34-3 Gastrointestinal Disorders

Acute gastroenteritis	Diverticulosis
Acute hepatitis	Esophagogastric varices
Appendicitis	Gastrointestinal bleeding
Bowel obstruction	Hemorrhoids
Cholecystitis	Pancreatitis
Chronic gastroenteritis	Peptic ulcer disease
Crohn's disease	Ulcerative colitis

MANAGEMENT OF THE PATIENT WITH AN ABDOMINAL EMERGENCY

Patients with acute abdominal pain or gastrointestinal bleeding cannot be managed effectively in the prehospital setting. The majority require extensive evaluation in the emergency department, including laboratory analysis, radiological imaging, fluid and medication therapy, and perhaps surgical intervention. The role of the paramedic is to support the patient's airway and ventilatory status; to perform and document an initial patient assessment, including a thorough history; to monitor vital signs and cardiac rhythm; to initiate intravenous therapy for fluid replacement or fluid resuscitation; and to transport the patient rapidly for physician evaluation (Box 34-2).

SPECIFIC ABDOMINAL EMERGENCIES

Abdominal emergencies can result from inflammation, infection, and obstruction. Some disorders may be associated with upper gastrointestinal bleeding. (Examples of such include lesions, peptic ulceration, and **esophagogastric varices.**) Some disorders may be associated with lower gastrointestinal bleeding. (Examples of such include colonic lesions, **diverticulosis,** and **hemorrhoids.**) Other disorders, such as pancreatitis and cholecystitis, more often are associated with acute abdominal pain in the absence of bleeding. Box 34-3 lists the specific gastrointestinal disorders discussed in this chapter.

Gastrointestinal Bleeding

Gastrointestinal bleeding is a common clinical problem seen by paramedics. It often requires hospitalization. It can vary from a chronic blood loss to a massive, life-threatening hemorrhage. The massive hemorrhage may be hard to stop or control. Many bleeding episodes resolve spontaneously. However, for a physician to identify the bleeding site is crucial to help prevent a recurrence. Bleeding from the gastrointestinal tract can be classified by site of origin as upper or lower gastrointestinal bleeding.

The most common causes of upper gastrointestinal bleeding are **peptic ulcer disease** and variceal rupture (e.g., esophageal varices that result from underlying chronic liver disease such as cirrhosis). Another cause of upper gastrointestinal bleeding is Mallory-Weiss syndrome. (This is an esophageal laceration that usually results from repeated vomiting or retching.) Other causes are tumors or cancers of the esophagus or stomach. Factors that may aggravate upper gastrointestinal bleeding include use of nonsteroidal antiinfammatory drugs such as ***aspirin*** and other antiarthritic drugs, chronic liver disease, blood-thinning medications (e.g., warfarin), and underlying medical conditions such as renal disease, hypertension, and cardiorespiratory diseases. Upper gastrointestinal bleeding accounts for more than 300,000 hospitalizations each year and has a mortality rate of about 10%.[2] Risk factors include increasing age, alcohol and tobacco use, and coexisting illness such as hypertension, diabetes, and cardiorespiratory disease.

The most common cause of lower gastrointestinal (colon) bleeding is diverticulosis. Other causes include colon cancers, colon polyps, and inflammatory bowel disorders such as ulcerative colitis and **Crohn's disease.** These conditions are described later in this chapter. Like upper gastrointestinal bleeding, lower gastrointestinal bleeding may be mild or may be brisk and difficult to control. Common complaints include cramping abdominal pain, diarrhea (which may be bloody), nausea, vomiting, and changes in the patient's stool and bowel habits.

Gastrointestinal bleeding depends on the acuteness and the source of the blood loss. Mild chronic gastrointestinal blood loss may present without any noticeable bleeding. It can result in an iron deficiency anemia. These patients often are unaware that they are bleeding and may or may not notice small amounts of blood with their bowel movements. Patients with severe cases of chronic or acute bleeding can have signs of anemia such as weakness, pallor, dizziness, shortness of breath, or angina. (The hematocrit of these patients may be within normal range in the early phase of their hemorrhage.)

More serious gastrointestinal bleeding may occur with hematemesis (bloody vomitus). Vomit may be red or have a dark, coffee ground–like appearance. Blood in the stool could present as bright red, dark and clotted, or black and tarry. Presentation depends on the location of the bleeding source. A black, tarry stool (melena) often indicates an upper gastrointestinal source of bleeding where blood has been digested partially. However, bleeding also could originate from the small intestine or right colon. Bright, red blood from the rectum (hematochezia) after a bowel movement usually signifies a bleeding source close to the rectal opening. Such bleeding often results from hemorrhoids. However, conditions such as rectal cancers, polyps, ulcerations or infections also can cause this type of bleeding.

Any source of gastrointestinal bleeding that is active or severe usually requires hospitalization. With hospitalization the hypovolemia can be managed with intravenously administered fluids or blood transfusions if needed. Attempts to identify and stop the source of hemorrhage may include the use of medications, diagnostic tests (e.g., barium gastrointestinal studies, nuclear scans, angiography, endoscopy, and colonoscopy), and other therapeutic measures such as gastric lavage, the placement of a Sengstaken-Blakemore tube (to tamponade bleeding in the esophagus), and in some cases, surgery. Prehospital care for patients with active and severe gastrointestinal bleeding includes provision of emotional support, administration of high-concentration oxygen, airway and ventilatory management, intravenous fluid bolus (20 mL/kg) fluid resuscitation (pneumatic antishock garment per protocol) as needed, and rapid transport for physician evaluation.

Acute Gastroenteritis

Acute gastroenteritis is inflammation of the stomach and intestines with an associated sudden onset of vomiting, diarrhea, or both. The condition is a common problem worldwide and is responsible for more than 4 million deaths per year in developing countries.[3] The condition may be caused by bacterial or viral infection, parasites (e.g., *Giardia,* responsible for "traveler's diarrhea, and *Cyclosporidium,* reported to be contracted in contaminated water), chemical toxins, and other conditions such as allergies, lactose intolerance, and immune disorders. The inflammation causes hemorrhage and erosion of the mucosal layers of the gastrointestinal tract. Inflammation also can affect the way in which water and nutrients are absorbed.

Infectious forms of acute gastroenteritis usually are caused by exposure to rotavirus, adenovirus, astrovirus, Norwalk virus, or from a group of Noroviruses. The condition often is called the "stomach flu," although it is not caused by the influenza viruses. Typically, children under 5 years of age are most vulnerable to rotaviruses. (These are the most common cause of watery diarrhea in children.) Adenoviruses and astroviruses cause diarrhea mostly in young children. Yet older children and adults also can be affected. The Norwalk virus and Noroviruses are more likely to cause diarrhea in older children and adults. Infectious acute gastroenteritis usually is transmitted through fecal-oral route and by ingestion of infected food or contaminated water. The condition is common in institutional settings (e.g., schools, day care centers, and nursing homes) and other group settings (e.g., banquet halls, cruise ships, dormitories, and campgrounds) where it can spread quickly. Infectious acute gastroenteritis also can arise among travelers in endemic areas. (Native populations in endemic areas generally are resistant.) Infectious acute gastroenteritis also can arise in populations in disaster areas where water supplies are contaminated. Bacteria that may be responsible for acute gastroenteritis include *Salmonella, Escherichia coli, Campylobacter,* and *Staphylococcus.* Contamination generally results from poor sanitation, the lack of safe drinking water, or contaminated food.

As the name implies, acute gastroenteritis is often abrupt and violent. It involves rapid loss of fluids and electrolytes from constant vomiting and diarrhea. Fluid loss and dehydration may be severe in pediatric patients, the elderly, and in those who are immunosuppressed. Hypokalemia and hyponatremia, acidosis, or alkalosis may develop. Treatment mainly is supportive, requiring intravenous fluid replacement, sedation, bed rest, and medications to control vomiting and diarrhea. Some forms of gastroenteritis can be treated with antibiotic therapy. Emergency medical services personnel who are working in disaster areas should observe the following guidelines[2]:

- Avoid patient contact if you are ill.
- Know the source of water supplies. Or drink hot beverages that have been boiled or disinfected.
- Avoid habits that aid fecal-oral/mucous membrane transmission.
- Observe body substance isolation precautions. Also observe good hand-washing procedures.

CRITICAL THINKING

What would be your main concern for a patient with a history of severe gastroenteritis?

Chronic Gastroenteritis

Chronic gastroenteritis results from inflammation of the stomach and intestines. This can produce long-term changes or damage to the gastric mucosa. The condition is usually due to microbial infection, hyperacidity, or the chronic use of alcohol, ***aspirin,*** and other nonsteroidal antiinflammatory medications. Chronic gastroenteritis commonly results from *Helicobacter pylori* infection but also may be caused by other bacteria such as *E. coli, Klebsiella pneumoniae, Enterobacter, Campylobacter jejuni, Vibrio cholerae, Shigella,* and *Salmonella.* With the exception of *Shigella* and *Salmonella,* many of the bacteria responsible for chronic gastroenteritis are part of the normal intestinal flora. Thus this precludes effective vaccination against these strains. Other causes of chronic gastroenteritis include the Norwalk virus and rotavirus and parasitic infection from protozoa such as *Giardia* and *Cryptosporidium parvum*. The pathogenic agents responsible for the disease may be contracted via fecal-oral transmission. They also may be contracted by contaminated food and water. Emergency medical services personnel should follow the same guidelines for personal safety as described previously.

NOTE *Helicobacter pylori* resides in the human stomach. The bacteria resides between the epithelial surface and the overlying mucosa. The bacteria is more prevalent in lower socioeconomic groups. The bacteria may be spread in adults and children through the fecal-oral route. The presence of *H. pylori* is believed to cause mucosal inflammation. This inflammation disrupts the normal defense mechanism of the stomach and can lead to ulceration.

Signs and symptoms of chronic gastroenteritis include epigastric pain, nausea and vomiting (which may be severe), fever, anorexia, mucosal bleeding (erosive gastritis), and epigastric tenderness on palpation. In severe cases the patient may have hypovolemia and shock. The condition is treated with diet regulation, medications (antibiotics, antacids), and fluid replacement or fluid resuscitation if hypovolemia or dehydration occurs.

Ulcerative Colitis

Ulcerative colitis also is known as colitis or proctitis. Ulcerative colitis is an inflammatory condition of the large intestine. The condition is classified as an inflammatory bowel disease. Ulcerative colitis is characterized by ulceration of the mucosa of the intestine. This usually occurs in the rectum and lower part of the colon but may affect the entire colon. The inflammation makes the colon empty often (causing diarrhea). In addition, the ulceration causes bleeding and produces pus. Ulcerative colitis can occur at any age. Yet most often ulcerative colitis starts between ages 15 and 30 or less often between ages 50 and 70. The condition affects men and women equally. A family history of the disease is present in 10% to 15% of cases. The cause of ulcerative colitis is unknown. However, the cause may be related to the immune system and the way it reacts to a virus or a bacterium that causes chronic inflammation in the intestinal wall. Other possible causes of the disorder include allergies to certain foods (e.g., lactose intolerance) and environmental and psychological factors.

The most common signs and symptoms of ulcerative colitis are fatigue, weight loss, anorexia, rectal bleeding, and the loss of body fluids and nutrients. Some patients have only mild symptoms. Other patients, however, experience frequent fever, bloody diarrhea, nausea, and severe abdominal cramping. Some patients with the disease have remissions that last for months or years; most patients' symptoms eventually return. After physician evaluation and stabilization, the condition usually is managed with steroids, electrolytes, antibiotics, and diet regulation. Few patients require surgery to manage ulcerative colitis; however, surgical removal of the diseased colon may be indicated in severe cases. Prehospital care is dictated by the severity of the patient's condition. The care may vary from providing only emotional support and transportation for physician evaluation to providing airway, ventilatory, and circulatory support to manage hypovolemia and shock.

NOTE In patients with acquired immunodeficiency syndrome, the chronic diarrhea and diffuse colonic involvement of Kaposi's sarcoma (described in Chapter 39) may mimic chronic ulcerative colitis. Undiagnosed signs of human immunodeficiency virus infection also may be the cause. At times, surgical bowel resection may be required in these patients.

Diverticulosis

A diverticulum is a sac or pouch that develops in the wall of the colon (Fig. 34-4). A diverticulum is a common development with advancing years and is associated with diets low in fiber. Diverticular outpouchings (a condition known as diverticulosis) tend to develop because of the high pressure within the contracting sigmoid colon that regulates movement of stool into the rectum. The outpouchings are most common at the weakest point in the colon wall. This is on the left side just above the rectum. As a diverticulum expands, it develops a thin wall compared to the rest of the colon. The thin wall may allow bacteria to seep through and cause infection. Often there is a small artery or arteri-

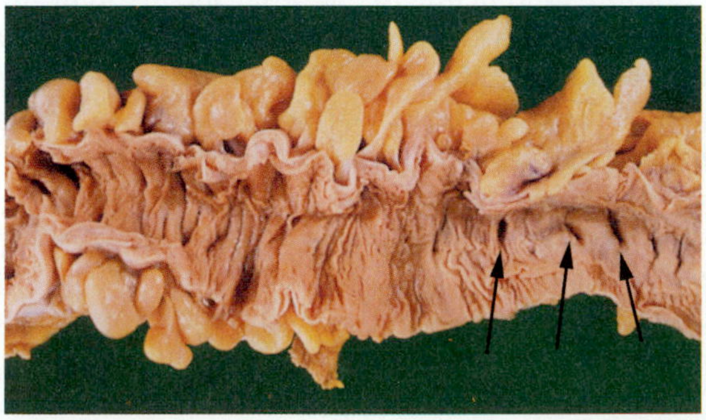

FIGURE 34-4 ■ Diverticular disease. In diverticular disease the outpouches *(arrows)* of mucosa seen in the sigmoid colon appear as slitlike openings from the mucosal surface of the opened bowel.

ole in the neck of the diverticulum from which subsequent bleeding may occur.

Most patients with diverticula are completely symptom free. However, up to 30% of these patients experience **diverticulitis** when one or more diverticula become obstructed with fecal matter. Mild complications of diverticulitis include irregular bowel habits (alternating constipation and diarrhea), fever, and lower left quadrant pain. Diverticulitis tends to reoccur within the first 5 years after the onset of symptoms. Definitive care for these patients includes diet regulation, a high-fiber diet to stimulate daily bowel movements, antibiotic therapy, and sometimes, surgical repair.

Serious complications of diverticular disease are associated with perforation of the bowel. These complications include massive bright red rectal bleeding (or dark stools if bleeding is from a diverticulum in the right colon). Hemorrhage from a diverticulum can occur rapidly, is often painless, and is the most common cause of massive rectal bleeding in older adults. If bacteria escape into the abdomen, peritonitis or an abscess may develop. The hemorrhage often ceases spontaneously. But if bleeding does not stop, emergency surgery may be necessary.

Appendicitis

Appendicitis is a common abdominal emergency. It occurs in 7% to 10% of the U.S. population. The condition may present at any age, but most patients are 8 to 25 years old; appendicitis rarely is seen in children less than 2 years of age.

Appendicitis occurs when the passageway between the appendix and the cecum is obstructed by fecal matter (fecalith). Appendicitis also may be due to an inflammation of the area from viral or bacterial infection. Obstruction of the passageway leads to distention of the appendix. Poor lymphatic and venous drainage allows bacterial infection to develop. If the condition continues, the inflamed organ eventually becomes gangrenous. Then the appendix ruptures into the peritoneal cavity. This results in peritonitis (which may progress to shock) or the development of abscesses.

Because of variations in the position of the appendix, age of the patient, and degree of inflammation, the clinical presentation of appendicitis is often inconsistent. (Many other disorders have similar signs and symptoms.) Young children and older adults also may have atypical illness because of reduced inflammatory response associated with extremes of age. This makes appendicitis more difficult to diagnose in these age groups. The classic presentation of appendicitis is abdominal pain or cramping, nausea, vomiting, chills, low-grade fever, and anorexia. At first, the pain is periumbilical and diffuse. Later the pain becomes intense and localized to the right lower quadrant just medial to the iliac crest *(McBurney point)*. If the appendix ruptures, the patient's pain diminishes before the development of peritoneal signs. The goal of definitive care for appendicitis is surgical appendectomy before rupture.

CRITICAL THINKING

What other illness presents similar signs or symptoms?

Peptic Ulcer Disease

Peptic ulcer disease results from a complex pathological interaction among the acidic gastric juice and proteolytic enzymes and the mucosal barrier. As described in Chapter 6, digestion occurs as food passes through the gastrointestinal tract. The stomach produces hydrochloric acid and an enzyme called pepsin to digest the food. From the stomach, food passes into the duodenum. In the duodenum, digestion and nutrient absorption continue. The stomach normally protects itself from the digestive fluids by producing mucus to shield stomach tissues. The stomach also produces bicarbonate to neutralize and break down digestive fluids into substances that are less harmful to stomach tissue. Blood circulation to the stomach lining, cell renewal, and cell repair also help protect the stomach.

Ulcers can form in the lining of the stomach or duodenum where acid and pepsin are present. These sores cause the disintegration and death of tissue as they erode the mucosal layers in the affected areas. If the sores are left untreated, massive hemorrhage or perforation may result. The three most common causes of peptic ulcer disease are *H. pylori* infection, nonsteroidal antiinflammatory drug use, and increased circulatory gastrin from gastrin-secreting tumors (Zollinger-Ellison syndrome),[1] all of which can cause the defense mechanisms of the stomach to fail. Ulcers can develop at any age. Yet they are rare among teenagers and even more uncommon in children. Duodenal ulcers occur for the first time usually between the ages of 30 and 50. They are more frequent in men than women.

The patient with a peptic ulcer usually is aware of the condition. The patient often uses over-the-counter antacids. The ulcer pain often is described as a burning or gnawing discomfort in the epigastric region or left upper quadrant (in the case of gastric ulcer). The discomfort develops before meals (classically, early morning) or during stressful periods, when the production of gastric acids increases. The pain usually is sudden in onset. Pain often is relieved by food intake, antacids, or vomiting. In addition to pain and vomiting of blood, the patient may experience melena as a result of blood passing through the gastrointestinal tract.

Prehospital care for patients with peptic ulcer disease includes obtaining a pertinent history, evaluating for hypotension, and providing circulatory support as needed. After physician evaluation, definitive care may involve antibiotics, antacids, H_2 receptor antagonists or other medications, and occasionally, diet regulation (the benefit of which is controversial). Some patients with acute peptic ulcer disease require hospitalization for fluid or blood replacement or for surgery if medications are not effective or blood loss is ongoing.

Bowel Obstruction

Bowel obstruction is an occlusion of the intestinal lumen. It results in blockage of normal flow of intestinal contents. Bowel obstruction may be caused by an ileus in which the bowel does not work properly. However, more commonly bowel obstruction results from mechanical obstruction such as adhesions, herniae (Box 34-4), fecal impaction, polyps, and tumors. Other causes of bowel obstruction are *intussusception* (telescoping of one portion of the intestine into another, which results in decreased blood supply of the involved segment), *volvulus* (twisting of the intestines), and ingested foreign bodies. Most bowel obstructions occur in the small bowel (accounting for 20% of all hospital admissions for abdominal complaints) and usually are caused by adhesions or herniae.[4] Large bowel obstructions most often result from tumors or fecal impactions.

NOTE Paralytic ileus can closely mimic bowel obstructions. (Paralytic ileus is a decrease or absence of intestinal peristalsis.) This pseudo-obstruction may result from a number of localized or systemic conditions such as medications (especially narcotics), intraperitoneal infection, complications of abdominal surgery, and metabolic disturbances (e.g., decreased potassium levels).

Signs and symptoms of intestinal obstruction include nausea and vomiting, abdominal pain, constipation, and abdominal distention. The speed of onset and degree of symptoms depend on the anatomical site of obstruction (small versus large bowel). The most significant danger is perforation of the bowel with generalized peritonitis and sepsis.

The patient with bowel obstruction often has abdominal pain; dehydration may result from vomiting, decreased intestinal absorption, and fluid loss into the lumen and interstitium (bowel wall edema). As the affected portion of the bowel distends, its blood supply is decreased. Then the segment becomes ischemic. The wall is weakened and perforates, producing peritonitis. If the intestine becomes strangulated, blood or plasma also may be lost from the affected intestinal segment. Definitive care involves fluid replacement, antibiotics, placement of a nasogastric tube for decompression, and frequently surgery to correct the obstructing lesion. (Nasogastric tube insertion is described in the appendix to this chapter.)

BOX 34-4 Hernia

A hernia is the protrusion of an organ from its normal position through a congenital or acquired opening. Herniation is most often through the musculature of the groin or abdominal wall. Increases in intraabdominal pressure can cause the peritoneum to push outward through such an opening. (Examples of such increases include those associated with straining, coughing, or lifting.) When this occurs, a sac is formed into which various organs within the peritoneal cavity may enter.

Most herniae are uncomplicated. Most herniae also can be placed back into the peritoneal cavity by a physician. If the herniae cannot be placed back, however, the trapped contents of the peritoneal sac (usually a portion of bowel) can become strangulated. These patients often have acute abdominal pain and systemic signs such as fever and tachycardia. Incarcerated or strangulated herniae can lead to serious complications, including intestinal obstruction, perforation, and peritonitis. Definitive care for complicated herniae is in-hospital observation, intravenous rehydration, pain medication, and surgical repair.

CRITICAL THINKING

Have you ever responded to a call for "constipation"? Did the paramedics consider this diagnosis a possibility? What was the attitude toward the patient?

Crohn's Disease

Crohn's disease is a chronic, inflammatory bowel disease that usually affects the ileum, the colon, or both structures. Crohn's disease may occur in persons of all ages but is primarily a disease of the young adult. (Most cases are diagnosed before age 30.) The disease is thought to be of autoimmune origin and tends to run in families and in certain ethnic groups. More than 20,000 cases are reported annually in the United States.[5] The incidence of Crohn's disease in the U.S. has been doubling every 10 years for the past 3 decades.[1]

The inflammation associated with Crohn' s disease may cause blockage of the intestine. Blockage occurs because the disease tends to thicken the intestinal wall with swelling and scar tissue, narrowing the passage. The disease also may cause ulcers that tunnel through the affected area into surrounding tissues such as the bladder, vagina, or skin. The areas around the anus and rectum often are involved. The tunnels, called fistulae, are a common complication and often become infected. Other complications associated with Crohn's disease include arthritis, skin problems, inflammation in the eyes or mouth, kidney stones, gallstones, or other diseases of the liver and biliary system.

Crohn's disease can be difficult to diagnose because its symptoms are similar to irritable bowel syndrome and ulcerative colitis. Crohn's disease is characterized by frequent attacks of diarrhea, severe abdominal pain, nausea, fever, chills, weakness, anorexia, and weight loss. (Patients with Crohn's and like diseases often suffer from depression because of the relentless and painful characteristics of

NOTE The term *irritable bowel syndrome* or spastic colon is used to describe abnormally increased motility of the small and large intestines. Unlike inflammatory bowel disease, the abdominal pain of irritable bowel syndrome generally is associated with emotional and physical stress. Pain generally is relieved by bowel movement as well.

these conditions.) The paramedic should suspect the disease in any patient with chronic inflammatory colitis and a history of rectal fistulae or abscesses. These patients frequently are hospitalized. Once patients are stabilized, the condition may be managed with antibiotics, steroids, antimotility agents to attempt to induce remission, and diet regulation.

Pancreatitis

As described in Chapter 6, the pancreas lies behind the stomach. The pancreas secretes digestive juices into the duodenum to help break down food into small molecules. These small molecules can be absorbed by the body. The gland also secretes insulin and glucagon into the bloodstream. These hormones help to maintain adequate glucose concentration. When the pancreas becomes inflamed (pancreatitis), it releases pancreatic enzymes into the blood, the pancreatic duct, and the pancreas itself. This causes further inflammation and autodigestion of the gland. Pancreatitis occurs in two stages: acute and chronic.

Acute pancreatitis occurs suddenly. It occurs soon after the pancreas becomes damaged or irritated by its own enzymes. Acute pancreatitis usually results from obstruction by gallstones in the bile duct or by alcohol abuse. Other less common causes of acute pancreatitis include elevated serum lipids, thromboembolism, drug toxicity, infection, and some surgeries. Acute pancreatitis affects about 80,000 Americans each year.[6]

Chronic pancreatitis begins as acute pancreatitis. It becomes chronic when the pancreas becomes scarred. This condition usually results from long-term and excessive alcohol consumption. However, chronic pancreatitis also may develop from other causes of pancreatitis. Chronic pancreatitis can lead to exocrine and endocrine failure. Rarely pancreatitis leads to pancreatic cancer.

Pancreatitis may cause severe epigastric pain. Pancreatitis often is associated with nausea, vomiting, and abdominal tenderness and distention. The abdominal pain often is described as severe, radiating from midumbilicus to the patient's back and shoulders. In severe cases the patient has fever, tachycardia, and signs of generalized sepsis and shock. These patients often are hospitalized. They are treated with intravenously administered fluids, pain medication, and placement of a nasogastric tube if the patient is vomiting.

Esophagogastric Varices

Esophagogastric varices are common with liver disease. They often result from portal hypertension caused by cirrhosis of the liver. Obstruction to blood flow in the liver, produced by the fibrosis in the liver, increases pressure. Obstruction also dilates vessels that drain into the liver. This subsequent dilation of thin-walled veins around the lower esophagus and upper end of the stomach produces esophagogastric varices. Varices can rupture. This results in life-threatening hemorrhage. Other causes of esophageal bleeding include esophagitis (associated with chronic use of alcohol and antiinflammatory nonsteroidal medications), malignancy, and episodes of prolonged, violent vomiting that produces a tear or laceration in the mucosa of the upper esophagus (Mallory-Weiss syndrome).

Clinically, a patient with esophageal bleeding has bright red hematemesis. This condition may be severe. If bleeding is profuse, melena may be evident. The patient may manifest the classic signs of shock as well. Variceal bleeding usually is massive and generally hard to control. Therapeutic intervention includes ensuring a patent airway and fluid resuscitation. (The placement of a nasogastric tube for gastric lavage is controversial.) Definitive care may include placement of a Sengstaken-Blakemore tube to tamponade bleeding vessels, surgical ligation of the bleeding varices, or transendoscopic injection of a sclerosing agent into the bleeding vessels. The mortality rate for patients with variceal bleeding is about 25%.[1]

Hemorrhoids

Hemorrhoids are swollen, distended veins. They are inside the anus (internal) or under the skin around the anus (external) (Fig. 34-5). Hemorrhoids are common during pregnancy. (They result from fetal pressure in the abdomen and hormonal changes that cause hemorrhoidal vessels to enlarge.) Hemorrhoids are present in 50% of all persons by age 50. Irritation of the distended veins is made worse by straining during bowel movements and by rubbing or cleaning around the anus, which may produce itching, bleeding, or both. As a rule, hemorrhoidal symptoms subside within a few days.

Pain from hemorrhoids is infrequent unless thrombosis, ulceration, or infection is present. Slight bleeding is the most common symptom. (Rarely do hemorrhoids cause significant hemorrhage.) The bleeding usually occurs during or after defecation. Blood dripping into the toilet after defecation or blood-streaked toilet tissue after wiping are common indications. Blood loss from hemorrhoids is usually slight. However, recurrent episodes of bleeding may be significant enough to produce anemia. Definitive care includes diet modification, stool softeners, tissue fixation techniques, and operative hemorrhoidectomy for severe cases.

Cholecystitis

Cholecystitis is inflammation of the gallbladder. The disease is common in the United States. Cholecystitis occurs in 15% to 20% of the population and is more common in women 30 to 50 years of age than in men. The disease becomes more common with age in both sexes. Risk factors for cholecystitis include female sex, oral contraceptive use, increasing age, obesity, diabetes mellitus, chronic alcohol ingestion, and African American or Asian ethnicity. The condition may be chronic with

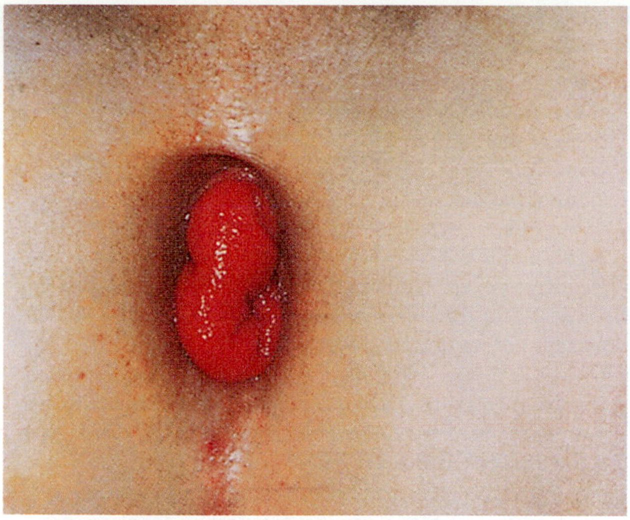

FIGURE 34-5 ■ Thrombosed external hemorrhoids.

recurrent subacute symptoms or acute because of gallstone obstruction.

In 90% of cases, acute cholecystitis is caused by gallstones (composed mainly of cholesterol) in the gallbladder. On occasion the gallstones totally obstruct the neck or cystic duct of the gallbladder. This leads to the common bile duct that empties into the small intestine. The trapped bile becomes concentrated. The bile causes irritation and pressure buildup in the gallbladder, which can lead to bacterial infection and perforation. The increased pressure causes a sudden onset of pain (biliary colic), which radiates to the right upper quadrant or right scapula. Patients with gallbladder disease commonly have their pain episodes at night. Generally, the episodes are associated with recent ingestion of fried or fatty foods. Severe illness, alcohol abuse and, rarely, tumors of the gallbladder also can cause cholecystitis.

Other associated hallmarks of cholecystitis include previous episodes, a family history of gallbladder disease, low-grade fever, nausea, vomiting that may be bile stained and described as bitter (variable), and pain and tenderness on palpation in the right upper quadrant. Passage of stones into the common bile duct with subsequent obstruction may cause shaking chills, high fever, jaundice, and acute pancreatitis. Treatment may include hospitalization, intravenous fluid therapy, antibiotics, and placement of a nasogastric tube. Definitive treatment is surgical removal of the gallbladder.

Acute Hepatitis

Hepatitis is inflammation of the liver. Hepatitis is the single most important cause of liver disease in the United States and worldwide (Box 34-5).

Acute hepatitis is associated with the sudden onset of malaise, weakness, anorexia, intermittent nausea and vomiting, and dull right upper quadrant pain. These signs usually are followed within 1 week by the onset of jaundice, dark urine, or both. Although many viruses can infect the liver, the three classes of viruses that are of main concern as causes of acute infectious hepatitis are hepatitis A virus, hepatitis B virus, and hepatitis C virus, formerly known as *non-A/non-B hepatitis virus*. All types produce similar pathological changes in the liver. These viruses also stimulate an antibody response that is specific to the type of virus causing the disease (Box 34-6). Many hepatitis infections are subclinical; they often present influenza-like symptoms.

The inflammation of hepatitis has many possible causes, including alcohol or other drug use, autoimmune disorders, and toxic bacterial, fungal, parasitic, and viral infections. Patients with hepatitis require a physician's evaluation and care. Proper immunization of paramedics is important. Observation of body substance isolation procedures also is crucial when paramedics are caring for these patients. Hepatitis is discussed in depth in Chapter 39.

CRITICAL THINKING

Why do you think a person would refuse the chance to be vaccinated against this deadly disease?

BOX 34-5 Hepatitis and Liver Diseases in the United States

- About 25 million Americans—one in every 10—are or have been afflicted with liver and biliary diseases.
- About 25,000 Americans die each year from chronic liver disease and cirrhosis; 300,000 persons are hospitalized each year because of cirrhosis.
- Alcoholic liver disease and chronic hepatitis C are the leading causes of cirrhosis.
- An estimated 40,000 persons were infected with the hepatitis C virus in 1998.
- An estimated 3.9 million persons are or have been infected with hepatitis C, 2.7 million of whom are infected chronically; about 70% of persons infected do not know they have the virus.
- From 8000 to 10,000 persons die of hepatitis C each year. The Centers for Disease Control and Prevention estimate that the number of annual deaths from hepatitis C will triple in the next 10 to 20 years.
- Hepatitis B is responsible for 5000 deaths annually, including 3000 to 4000 from cirrhosis and 1000 to 1500 from primary liver cancer.
- One out of every 250 persons is a carrier of hepatitis B and can pass it on to others, often unknowingly.
- About 80,000 new infections of hepatitis B were estimated to have occurred in the United States in 1999.
- Up to 90% of pregnant women who are carriers of the hepatitis B virus could transmit the virus to their children. Vaccinations of the newborns would prevent the newborns from becoming carriers.
- Because of the screening of pregnant women for hepatitis B virus and vaccinations of newborns with the hepatitis B vaccine, the number of infected newborns has declined.
- Hepatitis B is 100 times more infectious than human immunodeficiency virus, the virus that causes acquired immunodeficiency syndrome. About 500 million hepatitis B viral particles are in 1 tsp of blood compared with 5 to 10 particles of human immunodeficiency virus.
- The estimated medical and work loss cost per year of hepatitis B is $700 million; the estimated medical and work loss cost per year of hepatitis C is $600 million.
- One out of every 20 persons will be infected with hepatitis B in his or her lifetime.
- About 5000 liver transplants were performed in 2000. Because of the shortage of organs, nearly 1700 prospective recipients are estimated to have died in 2001 while waiting for a liver for transplantation. Currently, more than 18,000 persons are waiting for a liver transplant.
- You are at a high risk of hepatitis C infection if you were notified that you received blood from a donor who later tested positive for hepatitis C; have ever injected illegal drugs, even if you experimented a few times many years ago; received a blood transfusion or solid organ transplant before July 1992; received a blood product for clotting problems produced before 1987; have ever been on long-term kidney dialysis; or have received a tattoo or body piercing (although considered to be of a lesser degree of risk, contamination of needles is possible).
- You are at a high risk of hepatitis B infection if you have sex with someone infected with the virus; have sex with more than one partner; are a man and have sex with a man; live in the same house with someone who has lifelong hepatitis B virus infection; have a job that involves contact with human blood; inject drugs; are a patient or work in a home for the developmentally disabled; have hemophilia; or travel to areas where hepatitis B is common.
- Non-Hispanic African Americans have the highest infection rate for hepatitis C; Asian and Pacific Islanders have the highest rate for hepatitis B infection.

Modified from American Liver Foundation. *Hepatitis and Liver Disease in the United States,* http://www.liverfoundation.org/db/articles/1008. Accessed Feb. 21, 2005.

BOX 34-6 Risk Factors for Hepatitis

Hepatitis A

Health care practice without body substance isolation precautions
Household or sexual contact with an infected person
Living in an area with hepatitis A virus outbreak
Traveling to developing countries
Engaging in sex with infected partners or multiple partners
Drug use by injection

Hepatitis B

Health care practice without body substance isolation precautions
Infant born to mother infected with hepatitis B virus
Engaging in sex with infected partners or multiple partners
Drug use by injection
Receiving hemodialysis

Hepatitis C

Health care practice without body substance isolation precautions
Receiving blood transfusion before July 1992
Engaging in sex with infected partners or multiple partners
Drug use by injection
Receiving hemodialysis

SUMMARY

- The major organs most commonly associated with the gastrointestinal system include the esophagus, stomach, small and large intestines, liver, gallbladder, and pancreas.
- After the initial survey, assessment of abdominal pain should begin with a thorough history. The physical examination may help to determine whether the pain is visceral, somatic, or referred.
- The most common treatment for abdominal pain occurs at the hospital. The paramedic should provide supportive treatment, manage life threats, and transport the patient to an appropriate facility.
- Gastroenteritis is inflammation of the stomach and intestines caused by infectious agents, chemicals or other conditions.
- Gastritis is acute or chronic inflammation of the gastric mucosa. Gastritis commonly results from hyperacidity, alcohol or other drug ingestion, bile reflux, and *H. pylori* infection.
- Colitis is an inflammatory condition of the large intestine. Colitis is characterized by severe diarrhea and ulceration of the mucosa of the intestine (ulcerative colitis).
- Diverticulosis may result in bright red rectal bleeding if perforation occurs.
- Diverticulitis results when a diverticulum becomes obstructed with fecal matter.
- Appendicitis occurs when the passageway between the appendix and cecum is obstructed by fecal material or by inflammation caused by infection.
- Peptic ulcer disease occurs when open wounds or sores develop in the stomach or duodenum.
- Bowel obstruction is an occlusion of the intestinal lumen. It results in blockage of the normal flow of intestinal contents.
- Crohn's disease is a chronic, inflammatory bowel disease. The disease is of unknown origin.
- Inflammation of the pancreas is called pancreatitis. It causes severe abdominal pain.
- Esophagogastric varices result from obstruction of blood flow to the liver as a result of liver disease.
- Hemorrhoids are distended veins in the rectoanal area.
- Cholecystitis is inflammation of the gallbladder. It most often is associated with the presence of gallstones.
- Hepatitis is characterized by the sudden onset of malaise, weakness, anorexia, intermittent nausea and vomiting, and dull right upper quadrant pain. These signs usually are followed within 1 week by the onset of jaundice, dark urine, or both.

REFERENCES

1. Rosen P, Barkin R: *Emergency medicine: concepts and clinical practice,* ed 4, St Louis, 1998, Mosby.
2. US Department of Transportation, National Highway Traffic Safety Administration: *EMT-Paramedic national standard curriculum,* Washington, DC, 1998, The Department.
3. emedicine.com, Frye R et al: *Gastroenteritis, bacterial,* http://www.edmedicine.com/med/topic855.htm. Accessed Feb. 21, 2005.
4. emedicine.com, Nobie et al: *Obstruction, small bowel,* http://www.emedicine.com/emerg/topic66.htm. Accessed Feb. 21, 2005.
5. Crohn's & Colitis Foundation of America: Crohn's disease. Retrieved February 10, 2005, from http://www.ccfa.org/research/info/aboutcd
6. American Gastroenterological Association: Pancreatitis. Retrieved February 10, 2005, from http://www.gastro.org/clinicalRes/brochures/pancreatitis.html

APPENDIX NASOGASTRIC TUBE INSERTION

Nasogastric intubation may be indicated when the patient's stomach is very distended. Intubation also may be indicated when the removal of gastric contents by lavage is needed. Nasogastric intubation should be attempted only in conscious patients with an intact gag reflex. Intubation also may be attempted in unconscious patients whose airway is protected with an endotracheal tube.

One should note that passage of a nasogastric tube is unpleasant under the most ideal of conditions and should be considered as a prehospital procedure only under unusual circumstances and under medical direction (Appendix Figs. 34-1 and 34-2).

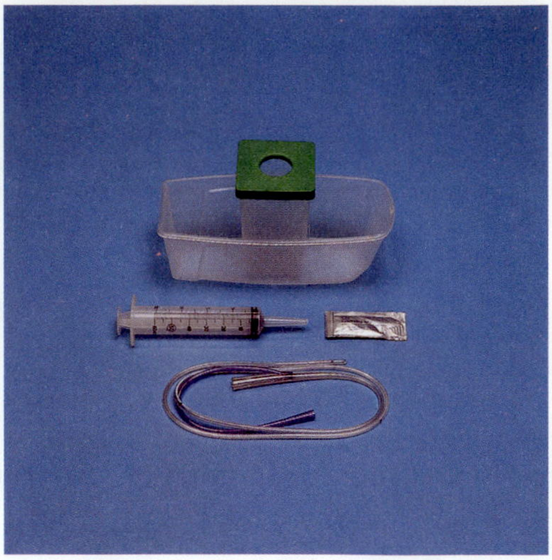

APPENDIX FIGURE 34-1 ■ Equipment for nasogastric tube insertion.

NECESSARY EQUIPMENT

- Personal protective equipment (gloves, mask, face shield)
- Double-lumen Levin tube (large enough to evacuate desired material)
- Water-soluble lubricant
- Tape
- 50-mL irrigation syringe
- Cup of water or ice chips
- Emesis basin
- Intermittent suction equipment

PROCEDURE

1. Explain the procedure to the patient.
2. Measure the length of tube to be inserted by placing the tip of the tube over the approximate area of the stomach and extending it to the patient's ear and from the ear to the tip of the nose. Note the marks on the tube used for measurement.
3. Lubricate the tip and the first 2 to 3 inches of the tube with a water-soluble lubricant.
4. Place the patient in a high Fowler's position, and instruct the patient to lean forward and to flex his or her neck.
5. Instruct the patient to suck on ice chips or to take small sips of water (if not contraindicated) and to swallow on command during the procedure. This assists passage of the tube.
6. Insert the tube along the floor of an unobstructed nostril. If the patient has a deviated septum choose the nostril with the most open channel.
7. Gently and slowly advance the tube. Do this while having the patient continue to swallow until the tube is at the level previously noted by the marks. Patients commonly choke and cough during the procedure. If this occurs, hold the tube in place and allow the patient to rest. If choking and coughing persist, remove the tube (it may have entered the trachea) and begin again.
8. After the tube has been inserted fully to its predetermined length, verify placement in the stomach by injecting 20 mL to 30 mL of air into the tube while auscultating the epigastric region for the sound of air movement. Leave the syringe attached to the tube until aspiration of stomach contents is initiated or intermittent suction is available.
9. Secure the tube with tape to the nose and forehead or cheek.
10. Lavage stomach contents by injecting 100-mL to 150-mL boluses of normal saline into the tube and allowing the return of gastric contents by aspiration or intermittent suction. Document the amount of fluid infused and returned by lavage.

POSSIBLE COMPLICATIONS

- Nasal hemorrhage
- Passage of the tube into the trachea
- Perforation of the esophagus
- Gastrointestinal bleeding
- Coiling of the tube in the posterior pharynx
- Obstruction of the passage resulting from septal deviation
- Passage of the tube intracranially (with cribriform plate fractures)

STEP-BY-STEP SKILL

APPENDIX FIGURE 34-2 ■ Nasogastric tube insertion.

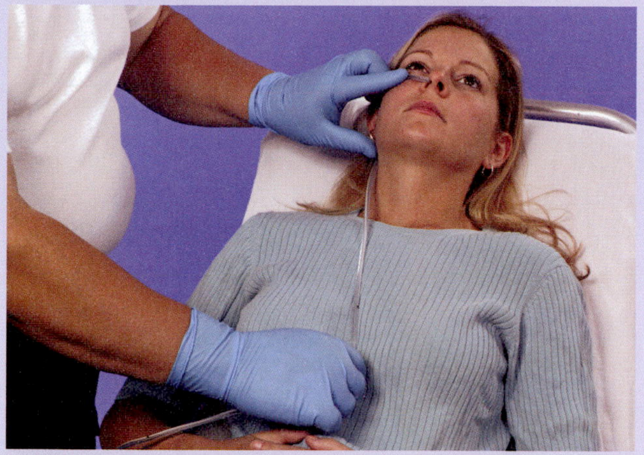

A ■ Measure the length of tube to be inserted by placing the tip of the tube over the approximate area of the stomach and extending it to the patient's ear and from the ear to the tip of the nose.

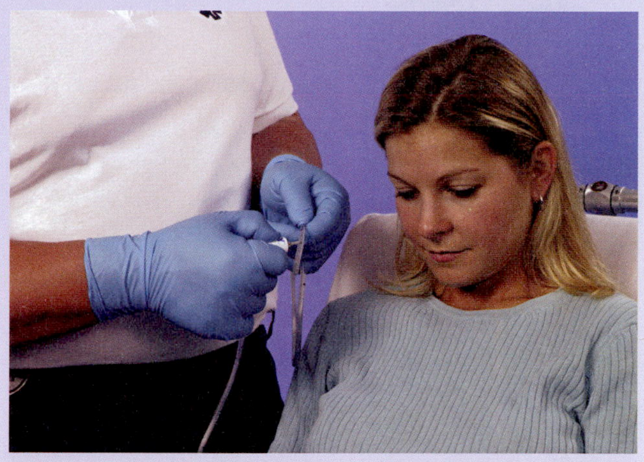

B ■ Lubricate the tip and the first 2 to 3 inches of the tube with a water-soluble lubricant.

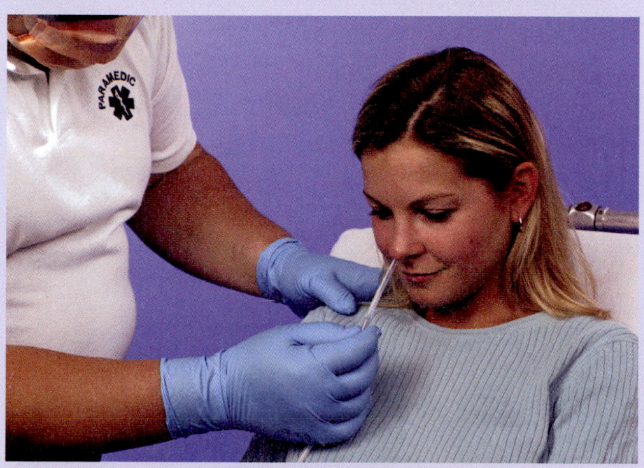

C ■ Place the patient in a high Fowler's position, and instruct the patient to lean forward and to flex his or her neck.

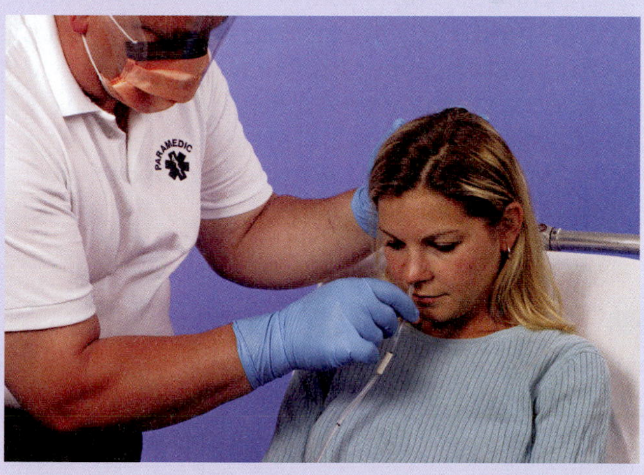

D ■ Gently and slowly advance the tube. Do this while having the patient continue to swallow until the tube is at the level previously noted by the marks.

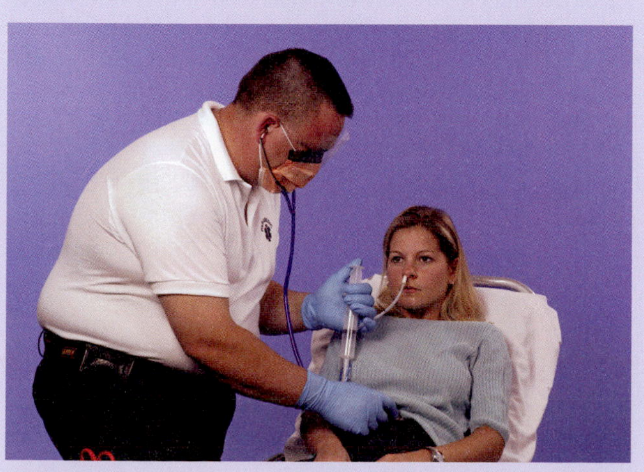

E ■ After the tube has been inserted fully to its predetermined length, verify placement in the stomach by injecting 20 mL to 30 mL of air into the tube while auscultating the epigastric region for the sound of air movement.

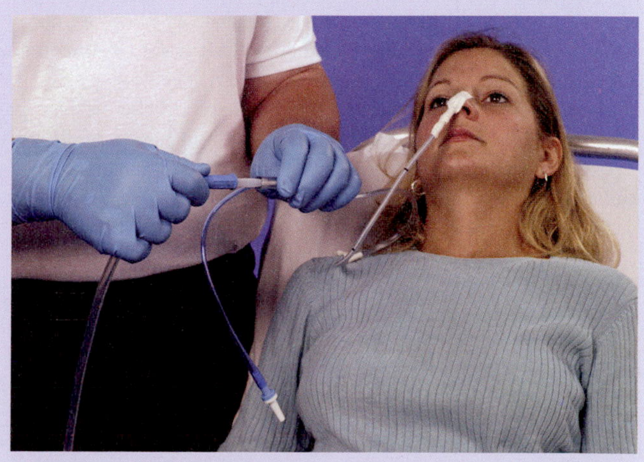

F ■ Lavage stomach contents by injecting 100-mL to 150-mL boluses of normal saline into the tube and allowing the return of gastric contents by aspiration or intermittent suction.

CHAPTER 35

Urology

OBJECTIVES

Upon completion of this chapter, the paramedic student will be able to:

1. Label a diagram of the urinary system.
2. Describe pathophysiology, signs and symptoms, assessment, and prehospital management of the patient with urinary retention, urinary tract infection, pyelonephritis, urinary calculus, epididymitis, and testicular torsion.
3. Outline the physical examination for patients with genitourinary disorders.
4. Discuss general prehospital management for the patient with a genitourinary disorder.
5. Distinguish between acute and chronic renal failure.
6. Describe the signs and symptoms of renal failure.
7. Describe dialysis and emergent conditions associated with it, including prehospital management.

KEY TERMS

acute renal failure: A clinical syndrome that results from a sudden and significant decrease in filtration through the glomeruli, leading to the accumulation of salt, water, and nitrogenous wastes within the body.

azotemia: The retention of excessive amounts of nitrogenous compounds in the blood.

chronic renal failure: A progressive, irreversible systemic disease caused by kidney dysfunction that leads to abnormalities in blood counts and blood chemistry levels.

dialysis: A technique used to normalize blood chemistry in patients with acute or chronic renal failure and to remove blood toxins in some patients who have taken a drug overdose.

disequilibrium syndrome: A group of neurological findings that sometimes occur during or immediately after dialysis; thought to result from a disproportionate decrease in osmolality of the extracellular fluid compared with that of the intracellular compartment in the brain or cerebral spinal fluid.

epididymitis: An inflammation of the epididymis, a tubular section of the male reproductive system that carries sperm from the testicle to the seminal vesicles.

peritoneal dialysis: A dialysis procedure that uses the peritoneum as a diffusible membrane; performed to correct an imbalance of fluid or electrolytes in the blood or to remove toxins, drugs, or other wastes normally excreted by the kidney.

pyelonephritis: An inflammation of the kidney parenchyma associated with microbial infection.

testicular torsion: A condition in which a testicle twists on its spermatic cord, disrupting its own blood supply.

uremia: The presence of excessive amounts of urea and other nitrogenous wastes produced in the blood.

urinary retention: The inability to urinate.

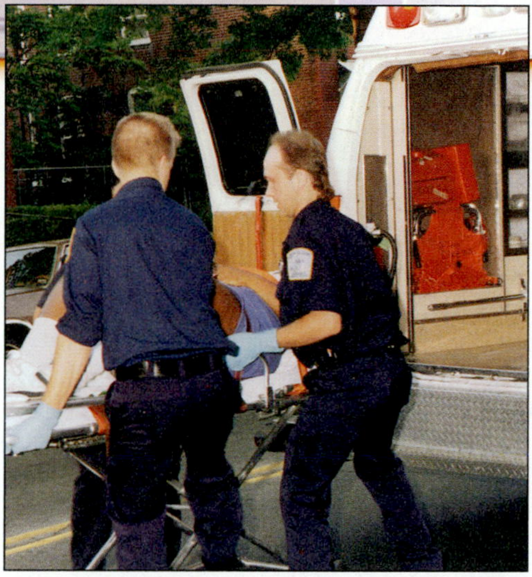

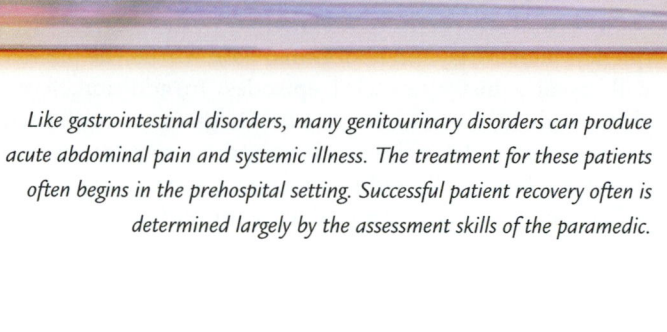

Like gastrointestinal disorders, many genitourinary disorders can produce acute abdominal pain and systemic illness. The treatment for these patients often begins in the prehospital setting. Successful patient recovery often is determined largely by the assessment skills of the paramedic.

ANATOMY AND PHYSIOLOGY REVIEW

As described in Chapter 6, the urinary system works with other body systems to maintain homeostasis. The urinary system does this by removing waste products from the blood. The system also helps to maintain a constant body fluid volume and composition. The urinary system is composed of the kidneys, the ureters, the urinary bladder, and the urethra (Fig. 35-1).

Renal and urinary tract diseases affect an estimated 20 million Americans. They directly cause more than 95,000 deaths per year.[1] Many types and causes of renal and urinary tract diseases exist. These range from mild to acute. Mild urinary tract infections are treatable with antibiotics. **Acute renal failure** requires kidney transplantation or renal **dialysis** to maintain life. Genitourinary disorders that may cause acute pain include **urinary retention,** urinary tract infection (UTI), **pyelonephritis,** urinary calculus, **epididymitis,** and **testicular torsion.** (Chapter 41 addresses other disorders specific to the female genitourinary system.) Like the pain associated with disorders of the abdomen, genitourinary disorders may produce visceral, somatic, and referred pain (see Chapter 34).

Urinary Retention

Urinary retention describes the inability to urinate. Possible causes include urethral stricture, an enlarged prostate (benign or malignant prostatic hypertrophy), central nervous system dysfunction, foreign body obstruction,

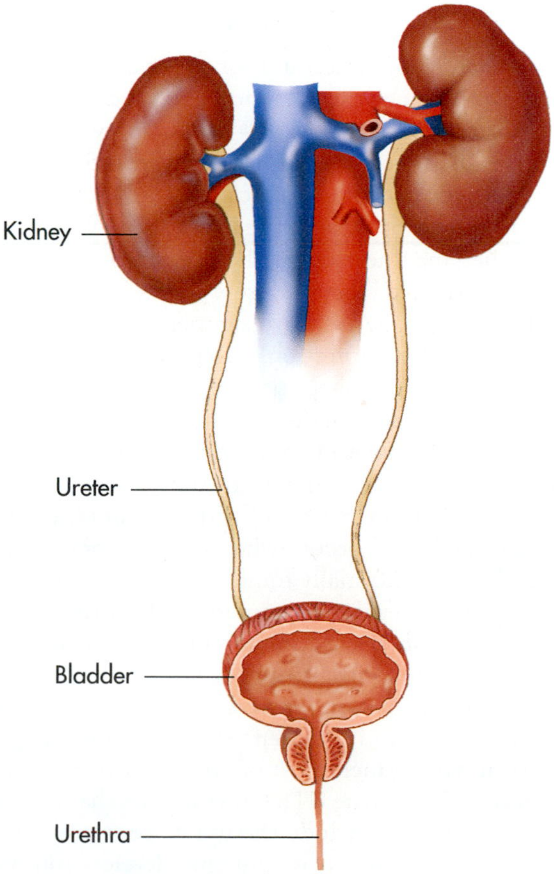

FIGURE 35-1 ■ Urinary system.

and use of certain drugs such as parasympatholytic or anticholinergic agents. Men are affected with urinary retention more often than are women. (This is most commonly due to an enlarged prostate.) However, other common causes can be found in both sexes.

The signs and symptoms of urinary retention include severe abdominal pain (except with central nervous system lesions) that is associated with an urgent need to urinate and a distended bladder. The distended bladder often is palpable. Patients with a progressive obstruction, such as prostatic hypertrophy, often have a history of urinary hesitancy, a poor urinary stream, a sense of incomplete emptying of the bladder, nocturia (excessive urination at night), and overflow incontinence (an overflow of urine from the bladder). In the emergency department, passage of a urethral catheter to empty the bladder often is required. Urinary retention is painful for the patient. The prehospital care mainly is supportive. The cause of the retention should be sought, and if it is not easily correctable following physician examination, the patient may require hospitalization.

CRITICAL THINKING

Have you ever been in a situation when you needed to urinate urgently but could not because of the circumstances? How did you feel?

Urinary Tract Infection

Urinary tract infections account for about 8 million physician office visits each year. They account for close to 2 million hospitalizations each year as well. Urinary tract infections are secondary only to respiratory tract infections as a problem seen by practicing physicians.[2] Urinary tract infections usually develop first in the lower urinary tract. (For instance, they may develop in the urethra or bladder.) If they are not treated, they progress to the upper urinary tract. (They may progress, for example, to the ureters or kidneys.) Upper tract infections often are associated with kidney infection (pyelonephritis, described later in this chapter) or abscesses that form within the kidney tissue. These conditions can lead to a reduced kidney function. They even can lead to death in untreated, severe cases.

The more common lower UTI of the urethra (urethritis) and bladder (cystitis) occurs when enteric flora (particularly *Escherichia coli* normally found in the bowel) enter the opening of the urethra and colonize the urinary tract. These infections are more common in women because the urethra is short and close to the vagina and rectum. The disease also occurs in men (as a result of urethritis, prostatitis, and cystitis) and children. However, urethritis and prostatitis in young men most often results from venereal disease rather than a true UTI. Other factors that may contribute to lower UTI include the use of contraceptive devices (women who use a diaphragm develop infections more often; condoms with spermicidal foam may cause the growth of *E. coli* in the vagina, which may enter the urethra), unsafe sexual practices, the presence of renal stones, bladder catheterization, and a suppressed immune system. In addition, men and women infected with *Chlamydia trachomatis* or *Mycoplasma hominis* can transmit the bacteria to their partner during sexual intercourse. These bacteria then could cause a UTI.

Signs and symptoms of UTI include dysuria, urinary frequency, hematuria, and abdominal pain. Often the patient will reveal a history of UTI episodes. In addition, fever, chills, and malaise may be present. Diagnosis is confirmed in the hospital through urinalysis and microscopic examination for blood cells, sediment, and bacteria. Urinary tract infections generally are treated with antibiotic therapy.

Pyelonephritis

Pyelonephritis is inflammation of the kidney parenchyma (upper urinary tract). Inflammation most often occurs as a result of lower UTI. The disease is associated with bacterial infection, particularly in the presence of occasional or persistent backflow (reflux) of infected urine from the bladder into the ureters or kidney pelvis. The bacterial infections may also be carried to one or both kidneys. They may be carried through the bloodstream or lymph glands from the infection that began in the bladder. Pyelonephritis is more common in adult women. Yet the condition can affect persons of any age and either sex. Acute episodes can be severe in the elderly and in persons who are immunosuppressed (e.g., those with cancer or acquired immunodeficiency syndrome).

The onset of signs and symptoms of pyelonephritis is usually abrupt. Pyelonephritis often is mistaken by the patient as resulting from straining the lower back. The condition may be complicated by systemic infection with signs and symptoms that include fever, chills, flank pain, cloudy or bloody urine, nausea, and vomiting. Left untreated, pyelonephritis can progress to a chronic condition. The condition can last for months or years. It may lead to scarring and possible loss of kidney function. Therapeutic intervention consists primarily of antibiotics, fluid replacement, and sometimes hospitalization.

CRITICAL THINKING

How will you examine the patient for flank pain?

Urinary Calculus

Urinary calculi (kidney stones) are pathological concretions that originate in the renal pelvis. They are one of the most painful and most common disorders of the urinary tract, accounting for about 250,000 hospitalizations each year.[3] An estimated 10% of persons in the United States will have a kidney stone at some point in their lives. Kidney stones result from supersaturation of the urine with insoluble salts. When the level of insoluble salts or uric acid in the urine is high; the urine lacks citrate (a chemical that normally inhibits the formation of stones); or insufficient water is present in the kidneys to dissolve waste products, kidney stones form. Kidney stones are most common in patients who are between the ages of 20 and 40. The disease is recurrent and is more common in men than in women. Associated risk factors for this condition include dehydration, central nervous system disorders (absent sensory/motor impulses), drug use (anesthetics, opiates, psychotropic agents, some herbal medicines), and surgery (a postoperative complication).

The chemical composition of the kidney stones depends on the chemical imbalance in the urine. The four most common types of stones are composed of calcium, uric acid, struvite, and cystine. Calcium stones are calcium compounds that are chemically bound to oxalate (most common) or phosphate; they account for about 85% of all kidney stones. Calcium stones typically occur in patients with metabolic (e.g., gout) or hormonal disorders (e.g., hyperparathyroidism). Stones composed of uric acid account for about 10% of kidney stones; their formation is more common in men. These stones may have a heritable component. Struvite stones (also known as infection stones) are more common in women. These stones often are linked to chronic bacterial UTI or frequent bladder catheterization. Cystine stones are the least common and result from a rare congenital condition in which there are large amounts of cystine (an amino acid in protein) in the urine. Cystine stones are difficult to treat and may require lifelong therapy.

Signs and symptoms of urinary calculus vary according to location. Most stones obstruct the ureter at points of ureteral narrowing in their passage from kidneys to bladder. This produces acute, excruciating pain. The pain originates in the flank area and radiates to the right or left lower abdominal quadrant, groin, and testes (in male patients). Renal or ureteral colic produces severe cyclical pain. This pain occurs as the ureter tries to use forceful contractions to push the stone into the bladder. This pain often has been described as having the same intensity as labor pain. The pain may be accompanied by restlessness, nausea and vomiting, urinary urgency or frequency, diaphoresis, low-grade fever, hematuria, dysuria, and increased blood pressure (because of the pain). Definitive care includes analgesics (anesthetics, opiates, psychotropics), fluid replacement, antiemetics, and possible hospital admission. If the calculus does not pass spontaneously, surgical intervention may be required (Box 35-1).

BOX 35-1 Prevention Strategies for Recurrent Renal Calculus

The composition of the stone determines what the patient can do to prevent another stone. Patients may be advised to do the following:

- Increase water consumption.
- Avoid foods containing calcium oxalate (e.g., chocolate, celery, grapes, strawberries, beans, and asparagus).
- Take daily supplements of vitamin B_6 and magnesium (to reduce the formation of oxalates).
- Avoid foods that raise uric acid levels (e.g., anchovies and sardines).
- Reduce uric acid by eating a low-protein diet.
- Limit salt intake to reduce the level of calcium oxalate in the urine.

CRITICAL THINKING

Have you cared for or known someone who had a urinary calculus? How did that person describe the pain? What was the level of discomfort?

Epididymitis

Epididymitis is inflammation of the epididymis. The epididymis is a tubular section of the male reproductive system. The organ carries sperm from the testicle to the seminal vesicles (see Chapter 6). Epididymitis often is caused by a bacterial infection that is associated with other structures of the genitourinary tract. Infection tends to occur in sexually active young men. The most common type of epididymitis in young men results from venereal disease.[2]

The signs and symptoms of epididymitis include a gradual onset of unilateral scrotal pain. This pain radiates to the spermatic cord. At times, tender swelling of the scrotum and testicle occurs. This swelling produces inflammation of one or both testes (orchitis). The patient may have a recent history of UTI, fever, and malaise as well. After physician evaluation, therapeutic intervention includes antibiotics, bed rest, analgesics, and elevation of the scrotum.

Testicular Torsion

Testicular torsion is a true urological emergency. In this condition, a testicle twists on its spermatic cord. This twisting disrupts the blood supply of the testicle. The condition may result from blunt trauma to the scrotal area. Yet it more often is spontaneous. The two peak periods in which torsion is likely to occur are the first year of life and at puberty, with a range in age from 5 months to 41 years, and an average of 16.2 years.[2]

Like epididymitis, testicular torsion results in a tender epididymis and painful swelling of the scrotal sac (Fig. 35-2). Unlike epididymitis, though, the patient usually is afebrile. The pain is sudden in onset. (Pain often is preceded by vigorous physical activity or an athletic event.) The pain is severe as well. (Pain sometimes radiates to the ipsilateral left quadrant.) In addition, the pain is unrelieved by rest or scrotal elevation. Pain often is associated with nausea and vomiting. Testicular torsion must be diagnosed and treated within 6 hours to prevent loss of the testis from ischemic infarction.[2] Therapeutic intervention includes the application of ice packs to the scrotum. Intervention also includes manual manipulation by a physician to reduce the torsion. The patient must undergo surgical repair within 4 to 6 hours of onset of the torsion. Thus rapid transport to the emergency department and early recognition are critical for treatment.

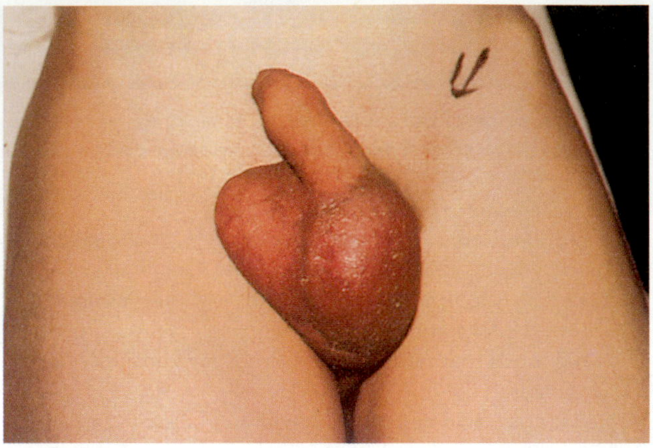

FIGURE 35-2 ■ Four-day old torsion of the left testis.

PHYSICAL EXAMINATION FOR PATIENTS WITH GENITOURINARY DISORDERS

As described in Chapter 11, an assessment of the abdomen and genitalia of either sex can be awkward. The assessment can be uncomfortable for the patient and the paramedic. The paramedic should protect the patient's privacy with the proper drapes. When possible, paramedics of the same sex as the patient should perform these examinations. If this is not possible, a chaperon should be present. The examiner should proceed with a calm, caring, and competent attitude. The paramedic should keep the patient and significant others informed of all actions. The examination is similar to that performed for abdominal pain (see Chapter 34) and should include the following:

- Initial assessment
- Focused history
  - OPQRST (*O*nset/origin, *P*rovokes, *Q*uality, *R*egion, *S*everity, *T*ime)
  - Previous history of similar event
  - Nausea or vomiting
  - Change in bowel habits or stool (constipation, diarrhea)
  - Change in urinary voiding pattern
  - Weight loss
  - Last oral intake
  - Last bowel movement
- Physical examination
  - Appearance
  - Posture
  - Level of consciousness
  - Apparent state of health
  - Skin color
  - Vital signs
  - Abdominal examination (inspection, auscultation, percussion, palpation)
  - Genitalia examination (if indicated)

MANAGEMENT AND TREATMENT PLAN

The paramedic should manage patients with genitourinary disorders as any other patient with acute pain, including providing airway, ventilatory, and circulatory support; administering high-concentration oxygen (if indicated); electrocardiogram and vital sign monitoring; and rapid, gentle transportation for physician evaluation in the patient's position of comfort. Patients should not be permitted to eat or drink because surgery may be indicated. The administration of analgesics generally is avoided in these patients. That way, the pain will not be masked. All patients who have had persistent genitourinary pain or discomfort for more than 6 hours should be transported for physician evaluation.

Renal Failure

The kidneys play a key role in maintaining homeostasis. They control extracellular fluid volume, maintain proper electrolyte composition and blood pH, and eliminate waste products. If this organ system malfunctions, serious systemic consequences develop. These include **uremia** (excessive amounts of urea and other nitrogenous waste products in the blood) with subsequent encephalopathy or pericarditis, hyperkalemia, acidosis, hypertension, and volume overload with subsequent congestive heart failure. The disease can be classified as *acute* or *chronic.* Classification depends on the duration of renal failure and on the potential for reversibility.

> **CRITICAL THINKING**
> Think about why a patient would develop the complications that were just described.

Acute Renal Failure

Acute renal failure (ARF) is a clinical syndrome that results from a sudden and significant decrease in filtration through the glomeruli that leads to the buildup of high levels of uremic toxins in the blood. Acute renal failure occurs when the kidneys are unable to excrete the daily load of toxins in the urine. Patients with ARF are separated into two groups based on the amount of urine excreted in 24 hours. One group is *oliguric.* (These patients excrete less than 500 mL/day.) The other is *nonoliguric.* (These patients excrete more than 500 mL/day.) Acute renal failure can threaten the life of a patient and carries a 50% mortality rate.[4] However, if ARF is recognized early and treated appropriately, it may be readily reversible. Causes of ARF are diverse and include trauma, shock, infection, urinary obstruction, and multisystem diseases.

The onset of ARF can occur within hours. As normal kidney function rapidly deteriorates, urine output frequently decreases (oliguria) or stops completely (anuria). This results in generalized edema from water and salt re-

TABLE 35-1 Classification of Acute Renal Failure

AREA OF DYSFUNCTION	POSSIBLE CAUSES
Prerenal	Hypovolemia
	Hemorrhagic blood loss (trauma, gastrointestinal bleeding, complications of childbirth)
	Loss of plasma volume (burns, peritonitis)
	Water and electrolyte losses (severe vomiting or diarrhea, intestinal obstruction, uncontrolled diabetes mellitus, inappropriate use of diuretics)
	Hypotension or hypoperfusion
	Septic shock
	Cardiac failure or shock
	Massive pulmonary embolism
	Stenosis or clamping of renal artery
Intrarenal	Acute tubular necrosis (postischemic or nephrotoxic)
	Glomerulopathies
	Malignant hypertension
	Coagulation defects
Postrenal	Obstructive uropathies (usually bilateral)
	Ureteral obstruction (edema, tumors, stones, clots)
	Bladder neck obstruction (enlarged prostate)

From McCance KL, Huether SE: *Pathophysiology: the biologic basis for disease in adults and children,* ed 4, St Louis, 2002, Mosby.

tention, acidosis from failure of the kidneys to rid the body of normal acidic products, high concentrations of nonprotein nitrogens (especially urea) from failure of the body to secrete metabolic end products, and high concentrations of other products of renal excretion (such as uric acid and potassium). The resulting condition often is termed *uremia.* If uremia is not recognized early and treated appropriately, renal dysfunction leads to the development of heart failure, volume overload, hyperkalemia, and metabolic acidosis. Acute renal failure may be classified as *prerenal, intrarenal,* or *postrenal* in origin (Table 35-1).

PRERENAL ACUTE RENAL FAILURE

Prerenal ARF results from inadequate perfusion of the kidneys. The damaged kidneys are unable to rid the blood of waste products such as urea and creatinine. This condition may be caused by hypovolemia or impaired cardiac output. Obstruction of renal arteries results in decreased blood flow to the kidneys and an increase in renal vascular resistance that effectively shunts blood away from the kidneys. Many patients with prerenal ARF are critically ill. They may have a number of preexisting medical conditions such as atherosclerosis, chronic liver disease, and heart failure. (Dehydration caused by diuretic use in patients with heart failure is a major cause of prerenal ARF.) In addition, perfusion often is poor within many organs. This may lead to multiple organ failure.

Signs and symptoms of prerenal ARF include dizziness, dry mouth, thirst, hypotension, tachycardia, and weight loss. The goal of treatment is to improve kidney perfusion and function by treating the underlying condition (e.g., infection, congestive heart failure, and liver failure). Fluids are administered intravenously to most patients to treat dehydration. After this, urine output generally increases and renal function improves.

INTRARENAL ACUTE RENAL FAILURE

Intrarenal ARF is also known as intrinsic ARF. It results from conditions that damage or injure both kidneys. Examples include glomerular and other microvascular diseases, tubular diseases, and interstitial diseases that cause direct damage to the kidney parenchyma. Nearly 90% of all cases are caused by ischemia or toxins. Both of these causes can lead to acute tubular necrosis (death of tubular cells).[5] Ischemic causes of intrarenal ARF are associated with renal hypoperfusion. These occur most often from hemorrhage, trauma, sepsis, and in patients undergoing cardiovascular surgery. Nephrotoxic causes of intrarenal ARF occur most often in the elderly and in patients with **chronic renal failure.** Drugs and other compounds that can trigger intrarenal ARF include antibiotics, nonsteroidal antiinflammatory drugs, anticancer drugs, radiocontrast dyes, alcohol and other drug use (e.g., cocaine). The condition also is associated with hypertension, autoimmune diseases (e.g., systemic lupus), and pyelonephritis.

Signs and symptoms of intrarenal ARF include fever, flank pain, joint pain, headache, hypertension, confusion, seizure, and oliguria. The goal of treatment is to restore adequate renal blood flow. This is done by resolving the underlying cause and its complications. In severe cases, renal dialysis (described later in this chapter) may be needed to manage the disease.

POSTRENAL ACUTE RENAL FAILURE

Postrenal ARF is caused by obstruction to urine flow to both kidneys. This form of renal failure may be caused by ureteral and urethral obstructions (bilateral calculi, prostatic enlargement, urethral strictures). The blockage of urine causes pressure to build in the renal nephrons and ultimately can cause the nephrons to shut down. The degree of renal failure corresponds directly with the degree of obstruction. Signs and symptoms of postrenal ARF include urine retention; distended bladder; gross hematuria; pain in the lower back, abdomen, groin, or genitalia; and peripheral edema. The condition is reversible by removing the obstruction to urine flow.

Chronic Renal Failure

Chronic renal failure (CRF) is a progressive, irreversible systemic disease. It develops over months to years as internal structures of the kidney are slowly damaged. Chronic renal

TABLE 35-2 Systemic Effects of Uremia

SYSTEM	MANIFESTATIONS	MECHANISMS	TREATMENT
Skeletal	Osteitis fibrosa (bone inflammation with fibrous degeneration); bone demineralization (principally subperiosteal loss of cortical bone in the fibers, lateral ends of the clavicles, and lamina dura of the teeth); spontaneous fractures, bone pain; osteomalacia (rickets) with end-stage renal failure	Bone resorption associated with hyperparathyroidism, vitamin D deficiency, and demineralization; lowered calcium and raised phosphate levels	Control of hyperphosphatemia to reduce hyperparathyroidism; administration of calcium and aluminum hydroxide antacids, which bind phosphate in the gut, together with a phosphate-restricted diet; vitamin D replacement; avoidance of magnesium antacids because of impaired magnesium excretion
Cardiopulmonary	Hypertension, pericarditis with fever, chest pain, and pericardial friction rub, pulmonary edema, Kussmaul respirations	Extracellular volume expansion as cause of hypertension; hypersecretion of rennin also associated with hypertension; fluid overload associated with pulmonary edema and acidosis leading to Kussmaul respirations	Volume reduction with diuretics that are not potassium sparing (to avoid hyperkalemia); angiotensin-converting enzyme (ACE) inhibitors; combination of propranolol, hydralazine, and minoxidil for those with high levels of reinin; bilateral nephrectomy with dialysis or transplantation
Neurologic	Encephalopathy (fatigue, loss of attention, difficulty problem solving); peripheral neuropathy (pain and burning in the legs and feet, loss of vibration sense and deep tendon reflexes); loss of motor coordination, twitching, fasciculations, stupor, and coma with advanced uremia	Uremic toxins associated with end-stage renal disease	Dialysis
Endocrine	Retarded growth in children	Decreased growth hormone	Exogenous recombinant human growth hormone
	Osteomalacia	Elevated parathyroid hormone levels	Same as for Skeletal above
	Higher incidence of goiter	Decreased thyroid hormone	Replacement when indicated
Hematologic	Anemia, usually normochromic normocytic; platelet disorders with prolonged bleeding times.	Reduced erythropoietin secretion associated with loss of renal mass, leading to reduced red cell production in the bone marrow; uremic toxins associated with shortened red cell survival	Dialysis; recombinant human erythropoietin and iron supplementation; conjugated estrogens; DDAVP (1-desamino-8-D-arginine vasopressin); transfusion
Gastrointestinal	Anorexia, nausea, vomiting; mouth ulcers, stomatitis, ruinous breath (uremic fetor), hiccups, peptic ulcers, gastrointestinal bleeding, and pancreatitis associated with end-stage renal failure	Retention of urea, metabolic acids, and other metabolic waste products, including methylguanidine	Protein-restricted diet for relief of nausea and vomiting
Integumentary	Abnormal pigmentation and pruritus	Retention of urochromes, contributing to sallow, yellow color; high plasma calcium levels associated with pruritus	Dialysis with control of serum calcium levels
Immunologic	Increased risk of infection that can cause death	Suppression of cell-mediated immunity; reduction in number and function of lymphocytes, diminished phagocytosis	Routine dialysis
Reproductive	Sexual dysfunction: menorrhagia, amenorrhea, infertility, and decreased libido in women; decreased testosterone levels, infertility, and decreased libido in men	Elevated hormones: luteinizing hormone (LH), follicle-stimulating hormone (FSH), prolactin, and LH-releasing hormone; decreased testosterone, estrogen, and progesterone	No specific treatment

From McCance KL, Huether SE: *Pathophysiology: the biologic basis for disease in adults and children,* ed 4, St Louis, 2002, Mosby.

failure may be caused by congenital disorders or prolonged pyelonephritis. In the industrialized world, though, CRF more often results from systemic diseases such as diabetes and hypertension and from autoimmune disorders. The kidneys try to make up for renal damage by hyperfiltration within the remaining working nephrons. Over time, hyperfiltration causes further nephron damage and loss of kidney function. Chronic loss of function causes generalized wasting and progressive scarring within all parts of the kidney. This damage results in a reduction in nephron mass and renal mass.

Like ARF, CRF results in the buildup of fluid and waste products in the body. This causes **azotemia.** (This is the retention of excessive amounts of nitrogenous compounds in the blood.) It also causes uremia. Most body systems are affected by CRF. Complications of the disease may include hypertension, congestive heart failure, anemia, electrolyte abnormalities, and others (Table 35-2). Chronic renal failure and end-stage renal disease affect more than 2 out of 1000 persons in the United States, and more than 50,000 Americans die each year from the disease.[6] Once CRF has been diagnosed and the cause has been identified, treatments are started to delay or possibly stop the progressive loss of kidney function. In its final stages, CRF often requires treatment with dialysis (hemodialysis or **peritoneal dialysis**) or a kidney transplant for the patient to survive. In addition to oliguria, the patient with CRF may exhibit the following six systemic manifestations:

1. Gastrointestinal manifestations
   a. Anorexia
   b. Nausea
   c. Vomiting
2. Cardiopulmonary manifestations
   a. Hypertension
   b. Pericarditis
   c. Pulmonary edema
   d. Peripheral, sacral, and periorbital edema
3. Nervous system manifestations
   a. Anxiety
   b. Delirium
   c. Progressive obtundation
   d. Hallucinations
   e. Muscle twitching
   f. Seizures
4. Metabolic or endocrine manifestations
   a. Glucose intolerance
   b. Electrolyte disturbances
   c. Anemia
5. Personality changes
   a. Fatigue
   b. Mental dullness
6. Signs of uremia
   a. Pasty, yellow skin discoloration and thin extremities from protein wasting
   b. Uremic frost caused by urea crystals that form on the skin (late finding)

Renal Dialysis

Dialysis is a technique used to normalize blood chemistry. Dialysis is used in patients with acute or chronic renal failure. Dialysis also removes blood toxins in some patients who have taken a drug overdose. The two types of dialysis are hemodialysis and peritoneal dialysis. Both of these bring the patent's blood into contact with a semipermeable membrane across which water-soluble substances diffuse into a dialyzing fluid (dialysate). Eventually electrolytes are balanced between the patient's blood and the dialysis fluid. Waste products are eliminated as well.

The amount of substance that transfers during dialysis depends on the difference in the concentrations of solutions on the two sides of the semipermeable membrane, the molecular size of the substance, and the length of time the blood and the dialysate remain in contact with the membrane. In patients with end-stage renal disease, hemodialysis usually is done 3 times a week. Each session may last 4 to 5 hours.

HEMODIALYSIS

In hemodialysis the patient's heparinized blood is pumped through a surgically constructed arteriovenous fistula. The fistula is a connection between an artery and a vein. An arteriovenous graft, which is a synthetic material grafted between the patient's artery and vein (Fig. 35-3), also can be used. These internal shunts usually are located in the inner aspect of the patient's forearm. Less often, they may be located in the medial aspect of the lower extremity. Some patients may have an external dialysis catheter or a small, button-shaped device (Hemasite). This device usually is located in the upper arm or proximal, anterior thigh. A Hemasite is similar to an arteriovenous graft. However, the Hemasite has an external rubber septum sutured to the skin. A dialysis catheter is inserted into this septum for treatment (see Chapter 48).

PERITONEAL DIALYSIS

In peritoneal dialysis the dialysis membrane is the patient's own peritoneum. The dialysate is infused into the peritoneal cavity by a temporary or permanently implanted catheter. Fluid and solutes diffuse from the blood in the peritoneal capillaries into the dialysate. After 1 to 2 hours, equilibration has occurred. At this point, the dialysate is drained and fresh fluid is infused. Peritoneal dialysis works much more slowly than hemodialysis. Over time, though, it is just as effective. In addition, peritoneal dialysis does not require chronic blood access. A major complication of peritoneal dialysis is peritonitis. This usually results when the proper aseptic technique is not used. Peritoneal dialysis may be carried out regularly in the home by the patient or by the family caregiver.

DIALYSIS EMERGENCIES

Emergencies the paramedic may encounter when caring for a patient with acute or chronic renal failure may result from the disease process itself. Such emergencies also may

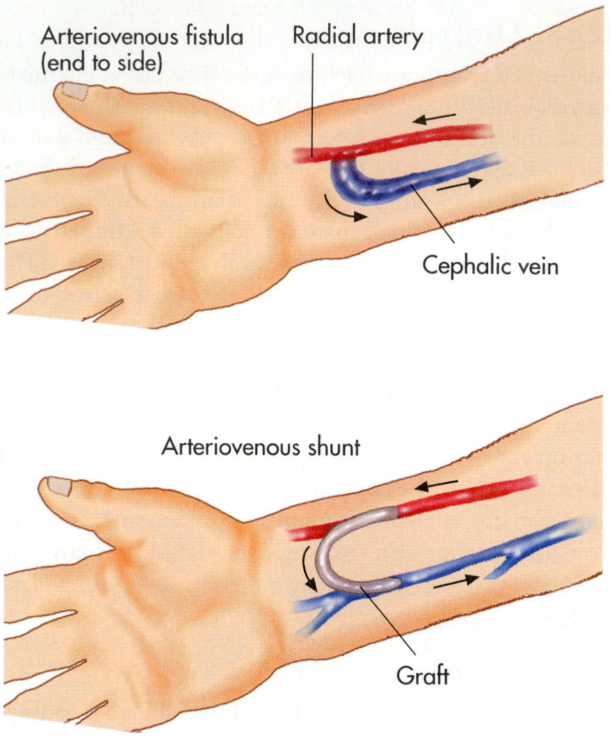

FIGURE 35-3 ■ Arteriovenous shunts.

result from complications of dialysis. For example, these patients may experience problems associated with vascular access, hemorrhage, hypotension, chest pain, severe hyperkalemia, **disequilibrium syndrome** (described hereafter), and the development of an air embolism. In addition, the paramedic should be aware of problems that may result from concurrent medical illness and its treatment. These problems include decreased ability to tolerate the stress of significant illness or trauma, inadvertent overadministration of intravenous fluid, and altered metabolism and unpredictable action of drugs.

CRITICAL THINKING

Which of these complications could cause an immediate life threat?

Vascular access problems. Problems associated with vascular access are bleeding at the site of puncture for dialysis, thrombosis, and infection. Bleeding from the fistula or graft usually is minimal. The bleeding usually can be controlled by direct pressure at the site. (Excessive pressure, though, can cause thrombosis in the graft or fistula.) A potential complication of an internal shunt is the development of a pseudoaneurysm. The aneurysm can rupture. In turn, this may cause a large hematoma and possible hypovolemia. If this occurs, the paramedic should apply direct pressure to the hematoma. The paramedic should assess and treat the patient for significant blood loss. This situation requires rapid transport for physician evaluation.

Fistulae and grafts that become occluded as a result of thrombus formation usually require surgical intervention or the administration of a thrombolytic agent to restore flow. Patients with a surgical anastomosis are instructed to check for the presence of a bruit or "thrill" periodically. The presence will verify unobstructed circulation. Attempts to clear the graft by irrigation or aspiration generally are not advised. If thrombosis occurs while the patient is undergoing dialysis, the dialysis should be stopped. Then intravenously administered fluids should be initiated in an alternative site. Decreased blood flow is a common trigger of thrombosis and is the main reason that one should not take the blood pressure in the arm with a vascular access.

An infection at the site of vascular access usually is the result of the puncture made during dialysis. Thus careful sterile technique is the rule when caring for these patients. Routine vascular access using the dialysis route should be discouraged. Vascular access infection should be considered when a dialysis patient has unexplained fever, malaise, or other signs of systemic infection.

NOTE When drawing blood or intravenously infusing fluids in a patient with a surgical anastomosis, the paramedic should choose an alternative site. The paramedic also should avoid taking blood pressure measurements and using tourniquets in an extremity with an arteriovenous fistula or graft. Rarely, medical direction may advise that the internal shunt be used to obtain vascular access. If so, the paramedic must be careful not to puncture the back wall of the vessel. The paramedic also must be sure to use careful aseptic technique during the procedure. Intravenous infusions must be monitored closely to avoid a "runaway IV." The intravenous catheter should be taped securely in place as well.

Hemorrhage. Patients who are receiving dialysis have an increased risk of hemorrhage. This risk arises from their regular exposure to anticoagulants during hemodialysis and from the decrease in their platelet function. Thus a patient who experiences hemorrhage from trauma or a medical condition (e.g., gastrointestinal bleeding) should be monitored closely for signs of hypovolemia. Most patients on dialysis have anemia. This lowers their ability to compensate for blood loss when they have acute hemorrhage. Any significant blood loss (whether external or internal) may produce dyspnea or angina. If hemorrhage from trauma occurs in an extremity with a fistula or graft, the paramedic should control the bleeding and immobilize the extremity. The paramedic should use special care to try to avoid obstructing circulation in the anastomosis.

Hypotension. Hypotension can occur with hemodialysis. This may result from the rapid reduction in intravascular volume, abrupt changes in electrolyte concentrations, or vascular instability that may occur during the procedure. In

> **BOX 35-2 Classic Signs of Congestive Heart Failure**
>
> Crackles
> Engorged neck veins
> Liver congestion and engorgement
> Pitting edema
> Pulmonary edema
> Shortness of breath

addition, the patient's mechanisms to cope with these physiological changes may be impaired. This may result in an inability to maintain normal blood pressure. Patients with hypotension caused by dialysis must be managed cautiously with the administration of volume-expanding fluids. The paramedic should be careful not to produce a fluid overload. This may manifest as hypertension and the classic signs of congestive heart failure (Box 35-2). Most patients respond to a small (200- to 300-mL) fluid challenge. If they do not, other potentially serious causes should be considered.

Chest Pain. The episodes of hypotension and mild hypoxemia that often occur during dialysis may result in myocardial ischemia and chest pain. The patient also may complain of other symptoms that are associated with decreased oxygen delivery. Examples of such symptoms include headache and dizziness. These complaints may indicate an evolving myocardial infarction. However, they often are relieved with the administration of oxygen, fluid replacement, and antianginal medications. Regardless, all patients with chest pain should be treated as though a myocardial infarction has occurred.

Dysrhythmias that result from myocardial ischemia also may be associated with dialysis. The most common ischemic rhythm disturbances are premature ventricular contractions. These generally respond well to supplemental oxygen and ***lidocaine.*** If dialysis is in progress, the procedure should be stopped. The paramedic should consult with medical direction.

Severe Hyperkalemia. Severe hyperkalemia is an emergency that poses a serious threat to life. It can occur rapidly in patients with acute renal failure. Severe hyperkalemia often results from poor dietary regulation and missed dialysis treatments. Patients with severe hyperkalemia may have weakness. Yet they often are asymptomatic. Typical electrocardiogram changes initially demonstrate a tall or tented T wave. As the potassium levels rise, conduction slows. This results in a prolonged P-R interval, depressed ST segments, and sometimes the loss of P waves. This may be followed by a widened QRS complex and delayed conduction in the interventricular conducting system. The electrocardiogram patterns resemble bundle branch blocks. Hyperkalemic disturbances may not become apparent until dangerous levels of potassium are present. Thus any patient with renal failure who is in cardiac arrest should be suspected of having severe hyperkalemia. Based on patient history, medical direction may recommend separate infusions of ***calcium*** and ***sodium bicarbonate*** during resuscitation.

> **NOTE** Dialysis patients who have chronic renal failure tolerate increased potassium levels better than do those patients with normal kidney function.

Disequilibrium Syndrome. *Disequilibrium syndrome* refers to a group of neurological findings that sometimes occur during or right after dialysis. These symptoms are usually mild (e.g., headache, restlessness, nausea, and fatigue). Yet they may be severe (including confusion, seizures, and coma). The syndrome is thought to result from a disproportionate decrease in osmolality of the extracellular fluid compared with that of the intracellular compartment in the brain or cerebrospinal fluid.[1] This results in an osmotic gradient between the blood and the brain. This in turn causes a movement of water into the brain and then cerebral edema and increased intracranial pressure. If seizures occur, an anticonvulsant may be indicated.

Air Embolism. Negative pressure on the venous side of the dialysis tubing or a malfunction in the machine can allow an air embolism to enter the patient's bloodstream. This is a rare occurrence. If air embolism occurs, the embolus may be carried to the right ventricle of the heart. In the heart the embolus may block the passage of blood to the left myocardium. The patient may experience severe dyspnea, cyanosis, hypotension, and respiratory distress. A patient with an air embolus requires high-concentration oxygen administration and rapid transport to a medical facility. In an effort to trap the embolism where it will be least likely to obstruct blood flow, the paramedic should position the patient on the left side. The patient should be transported in the modified Trendelenburg's position.

MANAGEMENT

To review, the prehospital management of patients with chronic or acute renal failure includes the following:

- Airway and ventilatory support with supplemental high-concentration oxygen administration
- Vascular access for fluid replacement, medication therapy (diuretics, antidysrhythmics, vasopressors), or fluid resuscitation if needed
- Meticulous aseptic technique if intravenous access is ordered by medical direction
- Electrocardiogram and other vital sign monitoring
- Rapid transport to an appropriate medical facility

SUMMARY

- The urinary system removes waste products from the blood. It helps to maintain a constant body fluid volume and composition as well.
- Urinary retention is the inability to urinate.
- Urinary tract infections can involve the upper or lower urinary tract.
- Pyelonephritis is inflammation of the kidney parenchyma.
- Urinary calculi are stones that originate in the kidney.
- Epididymitis is inflammation of the epididymis. The epididymis is the tube that carries sperm from the testicle to the seminal vesicles.
- Testicular torsion is a true emergency. In this condition a testicle twists on its spermatic cord. This disrupts the blood supply to the testicle.
- The physical examination for a patient with a urinary tract problem is similar to that performed for abdominal pain. Patients with genitourinary pain should be managed as any other patient with acute pain.
- Renal failure may result in uremia, hyperkalemia, acidosis, hypertension, and volume overload with congestive heart failure. Renal failure can be classified as acute or chronic. Classification depends on the duration and on the potential for reversibility.
- Dialysis is a technique used to normalize blood chemistry. Dialysis is used in patients who have acute or chronic renal failure. Dialysis also is used to remove blood toxins. The two dialysis techniques are hemodialysis and peritoneal dialysis. Dialysis emergencies may include problems with vascular access, hemorrhage, hypotension, chest pain, severe hyperkalemia, disequilibrium syndrome, and air embolism.

REFERENCES

1. http://www.kidneywa.org/PublicInformation/ *Urinary tract disease,* Accessed May 19, 2003, UrinaryTractDisease.htm. Site is now down.
2. Rosen P, Barkin R: *Emergency medicine: concepts and clinical practice,* ed 4, St Louis, 1998, Mosby.
3. *Kidney stones in adults,* National Kidney and Urologic Disease Clearinghouse (NKUDIC), http://kidney.niddk.nih.gov/kudiseases/pubs/stonesadults/index.htm. Accessed May 19, 2004.
4. US Department of Transportation, National Highway Traffic Safety Administration: *EMT-Paramedic national standard curriculum,* Washington, DC, 1998, The Department.
5. Nephrology channel, *Chronic renal failure,* http://www.nephrologychannel.com/crf/. Accessed May 21, 2004.
6. Medline Plus: Chronic renal failure. Retrieved May 21, 2003, from http://www.nlm.nih.gov/medlineplus/ency/article/000471.htm.

CHAPTER

36

Toxicology

OBJECTIVES

Upon completion of this chapter, the paramedic student will be able to:

1. Define poisoning.
2. Describe general principles for assessment and management of the patient who has ingested poison.
3. Describe the causative agents and pathophysiology of selected ingested poisons and management of patients who have taken them.
4. Describe how physical and chemical properties influence the effects of inhaled toxins.
5. Distinguish among the three categories of inhaled toxins: simple asphyxiants, chemical asphyxiants and systemic poisons, and irritants or corrosives.
6. Describe general principles of managing the patient who has inhaled poison.
7. Describe the signs, symptoms, and management of patients who have inhaled cyanide, ammonia, or hydrocarbon.
8. Describe the signs, symptoms, and management of patients injected with poison by insects, reptiles, and hazardous aquatic creatures.
9. Describe the signs, symptoms, and management of patients with organophosphate or carbamate poisoning.
10. Outline the general principles of managing patients with drug overdose.
11. Describe the effects, signs and symptoms, and specific management for selected drug overdose.
12. Describe the short- and long-term physiological effects of ethanol ingestion.
13. Describe signs, symptoms, and management of alcohol-related emergencies.
14. Identify general management principles for the most common toxic syndromes based on a knowledge of the characteristic physical findings associated with each syndrome.

KEY TERMS

botulism: An often fatal form of food poisoning caused by the bacillus *Clostridium botulinum*.

delirium tremens: An acute and sometimes fatal psychotic reaction caused by cessation of excessive intake of alcohol over a long period of time; also known as DTs.

envenomation: the injection of snake, arachnid, or insect venom into the body.

gastric lavage: Irrigation of the stomach with sterile water or normal saline.

Korsakoff's psychosis: A form of amnesia often seen in alcoholics, characterized by a loss of short-term memory and an inability to learn new skills.

Lyme disease: An acute, recurrent inflammatory infection transmitted by a tick.

nematocyst: A capsule containing threadlike, venomous stinging cells found in some coelenterates.

nystagmus: Involuntary rhythmic movements of the eyes.

poison: Any substance that produces harmful physiological or psychological effects.

Rocky Mountain spotted fever: A serious tick-borne infectious disease, characterized by chills, fever, severe headache, mental confusion, and rash.

tick paralysis: A rare, progressive, reversible disorder caused by several species of ticks that release a neurotoxin that causes weakness, incoordination, and paralysis.

West Nile virus: A potentially serious mosquito-borne illness that affects the central nervous system.

Our environment has a large number of potentially harmful substances. (These substances are natural and synthetic.) They can be accidentally or deliberately absorbed, ingested, inhaled, or injected.

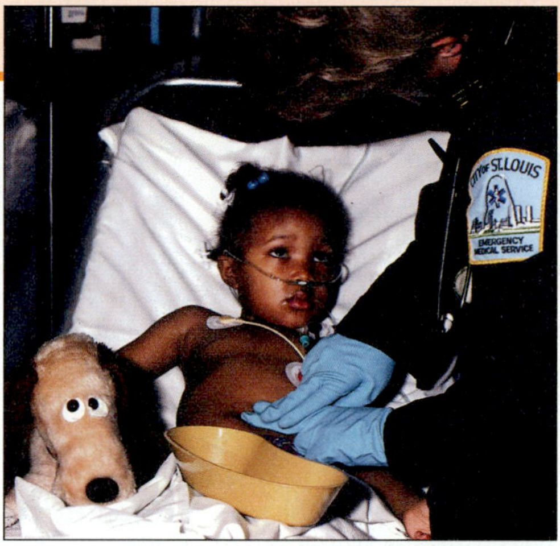

SECTION ONE

POISONINGS

A **poison** can be defined as any substance that produces harmful physiological or psychological effects. Emergencies that involve poisons are a major cause of morbidity and mortality in the United States. Poisons are responsible for 10% of all emergency department visits. They are the cause of 9% of all ambulance transports. Finally, they are responsible for 5% to 10% of all medical admissions to hospitals. According to the National Safety Council, poisoning by solids and liquids was the third leading cause of accidental death in the United States in 1999 and the second leading cause of unintentional death for persons aged 19 to 57.[1]

CRITICAL THINKING

How many substances that fit the definition of a poison are there in or around your home?

POISON CONTROL CENTERS

More than 60 poison control centers exist across the United States. These centers help to treat poisoning emergencies. Most centers are based in major medical centers or teaching hospitals. Each one belongs to regional poison control centers designated by the American Association of Poison Control Centers. Regional centers are staffed by medical professionals (1-800-222-1222). They offer 24-hour telephone access to population bases of at least 1 million. Each year, an estimated 4.7 million poisonings are reported to poison control centers throughout the United States. More than 90% of these poisonings happen in the home; 51% percent of poisoning victims are children younger than 6 years of age.[2] By helping persons manage emergencies at home, these centers prevent about 1.6 million hospitalizations and visits to doctors' offices each year.[3]

By request, information and treatment advice is given immediately by the poison control center. They provide this information through a large library of references on more than 350,000 toxic substances. These substances include drugs (legal, illicit, foreign, and veterinary), chemicals, plants, animals, insects, fish, snakes, cosmetics, and hazardous materials. Each request for information is followed up to determine the effectiveness and outcome of the treatment. In addition, the centers are responsible for the following six elements of an organized poison system:

1. Treatment information and toxicological consultation with health care providers (e.g., hospitals, physicians, emergency medical services [EMS] agencies), and the public, using a toll-free number with linkage into various 911 systems
2. Professional education to train those involved in care of poisoned patients
3. Data collection on all poisonings in the region for epidemiological and evaluation purposes
4. Public education and prevention
5. Research
6. Regional EMS poison system development (e.g., patient classification criteria, triage and management protocols, and regional transfer agreements)

Use by Emergency Medical Services Agencies

Regional poison control centers are a ready source of information for any toxicological emergency. Depending on local communications protocol, poison control centers may be contacted directly by EMS providers (and other emergency personnel) through telephone, cellular phone, a dispatching center, or medical direction. The immediate determination of potential toxicity is based on the specific agent or agents. It also is based on the amount ingested; the time of exposure; the weight and medical condition of the patient; and any treatment given before the arrival of EMS. The poison center also can coordinate treatment protocol by notifying the receiving hospital while the patient is en route to the emergency department.

GENERAL GUIDELINES FOR MANAGING A POISONED PATIENT

Poisons may enter the body through ingestion, inhalation, injection, and absorption. Box 36-1 lists three types of toxicological emergencies that may result in poisoning. Most poisoned patients require only supportive therapy to recover. (There are a few exceptions. An example of additional treatment is the use of lifesaving antidotes.) The poisoned patient often can be managed properly in the prehospital setting using the following guidelines:

1. Ensure adequate airway, ventilation, and circulation. Take action to prevent or reduce the risk of aspiration by carefully watching the patient's airway.
2. Obtain a thorough history, and perform a focused physical examination.
3. Consider hypoglycemia in an unconscious or convulsing patient.
4. Administer ***naloxone*** or ***nalmefene*** to a patient with respiratory depression.

BOX 36-1 Types of Toxicological Emergencies

Unintentional Poisoning
Childhood poisoning
Dosage errors
Environmental exposure
Idiosyncratic reactions
Occupational exposure

Drug and Alcohol Abuse

Intentional Poisoning/Overdose
Assault/homicide
Chemical warfare
Suicide attempts

5. If overdose is suspected, obtain an overdose history from the patient, family, or friends.
6. Consult with medical direction or a poison control center for specific management to prevent further absorption of the toxin (or antidote therapy).
7. Frequently reassess the patient; monitor vital signs and electrocardiogram.
8. Safely obtain any substance or substance container of a suspected poison. Transport it along with the patient. The paramedic should collect a sample of the patient's vomitus (if present) for laboratory analysis.
9. Transport the patient for physician examination.

When one is caring for a patient who has been poisoned, personal safety is the top priority. A toxicological emergency response may involve hazardous materials. It also may involve patient behavior that is unpredictable or violent. If the scene is not safe, the paramedic crew should retreat to a safe staging area. They should wait there until the scene has been secured by the proper personnel.

POISONING BY INGESTION

About 80% of all accidental ingestion of poisons occurs in children 1 to 3 years of age. These children eat or swallow a poisonous liquid or solid. The most common poison exposures in this group result from household products. Such products include petroleum-based agents, cleaning agents, and cosmetics; medications; toxic plants; and contaminated foods. Poisoning in adults, however, usually is intentional. (Yet unintentional poisoning from exposure to chemicals in the workplace also occurs.) Deliberate poisonings often are an attempt at suicide. They also may be the result of recreational or experimental drug abuse. Intentional poisonings may result from chemical warfare or acts of terrorism as well. They even may be a factor in assault and homicide.

The toxic effects of ingested poisons may be immediate or delayed, depending on the substance that was ingested. For example, corrosive substances such as strong acids and alkalis may produce immediate tissue damage. This is evidenced by burns to the lips, tongue, throat, and upper gastrointestinal tract. Other substances, such as medications and toxic plants, usually require absorption and distribution through the bloodstream (and alterations by different organs) to produce toxic effects. Only minimal absorption occurs in the stomach. Thus poisons may take several hours to enter the bloodstream through the small intestine. Therefore early management of the ingested poisoning focuses on treating the patient's symptoms. Management also includes removing the toxin from the stomach or binding it to prevent absorption before the poison enters the intestines.

Assessment and Management

The initial assessment and management of a poisoned patient is the same as for any other patient. First, the paramedic should ensure his or her personal safety. Then the paramedic should manage immediate threats to the patient's life. During scene size-up, the paramedic crew should be alert for specific clues or details that suggest a toxic emergency. Examples include open medication bottles, scattered pills, vomitus, and open containers of household products. Patient findings that may suggest poisoning include a decreased level of consciousness, airway compromise/injury (e.g., vomitus or pills in the mouth, burns in the oral cavity), abnormal respiratory patterns, and dysrhythmias such as tachycardia and bradycardia.

> ▶**NOTE** The paramedic must consider the possibility of poisoning whenever the patient's signs and symptoms cannot be attributed to other explainable conditions (e.g., hypoglycemia/hyperglycemia or cardiac dysfunction).

The main goal of physical assessment of poisoned patients is to identify effects on the respiratory system, the cardiovascular system, and the central nervous system. These effects are most likely to produce immediate threats to life. A detailed history of the event and any significant medical or psychiatric history also are important. This information may help to direct treatment in the field or in the emergency department. For example, preexisting cardiac, liver, or renal disease and some psychiatric illnesses may be worsened by a toxic ingestion. These conditions may require care in addition to treating the toxic ingestion.

RESPIRATORY COMPLICATIONS

The first priority in managing a poisoned patient after ensuring scene safety is to secure a patent airway. The paramedic should provide adequate ventilatory support as it is needed. This includes providing high-concentration oxygen. Treatment also includes possibly more advanced airway management to protect the airway and prevent aspiration (see Chapter 19). Other respiratory complications that may be associated with poisoning include the early development of noncardiogenic pulmonary edema or the later development of adult respiratory distress syndrome (see Chapter 30). Bronchospasm may result from direct or indirect toxic effects.

CARDIOVASCULAR COMPLICATIONS

The most common cardiovascular complication of poisoning by ingestion is cardiac dysrhythmias. Thus the paramedic should assess the patient's circulatory status and continually monitor it by electrocardiogram. The paramedic also should check the patient's blood pressure frequently. The presence of tachydysrhythmias or bradydysrhythmias may indicate serious disorders such as hypoxia and acidosis. Another cardiovascular complication is the development of hypotension. (This is associated with decreased vascular tone.) Rarely, hypertension develops. Hypertension may lead to cerebral vascular hemorrhage. (Toxicology in emergency cardiac care is covered in the appendix at the end of this chapter.)

NEUROLOGICAL COMPLICATIONS

The paramedic should perform and record a baseline neurological examination. Deviations from a normal sensorium may range from mild drowsiness and agitation to hallucinations, seizures, coma, and death. Neurological complications may result from the toxin itself. (An example of such is lead poisoning in children who have ingested paint chips.) Or the complications may result from a metabolic or perfusion disorder. (For example, this may be poor cardiac output because of cardiac dysrhythmias.)

HISTORY

The paramedic should obtain a thorough history of the exposure and any significant medical history from the patient, family members, or bystanders. This information may be unreliable (as in cases involving pediatric patients, drug abuse, or suicide attempts). However, the paramedic should determine the following if possible:

- What was ingested? (Obtain the poison container and remaining contents unless doing so poses a threat to rescuer safety.)
- When was the substance(s) ingested? (This may affect the decision to use ***activated charcoal*** or **gastric lavage,** to induce emesis, or to administer an antidote.)
- How much of the substance was ingested?
- Was an attempt made to induce vomiting? Did the patient vomit?
- Has an antidote or ***activated charcoal*** been administered?
- Does the patient have a psychiatric history pertinent to suicide attempts? Has the patient had episodes of recent depression?

Gastrointestinal Decontamination

The goal of managing serious poisonings that occurred by ingestion is to prevent the toxic substance from reaching the small intestine. This then limits its absorption. This task may be accomplished by gastrointestinal decontamination through the use of ***activated charcoal,*** and sometimes gastric lavage or ***syrup of ipecac.*** (Use of ***activated charcoal*** alone for removing poison from the gastrointestinal tract is considered equivalent or superior to other methods. It also has fewer complications.) Before attempting to remove poison from the gastrointestinal tract, the paramedic should consult with medical direction or a poison control center.

ACTIVATED CHARCOAL

Activated charcoal is an inert, nontoxic product of wood material. The wood has been heated to a high temperature. ***Activated charcoal*** is able to *adsorb* (collect in a condensed form) molecules of many chemical toxins while in the intestinal tract. The charcoal reduces absorption of the poison by as much as 50% and prevents it from being absorbed into the body systems.

Activated charcoal is a safe and effective treatment for most toxic ingestions (Box 36-2). The charcoal is administered in nearly all cases except when strong acid, strong alkali, or ethanol is the toxicant. Other agents not well adsorbed by activated charcoal include cyanide, ferrous sulfate, and methanol. If these substances have been ingested, activated charcoal probably should not be given. The paramedic should consult with medical direction or a poison control center. Activated charcoal also may be withheld when specific oral antidotes (e.g., *N*-acetylcysteine for acetaminophen overdose) are available. Activated charcoal also is withheld when the ingestion occurred 1 or more hours before the arrival of EMS. (Activated charcoal is most effective within the first hour after the ingestion of the toxic substance. After 1 hour, the toxin most likely will have passed from the stomach into the small intestine.)

Activated charcoal comes mixed in an aqueous solution with or without a cathartic. (A cathartic is an agent that causes bowel evacuation.) A cathartic (most commonly sorbitol) decreases the transit time and expels the charcoal within a short period. One complication of this therapy is poor patient acceptance in consuming the charcoal. (This may be especially the case in children.) Another complication is vomiting. Emergency medical services personnel should protect themselves, the patient, and the immediate area from being stained by the activated charcoal. The paramedic also should use personal protective measures when administering this agent.

CRITICAL THINKING

Why might a patient be reluctant to take activated charcoal?

BOX 36-2 Dosage of Activated Charcoal

1 to 2 g/kg body mass
30 to 100 g in adults
15 to 30 g in children
Prepared in a slurry and administered orally or by gastric tube

GASTRIC LAVAGE

Gastric lavage is a method of gastrointestinal decontamination. It has the advantage of immediate recovery of a portion of gastric contents. (This is the case, at least, if gastric lavage is done within 1 hour after ingestion while the contents are still in the stomach.) Gastric lavage offers a method for the administration of ***activated charcoal*** as well.

NOTE The first dose of activated charcoal sometimes is given via a nasogastric tube before actual lavage is begun. This allows for the immediate adsorption of toxins before they can pass through the stomach into the duodenum. In this case, lavage is continued until charcoal is no longer seen in the stomach contents (usually 2 to 3 L of fluid is needed to reach this point).

Gastric lavage generally is performed by using a large-bore orogastric tube (36 to 40 French in adults, 24 to 28 French in children) rather than a smaller nasogastric tube. The smaller tube may be too narrow to empty the stomach if large particles or pill fragments are present. These large tubes rarely should be inserted nasally because they may damage the mucosa or inside of the nose and result in epistaxis. The procedure for gastric lavage is as follows:

1. Place the conscious patient in a left lateral Trendelenburg (swimmer's) position. This will minimize the chance of aspiration in case of emesis. Endotracheal intubation should precede gastric lavage in patients with a depressed level of consciousness or in those without an intact gag reflex.
2. Insert the tube through the mouth into the patient's esophagus. Continue to advance the tube until it is placed in the stomach. If the paramedic notices resistance to passage, the procedure must cease.
3. Check the tube placement before lavage by air insufflation into the stomach with a large syringe. Auscultate over the patient's epigastrium.
4. Aspirate gastric contents to confirm correct placement.
5. Infuse tap water or normal saline in amounts not to exceed 150- to 200-mL aliquots in adults. These amounts should not exceed 50- to 100-mL aliquots in patients younger than 5 years of age. *Note:* To prevent water absorption and resultant fluid-electrolyte derangements in pediatric patients, only normal saline should be infused.
6. Continue gastric lavage until the return fluid appears clear. The return fluid should be about the same amount as the fluid administered.

Gastric lavage is contraindicated in patients who cannot protect their airway and who have an altered level of consciousness. Gastric lavage also is contraindicated in those who have ingested low-viscosity hydrocarbons (e.g., gasoline, kerosene, furniture polish, or mineral spirits) or caustic agents, where the risk of aspiration is increased. Gastric lavage can be performed in patients with an altered level of consciousness. However, the airway should be protected with endotracheal intubation before the procedure. Potential complications include agitation of the patient (produced by the procedure), inadvertent tracheal intubation, esophageal perforation, aspiration pneumonitis, and as previously stated, fluid and electrolyte imbalances in pediatric patients.

NOTE Gastric lavage is recommended only for patients who have ingested a potentially lethal amount of drug or toxin. The patient should have ingested the poison within the last hour. In obtunded or comatose patients, tracheal intubation (including rapid sequence intubation as indicated) should be performed before gastric lavage to prevent aspiration pneumonia.[4]

SYRUP OF IPECAC

Syrup of ipecac was once the treatment of choice in preventing the absorption of poisons. Yet studies have shown that ipecac-induced emesis reduces absorption by only about 30%. Studies also show that use of ipecac may interfere with the effectiveness of other methods of decontamination, such as ***activated charcoal. Syrup of ipecac*** also increases the risk of aspiration if the patient has decreasing or altered mental status. The drug is not recommended for routine use in the out-of-hospital setting. If administered, the syrup should be given within the first 30 minutes after the ingestion of a poison. It should be given only to patients who are alert and who have a gag reflex (Box 36-3). Potential complications of ipecac-induced emesis include Mallory-Weiss tear of the esophagus, pneumomediastinum, fatal diaphragmatic or gastric rupture, and aspiration pneumonitis. Contraindications include the following:

- Altered level of consciousness
- Ingestion of caustic substances (the esophagus would be exposed to the agent twice)
- Loss of gag reflex
- Seizures
- Pregnancy
- Acute myocardial infarction
- Ingestion of the following:
  - Acids
  - Alkalis
  - Ammonia
  - Nontoxic agents
  - Petroleum distillates (unless advised otherwise by medical direction or poison control)
  - Rapidly acting central nervous system (CNS) depressants (e.g., cyanide, tricyclic antidepressants)
  - Rapidly acting CNS irritants (e.g., strychnine)
  - Hydrocarbons (controversial)

BOX 36-3 Dosage of Ipecac

Patients 1 to 12 years
Contraindicated for patients less than 1 year old
15 mL of ipecac followed by two to three glasses of water
May be repeated in 20 minutes if vomiting does not occur

Patients Older than 12 years
30 mL of ipecac followed by two to three glasses of water
May be repeated in 20 minutes if vomiting does not occur

TABLE 36-1 Antidotes to Common Toxins

TOXIN	ANTIDOTE
Acetaminophen	*N*-acetylcysteine
Anticholinergic agents	Physostigmine
Benzodiazepines	Flumazenil
Beta-blockers	Glucagon
Calcium channel blockers	Calcium
Cyanide	Amyl nitrate, sodium nitrate, sodium thiosulfate
Cyclic antidepressants	Bicarbonate
Digoxin	Digoxin immune Fab
Iron	Deferoxamine
Methanol	Ethanol
Opiates	Naloxone
Organophosphates	Atropine, pralidoxime

Note: See the *Emergency Drug Index.*

Management of Specific Ingested Poisons

Specific ingested poisons discussed in this section include strong acids and alkalis, hydrocarbons, methanol, ethylene glycol, isopropanol, metals (iron, lead, and mercury), and poisons from food and plants. Few effective antidotes are available for ingested poisons. Thus managing the patient's symptoms and preventing absorption are the main goals in caring for the poisoned patient (Table 36-1).

STRONG ACIDS AND ALKALIS

Strong acids and alkalis include those found in toilet bowl cleaners, rust remover, ammonia, and most liquid drain cleaners (Box 36-4). These acids and alkalis may cause burns to the mouth, pharynx, esophagus, and sometimes the upper respiratory and gastrointestinal tracts. Perforation of the esophagus or stomach may result in vascular collapse, mediastinitis (inflammation of the mediastinum), or pneumoperitoneum (air or gas in the peritoneal cavity of the abdomen). The frequency of caustic ingestions (most commonly lye) is highest in small children, accounting for 5000 to 8000 accidental exposures each year.[1]

The ingestion of caustic and corrosive substances generally produces immediate damage to the mucous membrane and the intestinal tract. Acids generally complete their damage within 1 to 2 minutes. Alkali, however, particularly solid alkali, may continue to cause liquefaction of tissue and damage for minutes to hours. Thus the prehospital care usually is limited to airway and ventilatory support, intravenous fluid replacement, and rapid transport to an appropriate medical facility.

BOX 36-4 Common Acid and Alkali Substances

Acids	Alkalis
Acetic acid	Ammonia
Battery acid	Bleach
Bleach disinfectants	Disk (button) batteries
Hydrochloric acid	Drain pipe and toilet bowl cleaners
Metal cleaners	Hair dyes and tints
Phenol	Jewelry cleaners
Sulfuric acid	Metal cleaners or polishes
Swimming pool cleaners	Paint removers
Toilet bowl cleaners	Sodium or potassium hydroxide (lye)
	Washing powders

In some cases, medical direction may recommend diluting the acid or alkali in a conscious patient. This would be done with the oral administration of milk or water. (In the adult, 200 to 300 mL would be used. In a child, 15 mL/kg would be the maximum.) Efforts to neutralize the ingested agent with other fluids such as fruit juice, lemon juice, or vinegar are contraindicated. These fluids have the potential to induce intense heat-releasing (exothermic) reactions. These reactions may produce severe thermal burns.

CRITICAL THINKING

What is a risk of administering milk or water to a patient with this type of ingestion?

HYDROCARBONS

Hydrocarbons are a group of saturated and unsaturated compounds. They are derived mainly from crude oil, coal, or plant sources. Mixtures vary in their viscosity. (This is their resistance to flow.) They vary in their volatility as well. (This is their ability to vaporize.) These two attributes, along with other factors, determine the toxic effects of these agents. (Some of these other factors include surface tension, the presence of other chemicals in the product, total amount, and route of exposure.)

Hydrocarbons are found in many household products. Examples include cleaning and polishing agents (mineral seal oil or signal oil), spot removers, paints, cosmetics, pesticides, and hobby and craft materials. Hydrocarbons also are found in petroleum distillates (turpentine, kerosene, gasoline, lighter fluids, and pine oil products). In addition, a large group of halogenated hydrocarbons (carbon tetrachloride, trichloromethane, trichloroethylene, methyl chloride) and aromatic hydrocarbons (toluene, xylene, benzene) exist. Hydrocarbon poisonings are common, accounting for 7% of all ingestions in children under 5 years of age.[1] Most ingestions occur between May and September. This is the time when home use of petroleum products allows children the greatest amount of exposure (e.g., cleaning and yard machinery).

The most important physical characteristic in the potential toxicity of ingested hydrocarbons is its viscosity. The lower the viscosity (the thinner the liquid), the higher the risk of aspiration and associated complications. For example, an ingested hydrocarbon product with a low viscosity, such as gasoline or turpentine, rapidly spreads over the surface of the mouth and throat. The more volatile components become gases on contact with the warm mucous membranes. This exposure causes irritation, coughing, and possible aspiration. If aspiration occurs, it may allow a toxic amount of hydrocarbons to enter the lungs. Hydrocarbons with high viscosity (e.g., asphalt, grease, tar) are not aspirated or absorbed in the gastrointestinal tract. Thus they do not have significant toxicity.

NOTE A mnemonic for remembering hydrocarbons for which gastric lavage may be indicated is CHAMP: *c*amphor, *h*alogenated hydrocarbons, *a*romatic hydrocarbons, (heavy) *m*etal-containing hydrocarbons, and *p*esticide-containing hydrocarbons.

The clinical features of hydrocarbon ingestion vary widely. These features depend on the type of agent involved (Box 36-5). If the patient is not displaying symptoms on EMS arrival, the chances of serious complications usually are low. These patients generally are observed in the emergency department for several hours. They often require no treatment. However, any patient suspected of hydrocarbon ingestion who coughs, chokes, cries, or has spontaneous emesis on swallowing should be assumed to have aspirated the hydrocarbon until proved otherwise. Hydrocarbon ingestion may involve the patient's respiratory, gastrointestinal, and neurological systems. The clinical features may be immediate or delayed. Emergency care for symptomatic patients who have ingested hydrocarbon products includes the following:

1. Ensure a patent airway. Provide adequate ventilatory and circulatory support as needed.
2. Identify the substance. Contact medical direction or a poison control center.
3. Decontamination of the stomach generally is avoided in these patients. This prevents potential aspiration pneumonitis. Decontamination also is contraindicated with ingestion of mineral seal oil, signal oil, or polishing oils because of their low viscosity and the likelihood of aspiration. Medical direction may recommend gastric emptying of a petroleum product containing significant amounts (greater than 1 mL/kg) of camphor, benzene and its derivatives, organophosphates, halogenated hydrocarbons, and heavy metals such as arsenicals, lead, and mercury. In these cases, the chance of systemic toxicity is greater than the risk of aspiration. (The use of ***activated charcoal*** or diluents has not been shown to be effective in managing hydrocarbon ingestion.)

BOX 36-5 Clinical Features of Hydrocarbon Ingestion

Immediate: Up to 6 Hours

Gastrointestinal System
Abdominal pain
Belching
Irritation
Mucous membrane hyperemia
Nausea and vomiting

Respiratory System
Cough and choking
Cyanosis
Dyspnea
Inspiratory stridor
Tachypnea

Neurological System
Coma
Fever
Lethargy
Malaise
Seizures
Systemic factors

Delayed: Days to Weeks

Gastrointestinal System
Diarrhea
Hepatic toxicity

Respiratory System
Atelectasis
Bacterial pneumonia
Dyspnea
Hemolytic and aplastic anemias
Pulmonary edema
Spontaneous hemorrhage
Sputum production
Systemic factors

4. Initiate intravenous fluid therapy.
5. Monitor cardiac rhythm.
6. Transport the patient for physician evaluation.

CRITICAL THINKING

Will the potential lethal effects of this ingestion always be visible on the scene?

METHANOL

Methanol (wood alcohol) is a common industrial solvent and is obtained from the distillation of wood. Methanol is a poisonous alcohol found in a variety of products. Some of these include gas line antifreeze, windshield washer fluid, paints, paint removers, varnishes, canned fuels such as Sterno, and many shellacs. Methanol is a colorless liquid. It has an odor that is distinct from that of ethanol, the form of alcohol in alcoholic beverages. Poisonings may result from intentional or unintentional ingestions, absorption through the skin, or inhalation. Examples include deliberate use of the agent by chronic alcoholics to maintain an inebriated state, unintentional ingestion resulting from misuse or distribution of methanol for ethanol (as in contraband liquor), and accidental ingestions in children.

Methanol itself is no more toxic than ethanol. However, its metabolites are extremely toxic. As the alcohol is absorbed, it rapidly is converted in the liver to formaldehyde. Then in minutes the formaldehyde is converted to formic acid, causing massive metabolic acidosis. The accumulation of formic acid in the blood results in a group of symptoms relating to the CNS (depression), the gastrointestinal tract (pain, nausea, vomiting), the eyes (as little as 4 mL can cause blindness), and the development of metabolic acidosis. The onset of symptoms after ingestion ranges from 40 minutes to 72 hours.

CRITICAL THINKING

Do you think this could have been the origin of the expression "blind drunk"?

The symptoms of methanol poisoning correlate with the degree of acidosis and may include the following:

- CNS depression
  - Lethargy
  - Confusion
  - Coma
  - Seizures
- Gastrointestinal tract
  - Nausea and vomiting
  - Abdominal pain
- Visual complaints
  - Photophobia
  - Blurred or indistinct vision
  - Pupils that are dilated and sluggish to react to light
  - "Spots before the eyes"
  - "Snow-filled vision"
  - Blindness
- Metabolic acidosis
  - Shortness of breath
  - Tachypnea
  - Shock
  - Multisystem failure
  - Death

Emergency care for methanol poisoning is as follows:

1. *Supportive care:* Secure a patent airway. Provide adequate ventilatory and circulatory support as needed. Adequate ventilation is essential to ensure adequate oxygenation, help correct the profound metabolic acidosis, and maximize respiratory excretion. Establish an intravenous line. The patient should be placed on a cardiac monitor to detect rhythm disturbances.
2. *Gastrointestinal decontamination:* If the patient is seen within 1 hour after ingestion, gastric lavage is indicated. The effectiveness of ***activated charcoal*** in adsorbing methanol is controversial. Consult with medical direction or a poison control center.
3. *Correction of metabolic acidosis:* Medical direction may recommend trying to correct the metabolic acidosis with ***sodium bicarbonate.*** Large or repeated doses may be necessary. Serum formic acid may be neutralized with bicarbonate administration. However, hemodialysis probably will be necessary to remove toxic levels of methanol and formate.
4. *Prevention of the conversion of methanol to formic acid:* The conversion of methanol to formic acid may be prevented

by the administration of ethanol. (Ethanol has 9 times greater affinity for the enzyme that converts methanol to formic acid.) If the patient is conscious, give 30 to 60 mL of 80-proof ethanol by mouth or gastric lavage tube. Unconscious patients should have their airway protected with an endotracheal tube before gastric tube administration of ethanol.

5. *Transport:* Rapidly transport the patient to a proper medical facility for definitive treatment.

ETHYLENE GLYCOL

Ethylene glycol is a colorless, odorless, water-soluble liquid. Ethylene glycol commonly is used in windshield deicers, detergents, paints, radiator antifreeze, and coolants. The accidental ingestion of ethylene glycol is common in young children because of the brilliant colors added to these preparations. Ingestion also is due to the widespread availability of products containing ethylene glycol and the warm, sweet taste. The agent also is commonly misused by alcoholics as a substitute for ethanol. As little as 60 mL has been reported to be lethal to an adult.[5]

Early signs and symptoms of CNS depression usually are caused by the ethanol-like effects of ethylene glycol. However, toxicity from ethylene glycol, as from methanol, is caused by the buildup of glycolic and oxalic acids after metabolism. This buildup occurs mainly in the liver and kidneys. These acids may affect the CNS and cardiopulmonary and renal systems. These acids also cause the development of hypocalcemia (from the precipitation of oxalic acid as calcium oxalate). The signs and symptoms of ethylene glycol poisoning generally occur in three stages:

1. *Stage one:* Central nervous system effects occurring 1 to 12 hours after ingestion
   Slurred speech
   Ataxia
   Somnolence
   Nausea and vomiting
   Focal or generalized convulsions
   Hallucinations
   Stupor
   Coma
2. *Stage two:* Cardiopulmonary system effects occurring 12 to 36 hours after ingestion
   Rapidly progressive tachypnea
   Cyanosis
   Pulmonary edema
   Cardiac failure
3. *Stage three:* Renal system effects occurring 24 to 72 hours after ingestion
   Flank pain
   Cluster of urological symptoms (oliguria, crystalluria, proteinuria, anuria, hematuria, uremia)

> **CRITICAL THINKING**
>
> For what could the effects in stage one of ethylene glycol poisoning be mistaken?

Emergency care for ethylene glycol poisoning is similar to that used for methanol poisoning. The care includes the following:

1. Ensure a patent airway and provide adequate ventilatory and circulatory support as needed. Monitor the patient for dysrhythmias.
2. Use gastric lavage if the patient is seen within 1 hour after ingestion. Administer ***activated charcoal***. It has been shown to decrease gastrointestinal absorption of ethylene glycol by 50%.
3. Initiate intravenous fluid therapy with a volume-expanding fluid. This will help to maintain adequate urine output.
4. Administer ***sodium bicarbonate*** intravenously (per protocol) to correct acidosis.
5. Administer 80-proof ethanol (30 to 60 mL) by mouth or gastric tube. This will block the conversion of ethylene glycol into toxic acids by metabolism. Unmetabolized ethylene glycol is excreted by the lungs and kidneys.
6. Rapidly transport the patient for definitive treatment. This may include hemodialysis and continued ethanol administration.

In addition, the paramedic should anticipate orders from medical direction or a poison control center for the following medications:

- ***Thiamine*** to degrade glycolic acid to nontoxic metabolites
- ***Calcium gluconate*** or ***calcium chloride*** to manage hypocalcemia
- ***Diazepam*** or ***lorazepam*** to control seizure activity

ISOPROPANOL

Isopropanol (isopropyl alcohol) is a volatile, flammable, colorless liquid. It has a characteristic odor and bittersweet taste. Rubbing alcohol is the most common household source of this agent. Isopropanol also is used in disinfectants, degreasers, cosmetics, industrial solvents, and cleaning agents. Common routes of toxic exposure to isopropanol include intentional ingestion as a substitute for ethanol, accidental ingestion, and inhalation of high concentrations of local vapor, as from alcohol sponging of febrile children (a harmful and inappropriate procedure). Isopropanol is more toxic than ethanol. Yet isopropanol is less toxic than methanol or ethylene glycol. A potentially lethal dose in adults is 150 to 240 mL.[5] In children, any amount of ingestion should be considered potentially toxic.

After ingestion, the majority of isopropanol (80%) is converted to acetone. The rest is excreted unchanged by the kidneys. The acetone is excreted by the kidneys and to a lesser extent by the lungs. Isopropanol poisoning affects several body systems, including the central nervous, gastrointestinal, and renal systems. The signs and symptoms often occur within 30 minutes after ingestion. They include CNS and respiratory depression (isopropanol is 2 to 3 times more potent a CNS depressant than ethanol), abdominal pain, gastritis, hematemesis, and hypovolemia. Isopropanol poisoning causes acids to build up in the blood (acetonemia) and ketones to build up in the urine (ketonuria). However, no associated metabolic acidosis usually occurs unless the patient develops hypotension.

Emergency care for isopropanol poisoning mainly is supportive. Care includes airway and ventilatory support to ensure adequate respiratory elimination of acetone, gastric lavage (isopropanol also is secreted by the salivary glands and stomach), fluid resuscitation as needed, and rapid transport to an appropriate medical facility, where dialysis may be necessary. Administration of ethanol does not prevent the buildup of acids from metabolism to the same degree as in methanol or ethylene glycol poisoning.

METALS

Infants and children are high-risk groups for unintentional iron, lead, and mercury poisoning. Their immature immune systems and increased absorption as a function of age contribute to this risk.

Iron Poisoning. About 10% of the ingested iron (mainly ferrous sulfate) is absorbed each day from the small intestine. After absorption, the iron is converted and is stored in iron storage protein. Then the iron is transported to the liver, spleen, and bone marrow for incorporation into hemoglobin. When ingested iron exceeds the ability of the body to store it, the free iron circulates in the blood. The iron then is deposited into other tissues. Most iron poisonings result from the ingestion of pediatric multivitamins by children under 6 years of age.[2]

Unintentional or intentional ingestion of iron may be fatal. Ingested iron is corrosive to the lining of the gastrointestinal tract. Iron may produce gastrointestinal hemorrhage, bloody vomitus, painless bloody diarrhea, and dark stools. Severe cases involve the ingestion of more than 20 mg/kg. In such cases, iron toxicity can produce cardiovascular collapse and death 12 to 48 hours after ingestion.

Prehospital care includes supportive measures and rapid transport for physician evaluation and possible gastrointestinal decontamination to prevent further absorption. The use of ***activated charcoal*** generally is not recommended because it adsorbs iron poorly. Most patients with iron poisoning survive the episode. The long-term prognosis is favorable.

Lead Poisoning. Metallic lead has been used by human beings for more than 5000 years. Yet lead was not widely recognized as a potential health hazard until 1978. At that time, lead was banned from household paints in the United States (Box 36-6). Children are the most common victims of lead poisoning; an estimated 889,000 children in the United States have levels of lead in their bloodstream of 10 mg/dL or greater.[6] Most pediatric poisonings result from ingestion of lead-based paint chips and contaminated house dust. Lead toxicity in adults most commonly results from exposure by inhalation. If not detected early, children with high levels of lead in their bodies can suffer from damage to the brain and nervous system, behavioral and learning problems, hyperactivity, slowed growth, hearing problems, and headaches. Even children who appear healthy can have dangerous levels of lead in their bodies. Adults can suffer from a number of problems including the following:

- Difficulties during pregnancy
- Reproductive problems
- Hypertension
- Gastrointestinal disorders
- Nerve disorders
- Memory and concentration problems
- Muscle and joint pain

Most lead poisoning is slow in onset (from chronic ingestion or inhalation), eventually resulting in toxicity. The metal is excreted by the body slowly. Lead tends to accumulate in body tissues (mainly bone). Lead causes the most significant pathophysiology in the hematopoietic, neurological, and renal systems; however, it also affects the reproductive, gastrointestinal, skeletal, hepatic, and cardiovascular systems. Signs and symptoms of chronic exposure generally are nonspecific. These may include malaise, mental disturbances, incoordination, abdominal pain, diarrhea, and vomiting. If the intoxication is acute, anemia, weakness or paralysis of the limbs, seizures, and death may result. (If symptoms progress to include seizure and coma, the risk of death is high. Patients who survive are likely to sustain brain damage.) Prehospital care is focused on recognizing the potential for lead poisoning and transporting the patient for physician evaluation.

Lead poisoning is diagnosed from the patient's condition and history, from blood tests to measure lead levels, from x-ray films of the bones and abdomen that may reveal lead deposits, and with urine tests to measure the level of lead breakdown products. Following gastrointestinal decontamination, whole bowel irrigation may be done. This is usually done after an acute lead ingestion when evidence exists of lead in the stomach or small bowel. Many adults

BOX 36-6 Places Where Lead Can Be Found

Homes in the city, country, or suburbs
Apartments, single-family homes, and private and public housing painted before 1978
Soil around a home (soil contaminated from exterior paint, or other sources such as past use of leaded gasoline in cars)
Painted windows and window sills
Doors and door frames
Stairs, railings, and banisters
Porches and fences
Paint surfaces that have been scraped, dry-sanded, or heated (lead dust)
Old painted toys and furniture
The air after vacuuming or sweeping contaminated surfaces
Food and liquid stored in lead crystal or lead-glazed pottery or porcelain
Lead smelters or other industries
Hobbies that use lead (e.g., making pottery or stained glass)
Folk remedies (greta or azarcon used to treat an upset stomach)

and children who have high lead levels from chronic exposure require in-hospital and outpatient chelation therapy. This therapy detoxifies the lead and helps the body excrete the metal at a faster rate. All patients must be discharged to a lead-free environment.

CRITICAL THINKING

Paramedics play a key role in the emergency management of lead poisoning. What other role can they play in the management of this problem?

Mercury Poisoning. Mercury is the only metallic element that is liquid at room temperature. Mercury is used in thermometers, sphygmomanometers, and dental amalgam (dental fillings). Various compounds of mercury also are used in some paints, pesticides, cosmetics, drugs, and in certain industrial processes. All forms of mercury (except dental amalgam) are poisonous. Some, though, are absorbed into the body more readily than are others. Thus these are more dangerous.

Liquid mercury is highly volatile. Mercury vapor readily is absorbed into the body via the lungs. Inhalation of mercury vapor is the most common route of this poisoning. It may cause shortness of breath and lung damage. Mercury may be absorbed through the skin (causing severe inflammation) or intestines after ingestion as well. This results in nausea, vomiting, diarrhea, and abdominal pain. After mercury enters the body, it passes into the bloodstream. Mercury later builds up in various organs (mainly the brain and kidneys). This causes a wide range of symptoms that may include the following:

- Malaise
- Incoordination
- Excitability
- Tremors
- Numbness in the limbs
- Vision impairment
- Nausea and emesis (symptoms of renal failure)
- Mental status changes

The prehospital care mainly is supportive. Following physician evaluation, patients are managed with gastrointestinal decontamination (if the ingestion was recent) and chelating agents. In severe cases, hemodialysis may be indicated.

FOOD POISONING

Food poisoning is a term used for any illness of sudden onset (usually associated with stomach pain, vomiting, and diarrhea) suspected of being caused by food eaten within the previous 48 hours. Food poisoning can be classified as *infectious.* This means it results from bacteria or virus. It also can be *noninfectious.* This means it results from toxins or pollutants. Some foods also can cause poisoning of either type. (For example, shellfish such as mussels, clams, and oysters may be contaminated by viruses or bacteria or by toxins or chemical pollutants in water.)

Infectious (Bacterial) Types. One of the common types of bacteria responsible for food poisoning is salmonella. This organism is found in many animals (especially poultry) and in human beings. Salmonella bacteria also may be transferred to food from the excrement of infected animals or human beings. The bacteria may be transferred by food handling by an infected person as well. Other bacteria (e.g., strains of staphylococcal bacteria) cause formation of toxins. These toxins may be hard to destroy even with thorough cooking. Other bacteria that commonly cause diarrhea are certain strains of *Escherichia coli* (traveler's diarrhea) and *Campylobacter* and *Shigella* organisms.

Botulism is a rare but life-threatening form of food poisoning. It may result from eating improperly canned or preserved food that is contaminated with the bacterium *Clostridium botulinum.* This organism is found in soil and untreated water in most parts of the world. It also is harmlessly present in the intestinal tracts of many animals, including fish. Its spore-forming properties resist boiling, salting, smoking, and some forms of pickling. This allows the bacterium to thrive in improperly preserved or canned foods.

Although botulism is rare, the disease is more common in the United States than elsewhere in the world. This is due to the popularity of preserving food in the home. Botulinal toxin also has the potential to be a biological weapon because it is made by a living organism. (See Chapter 54.) Botulism is associated with severe CNS symptoms. These symptoms appear in a characteristic head-to-toe progression: headache, blurred or double vision, dysphagia, respiratory paralysis, and quadriplegia. Death from respiratory failure occurs in about 70% of untreated cases. *Pseudomembranous colitis* (associated with long-term administration of certain antibiotics) is another life-threatening form of diarrhea. It often is caused by *C. difficile.*

Infectious (Viral) Types. Two viruses most often cause food poisoning. One of these is the Norwalk virus. It is a common contaminant of shellfish. The other one is rotavirus. These agents may be responsible for illness when raw or partly cooked foodstuffs have been in contact with water contaminated by human excrement.

Noninfectious Types. Noninfectious types of food poisoning may result from consuming mushrooms and toadstools. Food poisoning also can result from eating fresh foods and vegetables that are accidentally contaminated with large amounts of insecticide. Chemical food poisoning may result from eating food stored in a contaminated container. (For example, this may be a container that previously was used to store poison.) Chemical food poisoning may result from improperly preparing and cooking various exotic foods as well. Drugs or medications also can cause diarrhea. Quinidine, certain antacids, some antibiotics, and stool softeners or laxatives may cause diarrhea.

Management Guidelines. The onset of signs and symptoms from food poisoning varies by cause and by how heavily the food was contaminated. As a rule, symptoms usually develop within 30 minutes in the case of chemical poisoning. They develop in 1 to 12 hours in the case of bacterial toxins. They develop in 12 to 48 hours with viral and bacterial infections. General principles of the management for patients with suspected food poisoning include the following:

- Use precautions to avoid contamination of self and equipment. (Wear gloves, a gown, or both if appropriate.)
- Ensure adequate airway, ventilatory, and circulatory support.
- Gather a complete history. This should include time and onset of symptoms, recent travel, the relation of symptoms to ingestion of a particular food, and effects on others who ate the same food. In addition, the paramedic should obtain information on the consistency, frequency, and odor of stool (including the presence of mucus or blood). Fever should be noted as well. Any patient history also should include significant medical history, allergies, and use of medications.
- Initiate intravenous therapy with a crystalloid solution. This will help to manage dehydration and electrolyte disturbances resulting from vomiting and diarrhea.
- Transport the patient for physician evaluation.

PLANT POISONING

Toxic plant ingestion is a frequently reported category of poisonings, second only to ingestion of cleaning substances.[1] The majority of these exposures occur in children under 6 years of age.

> **CRITICAL THINKING**
>
> What features of a plant would make it attractive for children to eat?

Signs and Symptoms. The signs of toxicity following the ingestion of major poisonous plants are predictable. They are categorized by the chemical and physical properties of the plant. Most signs and symptoms tend to be consistent with the type of major toxic chemical component in the plant. However, some differences exist. For example, anticholinergic crisis may result from ingestion of plants with certain alkaloid components (Jimson weed and lantana). This produces tachycardia; dilated pupils; hot, dry skin; decreased bowel sounds; altered vision; and abnormal mental status. Cholinergic symptoms may result from the ingestion of certain mushroom species. This produces bradycardia, miosis, salivation, hyperactive bowel sounds, and diarrhea. Nicotinic alkaloids (poison hemlock and delphinium) may at first act as stimulants. Yet this usually is soon followed by depression and weakness. Most signs and symptoms appear within several hours after ingestion, but some symptoms may be delayed 1 to 3 days. Box 36-7 lists common poisonous plants. Paramedics should be familiar with common poisonous plant life in their response area.

Management. Several hundred species of green plants in the United States contain toxic compounds. In addition, more than 100 varieties of mushrooms in the United States contain toxic compounds. Many similar species of plants and mushrooms have widely varying potencies. They also have widely varying combinations of toxins. In addition, such factors as the age of the plant and soil conditions may influence the severity of toxic symptoms. Thus management guidelines should be customized to the patient's symptoms rather than to one type of ingestion. Identification of the plant is crucial if possible. However, the inability to do so should not delay management. As always, the paramedic should consult with medical direction or a poison control center regarding appropriate emergency care. Principles in the management of toxic plant ingestion generally include the following:

1. Ensure adequate airway, ventilatory, and circulatory support.
2. In patients with a depressed gag reflex, unresponsiveness, or seizures, secure the airway with an endotracheal tube. Then use gastrointestinal decontamination. Medical direction or a poison control center may recommend administration of ***activated charcoal*** in place of gastric emptying or after it.
3. Initiate intravenous fluid therapy with a volume-expanding solution.
4. Monitor the patient's vital signs and cardiac rhythm.
5. Obtain a sample of the suspected plant or mushroom (if possible).
6. Transport the patient for physician evaluation. Most patients are hospitalized for observation and treatment as indicated for the toxin involved. Dialysis has not been shown to be effective in removing most plant toxins.

BOX 36-7 Common Poisonous Plants, Trees, and Shrubs

House Plants
Dieffenbachia
Hyacinth
Mistletoe
Narcissus
Oleander
Poinsettia

Flower-Garden Plants
Daffodil
Foxglove
Iris
Larkspur
Lily of the valley

Ornamental Plants
Azaleas
Daphne
Jasmine
Rhododendron
Wisteria

Other Plants
Buttercups
Jack-in-the-pulpit
Mayapple
Nightshade
Water and poison hemlock

Trees and Shrubs
Elderberry
Oaks
Wild and cultivated cherries

POISONING BY INHALATION

The unintentional or intentional inhalation of poisons can lead to a life-threatening emergency. The type and location of injury caused by toxic inhalation depend on the specific actions and behaviors of the chemical involved.[7] Respiratory difficulty may not appear for several hours after exposure to toxic fumes and smoke. All patients should be encouraged to be evaluated by a physician. This includes even those who are asymptomatic.

Physical Properties

The concentration of a chemical in the air helps to determine the severity of inhalation injury. The duration of exposure helps to determine this as well. At low concentrations and with brief exposure, the chemical may be removed from the air before reaching the lungs. In contrast, large concentrations or prolonged exposure are more likely to cause contact with the lungs. This in turn is more likely to cause damage to lung tissue. As a rule, increasing the concentration of the chemical or the length of exposure increases the dose received.

Solubility of the inhaled chemical affects the amount of inhalation injury. For example, water-soluble chemicals such as chlorine and anhydrous ammonia can be converted to hydrochloric acid and ammonium hydroxide, respectively, when they contact moisture in the respiratory tract. This produces injury in the nasopharynx, oropharynx, and conducting airways. In contrast, water-insoluble chemicals such as phosgene and nitrogen dioxide may have little effect on the upper airways. However, they can produce severe damage to the alveoli and respiratory bronchioles.

Chemicals may be inhaled as gases and vapors, mists, fumes, or particles. Gases and vapors mix with air and distribute themselves freely throughout the lung and its airways. Mists are liquid droplets dispersed in air. Their toxic effects depend on droplet size (the larger the size, the greater the exposure). Fumes contain fine particles of dust dispersed in air. Large particles are likely to be trapped in the nasopharynx and conducting airways, whereas small particles (1 to 5 μm) are more likely to penetrate the lower airways.

Chemical Properties

The ability of a chemical to interact with other chemicals and body tissue is called its *reactivity*. As a rule, highly reactive chemicals cause more severe and rapid injury than less-reactive chemicals. Four potential properties of chemicals that determine reactivity are the following:

1. *Chemical pH:* The likelihood for severe injury from alkaloid or acid exposure increases as the pH approaches its extremes: a pH of less than 2 for acidic substances and greater than 11.5 for alkaline substances.
2. *Direct-acting potential of chemicals:* Direct-acting chemicals are capable of producing injury without first being transformed or changed. An example is hydrofluoric acid. It causes severe corrosive burns on contact with mucous membranes of the upper airways.
3. *Indirect-acting potential of chemicals:* Indirect-acting chemicals must be transformed before they can produce injury. An example is phosgene. This is a gas that may cause acidic burns of the alveolar membranes after conversion to hydrogen chloride. (This process may take up to several hours.)
4. *Allergic potential of chemicals:* Some reactive chemicals bind with proteins to form structures that stimulate allergic reactions. For example, formaldehyde can cause severe asthmatic and anaphylactic reactions after even a small exposure. In general, the allergic potential of a chemical is related to its reactivity.

CRITICAL THINKING

Do you think that situations involving toxic gas inhalation are likely to involve one patient or multiple patients? Why?

CLASSIFICATIONS

Toxic gases can be classified in three categories: simple asphyxiants, chemical asphyxiants, and irritants/corrosives. Simple asphyxiants (methane, propane, and inert gases) cause toxicity by displacing or lowering the amount of oxygen in the air. Chemical asphyxiants (carbon monoxide and cyanide) possess built-in systemic toxicity. This appears after absorption into the circulation. Irritants/corrosives (chlorine and ammonia) cause cellular destruction and inflammation as they come into contact with moisture. Table 36-2 provides an overview of toxic gases and their clinical features.

General Management

The general principles of managing patients who have inhaled poisons are the same as for any other hazardous materials incident (see Chapters 53 and 54). These principles include the following:

1. Scene safety
2. Personal protective measures (protective clothing and appropriate respiratory protective apparatus)
3. Rapid removal of the patient from the poison environment
4. Surface decontamination
5. Adequate airway, ventilatory, and circulatory support
6. Initial assessment and physical examination
7. Irrigation of the eyes (as needed)
8. Intravenous line with a saline solution
9. Regular monitoring of vital signs and cardiac rhythm by electrocardiogram
10. Rapid transport to an appropriate medical facility

Management of Specific Inhaled Poisons

The specific inhaled poisons discussed in this section include cyanide, ammonia, and hydrocarbons. Carbon monoxide poisoning is described in Chapter 23. Other gases associated with atmospheres with low oxygen levels

TABLE 36-2 Clinical Features of Toxic Gases and Fumes

CLASS OF TOXIN	TOXIN	SOURCE	CLINICAL FEATURES	MANAGEMENT
Simple asphyxiants	Propane Methane Carbon dioxide Inert gases (nitrogen, argon)	Cooking gas Cooking gas All fires Industry (especially welding)	Displacement of normal air and lower fractional inspired oxygen concentration, symptoms of hypoxemia without airway irritation	Remove patient from source; give oxygen.
Chemical asphyxiants	Carbon monoxide	Fires	Formation of carboxyhemoglobin; inhibition of oxygen transport (Headache is earliest symptom.)	Give 100% oxygen.
	Hydrocyanic acid	Industry, burning plastics, furniture, fabrics	Highly toxic cellular asphyxiant	Use cyanide antidote.
	Hydrogen sulfide	Liquid manure pits, decaying organic materials	Highly toxic cellular asphyxiant similar to cyanide; sudden collapse; ability to smell characteristic odor of rotten eggs; rapid fatigue	Use sodium nitrite for cyanide (makes sulfmethemoglobin). Do not use thiosulfate.
Irritants High solubility in water	Chlorine gas Hydrochloric acid	Industry, swimming pool chemicals, bleach mixed with acid at home	Early onset of lacrimation, sore throat, stridor, tracheobronchitis; with heavy exposure, pulmonary edema in 2 to 6 hours	Use humidified oxygen, bronchodilators, and airway management.
	Ammonia	Industry, burning fabrics		
Low solubility in water	Nitrogen dioxide	Burning cellulose, fabrics Grain silos (acrid red gas)	Sweet "electric" smell; delayed onset (12-24 hours) of tracheobronchitis, pneumonitis, and pulmonary edema; late chronic bronchitis	Give oxygen: observe for 24 to 48 hours; give steroids (controversial).
	Ozone	Inert gas arc welding, industry		
	Phosgene	Burning of chlorinated organic material		
Allergenic	Toluene diisocyanate	Manufacture of polyurethanes	Reactive bronchoconstriction; possible long-term effects (chronic obstructive pulmonary disease) in susceptible persons	Use bronchodilators.
Metal fumes	Zinc Copper Tin Teflon	Welding (especially galvanized metal welding)	"Metal fumes fever"; chills, fever, myalgias, headache, nonproductive cough, leukocytosis 4 to 8 hours after exposure	Self-limited (12-24 hours)
	Arsine	Burning arsenic-containing ores, electronics industry	Highly toxic effect; hemolysis, pulmonary edema, renal failure; chronic arsenic toxicity	Perform exchange transfusion; use dimercaprol (BAL) for chronic arsenic toxicity only.
	Mercury Lead	Industry, welding	See specific metals	

From Ho MT: *Current emergency diagnosis and treatment,* ed 3, Norwalk, Conn, 1990, Appleton & Lange.

and chemical and biological warfare are discussed in Chapters 53 and 54.

CYANIDE

Cyanide refers to any of a number of highly toxic substances that contain the cyanogen chemical group. Because of its toxicity, cyanide has few applications. The agent sometimes is used in industry in electroplating, ore extraction, fumigation of buildings, and as a fertilizer. Cyanide has been used in gas chambers as a means of execution. Cyanide is one of the products of combustion from burning nylon and polyurethane. Thus cyanide is a potential hazard in fire environments.

Cyanide poisoning may result from the inhalation of cyanide gas; ingestion of cyanide salts, nitriles, or cyanogenic

BOX 36-8 Early and Advanced Signs and Symptoms of Cyanide Poisoning

Early Effects	Advanced Effects
Agitation	Acidosis
Anxiety	Dysrhythmias
Confusion	Hypotension
Dyspnea	Intractable hypotension
Hypertension with reflex bradycardia	Lactic acidosis
	Pulmonary edema
	Seizures
	Coma

glycosides (e.g., amygdalin, a substance found in the seeds of cherries, apples, pears, and apricots, and the principal constituent of Laetrile); or the infusion of nitroprusside. Cyanide also can be absorbed across the skin. Regardless of the route of entry, cyanide is a rapidly acting poison. It combines and reacts with ferric ions (Fe^3) of the respiratory enzyme cytochrome oxidase to inhibit cellular oxygenation. The cytotoxic hypoxia produces a rapid progression of symptoms from dyspnea to paralysis, unconsciousness, and death (Box 36-8). Large doses usually are fatal within minutes from respiratory arrest.

After ensuring personal safety, emergency care for a patient with cyanide poisoning begins with securing an open airway and providing adequate ventilatory support with high-concentration oxygen. Oxygen displaces cyanide from cytochrome oxidase and increases the effectiveness of drug administration. After these measures, the principal treatment of cyanide poisoning is to convert (oxidize) ferrous ions in hemoglobin (Fe^2) to ferric ions (Fe^3). This forms methemoglobin, hemoglobin with ferrous ion in the oxidized (Fe^3) state. Cyanide, which has a greater attraction to iron in the ferric state, is released from the cytochrome oxidase and combines with methemoglobin. This allows cytochrome oxidase to resume its function in normal cellular respiration. Cyanide antidotes, such as those found in the Pasadena cyanide antidote kit (formerly the *Lilly Cyanide Poison Kit*), are thought to be effective because they induce methemoglobin (Box 36-9).

Methemoglobin cannot transport oxygen. Therefore it must be reconverted to hemoglobin by administration of the drug sodium thiosulfate. This is accomplished in a three-step process. This process includes administration of (1) ***amyl nitrite*** by inhalation (converting about 5% of hemoglobin to methemoglobin); (2) sodium nitrite, which results in methemoglobinemia approaching 25% to 30%; and (3) sodium thiosulfate.

Prehospital care for patients with cyanide poisoning is as follows:

1. Don personal protective equipment as needed. This will help to prevent rescuer contamination.
2. Remove the patient from the cyanide source. Rapid decontamination and removal of the patient's contaminated clothing is key.
3. Ensure a patent airway and provide adequate ventilatory support.
4. Administer high-concentration oxygen.
5. If using the Pasadena cyanide antidote kit, consult with medical direction or a poison control center. Also, follow the instructions provided by the manufacturer.
6. If an antidote kit is not available, the paramedic should crush a pearl of ***amyl nitrite.*** The paramedic then can hold the amyl nitrite under the patient's nose for 15 of every 30 seconds. This should be followed by continuation of supplemental oxygen. If the patient's respirations are being assisted, place the crushed pearl under the intake valve of a bag-valve device.
7. Initiate intravenous fluid therapy with a volume-expanding solution.
8. Monitor cardiac rhythm by electrocardiogram.
9. Rapidly transport the patient for physician evaluation.

BOX 36-9 Cyanide Antidote Kit

Two Amyl Nitrite Inhalants in Gauze

Administer by inhalation 15 of every 30 seconds.

3% Sodium Nitrite (Stop Amyl Nitrite)

Adults: 10-mL slow intravenous administration over 2 to 4 minutes

Children: 0.2 mL/kg (up to 10 mL) slow intravenous administration over 5 minutes

Note: If hypotension develops, stop nitrite, treat for shock, and consider administration of *dopamine* (per medical direction).

25% Sodium Thiosulfate

Adults: 50-mL intravenous bolus

Children: 5 mL sodium thiosulfate per 1 mL sodium nitrite given

NOTE Hypotension should be anticipated as a side effect of antidote therapy. The patient should remain lying down, if possible. The blood pressure must be monitored closely as well. If hypotension develops, medical direction may recommend the administration of vasopressors.

AMMONIA INHALATION

Ammonia is a toxic irritant. It causes local pulmonary complications after inhalation. Exposure to ammonia vapors results in inflammation and irritation. In severe cases, exposure results in destruction of the mucosal tissue of all respiratory structures. This occurs as the ammonia vapor combines with water. As the two combine, a highly caustic alkaline compound is produced. Patients usually develop coughing, choking, congestion, burning, and tightness in the chest and a feeling of suffocation. These respiratory symptoms often go together with burning eyes and tearing. In severe cases, bronchospasm and pulmonary edema may develop. In addition to the general management principles, emergency care may include positive-pressure ventilation and the administration of diuretics and bronchodilators.

HYDROCARBON INHALATION

The hydrocarbons that pose the greatest risk for injury have low viscosity, high volatility, and high surface tension or adhesion of molecules along a surface. These characteristics allow hydrocarbons to enter the pulmonary tree. This causes aspiration pneumonitis. Inhalation of hydrocarbons creates the potential for systemic effects as well. Examples of such include CNS depression and liver, kidney, or bone marrow toxicity.

Most hydrocarbon inhalations result from "recreational use" of halogenated hydrocarbons (e.g., carbon tetrachloride and methylene chloride) or aromatic hydrocarbons (e.g., benzene and toluene). These agents may produce a state of inebriation or euphoria through "sniffing" or "huffing." (These involve placing the solvent on a rag and inhaling the vapors through a plastic bag.) The onset of these effects usually is rapid (typically occurring within seconds). It may be followed by CNS depression, respiratory failure, or cardiac dysrhythmias. Other signs and symptoms of hydrocarbon inhalation include the following:

- Burning sensation on swallowing
- Nausea and vomiting
- Abdominal cramps
- Weakness
- Anesthesia
- Hallucinations
- Changes in color perception
- Blindness
- Seizures
- Coma

Emergency care for hydrocarbon inhalation generally is supportive and includes airway, ventilatory, and circulatory support; intravenous fluid therapy; vital sign and electrocardiogram monitoring; and transport for physician evaluation.

POISONING BY INJECTION

Human poisonings from injection may result from drug misuse or abuse (described later in this chapter.) They also may result from arthropod bites and stings, reptile bites, and hazardous aquatic life. In contrast to most chemical compounds previously described, injected poisons are mixtures of many different substances. These mixtures may produce several different toxic reactions in human beings. Thus the paramedic must be prepared to manage reactions in many organ systems at the same time.

Arthropod Bites and Stings

Arthropods are invertebrate animals with jointed legs, a segmented body, and an exoskeleton. About 900,000 species of arthropods exist throughout the world. Some arthropods bite, some sting, and a few bite and sting. Arthropod venoms are complex and diverse in their chemistry and pharmacology. They may produce major toxic reactions in sensitized persons. Such reactions include anaphylaxis and upper airway obstruction. The various reactions to venoms are classified as local, toxic, systemic, and delayed[8] (Boxes 36-10 and 36-11).

HYMENOPTERA (WASPS, BEES, ANTS)

Hymenoptera is the name of a large, highly-specialized order of insects. The order includes wasps, bees, and ants. Hymenoptera venom is used for defense and subjugation of prey. Medically important venoms are mixtures of protein or polypeptide toxins, enzymes, and other compounds such as histamines, serotonin, acetylcholine, and dopamine. Hymenoptera stings most commonly are inflicted on the head and neck. The next most common sites are the foot, leg, hand, and arm. The mouth, pharynx, and esophagus may be stung when bees or yellow jackets in soft drink or beer containers are swallowed accidentally.

A single wasp, bee, or ant sting in an unsensitized person usually causes instant pain. This is followed by a wheal-and-flare reaction with variable edema. Large local reactions can spread more than 15 cm beyond the sting site. They also can persist for more than 24 hours. Anaphylaxis is the most serious complication of hymenoptera stings. An estimated 0.4% of the U.S. population has some degree of chemical allergy to insect venoms; 40 to 100 deaths caused by anaphylaxis from hymenoptera stings are reported annually.[5] Persons with a history of allergic reactions to stings often wear medical alert identification. These persons also often carry an emergency kit that contains a preloaded syringe of ***epinephrine*** (Epi-Pen).

The ant species of greatest concern in the United States is the imported fire ant. The venom of this ant is mainly an alkaloid. The fire ant is the only hymenopteran species with venom that results in necrotic activity. Sterile pustules at the sting site are not uncommon. Stings or bites from fire ants may produce systemic reactions. These stings or bites are managed like other hymenoptera stings. Secondary infection may occur (requiring antibiotic therapy), and extensive scarring may require skin grafts (rare).

Management. The prehospital care for mild hymenoptera stings should include close watching for signs or symptoms of an allergic reaction. If an extremity is involved, immobilization and elevation of the affected extremity may shorten the duration of the reaction. If physician evaluation is needed, because of signs of anaphylaxis or a severe local reaction, an antihistamine may be prescribed.

Honey bees (and other hymenoptera) often leave their stingers in the wound. If a stinger is present, it should be scraped or brushed off. Stingers should not be removed with forceps. This is because squeezing the attached venom sac may worsen the injury. Severe allergic reactions should be managed as described in Chapter 33. Hypovolemia (if present) should be treated in the conventional manner with a volume-expanding crystalloid infusion.

BOX 36-10 Types of Reactions to Venoms

Local Reaction
- Marked and prolonged edema at the sting site
- Possible involvement of one or more neighboring joints
- Possible occurrence in the mouth or throat, producing airway obstruction
- Severe local reactions that may increase the likelihood of future systemic reactions (controversial)
- Symptoms that usually subside within 24 hours

Toxic Reaction*
- Gastrointestinal disturbances
  - Diarrhea
  - Light-headedness
  - Vomiting
- Other symptoms
  - Convulsions (rare)
  - Edema without urticaria
  - Fever
  - Headache
  - Involuntary muscle spasms
  - Symptoms that usually subside within 48 hours
  - Syncope (common finding)

Systemic (Anaphylactic) Reaction†
- Reactions that can progress to death within minutes
- Immediate symptoms
  - Facial flushing
  - Generalized urticaria
  - Itching eyes or generalized itching

Systemic (Anaphylactic) Reaction†, cont'd
- Subsequent symptoms
  - Bloody and frothy sputum production
  - Chest or throat constriction or both
  - Chills and fever
  - Cyanosis
  - Dyspnea
  - Hypotension
  - Laryngeal stridor
  - Loss of bowel or bladder control
  - Loss of consciousness
  - Nausea and vomiting
  - Respiratory failure, cardiovascular collapse, or both
  - Shock
  - Wheezing

Delayed Reaction‡
- Serum sickness symptoms
  - Fever
  - Headache
  - Malaise
  - Polyarthritis
  - Urticaria

* Should be considered with a history of 10 or more stings.
† May occur in response to single or multiple stings.
‡ Usually occurs 10 to 14 days after a sting.

BOX 36-11 West Nile Virus

Mosquitoes are insects of the order Diptera (two-winged flies). Although they have long been associated with the spread of some diseases (e.g., malaria), some species recently have gained notoriety for spreading the West Nile virus. Mosquitoes become carriers of West Nile virus when they feed on infected birds. The mosquitoes then spread the virus to human beings and other animals when they bite.

West Nile virus was first isolated in Uganda in 1937. The virus was first reported in the United States (in Queens, New York) in 1999. Since then, more than 1600 cases and 56 deaths in the United States have been documented by the Centers for Disease Control and Prevention.[9]

West Nile virus is a potentially serious illness. It affects the central nervous system. The virus was a major cause of illness in the United States in 2002 and 2003. The symptoms (if present) usually develop within 3 to 14 days after being bitten by an infected mosquito. Most patients (about 80%) are asymptomatic after being bitten. About 20% of infected patients develop mild symptoms that include fever, headache, body aches, nausea and vomiting, and skin rash that lasts from a few days to several weeks. About 1 in 150 infected persons develop serious illness that can lead to seizures, coma, vision loss, numbness, paralysis, and other clinical manifestations such as West Nile fever, West Nile encephalitis, and West Nile meningitis. The neurological effects of the disease may be permanent.[10]

No specific treatment exists for West Nile virus. Care is mainly supportive. Prevention of the disease is best achieved by avoiding mosquito bites, applying insect repellent containing *N,N*-diethyl-meta-toluamide (DEET) to exposed skin when outdoors during peak mosquito hours (evening and early morning) and participating in community mosquito control programs.

[9]Centers for Disease Control and Prevention: West Nile virus: statistics, surveillance, and control. http://www.cdc.gov/ncidod/dvbid/westnile/surv&controlCaseCount04_detailed.htm. Accessed September 28, 2004.
[10]Centers for Disease Control and Prevention: West Nile virus: what you need to know. http://www.cdc.gov/ncidod/dvbid/westnile/wnv_factsheet.htm. Accessed September 28, 2004.

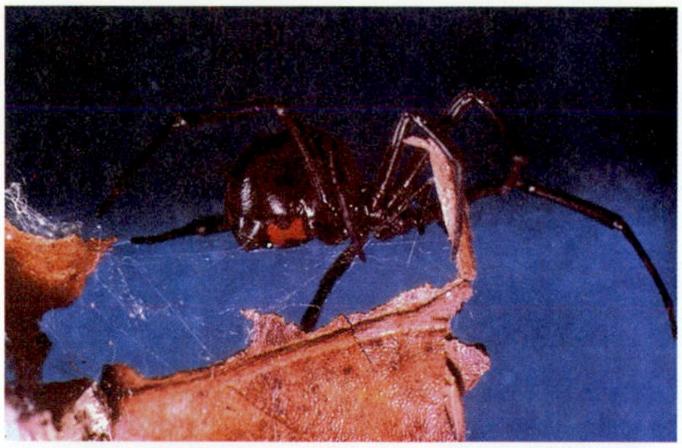

FIGURE 36-1 ■ Black widow spider.

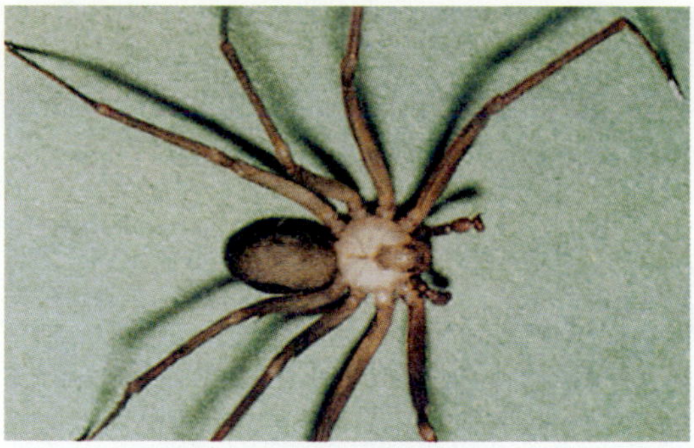

FIGURE 36-2 ■ Brown recluse spider.

ARACHNIDA (SPIDERS, SCORPIONS, TICKS)

Arachnida is a large class of arthropods. These organisms usually have four pairs of legs and a body divided into a cephalothorax (a combined head and thorax) and abdomen. Eleven types of Arachnida exist. This discussion, though, is limited to spiders, scorpions, and ticks.

Spider Bites. About 20,000 species of spiders are found in the United States. All of these, with the exception of two small groups, have venom glands. Two major types of reactions occur from spider venom. These are neurotoxic reactions resulting from the black widow bite and local tissue necrosis from the bites of most other spiders.

Black Widow Spider. The black widow is the most notorious spider in North America. A number of variations exist in the species. However, the typical mature female (who often devours her mate, thus the name *black widow*) is shiny and black with a red hourglass marking on the undersurface of the abdomen (Fig. 36-1). The size of the female varies with age but rarely exceeds 2.5 cm overall. (The male is about half the size of the female, brown, and nonvenomous to human beings.) The spider generally is found in undisturbed areas (under stones, logs, and clumps of vegetation). They rarely inhabit occupied dwellings. Most black widow bites occur in rural and suburban areas of southern and western states between April and October.

The bite of a black widow usually occurs when the spider has been disturbed. The bite generally is described by patients as a slight pinprick that is initially painless. As a rule, the only physical findings are two small fang marks. These are about 1 mm apart and surrounded by a small papule. Multiple bites usually rule out any type of spider **envenomation** because spiders rarely bite more than once. Within 1 hour of envenomation, the neurotoxin produces characteristic muscle spasms and cramps. These may result in abdominal rigidity (in the absence of palpable tenderness) and intense pain.

Abdominal rigidity in the absence of palpable tenderness is a crucial finding that helps distinguish envenomation from an acute abdominal condition. Associated symptoms include paresthesia (frequently described as a burning sensation in the soles of the feet or entire body); pain in the muscles of the shoulders, back, and chest; headache; dizziness; nausea and vomiting; edema of the eyelids; and increased perspiration and salivation. Emergency care for a patient with a black widow bite mainly is supportive. Care includes the following:

1. Ensure adequate airway, ventilatory, and circulatory support.
2. Clean the affected area with saline. Cover it with a sterile dressing. Intermittently apply ice to it. Obstruction tourniquets or suction devices do not help to delay absorption. A commercially prepared antivenin is available, but the antivenin should be administered only in the emergency department and only after appropriate sensitivity testing.
3. Moderate to severe symptoms require aggressive management. Per medical direction, muscle spasm, severe headache, vomiting, and paresthesia may be managed with ***diazepam*** or ***lorazepam*** and pain medication (e.g., ***morphine***). Severe hypertension may be managed with antihypertensive agents.
4. Transport the patient for physician evaluation. Most patients recover fully within 36 to 72 hours. Those at greatest risk for morbidity are the very young, older adults, and those with underlying hypertension or other medical problems.

Brown Recluse Spider. The brown recluse spider is also known as the fiddle-back spider. The spider is most prevalent in the Mississippi-Ohio-Missouri river basin and the southwestern United States. The species prefers hot, dry, and abandoned environments such as vacant buildings. The spider often is found in clothing closets. The spider is fawn to dark brown and is between 1 and 2 cm long (Fig. 36-2). Identifying characteristics of the brown recluse are six white eyes arranged in a semicircle on the head (versus the usual eight eyes of most other spiders) and the presence of a dark, violin-shaped marking on the top of the cephalothorax . The brown recluse is considered shy. It generally does not attack unless threatened. Like black widows, these spiders are most active from April to October.

The venom of the brown recluse manifests in a broad spectrum of reactions. Initially the bite causes little pain and often is overlooked by the victim. Some 1 to 2 hours later, localized pain and erythema develop (Fig. 36-3). This transient irritation often is followed within 1 to 2 days by a blister or

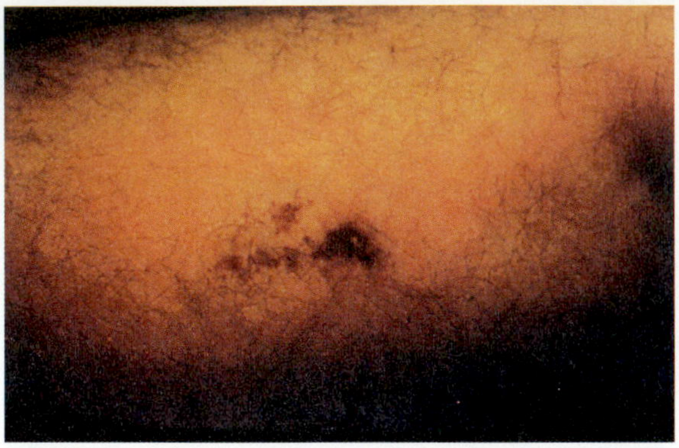

FIGURE 36-3 ■ Brown recluse spider bite at about 6 hours, with central hemorrhagic vesicle and gravitational pattern of venom spread.

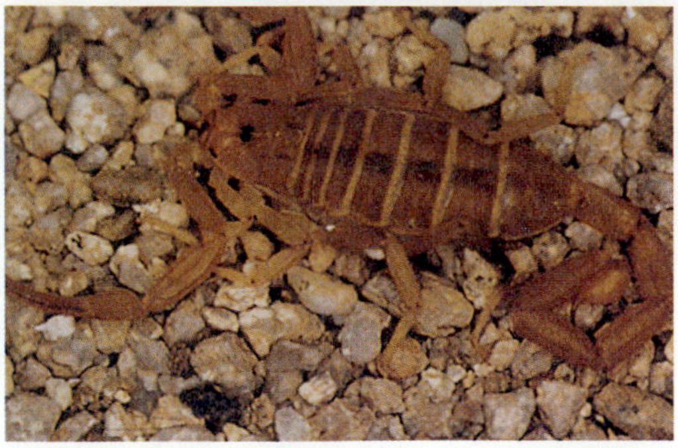

FIGURE 36-4 ■ The sculptured scorpion commonly found in the deserts of Arizona, New Mexico, and California.

vesicle. The lesion may be surrounded by an ischemic ring that is outlined further by an irregular red halo (erythematous). This produces the classical bull's-eye appearance. Over the next 24 to 72 hours, the area often becomes larger. Necrosis also may occur, and the center of the lesion may become purple or develop a black eschar. The eschar eventually sloughs within 2 to 5 weeks, leaving an ulcer of variable size and depth. The tissue defect may extend to include underlying muscle. The wound typically is slow to heal (often visible for months to years after the bite). Occasionally, excision and skin grafting are necessary. Systemic involvement may occur with signs and symptoms that include fever, chills, malaise, nausea and vomiting, generalized rash, and the development of hemolytic anemia, hemoglobinuria, and hypotension. Death occasionally occurs, usually from disturbance of the coagulation system or hepatic injury.

Emergency care for patients with a brown recluse bite mainly is supportive. Cold compresses and sterile dressings should be applied to the lesion. The patient should be transported for physician evaluation. As a rule, pharmacological therapy is not indicated in the prehospital setting. In-hospital therapy may include ice, antibiotics, and consideration of dapsone, a leukocyte inhibitor (controversial). An antivenin has been used in research. However, it is not widely clinically available. Most patients do well with treatment on an outpatient basis.

CRITICAL THINKING

For which type of spider bite is a patient most likely to call an ambulance? Why?

Scorpion Stings. More than 650 species of scorpions exist. Only a few, though, produce human envenomation. In North America the sculptured or bark scorpion is the only species that is dangerous to human beings. This scorpion is found in the southwestern United States and Mexico. The scorpion is nocturnal. It favors wooded areas along the edges of desert washes, where generally it clings upside down in its hideouts. It may be found under the bark of the eucalyptus and cottonwood trees. Occasionally the scorpion invades homes, especially adobe houses. The sculptured scorpion is small (2 to 7.5 cm) and yellow to brown, and some have tail stripes (Fig. 36-4). The species is most active from April to August, hibernating during the winter.

The venom of the scorpion is delivered by a stinger on the telson. The venom is used for defense and the acquisition of food. The venom is a mixture of proteins with complex effects on cellular sodium channels. It acts at the presynaptic terminal of the neuromuscular junction, releasing acetylcholine. This results in depolarization of the junction. The venom also stimulates sympathetic nerves and directly stimulates the CNS, causing hyperactivity. This particular scorpion venom does not contain enzymes that cause tissue destruction. Thus local inflammation is not a feature. If swelling, ecchymosis, or redness is present, the scorpion was not of the neurotoxic type. Box 36-12 lists the signs and symptoms of sculptured scorpion stings.

Despite the potential for life-threatening systemic effects, the vast majority of scorpion stings, especially in adults, produce symptoms that reach maximum severity within 5 hours. As a rule, mild analgesics, cool compresses, and in-hospital observation are all that are required for these patients. The use of antivenin for scorpion bites is reserved for severe cases. The prehospital care is supportive; airway control is the highest priority. The patient should be transported for physician evaluation.

Tick Bites. Tick bites seldom require emergency care. However, ticks are capable of causing human disease. They can transmit microorganisms or secrete toxins or venoms. In North America, hard ticks are the most familiar type, although soft ticks also are common to western states. Hard ticks have a leathery exterior. This makes them resistant to environmental stresses. They are relatively free of natural enemies. They can regenerate lost parts and have been known to survive without feeding for more than 4 years.[8] Local reactions to tick bites vary from the formation of a small pruritic nodule to development of extensive areas of ulceration that may be accompanied by fever, chills, and malaise unrelated to infection. Some of the more important diseases for which ticks are vectors include **Rocky Mountain spotted fever, Lyme disease,** and **tick paralysis.**

BOX 36-12 Signs and Symptoms of Scorpion Envenomation

- Hyperesthesia at the site of bite
- Pain, tingling, and a burning sensation radiating along the nerves at the location of the bite
- SLUDGE: *s*alivation, *l*acrimation, *u*rination, *d*efecation, *g*astrointestinal upset, and *e*mesis
- Initial bradycardia followed by tachycardia
- Cardiac dysrhythmias
- Muscle twitching
- Convulsions
- Roving eye movements (cranial nerve dysfunction)

Rocky Mountain Spotted Fever. Rocky Mountain spotted fever is an infectious disease transmitted from rabbits and other small mammals to human beings by the bites of the wood tick and dog tick. The disease occurs more commonly on the Atlantic seaboard and accounts for more than 40 deaths in the United States each year. Signs and symptoms usually develop within 5 to 7 days of the tick bite and include headache, high fever, and loss of appetite. Usually within 2 to 3 days after the onset of symptoms, small pink spots appear on the wrists and ankles. Eventually the rash spreads over the entire body, and the spots darken and enlarge and become petechial. In mild cases, recovery occurs within 20 days. The mortality rate, if untreated, is between 8% and 25%.

Lyme Disease. Lyme disease is the most commonly reported tick-borne disease in the United States. The disease is caused by a spirochete transmitted by the bite of an *Ixodes* tick known to infect deer and dogs. The course of the disease follows several stages. Initially a red dot appears at the site of the tick bite. This gradually expands into a reddened annular rash, often with central clearing. During this stage, fever, lethargy, muscle pain, and general malaise may develop. This stage may be followed by a second stage about 4 to 6 weeks later. The second stage is manifested by cardiac abnormalities (including various atrioventricular blocks) and neurological effects (including cranial nerve palsies). About 10% of infected patients go on to the second stage. Still later, a third stage may develop, with arthritis as the primary symptom. Unless the disease is diagnosed and treated, symptoms may continue for several years, gradually declining in severity.

Tick Paralysis. Tick paralysis results from a prolonged bite by a female wood tick. The disease occurs sporadically during the spring and summer months. Tick paralysis is caused by a neurotoxin secreted from the salivary glands of the tick during a bite. Tick paralysis develops in human beings within 6 days after the tick attaches to the host. At first the patient is restless and complains of paresthesia in the hands and feet. Over the next 24 to 48 hours, a flaccid paralysis may develop with loss of deep tendon reflexes. The paralysis begins at the feet and works its way up the body. Paralysis affects both sides of the body. In severe cases, death may result from respiratory paralysis. Removal of the tick usually results in rapid improvement and complete resolution within several days. If undiagnosed, the disease may be fatal, especially in young and older patients.

CRITICAL THINKING

How can you distinguish tick paralysis from other conditions that cause progressive paralysis?

Management. The principal treatment of tick bites is proper removal of the tick. The paramedic should grasp the tick as close to the skin surface as possible with forceps, tweezers, or protected fingers and pull it out with steady pressure. The paramedic should take care not to crush or squeeze the body of the tick, which can transmit disease from infective tick fluid. Other methods of tick removal, such as applying fingernail polish, isopropanol, or a hot match head, should be avoided. These traditional methods are ineffective and may induce the tick to salivate or regurgitate into the wound. After removal, the bite should be disinfected with soap and water and should be covered with a sterile dressing.

Reptile Bites

The American Association of Poison Control Centers National Data Collection System listed a total 6266 bites from poisonous and nonpoisonous snakes in 2001.[2] Of these exposures, 2223 were known to be poisonous, and the rest were from unidentified snakes. According to these records, three deaths were reported. This reflects the high morbidity and low mortality rates associated with snake venom poisoning. Of the 115 species of snakes in the United States, only 19 are venomous. The two main families of venomous snakes indigenous to the United States are pit vipers and coral snakes.

PIT VIPERS

The pit viper family that inhabits the United States consists of rattlesnakes (15 species), the cottonmouth (water) moccasin, the copperhead, the pigmy rattlesnake, and the Massasauga rattlesnake. The vast majority of snakebites in the United States are caused by the rattlesnake family.

The general term *pit viper* is derived from a depression or pit in the maxillary bone of these snakes (Fig. 36-5). This pit is believed to be a heat-sensing organ that detects warm-blooded prey or enemies. The pit guides the direction of the strike. The pit possibly determines the amount of venom released, based on the size and heat emission of the prey. Another identifying characteristic of the pit viper is its vertical elliptical pupils. The snake also has a triangular head that is distinct from the rest of the body. The rattlesnake is characterized further by rattles. (These are interlocking horny segments formed on the tail.) These sometimes vibrate in direct relation to environmental temperatures.

The venom apparatus of pit vipers consists of a gland and a duct. These are connected to one or more elongated hollow fangs on each side of the head. The venom is com-

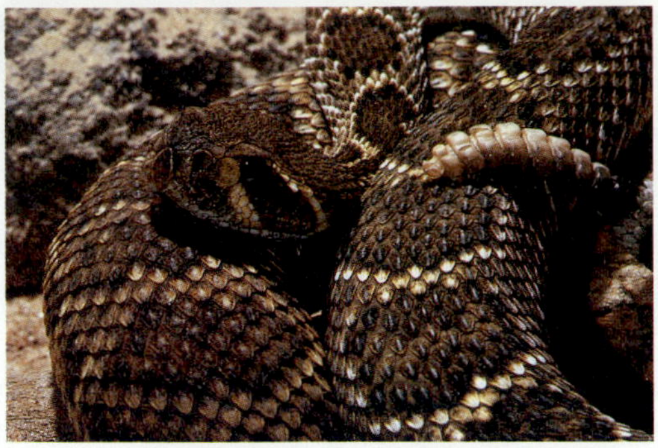

FIGURE 36-5 ■ Pit viper.

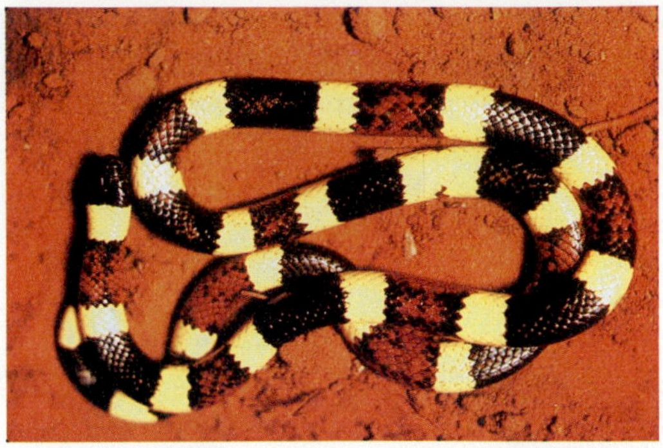

FIGURE 36-6 ■ Coral snake.

BOX 36-13 Signs and Symptoms of Pit Viper Envenomation

Mild Envenomation
Presence of one or more fang marks
Local swelling and pain
Lack of systemic symptoms

Moderate Envenomation
Presence of one or more fang marks
Pain and edema beyond the site
Systemic signs and symptoms
Weakness
Diaphoresis
Nausea and vomiting
Paresthesias

Severe Envenomation
Presence of one or more fang marks
Massive edema
Subcutaneous ecchymosis
Severe systemic symptoms
Shock

posed of a variety of proteins. These are designed to immobilize, kill, and digest prey. Depending on the species and the amount of venom injected, these proteins may be capable of producing various toxic effects on blood and other tissues, including hemolysis, intravascular coagulation, convulsions, and acute renal failure (Box 36-13). Bleeding caused by coagulation defects and massive swelling can lead to hypovolemic shock. On any given strike the snake may release a quantity of venom varying from little or none to almost the entire content of the glands. (A total of 20% of bites do not result in envenomation.[8])

CORAL SNAKES

Two members of the coral snake family are found in the United States: the Arizona coral snake and the Eastern coral snake. In contrast to the pit viper, the coral snake has round pupils and small, fixed fangs located near the anterior end of the maxilla. Most coral snakes have a three-color pattern with red, black, and yellow or white bands that completely encircle the body, along with a black snout (Fig. 36-6). Many nonpoisonous snakes in the United States mimic the appearance of the coral snake. The coral snake is identified by the sequence of colors: red bands bordered by yellow indicate a venomous species. Thus "red on yellow, kill a fellow; red on black, venom lack."

Most coral snakes are shy and docile and seldom bite unless threatened. The small mouth and fangs of the snake make it hard to bite anything larger than a finger, toe, or fold of skin. The coral snake tends to hang on and chew rather than to strike and release like the pit viper. The venom of the coral snake mainly is neurotoxic. The venom has a blocking action on acetylcholine receptor sites. The bite generally produces little or no pain and no necrosis or edema. Early signs and symptoms of a coral snake bite are slurred speech, dilated pupils, and dysphagia (usually delayed several hours after the bite). If untreated, the venom produces flaccid paralysis and death (within 8 to 24 hours) by respiratory failure, following nervous system dysfunction.

MANAGEMENT OF SNAKE ENVENOMATION

Venom, like any drug or toxin, has absorption, distribution, and elimination phases. Tissue damage increases as venom spreads into the lymphatics and blood. Thus emergency care is directed at retarding the systemic spread of the venom. Prehospital management of snake bites includes the following:

1. Stay clear of the striking range of the snake (about the length of the snake), and move the patient to a safe area. If the snake has been killed before EMS arrival, it should be transported in a closed container to the emergency department with the patient. Emergency medical services personnel should make no attempt to capture or kill the snake; doing so may result in a paramedic being bitten. Identification of the snake is not absolutely necessary to manage the patient appropriately.
2. Provide adequate airway, ventilatory, and circulatory support to the patient as needed. Continually monitor vital signs and the electrocardiogram. Also establish an intravenous line in an unaffected extremity with a volume-expanding fluid.

3. When practical, immobilize the bitten extremity in a neutral position. Immobilization by splinting may delay systemic absorption and may diminish local tissue necrosis. Every effort should be made to keep the patient at rest.
4. Prepare the patient for immediate transport to a proper medical facility.
5. Additional management of snakebites, such as incision and suction or use of a lymphatic-venous constriction band or pressure device, are controversial and potentially harmful. The paramedic should consult with medical direction and follow local protocol. Application of ice or chemical cold packs should be avoided. Their use may further damage tissue. In severe cases, administration of antivenin to neutralize the venom may be required. This is done in the hospital after the patient has been tested for allergies to the antivenin.

CRITICAL THINKING

What strategies can you use to calm the emotional state of a patient who has sustained a snake bite?

Hazardous Aquatic Life

The marine animals most likely to be involved in human poisonings in U.S. coastal waters are the coelenterates, echinoderms, and stingrays. The specialized venom apparatuses of these animals are used for defense and for capturing prey. In addition to venom produced by the animal, aquatic life may contain other poisonous substances as a result of toxic ingestions. Exposures to hazardous aquatic life result from recreational, industrial, scientific, and military oceanic activities.

COELENTERATES (JELLYFISH, SEA ANEMONES, FIRE CORAL)

Coelenterates are a group of more than 9000 species that may be encountered in the ocean (Fig. 36-7). Those species that carry venomous stinging cells (nematocysts) are known as Cnidaria. The **nematocyst** is venom filled and contains a long, coiled, hollow, threadlike tube that serves as a tiny hypodermic needle. Many types of nematocysts exist; an individual coelenterate may have more than one type. The severity of envenomation is related to the toxicity of the venom (which may contain various fractions), the number of nematocysts discharged, and the physical condition of the victim.

Jellyfish occur throughout the Atlantic and Pacific oceans. The Portuguese man-of-war is the largest jellyfish. Most jellyfish usually are found near the coastline. Their nematocyst-bearing tentacles may be up to 100 feet long. A single envenomation may involve several hundred thousand nematocysts. A swimmer who comes into contact with the tentacles of the jellyfish may suffer enough envenomation to produce systemic signs and symptoms. Nematocysts often remain embedded in the tissues of the victim. Detached tentacle fragments can retain their potency for months.

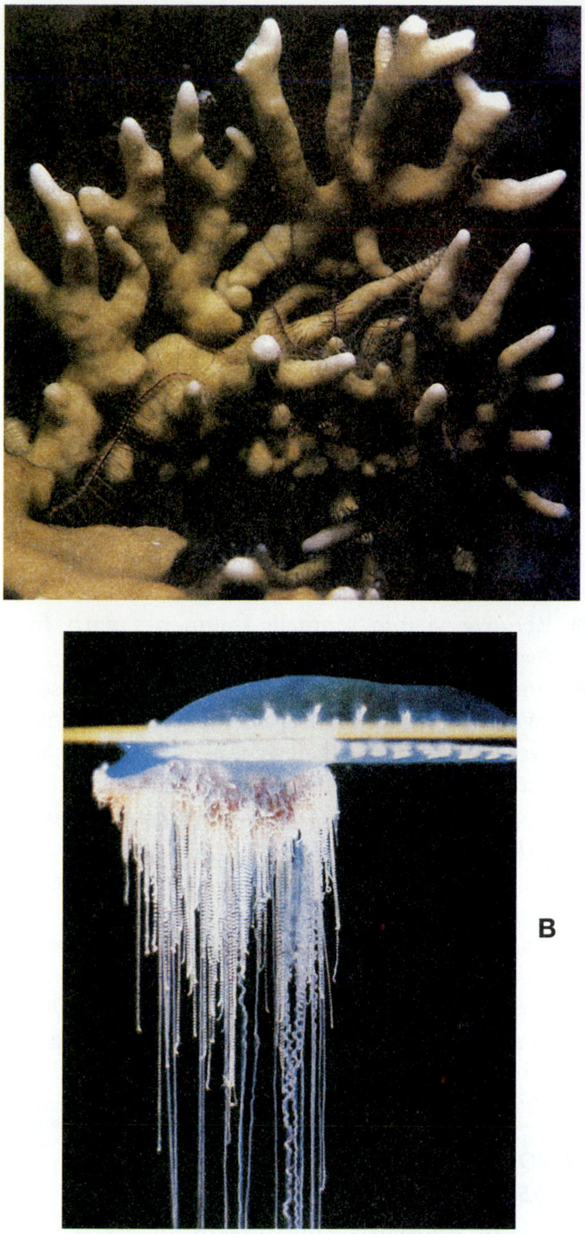

A

B

FIGURE 36-7 ■ Coelenterates. **A,** Fire coral. **B,** Man-of-war.

Sea anemones are colorful bottom dwellers. (They sometimes are found in tidal pools.) They have a flowerlike appearance. They possess slender projections. These are used to sting and paralyze passing fish. Their modifications of nematocysts are capable of producing mild to moderate pain in human beings.

Fire corals are not true (stony) corals but rather ocean-bottom dwellers. They are distributed widely in tropical waters. They often are mistaken for seaweed because they often are found attached to rocks, shells, and corals. These stinging corals may grow to 2 m in height and have a razor-sharp exoskeleton with thousands of protruding nematocyst-bearing tentacles.

Management. Coelenterate envenomation ranges in severity from irritant dermatitis to excruciating pain, respiratory depression, anaphylaxis, and life-threatening cardiovascular collapse. Envenomation most often is mild and usually is characterized by stinging, paresthesias, pruritus, and reddish-brown linear wheals or "tentacle prints." If a potent venom or a large body surface area is involved, systemic symptoms may include nausea, vomiting, abdominal pain, headache, bronchospasm, pulmonary edema, hypotension, and respiratory arrest. Emergency care is directed at stabilizing the patient and neutralizing the effects of the venom.

1. Stabilize the patient.
   - Provide adequate airway, ventilatory, and circulatory support as needed.
   - Continually monitor the patient's vital signs and electrocardiogram. Be prepared to provide advanced airway management if systemic reactions develop.
2. Counteract effects of the venom.
   - Remove visible tentacle fragments with forceps. Avoid touching the tentacles.
   - Immediately rinse the patient's wound with seawater. (Wet sand or freshwater usually causes the nematocysts to discharge their venom. Thus these are contraindicated.)
   - Apply copious amounts of isopropanol and then a baking soda paste to inactivate the nematocysts. (Isopropanol "fixes" nematocysts from firing. Baking soda helps remove them.)
   - Apply a lather of shaving cream. Gently shave the affected area to remove invisible nematocysts.
   - Rinse again until the pain is largely alleviated. If needed, consult medical direction regarding the administration of analgesics.
   - Transport the patient for physician evaluation.

ECHINODERMS (SEA URCHINS, STARFISH, SEA CUCUMBERS)

Echinoderms are marine animals with a water-vascular system. They usually have a hard, spiny skeleton and radial body (Fig. 36-8).

Sea urchins have a globular, dome-shaped body and are found on rocky bottoms or burrowed in sand or crevices. These animals have tiny spines, some of which are venomous. Between the spines of some sea urchins are small pincerlike organs that also are thought to discharge a poisonous substance. The spines are dangerous to handle and may break off easily in the flesh, lodging deeply and making removal difficult.

Some starfish are covered with thorny spines of calcium carbonate crystals that secrete toxins. As the spine enters the skin, it carries venom into the wound with immediate pain, copious bleeding, and mild edema. Multiple puncture wounds may result in acute systemic reactions.

Sea cucumbers are sausage-shaped animals. They are found in shallow and deep water. They produce a liquid toxin in a tentacle-shaped organ. This organ can be projected and extended anally. Generally the liquid is secreted into the surrounding ocean. It usually produces only a minor dermatitis or conjunctivitis in swimmers and divers.

Management. Emergency management for echinoderm envenomation usually involves caring for puncture wounds caused by spines and inactivating the venom. The paramedic should remove embedded spines with forceps. The paramedic should wear protective gloves and should be careful to avoid self-contamination. Larger spines may require surgical removal by a physician.

Echinoderm toxins may cause immediate intense pain, swelling, redness, aching in the affected extremity, and nausea. Delayed toxic effects may include respiratory distress, paresthesia of the lips and face, and in severe cases, respiratory paralysis and complete atonia. The paramedic must be prepared to deal with a variety of physical reactions.

Most marine venoms lose their toxicity when exposed to changes in temperature or humidity. The recommended management for stable patients is to immerse the affected area (usually the foot or hand) in warm water before and during transport. The water should be as hot as can be tolerated without scalding (no warmer than 45° C [113° F]). As a safety precaution, it generally is recommended that both hands or feet not be immersed at the same time. This protects against thermal injury that may go unnoticed by the patient because of numbness or pain in the affected part.

STINGRAYS

Stingrays are responsible for about 1800 injuries each year in the United States. These marine animals vary in size from 2 inches to 14 feet. They often are found half-buried in mud or sand in shallow water (Fig. 36-9). The venom organ of stingrays consists of two to four venomous barbs on the dorsum of a whiplike tail. Envenomation generally occurs from stepping on the sand-buried ray. This causes the tail to thrust up and forward, driving the barb into the victim's leg or foot. The barb (which is purely defensive) produces a large, severe laceration that may be more than 15 to 20 cm long. In addition to injecting venom into the wound, the entire barb tip of the venom apparatus sometimes is broken off and embedded in the tissue.

Stingray venom has local and systemic complications. Locally, the venom produces a traumatic injury that causes immediate, intense pain; edema; variable bleeding; and necrosis. Systemic manifestations include weakness, nausea, vomiting, diarrhea, vertigo, seizures, cardiac conduction abnormalities, paralysis, hypotension, and death.

Management. Prehospital care is directed to life support, alleviation of pain, inactivation of venom, and prevention of infection.

1. Ensure adequate airway, ventilatory, and circulatory support. Continually monitor the patient's vital signs and electrocardiogram.
2. Copiously irrigate the wound with normal saline or freshwater. If the venom apparatus is visible, it should be removed. Avoid coming in contact with it.

A

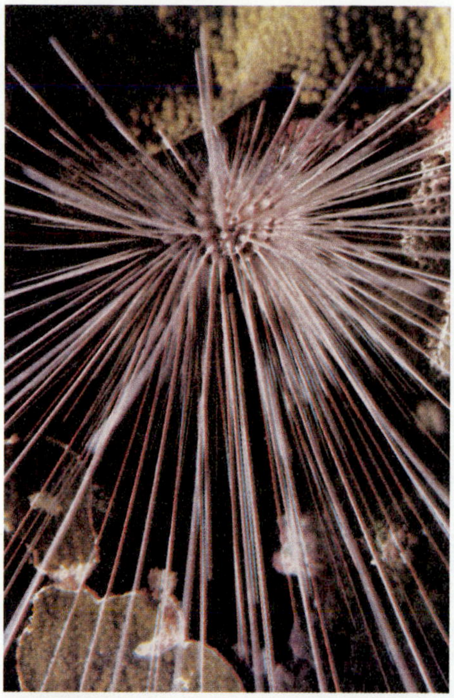

B

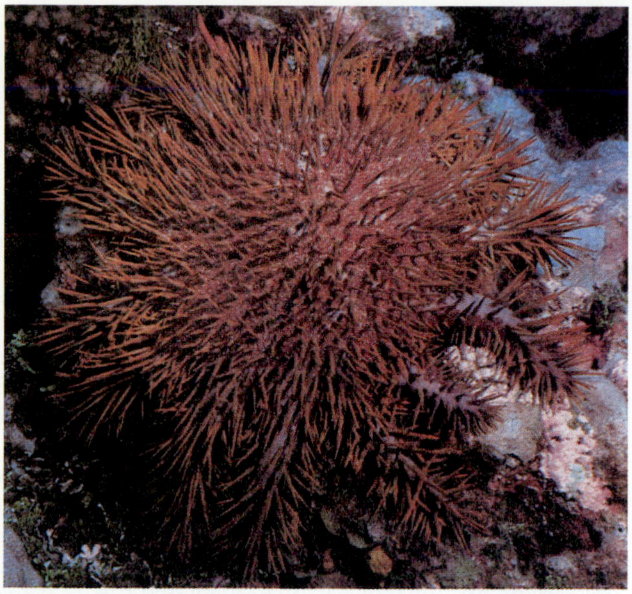

C

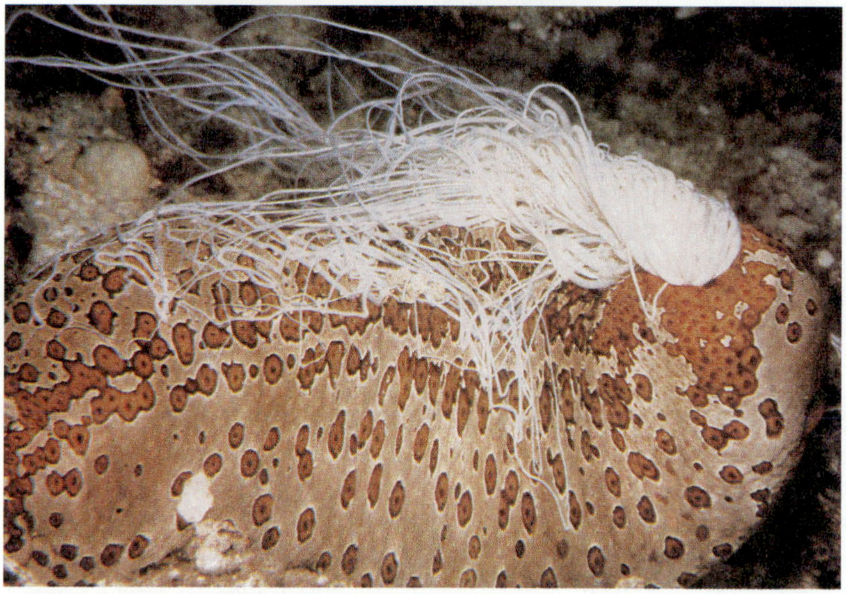

FIGURE 36-8 ■ Echinoderms. **A,** Black sea urchin. **B,** Crown-of-thorns starfish. **C,** Sea cucumber with extended tentacles.

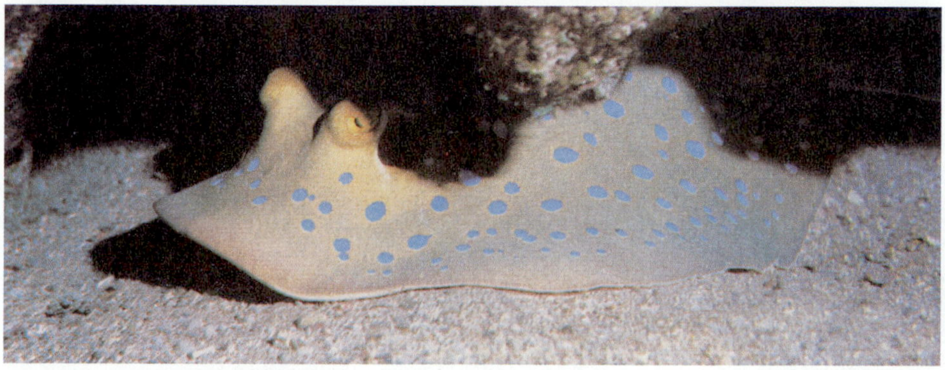

FIGURE 36-9 ■ Stingray.

3. Immerse the affected part in warm water as described before. Immersion should continue until the pain subsides or until the patient reaches the emergency department.
4. Medical direction may recommend the administration of analgesics.
5. Transport the patient for physician evaluation.

POISONING BY ABSORPTION

Many poisons can be absorbed through the skin. Two compounds, organophosphates and carbamates, are responsible for a large number of skin-absorbed poisonings each year. Organophosphates and carbamates are commonly available for commercial and public use in the form of pet, home, and commercial insecticides. Organophosphates also are used in the development of military nerve agents such as sarin and soman. (See Chapter 54.) Because of the widespread availability of insecticides that contain organophosphate/carbamate compounds, paramedics must be aware of the nature of these chemicals, necessary precautions for personal safety, and the immediate management that may be required before symptoms or signs of illness occur.

Organophosphates and carbamates are highly toxic. In addition, they are well absorbed by ingestion, inhalation, and dermal routes. Both classes have similar pharmacological actions, inhibiting the effects of acetylcholinesterase, an enzyme that degrades acetylcholine at nerve terminals. To review, acetylcholine is a cholinergic neurotransmitter for preganglionic autonomic fibers, somatic nerves to skeletal muscle, and many synapses in the CNS. When acetylcholinesterase is inhibited, acetylcholine accumulates at the synapses. This results in a cholinergic "overdrive." The signs and symptoms resulting from cholinergic overdrive are seen in organophosphate and carbamate poisoning.

Signs and Symptoms

Early signs and symptoms of organophosphate or carbamate poisoning may be nonspecific, including headache, dizziness, weakness, and nausea. As overstimulation and disruption of transmission in the central and peripheral nervous systems occur, signs and symptoms begin to develop. These signs and symptoms result from a wide range of physiological and metabolic problems (Box 36-14). The rapidity and sequence in which these signs and symptoms develop depend on the particular compound and on the amount and route of exposure. The onset of symptoms is probably quickest after inhalation. Onset is slowest (possibly delayed for several hours) after a primary skin exposure. A helpful mnemonic to recognize the signs of poisoning is *SLUDGE*. (This stands for *s*alivation, *l*acrimation, *u*rination, *d*efecation, *g*astrointestinal upset, and *e*mesis.)

CRITICAL THINKING

Consider a person who does not suspect poisoning. What condition might that person think he or she is suffering from with this clinical presentation?

BOX 36-14 Signs and Symptoms of Organophosphate or Carbamate Poisoning

Cardiovascular System
Bradycardia
Variable blood pressure (usually hypotensive)

Respiratory System
Bronchoconstriction
Dyspnea
Rhinorrhea
Wheezing

Gastrointestinal System
Blurred vision
Cramps
Defecation
Emesis
Increased bowel sounds
Lacrimation
Miosis
Rapidly changing pupil size

Central Nervous System
Anxiety
Coma
Convulsions
Dizziness
Respiratory depression

Musculoskeletal System
Fasciculations
Flaccid paralysis

Skin
Diaphoresis

Other
Salivation
Urination

Rapidly changing pupils with miosis are common with vapor exposure of organophosphates. Muscle twitching (fasciculations) can follow rapidly. Individual muscle twitching can result from liquid contact and local skin absorption at the site.

Management

Emergency care begins with scene safety, personal protection, and decontamination procedures. The scene should be secured by qualified personnel. Personal protective actions include wearing protective clothing and using respiratory protection. The patient should be removed safely from the contaminated area as soon as possible. That way, the decontamination procedures can begin. (See Chapter 53.) After these measures, patient care can be started. The general principles of management for poisoning by absorption include respiratory support, drug administration, and electrocardiogram monitoring. Organophosphates and carbamates produce similar physiological effects. However, carbamates have a shorter duration of action. Thus they have a more rapid decrease in their effect.

RESPIRATORY SUPPORT

Respiratory tract symptoms usually are first to appear after exposure to organophosphates or carbamates. In addition, respiratory paralysis may occur suddenly without warning. The need for advanced airway management and ventilatory support should be anticipated. Copious bronchial secretions may require suctioning. Bronchoconstriction also may necessitate positive-pressure ventilation and positive end-expiratory pressure.

DRUG ADMINISTRATION

Drug therapy in organophosphate or carbamate poisoning is directed at blocking the effects of acetylcholine, separating cholinesterase from the chemical compound, and suppressing seizure activity (if present). The drugs currently used as antidotes include ***atropine, pralidoxime chloride,*** and ***diazepam*** or ***lorazepam.***

Drug therapy should be started only if the patient has two or more signs or symptoms of poisoning and/or respiratory distress is present. Drug therapy also should be started only after consulting with medical direction or a poison control center.

Atropine reverses the muscarinic effects (bradycardia, bronchoconstriction, respiratory secretions, and miosis) of moderate to severe organophosphate or carbamate poisoning. The drug competitively antagonizes the actions of acetylcholine. This results in a decrease in the hyperactivity of smooth muscles and glands. The drug is indicated to dry the patient's secretions. It also helps to decrease pulmonary resistance to ventilation. Potentially hypoxic patients may require the administration of large doses of ***atropine*** (See the *Emergency Drug Index*). The electrocardiogram should be monitored for dysrhythmias (other than tachycardia). Supplemental oxygen should be given to minimize the risk of ventricular fibrillation. ***Atropine*** is the drug of choice for carbamate poisonings.

> **NOTE** As a rule, cholinergic poisoning causes the patient to be "wet." (This is manifested by profuse sweating, lacrimation, salivation, vomiting, diarrhea, and incontinence.) However, anticholinergic poisoning generally causes the patient to be "dry." (This is manifested by dry, flushed skin; elevated temperature; and urinary retention.) Being keen to this "wet vs. dry" symptomatology can be lifesaving for the poisoned patient. The wet-appearing patient will require atropine.

Pralidoxime is the treatment of choice for organophosphate poisoning after the administration of ***atropine***. ***Pralidoxime*** should be used for nearly all patients with significant exposures, particularly those with muscular twitching and weakness. ***Pralidoxime*** has the primary effect of reactivating acetylcholinesterase. The adult and pediatric doses for ***pralidoxime*** can be found in the *Emergency Drug Index*.

Diazepam or ***lorazepam*** may be indicated if seizures are present. The need for seizure control may arise before decontamination is complete. In this case, the drugs can be administered intramuscularly to control seizure activity. (See the *Emergency Drug Index*.) (Intravenous therapy should not be initiated in a patient in a contaminated area.) The paramedic should be alert to the risk for respiratory and CNS depression.

> **CRITICAL THINKING**
> Consider that you give diazepam or lorazepam for seizures in this case. Will that eliminate the need for atropine?

ELECTROCARDIOGRAM MONITORING

Electrocardiogram monitoring may reveal a variety of abnormalities, including idioventricular rhythms, multifocal premature ventricular contractions, ventricular tachycardia, torsades de pointes, ventricular fibrillation, complete heart block, and asystole (see the appendix at the end of this chapter). These dysrhythmias usually occur in two phases. The first phase begins with a transient episode of intense sympathetic tone. This results in sinus tachycardia. This phase is followed by a period of extreme parasympathetic tone. It may manifest as sinus bradycardia, atrioventricular block, and ST segment and T wave abnormalities. Slow ventricular dysrhythmias that do not respond to the usual therapy may need to be treated with overdrive pacing (see Chapter 29).

SECTION TWO
DRUG ABUSE

The term *drug abuse* refers to the use of prescription drugs for nonprescribed purposes. It also refers to the use of drugs that have no prescribed medical use (Box 36-15). Emergencies that result from drug abuse include adverse effects caused by the drug or impurities or contaminants mixed with the drug, life-threatening infections from intravenous or intradermal injection of drugs with unsterile equipment, injuries during intoxication, and drug dependence or withdrawal syndrome resulting from the habit-forming potential of many drugs (see Chapter 17).

No single cause or set of conditions clearly leads to drug abuse. It is widespread. Moreover, drug abuse is common among all socioeconomic, cultural, and ethnic groups. Drug abuse is a major medical, social, and interpersonal problem. It affects persons from all backgrounds and of all ages (Box 36-16). Because of the widespread use and misuse of drugs, the paramedic should maintain a high degree of suspicion. The paramedic should consider the possibility for a drug-related problem in any patient who has seizures, behavioral changes, or decreased level of consciousness. In addition, consideration of the visibility, accessibility, and careful handling of all medications carried on an EMS vehicle should be a part of any EMS policy and procedure.

> **CRITICAL THINKING**
> Why might a patient (or their friends) delay calling for help in a situation involving drug overdose?

TOXIC EFFECTS OF DRUGS

Emergency medical services personnel often encounter persons who are suffering from the toxic effects of drugs. Toxicity may be the result of an overdose, a potential sui-

BOX 36-15 Drug Abuse Terminology

Drug abuse: Self-medication or self-administration of a drug in chronically excessive amounts, resulting in psychological and/or physical dependence, functional impairment, and deviation from approved social norms

Drug dependence: Condition marked by an overwhelming desire to continue taking a drug for its desired effect, usually an altered mental activity, attitude, or outlook

Physical dependence: An adaptive physiological state occurring after prolonged use of many drugs (discontinuation causes withdrawal syndromes that are relieved by readministering the same drug or a pharmacologically related drug).

Psychological dependence: Emotional reliance on a drug (Manifestations range from a mild desire for a drug to craving and drug-seeking behavior to repeated compulsive use of a drug for its subjectively satisfying or pleasurable effects.)

Tolerance: A tendency to increase drug dosage to experience the same effect formerly produced by a smaller dose

Withdrawal syndrome: A predictable set of signs and symptoms that occurs after a decrease in the amount of the usual dose of a drug or its sudden cessation

BOX 36-16 Illicit Drug Use in the United States

A survey conducted by the Health and Human Services Substance Abuse and Mental Health Administration in 2002 revealed the following statistics:

- Almost 17 million Americans abused or were dependent on illicit drugs or alcohol in 2001; more than 2 million abused or were dependent on alcohol and illicit drugs.
- An estimated 28 million Americans used illicit drugs in 2001; of these
  - 450,000 had used heroin.
  - 4 million had used cocaine.
  - 8 million had used prescription pain medicines for nonmedical purposes.
  - 21 million had used marijuana.
  - 1.5 million began using hallucinogens.
  - 1.3 million began using Ecstasy (methylenedioxymethamphetamine).
  - 979,000 began using inhalants.
  - 973,000 began using tranquilizers.
  - 344,000 began using methamphetamine.
- More than 6 million children lived with at least one parent who abused or was dependent on alcohol or illicit drugs in 2001; about 10% of these children are 5 years old or younger.

From Health and Human Services News: Summary findings from the 2002 national household survey on drug abuse, US Department of Health and Human Services. http://www.samsha.gov. Accessed Sept. 29, 2004.

cide, polydrug administration, or an accident (accidental ingestion, miscalculation, changes in drug strength). Box 36-17 lists the drugs discussed in this chapter.

Common drugs of abuse (along with their names and uses) vary widely in different geographical areas. Also, the drugs of abuse often change over time. Table 36-3 is a partial list of common drugs of abuse, their street names, and miscellaneous terminology relating to drug use.

General Management Principles

The following are general principles for managing drug abuse and the overdose that may result:

1. Ensure that the scene is safe. Be prepared for unpredictable behavior from the patient as well. (Consider the need for help from law enforcement.)
2. Ensure adequate airway, ventilatory, and circulatory support as needed.
3. Obtain a history of the event. (This should include the self-administration of other drugs that may have been taken by another route.) Obtain any significant medical or psychiatric history as well.
4. Identify the substance. Consult with medical direction or a poison control center.
5. Perform a full, focused physical examination. Continually monitor the patient's vital functions and electrocardiogram.
6. Start intravenous therapy. Draw a blood sample for laboratory analysis. Also administer the proper drug antidotes. For instance, this may include ***naloxone*** if an opiate overdose is suspected. Pay special attention to the use of personal protective gear because many of these patients are at high risk of having an infectious disease.

BOX 36-17 Common Agents Involved in Poisoning

Acetaminophen	Nonprescription pain medicines
Cardiac medications	Opioids
Drugs abused for sexual purposes/sexual gratification	Phencyclidine
Hallucinogens	Salicylates
Lithium	Sedatives-hypnotics
Metals (iron, lead, and mercury)	Stimulants
Monoamine oxidase inhibitors	Tricyclic antidepressants

7. Prevent further absorption of an orally administered drug by the administration of ***activated charcoal*** (per protocol).
8. Rapidly transport the patient for physician evaluation.

When examining any patient suspected of abusing drugs, the paramedic should always look for track marks. (These may be in the antecubital space, under the tongue, or on top of the feet.) "Body packing" is concealing packets of drugs in body cavities of the stomach, rectum, and vagina. "Body stuffing" is swallowing drugs to avoid arrest. The possibility of these also should be considered

TABLE 36-3 Commonly Abused Drugs and Their Street Names

SUBSTANCE	EXAMPLES OF PROPRIETARY OR STREET NAMES	MEDICAL USES	ROUTE OF ADMINISTRATION	DEA SCHEDULE*	PERIOD OF DETECTION
Stimulants					
Amphetamine	Biphetamine, Dexedrine; black beauties, crosses, hearts	Attention deficit hyperactivity disorder (ADHD), obesity, narcolepsy	Injected, oral, smoked, sniffed	II	1-2 days
Cocaine	Coke, crack, flake, rocks, snow	Local anesthetic, vasoconstrictor	Injected, smoked, sniffed	II	1-4 days
Methamphetamine	Desoxyn; crank, crystal, glass, ice, speed	ADHD, obesity, narcolepsy	Injected, oral, smoked, sniffed	II	1-2 days
Methylphenidate	Ritalin	ADHD, narcolepsy	Injected, oral	II	1-2 days
Nicotine	Habitrol patch, Nicorette gum, Nicotrol spray, Prostep patch; cigars, cigarettes, smokeless tobacco, snuff, spit tobacco	Treatment for nicotine dependence	Smoked, sniffed, oral, transdermal	Not scheduled	1-2 days
Hallucinogens and Other Compounds					
LSD[†]	Acid, microdot	None	Oral	I	8 hours
Mescaline	Buttons, cactus, mesc, peyote	None	Oral	I	2-3 days
Phencyclidine and analogs	PCP; angel dust, boat, hog, love boat	Anesthetic (veterinary)	Injected, oral, smoked	I, II	2-8 days
Psilocybin	Magic mushroom, purple passion, shrooms	None	Oral	I	8 hours
Amphetamine variants	DOB, DOM, MDA, MDMA; adam, Ecstasy, STP, XTC	None	Oral	I	1-2 days
Marijuana	Blunt, grass, herb, pot, reefer, sinsemilla, smoke, weed	None	Oral, smoked	I	1 day-5 weeks
Hashish	Hash	None	Oral, smoked	I	1 day-5 weeks
Tetrahydrocannabinol	Marinol, THC	Antiemetic	Oral, smoked	I, II	1 day-5 weeks
Anabolic steroids	Testosterone (T/E ratio), stanozolol, nandrolone	Hormone replacement therapy	Oral, injected	III	Oral: up to 3 weeks (for testosterone and others); injected: up to 3 months (Nandrolone up to 9 months)

*Drug Enforcement Administration (DEA) Schedule I and II drugs have a high potential for abuse. They require greater storage security and have a quota on manufacture among other restrictions. Schedule I drugs are available for research only and have no approved medical use. Schedule II drugs are available only through prescription, cannot have refills, and require a form for ordering. Schedule III and IV drugs are available with prescription, may have five refills in 6 months, and may be ordered orally. Most Schedule V drugs are available over the counter.

From National Institutes of Health. http://www.nih.gov/. For additional information about National Institute on Drug Abuse, send e-mail to Information@lists.nida.nih.gov. This page last updated Wednesday, September 29, 1999.

The National Institute on Drug Abuse is part of the National Institutes of Health, the principal biomedical and behavioral research agency of the U.S. government. The National Institutes of Health is a component of the U.S. Department of Health and Human Services.

[†] *LSD,* Lysergic acid diethylamide; *DOB,* 1-(2,5-dimethoxy-4-bromophenyl)-2-aminopropane; *DOM,* dimethoxymethylamphetamine; *MDA,* 3,4-methylenedioxyamphetamine; *MDMA,* methylenedioxymethamphetamine; *THC,* tetrahydrocannabinol.

Continued

TABLE 36-3 Commonly Abused Drugs and Their Street Names, cont'd

SUBSTANCE	EXAMPLES OF PROPRIETARY OR STREET NAMES	MEDICAL USES	ROUTE OF ADMINISTRATION	DEA SCHEDULE*	PERIOD OF DETECTION
Opioids and Morphine Derivatives					
Codeine	Tylenol w/Codeine, Robitussin A-C, Empirin w/Codeine, Fiorinal w/Codeine	Analgesic, antitussive	Injected, oral	II, III, IV	1-2 days
Heroin	Diacetylmorphine; horse, smack	None	Injected, smoked, sniffed	I	1-2 days
Methadone	Amidone, Dolophine, Methadose	Analgesic, treatment for opiate dependence	Injected, oral	II	1 day-1 week
Morphine	Roxanol, Duramorph	Analgesic	Injected, oral, smoked	II, III	1-2 days
Opium	Laudanum, paregoric; Dover's powder	Analgesic, antidiarrheal	Oral, smoked	II, III, V	1-2 days
Depressants					
Alcohol	Beer, wine, liquor	Antidote for methanol poisoning	Oral	Not scheduled	6-10 hours
Barbiturates	Amytal, Nembutal, Seconal, phenobarbital; barbs	Anesthetic, anticonvulsant, hypnotic, sedative	Injected, oral	II, III, IV	2-10 days
Benzodiazepines	Ativan, Halcion, Librium, Rohypnol, Valium, Xanax; roofies, tranks	Antianxiety, anticonvulsant, hypnotic, sedative	Injected, oral	IV	1-6 weeks
Methaqualone	Quaalude, ludes	None	Oral	I	2 weeks

*Drug Enforcement Administration (DEA) Schedule I and II drugs have a high potential for abuse. They require greater storage security and have a quota on manufacture among other restrictions. Schedule I drugs are available for research only and have no approved medical use. Schedule II drugs are available only through prescription, cannot have refills, and require a form for ordering. Schedule III and IV drugs are available with prescription, may have five refills in 6 months, and may be ordered orally. Most Schedule V drugs are available over the counter.

From National Institutes of Health. http://www.nih.gov/. For additional information about National Institute on Drug Abuse, send e-mail to Information@lists.nida.nih.gov. This page last updated Wednesday, September 29, 1999.}

The National Institute on Drug Abuse is part of the National Institutes of Health, the principal biomedical and behavioral research agency of the U.S. government. The National Institutes of Health is a component of the U.S. Department of Health and Human Services.

† *LSD,* Lysergic acid diethylamide; *DOB,* 1-(2,5-dimethoxy-4-bromophenyl)-2-aminopropane; *DOM,* dimethoxymethylamphetamine; *MDA,* 3,4-methylenedioxyamphetamine; *MDMA,* methylenedioxymethamphetamine; *THC,* tetrahydrocannabinol.

when a person who abuses drugs appears ill for no apparent reason.

CRITICAL THINKING

For what illnesses is the patient who uses intravenous narcotics at risk?

Opioid Overdose

Heroin accounts for about 90% of the opioid abuse in the United States. Pure heroin is a bitter-tasting white powder. Heroin usually is adulterated or "cut" for street distribution. Heroin is cut with various agents such as lactose, sucrose, baking soda, powdered milk, starch, magnesium silicate (talc), procaine, quinine, and recently with scopolamine. A typical "bag" is the single-dose unit of heroin and may weigh 100 mg. On average, heroin is only 20% to 30% pure. Other opioid drugs include ***morphine,*** hydromorphone, methadone, ***meperidine,*** codeine, oxycodone, propoxyphene, and "designer opiates" that have been chemically modified such as alpha-methyl fentanyl ("China white").

Depending on the preparation, these drugs may be taken orally, injected intradermally ("skin popping") or intravenously ("mainlining"), taken intranasally ("snorted"), or smoked. All opioids are CNS depressants. They can cause life-threatening respiratory depression. In severe intoxication, hypotension, profound shock, and pulmonary edema may be present. Signs and symptoms of narcotic/opiate overdose include the following:

- Euphoria
- Arousable somnolence ("nodding")
- Nausea
- Pinpoint pupils (except with ***meperidine,*** hypoxia, or in combination with other types of drugs)
- Coma
- Seizures

ANTIDOTE THERAPY

As described in Chapter 17, ***naloxone*** is a pure opioid antagonist effective for virtually all opioid and opioid-like substances. The drug reverses the three major symptoms of opioid overdose (respiratory depression, coma, and miosis). Its use should be considered when opioid intoxication is suspected. ***Naloxone*** also is indicated for use when a coma of unknown origin is present. The EMS crew should be prepared to restrain the patient. The patient's behavior may be unpredictable when the effects of the drug are reversed and the patient experiences withdrawal symptoms. Medical direction may recommend that the ***naloxone*** be given in small amounts. The amount should be enough to keep the patient responsive and free from respiratory depression but somewhat docile during transport. (*Note:* In the absence of respiratory depression, the use of ***naloxone*** is controversial; seizure activity is a possible side effect of the drug.)

> **NOTE** Two other pure opioid antagonists are available. ***Naltrexone*** is an oral medication used in long-term programs for opioid addiction. ***Nalmefene*** appears to be as effective as ***naloxone*** in acute opioid intoxications. Moreover, nalmefene has a longer duration of action (4 to 8 hours) than naloxone.

Some opiates (e.g., heroin) have a longer duration than ***naloxone.*** Thus the patient must be monitored closely during antidote therapy. Repeated doses of ***naloxone*** may be needed as well. In communities where abuse of naloxone-resistant opiates or the use of China white is common, larger initial doses of ***naloxone*** may be needed. The desired signs of reversal of opiate intoxication are adequate airway reflexes and ventilations, not complete arousal.

Naloxone can cause a withdrawal syndrome in opioid-dependent patients. This is seldom life threatening. Withdrawal usually can be managed by symptomatic and supportive care. Box 36-18 lists signs and symptoms of opioid withdrawal.

BOX 36-18 Signs and Symptoms of Opioid Withdrawal

Abdominal cramps	Gooseflesh
Anorexia	Insomnia
Cold sweats or chills	Irritability
Diaphoresis	Nausea and vomiting
Diarrhea	Tachycardia
Fever	Tremors
General malaise	

Sedative-Hypnotic Overdose

Sedative-hypnotic agents include benzodiazepines and barbiturates. These drugs usually are taken orally. Yet they may be diluted and injected intravenously. Taking these drugs with alcohol greatly increases their effects. Sedative-hypnotic drugs commonly are known as *downers.*

Benzodiazepines are among the best-known and most widely prescribed drugs used to control symptoms of anxiety, stress, and insomnia. These drugs sometimes are used to manage alcohol withdrawal and to control seizure disorders as well. They promote sleep and relieve anxiety by depressing brain function. Often they are abused for their sedative effects. Individually, these drugs are somewhat nontoxic. They may accentuate the effects of other sedative-hypnotic agents. Common benzodiazepines are ***diazepam*** and chlordiazepoxide.

Barbiturates are general CNS depressants that inhibit impulse conduction in the brainstem. These drugs once were widely used to treat anxiety and insomnia. Their addictive properties and potential for abuse have led to their replacement by benzodiazepines and other nonbarbiturate drugs. Barbiturates that commonly are abused include phenobarbital, amobarbital, and secobarbital.

Signs and symptoms of sedative-hypnotic overdose chiefly are related to the central nervous and cardiovascular systems. Adverse effects include excessive drowsiness, staggering gait, and in some cases, paradoxical excitability. In cases of severe toxicity the patient may become comatose, with respiratory depression, hypotension, and shock. The pupils may be constricted. More often, though, they become fixed and dilated even in the absence of significant brain damage. Airway control and ventilatory management are the most important actions in managing significant sedative-hypnotic overdose. ***Flumazenil*** is a benzodiazepine antagonist. It can be used to reverse the effects of benzodiazepines. The drug, however, can produce seizure activity. ***Flumazenil*** is contraindicated in patients who are prone to seizures and in those with tricyclic antidepressant overdose.

Stimulant Overdose

Commonly abused stimulant drugs are those of the sympathomimetic family (e.g., amphetamine sulfate, dextroamphetamine, cocaine, methamphetamine) (Box 36-19).

Sympathomimetic drugs often are used to produce general mood elevation, improve task performance, suppress appetite, and prevent sleepiness. Structurally, the amphetamines are similar to catecholamines (epinephrine and norepinephrine). Yet they differ in their more pronounced effects on the CNS. Adverse effects include tachycardia, increased blood pressure, tachypnea, agitation, dilated pupils, tremors, and disorganized behavior. In severe intoxication the patient may exhibit psychosis and paranoia and may experience hallucinations. Sudden withdrawal or cessation of amphetamine use may result in a "crash" stage. In this stage the patient becomes depressed, suicidal, incoherent, or near coma. As a rule, these drugs are taken orally. They also may be smoked or injected for a more rapid onset of action. Amphetamines commonly are known as *speed* or *uppers.*

COCAINE

Cocaine is one of the most popular illegal drugs in the United States. Cocaine is a fine, white crystalline powder. Like heroin, street forms of cocaine usually are adulterated.

BOX 36-19 Methamphetamine

Methamphetamine is a synthetically manufactured central nervous system stimulant. Methamphetamine is legally manufactured for medicinal purposes (Methedrine and Desoxyn). Yet illicit production of methamphetamine as a street drug in the United States is on the rise. Common names for methamphetamine include meth, speed, crank, crystal, water, or ice.

Illegal methamphetamine can be produced inexpensively in clandestine meth labs with common chemical methods (hydriodic acid, phenyl-2-propane, sodium ammonia, thionychloride). The drug then can be smoked, injected, snorted, or taken orally. Once methamphetamine enters the body, it can produce skeletal muscle tremors, sleeplessness, and euphoria that can last up to 10 days. During these drug-induced sleepless "binges," users may become hostile and paranoid. This is followed by a "crash" (an emotionally depressed state) that can last for several days.

In addition to ensuring personal safety when dealing with these patients, the paramedic crew should be keenly aware of potential hazards associated with clandestine labs. These hazards include the production of highly explosive toxic gases (e.g., phosphine) that can be absorbed readily through the skin in quantities that can be fatal; an oxygen-depleted environment; the use of toxic solvents that can lead to lab explosions; and exposure to other dangerous chemicals. Any time a meth lab is suspected, the emergency medical services crew should withdraw. Patients and bystanders should be evacuated. Law enforcement and specialized hazardous materials personnel should be summoned to the scene. Drug-making paraphernalia that should alert the paramedic to the presence of a meth lab include the following*:

- Amber stains on walls, furniture, and counters
- Equipment that has a red or amber color
- Two large, round-bottom flasks (with stoppers) connected by a hose
- Pyrex-type meatloaf container
- Various measuring and funnel devices
- A heat source

*From Goss J: Meth labs, *J Emerg Med Serv JEMS* 23:1, 1998.

They vary in purity from 25% to 90%; doses vary from near 0 to 200 mg. This form of cocaine generally is taken intranasally by snorting a "line" containing 10 to 35 mg of the drug (depending on purity). After absorption through the mucous membranes, the effects of the drug begin within minutes. Peak effects occur 15 to 60 minutes after use, with a half-life of 1 to 2½ hours. Cocaine also is used parenterally by the subcutaneous, intramuscular, and intravenous routes; the intravenous route provides immediate absorption and intense stimulation (peak occurs within 5 minutes with a half-life of about 50 minutes). *Speed-balling* refers to an injection of a cocaine-heroin combination.

Freebase or "crack" cocaine is a more potent formulation of the drug. Crack is prepared by mixing powdered street cocaine with an alkaline solution and then adding a solvent such as ether. The combination separates into two layers. The top layer contains the dissolved cocaine. Evaporation of the solvent results in pure cocaine crystals, which are smoked and absorbed via the pulmonary route. Cocaine in this form is called *rock* or *crack* because of the popping sound produced when the crystals are heated. Freebase cocaine generally is combined with marijuana or tobacco and is smoked in a pipe or a cigarette. The reactions are similar to those experienced in intravenous use, with equal intensity and effects.

Cocaine is a major CNS stimulant. It causes profound sympathetic discharge. The increased levels of circulating catecholamines result in excitement, euphoria, talkativeness, and agitation. The effects of the drug can cause significant cardiovascular and neurological complications such as cardiac dysrhythmias, myocardial infarction, seizures, intracranial hemorrhage, hyperthermia, and psychiatric disturbances. Cocaine overdose can occur with any form of the drug and any route of administration. The adult fatal dose is thought to be about 1200 mg (1.2 g), but fatalities from cocaine-induced cardiac dysrhythmias have been reported with single doses of as little as 25 to 30 mg.[5]

Prehospital management of the cocaine-intoxicated patient may be difficult. Cocaine toxicity may range from minor symptoms to life-threatening overdose. Emergency care may require a full spectrum of basic and advanced life-support measures, including aggressive airway management, ventilatory and circulatory support, drug therapy (benzodiazepines are the mainstay of treatment initially in cocaine toxicity), and rapid transport to an appropriate medical facility (see the appendix at the end of this chapter).

PHENCYCLIDINE OVERDOSE

Phencyclidine (PCP) is a dissociative analgesic. (Originally it was used as a veterinary tranquilizer.) The drug has sympathomimetic and CNS stimulant and depressant properties. Phencyclidine is a potent psychoactive drug illegally sold in liquid, tablet, or powder form to be taken orally, intranasally, intravenously/intramuscularly, or with other drugs to be smoked (a "Sherman"). Most tablets contain about 5 mg of PCP. As a rule, PCP in its powder form is purer (50% to 100% PCP). Chronic use can result in permanent memory impairment and loss of higher brain functions. The pharmacological effects are dose related. They can be divided into low-dose and high-dose toxicity. Ketamine is a derivative of PCP and has identical actions.

Low-dose Toxicity. In low doses (less than 10 mg), PCP intoxication produces an unpredictable state that can resemble drunkenness. The user may have a sense of euphoria or confusion, disorientation, agitation, or sudden rage. An intoxicated patient often has a blank stare and a stumbling gait. The patient often is in a dissociative state. The patient's pupils generally are reactive. The patient may experience flushing, diaphoresis, facial grimacing, hypersalivation, and vomiting. **Nystagmus** with a burstlike quality is characteristic of low-dose PCP use. In this range of toxicity, death usually is related to behavioral disturbances resulting from spatial disorientation, drug-induced immobility, and insensitivity to pain. This insensitivity to pain leads to bold acts of strength. This is because the normal muscle activity limitation resulting from pain is inhibited.

CRITICAL THINKING

Why does this type of drug intoxication put the patient at a high risk for injury?

In low-dose toxicity sensory stimulation should be avoided. (Verbal and physical stimuli will make the clinical symptoms worse.) Violent and combative patients require protection from self-injury. Safeguards also must be provided for the emergency crew and bystanders. The paramedic should monitor the patient's vital signs and level of consciousness closely. The paramedic should observe the patient for increasing motor activity and muscle rigidity as well. These may precede seizures.

High-dose Toxicity. Patients with high-dose PCP intoxication (more than 10 mg) may be in a coma. (The coma may last from hours to several days.) These patients often are unresponsive to painful stimuli. Respiratory depression, hypertension, and tachycardia also may be present, depending on the dosage. In severe cases a hypertensive crisis causing cardiac failure, hypertensive encephalopathy, seizures, and intracerebral hemorrhage may result. Prehospital care is directed at managing respiratory and cardiac arrest and status epilepticus and rapidly transporting the patient for physician evaluation.

PHENCYCLIDINE PSYCHOSIS

Phencyclidine psychosis is a true psychiatric emergency. It may mimic schizophrenia. The psychosis usually is of acute onset. It may not become apparent until several days after drug ingestion. Psychosis can occur after a single low-dose exposure to PCP. Psychosis also may last from several days to weeks. Signs and symptoms may range from a catatonic and unresponsive state to bizarre and violent behavior. The patient often appears agitated and suspicious. The patient often experiences auditory hallucinations and paranoia. Appropriate management usually requires involuntary hospitalization, control of violent behavior, and administration of antipsychotic agents. When dealing with these patients in the prehospital setting, personal safety is of prime importance; law enforcement should be called upon for assistance.

Hallucinogen Overdose

Hallucinogens are substances that cause perceptual distortions. The most common hallucinogen in use today is lysergic acid diethylamide (LSD). Other hallucinogens include mescaline, found in the buttons of peyote cactus, which can be used legally in some religious settings; psilocybin mushrooms, found in the United States and Mexico; marijuana, the active agent of the plant *Cannabis sativa;* morning glory plant; nutmeg; mace; and some amphetamines, such as methylenedioxymethamphetamine (Ecstasy) and 3, 4-methylenedioxyamphetamine (MDEA Eve).

BOX 36-20 Five Signs of Major Tricyclic Antidepressant Toxicity

Cardiac dysrhythmias
Coma
Gastrointestinal disturbances
Hypotension or hypertension
Respiratory depression

Depending on the agent, the effects of hallucinogens may range from minor visual to more serious complications (associated with lysergic acid diethylamide use). The more serious effects include respiratory and CNS depression (rare). Prehospital management usually is limited to supportive care, minimal sensory stimulation, calming measures, and transportation to a medical facility. After arrival at the emergency department, these patients generally are placed in a quiet environment for observation.

Tricyclic Antidepressant Overdose

Tricyclic antidepressants often are prescribed to help manage depression and certain pain syndromes. These drugs work by blocking the uptake of norepinephrine and serotonin into the presynaptic neurons. They also alter the sensitivity of brain tissue to the actions of these chemicals. Serious tricyclic antidepressant toxicity results from sodium-channel blockade in the myocardium. Other toxicities include potassium efflux blockade and blockade of blood vessels, anticholinergic effects, and seizures. Commonly prescribed antidepressant drugs include the tricyclic antidepressants amitriptyline, imipramine, and nortriptyline. The newer *selective serotonin reuptake inhibitors* such as fluoxetine, sertraline, and paroxetine are chemically unrelated to tricyclic antidepressants. These are considered safe and effective compared with tricyclic antidepressants.

Early symptoms of tricyclic antidepressant overdose are dry mouth, blurred vision, confusion, inability to concentrate, and occasionally visual hallucinations. More severe symptoms include delirium, depressed respirations, hypertension, hypotension, hyperthermia, hypothermia, seizures, and coma (Box 36-20). Cardiac effects may range from tachycardia to bradycardia and various dysrhythmias caused by atrioventricular block. A prolonged QRS complex, a Glasgow Coma Scale less than 8, or both are characteristic findings that should alert the paramedic to a major toxicity with potentially serious complications. Sudden death from a cardiac arrest may occur several days after an overdose.

Prehospital management for major toxicity of a tricyclic antidepressant overdose is basic supportive care for the patient and rapid transport. Twenty-five percent of patients who ultimately die as a result of the overdose are alert and awake, and 75% have normal sinus rhythm when EMS personnel arrive.[2] Tachycardia, especially with a wide QRS complex greater than 100 ms, is an early sign of toxicity. ***Sodium bicarbonate,*** per medical direction, may begin to reverse cardiac toxicity. Any patient with a history of tricyclic antidepressant ingestion should receive airway, ventilatory, and circulatory support; intravenous access; electrocardiogram monitoring; and rapid transport for physician evaluation. Treatment for specific problems (e.g., seizures and ventricular dysrhythmias) is complex, using a combination of alkalinization and anticonvulsants. Rapid transport to the emergency department is the most prudent course of action.

CRITICAL THINKING

How can you ensure rapid transport of these patients?

Lithium

Lithium is a mood-stabilizing drug. At times lithium is prescribed for the management of bipolar disorders (see Chapter 40). The drug has a narrow dosage range (low toxic-to-therapeutic dose ratio). Thus lithium overdose is common. Patients who are prescribed lithium have frequent blood tests to monitor the level of lithium in the body.

Lithium helps to prevent mood swings. It does this by interfering with hormonal responses to cyclic adenosine monophosphate and by increasing the reuptake of norepinephrine. (This produces an antiadrenergic effect.) As a result of these actions, lithium has many effects on the body. These include muscle tremor, thirst, nausea, increased urination, abdominal cramping, and diarrhea. With toxic ingestion, signs and symptoms may include the following:

- Muscle weakness
- Slurred speech
- Severe trembling
- Blurred vision
- Confusion
- Seizure
- Apnea
- Coma

Prehospital care for patients with suspected lithium overdose should focus on airway management, ventilatory and circulatory support, and the control of seizure activity (if present). (***Activated charcoal*** does not effectively bind lithium.) In-hospital care may include restoring intravascular volume, maintaining urine output, correcting hyponatremia, and sometimes dialysis.

Cardiac Medications

Cardiac drugs are a common cause of poisoning deaths in children and adults. The drugs responsible for the majority of these fatalities are ***digoxin***, beta-blockers, and calcium channel blockers (Box 36-21; also see the appendix at the end of this chapter). As in all other cases of poisoning, patients with toxic ingestion of cardiac drugs require high-concentration oxygen administration, intravenous access, and careful monitoring of vital signs and electrocardiogram.

BOX 36-21 Toxic Effects of Common Cardiac Drugs

Digoxin
Atrial fibrillation
Atrial tachycardia
Bigeminal and multifocal premature ventricular contractions
First- and second-degree atrioventricular block
Sinus bradycardia
Ventricular tachycardia/ventricular fibrillation

Beta-Blockers
Bradycardia
Hypotension
Respiratory arrest
Seizure
Unconsciousness
Ventricular tachycardia/ventricular fibrillation (rare)

Calcium Channel Blockers
Acute respiratory distress syndrome
Asystole
Atrioventricular dissociation
Coma
Confusion
Hypotension
Lactic acidosis
Mild hyperglycemia/hyperkalemia
Pulmonary edema
Respiratory depression
Sinus arrest
Sinus bradycardia
Slurred speech

Digoxin exerts direct and indirect effects on sinoatrial and atrioventricular nodal fibers. At toxic levels the drug can halt impulses in the sinoatrial node, depress conduction through the atrioventricular node, and increase sensitivity of the sinoatrial and atrioventricular nodes to catecholamines.[5] ***Digoxin*** affects the Purkinje fibers as well. It decreases the resting potential and action potential duration of the heart. ***Digoxin*** also increases automaticity. This can cause an increase in premature ventricular contraction formation. Unlike most cardiovascular drugs, ***digoxin*** can produce almost any dysrhythmia or conduction block. In addition to dysrhythmias, common signs and symptoms of ***digoxin*** toxicity include nausea, anorexia, fatigue, visual disturbances, and a variety of disorders of the gastrointestinal, ophthalmological, and neurological systems. Oral overdoses generally are managed with ***activated charcoal*** and drugs to treat life-threatening dysrhythmias. Severe overdoses are managed with intravenous digoxin-specific Fab. This is a drug that decreases the morbidity and mortality associated with ***digoxin*** overdose.

CRITICAL THINKING

Why is it possible that this type of overdose would not be noticed immediately?

Beta-blockers are absorbed rapidly after ingestion. Toxicity impairs sinoatrial and atrioventricular node function. This leads to bradycardias and atrioventricular blocks. The associated depression in ventricular conduction and sodium channel blockade may cause the QRS complex to widen. Occasionally, patients become susceptible to ventricular dysrhythmias (rarely ventricular tachycardia or ventricular fibrillation). Other signs and symptoms include CNS and respiratory depression, hypotension, and seizures. Treatment for patients with beta-blocker overdose includes administration of ***activated charcoal*** and drugs to manage hypotension and dysrhythmias. The in-hospital care may include infusions of ***glucagon*** and various catecholamines. Hemodialysis may be necessary, depending on the particular agent involved.

Toxic ingestion of calcium channel blockers can lead to myocardial depression and peripheral vasodilation with negative inotropic, chronotropic, dromotropic, and vasotropic effects. Hypotension and bradycardia are early signs of toxicity. Overdose may result in serious dysrhythmias that include atrioventricular block of all degrees, sinus arrest, atrioventricular dissociation, junctional rhythm, and asystole. (Calcium channel blockers have little effect on ventricular conduction; ventricular dysrhythmias are uncommon.) Other signs and symptoms of calcium channel toxicity include nausea and vomiting, hypotension, and CNS and respiratory depression. In addition to airway, ventilatory, and circulatory support, emergency care may include the use of antidysrhythmics, vasopressors, and ***activated charcoal***.

Monoamine Oxidase Inhibitors

As described in Chapter 17, monoamine oxidase inhibitors block the breakdown of monoamines (norepinephrine, dopamine, serotonin). These CNS transmitters are distributed throughout the body. The highest concentration is in the brain, liver, and kidneys. Monoamine oxidase inhibitors are prescribed as antidepressants, antineoplastics, antibiotics, and antihypertensives. Some monoamine oxidase inhibitors (e.g., the antidepressants phenelzine and tranylcypromine) have active metabolites. Signs of monoamine oxidase inhibitor toxicity usually are delayed. (They may present 6 to 24 hours after ingestion.) The duration of effects also may last for several days (Box 36-22). These effects include CNS depression and various neuromuscular and cardiovascular system manifestations.

BOX 36-22 Effects of Monoamine Oxidase Inhibitor Toxicity

- Agitation
- Bradysystolic rhythms
- Cardiovascular system manifestations
- Central nervous system depression
- Hallucinations
- Hyperreflexia
- Hypertension
- Hypotension with vascular collapse
- Neuromuscular system manifestations
- Nystagmus
- Rigidity
- Seizure
- Sinus tachycardia

The prehospital care is mainly supportive. Care includes airway, ventilatory, and circulatory support; cardiac medications as needed; and rapid transport for physician evaluation. ***Activated charcoal*** is recommended for all patients if they are awake.

Nonsteroidal Antiinflammatory Drugs

Nonsteroidal antiinflammatory drugs are a group of drugs that have an analgesic and antipyretic action. They also reduce inflammation of joints and soft tissues, such as muscles and ligaments. They work by blocking the production of prostaglandins, which are chemicals that cause inflammation and trigger transmission of pain signals to the brain. Nonsteroidal antiinflammatory drugs are used widely to relieve symptoms caused by types of arthritis (rheumatoid arthritis, osteoarthritis, gout) and to treat back pain, menstrual pain, headaches, minor postoperative pain, and soft tissue injuries. Common nonsteroidal antiinflammatory drugs include diflunisal, fenoprofen, ibuprofen, and naproxen. Ibuprofen and naproxen are available over the counter. They are promoted as safer and more effective than ***aspirin*** and acetaminophen in the management of fever and mild to moderate pain.

IBUPROFEN OVERDOSE

Ibuprofen is the most commonly ingested nonsteroidal antiinflammatory drug in overdose. The effects usually are reversible and are seldom life threatening. (However, significant toxicity may result in coma, seizure, hypotension, and acute renal failure.) Chronic and acute ingestion is usually more than 300 mg/kg. In such an ingestion, common symptoms include mild gastrointestinal and CNS disturbances. These usually resolve within 24 hours after ingestion. Other less common effects include mild metabolic acidosis, muscle fasciculations, chills, hyperventilation, hypotension, and asymptomatic bradycardia. Emergency care for patients who have ingested toxic amounts of ibuprofen consists of gastric decontamination with ***activated charcoal,*** and careful monitoring for secondary complications such as hypotension and dysrhythmias.

SALICYLATE OVERDOSE

Salicylates are widely available in prescription and over-the-counter products such as acetylsalicylic acid ***(aspirin)***, many cold preparations, and oil of wintergreen (methyl sal-

NOTE At one time, the ingestion of colorful and tasty children's aspirin was the most common cause of pediatric poisoning. In response to this problem, the number of tablets now is limited to 36 per container. Because of the association of aspirin with Reye's syndrome, aspirin is not recommended for children younger than 16 years of age who have viral symptoms.

TABLE 36-4 Toxicity Guidelines to Salicylate

TOXICITY	AMOUNT INGESTED
Mild	Less than 150 mg/kg
Moderate to severe	150 to 300 mg/kg
Severe	More than 300 mg/kg
Fatal	More than 500 mg/kg

From Clark J: *Pharmacological basis of nursing*, ed 4, St Louis, 1993, Mosby.

icylate) and in combination with some analgesics such as propoxyphene and oxycodone. Table 36-4 contains general guidelines for salicylate toxicity.

The process of toxicity with salicylate poisoning is complex. Toxicity includes direct CNS stimulation, interference with cellular glucose uptake, and inhibition of Krebs cycle enzymes that affect energy production and amino acid metabolism. The volume of distribution is dose dependent and usually small. With toxic ingestion, however, redistribution of the drug into the CNS occurs. This prolongs elimination of the drug from the body. Complications that may result from chronic or acute ingestion of salicylates include CNS stimulation, gastrointestinal irritation, glucose metabolism, fluid and electrolyte imbalance, neurological symptoms, and coagulation defects.

Central Nervous System Stimulation. First, salicylates produce direct stimulation of the respiratory center in the CNS. This causes an increased rate and depth of respiration. This early respiratory alkalosis is followed by a compensatory elimination of bicarbonate ions by the kidneys. This produces a compensatory metabolic acidosis. Acids continue to build up from metabolism. This leads to profound metabolic acidosis. Confusion, lethargy, convulsions, respiratory arrest, coma, and brain death can occur in severe salicylate poisoning.

CRITICAL THINKING

Would you predict a tachypnea or bradypnea in these patients? Why?

Gastrointestinal Irritation. Salicylates have irritant effects on the lining of the stomach. This can lead to nausea, vomiting, and hematemesis. They also can cause pylorospasm. These spasms delay gastric emptying.

Glucose Metabolism. Interference with glucose uptake by the cells causes a buildup of serum glucose. Eventually, glucose in the cells is depleted. The patient shows signs of hypoglycemia (particularly in CNS tissue). Patients who die from salicylate poisoning often have primary CNS tissue toxicity and severe cerebral edema.

Fluid and Electrolyte Imbalance. The total amount of body fluids is affected adversely by hypermetabolism. Fluid and electrolyte losses occur via gastrointestinal fluids, emesis, and renal clearance. Acid-base disturbances may result in hypokalemia and hyperchloremia. Cardiac dysrhythmias, including premature ventricular contractions, ventricular tachycardia, and ventricular fibrillation, are possible.

Neurological Symptoms. Mild neurological effects are common. One example is tinnitus. (This is a symptom of salicylism on the cranial nerve VIII.) Another common effect is lethargy. Severe intoxication may result in hallucination, seizure, and coma.

Coagulation Effects. Salicylates alter normal platelet function. When taken in toxic amounts, they often lead to coagulation disorders. Thus these patients are at an increased risk of significant bleeding. Patients who take anticoagulants are at even greater risk for hemorrhage after salicylate ingestion.

In addition to general supportive measures, prehospital care for salicylate poisoning may include the administration of ***activated charcoal*** for decontamination of the gastrointestinal tract. Treatment also may include intravenously administered glucose to manage hypoglycemia. Salicylates are weak acids. They can be excreted by the kidney. Thus medical direction may recommend the administration of ***sodium bicarbonate*** in an effort to produce alkaline urine. Definitive care includes in-hospital intensive care observation, continued support of vital functions, and perhaps hemodialysis.

ACETAMINOPHEN OVERDOSE

Acetaminophen is a commonly prescribed analgesic and antipyretic agent. Acetaminophen is available in many prescription and nonprescription preparations (e.g., Tylenol and Panadol). The widespread availability of acetaminophen accounts for its high incidence in unintentional and intentional poisoning. Acetaminophen is 1 of 10 most commonly used drugs for intentional self-poisoning and is associated with significant morbidity and mortality.[5] Acetaminophen overdose can cause life-threatening liver damage from toxic metabolites if it is not managed within 16 to 24 hours of ingestion. As few as 30 standard-size (325-mg) acetaminophen tablets are toxic in an average adult. Acetaminophen also is present in many drug combinations including Darvocet-N, Excedrin, and Sinutab.

Acute acetaminophen ingestion is doses of 140 mg/kg or greater. The toxic effects of such an ingestion can be classified in four stages (Box 36-23). The course of toxicity begins with mild symptoms that may be overlooked or masked by more dramatic effects of other agents followed by temporary clinical improvement and finally peak liver damage. (If acetaminophen was the only drug taken and a dangerously high dose was ingested, the first two stages may be asymptomatic.) If antidote management is started within 8 hours of ingestion, full recovery should occur.

CRITICAL THINKING

Do you think most laypersons realize that acetaminophen overdose can be fatal?

Emergency care includes respiratory, cardiac, and hemodynamic support in critically ill patients. If ingestion is recent

BOX 36-23 Stages of Acetaminophen Poisoning

Stage I: Gastrointestinal Irritability (0 to 24 hours)
Anorexia
Diaphoresis
General malaise
Nausea
Pallor
Vomiting

Stage II: Abnormal Laboratory Findings (24 to 48 hours)
Possible abdominal pain and tenderness in the right abdominal quadrant
Resolution of stage I symptoms

Stage III: Hepatic Damage (72 to 96 hours)
Dysrhythmias
Hepatotoxicity with significant increase in hepatic enzymes
Hypoglycemia
Jaundice
Lethargy
Vomiting

Stage IV: Recovery (4 to 14 days) or Progressive Hepatic Failure
Resolution of hepatic dysfunction
Lack of permanent effects in patients who recover

Note: The percentage of patients who recover in stage IV depends on the amount of acetaminophen ingested and whether effective therapy (activated charcoal, acetylcysteine, or both) was given. Patients with serum levels in the hepatotoxic range have mortality rates up to 25% if untreated.

(within 1 hour) and the patient is alert, medical direction may recommend the administration of ***activated charcoal.*** Patients with progressive acetaminophen toxicity require in-hospital administration of the antidote, *N*-acetylcysteine.

Drugs Abused for Sexual Purposes/Sexual Gratification

Some drugs are abused for sexual purposes or for sexual gratification. These drugs commonly are classified by users as "uppers," "downers," and "all-arounders" (those that have more than one primary effect). Box 36-24 gives a sampling of these drugs. As described before, uppers are CNS stimulants. Downers are CNS depressants. The third category encompasses drugs such as anesthetics and mood-altering agents. They generally are taken alone or in combination to produce one or more of the following effects:

- A sense of euphoria
- Excitation ("rush")
- Relaxation ("blissed out")
- A loss of inhibition

Each of these drugs has different chemical structures, mechanisms of action, and side effects. So the problems associated with their use can vary greatly. Signs and symptoms of abuse can range from mild nausea and vomiting to life-threatening respiratory depression, hypotension, methemoglobinemia, coma, and death. The emergency care for these patients mainly is supportive. Care includes airway, ventilatory, and circulatory support, and rapid transport for physician evaluation. As with all other cases of patients who use mood-altering agents, personal safety is of primary importance.

BOX 36-24 Uppers, Downers, and All-Arounders

Uppers
Anabolic steroids
Coke/crack
Ecstasy
Speed/meth/crystal

Downers
Alcohol
Benzodiazepines (diazepam, temazepam, Rohypnol)
Gamma hydroxybutyrate (GHB)
Heroin

All-Arounders
Cannabis/skunk
Ketamine
Lysergic acid diethylamide (LSD)
Poppers (alkyl nitrates)

SECTION THREE ALCOHOLISM

Alcohol and related illness continue to be a major problem in the United States. In 2001, 109 million Americans (48.3% of the population) age 12 years and older reported current use of alcohol; 46 million (20.6% of the population) admitted to binge drinking; and 12.6 million (5.6% of the population) reported drinking five or more drinks per occasion on 5 or more days per month.[12] In addition, alcohol is a key factor in 40% of vehicle fatalities, 68% of manslaughters, 62% of assaults, 54% of murder attempts, and 48% of robberies. The economic cost of alcohol and other drug-related crime is $61.8 billion annually.[1]

CRITICAL THINKING
How many calls have you been on that involved patients intoxicated with alcohol? What kinds of calls were they?

ALCOHOL DEPENDENCE

Alcohol dependence is a disorder characterized by chronic, excessive consumption of alcohol that results in injury to health or in inadequate social function and the development of withdrawal symptoms when the patient stops drinking suddenly. An estimated 5 million alcohol-dependent persons live in the United States (that equals 1 in 50). Another 7 million have a hard time controlling their consumption of the drug. Alcohol dependence should be considered a chronic, progressive, potentially fatal disease characterized by remissions, relapses, and cures.

No single cause of alcohol dependence exists. Yet three causative factors are believed to interact in development of the illness. These are personality, environment (widespread social acceptance and availability of alcohol), and the addictive nature of the drug. In some cases, genetic and hormonal factors also may play a role in causing dependence. However, it generally is believed that any person, regardless of environment, genetic background, or personality traits, can become chemically dependent on alcohol when the drug is consumed for long periods.

The development of alcohol dependence can be divided into four main stages. These stages merge imperceptibly. The time frame of these stages may range from 5 to 25 years, but the average is about 10 years. In the first stage, tolerance of the drug develops in the heavy social drinker. This allows a person to consume larger quantities of alcohol before experiencing its ill effects. On entering the second stage, the drinker experiences memory lapses relating to events occurring during the drinking episodes. The third stage is characterized by loss or lack of control over alcohol; the drinker can no longer be certain of discontinuing alcohol consumption at will. The final stage begins with prolonged binges of intoxication. This is associated with mental and physical complications. Some drinkers halt their consumption for a brief time or permanently during one of the first three stages.

ETHANOL

The active ingredient in all alcoholic beverages is ethanol, a colorless, flammable liquid produced from the fermentation of carbohydrates by yeast. All alcoholic drinks are rated based on their ethanol percentage. The alcohol content of beer and wine is measured as a percentage by weight or volume. United States beers contain 2.3% to 5.1% alcohol by volume. Wines vary in ethanol content up to 14% to 16%. Distilled liquors are subjected to a rating process called *proof* (Box 36-25).

BOX 36-25 Alcohol "Proof"

Proof initially was based on a test in which gunpowder moistened with a distilled product was ignited. Ignition was "proof" that the alcohol content of the product was at least 50%. Although the ignition test has been replaced with modern techniques to determine alcohol percentage, the term has been retained. A product containing 50% alcohol is considered 100 proof.

Metabolism

Eighty percent to 90% of ingested alcohol is absorbed within 30 minutes. (Twenty percent is absorbed in the stomach, the rest in the small intestine.) Once absorbed, the drug is distributed rapidly throughout the vascular space. Alcohol reaches virtually every organ system. About 3% to 5% of alcohol is excreted unchanged via the lungs and kidneys; the rest is metabolized in the liver to carbon dioxide and water. The actual rate at which alcohol is metabolized depends on individual variation (e.g., physical and mental state, body weight, and size). Metabolism also depends on whether the drinker is alcohol dependent. Alcohol generally is metabolized at a constant rate of about 20 mg/dL per hour (in nonalcoholics). (This is regardless of its concentration.) The rate of metabolism may be increased in alcoholics.

Blood Alcohol Content

The alcohol content of blood is measured in terms of mass (milligrams) of alcohol per given volume of blood (deciliter). The time it takes for the alcohol concentration to peak in the blood depends on a number of factors. These include the rate at which the alcohol is consumed, the amount of food present in the stomach before drinking, and physical characteristics of the drinker. Blood alcohol content is used widely to evaluate the CNS status of an intoxicated person. Yet individuals differ greatly in how blood alcohol content relates to the degree of intoxication. In many states the legal limit of intoxication is 100 mg/dL. (This is equivalent to 0.10%.)

Some states have laws that allow paramedics to assist in conducting breathalyzer or blood tests. These tests detect alcohol or drug intoxication. Emergency medical services personnel should be well versed in the laws of their state before assisting with these tests. In addition, they should follow established protocols carefully.

CRITICAL THINKING

Can you use an alcohol prep to prepare the site before drawing a blood alcohol specimen? Why?

MEDICAL CONSEQUENCES OF CHRONIC ALCOHOL INGESTION

Alcohol affects nearly every organ system of the body. Thus persons who consume large amounts of alcohol are at risk for a number of physical and mental disorders. Through a variety of direct and indirect mechanisms, alcohol causes multiple systemic effects, including neurological disorders, nutritional deficiencies, fluid and elec-

TABLE 36-5 Alcohol Intake and Its Behavioral Effects

ALCOHOL CONTENT (OZ)	BEVERAGE INTAKE IN 1 HOUR*	BLOOD ALCOHOL LEVEL (MG/DL) IN A 150-LB MAN	BEHAVIORAL EFFECTS
½	1 oz 100-proof spirits 1 glass wine 1 can beer	0.025	No noticeable effect
1	2 oz 100-proof spirits 2 glasses wine 2 cans beer	0.050	Lower alertness, impaired judgment, good feeling, and less inhibition
2	4 oz 100-proof spirits 4 glasses wine 4 cans beer	0.100	Slow reaction time, impaired motor function, and less cautious; should not drive; may activate vomiting reflex
3	6 oz 100-proof spirits 6 glasses wine 6 cans beer	0.150	Large increase in reaction times
4	8 oz 100-proof spirits 8 glasses wine 8 cans beer	0.200	Marked depression of sensory and motor abilities
5	10 oz 100-proof spirits 10 glasses wine 10 cans beer	0.250	Severe depression of sensory and motor abilities
6	12 oz 100-proof spirits 12 glasses wine 12 cans beer	0.300	Stuporous and unconscious of surroundings
7	14 oz 100-proof spirits 14 glasses wine 14 cans beer	0.350	Unconscious
8	16 oz 100-proof spirits 16 glasses wine 16 cans beer	0.400	Lethal dose in 50% of the population
12	24 oz 100-proof spirits 24 glasses wine 24 cans beer	0.600	Lethal dose in 95% of the population

*Because only ¼ to ⅓ oz of alcohol is metabolized each hour, alcohol rapidly accumulates.

trolyte imbalances, gastrointestinal disorders, cardiac and skeletal muscle myopathy, and immune suppression. In addition, alcohol may affect a patient's ability to tolerate traumatic injury.

Neurological Disorders

Alcohol is a potent CNS depressant. When consumed in moderate amounts, the drug reduces anxiety and tension. Alcohol gives most drinkers a feeling of relaxation and confidence. The clinical effects of alcohol depend on the dose. They progress predictably as the level of consumption increases and blood alcohol content rises (Table 36-5). Initial feelings of well-being give way to impaired judgment and discrimination, prolonged reflexes, and incoordination and drowsiness. This ultimately may progress to stupor and coma. The long-term neurological effects of chronic alcohol abuse are similar to those of the aging process. They include short-term memory deficit, problems with coordination, and difficulty with concentration and abstraction.

Nutritional Deficiencies

Alcohol can satisfy the caloric requirements of the body for a brief time. It also decreases a drinker's appetite through an irritant effect on the stomach. Alcohol does satisfy the feeling of hunger. Yet it does not have essential vitamins, proteins, or fats. Thus alcohol-dependent persons may have a decreased dietary intake and malabsorption. This leads to multiple vitamin and mineral deficiencies. Clinical manifestations associated with these deficiencies include the following:

- Altered immunity
- Anorexia
- Cardiac dysrhythmias
- Coma
- Irritability and disorientation

- Muscle cramps
- Paresthesias
- Poor wound healing
- Seizures
- Tremor and ataxia

WERNICKE-KORSAKOFF SYNDROME

Alcohol-dependent persons are at particular risk of developing Wernicke-Korsakoff syndrome. This is a disease that results from chronic thiamine (vitamin B_1) deficiency. Some persons may have an inability to use thiamine because of an inherited disorder, whereas others may suffer from a reduction in intestinal absorption and metabolism of thiamine caused by alcohol. The disease affects the brain and nervous system. The syndrome disrupts central and peripheral nerve function. The disease may consist of two stages: Wernicke's encephalopathy and **Korsakoff's psychosis,** or a combination of the two.

Wernicke's encephalopathy usually develops suddenly with the clinical manifestations of ataxia, ocular changes (nystagmus), disturbances of speech and gait, signs of neuropathy (paresthesias, impaired reflexes), stupor, or coma (rare). Because the body needs thiamine to metabolize sugar, the syndrome may be caused by the intravenous administration of glucose or glucose-containing fluids in the malnourished patient. Wernicke's encephalopathy also is the cause of coma in 1% of all alcoholics. Therefore medical direction may recommend the intravenous administration of ***thiamine*** before intravenous administration of glucose in patients with altered mental status or coma of unknown origin.

> **CRITICAL THINKING**
>
> Why do you think recognizing this syndrome is delayed in alcoholic patients?

After administration of ***thiamine,*** patients with Wernicke's encephalopathy usually become more alert and attentive. But gait and mental difficulties often persist for days or months. In fact, fewer than half of the affected patients recover fully. Many chronic alcoholic patients also display signs of Korsakoff's psychosis. This is a mental disorder often found with Wernicke's encephalopathy. These signs include apathy, poor retentive memory, retrograde amnesia, confabulation (invention of stories to make up for gaps in memory), and dementia. Korsakoff's psychosis usually is considered irreversible. It leaves the patient permanently handicapped by memory loss. The patient also needs continual supervision.

Fluid and Electrolyte Imbalances

Urinary output increases after ingesting alcohol. (It increases over and above that expected from the amount of fluid ingested.) This diuresis results because alcohol blocks the secretion of antidiuretic hormone. This can lead to dehydration and electrolyte imbalances.

Gastrointestinal Disorders

The effects of alcohol on the gastrointestinal system can produce several types of alcohol-related illnesses and diseases. The alcohol-related gastrointestinal disorders most likely to initiate an EMS response include gastrointestinal hemorrhage, cirrhosis, and acute or chronic pancreatitis.

GASTROINTESTINAL HEMORRHAGE

Four primary causes of gastrointestinal hemorrhage in patients who drink alcohol are gastritis, ulcer formation, esophageal tear (Mallory-Weiss syndrome), and variceal hemorrhage. (See Chapter 34.) Gastritis results from the toxic effects of ethanol on the gastric mucosa. This leads to diffuse or localized areas of erosion. In the chronic form of gastritis, blood may ooze continually from the mucosal lining, and ulcers may develop.

Esophageal tears of the gastroesophageal junction, stomach, or esophagus usually follow severe or protracted vomiting or retching. The injury results when gastric contents are forced against an unrelaxed gastroesophageal junction. This produces a sudden increase in pressure and a mucosal tear with subsequent bleeding. The bleeding can be worsened by clotting abnormalities. Such abnormalities are common in patients with alcoholic liver disease.

Varices are a result of portal hypertension caused by cirrhosis. Any of these thin-walled, blood-engorged veins are subject to rupture and hemorrhage. But the most common site is the varices of the esophagus. Bleeding esophagogastric varices remain one of the most difficult conditions to manage. Severe blood loss through vomiting requires aggressive supportive care with large-bore intravenous lines and fluid resuscitation.

CIRRHOSIS

Cirrhosis of the liver is caused by chronic damage to liver cells. This chronic damage results in inflammation and eventually necrosis. In the disease process, bands of fibrosis (scar tissue) develop and break up the normal structure of the liver. The distortion and fibrosis of the liver lead to portal hypertension. This results in complications such as ascites, splenomegaly, and bleeding esophageal and gastric varices. In addition, cirrhosis may lead to hepatic encephalopathy. This is caused by the buildup of toxic metabolic waste products. These waste products normally would be detoxified by a healthy liver. One in 70 Americans is estimated to die as a direct result of chronic liver disease and cirrhosis. This accounts for 25,000 deaths each year.

ACUTE OR CHRONIC PANCREATITIS

Alcohol is the most common cause of acute and chronic pancreatitis. The exact mechanism by which alcohol produces pancreatic inflammation is not clear. However, pancreatitis may be caused at least in part by activation of pancreatic proenzymes, obstruction of pancreatic ducts, and stimulation of enzymatic secretion. A direct toxic effect may result, as has been demonstrated for the liver. Chronic pancreatitis usually produces the same symptoms as the acute form (described in Chapter 34). The pain, however, may last from several hours to several days. The attacks also become more frequent as the condition progresses. Other effects of chronic pancreatitis include malabsorption (a result of a deficiency of pancreatic enzymes), electrolyte imbalances such as hypocalcemia, and diabetes mellitus (caused by insufficient insulin production). Complications of pancreatitis are hemorrhagic pancreatitis, sepsis, and pancreatic abscess. These complications are associated with high mortality.

Cardiac and Skeletal Muscle Myopathy

Cardiac and skeletal muscle damage is thought to result from a direct toxic effect of alcohol or its metabolites. The pathological changes associated with these alcoholic muscle syndromes include intracellular edema, formation of lipid droplets, excessive cellular glycogen, and deranged sarcoplasmic reticula and mitochondria. In heart muscle, these changes result in a decreased force of contraction (negative inotropic effect), dysrhythmias, and a tendency to develop congestive heart failure. In skeletal muscle the major symptoms are weakness and muscle wasting.

Immune Suppression

Long-term alcohol abuse renders the immune system less effective. Alcohol abuse suppresses bone marrow production of white blood cells. In addition, red blood cells and platelet production are often decreased. Alcohol has direct, specific effects on lung tissue. These effects may impair macrophage mobilization and mucociliary function. As a result, the ability of the body to fight pulmonary infection is lowered. This makes the alcoholic more susceptible to viral and bacterial pneumonia. These infections may result from aspiration during alcoholic stupor or for other reasons. Although the exact cause is unknown, the incidence of cancer is increased in alcoholic patients. This also may be related to immune suppression.

CRITICAL THINKING

For what other pulmonary disease is the immune-suppressed alcoholic patient at risk?

Trauma

Alcohol suppresses clotting factors that are produced in the liver. This blood-clotting deficiency makes alcoholics prone to bruising and internal hemorrhage. The deficiency also adds to the frequency of subdural bleeding, even after relatively minor head trauma.

ALCOHOL EMERGENCIES

Several other conditions caused by consumption or abstinence from alcohol may require emergency care. These include acute alcohol intoxication, alcohol withdrawal syndromes, and disulfiram-ethanol reaction. Alcohol-induced ketoacidosis and hypoglycemia are discussed in Chapter 32.

Acute Alcohol Intoxication

The ingestion of alcohol may cause acute poisoning. This may occur if alcohol is consumed in large amounts over a short period. The clinical features are similar to those induced by sedative-hypnotic agents. The features can be correlated to a degree with blood alcohol content. At toxic levels, hypoventilation (including respiratory arrest), hypotension, and hypothermia may develop. The patient who has signs and symptoms of acute alcohol intoxication should be considered carefully for occult trauma and coexisting medical conditions such as hypoglycemia, cardiac myopathy and dysrhythmias, gastrointestinal bleeding, polydrug abuse, and ethylene glycol or methanol ingestion. Because the patient is prone to injury and usually has other medical problems, the paramedic should never assume that an intoxicated patient is merely inebriated.

MANAGEMENT

A patient who is mildly intoxicated should be transported for physician evaluation. In most cases, management requires patient observation in the emergency department only until the patient is sober. The paramedic should monitor the patient's vital signs and level of consciousness carefully en route. A thorough physical examination is warranted to rule out illness or injury masked by alcohol ingestion.

Care of the acutely intoxicated patient is aimed at protecting the patient from further injury and maintaining vital functions. If the patient is conscious and agitated, restraints may be necessary. This will protect the patient and any health care providers from harm. If physical restraint becomes necessary, the police should be summoned. After scene safety has been established, initial assessment and resuscitation should include the following:

1. Rapidly evaluate airway patency with spinal precautions. Assess the patient's ventilatory and hemodynamic status while obtaining a history. The patient's account of the event may be unreliable because of the alcohol ingestion.
2. Initiate intravenous therapy. Draw blood samples for laboratory analysis. Per protocol, administer ***thiamine, dextrose 50%*** (if hypoglycemia is likely or confirmed), and ***naloxone,*** if opiate overdose is suspected.
3. Continually monitor the patient's airway and provide adequate ventilatory and circulatory support as needed. Be prepared to provide suction and aggressive airway management.
4. Monitor electrocardiogram for dysrhythmias.
5. Rapidly transport the patient for physician evaluation.

Alcohol Withdrawal Syndromes

A period of relative or full abstinence from alcohol may cause withdrawal in an alcoholic. The severity of these syndromes depends on the magnitude of blood alcohol content (serum ethanol level), the length of time the level was maintained, the abruptness of cessation, the tissue tolerance to alcohol, and the general physical and psychological condition of the patient. The cause of alcohol withdrawal remains largely unknown. However, withdrawal is thought to result from CNS hyperexcitability (as the CNS depressant is removed). Biochemical changes such as respiratory alkalosis and hypomagnesemia can play a role also. Alcohol withdrawal syndromes can be divided into four general categories: minor reactions, hallucinations, alcohol withdrawal seizures, and **delirium tremens.**

MINOR REACTIONS

Minor reactions begin about 6 to 8 hours after cessation or reduction of alcohol intake. These symptoms peak within 24 to 36 hours. They may persist for 10 to 14 days. When alcohol withdrawal is confined to minor reactions, the prognosis for full recovery is excellent with the proper management. Minor reactions include the following:

- Sudden and unexpected startle
- Flushed face and diaphoresis
- Anorexia
- Nausea and vomiting
- Insomnia
- General muscle weakness
- Slight disorientation
- Generalized tremor (worsened by agitation)
- Mild tachycardia, hypertension, and hyperreflexia

> **CRITICAL THINKING**
> What kinds of feelings do you think the patient and the patient's family may be having during withdrawal reactions?

HALLUCINATIONS

Hallucinations usually occur 24 to 36 hours after stopping the drinking of alcohol. Disorders of perception are common. They may vary from auditory and visual illusions to frank hallucinations. The latter can produce agitation, fear, and panic. During this period, the patient may show signs of suicidal and homicidal tendencies, and minor reactions may be more pronounced. The prognosis for hallucinations is the same as for minor reactions with appropriate care.

ALCOHOL WITHDRAWAL SEIZURES

Alcohol withdrawal seizures (or "rum fits") usually occur 7 to 48 hours after ethanol cessation. These seizures may occur singly or in groups of two to six. They most often are grand mal of short duration; status seizures are rare. Alcohol withdrawal seizures are associated with varying degrees of tremor, anorexia, hallucinations, and autonomic hyperactivity. This category of withdrawal may be self-limiting or may progress to delirium tremens with or without a lucid interval.

Because of the high drug tolerance level of the alcoholic patient, seizure activity may require intravenous administration of large doses of ***diazepam*** or ***lorazepam.*** These drugs may synergistically interact with any ethanol still in the patient's system. Thus vital signs, respirations, and mental status should be monitored closely.

DELIRIUM TREMENS

Delirium tremens is the most dramatic and serious form of alcohol withdrawal. It affects about 5% of all alcoholics hospitalized for withdrawal. Delirium tremens usually occurs 72 to 96 hours after cessation of alcohol. Yet it may be delayed up to 14 days. The syndrome is characterized by psychomotor, speech, and autonomic hyperactivity; profound confusion; disorientation; delusion; vivid hallucinations; tremor; agitation; and insomnia. A single episode may last 1 to 3 days and, with multiple recurrences, may last up to 1 month.

Autonomic hyperactivity is the most distinguishing feature of delirium tremens. Delirium tremens is characterized by tachycardia, fever, hypertension, dilated pupils, and profuse diaphoresis. In severe cases, cardiovascular collapse may be present. Delirium tremens is a true medical emergency. It has a mortality rate as high as 15%. Associated alcohol-related illnesses such as pneumonia, pancreatitis, and hepatitis are frequent contributing causes of death.

MANAGEMENT

The care for patients with alcohol withdrawal syndromes mainly is supportive. After scene safety is ensured, the paramedic should monitor the patient's airway, ventilatory, and circulatory status carefully. Intravenous therapy should be started with a saline solution for rehydration. Pharmacological therapy may be indicated for an altered level of consciousness, dysrhythmias, or seizure activity. In addition, these patients need calm reassurance and frequent reorientation to the present. All patients with signs and symptoms of alcohol withdrawal syndrome require physician evaluation.

Disulfiram-Ethanol Reaction

Disulfiram (tetraethylthiuram disulfide [Antabuse]) is a medication prescribed to some alcoholic patients to help them abstain. The drug works by inhibiting ethanol metabolism. The drug also allows for the accumulation of the metabolite acetaldehyde. Acetaldehyde produces ill effects on the gastrointestinal, cardiovascular, and autonomic nervous systems. Acetaldehyde is the metabolic product that is thought to be responsible for the common "hangover." Patients who take disulfiram and then drink alcohol experience an unpleasant and potentially life-threatening physiological response. A disulfiram-like reaction also can occur in patients taking metronidazole for *Trichomonas* and other types of infection.

The disulfiram-ethanol reaction begins 15 to 30 minutes after the ingestion of two to five alcoholic drinks. The reaction continues for 1 to 2 hours. The reaction causes the patient to experience vertigo, headache, vomiting, flushing (which may give the skin a "lobster-red" appearance), dyspnea, diaphoresis, abdominal pain, and sometimes chest pain. More serious reactions include hypotension, shock, and dysrhythmias. Sudden death, myocardial and cerebral infarction, and cerebral hemorrhage also have been reported after as little as one drink of ethanol in patients taking disulfiram.

MANAGEMENT

Prehospital care for a disulfiram-ethanol reaction involves airway, ventilatory, and circulatory support; the administration of intravenous fluids to manage hypotension; pharmacological therapy as needed to manage dysrhythmias; and rapid transport for physician evaluation. Most patients recover from these episodes. Supportive care and in-hospital observation are usually all that are required.

SECTION FOUR
MANAGEMENT OF TOXIC SYNDROMES

GENERAL MANAGEMENT PRINCIPLES FOR TOXIC SYNDROMES

As stated before, most poisoned patients require only supportive therapy to recover (Box 36-26). (This is regardless of the toxic agent.) Grouping toxic agents and physical findings into toxic syndromes, however, can give the paramedic important clues to what type of poison or toxin is involved. This will aid the paramedic in remembering assessment and management strategies as well (Table 36-6). The five toxic syndromes presented in this chapter are the following[2,13]:

1. Cholinergic
2. Anticholinergic
3. Hallucinogenic
4. Opiate
5. Sympathomimetic

NOTE Toxic syndrome classification does not consider how or why the toxin was introduced into the body. Thus the paramedic should consider route of entry in addition to specific treatments.

BOX 36-26 General Management Guidelines for the Poisoned Patient

1. Ensure scene and personal safety.
2. Provide adequate airway, ventilation, and circulation.
3. Obtain a thorough history, and perform a focused physical examination.
4. Consider hypoglycemia in an unconscious or convulsing patient.
5. Administer naloxone or nalmefene to a patient with respiratory depression and suspected opioid ingestion.
6. If overdose is suspected, obtain an overdose history from the patient, family, or friends.
7. Consult with medical direction or a poison control center for specific treatment to prevent further absorption of the toxin (or antidote therapy).
8. Frequently monitor vital signs and electrocardiogram.
9. Safely obtain any substance or substance container of a suspected poison. Transport it with the patient.
10. Transport the patient for physician evaluation.

Cholinergics

Exposure to cholinergics is uncommon. However, it is important to recognize cholinergic poisoning so that lifesaving care can be started. Causative agents include pesticides (organophosphates, carbamates) and nerve agents (e.g., sarin and soman). Assessment findings include headache, dizziness, weakness, bradycardia, nausea, and a "wet" presentation manifested by profound *s*alivation, *l*acrimation, *u*rination, *d*efecation, *g*astrointestinal upset, and *e*mesis (SLUDGE). In severe cases, coma and convulsions may be present. In addition to airway, ventilatory, and circulatory support and decontamination, drug therapy may include administration of ***atropine, pralidoxime, diazepam*** or ***lorazepam,*** and ***activated charcoal.***

Anticholinergics

Exposure to anticholinergics is fairly common because so many medications and plants have anticholinergic properties. The signs and symptoms include tachycardia; dry, flushed skin; dilated pupils; and facial flushing. This "dry" patient presentation usually is managed with airway, ventilatory, and circulatory support, and rarely with the administration of physostigmine in the absence of tricyclic antidepressant overdose.

Hallucinogens

Common hallucinogens include lysergic acid diethylamide, PCP, peyote, mushrooms, and mescaline. Depending on the agent and dose, signs and symptoms may include CNS stimulation and/or depression, behavioral disturbances, delusions, hypertension, chest pain, tachycardia, seizures, and respiratory and cardiac arrest. Prehospital care for these patients is focused on ensuring personal safety and providing airway, ventilatory, and circulatory support.

Opiates

The opiate syndrome carries a hallmark triad of depressed level of consciousness, respiratory depression, and pinpoint pupils. Common causative agents include heroin, ***morphine,*** codeine, ***meperidine,*** propoxyphene, and fentanyl. Drugs in this class often are mixed with alcohol or other drugs (e.g., benzodiazepines). This leads to increased respiratory depression, hypotension, and bradycardia. Other signs and symptoms may include euphoria, nausea, pinpoint pupils, and seizures. In addition to ensuring airway, ventilatory, and circulatory support, drug therapy may in-

TABLE 36-6 Toxicological Syndromes

COMMON SIGNS	CAUSATIVE AGENTS	SPECIFIC TREATMENT
Cholinergic ("Wet" Patient Presentation)		
Confusion, central nervous system depression, weakness, SLUDGE (salivation, lacrimation, urination, defecation, gastrointestinal upset, emesis), bradycardia, wheezing, bronchoconstriction, miosis, coma, convulsion, diaphoresis, seizures	Organophosphate and carbamate insecticides, nerve agents, some mushrooms	***Atropine, pralidoxime*** (2-PAM chloride), ***diazepam*** (Valium), ***activated charcoal***
Anticholinergic ("Dry" Patient Presentation)		
Delirium, tachycardia, dry, flushed skin, dilated pupils, seizures, and dysrhythmias (in severe cases)	Antihistamines, antiparkinson medications, atropine, antipsychotic agents, antidepressants, skeletal muscle relaxants, many plants (e.g., Jimson weed and *Amanita muscaria*)	***Diazepam*** (Valium), *activated charcoal,* rarely physostigmine (Antilirium)
Hallucinogen		
Visual illusions, delusions, bizarre behavior, flashbacks, respiratory and central nervous system depression	LSD, PCP,* mescaline, some mushrooms, marijuana, Jimson weed, nutmeg, mace, some amphetamines	Minimal sensory stimulation and calming measures, ***diazepam*** (Valium) if necessary
Opioids		
Euphoria, hypotension, respiratory depression/arrest, nausea, pinpoint pupils, seizures, coma	Heroin, ***morphine,*** codeine, ***meperidine*** (Demerol), propoxyphene, fentanyl	***Naloxone*** (Narcan), ***nalmefene*** (Revex)
Sympathomimetic		
Delusions, paranoia, tachycardia or bradycardia, hypertension, diaphoresis; seizures, hypotension, and dysrhythmias in severe cases	Cocaine, amphetamine, methamphetamine, over-the-counter decongestants	Minimal sensory stimulation and calming measures, ***diazepam*** (Valium) if necessary

**LSD,* Lysergic acid diethylamide; *PCP,* phencyclidine.

clude the administration of ***naloxone*** or another opiate-specific antidote agent.

Sympathomimetics

The sympathomimetic syndrome usually results from acute overdose of amphetamines or cocaine. Signs and symptoms include elevated blood pressure, tachycardia, dilated pupils, and altered mental status (including paranoid delusions). In severe cases, cardiovascular collapse can occur. Management consists of ensuring personal safety and providing airway, ventilatory, and circulatory support.

CRITICAL THINKING

Why is it important to be able to identify these toxic syndromes?

SUMMARY

- A poison is any substance that produces harmful physiological or psychological effects.
- The toxic effects of ingested poisons may be immediate or delayed. This depends on the substance that is ingested. The main goal is to identify effects on the three vital organ systems most likely to produce immediate morbidity and mortality. These are the respiratory system, the cardiovascular system, and the CNS. The goal of managing serious poisonings by ingestion is to prevent the toxic substance from reaching the small intestine. This limits its absorption.
- Strong acids and alkalis may cause burns to the mouth, pharynx, esophagus, and sometimes the upper respiratory and gastrointestinal tracts. Prehospital care usu-

ally is limited to airway and ventilatory support, intravenous fluid replacement, and rapid transport to the appropriate medical facility.

- The most important physical characteristic in the potential toxicity of an ingested hydrocarbon is its viscosity. The lower the viscosity, the higher the risk of aspiration and associated complications. Hydrocarbon ingestion may involve the patient's respiratory, gastrointestinal, and neurological systems. The clinical features may be immediate or delayed.
- Methanol is a poisonous alcohol found in a number of products. Methanol itself is no more toxic than ethanol. Yet its metabolites (formaldehyde and formic acid) are toxic. Ingestion can affect the CNS, the gastrointestinal tract, and the eyes. Methanol also can cause the development of metabolic acidosis.
- Ethylene glycol toxicity is caused by the buildup of toxic metabolites, especially glycolic and oxalic acids after metabolism. This occurs mainly in the liver and kidneys. This toxicity may affect the CNS and cardiopulmonary and renal systems and may result in hypocalcemia.
- The majority of isopropanol (isopropyl alcohol) is metabolized to acetone after ingestion. Isopropanol poisoning affects several body systems, including the central nervous, gastrointestinal, and renal systems.
- Infants and children are high-risk groups for accidental iron, lead, and mercury poisoning. Their immature immune systems and increased absorption as a function of age contribute to this risk. Ingested iron is corrosive to gastrointestinal tract mucosa. Iron may produce lethal gastrointestinal hemorrhage, bloody vomitus, painless bloody diarrhea, and dark stools.
- *Food poisoning* is a term used for any illness of sudden onset (usually associated with stomach pain, vomiting, and diarrhea) suspected of being caused by food eaten within the previous 48 hours. Food poisoning can be classified as infectious. This results from a bacterium or virus. Food poisoning also can be classified as noninfectious. This results from toxins and pollutants.
- The toxic effects of major poisonous plant ingestions are predictable. They are categorized by the chemical and physical properties of the plant. Most responses are consistent with the type of major toxic chemical component in the plant.
- The concentration of a chemical in the air helps to determine the severity of an inhalation injury. The duration of exposure helps to determine this as well. Solubility also influences the extent of an inhalation injury. Highly reactive chemicals cause more severe and rapid injury than less reactive chemicals. Properties that determine chemical reactivity are chemical pH; direct-acting potential of chemicals; indirect-acting potential of chemicals; and allergic potential of chemicals.
- Cyanide refers to any of a number of highly toxic substances that contain the cyanogen chemical group. Regardless of the route of entry, cyanide is a rapidly acting poison. It combines and reacts with ferric ions of the respiratory enzyme cytochrome oxidase. This combination inhibits cellular oxygenation. This produces a rapid progression from dyspnea to paralysis, unconsciousness, and death.
- Ammonia is a toxic irritant that causes local pulmonary complications after inhalation. In severe cases, bronchospasm and pulmonary edema may develop.
- Hydrocarbon inhalation may cause aspiration pneumonitis. It also has the potential for systemic effects such as CNS depression and liver, kidney, or bone marrow toxicity.
- Simple asphyxiants cause toxicity by lowering ambient oxygen concentration. Chemical asphyxiants possess intrinsic systemic toxicity. This toxicity occurs after absorption into the circulation. Irritants or corrosives cause cellular destruction and inflammation as they come into contact with moisture in the respiratory tract.
- The general principles of managing inhaled poisons are the same as for any other hazardous materials incident.
- Hymenoptera and Arachnida cause the highest incidence of need for emergency care. Arthropod venoms are complex and diverse in their chemistry and pharmacology. They may produce major toxic reactions in sensitized persons. Such reactions include anaphylaxis and upper airway obstruction.
- The two main families of venomous snakes indigenous to the United States are pit vipers and coral snakes. Pit viper venom can produce various toxic effects on blood and other tissues. These effects include hemolysis, intravascular coagulation, convulsions, and acute renal failure. The venom of the coral snake is mainly neurotoxic. Signs and symptoms range from slurred speech, dilated pupils, and dysphagia to flaccid paralysis and death.
- The marine animals most likely to be involved in human poisonings in U.S. coastal waters are coelenterates, echinoderms, and stingrays. Coelenterate envenomation ranges in severity from irritant dermatitis to excruciating pain, respiratory depression, and life-threatening cardiovascular collapse. Echinoderm toxins may cause immediate intense pain, swelling, redness, aching in the affected extremity, and nausea. Delayed effects may include respiratory distress, paresthesia of the lips and face, and in severe cases, respiratory paralysis and complete atonia. Locally, stingray venom produces a painful traumatic injury. It may cause bleeding and necrosis. Systemic manifestations range from weakness and nausea to seizures, paralysis, hypotension, and death.

Continued

- Organophosphates and carbamates inhibit the effects of acetylcholinesterase. A mnemonic aid that may help the paramedic to recognize this type of poisoning is *SLUDGE*. (This stands for *s*alivation, *l*acrimation, *u*rination, *d*efecation, *g*astrointestinal upset, and *e*mesis.) The most specific findings, however, are miosis, rapidly changing pupils, and muscle fasciculation.
- General principles for managing drug abuse and overdose include scene safety; ensuring adequate airway, breathing, and circulation; history; substance identification; focused physical exam; initiation of an intravenous line; administration of an antidote if needed; prevention of further absorption; and rapid transport.
- Narcotics are CNS depressants. They can cause life-threatening respiratory depression. In severe intoxication, hypotension, profound shock, and pulmonary edema may be present. Naloxone is a pure narcotic antagonist effective for virtually all narcotic and narcotic-like substances.
- Sedative-hypnotic agents include benzodiazepines and barbiturates. Signs and symptoms of sedative-hypnotic overdose are related chiefly to the central nervous and cardiovascular symptoms. Flumazenil (Romazicon) is a benzodiazepine antagonist useful in reversing the effects of these agents.
- Commonly used stimulant drugs are those of the amphetamine family. Adverse effects include tachycardia, increased blood pressure, tachypnea, agitation, dilated pupils, tremors, and disorganized behavior. With sudden withdrawal, the patient becomes depressed, suicidal, incoherent, or near coma.
- Phencyclidine is a dissociative analgesic with sympathomimetic and CNS stimulant and depressant effects. In low doses, PCP intoxication produces an unpredictable state that can resemble drunkenness (and rage). High-dose intoxication may cause coma. This may last from several hours to days. Respiratory depression, hypertension, and tachycardia may be present. Phencyclidine psychosis is a psychiatric emergency. It may mimic schizophrenia.
- Hallucinogens are substances that cause distortions of perceptions. Depending on the agent, overdose may range from visual hallucinations and anticholinergic syndromes to more serious complications, including psychosis, flashbacks, and respiratory and CNS depression.
- Tricyclic antidepressant toxicity is thought to result from central and peripheral atropine-like anticholinergic effects and direct depressant effects on myocardial function. A prolonged QRS complex, a Glasgow Coma Scale score less than 8, or both, should alert the paramedic to a major tricyclic antidepressant toxicity.
- Lithium is a mood-stabilizing drug. Toxic ingestion can include CNS effects that can range from blurred vision and confusion to seizure and coma.
- Cardiac drugs are a common cause of poisoning deaths in children and adults. The drugs responsible for the majority of these fatalities are digitalis, beta-blockers, and calcium channel blockers.
- Monoamine oxidase inhibitors block or diminish the activity of the monoamines (norepinephrine, dopamine, serotonin). Toxic effects include CNS depression and various neuromuscular and cardiovascular system manifestations.
- Nonsteroidal antiinflammatory drugs work by blocking the production of prostaglandins. The effects of overdose of ibuprofen are usually reversible, are seldom life-threatening, and include mild gastrointestinal and CNS effects. Salicylate poisoning may cause CNS stimulation, gastrointestinal irritation, glucose metabolism, fluid and electrolyte imbalance, and coagulation defects.
- Acetaminophen overdose may cause life-threatening liver damage. This results from formation of a hepatotoxic intermediate metabolite if it is not managed within 16 to 24 hours of ingestion.
- Some drugs are abused for sexual purposes or for sexual gratification. These drugs commonly are classified by users as "uppers," "downers," and "all-arounders" (those that have more than one primary effect). Problems associated with their use vary widely.
- Alcohol dependence is a disorder characterized by chronic, excessive consumption of alcohol that results in injury to health or in inadequate social function and the development of withdrawal symptoms when the patient stops drinking suddenly. Alcohol causes multiple systemic effects. These include neurological disorders, nutritional deficiencies, fluid and electrolyte imbalances, gastrointestinal disorders, cardiac and skeletal muscle myopathy, and immune suppression. Several conditions caused by consumption or abstinence from alcohol that may require emergency care are acute alcohol intoxication, alcohol withdrawal syndromes, and disulfiram-ethanol reaction.
- The most common toxic syndromes are cholinergic, anticholinergic, hallucinogen, opiate, and sympathomimetic. Using these classifications allows the paramedic to group similar toxic agents together. Such classification allows the paramedic to remember more easily how to assess and treat the poisoned patient.

REFERENCES

1. National Safety Council: *Injury facts,* Chicago, 2002, The Council.
2. Litovitz TL et al: 2001 annual report of the American Association of Poison Control Centers Toxic Exposure Surveillance System, *Am J Emerg Med* 15:447, 1997.
3. National Household Survey on Drug Abuse, 2000. http://www.samhsa.gov/oas/NHSDA/2kNHSDA/chapter3.htm. Accessed August 8, 2004.
4. American Heart Association: Guidelines 2000 for cardiopulmonary resuscitation and emergency cardiovascular care, International Consensus on Science, *Circulation* 102(8):223, 2000.
5. Rosen P, Barkin R: *Emergency medicine: concepts and clinical practice,* ed 4, St Louis, 1998, Mosby.
6. American Academy of Pediatrics: *Handbook of pediatric environmental health: reducing risk at home, school, and play!* Washington, DC, 1999, The Academy.
7. Borak J et al: *Hazardous materials exposure,* Englewood Cliffs, NJ, 1991, Brady.
8. Auerbach PS, editor: *Wilderness medicine,* ed 3, St Louis, 1995, Mosby.
9. Centers for Disease Control and Prevention: West Nile virus: statistics, surveillance, and control. http://www.cdc.gov/ncidod/dvbid/westnile/surv&controlCaseCount04_detailed.htm. Accessed September 28, 2004.
10. Centers for Disease Control and Prevention: West Nile virus: what you need to know. http://www.cdc.gov/ncidod/dvbid/westnile/wnv_factsheet.htm. Accessed September 28, 2004.
11. US Department of Health and Human Services: 1998 annual national drug survey results, SAMHSA Press Office. http://wasigate.hhs.gov/cgi-bin. Accessed September 2, 2004.
12. National Clearinghouse for Alcohol and Drug Information: Violence and crime and alcohol and other drugs. http://www.health.org/makelink/ml-violc.htm. Accessed September 2, 2004.
13. US Department of Transportation, National Highway Traffic Safety Administration: *EMT-Paramedic national standard curriculum,* Washington, DC, 1998, The Department.

APPENDIX TOXICOLOGY IN EMERGENCY CARDIAC CARE

The American Heart Association has developed guidelines for the management of severe poisonings when standard emergency cardiac care guidelines may not be optimum or appropriate.[4] The following summarizes the American Heart Association guidelines. The paramedic should follow established protocol and should provide care to these patients with the advice of medical direction or a poison control center (Appendix Tables 1 and 2).

GUIDELINES FOR SEVERE POISONING

Drug-Induced Hemodynamically Significant Bradycardia

- ***Atropine*** is seldom helpful, but it is not harmful.
- ***Atropine*** (starting dose of 2 to 4 mg for adults) is lifesaving in organophosphate or carbamate poisoning.
- ***Isoproterenol*** may induce or aggravate hypotension and ventricular dysrhythmias and should not be given unless there is a massive beta-blocker poisoning (in which cases high doses of ***isoproterenol*** may be effective).
- Electrical cardiac pacing is often effective in cases of mild to moderate drug-induced hemodynamically significant bradycardia.
- Hemodynamically significant bradycardia that is resistant to atropine and pacing should be managed with vasopressors with greater beta-agonist activity.

Drug-Induced Hemodynamically Significant Tachycardia

- Hemodynamically significant tachycardia may induce myocardial ischemia, myocardial infarction, or ventricular dysrhythmias and may lead to high-output heart failure and shock.
- Avoid routine therapy with ***adenosine*** and synchronized cardioversion (tachycardia is likely to recur or to be refractory).
- ***Diltiazem*** and ***verapamil*** are relatively contraindicated in patients with borderline hypotension because they may cause more severe shock.
- Drug therapy is preferred when rate control is necessary.
- ***Diazepam*** or ***lorazepam*** in doses that do not produce a decreased level of consciousness or respiratory depression are generally safe and effective in patients with hemodynamically significant tachycardia.
- Cautious use of nonselective beta-blockers (e.g., ***propranolol***) may be effective when hemodynamically significant tachycardia is due to sympathomimetic poisoning.

Drug-Induced Hypertensive Emergencies

- Drug-induced hypertensive emergencies are often short-lived and do not require aggressive therapy (important because hypertension may occur in later cases of severe stimulant poisoning).
- Benzodiazepines are first-line therapy; short-acting agents (e.g., nitroprusside) are second-line therapy; carefully titrated doses of ***labetalol*** are third-line therapy (effective with sympathomimetic poisoning).
- ***Propranolol*** may block $beta_2$-receptors (leaving alpha-adrenergic stimulation unopposed and worsening hypertension) and is contraindicated.

Drug-Induced Acute Coronary Syndromes

- Treatment is similar to drug-induced hypertensive emergencies.
- Benzodiazepines and ***nitroglycerin*** are first-line agents; phentolamine is a second-line agent; ***propranolol*** is contraindicated.
- Fibrinolytics are contraindicated with uncontrolled, severe drug-induced hypertension.

Drug-Induced Ventricular Tachycardia and Ventricular Fibrillation

- Drug-induced ventricular tachycardia may be difficult to distinguish from drug-induced impaired conduction (wide complex).
- Drug-induced ventricular tachycardia is likely and should be cardioverted when a sudden conversion to wider-complex rhythm occurs with hypotension.
- Antidysrhythmics are indicated in hemodynamically stable drug-induced ventricular tachycardia.
- ***Procainamide*** is contraindicated in tricyclic antidepressant poisoning and in poisonings with drugs that have similar antidysrhythmic properties.
- ***Lidocaine*** is safe and effective in cases of cocaine poisoning and is the drug of choice in monomorphic ventricular tachycardia or ventricular fibrillation.
- ***Magnesium*** may be effective in some cases of drug-induced ventricular tachycardia but also may aggravate drug-induced hypotension.
- Correctable factors (hypoxemia, hypokalemia, hypomagnesemia) should be considered in the presence of torsades de pointes; the rhythm may respond to electrical and pharmacological therapy: ***magnesium***, ***lidocaine;*** electrical or pharmacological overdrive pacing; and perhaps potassium supplementation.

APPENDIX TABLE 1 Sympathomimetic and Cardiotoxic Drugs

DRUG CLASS	CARDIOVASCULAR SIGNS OF TOXICITY*	THERAPY TO CONSIDER
Stimulants, Sympathomimetic		
Amphetamines	Tachycardia	Alpha-blockers
Methamphetamine	Supraventricular and ventricular arrhythmias	Benzodiazepines
Cocaine	Impaired conduction	Lidocaine
Phencyclidine	Hypertensive emergencies	Sodium bicarbonate
	Acute coronary syndromes	
	Shock, cardiac arrest	
Calcium Channel Blockers		
Verapamil	Bradycardia	Mixed alpha- and beta-agonists
Nifedipine	Impaired conduction	Pacemakers
Diltiazem	Shock	Calcium infusions
	Cardiac arrest	Insulin euglycemia
Beta-Adrenergic Receptor Antagonists		
Propranolol	Bradycardia	Pacemakers
Atenolol	Impaired conduction	Mixed alpha- and beta-agonists
	Shock	Glucagon, insulin
	Cardiac arrest	Insulin euglycemia
Tricyclic Antidepressants		
Amitriptyline	Tachycardia	Sodium bicarbonate
Desipramine	Bradycardia	Mixed alpha- and beta-agonists or alpha-agonists
Nortriptyline	Ventricular arrhythmia	Lidocaine
	Impaired conduction	Procainamide is contraindicated
	Shock, cardiac arrest	
Cardiac Glycosides		
Digoxin	Bradycardia	Digoxin-specific Fab fragments
Digitoxin	Supraventricular and ventricular arrhythmias	(Digibind)
Foxglove	Impaired conduction	Magnesium
Oleander	Shock, cardiac arrest	Pacemakers
Anticholinergics		
Diphenhydramine	Tachycardia	Physostigmine
Doxylamine	Supraventricular and ventricular arrhythmias	
	Impaired conduction	
	Shock	
	Cardiac arrest	
Cholinergics		
Carbamates	Bradycardia	Atropine
Nerve agents	Ventricular arrhythmias	Decontamination
Organophosphates	Impaired conduction, shock	Pralidoxime
	Pulmonary edema, bronchospasm	Obidoxime
	Cardiac arrest	
Opiates		
Heroin	Hypoventilation (slow, shallow respirations)	Naloxone
Fentanyl	Bradycardia, hypotension	Nalmefene
Methadone		
Isoniazid	Lactic acidosis with or without seizures	Pyridoxine (vitamin B_6)
	Tachycardia or bradycardia	
	Shock, cardiac arrest	

*Unless stated otherwise, assume that all altered vital signs (bradycardia, tachycardia, tachypnea) are hemodynamically significant.

Continued

APPENDIX TABLE 1 Sympathomimetic and Cardiotoxic Drugs, cont'd

DRUG CLASS	CARDIOVASCULAR SIGNS OF TOXICITY*	THERAPY TO CONSIDER
Sodium Channel Blockers		
Type 1a antiarrhythmics, propranolol, verapamil, tricyclic antidepressants	Impaired conduction	Sodium bicarbonates
	Bradycardia	Pacemakers
	Ventricular arrhythmias	Alpha- and beta-agonists; high dose if necessary
	Seizures	
	Shock, cardiac arrest	Hypertonic saline

*Unless stated otherwise, assume that all altered vital signs (bradycardia, tachycardia, tachypnea) are hemodynamically significant.

APPENDIX TABLE 2 Drug-Induced Cardiovascular Emergencies and Altered Vital Signs

DRUG-INDUCED EMERGENCY	INDICATED	CONTRAINDICATED
Bradycardia*	Pacemaker (transcutaneous, intravenous) Mixed alpha- and beta-agonists For overdose of calcium channel blocker: calcium For overdose of beta-blocker: glucagon or beta-agonist	Isoproterenol if hypotensive Prophylactic transvenous pacing
Tachycardia	Benzodiazepines Selective $beta_1$-blockers Mixed alpha- and beta-blockers	Cardioversion Adenosine, verapamil, diltiazem For overdose of tricyclic antidepressant: physostigmine
Impaired conduction, ventricular arrhythmias	Sodium bicarbonate Lidocaine	For overdose of tricyclic antidepressant: type 1A antiarrhythmics (procainamide)
Hypertensive emergency	Benzodiazepines Mixed alpha- and beta-blockers Nitroprusside	Nonselective beta-blockers (propranolol)
Acute coronary syndrome	Benzodiazepines Nitroglycerin Alpha-blocker	Nonselective beta-blockers (propranolol)
Shock	Mixed alpha- and beta-agonists (high dose if necessary) For overdose of calcium channel blocker: calcium, insulin† For overdose of beta-blocker; glucagon, insulin† If refractory to maximal medical therapy: circulatory assist devices	Isoproterenol
Acute cholinergic syndrome	Atropine Pralidoxime/obidoxime	Succinylcholine
Acute anticholinergic syndrome	Physostigmine	Antipsychotics or other anticholinergics
Opiate poisoning	Naloxone Nalmefene	

*Unless stated otherwise, assume all altered vital signs (bradycardia, tachycardia, tachypnea) are hemodynamically significant.
†Administer to achieve euglycemia.

Drug-Induced Impaired Conduction

- Prolonged ventricular conduction predisposes the heart to monomorphic ventricular tachycardia.
- Hypertonic saline and systemic alkalinization can reverse adverse electrophysiological effects, preventing or terminating ventricular tachycardia caused by poisoning from sodium channel-blocking agents (hypertonic ***sodium bicarbonate*** is particularly valuable).
- Respiratory alkalosis can be a temporary measure until the appropriate degree of metabolic alkalosis can be achieved with ***sodium bicarbonate*** (repeat boluses of 1 to 2 mEq/kg for a goal arterial pH of 7.50 to 7.55).

Drug-Induced Shock

- Drug-induced shock usually results when the drug induces decreases in intravascular volume, falls in systemic vascular resistance, diminished myocardial contractility, or a combination of these factors.
- For drug-induced hypovolemic shock, give fluid challenge to correct hypovolemia and optimize preload; if ineffective give ***dopamine*** and then high-dose vasopressors (with central hemodynamic monitoring) if needed.
- For drug-induced distributive shock, potent vasoconstrictors (e.g., ***norepinephrine*** may be needed); ***dobutamine*** and ***isoproterenol*** decrease systemic vascular resistance and are contraindicated; high-dose vasopressors should be given until shock is treated adequately or adverse effects (e.g., ventricular dysrhythmias) develop.
- For drug-induced cardiogenic shock, inotropic agents (e.g., ***calcium, amrinone, glucagon, insulin, isoproterenol,*** and ***dobutamine*** often are required (sometimes in combination); concomitant use of a vasopressor may be needed.

Drug-Induced Cardiac Arrest

- Electrical cardioversion or defibrillation is appropriate for pulseless drug-induced ventricular tachycardia/ventricular fibrillation.
- The cost-benefit ratio of ***epinephrine*** in sympathomimetic poisoning with refractory ventricular fibrillation is unknown; if used, increase the interval between standard-amount doses (avoid high-doses of ***epinephrine***); ***propranolol*** is contraindicated in sympathomimetic poisoning.
- Resuscitation usually is terminated after 20 to 30 minutes of advanced cardiac life support unless there are signs that the CNS is viable; prolonged resuscitation and cardiopulmonary resuscitation (sometimes up to 3 to 5 hours) have been associated with good recovery and may be warranted in some poisoned patients.
- When resuscitation is unsuccessful, organ donation still may be an option.

CHAPTER

37

Hematology

OBJECTIVES

Upon completion of this chapter, the paramedic student will be able to:

1. Describe the physiology of blood and its components.
2. Discuss pathophysiology and signs and symptoms of specific hematological disorders.
3. Outline general assessment and management of patients with hematological disorders.

KEY TERMS

anemia: A decrease in blood hemoglobin.

hematology: The scientific study of blood and blood-forming organs.

hemophilia: A group of hereditary bleeding disorders in which one of the factors necessary for blood coagulation is deficient.

Hodgkin's disease: A malignant disorder characterized by pain and progressive enlargement of lymphoid tissue.

lymphoma: A group of diseases that range from slowly growing chronic disorders to rapidly evolving acute conditions.

multiple myeloma: A malignant neoplasm of the bone marrow.

polycythemia: A condition characterized by an unusually large number of red cells in the blood as a result of their increased production by the bone marrow.

sickle cell disease: A debilitating and unpredictable recessive genetic illness that produces an abnormal type of hemoglobin with an inferior oxygen-carrying capacity.

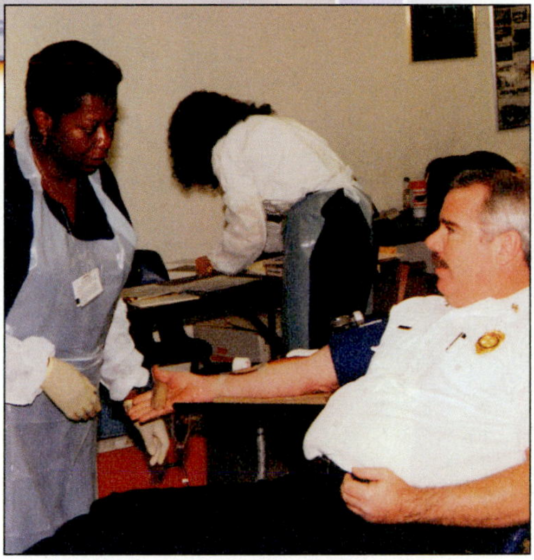

Hematology is the study of blood and blood-forming organs. Dysfunction in the hematological system can affect other body systems. This results in a variety of clinical manifestations that characterize hematological disorders. Prehospital care for most patients with hematological disorders is mainly supportive. However, the paramedic's knowledge of these diseases enhances assessment skills. It also provides an understanding of the treatment these patients need.

BLOOD AND BLOOD COMPONENTS

As described in Chapter 6, blood is composed of cells and formed elements surrounded by plasma. About 95% of the volume of formed elements consists of red blood cells (RBCs; erythrocytes). The remaining 5% consists of white blood cells (WBCs; leukocytes) and cell fragments (platelets) (Fig. 37-1 and Table 37-1). The continuous movement of blood keeps the formed elements dispersed throughout the plasma, where they are available to carry out their chief functions[1]: (1) delivery of substances needed for cellular metabolism in the tissues; (2) defense against invading microorganisms and injury; and (3) acid-base balance.

All types of blood cells are formed within the red bone marrow, which is present in all tissues at birth. In the adult the red bone marrow primarily is found in membranous bone such as the vertebrae, pelvis, sternum, and ribs. Yellow marrow produces some white cells but is composed mainly of connective tissue and fat. Other blood-forming organs include the following:

- Lymph nodes, which produce lymphocytes and antibodies
- The spleen, which stores large quantities of blood and produces lymphocytes, plasma cells, and antibodies
- The liver, a blood-forming organ only during intrauterine life, which plays an important role in the coagulation process

Plasma

Plasma, the clear portion of blood, is about 92% water. It contains three important proteins: albumin, globulins, and fibrinogen. Albumin is the most plentiful protein. Albumin is similar to egg white and gives blood its gummy texture. These large proteins keep the water concentration of blood low so that water diffuses readily from tissues into the blood. The globulins (alpha, beta, and gamma) transport other proteins and provide immunity to disease. Fibrinogen is responsible for blood clotting. Plasma proteins perform various functions that include maintaining blood pH (acting as either an acid or a base); transporting fat-soluble vitamins, hormones, and carbohydrates; and allowing the body to digest them temporarily for food. Plasma also contains salts, metals, and inorganic compounds.

Red Blood Cells

Red blood cells are the most abundant cells in the body. They are primarily responsible for tissue oxygenation. They appear as small rounded disks with nearly hollowed-out centers (Fig. 37-2). They are comprised mainly of water and the red protein hemoglobin. Red blood cell production continues throughout life to replace blood cells that grow old and die, are killed by disease, or are lost through bleeding. After RBC production occurs in the bone marrow, the new cell divides until there are 16 RBCs. The cells produce hemoglobin protein until the concentration of the protein becomes 95% of the dry weight of the cell. At this time, the cell expels its nucleus, giving the cell its characteristic pinched look. The new shape of the RBC increases the surface area of the cell and thus its oxygen-carrying potential. Red blood cells have a life span of about 120 days. As the cells age, their internal chemical machinery weakens; they lose elasticity; and they become trapped in small blood vessels in the bone marrow, liver, and spleen. They then are destroyed by specialized WBCs (macrophages). Most components of de-

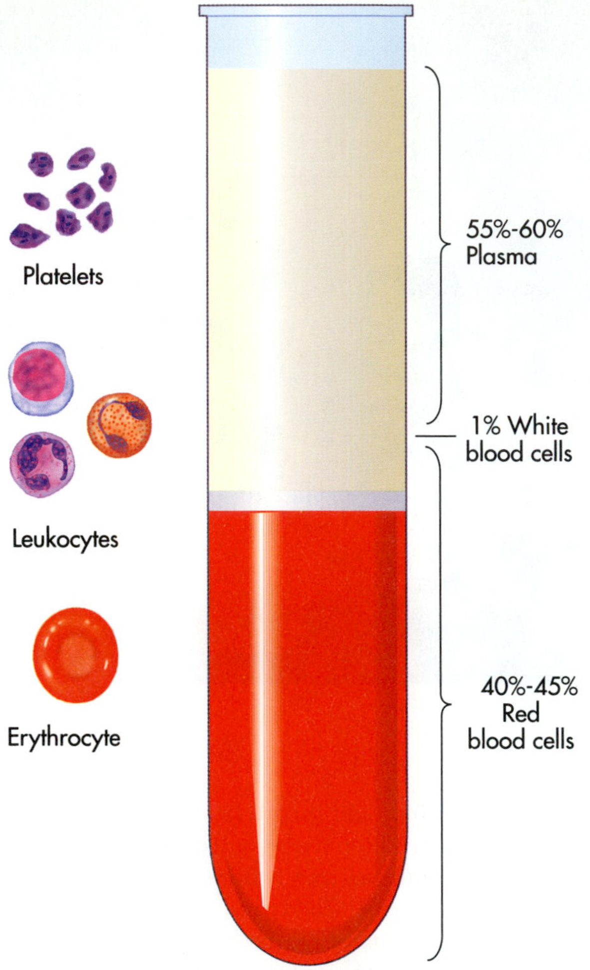

FIGURE 37-1 ■ Blood will settle into three distinct, proportional layers when treated with salt. The transparent yellow layer at the top is plasma, the liquid portion of blood through which solid elements travel. White blood cells (WBCs) settle in the narrow white band in the center, and red blood cells (RBCs), which give blood its crimson color, fall to the bottom of the flask. Red blood cells outnumber white blood cells 600 to 1.

stroyed hemoglobin molecules are used again. However, some are broken down to the waste product bilirubin.

Each RBC contains about 270 million hemoglobin molecules. Each hemoglobin molecule carries 4 oxygen molecules as well. The normal amount of hemoglobin in blood is about 15 g/100 mL. This normally is a little higher in males than in females. The number of RBCs is about 4.2 to 6.2 million cells/mm^3 (Box 37-1).

White Blood Cells

As described in Chapter 7, WBCs arise from the bone marrow and are released into the bloodstream. White blood cells destroy foreign substances (e.g., bacteria and viruses) and clear the bloodstream of debris. Leukocyte production increases in response to infection. This causes an elevated WBC count in the blood. Chapters 7, 33, and 39 provide a discussion of blood groups, the inflammatory process, and the immune response.

The bone marrow and lymph glands continually produce and maintain a reserve of WBCs. However, there are not many WBCs in the healthy bloodstream. The normal WBC count is about 5000 to 10,000 cells/mm^3. Monocytes make up about 5% of the total WBC count and increase with chronic infections. Lymphocytes account for about 27.5%, neutrophils about 65%, and eosinophils and basophils together about 2.5% of the total WBC count. A rise in the number of WBCs aids in the diagnosis of some diseases. An increased WBC count is specific for various illnesses such as bacterial infection, inflammation, leukemia, trauma, and stress.

The *differential count* (also called the *diff*) identifies the different types of leukocytes (WBCs) present in blood. The test is performed by spreading a drop of blood on a microscope slide; staining the slide; and examining it under a microscope. Cells are identified by the shape and appearance of the nucleus, the color of cytoplasm (the background of the cell), and the presence and color of granules. The percentage of each cell type is reported. At the same time, red cells and platelets are examined for abnormalities in appearance.

CRITICAL THINKING

What body functions are impaired if the white blood cell number or function is diminished?

Platelets

Platelets (thrombocytes) are small, sticky cells. They play an important role in blood clotting. When a blood vessel is cut, platelets travel to the site and swell into odd, irregular shapes and adhere to the damaged vessel wall. Platelets plug the leak and allow other cells to stick to them and to form a clot. However, if the damage to the vessel is too great, the platelets chemically signal the complex clotting process, the clotting cascade (described in Chapter 22). Platelets repair millions of ruptured capillaries each day. They often make the rest of the clotting cascade unnecessary (Box 37-2).

SPECIFIC HEMATOLOGICAL DISORDERS

Hematological disorders presented in this chapter are anemia, leukemia, lymphomas, polycythemia, disseminated intravascular coagulopathy, hemophilia, sickle cell disease, and multiple myeloma.

Anemia

Anemia is a condition in which the amount of hemoglobin or erythrocytes in the blood is below normal. Precipitating causes of anemia include chronic or acute blood loss, decreased production of erythrocytes, and increased destruction of erythrocytes.[2] One should note that anemia is not a disease. Rather, anemia is a symptom of a disease. Those at greatest risk are persons with chronic kidney disease, diabetes, heart disease, and cancer; chronic inflammatory con-

TABLE 37-1 Cellular Components of the Blood

CELL	STRUCTURAL CHARACTERISTICS	NORMAL AMOUNTS OF CIRCULATING BLOOD	FUNCTION	LIFESPAN
Erythrocyte (red blood cell)	Nonnucleated cytoplasmic disk containing hemoglobin	4.2-6.2 million/mm^3	Gas transport to and from tissue cells and lungs	80-120 days
Leukocyte (white blood cell)	Nucleated cell	5000-10,000/mm^3	Bodily defense mechanisms	See following times.
Lymphocyte	Mononuclear immunocyte	25% to 33% of leukocyte count (leukocyte differential)	Humoral and cell-mediated immunity	Days or years depending on type
Monocyte and macrophage	Large mononuclear phagocyte	3% to 7% of leukocyte differential	Phagocytosis; mononuclear phagocyte system	Months or years
Eosinophil	Segmented polymorpho-nuclear granulocyte	1% to 4% of leukocyte differential	Phagocytosis, antibody-mediated defense against parasites, allergic reactions, associated with Hodgkin disease, recovery phase of infection	Unknown
Neutrophil	Segmented polymorpho-nuclear granulocyte	57% to 67% of leukocyte differential	Phagocytosis, particularly during early phase of inflammation	4 days
Basophil	Segmented polymorpho-nuclear granulocyte	0% to 0.75% of leukocyte differential	Unknown, but associated with allergic reactions and mechanical irritation	Unknown
Platelet	Irregularly shaped cyto-plasmic fragment (not a cell)	140,000 to 340,000/mm^3	Hemostasis after vascular injury; normal coagulation and clot formation/retraction	8-11 days

From McCance KL, Huether SE: *Pathophysiology: the biologic basis for disease in adults and children*, ed 3, St Louis, 1998, Mosby.

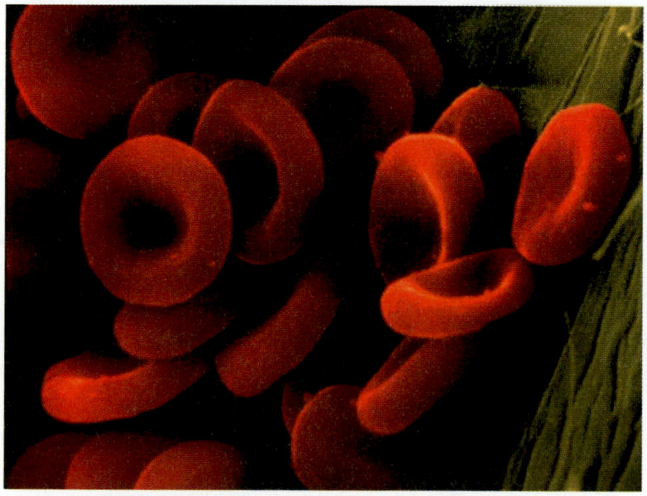

FIGURE 37-2 ■ Mature erythrocytes.

BOX 37-1 Laboratory Tests

Hematocrit is the fraction of the total volume of blood that consists of red blood cells (RBCs), normally about 45%. For example, a value of 46% implies that there are 46 mL of RBCs in 100 mL of blood. The normal hematocrit for males is 40% to 54%. In females a normal hematocrit is 38% to 47%. A low hematocrit indicates anemia that may result from trauma, surgery, internal bleeding, nutritional deficiency (e.g., iron or vitamin B_{12}), bone marrow disease, or sickle cell disease. A high hematocrit may be caused by dehydration, lung disease, certain tumors, and disorders of the bone marrow.

Hemoglobin is reported in grams per 100 mL of blood. The normal hemoglobin for males is 13.5 to 18 g/100 mL. In women a normal hemoglobin is 12 to 16 g/100 mL.

Reticulocyte count offers details about the rate of RBC production. A reticulocyte count of less than 0.5% of the RBC count usually indicates a slowdown in the process of RBC formation. A reticulocyte count greater than 1.5% usually indicates an acceleration of RBC formation.

BOX 37-2 Clotting Measurements

Clotting time is normally 7 to 10 minutes. The patient bleeds if the clotting time is prolonged. The patient develops intravascular clots if the clotting time is less than normal. Prothrombin (PT) time measures the clotting time of plasma (the intrinsic clotting cascade). The PT test is used to monitor patients taking certain medications and to diagnose clotting disorders. The PT test specifically evaluates the presence of factors VIIa, V, and X and of prothrombin and fibrinogen. A drop in the concentration of any of these factors will cause the blood to take longer to clot. A prolonged PT time is considered abnormal. The PT test is used in combination with the partial thromboplastin time (PTT) to screen for hemophilia and other hereditary clotting disorders.

The PTT uses blood to which a chemical has been added to prevent cotting before the test begins. The PTT measures the integrity of the extrinsic clotting cascade, which is affected by blood-thinning medications (e.g., heparin and warfarin). The PTT time can help determine a possible cause of abnormal bleeding or bruising. Increased PTT time in a person with a bleeding disorder may indicate that a clotting factor is missing or defective.

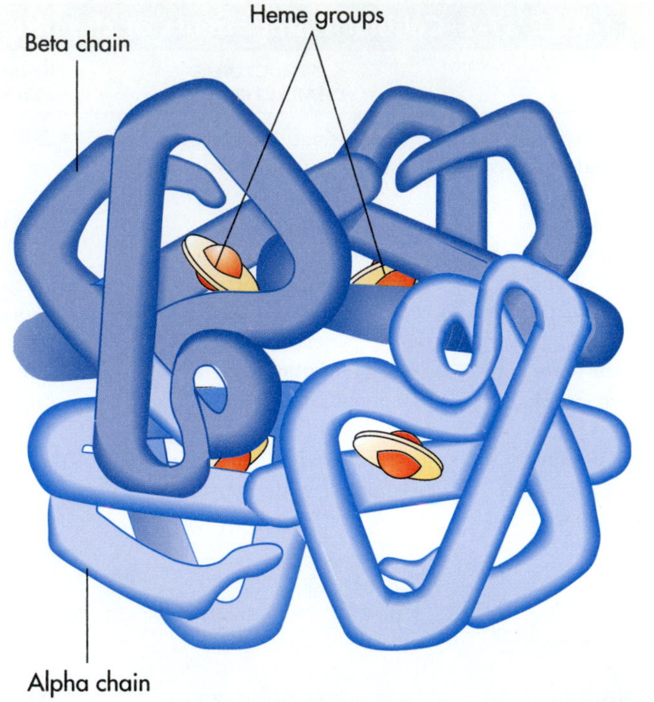

FIGURE 37-3 ■ The four-chained hemoglobin molecule is made from more than 10,000 atoms. Yet when fully laden, the molecule will carry only 4 pairs of oxygen atoms. Hemoglobin is built around 4 atoms of iron that act like oxygen magnets. Each red blood cell holds 300 million of these vital protein molecules.

ditions such as rheumatoid arthritis or inflammatory bowel disease; and persistent infections such as human immunodeficiency virus (HIV). These conditions can cause anemia by interfering with the production of oxygen-carrying RBCs. In the case of cancer and chemotherapy, anemia sometimes can be caused by the treatment itself. Two common forms of anemia are iron deficiency anemia and hemolytic anemia.

IRON DEFICIENCY ANEMIA

Iron is the critical part of a hemoglobin molecule, giving it the ability to bind oxygen (Fig. 37-3). The lack of iron in iron deficiency anemia prevents the bone marrow from making enough hemoglobin for the RBCs. The RBCs produced are small and have a pale center. They also have a reduced oxygen-carrying capacity. The most common cause of iron deficiency anemia in adults is blood loss from menstrual bleeding or intestinal bleeding.[3] A diet that is low in iron usually is the cause of iron deficiency anemia in children. Vitamin deficiencies also can produce anemia. Lack of folic acid (one of the B vitamins) is the most common form of vitamin-deficiency anemia.

CRITICAL THINKING

Can you predict the signs and symptoms of anemia?

HEMOLYTIC ANEMIA

Premature destruction of RBCs in the blood (hemolysis) causes hemolytic anemia. This destruction can result from an inherited disorder inside the RBC. It also can result from a disorder outside the cell. The condition usually is acquired later in life.

Inherited Disorders. Hemolysis can occur as a result of abnormal rigidity of the cell membrane. This rigidity causes the cell to become trapped at an early stage of its life span in the smaller blood vessels (usually of the spleen). In these smaller blood vessels the RBC is destroyed by macrophages. This type of anemia can occur from a genetic defect in the hemoglobin within the cell (e.g., sickle cell anemia and thalassemia). It also can occur from a defect in one of the enzymes in the cell that helps protect the cell from chemical damage during infectious illness. A deficiency of one of the enzymes, glucose-6-phosphate dehydrogenase, is common in African-Americans.

Acquired Disorders. Acquired hemolytic anemia results from one of three conditions:

1. Disorders in which normal RBCs are disrupted as a result of mechanical forces (e.g., abnormal blood vessel linings or blood clots)
2. Autoimmune disorders, which can destroy RBCs with antibodies that are produced by the immune system (e.g., an incompatible blood transfusion)
3. Conditions that can cause hemolytic anemia when RBCs are destroyed by microorganisms in the blood (e.g., malaria).

SIGNS AND SYMPTOMS OF ANEMIA

All forms of anemia share signs and symptoms. These signs and symptoms include fatigue and headaches, sometimes a sore mouth or tongue, brittle nails, and in severe cases, breathlessness and chest pain (Table 37-2). Other patient complaints are related to an abnormal decrease in the num-

TABLE 37-2 Causes, Signs and Symptoms, and Treatment for Specific Forms of Anemia

FORM OF ANEMIA	CAUSES	SIGNS AND SYMPTOMS	TREATMENT
Iron deficiency anemia	Insufficient intake of iron Gastrointestinal disorders (e.g., ulcer disease) External and/or internal bleeding Prolonged aspirin or NSAID therapy Gastrectomy (surgical removal of part or all of the stomach)	Those related to the underlying cause (e.g., bleeding) Those common to all forms of anemia	Correction of the underlying cause Supplemental iron tablets or injections
Hemolytic anemia	Genetic red blood cell disorder Autoimmune disorders Malaria and other infections	Jaundice Those common to all forms of anemia	Splenectomy Immunosuppressant drugs Avoidance of drugs or foods that precipitate hemolysis Antimalarial drugs Blood transfusions

NSAID, Nonsteroidal antiinflammatory drug.

ber of WBCs (leukopenia) or a reduction in platelets (thrombocytopenia) and may include the following:

- Bleeding from mucous membranes
- Cutaneous bleeding
- Fatigue
- Fever
- Lethargy

DIAGNOSIS AND TREATMENT

The patient's signs and symptoms, patient history, and examination of the patient's blood through blood tests and bone marrow biopsy indicate a diagnosis of most forms of anemia. For example, iron deficiency anemia usually reveals RBCs that are smaller than normal. Hemolytic anemia shows RBCs that are immature and abnormally shaped. Treatment should be indicated to correct, modify, or diminish the mechanism or process that is leading to defective RBC production or reduced RBC survival.

▶NOTE A bone marrow biopsy specimen taken from the sternum or pelvis offers details about the various parts of blood. The specimen also provides information about the presence of cells foreign to the marrow. Bone marrow biopsy is useful in diagnosing many hematological disorders such as anemia, leukemia, and certain infections. A bone marrow transplant sometimes is used to treat these and other diseases.

Leukemia

Leukemia refers to any of several types of cancer in which an abnormal proliferation of WBCs usually occurs in the bone marrow (Fig. 37-4). The proliferation of leukemic cells crowds and impairs the normal production of RBCs, WBCs, and platelets. Leukemia is more common in males than in females. Leukemia is also more common in Caucasians than in African-Americans. About 30,000 cases are diagnosed in the United States each year.[4]

The exact cause of leukemia is not known; however, genetics may play a role. Abnormal chromosomes associated with congenital disorders (e.g., Down's syndrome) and HIV-type viruses are associated with a rare form of this disease. Other factors that may play a role in the development of leukemia include exposure to radiation, viral infections, immune defects, and various chemicals in home and work environments.[2]

CLASSIFICATIONS

Leukemia is classified as *acute* or *chronic.* Cancer cells in acute leukemia begin proliferating at an early stage of their development (arrested as immature cells). Chronic leukemia implies an abnormal proliferation of more mature but not fully differentiated cells. Leukemias are classified further according to the type of WBC involved. Two common forms of leukemia are *acute lymphoblastic leukemia* and *acute myeloblastic leukemia.* The first affects mostly children. (It sometimes is called *childhood leukemia.*) The latter affects mostly middle-aged adults. Acute myeloblastic leukemia is one of the most intractable blood cancers. In both types, abnormal WBCs are produced in such large amounts that they eventually accumulate in the vital organs (liver, spleen, lymph, and brain). This impedes the function of these organs and leads to death. Chronic forms of leukemia can develop slowly, often over many years. Cases of disease often are discovered by chance during routine blood analysis.

SIGNS AND SYMPTOMS

The proliferation of leukemic cells or the resulting inadequate production of other normal blood cells makes the patient highly susceptible to serious infections, anemia, and bleeding episodes. Signs and symptoms of leukemia include the following:

- Abdominal fullness
- Bleeding
- Bone pain
- Elevated body temperature and diaphoresis
- Enlargement of lymph nodes
- Enlargement of the liver, spleen, and testes

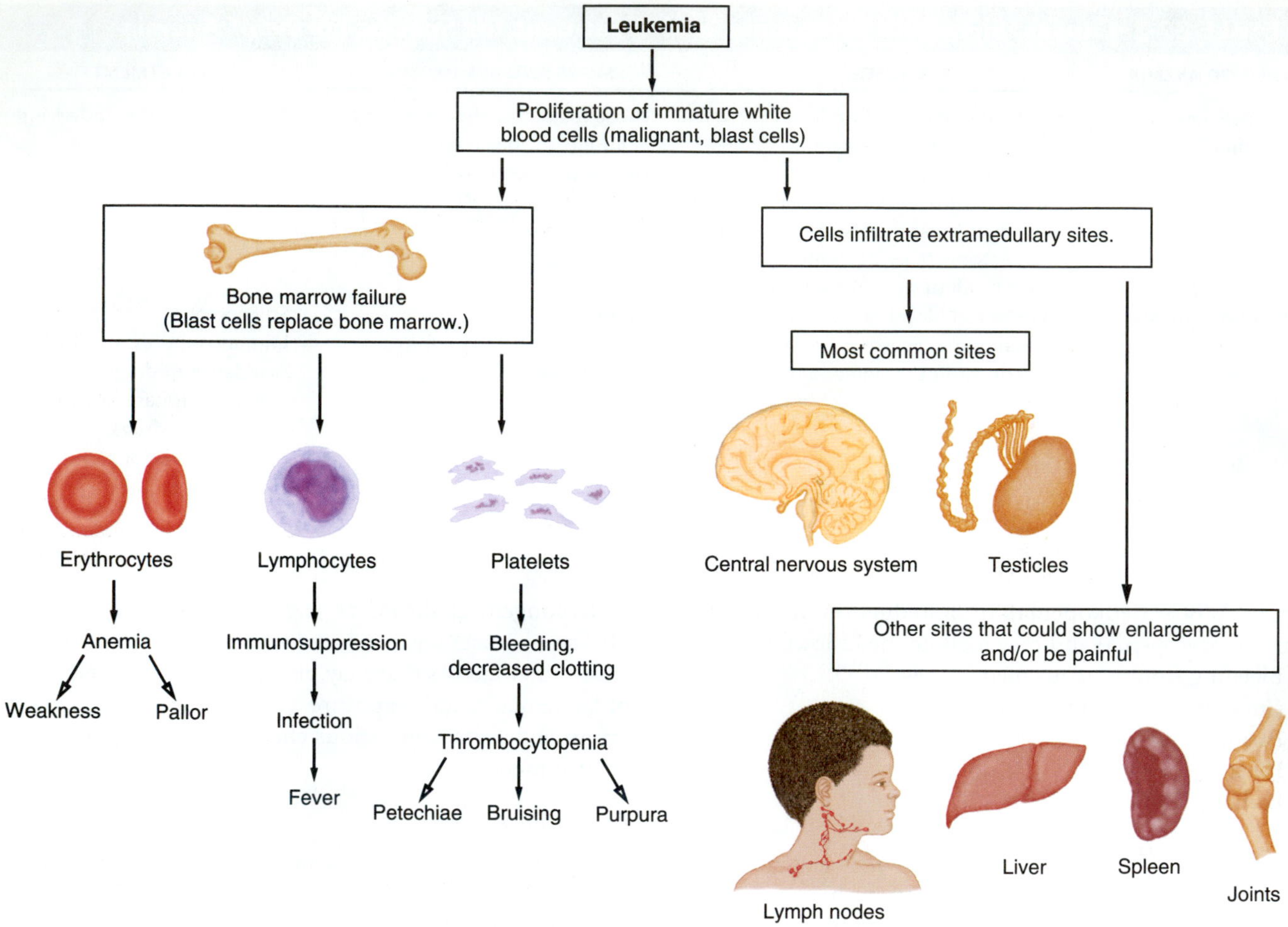

FIGURE 37-4 ■ Pathophysiology of leukemia.

- Fatigue
- Frequent bruising
- Headache
- Heat intolerance
- Night sweats
- Weight loss

CRITICAL THINKING

If a child has a lot of odd bruises, what would you suspect if a diagnosis of leukemia is not known?

DIAGNOSIS AND TREATMENT

The diagnosis of leukemia is confirmed by bone marrow biopsy. The severity of the disease is assessed by the degree of liver and spleen enlargement, anemia, and lack of platelets in the blood. Treatment for acute leukemia can include the transfusion of blood and platelets, antibiotic therapy to manage anemia and infection, and the use of anticancer drugs and sometimes radiation to destroy the leukemic cells. In some cases the leukemia is treated with a bone marrow transplant (Box 37-3). Patients with chronic leukemia can be managed effectively with medication. Many patients require no treatment in its early stages.

Lymphomas

Lymphoma is a general term applied to any neoplastic disorder of the lymphoid tissue. **Hodgkin's disease** is one type; all others, despite their diversity, are called *non-Hodgkin's lymphomas.* All lymphomas are malignant.

HODGKIN'S DISEASE

Hodgkin's disease is characterized by painless, progressive enlargement of lymphoid tissue found mainly in the lymph nodes and spleen (Fig. 37-5). Left unchecked, these cancer cells multiply and eventually displace healthy lymphocytes, suppressing the immune system. Signs and symptoms include swollen lymph nodes in the neck, armpits, or groin; fatigue; chills; and night sweats. Some patients also experience severe itching, persistent cough, weight loss, shortness of breath, and chest discomfort.

Hodgkin's disease is a rare cancer of unknown cause that may have a heritable component. The disease is more common in males than in females, with a peak incidence in persons in their 20s and in persons between 55 and 70

BOX 37-3 Blood and Marrow Stem Cell Transplantation

A *stem cell* is a cell the daughter cells of which may give rise to other cell types. Some cells can develop into several different types of mature cells, including lymphocytes, granulocytes, thrombocytes, and erythrocytes. Stem cells reside in marrow and also circulate in the blood. They also circulate in large numbers in fetal blood. They can be recovered from umbilical cord and placental blood after childbirth. Stem cells can be harvested, frozen, and stored for future transplantation.

Stem cell transplantation is standard therapy for selected patients with leukemia, lymphoma, and myeloma. The two major types of stem cell transplants are *autologous* and *allogenic.* An autologous transplant uses the patient's own marrow. The marrow is collected while the patient is in remission. The marrow may be treated with chemotherapy agents or antibodies to cleanse it of cancer cells that may be present in the marrow before it is given back to the patient. An allogenic transplant uses marrow from a donor. The donor is usually a brother or sister with the same tissue type. If a sibling is not available, a search of bone marrow registries for tissue-typed volunteers can be made for an unrelated donor. In addition to treating some cancers and other blood disorders, stem cells may play a key role in the future in treating diseases such as Alzheimer's, Parkinson's, and heart disease.

Adapted from The Leukemia and Lymphoma Society: Blood and marrow stem cell transplantation. http://www.leukemia-lymphoma.org/all_page?item_id=5965 Accessed January 11, 2004.

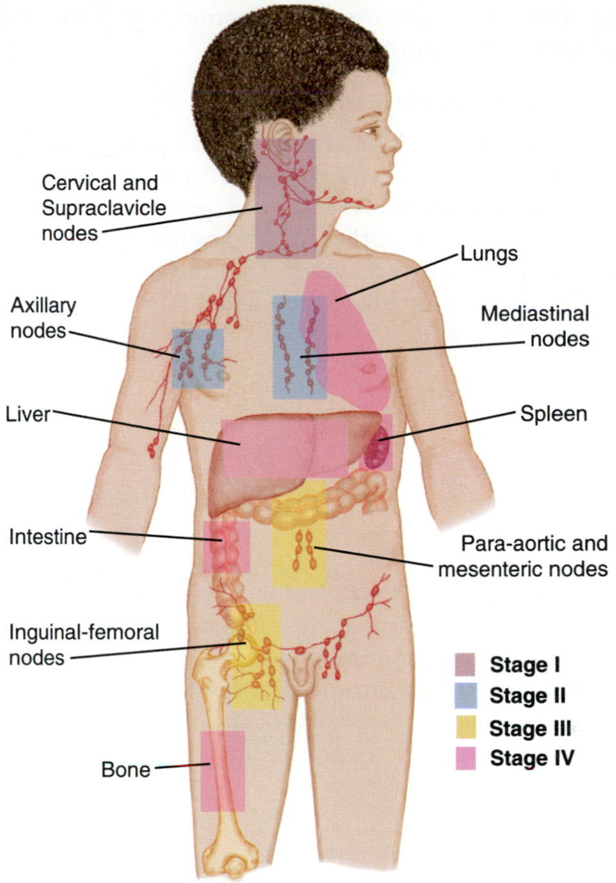

FIGURE 37-5 ■ Pathophysiology of Hodgkin's disease.

years of age.[1] The disease is confirmed by the identification of Reed-Sternberg cells in lymph nodes or organs affected by the cancer. Treatment depends on the level of lymph node and organ system involvement (the *stage* of the disease) and can consist of radiation and chemotherapy with anticancer drugs. Hodgkin's disease is one of the most curable cancers.

NON-HODGKIN'S LYMPHOMAS

Non-Hodgkin's lymphomas vary in their malignancy according to the nature and activity of the abnormal cells. At least 10 types of non-Hodgkin's lymphoma have been identified. Each type is ranked as low, intermediate, or high grade. This ranking is based on how aggressively the disease behaves. Low-grade diseases usually progress slowly. They also tend not to spread beyond the lymphatic system. High-grade diseases can spread to distant organs within a few months. Signs and symptoms include painless swelling of one or more groups of lymph nodes; enlargement of the liver and spleen; fever; and in rare cases, abdominal pain and gastrointestinal bleeding.

The cause of these cancers is largely unknown. One form, Burkitt's lymphoma, is strongly associated with infection by Epstein-Barr virus. This virus commonly is found in Africa. Other types have been linked to infection by HIV-type viruses and other conditions that affect the immune system (e.g., organ transplantation, radiation and chemotherapy, lupus, and rheumatoid arthritis). Treatment consists of radiation therapy, anticancer drugs, and sometimes bone marrow transplantation.

Polycythemia

Polycythemia is an increase in the total RBC mass of the blood. The condition may be a natural response to hypoxia (secondary polycythemia). Polycythemia also may occur for unknown reasons (primary polycythemia). Polycythemia also can result from dehydration (apparent polycythemia). In this instance, the RBC production does not exceed the upper limits of normal.

SECONDARY POLYCYTHEMIA

Secondary polycythemia can be naturally present in persons who live in or visit areas of high altitude. Polycythemia is due to reduced air pressure and low oxygen. When the oxygen supply to the blood is reduced, the kidneys produce the hormone *erythropoietin.* This hormone stimulates RBC production in the bone marrow to make up for the reduced oxygen supply. The result is an increase in the oxygen-carrying efficiency of the blood. The RBC numbers return to normal when the person returns to sea level. Secondary polycythemia also can be present in heavy smokers. The disease can be caused by chronic bronchitis and conditions that increase erythropoietin production (e.g., liver cancer and some kidney disorders).

PRIMARY POLYCYTHEMIA

Primary polycythemia is also known as *polycythemia vera.* Primary polycythemia is a rare disorder of the bone marrow. In this disorder the increased production of RBCs causes the blood to thicken. This condition primarily develops in persons over 50 years of age[2] and can lead to several physiological problems that include the following:

- Blurred vision
- Dizziness
- Generalized itching
- Headache
- Hypertension
- Red hands and feet; red-purple complexion
- Splenomegaly

Other complications associated with primary polycythemia include platelet disorders, which cause bleeding or clot formation; stroke; and the development of other bone marrow diseases (e.g., leukemias). Treatment consists of phlebotomy. (This is the slow removal of blood through a vein.) Treatment also consists of anticancer drug therapy. The therapy controls the overproduction of RBCs in the marrow.

Disseminated Intravascular Coagulopathy

Disseminated intravascular coagulopathy (described in Chapter 21) is a complication of severe injury, trauma, or disease. Disseminated intravascular coagulopathy is a common abnormal clotting disorder. The disease most often is seen in the critical care setting. It disrupts the balance among procoagulants, inhibitors, thrombus formation, and lysis. Signs and symptoms of disseminated intravascular coagulopathy include dyspnea, bleeding, and those associated with hypotension and hypoperfusion.

Disseminated intravascular coagulopathy occurs in two phases.[2] The first phase is characterized by free thrombin in the blood, fibrin deposits, and aggregation of platelets. The second phase is characterized by hemorrhage caused by the depletion of clotting factors. The clinical consequences of these processes predispose the patient to multiple-system organ failure from bleeding and coagulation disorders caused by the following:

- Loss of platelets and clotting factors
- Fibrinolysis
- Fibrin degradation interference
- Small vessel obstruction, tissue ischemia, RBC injury, and anemia from fibrin deposits

Disseminated intravascular coagulopathy is confirmed through laboratory tests. Then the treatment is aimed at reversing the underlying illness or injury that triggered the event. In an effort to control the depletion of clotting factors, in-hospital care includes the replacement of platelets, coagulation factors, and blood. At the same time, attempts are made to manage the primary process.

BOX 37-4 Hereditary Characteristics of Hemophilia

Chromosomes from the mother link with an equal number from the father, and each pair determines the type of information that genes carry. Females have two X chromosomes. Males have an X and a Y chromosome. The mother passes on the X chromosome to her child, and the father passes on an X or a Y. Two X chromosomes produce a female child; an X and a Y produce a male child.

Hemophilia stems from an abnormal gene on the X chromosome. A female with an abnormal X chromosome usually is spared the disease because, although she received one abnormal X chromosome from one parent, the normal X chromosome passed on from her other parent counteracted the abnormal gene. However, she is a carrier of the disease and can pass it on to her children. A woman can have hemophilia only if her mother is a carrier and her father has hemophilia, which is rare. Affected males do not pass the defective gene to sons, but they pass it on to all of their daughters. A male, however, receives only one X chromosome. If his mother is a carrier, the male child will have a 50% chance of having hemophilia.

Hemophilia

Hemophilia means "love of blood." Hemophilia is a group of inherited bleeding disorders (Box 37-4). Hemophilia A is due to a deficiency in factor VIII. This factor is essential to the process of blood clotting (Table 37-3). Another less common form of hemophilia, caused by a deficiency of factor IX, is known as *hemophilia B.* This hemophilia also is known as *Christmas disease* (named for a man first diagnosed with the disease in 1952). All types of hemophilia present with similar problems. Yet the specific factor involved determines the severity of bleeding.

Bleeding from hemophilia can occur spontaneously. It can occur even after minor injury. It also can occur during some medical procedures (e.g., tooth extraction). Hemorrhage can occur anywhere in the body. However, bleeding into joints, deep muscles, the urinary tract, and intracranial sites is the most common. Head trauma is potentially life threatening. Central nervous system bleeding is the major cause of death for patients with hemophilia in all age groups.[4]

Hemophilia is controlled by infusions of concentrates of factor VIII. These infusions can be administered by the patient. However, serious or unusual bleeding often calls for hospitalization. Persons with hemophilia are advised to avoid activities that may increase their risk of injury. These include, for example, contact sports. Most patients with hemophilia are knowledgeable about their disease. Most seek emergency care only when problems and trauma-related issues arise.

TABLE 37-3 Clotting Factors and Synonyms

FACTOR	SYNONYMS
I	Fibrinogen
II	Prothrombin
III	Thromboplastin
IV	Calcium
V	Proaccelerin
VI	None in use
VII	Serum prothrombin conversion accelerator
VIII	Antihemophilic globulin Antihemophilic factor
IX	Plasma thromboplastin component Christmas factor
X	Stuart factor
XI	Plasma thromboplastin antecedent
XII	Hageman factor
XIII	Fibrin-stabilizing factor

CRITICAL THINKING

Imagine that you are caring for a patient with hemophilia who has fallen 15 feet from a ladder. This patient refuses care and transportation. What should you do?

NOTE Factor VIII is made from large pools of donor blood. During the first few years of the acquired immunodeficiency syndrome epidemic, many persons with hemophilia and their sexual partners became infected with human immunodeficiency virus through factor VIII infusions. There are careful screening protocols for blood now. However, infusions still carry a minute risk of transmitting hepatitis B virus, hepatitis C virus, and human immunodeficiency virus to factor VIII recipients. Another factor VIII product, recombinant factor VIII (Recombinate), is produced by inserting cloned factor VIII into animal tissues. Recombinate is not made from human plasma, is the purest form of factor VIII, does not transmit viral contamination, and is as effective as plasma-derived factor VIII.[5]

Sickle Cell Disease

Sickle cell disease is also known as *sickle cell anemia.* Sickle cell disease is a debilitating and unpredictable recessive genetic illness. It affects persons of African descent. (Less often, it affects persons of Mediterranean origin.) One in 12 African-Americans and more than 70,000 Americans of different ethnic origins are estimated to suffer from sickle cell disease. About 1 in 12 African-Americans has *sickle cell trait* (Box 37-5). Signs and symptoms of sickle cell disease include the following:

- Delayed growth, development, and sexual maturation in children
- Jaundice
- Priapism in adolescent and adult males
- Splenomegaly
- Stroke

BOX 37-5 Characteristics of Sickle Cell Trait

A person must inherit two sickle cell genes—one from each parent—to develop sickle cell disease. When only one gene is present, the condition is known as a *sickle cell trait.* Persons with sickle cell trait usually do not experience symptoms except occasionally under low-oxygen conditions (e.g., scuba diving or traveling at high altitudes). However, these persons can pass the gene, and possibly the disease, on to their children. If both parents have sickle cell trait, the child has a 25% chance of developing the disease, a 50% chance of having sickle cell trait, and a 25% chance of having neither. Genetic counseling should be considered for carriers of the disease who plan to become parents. Many states require sickle cell screening of newborns.

PATHOPHYSIOLOGY

Sickle cell disease produces an abnormal type of hemoglobin called *hemoglobin S.* This abnormal type has an inferior oxygen-carrying capacity. When hemoglobin S is exposed to low oxygen states, it crystallizes. This distorts the RBCs into a sickle shape (Fig. 37-6). The sickle-shaped cells are fragile and easily destroyed. They also are unable to pass easily through tiny blood vessels and block flow to various organs and tissues. This causes a vasoocclusive sickle cell crisis that can be life threatening. As fewer RBCs pass through congested vessels, tissues and joints become starved for oxygen and other nutrients. This causes excruciating pain. Other signs and symptoms of sickle cell disease are increased weakness, aching, chest pain with shortness of breath, sudden and severe abdominal pain, bony deformities, icteric (jaundice) sclera (Fig. 37-7), fever, and arthralgia (joint pain) (Fig. 37-8).

CRITICAL THINKING

How do you think a patient with such chronic pain must feel at the beginning of a sickle cell crisis?

Sickle cell crisis can occur in any part of the body and can vary in intensity from one person to the next and from one crisis to the next. Over time the crises can destroy the spleen, kidneys, gallbladder, and other organs. Sickle cell crisis may occur for no apparent reason. It also may be triggered by conditions such as the following:

- Dehydration
- Exposure to extremes in temperature
- Infection
- Lack of oxygen

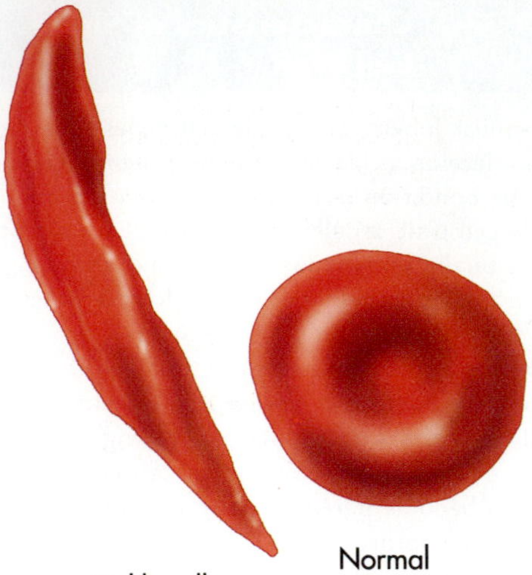

FIGURE 37-6 ■ Sickle cell versus normal erythrocyte.

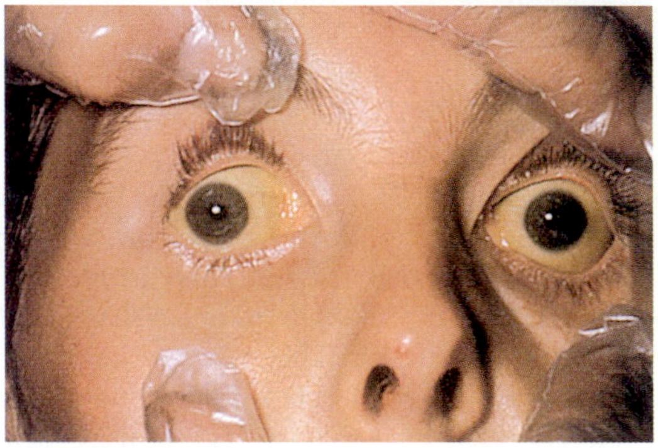

FIGURE 37-7 ■ Jaundice of the sclera.

- Strenuous physical activity
- Stress
- Trauma

Three less common types of sickle cell crisis are aplastic, hemolytic, and splenic sequestration. In aplastic crisis the bone marrow temporarily stops producing RBCs. In hemolytic crisis the RBCs break down too rapidly to be replaced adequately. Splenic sequestration usually is a childhood difficulty that occurs when blood becomes trapped in the spleen. This causes the organ to enlarge and possibly may lead to death.

MANAGEMENT

At this time, no cure exists for sickle cell disease. Because of the eventual damage that occurs to the spleen, patients with sickle cell disease are at increased risk for septicemia if infected by certain types of bacteria. Children with the disease should be current with all immunizations. When in crisis, these patients require prompt treatment with oxygen, intravenous therapy to manage dehydration, antibiotics to manage infection, and analgesics to manage pain. In severe cases a blood transfusion may be indicated to effect a temporary replacement of hemoglobin S. Blood transfusions also can be advised during pregnancy to reduce the risk of a crisis. A crisis can be fatal to the mother and fetus. Transfusions also may be advised before surgery because anesthesia can be hazardous to those with the disease.

Multiple Myeloma

Multiple myeloma is a malignant neoplasm of the bone marrow. The tumor, composed of plasma cells, destroys bone tissue (especially in flat bones). This causes pain, fractures, hypercalcemia, and skeletal deformities. In myeloma the neoplastic cells produce large amounts of protein (M protein) that affect the viscosity of the blood. Masses of coagulated protein can build up within the tissues and impair function. Some patients with this disease die of kidney failure. The kidneys fail because of the buildup of proteins that infiltrate the kidneys and block the renal tubules. In many ways, multiple myeloma resembles leukemia. However, the plasma cell proliferation generally is confined to the bone marrow.

CRITICAL THINKING

Which are the flat bones?

Other disorders associated with multiple myeloma include proteinuria, anemia, weight loss, pulmonary complications from rib fracture, and recurrent infections from suppression of the immune system. Patient complaints associated with multiple myeloma may include weakness, skeletal pain, hemorrhage, hematuria, lethargy, weight loss, and frequent fractures.

Multiple myeloma occurs rarely before 40 years of age and then occurs increasingly with age. The disease is more common in males than in females and may have a heritable component.[1] Multiple myeloma is diagnosed through x-ray films, blood studies, and tumor biopsy. Treatment consists of chemotherapy with anticancer drugs, radiation, plasma exchange, and bone marrow transplantation.

GENERAL ASSESSMENT AND MANAGEMENT OF PATIENTS WITH HEMATOLOGICAL DISORDERS

As stated previously, most patients with hematological disorders are knowledgeable about their disease. Often they call emergency medical services to help manage a "change" in their condition. They also may call to arrange for transportation to an emergency department for physician evaluation. The situations that invoke a call for emergency care vary by patient and disease. Common chief complaints can be classified by body system (Table 37-4).

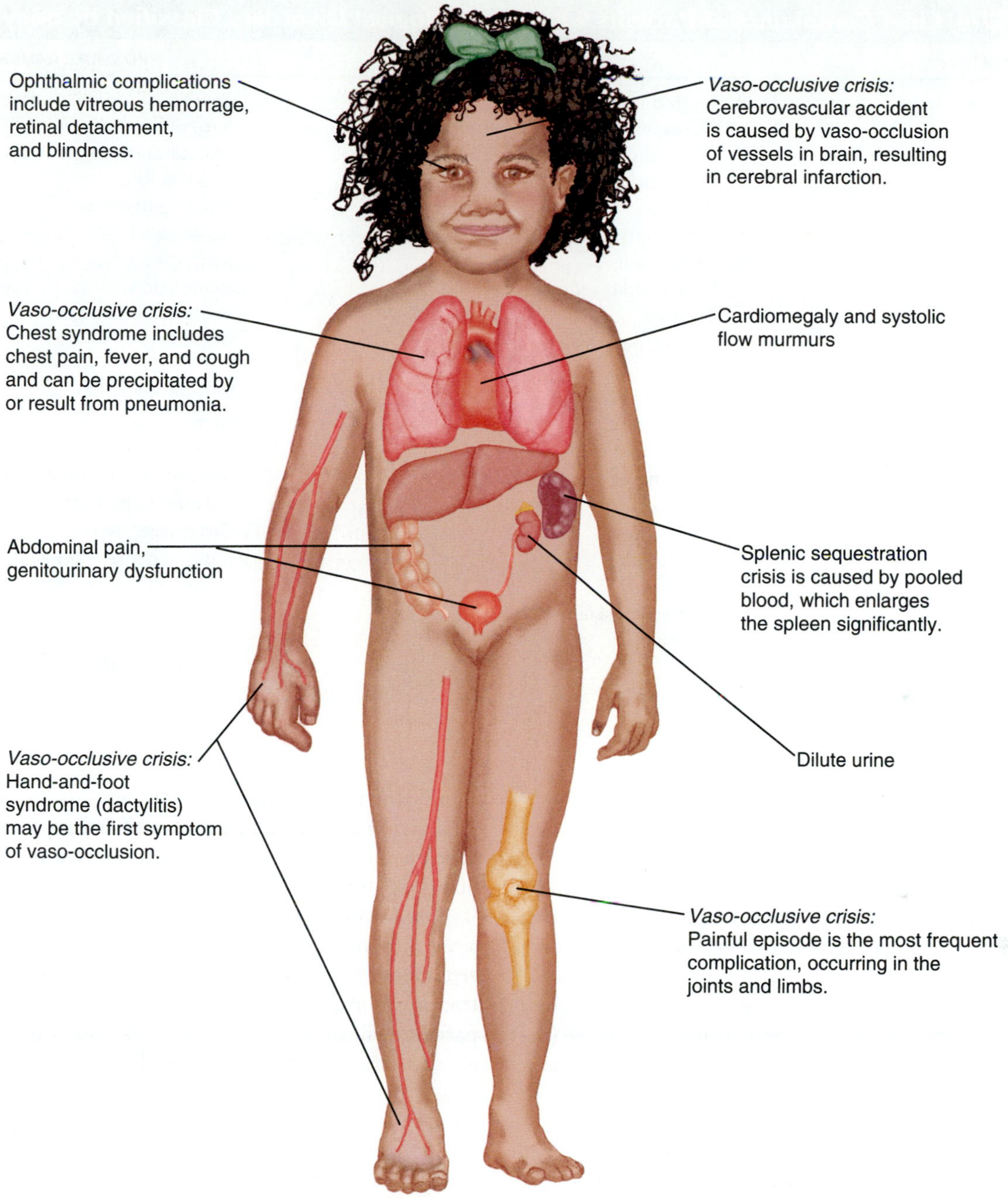
Ophthalmic complications include vitreous hemorrage, retinal detachment, and blindness.
Vaso-occlusive crisis: Cerebrovascular accident is caused by vaso-occlusion of vessels in brain, resulting in cerebral infarction.
Vaso-occlusive crisis: Chest syndrome includes chest pain, fever, and cough and can be precipitated by or result from pneumonia.
Cardiomegaly and systolic flow murmurs
Abdominal pain, genitourinary dysfunction
Splenic sequestration crisis is caused by pooled blood, which enlarges the spleen significantly.
Dilute urine
Vaso-occlusive crisis: Hand-and-foot syndrome (dactylitis) may be the first symptom of vaso-occlusion.
Vaso-occlusive crisis: Painful episode is the most frequent complication, occurring in the joints and limbs.

FIGURE 37-8 ■ Pathophysiology of sickle cell disease.

Prehospital Care

In many cases the prehospital care for a patient with a hematological disorder will be mainly supportive. But as with any other patient care encounter, the paramedic should perform a general assessment, a focused history, and focused physical examination. These measures will guide patient care. They also will help to determine the appropriateness of emergency transport. Some patients with hematological disorders will have complex medical histories. When possible, these patients should be transported to their primary hospital. (This is the hospital where they usually receive their medical care.)

As referenced in Table 37-4, a patient with a hematological disorder may have a variety of complaints and physical findings. Some patient complaints may be vague as well. (Examples include fever, fatigue, and headache.) This can complicate the paramedic's assessment further. After ensuring adequate airway, ventilatory, and circulatory status, the paramedic should assess vital signs and perform a physical examination. The paramedic should assess the patient's skin for color and turgor. The paramedic should note any cyanosis or jaundice, warmth or coolness, bruising, edema, or ulcerations. The paramedic also should ascertain any new onset of fever, weakness, cough, rash,

TABLE 37-4 Chief Complaints of Patients with Hematological Disorders Classified by Body System

BODY SYSTEM	COMPLAINTS	POSSIBLE CAUSES
Central nervous system	Altered level of consciousness	Anemia, sickle cell disease
	Increased weakness, numbness	Autoimmune disease
	Visual disturbances/loss of vision	Unilateral sensory deficits
Cardiorespiratory	Dyspnea/crackles	Heart failure
	Anemia	Bleeding disorders
	Pulmonary edema	Hemoptysis
	Chest pain	Tachycardia
Integumentary	Prolonged bleeding	Hemolytic anemia; polycythemia
	Bruising	Sickle cell disease; liver disease
	Itching/petechiae	Jaundice
	Pallor	
Musculoskeletal	Bone or joint pain	Autoimmune disease
	Fracture	Hemophilia
Gastrointestinal	Abdominal pain	Hemolytic anemia, viral disease
	Bleeding of the gums/gingivitis	Blood-clotting abnormalities
	Epistaxis	Autoimmune disease
		Generalized sepsis
	Ulceration	Melena/hematemesis
Genitourinary	Hematuria	Sickle cell disease, bleeding disorders
	Menorrhagia/amenorrhagia	
	Priapism	Infection
		Sexually transmitted disease

spontaneous bleeding (e.g., bleeding gums, epistaxis), vomiting, or diarrhea. Some hematological disorders can involve the ability of the blood to deliver enough oxygen to tissues. Thus the paramedic should question all patients with hematological disorders specifically about recent dizziness, syncope, difficulty breathing, and heartbeat irregularities.

Other key elements of the patient assessment and history include identifying existing hematological disease (including any family history of hematological disease), any significant medical history or recent injury, the patient's medication use (prescriptions and over-the-counter medications, herbal supplements), allergies, and alcohol or illicit drug use.

Based on the patient's condition, prehospital care measures may include oxygen administration, intravenous fluid replacement, the use of antidysrhythmics, and the administration of analgesics for pain management. Some of these patients will be gravely ill; calming and comfort measures for the patient and family should be provided.

SUMMARY

- Blood is composed of cells and formed elements surrounded by plasma. About 95% of the volume of formed elements consists of RBCs (erythrocytes). The remaining 5% consists of WBCs (leukocytes) and cell fragments (platelets).
- Anemia is a condition in which the amount of hemoglobin or erythrocytes in the blood is below normal. Two common forms of anemia are iron deficiency anemia and hemolytic anemia. All forms of anemia share signs and symptoms. These signs and symptoms include fatigue and headaches, sometimes a sore mouth or tongue, brittle nails, and in severe cases, breathlessness and chest pain. Diagnosis is made by history and from blood tests and bone marrow biopsy.
- *Leukemia* refers to any of several types of cancer in which an abnormal proliferation of WBCs usually occurs in the bone marrow. The proliferation of leukemic cells crowds and impairs the normal production of RBCs, WBCs, and platelets. Leukemia is classified as acute or chronic. The proliferation of leukemic cells makes the patient highly susceptible to serious infections, anemia, and bleeding episodes. The diagnosis is confirmed by bone marrow biopsy.
- *Lymphoma* refers to a group of diseases that range from slowly growing chronic disorders to rapidly evolving acute conditions. Hodgkin's disease is one type; all others are called *non-Hodgkin's lymphomas.*

- Polycythemia is characterized by an unusually large number of RBCs in the blood as a result of their increased production by the bone marrow. Polycythemia may be a natural response to hypoxia. (This is known as secondary polycythemia.) Polycythemia also may occur for unknown reasons. (This is known as primary polycythemia.)
- Disseminated intravascular coagulopathy is a complication of severe injury, trauma, or disease. It disrupts the balance among procoagulants, thrombin formation, inhibitors, and lysis. Signs and symptoms of disseminated intravascular coagulopathy include dyspnea, bleeding, and those associated with hypotension and hypoperfusion. The treatment is aimed at reversing the underlying illness or injury that triggered the event.
- Hemophilia A is caused by a deficiency of a blood protein called *factor VIII.* Hemophilia B is caused by a deficiency of factor IX. Bleeding from hemophilia can occur spontaneously, after even minor injury, or during some medical procedures.
- Sickle cell disease is a debilitating and unpredictable recessive genetic illness. It affects persons of African descent. Less often, it affects persons of Mediterranean origin. Sickle cell anemia produces an abnormal type of hemoglobin. This is called *hemoglobin S.* This abnormal type has an inferior oxygen-carrying capacity. Complications of sickle cell disease include episodes of severe pain, fatigue, pallor, jaundice, stroke, delayed growth, hematuria, priapism, and splenomegaly.
- Multiple myeloma is a malignant neoplasm of the bone marrow. The tumor destroys bone tissue (especially flat bones). This causes pain, fractures, hypercalcemia, and skeletal deformities.
- In many cases of hematological disorders, the prehospital treatment is supportive. Treatment includes ensuring adequate airway, ventilatory, and circulatory support.

REFERENCES

1. McCance KL, Huether SE: *Pathophysiology: the biologic basis for disease in adults and children,* ed 3, St Louis, 1998, Mosby.
2. US Department of Transportation, National Highway Traffic Safety Administration: *EMT-Paramedic national standard curriculum,* Washington, DC, 1998, The Department.
3. Rosen P, Barkin R: *Emergency medicine: concepts and clinical practice,* ed 4, St Louis, 1998, Mosby.
4. *The medical advisor,* Alexandria, Va, 1996, Time-Life Books.
5. Hemophilia Health Services: *About hemophilia,* http://www.accredohealth.net/hhs/hc_pros/about_bleeding/hemophilia.htm. Accessed Feb. 22, 2005.

CHAPTER

38

Environmental Conditions

OBJECTIVES

Upon completion of this chapter, the paramedic student will be able to:

1. Describe the physiology of thermoregulation.
2. Discuss the risk factors, pathophysiology, assessment findings, and management of specific hyperthermic conditions.
3. Discuss the risk factors, pathophysiology, assessment findings, and management of specific hypothermic conditions and frostbite.
4. Discuss the risk factors, pathophysiology, assessment findings, and management of submersion and drowning.
5. Identify the mechanical effects of pressure on the body based on a knowledge of the basic properties of gases.
6. Discuss the risk factors, pathophysiology, assessment findings, and management of diving emergencies and high-altitude illness.

KEY TERMS

acute mountain sickness: A common high-altitude illness that results when an unacclimatized person rapidly ascends to high altitudes.

core body temperature: The temperature of deep structures of the body as compared with the temperatures of peripheral tissues.

decompression sickness: A multisystem disorder that results when nitrogen in compressed air converts back from solution to gas, forming bubbles in the tissues and blood.

drowning: A mortal event in which a submersion victim is pronounced dead at the scene of the attempted resuscitation or within 24 hours after arrival in the emergency department or hospital.

frostbite: A localized injury that results from environmentally induced freezing of body tissues.

heat cramps: Brief, intermittent, and often severe muscular cramps that frequently occur in muscles fatigued by heavy work or exercise.

heat exhaustion: A form of heat illness characterized by minor aberrations in mental status, dizziness, nausea, headache, and a mild to moderate increase in the core body temperature.

heat stroke: A syndrome that occurs when the thermoregulatory mechanisms normally in place to meet the demands of heat stress break down entirely. As a result, the body temperature increases to extreme levels. Multisystem tissue damage and physiological collapse also occur.

high-altitude cerebral edema: The most severe form of acute high-altitude illness. It is characterized by a progression of global cerebral signs in the presence of acute mountain sickness.

high-altitude pulmonary edema: A high-altitude illness thought to be caused at least partly by an increase in pulmonary artery pressure that develops in response to hypoxia.

nitrogen narcosis: An illness associated with scuba diving in which nitrogen becomes dissolved in solution as a result of greater than normal atmospheric pressure; also known as rapture of the deep.

submersion: An incident in which a person experiences some swimming-related distress that is sufficient to require support in the prehospital setting and transportation to a medical facility for further observation and treatment.

thermogenesis: The production of heat, especially by the cells of the body.

thermolysis: The dissipation of heat by means of radiation, evaporation, conduction, or convection.

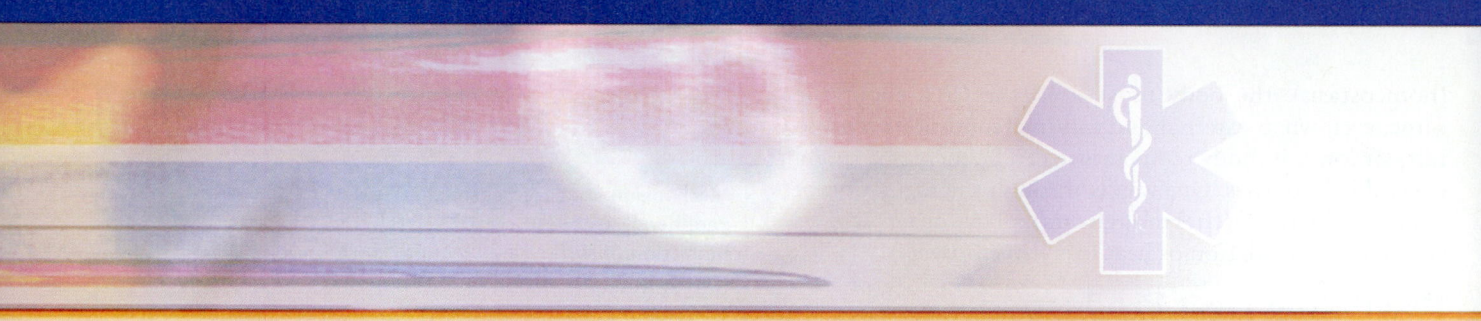

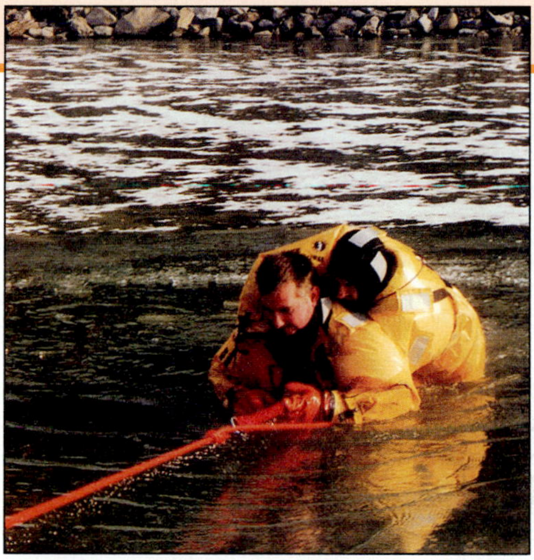

Exposure to elements in the environment can produce many types of emergencies. Paramedics must be ready to recognize and manage these conditions. They can do this by becoming knowledgeable about the causative factors and by learning the pathophysiology of specific disorders.

THERMOREGULATION

A temperature center in the brain regulates body temperature. This center is located in the posterior hypothalamus. It receives information from other areas of the brain (central thermoreceptors). It also receives information from the skin and some mucous membranes (peripheral thermoreceptors). Peripheral thermoreceptors are nerve endings usually categorized as cold receptors and warm receptors. Cold receptors are stimulated by low skin temperatures. Warm receptors are stimulated by high skin temperatures. Information from these receptors is transmitted by the spinal cord to the posterior hypothalamus. The posterior hypothalamus responds with appropriate signals to help the body reduce heat loss and increase heat production (cold receptor stimulation) or increase heat loss and reduce heat production (warm receptor stimulation).

CRITICAL THINKING

The body has many more cold receptors than heat receptors. Why do you think this is so?

Central thermoreceptors are neurons that are sensitive to changes in temperature. These neurons react directly to changes in the temperature of the blood. They send messages to the skeletal muscle through the central nervous system (CNS). They affect vasomotor tone, sweating, and the metabolic rate through sympathetic nerve output to skin arterioles, sweat glands, and the adrenal medulla.

As discussed in Chapter 11, the thermoregulatory center has a built-in set point. This maintains a relatively constant **core body temperature** (CBT) of 98.6° F (37° C). To maintain the best environment for normal cell metabolism (homeostasis), the body must keep the CBT about the same, even when external and internal conditions tend to raise or lower it. Body temperature can be increased or decreased in two ways. One way is through the regulation of heat production **(thermogenesis).** The other way is through the regulation of heat loss **(thermolysis).**

Regulating Heat Production

The body can generate heat in response to cold. It does this through mechanical, chemical, metabolic, and endocrine activities. Several physiological and biochemical factors affect the direction and magnitude of these compensatory responses. Such factors include the person's age, general health, and nutritional status.

Heat is produced by cellular metabolism (oxidation of energy sources). Every tissue contributes to this type of heat production. Skeletal muscles produce the largest amount of heat, particularly when shivering occurs. Shivering is often associated with chattering of the teeth. Along with shivering, vasoconstriction occurs to conserve as much heat as possible. Shivering is the body's best defense against cold. It can increase heat production by as much as 400%.

CRITICAL THINKING

What fuels does the body need to increase heat production through the mechanism of shivering?

Endocrine glands also regulate heat production. They do this through the release of hormones from the thyroid gland and adrenal medulla. An increase in the activity of sympathetic nerves that lead to adipose tissue increases the basal metabolic rate. This results in an increase in heat production. Box 38-1 presents examples of ways the body regulates heat production.

BOX 38-1 Compensatory Mechanisms for Regulating Heat Production

Mechanisms that Decrease Heat Loss
Peripheral vasoconstriction
Reduction of surface area by body position (or clothing)
Piloerection (not effective in humans)

Mechanisms that Increase Heat Production
Shivering
Increased voluntary activity
Increased hormone secretion
Increased appetite

Regulating Heat Loss

Heat is lost from the body to the external environment through the skin, lungs, and excretions. The skin is the most important of these in regulating heat loss. Radiation, conduction, convection, and evaporation are the major mechanisms of heat loss (Fig. 38-1).

The surface of the human body constantly emits heat in the form of infrared rays. If the surface of the body is warmer than the environment, heat is lost through *radiation* (thermal gradient).

Conduction is the exchange of heat that occurs simply by transfer. Heat moves from a higher temperature to a lower temperature. Thus the body surface loses or gains heat by direct contact with cooler or warmer surfaces, including air. If the ambient air temperature is lower than the skin temperature, body heat is lost to the surrounding air by conduction.

Convection is the process by which air or water next to the body is heated, moves away, and is replaced by cool air or water. The cool air or water repeats the process. Convection can be greatly aided by external forces such as wind or fans. It promotes conductive heat exchange by continuously maintaining a supply of cool air. Factors that contribute to the cooling effects of convection are the velocity of air currents and the temperature of the air. The windchill chart (Table 38-1) calculates the cooling effects of the ambient temperature based on thermometer readings and wind speed.

CRITICAL THINKING

How does wearing the fully enclosed hazardous materials suit affect your body's ability to regulate temperature?

When fluid evaporates, it absorbs heat from surrounding objects and air. The temperature of the surrounding air and the relative humidity greatly affect the amount of heat lost as a result of *evaporation* of moisture from the skin or the respiratory tract. The relative humidity is 100% when the air is fully saturated with moisture. Sweating can markedly increase evaporative heat loss so long as the humidity is low enough to allow the sweat to evaporate. At humidity levels above 75%, evaporation decreases. At levels approaching 90%, evaporation essentially ceases. Box 38-2 presents other examples of ways the body regulates heat loss.

External Environmental Factors

Some factors in the environment contribute to a medical emergency. They also may affect rescue and transport. These elements include the climate, season, weather, atmospheric pressure, and terrain. When the potential for an environmental emergency exists, the paramedic must consider the following factors:

- Localized prevailing weather norms and any deviations
- Characteristics of seasonal variation in climate
- Weather extremes (wind, rain, snow, humidity)
- Barometric pressure (e.g., at altitude or under water)
- Terrain that can complicate injury or rescue

The patient's health also is a factor related to environmental stressors. It can make other medical or traumatic conditions worse. Examples include the patient's age, predisposing medical conditions, use of prescription and over-the-counter medications, use of alcohol or recreational drugs, and previous rate of exertion.

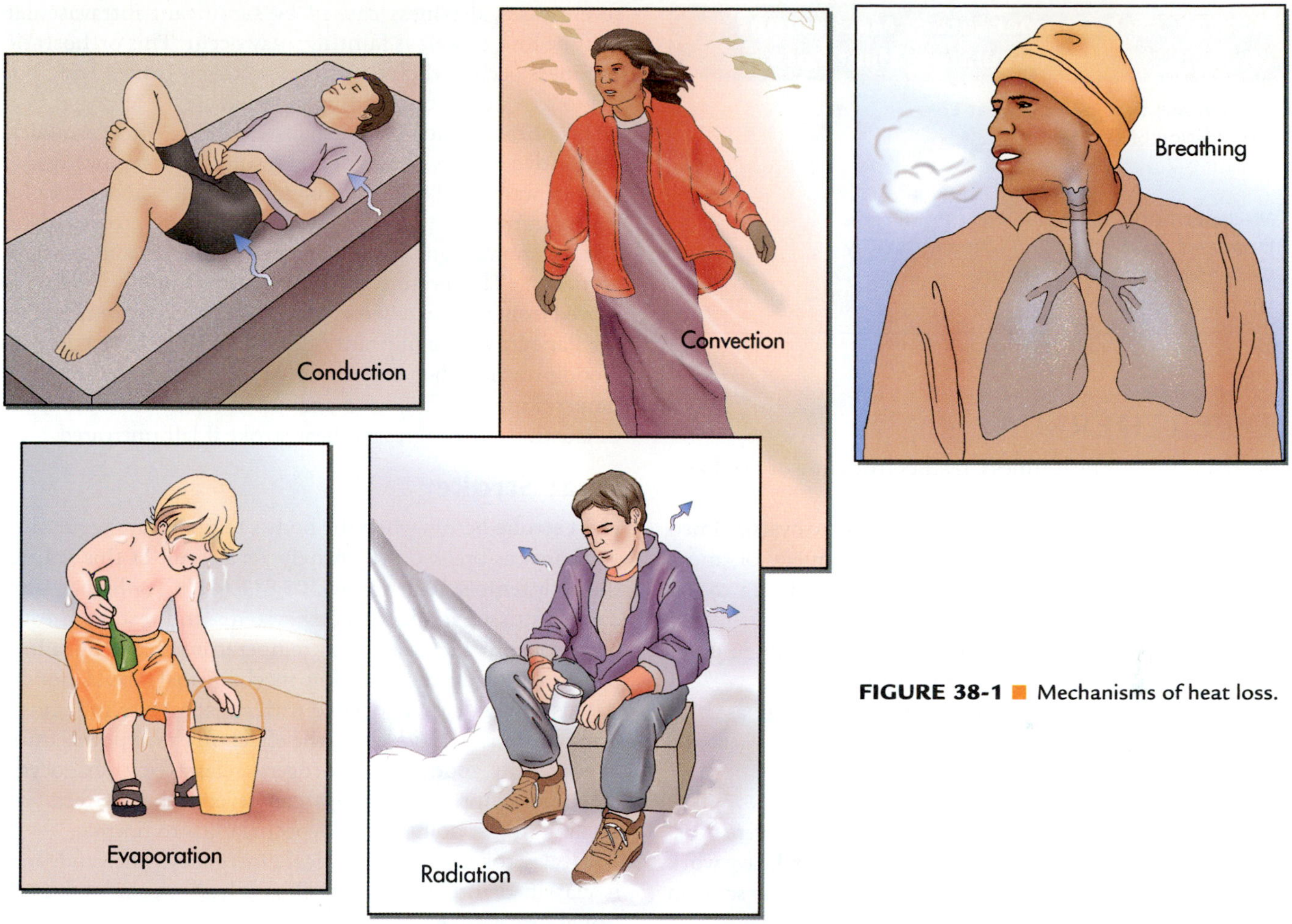

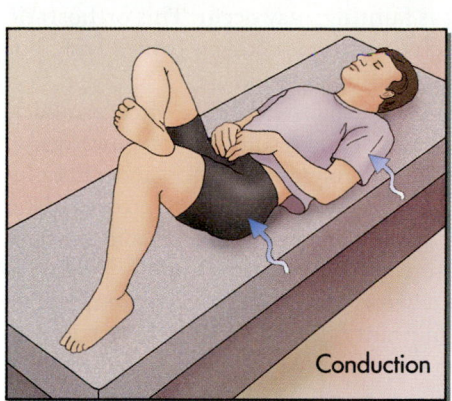

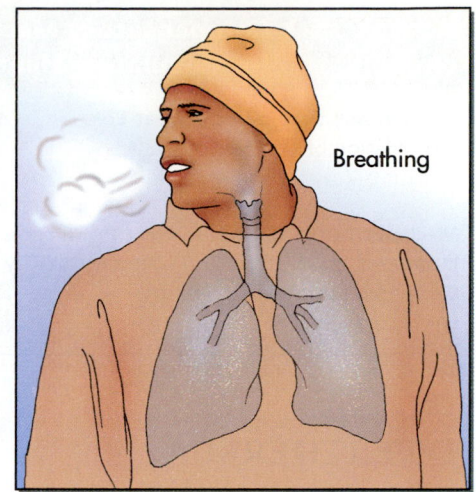

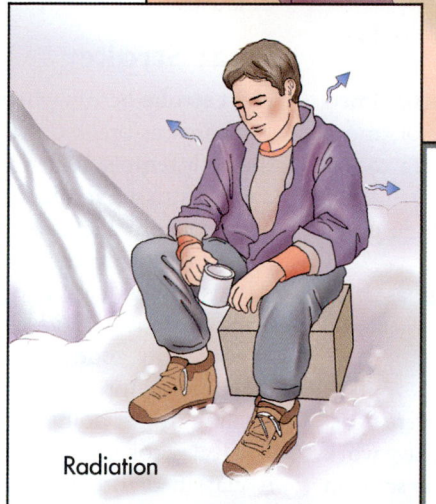

FIGURE 38-1 ■ Mechanisms of heat loss.

TABLE 38-1 Cooling Power of Wind on Exposed Flesh Expressed as an Equivalent Temperature (under Calm Conditions)

ESTIMATED WIND SPEED (MPH)	ACTUAL THERMOMETER READING (°F) 50	40	30	20	10	0	−10	−20	−30	−40	−50	−60
	EQUIVALENT WINDCHILL TEMPERATURE (°F)											
Calm	50	40	30	20	10	0	−10	−20	−30	−40	−50	−60
5	48	37	27	16	6	−5	−15	−26	−36	−47	−57	−68
10	40	28	16	4	−9	−24	−33	−46	−58	−70	−83	−95
15	36	22	9	−5	−18	−32	−45	−58	−72	−85	−99	−112
20	32	18	4	−10	−25	−39	−53	−67	−82	−96	−110	−124
25	30	16	0	−15	−29	−44	−59	−74	−88	−104	−118	−133
30	28	13	−2	−18	−33	−48	−63	−79	−94	−109	−125	−140
35	27	11	−4	−21	−35	−51	−62	−82	−98	−113	−129	−145
40	26	10	−6	−21	−37	−53	−69	−85	−100	−116	−132	−148
Winds speeds >40 mph have little additional effect.	Little danger. In >5 hours with dry skin. Most serious danger is false sense of security.				Increasing danger. Exposed flesh may freeze within 1 minute.			Great danger. Flesh may freeze within 30 seconds.				
	Trench foot and immersion foot can occur at any point on this chart.											

From Sheehy S: *Emergency nursing,* ed 3, St Louis, 1992, Mosby.
Measure local temperature and wind speed if possible. If not, *estimate.* Enter table at closest 5° interval along the top and at appropriate wind speed along the left side. The intersection of these two values gives the approximate equivalent chill temperature (i.e., the temperature that would cause the same rate of cooling under calm conditions). Note that regardless of the cooling rate, the body does not cool below the actual air temperature unless the person is wet.

BOX 38-2 Compensatory Mechanisms for Regulating Heat Loss

Mechanisms that Increase Heat Loss
Vasodilation of skin vessels
Sweating

Mechanisms that Decrease Heat Production
Decreased muscle tone and voluntary activity
Decreased hormone secretion
Decreased appetite

HYPERTHERMIA

Hyperthermia, or heat illness, results from one of two basic causes:

1. Temperature-regulating mechanisms are overwhelmed by high temperatures in the environment or, more commonly, by excessive exercise in moderate to extremely high temperatures.
2. Temperature-regulating centers fail, usually in older adults or in ill or incapacitated patients.

Either cause can result in heat illness such as heat cramps, heat exhaustion, and heat stroke.

Heat Cramps

Heat cramps are brief, intermittent, and often severe muscular cramps that occur in muscles fatigued by heavy work or exercise. The primary cause of these cramps is sodium and water loss.

People who suffer from heat cramps sweat profusely and drink water without adequate salt. During times of high environmental temperatures, 1 to 3 L of water per hour can be lost through sweating. Each liter contains 30 to 50 mEq of sodium chloride. The water and sodium deficiency together cause muscle cramping. This normally occurs in the most heavily exercised muscles, including the calves and arms, although any muscle can be involved. The patient is usually alert, has hot, sweaty skin, tachycardia, and a normal blood pressure. The CBT is normal.

Heat cramps are easily managed. The patient should be removed from the hot environment. Also, sodium and water should be replaced. In more serious cases, medical direction may recommend intravenous (IV) infusion of a balanced sodium chloride solution. Oral salt additives (e.g., salt tablets) can cause gastrointestinal irritation, ulceration, and vomiting. This worsens the electrolyte imbalance. Paramedics should follow local protocol with regard to providing a salt-containing beverage (e.g., Gatorade and PowerAde) to help rehydrate patients.

Heat Exhaustion

Heat exhaustion is a more severe form of heat illness. It is characterized by changes in mental status (e.g., irritability and poor judgment), dizziness, nausea, headache, and mild to moderate elevation of the CBT (up to 103° F [39° C]). In severe cases, dizziness caused by significant intravascular volume loss, as well as fainting, may occur. This orthostatic dizziness occurs when the patient changes from a lying position to a sitting or standing position.

Like heat cramps, heat exhaustion more often is associated with a hot environment and results in profuse sweating. Loss of water and salt, electrolyte imbalance, and difficulty maintaining blood pressure contribute to the problem. The patient shows signs of inadequate peripheral and cerebral perfusion. The person usually recovers rapidly when removed from the hot environment and given replacement fluids. Patients with significant fluid loss or who show a drop in blood pressure when they sit up or stand may require IV administration of a balanced sodium chloride solution. Heat exhaustion can progress to heat stroke if left untreated.

Heat Stroke

Heat stroke occurs when the body's temperature-regulating mechanisms break down entirely. As a result of this failure, the body temperature rises to 105.8° F (41° C) or higher. This damages tissue in all the body systems and results in total body collapse. Increased body temperature caused by failure of the temperature-regulating mechanisms should not be confused with fever associated with a response to inflammation or infection. With fever, the effect on the hypothalamus is caused by endogenous pyrogens released by phagocytic leukocytes. Antipyretic drugs can reverse these effects, returning the set point of the hypothalamus to normal.

Heat stroke is a true medical emergency. The syndrome is classified into two types: classic heat stroke and exertional heat stroke.

Classic heat stroke occurs during periods of sustained high ambient temperatures and humidity. The illness commonly affects the young, older adults, and those who live in poorly ventilated homes without air conditioning. An example is a young child left in an enclosed car on a hot afternoon. Another example is an older person confined to a hot room during a heat wave. Victims of classic heat stroke also often suffer from chronic diseases. Some of these include diabetes, heart disease, alcoholism, or psychiatric disorders. These diseases predispose the individual to the syndrome. Many patients who are susceptible to classic heat stroke take prescribed medications for other conditions. These may include diuretics, antihypertensives, psychotropics (antipsychotics, antihistamines, phenothiazines), and anticholinergics. These drugs further impair a person's ability to tolerate heat stress. In these patients the illness develops from poor dissipation of environmental heat.

NOTE The autoimmune neuropathy associated with diabetes can interfere with vasodilation, perspiration, and thermoregulatory input. Some cardiac drugs (e.g., diuretics and beta blockers) can predispose a patient to dehydration, can interfere with vasodilation, and can reduce the body's ability to increase the heart rate in response to a volume loss.

In contrast to patients with classic heat stroke, patients with *exertional heat stroke* are usually young and healthy.

Athletes and military recruits who exercise in the heat and humidity often are affected. In these situations, heat builds up more rapidly in the body than it can be dispersed into the environment. Preventive measures to reduce the risk of exertional heat illness for all age groups include the following:

- Avoiding or limiting exercise in hot environments
- Maintaining an adequate fluid intake
- Achieving acclimatization, which results in more perspiration with a lower salt concentration, thereby increasing fluid volume in the body

CLINICAL MANIFESTATIONS

As described previously, the temperature-regulating centers in the brain receive their information largely from the temperature of circulating blood in the deep and superficial veins and from the skin. In response to hypothalamic stimulation, a number of physiological events occur: (1) the respiratory rate quickens to increase heat loss through exhaled air; (2) cardiac output increases to provide more blood flow through skin and muscle to enhance heat radiation; and (3) sweat gland activity increases to enhance evaporative heat loss. These compensatory mechanisms require a normally functioning CNS to properly respond to the temperature extreme. They also require a working cardiovascular system to move excess heat from the core to the surface of the body. Problems in either or both of these systems lead to a rapidly increasing CBT.

Central Nervous System Manifestations. The CNS manifestations of heat stroke vary. Some patients may be in frank coma. Others may show confusion and irrational behavior before collapse. Convulsions are common. They can occur early or late in the course of the illness. Because the brain stores little energy, it depends on a constant supply of oxygen and glucose. Decreased cerebral perfusion pressure results in cerebral ischemia and acidosis. Increased temperatures markedly increase the metabolic demands of the brain as well. The extent of brain damage depends on the severity and duration of the hyperthermic episode. Fever from illness (e.g., infection) and an increased CBT from heat stroke produce similar symptoms, especially in the central nervous system. The paramedic should obtain a thorough history (if available) so as to distinguish between the two syndromes. If unsure of the cause, the paramedic should treat the patient for heat stroke.

> **CRITICAL THINKING**
>
> What other conditions can demonstrate the types of mental status changes seen with heat stroke?

Cardiovascular Manifestations. A rise in skin temperature reduces the thermal gradient between the core and the skin. This causes an increase in skin blood flow (peripheral vasodilation), which gives the skin a flushed appearance. About 25% of victims of exertional heat stroke have persistent sweating, which results from increased release of catecholamines. In classic heat stroke, sweating usually is absent. This is due to dehydration, drug use that impairs sweating, direct thermal injury to sweat glands, or sweat gland fatigue. Therefore the presence of sweating does not rule out the diagnosis. Also, the cessation of sweating is not the cause of heat stroke.

Peripheral vasodilation results in decreased vascular resistance and shunting as the illness progresses. High-output cardiac failure is common. It is manifested by extreme tachycardia and hypotension. Cardiac output initially can be four to five times normal. However, as temperatures continue to rise, myocardial contractility begins to decrease. Also, the central venous pressure rises. In any age group, the presence of hypotension and decreased cardiac output points to a poor prognosis.

Other Systemic Manifestations. Other systemic manifestations associated with heat stroke include pulmonary edema (accompanied by systemic acidosis, tachypnea, hypoxemia, and hypercapnia), myocardial dysfunction, gastrointestinal bleeding, a reduction in renal function (secondary to hypovolemia and hypoperfusion), hepatic injury, clotting disorders, and electrolyte abnormalities.

MANAGEMENT

Heat stroke almost invariably leads to death if left untreated. The factors most important to a successful outcome are initiation of basic life support (BLS) and advanced life support (ALS) measures, rapid recognition of the heat illness, and rapid cooling of the patient. After ensuring an adequate airway and ventilatory and circulatory support, the paramedic should manage the patient with heat stroke as follows:

1. Move the patient to a cool environment. Remove all the patient's clothing. If available, use hyperthermic thermometers (e.g., rectal probes) to monitor the CBT. Take and record the temperature at least every 5 minutes during the cooling process. This ensures adequate rates of cooling. It also helps to prevent inadvertent (rebound) hypothermia. Rebound hypothermia can best be avoided by stopping the cooling measures when the patient's CBT reaches about 102° F (39° C).
2. Begin cooling by fanning the patient while keeping the skin wet. Continue lowering the body temperature by this method en route to the hospital. If transport is delayed, complete immersion or spraying tepid water (60° F [16° C]) over the body surface is recommended. Avoid submersion in ice water or cold water cooling. These methods can lead to shivering, frank shaking, peripheral vasoconstriction, and convulsions, which act to increase the CBT as the body temperature is lowered.
3. If hypovolemia is present, give the patient an initial fluid challenge of 500 mL over 15 minutes. In most patients the blood pressure rises to a normal range during the cooling process. This occurs as large volumes of blood from the skin move back to the central circulation. Rapid cooling directly improves cardiac output. Be very cautious with fluid replacement. Also, closely monitor the patient for signs of fluid overload. The administra-

tion of too much fluid can cause pulmonary edema, especially in older adults.

4. Administer medications as prescribed by medical direction. Depending on the patient's status and response to cooling methods, these drugs may include ***diazepam*** or ***lorazepam*** for sedation and seizure control, ***mannitol*** to promote renal blood flow and diuresis, and glucose to manage hypoglycemia.

HYPOTHERMIA

Hypothermia (CBT less than 95° F [35° C]) can result from a decrease in heat production, an increase in heat loss, or a combination of these two processes.

Hypothermia can have metabolic, neurological, traumatic, toxic, and infectious causes. However, it most often is seen in cold climates and in exposure to extremely cold conditions in the environment. Failure to recognize and properly treat hypothermia can increase the rate of morbidity and mortality.

Pathophysiology

Exposure to cold produces a chain of events in the body aimed at conserving core heat. Initially, immediate vasoconstriction in the peripheral vessels occurs. At the same time, the rate of metabolism by the CNS increases. The blood pressure and the heart and respiratory rates also increase dramatically. As cold exposure continues, muscle tone increases. The body generates heat in the form of shivering. Shivering continues until the CBT reaches about 86° F (30° C), glucose or glycogen is depleted, or insulin is no longer available for glucose transfer. When shivering stops, cooling is rapid. A general decline then begins in the function of all body systems.

With continued cooling, respirations decline slowly; the pulse rate and blood pressure decrease; the blood pH drops; and significant electrolyte imbalances emerge. Hypovolemia can develop from a shift of fluid out of the vascular space, with increased loss of fluid through urination (cold diuresis). After early tachycardia, progressive bradycardia develops. This often does not respond to ***atropine.*** Significant electrocardiograph (ECG) changes occur. These include prolonged PR, QRS, and QT intervals; obscure or absent P waves; and ST-segment and T-wave abnormalities. In addition, the J point (Osborn wave) may be present at the junction of the QRS complex and ST segment (see Chapter 29) (Fig. 38-2). These events generally are followed by cardiac and respiratory arrest as the CBT approaches 68° F (20° C).

The progression of clinical signs and symptoms of hypothermia is divided into three classes based on the CBT[1]: mild, moderate, and severe. Mild hypothermia is classified as a CBT between 93.2° and 96.8° F (34° and 36° C); moderate hypothermia as a CBT between 86° and 93° F (30° and 34° C); and severe hypothermia as a CBT below 86° F (30° C). The signs and symptoms of the three classes of hypothermia are listed in Table 38-2.

Those at increased risk for developing accidental hypothermia are outdoor enthusiasts (e.g., campers, hikers, hunters, and fishermen), older adults, the very young, and individuals with concurrent medical or psychiatric illness. Thermoregulatory mechanisms also can be impaired by

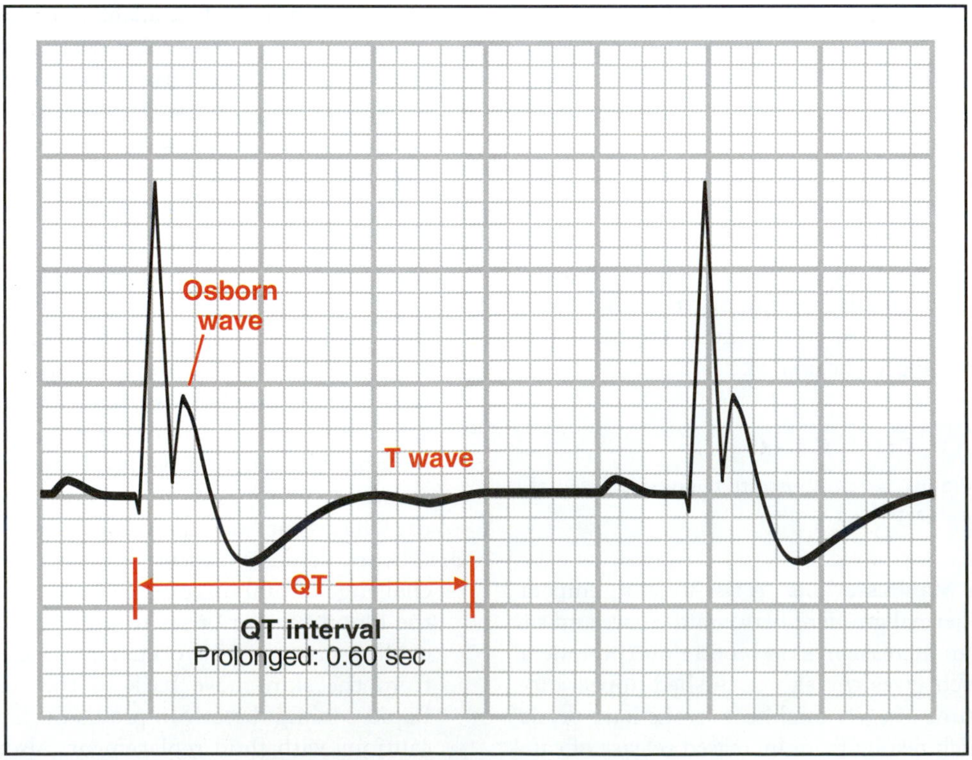

FIGURE 38-2 ■ Osborn wave of hypothermia.

brain damage caused by trauma, hemorrhage, hypoxia, and CNS depression from drug overdose or intoxicants. Drugs known to impair thermoregulation include alcohol, antidepressants, antipyretics, phenothiazines, sedatives, and various pain medicines (including ***aspirin***, acetaminophen, and nonsteroidal antiinflammatory drugs [NSAIDs]). Acid-base imbalances, such as those that occur during ketoacidosis, also can affect the body's ability to stabilize body temperature. This occurs when the imbalances cause a decrease in heat production or an increase in heat loss.

CRITICAL THINKING

What group of people is especially vulnerable to hypothermia as a result of their environmental, medical, and social situation?

Management

The first step in managing hypothermia is to maintain a high degree of suspicion for its presence. When the exposure is obvious (e.g., a victim involved in an avalanche or cold water immersion), diagnosis is simple. However, in some situations the signs and symptoms may be subtle (e.g., hunger, nausea, chills, and dizziness). When hypothermia is suspected, the paramedic's first action is to extricate and evacuate the patient to a site of warm shelter. Then, the paramedic should remove any cold, wet clothing the patient may be wearing; prevent any further drop in the CBT; survey for traumatic injuries; cover the patient with warm blankets and raise the temperature in the ambulance; and rapidly transport the patient for definitive care. Fig. 38-3 presents a treatment algorithm for hypothermia.

MILD TO MODERATE HYPOTHERMIA

In mild to moderate cases of hypothermia, removal of the victim from the cold environment and passive rewarming may be all that is needed to manage the cold exposure. The paramedic can accomplish this by removing wet clothing. (Wet clothes allow five times as much heat loss as dry clothes.) The paramedic then should wrap the victim in a dry blanket to prevent further chilling and to help retain body heat. If the victim is conscious, warm drinks and sugar sources can support a gradual rise in the CBT. These also can help correct any dehydration. The patient should not be given any alcoholic beverages. Alcoholic beverages cause peripheral vasodilation and increase heat loss from the skin. Beverages with caffeine also should not be given, because they cause vasoconstriction and diuresis. Patients with mild to moderate hypothermia may be lethargic and somewhat dulled mentally. Generally, though, they are oriented and show no marked mental derangements.

These patients can be safely and effectively rewarmed with hot packs. The packs should be covered with towels to prevent burns. They then can be applied to the neck, armpits, and groin. IV fluid therapy may be warranted to correct a drop in blood pressure caused by heat-stimulated peripheral vasodilation. If possible, the paramedic should administer heated, humidified oxygen. Patients with mild to moderate hypothermia usually improve rapidly with proper treatment. However, close monitoring and transport to the hospital for evaluation by a physician are indicated.

MODERATE TO SEVERE HYPOTHERMIA

With moderate to severe hypothermia (a CBT below 90° F [32° C]), changes in consciousness are almost always present. They include disorientation, confusion, and lethargy proceeding to stupor and coma. Patients with moderate to severe hypothermia usually have lost the ability to shiver. The loss of muscle coordination makes them unable to perform important tasks.

The management of patients with moderate to severe hypothermia begins with ensuring an adequate airway, providing ventilatory and circulatory support, and maintaining body temperature. These patients should not be allowed to move about independently. They also should be not allowed to exert themselves physically. Even minor physical activity can bring about dysrhythmias, including ventricular fibrillation. Moderate hypothermia is managed with external heat application (e.g., heat packs, heat guns, and heat lights); administration of heated, humidified oxygen; IV fluid therapy (warmed, if possible); and rapid, gentle transport for definitive care. Careful monitoring of the patient's mental status, ECG, and vital functions is imperative. Low-reading thermometers (e.g., tympanic membrane sensors, rectal probes), if available, can be used to

TABLE 38-2 Progression of Clinical Signs and Symptoms of Hypothermia

CLASSIFICATION	CORE BODY TEMPERATURE	SIGNS AND SYMPTOMS
Mild	96.8° F (36° C) 93.2° F (34° C)	Increased metabolic rate, maximum shivering, thermogenesis Impaired judgment, slurred speech
Moderate	86° F (30° C)	Respiratory depression, myocardial irritability, bradycardia, atrial fibrillation, Osborn waves
Severe	<86° F (<30° C)	Basal metabolic rate 50% of normal, loss of deep tendon reflexes, fixed and dilated pupils, spontaneous ventricular fibrillation

Often no reliable correlation is seen between clinical signs and symptoms and a specific core body temperature.

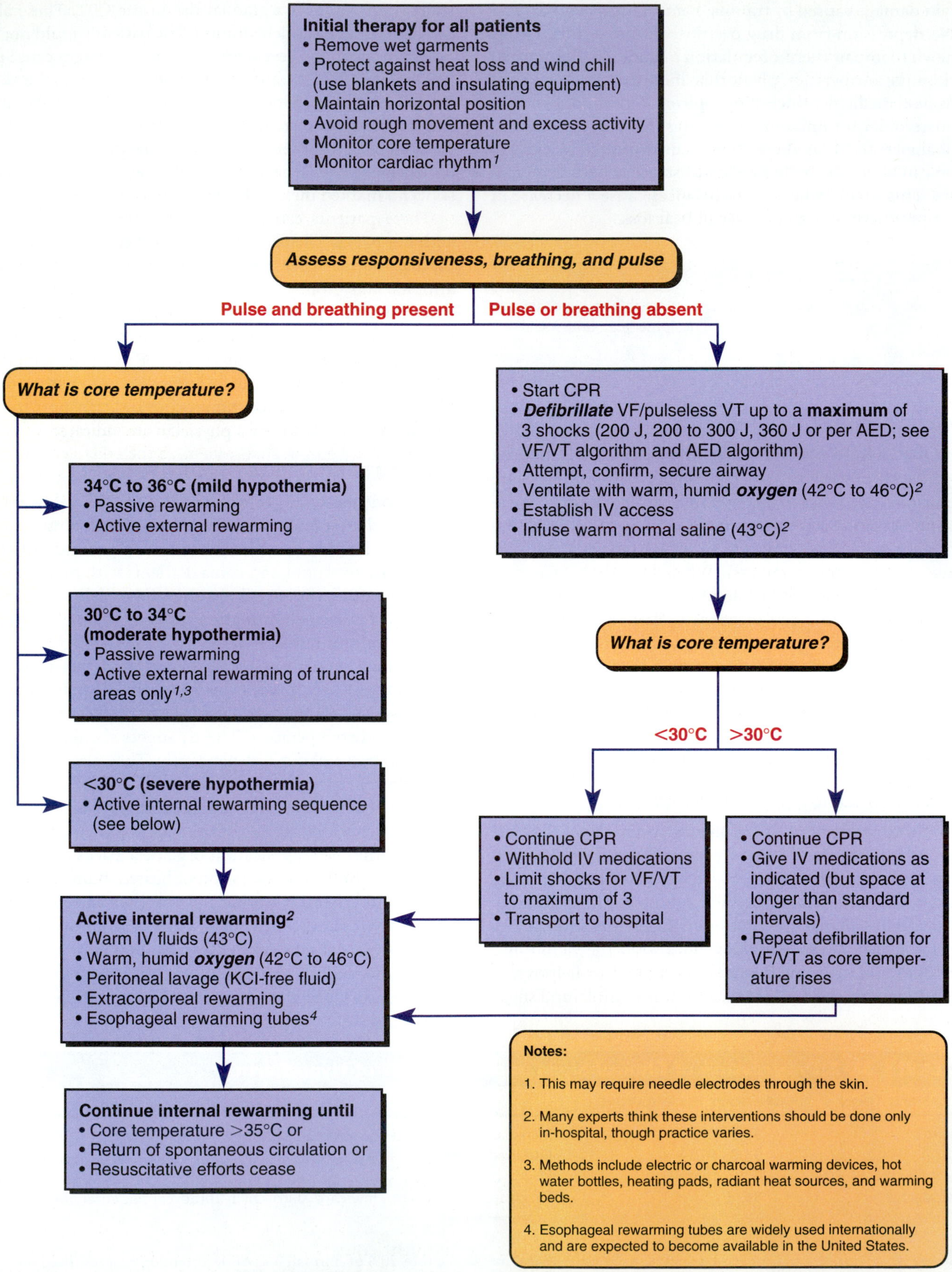
Initial therapy for all patients
• Remove wet garments
• Protect against heat loss and wind chill (use blankets and insulating equipment)
• Maintain horizontal position
• Avoid rough movement and excess activity
• Monitor core temperature
• Monitor cardiac rhythm[1]
Assess responsiveness, breathing, and pulse
Pulse and breathing present
Pulse or breathing absent
What is core temperature?
34°C to 36°C (mild hypothermia)
• Passive rewarming
• Active external rewarming
30°C to 34°C (moderate hypothermia)
• Passive rewarming
• Active external rewarming of truncal areas only[1,3]
<30°C (severe hypothermia)
• Active internal rewarming sequence (see below)
• Start CPR
• Defibrillate VF/pulseless VT up to a maximum of 3 shocks (200 J, 200 to 300 J, 360 J or per AED; see VF/VT algorithm and AED algorithm)
• Attempt, confirm, secure airway
• Ventilate with warm, humid oxygen (42°C to 46°C)[2]
• Establish IV access
• Infuse warm normal saline (43°C)[2]
What is core temperature?
<30°C
>30°C
• Continue CPR
• Withhold IV medications
• Limit shocks for VF/VT to maximum of 3
• Transport to hospital
• Continue CPR
• Give IV medications as indicated (but space at longer than standard intervals)
• Repeat defibrillation for VF/VT as core temperature rises
Active internal rewarming[2]
• Warm IV fluids (43°C)
• Warm, humid oxygen (42°C to 46°C)
• Peritoneal lavage (KCl-free fluid)
• Extracorporeal rewarming
• Esophageal rewarming tubes[4]
Continue internal rewarming until
• Core temperature >35°C or
• Return of spontaneous circulation or
• Resuscitative efforts cease
Notes:
1. This may require needle electrodes through the skin.
2. Many experts think these interventions should be done only in-hospital, though practice varies.
3. Methods include electric or charcoal warming devices, hot water bottles, heating pads, radiant heat sources, and warming beds.
4. Esophageal rewarming tubes are widely used internationally and are expected to become available in the United States.

FIGURE 38-3 ■ Algorithm for the treatment of hypothermia.

measure the patient's CBT. This should be done every 5 minutes.

When a person's CBT is below 82.4° F (28° C), the individual usually is unconscious. Such a patient should be gently moved to a warm environment if vital signs are present. The paramedic should institute passive external rewarming during transport. Heated, humidified oxygen can be administered as well. Airway management should begin with basic manual procedures (head-tilt chin-lift) and slow ventilatory assistance. The use of oral or nasal airways, including intubation, can induce ventricular dysrhythmias. Therefore, if these procedures must be used, the most experienced paramedic should perform them. Overzealous ventilatory assistance can induce hypocapnia and resultant ventricular irritability.[1] However, when these procedures are indicated, they should not be withheld. Medical direction may recommend the administration of ***thiamine, 50% dextrose,*** and ***naloxone,*** as well as an initial fluid challenge of 250 to 500 mL of 5% dextrose in water (D_5W) or normal saline. Lactated Ringer solution should not be used. This is because the cold liver may not be able to metabolize the lactate.

Severely hypothermic patients have no vital signs, including respiratory effort, pulse, or blood pressure. Depending on the core temperature, cyanosis; fixed, dilated pupils; and stiff, rigid muscles (simulating rigor mortis) may be present. Prolonged resuscitation attempts can be beneficial in severely hypothermic patients. Cardiopulmonary resuscitation (CPR) is indicated even if signs of death are present. Hypothermic patients cannot be presumed dead until a CBT of 94° to 95° F (34° to 35° C) is reached and resuscitation efforts are still unsuccessful. The paramedic should confirm a nonperfusing rhythm (ventricular fibrillation [VF], pulseless ventricular tachycardia [VT], or asystole) by ECG monitor for a minimum of 30 to 45 seconds. CPR should be instituted only if absolutely no vital signs are detected.

Endotracheal (ET) intubation is required if the hypothermia victim is unconscious or if ventilation is inadequate. Intubation serves two purposes: (1) it allows effective ventilation with warm, humidified oxygen; and (2) it isolates the airway, reducing the likelihood of aspiration.[1] Resuscitation in the prehospital setting may be withheld if the victim has obvious lethal injuries or if the body is frozen so completely that chest compression is impossible and the nose and mouth are blocked with ice.[1]

If a patient in cardiac arrest with a shockable rhythm fails to respond to three defibrillation attempts, the paramedic should lengthen the interval between further attempts. This is also true for the administration of drugs. Additional defibrillation attempts and drug therapy can begin once the patient has been rewarmed in the emergency department (ED). Medications, including ***epinephrine, lidocaine,*** and ***procainamide,*** can accumulate to toxic levels in the peripheral circulation if they are administered repeatedly in a severely hypothermic patient. For these reasons, IV drugs often are withheld when the CBT is lower than 86° F (30° C). If the CBT is above 86° F (30° C), IV drugs may be given, but with longer intervals between doses.[1] IV drug therapy in these patients should be guided by medical direction.

Cardiac arrest in the patient with severe hypothermia requires rapid transport to the hospital. The hospital should be equipped to provide internal core rewarming. In patients with vital signs, the rewarming technique of choice involves placing the patient on cardiopulmonary bypass (active core rewarming). This sustains perfusion while the patient is being rewarmed. Peritoneal and pleural lavage and esophageal rewarming techniques also have been used successfully to treat patients with extreme hypothermia and cardiac arrest.

Most authorities agree that active rewarming methods other than the administration of heated, humidified oxygen are inappropriate field care for severe hypothermia.[1] Rewarming methods such as hot water immersion can cause hypotension from peripheral vasodilation (rewarming shock). Acidosis can result from the sudden return of cold, acidotic blood and waste products to the body's core (afterdrop phenomenon). Therefore active field rewarming techniques generally are avoided. They generally are not used unless patient transport is delayed.

FROSTBITE

Frostbite is a localized injury. It results from environmentally induced freezing of body tissues. It often occurs in the lower extremities, particularly the toes and feet. Less often it occurs in the upper extremities (the fingers and hands). Frostbite also occurs on the ears, nose, and other body areas not protected from environmental extremes.

Pathophysiology

Frostbite occurs as ice crystals form in tissue. This produces macrovascular and microvascular damage and direct cellular injury. The freezing depth depends on the intensity and duration of cold exposure. Severe freezing can also occur in tissue exposed to volatile hydrocarbons at low temperatures.

Under most conditions of frostbite, ice crystals form in the extracellular tissue. This draws water out of the cells and into the extravascular spaces. As a result, the electrolyte concentration in the cell can reach toxic levels. The ice crystals can also expand and cause direct mechanical destruction of tissue. This leads to damage to blood vessels (particularly the endothelial cells), partial shrinkage and collapse of the cell membrane, loss of vascular integrity, local edema, and disruption of nutritive blood flow. Ischemia often produces the most damaging effects of frostbite.

When frozen tissue thaws, blood flow through the capillaries is initially restored. However, blood flow declines within minutes after thawing. This occurs as the arterioles and venules constrict and release emboli, which travel through the small vessels. Progressive tissue loss results from thrombosis and hypoxia. The endothelium is damaged. This further damages the small vessels and causes the skin to die. The process of thawing and refreezing is more harmful to tissue than allowing the frostbitten part to remain frozen until it can be warmed with minimal risk of refreezing. In addition to extreme temperature, wind, and humidity, predisposing factors for frostbite include the following:

- Lack of protective clothing
- Poor nutrition
- Preexisting injury or medical or psychiatric illness
- Fatigue
- Decrease in local tissue perfusion
- Tobacco use
- Atherosclerosis
- Tight, constrictive clothing
- Increased vasodilation
- Alcohol consumption
- Use of medications
- History of previous cold injury

Classifications and Symptoms

Cold injury can be subdivided into a number of classifications. For example, cold injury commonly is divided into two categories: superficial frostbite (also known as *frostnip*) and deep frostbite. Superficial frostbite involves some minimal tissue loss. With deep frostbite, significant tissue loss occurs even with proper therapy. Superficial frostbite usually involves the dermis and shallow subcutaneous layers. Deep frostbite is associated with the subdermal layers and deep tissues.

Initial evaluation of the severity of the frostbite is difficult. This is because the injury does not always reflect the underlying vascular changes. Regardless of the depth of injury, the area may appear to be frozen. Palpation may help the paramedic to distinguish between superficial and deep injury. With superficial injury, the underlying tissue springs back on compression. With deep injury, the underlying tissue is hard and cannot be compressed.

SUPERFICIAL FROSTBITE

In most patients with superficial frostbite, the initial symptoms are coldness and numbness in the affected area. These symptoms are followed by extreme pain (tingling and throbbing) during rewarming. After rewarming, edema usually appears within 3 hours. This is followed by the formation of vesicles within 3 to 24 hours (Fig. 38-4). The blisters begin to resolve within 1 week, after which the skin blackens into a hard eschar. Eventually the blackened tissue peels away (demarcation). This reveals shiny, red skin beneath. This tissue is sensitive to heat and cold. Also, for unknown reasons, the tissue remains unusually susceptible to repeated frostbite injury.

▶ **NOTE** Trench foot (immersion foot) is similar to frostbite. However, it occurs at temperatures above freezing. The signs and symptoms of this condition are similar to those of frostbite. They include pain and the formation of blisters with rewarming. The paramedic should cover the affected area with sterile dressings and keep it dry and warm.

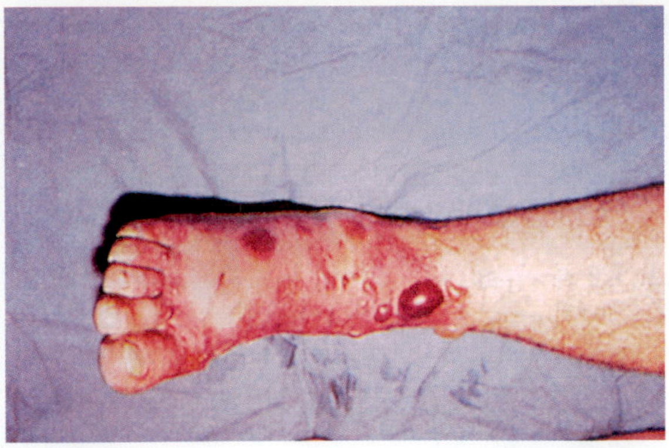

FIGURE 38-4 ■ Edema and blister formation 24 hours after frostbite injury in an area covered by a tightly fitting boot.

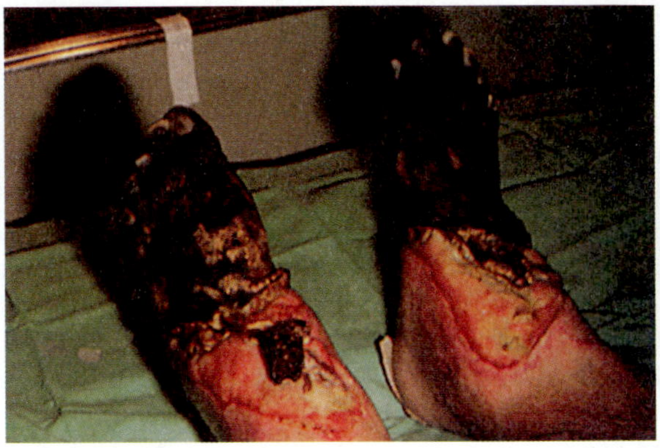

FIGURE 38-5 ■ Gangrenous necrosis 6 weeks after a frostbite injury.

DEEP FROSTBITE

In deep frostbite the disrupted nutritional capillary flow is never restored to the damaged tissue. The affected area remains cold, mottled, and blue or gray after rewarming. During the first 9 to 15 days, severely frostbitten skin forms a black, hard eschar. In contrast to superficial frostbite, edema is slow to develop. Deep blisters with purple, blood-containing fluid may appear within 1 to 3 weeks. Within 22 to 45 days, definite lines of demarcation develop between the eschar and viable tissue. In time, nonviable skin and deep structures mummify and slough (Fig. 38-5).

Management

Prehospital care for frostbite is limited to supporting the patient's vital functions, elevation and protection of the affected extremity (jewelry should be removed), pain management, and rapid transport to a medical facility. Vigorous rubbing or massage is ineffective. It also is potentially harmful. Partial, slow rewarming with blankets or other warm objects can worsen the injury. If the frostbite involves the patient's lower extremities, the person should not be allowed to walk. During transport, all restrictive and wet clothing should be removed from the patient. These should be replaced with warm, dry clothing and blankets to guard against hypothermia. The paramedic should not allow the patient to consume alcohol or smoke tobacco. Rapid rewarming of the frozen part by immersion in hot water (maximum of 104° F [40° C]) is the most effective therapeutic measure for preserving viable tissue. However, because of the risk of refreezing, this method of rewarming is not recommended in the prehospital setting.

SUBMERSION

Drowning was the fifth leading cause of unintentional death in the United States in 2001. It was the second leading cause of unintentional injury death among children and youths. Also, about 80,000 submersion incidents are reported each year. Of these, 85% of the victims are male, and two thirds of the victims are nonswimmers.[2]

Classifications

Submersion incidents can be classified in different ways. This text defines **submersion** as an incident in which a person experiences some swimming-related distress that is sufficient to require treatment by emergency medical services (EMS). It also requires transport to a medical facility for further observation and treatment. **Drowning** is defined as a "mortal" event. The victim is pronounced dead at the scene or within 24 hours after arrival in the ED. If death occurs after 24 hours, it is considered a *drowning-related death.*[3] Victims of submersion incidents usually fall into one of two categories:

- Conscious patients, such as nonswimmers, exhausted swimmers, river canoeists who become trapped by roots or strong currents, individuals who fall overboard or off a dock, and motor vehicle crash victims who are trapped in submerged vehicles
- Unconscious patients, such as those who suffer a stroke or cardiac arrest while swimming, and those who fall into water and die as a result of hypothermia

Pathophysiology

Drowning begins with intentional or unintentional submersion. After submersion, the victim realizes he or she is in distress. An example of this is a nonswimmer who panics or a swimmer who tires out. Drowning begins with the conscious victim taking in several deep breaths. This is an attempt to store oxygen before breath-holding (Fig. 38-6). The victim holds the breath until breathing reflexes override the breath-holding effort. As water is aspirated, laryngospasm occurs. Laryngospasm and aspiration produce severe hypoxia. This results in serious hypoxemia and acidosis, which lead to cardiac dysrhythmias and loss of oxygen to the CNS. In 15% of drownings, the laryngospasm is severe enough that very little fluid is aspirated *(dry drowning).* In the remaining 85% of drownings, fluid enters the lungs *(wet drowning).* The physiological events that follow are partly determined by the type and amount of water aspirated. Regardless of the type of water aspirated, the pathophysiology of drowning is characterized by hypoxia, hypercapnia, and acidosis, which result in cardiac arrest.

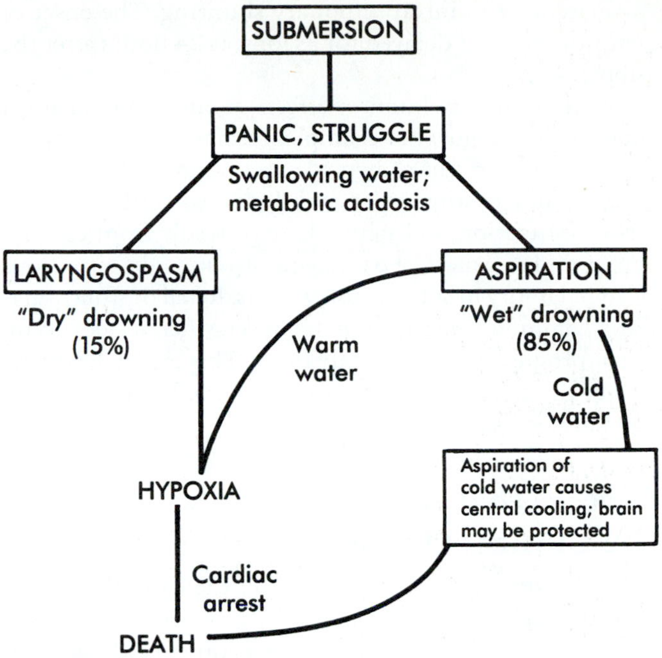

FIGURE 38-6 ■ Progression of the drowning incident.

CRITICAL THINKING

Do other swimmers or onlookers often "hear" a person who is drowning?

Drowning can occur in almost any type of water. Victims of submersion aspirate salt water or fresh water, tap water, or contaminated water (such as water containing sewage, chemicals, algae, bacteria, or sand). In theory, different fluids have different effects. However, these differences are not clinically significant in prehospital care. They should not be considered in the initial management of submersion patients. The single most important factor is the duration of submersion and the duration and severity of hypoxia.[3]

Pulmonary Pathophysiology Secondary to Near Drowning

Respiratory failure, lack of oxygen to the brain, and acidosis are the life-threatening complications of submersion. Hypoxia can result from the following factors:

- Fluid in the alveoli and interstitial spaces
- Loss of surfactant
- Contaminant particles in the alveoli and tracheobronchial tree
- Damage to the alveolar-capillary membrane and vascular endothelium

Poor perfusion and hypoxemia lead to metabolic acidosis in most patients. In those who survive the incident, acute respiratory failure may occur. This includes the development of adult respiratory distress syndrome (ARDS). ARDS (described in Chapter 30) reduces lung compliance and increases ventilation-perfusion mismatches and intrapulmonary shunting. The onset of symptoms can be delayed for as long as 24 hours after the submersion.

In addition to pulmonary effects, submersion can affect other body systems. For example, cardiovascular problems can occur as a result of hypoxia and acidosis. These problems include dysrhythmias and decreased cardiac output. CNS dysfunction and nerve damage result from cerebral edema and anoxia. The paramedic also must be suspicious of spinal injury in submersion victims. Renal dysfunction is not a common complication. However, when it does occur, it can progress to acute renal failure. This is usually the result of hypoxic injury or hemoglobinuria, leading to acute tubular necrosis.

Factors that Affect the Clinical Outcome

The following four factors can affect the clinical outcome of a submersion incident.

1. *Temperature of the water.* Submersion in cold water can have beneficial and negative effects. The rapid onset of hypothermia can serve a protective function. This is especially the case with brain viability in patients who have undergone prolonged submersion. An incident in which a child was submerged for 66 minutes in a creek with a water temperature of 37° F (5° C) is the longest documented submersion with a good neurological outcome.[4] This phenomenon is not fully understood. A contributing factor may be the *mammalian diving reflex*. This is a reflex stimulated by cold water. It shunts blood to the brain and heart from the skin, gastrointestinal tract, and extremities. This reflex occurs in seals and lower mammals. It also occurs in humans to some extent. Hypothermia may be organ protective. It also contributes to neurological recovery after prolonged submersion. It probably does this by reducing the metabolic needs of the brain. (Hypothermia also may develop secondary to submersion and later heat loss through evaporation during attempts at resuscitation. In these cases, the hypothermia is not protective.) The relative contributions of the diving reflex and hypothermia are not clear. The adverse effects of submersion in cold water include severe ventricular dysrhythmias.
2. *Duration of submersion.* The longer the time submersed, the less likely the patient is to survive. When rescue takes longer than 30 minutes, victims rescued from warm water in summer months or in warm southern waters usually do not survive. Submersion in cold water for up to 60 minutes has been associated with survival, including intact brain function. Therefore most patients rescued from cold water should receive resuscitation. Resuscitation is indicated unless physical evidence of death is present (e.g., putrefaction, dependent lividity, and rigor mortis). Submersion victims who have spontaneous circulation and breathing when they reach the hospital usually recover, with good outcomes.[3]
3. *Cleanliness of the water.* Contaminants in water have an irritant effect on the pulmonary system. This may lead to bronchospasm. It also may lead to poor gas exchange. These can cause a secondary pulmonary infection with delayed severe respiratory compromise.
4. *Age of the victim.* The younger the patient or victim, the better the chance for survival.

Management

At the site of a submersion incident, the safety of the EMS crew is paramount. Only personnel trained in water rescue should try to intervene (see Chapter 51). Depending on the type and duration of submersion, the patient's symptoms may vary. The person may have no symptoms or may be in cardiac arrest. After gaining access to the victim, the paramedic should take spinal precautions while the victim is still in the water (see Chapter 22). The paramedic should begin rescue breathing (if needed) as soon as possible. The use of subdiaphragmatic thrusts to remove water from the airways is controversial and generally is not recommended unless foreign body airway obstruction is suspected.[3] Chest thrusts can be used as an alternative to the Heimlich maneuver.

After removing the patient from the water, the paramedic should evaluate the person. An adequate airway should be ensured, and ventilatory and circulatory support should be provided as needed. Other forms of initial patient care include administration of high-concentration oxygen, ECG monitoring, and establishment of an IV line. Patients who are in cardiac arrest should be managed with standard BLS and ALS protocols. They also should be rapidly transported to the hospital.

Victims of submersion incidents often are at risk from immersion hypothermia; heat loss in water can be up to 32 times greater than in air. Hypothermia can make resuscitation more difficult. It calls for special consideration with regard to gentle handling, the administration of drugs, and defibrillation. As with all other victims of hypothermia, the paramedic should remove the patient's wet clothing. The patient then should be dried and wrapped in blankets to conserve body heat. External warming and the administration of heated, humidified oxygen at the scene and during transport should be considered. All patients suspected of having hypothermia should be managed as described before and as outlined in Fig. 38-3.

Even patients with no symptoms require transport for evaluation by a physician. They should be given oxygen. Paramedics also should monitor these patients carefully so as to recognize the aspiration pneumonia and hypoxia that can result from submersion. Oxygen is the most important treatment needed by submersion victims.

CRITICAL THINKING

What are the risks to rescuers on a call involving submersion victims?

DIVING EMERGENCIES

The United States has more than 4 million recreational scuba divers, and more than 400,000 new sport divers are certified each year.[5] Emergencies unique to pressure-related diving include those caused by the mechanical effects of pressure (barotrauma), air embolism, and the breathing of compressed air (**decompression sickness** and **nitrogen narcosis**).

> **NOTE** The term *scuba* is actually an acronym. It stands for self-contained underwater breathing apparatus. This equipment allows divers to breathe underwater. Scuba gear typically consists of one or two compressed air tanks. These are strapped to the diver's back and connected by a hose to a mouthpiece.

Basic Properties of Gases

The weight of the atmosphere exerts a pressure of 14.7 pounds per square inch (psi) of force at sea level. This means that a 1-inch column of air as tall as the atmosphere would weigh 14.7 pounds. This weight is commonly referred to as *1 atmosphere of pressure* (1 atm). Water weighs considerably more than air and can exert much more pressure. For example, a 1-inch column of seawater needs to be only 33 feet tall to weigh 14.7 pounds. This means that at a depth of 33 feet, the total pressure is 29.4 psi, or 2 atm of pressure (1 atm from the air and 1 atm from the 33 feet of water). This is referred to as *ambient pressure* or *absolute pressure.* Every additional 33 feet of seawater adds another 14.7 pounds of pressure, or another 1 atm.

LAWS PERTAINING TO GASES

Three laws of the properties of gases underpin all pressure diving-related emergencies (and some high-altitude illnesses). These are Boyle's law, Dalton's law, and Henry's law. The following properties of gases can aid comprehension of these laws: increased pressure dissolves gases into the blood; oxygen metabolizes, and nitrogen dissolves.

Boyle's Law. Boyle's law states that, if temperature remains constant, the volume of a given mass of gas is inversely proportional to the absolute pressure; that is, when the pressure is doubled, the volume of gas is halved (compressed into a smaller space), and vice versa. This can be expressed by the equation $PV = K$, in which *P* is pressure; *V* is volume; and *K* is a constant. Boyle's law explains the "popping" or "squeezing" sensation in the ears that a person may feel when traveling by air. It is the basic mechanism for all types of barotrauma: *trapped gases expand as pressure decreases.* For example, when a diver uses a scuba tank of pressurized air, the lung volumes remain constant at various depths. If the diver ascends but does not exhale, water pressure decreases and the gas in the lungs expands. This greatly increases the pressure in the lungs.

> **NOTE** Gas expands as pressure decreases. This fact applies to increases in altitude that occur during air transportation. For example, in a patient transported by air, gas can expand in the respiratory system, gastrointestinal system, or sinuses as altitude increases and pressure decreases. Medical equipment also can be affected by a increase in air volume. Examples of such include endotracheal tube cuffs and the pneumatic antishock garment (PASG).

Dalton's Law. Dalton's law states that the pressure exerted by each gas in a mixture of gases is the same pressure that the gas would exert if it alone occupied the same volume. On the other hand, the total pressure of a mixture of gases equals the sum of the partial pressures that make up the mixture. This law is expressed by the equation $Pt = Po_2 + PN_2 + Px$, where *Pt* is the total pressure; Po_2 is the partial pressure of oxygen; PN_2 is the partial pressure of nitrogen; and *Px* is the partial pressure of the remaining gases in the mixture.

To simplify, the air we breathe is about 80% nitrogen and 20% oxygen; that is, about 80% of the pressure of the air (i.e., the gas mixture) is exerted by the nitrogen in the mixture. About 20% of the pressure is exerted by the oxygen in the mixture. This means that at sea level, the pressure exerted on us by the nitrogen in the air is 80% of 14.7, or 11.76 psi; the pressure from the oxygen is 20% of 14.7, or 2.94 psi. Together, these account for the 14.7 psi of pressure at the surface. Even though the gas mixtures remain with normal percentages of nitrogen and oxygen, the partial pressures of these gases change at different altitudes above sea level or at depths below sea level. The principles of this law explain problems that can arise from the breathing of compressed air: *gas expansion causes the partial pressure of oxygen to drop as gas molecules move farther apart, reducing the available oxygen.*

Henry's Law. Henry's law states that, at a constant temperature, the solubility of a gas in a liquid solution is proportionate to the partial pressure of the gas. This means that more gas can be dissolved into a liquid at a higher pressure, and less gas can be dissolved into the liquid when that pressure is released. For example, when a container of a carbonated beverage (pressurized with dissolved carbon dioxide gas) is opened, a "pop" is heard and bubbles form on the liquid. This occurs because the pressure in the container is no longer great enough to hold the dissolved gas inside. Henry's law is expressed by the equation $\%X = Px/Pt \times 100$, where *%X* is the amount of gas dissolved in a liquid; *Px* is the partial pressure of the gas; and *Pt* is the total atmospheric pressure. This law explains why more nitrogen, which makes up almost 80% of air, dissolves in a diver's body as ambient pressure increases with descent. This dissolved nitrogen is released from the tissues on ascent as pressure decreases.

Barotrauma

Barotrauma is tissue damage. It results from compression or expansion of gas spaces when the gas pressure in the body or its compartments differs from the ambient pressure. The type of barotrauma depends on whether the diver is in descent or ascent. Barotrauma is the most common injury of scuba divers.

BAROTRAUMA OF DESCENT

Barotrauma of descent (also known as *squeeze*) results from the compression of gas in enclosed spaces as the ambient pressure increases with descent under water. Air trapped in noncollapsible chambers is compressed. This leads to a vacuum-type effect that results in severe, sharp pain caused by the distortion; vascular engorgement; edema; and hemorrhage of the exposed tissue (Box 38-3). As a rule, squeeze usually results from a blocked eustachian tube or from failure of the diver to clear (open) the eustachian tube with exhalation during descent. The ears and paranasal sinuses are most likely to be affected. Squeeze occurs in the ears, sinuses, lungs and airways, gastrointestinal tract, thorax, teeth (pulp decay, recent extraction sockets or fillings), or added air spaces (face mask or diving suit).

The management of barotrauma of descent involves slowly returning the diver to shallower depths. Prehospital care is mainly supportive. After the patient has been evaluated by a physician, definitive care may include bed rest with the head elevated, avoidance of strain and strenuous activity, use of decongestants and possibly antihistamines and antibiotics, and perhaps surgical repair.

> **CRITICAL THINKING**
> What preexisting illness can make a diver more susceptible to squeeze?

BOX 38-3 Signs and Symptoms of Diving-Related Conditions

Squeeze
- Pain
- Sensation of fullness
- Headache
- Disorientation
- Vertigo
- Nausea
- Bleeding from the nose or ears

Pulmonary Overpressurization Syndrome (POPS)
- Gradually increasing chest pain
- Hoarseness
- Neck fullness
- Dyspnea
- Dysphagia
- Subcutaneous emphysema

Air Embolism
- Focal paralysis or sensory changes (strokelike symptoms)
- Aphasia
- Confusion
- Blindness or other visual disturbances
- Convulsions
- Loss of consciousness
- Dizziness
- Vertigo
- Abdominal pain
- Cardiac arrest

Decompression Sickness
- Shortness of breath
- Itch
- Rash
- Joint pain
- Crepitus
- Fatigue
- Vertigo
- Paresthesias
- Paralysis
- Seizures
- Unconsciousness

Nitrogen Narcosis
- Impaired judgment
- Sensation of alcohol intoxication
- Slowed motor response
- Loss of proprioception
- Euphoria

BAROTRAUMA OF ASCENT

Barotrauma of ascent occurs through the reverse process of descent ("reverse squeeze"). Assuming that the air-filled cavities of the body have equalized pressure during the diver's descent, the volume of air trapped in this pressurized space expands as ambient pressure decreases with ascent (Boyle's law). If air is not allowed to escape because of obstruction (e.g., breath-holding, bronchospasm, or mucus plug), the expanding gases distend the tissues surrounding them. The most common cause of this type of barotrauma is breath-holding during ascent. Divers hold their breath because they are running out of air or because they panic. Making stops during the ascent allows more time for safe *off-gassing.* Many hyperbaric professionals advise a 3- to 5-minute safety stop at 15 to 20 feet for any dive. For dives below 60 feet, another safety stop at 30 feet may be of value. If possible, the paramedic should ask the diver about safety stops during ascent.

> **NOTE** Compressed gas at 33 feet (2 atmospheres) doubles in volume when the diver moves to the surface (1 atmosphere). This is because the pressure is half of 33 feet. The last 6 feet of ascent have the greatest potential for volume expansion. This is considered the most dangerous depth.

Problems from reverse squeeze are rare. However, pulmonary overpressurization syndrome (POPS) can occur as a result of expansion of trapped air in the lungs. POPS can lead to alveolar rupture. It also can lead to leakage of air into areas outside the alveoli. The clinical syndromes associated with barotrauma of ascent include pneumomediastinum, subcutaneous emphysema, pneumopericardium, pneumothorax, pneumoperitoneum, and systemic arterial air embolism. Except for tension pneumothorax (a rare complication that may require needle or tube decompression) and air embolism, which may require hyperbaric recompression therapy, POPS usually requires only administration of oxygen, observation, and transport for evaluation by a physician.

AIR EMBOLISM

Air embolism is the most serious complication of pulmonary barotrauma. It is a major cause of death and disability among sport divers. Divers risk this condition when they ascend too rapidly or hold their breath during ascent.

Air embolism results as the expanding air disrupts tissues and air is forced into the circulatory system. The air bubbles pass through the left side of the heart and become lodged in small arterioles. This occludes distal circulation. The syndrome usually manifests as the diver surfaces and exhales. Exhaling releases the high intrapulmonic pressure that resulted from lung overexpansion. With the decrease in intrathoracic pressure, bubbles advance into the left side of the heart and enter the systemic arterial supply. This results in a dramatic presentation. The clinical manifestations depend on the site of systemic arterial occlusion. The most common presentation of air embolism is similar to that of stroke. It includes vertigo, confusion, loss of consciousness, visual disturbances, and focal neurological deficits.

Air embolism should be suspected if a diver suddenly loses consciousness right after surfacing. Paramedics should begin BLS and ALS measures, and the patient should be rapidly transported for recompression treatment. If endotracheal intubation is required, the balloon cuff of the ET tube should be filled with normal saline instead of air. This prevents inadvertent extubation during recompression. Also, the patient should be thoroughly evaluated for signs of POPS, such as a pneumothorax.

A patient suspected of having an air embolism should be transported in the left lateral recumbent position. If not contraindicated by injury, the thorax should be elevated 15 degrees. Some medical direction agencies advise transporting the patient in a supine position. This helps to avoid aggravating cerebral edema that may develop. (The paramedic should always follow local protocol.) If air transport is to be used, the patient should be transported by an aircraft that is pressurized to sea level. The patient also can be transported by a rotary wing aircraft that flies at low altitude. This prevents existing intraarterial air bubbles from expanding further. The flight altitude must be as low as possible if the internal cabin pressure cannot be maintained at sea level. Ideally, it should never be over 1000 feet above sea level.

Recompression. Management of a patient with an air embolism consists of rapidly increasing the ambient pressure (recompression). This is done in a hyperbaric oxygen chamber (Fig. 38-7) (Box 38-4). Hyperbaric chambers allow for the delivery of oxygen at a higher than normal atmospheric pressure. The process is used to overcome the natural limit of oxygen solubility in blood. It thus reduces the intravascular bubble volume and restores tissue perfusion. Slow decompression helps to prevent bubbles from reforming. Paramedics should know the location of the nearest hyperbaric treatment facility and should follow the protocol established by medical direction.

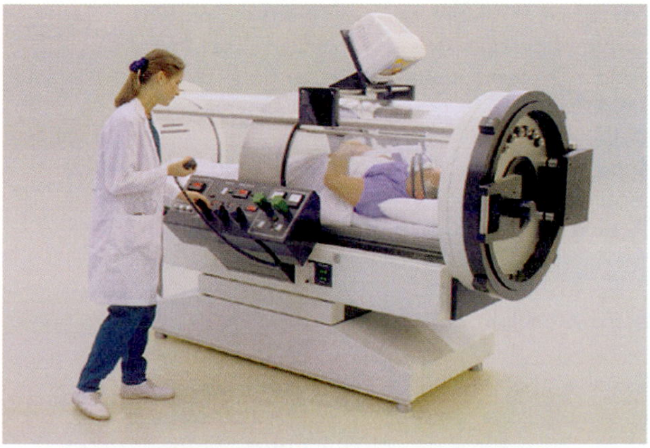

FIGURE 38-7 ■ Hyperbaric oxygen chamber.

CRITICAL THINKING

Where is the nearest hyperbaric chamber in your area?

NOTE The Diver's Alert Network, a nonprofit organization operated by Duke University Medical Center, specializes in diving-related illnesses. It offers consultation and referral services. The telephone number is 1-800-446-2671.

DECOMPRESSION SICKNESS

Decompression sickness is also known as *the bends, dysbarism, caisson disease*, and *diver's paralysis*. It is a multisystem disorder. It results when nitrogen in compressed air (dissolved into tissues and blood from the increase in the partial pressure of the gas at depth) converts back from solution to gas. This results in the formation of bubbles in the tissues and blood. The syndrome occurs when the ambient pressure decreases (Henry's law). The cause is an ascent that is too rapid. In such an ascent, the balance between the dissolved nitrogen in tissue and blood and the partial pressure of nitrogen in the inspired gas cannot be reached.

The most significant effect of the nitrogen bubbles is occlusion of blood vessels, which impairs arterial venous flow. Because the bubbles can form in any tissue, *lym-*

BOX 38-4 Hyperbaric Oxygen Therapy

Altering the surrounding air pressure for medical treatment is a practice that dates back to the seventeenth century. At that time, "fevers and inflammations" were treated in crude chambers that were pressurized using hand bellows. Today, hyperbaric oxygen therapy (HBOT) is carried out in single-person chambers. These are monoplace chambers. The treatment also can be done in larger multiplace chambers, which can house several patients and the attending hyperbaric health care workers. HBOT has proved to be effective in the treatment of a wide variety of medical disorders. These include air embolism and decompression sickness; carbon monoxide poisoning and smoke inhalation; carbon monoxide poisoning complicated by cyanide poisoning; clostridial myonecrosis (gas gangrene); crush injury, compartment syndrome, and other acute traumatic ischemias; intracranial abscesses; and thermal burns. It also has been shown to enhance the healing of certain problem wounds.

phedema (the accumulation of lymph in soft tissues), cellular distention, and cellular rupture also can occur. The net effect of all these processes is poor tissue perfusion and ischemia. The joints and the spinal cord are most often affected.

The paramedic should suspect decompression sickness in any patient who has symptoms within 12 to 36 hours after a scuba dive. These will be symptoms that cannot be explained by other conditions. (An example is a patient with unexplained joint pain who had been diving within the previous 24 hours.) Prehospital care includes support of vital functions, administration of high-concentration oxygen, fluid resuscitation, and rapid transportation for recompression. The patient transport and air evacuation guidelines described for air embolism should also be used with these patients.

NITROGEN NARCOSIS

Nitrogen narcosis ("rapture of the deep") is a condition in which nitrogen becomes dissolved in the blood. This is caused by a higher than normal partial pressure of nitrogen. Dissolved nitrogen crosses the blood-brain barrier. It produces depressant effects similar to those of alcohol. This can seriously impair the diver's thinking. It also can lead to lethal errors in judgment. Symptoms of nitrogen narcosis usually become evident at depths of 75 to 100 feet. At depths below 300 feet, with standard air (an oxygen-nitrogen mixture), the diver losses consciousness. Nitrogen narcosis affects all divers. However, experienced divers tolerate it better. Helium-oxygen mixtures are used for deep dives to improve the nitrogen complication. The narcotic effects of nitrogen are reversed with ascent.

Nitrogen narcosis is a common factor in diving accidents, and it may be responsible for memory loss. Prehospital care is mainly supportive. The paramedic should assess the patient for injuries that may have occurred during the dive, and the patient should be transported for evaluation by a physician.

NOTE Less common diving-related illnesses may result from oxygen toxicity (usually seen with prolonged exposure to oxygen or exposure to excessive concentrations of oxygen), breathing of contaminated gases, hypercapnia, and hyperventilation.

HIGH-ALTITUDE ILLNESS

High-altitude illness principally occurs at altitudes of 8000 feet or more above sea level.[6] It is attributed directly to exposure to reduced atmospheric pressure (described previously), which results in hypobaric hypoxia. Activities associated with these syndromes include mountain climbing, aircraft or glider flight, riding in hot air balloons, and the use of low-pressure or vacuum chambers.

The high-altitude syndromes discussed in this chapter are **acute mountain sickness** (AMS), **high-altitude pulmonary edema** (HAPE), and **high-altitude cerebral edema** (HACE). Emergency care for all forms of high-altitude illness includes airway, ventilatory, and circulatory support and descent to a lower altitude. In addition, a physician should evaluate all patients with high-altitude illness. Strategies for preventing high-altitude illness include the following:

1. Gradual ascent (days)
2. Limited exertion
3. Decreased sleeping at altitude
4. High-carbohydrate diet
5. Medications (all are controversial)
   - Acetazolamide (to speed acclimatization and reduce the incidence of AMS)
   - Nifedipine (used solely by those with a history of HAPE to prevent recurrence upon ascent)
   - Steroids

Exposure to high altitude can worsen chronic medical conditions. This is the case even without apparent altitude sickness. (Examples of such conditions include angina pectoris, congestive heart failure [CHF], chronic obstructive pulmonary disease [COPD], and hypertension.) These conditions can worsen as a result of a low partial pressure of oxygen. A low partial pressure of oxygen means that less oxygen is inhaled with each normal respiratory volume.

Acute Mountain Sickness

AMS is a common high-altitude illness. It results when an unacclimatized person ascends rapidly to high altitudes. The illness usually develops within 4 to 6 hours of reaching a high altitude and reaches maximum severity within 24 to 48 hours (Box 38-5). It abates on the third or fourth day after exposure with gradual acclimatization.

BOX 38-5 Signs and Symptoms of High-Altitude Illness

Acute Mountain Sickness (AMS)
Headache (most common symptom) attributed to subacute cerebral edema or to spasm or dilation of cerebral blood vessels secondary to hypocapnia or hypoxia
Malaise
Anorexia
Vomiting
Dizziness
Irritability
Impaired memory
Dyspnea on exertion

High-Altitude Pulmonary Edema (HAPE)
Shortness of breath
Dyspnea
Cough (with or without frothy sputum)
Generalized weakness
Lethargy
Disorientation

High-Altitude Cerebral Edema (HACE)
Headache
Ataxia
Altered consciousness
Confusion
Hallucinations
Drowsiness
Stupor
Coma

The physical findings with AMS vary. They include tachycardia, bradycardia, postural hypotension, and ataxia (impaired ability to coordinate movement). Ataxia is a key sign of the progression of the illness. As AMS becomes severe, the victim may experience alterations in consciousness, disorientation, and impaired judgment. Coma may occur within 24 hours after the onset of ataxia. Emergency care includes administration of oxygen. It also includes descent to as low an altitude as needed to achieve relief. Definitive treatment after evaluation by a physician may involve the use of diuretics to treat fluid retention associated with AMS, steroids to reduce associated cerebral edema, and hyperbaric therapy.

High-Altitude Pulmonary Edema

HAPE is caused at least partly by increased pulmonary artery pressure that develops in response to hypoxia. The increased pressure results in the release of leukotrienes. These increase the permeability of pulmonary arterioles. The increased pressure also results in the leakage of fluid into extravascular space. The initial symptoms of HAPE usually begin 24 to 72 hours after the exposure to high altitudes. The symptoms often are preceded by vigorous exercise.

Physical findings in patients with HAPE include hyperpnea, crackles, rhonchi, tachycardia, and cyanosis. Emergency care includes administration of oxygen to increase arterial oxygenation and reduce pulmonary artery pressure. It also includes descent to a lower altitude. After evaluation by a physician, the patient may be hospitalized for observation.

Portable hyperbaric chambers (e.g., the Gamow bag and Gamow tent) are commercially available. These reverse the effects of high-altitude pulmonary and cerebral edema. They are used by some EMS agencies in high-risk areas.

High-Altitude Cerebral Edema

HACE is the most severe form of acute high-altitude illness. It is characterized by a progression of global cerebral signs in the presence of AMS. These signs probably are related to an increase in intracranial pressure caused by cerebral edema and swelling. Therefore the distinctions between AMS and HACE are inherently blurred. The progression from mild AMS to unconsciousness associated with HACE can occur quickly (i.e., within 12 hours). However, it usually requires 1 to 3 days of exposure to high altitudes.

HACE must be managed promptly, because without treatment the syndrome rapidly progresses to stupor, coma, and death. As with other forms of high-altitude illness, emergency care focuses on airway, ventilatory, and circulatory support and descent to a lower altitude.

SUMMARY

- Body temperature is governed by a thermoregulatory center in the posterior hypothalamus. Body temperature can be raised or lowered in two ways: through the regulation of heat production (thermogenesis) and through the regulation of heat loss (thermolysis).
- Heat illness results from one of two basic causes. First, the normal temperature-regulating functions can be overwhelmed by conditions in the environment. These conditions can include heat stress. More often they involve excessive exercise in moderate to extreme environmental conditions. Second, the body's thermoregulatory mechanism can fail. This may occur in older adults or ill or debilitated individuals. Heat cramps are brief, intermittent, and often severe. They are muscular cramps that occur in muscles fatigued by heavy work or exercise. Heat exhaustion is characterized by minor aberrations in mental status, dizziness, nausea, headache, and a mild to moderate rise in the CBT (up to 103° F [39° C]). Heat stroke occurs when the temperature-regulating functions break down entirely, and the body temperature rises to 105.8° F (41° C) or higher. Temperatures this high damage all tissues and lead to collapse.
- Hypothermia (a CBT lower than 95° F [35° C]) can result from a decrease in heat production, an increase in heat loss, or a combination of these two factors. The progression of clinical signs and symptoms of hypothermia is divided into three classes based on the CBT: mild (CBT of 93.2° to 96.8° F [34° to 36° C]), moderate (CBT of 86°° to 93° F [30° to 34° C]), and severe (CBT below 86° F [30° C]). Severely hypothermic patients have no vital signs, including respiratory effort, pulse, and blood pressure.
- Frostbite is a localized injury. It results from environmentally induced freezing of body tissues. This freezing leads to damage to blood vessels. Ischemia often produces the most damaging effects of frostbite. In deep frostbite this can include mummification and sloughing of nonviable skin and deep structures.
- Drowning is an event in which a submersion victim is pronounced dead at the scene of the attempted resuscitation or within 24 hours after arrival in the ED or hospital. Near drowning is submersion with survival at least for a period of time. Regardless of the type of water aspirated, the pathophysiology of drowning is characterized by hypoxia, hypercapnia, and acidosis, which result in cardiac arrest.

- The three laws of the basic properties of gases that are involved in all pressure-related diving emergencies are Boyle's law, Dalton's law, and Henry's law. Increased pressure dissolves gases into blood; oxygen metabolizes, and nitrogen dissolves.
- Barotrauma is tissue damage. It results from compression or expansion of gas spaces when the gas pressure in the body differs from the ambient pressure. The type of barotrauma depends on whether the diver is in descent or ascent. Air embolism is the most serious complication of pulmonary barotrauma. It is a major cause of death and disability among sport divers.
- High-altitude illness results from exposure to reduced atmospheric pressure, which results in hypoxia. Forms of high-altitude illness include acute mountain sickness, high-altitude pulmonary edema, and high-altitude cerebral edema.

REFERENCES

1. American Heart Association: Guidelines 2000 for cardiopulmonary resuscitation and emergency cardiovascular care, International Consensus on Science, *Circulation* 102 (8):229-232, 2000.
2. National Safety Council: *Injury facts*, Itasca, Ill, 2002, The Council.
3. American Heart Association: Guidelines 2000 for cardiopulmonary resuscitation and emergency cardiovascular care, International Consensus on Science, *Circulation* 102(8):233-236, 2000.
4. Callaham M: *Current practice of emergency medicine,* ed 2, Philadelphia, 1991, BC Decker.
5. Auerbach PS: *Wilderness medicine,* ed 3, St Louis, 1995, Mosby.
6. U.S. Department of Transportation, National Highway Traffic Safety Administration: *EMT-paramedic national standard curriculum,* Washington, DC, 1998, The Department.

CHAPTER 39

Infectious and Communicable Diseases

OBJECTIVES

Upon completion of this chapter, the paramedic student will be able to:

1. Identify general public health principles related to infectious diseases.
2. Describe the chain of elements necessary for an infectious disease to occur.
3. Explain how internal and external barriers affect susceptibility to infection.
4. Differentiate the four stages of infectious disease: the latent period, the incubation period, the communicability period, and the disease period.
5. Describe the mode of transmission, pathophysiology, prehospital considerations, and personal protective measures to be taken for the human immunodeficiency virus (HIV), hepatitis, tuberculosis, meningococcal meningitis, and pneumonia.
6. Describe the mode of transmission, pathophysiology, signs and symptoms, and prehospital considerations for patients who have rabies or tetanus.
7. List the signs, symptoms, and possible secondary complications of selected childhood viral diseases.
8. List the signs, symptoms, and possible secondary complications of influenza, severe acute respiratory syndrome (SARS), and mononucleosis.
9. Describe the mode of transmission, pathophysiology, prehospital considerations, and personal protective measures for sexually transmitted diseases.
10. Identify the signs and symptoms and prehospital considerations for lice and scabies.
11. Outline the reporting process for exposure to infectious or communicable diseases.
12. Discuss the paramedic's role in preventing disease transmission.

KEY TERMS

communicability period: A stage of infection that begins when the latent period ends and continues as long as the agent is present and can spread to other hosts.

communicable disease: An infectious disease that can be transmitted from one person to another.

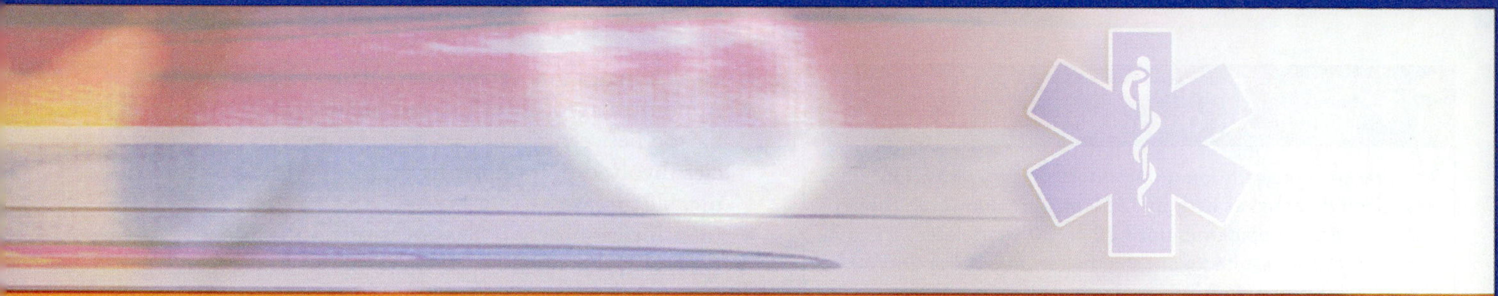

complement system: A group of proteins that coat bacteria and help to kill them directly or assist in having them taken up by neutrophils in the blood or by macrophages in the tissues.

designated officer (DO): A person who serves as a liaison between the public safety agency and community health agencies involved in monitoring and responding to communicable diseases.

disease period: A stage of infection that follows the incubation period; the duration of this stage varies with the disease.

exposure incident: Any specific contact of the eyes, the mouth, other mucous membranes, or nonintact skin, or any parenteral contact, with blood, blood products, bloody body fluids, or other potentially infectious materials.

incubation period: The stage of infection during which an organism reproduces; it begins with invasion of the agent and ends when the disease process begins.

infectious disease: Any illness caused by a specific microorganism.

latent period: A stage of infection that begins when a pathogenic agent invades the body and ends when the agent can be shed or communicated.

Emergencies that involve infectious and communicable diseases are common in the prehospital setting. They can pose a significant health risk to emergency medical services (EMS) providers. This chapter addresses the duties of the paramedic and EMS agencies in ensuring personal protection. It also presents the causes of infectious and communicable diseases, as well as special aspects of providing care for these conditions.

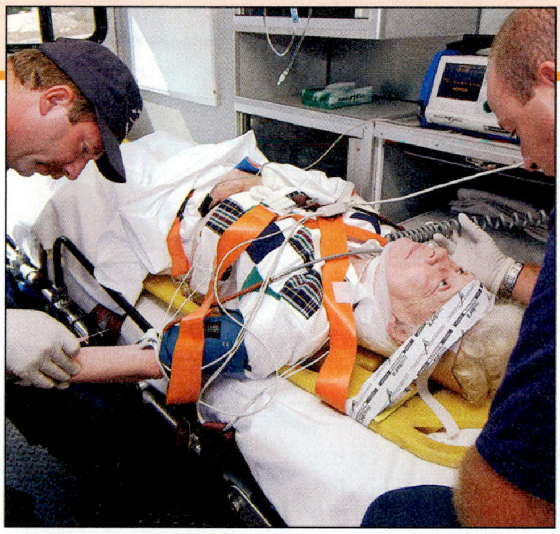

PUBLIC HEALTH PRINCIPLES RELATED TO INFECTIOUS DISEASES

An **infectious disease** is any illness caused by a specific germ. A **communicable disease** is an infectious disease that can be passed from one person to another. Infectious (communicable) diseases affect entire groups of people. These groups are defined by location, age, and socioeconomic status. They also are defined by the relationships between the groups. Groups can display varying susceptibilities (and varying degrees of susceptibility) to infection. In addition to demographics, other factors can affect the life cycle of an infectious agent within a group. One of these is the ability of a group to migrate or to move internationally. Another factor is genetics. A third factor is the effectiveness of treatment once the infection has occurred in the group (Box 39-1).

When a disease outbreak occurs, local, state, private, and federal health agencies and other organizations become involved in prevention and management. Local agencies usually are the first line of defense in disease surveillance and outbreak. They include municipal, city, and county agencies such as health departments, fire departments, and EMS agencies.

State agencies often are involved in the regulation and enforcement of federal guidelines. They frequently are required by statute or public law to meet or exceed federal guidelines and recommendations for prevention and management of disease outbreaks.

The private sector is composed of regional and national health care providers, local and national health maintenance organizations, laboratories (hospital and private), infection control and disease specialists, and others. These groups influence protocols and guidelines for tracking diseases and responding to outbreaks.

Federal and national organizations include Congress, which plays an integral role in national health policy by passing public laws and drafting the federal budget; the U.S. Department of Labor's Occupational Safety and Health

BOX 39-1 The Emergence of AIDS: An Outbreak of Disease

The presence of the human immunodeficiency virus (HIV) may have been detected as early as 1959 in Zaire. However, the virus did not become epidemic until 20 to 30 years later. The outbreak may have resulted from the migration of poor and young sexually active people from rural areas to urban centers in developing countries. This group often returned to rural areas or moved internationally because of civil wars, tourism, business travel, and the drug trade.

Acquired immunodeficiency syndrome (AIDS) was first identified in the United States in 1981. Young, previously healthy homosexual men in New York and California were found to have an unusual clustering of rare diseases (most notably Kaposi sarcoma, Pneumocystis carinii pneumonia, and unexplained persistent lymphadenopathy). A review of laboratory tests from that time for antibodies to HIV suggests that the virus entered the U.S. population in the late 1970s. To date, an estimated 850,000 to 950,000 persons in the United States are living with human immunodeficiency virus (HIV), including 180,000 to 280,000 who do not know they are infected. It is estimated that more than 38 million people worldwide are living with HIV infection or AIDS, and more than 45 million new infections are projected to occur this decade. Since the epidemic began in 1981, more than 20 million people have died of AIDS.

UNAIDS 2004 Report on the Global AIDS Epidemic - Executive Summary, http://www.unaids.org/bankok2004/GAR2004_html/ExecSummary_en/ExecSumm_en.htm#P15_98. Accessed Feb. 22, 2005.

Administration (OSHA); and agencies under the U.S. Department of Health and Human Services, such as the Centers for Disease Control and Prevention (CDC) and the National Institute for Occupational Safety and Health (NIOSH). Other federal and national organizations involved in the prevention and management of disease outbreaks include the U.S. Department of Defense, Federal Emergency Management Agency (FEMA), the National Fire Protection Association (NFPA), the U.S. Fire Protection Administration (USFPA), and the International Association of Firefighters (IAFF).

CRITICAL THINKING

Have you had an outbreak of a communicable disease in your region? How was it controlled?

Agency Responsibility in Infectious Agent Exposure

National concerns regarding communicable disease and infection control have resulted in public law, guidelines, standards, and recommendations to protect health care providers and emergency responders from infectious diseases. The components of a health care agency's exposure control plan include the following[1]:

- Health maintenance and surveillance
- Appointment of a **designated officer (DO)** to serve as a liaison between the agency and community health agencies involved in monitoring and responding to communicable diseases
- Identification of job classifications and, in some cases, specific tasks when exposure to blood-borne pathogens is possible
- A schedule detailing when and how the provisions of blood-borne pathogen standards will be implemented
- Personal protective equipment (PPE)
- Body substance isolation (BSI)
- Procedures for evaluating exposure and postexposure counseling (e.g., the Ryan White Act)
- Notifying and working with local health authorities and state and federal agencies regarding exposures
- Personal, building, vehicle, and equipment disinfection and storage
- Education of employees regarding disinfection agents
- After-action analysis of the agency's response
- Correct disposal of needles and sharps in appropriate containers
- Correct handling of linens and supplies that become contaminated with body fluids during patient care
- Identification of agency and/or contracted personnel for counseling, authorization of acute medical care, and documentation

GUIDELINES, RECOMMENDATIONS, STANDARDS, AND LAWS

To protect health care workers against the spread of infection, OSHA requires that personal protective equipment be made available to all employees considered at high risk for exposure to infectious diseases. It also requires that all employees be offered preexposure prophylaxis against hepatitis through inoculation with hepatitis vaccines.[2] The CDC and NFPA have established similar guidelines, recommendations, and standards regarding the protection of health care workers and emergency providers from blood-borne pathogens. This includes regular testing for tuberculosis. It also includes vaccination for measles in individuals who do not have immunity (Box 39-2).

The *Ryan White Comprehensive AIDS Resources Emergency Act* (PL 101-381), passed in 1990, requires notification of emergency responders if they have been exposed to infectious diseases. It also requires that employers name a DO to direct communications between the hospital and emergency service in case of an exposure. Notification must be made within 48 hours of determination of the presence of the disease.

The CDC has classified infectious disease into two types: airborne and blood-borne. The primary airborne disease is infectious tuberculosis. The primary blood-borne diseases spread by pathogens are the hepatitis B and C viruses and HIV. The CDC also lists less common infectious diseases.

BOX 39-2 Recommended Immunizations for Emergency Medical Services Providers*

Hepatitis B†	Mumps
Diphtheria	Rubella
Influenza	Tetanus
Measles	Polio

*Testing for tuberculosis (TB) is required at the time of initial employment and annually thereafter.
†This vaccination is required by the federal Occupational Safety and Health Administration.

These include diphtheria, hemorrhagic fevers, meningococcal disease, plague, and rabies.

Currently, medical facilities are not required to test patients for any infectious disease. If paramedics suspect a possible exposure, they may submit a written notice to the DO. The DO, in turn, must submit a written request for a determination to the medical facility that treated the patient. The medical facility must try to identify the patient in question. It must review the results of diagnostic tests performed. It also must review any signs and symptoms the patient may have had that correspond to the CDC list of infectious diseases. After determining whether a paramedic may have been exposed to an infectious disease, the medical facility must notify the DO within 48 hours of receiving the request.

CRITICAL THINKING

What rights do you think paramedics had to obtain infectious disease information before the Ryan White law was passed?

Personal Responsibilities in Infectious Agent Exposure

Paramedics should familiarize themselves with the laws, regulations, and national standards regarding infectious disease. They should take personal protective measures against exposure to these pathogens. At times all paramedics will provide patient care to a person with an infectious disease. They must be aware of the potential consequences of the disease for public health and through contact with family members and friends. Table 39-1 and Box 39-3 provide an overview of CDC guidelines. These are designed to help prevent the spread of infectious disease to public safety and emergency response workers. Paramedics should follow local protocol regarding similar or additional precautions for personal protection and should be aware of their individual responsibilities, including the following[1]:

- A proactive attitude toward infection control
- Maintenance of personal hygiene and prevention of offensive body odors (esthetics of patient care)
- Attention to wounds and maintenance of the skin (the external barrier to infection)
- Effective hand washing after every patient contact using warm water and antiseptic cleanser or waterless antiseptic cleanser when portable water is unavailable
- Washing or disposing of work garments before entering the home
- Handling uniforms in accordance with the agency's definition of PPE
- Proper handling and laundering of work clothes soiled with body fluids, with consideration for bathing and showering after the work shift and before returning home
- Preparing food and eating in appropriate areas
- Maintenance of general physiological and psychological health to prevent distress, which can compromise the immune system of a healthy individual
- Proper disposal of needles and sharps in appropriate containers
- Proper disposal of body fluid–tinged linens and supplies
- Awareness and avoidance of tendencies to wipe the face and/or rub the eyes, nose, or mouth with gloved hands
- Knowledge of general classifications of exposure to determine the extent of infection control measures applied to the health care worker

BODY SUBSTANCE ISOLATION

In 1987 the CDC published the *Recommendations for Prevention of HIV Transmission Guidelines in Health-Care Settings*, which recommended that body fluid precautions (the universal [standard] precautions recommended by the CDC in 1983) be extended and used for all patients, regardless of their bloodborne infection status.[3] Since then, the U.S. Food and Drug Administration (FDA) and the CDC have worked together to identify further the body fluids to which universal precautions apply (Box 39-4).

The universal/standard precautions (mainly applicable to clinical and research facilities) for EMS personnel are superseded by body substance isolation (BSI) guidelines. These are an enhanced version of the universal/standard precautions. BSI is based on the premise that *all* exposures to body fluids, under any circumstances, are potentially infectious.[1]

DECONTAMINATION METHODS AND PROCEDURES

Guidelines for cleaning, disinfecting, and sterilizing patient care equipment have been established by the CDC, OSHA, the Environmental Protection Agency (EPA), USFA, and other agencies and organizations. These guidelines are part of an EMS agency's protocols and standard operating procedures. The following is a brief description of these decontamination methods and procedures.[4]

Sterilization destroys all forms of microbial life. It is used for instruments that penetrate the skin or come in contact with normally sterile parts of the body (e.g., scalpels and needles). Methods that may be used for sterilization include steam under pressure (autoclave), gas (ethylene oxide), dry heat, and immersion in EPA-approved chemical sterilant.

BOX 39-3 Guidelines for Prevention of Transmission of the Human Immunodeficiency Virus (HIV) and Hepatitis B Virus to Health Care and Public Safety Workers

These general principles have been developed from existing principles of occupational safety and health. They have been developed in conjunction with data from studies of health care workers in hospitals. The basic premise is that workers must be protected from exposure to blood and other potentially infectious body fluids in the course of their work. However, data concerning the risks these worker groups face are lacking. This complicates the development of control principles. Thus the guidelines here are based on principles of prudent public health practice.

Fire and emergency medical services personnel provide medical care in the prehospital setting. The following guidelines can help rescue personnel make decisions on the use of personal protective equipment and resuscitation equipment. They also are meant to help them make decisions regarding documentation, disinfection, and disposal procedures.

Personal Protective Equipment

The proper personal protective equipment should be made available by the employer. This reduces the risk of exposure. For many situations, the rescuer's chance of being exposed to blood and other body fluids to which universal precautions apply can be determined in advance. If the chance of exposure is high, the worker should put on protective attire before beginning patient care. (Examples of high-risk situations include cardiopulmonary resuscitation, intravenous line insertion, trauma, and childbirth.) (This list is not intended to be all-inclusive.) Important pieces of protective gear include the following:

1. *Gloves.* Disposable gloves should be a standard part of emergency response equipment. All personnel should put them on before giving any care that involves exposure to blood or other body fluids to which universal precautions apply. Extra pairs should always be available. No single type or thickness of glove offers the best protection in all situations. Considerations in the choice of disposable gloves should include dexterity, durability, fit, and the task to be performed. When large amounts of blood are likely, the gloves must fit tightly at the wrist. This prevents contamination of the hands around the cuff. For care of several trauma victims, gloves should be changed between patients if the situation allows.

   More extensive personal protective measures are indicated when broken glass and sharp edges are likely to be encountered. Such a situation might include extricating a person from a car wreck. Structural firefighting gloves that meet the requirements of the federal Occupational Safety and Health Administration for firefighter gloves* should be worn in any situation in which sharp or rough surfaces are likely to be encountered.

   While wearing gloves, paramedics should avoid handling personal items (e.g., combs, pens) that could become soiled or contaminated. Gloves that have become contaminated with blood or other body fluids should be removed as soon as possible. In doing so, paramedics should take care to avoid skin contact with the exterior surface of the gloves. Contaminated gloves should be placed and transported in bags that prevent leakage. They should be disposed of properly or, in the case of reusable gloves, cleaned and disinfected as required.
2. *Mask, eyewear, and gowns.* Masks, eyewear, and gowns should be kept on all emergency vehicles that respond or may respond to medical emergencies or victim rescues. This barrier equipment should be used in accordance with the level of exposure encountered. Minor cuts or small amounts of blood do not merit the same degree of barrier use as that needed for victims with massive blood loss. Management of the patient who is not bleeding and who has no body fluids present should not routinely require the use of barrier precautions. Masks and eyewear (e.g., safety glasses) should be worn together or a face shield should be used by all personnel for any situation that is likely to involve splashes of blood or other body fluids to which universal precautions apply. Gowns or aprons should be worn to protect clothing from blood splashes. If large splashes or amounts of blood are present or anticipated, nonpermeable gowns or aprons should be worn. An extra change of work clothing should be available at all times.
3. *Resuscitation equipment.* No transmission of hepatitis B virus or HIV infection during mouth-to-mouth resuscitation has been documented. However, because of the risk of transmission of other infectious diseases through saliva, disposable airway equipment or resuscitation bags should be used. Diseases that can be spread in saliva include herpes simplex infection and *Neisseria meningitidis.* Theoretically, a risk exists of HIV and hepatitis B virus transmission during artificial ventilation of trauma victims. Disposable resuscitation equipment and devices should be used once and then discarded. If reusable, this equipment should be thoroughly cleaned and disinfected after each use according to the manufacturer's recommendations.

   Mechanical respiratory assist devices (e.g., bag-valve-masks, oxygen demand-valve resuscitators) should be available on all emergency vehicles. They also should be available to all emergency response personnel who respond to medical emergencies or victim rescues.

   Pocket mouth-to-mask resuscitation masks are designed to prevent personnel from coming in contact with victims' blood and blood-contaminated saliva, respiratory secretions, and vomitus. These should be provided to all personnel who provide or may provide emergency treatment.

Modified from US Department of Health and Human Services, Centers for Disease Control and Prevention, National Institute of Occupational Safety and Health: *Guidelines for prevention of transmission of human immunodeficiency virus and hepatitis B virus to health-care and public-safety workers,* Washington, DC, 1989, DHHS, CDC, NIOSH.

*Standards are presented in 29 Code of Federal Register (CFR) 1910.156 and in National Fire Protection Association Standard 1973, Gloves for Structural Fire Fighters.

TABLE 39-1 Personal Equipment for Protection against Transmission of Human Immunodeficiency Virus (HIV) and Hepatitis B Virus

ACTIVITY	DISPOSABLE GLOVES	GOWN	MASK	PROTECTIVE EYEWEAR
Bleeding control (spurting blood)	Yes	Yes	Yes	Yes
Bleeding control (minimal blood)	Yes	No	No	No
Emergency childbirth	Yes	Yes	Yes*	Yes*
Intravenous therapy	Yes	No	No	No
Endotracheal intubation	Yes	No	Yes*	Yes*
Oral or nasal suctioning	Yes	No	No	No
Administration of an injection	No	No	No	No

Modified from Centers for Disease Control: *Examples of recommended personal protective equipment for worker protection against HIV and HBV transmission in prehospital setting,* February 1989.
*If splashing is likely.

BOX 39-4 Clarification of Use of Universal Precautions*

Body Fluids to Which Universal Precautions Apply
- Blood and other body fluids containing visible blood
- Semen and vaginal secretions
- Human tissue
- Human fluids (cerebrospinal fluid, synovial fluid, pleural fluid, peritoneal fluid, pericardial fluid, amniotic fluid)

Body Fluids to Which Universal Precautions Do Not Apply (in the Absence of Blood)
- Feces
- Nasal secretions
- Sputum
- Sweat
- Tears
- Urine
- Vomitus

Precautions for Other Body Fluids In Special Settings
- Human breast milk in mothers infected with the hepatitis B virus (HBV) (e.g., milk banking procedures)
- Saliva in some individuals infected with HBV or the human immunodeficiency virus (HIV) (e.g., human bites [remote], dental procedures)

Modified from Perspectives in disease prevention and health promotion update: universal precautions for prevention of transmission of human immunodeficiency virus, hepatitis B virus, and other bloodborne pathogens in health-care settings, *MMWR Morb Mortal Wkly Rep* 37(24):377, 1988.
*Established by the Centers for Disease Control and Prevention and the U.S. Food and Drug Administration.

High-level disinfection destroys all forms of microbial life *except* high numbers of bacterial spores. It is used for reusable instruments that come into contact with mucous membranes (e.g., laryngoscope blades, endotracheal tubes). Methods that may be used for high-level disinfection include hot water pressurization and exposure to an EPA-registered chemical sterilant.

Intermediate-level disinfection destroys *Mycobacterium tuberculosis,* most viruses, vegetative bacteria, and most fungi, but not bacterial spores. It is used for surfaces that come in contact with intact skin (e.g., stethoscopes, blood pressure cuffs, splints). It also is used for surfaces that have been visibly contaminated with blood or body fluids. (Surfaces must be cleaned of visible material before disinfection.) Methods that may be used for intermediate-level disinfection include use of EPA-registered "hospital disinfectant" chemical germicides that claim to be tuberculocidal on the label, hard surface germicides, and solutions containing at least 550 parts per million (ppm) free available chlorine (1:100 dilution of common household bleach; approximately ¼ cup of bleach per 1 gallon of water).

Low-level disinfection destroys some viruses, most bacteria, and some fungi, but not *M. tuberculosis* or bacterial spores. It is used for routine housekeeping. It also is used to clean up soiling when no blood is visible. Methods that may be used for low-level disinfection include use of EPA-registered "hospital disinfectants." (The label carries no claim of tuberculocidal activity.)

Environmental disinfection cleans soiled surfaces in the environment, such as floors, ambulance seats, and counter tops. Such surfaces should be disinfected with cleaners or disinfectant agents.

PATHOPHYSIOLOGY OF INFECTIOUS DISEASE

Infectious (communicable) disease is the fifth most common cause of death in the United States.[5] The development and/or manifestations of clinical disease depend on several factors, including the virulence (degree of pathogenicity) of the infectious agent, the number of infectious agents (dose), the resistance (immune status) of the host, and the correct mode of entry.[6] These factors all rely on an intact chain of elements to produce an infectious disease (Fig. 39-1). The elements of the chain include the following[7]:

- The pathogenic agent
- A reservoir
- A portal of exit from the reservoir
- An environment conducive to transmission of the pathogenic agent

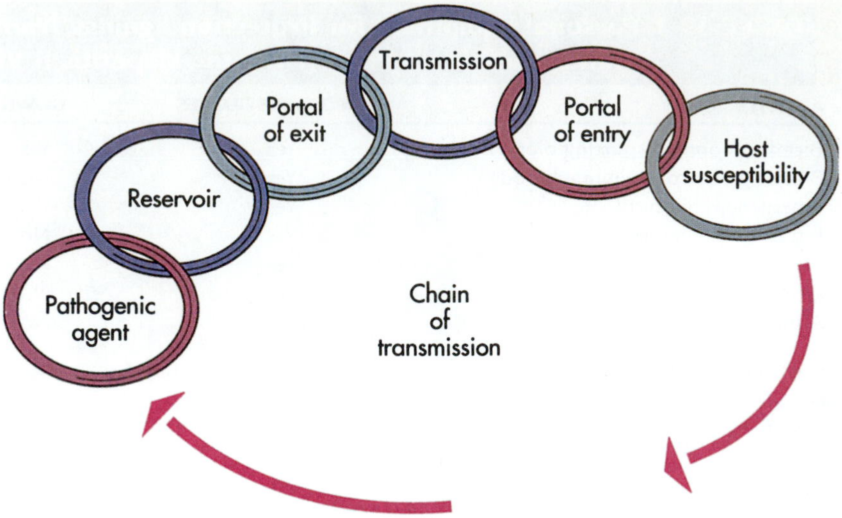

FIGURE 39-1 ■ Chain of transmission for infection. The chain must be intact for an infection to be transmitted to another host. Transmission can be controlled by breaking any link in the chain.

BOX 39-5 Review of Infectious Agents and Their Properties

Bacteria
- Bacteria are *prokaryotic* (i.e., the nuclear material is not contained within a distinctive envelope).
- They can self-reproduce without a host cell.
- Signs and symptoms depend on the cells and tissues affected.
- Bacteria produce toxins (these are often more lethal than the bacterium itself).
- Endotoxins (chemicals, usually proteins) are integral parts of a bacteria's outer membrane and are constantly shed from living bacteria.
- Exotoxins (proteins released by bacteria that can cause disease symptoms by acting as neurotoxins or enterotoxins)
- Lysis of bacteria may result in the release of endotoxins.
- Bacteria can cause localized or systemic infection.

Viruses
- Viruses are living organisms without a nucleus.
- They must invade host cells to reproduce.
- Many cannot survive outside a host cell.
- Viruses may contain other microorganisms.

Fungi
- Fungi are *eukaryotic* (i.e., the nuclear material is contained within a distinct envelope).
- A protective capsule surrounds the cell wall to protect the organism from phagocytes.

Protozoa
- Protozoa are single-celled microorganisms.
- They are more complex than bacteria.

Helminths (Worms [Including Tapeworms], Roundworms)
- Helminths are pathogenic parasites.
- They are not necessarily microorganisms.

- A portal of entry into the new host
- Susceptibility of the new host to the infectious disease

Even if all these elements are present, exposure does not necessarily mean that a person will become infected.

Pathogenic Agent

As described in Chapter 7, pathogens are organisms that can cause disease in the human host. They are classified according to shape (morphology), chemical composition, growth requirements, and viability. Pathogens rely on a host to supply their nutritional needs.

Some pathogens (e.g., certain bacteria) are metabolically equipped to survive outside a host. In contrast, others (e.g., certain viruses) can survive only in the human cell (Box 39-5). Some viruses, such as HIV and the hepatitis B virus (HBV), can survive for several hours outside a host. This is why blood products can be infectious.

Most bacteria are susceptible to certain drugs (antibiotics). These drugs either kill the bacteria or inhibit their growth. Viruses, however, are more difficult to treat because they reside in cells for most of their life cycle and become intricately enmeshed in the host cell's deoxyribonucleic acid (DNA). Factors that affect a pathogen's ability to cause disease include the following:

- The ability to invade and reproduce in a host and the mode by which it does so
- The speed of reproduction, the ability to produce a toxin, and the degree of tissue damage that results
- Potency
- The ability to induce or evade an immune response in the host

Reservoir

Pathogens may live and reproduce in humans or other animal hosts. They also may live and reproduce in an arthropod, a plant, soil, water, food, or some other organic substance, or a combination of these reservoirs. When infected, the human host may show signs of clinical illness. However, the host may be an *asymptomatic carrier* (i.e., a person who can pass the pathogen to others without showing signs of illness). The life cycle of the infectious agent depends on three factors: the demographics of the host, genetic factors, and the efficacy of therapeutic interventions once infection has been established.

Portal of Exit

The method by which a pathogenic agent leaves one host to invade another involves a portal of exit. The portal of exit from the human host depends on the agent. The portal may be single or multiple, involving the genitourinary (GU) tract, intestinal tract, oral cavity, respiratory tract, an open lesion, or any wound through which blood escapes. The time during which an actively infectious pathogen escapes to produce disease in another host coincides with the period of communicability (described later in this chapter). This period varies with each disease.

Transmission

The portal of exit and the portal of entry determine the mode of transmission. This mode may be direct or indirect. Direct transmission results from physical contact between the source and the victim. Examples of direct transmission include oral transmission and transmission by airborne mucus droplets, fecal contamination, and sexual contact.

In indirect transmission, the organism survives on animate or inanimate objects for a time without a human host. Diseases can be transmitted indirectly by air, food, water, soil, or biological matter.

Portal of Entry

The portal of entry is the means by which the pathogenic agent enters a new host. It may be ingestion, inhalation, percutaneous injection, crossing of a mucous membrane, or crossing of the placenta. The time it takes for the infectious process to begin in a new host varies with the disease and host susceptibility. Diseases differ in how long the exposure must be and how many germs are required to invade the new host. Exposure to an infectious agent does not always produce infection (Box 39-6).

BOX 39-6 Methicillin-Resistant *Staphylococcus aureus* (MRSA)

Staphylococcus aureus (often referred to as *staph*), is a bacterium commonly carried on the skin and in the nose of healthy people. Sometimes staph can cause infection. Staph bacteria are one of the most common causes of skin infections in the United States.[5] Most infections are minor (e.g., pimples and boils). Most of these can be managed without antibiotics. However, some infections are serious. These include surgical wound infections, bone infections, pneumonia, septicemia, and others, which may be resistant to penicillin-related antibiotics.

MRSA occurs more often in patients in hospitals and other health care facilities who are elderly or very sick; who have an open wound (e.g., bed sore) or an indwelling urinary catheter; or who are receiving intravenous (IV) therapy. Staphylococci and MRSA most often are spread by direct physical contact and not by airborne transmission. Spread may also occur through indirect contact by the touching of objects (e.g., towels, sheets, wound dressings, clothes) contaminated by the infected skin of a person with MRSA or staph bacteria. It is important for all health care providers to (1) use universal precautions; (2) practice good hand washing before and after each patient encounter; and (3) avoid contact with open wounds or material contaminated by wounds.

CRITICAL THINKING

Think of a precaution or intervention that could break each of the links in the chain of disease transmission.

Host Susceptibility

Host susceptibility is influenced by a person's immune response (described in Chapters 7 and 33). It also is influenced by several other factors. Some of these factors include the following:

1. Human characteristics
   - Age
   - Gender
   - Ethnic group
   - Heredity
2. General health status
   - Nutrition
   - Hormonal balance
   - Presence of concurrent disease
   - History of previous disease
3. Immune status
   - Prior exposure to disease (conferring resistance)
   - Effective immunization against disease (conferring host immunity)
4. Geographical and environmental conditions
5. Cultural behaviors
   - Eating habits
   - Personal hygiene
   - Sexual behaviors

PHYSIOLOGY OF THE HUMAN RESPONSE TO INFECTION

The human body is regularly exposed to pathogens that can cause illness. Even so, most people do not succumb to infectious disease. This protection is provided by external and internal barriers. These barriers act as lines of defense against infection.

External Barriers

The first line of defense against infection is the surface of the body, which is exposed to the environment. This includes the skin and the mucous membranes of the diges-

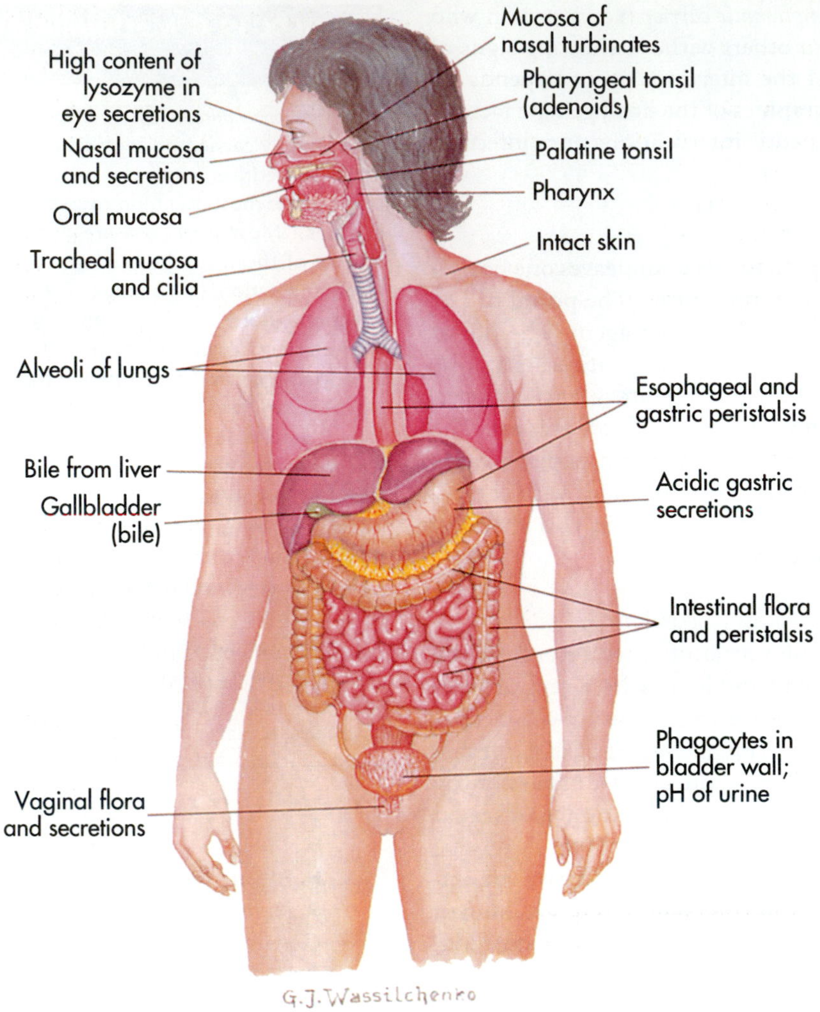

FIGURE 39-2 ■ First line of defense: external barriers.

tive, respiratory, and GU tract. These areas are inhabited by an indigenous flora (agents that could produce disease if allowed access to the interior of the body). The surface of the body forms a continuous closed barrier between the internal organs and the environment (Fig. 39-2).

FLORA

Nearly the whole body surface is inhabited by normal microbial flora. The flora enhance the effectiveness of the surface barrier. They do this by interfering with the establishment of pathogenic agents in several ways. Indigenous flora compete with pathogens for space and nutrients. They maintain a pH optimal for their own growth. This pH can be incompatible with that needed for many pathogenic agents to survive. Some flora also secrete germicidal substances. The flora are also thought to stimulate the immune system.

Resident (normal) flora play a key role in the body's defense. However, some indigenous flora can be pathogenic under certain conditions. For example, flora can cause infection when the skin or mucous membranes are interrupted. They also can cause infection when flora are displaced from their natural habitat to another area of the body. (This is a common cause of urinary tract infection after catheterization of the bladder.)

SKIN

Intact skin defends against infection. It does this in two ways. First, it prevents penetration. Second, it maintains an acidic pH level that inhibits the growth of pathogenic bacteria. In addition, microbes are sloughed from the skin's surface with dead skin cells, and oil and sweat wash microorganisms from the skin's pores.

GASTROINTESTINAL SYSTEM

The normal bacteria in the gastrointestinal (GI) system provide competition between colonies of microorganisms for nutrients and space. Normal bacteria help prevent the growth of pathogenic organisms. In addition, stomach acid may destroy some microorganisms. It also may deactivate their toxic products. The digestive system eliminates pathogens through feces.

UPPER RESPIRATORY TRACT

The sticky membranes of the upper airway protect against pathogens. They do this by trapping large particles. These particles may then be swallowed or expelled by coughing or sneezing. Coarse nasal hairs and cilia also trap and filter foreign substances in inspired air. They prevent the pathogens from reaching the lower respiratory tract. In addition, the lymph tissues of the tonsils and adenoids allow a rapid local immunological response to pathogenic organisms that may enter the respiratory tract.

GENITOURINARY TRACT

The natural process of urination and urine's ability to kill bacteria help prevent infections in the GU tract. Antibacterial substances in prostatic fluid and the vagina also help prevent infection in the GU system.

Internal Barriers

Internal barriers protect against germs when the external lines of defense cannot. Internal barriers include the inflammatory response and the immune response. These share many of the same processes and cellular components.

INFLAMMATORY RESPONSE

Inflammation (described in Chapter 7) is a local reaction to cellular injury. It occurs in response to a microbial infection. When invasion occurs, this line of defense is activated. It works to prevent further invasion of the pathogen by isolating, destroying, or neutralizing the microorganism (Fig. 39-3).

The inflammatory response usually is protective and beneficial. However, it may initiate destruction of the body's own tissue. It may be destructive if the response is sustained or directed against the host's own antigens. To review, the inflammatory response may be divided into three separate stages: first, cellular response to injury; second, vascular response to injury; and third, phagocytosis.

Cellular Response to Injury. As described in Chapter 7, the body mounts various types of cellular response to injury. The processes responsible for the cellular injury also are complex. Some cells are the targets of specific inflammatory mediators (e.g., leukotrienes, histamine). When these cells are injured, the cell's metabolism is damaged. This leads to decreasing energy reserves in the cells. When the energy reserves are depleted, a buildup of sodium ions causes the cell to swell. Along with increasing acidosis, this swelling further impairs the cell's ability to function. It leads to deterioration of the cell membranes. Eventually, the membranes of the cells begin to leak. This contributes to cellular destruction, autolysis, and stimulation of the inflammatory response in surrounding tissues.

Vascular Response to Injury. Localized hyperemia (an increase in blood in the area) develops after cellular injury. This produces edema. Leukocytes collect inside the vessels. There they release chemotactic factors (chemicals that attract more leukocytes to the area). These factors eventually migrate to the injured tissue.

Phagocytosis. Through phagocytosis, leukocytes engulf, digest, and destroy the invading pathogens. Circulating macrophages clear the area of dead cells and other debris. The ingestion of bacteria and dead cells (internal phagocytosis) releases chemicals that destroy leukocytes.

IMMUNE RESPONSE

The first two lines of defense against infection use the same mechanism to respond to all pathogens. However, the immune response is specific to individual pathogens. The immune system has four unique characteristics:

1. It has "self-nonself" recognition; therefore it usually responds only to foreign antigens.
2. It produces antibodies that are antigen specific. That is, new antibodies can be produced in response to new antigens.
3. Some of the antibody-producing lymphocytes become *memory cells*. These cells allow for a more rapid response to repeat invasions by the same antigen.
4. The immune system is self-regulated. It activates only when a pathogen invades. This ability prevents healthy tissues from being destroyed. When this function goes awry, autoimmune disease can occur (e.g., rheumatoid arthritis, active glomerulonephritis, and systemic lupus erythematosus). The immune system may require extrinsic regulation with drugs in patients with transplanted organs or severe autoimmune diseases.

CRITICAL THINKING

Why would a person's internal defenses be weakened after removal of the spleen?

The body's immune response to an invading pathogen depends partly on the size of the pathogen. It also depends on the pathogen's ability to produce an antibody. Often, peripheral phagocytic cells encounter a pathogen first. However, circulating B and T cells (described in Chapter 6) also are scouting for pathogens (Box 39-7). Complex interactions occur among neutrophils, macrophages, and B and T cells. These cells assist each other in processing antigens that can recognize and destroy the invading pathogens.

The B cell's role is to produce antibody (humoral immunity). This antibody coats the pathogen and facilitates phagocytosis. Antibody can also fix *complement*. The **complement system** is a group of proteins that coat bacteria and help to kill them directly. Or the proteins can have the bacteria taken up by neutrophils in the blood or by macrophages in the tissues. T cells not only process antigen for the B cells, they also include a subpopulation of "killer cells." These cells play a major role in cell-mediated immunity (Fig. 39-4).

Both the humoral and cell-mediated types of immunity take time to work. Both require previous exposure to mobilize specialized white cells. In time, these white cells differentiate between antibodies. They then organize an attack

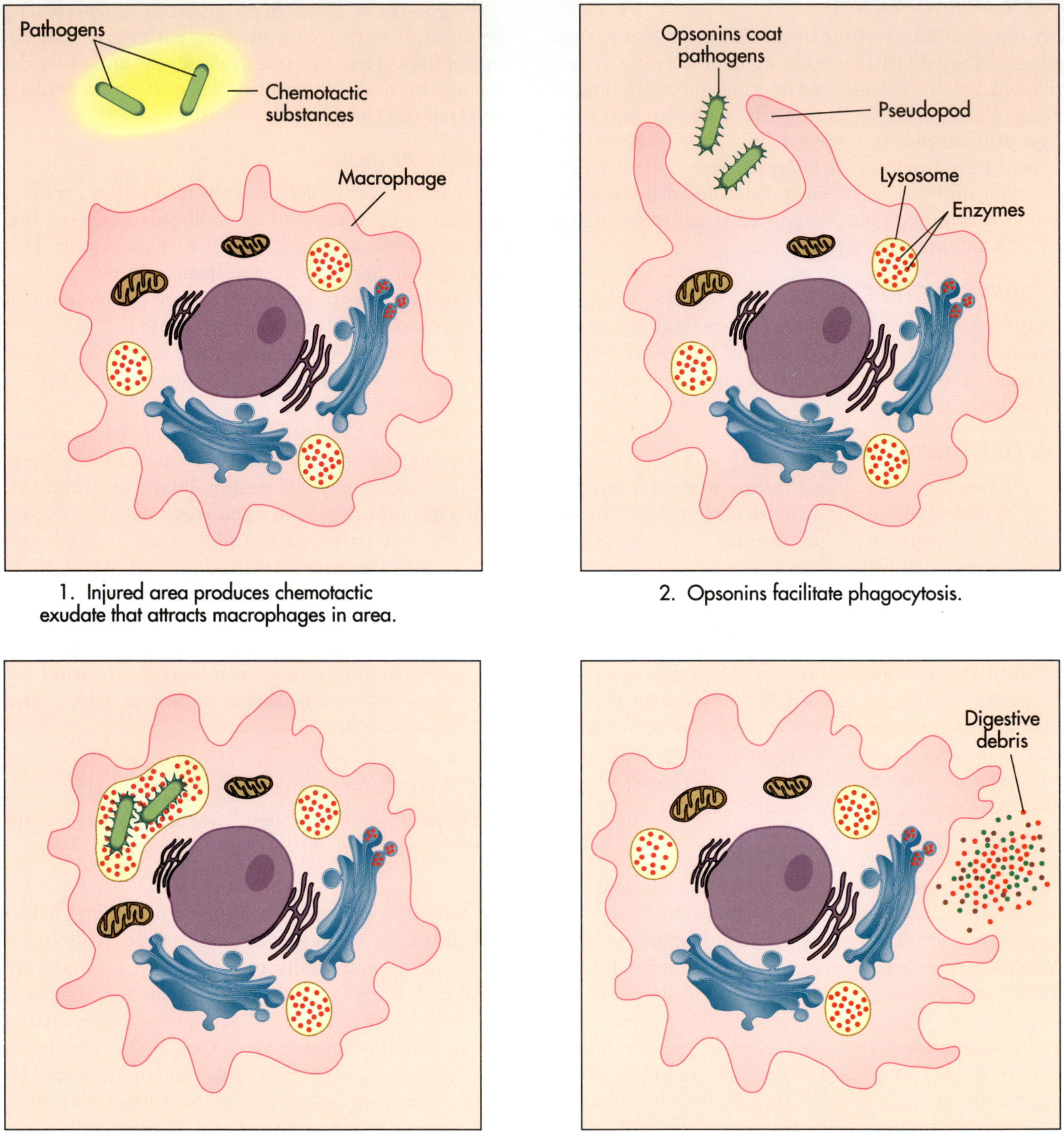

1. Injured area produces chemotactic exudate that attracts macrophages in area.

2. Opsonins facilitate phagocytosis.

3. The engulfed pathogen becomes digested by enzymes in the lysosomes.

4. The macrophage expels debris after digestion is complete, including prostaglandins, interferon, and complement components. These elements continue the immune response.

FIGURE 39-3 ■ Second line of defense: inflammatory response.

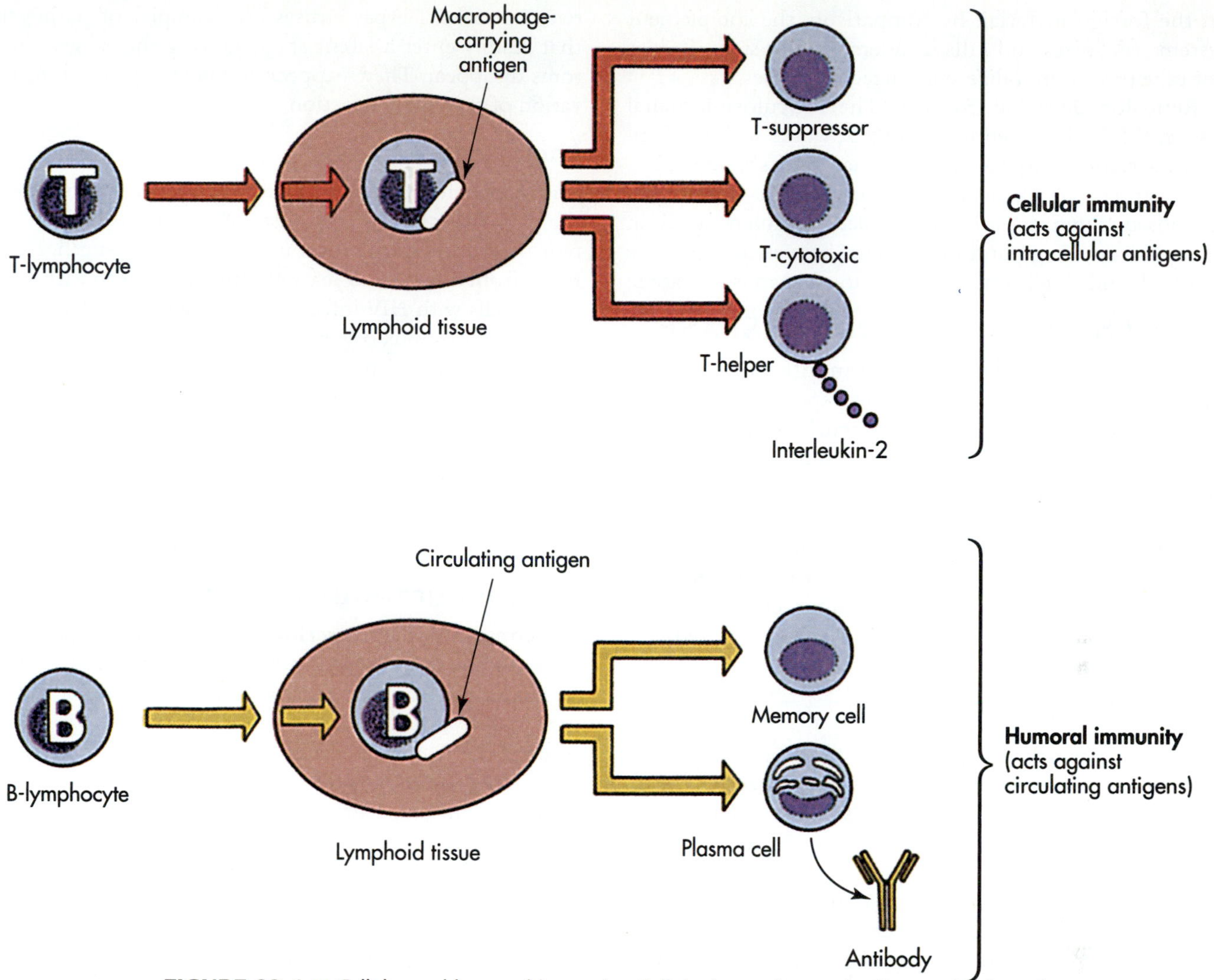

FIGURE 39-4 ■ Cellular and humoral immunity. Cellular immunity results from activation of T cells through contact with intracellular organisms. Activated T cells differentiate and proliferate. Humoral (antibody-mediated) immunity results from the activation of B cells.

BOX 39-7 Types of T Cells

Sensitized T cells develop into distinct groups. Each group has a specific set of functions that coordinate the activity of other components of the immune system.

- *Killer T cells* (like B cells) are sensitized and stimulated to multiply by the presence of antigens on abnormal body cells. Unlike B cells, killer T cells do not produce antibodies.
- *Helper T cells* "turn on" the activities of killer (cytotoxic) cells. They also control other aspects of the immune response.
- *Suppressor T cells* "turn off" the action of the helper and killer T cells. This prevents them from causing harmful immune reactions.
- *Inflammatory T cells* stimulate allergic reactions, anaphylaxis, and autoimmune reactions.

on the foreign material. By comparison, the complement system recognizes and kills invaders on first sight. It does not take time to mobilize specialized responses.

Reticuloendothelial System. The reticuloendothelial system (RES), described in Chapter 7, works with the lymphatic system to dispose of debris that results from the immune system attack on invading organisms. The RES is composed of immune cells in the spleen, lymph nodes, liver, bone marrow, lungs, and intestines. These structures store mature B and T cells until the immune system is activated.

STAGES OF INFECTIOUS DISEASE

The progression from exposure to an infectious agent to the onset of clinical disease follows specific stages. The duration of each stage and the potential outcomes vary, depending on the infectious agent and individual host factors. These stages are the latent period, the incubation period, the communicability period, and the disease period (Table 39-2). The risk of infection may be *theoretical*. That is, transmission is acknowledged to be possible but has not actually occurred. The risk of infection is considered *measurable* when infection is confirmed or deduced from reported data.

Latent Period

The **latent period** begins when the pathogen invades the body. During this period, infection has occurred but the infectious agent cannot be passed (or "shed") to someone else or cause clinically significant symptoms. In some diseases (e.g., HIV), the latent period is quite stable and can last several years. In others (e.g., influenza), the latent period may last only 24 to 72 hours. The latent period as a stage of infectious disease is distinct from a latent infection. A *latent infection* is an inactive infection that can still shed and produce symptoms; a *latent disease* is characterized by periods of inactivity either before signs and symptoms appear or between attacks. Herpes viruses are examples of pathogens that readily enter a latent stage. During this stage, symptoms disappear. They reappear at a later time upon reactivation of the latent infection.

TABLE 39-2 Stages of Infectious Disease

STAGE	BEGINS	ENDS
Latent period	With invasion	When the agent can be shed
Incubation period	With invasion	When the disease process begins
Communicability period	When the latent period ends	Continues as long as the agent is present and can spread to others
Disease period	Follows incubation period	Variable duration

Incubation Period

The **incubation period** is the interval between exposure to the pathogen and the first onset of symptoms. Like the latent period, the incubation period varies in length. It can range from hours to 15 years or longer, as is seen with some individuals with HIV infection. During the incubation period, the infectious organism reproduces in the host. The body is stimulated to produce antibodies specific for the disease or antigen. A person's blood may test positive (seroconversion) for exposure to the disease. A *window phase*, however, follows infection. In this phase, the antigen is present but there is no detectable antibody. A person whose blood is tested for disease-specific antibodies in the window phase may test negative, even when infection is present.

Communicability Period

The **communicability period** follows the latent period. It lasts as long as the agent is present and can spread to other hosts. (Clinically significant symptoms from the infection may manifest during this period.) This stage is variable. It often is the major determining factor in ease of transmission. The communicability period and the method of transmission can be altered in some diseases (e.g., tuberculosis, syphilis, gonorrhea). This depends on the stage of the disease and the primary site of infection.

Disease Period

The **disease period** follows the incubation period. It varies in duration, depending on the specific disease. This stage may be free of symptoms or it may produce overt symptoms. These symptoms can arise directly from the invading organism or from the body's response to the disease. During the disease period, the body may be able to rid itself of the disease entirely. On the other hand, the organism may become incorporated and lie inactive inside certain cells (a latent disease). Several viruses (e.g., HIV and hepatitis) can lead to latent infection. The resolution of symptoms does not mean the infectious agent has been destroyed.

CRITICAL THINKING

Which of the four stages of infectious disease can overlap? What problems can the overlap (or overlaps) pose?

HUMAN IMMUNODEFICIENCY VIRUS

HIV is present in the blood and serum-derived body fluids (semen, vaginal or cervical secretions) of people infected with the virus. The disease is directly transmitted person to person. It is passed through anal or vaginal intercourse, across the placenta, or by contact between infected blood or body fluids and mucous membranes or open wounds. It also can be transmitted indirectly. This occurs through transfusion with contaminated blood or blood products, transplantation of tissues and organs, and the use of contaminated needles or syringes. The incidence of HIV is highest in people with the following risk factors:

- High-risk sexual behavior
- Intravenous drug abuse
- Transfusion recipient between 1978 and 1985
- Hemophilia or other coagulation disorders requiring blood products
- Infant born to an HIV-positive mother

Other factors that may affect susceptibility to HIV include concurrent sexually transmitted diseases (STDs), especially those that cause skin ulcerations. Also, retention of the penile foreskin may increase susceptibility to HIV. Race and gender do not appear to be risk factors.[1]

Pathophysiology

HIV infection results from one of two retroviruses that convert genetic ribonucleic acid (RNA) to DNA after entering the host cell. The two types are known as *HIV-1* and *HIV-2*. Once the retrovirus is inside the cell, the cell's genetic material is altered into a hybrid of part virus and part cell. The virus basically takes over the cell to make more viral particles. When enough of the viral particles have been produced, the host cell ruptures. This destroys the cell and releases the virus into the blood to seek new target cells. The cell receptor sought by HIV is a T cell that has molecules called CD4 on its surface (CD4 T cell). When HIV attaches itself to the CD4 molecule, it allows the virus to enter and infect the cells, damaging them in the process. The CD4 T cell count is used to determine how active the disease is; a very low count suggests severe disease. These CD4 molecules are also found on the surface of certain nerve cells, and monocytes and phagocytes, which probably carry the disease to other parts of the body. Even though the body develops antigen-specific antibodies to HIV, these antibodies do not protect against HIV. Secondary complications generally are caused by opportunistic infections that develop as the immune system deteriorates. These infections include the following:

- Pulmonary tuberculosis
- Recurrent pneumonia
- *Pneumocystis carinii* pneumonia
- Kaposi sarcoma
- Wasting syndrome
- HIV dementia
- Sensory neuropathy
- Toxoplasmosis of the central nervous system

NOTE The two types of HIV (HIV-1 and HIV-2) are serologically and geographically distinct. However, they have similar epidemiological characteristics. HIV-1 is much more pathogenic than HIV-2. Most cases worldwide and in the United States are caused by HIV-1. HIV-2 seems to be more restricted to West Africa.[1] Some blood screening procedures test only for HIV-1.

Classification and Categories

The average interval from transmission of HIV to the development of serious complications is about 10 years if the condition goes untreated. However, this time frame can vary greatly (Table 39-3).

The CDC has devised a classification system for HIV (revised in 1993) with three categories based on the CD4 T-cell count[8]:

Category 1: Cell count of 500/mL or higher
Category 2: Cell count of 200 to 499/μL
Category 3: Cell count below 200/μL

As the number of CD4 T cells decreases, the risk and severity of opportunistic illness increase. After viral transmission, the progression of HIV in adolescents and adults can be divided into three clinical categories: A, B, and C.

CATEGORY A

- *Acute retroviral infection:* This syndrome generally occurs 2 to 4 weeks after exposure. Clinical features include an infectious mononucleosis–like illness with fever, adenopathy, and sore throat. The febrile illness is self-limited. It usually lasts 1 to 2 weeks. During this stage, a transient decrease is observed in the CD4 T-cell count.
- *Seroconversion:* The serological response with antigen-specific antibodies to HIV generally occurs 6 to 12 weeks after transmission. During this stage, the CD4 T-cell count returns to normal.

CRITICAL THINKING

What will probably happen if a sample is drawn for a blood test for HIV antibodies during the third week after exposure?

- *Asymptomatic infection:* The individual with HIV may have persistent generalized lymphadenopathy (enlarged lymph nodes involving two noncontiguous sites other than inguinal nodes) and a gradual decline in the CD4 T-cell count.

CATEGORY B

- *Early symptomatic HIV:* The usual CD4 T-cell count in this group is 100 to 300/μL. At this stage, common complications include localized candidal infections (thrush, *Candida esophagitis, Candida vaginitis*), oral lesions, shingles, pelvic inflammatory disease, peripheral neuropathy, and constitutional symptoms such as fever or diarrhea that last longer than 1 month.

TABLE 39-3 Incubation and Communicability Periods of Various Infectious Diseases

INCUBATION PERIOD	COMMUNICABILITY PERIOD
Childhood Diseases	
Chickenpox	
2 to 3 weeks (average 13 to 17 days)	Occurs 1 or 2 days before the onset of rash and until lesions have crusted over and not more than 6 days after the appearance of vesicles
Mumps	
2 to 3 weeks (average 18 days)	Occurs 6 days before parotid symptoms to 9 days after; disease is most communicable 48 hours after parotid swelling develops
Pertussis	
7 to 14 days, commonly 7 to 10 days	Occurs 7 days after exposure and lasts 3 weeks after onset; highly communicable in early stage before cough; not communicable after 3 weeks, although cough may be present
Rubella	
14 to 23 days (average 16 to 18 days)	Occurs from 1 week before to 4 days after appearance of rash; infants with congenital rubella syndrome may shed virus for months after birth
Rubeola	
Commonly 10 days, 8 to 13 days until fever, 14 days until rash	Occurs a few days before the fever to 5 to 7 days after appearance of rash
Hantavirus	
3 days to 6 weeks	No known human-to-human transmission
Hepatitis Virus	
Hepatitis A Virus (HAV)	
15 to 50 days (average 28 to 30 days)	Usually occurs in latter half of incubation period and continues for several days after onset of jaundice
Hepatitis B Virus (HBV)	
45 to 180 days (average 60 to 90 days)	Occurs during incubation period and lasts throughout clinical course (carrier state may persist for years)
Hepatitis C Virus (HCV)	
2 weeks to 6 months (average 6 to 9 weeks)	Occurs 1 or more weeks before onset of symptoms and indefinitely during chronic and carrier states
Human Immunodeficiency Virus (HIV)	
Varies: 6 to 12 weeks from exposure to seropositivity, up to 20 years for symptomatic immune suppression and to diagnosis of acquired immunodeficiency syndrome (AIDS)	Is lifelong from presence of HIV in serum until death; degree of communicability may vary during course of HIV infection
Influenza	
24 to 72 hours	Occurs 3 days after onset of symptoms; infection produces immunity to specific strain of virus, but duration of immunity varies
Meningitis	
2 to 10 days	Varies; lasts as long as infectious agents remain in nasal and oral secretions; microorganisms disappear from upper respiratory tract within 24 hours of antibiotic therapy
Mononucleosis	
4 to 6 weeks	Prolonged; pharyngeal excretion may last for years; 15% to 20% of adults are carriers

TABLE 39-3 Incubation and Communicability Periods of Various Infectious Diseases, cont'd

INCUBATION PERIOD	COMMUNICABILITY PERIOD
Pneumonia	
1 to 3 days	Occurs until organisms have been eliminated from respiratory discharges (24 to 48 hours after antibiotic treatment)
Rabies	
Usually 2 to 16 weeks	Human-to-human transmission by bite, scratch, or aerosolization has not been documented; theoretical transmission from contact with secretions of infected person
Severe Acute Respiratory Syndrome (SARS)	
10 days	Information to date suggests that people are most likely to be infectious when they have symptoms, such as fever or cough. However, it is not known how long before or after symptoms appear that the disease can be transmitted.
Sexually Transmitted Diseases	
Chlamydia	
5 to 10 days	Unknown
Gonorrhea	
2 to 7 days	Occurs for months if disease goes untreated
Herpes simplex virus (HSV)	
HSV-1 2 to 12 days	Occurs when lesions are present; virus is found in saliva as long as 7 weeks after recovery from lesions; transient shedding of virus is common
HSV-2 2 to 12 days (average 6 days)	Occurs in 7 to 12 days with lesion; transient shedding of virus in the absence of lesions probably occurs
Syphilis	
10 days to 10 weeks (average 3 weeks)	Varies; occurs during primary and secondary stages and in mucocutaneous recurrences (2 to 4 years if disease goes untreated)
Tetanus	
3 to 21 days, commonly 10 days	Not directly transmitted; recovery from tetanus does not confer permanent immunity
Tuberculosis (TB)	
4 to 12 weeks after exposure or any time the disease is in a latent stage	Occurs as long as bacilli are present in sputum, sometimes intermittently for years

CATEGORY C

- *Late symptomatic HIV:* This stage represents all acquired immunodeficiency syndrome (AIDS)-defining diagnoses found primarily with CD4 T-cell counts of 0 to 200/μL, including severe opportunistic infections; bacterial pneumonia (e.g., *P. carinii* pneumonia); pulmonary tuberculosis; debilitating diarrhea; tumors in any body system, including Kaposi sarcoma (Fig. 39-5, 39-6); HIV-associated dementia; and neurological manifestations.
- *Advanced HIV:* In this stage, the person has a CD4 T-cell count of 0 to 50/μL. These patients have a limited life expectancy, and most of them die of AIDS-related complications.

Personal Protection

Strict compliance with universal precautions is the only preventive measure health care workers can take against HIV. However, the chance of EMS personnel acquiring the infection through exposure to infected blood appears to be low (0.2% to 0.44%).[1] HBV exposure is a much greater occupational hazard.[9] The risk to health care workers increases under the following circumstances:

1. The exposure involves a large amount of blood. This can occur when a piece of equipment is visibly contaminated with blood; when care of the patient involves placing a needle in a vein or an artery; and when the patient has deep injuries. The needle size and type (hollow bore or suture) and the depth of penetration influence the volume transferred to the skin. Health care workers suffer 600,000 to 1 million injuries from conventional needles and sharps each year.[10]

CRITICAL THINKING

Why would testing within 2 to 3 weeks of exposure be needed?

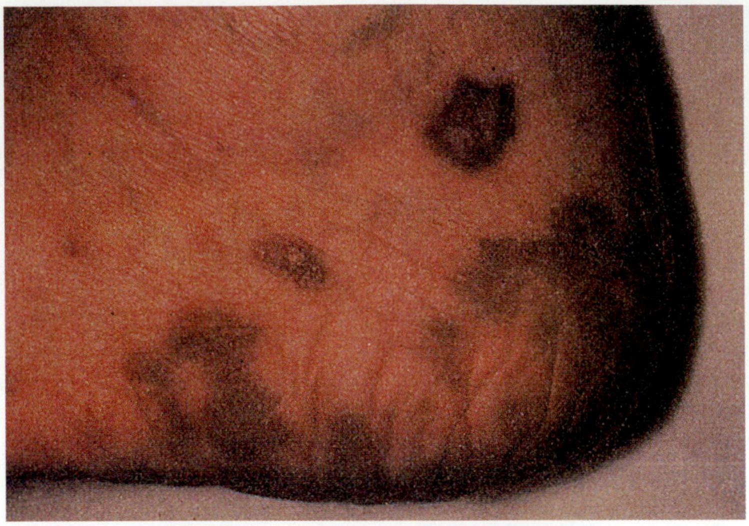

FIGURE 39-5 ■ Kaposi sarcoma of the heel and lateral foot.

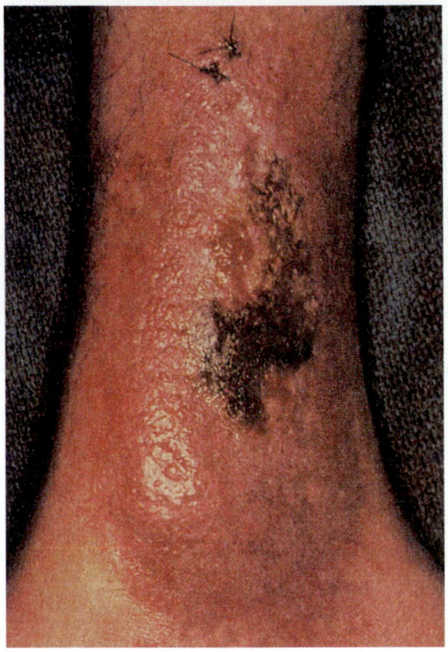

FIGURE 39-6 ■ Kaposi sarcoma of the distal leg and ankle.

2. The exposure involves a patient with a terminal illness, possibly reflecting a higher dose of HIV in the late course of AIDS. The risk of exposure must be understood in terms of how the exposure occurred and what factors were involved. Although the potential may appear high, the probability actually may be quite low. Paramedics should follow agency protocol for notification and reporting of significant exposures to any infectious disease.

Postexposure Prophylaxis

If exposure is confirmed or suspected, the paramedic should immediately notify the DO (per protocol). This allows elective postexposure prophylaxis (PEP) to begin. Information on primary HIV indicates that systemic infection does not occur immediately; this leaves a narrow window of opportunity in which postexposure antiretroviral intervention may modify viral replication.[11] Several antiretroviral agents from at least four classes of drugs are available for the treatment of HIV. Examples include fusion inhibitors, the nucleoside/nucleotide reverse transcriptase inhibitors (NRTIs), nonnucleoside reverse transcriptase inhibitors (NNRTIs), and protease inhibitors (PIs). After PEP, testing for HIV is performed 2 to 3 weeks after the exposure. It is performed again at 6 weeks, 3 months, 6 months, and 1 year.

NOTE An important goal of PEP is to encourage and facilitate compliance with a 4-week PEP regimen of two drugs used for most HIV exposures. (These include zidovudine [ZDV] and lamivudine [3TC]; 3TC and stavudine [d4T]; or didanosine [ddI] and d4T.) Moreover, an expanded regimen that includes the addition of a third drug is used for cases of HIV exposures that have an increased risk of transmission. When the patient's virus is known or suspected to be resistant to one or more of the drugs considered for the PEP regimen, the selection of drugs to which the virus is unlikely to be resistant is recommended.[12] All antiretroviral drugs have been associated with side effects (mainly gastrointestinal). In addition, some of these drugs (especially protease inhibitors) cause potentially serious drug interactions. Paramedics should receive counseling regarding evaluation and treatment after an exposure.

Psychological Reactions to HIV

HIV is almost always a progressive disease with morbid late consequences. Throughout the course of the infection, patients are likely to feel and express anger about many aspects of their illness. These include pain, dying prematurely and without dignity, and the social rejection and prejudice that the person may experience. Patient care should include helping these patients feel that they can obtain acceptance and compassion from health care workers.

Although no vaccine exists for HIV, many clinical trials are underway. Despite current limitations, the progression of the illness can be delayed with drug therapy and other strategies. This allows time for access to new therapeutic options.

HEPATITIS

As described in Chapter 34, hepatitis is a viral disease that produces pathological changes in the liver. The hepatitis viruses are divided into three main classes: hepatitis A (viral hepatitis), HBV (serum hepatitis), and hepatitis C (non-A/non-B hepatitis) (Table 39-4).

> **NOTE** Hepatitis non-ABC is a fourth class of hepatitis caused by infection with the hepatitis D virus and the newer hepatitis viruses (E and G). The routes of transmission for these viruses are similar to those for the hepatitis B virus (HBV). They often are mistaken for HBV.

Hepatitis A Virus

Hepatitis A (HAV) is the most common type of viral hepatitis in the United States. The disease is acquired by ingesting HAV-contaminated food or drink. It also is acquired by the fecal/oral route. The virus localizes in the liver, reproduces, enters the bile, and is carried to the intestinal tract. From there it is shed in the feces. (Fecal shedding usually occurs before the onset of clinical symptoms.) Antibodies (anti-HAV) develop during acute disease. They also develop late in convalescence. Once infected, the person is immune to HAV for life. Hepatitis A is the only hepatitis virus that does not lead to chronic liver disease or a chronic carrier state. Many HAV infections are subclinical. They often manifest with influenza-like symptoms. About 1 in 100 patients with HAV suffers from a fulminant infection that may require a liver transplant.[13]

Immune globulin (IG) can provide temporary immunity to the virus (i.e., 2 to 3 months). It must be given before exposure to HAV or within 2 weeks after contact. Hepatitis A vaccines approved for people 2 years of age or older are recommended for the following groups:

- People who have close physical contact with those who live in areas with poor sanitary conditions or who are traveling or working in developing countries
- Men who have sex with other men
- Users of illicit drugs
- Children in populations that have repeated epidemics of hepatitis A (Native Alaskans, Native Americans, Pacific Islanders, and certain closed religious communities)
- People who have chronic liver disease or clotting factor disorders

The safety of the vaccine during pregnancy has not been determined.

Hepatitis B Virus

Infectious HBV particles are found in blood and in secretions containing serum (e.g., oozing, cutaneous lesions). They also are found in secretions derived from serum (e.g., saliva, semen, vaginal secretions). Like other viral types of hepatitis, HBV affects the liver and causes the signs and symptoms described previously. The virus may produce chronic infection. This can lead to cirrhosis and other complications. Although HBV usually lasts less than 6 months, the carrier state may persist for years.

The effects of HBV vary. Only a low-grade fever and malaise (influenza-like illness) may occur, with complete resolution of symptoms. On the other hand, extensive liver necrosis may develop that can lead to death. Other complications associated with HBV include coagulation defects, impaired protein production, impaired bilirubin elimination, pancreatitis, and hepatic cancer. Exposure generally occurs in one of five ways:

1. Direct percutaneous inoculation of infectious serum or plasma by needle or transfusion of infected blood or blood products
2. Indirect percutaneous introduction of infective serum or plasma (e.g., skin cuts or abrasions, tattoo/body piercing)
3. Absorption of infective serum or plasma through mucosal surfaces (e.g., the eyes or mouth), transplacentally, or through contamination from the mother's infective blood at birth
4. Absorption of infective secretions (e.g., saliva or semen) through mucosal surfaces, as might occur during vaginal, anal, or oral sexual contact (but never fecal transmission)
5. Transfer of infective serum or plasma via inanimate environmental surfaces

HBV is stable on environmental surfaces and can remain infective in visible blood for longer than 7 days.[1]

> **CRITICAL THINKING**
> Why is information about exposure risks important to paramedics?

PREEXPOSURE PROPHYLAXIS

With regulatory and legislative efforts and the publication of OSHA's *Bloodborne Pathogen Standard,* cases of HBV in health care workers have dropped from 17,000 annually to about 400 annually.[14] (The exposure risk for health care providers working with HBV-positive patients is estimated to be 2% to 40%.) Yet, even with this decline, HBV is a serious concern to all health care workers. The CDC recommends and OSHA requires that HBV vaccines be offered to all health care workers. The vaccine sometimes is given to newborns. Several states now require immunization of children who are middle school age.

Blood is the most important potential source of HBV in the workplace. The risk of infection is directly proportional to the probability that the blood contains HBV, the recipient's immunity status, and the efficacy of transmission. HBV vaccinations are available that provide protection for 18 years in those who respond to the inoculation.[11] The HBV vaccination schedule generally requires three doses over 6 months. These are intramuscular (deltoid) doses. For the best protection against HBV, the series should be completed before an exposure occurs. Vaccinations currently available include Recombivax HB and Engerix-B.

TABLE 39-4 The ABCs of Hepatitis

	HEPATITIS A (HAV)	HEPATITIS B (HBV)	HEPATITIS C (HCV)	HEPATITIS D (HDV)	HEPATITIS E (HEV)
Description	HAV is a virus that causes inflammation of the liver. It does not lead to chronic disease.	HBV is a virus that causes inflammation of the liver. It can damage liver cells, leading to cirrhosis and cancer.	HCV is a virus that causes inflammation of the liver. It can damage liver cells, leading to cirrhosis and cancer.	HDV is a virus that causes inflammation of the liver. It infects only people with HBV.	HEV is a virus that causes inflammation of the liver. It is rare in the United States. There is no chronic state.
Incubation period	2 to 7 weeks (average 4 weeks)	6 to 23 weeks (average 17 weeks)	2 to 25 weeks (average 7 to 9 weeks)	2 to 8 weeks	2 to 9 weeks (average 40 days)
Transmission	By fecal/oral route, through close person-to-person contact or ingestion of contaminated food and water	Contact with infected blood, seminal fluid, vaginal secretions, and contaminated needles, including tattoo and body-piercing tools; infected mother to newborn; human bite; sexual contact	Contact with infected blood, contaminated intravenous (IV) needles, razors, and tattoo or body-piercing tools; infected mother to newborn; *not* easily spread through sexual contact	Contact with infected blood, contaminated needles; sexual contact with HDV-infected person	By fecal/oral route; in other countries, outbreaks associated with contaminated water supply
Symptoms	May have none; otherwise, the person may have light stools, dark urine, fatigue, fever, nausea, vomiting, abdominal pain, and jaundice	May have none; some people have mild, flulike symptoms, dark urine, light stools, jaundice, fatigue, and fever	Same as for HBV	Same as for HBV	Same as for HBV
Treatment of chronic disease	Not applicable	Interferon and lamivudine, with varying success	Interferon and combination therapies, with varying success	Interferon, with varying success	Not applicable
Vaccine	Two doses may be given to anyone over 2 years of age.	Three doses may be given to individuals of any age.	None	HBV vaccine prevents infection with HDV.	None
People at risk	Household members or those who have sexual contact with an infected person; those who live in an area where an HAV outbreak has occurred; travelers to developing countries; people who engage in anal/oral sex; injection drug users.	Infants born to an infected mother; those who have sex with an infected person or multiple partners; injection drug users; emergency responders; health care workers; people who engage in anal/oral sex; hemodialysis patients	People who received a blood transfusion before 1992; health care workers; injection drug users; hemodialysis patients; infants born to infected mothers; those who have sex with multiple partners	Injection drug users; people who engage in anal/oral sex; people who have sex with an HDV-infected person	Travelers to developing countries, especially pregnant women
Prevention	Administration of immune globulin within 2 weeks of exposure; vaccination; washing hands with soap and water after using the toilet; using household bleach (10 parts water to 1 part bleach) to clean surfaces contaminated with feces, such as changing tables; practicing safe sex	Administration of immune globulin within 2 weeks of exposure; vaccination (provides protection for 18 years); cleaning up infected blood with household bleach; wearing protective gloves when touching blood; no sharing of razors, toothbrushes, or needles; practicing safe sex	Cleaning up spilled blood with household bleach; wearing protective gloves when touching blood; no sharing of razors, toothbrushes, or needles; practicing safe sex	Administration of HBV vaccine to prevent HBV infection; practicing safe sex	Avoiding drinking or using water that may be contaminated

From Hepatitis Foundation International On-Line. http://hepfi.org.

BOX 39-8 Antiviral Therapy with Interferons

Interferons are proteins produced naturally by body cells in response to viral infection and other stimuli. Interferon alpha (Intron A and others) is effective at controlling the spread of common colds caused by rhinoviruses. It may be effective at treating chronic infections caused by the hepatitis B and C viruses (HBV and HCV) and the human immunodeficiency virus (HIV). The U.S. Food and Drug Administration (FDA) has approved combination therapy with Pegasys (peginterferon alfa-2a), and Copegus (ribavirin) for the treatment of adults with chronic hepatitis C who have compensated liver disease and have not previously been treated with interferon alpha.

Interferons work by attaching to the membranes of host cells and stimulating the host cells to attack the virus. If a virus invades a cell primed by interferon, enzymes are produced that impair viral copying. This nullifies the virus. Interferons also increase the activity of natural killer cells to stop or shorten the effects of the virus. Side effects of interferon include fever, malaise, headache, fatigue, hair loss, and bone marrow suppression.

POSTEXPOSURE PROPHYLAXIS

Postexposure prophylaxis may be indicated if an unvaccinated person or a person who has not completed the vaccination schedule is exposed to HBV. Before treatment, a blood test is performed to determine immunity to HBV. People who are not immune generally receive the HBV vaccine and hepatitis B immune globulin. (This is an antibody used in postexposure treatment to provide passive immunity to HBV.)

Hepatitis C Virus

Hepatitis C virus (HCV) is a blood-borne virus. It causes a disease similar to HBV. The virus was associated with receipt of contaminated blood during transfusion before 1992. (It accounts for more than 90% of posttransfusion hepatitis in the United States.) Currently, about 4 million Americans are believed to be infected with the virus. Hepatitis C is the infection that most often results from needle-stick and sharps injury.[15] Of health care workers who become infected, 85% become chronic carriers. About one half to two thirds of those infected with HCV develop chronic hepatitis; one in five suffers severe liver disease, such as cirrhosis and liver cancer. No vaccine is available for HCV.

Although HCV is transmitted in the same manner as other forms of hepatitis, it is not easily spread through sexual contact. Signs and symptoms of the disease, when they occur, are similar to those of other types of hepatitis. Most people infected with HCV are asymptomatic.

Signs and Symptoms

Infection with any of the causative viruses may be symptomless. On the other hand, it may cause a typical hepatitis with an abrupt onset of flulike illness that is followed by jaundice or dark urine, or both. A patient is most infectious during the first week of symptoms (see Table 39-3). Within 2 to 3 months of infection, the patient usually develops nonspecific symptoms. These may include anorexia, nausea and vomiting, fever, joint pain, and generalized rashes. About 1% of patients hospitalized with HBV develop full-blown liver crisis and die (Box 39-8).

Patient Management and Protective Measures

The management of patients out of the hospital is mainly supportive. The goal is to maintain circulatory status and prevent shock. All health care workers involved in the patient's care must follow careful personal protective measures. This includes effective hand washing. It also involves proper care in the use of diagnostic and therapeutic equipment (e.g., high-level disinfection of laryngoscope blades) and appropriate disposal of sharps.

TUBERCULOSIS

Each year, 8 million new cases of tuberculosis (TB) occur worldwide, and 3 million people die of the disease.[16] Reports of TB in the United States had declined continually since the turn of the twentieth century. However, in 1985 this trend reversed. The reversal is attributed to the epidemic of HIV. The incidence of tuberculosis (TB) among patients with HIV is 40 times the incidence among people who are not infected with HIV.[17] Other factors include:

- Immigration of people from areas with a high prevalence of TB
- Transmission of TB in high-risk environments, such as correctional facilities, homeless shelters, hospitals, and nursing homes
- Deterioration of the TB public health care infrastructure

CRITICAL THINKING

Why is TB more prevalent in patients with HIV?

Pathophysiology

As described in Chapter 30, TB is a chronic pulmonary disease. It is acquired through inhalation of a dried-droplet nucleus containing tubercle bacilli (*Mycobacterium tuberculosis, Mycobacterium bovis*, or a variety of atypical mycobacteria). TB is passed mainly by infected persons coughing or sneezing the bacteria into the air. It can also be passed through contact with the sputum of an infected person. People who share the same air space as those with infectious TB are at highest risk for infection. Transmission also may occur by ingestion or through the skin or mucous membranes. However, this is less common.

The pathology of TB is related to the production of inflammatory lesions throughout the body. It also is related to the ability of the TB bacillus to break through the body's natural defenses. This leads to the formation of caseating granulomas (necrotic inflammatory cells) and TB cavities.

These may cause chronic and debilitating lung disease. Susceptibility to mycobacterial infection generally is highest in children younger than 3 years of age; in adults older than 65; and in chronically ill, malnourished, and immunosuppressed or immunocompromised individuals. The infection may remain dormant for an indefinite time, often not causing disease. On the other hand, it may lead to active, contagious disease.

Tuberculosis is characterized by stages of early infection (frequently asymptomatic), latency, and a potential for recurrent postprimary disease (see Table 39-3). Signs and symptoms of TB include cough, fever, night sweats, weight loss, fatigue, and hemoptysis. The organ systems affected and the associated complications include the following:

1. Cardiovascular system
   - Pericardial effusions
   - Lymphadenopathy (cervical lymph nodes are usually involved)
2. Skeletal system
   - Intervertebral disk deterioration
   - Chronic arthritis of one joint
3. Central nervous system (CNS)
   - Subacute meningitis
   - Brain granulomas
4. Systemic miliary TB (extensive dissemination by the bloodstream of tubercle bacilli)

In the United States, an estimated 10 million to 15 million people are infected with *M. tuberculosis*. Without intervention, approximately 10% of these people will develop TB disease at some point in their lives.[14] Paramedics should maintain a high degree of suspicion for TB in individuals with undiagnosed lung disease, especially patients who are HIV positive.

Tuberculosis Testing

The signs and symptoms of initial infection may be minimal. However, early infection can be detected using the Mantoux tuberculin skin test (purified protein derivative [PPD]). A positive reaction to the PPD test indicates past infection and the presence of antibodies. Patients with positive test results usually have a chest x-ray and an acid-fast bacilli (AFB) sputum culture before treatment. Counseling and HIV antibody testing should be offered to all people infected with TB. This is because medical management may be altered if HIV is present. By law, every state is required to report cases of TB. A negative TB skin test result does not fully rule out TB infection. This is especially the case in people with TB-like symptoms, HIV, or AIDS. In these cases, a repeat skin test may be warranted 10 weeks after exposure.

Because identification and early treatment of TB are important, all health care workers should receive a routine evaluation consisting of PPD and, in some cases, a chest x-ray and AFB culture.[1] A negative immune response does not preclude reinfection with subsequent exposure.

Patient Care and Protective Measures

Paramedics should be aware of areas with a high incidence of active TB in their service region. (This information is reported by the local health authorities.) Prehospital care for patients with infectious TB is mainly supportive. As with any other infectious disease, universal precautions should be taken during patient care. This includes respiratory barriers for the patient and the paramedic. Surgical masks are insufficient for preventing inhalation of tuberculosis bacteria. However, they do reduce the number of droplet nuclei escaping from the patient. Therefore they should be placed on the patient during transport. NIOSH recommends that health care workers use particulate filter respirators (N-type respirators) when caring for patients with tuberculosis (Fig. 39-7 and Box 39-9). Ambulance ventilation systems that include high-efficiency particulate air (HEPA) filtration and a nonrecirculating ventilation cycle are another measure for preventing exposure to TB during patient transport. After each call, disinfection of all patient care equipment should be performed.

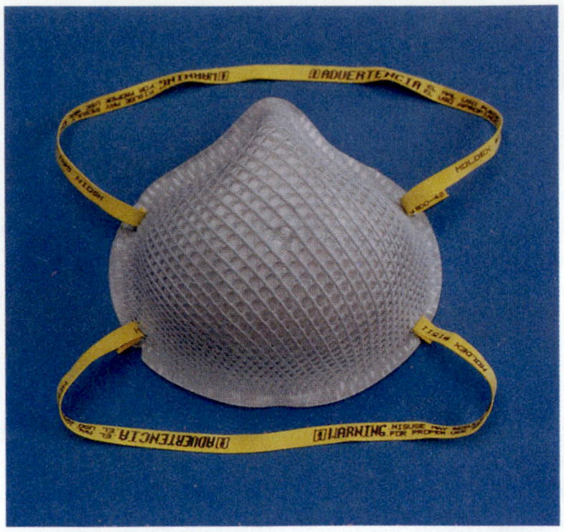

FIGURE 39-7 ■ High-efficiency particulate air (HEPA) respirator.

Treatment

If effective treatment is begun without delay, TB is usually curable. Multidrug-resistant TB is on the rise (Box 39-10). For this reason, most patients with TB are started on a lengthy, four-drug regimen of isoniazid (INH), rifampin (RIF), pyrazinamide (PZA), and ethambutol (EMB) or streptomycin (SM) until the drug susceptibility results are known. (Patients who undergo preventive therapy should be monitored for drug side effects. They should be watched especially for signs and symptoms of hepatitis.) Sputum and cultures usually become negative 3 to 8 weeks after the start of therapy.

PROPHYLACTIC ISONIAZID

For individuals younger than 35 years of age who have a positive result on a PPD skin test and who have not previously been treated, administration of INH is recommended. Isoniazid is not routinely recommended for those younger than 35 years old because it may damage the liver. However, the drug is used if one or more of the following factors[1] is present:

- Recent infection, as evidenced by PPD skin test conversion
- Close or household contact with a known case of infectious TB

BOX 39-9 Tuberculosis-Protective Respirators

The federal Occupational Safety and Health Administration (OSHA), in conjunction with guidelines established by the Centers for Disease Control and Prevention (CDC), currently requires the use of respirators. OSHA is enforcing their use while developing specific standards for preventing the exposure of health care workers to tuberculosis (TB) . The required respirator certified by the National Institute for Occupational Safety and Health (NIOSH) must have a disposable (or replaceable) high-efficiency particulate air (HEPA) filter capable of trapping airborne particles. Whenever respirators (including disposables) are required, a complete respiratory protection program must be implemented in accordance with federal regulations.* Elements of the required respiratory protection program include the following:

1. Permissible practices for respirator use
2. Respirator program administration
3. Selection of respirators
4. Inspection of respirators
5. Cleaning and maintenance of respirators
6. Storage of respirators
7. Training in respiratory protection
8. Fit testing of respirators (to ensure accurate sizing)
9. Respirator program evaluation
10. Medical surveillance of respirator users

Modified from US Department of Health and Human Services, National Institute of Occupational Safety and Health: *NIOSH guide to the selection and use of particulate respirators,* certified under 42 CFR 84, DHHS (NIOSH) Washington, DC. Publication No. 96-101, 1996.

*These specifications are found in 29 Code of Federal Register (CFR) 1910.134.

BOX 39-10 Multidrug-Resistant Tuberculosis

During the resurgence of tuberculosis (TB) in the United States that began in 1985, outbreaks of multidrug-resistant TB (MDR-TB) occurred in hospitals and prisons. This resulted in high death rates. It also resulted in transmission to health care workers.

MDR-TB is resistant to conventional drugs (isoniazid and rifampin). It is a very serious form of TB, because preventive therapy is limited. People at high risk for MDR-TB include the following:

- Those recently exposed to MDR-TB (especially if they are immunocompromised)
- TB patients who fail to take medications as prescribed
- TB patients who were prescribed an ineffective treatment regimen
- Patients previously treated for TB

A major cause of treatment failure and drug-resistant TB is failure to follow the treatment regimen. This threatens the health of TB patients and poses a serious public health risk. It also leads to prolonged infectivity and the spread of TB in the community.

- Abnormal chest x-ray
- Prolonged therapy with immunosuppressive drugs
- HIV or other immunosuppressive disease

Patients who are receiving INH should avoid alcohol. This reduces the chance for chemical- or drug-induced hepatitis. (Patients who are receiving INH should also avoid pregnancy.) Side effects of INH include paresthesias, seizures (toxic reaction), orthostatic hypotension, nausea and vomiting, hepatitis, and hypersensitivity to the drug.

MENINGOCOCCAL MENINGITIS

Meningococcal meningitis is also known as *spinal meningitis.* It is inflammation of the membranes that surround the spinal cord and brain. Meningococcal meningitis can be caused by a variety of different bacteria, viruses, and other microorganisms (see Table 39-3). A major cause of bacterial meningitis is *Neisseria meningitidis.* Like *M. tuberculosis,* it is spread by airborne pathogens. The usual mode of transmission is prolonged, direct contact with upper respiratory secretions (discharge from the nose and throat) from an infected person or carrier. Once inhaled, the bacteria invade the respiratory passages. They travel by way of the blood to the brain and spinal cord. As the infecting agent spreads to more organs, it causes toxic effects in the involved organ system.

An estimated 2% to 10% of the population may carry meningococci at any one time.[1] The throat's epithelial lining generally prevents the germ from invading the meninges and the cerebrospinal fluid. Although the conversion from carrier to clinical disease is rare in developed countries, outbreaks of disease in the United States have increased since the 1990s, partly because of increased rates of disease in people who may have a common organizational affiliation or who live in the same community.[18]

Other Infectious Agents Known to Cause Meningitis

Other common pathogens that cause meningitis include *Streptococcus pneumoniae* and *Haemophilus influenzae* type b (Hib), and some viruses. *S. pneumoniae* is the second most common cause of bacterial meningitis in adults, the most common cause of pneumonia in adults, and the most common cause of otitis media (middle ear infection) in children. This bacteria is spread by droplets, prolonged personal contact, or extended contact with linen soiled with respiratory discharges.

H. influenzae has the same mode of transmission as *N. meningitidis*. Vaccines for children were introduced in 1981. Before that time, *H. influenzae* was the leading cause of bacterial meningitis in children 6 months to 3 years of age. (This bacteria is also responsible for conditions such as pediatric epiglottitis, septic arthritis, and generalized sepsis.) This type of meningitis can be treated with antibiotics. However, 50% of infected children have lasting damage to the nervous system.

Fortunately, none of the bacteria that cause meningitis is as contagious as the common cold or flu. In addition, they are not spread by casual contact or by simply breathing the air where a person with meningitis has been.[18]

Viral meningitis (aseptic meningitis) is a syndrome generally associated with an existing systemic viral disease (e.g., enteroviral infection, herpes virus infection, mumps and, less commonly, influenza). Symptoms are similar to those of bacterial meningitis (described below). However, they are usually less severe. In most cases viral meningitis is self-limited, and the patient recovers fully. The patient may experience muscle weakness and malaise during prolonged convalescence. Viral meningitis is not believed to be communicable.

Signs and Symptoms

The signs and symptoms of meningitis depend on the patient's age and general health. In infants, for example, signs of meningeal irritation may be absent. On the other hand, they may include only irritability, poor feeding or vomiting, a high-pitched cry, and fullness of the fontanelle. (Maternal antibodies generally protect neonates to 6 months of age.) In older infants and children, signs of meningitis may include malaise, low-grade fever, projectile vomiting, petechial rash (Fig. 39-8), headache, and stiff neck from meningeal irritation (nuchal rigidity). Diagnostic signs of meningitis in older children include the *Brudzinski sign* (involuntary flexion of the arm, hip, and knee when the neck is passively flexed) and the *Kernig sign* (loss of the ability in a seated or supine patient to completely extend the leg when the thigh is flexed on the abdomen; the patient usually can extend the leg completely when the thigh is not flexed on the abdomen).

CRITICAL THINKING
What does a petechial rash look like?

The risk of bacterial meningitis is most significant in neonates and in children 6 months to 2 years of age. However, infection should be suspected in any patient with fever, headache, stiff neck, altered mental status, or underlying health problems (e.g., recent neurosurgery, trauma, or immunocompromise). If extensive meningeal involvement develops in a toxic or debilitated patient, the illness may be accompanied by acute adrenal insufficiency, convulsions, coma, and disseminated intravascular coagulation (Waterhouse-Friderichsen syndrome). In this case, death can occur in 6 to 8 hours. Other conditions and long-term complications associated with severe meningitis include blindness and deafness (from cranial nerve damage), arthritis, myocarditis, and pericarditis. Death can follow overwhelming infection.

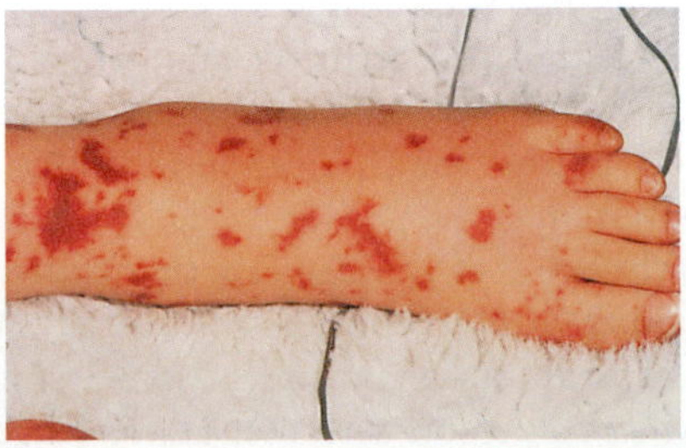

FIGURE 39-8 ■ Petechial rash in meningococcal infection.

Immunization and Control Measures

Vaccines are available for Hib, some strains of *N. meningitidis,* and many types of *S. pneumoniae*. The vaccines against Hib are very safe and highly effective. By 6 months of age, infants should have received at least three doses of Hib vaccine; a fourth dose ("booster") is recommended between 12 and 18 months of age. Vaccine against some strains of *N. meningitidis* is not routinely used in the United States and is not effective in children under 18 months of age.[17] However, the vaccine is sometimes used to control outbreaks of some types of meningococcal meningitis. Vaccines to prevent meningitis caused by *S. pneumoniae* also can prevent other forms of infection arising from the bacterium. This vaccine is ineffective for children under 2 years of age. However, it is recommended for all people over age 65. It also is recommended for younger people with certain chronic medical problems. Vaccines against meningitis have been instrumental in preventing outbreaks of the disease among military recruits in the United States. Before 1971, such outbreaks were a common occurrence.[1]

Patient Management and Protective Measures

Patient management focuses on ensuring an adequate airway and ventilatory and circulatory support. The paramedic must take protective measures when caring for patients who have signs and symptoms of meningitis. Universal and BSI precautions (with surgical masks on the patient) should be used during care and transport. The EMS agency should have an exposure control plan for meningitis.

Early diagnosis and treatment of bacterial meningitis are essential. The diagnosis usually is confirmed by finding the bacteria in a sample of the patient's spinal fluid. This is obtained through a spinal tap (lumbar puncture). The disease is then treated using several antibiotics. Drugs to prevent the disease are available for those who may have intimate contact with the patient (e.g., family members).

NOTE Meningitis is a true medical emergency. A chief goal of emergency care is administration of a proper antibiotic. The drug should be given 30 to 60 minutes after arriving at the emergency department.

PNEUMONIA

As described in Chapter 30, pneumonia is an acute inflammation of the bronchioles and alveoli. It can be spread by droplets and by direct and indirect contact with respiratory secretions (see Table 39-3). Etiologic agents responsible for this disease may be bacterial *(S. pneumoniae, M. pneumoniae, Staphylococcus. aureus, H. influenzae, Klebsiella pneumoniae, Moraxella catarrhalis, Legionella sp.),* viral, or fungal. These organisms may affect several body systems. They include the respiratory system (pneumonia); the CNS (meningitis); and the ears, nose, and throat (otitis, pharyngitis media). The signs and symptoms of pneumonia include the following:

- Sudden onset of chills, high-grade fever, chest pain with respirations, and dyspnea
- Tachypnea and chest retractions (an ominous sign in children)
- Congestion caused by the development of purulent alveolar exudates in one or more lobes
- A productive cough with yellow-green phlegm

Susceptibility and Resistance

Susceptibility to pneumonia is increased by processes such as smoking, pulmonary edema, influenza, exposure to inhaled toxins, chronic lung disease, and aspiration of any form (postalcohol ingestion, near drowning, regurgitation caused by gastric distention from bag-valve-mask ventilation). Extremes of age also appear to increase susceptibility to the disease (e.g., elderly individuals and infants with a low birth weight and/or malnourishment). Other high-risk groups for pneumonia include people with the following conditions:

- Sickle cell disease
- Cardiovascular disease
- Asplenia (congenital absence or surgical removal of the spleen)
- Diabetes
- Chronic renal failure (or other kidney disease)
- HIV
- Organ transplantation
- Multiple myeloma, lymphoma, or Hodgkin disease

Patient Management and Protective Measures

Prehospital care for patients with pneumonia includes providing airway support, oxygen, ventilatory assistance (as needed), intravenous (IV) fluids, cardiac monitoring, and transport for evaluation by a physician. Bacterial pneumonia is usually managed with analgesics, decongestants, expectorants, and antibiotic therapy. Patients generally do not need to be isolated from others. In hospitals, pneumonia patients may be isolated from other patients who may be more susceptible to infection.

CRITICAL THINKING

Which locations in your area are at high risk for influenza outbreaks?

Measures for protecting health care workers include BSI precautions and effective hand washing. Airway barriers should be used if TB is suspected. Immunizations exist for some causes of pneumonia. However, they generally are not recommended for people who come in contact with patients who have the disease.

TETANUS

Tetanus is a serious, sometimes fatal, disease of the central nervous system. It is caused by infection of a wound with spores of *Clostridium tetani.* Tetanus spores live mainly in soil and manure. However, they are also found in the human intestine. If the spores enter tissue (e.g., through a puncture wound or burn), they multiply and produce a toxin that acts on the nerves controlling muscular activity. (Dead or necrotic tissue is a favorable environment for *C. tetani.*) About 500,000 cases of tetanus occur worldwide each year, with a mortality rate of 45%. These deaths often occur from wounds that appear too trivial for medical evaluation. Only about 100 cases of tetanus are reported annually in the United States. They occur most often in patients 50 years of age or older. The relatively low number of tetanus cases in the United States is a result of immunization of the general population with tetanus vaccines.[19]

Signs and Symptoms

The most common symptom of tetanus is *trismus* (stiffness of the jaw); it is also known as *lockjaw* because of the accompanying difficulty in opening the mouth (Fig. 39-9). Other symptoms include the following:

- Muscular tetany (muscle spasms and twitching)
- Painful muscular contractions in the neck, moving to the trunk
- Abdominal rigidity (often the first sign in pediatric patients)
- Painful spasms (contortions) of the face *(risus sardonicus),* which produce a grotesque smile
- Respiratory failure

Patient Management and Protective Measures

The prehospital care goals are to support vital functions. This may include aggressive airway management (intubation and surgical or needle cricothyrotomy). Muscle spasms should be treated with ***diazepam*** or ***lorazepam,*** ben-

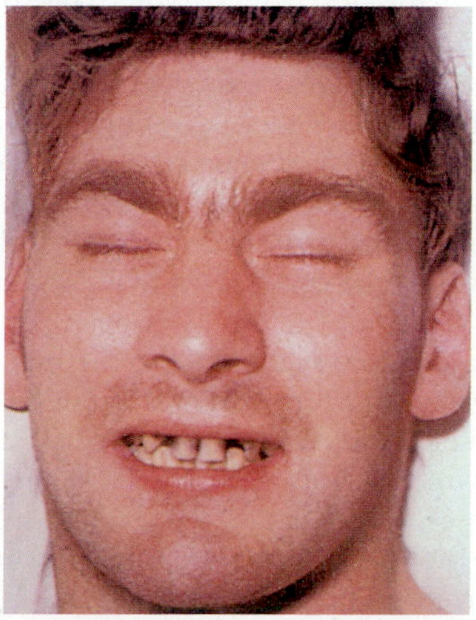

FIGURE 39-9 ■ Trismus as a result of mild tetanus that developed 10 days after the individual received a benign-looking leg wound.

zodiazepines, or paralytic agents (per medical direction). Other drugs that may be indicated include IV fluids, ***magnesium sulfate,*** narcotics, and antidysrhythmics. After evaluation by a physician and stabilization of the patient's condition, care for individuals with tetanus includes administration of antitoxin (tetanus immune globulin [TIG]) to provide postexposure passive immunity, treatment to eliminate the toxin, active immunization with tetanus toxoid, and wound care. Most patients recover fully if they receive prompt treatment.

CRITICAL THINKING

When a patient with an open skin wound refuses care, do you ever explain the risks of tetanus infection?

Immunization

Immunization against tetanus usually is started in children. It is achieved using diphtheria-pertussis-tetanus (DPT) vaccination. This is a combined immunization against diphtheria (laryngitis, pharyngitis with discharge), pertussis (whooping cough), and tetanus. After the initial immunization, children receive a booster shot before starting elementary school. After that, a booster shot is recommended every 10 years.

Patients who have a recent wound should be counseled about postinjury tetanus prophylaxis. They also should be counseled on effective wound care. All patients should be questioned about their tetanus immunization status. (Boosters should be given every 10 years; 5 years for a "dirty" wound.) Recovery from infection does not confer immunity.

RABIES

Rabies *(hydrophobia)* is an acute viral infection of the central nervous system. The disease mainly affects animals. However, it can be transmitted from an infected animal to a human through virus-laden saliva (e.g., by a bite or scratch). (Transmission from person to person is theoretical but has never been documented.[1]) In the United States, wildlife rabies is common in skunks, raccoons, bats, foxes, dogs, wolves, jackals, mongooses, and coyotes. Healthy wild animals (e.g., skunks) are seldom seen by casual observance. A high degree of suspicion for rabies is indicated for all animals found outside their natural habitat. Hawaii is the only rabies-free state in the United States.

Humans are highly susceptible to the rabies virus after exposure to saliva in a bite or scratch from an infected animal. Several factors govern the severity of infection, including the following:

- Severity of the wound
- Richness of nerve supply close to the wound
- Distance from the wound to the CNS
- Amount and strain of the virus
- Degree of protection provided by clothing

Signs and Symptoms

The incubation period between a bite and the appearance of symptoms ranges from 9 days to 7 years[1] (see Table 39-3). Initial symptoms include low-grade fever, headache, loss of appetite, hyperactivity, disorientation and, in some cases, seizures. Often the patient has an intense thirst, but attempts to drink result in violent, painful spasms in the throat (hence the name *hydrophobia*). Eye and facial muscles may become paralyzed as the disease progresses. Without medical intervention, the disease lasts 2 to 6 days, often resulting in death secondary to respiratory failure.

Patient Management and Protective Measures

Physicians treat the signs and symptoms of the disease and provide respiratory and cardiovascular support (as needed). Patients also are treated with sedatives and analgesics. Thorough debridement of the wound without sutures (if possible) is indicated. This allows free bleeding and drainage. Human rabies immune globulin may be given to provide passive immunization. Also, a rabies vaccine (Human Diploid Rabies Vaccine, Rabies Vaccine) is given by injections spread over several weeks. (Injections are no longer given in the stomach.) Tetanus prophylaxis and antibiotics may be indicated for treatment of the bite wound.

CRITICAL THINKING

Has a case of rabies ever occurred in your community? What animal was implicated?

Most cases of rabies in humans are the result of a bite from a rabid dog. However, the possibility of rabies must be considered with *all* mammal bites. Scene safety and use of BSI precautions during wound management are paramount. Law enforcement personnel and animal control authorities should be contacted to assist in scene control.

If given within 2 days of the bite, immunizations almost always prevent rabies. Immunizations should be given for contact with open wounds or for exposure of mucous membranes to saliva. Immunizations also should be given to people with a high probability of contact with animal reservoirs (e.g., animal care workers, animal shelter personnel, and outdoor workers). If an animal is suspected of being rabid, it should be killed by the proper authorities and its brain should be examined for rabies inclusion bodies. If no inclusion bodies are found, the patient's rabies treatment is stopped.

HANTAVIRUS

Hantavirus was previously known to be associated with hemorrhagic fever with renal syndrome that occurs in Asia. Hantaviruses also are associated with a syndrome of severe respiratory distress and shock. This syndrome has occurred in several areas of the United States.[18] The virus is carried by rodents. It is transmitted by inhalation of aerosol material contaminated with rodent urine and feces (see Table 39-3). Many forms of this disease occur in specific geographical areas.

Hantavirus can cause significant disease in humans. Patients are usually healthy adults who experience an onset of fever and malaise. This is followed several days later by respiratory distress. (The severity of the illness is determined by the strain of the virus.) Other signs and symptoms may include fever, chills, headache, and GI upset, and capillary hemorrhage. With severe infection, oliguria, kidney failure, and hypotension occur. Death typically results from decreased cardiac output and eventual cardiovascular collapse. Treatment is supportive and guided by medical direction. Body substance isolation precautions are indicated because of the infectious nature of these viruses.

VIRAL DISEASES OF CHILDHOOD

The childhood infectious diseases presented in this chapter include rubella (German measles), rubeola (red measles or hard measles), mumps (parotitis), chickenpox (varicella), and pertussis (whooping cough). These infectious diseases are preventable with immunization for chickenpox and with the triple immunization measles, mumps, and rubella (MMR) vaccine. The incidence of these childhood diseases has declined because of widespread immunization of children. Immunization provides long-lasting immunity. It is known to be 98% to 99% effective.

All health care workers should use personal protective measures when caring for children with viral infections. Protective immunization, effective hand washing, BSI (including the use of surgical masks for both the paramedic and the patient), and careful handling of linens, supplies, and equipment that may be contaminated are important in preventing the spread of these diseases.

Rubella

Rubella is a mild, febrile, and highly communicable viral disease caused by the rubella virus. It is characterized by a diffuse, punctate, macular rash (Fig. 39-10). The disease usually is transmitted by direct contact with nasopharyngeal secretions or droplet spray from an infected person. It also may be passed transplacentally (producing active infection in the fetus) and by contact with articles contaminated with blood, urine, or feces. After inoculation, the virus invades the lymph system. From there it enters the blood and produces an immune response. The subsequent rash spreads from the forehead to the face to the torso to the extremities (lasting 3 days). (A rash that lasts longer than 3 days indicates the presence of rubeola.) Maximal communicability appears to be the first few days before and 5 to 7 days after the onset of the rash. Complications from the disease are rare. However, young females sometimes develop a self-limiting arthritis (see Table 39-3).

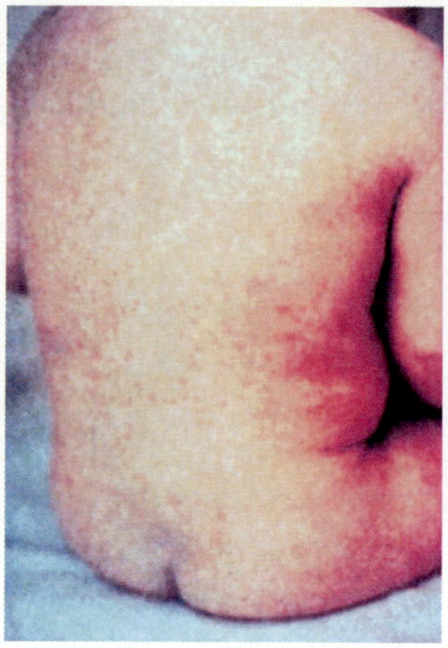

FIGURE 39-10 ■ Acquired rubella (German measles) in an 11-month-old infant.

> **CRITICAL THINKING**
>
> Is there any way a paramedic can avoid rubella other than being immunized for it?

Congenital rubella syndrome (CRS) affects approximately 90% of infants born to women who were infected with rubella during the first trimester of pregnancy.[1] The disease is associated with multiple congenital anomalies, mental retardation, deafness, and an increased risk of death from congenital heart disease and sepsis during the first 6 months of life. Infants with CRS shed large numbers of the virus in their secretions. The CDC recommends that all health care providers receive immunization if they are not immune from previous rubella infection. This helps to reduce the risk of exposure to themselves and those they treat. Immunization is not recommended for pregnant women. This is due to the theoretical risk that the vaccine could cause developmental defects. As a precaution, pregnant EMS providers should not be exposed to patients with rubella.

Rubeola

Rubeola is an acute, highly communicable viral disease. It is caused by the measles virus. It is characterized by fever, conjunctivitis, cough, bronchitis, and a blotchy red rash (Fig. 39-11). The virus is found in the blood, urine, and pharyngeal secretions. It usually is passed directly or indirectly through contact with infected respiratory secretions. With exposure, the virus invades the respiratory epithelium. It spreads via the lymph system. Rubeola may predispose a person to secondary bacterial complications such as otitis media, pneumonia, and myocarditis. The most serious life-threatening complication is subacute sclerosing panencephalitis. (This is a slowly progressing neurological disease. It is marked by loss of mental capacity and muscle coordination.)

Early (prodromal) symptoms that mark the onset of disease include high fever, nasal discharge, conjunctivitis,

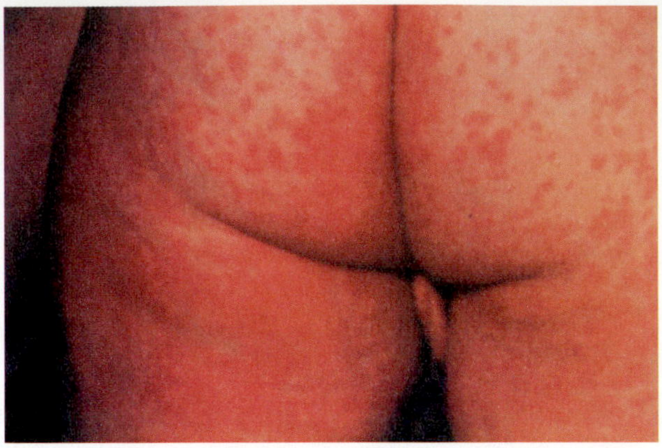

FIGURE 39-11 ■ Rubeola (measles) rash on the third day.

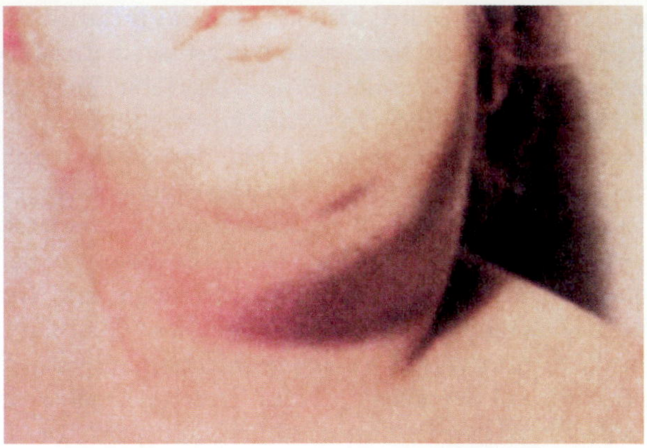

FIGURE 39-12 ■ Submaxillary mumps in an infant.

photophobia, and cough (see Table 39-3). One or 2 days before the rash emerges, white spots are usually noted on the inside of the cheek (Koplik spots). The dermal rash begins a few days after respiratory tract involvement. The rash is red and maculopapular. It spreads from the forehead to the face, neck, and torso and eventually to the feet, usually by the third day. (The onset of the rash coincides with the production of serum antibodies.) Uncomplicated cases of rubeola usually last 6 days. Recovery from the illness confers lifelong immunity.

Mumps

Mumps is an acute, communicable systemic viral disease caused by the mumps virus. It is characterized by localized edema of one or more of the salivary glands (usually the parotid). The swelling may affect both or only one side of the neck (Fig. 39-12). In some cases involvement of other glands also occurs. The virus is passed through direct contact with the saliva droplets of an infected person (see Table 39-3).

The virus invades and multiplies in the parotid gland or the upper respiratory passages. From there it enters the bloodstream and localizes in glandular or nervous tissue. The parotid, testes, and pancreas are the most frequently involved glands. When mumps occurs after the onset of puberty, it may cause a painful inflammation of the testicle (orchitis) and testicular atrophy; however, sterility is rare. The intensity of symptoms in mumps varies; 30% of infections are asymptomatic. Immunity after recovery is lifelong. Placental transfer of antibodies sometimes occurs.

CRITICAL THINKING

Why are some viral diseases of childhood still seen despite widespread immunization?

Chickenpox

Chickenpox is a common childhood disease caused by the varicella-zoster virus. (Varicella-zoster is a member of the herpes virus family.) The virus is passed by direct and indirect contact with droplets (mainly airborne) from the respiratory passages of an infected person. Exposure to linen tainted with vesicular or mucous membrane discharges of infected people has been implicated.[1]

Chickenpox is highly communicable (see Table 39-3). It is characterized by a sudden onset of low-grade fever, mild malaise, and a skin eruption that is maculopapular for a few hours and vesicular for 3 to 4 days, leaving a granular scab (Fig. 39-13). At first, the skin lesions appear on the trunk. They usually progress to the extremities. The crops of skin eruptions (each associated with itching) usually are more abundant on covered areas of the body. The scalp, conjunctivae, and upper respiratory tract may also be affected. The appearance of crops of vesicles (fresh vesicles appearing while other lesions are scabbed) differentiates chickenpox from smallpox. (Smallpox has vesicles of the same age.) Treatment is symptomatic. Moreover, the disease is self-limited. Complications may include secondary bacterial infections, aseptic meningitis, mononucleosis, and Reye syndrome. Children with chickenpox should be isolated from schools, medical offices, emergency departments, and public places until all lesions are crusted and dry.

After recovery, the virus is thought to remain in the body in an asymptomatic latent stage. (It is possibly localized in the dorsal root ganglia.) The virus may reactivate during periods of stress or immunosuppression. During these periods, it may produce an illness known as *shingles*. The vesicles associated with shingles appear on the skin area supplied by the sensory nerves of a single group or associated groups of dorsal root ganglia (Fig. 39-14). Unlike chickenpox, shingles is not passed through respiratory droplets. However, it can cause chickenpox in susceptible individuals who come in contact with open skin lesions (lesions that are not yet scabbed).

Antiviral drugs may shorten the duration of symptoms and pain in older patients. EMS workers who have not had chickenpox should consider getting the vaccine. Data indicate that adult antibody production occurs in 82% of patients after one dose. It occurs in 92% of patients after two doses. (The vaccine should not be given to people who re-

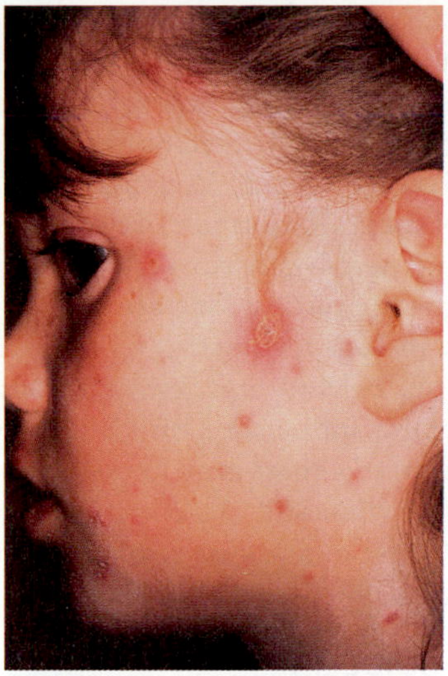

FIGURE 39-13 ■ Chickenpox skin lesions.

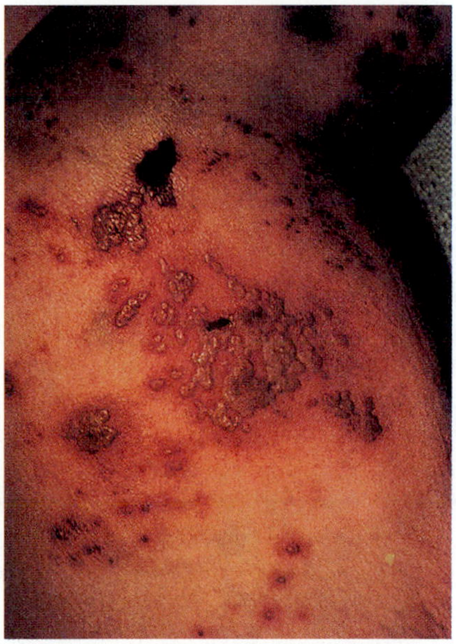

FIGURE 39-14 ■ Vesicles associated with shingles.

ceived high doses of systemic steroids in the previous month.) About 5% of those who receive the vaccine develop a rash. Some develop frank chickenpox, which is very debilitating in adults. To protect the fetus, varicella-zoster immune globulin (VZIG) is recommended for pregnant women with significant exposure to chickenpox who do not have a history of previous exposure.

Pertussis

Pertussis is an infectious disease that mainly affects infants and young children (see Table 39-3). It is caused by *Bordetella pertussis* and is spread by direct contact with discharges from mucous membranes contained in airborne droplets. The disease causes inflammation of the entire respiratory tract. It also causes a subtle onset of cough that becomes paroxysmal in 1 to 2 weeks. This cough can last 1 to 2 months. The coughing episodes are violent (sometimes without an intervening inhalation), causing the high-pitched inspiratory "whoop," and end with expulsion of clear mucus and vomiting. (The whoop often is not present in children younger than 6 months of age.) Before the introduction of a vaccine against pertussis in the 1950s, the disease killed more children in the United States than all other infectious diseases combined.[20] Pertussis vaccine usually is given in combination with diphtheria and tetanus (DPT) vaccines to children at 2, 4, and 6 months of age; a booster dose is given at age 5.

The ability to spread pertussis is thought to be greatest before the onset of paroxysmal coughing. (This explains the need for BSI and surgical mask protection for the paramedic and the patient.) Erythromycin is known to shorten the communicability period, but it can reduce symptoms only if given during the incubation period. (This is before the onset of paroxysmal cough.) Infection with pertussis usually provides immunity. However, attacks after immunization in older children and adults indicate that immunity may diminish over time.

OTHER VIRAL DISEASES

Other viral diseases easily transmitted during the course of patient care include influenza, severe acute respiratory syndrome (SARS), mononucleosis, and herpes simplex type 1 (HSV-1) infection (described later in this chapter). As with all other contacts with patients who may have infectious disease, BSI precautions are indicated during patient care.

Influenza

As described in Chapter 30, influenza is a respiratory infection. It is spread by influenza viruses A, B, and C (see Table 39-3). The disease is popularly known as "the flu." It is spread by virus-infected droplets that are coughed or sneezed into the air. Influenza usually occurs in small outbreaks or, every few years, in epidemics. Resistance is normally conferred after recovery. However, this resistance is only to the specific strain or variant (Box 39-11).

Signs and symptoms typically include chills, fever, headache, muscular aches, loss of appetite, and fatigue. These symptoms are followed by upper respiratory infection and a cough (often severe and drawn out) that lasts for 2 to 7 days. Patient management is mainly supportive. Mild cases of viral infection usually are not treated.

Severe cases (especially in the elderly and those with lung or heart disease) may result in secondary bacterial infection (e.g., *S. pneumoniae*). These cases can be fatal. Other viral respiratory diseases that can lead to bacterial complications include acute afebrile viral respiratory disease (excluding influenza) and acute febrile respiratory disease. Both diseases may cause illnesses in the upper and lower respiratory tract. These illnesses include pharyngitis, laryngitis, croup, bronchitis, and bronchiolitis.

BOX 39-11 Influenza Virus Types A, B, and C

People infected with certain strains of influenza type A or type B acquire immunity to that strain. However, the type A and type B viruses occasionally alter to produce new strains. This leads to a new infection. Type B virus is relatively stable. However, it occasionally alters to overcome resistance and may lead to small outbreaks of infection. Type A virus is highly unstable. It has caused worldwide flu epidemics. These variants are named for the geographical site and year of isolation (e.g., the Spanish flu in 1918, Asian flu in 1957, and Hong Kong flu in 1968) and the culture number (e.g., A/Japan/305/57).

Type C virus stimulates antibodies that provide immunity for life.

Flu vaccines contain killed strains of type A and type B virus that are known to be currently in circulation. These vaccines may help prevent infection. A nasal spray flu vaccine, FluMist (virus vaccine live, intranasal), has also been approved for protection against influenza A and B viruses in healthy people between 5 and 49 years of age. However, immunity does not last long. Therefore the vaccine must be repeated each year just before the start of the flu season (November to March in the United States). Health care workers should be immunized in the fall of each year with the current vaccine.

Amantadine, rimantadine, or zanamivir may be given to hospitalized patients to protect against influenza A. Despite advances in prevention and treatment, about 36,000 people die each year in the United States from influenza and its complications.

CRITICAL THINKING

Will you get the influenza vaccine? What influenced your decision?

Severe Acute Respiratory Syndrome

As described in Chapter 30, severe acute respiratory syndrome emerged as a disease in China in November 2003. It has made thousands of people sick worldwide. SARS is caused by a new member of the coronavirus family (SARS coronavirus [SARS CO-V]). It appears to be spread by close person-to-person contact. This type of contact results in exposure to infectious droplets. It also is possible that SARS can be spread more broadly through the air or by other ways that are currently not known.

The illness usually begins with a fever over 100.4° F (38° C). The fever is sometimes associated with chills or other symptoms. These include headache, a general feeling of discomfort, and body aches. Some people also experience mild respiratory symptoms at the outset. After 2 to 7 days, SARS patients may develop a dry, nonproductive cough. This cough might be accompanied by or progress to hypoxemia. In 10% to 20% of cases, patients require mechanical ventilation; the mortality rate for the disease is about 8%.[21] Most cases of SARS in the United States have occurred among travelers returning to the United States from other parts of the world affected by SARS. Very few cases have resulted from spread of the condition to close contacts such as family members and health care workers.

Initial diagnostic testing for patients suspected of having SARS may include a chest x-ray, pulse oximetry, blood cultures, sputum culture, and testing for viral respiratory pathogens, notably influenza A and B and respiratory syncytial virus. Currently, there is no known cure or vaccine for the disease. More than 80% of patients with SARS improve on their own. Strict quarantine remains the most effective means of control.

TRANSPORT GUIDELINES FOR POSSIBLE SARS PATIENTS

The transport guidelines for patients who may have SARS (Box 39-12) have been adapted from currently recommended infection control measures for hospitalized patients with SARS.[22]

Mononucleosis

Mononucleosis is often referred to as "mono." It is caused either by the Epstein-Barr virus (EBV) or by cytomegalovirus (CMV). Both of these are members of the herpes virus family (see Table 39-3). Mononucleosis is spread from person to person via the oropharyngeal route and saliva (hence the name *kissing disease*). Blood transfusions also can be a mode of transmission. However, resultant clinical disease is rare. Most people with a healthy immune system are able to fend off the infection even after significant exposure. Transmission from care providers to young children is common.[1] About 90% of people over age 35 have antibodies to CMV or EBV. This is probably the result of mild, childhood infection, often passed off as a common cold or the flu. Previous infection with EBV generally confers a high degree of resistance to future exposures.

Signs and symptoms appear gradually. They are characterized by fever (which may last for weeks), sore throat, oropharyngeal discharges, lymphadenopathy (especially posterior cervical), and splenomegaly with abdominal tenderness. About 10% of people also develop a generalized rash or darkened areas in the mouth that resemble bruises. Recovery usually occurs in a few weeks. However, some people take months to regain their former level of energy. The patient may remain a carrier for several months after symptoms disappear. No immunization is available for mononucleosis.

SEXUALLY TRANSMITTED DISEASES

Sexually transmitted diseases are diseases that can be passed from person to person through sexual activity. They may be transmitted to another person even when the infected person has no symptoms. More than 20 pathogens have been identified as belonging to this group of diseases

BOX 39-12 Guidelines for the Transport of Patients with Severe Acute Respiratory Syndrome (SARS)

Emergency Medical Ground Transport of Possible SARS Patients—General Considerations

- Patients suspected of having SARS should be transported using the minimum number of emergency medical services (EMS) personnel. No patients without SARS and no passengers should be in the vehicle.
- Hospitals must be notified before the arrival of possible SARS patients. This helps the hospital to use the proper infection control procedures and to prepare the facilities.
- Concerns about the movement of possible SARS patients in the United States should be discussed with the proper local, state, and federal health authorities, including the Centers for Disease Control and Prevention (CDC). The CDC's 24-hour response telephone number is 1-770-488-7100.

Infection Control—General

- In addition to respiratory droplet and possible airborne spread, SARS may be transmitted if residual infectious particles on environmental surfaces are brought into direct contact with the eyes, nose, or mouth (e.g., by unwashed hands). Hand hygiene, therefore, is of prime importance for all personnel working with possible SARS patients.
- Protective equipment should be used throughout transport of a possible SARS patient.
- No personal activities should be performed during transport of a possible SARS patient. This includes eating, drinking, applying cosmetics, and handling contact lenses.

Protective Equipment and Procedures

- Disposable, nonsterile gloves must be worn for all patient contact.
- Gloves should be removed and discarded in biohazard bags after patient care is complete (e.g., between patients). This should also be done when gloves become soiled or are damaged.
- The hands must be washed or disinfected with a waterless hand sanitizer immediately after removal of the gloves.
- Disposable, fluid-resistant gowns should be worn for all direct patient care.
- Gowns should be removed and discarded in biohazard bags after patient care is complete or when they become soiled or are damaged.
- Eye protection must be worn in the patient care compartment. It also must be worn when the paramedic is working within 6 feet (2 m) of the patient. Corrective eyeglasses alone are not appropriate protection.
- N-95 (or greater) respirators should be worn by personnel in the patient care compartment during transport of a possible SARS patient; personnel wearing respirators should be fit tested.
- The door or window between the driver and patient compartments should be closed before a possible SARS patient is brought onboard. N-95 (or greater) respirators should be worn by the driver if the driver's compartment is open to the patient care compartment. Drivers that provide direct patient care (including moving patients on stretchers) should wear a disposable gown, eye protection, and gloves as described above during patient care activities. Gowns and gloves are not required for personnel whose duties are strictly limited to driving.
- Vehicles that have separate driver and patient compartments and separate ventilation to those areas are preferred for transport of possible SARS patients. If a vehicle without separate compartments and ventilation must be used, the outside air vents in the driver compartment should be open. Also, the rear exhaust ventilation fans should be turned to the highest setting during transport. This provides relative negative pressure in the patient care compartment.
- Nonrebreather face masks may be used to provide the patient with oxygen support during transport.
- If possible, the patient may wear a paper surgical mask to reduce droplet production.
- Positive-pressure ventilation should be performed using a resuscitation bag-valve-mask. A model that can provide high-efficiency particulate air (HEPA) or equal filtration of expired air is preferred.
- Procedures that may cause the patient to cough should be avoided (e.g., nebulizer treatments).

Mechanically Ventilated Patients

- EMS agencies should consult the manufacturer of the ventilators they use to confirm proper filtration capability and the effect of filtration on positive-pressure ventilation.
- Mechanical ventilators for the transport of possible SARS patients should provide HEPA or equal filtration of airflow exhaust.

Clinical Specimens

- Standard precautions must be used in collecting and transporting clinical specimens.
- Clinical specimens should be labeled with the proper patient information. They should be placed in a clean, self-sealing bag for storage and transport.

Waste Disposal

- Dry solid waste (e.g., used gloves, dressings) should be collected in biohazard bags. It should be disposed of as regulated medical waste. Disposal should be done in accordance with local requirements at the destination hospital.
- Waste that is saturated with blood, body fluids, or excreta should be collected in leak-proof biohazard bags or containers for disposal as regulated medical waste in accordance with local requirements at the destination hospital.
- Sharp items such as used needles or scalpel blades should be collected in puncture-resistant sharps containers. They should be disposed of as regulated medical waste. Disposal should be done in accordance with local requirements at the destination hospital.
- Suctioned fluids and secretions should be stored in sealed containers. These should be disposed of as regulated medical waste. Disposal should be done in accordance with local requirements at the destination hospital. Handling that might result in splashes or aerosols during transport should be avoided.
- Suction devices should be fitted with in-line HEPA or equal filters in accordance with the manufacturer's recommendations.

Continued

BOX 39-12 Guidelines for the Transport of Patients with Severe Acute Respiratory Syndrome (SARS), cont'd

Cleaning and Disinfection after Transport of a Possible SARS Patient

- Compressed air that might cause infectious material to become airborne should not be used for cleaning the vehicle or reusable equipment.
- Non-patient care areas of the vehicle should be cleaned and maintained according to the vehicle manufacturer's recommendations.
- Personnel doing the cleaning should wear nonsterile gloves, disposable gowns, and eye protection while cleaning the patient care compartment.
- Patient care compartments (including stretchers, railings, medical equipment, control panels, and adjacent flooring, walls, and work surfaces likely to be directly contaminated during care) should be cleaned using a hospital disinfectant approved by the Environmental Protection Agency (EPA) in accordance with the manufacturer's recommendations.
- Spills of body fluids during transport should be cleaned up by placing absorbent material over the spill. The used cleaning material should be collected in a biohazard bag. The area of the spill should be cleaned using an EPA-registered hospital disinfectant. Cleaning personnel should be notified of the spill location and the initial clean-up that was done.
- Contaminated reusable equipment should be cleaned and disinfected right after use and before it is returned to service.
- Personnel should wear nonsterile gloves, disposable gowns, and face shields while cleaning reusable equipment.
- Reusable equipment should be cleaned and disinfected according to the manufacturer's instructions.

Follow-Up of EMS Personnel Who Transport Possible SARS Patients

- Personnel who have transported a possible SARS patient and who develop symptoms of SARS within the 10-day postexposure period should be examined by a physician. They also should be reported to the state health department and to the CDC at the 24-hour response number listed above.
- Personnel may continue working during the 10-day postexposure period if they have no symptoms of fever or respiratory illness.

National Council of State EMS Training Coordinators Executive Committee of the National Association of State EMS Directors (NASEMSD), Centers for Disease Control and Prevention: *Updated interim guidance: prehospital emergency medical care and ground transport of suspected severe acute respiratory syndrome patients,* Atlanta.[22]

(including HBV and HIV). Other common STDs are syphilis, gonorrhea, chlamydia, and herpes virus infections.

Several pathogenic agents are responsible for the host of STDs. These include bacteria, viruses, protozoa, fungi, and ectoparasites. These pathogens can produce multiple disease syndromes. Also, patients with STD syndromes often have multiple STDs. These infections usually cause a short-lived cellular immune response. They also can produce longer-lasting humoral antibody response. Neither of these protects against future exposures.

Syphilis

Syphilis is a systemic disease. It is characterized by a primary lesion, a secondary eruption involving the skin and mucous membranes, long latency periods, and late, seriously disabling lesions of the skin, bones, viscera, CNS, and cardiovascular system. The disease results from penetration of the skin, whether intact or broken, by the bacteria *Treponema pallidum.* Common modes of transmission include direct contact with fluid or pus from lesions on the skin and mucous membranes, blood transfusions or needle sticks (rare), and congenital transmission. After penetration, the organisms travel (within hours) to the lymph nodes. From there they are carried throughout the body. After the initial infection, syphilis follows well-defined stages of disease (see Table 39-3). It can be treated with antibiotic therapy. No immunization is available. It is estimated that 30% of exposures result in infection.

PRIMARY STAGE

Within 10 to 90 days of exposure, a primary lesion, or *chancre,* develops at the site of initial invasion (Fig. 39-15). The surface of the chancre is usually crusted or ulcerated. It varies in size from 1 to 2 cm in diameter. The lesion usually is single and painless. In addition, it generally heals spontaneously within 1 to 5 weeks. Syphilis is highly communicable during this stage.

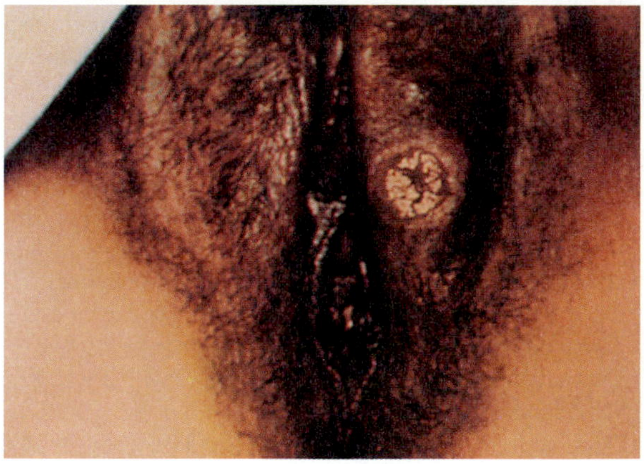

FIGURE 39-15 ■ Primary syphilis chancre on the labia.

SECONDARY STAGE

The secondary stage begins about 2 to 10 weeks after the appearance of the primary lesion. This stage lasts for 2 to 6 weeks. It is heralded by systemic symptoms. These include headache, malaise, anorexia, fever, sore throat, lymphadenopathy, and bald spots in the area of infection. In addition, the patient may develop a rash, which usually is bilaterally symmetrical and often involves the palms and soles. Painless, wartlike regions *(condylomata lata),* which are extremely infectious, may also be found in moist, warm sites (e.g., the inguinal area). The CNS, eyes, bones, joints, or kidneys may be affected during this stage.

CRITICAL THINKING

Why do you think a patient in the secondary stage of syphilis would call EMS?

LATENCY

A latency period follows the secondary stage in untreated individuals. (This may range from 1 to 40 years or more.) During this period, recurrent episodes of secondary stage symptoms with subclinical infection may occur. This happens in about 25% of cases. About 33% of these patients progress to tertiary syphilis; the remainder remain free of symptoms. Tertiary syphilis is infectious involvement of the skin, CNS, and cardiovascular systems and may include the following manifestations:

1. Skin
   - Granulomatous lesions (gummas) on skin (painless) and bone (painful)
2. Central nervous system
   - Paresis
   - *Tabes dorsalis* (spinal column degeneration characterized by a wide gait and ataxia ["syphilitic shuffle"])
   - Loss of reflexes, pain, and temperature sensation
   - Meningitis
   - Psychosis
3. Cardiovascular
   - Cerebrovascular occlusion
   - Dissecting aneurysm of the ascending aorta
   - Myocardial insufficiency; aortic necrosis (which can lead to aortic rupture and death)

Gonorrhea

Gonorrhea is caused by the bacterium *Neisseria gonorrhoeae.* It is transmitted between individuals by fluids and pus from infected mucous membranes. It can also be spread from an infected mother to her baby during pregnancy and delivery. The disease occurs in both men and women. However, it differs in course, severity, and ease of recognition. Gonorrhea often is treatable with antibiotics. However, some strains brought into the United States from other countries are resistant to the usual antibiotic therapy. Immunization is not available. Antibodies develop after exposure, but the antibodies are specific to the strain of gonorrhea that caused the infection. Consequently, future reinfection with other strains can occur.

Affected areas of the male anatomy are the urethra, Littre gland, Cowper gland, prostate gland, seminal vesicles, and epididymis. A sudden onset of dysuria, urgency, and frequency is seen several days after exposure (see Table 39-3). The associated urethral discharge rapidly becomes purulent and profuse. Direct spread of the infection may result in prostatitis, epididymitis, and seminal vesiculitis. Primary gonorrheal infections may also affect the pharynx, conjunctivae, and anus.

Affected areas of the female anatomy are the Bartholin glands, Skene glands, urethra, cervix, and fallopian tubes. More than 50% of infected women remain free of symptoms; others have a mucopurulent discharge that varies from scant to profuse. Contiguous spread of the disease may lead to endometritis, salpingitis, and parametritis (pelvic inflammatory disease) and the formation of tuboovarian abscesses. Complete or partial occlusion of the fallopian tubes may result in sterility and increased risk for ectopic pregnancy.

Between 1% and 3% of gonococcal infections become disseminated in the blood. This extension of the disease may produce septicemia, arthritis, endocarditis, meningitis, and skin lesions. In the bacteremic stage, the patient may complain of fever, chills, and malaise. Erythematous lesions are common, especially on the extremities. They may occur in clusters or singly.

Chlamydia

Chlamydia trachomatis is a major cause of sexually transmitted nonspecific urethritis (NSU) or nongonococcal genital infection. The disease is the most common sexually transmitted disease in the United States. (An estimated 25% of men are carriers.) It is a leading cause of preventable blindness. The signs and symptoms are similar to those of gonorrhea. This makes differentiation difficult. No immunization is available.

In men, NSU may cause a penile discharge. It also may cause complications such as swelling of the testes, which, if untreated, may lead to infertility. In women, NSU usually is symptomless. However, it may cause a vaginal discharge or pain with urination, salpingitis, and cervicitis. Transmission occurs secondary to direct contact with exudates, either sexually or during birth (Fig. 39-16; also see Table 39-3). Chlamydial infections are treated with antibiotics.

Herpes Virus Infections

Four herpes viruses have been described. One is the herpes simplex virus. The others are CMV, which is associated with mononucleosis, hepatitis, and severe systemic disease in the immunosuppressed host; EBV, which causes mononucleosis; and varicella-zoster virus, which causes chickenpox and shingles. This section of the text addresses only the herpes viruses associated with STDs.

HERPES SIMPLEX VIRUS

The two antigenically distinct herpes simplex viruses responsible for STDs are HSV-1 and herpes simplex virus type 2 (HSV-2). Both pathogens can cause herpes infection. Also, both can cause infection anywhere in the body. As a rule, HSV-1 most often is associated with herpes above the waist. In contrast, HSV-2 generally is associated with genital herpes. However, either type can cause disease in the genital area. Immunization is not available for either virus.

HSV is common in the United States. It causes 300,000 to 500,000 new infections each year. It is estimated that 70% to 90% of adults have antibodies against HSV-1. The mode

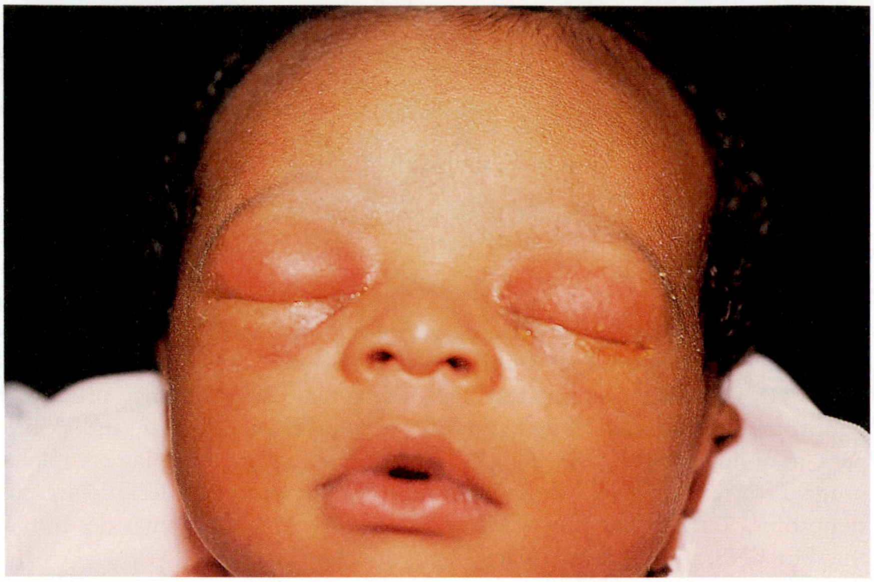

FIGURE 39-16 ■ Conjunctivitis from a chlamydial infection in an 8-day-old infant.

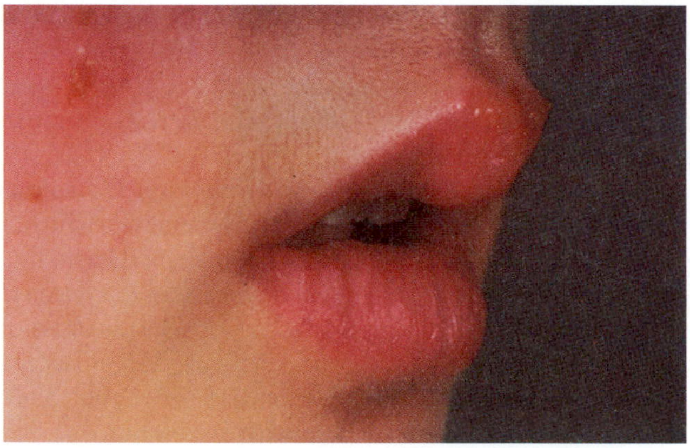

FIGURE 39-17 ■ "Fever blister" caused by the herpes simplex virus.

of transmission for HSV is strictly skin-to-skin contact with an infected area of the body. The virus enters through a break in the skin or through mucous membranes. Sexual contact is not required for transmission. For example, touching the herpes virus may result in finger infection (herpetic whitlow). Many young children who develop oral herpes (HSV-1) probably contract the virus through a casual kiss from a parent or relative. The virus also may be spread to other external body sites by autoinoculation (e.g., it may be spread from lip to finger to genitalia). Initial HSV-1 transmission usually occurs by 4 years of age. It is manifested by gingivostomatitis ("cold sores" or "fever blisters") (Fig. 39-17). Initial HSV-2 infection generally results from sexual activity. It is manifested by painful vesicular lesions of the cervix, vulva, penis, rectum, anus, and mouth (depending on sexual practices).

Once present in tissue, HSV produces an acute infection, with tissue destruction limited to one site. This primary infection produces a vesicular lesion (blister). The lesion heals spontaneously from the outside in without lasting scarring. However, the virus remains alive in the body despite circulating antibodies (see Table 39-3).

After the primary infection, the HSV enters the central nervous system nearest to the site of initial infection. It travels along sensory nerve pathways to a sensory nerve ganglion. There it remains in a latent stage until reactivated. When triggered by another infectious disease, menstruation, emotional stress, trauma, or immunosuppression, the virus reaches the epidermis by way of peripheral nerves. It reproduces a recurrent infectious disease state. This state usually lasts 4 to 10 days. The lesions usually appear in the area of initial inoculation. The number of lesions a person might experience during any given episode varies considerably.

HSV can remain inactive for a long time. It is unknown why many infected people never develop the disease, whereas others experience a lifetime of periodic outbreaks. Antiviral agents such as acyclovir may shorten the duration of an outbreak. They also may be used as prophylactic agents in instances of frequent recurrence.

CRITICAL THINKING

Why do you think the incidence of herpetic whitlow in health care workers has declined over the last 10 years?

LICE AND SCABIES

Lice and scabies are potential health hazards for all health care providers. Both can transmit communicable skin diseases and systemic illness, as well as dermatitis and discomfort. (Other vector-borne illnesses [e.g., Lyme disease] are described in Chapter 36.)

A

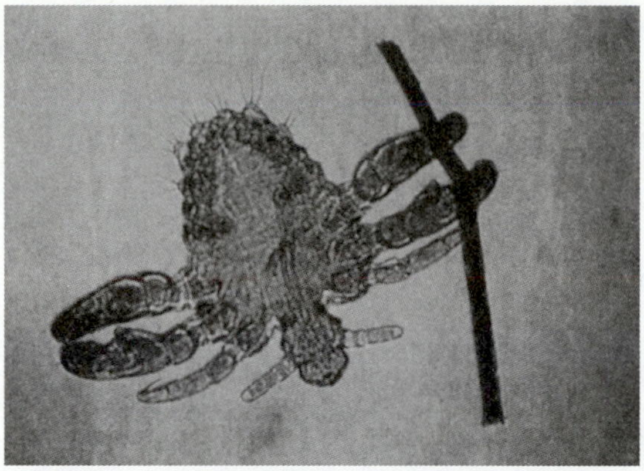

B

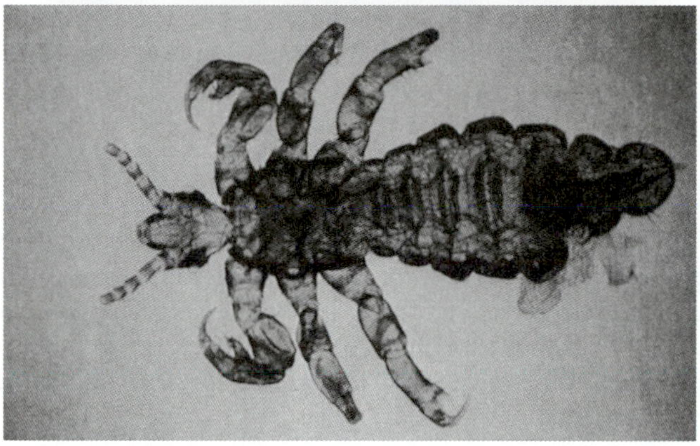

FIGURE 39-18 ■ **A,** The pubic, or crab, louse. **B,** Male of the human head louse.

Lice

Lice are small, wingless insects that are ectoparasites of birds and mammals. Most are host specific. Two of the species are human parasites. One is *Phthirus pubis,* the pubic, or crab, louse. The other is *Pediculus humanus,* which has two forms: *Phthirus capitis* (the head louse) and *Phthirus corporis* (the body louse, which was involved in outbreaks of epidemic typhus and trench fever in World War I) (Fig. 39-18). Lice have a three-stage life cycle. The eggs hatch in 7 to 10 days; the nymph stage lasts 7 to 13 days; and the egg-to-egg cycle lasts about 3 weeks.

Lice subsist on blood from the host and have mouths modified for piercing and sucking. During biting and feeding, secretions from the louse cause a small, red macule and pruritus. Long infestation periods may result in a decrease in pruritus and often a thick, dry, scaly appearance to the skin. In severe cases, oozing and crusting may be present. If sensitization to lice saliva and feces occurs, inflammation may develop. Secondary infection may result from scratching of lesions. Lice spread through close personal contact, and sharing of clothing and bedding may result in outbreaks (e.g., at school, day care facilities, and in families).

Pubic lice have a distinctive appearance. They are suggestive of miniature crabs. Gray-blue spots may be observed on the abdomen and thighs of infested patients. The eggs (*nits* or *ova*) often are evident on the shaft of pubic hairs. They are sometimes seen in the eyelashes, eyebrows, and axillary hairs. Pubic lice usually are acquired during sexual activity or from unchanged bedding in which egg-infested pubic hairs have been shed. Although primary bite lesions seldom are evident, the patient normally complains of intense pruritus and pubic scratching.

Head lice have an elongated body with a head that is slightly narrower than the thorax. Each louse has three pairs of legs, which possess delicate hooks at the distal extremities. The white ova of head lice (usually one nit to a shaft) are easily mistaken for dandruff, but the nits cannot be brushed out. These parasites most frequently affect children.

Body lice are slightly larger than head lice and concentrate around the waist, shoulders, axillae, and neck. Body lice and their nits usually are found in seams and on the fibers of clothing. The lesions from their bites begin as small, noninflammatory red spots, which quickly become papular wheals that resemble linear scratch marks (parallel scratch marks on the shoulders are a common finding). Head lice and body lice interbreed.

The treatment for all types of lice is designed to eradicate the parasites and nits and to prevent reinfestation. Patients usually are advised to wash all clothing, bedding, and personal articles thoroughly in hot water. They also are advised to wash the infected body area with gamma benzene hexachloride shampoo (Kwell), crotamiton (Eurax), Rid, or Nix. (Overtreatment should be avoided to prevent toxicity.)

Scabies

The human scabies mite (*Sarcoptes scabiei* var. *hominis*) is a parasite. It completes its entire life cycle in and on the epidermis of its host. Scabies infestation resembles a lice infestation. However, scabies bites generally are concentrated around the hands and feet, especially in the webs of the fingers and toes (Fig. 39-19). Other common infestation areas include the face and scalp of children, the nipples in females, and the penis in males. The scabies mite usually is passed by intimate contact or acquired from infested bedding, furniture, and clothing. The mite can burrow into the skin within 2½ minutes.[1]

Scabies infestation often is manifested by severe nocturnal pruritus. However, it takes 4 to 6 weeks for sensitization to develop and itching to begin. The adult female mite is responsible for symptoms. After impregnation, she burrows into the epidermis to lay her eggs. She remains in the burrow for a life span of about 1 month. Although vesicles and papules form at the surface, they often are disguised by the results of scratching. In severe cases (e.g., Norwegian scabies), oozing, crusting, and secondary infection may result. Susceptibility is general. However, people with a previous exposure usually develop fewer mites on later exposures and experience symptoms earlier (within 1 to 4 days).

The treatment is similar to that prescribed for lice infestation. Symptoms may persist for longer than 1 month until the mite and mite products are shed with the epidermis. (Mites are communicable until all mites and eggs have been destroyed.) Reinfestation is common, therefore the patient

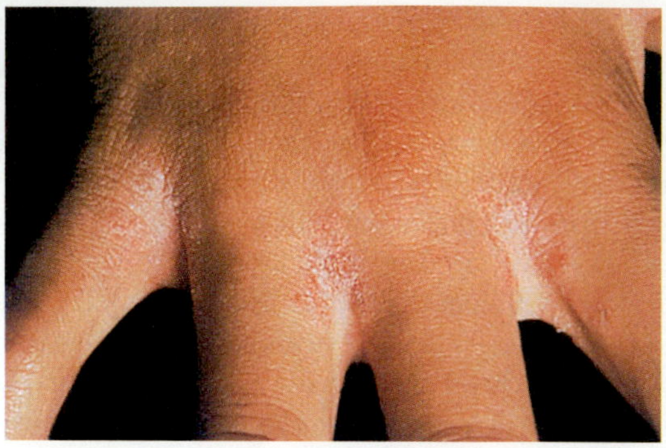

FIGURE 39-19 ■ Common site of burrows in scabies.

> **BOX 39-13 Protective Measures against Lice and Scabies**
>
> 1. Observe body substance isolation (BSI) and bag linen separately.
> 2. Spray the patient compartment of the ambulance with an effective insecticide. (Most commercial sprays contain effective pyrethrins, malathion, or carbamates.)
> 3. Spray the floor, gurney, and immediate areas where the patient's head was positioned (lice do not jump great distances).
> 4. Remove all insecticide residues with an appropriate solution.
> 5. Wear gloves during all steps and wash hands thoroughly when finished.
> 6. To treat a lice or scabies infestation:
>   - Use an appropriate body or hair pediculicide; repeat in 7 to 10 days.
>   - Launder personal clothing in hot water in a washer and dry on high heat in the dryer (of questionable benefit).

should be reexamined if the itching has not abated after several weeks. Antibiotic therapy may be needed to treat secondary bacterial infection. Immunization is not available. Protective measures against lice and scabies infestation are presented in Box 39-13.

REPORTING AN EXPOSURE TO AN INFECTIOUS OR A COMMUNICABLE DISEASE

An **exposure incident** (significant exposure) is any specific contact of the eyes, the mouth, other mucous membranes, or nonintact skin, or parenteral contact, with blood, blood products, bloody body fluids, or other potentially infectious materials. Exposures and all suspected exposures to an infectious or communicable disease must be reported to the DO. Reporting a possible exposure is important for the following reasons[1]:

1. It permits immediate medical follow-up. This allows identification of infection and immediate intervention.
2. It enables the DO to evaluate the circumstances of the incident. It also allows the DO to determine what changes to make to prevent future exposures.
3. It aids follow-up testing of the source person if permission for testing can be obtained.

Reporting also ensures that if the health care worker is infected, it has been documented that the disease occurred from a work-related exposure.

> **NOTE** Under provisions of the Ryan White Act, an exposed employee has the right to request the infection status of the source patient from the patient's health care provider. Neither the agency nor the employee, however, can force testing of the source patient. As part of a good exposure control plan, employees must know what to do if an exposure incident occurs.

Submitting the Report

The Ryan White Act requires employers to appoint someone in the organization to whom an exposed employee can report. That person or officer follows the exposure control plan. The plan must comply with standards and guidelines relative to the exposure and must meet any local reporting requirements.

Medical Evaluation and Follow-Up

By law, employers must provide free medical evaluation and treatment to exposed employees. This would include the following:

- Counseling regarding the risks, signs and symptoms, probability of developing clinical disease, and how to prevent future spread of the potential infection
- Appropriate treatment in line with current U.S. Public Health Service recommendations
- A discussion of medications offered and their side effects and contraindications
- Evaluation of any reported illness to determine whether the symptoms are related to HIV or hepatitis

STEPS INVOLVED

Blood tests of exposed employees are always contingent on employee agreement. Employees have the option to provide blood samples. However, they can refuse permission for HIV testing at the time the sample is drawn. The employer must maintain the blood samples for 90 days in case employees change their mind regarding testing if HIV- or hepatitis-like symptoms develop.

> **CRITICAL THINKING**
> How do you think you would feel if you were stuck by a contaminated needle and the patient refused HIV testing?

As an agent of the employer, a health care provider must take the following steps: (1) provide counseling to the employee based on test results; (2) provide informed consent regarding prophylaxis and therapeutic regimens; and (3) implement those regimens after receiving approval from the employee. Vaccines also should be made available to all employees who are exposed to blood and other potentially infectious materials during their work.

Written Report and Confidentiality

The health care provider will send a written report to the DO of the employer. This states whether vaccination was offered to the exposed employee. It also states whether the employee received it. The written report also must note that the employee was informed of the results of the evaluation and told of any medical conditions resulting from the exposure that may require further evaluation or treatment. A copy of this report must be provided to the employee and to the DO for the agency's files.

All other elements of the employee's medical record are confidential. They cannot be supplied to the employer. The employee must give written consent for anyone to view the records. The records must be maintained for the duration of employment plus 30 years. This complies with OSHA standards regarding access to employee exposure and medical records.

PARAMEDIC'S ROLE IN PREVENTING DISEASE TRANSMISSION

Paramedics will have to deal with patients who have infectious diseases. It is important for them to be vigilant about the consequences to themselves and to their patients and co-workers. Part of this professional duty in preventing the spread of disease is knowing when *not* to go to work. A health care worker should not go to work if the following conditions are present:

- Fever
- Diarrhea
- Draining wound or any type of wet lesion
- Jaundice
- Mononucleosis
- Treatment with a medication and/or shampoo for lice or scabies
- Strep throat (unless antibiotics have been taken for longer than 24 hours)
- Cold (unless the paramedic wears a surgical mask)

Health care workers also should ensure that their personal immunization status is current for MMR, hepatitis, DPT, polio, chickenpox, and influenza.

> **CRITICAL THINKING**
> Have you come to school or work with any of these conditions?

Other Considerations in Disease Prevention

When called to provide emergency care, paramedics should always approach the scene with caution. They must keep in mind that an uncontrolled scene increases the likelihood of transmission of body fluids. Body substance isolation guidelines should be observed at all times. These include wearing gloves, protective eyewear, a face shield, and a gown (if splash or spray is possible) and wearing an appropriate particulate mask when airborne disease is suspected. As mentioned before, BSI is based on the premise that all body fluids, in any situation, may be infectious.

As a rule, if a patient has a cough, headache, general weakness, recent weight loss, nuchal rigidity, or high fever, the paramedic should immediately suspect an infectious process. Regardless of the patient's infectious status, however, the paramedic should do the following:

- Provide the same level of care to all patients.
- Disinfect equipment and the patient compartment with the proper disinfectant solution.
- Practice effective hand washing.
- Report any infectious exposure to the agency's DO.

> **CRITICAL THINKING**
> Imagine that you are on a call and get a small splash of blood in your eyes. What do you think would prevent you from reporting it immediately so that your postexposure care could begin?

SUMMARY

- National concerns about communicable disease and infection control have resulted in public law, standards, guidelines, and recommendations to protect health care providers and emergency responders against infectious diseases. Paramedics must be familiar with these guidelines. They also must take personal protective measures against exposure to these pathogens.
- The chain of elements needed to transmit an infectious disease includes the pathogenic agent, a reservoir, a portal of exit from the reservoir, an environment conducive to transmission of the pathogenic agent, a portal of entry into the new host, and susceptibility of the new host to the infectious disease.

Continued

- The human body is protected from infectious disease by external and internal barriers. These serve as lines of defense against infection. External barriers include the skin, GI system, upper respiratory tract, and genitourinary tract. Internal barriers include the inflammatory response and the immune response.
- The progression of infectious disease from exposure to the onset of symptoms follows four stages. These are the latent period, the incubation period, the communicability period, and the disease period.
- The human immunodeficiency virus is directly transmitted person to person. This occurs through anal or vaginal intercourse, across the placenta, by contact with infected blood or body fluids on mucous membranes or open wounds, through blood transfusion or tissue transplant, or by the use of contaminated needles or syringes. The virus affects the CD4 T cells. Secondary complications are usually related to opportunistic infections that arise as the immune system deteriorates. Progression of the disease can be divided into category A (acute retroviral infection, seroconversion, and asymptomatic infection); category B (early symptomatic HIV); and category C (late symptomatic HIV and advanced HIV). Paramedics should observe strict compliance with universal precautions for protection against HIV. Patient care should include helping these patients feel that they can obtain acceptance and compassion from health care workers.
- Hepatitis is a viral disease. It produces pathologic changes in the liver. The three main classes of hepatitis virus are hepatitis A, hepatitis B, and hepatitis C.
- Tuberculosis is a chronic pulmonary disease. It is acquired through inhalation of tubercle bacilli. The infection is passed mainly when infected people cough or sneeze the bacteria into the air or by contact with sputum that contains virulent TB bacilli. The infection is characterized by stages of early infection (frequently asymptomatic), latency, and a potential for recurrent postprimary disease.
- Meningococcal meningitis is an inflammation of the membranes that surround the spinal cord and brain. It can be caused by bacteria, viruses, and other microorganisms.
- Pneumonia is an acute inflammatory process of the respiratory bronchioles and alveoli. Bacteria, viruses, and fungi can cause this disease.
- Tetanus is a serious, sometimes fatal, disease of the CNS. It is caused by infection of a wound with spores of the bacterium *C. tetani*. The most common symptom is trismus (difficulty opening the mouth).
- Rabies is an acute viral infection of the CNS. Humans are highly susceptible to the rabies virus after exposure to saliva from the bite or scratch of an infected animal.
- Hantaviruses are carried by rodents. They are transmitted through inhalation of material contaminated with rodent urine and feces. Many forms of this disease occur in specific geographical areas.
- Rubella is a mild, febrile, highly communicable viral disease. It is characterized by a diffuse, punctate, macular rash. The CDC recommends that all health care providers receive immunization if they are not immune as a result of previous rubella infection.
- Rubeola is an acute, highly communicable viral disease caused by the measles virus. It is characterized by fever, conjunctivitis, cough, bronchitis, and a blotchy red rash.
- Mumps is an acute, communicable systemic viral disease. It is characterized by localized unilateral or bilateral edema of one or more of the salivary glands. Occasionally other glands are also involved.
- Chickenpox is highly communicable. It is characterized by a sudden onset of low-grade fever, mild malaise, and a maculopapular skin eruption that lasts for a few hours. This is followed by a vesicular eruption that lasts for 3 to 4 days, leaving a granular scab. The virus may reactivate during periods of stress or immunosuppression. At that time, it may cause an illness known as *shingles*.
- Pertussis is an infectious disease that leads to inflammation of the entire respiratory tract. It causes an insidious cough. The cough becomes paroxysmal in 1 to 2 weeks and lasts 1 to 2 months.
- Influenza is mainly a respiratory infection. It is spread by influenza viruses A, B, and C.
- Severe acute respiratory syndrome (SARS) is a viral illness first detected in 2003. It is spread by exposure to infected droplets. The illness begins with a fever and mild respiratory symptoms. It can progress to respiratory failure and death.
- Mononucleosis is caused either by the Epstein-Barr virus or by cytomegalovirus. Both of these are members of the herpes virus family.
- Syphilis is a systemic disease. It is characterized by a primary lesion; a secondary eruption involving skin and mucous membranes; long latency periods; and eventually by seriously disabling lesions of the skin, bone, viscera, CNS, and cardiovascular system.
- Gonorrhea is caused by the sexually transmitted bacterium *N. gonorrhoeae*. Gonorrhea can be treated with antibiotics. However, some strains brought into the United States from other countries do not respond to the usual antibiotic therapy.
- Chlamydia is a major cause of sexually transmitted nonspecific urethritis or genital infection. Signs and symptoms are similar to those of gonorrhea.

- Herpes simplex virus is transmitted by skin-to-skin contact with an infected area of the body. The primary infection produces a vesicular lesion (blister). This lesion heals spontaneously. After the primary infection, the virus travels to a sensory nerve ganglion. It remains there in a latent stage until reactivated.
- Lice are small, wingless insects that are ectoparasites of birds and mammals. During biting and feeding, lice secrete a substance that causes small, red macules and pruritus.
- The human scabies mite is a parasite. It completes its life cycle in and on the epidermis of the host. Scabies bites are usually concentrated around the hands and feet, especially in the webs of the fingers and toes.
- Reporting a possible communicable disease exposure permits immediate medical follow-up. It also enables the DO to make changes that might prevent exposures in the future. Moreover, it helps employees to obtain the proper evaluation and testing.
- Part of the paramedic's professional duty with regard to infectious disease transmission is to know when not to go to work. Paramedics also have a duty to use the proper BSI precautions at all times.

REFERENCES

1. US Department of Transportation National Highway Traffic Safety Administration: *EMT-paramedic national standard curriculum,* Washington, DC, 1998, The Department.
2. Centers for Disease Control: *Final rule on protecting health care workers from occupational exposure to bloodborne pathogens* (29 CFR 1910.1030), Atlanta, March 1993.
3. Centers for Disease Control: Perspectives in disease prevention and health promotion update: universal precautions for prevention of transmission of immunodeficiency virus, hepatitis B virus, and other bloodborne pathogens in health care settings, *MMWR Morb Mortal Wkly Rep* 37(24):377, 1988.
4. US Department of Health and Human Services, Centers for Disease Control: *A curriculum guide for public-safety and emergency response workers,* Atlanta, 1989, DHHS, CDC.
5. Centers for Disease Control: *MRSA fact sheet.* www.cdc.gov/ncidod/hip/Aresist/mrsafaq.htm. Accessed October 2, 2004.
6. McCance K, Huether S: *Pathophysiology: the biologic basis for disease in adults and children,* ed 4, St Louis, 2002, Mosby.
7. Grimes D: *Infectious diseases,* St Louis, 1991, Mosby.
8. National Center for Infectious Diseases of HIV/AIDS: 1993 revised classification system for HIV infection and expanded surveillance case definition for AIDS among adolescents and adults. http://aepo-xdv-www.epo.cdc.gov. Accessed October 24, 2004.
9. Recommendations for preventing transmission of human immunodeficiency virus and hepatitis B virus to patients during exposure-prone invasive procedures, *MMWR Morb Mortal Wkly Rep* 40 (RR08):1, 1991.
10. Evaluation of safety devices for preventing percutaneous injuries among health care workers during phlebotomy procedures, *MMWR Morb Mortal Wkly Rep* 46:21, 1997.
11. Public health service guidelines of the management of health care worker exposures to HIV and recommendations for postexposure prophylaxis, *MMWR Morb Mortal Wkly Rep* 47:1, 1998.
12. Updated US Public Health Service guidelines for the management of occupational exposures to HBV, HCV, and HIV and recommendations for postexposure prophylaxis, *MMWR Morb Mortal Wkly Rep* 50(RR-11):1, 2001.
13. Hepatitis International On-line. http://hepfi.org.
14. Mahoney F et al: Progress toward the elimination of hepatitis B virus transmission among health care workers in the United States, *Arch Intern Med* 157:2601, 1997.
15. Recommendations for prevention and control of hepatitis C virus (HCV) infection and HCV-related chronic disease, *MMWR Morb Mortal Wkly Rep* 47:1, 1998.
16. Centers for Disease Control and Prevention: *TB facts for health care workers: tuberculosis—yes, it's still a problem,* Atlanta, 1999, the CDC.
17. *TB (tuberculosis), New Mexico AIDS InfoNet fact sheet* (No. 515), New Mexico AIDS Education and Training Center, National Library of Medicine and New Mexico Department of Health, Albuquerque, October 10, 1998.
18. Control and prevention of meningococcal disease and control and prevention of serogroup C meningococcal disease: evaluation and management of suspected outbreaks: recommendations of the advisory committee on immunization practices (ACIP), *MMWR Morb Mortal Wkly Rep* 46(RR-5):13, 1997.
19. Marx J, Hochberger R, Walls R: *Emergency medicine: concepts and clinical practice,* ed 5, St Louis, 2002, Mosby.
20. American Medical Association: *Home medical encyclopedia,* New York, 1989, Random House.
21. Centers for Disease Control and Prevention: *Severe acute respiratory syndrome (SARS).* www.cdc.gov/niosh/topics/sars. Accessed November 14, 2004.
22. National Council of State EMS Training Coordinators Executive Committee of the National Association of State EMS Directors (NASEMSD), Centers for Disease Control and Prevention: *Updated interim guidance: prehospital emergency medical care and ground transport of suspected severe acute respiratory syndrome patients,* Atlanta.

CHAPTER 40

Behavioral and Psychiatric Disorders

OBJECTIVES

Upon completion of this chapter, the paramedic student will be able to:

1. Explain what constitutes a behavioral emergency.
2. Identify potential causes for behavioral and psychiatric illness.
3. List three critical principles that should be considered in the prehospital care of a patient with a behavioral emergency.
4. Outline key elements of the prehospital patient examination during a behavioral emergency.
5. Describe effective techniques for interviewing a patient during a behavioral emergency.
6. Differentiate key symptoms and management techniques for selected behavioral and psychiatric disorders.
7. Identify factors the paramedic must consider when assessing a suicide risk.
8. Formulate appropriate interview questions for determining suicidal intent.
9. Explain prehospital management techniques for a patient who has attempted suicide.
10. Describe the assessment of a potentially violent patient.
11. Outline measures that may be used to try to safely diffuse a potentially violent patient situation.
12. List situations in which patient restraint can be used.
13. Discuss the key principles of patient restraint.
14. Describe safety measures that should be taken when patient violence is anticipated.
15. Explain variations in approach to behavioral emergencies in children.

KEY TERMS

affect: An outward manifestation of a person's feelings or emotions.

anxiety: A state or feeling of apprehension, uneasiness, agitation, uncertainty, and fear resulting from the anticipation of some threat or danger.

behavioral emergency: A change in mood or behavior that cannot be tolerated by the involved person or others and that requires immediate attention.

delusions: Persistent beliefs or perceptions held by a person despite evidence that refutes them (i.e., false beliefs).

depression: A mood disturbance characterized by feelings of sadness, despair, and discouragement.

dyskinesia: An impairment of the ability to execute voluntary movements; often an adverse effect of prolonged use of antipsychotic medications.

hallucinations: The apparent perception of sights, sounds, and other sensory phenomena that are not actually present.

mania: A mood disorder characterized by extreme excitement, hyperactivity, agitation, and sometimes violent and self-destructive behavior.

mental status examination: An evaluation tool that includes an assessment of appearance and behavior, speech and language, emotional stability, and cognitive abilities.
paranoia: A condition characterized by an elaborate, overly suspicious system of thinking.
psychosis: Maladaptive behavior involving major distortions of reality.
schizophrenia: A group of disorders characterized by recurrent episodes of psychotic behavior.

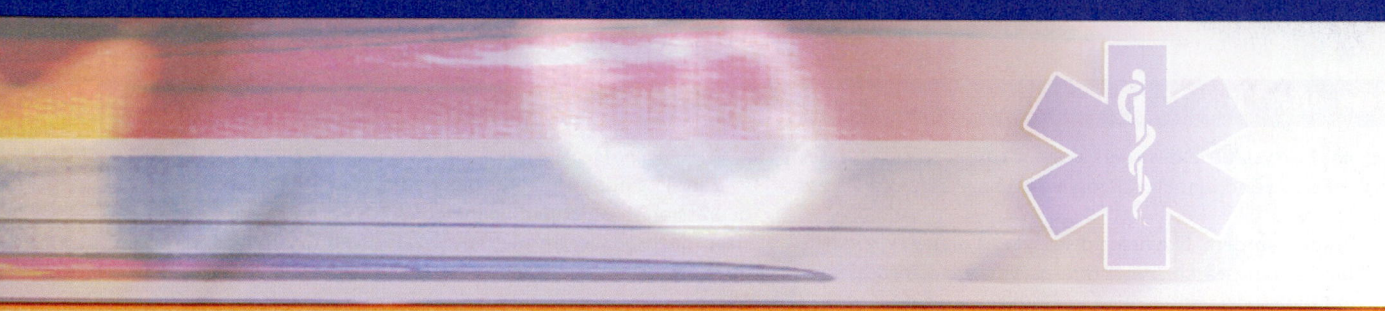

Behavioral and psychiatric emergencies call for an approach that is different from those used for emergency medical or trauma calls. The paramedic has no scientific tools to use in assessing the situation. Also, no firm protocols can guarantee a positive outcome. Fortunately, most behavioral emergencies require only strong communication skills and supportive measures. These measures can prevent the crisis from escalating. The paramedic's chief role often is to provide understanding, compassion, and direction for people who are temporarily in turmoil. Emergency medical services (EMS) personnel must focus on helping and protecting these patients. They do so until the patient is able to gain control or other therapeutic skills can be applied.

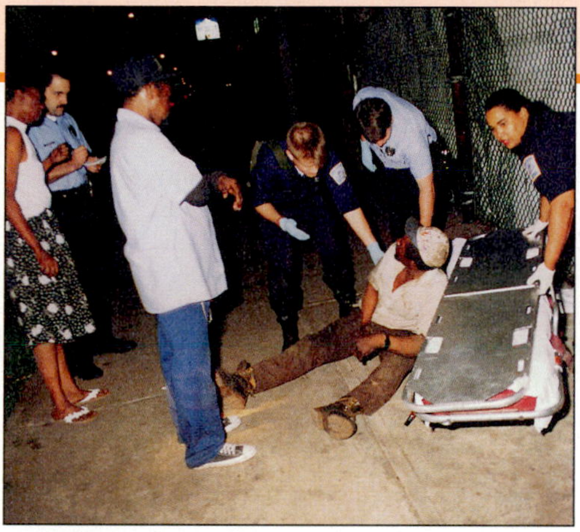

UNDERSTANDING BEHAVIORAL EMERGENCIES

The proportion of the U.S. population that has some form of mental health problem has been estimated to be as high as 20%. It also has been estimated that one in seven individuals will need treatment at some point in life for an emotional disturbance. Mental health problems incapacitate more people in the United States than all other health problems combined.[1]

There is no clear agreement on or ideal model for "normal" behavior. It generally is considered to be adaptive behavior that is accepted by society. (This can vary by culture and ethnic group.) The concept of abnormal (maladaptive) behavior also is defined by society as behavior that

- Deviates from society's norms and expectations
- Interferes with well-being and ability to function
- Harms the individual or group

CRITICAL THINKING

Can you think of a time in your life when you, a family member, or a close friend had a behavior that fit the definition of abnormal behavior? How did it make you feel?

A **behavioral emergency** can be defined as a change in mood or behavior that cannot be tolerated by the involved person or others and that requires immediate attention. Behavioral emergencies may range from a brief inability to cope with stress or **anxiety** to more intense situations in which patients may be dangerous to themselves and others. However, most people with mental illness function well on a daily basis. Common conditions such as depression, anxiety disorders, and mild personality disorders often are effectively managed with medication and counseling in outpatient mental health centers. Ten common myths about mental illness are listed in Box 40-1. Most behavioral emergencies have a biological, psychosocial, or sociocultural cause. In fact, mental illness may be the result of more than one of these factors (Fig. 40-1).

Biological Causes

Physical or biochemical disturbances in the brain may be inherited. These disturbances can result in major changes in behavior. In mental health care, biological disturbances are mental disorders that result from a physical (biochemical and organic) rather than a purely psychological cause. Examples include genetic factors, prenatal and postnatal factors (including infection, and endocrine, metabolic, and

BOX 40-1 Top 10 Myths about Mental Illness

Myth no. 1: Psychiatric disorders are not true medical illnesses like heart disease and diabetes. People who have a mental illness are just "crazy."

Fact: Brain disorders, like heart disease and diabetes, are true medical illnesses. Research shows that psychiatric disorders have genetic and biological causes. Also, these diseases can be treated effectively.

Myth no. 2: People with a severe mental illness, such as schizophrenia, are usually dangerous and violent.

Fact: Statistics show that the incidence of violence among people who have a brain disorder is not much higher than it is in the general population. Individuals suffering from a psychosis such as schizophrenia are more often frightened, confused, and despairing than violent.

Myth no. 3: Mental illness is the result of bad parenting.

Fact: Most experts agree that genetic factors, along with other risk factors, lead to psychiatric disorders. In other words, mental illnesses have a physical cause.

Myth no. 4: Depression results from a personality weakness or character flaw. People who are depressed could just snap out of it if they tried hard enough.

Fact: Depression has nothing to do with being lazy or weak. It results from changes in brain chemistry or brain function. Medication and/or psychotherapy often help people to recover.

Myth no. 5: Schizophrenia means that the person has a split personality, and there is no way to control it.

Fact: Schizophrenia is often confused with multiple personality disorder. Actually, schizophrenia is a brain disorder that robs people of their ability to think clearly and logically. An estimated 2.5 million Americans have schizophrenia. Their symptoms range from social withdrawal to hallucinations and delusions. Medication has helped many of these people to lead fulfilling, productive lives.

Myth no. 6: Depression is a normal part of the aging process.

Fact: It is not normal for older adults to be depressed. Signs of depression in older people include a loss of interest in activities, sleep disturbance, and lethargy. Depression in the elderly often goes undiagnosed. Older adults and their family members need to recognize the problem and seek professional help.

Myth no. 7: Depression and other illnesses, such as anxiety disorders, do not affect children or adolescents. Any problems they have are just a part of growing up.

Fact: Children and adolescents can develop severe mental illnesses. In the United States, 1 in 10 children and adolescents has a mental disorder severe enough to cause impairment. Yet only about 20% of these children receive treatment. Left untreated, these problems can get worse. *Anyone who talks about suicide should be taken very seriously.*

Myth no. 8: If you have a mental illness, you can will it away. Being treated for a psychiatric disorder means an individual has in some way "failed" or is weak.

Fact: A serious mental illness cannot be willed away. Ignoring the problem does not make it go away, either. It takes courage to seek professional help.

Myth no. 9: Addiction is a lifestyle choice and shows a lack of willpower. People with a substance abuse problem are morally weak or "bad."

Fact: Addiction is a disease that generally results from changes in brain chemistry. It has nothing to do with being a "bad" person.

Myth no. 10: Electroconvulsive therapy (ECT), formerly known as "shock treatment," is painful and barbaric.

Fact: ECT has given a new lease on life to many people who suffer from severe and debilitating depression. It is used when other treatments such as psychotherapy or medication fail or cannot be used. Patients who receive ECT are asleep and under anesthesia, therefore they do not feel anything.

"Top 10 myths about mental illness based on a nationwide survey" NARSD From National Alliance for Research on Schizophrenia and Depression. Great Neck, NY, 2003.

vascular disorders), an imbalance in brain chemistry, and alterations in neurotransmission. An example of a biological mental illness is schizophrenia (described later in this chapter). In this illness, specific genes have been identified that may influence the balance of chemicals in the brain. These chemicals are called *neurotransmitters.* They are responsible for communication among the brain cells.

Organic causes of behavioral emergencies that have been discussed throughout this text include substance abuse, trauma, illness (e.g., diabetes, electrolyte imbalance), infections, tumors, and dementia (Box 40-2). It is important that the paramedic consider the possibility of these medical conditions in all behavioral emergencies.

Psychosocial Causes

Psychosocial mental illness may have many causes. It often is related to an individual's personality type. It also may be related to the person's ability to resolve situational conflict in life. For example, psychosocial mental illness may result from childhood trauma, child abuse or neglect, or a dysfunctional family structure that affects relationships with parents and siblings. Biological disorders (e.g., genetic factors and chemical imbalance) may contribute to psychosocial causes of mental illness.

Sociocultural Causes

Sociocultural causes of mental illness are related to the way a person balances emotions, thoughts, and interactions in society. When this balance shifts rapidly, a person may experience emotional turmoil. This turmoil may result in crisis. Factors that may be related to sociocultural causes of behavioral emergencies include personal relationships, family stability, economic status, social cohesion, work environment, and personal belief systems and values. Changes in behavior caused by personal or situational stress often are linked to a specific event or series of events. Examples include environmental violence (e.g., war, riots, rape, assault), the death of a loved one, ongoing discrimination or prejudice, and economic and employment problems.

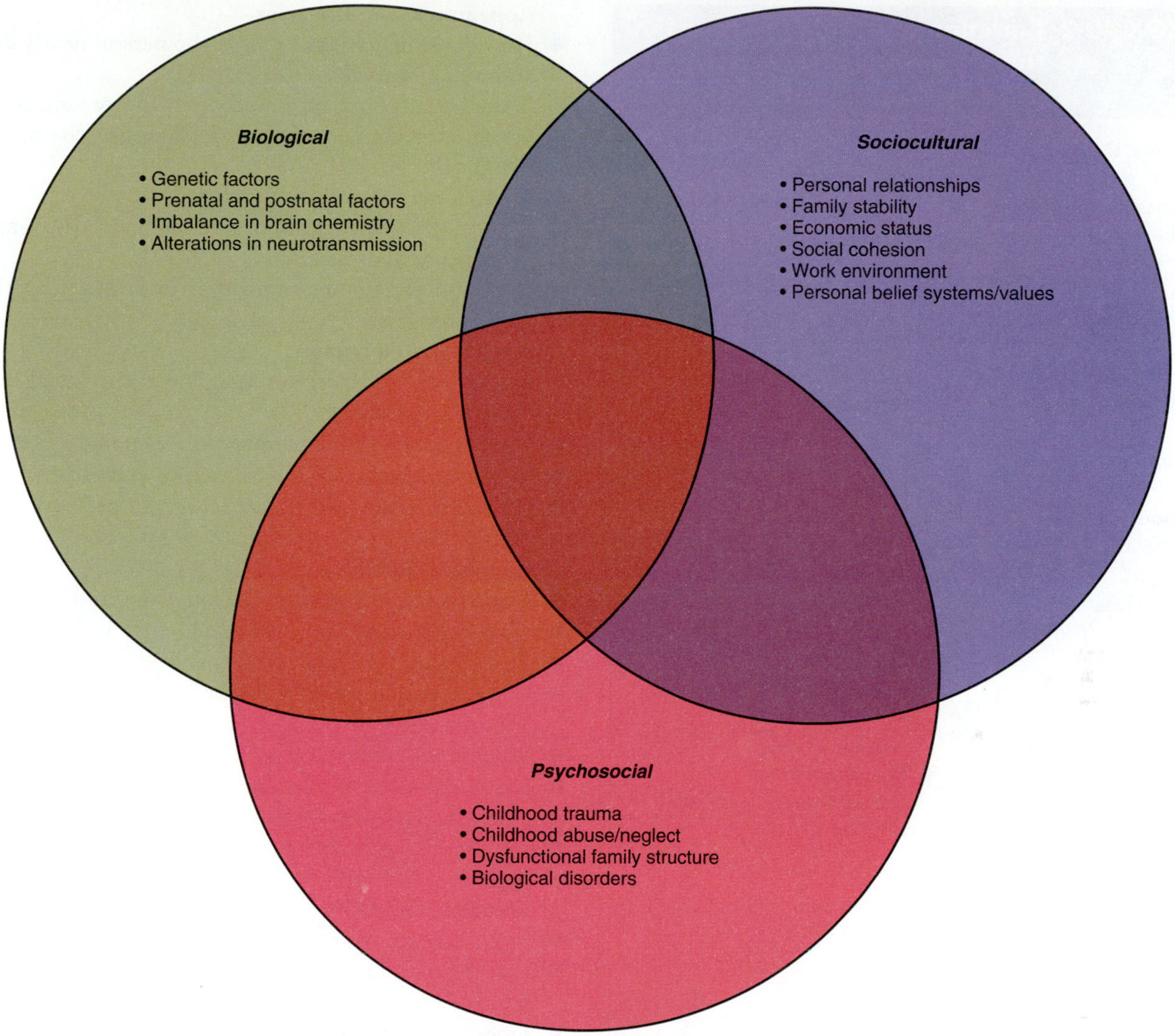

FIGURE 40-1 ■ Common causes of behavioral emergencies.

ASSESSMENT AND MANAGEMENT OF BEHAVIORAL EMERGENCIES

The initial assessment and management of a patient with a behavioral emergency are similar to those used in any other EMS response. These steps include ensuring scene safety, containing the crisis, giving proper emergency medical care, and transporting the patient to an appropriate health care facility. In addition, most EMS services have protocols that call for the police to evaluate the scene for possible danger and to control any acts of aggression by the patient.

Assessment

Paramedics should begin the assessment by creating a rapport with the patient. They can do this while gathering information needed for immediate management of life-threatening conditions. On arrival, paramedics should survey the scene for any relevant details. These may include evidence of substance abuse, a suicide attempt, or other clues that may shed light on the patient's state. The patient should be observed for emotional response, such as fear, anger, confusion, or hostility. While providing patient care, the paramedic should focus the evaluation on the patient's level of cognitive functioning. This includes alertness, orientation, speech patterns, **affect,** and the way in which the patient interacts with friends, loved ones, and family members. When possible, the number of people around the patient should be limited. This helps to control the scene. Anyone who interferes with the scene or the patient assessment or who adversely affects the patient's condition should be removed from the area.

Other information can be volunteered by the patient, obtained from the patient interview, or provided by family members, bystanders, and first responders. The patient's family or caregiver should be interviewed about the patient's usual level of functioning, about recent stress in the patient's life, and about approaches that may help the paramedic to gain the patient's trust and cooperation. Information that should be obtained for a full background and history of the event include significant past medical history, medications the patient has taken (Table 40-1), past psychiatric problems, and any precipitating factors that may have contributed to the behavioral emergency.

BOX 40-2 Common Medical Conditions that Manifest as Behavioral Disorders

Metabolic Disorders
Glucose, sodium, calcium, or magnesium imbalance
Acid-base imbalance
Acute hypoxia
Renal failure
Hepatic failure

Endocrine Disorders
Thyroid disease
Parathyroid disease
Adrenal hormone imbalance

Infectious Diseases
Encephalitis
Meningitis
Brain abscess
Severe systemic infection

Trauma
Concussion
Intracranial hematoma (especially subdural hematoma)

Cardiovascular Disorders
Cardiac dysrhythmia
Hypotension
Transient ischemic attack
Cerebrovascular accident (or stroke)
Hypertensive encephalopathy

Neoplastic Diseases
Central nervous system tumors or metastases

Degenerative Diseases
Dementia of the Alzheimer's type
Other dementias

Drug Abuse
Alcohol
Barbiturates
Narcotics
Sedative-hypnotics
Amphetamines and other stimulants
Hallucinogens

Drug Reactions
Beta-adrenergic blockers
Antihypertensives
Cardiac drugs
Bronchodilators
Beta-adrenergic agonists
Anticonvulsants

Interview Techniques

After managing any life-threatening illness or injury, the paramedic should interview the patient if possible. The paramedic should not ask for more details than are needed. A limited and supportive interview strengthens the paramedic's rapport with the patient. It also can help to establish and maintain a relationship during the provision of patient care. Effective interview techniques include active listening, showing support and empathy, preventing interruptions, and respecting the patient's personal space by limiting physical touch (Box 40-3).

MENTAL STATUS EXAMINATION

A **mental status examination** (MSE) is an evaluation tool. It can help the paramedic during the patient assessment. Although many variations of an MSE are available, most include an assessment of appearance and behavior, speech and language, cognitive abilities, and emotional stability.[2] The following factors should be assessed in each of these areas.

Appearance and Behavior
- How does the patient look? Is the person neatly dressed and well groomed?
- Is the patient pleasant and cooperative or agitated?
- Is the patient's behavior appropriate for the particular situation?
- What is the patient's body language?
- Do body movements or posture suggest tension, anxiety, hostility, or aggression?
- Does the patient maintain eye contact during the patient interview?

Speech and Language
- Is the patient's speech intelligible and normal in tone, volume, and rate?
- Does the tone of the patient's voice change?
- Is speech spontaneous, with ease of expression?
- Do the patient's words and sentences proceed in an orderly fashion?

Cognitive Abilities
- Is the patient oriented to person, time, and place?
- Does the patient know who and where he or she is?
- Does the patient know who you are?
- Can the patient remain focused on your questions and conversation?
- What is the patient's attention span?
- Can the patient follow a series of short commands?
- Does the patient respond to directions appropriately?
- Are the patient's comments logical and presented in an organized fashion?

Emotional Stability
- Is the patient aware of his or her environment?
- Can the patient describe or rate his or her mood using a scale of 1 to 10?
- Does the patient appear happy, sad, depressed, or angry?
- Is the patient's mood appropriate for the specific situation?
- Does the patient show mood swings or behaviors that indicate anxiety, depression, anger, or hostility?
- Does the patient stay focused during the interview or stray quickly to related topics?
- Is the patient experiencing perceptual distortions or hallucinations?

CRITICAL THINKING

Think about interviewing techniques that you've seen EMS crews use when caring for patients with behavioral emergencies. Were the techniques effective? Could the paramedics have improved their patient care by using any of the techniques listed in Box 40-3?

DIFFICULT PATIENT INTERVIEWS

Some patients with behavioral or psychiatric disorders are difficult to interview. For example, a patient may refuse to talk to the paramedic. (This may be the case especially if the family requested EMS assistance without the patient's consent.) A patient may be extremely talkative and have disor-

TABLE 40-1 Examples of Drugs Used to Treat Psychiatric Disorders

TRADE NAME	GENERIC NAME	DRUG CLASS
Akineton	Biperiden	Antiparkinson agent
Anafranil:	Clomipramine	Antidepressant
Asendin	Amoxapine	Antidepressant
Aventyl	Nortriptyline	Antidepressant
Thorazine, Largactil, Chlorpromanyl, Novo-Chlorpromazine	Chlorpromazine	Antipsychotic
Clozaril	Clozapine	Antipsychotic
Cogentin, Apo-Benztropine, PMS Benztropine	Benztropine mesylate	Antiparkinson agent
Desyrel	Trazodone	Antidepressant
Elavil, Levate, Apo-Amitriptyline, Novotriptyn, PMS Amitripyline	Amitriptyline	Antidepressant
Eldepryl, SD Deprenyl	Selegiline	Antiparkinson agent
Fluanxol	Flupenthixol dihydrochloride	Antipsychotic
Modecate, Apo-Fluphenazine, Permitil, Moditen	Fluphenazine	Antipsychotic
Haldol, Apo-Haloperidol, Novo Peridol, Peridol, PMS Haloperidol	Haloperidol	Antipsychotic
Kemadrin, PMS Procyclidine, Procyclid	Procyclidine	Antiparkinson agent
Lithium, Lithane, Carbolith, Duralith, Lithane, Lithizine	Lithium carbonate	Antipsychotic
Luvox	Fluvoxamine maleate	Antidepressant
Marplan	Isocarboxazid	Antidepressant
Mellaril, Apo-Thioridazine, Novo Ridazine, PMS Thioridazine	Thioridazine	Antipsychotic
Nardil	Phenelzine	Antidepressant
Neuleptil	Pericyazine	Antipsychotic
Norpramin, Pertofrane	Desipramine	Antidepressant
Nozinan	Methotrimeprazine	Antipsychotic
Orap	Pimozide	Antipsychotic
Parnate	Tranylcypromine	Antidepressant
Parsitan, Profenamine	Ethopropazine	Antiparkinson agent
Piportil L4	Pipotiazine	Antipsychotic
Promazine	Promazine	Antipsychotic
Prozac	Fluoxetine	Antidepressant
Ritalin	Methylphenidate	Cerebral stimulant
Risperdal	Risperidone	Antipsychotic
Serentil	Mesoridazine	Antipsychotic
Sinequan, Novo-Doxepin, Triadapin	Doxepin	Antidepressant
Stelazine, Apo-Trifluoperazine, PMS Trifluoperazine, Terfluzine, Novo Flurazine, Solazine	Trifluoperazine	Antipsychotic
Stemetil, Prorazin, PMS Prochlorperazine	Prochlorperazine	Antipsychotic
Surmontil, Apo-Trimip, Novo-Trimpramine, Rhotrimine	Trimipramine	Antidepressant
Tegretol, Apo-Carbamazepine, Mazepine, Novocarbamaz PMS	Carbamazepine	Antipsychotic
Tofranil, Apo-Imipramine, Impril, Novopramine, PMS Imipramine	Imipramine	Antidepressant
Trilafon, Apo-Perphenazine, PMS Perphenazine	Perphenazine	Antipsychotic
Triptil	Protriptyline	Antidepressant
Valium, Apo-Diazepam, Diazemuls, Novodipam, PMS Diazepam, Vivol	Diazepam	Antianxiety
Xanax, Apo-Alpraz, Novo Alprazol, Nu-Alpraz	Alprazolam	Antianxiety
Zoloft	Sertraline	Antidepressant

ganized speech. In addition, a patient may be confrontational. If a patient refuses to be interviewed, paramedics should speak to the patient in a quiet voice. They should avoid questions that the patient may see as an "interrogation." Also, paramedics should allow the patient extra time to respond. Patients who are too talkative need to have their attention focused on the interview. To do this, the paramedic can raise a hand or call the person's name. With a confrontational patient, additional help may be required to ensure scene safety.

Other Patient Care Measures

After the initial assessment and history taking, the rest of the examination is determined by the patient; specifically, this means by the person's overall condition and the nature of the psychiatric problem. There may be a good reason to suspect an organic cause for the patient's condition. If so, a physical examination should be performed. Otherwise, patient care for a person with a behavioral emergency may be limited to maintaining an effective rapport with the patient during transfer to the hospital.

BOX 40-3 Ten Useful Interviewing Skills for Behavioral Emergencies

1. Listen to the patient in a caring, concerned, and receptive manner. Be aware of nonverbal cues. Examples of such are eye contact, facial expression, and posture. These can reassure the patient that you are responding with empathy.
2. Elicit feelings as well as facts to help develop a more accurate impression of the patient. If the patient is anxious, encourage the person to share details relevant to that feeling.
3. Respond to the patient's feelings by acknowledging and labeling them. (For example, you might say, "You seem angry.") This may help validate and legitimize the patient's intense and sometimes overwhelming feelings.
4. Correct cognitive misconceptions or distortions. If a distorted sense of reality is producing fear or anxiety, offer a simple and correct explanation.
5. Explain to the patient the care the person can expect to receive upon arrival at the hospital.
6. Offer honest and realistic reassurance and support. Providing this support helps calm the patient and establishes rapport.
7. Ask effective questions. Ask closed-ended questions if you are seeking immediate information. For example, "Are you thinking of hurting yourself?" and "What medicines did you take?" Open-ended questions are appropriate after you have identified problems that require immediate attention. Such questions allow the patient to develop answers that usually help the paramedic more fully understand the problem.
8. Avoid questions that may lead the person to say things he or she did not intend.
9. Structure the interview to develop a pattern rather than allowing a natural flow of details. Histories or sequences of events in chronological order usually allow for a fuller understanding of the patient's problem. (This is particularly true for causal relationships.) This order also helps the patient to organize thoughts. Keep the patient's responses focused. This can be done by using comments such as "What happened next?" and "Was that before or after what you were just telling me about?"
10. Conclude the interview. After getting the relevant information, encourage the patient to describe other important events or feelings.

Modified from Bassuk EL: *Behavioral emergencies: a field guide for EMTs and paramedics,* Boston, 1983, Little, Brown.

SPECIFIC BEHAVIORAL AND PSYCHIATRIC DISORDERS

More than 250 psychiatric conditions have been noted by mental health workers. In addition, some patients may have symptoms that are associated with more than one condition. The following are common classifications of mental disorders discussed in this chapter[1]:

- Cognitive disorders
- Schizophrenia
- Anxiety disorders
- Mood disorders
- Substance-related disorders
- Somatoform disorders
- Factitious disorders
- Dissociative disorders
- Eating disorders
- Impulse control disorders
- Personality disorders

NOTE The American Psychiatric Association (APA) also has identified major classes of psychiatric disorders. These are known as *DSM-IV-TR* groups.[3] (DSM-IV-TR refers to the APA's *Diagnostic and Statistical Manual of Mental Disorders,* edition 4, text revision, which was published in 2000.) Many mental health professionals use these classifications for diagnostic purposes. In addition to the disorders listed in the text, other DSM-IV classes of psychiatric disorders include the following:

- Disorders first diagnosed in infancy, childhood, and adolescence
- Delirium, dementia, amnesia, and other cognitive disorders
- Psychotic disorders other than schizophrenia
- Mental disorders caused by a general medical condition
- Sexual and gender identity disorders
- Sleep disorders
- Adjustment disorders
- Other conditions that may be the focus of clinical attention

Patient care for most behavioral emergencies is mainly supportive. It usually involves providing emotional support, assessing and managing coexisting emergency medical problems, and transporting the patient for evaluation by a physician. In some cases paramedics may need to take measures to protect the patient and others from harm. This includes the possible use of physical and chemical restraint (described later in this chapter).

Cognitive Disorders

Cognitive disorders may have an organic cause (e.g., a disease process). They also may be a result of physical or chemical injury, such as trauma or drug abuse. All cognitive disorders result in a disturbance of cognitive functioning. This may manifest as delirium or dementia (see Chapter 45).

DELIRIUM

Delirium is an abrupt disorientation of time and place. It usually involves **delusions** (false beliefs) and **hallucinations** (the individual appears to perceive sights, sounds, and other sensory phenomena that are not actually present). The symptoms vary according to an individual's personality, the environment, and the severity of the illness. Common signs and symptoms of delirium include inattention, memory impairment, disorientation, clouding of consciousness, and vivid visual hallucinations. Treatment of delirium is aimed at correcting the underlying physical disorder to reduce anxiety. Sedatives may be required to manage the patient. The exact occurrence rate of delirium is unknown, because it often is overlooked. However, some groups of people are more sus-

BOX 40-4 Some Causes of Dementia

Degenerative Diseases
Huntington disease
Parkinson disease (not in all cases)
Cerebellar degenerations
Amyotrophic lateral sclerosis (not in all cases)
Rare genetic and metabolic diseases

Vascular Dementia
Multiinfarct dementia
Microinfarct dementia
Large infarct dementia
Cerebral embolic disease

Anoxic Dementia
Cardiac arrest
Cardiac failure (severe)
Carbon monoxide poisoning

Traumatic Dementia
Dementia pugilistica (boxer's dementia)
Head injury (open or closed)

Infectious Dementia
Acquired immunodeficiency syndrome (AIDS) dementia
Opportunistic infection

Infectious Dementia, cont'd
Postencephalitic dementia
Herpes dementia
Fungal meningitis or encephalitis
Bacterial meningitis or encephalitis
Parasitic encephalitis
Brain abscess
Neurosyphilis (general paresia)

Space-Occupying Lesions
Chronic or acute subdural hematoma
Primary brain tumor
Metastatic tumor

Autoimmune Disorders
Disseminated lupus erythematosus
Vasculitis

Toxic Dementia
Alcohol
Metals (e.g., lead, mercury, arsenic)
Organic poisons (e.g., solvents, some insecticides)

From FYI: *Disorders causing dementia,* Alzheimer's Association, Northern Virginia Chapter. www.alz-nova.org/fyi.htm. Accessed October 30, 2004.

BOX 40-5 Facts about Schizophrenia

- More than 2 million adult Americans are affected by schizophrenia.
- In men, schizophrenia usually appears in the late teens or early 20s.
- In women, schizophrenia usually appears in the 20s to early 30s.
- Schizophrenia affects men and women with equal frequency.
- Most people with schizophrenia suffer chronically throughout their lives.
- One in 10 people with schizophrenia eventually commits suicide.
- Schizophrenia costs the United States more than $48 billion annually.

ceptible to delirium than others. These groups include the following:

- Older adults
- Children
- Burn patients
- Patients who have had major heart surgery
- Patients who have had a previous brain injury (e.g., stroke)
- Patients with acquired immunodeficiency syndrome (AIDS)

DEMENTIA

Dementia is a clinical state characterized by loss of function in multiple cognitive domains. It is a slow, progressive loss of awareness of time and place. It usually involves an inability to learn new things or to remember recent events. About 75 types of dementia have been identified (Box 40-4). However, most cases result from cerebrovascular disease (including stroke) and Alzheimer disease (an irreversible, gradual loss of brain cells and shrinkage of brain tissue). Dementia is a major health problem in the United States because of Americans' long life spans. The disorder affects about 10% of those over age 65 and 20% of those over age 75. The personal habits of patients with dementia often deteriorate. Speech may become incoherent. Also, many of these patients may enter a "second childhood." These patients need total care for feeding, toileting, and physical activities. Treatment of certain illnesses may help to slow the mental decline associated with this disease.

Delirium and dementia may be difficult to differentiate. This is because both may cause disorientation and impaired memory, thinking, and judgment. Dementia usually occurs in people without diminished alertness. Dementia appears slowly and worsens over time. Sleeping and waking problems occur less often in people with dementia than in those with delirium. People with dementia may have difficulty with short- and long-term memory, as well as impairment of judgment and abstract thinking. Delirium sometimes may occur at the same time as dementia. This is especially the case in older adults or people with chronic illnesses.

CRITICAL THINKING

Besides auditory hallucinations, think of other sensory hallucinations that can occur in these patients.

Schizophrenia

Schizophrenia is a group of disorders. It is characterized by recurrent episodes of psychotic behavior. Although the exact cause of the disease has not yet been identified, it may result from a combination of genetics (a family history of schizophrenia often exists), chemical and hormonal changes, autoimmune illness, viral infection, and other stress factors.[4] Schizophrenia usually becomes apparent during adolescence or early adulthood (Box 40-5).[5] Signs and symptoms of the illness appear slowly over time. They become more pronounced and bizarre as the disease progresses. These patients often develop abnormalities of thought processing, thought content, perception, and judgment. Hallmarks of the disease are **para-**

BOX 40-6 Responding to Paranoia, Delusions, and Hallucinations

1. First, assess whether the problem is troublesome or frightening to the person experiencing it. If not, ignoring it may be the best approach.
2. If a person seems to be hallucinating, leave the individual alone or approach slowly so as not to frighten the person. Respond with caution.
3. Don't try to argue or rationalize. Realize that hallucinations and delusions seem very real to the person who is experiencing them. Arguing does not build trust.
4. Offer reassurance and validation. You might say, "I know this is troubling for you. Let me see if I can help."
5. Check out the reality of the situation; maybe what the person sees or thinks is true.
6. Sometimes things in the environment may be misinterpreted (i.e., a glare or shadow in the window, a noisy furnace). These may be frightening. Explain the potential or actual misinterpretation (e.g., that the noise is the furnace turning on).
7. Modify the environment if necessary. (A mirror may become distracting or confusing; adding more lights may be helpful at night.)
8. Assess whether the person is having problems with hearing or vision. Resolving such problems can reduce the degree of disability.
9. Recall that whispering or laughing around the person may be misinterpreted.
10. Do not take any accusations personally.
11. Use distraction to try to pull the person's focus from the delusion or hallucination.
12. If the person asks you directly whether you see or hear something, be honest. However, don't struggle to convince or reason with the individual about what is real.
13. Try to respond to what the person may be feeling: insecurity, fear, and confusion.
14. Rule out any illnesses or the use of any medicines that could be contributing to the problem.
15. Use tact and firmness in persuading a patient to be transported to the hospital.

Modified from the Alzheimer's Association handout: *Hallucinations and delusions and understanding difficult behaviors;* Anne Robinson, Beth Spencer, Laurie White (1989), Eastern Michigan University, Ypsilanti, Mich.

noia, delusions, and auditory hallucinations (e.g., hearing voices that insult or make demands) (Box 40-6.)

Many patients with schizophrenia function quite well with drug therapy. Others function poorly between frank psychotic episodes. (These episodes often are the result of failure to comply with drug therapy.) Most patients must take antipsychotic drugs and agents that block the action of dopamine for the rest of their lives. If the person takes these medications regularly, the obvious symptoms usually are controlled. However, the drugs may produce side effects, especially **dyskinesia** (abnormal muscular movements) and tremor.

Anxiety Disorders

A certain amount of anxiety is useful. In fact, it is necessary for adapting constructively to stress (see Chapter 2). However, a patient who suffers from an anxiety disorder has a persistent, fearful feeling that cannot be consciously related to reality (Box 40-7).[5] This type of illness can be disabling. The patient may withdraw from daily activities. This is usually an unsuccessful attempt to avoid the episodes of intense activity. Severe anxiety disorders may manifest in a panic disorder ("panic attack") with the following signs and symptoms (Box 40-8)[5]:

- Hyperventilation
- Feeling of breathlessness or smothering
- Blurred vision
- Perioral and hand and foot paresthesias
- Fear of losing control
- Fear of dying
- Somatic complaints
- Chest discomfort
- Palpitations or tachycardia
- Dyspnea
- Choking
- Faintness
- Syncope
- Vertigo
- Trembling and sweating
- Urinary frequency and diarrhea

Patient management is mainly supportive. The paramedic should assure these patients that although they may feel as if they are dying, they are not. Also, the paramedic should assure them that effective treatment is available. Panic attacks may mimic a number of medical emergencies, including myocardial infarction. Therefore any patient who shows the signs and symptoms described before should be fully assessed at the scene and transported for evaluation by a physician. (Sedation may be required.) Patients with anxiety disorders should not be left alone.

PHOBIA

A *phobia* is a type of anxiety disorder. A person with a phobia has transferred anxiety onto a situation or an object in the form of an irrational, intense fear, such as a fear of heights, closed spaces, water, or other people. As the object or situation comes closer, the person's anxiety increases. If the crisis is allowed to continue, the patient's anxiety may escalate into a panic attack. These patients usually recognize that their fear is unreasonable. However, they cannot overcome the phobia. In some cases the phobia does not

CRITICAL THINKING

Do you know someone with an intense fear of a situation or object? How does this person behave when subjected to the object of the phobia?

BOX 40-7 Facts about Anxiety Disorders

- More than 16 million adults between the ages of 18 and 54 in the United States suffer from anxiety disorders.
- Anxiety disorders often are complicated by depression, eating disorders, or substance abuse.
- Anxiety disorders cost the nation more than $46 billion each year.

BOX 40-8 Facts about Panic Disorders

- Panic disorders affect about 2.4 million people in the United States each year.
- Panic disorders usually strike in young adulthood; about half of those affected develop the condition before age 24.
- Women are twice as likely as men to develop a panic disorder.
- People with a panic disorder also may suffer from depression and substance abuse. About 30% of people with panic disorder abuse alcohol; 17% abuse other drugs (e.g., cocaine, marijuana).
- About one third of those with a panic disorder develop agoraphobia.

BOX 40-9 Facts about Obsessive-Compulsive Disorder

- About 3.3 million American adults have obsessive-compulsive disorder (OCD) in a given year.
- OCD affects men and women with equal frequency.
- The nation's social and economic losses caused by OCD total more than $8 billion each year.

BOX 40-10 Facts about Posttraumatic Syndrome

- About 5.2 million people in the United States have posttraumatic syndrome during the course of a given year.
- Posttraumatic syndrome can develop at any age, including childhood.
- Posttraumatic syndrome is more common in women than men.
- About 30% of men and women who have spent time in a war zone experience this disorder.
- Posttraumatic syndrome often occurs after violent personal assaults, such as rape, mugging, or domestic violence; terrorism; natural or human-caused disasters; and accidents.
- Depression, alcohol or other substance abuse, or another anxiety disorder often accompanies posttraumatic syndrome.

initiate the EMS response but becomes a secondary complication in emergency care. An example is a person who is phobic of water being trapped in a submerged car.

When caring for patients with a phobia, the paramedic should take care to explain each step of an emergency or rescue procedure. The key is a careful rehearsal with the patient, in which the paramedic explains exactly what care will be given and how it will be performed. In addition, the EMS crew should show patience and understanding of the phobia. They should assure the patient that no forceful steps will be taken to place the person into a position unwillingly.

OBSESSIVE-COMPULSIVE DISORDER

Obsessive-compulsive disorder (OCD) is a psychiatric disorder in which a person feels stress or anxiety about thoughts or rituals over which the individual has little control (Box 40-9).[5] The disorder can take many forms. These include excessive hand washing or showering, or upsetting thoughts (e.g., violence, vulgarities, harm to oneself or others). Obsessions may also involve special numbers, colors, single words or phrases, and sometimes melodies.

Although most adults realize to some degree that these obsessions and compulsions are senseless, they have great difficulty stopping them. Children with OCD may not realize that their behavior is unusual. OCD affects men and women equally, can start at any age, and may have a heritable component. People with OCD often cleverly hide their condition from family, friends, and co-workers. Medications and behavior therapy are often effective in controlling the symptoms of this disorder.

POSTTRAUMATIC SYNDROME

Posttraumatic syndrome (posttraumatic stress disorder) is an anxiety reaction to severe psychosocial events (Box 40-10).[5] These events often are life-threatening. (Examples include events associated with military service or rape.) The events often result in repetitive, intrusive memories. Manifestations of this illness may include depression, sleep disturbances, nightmares, and survivor guilt. The syndrome often is complicated by substance abuse.

EMS personnel and other emergency responders may be subject to this syndrome as a result of their work. Examples include responding to major incidents with a large number of injured people, the death of a co-worker, a sudden infant death syndrome (SIDS) death, and the stress associated with responding to emergency calls (see Chapter 2).

Mood Disorders

The term *mood disorder* is used to describe changes in emotions that a person experiences in life. (For example, these may include happiness, depression, fear, and anxiety.) Two conditions commonly associated with mood disorders are depression and bipolar disorder, both of which are associated with an increased risk of suicide.[1]

DEPRESSION

Depression is a mood disturbance. It is characterized by feelings of sadness, despair, and discouragement. It is one of the most prevalent major psychiatric conditions, affecting 10% to 15% of the general population (Box 40-11).[1,5] Depression is usually episodic (episodes usually last longer than 1 month) with periods of remission. It is known to have either a gradual or rapid onset and, at times, a clustering of episodes. The depressed patient may show feelings of hopelessness, extreme isolation, tenseness, and irritability. In severe cases the depression may be followed by *anhedonia* (the inability to feel pleasure or happiness from experiences that ordinarily are pleasurable), insomnia or hypersomnia, weight loss (from diminished appetite) or gain, decreased libido, and deep feelings of worthlessness and guilt. The mnemonic *in sad cages* identifies the major features of depression[6]:

Interest
Sleep
Appetite
Depressed mood
Concentration
Activity
Guilt
Energy
Suicide

Depression is common in the elderly. It also is associated with an increased risk of suicide for all age groups (described later in this chapter). Care for depressed patients is directed at quietly talking to the patient about things that appear to be of interest and trying to gain responsiveness. Depression may be treated with antidepressant drug therapy (see Chapter 17), counseling, psychotherapy and, in a small number of cases, electroconvulsive therapy (ECT).

BIPOLAR DISORDER

Bipolar disorder is a biphasic emotional disorder in which depressive and manic episodes alternate (Fig. 40-2). **Mania** is characterized by excessive elation, talkativeness, flight of ideas, motor activity, irritability, accelerated speech and, often, delusions that center around personal grandeur. Bipolar disorders sometimes develop slowly over time. However, they may occur abruptly and may be brought on by a single event. The manic phase can be very brief or can last weeks to months. Compared with depression, mania is rare. The most frequent age for initial episodes is 20 to 35 years, with initial attacks of depression occurring about 10 years later (Box 40-12).[5] Many patients with bipolar disorder are treated with lithium. As described in Chapter 17, lithium has a narrow therapeutic index; a common illness, such as influenza with diarrhea and or vomiting, can result in lithium toxicity.

Emergency care should consist of calm, firm emotional support. It also should include transport for evaluation by a physician. If this is the patient's first manic episode, the paramedic should consider the possibility of drug abuse. It usually is a good idea to keep sensory stimulation to a minimum. If the patient's condition allows, EMS transport should proceed without using the lights and sirens.

BOX 40-11 Facts about Depression

- More than 19 million adult Americans suffer from depression each year. Many are unnecessarily unable to function normally for weeks or months because their illness goes untreated.
- Almost twice as many women (12%) as men (7%) are affected by depressive illness each year.
- Depression is a frequent and serious complication of heart attack, stroke, diabetes, and cancer.
- Depression increases the risk of heart attack.
- Depression costs the nation more than $30 billion a year in direct and indirect costs.
- Major depression is the leading cause of disability worldwide.

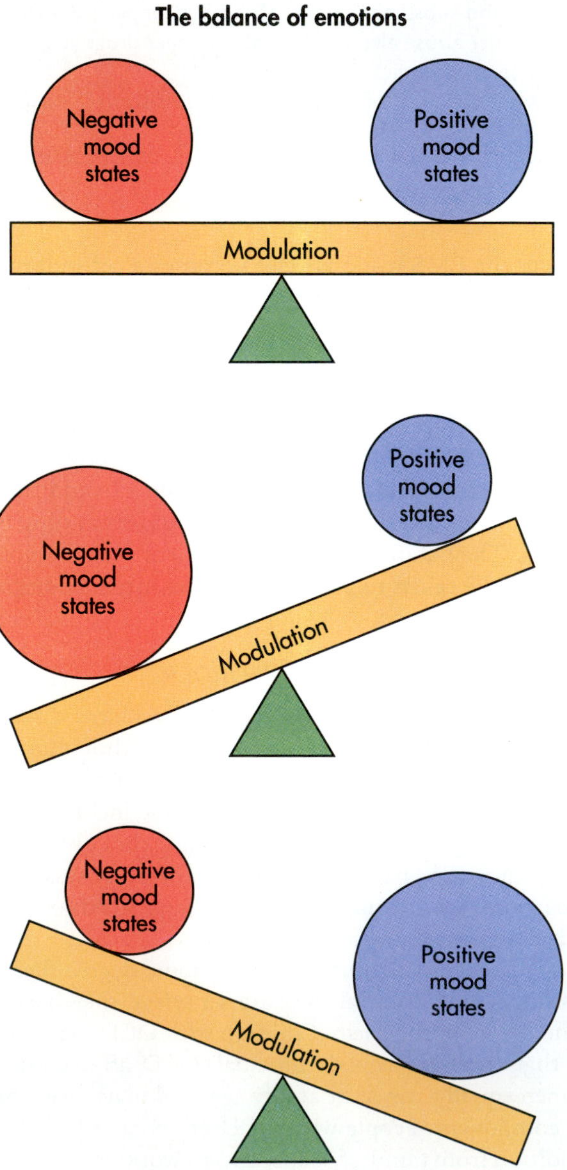

FIGURE 40-2 ■ Bipolar disorder.

CRITICAL THINKING

Do you think patients would be at higher risk for suicide during the depressive or the manic phase of bipolar disorder? Why?

SUICIDE AND SUICIDE THREATS

A threat of suicide is a sign that a patient has a serious crisis that calls for immediate intervention. In many cases suicide attempts are a cry for help. They also may be a form of direct or indirect communication. (They may be saying, "I don't want to live" or "I am angry with you.") Other suicide attempts are an effort by the patient to manipulate relationships so that the patient is surrounded by people who are ready and willing to provide advice and support (Box 40-13). In assessing the risk of suicide, the paramedic should consider these seven facts:

1. Suicide is the third leading cause of death in people 15 to 25 years of age. It is the fourth leading cause of death in people 25 to 45 years of age.
2. In the United States, white men over age 85 have the highest suicide rate.
3. Women attempt suicide more often than men do.
4. Men commit suicide more often than women do.
5. Men use more violent means (guns, knives) than women (pills, razor blades).
6. About 60% of those who successfully commit suicide have a history of a previous attempt.
7. The more specific and detailed the suicide plan, the greater the suicide potential.

Other factors associated with suicide threats include the recent death of a loved one or loss of a significant relationship, a financial setback or job loss, chronic or debilitating illness, social isolation, alcohol or other drug abuse, depression, and schizophrenia. If a suicide attempt is suspected, the paramedic should discuss these intentions with the patient. Questions such as, "Do you have thoughts

BOX 40-12 Facts about Bipolar Disorder

- More than 23 million Americans age 18 or older suffer from bipolar disorder. (This is about 1% of the U.S. population.)
- As many as 20% of people with bipolar disorder die by suicide.
- Men and women are equally likely to develop bipolar disorder.

BOX 40-13 Myths about Suicide

Myth: People who talk about killing themselves rarely commit suicide.

Fact: Most people who commit suicide have given some clue or warning of their intent. *Suicidal threats and attempts should always be treated seriously.*

Myth: The tendency to commit suicide is inherited. It is passed from generation to generation.

Fact: Suicide does tend to run in families. However, the tendency does not appear to be transmitted genetically.

Myth: All suicidal people are deeply depressed.

Fact: Depression is often associated with suicidal feelings. However, not all people who kill themselves are obviously depressed. In fact, some suicidal people appear to be happier than they have been in quite a while because they have decided to "resolve" all their problems at the same time.

Myth: There is a very low correlation between alcoholism and suicide.

Fact: Alcoholism and suicide often go hand in hand. Alcoholics are prone to suicide. Even people who do not normally drink often ingest alcohol shortly before killing themselves.

Myth: Suicidal people are mentally ill.

Fact: Many suicidal people are depressed and distraught. However, most of them would not be diagnosed as mentally ill.

Myth: If a person attempts suicide, that individual will always entertain thoughts of suicide.

Fact: Most people who are suicidal are that way for only a brief period in their lives. An attempter who receives the proper assistance and support probably will never be suicidal again. Only about 10% of attempters later complete the act.

Myth: Asking a person about his or her suicidal intentions encourages the individual to act.

Fact: Actually, the opposite is true. Asking a person directly about suicidal intent often lowers the individual's anxiety level. In fact, it often acts as a deterrent to suicidal emotions.

Myth: Suicide is more common among the lower classes.

Fact: Suicide occurs in all socioeconomic groups. No one class is more susceptible to it than another.

Myth: Suicidal people rarely seek medical attention.

Fact: Research has consistently shown that about 75% of suicidal people visit a physician within 3 months of killing themselves.

Myth: Suicide is basically a problem limited to young people.

Fact: The suicide rate rises with age and reaches a peak among older white men.

Myth: Professional people do not kill themselves.

Fact: Physicians, lawyers, dentists, and pharmacists may have high suicide rates.

Myth: When a person's depression lifts, the danger of suicide disappears.

Fact: The greatest danger of suicide exists during the first 3 months after a person recovers from a deep depression.

Myth: Suicide is a spontaneous activity that occurs without warning.

Fact: Most people plan their self-destruction. Then they give clues that they have become suicidal.

Myth: Because it includes the Christmas season, December has a high suicide rate.

Fact: No rash of suicides occurs at Christmas. In fact, December has the lowest rate of any month.

From Suicide Prevention Allied Regional Effort (SPARE): *The mythology of suicide,* Denver, 1987.

about killing yourself or others?" or "Have you ever tried to kill yourself?" are appropriate; many depressed patients are willing to discuss their suicidal (or homicidal) thoughts. During the patient interview, the paramedic should try to determine three important factors: (1) whether the patient has a plan (how and when the suicide will be done); (2) whether the plan is intended to be successful; and (3) whether the patient has the means or method to follow through with the plan.

> **CRITICAL THINKING**
>
> How would you feel about asking a patient, "Have you ever thought about killing yourself?"

When responding to a suicide attempt, paramedics should request police protection before approaching the scene. (Armed patients must be considered homicidal as well as suicidal.) After scene safety has been ensured and paramedics have gained access to the patient, the scene should be checked for the presence of dangerous objects (see Chapter 52).

The first priority in patient management is medical care. Unconscious patients should be managed with airway, ventilatory, and circulatory support and rapid transport. If the patient is conscious, creating rapport as soon as possible is essential. The paramedic should conduct a brief interview to assess the situation and determine the need for and direction of further action. To help reduce the potential for suicide, paramedics can take the following six steps:

1. Provide support and honest assurance about the patient's well-being.
2. Provide for physical safety as well as emotional security. Establish protective limits and measures. This helps to prevent injury to the patient or others. It also conveys to these patients that the paramedic will help them control their behavior until they can gain self-control.
3. Listen to the person, even if the speech seems bizarre, inappropriate, or unrealistic. Do not feel that every statement must be answered or that advice or opinions must be given. During the interview, acknowledge the patient's feelings; do not argue with the patient's wish to die. Explain alternatives to suicide that the patient may not have considered.
4. Determine the patient's support system or significant others when possible. Others may be better able to communicate with and calm the patient.
5. Encourage and reassure the patient during the crisis.
6. Transport the patient to the proper facility for emergency intervention.

Substance-Related Disorders

Some patients with a behavioral emergency may also be using alcohol or illegal drugs. This may cause difficulties during the physical examination. (Substance-related disorders are described in Chapter 36.) Often these patients are trying to "self-medicate." They are trying to improve their mood or lessen the anxiety associated with mental illness. Other patients self-medicate before receiving a diagnosis for their illness or before seeking professional help. Signs that may indicate alcohol or illicit drug use include a breath odor of alcohol, the presence of drug paraphernalia, and needle tracks on the extremities.

PATIENTS WITH A DUAL DIAGNOSIS

Some people struggle both with serious mental illness and substance abuse. This *dual diagnosis* may be difficult to identify, because one disorder may mimic the symptoms of the other (Box 40-14).[5] It therefore is easy to attribute the patient's symptoms to only one of the two afflictions. It is estimated that as many as 50% of mentally ill individuals have a substance abuse problem.[7]

The drug most often used is alcohol. The next most commonly used drugs are marijuana and cocaine. Prescription drugs such as tranquilizers and sleeping medicines may also be abused. Factors associated with a dual diagnosis include the following:

- Recreational use of alcohol or other drugs
- Misguided attempts to self-medicate to relieve anxiety or depression
- Susceptibility to mental illness *and* substance abuse
- Environmental and social influences

Patients who have a dual diagnosis may go back and forth between requesting EMS assistance for mental illness and for substance abuse. Most psychiatric and drug counseling organizations agree that the two disorders must be treated at the same time.

Somatoform Disorders

Somatoform disorders are conditions in which no physical cause can be found for the patient's symptoms. Strong evidence indicates that the underlying cause is psychological. Two of the most common disorders in this group are somatization disorder and conversion disorder. Both are associated with anxiety, depression, and threats of suicide. Treatment for both disorders often requires psychotherapy, which can address the emotional conflicts that manifest in these illnesses.

> **BOX 40-14 Facts About Dual Diagnosis**
>
> - About 7.2 million people between the ages of 18 and 54 suffer from both a substance abuse problem and a mental illness.
> - About 37% of alcohol abusers and 53% of drug abusers also have at least one serious mental illness.
> - Of all people diagnosed as mentally ill, 29% abuse either alcohol or other drugs.
> - A patient with schizophrenia has a 10% higher than average risk of being an alcoholic or a drug abuser.

SOMATIZATION DISORDER

Somatization disorder is a condition in which an individual has complaints (lasting several years) of various physical problems for which no physical cause can be found (Box 40-15).[8] The condition is more common in women than men. It sometimes results in unnecessary surgery and other treatments. These patients most often complain of neurological symptoms (double vision, seizure, weakness), gynecological symptoms (painful menstruation, painful intercourse), and gastrointestinal symptoms (abdominal pain, nausea).

CONVERSION DISORDER

Conversion disorder is a mental illness in which painful emotions are repressed and unconsciously converted into physical symptoms (Box 40-16).[9] A loss of sensory or motor capabilities or of special senses may occur. For example, the person suddenly may not be able to speak, hear, see, or feel, or an arm or a leg may be paralyzed. In many cases the areas of the body affected do not correspond to the actual arrangement of neural pathways. The symptoms also may come and go or may appear at different times and in different areas of the body.

MANAGEMENT

Paramedics should manage symptoms of somatoform disorders as if they are real, because differentiating these disorders from an organic ailment may be difficult. The paramedic should recognize that these patients are not "faking"; they believe their illness or loss of function to be factual. These patients require evaluation by a physician.

Factitious Disorders

Factitious disorders are a group of disorders in which symptoms mimic a true illness. However, the symptoms have actually been invented. The symptoms are under the control of the patient, who is attempting to gain attention. The most common disorder in this group is Munchausen syndrome. With this disorder, the patient makes routine pleas for treatment and hospitalization for a symptomatic, but imaginary, acute illness. Other complaints that may be associated with factitious disorders include bereavement, Cushing syndrome, dental problems, infection with the human immunodeficiency virus (HIV), hypoglycemia, stroke, and Munchausen syndrome by proxy, in which a person injures or induces illness in others (usually children) in order to gain sympathy.

The symptoms of a factitious disorder are often dramatic but plausible. They usually resolve with treatment. After the treatment, the person seeks treatment for another invented disease. Once the factitious disorder is diagnosed, treatment is aimed at protecting these people from surgeries and treatments they do not need.

Dissociative Disorders

Dissociative disorders are a group of psychological illnesses. In these illnesses, a particular mental function is separated (dissociated) from the mind as a whole. These disorders include the following:

- *Dissociative amnesia:* A disorder characterized by the blocking out of critical personal information, usually of a traumatic or stressful nature. Dissociative amnesia, unlike other types of amnesia, does not result from other medical trauma.
- *Dissociative fugue:* A rare disorder in which an individual suddenly and unexpectedly takes physical leave of the surroundings.
- *Dissociative identity disorder:* A disorder that has been called "multiple personality disorder."
- *Depersonalization disorder:* A condition marked by a feeling of detachment or distance from one's own experience, body, or self.

Dissociative disorders usually are associated with emotional conflicts. These conflicts are so repressed that a split in the personality occurs. This results in an altered state of consciousness or a confusion in identity. The condition also may be caused by an inability to cope with severe stress or conflict; dissociation occurs soon after a catastrophic event (e.g., the

BOX 40-15 Facts about Somatization Disorders

- The lifetime prevalence rate for somatization disorder is 0.2% to 2% of the U.S. population.
- Somatization disorders are rare in men.
- Somatization disorders tend to run in families. They occur in 10% to 20% of the primary female relatives of somatization disorder patients.
- Most somatization disorders begin in adolescence or early adulthood. Most are chronic in nature.
- The symptoms sometimes increase and decrease in severity over time. Usually, though, the individual has a few symptom-free episodes.
- Anxiety and depression often accompany the disorder.
- Suicide threats are common in these patients, but suicide is rarely carried out.

BOX 40-16 Facts About Conversion Disorder

- True conversion disorder is rare in the United States.
- The disorder is seen more often in lower socioeconomic groups. It may be more common in military personnel exposed to combat.
- Conversion disorder may appear at any age. However, it is rare before age 10 or after age 35.
- In pediatric patients, the incidence of conversion is higher after physical or sexual abuse. The incidence also rises among children whose parents are very ill or have chronic pain.
- About 64% of adult patients with conversion disorder have evidence of organic brain disorder.

BOX 40-17 Facts about Eating Disorders

- More than 5 million Americans suffer from eating disorders.
- Anorexia, bulimia, and binge eating disorders are diseases that affect the mind and body at the same time.
- Three percent of adolescent and adult women have an eating disorder. One percent of men have an eating disorder.
- A young woman with anorexia is 12 times more likely to die than another woman her age without anorexia.
- Fifteen percent of young women have substantially poor eating attitudes and behaviors.

traumatic death of a child or spouse). People with dissociative disorders often are unable to remember their names or personal histories. However, they can still speak, read, and learn new material. Treatment may include antianxiety medications, hypnosis, and psychotherapy.

Eating Disorders

The two most common eating disorders considered to be forms of psychiatric illness are anorexia nervosa and bulimia nervosa (Box 40-17).[10] Both of these eating disorders can lead to serious dehydration, starvation, and electrolyte imbalances. They also may cause critical illness or death. The disorders are best managed with supervision and regulation of eating habits, psychotherapy and, sometimes, antidepressants. Most patients require hospitalization.

ANOREXIA NERVOSA

Anorexia nervosa is an eating disorder characterized by an intense fear of being obese, severe weight loss, malnutrition and, eventually, amenorrhea. A patient feels intensely hungry, even though hunger pains are denied. Signs and symptoms include weight loss, obsession with exercise, fatigue, binge eating, induced vomiting, and use of laxatives to promote weight loss. The condition mainly is seen in adolescents, mostly girls. It usually is associated with emotional stress or conflict. It often is difficult to identify an exact underlying cause for this disease.

BULIMIA NERVOSA

Bulimia nervosa is sometimes considered a form of anorexia. It is an insatiable craving for food. This craving often results in episodes of binge eating followed by purging (through self-induced vomiting or use of laxatives), depression, and self-deprivation. Like anorexia, bulimia is most common in adolescent girls and young women. Anorexic and bulimic patients often worry about their compulsive behavior. As a result, they may become depressed and suicidal.

Impulse Control Disorders

Impulse control disorders are a group of psychiatric conditions. They are characterized by the inability to resist an impulse or a temptation to perform some act that is unlawful, socially unacceptable, or self-harmful. Disorders in this category include the following:

- *Intermittent explosive disorder:* A condition marked by frequent and often unpredictable episodes of extreme anger or physical outbursts. Between episodes there is usually no evidence of violence or physical threat.
- *Kleptomania*: The failure to resist impulses to steal things that are not needed for either personal use or for their monetary value.
- *Pathological gambling:* A persistent and maladaptive pattern of gambling that causes difficulties with interpersonal, financial, and vocational functioning.
- *Pyromania:* Deliberate and purposeful fire setting for nonmonetary gain. This condition typically is associated with tension or heightened arousal before the act and with gratification or relief afterward.
- *Trichotillomania:* The recurrent pulling out of one's own hair, which results in significant hair loss.

Impulse control disorders often are difficult to treat. Most are managed with behavior modification and drug therapy. Failure to control these disorders may result in violent behavior or unlawful activities (e.g., road rage). Therefore many patients may end up incarcerated.

PERSONALITY DISORDERS

Personality disorders are a large group of conditions distinguished by a failure to learn from experience or to adapt appropriately to changes. This failure results in personal distress and impairment of social functioning. These disorders may have an environmental component. They may also be genetic. Personality disorders become especially obvious during times of stress.

The symptoms of a personality disorder usually are first recognized in early adolescence. They continue throughout the person's life. The symptoms may vary in frequency and intensity. Generally, however, they are relatively constant. They usually affect most aspects of a patient's life. This includes thoughts, emotions, relationships and interpersonal skills, and impulse control. Personality disorders have been classified in a variety of ways. However, the following are three common disorders:

- *Antisocial personality disorder:* A long-standing pattern (after the age of 15) of disregard for the rights of others. It is often associated with irresponsible behavior and a lack of remorse for wrongdoing.
- *Borderline personality disorder:* A pattern of unstable relationships, poor or negative self-image, mood swings, and poor impulse control. It may be associated with destructive and self-harming behaviors (e.g., suicide attempts, self-mutilation), an intense fear of abandonment, and displays of sudden anger.
- *Narcissistic personality disorder:* A pattern of grandiosity, need for admiration, and sense of entitlement. It often is associated with exaggerated achievements and fantasies about unlimited success, power, love, or beauty.

Many factors are associated with the development of a personality disorder. These may include unstable relationships during childhood, family violence, and childhood abuse or neglect. Treatment involves behavior modification techniques, counseling, drug therapy, and individual psychotherapy.

SPECIAL CONSIDERATIONS FOR PATIENTS WITH BEHAVIORAL PROBLEMS

In addition to caring for the immediate needs of patients with behavioral problems, paramedics may have to deal with complications arising from the situation or other factors affecting the patient. Among these factors are the patient's age and the possibility of violent behavior. This section presents special considerations for pediatric patients, elderly patients, and the potentially violent patient.

CRITICAL THINKING

When responding to a behavioral emergency that involves a child or an adolescent, do you use the same safety guidelines that you use with an adult?

Behavioral Problems in Children

Young children who are victims of emotional crisis need to be managed with techniques that are different from those used to care for older children and adults. The following suggestions may be helpful to the paramedic in dealing with some children:

1. Gain the child's trust and try to convince the child that you are a friend who can help.
2. Make it clear that you are strong enough to be in control but will not hurt the child.
3. Keep the interview questions brief; the child's attention span may be extremely short.
4. Never lie; be honest.
5. Use all available resources to communicate (e.g., drawing pictures, telling stories).
6. Involve parents or caregivers in the interview or examination if appropriate.
7. Take any threat of violence seriously.

If the child's behavior or physical condition makes restraint necessary, the paramedic should use only reasonable force (with sufficient help) to ensure the patient's safety and the safety of the EMS crew. Calming measures may fail to work. If so, wrapping the child in a full body blanket secured to the stretcher with straps often is sufficient during transport for evaluation by a physician. As with any method of restraint, the paramedic should monitor the child's airway and circulation and make sure that they are not compromised. Documentation should be thorough and complete.

Behavioral Problems in Elderly Patients

An estimated 15% to 25% of elderly people in the United States suffer from significant symptoms of mental illness. More than 5 million elderly individuals are clinically depressed.[11] Most of these disorders can be diagnosed and treated successfully. However, many of these people do not seek care. Problem behavior in an elderly patient can be a sign of a long-standing psychiatric disorder; a newly emerging psychiatric problem; a medical illness; substance abuse; drug noncompliance or drug interactions; and other factors (see Chapter 45). The following suggestions may be helpful to the paramedic in communicating with some elderly patients:

1. Identify yourself and speak at eye level to make sure the patient can see you.
2. Address the patient by surname (e.g., "Mr. Jones" or "Miss [or Mrs.] Smith") unless directed otherwise.
3. Speak slowly, distinctly, and respectfully.
4. Ask one question at a time and allow time for complete answers.
5. Listen closely.
6. Explain what you are doing and why.
7. Provide reassuring physical touch.
8. Be patient.
9. Permit family members and caregivers to remain with the patient if appropriate.
10. Preserve the patient's dignity.

Assessing the Potentially Violent Patient

Only a small number of people with mental health problems are potentially violent. Nonetheless, assessment and management of the potentially violent patient should be part of an EMS protocol. The following four factors may help the paramedic determine the potential for a violent episode[12]:

1. Past history (Has the patient previously shown hostile, aggressive, or violent behavior?)
2. Posture (Is the patient sitting or standing? Does the patient appear to be tense or rigid?)
3. Vocal activity (Loud, obscene, and erratic speech indicates emotional distress.)
4. Physical activity (Is the patient pacing or agitated or protecting his or her physical boundaries?)

If any of these signs of potentially violent behavior are present, paramedics should try to reduce the effect of the stress. However, they should avoid confrontation. Paramedics should prepare a way to cope with the crisis. This plan should reduce the potential for a life-threatening inci-

NOTE Paramedics should retreat from the scene in certain situations; for example, if they anticipate violence that would threaten their personal safety or the safety of the crew. They should wait for law enforcement personnel to ensure that the scene is safe.

dent. It also should reduce the chance for psychologically damaging consequences.

CONTROLLING VIOLENT SITUATIONS

Severely disturbed patients who pose a threat to themselves or others may need to be restrained, transported, and hospitalized against their will. Each state has a law setting out the criteria for involuntary commitment. The paramedic should be familiar with all relevant laws. The premise on which most state laws are based suggests that one person may restrain another to protect life or prevent injury.

When a psychiatric patient refuses care, EMS personnel should consult with medical direction. The decision to restrain, treat, or release the patient is a medical direction decision. If violent behavior must be contained, "reasonable force" should be used to restrain the patient. It should be used as humanely as possible and with respect for the patient's dignity. In most cases the restraint duty (if needed) should be given to law enforcement personnel. As in all other aspects of health care, details of the incident should be carefully recorded for future reference. When dealing with a patient who may require restraint, the paramedic should do the following:

1. Provide a safe environment.
2. Gather a significant medical and psychiatric history.
3. Attempt to gain the patient's cooperation.
4. Be confident but not confrontational.

> **CRITICAL THINKING**
>
> Have you ever seen an EMS crew member or a police officer lose control of his or her own behavior when dealing with a violent patient? How did it affect the patient's physical or psychological state?

RESTRAINT GUIDELINES

The following guidelines can help paramedics to use restraint appropriately:

- If the patient is homicidal, do not attempt restraint without assistance from law enforcement personnel. If the patient is armed, move everyone out of range and retreat from the scene. Wait for law enforcement personnel.
- Remember that the patient may not be responsible for his or her actions.
- When planning the restraining action, include a backup plan in case the initial attempt fails.
- Make sure that adequate help is available. This means that at least four capable people should be available to help restrain an adult patient.
- Keep in mind that the potential for personal injury and legal liability is always present.

RESTRAINT METHODS

A number of restraint methods can be used to manage a violent patient. A gentle, nonthreatening, low-profile technique should be attempted first. The approach should move to more direct intervention as needed. The options of physical restraint should always be explained to the patient before force is applied. If still unwilling to cooperate, the patient should be informed that restraint is required to protect against injury and to ensure the safety of others.

Before approaching a violent patient, the paramedic should be aware of the patient's surroundings. Seemingly harmless items should be noted, such as ashtrays, lighted cigarettes, hot coffee, letter openers, soda bottles, cans, and furniture. No attempt should be made to enter the patient's physical space until the other members involved in the restraint action are ready to proceed. (The patient's physical space usually is considered to be one arm's length.)

The patient's muscle groups and potential range of motion should be considered before restraint is initiated. The paramedic should plan to position the patient in a way that limits strength and range of motion. Each member of the restraint team should be assigned a specific body part or responsibility before the actual restraint procedure is started.

Paramedics must be familiar with the restraint devices available. They also should be able to improvise if the need arises. The preferred method is to use commercially manufactured wrist/waist/ankle padded leather or Velcro straps, or full jacket restraints (Fig. 40-3). Effective restraints also may be improvised using common materials such as the following:

- Small towels that can be wrapped around the patient's wrists and ankles and secured with tape to the stretcher
- Cravats
- Webbed straps ordinarily used to secure patients to spine boards
- Roller bandage
- Blanket roll

Regardless of the types used, restraints should be strong enough to achieve the desired effect. However, they should not compromise circulatory or respiratory status.

SEQUENCE OF RESTRAINT ACTIONS

Trained personnel can use many restraint techniques. The following sequence is an example of a restraint action that may be used to contain violent behavior.

1. The paramedic offers the patient one final chance to cooperate.
2. If the patient does not respond, at least two rescuers move swiftly toward the person. They position themselves close to and slightly behind the patient. Each rescuer should then position an inside leg in front of the patient's leg to force the patient to the ground if necessary (Fig. 40-4). Swift movement by two or more rescuers minimizes the patient's ability to focus on restraint actions. It also reduces the accuracy of kicks or blows. During the restraint procedure, the patient should be continually reassured by a rescuer not involved in the physical maneuver.
3. If the patient calms and agrees to be transported without restraints, the paramedic positions the patient lat-

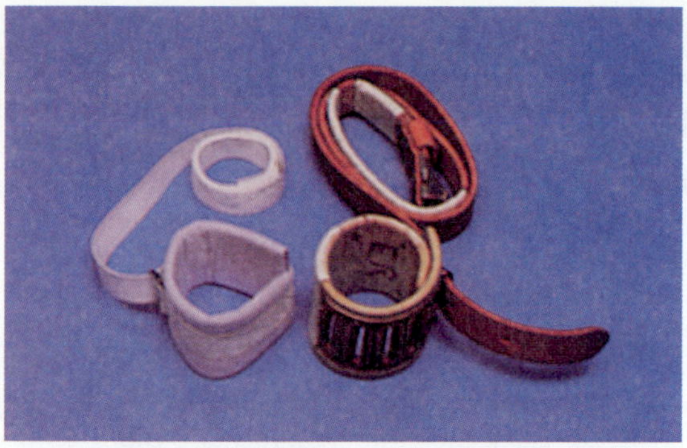

FIGURE 40-3 ■ Restraint devices.

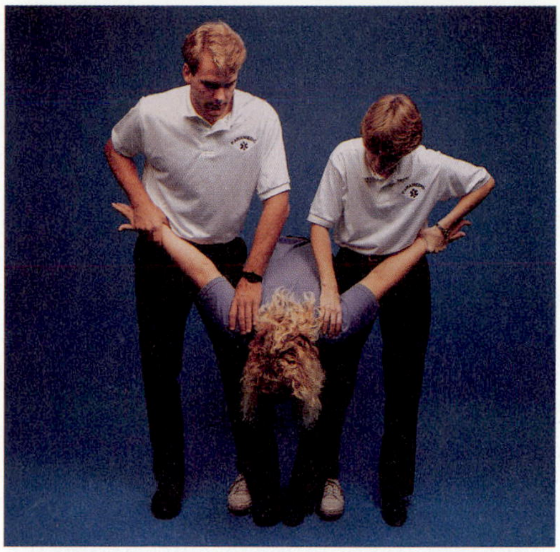

FIGURE 40-4 ■ Control position. Rescuers face the same direction. The rescuers' inside legs are placed in front of the patient. The rescuers' outside hands hold the patient's wrists. The rescuers' inside hands form a C on the patient's shoulders.

eral or supine on a stretcher (if not contraindicated by the mechanism of injury or medical condition). The paramedic secures the patient with straps to limit range of motion (Fig. 40-5). If the patient becomes dangerous en route to the hospital, restraints should be used.

4. Once applied, restraints should not be removed until the patient is delivered to the emergency department. Alternatively, they can be removed if adequate resources are available to control the situation. The patient's respiratory and circulatory status should be assessed frequently and documented. This ensures that the restraint action has not compromised vital functions. If a change in the restraints is required, adequate assistance must be available. Also, only one limb should be repositioned at a time.

Restraint procedures should be fully documented on the patient care report. Any attempts at negotiation and a description of the patient's behavior before the person was restrained should be clearly described. Paramedics should document that circulatory evaluation and continued monitoring of the patient were performed after restraint.

Again, physical restraint is advised only when all verbal and nonverbal techniques have been exhausted and only when a person presents a danger to self or others.

PERSONAL SAFETY

Paramedics' personal safety should be considered in any emergency response. However, behavioral emergencies are more likely to require that paramedics protect themselves and the crew from hostile injury. The following measures for preventing personal injury should be considered:

- When possible, remain a safe distance from the patient.
- Do not allow the patient to block the exit.
- Keep large furniture between you and the patient. Do not allow a single paramedic to remain alone with the patient.
- Do not make statements that the patient might perceive as threatening.
- Use folded blankets or cushions to absorb the impact of thrown objects.

Various training programs have been developed to provide safety and security to the rescuer and the violent patient. Paramedics should learn nonviolent personal protection maneuvers. They also should practice these maneuvers under the supervision of someone trained in them.

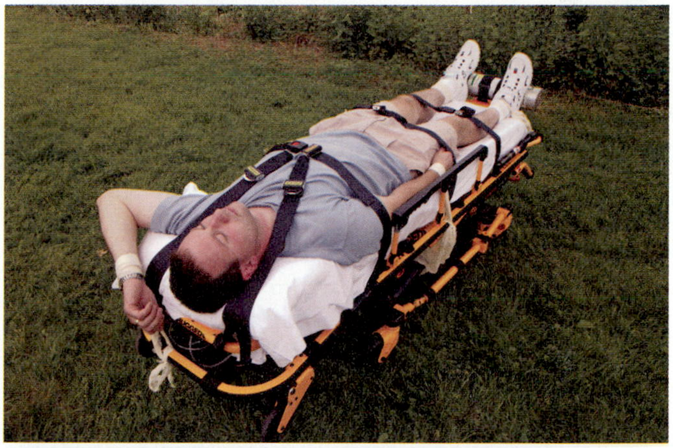

FIGURE 40-5 ■ Patient restrained in supine position.

CHEMICAL RESTRAINT

The term *chemical restraint* refers to the use of drugs to control behavior. Drug treatment varies. However, it generally is intended to provide sedation. Two groups of drugs that are effective for chemical restraint are benzodiazepines and antipsychotics (see Chapter 17).

Benzodiazepines bind to specific receptors in the cerebral cortex and limbic system (a major integrating system that governs emotional behavior). These drugs are popular because of their very high therapeutic index. They have four main actions: anxiety reducing, sedative-hypnotic, muscle relaxing, and anticonvulsant. Benzodiazepines commonly used for chemical restraint include ***diazepam, midazolam,*** and ***lorazepam.***

Antipsychotics block dopamine receptors in specific areas of the central nervous system. These drugs are primarily used to treat schizophrenia. They also are used to treat other conditions that produce disturbed behavior (e.g., Tourette syndrome and senile dementia associated with Alzheimer disease). Two well-known antipsychotics used for chemical restraint are ***droperidol*** and ***haloperidol***. Short-term use of antipsychotics rarely produces extrapyramidal reactions (e.g., pseudoparkinsonism, akathisia, dystonias, tardive dyskinesia). However, if such reactions occur, administration of ***diphenhydramine*** may reverse these side effects.

Benzodiazepines and antipsychotics can be very effective at controlling hostile or combative patients. As with all other restraint methods, paramedics should consult with medical direction, follow protocol, and carefully document the event.

NOTE As described in Chapter 17, extrapyramidal reactions are neuromuscular effects that can be caused by some antipsychotic medications. These effects include parkinson-like symptoms (e.g., tremor, muscle rigidity, pill-rolling motion, shuffling gait), akathisia (abnormal restlessness, agitation), dystonias (abnormal muscle tone or posturing), and tardive dyskinesia (involuntary, repetitious movement). The occurrence and severity of extrapyramidal reactions frequently are dose related. They often subside when the dose is reduced or the drug is halted. However in some patients, tardive dyskinesia persists even after drug therapy is stopped. (This is especially the case for patients on long-term drug therapy.) These rhythmical, involuntary movements are most evident in the tongue, face, mouth, or jaw. They are characterized by protrusion of the tongue, puffing of the cheeks, puckering of the mouth, chewing movements, and sometimes involuntary movements of the extremities.

SUMMARY

- A behavioral emergency is a change in mood or behavior. This change cannot be tolerated by the involved person or others. It calls for immediate attention.
- Physical or biochemical disturbances can result in significant changes in behavior. Psychosocial mental illness is often the result of childhood trauma, parental deprivation, or a dysfunctional family structure.
- Changes in behavior caused by interpersonal or situational stress are often linked to specific incidents, such as environmental violence, the death of a loved one, economic or employment problems, or prejudice and discrimination.
- When dealing with behavioral emergencies, paramedics should contain the crisis. They also should provide the proper emergency care and transport the patient to an appropriate health care facility.
- During the patient assessment, an attempt should be made to determine the patient's mental state, name and age, significant past medical history, medications (and compliance), and past psychiatric problems, as well as the precipitating situation or problem.
- Effective interviewing techniques include active listening, being supportive and empathetic, limiting interruptions, and respecting the patient's personal space.
- All cognitive disorders result in a disturbance in thinking that may manifest as delirium or dementia.
- Schizophrenia is characterized by recurrent episodes of psychotic behavior. This behavior may include abnormalities of thought process, thought content, perception, and judgment.
- Anxiety disorders may cause a panic attack. Anxiety disorders include phobias, obsessive-compulsive disorders, and posttraumatic syndrome.
- Depression is an impairment of normal functioning. A person with depression may have feelings of hopelessness, worthlessness, and guilt, as well as loss of appetite and diminished libido.
- Bipolar disorder is a manic-depressive illness. In this illness, depressive and manic episodes alternate.
- Somatoform disorders are marked by the presence of physical symptoms for which no physical cause can be found. The cause is thought to be psychological. These disorders include somatization disorder and conversion disorder.
- Factitious disorders are disorders in which symptoms mimic a true illness. However, the symptoms have been invented. They are under the patient's control.
- Dissociative disorders are a group of psychological illnesses. In these disorders, a particular mental function is separated from the mind as a whole.
- The most common eating disorders considered to be forms of psychiatric illness are anorexia nervosa and bulimia nervosa.
- Impulse control disorders are characterized by the inability to resist an impulse or a temptation to do some act that is unlawful, socially unacceptable, or self-harmful.
- Personality disorders are conditions characterized by failure to learn from experience or to adapt appropriately to changes. This results in personal distress and impairment of social functioning.
- A threat of suicide is an indication that a patient has a serious crisis. This crisis requires immediate intervention.
- Questions that determine the patient's plan, intent, and means to commit suicide should be asked.

- With a suicide attempt, the first step is to ensure the safety of the scene. The first priority in patient management is medical care. If the patient is conscious, it is crucial that paramedics develop a rapport with the individual as soon as possible.
- Assessment of a potentially violent patient should include past history of violence, posture, vocal activity, and physical activity.
- When trying to defuse a situation involving a potentially violent patient, the paramedic should ensure a safe environment, gather the patient's history, try to gain the patient's cooperation, avoid threats, and explain the paramedic's role in providing care.
- Severely disturbed patients who pose a threat to themselves or others may need to be restrained.
- Reasonable force to restrain a patient should be used as humanely as possible. An adequate number of personnel is needed to ensure patient and rescuer safety during restraint. The risk of personal injury and legal liability is always present.
- Personal safety measures taken during a response to a behavioral emergency should include not allowing the patient to block the exit, keeping large furniture between the paramedic and the patient, working as a team, avoiding threatening statements, and using soft materials to absorb the impact of thrown objects.
- When caring for children with behavioral emergencies, the paramedic should attempt to gain their trust, tell them they won't be hurt, keep questions brief, be honest, involve the parents if appropriate, and take threats of violence seriously.

REFERENCES

1. US Department of Transportation, National Highway Traffic Safety Administration: *EMT-paramedic national standard curriculum,* Washington, DC, 1998, The Department.
2. Seidel HM et al: *Mosby's guide to physical examination,* ed 5, St Louis, 2002, Mosby.
3. American Psychiatric Association: *Diagnostic and statistical manual of mental disorders-IV,* text revision, Washington, DC, 2000, The Association.
4. American Psychiatric Association: www.psych.org/public_info/schizo.cfm. Accessed September 28, 2004.
5. National Institute of Mental Health: *The numbers count: mental illness in America,* NIH Publication No. NIH 99-4584, Bethesda, MD, National Institute of Mental Health, 2001.
6. Salerno M: Psychosocial disorders. In Millonig VL, editor: *Adult nurse practitioner certification review guide,* ed 2, Potomac, MD, 1994, Health Leadership Associates.
7. National Alliance for the Mentally Ill: Helpline fact sheet: *Dual diagnosis: mental illness and substance abuse,* Arlington, VA. web.nami.org/helpline/dualdiagnosis.htm.
8. Vanderbilt Medical Center: *Conversion and somatization disorders.* www.mc.vanderbilt.edu. Accessed October 3, 2004.
9. Dufel S: *Conversion disorder.* www.emedicine.com/emerg/topic112.htm.
10. Harvard Eating Disorders Center: *Facts about eating disorders.* www.hedc.org/info.html. Accessed November 5, 2004.
11. American Psychiatric Association: *Mental health of the elderly.* www.psych.org/public_info/elderly.cfm.
12. Judd R, Peszke M: Psychological and behavioral emergencies, *Top Emerg Med* 4(4):7, 1983.

CHAPTER

41

Gynecology

OBJECTIVES

Upon completion of this chapter, the paramedic student will be able to:

1. Describe the physiological processes of menstruation and ovulation.
2. Describe the pathophysiology of the following nontraumatic causes of abdominal pain in females: pelvic inflammatory disease, ruptured ovarian cyst, cystitis, dysmenorrhea, mittelschmerz, endometriosis, ectopic pregnancy, vaginal bleeding.
3. Describe the pathophysiology of traumatic causes of abdominal pain in females, including vaginal bleeding and sexual assault.
4. Outline the prehospital assessment and management of the female with abdominal pain.
5. Outline specific assessment and management for the patient who has been sexually assaulted.
6. Describe specific prehospital measures to preserve evidence in sexual assault cases.

KEY TERMS

cesarean delivery: A surgical procedure in which the abdomen and uterus are incised and the baby is delivered transabdominally.

dilation and curettage: A gynecological procedure that refers to widening of the uterine cervix and scrapping away of the endometrium of the uterus.

endometrium: The mucous membrane lining of the uterus, which changes in thickness and structure with the menstrual cycle.

hysterectomy: The surgical removal of the uterus.

menarche: The first menstruation and commencement of the cyclic menstrual function.

menopause: The cessation of menses.

menstruation: The periodic discharge through the vagina of a blood secretion containing tissue debris from the shedding of the endometrium from the nonpregnant uterus.

ovulation: The release of an ovum or secondary oocyte from the vesicular follicle.

sexual assault: The forcible perpetration of an act of sexual contact on the body of another person, male or female, without his or her consent.

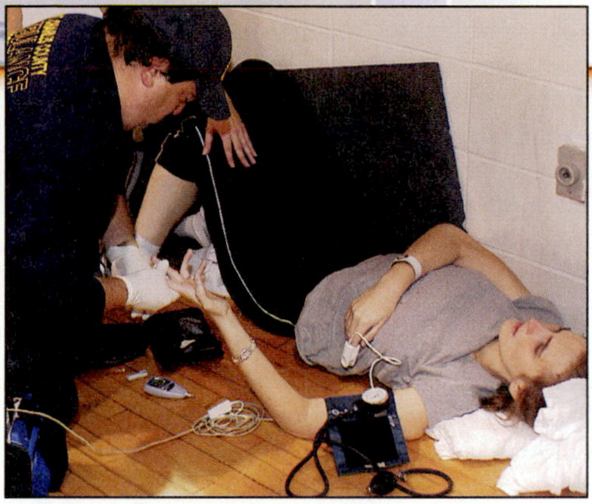

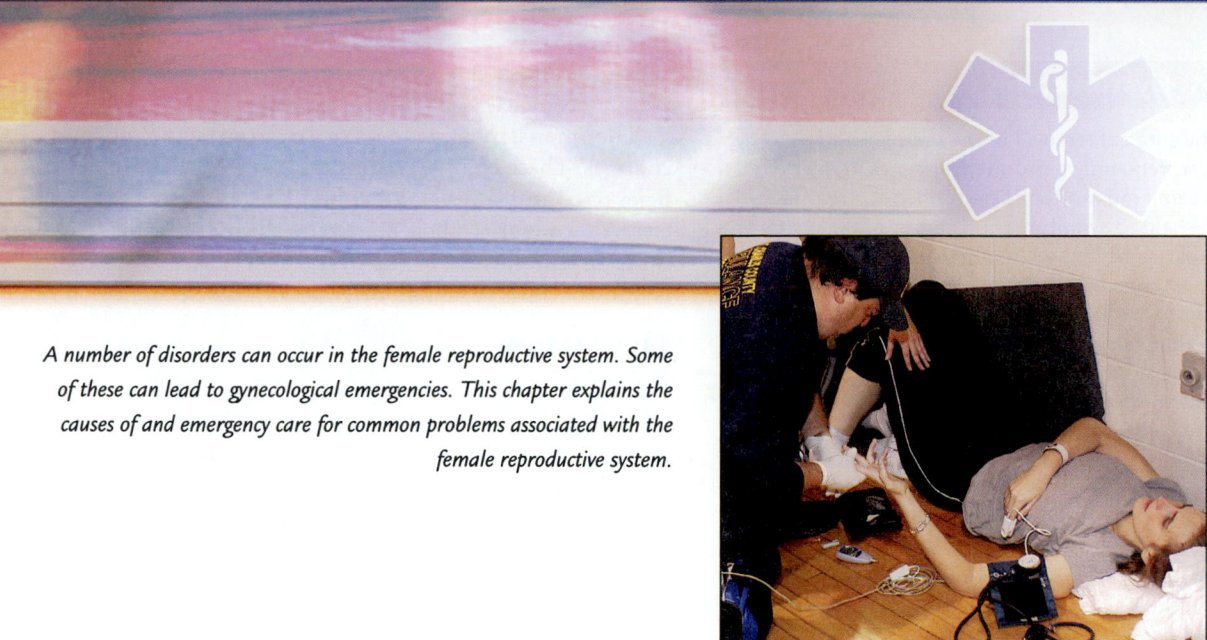

A number of disorders can occur in the female reproductive system. Some of these can lead to gynecological emergencies. This chapter explains the causes of and emergency care for common problems associated with the female reproductive system.

ORGANS OF THE FEMALE REPRODUCTIVE SYSTEM

The female reproductive organs were illustrated and described in Chapter 6. They include the ovaries, fallopian tubes, uterus, vagina, external genital organs, and mammary glands. (Fig. 41-1 provides a review of these structures.)

MENSTRUATION AND OVULATION

Menstruation

Menstruation is the normal, periodic discharge of blood, mucus, and cellular debris from the uterine mucosa. The normal menstrual cycle lasts about 28 days. It occurs at more or less regular intervals from puberty to **menopause** (except during pregnancy and lactation). The average menstrual flow is 25 to 60 mL. The flow usually lasts 4 to 6 days and is fairly constant from cycle to cycle. The onset of menses **(menarche)** generally begins between ages 12 and 13. Menstruation ends permanently (menopause) at an average age of 47 years. However, depending on the person, normal menopause age may vary from ages 35 to 60 years (Box 41-1).

Follicle and Oocyte Development

By the fourth prenatal month, the ovaries contain about 5 million cells. From these cells, oocytes (immature ova) develop. At birth, there are about 2 million primary oocytes. These decline in number to 300,000 to 400,000 at puberty. Of these primary oocytes, only about 400 eventually are released from the ovary. Oocytes are surrounded by a layer of

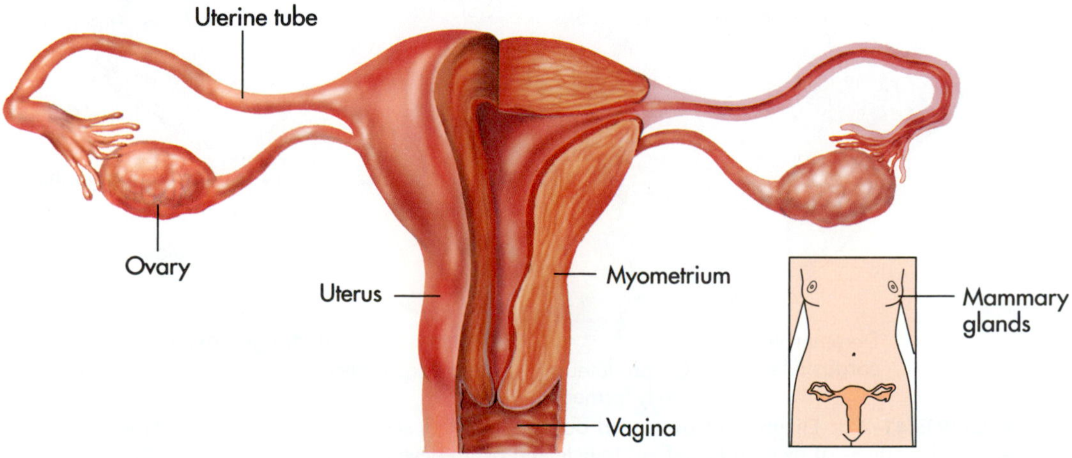

FIGURE 41-1 ■ Female organs.

BOX 41-1 Hysterectomy

Hysterectomy is the surgical removal of the uterus. Hysterectomy is one of the most frequently performed surgeries in the United States. Hysterectomy most often is performed to treat fibroid tumors that have caused symptoms and cancer of the uterus or cervix. Other indications for the surgery include heavy menstrual bleeding, endometriosis, pelvic inflammatory disease, and the removal of a prolapsed uterus. Depending on the type of hysterectomy, the surgery may be performed through the abdomen or vagina or laparoscopically.

In a *subtotal hysterectomy,* only the upper part of the uterus is removed; the cervix is not. (The fallopian tubes and ovaries may or may not be removed.) In a *total hysterectomy* (also called a complete hysterectomy), the body of the uterus, the cervix, the fallopian tubes, and the ovaries are removed. If cancer is present or in an advanced stage, a *radical hysterectomy* may be required in which the pelvic lymph nodes and lymph channels also are removed. After a hysterectomy, women are unable to bear children, do not menstruate, and need no contraception.

Serious complications can occur from the surgery. These include blood clots, infection, adhesions, postoperative hemorrhage, bowel obstruction, or injury to the urinary tract. In addition to the direct surgical risks, there may be long-term physical and psychological effects. Examples of such include depression and loss of sexual pleasure. If the ovaries are removed along with the uterus before menopause, the risk of developing osteoporosis and heart disease may be increased.

cells (granulosa cells). The entire structure is known as a primary follicle (Fig. 41-2).

The menstrual cycle is associated with hormonal changes. These changes stimulate some of the primary follicles to continue development and become secondary follicles. A secondary follicle continues to enlarge. This forms a lump on the surface of the ovary. The fully mature follicle is known as the vesicular, or graafian, follicle.

Ovulation

Cellular secretions of the graafian follicle cause it to swell more rapidly than can be accommodated by follicular growth. The follicle expands and ruptures. This forces a small amount of blood and follicular fluid out of the vesicle. Shortly after this initial burst of fluid, an oocyte escapes from the follicle. The release of this secondary oocyte is termed **ovulation.**

After ovulation the follicle is transformed into a yellow glandular structure. This structure is called the corpus luteum. The cells of this structure secrete large amounts of progesterone and some estrogen. If pregnancy occurs, the fertilized oocyte (zygote) begins releasing a hormonelike substance (chorionic gonadotropin). This substance keeps the corpus luteum from degenerating. As a result, blood levels of estrogen and progesterone do not decrease. Moreover, the menstrual period does not occur. In the absence of preg-

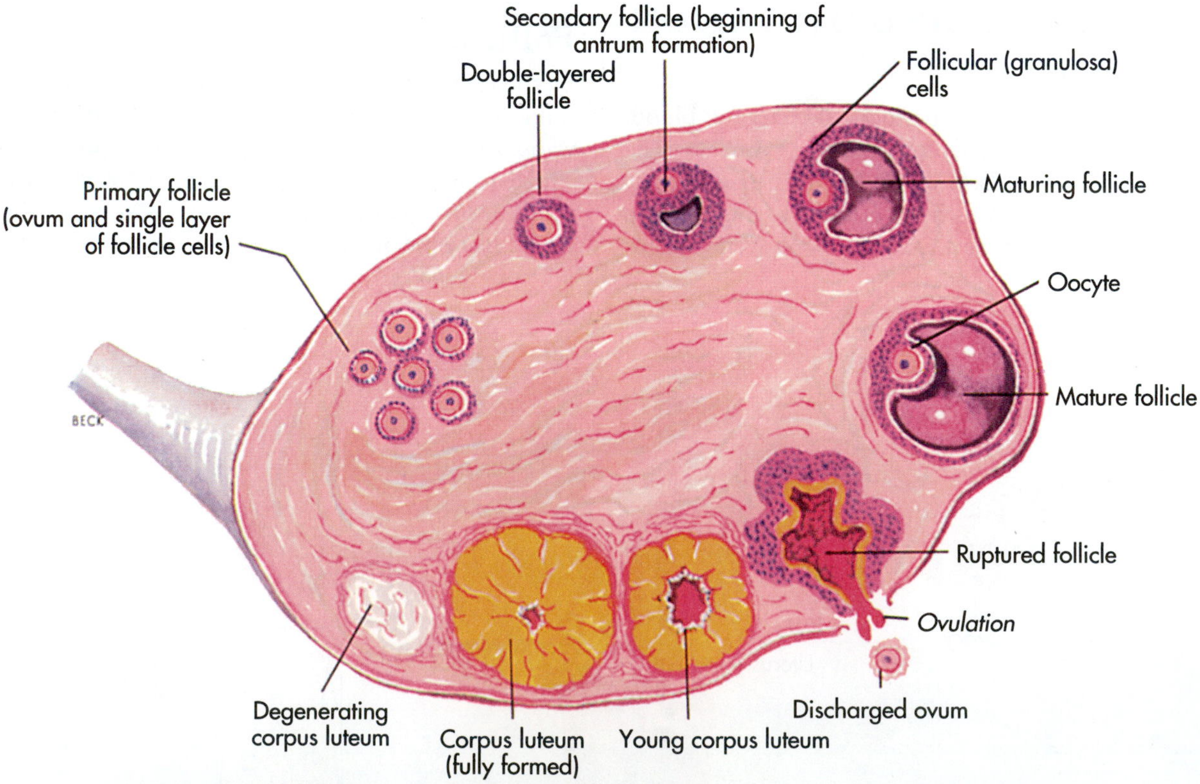

FIGURE 41-2 ■ Diagram of ovary and oogenesis. Cross section of mammalian ovary shows successive stages of ovarian (graafian) follicle and ovum development. Begin with the first stage (primary follicle) and follow around clockwise to the final stage (degenerating corpus luteum).

nancy the corpus luteum degenerates. The secondary oocyte passes out of the system with the menstrual flow.

Hormonal Control of Ovulation and Menses

Hormones released from the hypothalamus and anterior pituitary control ovulation and menses. Follicle-stimulating hormone stimulates development of the follicle. Follicle-stimulating hormone also stimulates the cells that produce estrogen. Before ovulation, these cells release estrogen. They cause a surge in the pituitary production of luteinizing hormone. This initiates the ovarian cycle (and leads to ovulation). This in turn regulates the uterine cycle (Fig. 41-3). Under the influence of the ovarian hormones, the lining of the uterus **(endometrium)** goes through two phases of development. These are the proliferative and secretory phases.

CRITICAL THINKING

What could happen to the menstrual cycle if the hormonal balance was off?

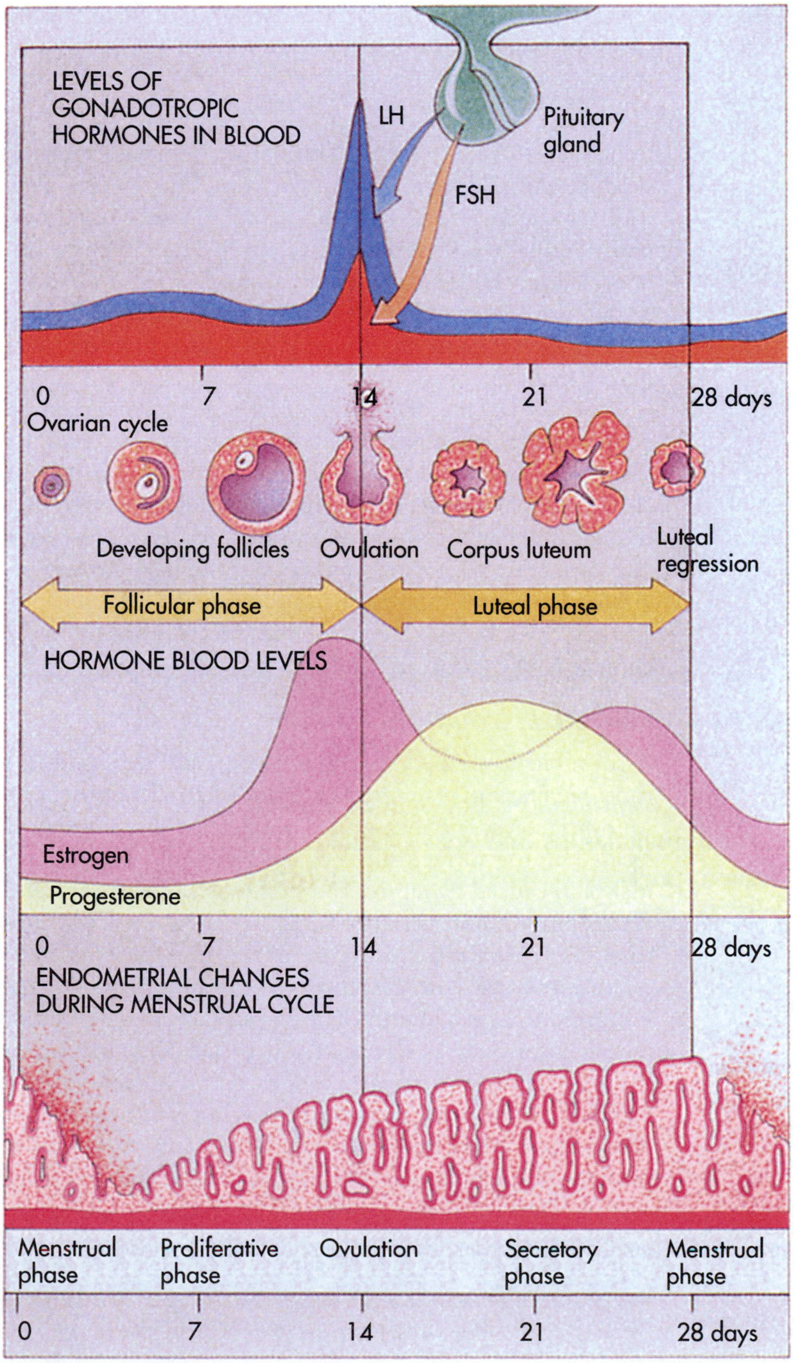

FIGURE 41-3 ■ Human menstrual cycle. The interrelationship of pituitary, ovarian, and uterine functions throughout the usual 28-day cycle. A sharp increase in luteinizing hormone levels causes ovulation, whereas menstruation (sloughing of the endometrial lining) is initiated by lower levels of progesterone.

The proliferative phase starts and is sustained by increasing amounts of estrogen. This estrogen is produced by the maturing follicle. Estrogen stimulates the endometrium to grow and increase in thickness. This prepares the uterus for implantation of a fertilized ovum. The secretory phase begins after ovulation. This phase is under the combined influence of estrogen and progesterone. During this phase, the endometrium is prepared for implantation of the fertilized ovum. Within 7 days after ovulation (about day 21 of the menstrual cycle), the endometrium is ready to receive the developing embryo if fertilization has occurred.

In the absence of fertilization, the ovum can survive only 6 to 24 hours. After this time the hormone levels drop and the endometrium is shed as menstrual flow. This process usually takes place on day 28 of the cycle. (This is about 14 days after ovulation.) The oocyte is capable of being fertilized for up to 24 hours after ovulation (see Chapter 42).

BOX 41-2 Classification of Gynecological Emergencies

Nontraumatic Abdominal Emergencies
Cystitis
Ectopic pregnancy
Endometriosis
Endometritis
Mittelschmerz
Pelvic inflammatory disease
Ruptured ovarian cyst
Vaginal bleeding

Traumatic Abdominal Emergencies
Vaginal bleeding

Sexual Assault

SPECIFIC GYNECOLOGICAL EMERGENCIES

Gynecological emergencies are classified into three groups: nontraumatic, traumatic, and **sexual assault** (Box 41-2). Regardless of the type of emergency, pregnancy should always be considered in any woman who is of the age to bear a child. Pregnancy should be a possibility until determined otherwise by a physician.

Nontraumatic Emergencies

In addition to gastrointestinal causes of abdominal pain (described in Chapter 34), acute or chronic infection involving a patient's uterus, ovaries, fallopian tubes, and adjacent structures may be a source of severe abdominal pain. The scope of abdominal pain associated with the female reproductive system may range widely. Pain may be simply minor episodes of difficult menstruation. But pain also can be from a hemorrhage from a ruptured ovarian cyst or ectopic pregnancy. These can pose a threat to life.

PELVIC INFLAMMATORY DISEASE

Pelvic inflammatory disease (PID) affects about 1 million women annually and is responsible for more than 250,000 hospitalizations each year.[1] The disease results from infection of the cervix, uterus, fallopian tubes, and ovaries and their supporting structures (Fig. 41-4). Pelvic inflammatory disease usually is caused by sexually transmitted bacteria. The most common are *Neisseria gonorrhoeae* and *Chlamydia trachomatis* (chlamydia). Staphylococci, streptococci, and other pathogens also may cause infection. However, these organisms usually are transmitted during medical procedures.

Infections from the vaginal area may travel up the vagina and infect the cervix (cervicitis). This can be followed by infection of the uterus proper (endometritis) and fallopian tubes (salpingitis). Finally, the supporting structures around the uterus and fallopian tubes (parametritis) may become infected. The infection is caused by many pathogens. Infection produces diffuse lower abdominal pain. This is associated with low-grade fever (variable), vaginal discharge, and dyspareunia (pain with sexual intercourse). The inflammation often follows the onset of menstrual bleeding by 7 to 10 days. At that time the reproductive organs are vulnerable to bacterial infection because the lining of the uterus has been shed during menstruation.

Pelvic inflammatory disease often is accompanied by pain on ambulation, with the patient bent forward; taking short, slow steps; and often guarding the abdomen (the "PID shuffle"). Consequences include secondary infertility, ectopic pregnancies, and tuboovarian abscesses. In severe cases the reproductive organs may need to be removed surgically. Definitive treatment usually consists of antibiotic therapy. This helps to control the infection and prevent damage to the fallopian tubes.

RUPTURED OVARIAN CYST

A ruptured ovarian cyst is a gynecological emergency. A ruptured cyst can result in significant internal hemorrhage. An ovarian cyst is a thin-walled, fluid-filled sac. The cyst is located on the surface of the ovary (Fig. 41-5). The abdominal pain caused by an ovarian cyst may result from rapid expansion, torsion that produces ischemia, or acute rupture. The type of cyst most prone to rupture is known as the *corpus luteum cyst.* This cyst forms as a result of hemorrhage in a mature corpus luteum. The corpus luteum develops after ovulation (day 14 of the 28-day cycle). Thus most ruptures occur about 1 week before menstrual bleeding is to begin. However, some patients with a ruptured ovarian cyst have vaginal bleeding or report a late or missed period at the time of rupture.

CRITICAL THINKING

Consider a patient who you suspect has a ruptured ovarian cyst. How will you assess for the possibility of bleeding?

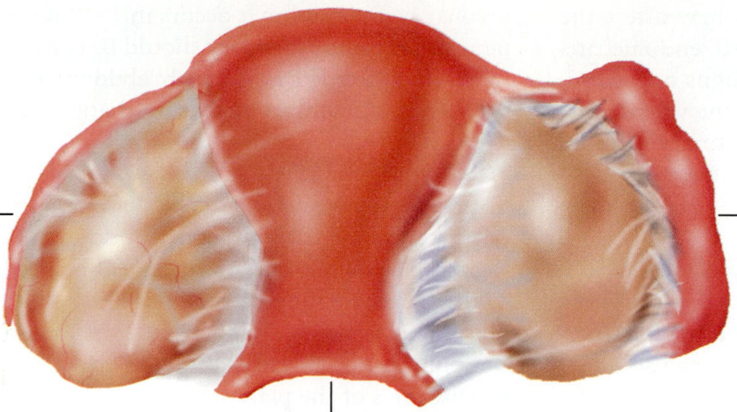

FIGURE 41-4 ■ Pelvic inflammatory disease.

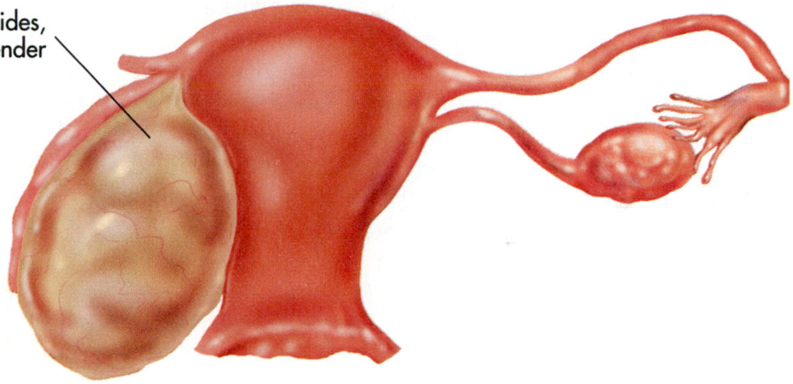

FIGURE 41-5 ■ Ovarian cyst.

A ruptured ovarian cyst can result in localized, one-sided lower abdominal pain. A ruptured cyst also can result in signs of peritonitis if massive hemorrhage has occurred. The onset of pain often is associated with minimal abdominal trauma, sexual intercourse, or exercise.

CYSTITIS

Cystitis is inflammation of the inner lining of the bladder. It usually is caused by a bacterial infection. Both sexes can develop infection. However, cystitis in women is more common. The main symptom of cystitis is a frequent urge to pass urine, with only a small amount of urine passed each time. Other signs and symptoms may include painful (burning) urination, fever, chills, and lower abdominal pain. The urine occasionally may be foul smelling or contain blood. Prompt treatment of cystitis with antibiotics usually settles the infection within 24 hours. Cystitis also can occur from structural abnormality of the ureters. (This is common in children.) Cystitis can occur from compression of the urethra as well (e.g., an enlarged prostate gland in men). Finally, it also can occur from indwelling urinary catheters.

DYSMENORRHEA AND MITTELSCHMERZ

Many women experience pain during menstruation. This is called dysmenorrhea. Dysmenorrhea also may include headache, faintness, dizziness, nausea, diarrhea, backache, and leg pain. In severe cases, chills, headache, diarrhea, nausea, vomiting, and syncope can occur. Dysmenorrhea occurs more often in women who are not sexually active and women who have not borne children. The lower abdominal pains associated with dysmenorrhea are thought to be related to muscular contraction of the myometrium (the muscular layer of the uterus). These muscle contractions are mediated by local prostaglandins. Other factors associated with dysmenorrhea include infection, inflammation, and the presence of an intrauterine contraceptive device.

Mittelschmerz is German for "middle pain." This pain may occur from the rupture of the graafian follicle and bleeding from the ovary during the menstrual cycle. Mittelschmerz is characterized by right or left lower quadrant abdominal pain. This pain occurs in the normal midcycle of a menstrual period (after ovulation). The pain lasts about 24 to 36 hours. The hormones produced by the ovary also may produce slight endometrial bleeding and low-grade fever. Dysmenorrhea and mittelschmerz do not pose a threat to life. However, physician evaluation is required to rule out more serious causes of menstrual pain. Evaluation also is required to differentiate the pain from that of appendicitis.

ENDOMETRITIS

Endometritis is inflammation of the uterine lining. It usually results from infection. Often, it occurs after childbirth or abortion and usually is caused by retained placental tissue. (The condition also is a feature of PID and other sexually transmitted infections.) Endometritis may affect the uterus and fallopian tubes. If left untreated, endometritis may result in sterility, sepsis, and death. Signs and symptoms of endometritis include fever, purulent vaginal discharge, and lower abdominal pain. The treatment includes removal of any foreign tissue and antibiotic therapy.

ENDOMETRIOSIS

Endometriosis is an abnormal gynecological condition. Endometriosis is characterized by endometrial tissue growing outside of the uterus. This may occur as a result of fragments of endometrium being regurgitated backward (during menstruation) through the fallopian tubes into the peritoneal cavity. There the fragments attach and grow as small cystic structures. The endometrial tissue of endometriosis functions cyclically. It undergoes periodic menstrual breakdown. This results in bleeding within cysts, stretching of the cyst wall, and pain.

Endometriosis is more common in women who defer pregnancy. The average age of women found to have endometriosis is 37 years. Characteristic symptoms of endometriosis are pain (particularly dysmenorrhea), painful defecation, and suprapubic soreness. Other common symptoms include vaginal spotting of blood before the start of a period and infertility. After physician evaluation, treatment may consist of drug therapy with analgesics or hormones. Sometimes it may include surgery.

CRITICAL THINKING

Why do you think these patients with endometriosis tend to be infertile?

ECTOPIC PREGNANCY

An ectopic pregnancy can be a life-threatening emergency. An ectopic pregnancy develops outside the uterus. (Most often it occurs in the fallopian tube. Sometimes, though, it may develop in the ovary or [rarely] the abdominal cavity or cervix.) Most ectopic pregnancies are discovered in the first 2 months. They often are found before the woman realizes she is pregnant. Signs and symptoms include severe abdominal pain and vaginal "spotting." If rupture occurs, internal hemorrhage, sepsis, and shock may develop. Once ectopic pregnancy is confirmed, it is treated with surgery. Surgery is performed to remove the developing fetus, placenta, and any damaged tissue at the site of the pregnancy. Ectopic pregnancy is common: it occurs in 19.7 of every 1000 pregnancies.[1] Ectopic pregnancy should be considered in any female of reproductive age with abdominal pain. (Ectopic pregnancy is described further in Chapter 42.)

NOTE Torsion of an ovary around its vascular pedicle (ovarian torsion) may produce severe, sudden pain. (This pain is usually on the right side.) Torsion also may produce a dull ache with sharp exacerbations. This condition may be associated with nausea, vomiting, and low-grade fever. Torsion often presents similarly to ectopic pregnancy, urinary tract infection, or appendicitis. Ovarian torsion is a surgical emergency. It can lead to infection and necrosis of the ovary. This may result in peritonitis and shock.

VAGINAL BLEEDING

Vaginal bleeding refers to the loss of blood from the uterus, cervix, or vagina. The most common source of nontraumatic vaginal bleeding is menstruation. (This bleeding rarely results in a request for emergency care.) Possible causes of serious nonmenstrual bleeding include the following:

- Spontaneous abortion
- Disorders of the placenta
- Hormonal imbalances (especially menopause)
- Lesions
- PID
- Onset of labor

The paramedic should never assume that vaginal hemorrhage is due to *normal* menstruation. Some causes of vaginal bleeding may be life threatening. They may even lead to hypovolemic shock and death. (The vaginal passage of clots usually indicates bleeding at a rate greater than menstrual flow.)

Traumatic Emergencies

Traumatic abdominal pain in a female patient usually is associated with vaginal bleeding or sexual assault.

VAGINAL BLEEDING

Traumatic causes of vaginal bleeding are described in Chapter 27. These causes include straddle injuries, blows to the perineum, and blunt forces to the lower abdomen. Other causes include foreign bodies inserted into the vagina, injury during intercourse, abortion attempts, and soft tissue injuries resulting from sexual assault. Complications of vaginal bleeding that results from trauma may cause pelvic organs to rupture. This can lead to life-threatening hypovolemia and shock. Treatment is the same as for other severe internal injuries. Treatment often requires surgical repair.

ASSESSMENT AND MANAGEMENT

Finding the cause of lower abdominal pain in females is difficult. Many gynecological conditions produce common characteristics. For example, ruptured ectopic pregnancy, ruptured ovarian cyst, and PID can have identical presentations (Table 41-1). The goal of prehospital care is to identify quickly the conditions that require aggressive therapy. The other goal is rapid transport for surgery. Prehospital care includes obtaining a history of the present illness (including a thorough gynecological history); providing airway, ventilatory, and circulatory support as needed; and transporting the patient for physician evaluation.

HISTORY OF PRESENT ILLNESS AND OBSTETRICAL HISTORY

The paramedic should obtain a history of the present illness. This will help the paramedic to better understand the patient's chief complaint (see Chapter 10). Important associated symptoms include the presence of fever, diaphoresis,

TABLE 41-1 Characteristics of Abdominal Pain in Gynecological Emergencies

ONSET	LOCATION	QUALITY	RADIATION	VAGINAL DISCHARGE	MENSTRUAL HISTORY
Ruptured Ectopic Pregnancy					
Rapid (can become generalized)	Unilateral (can generalize)	Cramplike, then steady	Shoulder (may indicate intraperitoneal bleeding)	Vaginal bleeding (75% of cases)	Amenorrhea, 6 weeks or more since last period
Ruptured Ovarian Cyst					
Sudden	Unilateral (can generalize)	Steady	Shoulder (may indicate intraperitoneal bleeding)	Possible vaginal bleeding	Usually 1 week before period
Pelvic Inflammatory Disease					
Gradual (can become generalized)	Diffuse, bilateral	Steady ache	Right upper quadrant	Water, foul-smelling discharge	Usually within 1 week after period

syncope, diarrhea, constipation, and abdominal cramping. The interview should include a thorough obstetrical history. The obstetrical history includes 10 components as follow[2] (see Chapter 42):

CRITICAL THINKING

Will the patient always give you accurate information about whether she is pregnant? Why?

1. *Pregnancy.* The paramedic should determine the total number of pregnancies (gravida) the patient has had. The paramedic also should determine the number of pregnancies that were carried to term (para).
2. *Previous cesarean deliveries.* A **cesarean delivery** is a surgical procedure. In a cesarean section the abdomen and uterus are incised. Then the baby is delivered through the abdomen. Cesarean delivery is usually done when maternal or fetal conditions might make vaginal delivery risky. A history of a previous cesarean delivery may indicate a high-risk pregnancy.
3. *Last menstrual period.* The paramedic should obtain information about the patient's last menstrual period. Questions to ask about the patient's last menstrual period include the following:
   - When did it start (the date)? When did it end (the duration)? Have the menstrual periods occurred regularly for the patient?
   - Was the last menstrual period normal for the patient? Was the menstrual flow heavier or lighter than other periods?
   - Was there any bleeding between periods?
4. *Possibility of pregnancy.* Some patients may hesitate to disclose a possible pregnancy. They may not answer honestly a direct question such as "Could you be pregnant?" If pregnancy is suspected (but not confirmed by the patient), the paramedic should ask specific questions about missed or late periods, breast tenderness, urinary frequency, morning sickness (nausea and/or vomiting), and unprotected sexual activity to determine the likelihood of a pregnancy.
5. *History of previous gynecological problems.* The paramedic should identify previous gynecological problems. Knowledge of these problems can be helpful to others who may be involved in the patient's care. Examples of previous gynecological problems that are important to obtain during the patient history include infections, bleeding, dyspareunia, miscarriage, abortion, the need for a **dilation and curettage,** and ectopic pregnancy.

NOTE Dilation and curettage is a gynecological procedure. It refers to widening of the uterine cervix and scraping away of the endometrium of the uterus. The procedure is used for a variety of conditions. These include diagnosing disease of the uterus, correcting heavy or prolonged vaginal bleeding, and emptying the uterus of the products of conception following delivery or abortion.

6. *Present blood loss.* If the patient is actively bleeding, the paramedic should ask questions about the color (bright versus dark red blood), the amount of blood loss (estimated by the number of pads/tampons soaked per hour), and the duration of the bleeding episode.
7. *Vaginal discharge.* If the patient has a discharge, the paramedic should question her about the color, amount, and odor of the discharge. These findings may indicate the presence of infection, venereal disease, or other illness.
8. *Use and type of contraceptive.* The use and type of contraception is a key part of the obstetrical history. For example, the use of birth control pills has been associated with hypertension and pulmonary embolus. Also, intrauterine devices can cause intrauterine bleeding and infection. Other methods of contraception include the

withdrawal or rhythm method (which may increase the likelihood of pregnancy), the use of spermicides and condoms, contraceptive systems (e.g., Norplant and Depo-Provera), and surgical tubal ligation.

9. *History of trauma to the reproductive system.* The paramedic should question all patients about any injury to the reproductive tract. Such an injury may be responsible for vaginal bleeding or discharge. The paramedic should ask a sexually active patient whether pain or bleeding has occurred during or after intercourse.
10. *Degree of emotional distress.* The paramedic should evaluate the patient's emotional distress. Factors that may be responsible for a patient's emotional distress include personal health issues, depression, an unwanted pregnancy, and financial worries.

PHYSICAL EXAMINATION

The paramedic should conduct a physical examination in a comforting and professional manner with consideration for the patient's modesty and privacy. The paramedic should be considerate of reasons for patient discomfort as well. When evaluating the potential for serious blood loss, the paramedic should assess the patient's skin and mucous membranes for color, cyanosis, or pallor. Vital sign assessment should include orthostatic measurements. If indicated, the vaginal area should be inspected for bleeding or discharge, noting the color, amount, and presence of clots and/or tissue. The paramedic should auscultate the abdomen (if time allows). The patient's abdomen should be palpated to assess for masses, areas of tenderness, guarding, distention, and rebound tenderness.

PATIENT MANAGEMENT

Management includes support of the patient's vital functions and administration of high-concentration oxygen during transport. Intravenous access usually is not needed unless the patient is demonstrating signs of impending shock or has excessive vaginal bleeding. Many patients prefer to be transported in a left-lateral recumbent, knee-chest position. Or they may prefer a hips-raised, knees-bent position for comfort. Vaginal bleeding should be controlled with the application of sanitary pads or trauma dressings. The vagina should never be packed with dressings or tampons. The paramedic should count the number of soaked pads and should record the number on the patient care report.

During transport, the paramedic should monitor the patient for the onset of serious bleeding. If this occurs or the patient's condition begins to deteriorate, the paramedic should establish one or two large-bore intravenous lines with normal saline or lactated Ringer's solution. At this point, electrocardiograph and pulse oximetry monitoring are indicated. Drug therapy (e.g., analgesics) may mask key symptoms. Thus drugs generally should not be given before physician evaluation.

Sexual Assault

Sexual assault is a crime of violence. It has serious physical and psychological implications. Anyone of either gender at any age can be sexually assaulted (see Chapter 46). However, women and girls are most often the victims. One estimate indicates that one in three women will be raped during their lifetimes and that only 16% of these crimes will be reported.[3] Often, the paramedic is first to encounter these patients. Tact, kindness, and sensitivity during the patient care episode are essential.

CRITICAL THINKING

How do you feel about rape, and how would you manage a patient who has been raped?

Initially, the paramedic should care for a victim of sexual assault like any other injured patient. The first priority is to manage any injury that poses a threat to life. After that, though, the approach should be modified in reference to history taking and the physical examination. Before taking a history or performing an examination, the paramedic should move the patient to a private area. If possible, the patient should be interviewed and examined by a paramedic of the same sex.

HISTORY TAKING

As a rule, victims of sexual assault should not be questioned in detail about the incident in the prehospital setting. The history should be limited to the elements needed to provide emergency care. For example, questions regarding penetration, sexual history, or practices are irrelevant to prehospital care. They only add to the patient's emotional stress. The patient should be allowed to speak openly and all information should be recorded accurately and thoroughly. Common reactions to sexual assault may range from anxiety to withdrawal and silence. Denial, anger, and fear also are normal behavior patterns.

ASSESSMENT

The physical examination should identify any physical trauma, outside the pelvic area, that needs immediate attention. To find facial fractures, human bites of the hands and breasts, long bone fractures, broken ribs, or trauma to the abdomen is not unusual. The paramedic should examine the genitalia only if severe injury is present or is suspected. When possible, the paramedic should explain all procedures before iniating them. All examination findings should be documented, including the patient's emotional state, condition of the patient's clothing, obvious injuries, and any patient care rendered. A nonjudgmental and professional attitude is important. Feelings and prejudices about the victim or the assault should not affect the delivery of care.

MANAGEMENT

After managing life-threatening injury, emotional support is the most important patient care procedure one can offer a victim of sexual assault. The paramedic should provide a safe environment for the patient and should respond appropriately to the victim's physical and emotional needs. Paramedics also should be aware of the need to preserve evidence from the crime scene (further described in Chapter 52). Special considerations include the following:

- Handle clothing as little as possible.
- Do not clean wounds unless absolutely necessary.
- Do not allow the patient to drink or brush teeth.
- Do not use plastic bags for blood-stained articles.
- Bag each clothing item separately.
- Ask the victim not to change clothes or bathe.
- Disturb the crime scene as little as possible.

SUMMARY

- Menstruation is the normal, periodic discharge of blood, mucus, and cellular debris from the uterine mucosa. Ovulation is the release of a secondary oocyte from the ovary.
- Pelvic inflammatory disease results from infection of the cervix, uterus, fallopian tubes, and ovaries and their supporting structures.
- Ruptured ovarian cyst occurs when a thin-walled, fluid-filled sac located on the ovary ruptures. This can cause internal hemorrhage.
- Cystitis is inflammation of the inner lining of the bladder. It usually is caused by a bacterial infection.
- Dysmenorrhea is characterized by painful menses. It may be associated with headache, faintness, dizziness, nausea, diarrhea, backache, and leg pain.
- *Mittelschmerz* is German for "middle pain." This pain may occur from the rupture of the graafian follicle and bleeding from the ovary during the menstrual cycle.
- Endometritis is inflammation of the uterine lining. Endometriosis is characterized by endometrial tissue growing outside of the uterus.
- An ectopic pregnancy is one that develops outside the uterus.
- Vaginal bleeding is the loss of blood from the uterus, cervix, or vagina.
- Traumatic causes of vaginal bleeding include straddle injuries, blows to the perineum, blunt forces to the lower abdomen, foreign bodies in the vagina, injury during intercourse, abortion attempts, and soft tissue injuries from sexual assault.
- The goal of prehospital care of lower abdominal pain in the female is to obtain a history (including a gynecological history); provide airway, ventilatory, and circulatory support as needed; and provide transport for physician evaluation.
- Sexual assault is a crime of violence. It can have serious physical and psychological effects.
- Paramedics should be aware of the need to preserve evidence from a sexual assault crime scene.

REFERENCES

1. Rosen P, Barkin R: *Emergency medicine: concepts and clinical practice,* ed 4, St Louis, 1998, Mosby.
2. US Department of Transportation, National Highway Traffic Safety Administration: *EMT-Paramedic national standard curriculum,* Washington, DC, 1998, The Department.
3. DC Rape Crisis Center: Rape and sexual assault fact sheet. http://www.dcrcc.org/facts.html. Accessed January 13, 2004.

CHAPTER

42

Obstetrics

OBJECTIVES

Upon completion of this chapter, the paramedic student will be able to:

1. Describe the organization and function of the specialized structures of pregnancy.
2. Outline fetal development from ovulation through adaptations at birth.
3. Explain normal maternal physiological changes that occur during pregnancy and how they influence prehospital patient care and transportation.
4. Describe appropriate information to be elicited during the obstetrical patient's history.
5. Describe specific techniques for assessment of the pregnant patient.
6. Describe general prehospital care of the pregnant patient.
7. Discuss the implications of prehospital care after trauma to the fetus and mother.
8. Describe the assessment and management of patients with preeclampsia and eclampsia.
9. Explain the pathophysiology, signs and symptoms, and management of the processes that cause vaginal bleeding in pregnancy.
10. Outline the physiological changes that occur during the stages of labor.
11. Describe the role of the paramedic during normal labor and delivery.
12. Compute an Apgar score.
13. Describe assessment and management of postpartum hemorrhage.
14. Discuss the identification, implications, and prehospital management of complicated deliveries.

KEY TERMS

abortion: The termination of pregnancy from any cause before 20 weeks' gestation.

abruptio placentae: A partial or full detachment of a normally implanted placenta at more than 20 weeks' gestation.

Apgar score: The evaluation of a newborn's physical condition, usually performed at 1 minute and 5 minutes after birth, including heart rate, respiratory effort, muscle tone, reflex irritability, and color.

crowning: The phase at the end of labor in which the fetal head is seen at the opening of the vagina.

eclampsia: A grave form of pregnancy-induced hypertension, characterized by convulsions, coma, proteinuria, and edema.

ectopic pregnancy: A pregnancy that occurs when a fertilized ovum implants anywhere other than the uterus.

gestation: The period from fertilization of the ovum until birth.

gravida: The number of all current and past pregnancies.

para: The number of past pregnancies that have remained viable to delivery.

parturition: The process by which an infant is born.

placenta: A highly vascular fetal-maternal organ through which the fetus absorbs oxygen, nutrients, and other substances and excretes carbon dioxide and other wastes.

placenta previa: Placental implantation in the lower uterine segment partially or completely covering the cervical opening.

preeclampsia: An abnormal disease of pregnancy characterized by the onset of acute hypertension after the twenty-fourth week of gestation.

uterine rupture: A spontaneous or traumatic rupture of the uterine wall.

Childbirth is common in the prehospital setting. Most often, emergency medical services personnel only assist in this natural process. They provide care for the mother and newborn. At times, though, obstetrical emergencies can develop suddenly. They can even become life-threatening. The paramedic must be prepared to recognize and manage these events. The paramedic also must be ready to assist in abnormal deliveries. This chapter presents the causes and treatment of obstetrical emergencies. It also discusses the normal and abnormal events associated with childbirth.

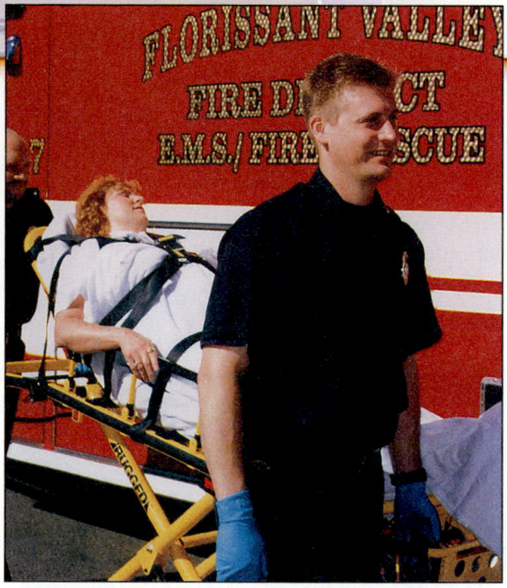

NORMAL EVENTS OF PREGNANCY

In a normal pregnancy, fertilization occurs in the fallopian tube. Fertilization takes place when the head of a sperm penetrates a mature ovum. After penetration the nuclei of the sperm and ovum fuse. At this time the newly fertilized ovum becomes a zygote. The zygote undergoes repeated cell divisions as it passes down the fallopian tube. After a few days of rapid cell division, a ball of cells called a *morula* is formed with cell differentiation between the inner layer of cells (blastocyst cells) and the outer layer of cells (trophoblast cells). Trophoblast cells attach to the endometrium lining of the uterus. Implantation begins within 7 days after fertilization. Implantation is completed when the trophoblast cells make contact with maternal circulation. (This is about day 12.) Trophoblast cells go on to make various life support systems for the embryo (**placenta,** amniotic sac, umbilical cord); blastocyst cells develop into the embryo itself (Fig. 42-1).

SPECIALIZED STRUCTURES OF PREGNANCY

Specialized structures of pregnancy include the placenta, the umbilical cord, and the amniotic sac and its fluid. These structures provide nutrients for the developing embryo. They are part of fetal circulation as well.

Placenta

The trophoblast cells continue to develop and form the placenta for about 14 days after ovulation. The placenta is a disklike organ composed of interlocking fetal and maternal tissues. The placenta is the organ of exchange between the mother and fetus and is responsible for the following five functions:

1. *Transfer of gases.* The diffusion of oxygen and carbon dioxide through the placental membrane is similar to the diffusion that occurs in the lungs. Dissolved oxygen in maternal blood passes through the placenta into fetal blood. This takes place as a result of the pressure gradient between the blood of the mother and fetus. However, as fetal carbon dioxide pressure (P_{CO_2}) builds up, a low pressure gradient of carbon dioxide develops across the placental membrane. The carbon dioxide then diffuses from fetal blood to maternal blood.

> **CRITICAL THINKING**
> What happens to diffusion of gases if the mother becomes hypoxic?

2. *Transport of nutrients.* Other metabolic substrates that the fetus needs diffuse into fetal blood in the same manner as oxygen. For example, glucose levels in fetal blood are about 20% to 30% lower than those in maternal blood. This results in a rapid diffusion of glucose to the fetus. Diffusion also transports other substrates. These include fatty acids, potassium, sodium, and chloride. The placenta also actively absorbs some nutrients from maternal blood.
3. *Excretion of wastes.* Waste products diffuse from fetal blood into maternal blood. Examples of such products

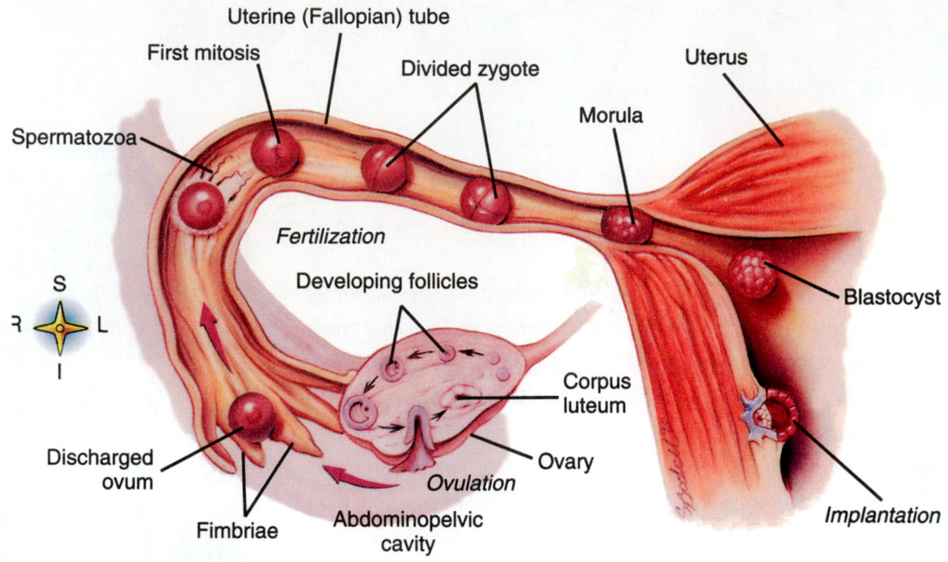

FIGURE 42-1 ■ Fertilization and implantation. At ovulation the ovary releases an ovum, which begins its journey through the uterine tube. While the ovum is in the tube, a sperm fertilizes the ovum to form the single-celled zygote. After a few days of rapid cell division, a ball of cells called a *morula* forms. After the morula develops into a hollow ball (blastocyte), implantation occurs.

are urea, uric acid, and creatinine. They are excreted with the waste products of the mother. Wastes transfer from fetal circulation to maternal circulation in the same manner as carbon dioxide does.

4. *Hormone production.* The placenta becomes a temporary endocrine gland. It secretes estrogen and progesterone. By the third month of fetal development the corpus luteum (described in Chapter 41) on the ovary no longer is needed to sustain the pregnancy. Estrogen, progesterone, and other hormones maintain the uterine lining, prevent the occurrence of menses, and stimulate changes in the pregnant woman's breasts, vagina, cervix, and pelvis that prepare her body for delivery and lactation.
5. *Formation of a barrier.* The placenta forms a barrier against some harmful substances and chemicals in the mother's circulation. Yet the placental barrier is incomplete; it is only partially selective. Thus the placental barrier does not fully protect the fetus. Certain medications easily cross the placenta. Among these are steroids, narcotics, anesthetics, and some antibiotics.

Umbilical Cord

Blood flows from the fetus to the placenta through two umbilical arteries. These arteries carry deoxygenated blood. Oxygenated blood returns to the fetus through the umbilical vein. This system is independent of and separated from the maternal circulation. Other structures unique to fetal circulation are the ductus venosus, the foramen ovale, and the ductus arteriosus. The ductus venosus is a continuation of the umbilical cord. It serves as a shunt to allow most blood returning from the placenta to bypass the immature liver of the embryo. The ductus venosus empties directly into the inferior vena cava. The foramen ovale and the ductus arteriosus allow blood to bypass the embryo's lungs. The lungs remain collapsed until birth.

The foramen ovale shunts blood from the right atrium directly into the left atrium. The ductus arteriosus connects the aorta and the pulmonary artery. Thus the well-oxygenated blood from the placenta enters the left side of the heart rather than the right side. The left ventricle pumps the oxygenated blood mainly into vessels of the head and forelimbs. The blood entering the right atrium from the superior vena cava progresses downward through the tricuspid valve into the right ventricle. Most of this blood is deoxygenated blood from the head region of the fetus. The blood is pumped by the right ventricle into the pulmonary artery. The deoxygenated blood passes from the pulmonary artery, through the ductus arteriosus, into the descending aorta, through the two umbilical arteries, and into the placenta for oxygenation. At birth the various arteriovenous shunts close in most infants (Fig. 42-2).

Amniotic Sac and Amniotic Fluid

The amniotic sac is a fluid-filled cavity. It completely surrounds and protects the embryo. Amniotic fluid originates from several fetal sources. These include fetal urine and secretions from the respiratory tract, skin, and amniotic membranes. The fluid builds up rapidly. It amounts to about 175 to 225 mL by the fifteenth week of pregnancy and about 1 L at birth. The rupture of the amniotic membranes produces the watery discharge at the time of delivery.

FETAL GROWTH AND DEVELOPMENT

The developing ovum is called an *embryo* during the first 8 weeks of pregnancy. After those first 8 weeks and until birth it is called a *fetus.* The period during which the fetus grows and develops within the uterus is known as **gestation.** It usually averages 40 weeks from the time of fertilization to delivery of the newborn. Gestation is divided into 90-day periods called trimesters. Conception occurs about 14 days after the first day of the last menstrual period. Thus the obstetrician can calculate fetal development with reasonable

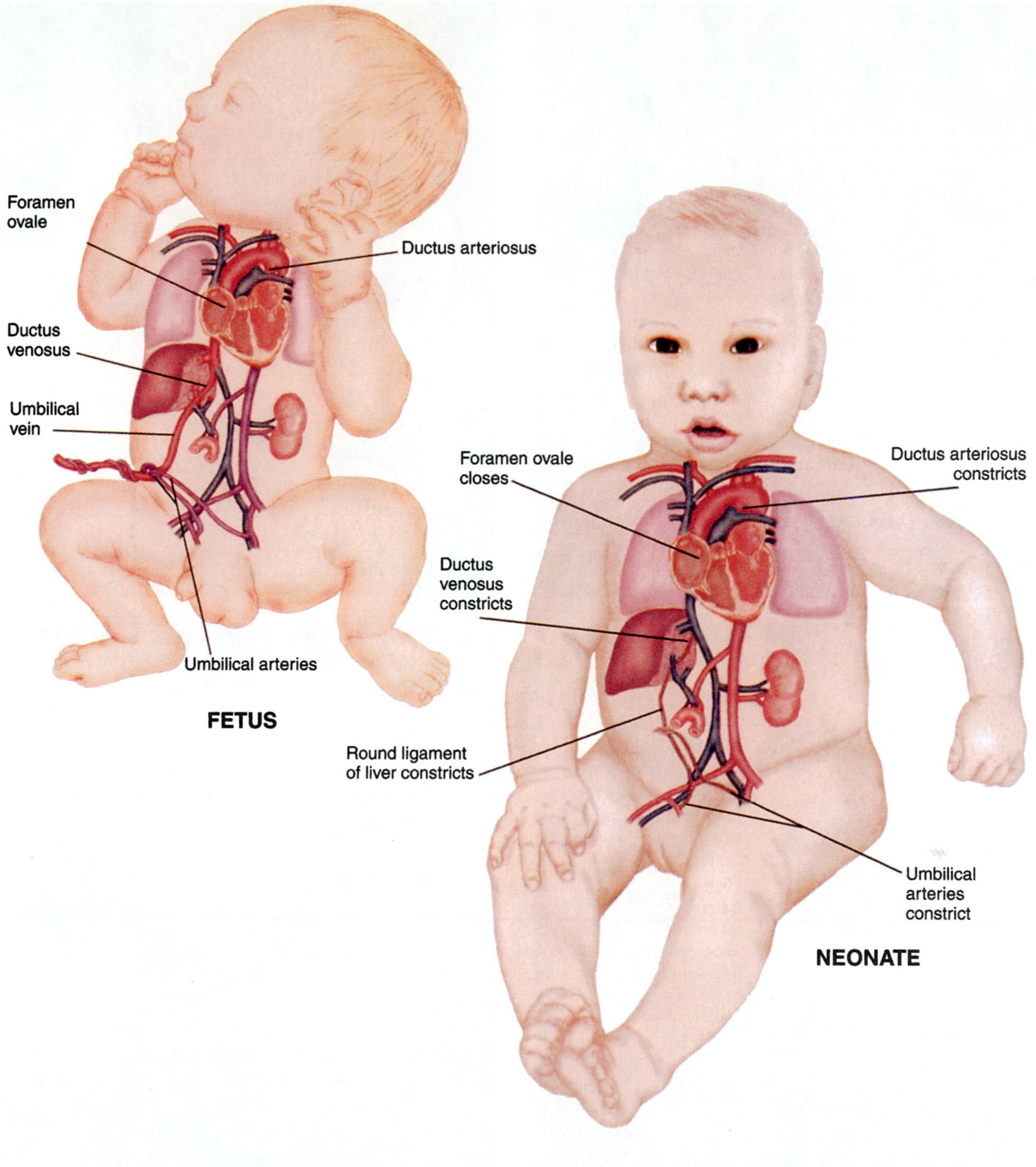

FIGURE 42-2 ■ Fetal circulation and changes in circulation after birth.

accuracy. The obstetrician also can calculate the estimated date of confinement. This also is known as the delivery date. Rapid fetal growth and development characterize the period of gestation (Fig. 42-3 and Box 42-1).

Adjustments of the Infant at Birth

Birth results in the infant's loss of the placental connection with the mother. Thus birth also results in loss of metabolic support. The infant's immediate need to obtain oxygen and excrete carbon dioxide is critical. This requires changes in the fetal circulation that permit adequate blood flow through the lungs.

After a normal delivery by a mother who is not depressed with anesthetics, a newborn usually begins to breathe spontaneously. This occurs when the chest exits the birth canal or with some external stimulation. At birth, surface tension of the viscid fluid that fills the alveoli holds the walls of the alveoli together. The newborn needs to cre-

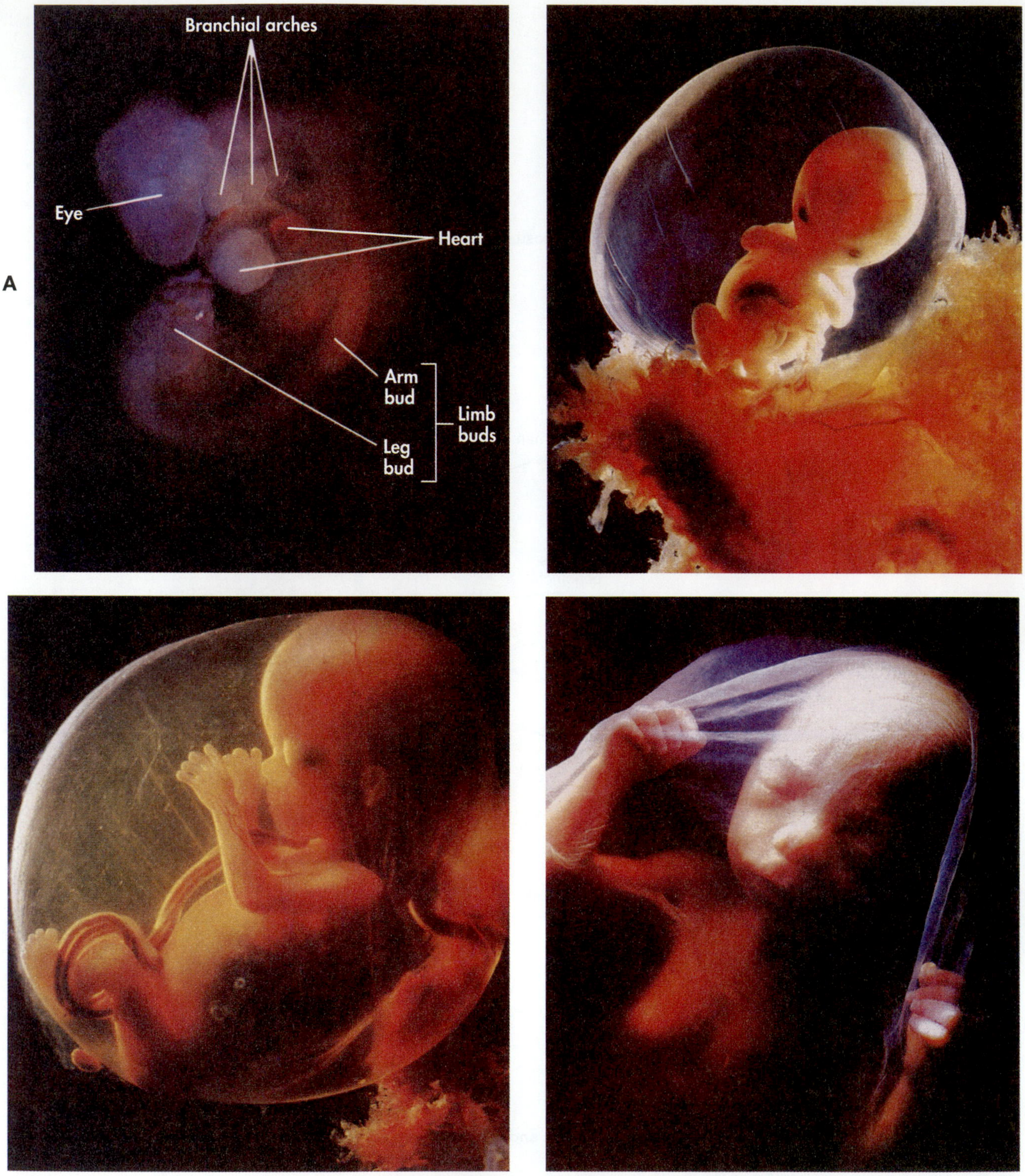

FIGURE 42-3 ■ Human embryos and fetuses. **A,** At 35 days. **B,** At 49 days. **C,** At the end of the first trimester. **D,** At 4 months.

ate more than 25 mm Hg of negative pressure to oppose the effects of this surface tension. This allows the alveoli to open for the first time. The first breaths of the newborn can create as much as 50 mm Hg of negative pressure in the intrapleural space. These powerful first breaths open the alveoli. They allow further respirations to occur with much less effort.

The ductus venosus, ductus arteriosus, and foramen ovale bypass the immature liver and nonfunctional lungs of the developing fetus. Blood flow through the placenta ceases at birth. At that point, pressure in the aorta, left ventricle, and left atrium increases. This results in an increase in systemic vascular resistance. Also, pressure in the lungs decreases as they expand. This reduces the pulmonary ar-

BOX 42-1 Embryo and Fetal Development in Utero for Each Lunar Month (28 days)

First Lunar Month
- Foundations form for the nervous system, genitourinary system, skin, bones, and lungs.
- Buds of arms and legs begin to form.
- Rudiments of eyes, ears, and nose appear.

Second Lunar Month
- The head is disproportionately large because of brain development.
- Gender differentiation begins.
- The centers of bones begin to ossify.

Third Lunar Month
- Fingers and toes are distinct.
- The placenta is complete.
- Fetal circulation is complete.

Fourth Lunar Month
- Gender is differentiated.
- Rudimentary kidneys secrete urine.
- Heartbeat is present.
- Nasal septum and palate close.

Fifth Lunar Month
- Fetal movements are felt by the mother.
- Heart sounds are perceptible with a fetoscope.

Sixth Lunar Month
- The skin appears wrinkled.
- Eyebrows and fingernails develop.

Seventh Lunar Month
- The skin is red.
- The pupillary membrane disappears from the eyes.
- If born, the infant cries and breathes but frequently dies.

Eighth Lunar Month
- The fetus is viable if born.
- The eyelids open.
- Fingerprints are set.
- Vigorous fetal movement occurs.

Ninth Lunar Month
- The face and body have a loose, wrinkled appearance because of subcutaneous fat deposits.
- Amniotic fluid decreases somewhat.

Tenth Lunar Month
- Skin is smooth.
- Eyes are uniformly slate colored.
- The bones of the skull are ossified and nearly together at sutures.

terial, right ventricular, and right atrial pressures. As a result of these changes in pressure, the arteriovenous shunts close normally within a few hours after birth. They eventually close completely and are covered with a growth of fibrous tissue.

CRITICAL THINKING

Do fetal heart tones sound normal if you auscultate them immediately after birth?

OBSTETRICAL TERMINOLOGY

Pregnant patients are described by their gravid and parous states. The term **gravida** refers to the number of all of the woman's current and past pregnancies; **para** refers only to the number of the woman's past pregnancies that have resulted in a live birth. For example, a woman who is pregnant for the first time is gravida 1, para 0 (Box 42-2).

BOX 42-2 Obstetrical Terminology

Antepartum: the maternal period before delivery
Grand multipara: a woman who has had seven deliveries or more
Multigravida: a woman who has had two or more pregnancies
Multipara: a woman who has had two or more deliveries
Nullipara: a woman who has never delivered
Perinatal: occurring at or near the time of birth
Postpartum: the maternal period after delivery
Prenatal: existing or occurring before birth
Primigravida: a woman who is pregnant for the first time
Primipara: a woman who has given birth only once
Term: a pregnancy that has reached 40 weeks' gestation

PATIENT ASSESSMENT

The paramedic must be familiar with the normal physiological changes that occur in the pregnant woman. This will help the paramedic to assess a pregnant patient.

Maternal Changes during Pregnancy

Menstruation ceases in the pregnant woman. The uterus also enlarges. The pregnant woman undergoes many other physical changes as well. These changes affect the genital tract, breasts, gastrointestinal system, cardiovascular system, respiratory system, and metabolism.

GENITAL TRACT

Uterus
- Uterine size increases from 70 g (nongravid) to 1000 g by term.
- The uterus triples in size and weight by the second month of pregnancy.
- The uterus occupies the entire pelvic cavity. It may be palpated suprapubically by the third month of pregnancy.
- The uterus becomes an abdominal organ and the top of the uterus (fundus) reaches the level of the umbilicus by the fourth month of pregnancy.

- The uterine fundus recedes a little when the fetus descends into the pelvis. This occurs in the last trimester.

Cervix

Increased uterine blood and lymphatic flow cause pelvic congestion and edema. This results in softening and bluish discoloration of the cervix (Chadwick's sign).

Vagina

- The vagina develops a violet color. This is due to increased vascularity.
- The vaginal walls prepare for labor. The vaginal mucosa increases in thickness.
- Vaginal secretions increase. The pH decreases to about 3.5; this is due to increased production of lactic acid from glycogen in the vaginal epithelium. Acidic pH helps keep the vaginal area fairly free of pathogens.

Bladder

Frequency of urination occurs from pressure of the expanding uterus on the bladder. Frequency disappears when the uterus rises out of the pelvis. It returns once again when the fetal head engages in the pelvis near term.

Breasts

- The breasts become tender in the early weeks of pregnancy.
- The breasts increase in size as a result of hypertrophy of the mammary alveoli by the second month of pregnancy.
- The nipples become larger, more deeply pigmented, and more erectile early in pregnancy.
- As breast glands proliferate, they begin to secrete a clear fluid by the tenth week of pregnancy.

GASTROINTESTINAL SYSTEM

- Morning sickness and nausea may occur at any time. They usually begin by the sixth and abate by the fourteenth week of pregnancy. The cause of morning sickness is related to the high serum levels of chorionic gonadotropin in early pregnancy.
- The enlarging uterus displaces the patient's stomach and intestines upward and laterally. This may cause indigestion. It can increase the risk for aspiration in unconscious patients.

> **CRITICAL THINKING**
>
> Consider an unconscious pregnant woman who has sustained trauma. What are problems associated with these gastrointestinal changes?

- The liver is displaced backward, upward, and to the right.
- The tone and motility of the gastrointestinal tract decrease, leading to prolonged gastric emptying and relaxation of the pyloric sphincter. Heartburn and constipation are common.

CARDIOVASCULAR SYSTEM

Heart

- Elevation of the diaphragm displaces the heart to the left and upward. Flat or negative T waves may be present in lead III on the electrocardiogram.
- Cardiac output increases by 30% by the thirty-fourth week of pregnancy.
- The pulse rate may increase 15 to 20 beats/min above baseline late in the third trimester (variable).
- Pulmonic systolic and apical systolic murmurs are common. This is because lowered blood viscosity and increased flow lead to turbulence in the great vessels.

Circulation

- Total blood volume increases by 30%. Plasma volume increases by 50%.
- Blood pressure decreases 10 to 15 mm Hg during the second trimester. This is because of the reduction in peripheral resistance. Blood pressure gradually increases to prepregnancy levels toward term.
- The enlarged uterus interferes with venous return from the legs.
- Hemorrhoids, slight edema of the ankles, and varicose veins may be present.
- The supine position may cause the uterus to compress the inferior vena cava. This can produce decreased cardiac filling and decreased cardiac output (supine hypotension syndrome). The patient may become faint and hypotensive while lying on her back after the first or second trimester.

Blood

- Increased plasma volume results in a decrease in hemoglobin and hematocrit concentrations.
- The leukocyte count increases.
- Fibrinogen levels increase by 50% because of the influence of estrogen and progesterone.

RESPIRATORY SYSTEM

- Tidal volume and minute ventilation increase by 30% to 40% in late pregnancy.
- Functional residual capacity decreases by about 25%.
- The respiratory rate may be normal. It also may increase because of elevation of the diaphragm by the enlarged uterus.
- P_{CO_2} normally decreases. This is because of an increased respiratory rate. P_{CO_2} changes from 40 torr to 30 torr to provide a gradient for fetal carbon dioxide. This may cause dizziness and a sensation of shortness of breath for the pregnant woman.

METABOLISM

- The mother experiences a normal weight gain of 9.1 kg (20 lb).
- Increased water retention produces an increase in pressure within the capillaries. This can result in edema.
- The metabolic rate and caloric demand (especially for protein) increase.
- Glucose escapes into the urine because of increased glomerular filtration.
- Maternal gestational diabetes mellitus (GDM) may result from an impaired ability to metabolize carbohydrates. This usually is caused by a deficiency of insulin. Gestational diabetes mellitus is further described later in this chapter.

- Fetal demands for calcium and iron may deplete maternal stores if the patient does not supplement them through diet.

History

When obtaining a history from an obstetrical patient, the paramedic first should gather details about the chief complaint. This complaint may not be related to the pregnancy. Paramedics should solicit information about the onset of signs and symptoms in confidence. Also, they should provide privacy for the physical examination. After ruling out life-threatening illness or injury, the paramedic should interview the patient to obtain relevant data, including the following eight points:

> **NOTE** Pregnancy may aggravate some preexisting medical conditions. Examples of such are diabetes, heart disease, hypertension, and seizure disorders. And some medications (e.g., anithypertensive agents and oral hypoglycemic drugs) used to manage these disorders cannot be taken by the mother during her pregnancy. This is due to the potential harm to the fetus. Thus a thorough patient history is key. The history will help the paramedic anticipate care that may be required at the scene and during patient transport.

1. Obstetrical history
   a. Length of gestation
   b. Parity and gravidity
   c. Previous cesarean delivery
   d. Maternal lifestyle (alcohol or other drug use, smoking history)
   e. Infectious disease status
   f. History of previous gynecological or obstetrical complications (e.g., **eclampsia,** GDM, premature labor, or ectopic pregnancy)
2. Presence of pain
   a. Onset (gradual or sudden)
   b. Character
   c. Duration and evolution over time
   d. Location and radiation
3. Presence, quantity, and character of vaginal bleeding
4. Presence of abnormal vaginal discharge
5. Presence of "show" (expulsion of the mucous plug in early labor) or rupture of membranes
6. Current general health and prenatal care (none, physician, nurse, midwife)
7. Allergies and medications taken (especially the use of narcotics in the last 4 hours)
8. Maternal urge to bear down or sensation of imminent bowel movement, indicating imminent delivery

Physical Examination

The patient's chief complaint determines the extent of the examination. The goal in examining an obstetrical patient is to identify acute life-threatening conditions rapidly. A part of this goal is to identify imminent delivery. If delivery is near, the paramedic must take the proper management steps.

The paramedic should assess the patient's general appearance and skin color. If she is very pale, the paramedic should suspect hemorrhage. Sunken cheeks, cracked lips, or hollow eyes with a history of vomiting indicate dehydration. The paramedic should monitor the patient's vital signs often during the care. Orthostatic vital signs may indicate the early presence of significant bleeding or fluid loss. The paramedic should recall that normal physiological changes in the pregnant patient can produce variations in vital signs. Examples of such are mild tachycardia, a slight fall in systolic and diastolic blood pressures, and an increase in respiratory rate.

The paramedic should examine the patient's abdomen for scars and gross deformities. The latter may be caused by a hernia or marked abdominal distention. Gentle palpation may reveal the presence of masses, enlarged organs, intestinal distention, or a distended bladder. In late pregnancy, though, these may be hard to recognize. During the examination, it may be possible to discern peritoneal irritation. Peritoneal irritation is diagnosed by the presence of tenderness, guarding, or rebound tenderness. If the patient is obviously pregnant, the paramedic may need to assess uterine size and monitor the fetus.

EVALUATION OF UTERINE SIZE

The uterine contour usually is irregular between 8 and 10 weeks' gestation. Thus early uterine enlargement may not be symmetrical. Moreover, the uterus may be deviated to one side. The uterus is above the symphysis pubis at 12 to 16 weeks' gestation. The uterus is at the level of the umbilicus at 24 weeks and near the xiphoid process at term. Figure 42-4 shows changes in fundal height at the various weeks of gestation.

FETAL MONITORING

Fetal heart sounds can be auscultated between 16 and 40 weeks' gestation. (They may be hard to hear in a noisy environment.) They can be auscultated by use of a stethoscope, fetoscope, or Doppler probe (Fig. 42-5). One benefit of fetal monitoring is determining whether the fetus has a heart beat. Another is providing baseline measurements for later use in case the fetus or the mother becomes distressed. The paramedic should monitor the fetal heart rate and maternal vital signs every 5 to 10 minutes.

When auscultating the fetal heart rate, the paramedic should position the high-intensity diaphragm of the stethoscope (the bell of the fetoscope or the microphone of the Doppler probe) firmly on the mother's abdominal wall. The paramedic then moves the diaphragm in a circular pattern of 6 to 8 inches in diameter around the woman's umbilicus. The paramedic moves the device until fetal heart tones can be heard (Fig. 42-6). Once the paramedic locates the tones, the paramedic measures fetal heart rate in beats per minute.

The normal fetal heart rate is 120 to 160 beats/min. A fetal heart rate that remains above 160 (fetal tachycardia) or

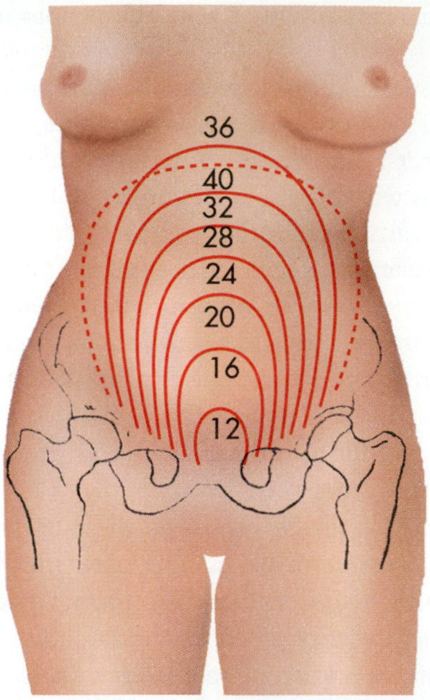

FIGURE 42-4 ■ Changes in fundal height during pregnancy. *Weeks 10 to 12:* The uterus is within the pelvis, and fetal heartbeat can be detected with a Doppler probe. *Week 12:* The uterus is palpable just above the symphysis pubis. *Week 16:* The uterus is palpable just between the symphysis pubis and umbilicus. *Week 20:* The uterine fundus is at the lower border of the umbilicus. A fetal heartbeat can be auscultated with a fetoscope. *Weeks 24 to 26:* The uterus becomes ovoid, and the fetus is palpable. *Week 28:* The uterus is about halfway between the umbilicus and xiphoid process, and the fetus is easily palpable. *Week 32:* The uterine fundus is just below the xiphoid. *Week 40:* Fundal height drops as the fetus begins to engage in the pelvis.

below 120 beats/min (fetal bradycardia) is an early sign of fetal distress. It also is a sign of fetal or maternal hypoxia. Intermittent, short-term increases or decreases in the fetal heart rate usually are normal. Variation can occur at any time. Short-term periodic changes in fetal heart rate are common during fetal sleep, fetal movement, and contractions associated with labor and delivery.

General Management of the Obstetrical Patient

If birth is not imminent, care for the healthy patient should be limited to basic treatment modalities (airway, ventilatory, and circulatory support) and transportation for physician evaluation. In the absence of distress or injury, the patient should be transported in a comfortable position. (This is usually left lateral recumbent.) The paramedic may need to monitor the electrocardiogram, administer high-concentration oxygen, and monitor the fetus based on patient assessment and vital sign determinations. Medical direction may advise intravenous (IV) access in some patients. Most drugs usually are inappropriate. They may mask symptoms of a worsening condition.

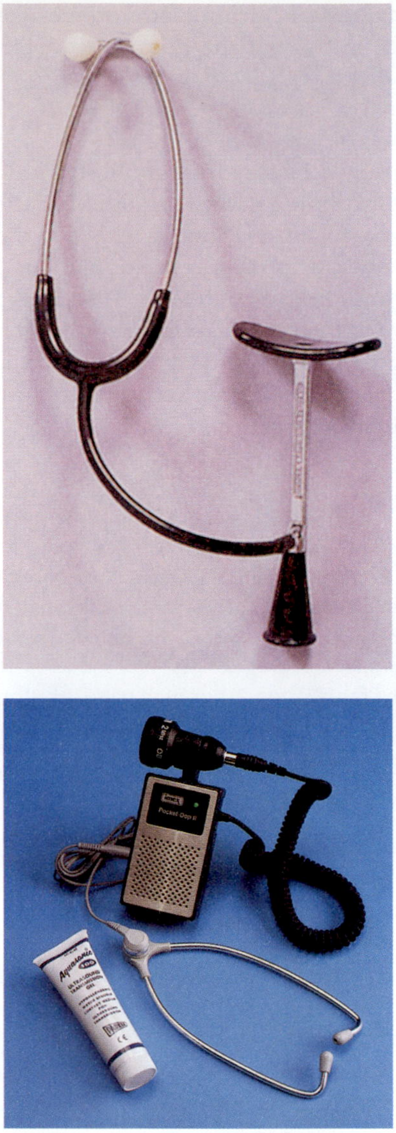

A

B

FIGURE 42-5 ■ **A,** Fetoscope. **B,** Doppler probe.

COMPLICATIONS OF PREGNANCY

Complications associated with pregnancy can result from trauma, medical conditions, prior disease processes that the pregnancy can aggravate or mask, the pregnancy itself (vaginal or intraperitoneal hemorrhage), spontaneous abortion, or problems associated with labor and delivery. Often the patient with gynecological or obstetrical complaints is embarrassed, apprehensive, and if pregnant, concerned about the unborn child. Tact, understanding, and a caring, supportive attitude from the paramedic are important when managing these patients.

Trauma during Pregnancy

When a pregnant woman is severely injured, the fetus is at high risk for death. When the mother sustains life-threatening injuries, 40.6% of fetuses die compared with only 1.6% in

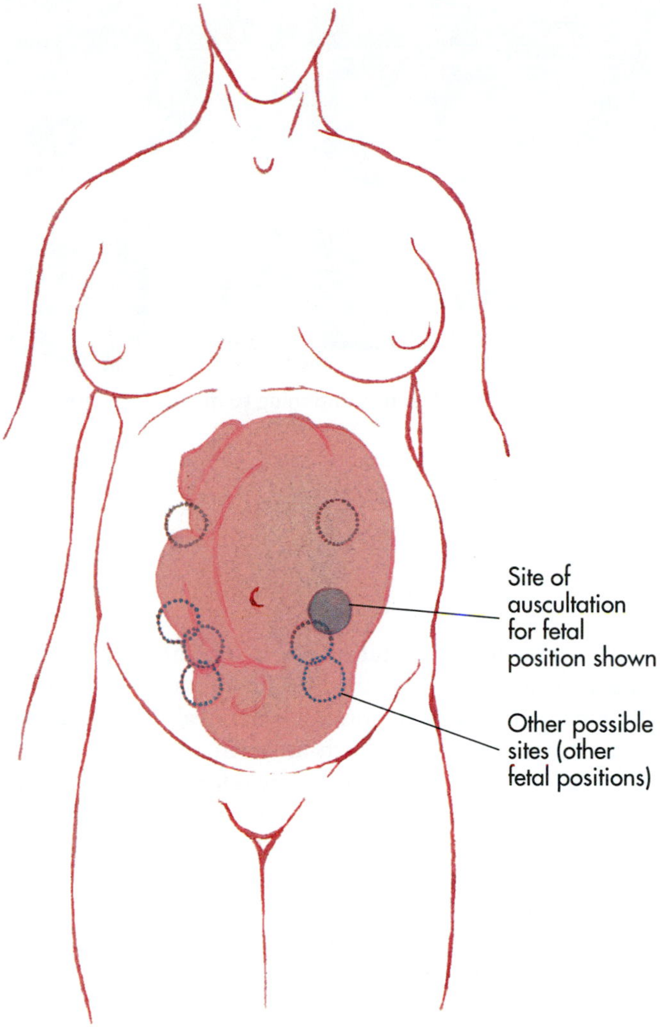

FIGURE 42-6 ■ Sites for auscultation of fetal heart tones.

non-life-threatening cases.[1] Mortality related to the pregnancy itself is rare, occurring in an estimated 1 of every 30,000 deliveries.[2] The anatomical and physiological changes of pregnancy can change the pregnant woman's response to injury. This may necessitate modified assessment, treatment, and transportation strategies.

MATERNAL INJURY

The causes of maternal injury in decreasing order of frequency are vehicular crashes, falls, and penetrating objects. These injuries can result in trauma to the gravid uterus. They also can cause trauma to the maternal bladder, liver, and spleen. In addition, an injury that results in a pelvic fracture can produce massive hemorrhage and damage to the fetal skull. As described in Chapter 20, the severity of any injury depends on many factors. The injury may involve multiple organ systems as well.

During pregnancy, the fetus is well protected within the uterus; amniotic fluid surrounds the fetus. This fluid serves as an excellent shock absorber. Because of this protection the fetus rarely experiences physical trauma except as a result of direct penetrating wounds or extensive blunt trauma to the maternal abdomen. The greatest risk of fetal death is from fetal distress and intrauterine demise caused by trauma to the mother or her death. Thus when dealing with a pregnant trauma patient, the paramedic promptly should assess and intervene on behalf of the mother. Severe abdominal injury can result in premature separation of the placenta, premature labor or abortion, rupture of the uterus, and fetal death. Causes of fetal death from maternal trauma include death of the mother, separation of the placenta, maternal shock, uterine rupture, and fetal head injury.

ASSESSMENT AND MANAGEMENT

The priorities in assessing and managing a pregnant trauma patient are the same as for a nongravid patient: adequate airway, ventilatory, and circulatory support with spinal precautions; hemorrhage control; and rapid assessment, stabilization, and rapid transportation to a medical facility. Resuscitating the mother is key to the survival of the mother and fetus. Thus during the first stages of assessing and managing, the mother's status should be the focus. Despite the severity, all pregnant trauma patients should be transported for physician evaluation.

The examination should be thorough. The paramedic must detect, identify, and manage injuries that contribute to hypovolemia or hypoxia. With the normal increase in maternal blood volume, the mother can tolerate more blood loss before showing signs and symptoms of shock. A 30% to 35% reduction in blood volume can produce minimal changes in blood pressure but reduce uterine blood flow by 10% to 20%.[1] Thus the mother may maintain adequate blood pressure at the expense of the fetus. The true amount of blood loss may be difficult to detect. Fetal monitoring is the best available indicator of fetal well-being after trauma. But patient transport should never be delayed to assess fetal heart rate.

Accelerations of fetal heart rate above baseline are associated with fetal movement and contractions. However, this also may be an early sign of fetal distress. Decreased fetal movement and increased fetal heart rate can indicate maternal shock.

Slow fetal heart rates (below the baseline) result from a decrease in cardiac output and hypoxia. A hypoxic fetus in metabolic acidosis cannot accelerate his or her heart rate. Thus the fetus becomes bradycardic (a heart rate of less than 120 beats/min). Sustained fetal bradycardia (lasting 10 minutes or more) may be a response to increased parasympathetic tone. The fetus can tolerate this only for a short time before becoming acidotic. Fetal bradycardia usually is a late sign of maternal hypoxia and decreased maternal circulating volume.

CRITICAL THINKING

How do you think the traumatized pregnant patient feels emotionally?

BOX 42-3 Causes of Cardiac Arrest Associated with Pregnancy

Events That Occur at the Time of Delivery
Amniotic fluid embolism
Drug toxicity (e.g., because of magnesium sulfate or epidural anesthetic)
Eclampsia

Events That Occur from Complex Physiological Changes Associated with Pregnancy
Aortic dissection
Congestive cardiomyopathy
Hemorrhage from a pregnancy-related pathological condition
Pulmonary embolism

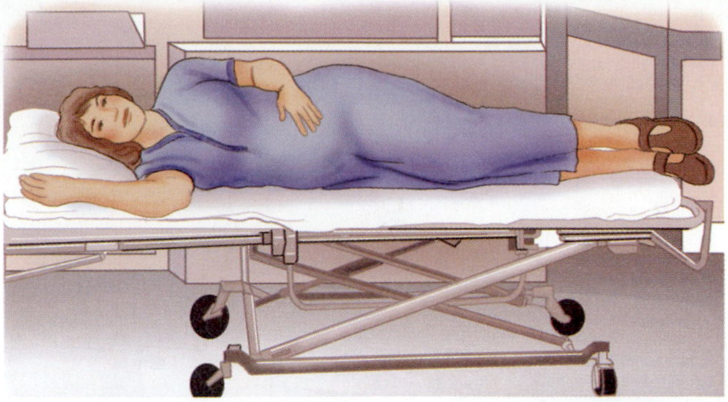

FIGURE 42-7 ■ Patient positioning to displace the uterus.

SPECIAL MANAGEMENT CONSIDERATIONS

Special considerations in managing the pregnant trauma patient include oxygenation, volume replacement, and hemorrhage control. Labor is a complication of trauma in pregnancy. The emergency medical services (EMS) crew should be ready to manage delivery or spontaneous abortion.

Cardiac arrest can occur in pregnant women from a number of causes (Box 42-3). However, many cardiovascular problems associated with pregnancy are related to changes in anatomy that produce a decrease in the return of venous blood.[2] Key interventions to prevent cardiac arrest in a distressed or compromised pregnant patient include placing the patient in the left lateral position or *manually* and *gently* displacing the uterus to the left, administering 100% oxygen, and giving a fluid bolus. The key to resuscitation of the child is resuscitation of the mother. The mother cannot be resuscitated until blood flow to her right ventricle is restored.

If cardiac arrest occurs, the paramedic should institute cardiopulmonary resuscitation with a few modifications[2]:

- Relieve pressure on the aorta and the inferior vena cava by manually repositioning the uterus. This also can be done by using wedge-shaped cushions, pillows, or overturned chairs to displace the uterus (Fig. 42-7).
- Generally perform chest compressions higher on the sternum (that ensures a palpable pulse wave) to adjust for the shifting of the pelvic and abdominal contents toward the head.
- Address the need for left lateral tilt of the torso to prevent compression or blockage of the vena cava. This can be achieved with wedge-shaped pillows that support the tilted torso during chest compression. It also can be achieved by using the angled backs of several chairs and the angled thighs of several rescuers to place the patient in the left lateral tilt position.

An aggressive resuscitation effort is justified in patients who are near term. This can allow for a cesarean delivery at the emergency department. Fetal survival is good if the time between maternal death and delivery is less than 5 minutes. Survival is poor if the time is longer than 20 to 25 minutes. Alerting the emergency department staff of the possibility of the need for an emergency cesarean section is critical to infant survival.

Oxygenation

- Adequate maternal airway maintenance and oxygenation are essential to prevention of fetal hypoxemia.
- Oxygen requirements are 10% to 20% greater than in the normal, nonpregnant patient. Fetal hypoxia may occur with even small changes in maternal oxygenation. The paramedic should administer high-concentration oxygen.
- If available, pulse oximetry should be used to monitor oxygen saturation.

Volume Replacement

- Signs and symptoms of hypovolemia may not be present until a blood loss is large.
- Blood is shunted preferentially from the uterus to preserve maternal blood pressure.
- Bleeding also may occur inside the uterus. The pregnant uterus can sequester up to 2000 mL of blood after separation of the placenta with little or no evidence of vaginal bleeding.[1]
- Crystalloid fluid replacement is indicated, even when blood pressure remains normal.
- Use of the pneumatic antishock garment is controversial. If the pneumatic antishock garment is to be applied, only the leg compartments should be inflated. This is because use of the abdominal compartment may increase blood loss from pelvic injury. The paramedic may inflate the abdominal compartment when maternal and fetal deaths are imminent and the paramedic is ordered to by medical direction. However, this is rarely done.

- Vasopressors generally are not recommended. They decrease uterine blood flow and fetal oxygen delivery.

Hemorrhage Control

- External hemorrhage should be controlled the same as in a nonpregnant patient.
- Vaginal bleeding may point to placental separation or uterine rupture.
- Avoid a vaginal examination. It may increase bleeding and bring on delivery. This may be the case especially if unsuspected placenta previa is present (described later in chapter).
- Document the amount and color of vaginal bleeding.
- Collect and transport any expelled tissue with the patient to the facility.

TRANSPORTATION PLANS

Pregnant patients after 3 to 4 months' gestation should not be transported in a supine position because of the potential for supine hypotension. In the absence of suspected spinal injury, the patient should be transported in a left lateral recumbent position. If spinal injury is suspected, the patient should be prepared for transportation in the following manner:

1. Fully immobilize the patient on a long spine board.
2. After immobilization, carefully tilt the board on its left side by logrolling the secured patient 10 to 15 degrees.
3. Place a blanket, pillow, or towel under the right side of the board to move the uterus to the left side.

CRITICAL THINKING

Are facilities in your community prepared to manage deliveries that are high risk?

Medical Conditions and Disease Processes

Pregnancy can mask or worsen some medical conditions and diseases. These include acute appendicitis, acute cholecystitis, hypertension, diabetes, infection, neuromuscular disorders, and cardiovascular disease. Two hypertensive disorders are specific to pregnancy. They are **preeclampsia** and eclampsia (toxemia of pregnancy). Hypertensive disorders occur in about 5% of pregnancies in the United States and increase the risk to the mother and the fetus.[1]

PREECLAMPSIA AND ECLAMPSIA

Preeclampsia is a disease of unknown origin. It mainly affects previously healthy, normotensive women in their first pregnancy. The disease occurs after 24 weeks' gestation, often near term. The pathophysiology of preeclampsia, which does not reverse until after delivery, is characterized by vasospasm, endothelial cell injury, increased capillary permeability, and activation of the clotting cascade. The signs and symptoms of preeclampsia result from hypoperfusion to the tissue or organs involved (Box 42-4). Eclampsia is characterized by the same signs and symptoms with the addition of seizures or coma.

BOX 42-4 Signs and Symptoms of Preeclampsia

Cerebrum
Headache
Hyperreflexia
Dizziness
Confusion
Seizures
Coma

Retina
Blurred vision
Diplopia

Gastrointestinal System
Nausea
Vomiting
Right upper quadrant or epigastric pain and tenderness

Renal System
Proteinuria
Azotemia
Oliguria
Anuria
Hematuria
Hemoglobinuria

Vasculature or Endothelium
Hypertension
Edema
Activation of the clotting cascade

Placenta
Abruptio placentae
Fetal distress

The criteria for diagnosis of preeclampsia are based on the presence of the classic triad, which includes hypertension (blood pressure greater than 140/90 mm Hg, an acute rise of 20 mm Hg in systolic pressure, or a rise of 10 mm Hg in diastolic pressure over prepregnancy levels), proteinuria, and excessive weight gain with edema.[3] In addition to nulliparity, factors predisposing to preeclampsia include advanced maternal age, chronic hypertension, chronic renal disease, vascular diseases such as diabetes and systemic lupus, and multiple gestation. Preeclampsia is a clinical diagnosis that can be confirmed by postpartum renal biopsy. When preeclampsia is suspected, most patients are hospitalized. If not, they are confined to bed rest at home until delivery.

Management. Not all hypertensive patients have preeclampsia. Also, not all preeclamptic patients have hypertension. The illness has many serious complications. Thus the paramedic should always suspect preeclampsia or eclampsia when hypertension is present in late pregnancy. If preeclampsia or eclampsia is suspected, prehospital care is directed at preventing or controlling seizures and treating hypertension.

Seizure activity in eclampsia is similar to generalized grand mal seizures of other causes. Seizure activity is characterized by tonic-clonic activity (described in Chapter 31). The seizure often begins around the mouth in the form of twitching. Eclampsia may be associated with apnea during the seizure. Labor can begin suddenly and progress rapidly. The regimen for managing severe preeclampsia is as follows:

1. Place the patient in a left lateral recumbent position. This will help to maintain or improve uteroplacental blood flow. It also will help to lessen the risk of insult to the fetus.
2. Handle the patient gently. Minimize sensory stimulation. (For example, darken the ambulance.) This will help to avoid seizures.

3. Administer high-concentration oxygen. Assist respirations as needed.
4. Initiate IV therapy per protocol.
5. Be prepared for seizures at any moment. Be prepared to provide airway, ventilatory, and circulatory support.
6. Be prepared to administer the following medications per medical direction and local protocol:
   a. ***Magnesium sulfate*** 10%. The antidote ***(calcium gluconate)*** should be close at hand to treat respiratory depression.
   b. ***Diazepam*** or ***lorazepam***
      (1) May precipitate a fall in blood pressure.
      (2) May jeopardize fetal circulation.
      (3) Closely monitor vital signs.
7. Gently transport the patient to a proper medical facility.

GESTATIONAL DIABETES MELLITUS

As stated before, GMD is caused by pregnancy. The condition occurs in about 4% of all pregnancies, affecting 135,000 women in the United States each year.[4] Gestational diabetes mellitus is thought to be related to an inability of the mother to metabolize carbohydrates. This may be caused by a deficiency of the mother's insulin or from placental hormones that block the action of the mother's insulin *(insulin resistance)*. As a result, the mother's body is not able to produce or use all of the insulin it needs during the pregnancy. Excessive amounts of her glucose are transmitted to the fetus where it is stored as fat. Treatment for GMD includes regular glucose monitoring, dietary modification, and exercise. In some cases, pregnant women will need insulin injections to manage the condition. Gestational diabetes mellitus usually subsides after pregnancy. However, it may return in later years or with future pregnancies.

Most women with GDM are aware of their condition through prenatal care. Most of these women have healthy pregnancies and healthy babies. Without treatment, however, mothers with GDM often have very large babies. This makes for a more difficult labor and delivery (with increased risk for fetal and maternal injury) and a longer recovery. In addition, children whose mothers had GDM are at higher risk for certain health problems. Examples of such are respiratory distress syndrome, obesity and related health issues as children or adults, and an increased risk for developing type 2 diabetes during their lifetime.

Management. Prehospital care for patients with GDM may include airway, ventilatory, and circulatory support; glucose testing; managing hypoglycemia with IV fluids and ***dextrose;*** or managing hyperglycemia with the administration of ***insulin.*** (See Chapter 32.)

VAGINAL BLEEDING

Vaginal bleeding during pregnancy can result from abortion (miscarriage), ectopic pregnancy, abruptio placentae, placenta previa, uterine rupture, or postpartum hemorrhage. Patients with vaginal bleeding have varying degrees of blood loss. Some require aggressive resuscitation.

BOX 42-5 Classifications of Abortion

Complete abortion: an abortion in which the patient has passed all of the products of conception
Criminal abortion: an intentional ending of any pregnancy under any condition not allowed by law
Incomplete abortion: an abortion in which the patient has passed some but not all of the products of conception
Induced abortion: an abortion in which the pregnancy is terminated intentionally
Missed abortion: the retention of the fetus in utero for 4 or more weeks after fetal death
Spontaneous abortion: an abortion that usually occurs before the twelfth week of gestation (the lay term is *miscarriage*). (Predisposing factors include acute or chronic illness in the mother, abnormalities in the fetus, and abnormal attachment of the placenta. Often the cause is unknown.)
Therapeutic abortion: a pregnancy legally terminated for reasons of maternal well-being.
Threatened abortion: an abortion in which a patient has some uterine bleeding with an intrauterine pregnancy in which the internal cervical os is closed. A threatened abortion may stabilize and end in normal delivery or progress to an incomplete or complete abortion.

CRITICAL THINKING

As the mother loses blood from vaginal hemorrhage, what effect does that have on the fetus?

Abortion. Abortion is the termination of pregnancy from any cause before 20 weeks' gestation. (After this time, it is known as a *preterm birth.*) Abortion is the most frequent cause of vaginal bleeding in pregnant women. It occurs in about 1 in 10 pregnancies. Box 42-5 lists common classifications of abortion.

Most abortions occur in the first trimester, usually before the tenth week. The patient often is anxious and apprehensive and complains of vaginal bleeding. This bleeding may be slight or profuse. In addition, the patient may have suprapubic pain. This pain is referred to the lower back and described as cramplike and similar to the pain of labor or menstruation. When obtaining a history, the paramedic should ascertain the time of onset of pain and bleeding, amount of blood loss (a soaked sanitary pad suggests 20 to 30 mL of blood loss), and whether the patient passed any tissue with the blood. If the patient passed tissue during bleeding episodes, the tissue should be collected and transported with the patient for analysis.

Management. The paramedic should watch all first-trimester emergencies closely for signs of significant blood loss and hypovolemia. The paramedic should measure vital signs (including orthostatic vital signs) often during transport. Depending on the patient's vital signs, IV fluid ther-

TABLE 42-1 Differentiation of Abruptio Placentae, Placenta Previa, and Uterine Rupture

HISTORY	BLEEDING	ABNORMAL PAIN	ABDOMINAL EXAMINATION
Abruptio Placentae			
Association with toxemia of pregnancy and hypertension of any cause	Single attack of scant, dark vaginal bleeding (often concealed) that continues until delivery	Present	Localized uterine tenderness Labor Absent fetal heart tones (often)
Placenta Previa			
Lack of association with toxemia of pregnancy	Repeated "warning" hemorrhages over days to weeks	Usually absent	Lack of uterine tenderness (usually) Labor (rare) Fetal heart tones (usually)
Uterine Rupture			
Previous cesarean section	Possible bleeding	Usually present and associated with sudden onset of nausea and vomiting	Diffuse abdominal tenderness Sudden cessation of labor Possible fetal heart tones

apy may be indicated. All patients with suspected abortion should receive oxygen, emotional support, and transportation for physician evaluation.

Ectopic Pregnancy. An ectopic pregnancy occurs when a fertilized ovum implants anywhere other than the uterus. Ectopic gestation occurs in 1 of every 200 pregnancies; it is the leading cause of first-trimester death and accounts for more than 11% of all maternal deaths in the United States.[1] Death from ectopic pregnancy usually results from hemorrhage.

Ectopic pregnancy has many causes. But most involve factors that delay or prevent the passage of the fertilized ovum to its normal site of implantation. Predisposing factors include pelvic inflammatory disease, adhesions from previous surgery, tubal ligation, previous ectopic pregnancy, and possibly the presence of intrauterine contraceptive devices. Thus obtaining a full gynecological history is key. Although the time from fertilization varies, most ruptures occur by 2 to 12 weeks' gestation.

The signs and symptoms of ectopic pregnancy often are difficult to distinguish from those of a ruptured ovarian cyst, pelvic inflammatory disease, appendicitis, or abortion (thus the name the *great imitator*). The classic triad of symptoms includes abdominal pain, vaginal bleeding, and amenorrhea (absence of menstruation); however, vaginal bleeding may be absent, spotty, or minimal, and amenorrhea may be replaced by oligomenorrhea (scanty flow). The variable presentation of this type of pregnancy is one reason for its high-risk profile. Other symptoms of ectopic pregnancy include signs of early pregnancy. These include referred pain to the shoulder, nausea, vomiting, syncope, and the classic signs of shock.

Management. A ruptured ectopic pregnancy is a true emergency. It calls for initial resuscitation measures. It requires rapid transport for surgery as well. The patient may become unstable quickly. If the paramedic suspects an ectopic pregnancy, the paramedic should manage the patient like any victim of hemorrhagic shock—with airway, ventilatory, and circulatory support and aggressive IV fluid resuscitation.

Third-trimester Bleeding. Third-trimester bleeding occurs in 3% of all pregnancies and is never normal. The majority of bleeding episodes are a result of abruptio placentae, placenta previa, or uterine rupture. Table 42-1 differentiates among abruptio placentae, placenta previa, and uterine rupture.

Abruptio Placentae. Abruptio placentae is partial or full detachment of a normally implanted placenta at more than 20 weeks' gestation. It occurs in up to 2% of all pregnancies and is severe enough to result in fetal death in 1 in 400 cases of abruption.[1] Predisposing factors to abruptio placentae include maternal hypertension, preeclampsia, multiparity, trauma, and previous abruption.

CRITICAL THINKING

Why is abruptio placentae associated with such a high fetal death rate?

The common presentation of abruptio placentae is sudden third-trimester vaginal bleeding and pain. The vaginal bleeding may be minimal. Bleeding often is out of proportion to the degree of shock because much of the hemorrhage may be concealed. The more extensive the separation, the greater the uterine irritability, resulting in a tender abdomen and rigid uterus. Contractions may be present. In severe abruptio placentae, fetal heart sounds are absent because fetal death is likely.

Placenta Previa. Placenta previa is placental implantation in the lower uterine segment partially or completely covering the cervical opening. It occurs in about 1 in 300 deliveries. The incidence is higher in preterm births. The condition is characterized by painless, bright red bleeding without uterine contraction. The bleeding may occur in episodes. It may be slight to moderate. In addition, bleeding may become more profuse if active labor begins. Fetal heart rate slows because of hypoxia.

Placenta previa is associated with increasing maternal age, multiparity, previous cesarean section, and previous placenta previa episodes. Recent sexual intercourse can lead to bleeding.

Uterine Rupture. Uterine rupture is a spontaneous or traumatic rupture of the uterine wall. It may result from reopening of a previous uterine scar (e.g., a previous cesarean section), a prolonged or obstructed labor, or direct trauma. Uterine rupture occurs in about 1 in 1400 deliveries and has a 5% to 15% maternal mortality rate and a 50% fetal mortality rate.[1]

Uterine rupture is characterized by sudden abdominal pain described as steady and "tearing," active labor, early signs of shock (complaints of weakness, dizziness, anxiety), and vaginal bleeding, which may not be visible. On examination, the abdomen usually is rigid. The patient complains of diffuse abdominal pain. Fetal parts may be felt easily through the abdominal wall.

Management. The prehospital management of a patient with third-trimester bleeding is aimed at preventing shock. The paramedic should not try to examine the patient vaginally; doing so may increase hemorrhage and bring on labor. Emergency care measures should include the following:

1. Provide adequate airway, ventilatory, and circulatory support as needed (with spinal precautions if indicated).
2. Place the patient in a left lateral recumbent position.
3. Begin transport immediately.
4. Initiate IV therapy with volume-expanding fluid.
5. Apply a fresh perineal pad. Note the time of application to assess bleeding during transport.
6. Check fundal height. Document it for baseline measurement.
7. Closely monitor the patient's vital signs en route to the facility.

LABOR AND DELIVERY

Parturition is the process by which the infant is born. Near the end of pregnancy the uterus becomes more and more irritable. It exhibits occasional contractions. These contractions become stronger and more frequent until parturition begins. During and as a result of these contractions, the cervix begins to dilate. As uterine contractions increase, complete cervical dilation occurs to about 10 cm; the amniotic sac ruptures; and the fetus, and shortly thereafter the placenta, are expelled from the uterus through the vaginal canal (Fig. 42-8).

Stages of Labor. Labor follows several distinct stages. The lengths of these stages vary. This depends on whether the mother is nullipara or multipara (Box 42-6). Thus the paramedic should use the stages only as a guideline in assessing labor progression in the average pregnancy. About 2 to 3 weeks before the onset of active labor, the cervix undergoes the process of softening, effacement (thinning), and dilation. At the same time, the uterus begins to become a contractile organ. Braxton-Hicks contractions refer to irregular tightening of the pregnant uterus. These begin in the first trimester (before 30 weeks' gestation). They are usually benign and painless. They often subside with walking or other exercise. Many patients are not aware of Braxton-Hicks contractions. They may perceive them as a slight uterine hardening. As the pregnancy continues, the contractions increase in frequency and duration. This heralds the onset of clinical labor. A great deal of individual variation exists in the perception and tolerance of uterine contractions. Some mothers experience somewhat painless contractions even with the onset of labor. However, others are uncomfortable from the earlier and less intense Braxton-Hicks contractions. In the former group, delivery may be more imminent than anticipated; members of the latter group may develop false labor several days to weeks before term.

Labor begins with the infant's descent into the birth canal. The fetal descent is characterized by a relief of pressure in the upper abdomen and a simultaneous increase in pressure in the pelvis. During this stage a mucous plug (sometimes mixed with blood, thus the name *bloody show*) is expelled from the dilating cervix and discharged from the vagina. The mother may not notice these early changes as a sign of labor.

The first stage of labor begins with the onset of regular contractions. It ends with full dilation of the cervix. The uterine contractions generally occur at 5- to 15-minute intervals. They are characterized by cramplike abdominal pains. These pains radiate to the small of the back. As the uterus contracts, the cervix becomes soft and thinned (effaced). The less muscular lower segment of the uterus is pulled upward over the presenting part. The first stage usually lasts 8 to 12 hours in the first-time mother. It usually lasts about 6 to 8 hours in the women who have had previous deliveries. In most pregnancies the amniotic sac ruptures (*rupture of membranes*) toward the end of the first stage of labor.

CRITICAL THINKING

What comfort measures can you use during transportation for the patient who is in the first stage of labor?

The second stage of labor is measured from full dilation of the cervix to delivery of the infant. During the second stage the fetal head enters the birth canal. The mother's pain and contractions become more intense and frequent (usually 2 to 3 minutes apart). Often the mother becomes diaphoretic and tachycardiac during this stage. She experiences an urge to bear down with each contraction. In addition, she may express the need to have a bowel movement. (This is a normal sensation caused by pressure of the fetal head against the mother's rectum.) The presenting part of the fetus (usually the head) emerges from the vaginal opening. This process, known as **crowning,** indicates that delivery is imminent. The second stage of labor usually lasts 1 to

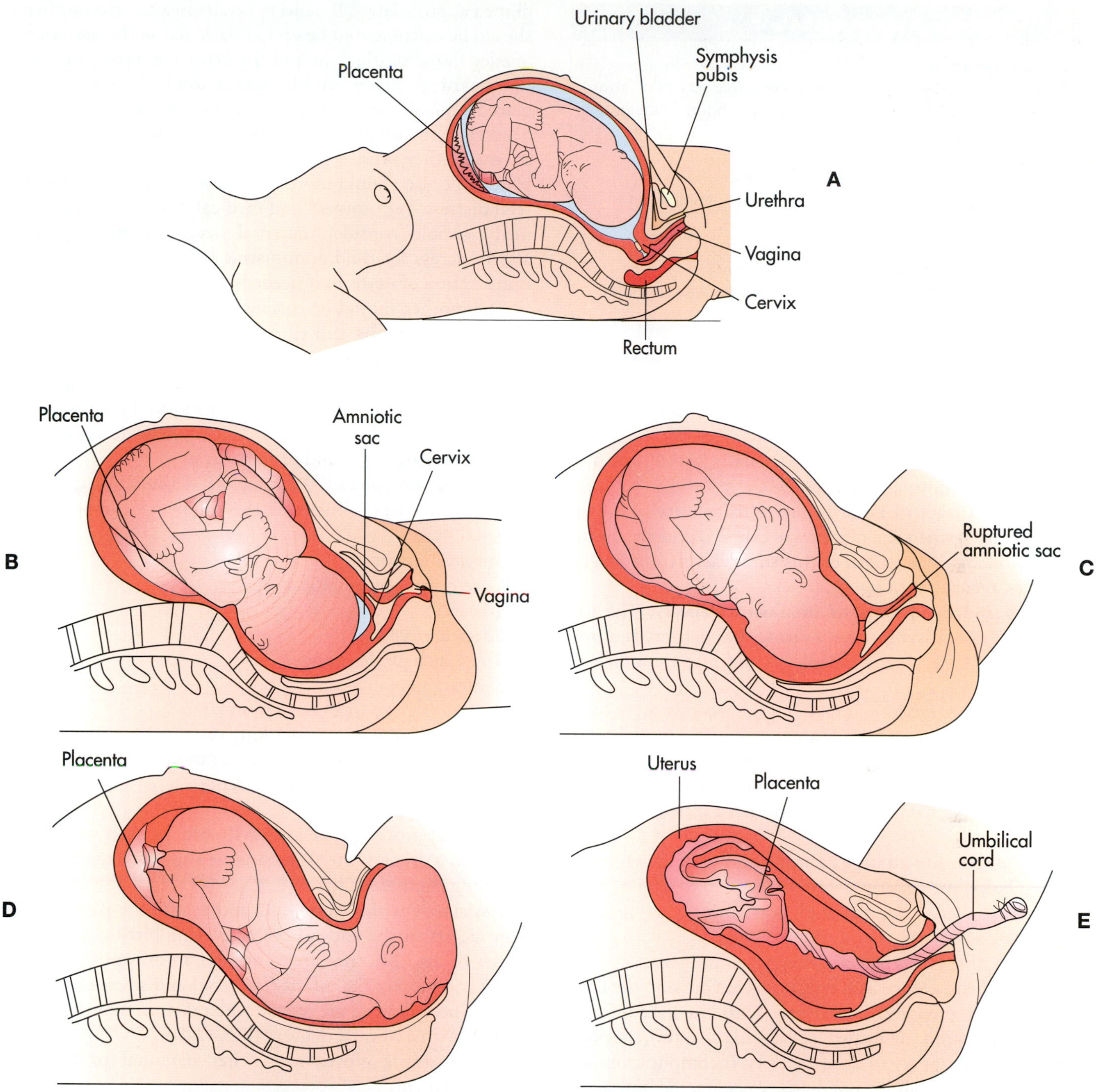

FIGURE 42-8 ■ Parturition. **A,** The relation of the fetus to the mother. **B,** The fetus moves into the birth canal. **C,** Dilation of the cervix is complete. **D,** The fetus is expelled from the uterus. **E,** The placenta is expelled.

BOX 42-6 Stages of Labor

Stage I (Dilation)
- Onset of regular contractions to complete cervical dilation
- Average time: 12½ hours in primipara, 7 hours in multipara

Stage II (Expulsion)
- Full dilation of cervix to delivery of the newborn
- Average time: 80 minutes in primipara, 30 minutes in multipara

Stage III (Placenta Delivery)
- Immediately after delivery of the infant until expulsion of the placenta
- Average time: 5 to 20 minutes

2 hours in the nullipara mother. It usually lasts 30 minutes or less in the multipara mother.

The third stage of labor begins with delivery of the infant and ends when the placenta is expelled and the uterus has contracted. The length of this stage varies from 5 to 60 minutes, regardless of parity.

Signs and Symptoms of Imminent Delivery. The following signs and symptoms indicate that delivery is imminent. With these, the paramedic should prepare for childbirth at the scene:

- Regular contractions last 45 to 60 seconds at 1- to 2-minute intervals. Intervals are measured from the beginning of one contraction to the beginning of the next. If contractions are more than 5 minutes apart, there generally is time to transport the mother to a receiving hospital.
- The mother has an urge to bear down or has a sensation of a bowel movement.
- There is a large amount of bloody show.
- Crowning occurs.
- The mother believes that delivery is imminent.

If any of these signs and symptoms are present, the EMS crew should prepare for delivery. With the exception of cord presentation (described later in this chapter), the paramedic should not try to delay delivery. If complications are anticipated or an abnormal delivery occurs, medical direction may recommend expedited transport of the patient to a medical facility.

Preparation for Delivery. When preparing for delivery, the paramedic should try to provide an area of privacy. The mother should be positioned on a bed, stretcher, or table. The surface should be long enough to project beyond the mother's vagina. The delivery area should be as clean as possible. It should be covered with absorbent material to guard against staining and contamination by blood and fecal material.

The mother should be placed on her back. Her knees should be flexed and widely separated (or in another position preferred by the mother). The vaginal area should be draped appropriately. If delivery occurs in a car, the mother should be instructed to lie on her back across the seat with one leg flexed on the seat and the other leg resting on the floorboard. A pillow or blanket, if available, should be placed beneath the mother's buttocks. This will aid in the delivery of the infant's head. The paramedic should evaluate the mother's vital signs for baseline measurements. The paramedic also should monitor fetal heart rate for signs of fetal distress. Per protocol and medical direction, the paramedic should consider maternal oxygen administration and IV access for fluid administration or postdelivery administration of ***oxytocin*** if needed.

The mother should be coached to bear down and push during contractions and to rest between contractions to conserve strength. If the mother finds it difficult to refrain from pushing, the paramedic should encourage her to breathe deeply or "pant" through her mouth between contractions. Deep breathing and panting help decrease the force of bearing down and promote rest.

Delivery Equipment. Prehospital delivery equipment ("OB kit") generally includes the following components (Fig. 42-9):

- Surgical scissors
- Cord clamps or umbilical tape
- Towels
- Surgical masks
- 4 × 4 inch gauze sponges
- Sanitary napkins
- Bulb syringe and DeLee suction kit
- Baby blanket and baby stocking cap
- Plastic bag for placental transportation
- Neonatal resuscitation equipment
- IV fluid supplies

Personal protective measures should be used when assisting in a delivery. Sterile technique should be used when handling equipment.

Assistance with Delivery. In most cases the paramedic only assists in the natural events of childbirth. The chief duties of the EMS crew are to prevent an uncontrolled delivery and protect the infant from cold and stress after the birth. The following are steps to be taken in assisting the mother with a normal delivery (Fig. 42-10):

1. Don sterile gloves and other personal protective equipment.
2. When crowning occurs, apply gentle palm pressure to the infant's head to prevent an explosive delivery and tearing of the perineum. If membranes are still intact, tear the sac with finger pressure to allow escape of amniotic fluid.
3. After delivery of the head, examine the infant's neck for a looped umbilical cord. If the cord is looped around the neck, gently slip it over the infant's head.
4. Suction the infant's mouth and nose with a bulb syringe to clear the airway. Perform suction after the head appears but before the next contraction. The next contraction delivers the shoulders and chest. The birth canal prevents chest expansion and minimizes the risk

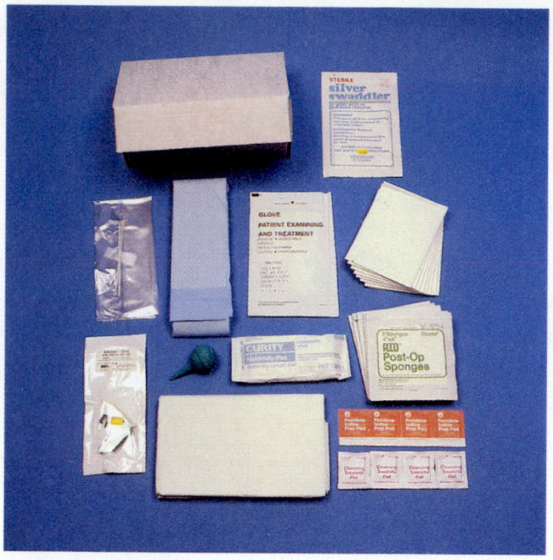

FIGURE 42-9 ■ Prehospital delivery equipment.

of aspiration if suction is performed well before the first breath, which usually occurs on delivery of the chest and shoulders.

5. Support the infant's head as it rotates for shoulder presentation. Most infants present face down. Then the infant rotates to the left so that the shoulders present in an anterior-posterior position.
6. With gentle pressure, guide the infant's head downward to deliver the anterior shoulder and then upward to release the posterior shoulder. The rest of the infant is delivered quickly by smooth uterine contraction.
7. Be careful to grasp and support the infant as he or she emerges. Use care because the infant is slippery. Hold the infant firmly with his or her head dependent to aid drainage of secretions. Maintain the infant's position at or slightly above the level of the mother's vagina. This will prevent overtransfusion or undertransfusion of blood from the umbilical cord.
8. Clear the infant's airway of any secretions with sterile gauze, and repeat suction of the infant's nose and mouth.
9. Dry the infant with sterile towels, and cover the infant (especially the head) to reduce heat loss.
10. Record the infant's gender and time of birth.

CRITICAL THINKING

How do you think you will feel after delivering a healthy infant?

Evaluation of the Infant. After delivery, the paramedic should dry and cover the newborn to prevent heat loss and should position the newborn on the side or with padding under the back, clear the airway, and provide tactile stimulation to initiate respirations. The paramedic should continue suction as necessary. If there is no need for resuscitation, the paramedic should assign an **Apgar score** at 1 minute and 5 minutes to evaluate in the infant (Table 42-2). Criteria for computing the Apgar score include *appearance* (color), *pulse* (heart rate), *grimace* (reflex irritability to stimulation), *activity* (muscle tone), and *respiratory effort.* Each criterion is rated from 0 to 2. The numbers are added for a total Apgar score. The paramedic should never delay or interrupt resuscitation efforts to assign an Apgar score.

An Apgar score of 10 indicates that the infant is in the best possible condition, 7 to 9 indicates that the infant is slightly depressed (near normal), 4 to 6 indicates that the infant is moderately depressed, and 0 to 3 indicates that the infant is severely depressed. Most newborns have an Apgar score of 8 to 10 at 1 minute after birth. Newborns with an Apgar score of less than 6 generally require resuscitation; however, *the paramedic should not use the Apgar score to determine the need for resuscitation.*[5] (Neonatal resuscitation is presented in Chapter 44.)

Cutting the Umbilical Cord. After the paramedic delivers and evaluates the infant, the paramedic should clamp (or tie with umbilical tape) and cut the umbilical cord (Fig. 42-11). The paramedic should take the following steps to manage the umbilical cord:

1. Clamp the cord about 4 to 6 inches away from the infant in two places. Do not strip or milk the cord; doing so may lead to red blood cell destruction, polycythemia, and hyperbilirubinemia.
2. Cut between the two clamps with sterile scissors or a scalpel.
3. Examine the cut ends of the cord to ensure that there is no bleeding. If the cut end attached to the infant is bleeding, clamp the cord proximal to the previous clamp and reassess for bleeding. Do not remove the first clamp.
4. Handle the cord carefully at all times because it can tear easily.

Delivery of the Placenta. The placenta normally is delivered within 20 minutes of the infant. Thus transport should not be delayed for placental delivery. Sometimes referred to as the fourth stage of labor, placental delivery is characterized by episodes of contractions, a palpable rise of the uterus within the abdomen, lengthening of the umbilical cord protruding from the vagina, and a sudden gush of vaginal blood.

As the placenta is delivered, the mother should be told to bear down with contractions. The paramedic should hold the placenta with both hands and twist the placenta gently as it is delivered to help it fully separate from the uterine wall. (Never pull on the umbilical cord to assist with placental delivery.) When the placenta is expelled, the paramedic should place it in a plastic bag or other container. The placenta should be transported with the mother and infant to the receiving hospital. At the hospital the placenta will be examined for abnormality and completeness. Pieces of placenta retained in the uterus can cause persistent hemorrhage and infection.

After the delivery of the placenta, the paramedic should assess the perineum for tears. If tears are present, the paramedic should manage them by applying sanitary napkins to the area and maintaining direct pressure. The paramedic

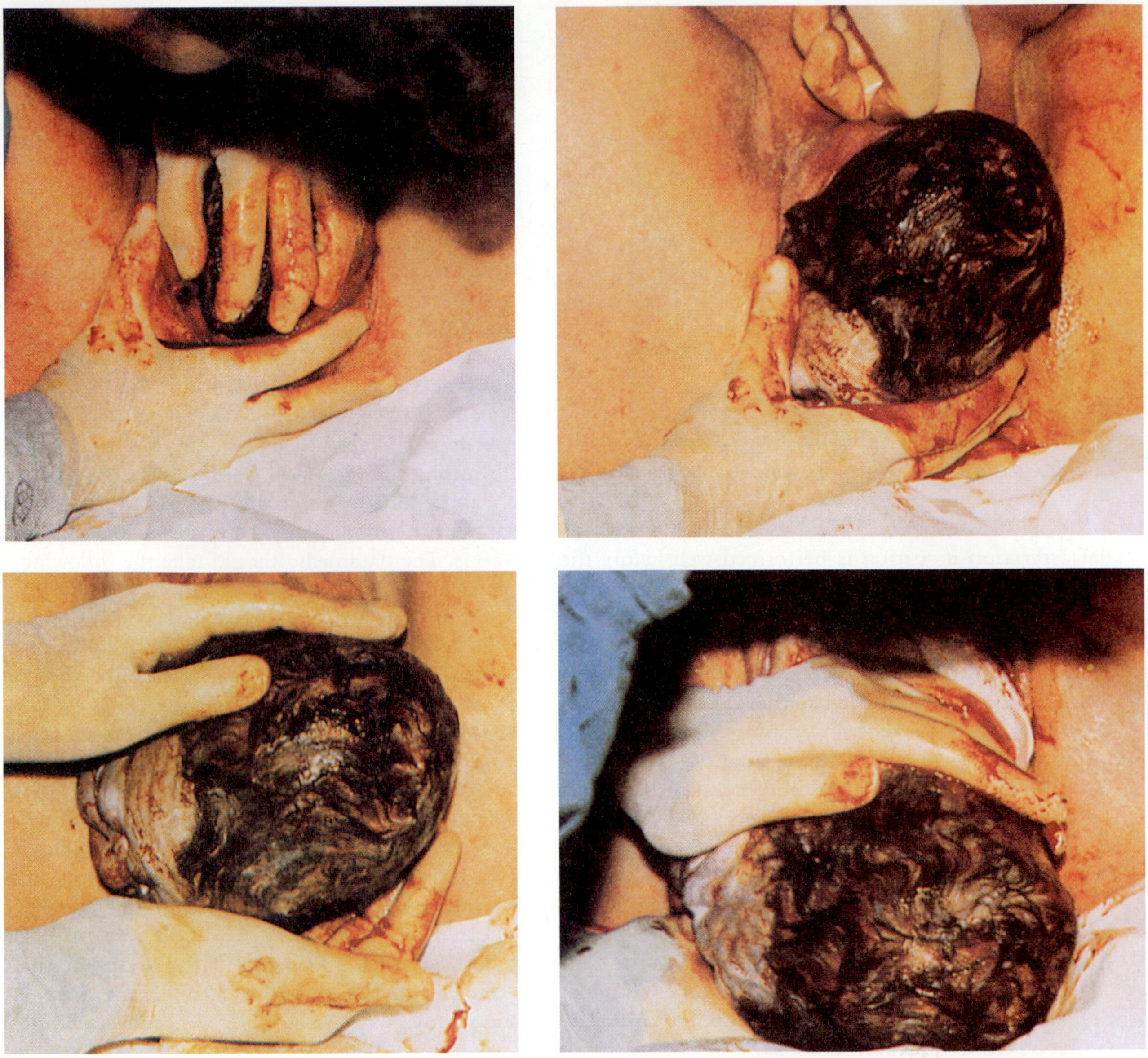

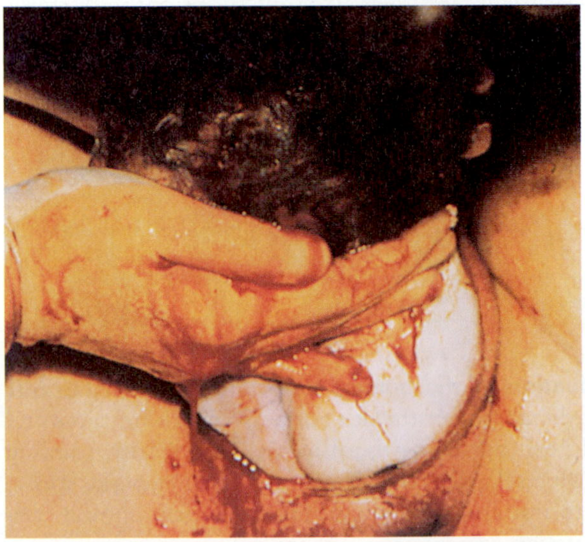

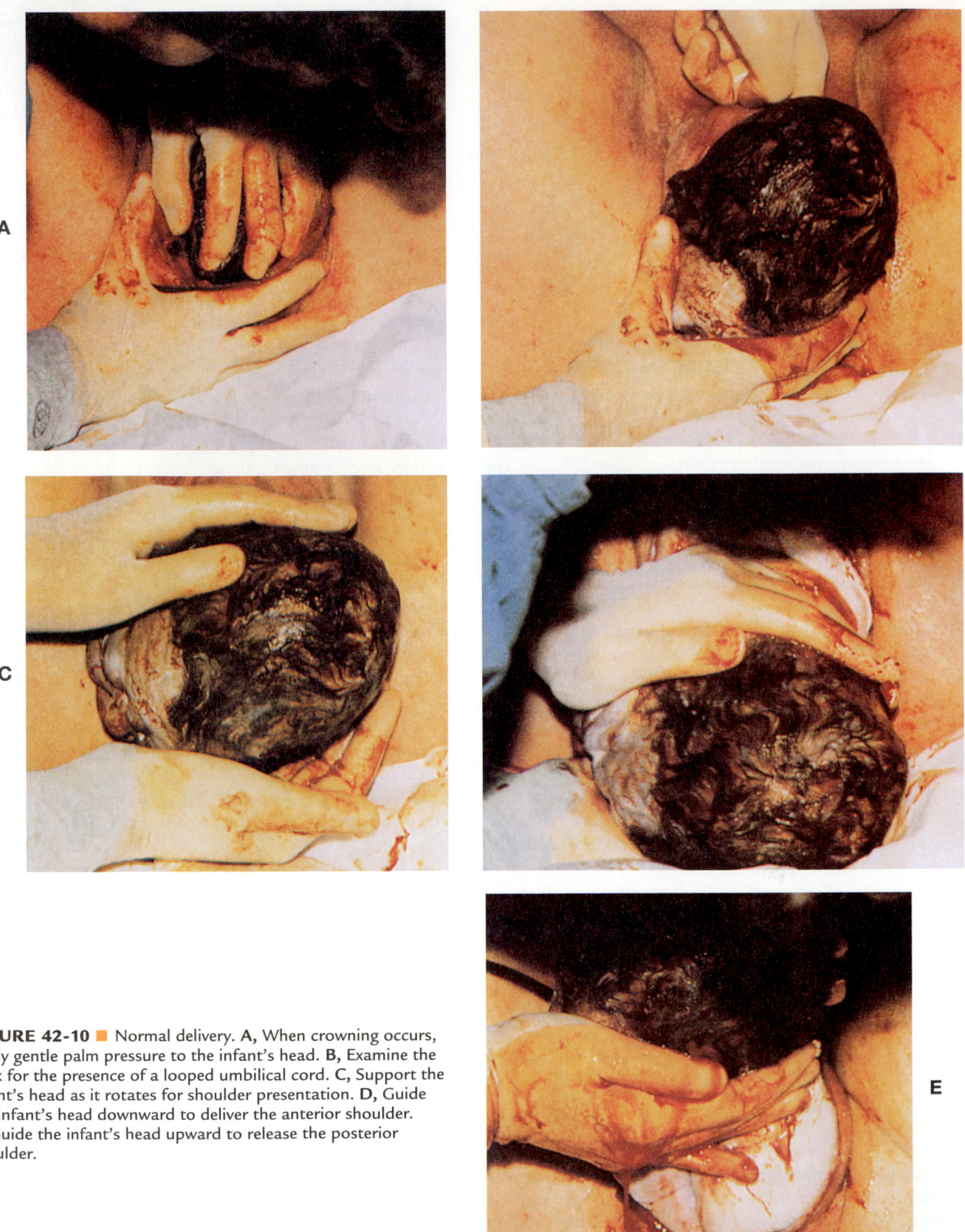

FIGURE 42-10 ■ Normal delivery. **A,** When crowning occurs, apply gentle palm pressure to the infant's head. **B,** Examine the neck for the presence of a looped umbilical cord. **C,** Support the infant's head as it rotates for shoulder presentation. **D,** Guide the infant's head downward to deliver the anterior shoulder. **E,** Guide the infant's head upward to release the posterior shoulder.

TABLE 42-2 The Apgar Scoring System

SIGN	0	1	2
Appearance (skin color)	Blue, pale	Body pink, blue extremities	Completely pink
Pulse rate (heart rate)	Absent	<100/minute	>100/minute
Grimace (irritability)	No response	Grimace	Cough, sneeze, cry
Activity (muscle tone)	Limp	Some flexion	Active motion
Respirations (respiratory effort)	Absent	Slow, irregular	Good, crying

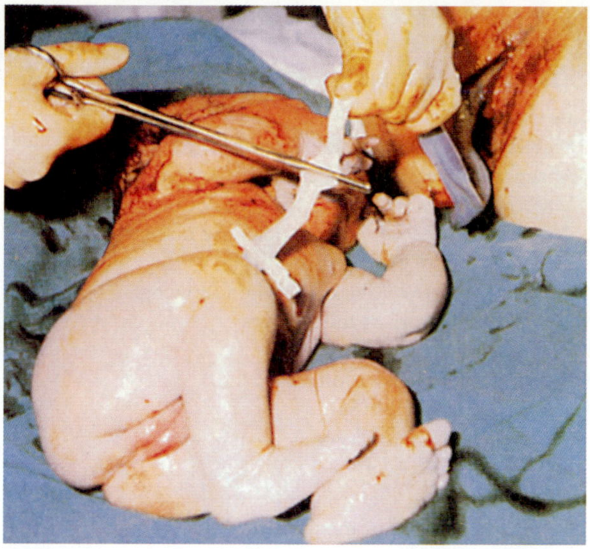

FIGURE 42-11 ■ After delivery and evaluation of the infant, the paramedic clamps and cuts the cord.

should monitor the mother closely during transport for signs of hemorrhage or shock and initiate fundal massage to promote uterine contraction. Medical direction may prescribe ***oxytocin*** to manage postpartum hemorrhage as well.

Postpartum Hemorrhage. Postpartum hemorrhage is characterized by more than 500 mL of blood loss after the delivery of the newborn. Hemorrhage often occurs within the first few hours after delivery. Yet it can be delayed up to 24 hours. Postpartum hemorrhage occurs in about 5% of all deliveries. Hemorrhage often results from ineffective or incomplete contraction of the interlacing uterine muscle fibers. Other causes of postpartum hemorrhage include retained pieces of placenta or membranes in the uterus. Hemorrhage also can be caused by vaginal or cervical tears during delivery (rare). Risk factors associated with postpartum hemorrhage include uterine atony (lack of tone) from prolonged or tumultuous labor, grand multiparity, twin pregnancy, placenta previa, and a full bladder.

Management. Postpartum hemorrhage can occur in the prehospital setting after a field delivery, home delivery, or delivery at an independent birthing center. The assessment and management are similar to those described for third-trimester bleeding. In addition, the paramedic should take the following six measures to encourage uterine contraction:

1. *Control external hemorrhage.* Manage external bleeding from perineal tears with firm pressure.
2. *Massage the uterus.* Palpate the uterus for firmness or loss of tone. If the uterus does not feel firm, apply fundal pressure by supporting the lower uterine segment with the edge of one hand just above the symphysis and massaging the fundus with the other hand. Continue massaging until the uterus feels firm. Reevaluate the patient every 10 minutes; note the location of the fundus in relation to the level of the umbilicus, the degree of firmness, and vaginal flow.
3. *Encourage the infant to breast-feed.* If the mother and infant are stable, place the newborn to her breast to encourage breast-feeding. Stimulation of the breasts may promote uterine contraction.
4. *Administer oxytocin.* Per medical direction and after ensuring that a second fetus is not present in the uterus, add 10 units of ***oxytocin*** to 1000 mL lactated Ringer's solution. Infuse at 20 to 30 drops/min via microdrip tubing (titrated to the severity of hemorrhage and uterine response or as ordered by medical direction). Continue with fluid resuscitation as indicated by the patient's vital signs.
5. Do not attempt a vaginal examination. Also, do not attempt vaginal packing to control hemorrhage.
6. Rapidly transport the patient for physician evaluation.

DELIVERY COMPLICATIONS

As stated before, most women have routine pregnancies. Prehospital deliveries seldom present any significant problems for the mother, newborn, or emergency crew. The delivery complications discussed in this chapter include cephalopelvic disproportion, abnormal presentation, premature birth, multiple gestation, precipitous delivery, uterine inversion, pulmonary embolus, and fetal membrane disorders. Box 42-7 lists factors that should alert the paramedic to anticipate an abnormal delivery.

Cephalopelvic Disproportion

Cephalopelvic disproportion is a condition in which the newborn's head is too large or the mother's birth canal is too small to allow normal labor or birth. The mother often is primigravida and having strong, frequent contractions for a prolonged period. This condition requires a cesarean delivery to be performed because rupture of the uterus and fetal death are possible. Prehospital care is limited to maternal oxygen administration, IV access for fluid resuscitation if needed, and rapid transport to the receiving hospital.

BOX 42-7 Factors Associated with High Risk of Abnormal Delivery

Maternal Factors

- Maternal age: very young or very old
- Absence of prenatal care
- Maternal lifestyle: alcohol, tobacco, or drug usage
- Preexisting maternal illness, including diabetes, chronic hypertension, or Rh sensitization
- Previous obstetrical history of the following:
  Premature delivery or miscarriage
  Perinatal loss
  Previous malformed neonate
  Previous multiple births
  Previous cesarean delivery
- Intrapartum disorders
  Preeclampsia
  Prolonged rupture of membranes
  Prolonged labor
  Abnormal presentation
  Abruptio placentae
  Placenta previa

Fetal Factors

- Lack of fetal well-being
  History of decreased fetal movement
  History of heart rate abnormalities
  Evidence of fetal distress
- Fetal immaturity: prematurity as established by dates, ultrasound, uterine size, amniocentesis
- Fetal growth: history of poor intrauterine growth or post-date delivery
- Specific fetal malformation detected by ultrasound: diaphragmatic hernia or omphalocele

Abnormal Presentation

Most infants are born head first (cephalic or vertex presentation). But sometimes a presentation is abnormal. These include a breech presentation, shoulder dystocia, shoulder presentation, and a cord presentation (prolapsed umbilical cord).

BREECH PRESENTATION

In breech presentations the largest part of the fetus (the head) is delivered last. Breech presentation occurs in 3% to 4% of deliveries at term. Breech presentation is more frequent with multiple births and when labor occurs before 32 weeks' gestation. Categories of breech presentation include the following (Fig. 42-12):

- *Front or frank breech.* The fetal hips are flexed and the legs extend in front of the fetus. The buttocks are the presenting part. Frank breech accounts for about 60% of breech presentations.
- *Complete breech.* The fetus has both knees and hips flexed. The buttocks are the presenting part. Complete breech accounts for about 5% of breech presentations.

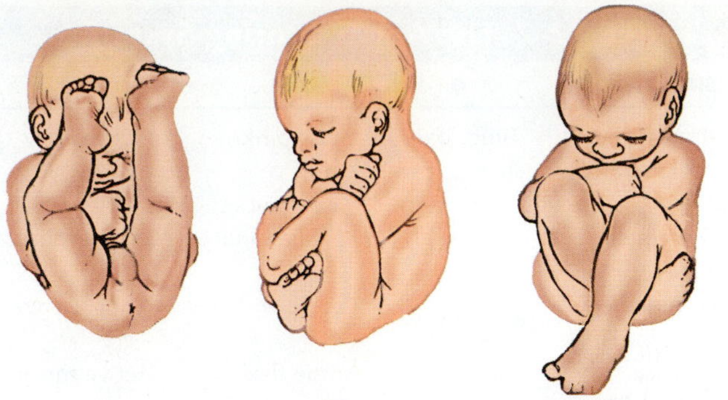

FIGURE 42-12 ■ Types of breech presentation. **A,** Front or back. **B,** Complete. **C,** Incomplete.

- *Incomplete breech.* The fetus has one or both hips incompletely flexed. This results in presentation of one or both lower extremities (often a foot). Incomplete breech accounts for about 30% of breech presentations.

CRITICAL THINKING

What resources can you use to assist in a delivery with an abnormal presentation?

Management. An infant in a breech presentation is best delivered in a hospital. In a hospital, emergency cesarean section is an alternative to vaginal delivery. Sometimes, however, the paramedic must assist in a breech delivery. If delivery is imminent, the EMS crew should proceed as follows:

1. Prepare the mother for delivery as described before.
2. Provide supplemental oxygen and IV access; continuously monitor the fetal heart rate.
3. Allow the fetus to deliver spontaneously up to the level of the umbilicus. If the fetus is in a front presentation, gently extract the legs downward after the buttocks are delivered.
4. After the infant's legs are clear, support his or her body with the palm of the hand and volar surface of the arm.
5. After the umbilicus is visible, gently extract a 4- to 6-inch loop of umbilical cord to allow delivery without excessive traction on the cord. Gently rotate the fetus to align the shoulders in an anterior-posterior position. Continue with gentle traction until the axilla is visible.
6. Gently guide the infant upward to deliver the posterior shoulder.
7. Gently guide the infant downward to deliver the anterior shoulder.
8. Ensure that the fetal face or abdomen is turned away from the maternal symphysis.
9. Be aware that the head often is delivered without difficulty after shoulder delivery. Be careful to avoid excessive head and spine manipulation or traction.

If the head does not deliver immediately, the paramedic must take action to prevent suffocation of the infant. The paramedic should place a gloved hand in the vagina. The palm should be toward the infant's face, forming a V with the index and middle fingers on either side of the infant's nose. The vaginal wall should be gently pushed away from the infant's face until the head is delivered. If the head does not deliver within 3 minutes, the paramedic should maintain the infant's airway with the V formation. The mother should be transported rapidly to the hospital.

SHOULDER DYSTOCIA

Shoulder dystocia occurs when the fetal shoulders are wedged against the maternal symphysis pubis. This blocks shoulder delivery. In this presentation the head delivers normally but then pulls back tightly against the maternal perineum. The incidence of shoulder dystocia is small. However, shoulder dystocia increases greatly with increasing birth weight. (Up to 10% incidence occurs with birth weights of 10 lb or more.) Complications include brachial plexus damage, fractured clavicle, and fetal anoxia from cord compression.

Management. Shoulder dystocia delivery calls for dislodging one shoulder and then rotating the fetal shoulder girdle at an angle into the wider part of the pelvic opening. Because the shoulder is pressing against the pelvis, there is a potential for cord compression. Thus the paramedic should deliver the anterior shoulder immediately after the head. (This should be done before suctioning of the nares and mouth.) Several maneuvers can help the paramedic successfully deliver an infant when shoulder dystocia arises. The following steps represent one approach to shoulder dystocia:

1. Position the mother on her left side in a dorsal-knee-chest position. This increases the diameter of the pelvis.
2. Try to guide the infant's head downward to allow the anterior shoulder to slip under the symphysis pubis. Avoid excessive force or manipulation.
3. Gently rotate the fetal shoulder girdle at an angle to the wider pelvic opening. The posterior shoulder usually delivers without resistance. Medical direction may recommend that the paramedic try to deliver the posterior shoulder first. The paramedic can achieve this by rotating the posterior shoulder downward and into the left posterior quadrant. The anterior shoulder usually follows.
4. After delivery, continue with resuscitative measures as needed.

SHOULDER PRESENTATION

Shoulder presentation (transverse presentation) results when the long axis of the fetus lies perpendicular to that of the mother. This position usually results in the fetal shoulder lying over the pelvic opening. The fetal arm or hand may be the presenting part. This abnormal delivery occurs in only 0.3% of deliveries but occurs in 10% of second twins.

Management. Normal delivery of a shoulder presentation is not possible. The paramedic should provide the mother with adequate oxygen, ventilatory and circulatory support, and rapid transport to the hospital. A cesarean section is required whether the fetus is viable or not.

CORD PRESENTATION

Cord presentation occurs when the cord slips down into or out of the vagina after the amniotic membranes have ruptured. The umbilical cord is compressed against the presenting part of the fetus. This diminishes fetal oxygenation from the placenta. A prolapsed cord occurs in about 1 in every 200 pregnancies. The paramedic should suspect a prolasped cord when fetal distress is present. Predisposing factors include breech presentation, premature rupture of membranes (described later), a large fetus, multiple gestation, a long cord, and preterm labor.

Management. Fetal asphyxia can ensue rapidly if circulation through the cord is not reestablished and maintained until delivery. If the paramedic can see or feel the umbilical cord in the vagina, the paramedic should take the following steps:

1. Position the mother with hips elevated as much as possible. The Trendelenburg or knee-chest position may relieve pressure on the cord.
2. Administer oxygen to the mother.
3. Instruct the mother to pant with each contraction to prevent bearing down.
4. If help is available, apply moist sterile dressings to the exposed cord. This will minimize temperature changes that may cause umbilical artery spasm.
5. With a gloved hand, gently push the infant back into the vagina. Elevate the presenting part to relieve pressure on the cord. The cord may retract spontaneously. However, the paramedic should not try to reposition the cord.
6. Maintain this hand position during rapid transport to the hospital. The definitive treatment is a cesarean section.

OTHER ABNORMAL PRESENTATIONS

Other abnormal presentations include face or brow presentation and occiput posterior presentation. In these presentations the infant's head is delivered face up instead of face down. Face-up presentations result in increased risks to the fetus because of difficult labor and delivery. Sometimes the fetus has other associated abnormalities. These presentations may require cesarean section. Thus early recognition of potential complications, maternal support and reassurance, and rapid transport for definitive care are the goals of prehospital management.

Premature Birth

A premature infant is born before 37 weeks' gestation. Low birth weight (less than 2.5 kg [5.5 lb]) also determines prematurity, although the conditions are not synonymous. Premature deliveries occur in 6% to 9% of all pregnancies. After a preterm labor the newborn is at increased risk for hypothermia because of a large surface/mass ratio and for cardiorespiratory distress because the cardiovascular system is premature. Therefore these infants require special care and observation. After delivery, prehospital management for a premature infant includes the following:

- Keep the infant warm. Dry the infant, wrap the infant in a warm blanket, place the infant on the mother's abdomen, and cover the mother and infant.

- Frequently suction secretions from the infant's mouth and nares.
- Carefully monitor the cut end of the umbilical cord for oozing. If bleeding is present, manage as described before.
- Administer humidified free-flow oxygen through a makeshift oxygen tent. Aim oxygen flow toward the top of the tent; do not allow it to flow directly into the infant's face.
- Protect the infant from contamination. Don a mask and gown and minimize family member and bystander contact with the infant.
- Gently transport the mother and infant to the receiving hospital.

One should note that *tocolytic agents* (drugs used to inhibit labor) are used widely today by some mothers who are at risk for a premature birth. These drugs may be administered in the home setting. They include magnesium sulfate, ritodrine, terbutaline, indomethacin, and others. The paramedic should ask the patient about any recent medication use, including the use of tocolytic agents.

Multiple Gestation

A multiple gestation is a pregnancy with more than one fetus. Twins occur in 1 in 80 to 90 births (Box 42-8), and triplets occur in 1 in 8000 births.[1] Multiple gestation places more stress on the maternal system. Multiple gestation also is accompanied by an increased complication rate. Associated complications include premature labor and delivery (30% to 50% of twin deliveries are premature), premature rupture of membranes, abruptio placentae, postpartum hemorrhage, and abnormal presentation. A mother who has not had prenatal care is often unaware of her multiple pregnancy.

CRITICAL THINKING

Do you have enough supplies on your ambulance to manage more than one delivery?

DELIVERY PROCEDURE

First-twin delivery is identical to single delivery with the same presentation. However, up to 50% of second-twin deliveries are not in a normal presentation position. Fetuses are smaller in multiple births. Thus the breech presentation of the second twin usually does not pose any serious delivery issues.

After the delivery of the first twin, the paramedic should cut and clamp (or tie) the umbilical cord as usual. Within 5 to 10 minutes after delivery of the first twin, labor begins again. The delivery of the second twin usually occurs within 30 to 45 minutes. Medical direction may recommend transport before the delivery of the second twin. Usually both twins are born before the delivery of the placenta.

Infants in multiple births often are smaller than infants in single term births. The paramedic should give special attention to keeping these infants warm, well oxygenated, and free from unnecessary contamination as described for premature infants. Postpartum hemorrhage may be more severe after multiple births. Hemorrhage may require fluid resuscitation, uterine massage, and ***oxytocin*** infusion to control bleeding.

BOX 42-8 Twin Terminology

Fraternal twins result from the fertilization of two ova by two spermatozoa. Each fraternal twin has a separate placenta. Each also is separated by individual amniotic membranes. Fraternal twins are not identical in appearance. They are often of different gender.

Identical twins result from the fertilization of a single ovum. They may share a common placenta and amniotic sac or have separate placental structures. Identical twins are less common than fraternal twins. (They occur in one out of three twin conceptions.) Unlike fraternal twins, identical twins look alike, are of the same gender, and are genetically identical.

Precipitous Delivery

A precipitous delivery is a rapid spontaneous delivery with less than 3 hours from onset of labor to birth. Delivery results from overactive uterine contractions and little maternal soft tissue or bony resistance. A precipitous delivery most often occurs in a mother who is grand multipara. It can be associated with soft tissue injury and uterine rupture (rare). Precipitous delivery has an increased perinatal mortality rate because of trauma and hypoxia. The main danger to the fetus during this kind of delivery is from cerebral trauma or tearing of the umbilical cord.

If the paramedic expects a precipitous delivery, the paramedic should try to prevent an explosive one. The paramedic can do this by providing gentle counterpressure to the infant's head; however, the paramedic should not attempt to detain fetal head descent. After the delivery the paramedic should keep the infant dry and warm to prevent heat loss and should examine the mother for perineal tears. These tears often accompany a rapid birth.

Uterine Inversion

Uterine inversion is an infrequent complication of childbirth. Yet uterine inversion is a serious condition. It occurs in about 1 in 2100 deliveries. With this condition the uterus turns inside out.

Uterine inversion may occur suddenly after a contraction. It also may appear with increased abdominal pressure caused by coughing or sneezing. However, uterine inversion more often is caused by medical personnel or a medical procedure (iatrogenic). It can result from excessive pulling on the umbilical cord and fundal massage. The risk is higher when the placenta has implanted high in the uterus. Uterine inversion is incomplete if the top of the uterus does not protrude through the cervix. Uterine inversion is complete if the entire uterus protrudes through the cervical opening. Signs and symptoms of uterine inversion include postpartum hemorrhage and sudden and severe lower abdominal pain. The hemorrhage may be profuse. Hypovolemic shock may develop quickly.

MANAGEMENT

Prehospital care for a patient with uterine inversion includes airway, ventilatory, and circulatory support and rapid transportation for physician evaluation. Medical direction may recommend that the paramedic attempt manual replacement of the uterus only if the cervix has not yet constricted. The technique for manual replacement is as follows:

1. Place the patient in a supine position.
2. Do not attempt to remove the placenta, which will increase hemorrhage.
3. Apply pressure with the fingertips and palm of a gloved hand and push the fundus upward and through the cervical canal. If this is ineffective, cover all protruding tissues with moist sterile dressings and rapidly transport the patient.

Manual replacement of the uterus may be painful to the patient. Medical direction may indicate the use of analgesics. The paramedic should explain the need for the procedure to the patient.

Pulmonary Embolism

The development of pulmonary embolism during pregnancy, labor, or the postpartum period is one of the most common causes of maternal death. The embolus often results from a blood clot in the pelvic circulation (venous thromboembolism). Embolus more often is associated with cesarean section than vaginal delivery. The patient often has classic signs and symptoms. These include sudden dyspnea; sharp, focal chest pains; tachycardia; tachypnea; and sometimes hypotension. If the embolism occurs in the prehospital setting, emergency care should be focused on airway, ventilatory, and circulatory support; electrocardiogram monitoring; and rapid transportation for physician evaluation (see Chapter 30).

Fetal Membrane Disorders

The fetal membrane disorders discussed in this chapter include premature rupture of membranes and amniotic fluid embolism. Another fetal membrane disorder, meconium staining, is described in Chapter 43.

PREMATURE RUPTURE OF MEMBRANES

Premature rupture of the membranes is a rupture of the amniotic sac before the onset of labor. The condition is termed *premature* regardless of fetal age. Premature rupture occurs in about 1 in 10 pregnancies. At term, 70% of patients are in labor within 12 hours of premature rupture of the membranes, and 85% are in labor within 24 hours.[1] Signs and symptoms include a history of a trickle or sudden gush of fluid from the vagina. The paramedic should transport patients for physician evaluation. The medical facility will prepare for delivery if the patient begins labor. Delivery is required if an infection of fetal membranes is diagnosed. (This is called chorioamnionitis.)

Chorioamnionitis is linked to premature rupture of membranes occurring 24 hours before labor begins. It also can occur with a prolonged labor. The infection generally is accompanied by maternal fever, chills, and uterine pain. Infection is treated with antibiotics. The best treatment for this infection is the delivery of the fetus.

AMNIOTIC FLUID EMBOLISM

When amniotic fluid enters the maternal circulation during labor or delivery or immediately after delivery, an amniotic fluid embolism can occur. Probable routes of entry include lacerations of the endocervical veins during cervical dilation, the lower uterine segment or placental site, and uterine veins at sites of uterine trauma. Particulate matter in the amniotic fluid (e.g., meconium, lanugo hairs, and fetal squamous cells) forms an embolus and obstructs the pulmonary vasculature. Amniotic fluid embolism is rare, occurring in 1 in 20,000 to 30,000 deliveries.[1] The condition most often is seen in multiparous women late in the first stage of labor. Other conditions that can increase the incidence of this severe complication are placenta previa, abruptio placentae, and intrauterine fetal death. The maternal mortality rate is near 90%.

The signs and symptoms of amniotic fluid embolism are the same as those described for pulmonary embolism. They may include cardiopulmonary arrest. These patients are managed with airway, ventilatory, and circulatory support; fluid resuscitation; and rapid transportation.

SUMMARY

- The placenta is a disklike organ. The placenta is composed of interlocking fetal and maternal tissues. The placenta is the organ of exchange between the mother and fetus. Blood flows from the fetus to the placenta through two umbilical arteries. These arteries carry deoxygenated blood. Oxygenated blood returns to the fetus through the umbilical vein. The amniotic sac is a fluid-filled cavity. It completely surrounds and protects the embryo.
- The developing ovum is known as an embryo during the first 8 weeks of pregnancy. After that time and until birth it is called a fetus. Gestation (fetal development) usually averages 40 weeks from the time of fertilization to the delivery of the newborn.
- The pregnant woman undergoes many physiological changes that affect the genital tract, breasts, gastrointestinal system, cardiovascular system, respiratory system, and metabolism.

Continued

- The patient history should include obstetrical history; presence of pain; presence, quantity, and character of vaginal bleeding; presence of abnormal vaginal discharge; presence of bloody show; current general health and prenatal care; allergies and medicines taken; and maternal urge to bear down.
- The goal in examining an obstetrical patient is to identify rapidly any acute life-threatening conditions. A part of this involves identifying imminent delivery. Then the paramedic must take the proper management steps. In addition to the routine physical examination, the paramedic should assess the abdomen, uterine size, and fetal heart sounds.
- If birth is not imminent, the paramedic should limit prehospital care for the healthy patient. Care should be limited to basic treatment modalities. It should include transport for physician evaluation as well.
- Causes of fetal death from maternal trauma include death of the mother, separation of the placenta, maternal shock, uterine rupture, and fetal head injury.
- Preeclampsia occurs after 20 weeks' gestation. The criteria for diagnosis include hypertension, proteinuria, and excessive weight gain with edema. Eclampsia is characterized by the same signs and symptoms with the addition of seizures or coma.
- Vaginal bleeding during pregnancy can result from abortion (miscarriage), ectopic pregnancy, abruptio placentae, placenta previa, uterine rupture, or postpartum hemorrhage. Abortion is the termination of pregnancy from any cause before 20 weeks' gestation. Ectopic pregnancy occurs when a fertilized ovum implants anywhere other than the uterus. Abruptio placentae is partial or complete detachment of the placenta at more than 20 weeks' gestation. Placenta previa is placental implantation in the lower uterine segment partially or completely covering the cervical opening. Uterine rupture is a spontaneous or traumatic rupture of the uterine wall.
- The first stage of labor begins with the onset of regular contractions. It ends with complete dilation of the cervix. The second stage of labor is measured from full dilation of the cervix to delivery of the infant. The third stage of labor begins with delivery of the infant and ends when the placenta is expelled and the uterus has contracted.
- One of the primary responsibilities of the EMS crew is to prevent an uncontrolled delivery. The other is to protect the infant from cold and stress after birth.
- Criteria for computing the Apgar score include appearance (color), pulse (heart rate), grimace (reflex irritability), activity (muscle tone), and respiratory effort.
- More than 500 mL of blood loss after the delivery of the newborn is called a postpartum hemorrhage. It often results from ineffective or incomplete contraction of the uterus.
- Paramedics should be alert to factors that point to a possible abnormal delivery.
- Cephalopelvic disproportion produces a difficult labor because of the presence of a small pelvis, an oversized uterus, or fetal abnormalities. Most infants are born head first (cephalic or vertex presentation). However, sometimes a presentation is abnormal. In breech presentation the largest part of the fetus (the head) is delivered last. Shoulder dystocia occurs when the fetal shoulders press against the maternal symphysis pubis. This blocks shoulder delivery. Shoulder presentation (transverse presentation) results when the long axis of the fetus lies perpendicular to that of the mother. The fetal arm or hand may be the presenting part. Cord presentation occurs when the cord slips down into the vagina or presents externally.
- A premature infant is born before 37 weeks' gestation.
- A multiple gestation is a pregnancy with more than one fetus. Mutiple gestation is accompanied by an increased complication rate.
- A precipitous delivery is a rapid, spontaneous delivery with less than 3 hours from onset of labor to birth. The main danger to the fetus is from cerebral trauma or tearing of the umbilical cord.
- Uterine inversion is a rare and serious complication of childbirth. With this condition the uterus turns inside out.
- The development of pulmonary embolism during pregnancy, labor, or the postpartum period is one of the most common causes of maternal death.
- Premature rupture of the membranes is a rupture of the amniotic sac before the onset of labor, regardless of gestational age.
- An amniotic fluid embolism may occur when amniotic fluid enters the maternal circulation during labor or delivery or immediately after delivery.

REFERENCES

1. Rosen P, Barkin R: *Emergency medicine: concepts and clinical practice,* ed 4, St Louis, 1998, Mosby.
2. American Heart Association: Guidelines 2000 for cardiopulmonary resuscitation and emergency cardiovascular care, International Consensus on Science, *Circulation* 102(8):247, 2000.
3. US Department of Transportation, National Highway Traffic Safety Administration: *EMT-Paramedic national standard curriculum,* Washington, DC, 1998, The Department.
4. National Institutes of Health, National Institute of Child Health and Infant Development: Are you at risk for gestational diabetes? http://www.nichd.nih.gov/publications/pubs/gest_diabetes.htm#Whatisges. Accessed November 6, 2004.
5. American Heart Association: *Pediatric advanced life support,* Dallas, 1997, The Association.

PART NINE

IN THIS PART

CHAPTER 43 Neonatology

CHAPTER 44 Pediatrics

CHAPTER 45 Geriatrics

CHAPTER 46 Abuse and Neglect

CHAPTER 47 Patients with Special Challenges

CHAPTER 48 Acute Interventions for the Home Health Care Patient

CHAPTER

43

Neonatology

OBJECTIVES

Upon completion of this chapter, the paramedic student will be able to:

1. Identify risk factors associated with the need for neonatal resuscitation.
2. Describe physiological adaptations at birth.
3. Outline the prehospital assessment and management of the neonate.
4. Describe resuscitation of the distressed neonate.
5. Discuss postresuscitative management and transport.
6. Describe signs and symptoms and prehospital management of specific neonatal resuscitation situations.
7. Identify injuries associated with birth.
8. Describe appropriate interventions to manage the emotional needs of the neonate's family.

KEY TERMS

antepartum: The period before labor and delivery.
apnea: An absence of spontaneous respirations.
congenital anomalies: Defects that occur during fetal development.
diaphragmatic hernia: A herniation in the diaphragm caused by the improper fusion of structures during fetal development.
intrapartum: The period during labor and delivery.
meconium staining: The inhalation of meconium by the fetus or newborn; this can block air passages and result in failure of the lungs to expand or cause other pulmonary dysfunction.
neonate: An infant in the first 28 days of life.
newborn: An infant in the first few hours of life.
preterm infant: An infant born before 37 weeks of gestation.

About 6% of infants born in U.S. hospitals require resuscitation immediately after birth, and this figure is believed be much higher in the prehospital setting.[1] This chapter addresses risk factors that may lead to the need for resuscitation in this patient group. It also describes initial patient care that may be required for the newborn and neonate.

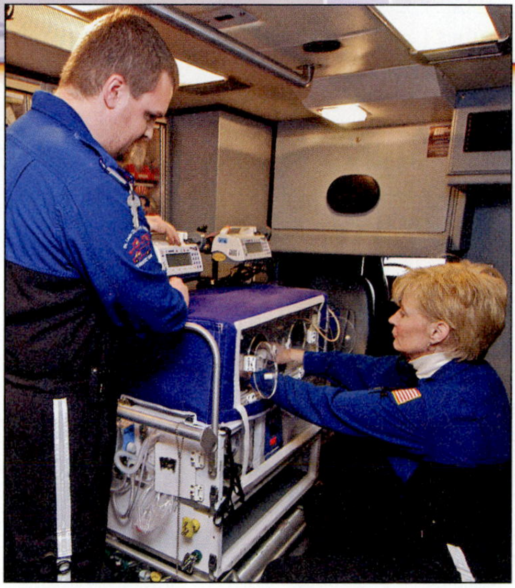

RISK FACTORS ASSOCIATED WITH THE NEED FOR RESUSCITATION

The vast majority of term newborns require no resuscitation beyond maintenance of temperature, suctioning of the airway, and mild stimulation.[2] The incidence of complications, however, increases as birth weight decreases. In fact, resuscitation is required for about 80% of the 30,000 babies who weigh less than 1500 g (3.12 lb) at birth.[3]

The average term **newborn** weighs about 3600 g (7.5 lb). The baby's birth weight depends on a number of factors. These include the size and racial origin of the parents. For example, small parents tend to have small babies. Also, Asian babies tend to be smaller than Caucasian babies. Newborn boys usually weigh about 8 oz more than do baby girls. Causes of low birth weight include premature birth, undernourishment in the uterus, and certain maternal factors. These factors include, for example, preeclampsia and cigarette smoking during pregnancy.

In addition to low birth weight, various **antepartum** (before labor and delivery) and **intrapartum** (during labor and delivery) risk factors may affect the need for resuscitation; these include the following[1] (the obstetric history is presented in Chapter 42):

- Antepartum
  - Multiple gestation
  - Inadequate prenatal care
  - Mother's age (less than age 16 or older than age 35)
  - History of perinatal morbidity or mortality
  - Postterm gestation
  - Drugs/medications
  - Toxemia, hypertension, diabetes
- Intrapartum
  - Premature labor
  - Meconium-stained amniotic fluid
  - Rupture of membranes greater than 24 hours before delivery
  - Use of narcotics within 4 hours of delivery
  - Abnormal presentation
  - Prolonged labor or precipitous delivery
  - Prolapsed cord
  - Bleeding

When any of the foregoing risk factors are present during delivery, the paramedic should prepare equipment and drugs that may be needed for neonatal resuscitation (Box 43-1). The paramedic also should advise medical direction of the situation so the appropriate destination hospital can be determined.

CRITICAL THINKING

Does your ambulance have the right size equipment for resuscitation of the newborn?

Congenital Anomalies

Congenital anomalies are defects that occur during fetal development. (They develop usually within the first trimester.) They are present in about 2% of all births. These defects are responsible for nearly half of all deaths in new-

BOX 43-1 Neonatal Resuscitation Equipment and Drugs

In addition to a standard obstetrics kit, neonatal resuscitation equipment should include the following:

- Endotracheal tube stylets
- Endotracheal tubes (2.5, 3.0, 3.5, 4.0)
- Meconium aspirator attachment
- Laryngoscope blades (straight, 0, and 1)
- Laryngoscope handles
- Face masks (premature, newborn, and infant sizes)
- Orogastric/nasogastric tubes
- Multiple blankets
- Medications and fluids
  - Dextrose 10%
  - Epinephrine 1:10,000
  - Naloxone
  - Sodium bicarbonate (0.5 mEq/mL; 4.2% solution)
  - Volume expanders (normal saline, lactated Ringer's solution)
- Self-inflating bag (450 mL to 750 mL)
- Umbilical vessel catheterization equipment
- Suction catheters (5, 8, and 10 French)
- Syringes (1, 3, 10, and 20 mL)
- Three-way stopcocks

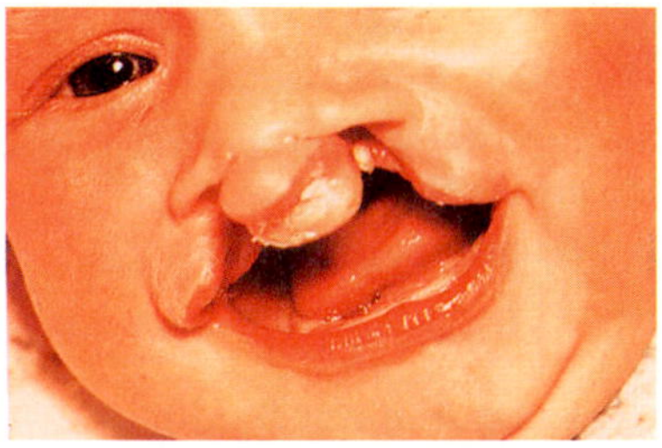

FIGURE 43-1 ■ Cleft lip.

borns. Thus the presence of congenital anomalies may be a factor in the need for neonatal resuscitation. Congenital anomalies may be associated with genetics, heredity, maternal infection, alcohol or other drug use during pregnancy, and other factors. Many types of congenital anomalies can occur. Some of the more common are the following:

Choanal atresia: A bony or membranous occlusion that blocks the passageway between the nose and pharynx; it can result in serious ventilation problems in the **neonate**

Cleft lip: One or more fissures that originate in the embryo; a vertical, usually off-center split in the upper lip that may extend to the nose (Fig. 43-1)

Cleft palate: A fissure in the roof of the mouth that runs along its midline; it may extend through the hard and soft palates into the nasal cavities

Diaphragmatic hernia: The protrusion of a part of the stomach through an opening in the diaphragm (described later in this chapter)

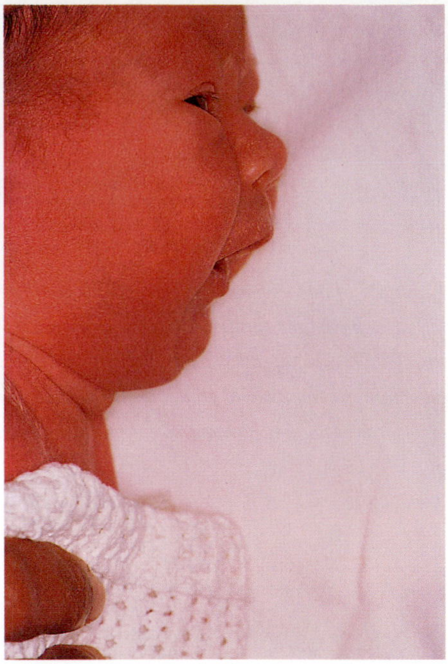

FIGURE 43-2 ■ Pierre Robin syndrome.

Pierre Robin syndrome: A complex of anomalies including a small mandible, cleft lip, cleft palate, other craniofacial abnormalities, and defects of the eyes and ears (Fig. 43-2).

PHYSIOLOGICAL ADAPTATIONS AT BIRTH

At birth, newborns make three major physiological adaptations necessary for survival: (1) emptying fluids from their lungs and beginning ventilation, (2) changing their circulatory pattern, and (3) maintaining body temperature.[4]

During vaginal delivery, the newborn's chest usually is compressed. This forces fluid from the lungs into the mouth and nose. As the chest wall recoils, air is drawn into the lungs. The newborn takes the first breath in response to chemical changes and changes in temperature.

When the cord is cut and placental circulation shuts down, the circulatory system must function on its own. This involves the immediate and permanent closure of the pathways that allowed the fetus to receive oxygen without the use of lungs (described in Chapter 42). As the lungs expand with initial breaths, the resistance to blood flow in the lungs decreases. At this time, the newborn's blood begins to be oxygenated.

Newborns are sensitive to hypoxia. Permanent brain damage will occur from prolonged hypoxemia. Causes of hypoxia include compression of the cord, difficult labor and delivery, maternal hemorrhage, airway obstruction, hypothermia, newborn blood loss, and immature lungs in the premature newborn.

Newborns are at great risk for rapidly developing hypothermia. Thus they should be delivered in a warm, draft-free area when possible. This risk factor is due to their larger body surface area, decreased tissue insulation, and immature temperature regulatory mechanisms. The cool, wet environment of birth also increases heat loss for the newborn. Newborns try to conserve body heat through vasoconstriction and increasing their metabolism. This places them at risk for hypoxemia, acidosis, bradycardia, and hypoglycemia.

ASSESSMENT AND MANAGEMENT OF THE NEONATE

The initial steps of neonatal resuscitation (with the exception of infants born through meconium, described below.[3] These steps enable the paramedic to recognize immediately an infant in need of resuscitation and leads to efficient and effective emergency care delivery (Fig. 43-3):

1. Prevent heat loss and avoid hypothermia.
2. Clear the airway by positioning and suctioning.
3. Provide stimulation by rubbing or patting the baby, and initiate breathing if needed.
4. Further evaluate the infant.

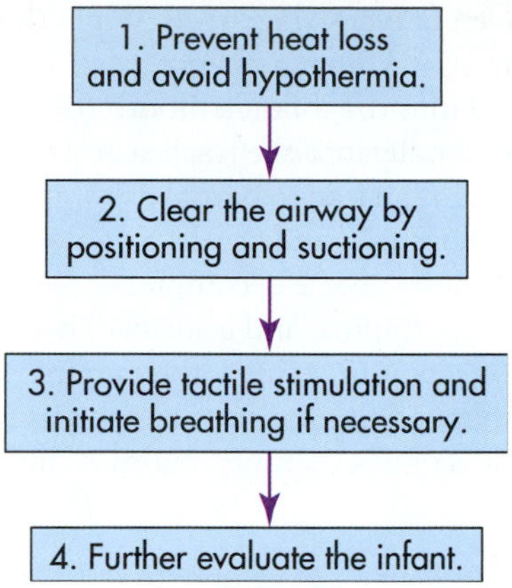
1. Prevent heat loss and avoid hypothermia.
2. Clear the airway by positioning and suctioning.
3. Provide tactile stimulation and initiate breathing if necessary.
4. Further evaluate the infant.

FIGURE 43-3 ■ Steps in neonatal resuscitation.

> **NOTE** Body substance isolation precautions should be used during delivery of a newborn. Gloves, gowns, and goggles should be worn when handling the newborn or contaminated equipment.

Prevention of Heat Loss and Hypothermia

Even healthy term newborns are limited in their ability to conserve heat when exposed to cold. They can develop hypothermia. Therefore immediately after delivery, the paramedic should dry the infant's body and head to prevent evaporative heat loss and metabolic problems that may be brought on by cold stress. (Cold stress can increase oxygen consumption and impede effective breathing.) Hypothermia can be associated with perinatal respiratory depression. The act of drying also provides gentle stimulation. Drying may initiate or help maintain respirations. The paramedic also should take care to remove any wet coverings from the infant and cover the infant with dry wrappings. The majority of heat loss can be prevented by covering the newborn's head. (The head accounts for 20% of the newborn's body surface area.)

> **CRITICAL THINKING**
> What other measures can you take to warm the infant?

Opening the Airway

After the newborn has been dried and covered, the next step is to establish an open airway. The paramedic opens the airway by correctly positioning the infant and suctioning secretions from the mouth and nose. The paramedic should place the neonate on the back or side. The head should be in a neutral (or slightly extended) position. The paramedic should take care to prevent hyperextension or underextension. These may compromise the airway. Placing a blanket or towel under the infant's shoulders (thereby elevating the torso ¾ to 1 inch) can help maintain the correct position.

> **CRITICAL THINKING**
> Do infants breathe through their noses or mouths?

Once the infant has been properly positioned, the paramedic should suction secretions from mouth and nose with a bulb syringe. The mouth should be suctioned first. This prevents aspiration in case the infant gasps when the nose is cleared of secretions. Each application of suction should last no more than 5 seconds to prevent hypoxia.

The paramedic should be careful to avoid deep or vigorous suctioning. Stimulation of the throat can produce a vagal response with resulting bradycardia, **apnea,** or both. The paramedic should monitor the newborn's heart rate during suctioning. The paramedic should provide time between suctioning attempts for spontaneous ventilation or assisted ventilation with 100% oxygen. Like drying, suctioning provides a degree of tactile stimulation that may initiate breathing.

MECONIUM STAINING

Meconium staining is the presence of fetal stool in the amniotic fluid. (It occurs in utero or intrapartum.) The condition occurs in about 12% of all deliveries. Meconium staining is more common in postterm and small-for-gestational-age newborns. It also is more common in those infants who develop fetal distress during labor and delivery. Meconium staining is associated with increased perinatal mortality, hypoxemia, aspiration pneumonia, pneumothorax, and pulmonary hypertension.

The appearance of meconium depends on the amount of meconium particles and amniotic fluid. Meconium staining may appear as only a slight yellow or light green staining that is thin and watery. Or it may have a thick pea soup appearance that is dark green or black (Fig. 43-4). When thick meconium is present in amniotic fluid, a chance exists that the particles will be aspirated into the infant's mouth (often with the first breath) and potentially into the trachea and lungs. Aspiration of thick meconium can lead to partial or complete obstruction of the airways, atelectasis, and the development of pneumothorax that may require needle decompression. Death can result from hypoxia, hypercapnia, and acidosis. Therefore when amniotic fluid is meconium stained, the paramedic should suction the mouth, pharynx, and nose as soon as the head is delivered (regardless of whether meconium is thin or thick).[6]

> **NOTE** Meconium can be used to test for maternal drug use. It has a greater sensitivity than urine and positive findings that persist longer. If time permits, a specimen should be collected and delivered to the emergency department.

After meconium is observed in the amniotic fluid, the goal is to prevent or lessen the risk of aspiration by the newborn. The presence of meconium can be determined only after the membranes have ruptured. Thus it is critical that the right equipment be available. The EMS crew must be organized to act instantly as well. Emergency care includes the following steps:

1. Prepare the necessary equipment (e.g., intubation equipment, bulb syringe and DeLee suction, 12 French or larger suction catheter, portable suction and irrigation solution, gauze pads, infant bag-valve device). Intubation equipment should include padding for patient positioning, stethoscope, number 0 and number 1 laryngoscope blades, endotracheal tubes (2.5, 3.0, 3.5, 4.0), stylet, meconium aspirator, and oxygen tubing. The procedure for endotracheal intubation is described in Chapter 19.
2. After the baby's head is delivered (and before shoulder delivery), clear the infant's airway. Thoroughly suction secretions from the nose, mouth, and pharynx before stimulating the infant to breathe.

> **CRITICAL THINKING**
> Why would you want to intubate and suction meconium before the infant's first breath?

3. After delivery of the infant, remove residual meconium in the hypopharynx by suction under direct visualization.
4. If the neonate is depressed (absent or depressed respirations, decreased muscle tone, heart rate less than 100 beats/min), quickly intubate the trachea. (This should be done preferably before the baby has taken a first breath.) Apply suction to the proximal end of the endotracheal tube while withdrawing the tube. During intubation and suction, aim 100% oxygen toward the infant's face. At the same time, monitor the fetal heart rate for bradycardia. If bradycardia develops, ventilate the infant using a bag-valve device after suctioning. This will help to prevent persistent bradycardia and hypoxia.

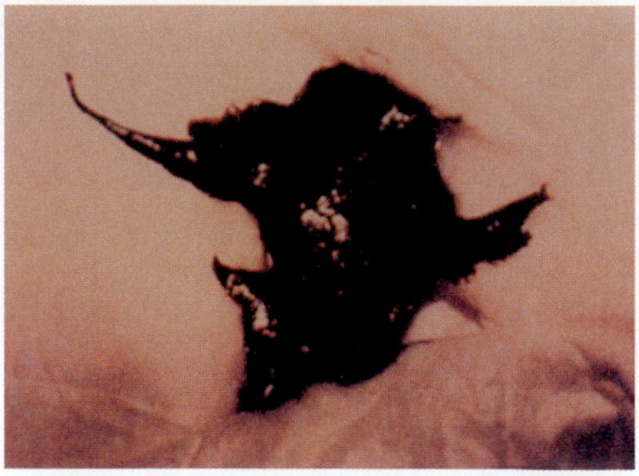

FIGURE 43-4 ■ Meconium-stained birth.

5. Repeat the intubation-suction-extubation cycle until no further meconium is suctioned. Do not ventilate between intubations.
6. After tracheal suction is complete, continue resuscitative measures as needed. If respirations are adequate, manage the infant's airway in the normal way. Medical direction may advise that an 8 French orogastric tube be inserted and left open to air. This may help prevent aspiration of gastric contents. Other considerations include preventing hypothermia, administering a fluid challenge to manage hypotension (if present), providing emotional support to the mother and family, and transporting the high-risk infant to an appropriate hospital.

Provision of Tactile Stimulation

If drying and suctioning do not induce breathing, the paramedic should provide more tactile stimulation. The two safe and proper ways of providing such stimulation are slapping or flicking the soles of the infant's feet and rubbing the infant's back. The infant still may not breathe after a brief time (5 to 10 seconds) of stimulation. In such a case, the paramedic should start positive-pressure ventilation immediately with a pediatric bag-valve device and supplemental oxygen (at 40 to 60 ventilations per minute).

Evaluation of the Infant

Drying, positioning, suctioning, and stimulating are necessary in every infant at birth. These actions help to clear the airway and initiate breathing. The next step in resuscitation depends on evaluation of the infant's respiratory effort, heart rate, and color. The following steps are suggested for monitoring and evaluating the newborn (Fig. 43-5):

1. Observe and assess the infant's respirations. If they are normal (e.g., crying), continue the evaluation. If breathing is poor or gasping is present, start positive-pressure ventilation immediately. If the respiratory response is slow or shallow, try a brief period of stimulation. At the same time, administer 100% oxygen. If no response is noted after 5 to 10 seconds of stimulation and oxygen, begin positive-pressure ventilation.
2. Evaluate the infant's heart rate by stethoscope, or palpate the pulse at the base of the umbilical cord. If the heart

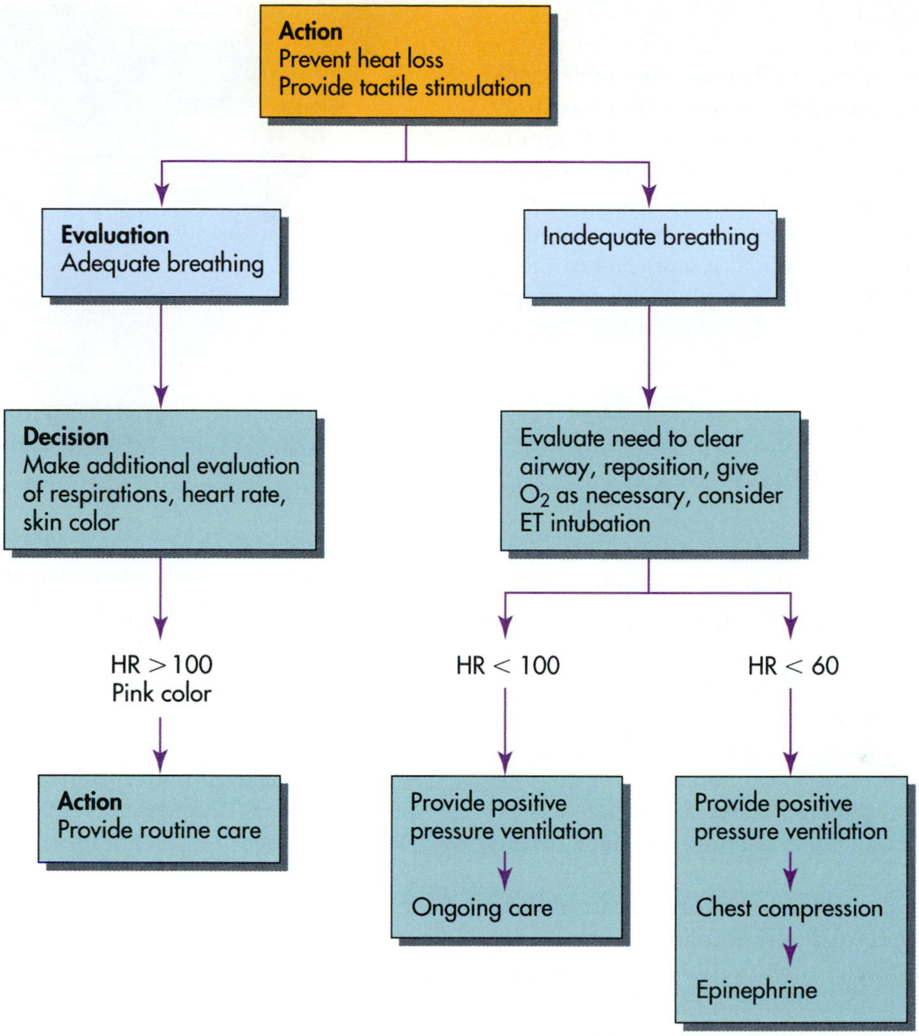

FIGURE 43-5 ■ Action-evaluation-decision cycle.

rate is greater than 100 beats/min, continue the evaluation. If the heart rate is less than 100 beats/min, begin positive-pressure ventilation. If the heart rate is less than 60 beats/min and does not increase despite 30 seconds of positive-pressure ventilation, coordinate chest compressions with ventilations at a ratio of 3:1 at a rate of 120 per minute. This will achieve about 90 compressions and 30 breaths per minute. Administer ***epinephrine*** if the heart rate remains 60 beats/min despite 30 seconds of assisted ventilations and chest compressions.[5]

> **NOTE** As described in Chapter 29, chest compression with two thumb-encircled hands is the preferred technique. This technique is used for chest compressions for newborn infants and older infants when size permits. Compressions should be performed on the lower third of the sternum. Depth of compression should be about one third of the anterior-posterior diameter of the chest and should be sufficiently deep to generate a palpable pulse.[5]

> **CRITICAL THINKING**
> Why would compressions be initiated when the infant still has a pulse?

3. Evaluate the infant's color. Peripheral cyanosis (acrocyanosis) is common in the first few minutes of life. Peripheral cyanosis is not indicative of hypoxemia. If, however, central cyanosis, bradycardia, or other signs of distress are present in a newborn infant with spontaneous respirations and an adequate heart rate, administer 100% oxygen while determining the need for more interventions. One hundred percent oxygen should be used. Potential long-term hazards, such as retinopathy, should not be a concern during this emergency. Free-flow oxygen can be given through a face mask and flow-inflating bag, an oxygen mask, or a hand cupped around oxygen tubing (held 2 inches from the infant's nose) using an oxygen flow rate of at least 5 L/min[5]. Give oxygen until the mucous membranes turn pink.

> **NOTE** Hypoxia is nearly always present in a newly born infant who requires resuscitation.[5]

APGAR SCORE

The Apgar score (described in Chapter 42) enables rapid evaluation of a newborn's condition at specific intervals after birth. The score routinely is assessed at 1 and 5 minutes of age. The Apgar score is a useful tool to evaluate the newborn. However, the Apgar score should not be used alone in determining the need for resuscitation. To review, an Apgar score of 7 to 10 is considered normal; a score of 4 to 6 identifies a moderately distressed infant who requires oxygen and stimulation; and a score less than 4 identifies a severely distressed infant who requires resuscitation.

RESUSCITATION OF THE DISTRESSED NEWBORN

As described before, risk factors associated with the need for resuscitation include premature delivery, maternal health problems, complicated pregnancies, and delivery complications. If with continued assisted ventilations the infant's condition continues to deteriorate or fails to improve, the infant may require endotracheal intubation and the administration of drugs (Fig. 43-6). Before the paramedic considers intubation or drug therapy, the paramedic should consider two aspects of the resuscitation process:

1. Is chest movement adequate? Check for the adequacy of chest expansion and auscultate for bilateral breath sounds.
   a. Is the bag-valve face mask seal tight? A relatively large mask should be turned upside down for a better fit.
   b. Is the airway blocked from improper head position or secretions in the nose, mouth, or pharynx? Reassess head position and reexamine the airway for the presence of secretions.
   c. Is adequate ventilatory pressure being used? A bag-valve-mask pop-off valve may need to be disabled to allow for higher inspiratory pressures, especially for premature or meconium-aspiration delivery.[2]
   d. Is air in the stomach interfering with chest expansion? Consider placing a nasogastric or orogastric tube per protocol.
2. Is 100% oxygen being administered?
   a. Is the oxygen tubing attached to the bag and flowmeter?
   b. If using a self-inflating bag, is the oxygen reservoir attached?

NOTE Endotracheal intubation may be indicated at several points during neonatal resuscitation.[5] These points include the following:

- When tracheal suctioning for meconium is required
- If bag-mask ventilation is ineffective or prolonged
- When chest compressions are performed
- When tracheal administration of medications is desired
- Special resuscitation circumstances (e.g., congenital diaphragmatic hernia or extremely low birth rate)

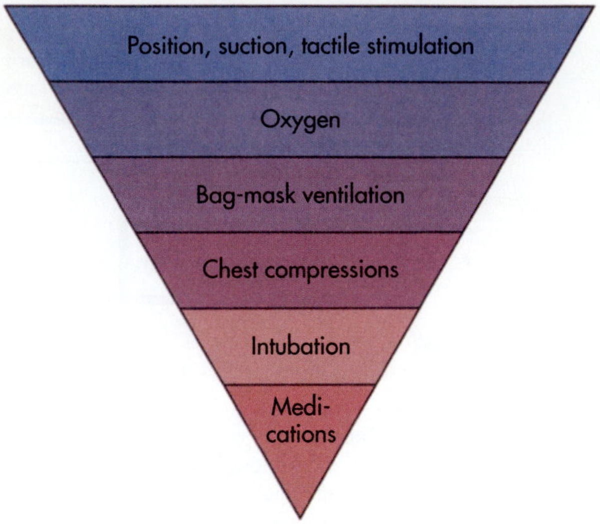

FIGURE 43-6 ■ Inverted pyramid reflecting the approximate relative frequency of neonatal resuscitative efforts. Note that a majority of infants respond to simple measures.

The paramedic should verify tube placement using primary and secondary confirmation methods. The laryngeal mask airway may be used to establish an airway in a newborn if bag-mask ventilation is ineffective or tracheal intubation has failed (Chapter 19).[5]

Routes of Drug Administration

Drugs rarely are indicated in the resuscitation of the newly born infant. As a rule, drugs should be administered only if the heart rate remains less than 60 beats/min despite adequate ventilation with 100% oxygen and chest compressions.[5] The tracheal route is usually the most rapidly accessible route during resuscitation; the umbilical vein is the most rapidly accessible venous route. Peripheral sites (scalp or peripheral vein) may be used. However, they are usually harder to cannulate. The intraosseous route is not used often in newborns. The umbilical vein is more accessible, the small bones are fragile, and the intraosseous space is small in a premature infant.

Accessing the Umbilical Vein

As described in Chapter 42, the umbilical cord contains three vessels: two arteries and one vein. The vein in the umbilical cord has a thin wall and is larger than the arteries. The arteries are thick walled and usually paired. To gain access to the umbilical vein, the paramedic should take the following steps (Fig. 43-7):

1. Set up intravenous (IV) fluid (per protocol) and tubing with a three-way stopcock.
2. Select a 3.5 or 5 French umbilical catheter.
3. Connect the catheter to the stopcock, and purge the air from the catheter.
4. Cleanse the umbilical stump and surrounding skin with antibacterial solution (per protocol).

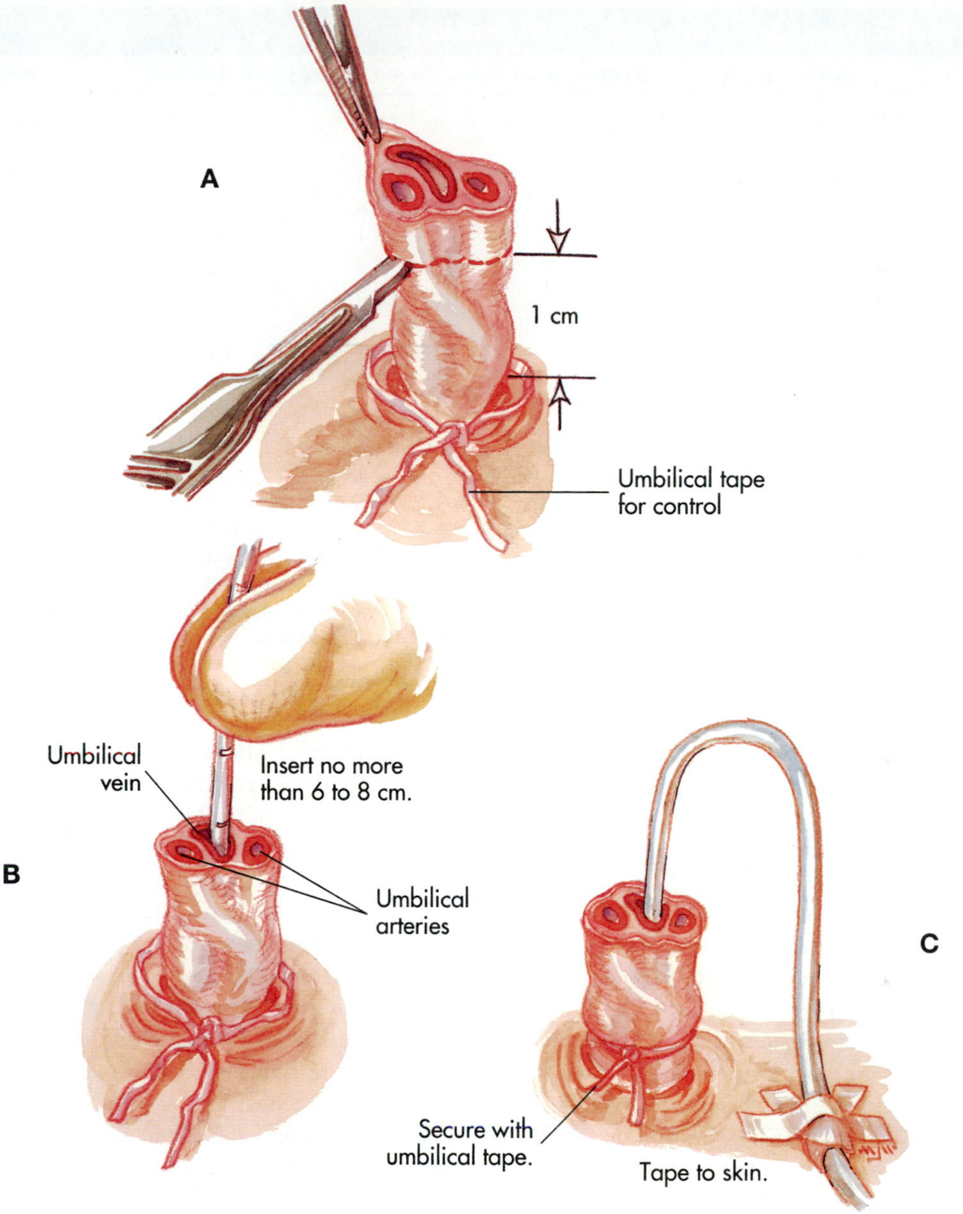

FIGURE 43-7 ■ Umbilical vein cannulation procedure. **A,** Identify the umbilical vein after trimming the cord. **B,** Insert the umbilical catheter or angiocatheter into the vein. **C,** Secure the base of the cord to hold the catheter in place and stabilize the catheter with tape.

5. Loosely tie umbilical tape around the cord near the body so that pressure can be applied to control bleeding.
6. Hold the umbilical stump firmly and trim (with a scalpel) the cord several centimeters above the abdomen.
7. Locate the umbilical vein and insert the catheter until blood is freely obtained. Do not insert the catheter more than 6 to 8 cm. If the catheter is inserted farther, there is a risk of infusing solutions directly into the liver rather than the systemic circulation. Take care to avoid introduction of air emboli into the umbilical vein.
8. Draw blood for a sample, if needed.
9. Start the infusion and regulate the fluid flow per medical direction.
10. Secure the catheter in place with tape and cover with a sterile dressing.
11. Document the procedure.

The umbilical cord also may be cannulated by using a typical IV catheter. Insert the catheter-over-needle through the side of the proximal end of the cord into the vein and advance it upward through the translucent wall. Start the infusion, adjust the fluid flow per medical direction, and secure the catheter in place with tape.

TABLE 43-1 Medications for Neonatal Resuscitation

MEDICATION	DOSE/ROUTE	CONCENTRATION	WEIGHT (KG)	TOTAL (ML)	PRECAUTIONS
Epinephrine	0.01-0.03 mg/kg IV or ET*	1:10,000	1	0.1-0.3	Give rapidly
			2	0.2-0.6	Repeat every 3-5 min.
			3	0.3-0.9	
			4	0.4-1.2	
Volume expanders	10 mL/kg IV over		1	10	Reassess after each bolus.
Normal saline	5-10 min		2	20	
Lactated Ringer's			3	30	
			4	40	
Naloxone	0.1 mg/kg IV, ET,	0.4 mg/mL	1	0.25	Repeat doses may be needed
	or IM/SQ if perfusion		2	0.50	to prevent apnea
	is adequate		3	0.75	
			4	1.00	
		1.0 mg/mL	1	0.1	Do not give if mother is
			2	0.2	suspected of abusing
			3	0.3	narcotics.
			4	0.4	

**Note:* The endotracheal tube dose may not result in effective plasma concentration of drug, so vascular access should be established as soon as possible. Drugs administered by endotracheal tube should be diluted to volume of 3 to 5 mL before instillation.
IM, Intramuscular; *ET,* endotracheal tube; *IV,* intravenous; *SQ,* subcutaneous.

Medications Used in Neonatal Resuscitation

Medications most frequently used during neonatal resuscitation are ***epinephrine,*** volume expanders, and ***naloxone***. (Table 43-1 lists the medications recommended by the American Heart Association and the American Academy of Pediatrics.) Important points to remember in neonatal resuscitation include the following:

- Prevent heat loss and avoid hypothermia.
- In the newly born infant with a heart rate greater than 100 beats/min and who is unresponsive to stimulation, the main concern is to ventilate the infant adequately.
- When meconium is observed in the amniotic fluid, deliver the head and suction the meconium from the hypopharynx on delivery of the head. If the neonate is distressed, perform direct tracheal suctioning to remove meconium from the airway.
- Provide chest compressions if the heart rate is absent or remains less than 60 beats/min despite adequate assisted ventilation with 100% oxygen for 30 seconds.
- Coordinate chest compressions with ventilations at a ratio of 3:1 and at a rate of 120 events per minute to achieve about 90 compressions and 30 breaths per minute.
- Administer epinephrine when the heart remains less than 60 beats/min despite 30 seconds of effective assisted ventilation and chest compressions.

POSTRESUSCITATION CARE

The three most common complications of the postresuscitation period are endotracheal tube migration (including dislodgment), tube occlusion by mucus or meconium, and pneumothorax.[2] These complications should be suspected in the presence of the following:

- Decreased chest wall movement
- Diminished breath sounds
- Return of bradycardia
- Unilateral decrease in chest expansion
- Altered intensity to pitch of breath sounds
- Increased resistance to hand ventilation

Corrective management in the field for these postresuscitative complications may include adjustment of the endotracheal tube (exhaled carbon dioxide devices are useful for monitoring tracheal tube placement), reintubation, and suction. Needle decompression to manage a suspected pneumothorax must be guided carefully by medical direction.

CRITICAL THINKING

How much movement would it take to dislodge an endotracheal tube from a neonate?

NEONATAL TRANSPORT

During transport of the neonate, it is important to maintain the infant's body temperature and prevent hypothermia. In addition, it is critical to maintain oxygen administration and to support the infant's ventilations. In the initial prehospital phase of care, transport strategies usually are limited to providing a warm ambulance, free-flow oxygen administration, covering the baby's head, and applying warm blankets to prevent hypothermic complications. Specialized transport equipment such as isolettes and radiant heating units often are used for interhospital

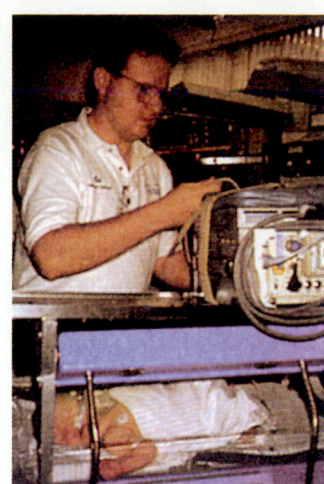

FIGURE 43-8 ■ Neonatal transport.

transfers. These devices require special training. Highly trained neonatal transport teams consisting of paramedics, nurses, respiratory therapists, and physicians are part of several well-organized regional referral systems throughout the United States (Fig. 43-8).

SPECIFIC SITUATIONS

Specific situations may call for advanced life support for the neonate. These situations include apnea, **diaphragmatic hernia,** bradycardia, prematurity, respiratory distress and cyanosis, hypovolemia, seizures, fever, hypothermia, hypoglycemia, vomiting and diarrhea, and common birth injuries. While providing advanced life support in these and other situations, the paramedic must consider the emotional needs of the mother and family. When possible, the paramedic should explain what is being done for the infant and why a procedure is necessary.

Apnea

Apnea is an absence of spontaneous respirations. *Primary apnea* is controlled by P_{CO_2} levels and is a self-limiting condition. Primary apnea is common right after birth. *Secondary apnea* is described as apnea that exceeds 20 seconds without spontaneous breathing occurring. This can lead to hypoxemia and bradycardia. Secondary apnea is common in the **preterm infant.** It often results from hypoxia or hypothermia. Secondary apnea also may be caused by conditions that include maternal use of narcotics or central nervous system depressants, prolonged or difficult labor and delivery, airway and respiratory muscle weakness, septicemia, metabolic disorders, and central nervous system disorders.

Emergency care for an infant with prolonged apnea begins with stimulating the infant to breathe. This is done by flicking the soles of the feet or rubbing the back. If needed, a bag-valve device (with a disabled pop-off valve) should be used. The paramedic should use the least amount of pressure that produces adequate chest rise. The paramedic should suction secretions from the infant's airway as needed and maintain the infant's body temperature to prevent hypothermia. Endotracheal intubation and circulatory support may be required if central cyanosis persists despite adequate ventilations. Drug therapy that may be appropriate in managing some infants with prolonged apnea includes ***dextrose*** (10% dextrose in water), if hypoglycemia is suspected or confirmed, and ***naloxone*** for reversal of respiratory depression in a newborn whose mother received narcotics within 4 hours of delivery.[5] (Narcotic antagonists should not be given to the infant if the mother is a drug abuser. Doing so may induce drug withdrawal in the neonate.) Apnea that is treated early and aggressively normally results in a good outcome.

Diaphragmatic Hernia

Diaphragmatic hernia is a rare condition. (It occurs in 1 of every 2200 live births.) Herniation is caused by a malformation of the diaphragm during fetal development. It may occur on the left, right, or both sides, but the left side is most common (90%). The hernia leaves a hole in the diaphragm muscle. This allows abdominal organs such as the stomach, bowels, kidney, liver, and spleen to enter into the thorax. The lung on the affected side cannot develop normally. This reduces lung capacity and can damage other organs, including the heart. Respiratory distress usually develops shortly after birth because the diaphragm cannot work properly. Crowding of the lungs by other organs also may cause the lungs to collapse. Diaphragmatic hernia is a true emergency that requires surgical repair. Newborns who do not survive usually die during the first days or weeks of life. (Survival for the infant who requires mechanical ventilation in the first 18 to 24 hours of life is about 50%. If there is no respiratory distress within the first 24 hours of life, survival approaches 100%.)[1] Assessment findings may include the following:

- Little to severe distress
- Cyanosis unresponsive to ventilations
- Scaphoid (flat) abdomen
- The presence of bowel sounds in the chest
- Displaced heart sounds

Prehospital care includes elevating the infant's head and thorax to assist with downward displacement of the abdominal organs, ensuring adequate oxygenation, providing ventilatory and circulatory support, and rapidly transporting the newborn to an appropriate hospital for definitive care. Medical direction may direct the placement of an orogastric tube, with low periodic suction to improve ventilations. In some cases, tracheal intubation may be needed. The use of a bag-valve device or aggressive positive pressure ventilation, however, may worsen the condition. It may cause gastric distention. Thus use of a bag-valve device is contraindicated.

Bradycardia

Bradycardia is described as a heart rate less than 100 beats/min. In the neonate, bradycardia most commonly is caused by hypoxia. It also may result from increased intracranial pressure, hypothyroidism, and acidosis. Other risk factors include prolonged suctioning and the use of airway or any invasive procedures during resuscitation. Bradycardia is a minimal risk to life in neonates if it is corrected quickly.

The initial management for a neonate with bradycardia is to assess for upper airway obstruction. Such obstruction may be caused by airway secretions, foreign body, or the position of the tongue or soft tissues of the neck. Prehospital care to improve ventilation may include airway positioning, suction, positive pressure ventilation with supplemental oxygen, and tracheal intubation. The paramedic should monitor ventilatory and circulatory status of the infant closely. This will determine the need for more advanced life support measures. Such measures may include chest compressions and drug therapy (described later in this chapter and in Chapter 44).

Prematurity

A **premature infant** refers to a baby who is born before 37 weeks of gestation. (The weight of these newborns often is between 0.6 to 2.2 kg ($1\frac{1}{2}$ to 5 lb). Healthy premature infants who weigh greater than 1700 g have a survivability and outcome about equal to that of full-term infants. The mortality rate decreases weekly with gestation beyond the onset of fetal viability (currently around 23 to 24 weeks of gestation).[1] Premature infants have an increased risk for respiratory depression, hypothermia, and brain injury from hypoxemia. They are also especially vulnerable to changes in blood pressure, intraventricular hemorrhage, and fluctuations in serum osmolarity. The degree of immaturity determines how the infant appears physically. However, most premature infants will have a large trunk, short extremities, less subcutaneous fat than full-term infants, and skin that appears translucent.

The prehospital care for premature infants is the same as for any other newborn. It may include airway, ventilatory, and circulatory support. *The paramedic should attempt resuscitation if the infant has any signs of life.* The paramedic must take special care to maintain the infant's body temperature and to prevent hypothermia. Transport to a facility with special services for low-birth-weight newborns may be indicated.

▶**NOTE** Concern for eye damage (retinopathy of prematurity) from long-term oxygen use in premature infants is not a factor in the emergency setting. Remember, hypoxemia causes irreversible brain damage in these newborns. High-concentration oxygen must be used.

Respiratory Distress and Cyanosis

Prematurity is the most common cause of respiratory distress and cyanosis in the neonate. These conditions occur most often in infants less than 1200 g ($2\frac{1}{2}$ lb) and 30 weeks of gestation. These problems may be related to the infant's immature central respiratory control center. The center is affected more easily by environmental and metabolic changes than that of the full-term infant. Other risk factors for respiratory distress and cyanosis in the neonate include multiple gestations, prenatal maternal complications, and infants born with the following conditions:

- Birth defects
- Central nervous system disorders
- Diaphragmatic hernia
- Lung immaturity
- Lung or heart disease
- Meconium or amniotic fluid aspiration
- Metabolic acidosis
- Mucous obstruction of nasal passages
- Pneumonia
- Primary pulmonary hypertension
- Shock and sepsis

Respiratory distress and cyanosis can lead to cardiac arrest in the neonate. The situation calls for immediate actions to improve breathing and support respirations. Assessment findings may include tachypnea, paradoxical breathing, intercostal retractions, nasal flaring, expiratory grunting, and central cyanosis. As described before, respiratory insufficiency in the neonate generally is managed with stimulation, positioning of the airway, prevention of heat loss and hypothermia, oxygenation and ventilation, suction, and intubation with ventilatory support (if needed).

Hypovolemia

Hypovolemia in infants may result from dehydration, hemorrhage, trauma, or sepsis. It also may be associated with myocardial dysfunction. Signs and symptoms of hypovolemia include mottled or pale color, cool skin, tachycardia, diminished peripheral pulses, and delayed capillary refill despite normal ambient temperature. Shock may be present despite a normal blood pressure. Prompt and effective treatment of early signs of compensated shock may prevent the development of hypotension (decompensated shock) and associated high morbidity and mortality.[2] Prehospital care is always directed at ensuring adequate airway, ventilatory, and circulatory support (including control of external hemorrhage) and providing rapid transport to an appropriate facility.

When signs of hypovolemia are present, the paramedic should give a fluid bolus (10 mL/kg over 5 to 10 minutes of isotonic crystalloid) immediately after obtaining IV access. The paramedic should reassess the infant. If signs of shock persist, the paramedic should give a second 10-mL/kg bolus. Further boluses should be given as needed and under the guidance of medical direction.

Seizures

Seizures occur in a small percentage of newborns. When present, they usually are a sign of an underlying abnormality (Box 43-2). Prolonged seizures or frequent seizures may result in metabolic changes and problems with breathing and heart rate.

BOX 43-2 Causes of Neonatal Seizures

- Developmental abnormalities
- Drug withdrawal
- Hypoglycemia
- Hypoxic-ischemic encephalopathy
- Intracranial hemorrhage
- Meningitis or encephalopathy
- Metabolic disturbances

TYPES OF SEIZURES

Seizures in neonates usually are fragmented and not well sustained. They have been classified as *subtle seizures, tonic seizures, multifocal seizures, focal clonic seizures,* and *myoclonic seizures.*[1]

Subtle seizures involve eye deviation, blinking, sucking, swimming movements of the arms, and peddling movements of the legs. Apnea may be present during subtle seizures. Tonic seizures usually involve extension of the limbs. Less often, they involve flexion of the upper extremities and extension of the lower extremities. This type of seizure is more common in infants who are premature. Tonic seizure is more common especially in infants with intraventricular hemorrhage. Multifocal seizures usually involve clonic activity in one extremity that may migrate randomly to another area of the body. This type of seizure mainly occurs in full-term infants. Focal clonic seizures involve clonic, localized jerking. They have been known to occur in full-term and premature newborns. Myoclonic seizures involve flexion and jerking of the upper or lower extremities. These seizures may occur singly. They also may occur in a series of repetitive jerking cycles.

Emergency care for managing neonatal seizures includes providing airway, ventilatory, and circulatory support and maintaining the infant's body temperature. Drug therapy that may be prescribed by medical direction includes ***dextrose*** to treat hypoglycemia, anticonvulsant agents, and perhaps benzodiazepines (for status epilepticus). Seizure activity is always considered pathological; rapid transport for physician evaluation is needed.

Fever

Fever in neonates is described as a rectal temperature greater than 100.4° F [38.0° C]). Fever in neonates usually is a cause for concern and often is a response to an acute viral or bacterial infection. Fever also may result from a change in the infant's limited ability to control body temperature. It also may be an effect of dehydration. The rise in core temperature increases oxygen demands and increases glucose metabolism. These increases may lead to metabolic acidosis. Assessment findings may include mental status changes (e.g., irritability and somnolence), a history of decreased intake, rashes and petechia, and warm or hot skin.

NOTE Term newborns produce beads of sweat on their brow but not over the rest of their bodies. Premature infants generally have no visible sweat.

The prehospital care for febrile infants mainly is supportive. As a rule, cooling procedures and the use of antipyretics will be delayed until the child has arrived at the hospital. Febrile seizures usually affect children between 6 months and 5 years of age. Generally they are not a concern in caring for the neonate (see Chapter 44). All febrile neonates require immediate transport for physician evaluation. These patients should be presumed to have systemic sepsis until it is proved otherwise.

Hypothermia

As described in Chapter 38, hypothermia is a core body temperature below 95° F (35° C). Hypothermia may result from a decrease in heat production, an increase in heat loss (through evaporation, conduction, convection, or radiation), or a combination of both. Neonates are sensitive to the effects of hypothermia because of their increased surface-to-volume ratio. This is especially the case when they are wet (e.g., after delivery). The associated increase in metabolic demand to maintain body temperature can cause metabolic acidosis, pulmonary hypertension, and hypoxemia. Hypothermia also may be a sign of sepsis in the neonate. Assessment findings may include the following:

- Pale color
- Cool skin (especially in the extremities)
- Respiratory distress
- Apnea
- Bradycardia
- Central cyanosis
- Acrocyanosis (cyanosis of the extremities)
- Irritability (initially)
- Lethargy (in the late stage)
- Absence of shivering (variable)

The prehospital care for these patients may include provision of basic and advanced cardiac life support. (This depends on the severity of hypothermia.) The care also consists of rapid transport to an appropriate facility. Other therapeutic measures include ensuring that the infant is dry and warm, warming the hands before touching the newborn, and perhaps the administration of ***dextrose*** to treat hypoglycemia and IV therapy with warm fluids. The patient should be transported in a heated ambulance (76° to 80° F [24° to 26.5° C]).

Hypoglycemia

A blood glucose measurement less than 40 mg/dL in the infant indicates hypoglycemia (described in Chapter 32).[5] The condition should be determined by blood glucose screening on all sick infants. Hypoglycemia may be due to inadequate glucose intake or increased use of glucose. Risk factors associated with hypoglycemia include asphyxia, toxemia, being the smaller twin, central nervous system hemorrhage, and sepsis. Assessment findings may include the following:

- Twitching or seizure
- Limpness
- Lethargy
- Eye rolling
- High-pitched crying
- Apnea
- Irregular respirations
- Cyanosis (possibly)

> **NOTE** Small infants and chronically ill children have limited glycogen stores. These may be depleted rapidly during stress events. If allowed to persist, hypoglycemia can depress myocardial function. Hypoglycemia may have catastrophic effects on the brain as well.

The prehospital care is directed at ensuring adequate airway, ventilatory, and circulatory support; maintaining body temperature; providing rapid transport; and perhaps IV administration of ***dextrose 10%*** (per medical direction) (Box 43-3). The paramedic should check the glucose level again if the infant fails to respond to initial resuscitative measures. All infants who do not respond normally and those who are hypoglycemic and fail to respond to the ***dextrose*** should be transported immediately to a medical facility.

Vomiting and Diarrhea

Occasional vomiting or diarrhea is not unusual in the neonate. For example, vomiting mucus (that may be streaked with blood) is common in the first few hours of life. Also, five to six stools per day is considered normal, especially if the infant is breast-feeding. Persistent vomiting and/or diarrhea, however, should be considered warning signs of serious illness.

VOMITING

Persistent vomiting in the first 24 hours of life suggests an obstruction in the upper digestive tract or perhaps increased intracranial pressure. Vomit that contains non–bile-stained fluid is a sign of anatomical or functional obstruction. This obstruction is at or above the first portion of the duodenum. Vomiting also may indicate gastroesophageal reflux. Bile-stained vomit may result from obstruction below the opening of the bile duct. Vomit that contains dark blood usually is a sign of life-threatening illness. Assessment findings may include a distended stomach and signs of infection, dehydration, and increased intracranial pressure. The paramedic also should consider that the vomiting may be a result of drug withdrawal (from the mother's drug use).

The prehospital care usually requires maintaining an airway that is clear of vomit and ensuring adequate oxygenation. In severe cases, medical direction may advise that IV fluid therapy be started before transport. Fluid therapy treats dehydration and any bradycardia that may develop from vagal stimulation. If possible, infants should be transported on their sides. This will help prevent aspiration.

BOX 43-3 Glucose Administration

Dose: 0.5 to 1.0 g/kg intravenously over 20 minutes

Preparation: Dilute dextrose 50% 1:1 with sterile water, resulting in 25% dextrose in water solution; administer 2 to 4 mL/kg.

or

Dilute dextrose 50% 1:4 with sterile water, resulting in 10% dextrose in water solution; administer 5 to 10 mL/kg.

Precautions: Hypertonic glucose is hyperosmolar and may sclerose peripheral veins.

Note: Some sterile water has preservatives containing alcohol. This solution should not be used. It can cause profound hypoglycemia and death when administered to infants.

DIARRHEA

Persistent diarrhea can lead to serious dehydration in the neonate. It can lead to electrolyte imbalances as well. The diarrhea often is associated with a bacterial or viral infection. Other possible causes include the following:

- Cystic fibrosis
- Gastroenteritis
- Lactose intolerance
- Neonatal abstinence syndrome (drug withdrawal)
- Phototherapy (a treatment for hyperbilirubinemia and jaundice in the newborn)
- Rotavirus
- Thyrotoxicosis

Assessment findings often include the presence of loose stools, decreased urinary output, and signs of dehydration. Treatment consists of supporting the infant's vital functions, IV fluid therapy (per medical direction), and rapid transport to the receiving hospital.

Common Birth Injuries

About 2% to 7% of every 1000 live births result in avoidable and unavoidable physical and anoxic trauma during labor and delivery. Of every 100,000 infants, 5 to 8 are estimated to die of birth trauma and 25 die of anoxic injuries (accounting for 2% to 3% of infant deaths).[1]

An uncontrolled, explosive delivery (described in Chapter 42) is the greatest risk factor for birth injuries. Cranial injuries may include molding of the head and overriding of the parietal bones, soft tissue injuries from forceps delivery, subconjunctival and retinal hemorrhage, subperiosteal hemorrhage, and skull fracture. Intracranial hemorrhage can occur from trauma or asphyxia. Spine and spinal cord injury can result from strong traction or a lateral pull during delivery. Other birth injuries include peripheral nerve injury, liver or spleen injury, adrenal hemorrhage, clavicle or extremity fracture, and brain or soft tissue injury from hypoxia-ischemia. The assessment findings vary by the nature of the injury. They may include the following:

- Diffuse, sometimes ecchymotic, edematous swelling of the soft tissues of the scalp
- Paralysis below the level of spinal cord injury

- Paralysis of the upper arm with or without paralysis of the forearm
- Paralysis of the diaphragm
- Movement on only one side of the face when the newborn cries
- Inability to move the arm freely on the same side of a fractured clavicle
- Lack of spontaneous movement of an injured extremity
- Hypoxia
- Shock

The goal of prehospital care for an infant with a birth injury is to support the newborn's vital functions. This can be done by ensuring adequate oxygenation, ventilation, and circulatory support and administering fluid or drug therapy (if indicated). These infants are high-risk newborns. They require rapid transport to a proper medical facility.

Neonatal Resuscitation, Postresuscitation, and Stabilization

A neonate's heart generally is healthy and strong. However, disorders in the conduction system of the heart can and do occur. Most often the disorders occur as a result of hypoxemia and respiratory arrest. The outcome for these infants is poor if interventions are not begun quickly. In addition, the likelihood for brain and organ damage is increased in infants who require resuscitation. The paramedic should continually assess and monitor neonates with respiratory distress for treatable causes of the distress.

Asystole and pulseless cardiac arrest are uncommon in the neonate. Like bradycardia, they usually are the result of hypoxia. Cardiac arrest also can be caused by primary and secondary apnea, unresolved bradycardia, and persistent fetal circulation (persistent pulmonary hypertension). Assessment findings may include peripheral cyanosis, inadequate respiratory effort, and ineffective or absent heart rate. Risk factors associated with cardiac arrest in the newborn include the following:

- Congenital malformations
- Congenital neuromuscular disease
- Drugs administered or taken by the mother
- Intrapartum hypoxemia
- Intrauterine asphyxia

Emergency care for neonates with asystole or pulseless arrest was described earlier in this chapter and includes airway, ventilatory, and circulatory support; pharmacological therapy; and rapid transport to an appropriate medical facility.

CRITICAL THINKING

How will you feel if you deliver a critically ill or dead infant?

PSYCHOLOGICAL AND EMOTIONAL SUPPORT

The paramedic must be aware of the normal feelings and reactions of parents, siblings, other family members, and caregivers while providing emergency care to an ill or injured child. (These events also are often highly charged and emotional for the emergency crew.) The paramedic should keep those at the scene abreast of all procedures being performed. The paramedic also should inform family members of the necessity of the procedures.

NOTE After delivery, the mother continues to be a patient herself. She still has certain physical and emotional needs.

As a rule, emergency responders should never discuss the infant's chances of survival with a parent or family member. They also should not give false hope about the infant's condition. The paramedic should assure the family that everything that can be done for the child is being done. The paramedic also should assure the family that their baby will receive the best possible care during transport and at the hospital. The hospital will have support personnel who can assist family members and loved ones.

SUMMARY

- When oxygenation and continued ventilations do not improve the infant's condition or the infant begins to deteriorate further, endotracheal intubation and administration of drugs may be required. The drugs most often used during neonatal resuscitation are epinephrine, volume expanders, and naloxone.
- Some of the more common congenital anomalies include choanal atresia, cleft lip, diaphragmatic hernia, and Pierre Robin syndrome.
- At birth, newborns make three major physiological adaptations necessary for survival: (1) emptying fluids from their lungs and beginning ventilation, (2) changing their circulatory pattern, and (3) maintaining body temperature.
- The initial steps of neonatal resuscitation (except for those born through meconium) are to prevent heat loss, clear the airway by positioning and suctioning, provide tactile stimulation and initiate breathing if necessary, and further evaluate the infant.

Continued

- The three most common complications during the postresuscitation period are endotracheal position change (including dislodgment), tube occlusion by mucus or meconium, and pneumothorax. During transport of the neonate, it is important to maintain body temperature, oxygen administration, and ventilatory support.
- Specific situations that may require advanced life support for the neonate include meconium staining, apnea, diaphragmatic hernia, bradycardia, premature infants, respiratory distress and cyanosis, hypovolemia, seizures, fever, hypothermia, hypoglycemia, and vomiting and diarrhea.
- Premature infants have an increased risk of respiratory suppression, hypothermia, and head and brain injury. In addition to low birth weight, various antepartum and intrapartum risk factors may affect the need for resuscitation.
- About 2% to 7% of every 1000 live births result in avoidable and unavoidable mechanical and anoxic trauma during labor and delivery.
- The paramedic should be aware of the normal feelings and reactions of parents, siblings, other family members, and caregivers while providing emergency care to an ill or injured child.

REFERENCES

1. US Department of Transportation, National Highway Traffic Safety Administration: *EMT-Paramedic national standard curriculum,* Washington, DC, 1998, The Department.
2. American Heart Association: *Pediatric advanced life support,* Dallas, 1997, The Association.
3. American Heart Association: *Textbook of neonatal resuscitation,* Dallas, 1995, American Academy of Pediatrics.
4. Eichelberger M et al: *Pediatric emergencies,* Englewood Cliffs, NJ, 1992, Prentice-Hall.
5. American Heart Association: Guidelines 2000 for cardiopulmonary resuscitation and emergency cardiovascular care, International Consensus on Science, *Circulation* 102(8):343, 2000.
6. Hoekelman R et al: *Primary pediatric care,* ed 3, St Louis, 1997, Mosby.

CHAPTER

44

Pediatrics

OBJECTIVES

Upon completion of this chapter, the paramedic student will be able to:

1. Identify the role of the Emergency Medical Services for Children program.
2. Identify modifications in patient assessment techniques that assist in the examination of patients at different developmental levels.
3. Identify age-related illnesses and injuries in pediatric patients.
4. Outline the general principles of assessment and management of the pediatric patient.
5. Describe the pathophysiology, signs and symptoms, and management of selected pediatric respiratory emergencies.
6. Describe the pathophysiology, signs and symptoms, and management of shock in the pediatric patient.
7. Describe the pathophysiology, signs and symptoms, and management of selected pediatric dysrhythmias.
8. Describe the pathophysiology, signs and symptoms, and management of pediatric seizures.
9. Describe the pathophysiology, signs and symptoms, and management of hypoglycemia and hyperglycemia in the pediatric patient.
10. Describe the pathophysiology, signs and symptoms, and management of infectious pediatric emergencies.
11. Identify common causes of poisoning and toxic exposure in the pediatric patient.
12. Describe special considerations for assessment and management of specific injuries in children.
13. Outline the pathophysiology and management of sudden infant death syndrome.
14. Describe the risk factors, key signs and symptoms, and management of injuries or illness resulting from child abuse and neglect.
15. Identify prehospital considerations for the care of infants and children with special needs.

KEY TERMS

bacterial tracheitis: A bacterial infection of the upper airway and subglottic trachea.

child abuse: The physical, sexual, or emotional maltreatment of a child.

shunt: A tube or device surgically implanted in the body to redirect body fluid from one cavity or vessel to another.

sudden infant death syndrome: The unexpected and sudden death of an apparently normal and healthy infant that occurs during sleep.

Emergencies involving pediatric patients account for about 10% or fewer of emergency medical services responses.[1] However, caring for these patients has unique challenges. The challenges are related to size, physical and intellectual maturation, and diseases specific to neonates, infants, and children. This chapter addresses the anatomical and physiological mechanisms of growth and development, medical emergencies common to children, and initial assessment and management strategies that often are critical in the patient's survival.

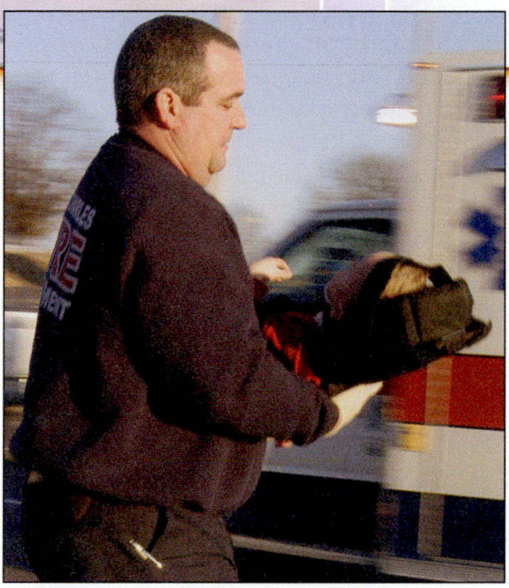

THE PARAMEDIC'S ROLE IN CARING FOR PEDIATRIC PATIENTS

Paramedics play an important role in the care of infants and children. This role involves the prehospital care and interfacility transfer. Emergency medical services personnel can help to reduce mortality and morbidity for children as well. They can become active participants in school, community, and parent education programs and provide thorough documentation appropriate for prehospital trauma registries, epidemiological research, and surveillance. (See Chapter 3.) For paramedics, improvement of their knowledge and clinical skills is important. They can do this through continuing education programs that are specific to the pediatric age group. A sampling of continuing education programs include the following:

- Advanced Pediatric Life Support
- Neonatal Resuscitation Program
- Pediatric Basic Trauma Life Support
- Pediatric Emergencies for Paramedics
- Pediatric Education for the Prehospital Professional
- Prehospital Pediatric Care
- Teaching Resources for Instructors of Prehospital Pediatrics

Other ways to enhance continuing education and clinical skills include reading textbooks and journals, Internet study, attending regional conferences and seminars, and working or volunteering at pediatric emergency departments, pediatric hospitals, or a pediatrician's office.

EMERGENCY MEDICAL SERVICES FOR CHILDREN

In 1985 the Emergency Medical Services for Children Demonstration Program was established through grants provided by the Maternal and Child Health Bureau of the U.S. Department of Health and Human Services and by the National Highway Traffic Safety Administration, a division of the U.S. Department of Transportation. This program, which was designed to enhance and expand emergency medical services for acutely ill and injured children, defined 12 basic components of an effective Emergency Medical Services for Children system[2]:

1. System approach
2. Education
3. Data collection
4. Quality improvement
5. Injury prevention
6. Access
7. Prehospital care
8. Emergency care
9. Definitive care
10. Rehabilitation
11. Finance
12. Continual health care from birth to young adulthood

CRITICAL THINKING

Are you familiar with any Emergency Medical Services for Children injury prevention programs that are in your area?

Emergency Medical Services for Children grants and the organizational efforts aimed at improving emergency care for children have resulted in specific programs targeted to prehospital care providers. These include continuing education programs, educational resources for instructors, equipment guidelines, protocols for prehospital management, quality improvement procedures for evaluating prehospital care for children, and designation of facilities with special capabilities for pediatric care. As stated in *Emergency Medical Service for Children: A Report to the Nation,* published in 1991 by the National Center for Education in Maternal and Child Health, "The lives of many infants, children, and young adults . . . can be saved through implementation of emergency medical services for children (EMSC). Outcomes for critically ill and injured children can be influenced by the provision of timely care by health care professionals who are well trained and equipped for pediatric emergency and critical care."[3]

GROWTH AND DEVELOPMENT REVIEW

As described in Chapter 8, children have unique anatomical, physiological, and psychological characteristics that change during their development. The following is a review of growth and development by age group. Special considerations and approach strategies that must be taken into account when caring for pediatric patients are provided in Box 44-1. (See Chapter 11.)

CRITICAL THINKING

How comfortable are you with the "normal" well child?

Newborn (First Few Hours of Life)

Assessment and care for the newborn is described in Chapter 43. The method most commonly used to evaluate the newborn is the Apgar score. Resuscitation of the newborn (if needed) should follow the recommendations established by the American Heart Association, including those found in the curriculum for the Neonatal Resuscitation Program. To review, the newborn's heart rate during the first 30 minutes of life is between 120 and 160 beats/min. Respirations at birth are usually between 40 and 60 breaths/min. They average 30 to 40 breaths/min within a few minutes after delivery (Table 44-1). The full-term newborn normally weighs 3 to 3.5 kg (about 6 to 8 lb).

Neonate (First 28 Days of Life)

Total body weight in the neonate may decrease 5% to 10% during the first few days of life because of the excretion of extracellular fluid. (This lost weight is regained by the second week of life and generally exceeds the newborn weight.) Most infants gain an average of 5 to 6 oz per week.

Neonates respond to a wide variety of stimuli. They also have a range of reflexes. Many of these reflexes are protective and include those associated with breathing, eating, and stress or discomfort. Neonates sleep an average of 16 to 18 hours per day, with sleep and wakefulness evenly distributed over 24 hours. Breathing occurs mainly through the nose during the first month of life. The horizontal position of the ribs produces the characteristic diaphragmatic breathing in this age group. Although crying is common in the neonate, the crying gradually decreases throughout infancy. Persistent crying may indicate physiological distress. Illnesses that may be encountered in this age group are those that cause respiratory problems, jaundice, vomiting, fever, sepsis, meningitis, and problems of prematurity.

Infant (2 to 12 Months)

Between 4 and 6 months of age, most infants have doubled their birth weight, tripling it within 9 to 12 months. In the first year of life the heart also doubles in size, the heart rate gradually slows, and weight and blood pressure begin to increase.

During infancy, major advances in physical and mental skills occur as the brain and nervous system gradually mature. By 12 months of age the development of mature nerves is nearly complete, and along with muscle strength, enables many infants to stand and walk with little or no assistance. (Muscle weight in infants is about 25% of the entire musculoskeletal system.) Common illnesses typically affect the respiratory, gastrointestinal, and central nervous system. They manifest themselves as respiratory distress; nausea, vomiting, and diarrhea; dehydration; and seizures, respectively. Other illnesses that may be encountered in this age group include sepsis, meningitis, and **sudden infant death syndrome** (SIDS). In addition, the older infant (6 to 12 months of age) may experience bronchiolitis, croup, foreign body airway obstruction, and physical injury from sexual abuse, neglect, falls, and motor vehicle crashes.

Toddler (1 to 3 Years)

Muscle mass and bone density increase during the toddler years. Most children gain an average of 2 kg (about 4 lb) each year. By age 2, much of the nervous system is fully developed. By this time, basic motor skills (e.g., balance and walking) and fine motor skills (e.g., stacking building blocks) also become visible. In addition, most children are capable of controlling bladder and bowel function by 2 to 3 years of age. By 2 years of age, toddlers have developed unique personality traits, moods, and specific likes and dislikes. Basic language skills are mastered by age 3. However, these skills continue to be refined through childhood. By 3 years of age toddlers and preschoolers also begin to recognize the difference between the sexes and start to model themselves after persons of their own gender. Illnesses in this age group may cause respiratory distress (e.g., from asthma, bronchiolitis, foreign body aspiration, or croup) vomiting and diarrhea with dehydration, febrile seizures, sepsis, and meningitis. Toddlers who are learning to walk are prone to falls. They also may find themselves in dangerous environments without proper supervision or barriers

BOX 44-1 Developmental Stages and Approach Strategies for Pediatric Patients

Infants

Major Fears

Separation and strangers

Approach Strategies

Provide consistent caretakers.
Reduce parents' anxiety, because it is transmitted to the infant.
Minimize separation from parents.

Toddlers

Major Fears

Separation and loss of control

Characteristics of Thinking

Primitive
Unable to recognize views of others
Little concept of body integrity

Approach Strategies

Keep explanations simple.
Choose words carefully.
Let toddler play with equipment (stethoscope).
Minimize separation from parents.

Preschoolers

Major Fears

Bodily injury and mutilation
Loss of control
The unknown and the dark
Being left alone

Characteristics of Thinking

Highly literal interpretation of words
Unable to abstract
Primitive ideas about the body (e.g., fear that all blood will "leak out" if a bandage is removed)

Approach Strategies

Keep explanations simple and concise.
Choose words carefully.
Emphasize that a procedure will help the child be healthier.
Be honest.

School-Age Children

Major Fears

Loss of control
Bodily injury and mutilation
Failure to live up to expectations of others
Death

School-Age Children, cont'd

Characteristics of Thinking

Vague or false ideas about physical illness and body structure and function
Able to listen attentively without always comprehending
Reluctant to ask questions about something they think they are expected to know
Increased awareness of significant illness, possible hazards of treatments, lifelong consequences of injury, and the meaning of death

Approach Strategies

Ask children to explain what they understand.
Provide as many choices as possible to increase the child's sense of control.
Reassure the child that he or she has done nothing wrong and that necessary procedures are not punishment.
Anticipate and answer questions about long-term consequences (e.g., what the scar will look like and how long activities may be curtailed).

Adolescents

Major Fears

Loss of control
Altered body image
Separation from peer group

Characteristics of Thinking

Able to think abstractly
Tendency toward hyperresponsiveness to pain (reactions not always in proportion to event)
Little understanding of the structure and workings of the body

Approach Strategies

When appropriate, allow adolescents to be a part of decision making about their care.
Give information sensitively.
Express how important their compliance and cooperation are to their treatment.
Be honest about consequences.
Use or teach coping mechanisms such as relaxation, deep breathing, and self-comforting talk.

TABLE 44-1 Average Vital Signs by Age Group

AGE	PULSE (PER MINUTE)	RESPIRATIONS (PER MINUTE)	BLOOD PRESSURE (MM HG)
Newborn	120-160	40-60	80/40
1 year	80-140	30-40	82/44
3 years	80-120	25-30	86/50
5 years	70-115	20-25	90/52
7 years	70-115	20-25	94/54
10 years	70-115	15-20	100/60
15 years	70-90	15-20	110/64

Note: Normal vital signs vary with age. Carry a reminder chart to ensure accuracy. Do not depend on your memory in an emergency. Blood pressure in a child over 1 year may be estimated with the following formula: (age in years × 2) + 70 = minimum systolic blood pressure. Example for a 3-year-old child: (3 × 2 = 6) + 70 = 76 mm Hg.

(e.g., baby gates). Physical injuries also occur from poisonings from accidental ingestions, physical/sexual abuse, drowning, and motor vehicle crashes.

Preschooler (3 to 5 Years)

During the preschool years, children experience advances in gross and fine motor skills. Peer relationships also begin to form with other children near the same age and level of maturity. These relationships often begin with play that involves acting out fantasies or using imagination for new situations; all of which can lead to problem-solving skills and cognitive development. Illnesses and injuries that may be encountered in this age group include those mentioned before for toddlers. In addition, preschoolers are more likely to experience injuries from thermal burns. They also are more likely to be victims of submersion incidents or drowning. Preschoolers are curious and often have an urge to explore. Many have a minimal concept of danger.

School Age (6 to 12 Years)

The growth of school-age children is slower and steadier than during the infancy, toddler, and preschooler years. Most children gain about 3 kg (6.6 lb) per year. They average a yearly gain in height of about 2½ inches (6 cm). Most bodily functions reach adult levels in this age group. Two key areas of development during the school-age years include an increased ability to concentrate and learn quickly and the onset of puberty. Psychosocial development of school-age children varies by individual. As a rule however, self-concept and moral traits and behavior begin to emerge during the school-age years. During these years, children spend more time with others outside their immediate family. Most illnesses in school-age children are caused by viral infection. Injuries become more common in this age group because of increased physical activity. These injuries include injuries from bicycle crashes, fractures from falls, and sport-related injuries.

▶**NOTE** About 40,000 to 50,000 children are estimated to be injured permanently each year, and at least 1 million seek medical care because of unintentional injuries.[4]

Adolescent (13 to 18 Years)

During adolescence, the final phase of change in growth and development occurs. Organs rapidly increase in size, blood chemistry values become nearly equal to adult levels, and growth of bone and muscle mass becomes nearly complete. Also in adolescence a person reaches reproductive maturity. With the development of secondary sex characteristics in both sexes comes a final period of rapid growth. Most boys gain an average of 8 inches in height before age 21 when growth usually stops. Growth in girls is less dramatic and is usually complete by age 18.

Along with the physical changes associated with adolescence, most teenagers begin to experiment with different identities. They begin to develop their personality into that of an adult. Many make dramatic moves away from parents and family members toward their peer groups. In their peer groups, they may experiment with alcohol and other drugs, sex, and extreme forms of behavior. In addition to those physical injuries mentioned for younger age groups, situations the paramedic may encounter in this age group (and that are not seen as often in other age groups) include behavioral emergencies associated with alcohol or other drugs use, eating disorders, depression, suicide and suicide gestures, sexually transmitted diseases, pregnancy, and sexual assault.

ANATOMY AND PHYSIOLOGY REVIEW

As stressed throughout this text, physical differences in infants and children set them apart from the adult patient. The following is a review of anatomy and physiology by body region. Also included are special emergency care implications for the pediatric patient.

Head

As mentioned before, a child's head is proportionally large. It accounts for about 25% of the total body weight in newborns. Children also have a larger occipital region and a face that is small compared with the size of the head. Because of these anatomical features, a high percentage of blunt trauma in children involves the head and face. When using spinal stabilization for a child less than 3 years of age, a thin layer of padding under the child's shoulders may be needed to obtain a neutral position. A folded sheet placed under the occiput of a severely ill child over 3 years of age (or under the shoulders of a child less than 3 years of age) can help establish a sniffing position needed to maintain the airway.

To accommodate for brain growth in the infant, the anterior fontanelle remains open for 9 to 18 months after birth. The anterior fontanelle is usually level or slightly below the surface of the skull. A tight or bulging fontanelle suggests increased intracranial pressure (ICP; as seen with meningitis); a sunken fontanelle indicates possible dehydration. The paramedic should assess the anterior fontanelle in infants and young children who are ill or injured. The fontanelle is best assessed when the child is upright and not crying.

Airway

The airway structures of children are narrower and less stable at all levels than those of adults. This makes the airways of pediatric patients more easily blocked by secretions, obstructions, and injury or inflammation. In addition, the larynx is higher (at the level of the cervical vertebrae C3 to C4) and more anterior, extending into the pharynx. The trachea is bifurcated at a higher level. The tracheal cartilage also is softer and smaller in length and diameter. The cricoid ring is the narrowest part of the airway in young children. The jaw is proportionally small, and the tongue is proportionally large. This increases the likelihood of airway obstruction by the tongue in the unconscious child. The epiglottis in infants is omega shaped and extends into the airway at a 45-degree angle. The epiglottic folds also have softer cartilage and can become "floppy," causing airway obstruction. As described in Chapter 19, and later in this chapter, management considerations for these patients include the following:

- Placing a thin layer of padding under the shoulders to maintain a neutral position of the airway structures in children less than 3 years of age
- Placing a folded sheet under the occiput to obtain a sniffing position in children over 3 years of age
- Avoiding hyperflexion or hyperextension of the neck, which can obstruct the airway
- Using suction to clear the airway of secretions and particulate matter
- Modifying tracheal intubation techniques by ensuring a gentle touch to the soft tissue of the airway, which is easily injured and inflamed; using a straight blade that lifts the epiglottis; choosing an appropriately sized endotracheal tube (uncuffed for children under 8 years of age); and constantly monitoring the airway for proper endotracheal tube placement

The paramedic also should remember that infants breathe mainly through the nose during the first month of life. Obstruction of the small nares by secretions can result easily in respiratory insufficiency. Thus assessment and suction of the nares as needed is important. This is especially important in infants less than 6 months of age.

Chest and Lungs

In infants and young children the chief support for the chest wall comes from muscles rather than bones. These chest muscles are immature. They can fatigue easily. The use of these muscles for breathing also requires higher metabolic and oxygen consumption rates than in older children and adults. This increases the pediatric patient's susceptibility to the buildup of lactic acid in the blood. The ribs of a child are more pliable and are positioned horizontally, and the mediastinum is more mobile. Therefore the chest wall offers less protection to internal organs. It allows for significant internal injury to occur without external signs of trauma (e.g., fractured ribs). Rib fractures are less common in children. Yet they can occur with **child abuse** and other forms of trauma.

The lung tissue of a pediatric patient is fragile. Because of this and the limited protection provided by the chest wall, pulmonary contusions from trauma and pneumothorax from barotrauma are common in this age group. When evaluating a pediatric patient who has suffered major trauma, the paramedic should remember that infants and children are diaphragmatic breathers and are prone to gastric distention; the mobile mediastinum may have a greater shift with a tension pneumothorax; and the thin chest wall easily transmits breath sounds which may complicate the assessment of a pneumothorax or endotracheal tube placement. As a result, auscultation of breath sounds from the axillary regions in addition to the anterior and posterior thorax often is helpful.

Abdomen

Like the chest wall, the immature muscles of the abdomen in a child offer less protection to internal organs. In addition, the abdominal organs are closer together. The liver and spleen are proportionally larger and more vascular, as well. These features allow for multiple organ injuries to be more common following abdominal trauma. The liver and spleen also are injured more often than in the adult patient.

Extremities

Bones in children are softer and more porous until adolescence. As long bones mature, hormones act on the cartilage in growing bones, replacing the soft cartilage with hard bones. The epiphyseal plate *(growth plate)* also lengthens as bones develop, and bones thicken as new layers of bone are deposited on existing bone.

Because of the soft composition of bones in pediatric patients, at first all strains and sprains should be considered a fracture. They should be managed with full immobilization of the extremity. In addition, paramedics should be wary of injuries to the growth plate that may disrupt bone growth. Careful technique during intraosseous infusion procedures is critical. This is because improper insertion into the growth plate can affect future bone growth. (See Chapter 18.)

Skin and Body Surface Area

The skin in children is thinner and more elastic than the skin of adults. In addition, the child has less subcutaneous fat. The child has a larger body surface area–to–body mass ratio as well. These factors can affect injury and illness in children in several ways. For example, the thinner skin of a child allows for deeper injury to occur from heat or cold exposure. The lack of subcutaneous fat and the larger body surface area–to–body mass ratio also increase a child's likelihood of hypothermia, hyperthermia, and dehydration from fluid loss.

Respiratory System

The tidal volume of infants and young children is proportionally smaller than that of adolescents and adults. The metabolic oxygen requirements for normal breathing are about double. Pediatric patients also have smaller functional residual capacity. Thus they have proportionally smaller oxygen reserves. Because of these factors, hypoxia can develop rapidly in infants and young children. The paramedic also should remember that muscles are the main support for the chest wall. These muscles can tire easily during respiratory distress. This in turn can lead quickly to respiratory arrest.

Cardiovascular System

Cardiac output is rate dependent in infants and small children. (The faster the heart rate, the greater the cardiac output.) Pediatric patients are not as able as adults to increase contractility of the heart or increase stroke volume. The circulating blood volume in pediatric patients is proportionally larger than in adults. Yet the child's absolute blood volume is smaller. The ability of children to use vasoconstriction to decrease size of the vessels allows them to maintain blood pressure longer than adults. However, early intervention is required to prevent irreversible or decompensated shock. Special considerations in managing these patients include the following:

- Cardiovascular reserve is vigorous, but limited.
- Loss of small volumes of fluid and blood can cause shock.
- A child may be in shock despite a normal blood pressure.
- Bradycardia is often a response to hypoxia.

As described in Chapter 21, hypotension is a late sign of shock in the pediatric patient. Thus the assessment of shock must be based on clinical signs of tissue perfusion (e.g., level of consciousness, skin color, and capillary refill). The paramedic should suspect shock in any ill or injured child who has tachycardia and evidence of decreased perfusion.

Nervous System

As described in Chapter 8, the nervous system develops throughout childhood. Developing neural tissue is fragile. In addition, the anterior and posterior fontanelles remain open for a period of time. As such, direct trauma to the head can lead to brain injuries that are more devastating in young children. The child's brain and spinal cord also are less well protected by the skull and spinal column. This allows for greater force to be transmitted to the brain and spinal cord with resultant injury, even in the absence of spinal column injury.

Metabolic Differences

The way in which children and adults expend energy differs in many ways. For example, infants and children have limited glycogen and glucose stores. Their blood glucose levels can drop quite low in response to illness or injury. This can occur even without a history of diabetes mellitus. Pediatric patients can experience significant volume loss from vomiting and diarrhea. Children are also prone to hypothermia because of their increased body surface area. Newborns and neonates also do not have the ability to shiver to maintain body temperature. For these reasons, it is important to assess a severely ill or injured child for hypoglycemia or hypoperfusion, to minimize heat loss, and to keep all children warm during treatment and transport.

CRITICAL THINKING

Why is it important to know what injuries and illnesses are commonly seen in specific age groups?

GENERAL PRINCIPLES OF PEDIATRIC ASSESSMENT

Initial patient evaluation for children should include observing the patient and involving the parent or guardian in the assessment (see Chapter 12). The parent or guardian often can help make the child more comfortable during the assessment. The parent also usually can offer key details about the child's medical history. The parent also may know whether aspects of the child's behavior or response are normal or abnormal.

Scene Size-up

As with all other patient care, the paramedic should begin the physical assessment with a quick scene survey. The paramedic should note any hazards or potential hazards. The paramedic also should note any visible mechanism of injury or illness. For example, the presence of pills, medicine bottles, or household chemicals may indicate the possibility of toxic ingestion. Injury and a history that does not match or fit the mechanism of injury also may indicate child abuse. In addition, the paramedic should observe the relationship between the parent, guardian, or caregiver and the child. The paramedic should determine the appropriateness of their interaction. For example, does the interaction demonstrate concern or is it angry or indifferent?

CRITICAL THINKING

Would you want to make a comment to the parents about an unsafe situation on the scene before transport? Why or why not?

Other important assessments the paramedic can make during the scene size-up include the orderliness, cleanliness, and safety of the home and the general appearance of other children in the family.

Initial Assessment

The initial assessment begins with the paramedic forming a general impression of the patient. This assessment should focus on the details most valuable for determining whether life-threatening conditions exist. The *pediatric assessment triangle* (Fig. 44-1) is a paradigm that can be used to quickly assess a child (as well as adults) and the need for immediate intervention. The assessment triangle has three components. The first one is appearance (mental status and muscle tone). The second one is work of breathing (respiratory rate and effort). And the third one is circulation (skin signs and skin color). If the child's condition is urgent, care should proceed with rapid assessment of airway, breathing, and circulation; management; and rapid transport. If the child's condition is not urgent, care can proceed with a focused history and detailed physical examination.

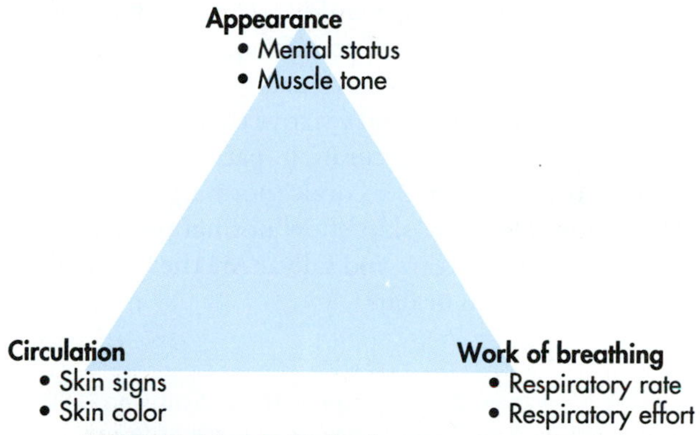

FIGURE 44-1 ■ Pediatric assessment triangle.

CRITICAL THINKING

Think about one abnormal finding in each area of the assessment triangle. Would that single finding influence your triage decision?

Vital Functions

The AVPU scale (*alert*; responds to *verbal* stimuli; responds to *painful* stimuli; *unresponsive*) or the Modified Glasgow Coma Scale (Table 44-2) can be used to determine the child's level of consciousness and to assess for signs of inadequate oxygenation.

TABLE 44-2 Pediatric Modification of Glasgow Coma Scale by Age of Patient*

GLASGOW COMA SCALE SCORE	PEDIATRIC MODIFICATION	
Eye Opening		
≥1 Year	*Birth to 1 Year*	
4 Spontaneously	4 Spontaneously	
3 To verbal command	3 To shout	
2 To pain	2 To pain	
1 No response	1 No response	
Best Motor Response		
≥1 Year	*Birth to 1 Year*	
6 Obeys	5 Localizes pain	
5 Localizes pain	4 Flexion withdrawal	
4 Flexion withdrawal	3 Flexion abnormal (decorticate)	
3 Flexion abnormal (decorticate)	2 Extension (decerebrate)	
2 Extension (decerebrate)	1 No response	
1 No response		
Best Verbal Response		
>5 Years	*Birth to 2 Years*	*2-5 Years*
5 Oriented and converses	5 Cries appropriately, smiles, coos	5 Appropriate words and phrases
4 Disoriented and converses	4 Cries	4 Inappropriate words
3 Inappropriate words	3 Inappropriate crying/screaming	3 Cries/screams
2 Incomprehensible sounds	2 Grunts	2 Grunts
1 No response	1 No response	1 No response

*The Glasgow Coma Scale score is the sum of the individual scores from eye opening, best verbal response, and best motor response, using age-specific criteria. A Glasgow Coma Scale score of 13 to 15 indicates mild head injury; a score of 9 to 12 indicates moderate head injury; and a score of 8 or lower indicates severe head injury.

AIRWAY AND BREATHING

The child's airway should be patent, and breathing should proceed with adequate chest rise and fall. Signs of respiratory distress include the following:

- Abnormal breath sounds
- Absent breath sounds
- Bradypnea
- Grunting
- Head bobbing
- Irregular breathing pattern
- Nasal flaring
- Tachypnea
- Use of accessory muscles

CIRCULATION

The paramedic assesses circulation by comparing the strength and quality of central and peripheral pulses, measuring blood pressure (in children over 3 years of age), evaluating skin color, temperature, moisture, and turgor and capillary refill, and looking for visible hemorrhage. Table 44-1 provides normal vital signs for each age group.

Transition Phase

The transition phase is included throughout assessment. This phase is used to allow the child to become more familiar with the paramedic crew and medical equipment (e.g., "get to know you" conversations and playing with stethoscope) (see Chapter 11). Use of this phase depends on the seriousness of the patient's condition. This phase is appropriate only for a conscious child who is not acutely ill. If the patient is unconscious or acutely ill, management should proceed quickly to emergency care and transport.

Focused History

When obtaining the focused history for an infant, a toddler, or a preschooler, the paramedic often must elicit information from the parent, guardian, or caregiver. School-age and adolescent patients can provide most information by themselves. The paramedic should question them in private (away from parents or family members) about sexual activity, pregnancy, alcohol or other drug use, or suspicion of child abuse (if appropriate for the complaint). The focused history can be obtained using the SAMPLE and OPQRST methods.* (These methods are described in Chapter 10.) The paramedic should use these methods as appropriate for the patient's age. Important elements of the focused history are as follows:

1. Chief complaint
   - Nature of illness or injury
   - The length (duration) of illness or injury
   - Last meal
   - Presence of fever
   - Effects on behavior
   - Vomiting or diarrhea
   - Frequency of urination
2. Medications and allergies
3. Medical history
   - Physician care
   - Chronic illnesses

* *SAMPLE* is *s*igns and symptoms, *a*llergies, *m*edications, *p*ast medical history, *l*ast meal or oral intake, *e*vents before the emergency; *OPQRST* is *o*nset/origin, *p*rovokes, *q*uality, *r*egion, *s*everity, *t*ime.

Detailed Physical Examination

The paramedic should perform a detailed physical examination as described in Chapter 12. The exam should proceed from head to toe in older children. It should proceed from toe to head in younger children (under 2 years of age). Depending on the patient's condition, some or all of the following assessments may be appropriate:

- Pupils: Are they equal and reactive to light?
- Capillary refill (most accurate in patients under 6 years of age): Is it less than 2 seconds (normal) or delayed?
- Hydration: Does the skin show normal resiliency (skin turgor)? Are there tears and saliva? Are the fontanelles in the infant sunken or flat?

> **NOTE** When assessing a pediatric patient who is ill, it is important to note the presence or absence of fever, nausea, vomiting, diarrhea, and frequency of urination.

If time allows and the patient's condition warrants, noninvasive monitoring of vital signs can provide more information. Examples include the use of pulse oximetry to measure perfusion and oxygen saturation, blood pressure assessment, and measurement of body temperature. In addition, all seriously ill or injured children should receive continuous electrocardiogram monitoring.

Ongoing Assessment

Ongoing assessment is appropriate for all patients. It should be performed throughout the patient care. The purpose of ongoing assessment is to monitor the patient for changes in respiratory effort, skin color and temperature, mental status, and vital signs (including pulse oximetry measurements). Measurement tools (e.g., blood pressure cuffs and electrodes) should be appropriate for the size of the child. A key point to remember is that a child's condition can change rapidly. Thus vital signs should be assessed every 15 minutes in a child who is not critical. They should be assessed every 5 minutes in a child who is seriously ill or injured.

> **CRITICAL THINKING**
> Why is ongoing assessment critical when caring for the young child?

GENERAL PRINCIPLES OF PATIENT MANAGEMENT

The principles of patient care depend on the patient's condition. These principles may include basic airway management, advanced airway management, circulatory support, pharmacological therapy, nonpharmacological therapy, transport considerations, and psychological support and communication strategies.

Basic Airway Management

Basic and advanced airway management procedures for the pediatric patient are presented in detail in Chapter 19. These procedures may include manual positioning of the airway, removal of foreign body airway obstruction with chest or abdominal thrusts, suctioning secretions from the airway, providing supplemental oxygen, using oral or nasal airway adjuncts, and assisting ventilation with a bag-valve device.

Advanced Airway Management

Advanced airway management procedures may be needed when caring for a child who is acutely ill or seriously injured. These techniques include removing foreign body airway obstruction under direct visualization with Magill forceps, endotracheal intubation (including rapid sequence intubation, and cricothyroidotomy (per medical direction) when other methods to maintain a patent airway have failed.

Circulatory Support

Circulatory support may be required in an ill or injured child. In addition to providing basic life support with cardiopulmonary resuscitation, vascular access may be required for drug therapy and fluid resuscitation. Methods to obtain vascular access in pediatric patients are described in Chapter 18 and later in this chapter. These methods may include peripheral venous cannulation and intraosseous infusion.

Pharmacological Therapy

At times, drug therapy will be required when caring for the pediatric patient. Examples include therapy for pain management; rapid sequence intubation; and patients with respiratory, cardiac, endocrinological, or neurological conditions. Drugs that are used in pediatric emergencies are described later in this chapter and in the *Emergency Drug Index*.

Additional Therapy

Additional therapies are indicated depending on the type of illness or injury. These include spinal immobilization for trauma patients, hemorrhage control and bandaging and splinting, and electrical therapy (described later in this chapter). In addition, lowering body temperature with cooling methods or maintaining body temperature with blankets and warm clothing may be needed.

Transport Considerations

As described in Chapter 20, some pediatric patients need transport to a specialty care medical facility. Examples of specialty care facilities are pediatric trauma centers, high-risk newborn care facilities, and pediatric burn centers. In addition to choosing a *proper facility,* the paramedic crew must consider the *proper mode* of caring for these patients. This includes deciding to provide rapid transport versus providing on-scene care. It also includes deciding on the use of ground or air ambulance.

Psychological Support

As described previously in this chapter and throughout this text, it is important for the paramedic to provide psychological support to the pediatric patient. The paramedic must provide support to the patient's family or caregivers as well. Pediatric emergencies often are emotionally charged events. Helpful strategies for approaching and communicating with pediatric patients and their caregivers are described in Chapter 9.

SPECIFIC PATHOPHYSIOLOGY, ASSESSMENT, AND MANAGEMENT

The conditions discussed in this section are respiratory compromise, shock, dysrhythmias, seizure, hypoglycemia and hyperglycemia, infection, poisoning and toxic exposure, trauma, SIDS, and child abuse and neglect.

Respiratory Compromise

Respiratory problems can be caused by many conditions that affect the upper and lower airways. These include upper and lower foreign body airway obstruction, upper airway disease (croup, epiglottitis, and **bacterial tracheitis**), and lower airway disease (asthma, bronchiolitis, and pneumonia). Most cases of cardiac arrest in children occur because of respiratory insufficiency.[5] For this reason, respiratory emergencies call for rapid assessment and management. The severity of respiratory compromise may be classified as respiratory distress, respiratory failure, and respiratory arrest.

▶**NOTE** The paramedic should try to calm and reassure a child with respiratory compromise. The paramedic should not agitate the conscious patient or lay the child down (supine). Doing so may aggravate the airway condition. It may even lead to life-threatening airway obstruction. When possible, allow the parent or other caregiver to stay with the child. The receiving hospital should be advised of the patient's status as soon as possible. That way, arrangements can be made for appropriate medical personnel.

Respiratory distress is the mildest form of respiratory compromise. Respiratory distress is evident by an increase in the rate and depth of breathing and by the use of accessory muscles to assist ventilation (Fig. 44-2). These changes cause a slight decrease in arterial carbon dioxide levels in the blood as respiratory rate increases. As respiratory distress increases, the patient becomes exhausted. The PCO_2 gradually increases as the patient's condition gets worse. Signs and symptoms of respiratory distress include the following:

- A change in mental status from normal to irritable or anxious
- Tachypnea
- Retractions (accessory muscle use)
- Nasal flaring (in infants)
- Poor muscle tone
- Tachycardia
- Head bobbing
- Grunting
- Cyanosis that improves with supplemental oxygen

If left untreated, respiratory distress may lead to respiratory failure.

Respiratory failure results from poor ventilation or lack of oxygenation. It occurs when the heart and lungs do not exchange enough oxygen and carbon dioxide. This causes a decrease in PO_2 and an increase in PCO_2 (leading to respiratory acidosis). Signs and symptoms of respiratory failure include the following:

- Irritability deteriorating to lethargy
- Marked tachypnea deteriorating to bradypnea
- Marked retractions deteriorating to agonal respirations
- Marked tachycardia deteriorating to bradycardia
- Central cyanosis

Respiratory failure in any patient is an ominous sign. Without immediate help, respiratory arrest can occur.

Respiratory arrest is the cessation of breathing. Good outcomes can be expected with early treatment. However, failure to treat respiratory arrest can lead to cardiopulmonary arrest. Signs and symptoms of respiratory arrest include the following:

- Unresponsiveness
- Apnea
- Absent chest wall movement
- Limp muscle tone
- Bradycardia deteriorating to asystole
- Profound cyanosis

Providing aggressive ventilatory and circulatory support for patients in respiratory distress is critical. Airway interventions may include bag-valve-mask ventilation, endotracheal intubation, gastric decompression (if abdominal distention is impeding ventilation), needle decompression for pneumothorax, and cricothyrotomy for complete upper airway obstruction that cannot be relieved by other means. The success of emergency care is indicated by an improvement in the patient's color and oxygen saturation, an improvement in the pulse rate, and an improved level of consciousness.

UPPER AND LOWER FOREIGN BODY AIRWAY OBSTRUCTION

Obstruction of the upper or lower airway by a foreign body may cause a partial or full obstruction. This usually occurs in toddlers and preschoolers (1 to 4 years of age). Obstruction often is caused by food (hard candy, nuts, seeds, hot dogs) or small objects (coins, balloons). The paramedic should suspect foreign body aspiration in an otherwise healthy child with sudden onset of respiratory compromise.

Signs and symptoms of airway obstruction include anxiety, inspiratory stridor, muffled or hoarse voice, drooling, pain in the throat, decreased breath sounds, rales, rhonchi, and wheezing. The child may have a history of choking (observed by an adult). If a full obstruction cannot be relieved with basic and advanced methods of clearing, tracheal intubation may be indicated. Full obstruction calls for immediate intervention to relieve the obstruction. Basic and advanced methods of clearing the airway are presented in Chapter 19.

If a child with a partial obstruction is conscious and has adequate movement of air, the paramedic should not agitate the child. Rather, the paramedic should provide continuous respiratory monitoring. Also, the child should be transported immediately to the hospital. Agitation or attempts to relieve a partial obstruction may cause the foreign body to move. This may lead to full obstruction.

CROUP

Croup (laryngotracheobronchitis) is a common, viral infection of the upper airway. It usually occurs in children between the ages of 6 months and 4 years. It often occurs during the late fall and early winter months. Croup usually is caused by the parainfluenza virus. However, respiratory syncytial virus, rubeola, and adenovirus also can cause croup. Croup may involve the entire respiratory tract. However, the symptoms are caused by inflammation in the subglottic region (at the level of the larynx extending to the cricoid cartilage) (Fig. 44-3).

A child with croup usually has a history of recent upper respiratory tract infection and a low-grade fever. The patient may have hoarseness, inspiratory stridor (from subglottic edema), and a barking cough. Wheezing may be present if the lower airways are involved. However, symptoms occur mainly on inspiration. Most often, the emergency episode occurs at night after the child has gone to bed. On the arrival of the paramedics, a patient with severe croup may have all the classic signs of respiratory distress. The child may be sitting upright and leaning forward to aid breathing (variable). Also, nasal flaring, intercostal retraction, and cyanosis (a late sign of respiratory insufficiency) may be present. Children with severe croup are at risk of serious airway obstruction from the narrowed diameter of the trachea.

Prehospital management of croup includes airway maintenance, administration of cool mist or humidified or nebulized oxygen, and transportation in a position of comfort. Symptoms may improve dramatically in patients with

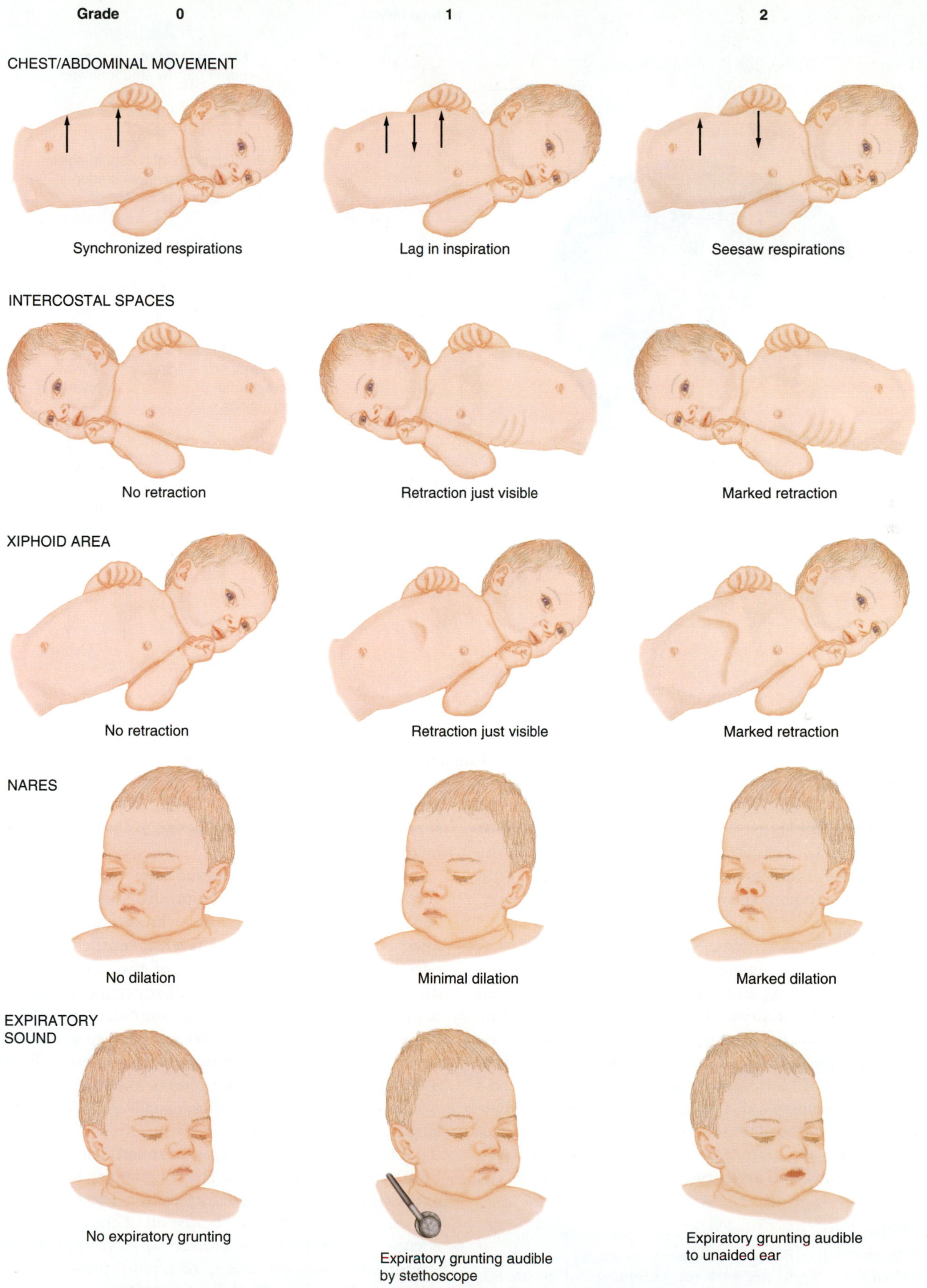

FIGURE 44-2 ■ Assessment of respiratory distress. The Silverman-Andersen index is used to score the infant's degree of respiratory difficulty. The score for individual criteria matches the grade, with a total possible score of 10 indicating severe distress.

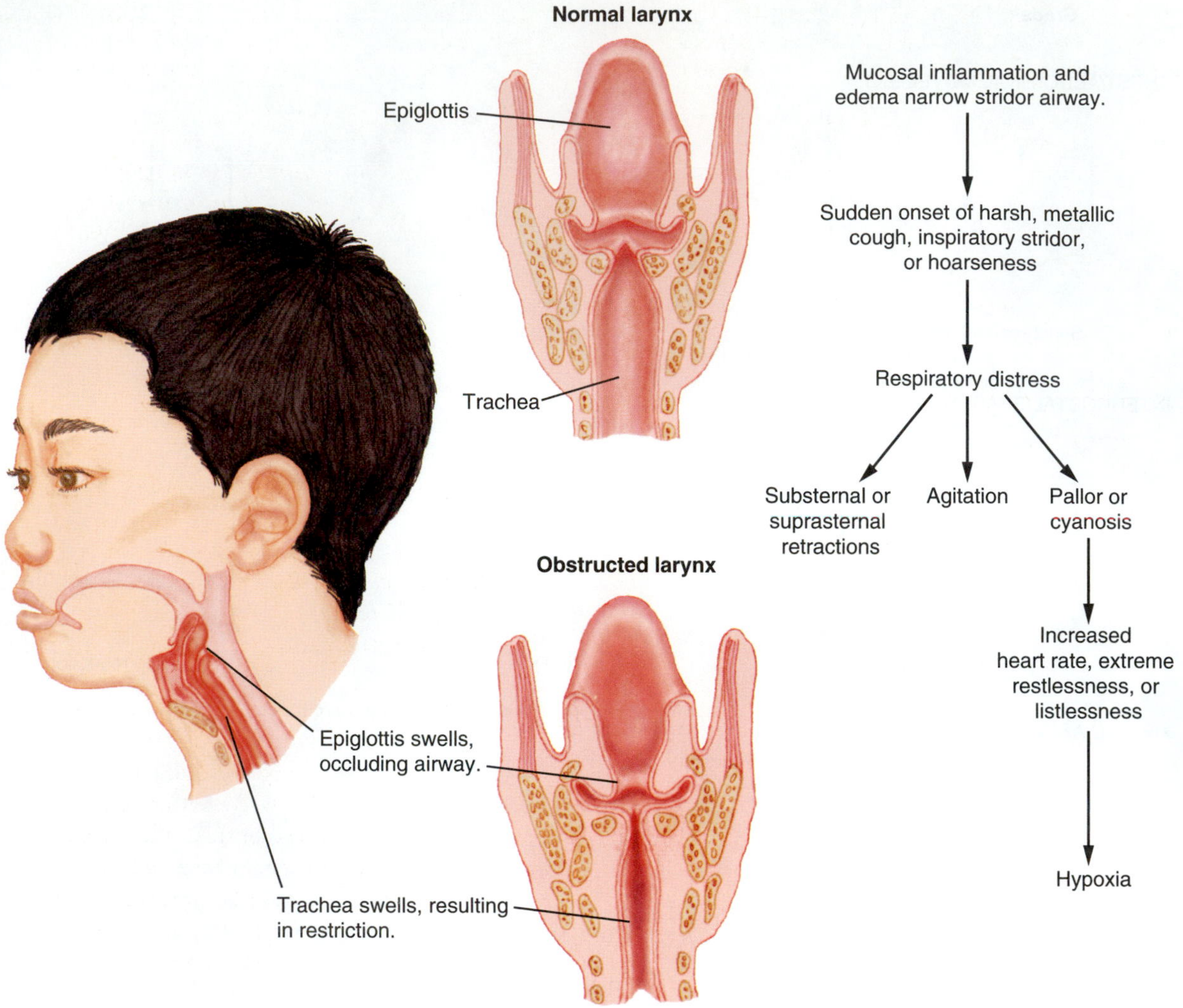

FIGURE 44-3 ■ Pathophysiology of croup.

croup after the child is exposed to cool, humidified air. (For example, this may occur after moving the patient from the residence to the emergency vehicle.) The paramedic should make all efforts to keep the child comfortable and at ease.

EPIGLOTTITIS

Although uncommon, epiglottitis can progress rapidly and become life threatening. Epiglottitis is caused by a bacterial infection of the upper airway. It most often affects children between 3 and 7 years of age. However, it can occur at any age. The disease usually is associated with *Haemophilus influenzae* type B, but *Streptococcus, Pneumococcus,* and *Staphylococcus* organisms also have been implicated. The bacterial infection causes edema and occlusion from swelling of the epiglottis and supraglottic structures (pharynx, aryepiglottic folds, and arytenoid cartilage). Epiglottitis is a true emergency. It requires prompt, expert airway management.

> **NOTE** The *Haemophilus influenzae* type B (Hib) vaccine has dramatically reduced the number of cases of epiglottitis in children.[4] See Appendix 44-1 for recommended childhood and adolescent immunizations.

Epiglottitis usually begins suddenly. Typically, the child goes to bed without any symptoms. But then the child wakes up complaining of a sore throat and pain on swallowing. The child may have fever, a muffled voice (from edema of the mucosal covering of the vocal cords), and drooling from the pooled saliva that occurs because of difficult and painful swallowing (an ominous sign of impending airway obstruction). Differentiating epiglottitis from croup in the prehospital setting may be difficult. Table 44-3 lists the different characteristics of these illnesses.

On arrival, the paramedics usually find a child with epiglottitis sitting upright (Fig. 44-4). Often the child is leaning forward with the head hyperextended. This position aids breathing (tripod position). The tongue may be protruding, or the child may have inspiratory stridor. These children usually do not cry or struggle because all of their attention and energy is being used to maximize air exchange. Inspiratory stridor with a characteristic rattle often is present. The child also may be gasping or gulping for air. Classic signs of respiratory distress usually are present. The definitive care for

TABLE 44-3 Comparison of the Symptoms of Croup and Epiglottitis

CHARACTERISTICS	CROUP	EPIGLOTTITIS
Occurrence	6 months to 4 years	3-7 years
Onset	Slow	Rapid
Comfortable position	Patient may lie down or sit upright	Patient prefers to sit upright
Cough	Barking cough	No barking cough; may have inspiratory stridor
Drooling	No drooling	Drooling, pain on swallowing
Temperature	Under 104° F	Over 104° F

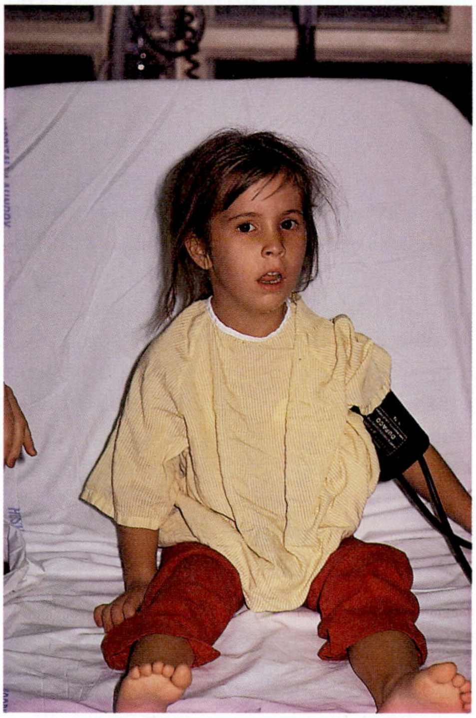

FIGURE 44-4 ■ Acute epiglottitis at presentation.

epiglottitis is in-hospital intubation and parenteral antibiotic therapy.

CRITICAL THINKING

What other childhood respiratory problems (traumatic and nontraumatic) can manifest with stridor?

Children with acute epiglottitis are in danger of full airway obstruction and respiratory arrest. Occlusion of the airway can occur suddenly. Occlusion may be caused by minor irritation of the throat, stress, and anxiety. For these reasons, gentle handling of a child suspected of having epiglottitis is essential. The following guidelines in prehospital management should be observed:

- Do not try to lay the child down or to change the position of comfort.
- Do not try to visualize the airway if the child is still ventilating adequately.
- Advise medical direction of the suspicion of epiglottitis. That way, the personnel and resources can be made available.
- Administer 100% humidified oxygen by mask unless it provokes agitation.
- Do not attempt vascular access.
- Have the correct-sized emergency airway equipment selected and ready.
- Transport the child to the hospital in the position of comfort.

If respiratory arrest occurs before arrival at the emergency department, the paramedic must attempt intubation. The paramedic should hyperventilate and preoxygenate the child's lungs with a bag-valve device before intubation. After the airway has been established, the paramedic should obtain intravenous (IV) access if time allows.

The paramedic should be prepared for a difficult intubation because the vocal cords are likely to be hidden by swollen tissues. An uncuffed endotracheal tube one to two sizes smaller than normal should be used. The paramedic should locate the laryngeal opening to the larynx by looking for mucus bubbles in the cleft between the edematous aryepiglottic folds and the swollen epiglottis. (Chest compressions during glottic visualization may produce a bubble at the tracheal opening.) In the rare instance that intubation cannot be achieved and the child cannot be ventilated adequately by a bag-valve device, medical direction may advise needle cricothyroidotomy. Often a child can be ventilated through the occlusive crisis of epiglottitis by bag-valve-mask ventilation using a tight facial seal. This may call for two persons—one to maintain the seal and the other to ventilate.

BACTERIAL TRACHEITIS

Bacterial tracheitis is an uncommon infection of the upper airway and subglottic trachea. It may occur after a viral illness. It generally occurs in infants and toddlers (1 to 5 years of age). However, bacterial tracheitis also can occur in older children. The signs and symptoms of bacterial tracheitis are those of respiratory distress or failure (depending on the severity) and may include the following:

- Agitation
- Cough that produces pus or mucus
- High-grade fever
- Hoarseness

- Inspiratory and expiratory stridor
- Throat pain

Emergency care is directed at providing airway, ventilatory, and circulatory support and rapid transport for evaluation by a physician. If airway obstruction, respiratory failure, or respiratory arrest develops, tracheal intubation is required with tracheal suction to remove mucus or pus. (Bag-valve-mask ventilation may require high pressures.) The hospital care includes intravenously administered antibiotics that are specific for the causative organism. These will be given after the child's airway has been stabilized.

ASTHMA

Asthma (described in Chapter 30) is characterized by inflammation, bronchoconstriction, and mucus production that obstruct the lower airways. Asthma results from autonomic dysfunction or exposure to sensitizing agents. The hallmarks of an acute exacerbation are anxiety, dyspnea, tachypnea, and audible expiratory wheezes with a prolonged expiratory phase. (A silent chest indicates impending respiratory failure.) Asthma is common among children over 2 years of age. It affects 5% to 10% of those under 10 years of age. An acute exacerbation may be triggered by infection, changes in temperature, physical exercise, and emotional response.

CRITICAL THINKING

What other signs or symptoms would lead you to believe that a child with asthma is decompensating?

The goals of prehospital management include ventilatory assistance (as needed), administration of humidified oxygen, reversal of the bronchospasm, and rapid transport for evaluation and treatment. Severe asthma may be life threatening. They can progress rapidly to respiratory failure. The paramedic should be ready to begin aggressive airway management along with ventilatory and circulatory support. Depending on local protocol, prior medication use, and the recommendations of medical direction, drug therapy may include aerosolized bronchodilators (***albuterol***, ***ipratropium***, ***terbutaline***), subcutaneously administered ***epinephrine*** or ***terbutaline*** with severe respiratory distress or failure, and sometimes corticosteroids (e.g., ***methylprednisolone***) during prolonged transports. (See the *Emergency Drug Index*.) If the patient requires tracheal intubation, medical direction may advise low tidal volumes (5 to 8 mL/kg) to reduce the potential for barotrauma.

BRONCHIOLITIS

Bronchiolitis is a viral disease often caused by respiratory syncytial virus infection of the lower airway. It usually affects children under 2 years of age. It often occurs in the winter months. Generally, bronchiolitis is associated with an upper respiratory infection. Bronchiolitis (like asthma) manifests with tachypnea and wheezing.

TABLE 44-4 Differentiation of Bronchiolitis and Asthma

CLINICAL FEATURES	BRONCHIOLITIS	ASTHMA
Occurrence	Usually <18 months	Any age
Season	Winter, spring	Any time
Family history of asthma	Usually absent	Usually present
Cause	Virus	Allergy, infection, exercise
Response to drugs	Some reversal of bronchospasm with beta-agonists	Reversal of bronchospasm

The illness is caused by infection and the inflammation of the distal airway. Bronchiolitis sometimes is unresponsive to therapy aimed at relieving bronchospasm. Table 44-4 lists key features that may aid in differential diagnosis.

Bronchiolitis generally is not serious and recovery is uneventful. However, sometimes it may become life threatening. Infants are at greater risk of developing respiratory failure from this condition because of the small diameter of the bronchioles. The prehospital care is aimed at providing ventilatory support with humidified oxygen. The patient should be transported rapidly for evaluation by a physician. A therapeutic trial of the administration of ***albuterol*** via nebulizer may reduce respiratory distress greatly.

PNEUMONIA

Pneumonia (described in Chapter 30) is an acute infection of the lower airway and lungs. It involves the alveolar walls or the alveoli. Pneumonia commonly is caused by a bacterial or viral infection. Children with pneumonia may have a history of recent airway infection. They also may have respiratory distress or failure (depending on the severity) and any of the following:

- Decreased breath sounds
- Fever
- Pain in the chest
- Rales
- Rhonchi (localized or diffuse)
- Tachypnea

Most children with pneumonia have only mild signs and symptoms. Most require no immediate treatment or airway support. However, when respiratory distress is present, stabilization of the airway is the highest priority. In severe cases, bronchodilators may be indicated. Assisted ventilations via bag-valve device or intubation of the trachea also may be required.

Shock

As described in Chapter 21, shock is an abnormal condition characterized by inadequate delivery of oxygen to meet the

BOX 44-2 Signs and Symptoms of Compensated and Decompensated Shock

Compensated (Reversible)
Cool, pale extremities
Decreased urinary output
Delayed capillary refill
Irritability or anxiety
Normal systolic blood pressure
Tachycardia
Tachypnea
Weak peripheral pulses/full central pulses

Decompensated (Often Irreversible)
Absent peripheral pulses/weak central pulses
Cool, pale, dusky, mottled extremities
Hypotension
Lethargy or coma
Marked tachycardia or bradycardia
Marked tachypnea or bradypnea
Significantly decreased urinary output
Significantly delayed capillary refill

metabolic demands of tissues. The condition may occur with increased, normal, or decreased blood pressure. Shock is categorized as *compensated* (shock without hypotension) or *decompensated* (shock with hypotension) (Box 44-2).

The paramedic must take into account a number of special considerations when caring for a child in shock. These include circulating blood volume, body surface area and hypothermia, cardiac reserve, respiratory fatigue, vital signs, and assessment.

CIRCULATING BLOOD VOLUME

In adults, blood volume accounts for 5% to 6% of total body weight, or 50 to 60 mL/kg of body weight; in children, blood volume accounts for 7% to 8% of total body weight, or 70 to 80 mL/kg of body weight. Although the percentage of circulating blood volume in a child is greater than that in an adult, a child's actual blood volume is considerably lower than an adult's. Therefore a relatively small loss of blood may be devastating. For example, a blood loss of 100 mL in an adult is a 2% loss; a 100 mL loss in an infant is a 15% to 20% loss, resulting in shock.

A child with a blood or fluid deficit will maintain stable hemodynamics until all compensatory mechanisms fail (i.e., the blood pressure may be normal or only slightly decreased) (Table 44-5). At that point, shock progresses rapidly, with serious deterioration. These efficient compensatory mechanisms can mask a potentially life-threatening condition. Thus the paramedic must hold a high degree of suspicion. The paramedic must actively search for shock as a cause of the patient's complaint or clinical presentation. Early recognition, stabilization (airway control, fluid replacement), and rapid transport to a proper facility are critical when caring for children in shock.

TABLE 44-5 Systolic Blood Pressure Characterizing Hypotension in the Pediatric Patient

AGE	SYSTOLIC BLOOD PRESSURE
Term neonates (0 to 28 days of age)	<60 mm Hg
Infants (1 month to 12 months)	<70 mm Hg
Children (1 year to 10 years)	<70 mm Hg (2 × age in years)
Beyond 10 years	<90 mm Hg

CRITICAL THINKING
How comfortable are you with starting an intravenous infusion on an infant or young child?

BODY SURFACE AREA AND HYPOTHERMIA

Young children have a large body surface area in proportion to body weight. Their compensatory mechanisms (e.g., shivering) also are not well developed. Children in shock quickly can develop hypothermia from exposure and concurrent metabolic acidosis, increased vascular resistance, respiratory depression, and myocardial dysfunction. Hypothermia makes resuscitation and drug therapy less effective. Thus the paramedic should maintain the patient's body temperature by using blankets, covering the child's head with towels, and using warming devices for IV fluids.

CARDIAC RESERVE

Infants and children already have high metabolic needs. As a result, they have less cardiac reserve than adults for stressful situations such as shock. An important step is to reduce the energy and oxygen requirements of a child in shock as much as possible. This can be done by providing ventilatory support, reducing anxiety, and maintaining moderate ambient temperatures.

RESPIRATORY FATIGUE

Respiratory muscle fatigue may lead to hypoventilation, hypoxemia, and respiratory failure or arrest. Like other compensatory mechanisms of the child, respiratory compensation generally is at a maximum until it is depleted. At that time, deterioration can be sudden. For this reason, airway control and supplemental oxygen are essential in all children who are seriously ill or injured.

VITAL SIGNS AND ASSESSMENT

The paramedic must consider many factors when evaluating a child's vital signs. For example, blood pressure and pulse rate vary greatly. They vary with age, body temperature, and degree of agitation. The paramedic should measure vital signs as baseline assessments; they may be of limited value in assessing the circulation of a child in shock. The most effective assessment is constant monitoring of the child's mental and physical status and the response to therapy. The following nine evaluation components should be noted when assessing a child in shock:

1. Level of consciousness
   Ability to make eye contact
   Ability to recognize family members
   Agitation
   Anxiety
2. Skin
   Capillary refill (in children under 6 years of age)
   Color
   Moisture
   Temperature
   Turgor
3. Mucous membranes
   Color
   Moisture
4. Nail beds
   Capillary refill (in children younger than 6 years of age)
   Color
5. Peripheral circulation
   Collapse
   Distention
6. Cardiac
   Electrocardiogram findings
   Location of pulses
   Quality of pulses
   Rate
   Rhythm
7. Respiration
   Depth
   Rate
8. Blood pressure (in children over 3 years of age)
9. Body temperature

> **NOTE** Sustained tachycardia in the absence of obvious causes such as fever, pain, and agitation may be an early sign of cardiovascular compromise. Bradycardia, however, may be a preterminal cardiac rhythm indicating advanced shock and often is associated with hypotension.[5]

HYPOVOLEMIA

One common cause of hypovolemia in children is dehydration resulting from vomiting and diarrhea. Another is blood loss resulting from trauma or internal bleeding. Children are also at risk of intravascular volume depletion as a result of burns. (See Chapter 23.)

Dehydration. Profound fluid and electrolyte imbalances can occur in children as a result of diarrhea, vomiting, poor fluid intake, fever, or burns. Dehydration compromises cardiac output and systemic perfusion. This occurs if the child loses the fluid equivalent of 5% or more of total body weight. For the adolescent, losses of 5% to 7% of total body weight can compromise perfusion (Fig. 44-5). If allowed to progress, dehydration can result in renal failure, shock, and death. The severity of the dehydration and fluid loss can be estimated from a history of the child's weight loss and the physical examination (Fig. 44-6). Table 44-6 provides signs and symptoms related to degrees of dehydration.

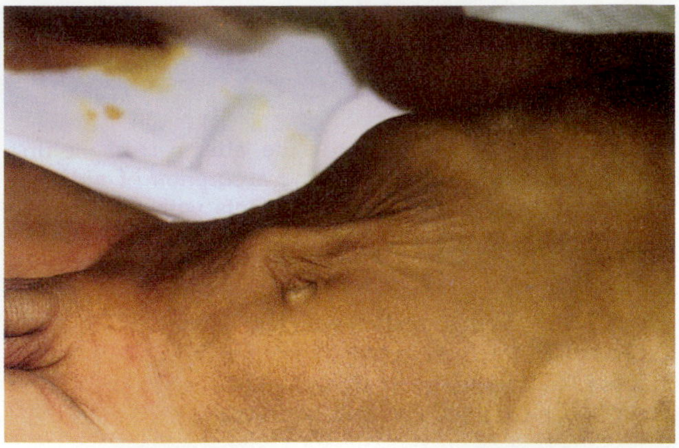

FIGURE 44-5 ■ Severe dehydration.

Airway and ventilatory support (if needed) are the initial steps in treatment for the dehydrated child. Next, treatment is directed at replacing and maintaining blood volume and perfusion. Intravenous therapy should be initiated (per medical direction) with isotonic crystalloids such as lactated Ringer's solution or normal saline. A fluid bolus of 20 mL/kg (administered in less than 20 minutes)[6] should be administered and may be repeated until the patient's systemic perfusion improves and an appropriate blood pressure has been obtained. After physician evaluation and initial shock resuscitation, the fluid administration rate and type of fluid replacement are determined by the volume and type of fluid deficit (isotonic, hypotonic, hypertonic) and the patient's response to therapy.

> **CRITICAL THINKING**
> What are some ways to determine the child's weight for fluid and drug dosing?

Blood Loss. As stated before, even a small amount of blood loss can be serious for the pediatric patient (Table 44-7). After the paramedic achieves control of external hemorrhage (if present), secures the patient's airway, and provides high-concentration oxygen, the child's circulatory status may require support with IV therapy (per medical direction).

As with other causes of hypovolemia, volume replacement is needed. Isotonic crystalloid solutions such as normal saline or lactated Ringer's solution should be used. The first bolus should be 20 mL/kg. If the volume loss is in the

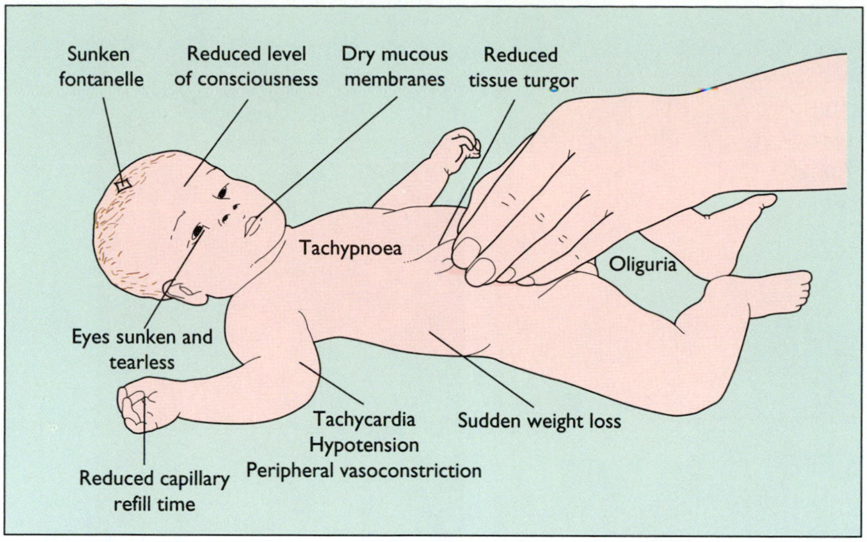

FIGURE 44-6 ■ Clinical features of dehydration in an infant.

TABLE 44-6 Assessment of Degree of Dehydration

CLINICAL PARAMETERS	MILD	MODERATE	SEVERE
Body weight loss	Infant: 5% (50 mL/kg)	10% (100 mL/kg)	15% (150 mL/kg)
Skin turgor	Slightly decreased	Moderately decreased	Greatly decreased
Fontanelle (infant)	Possibly flat or depressed	Depressed	Significantly depressed
Mucous membranes	Dry	Very dry	Parched
Skin perfusion	Warm with normal color	Cool (extremities) Pale	Cold (extremities) Mottled or gray
Heart rate	Mildly tachycardic	Moderately tachycardic	Extremely tachycardic
Peripheral pulses	Normal	Diminished	Absent
Blood pressure	Normal	Normal	Reduced
Sensorium	Normal or irritable	Irritable or lethargic	Unresponsive

TABLE 44-7 Classification of Hemorrhagic Shock in Pediatric Trauma Patients Based on Systemic Signs

SYSTEM	VERY MILD HEMORRHAGE*	MILD HEMORRHAGE†	MODERATE HEMORRHAGE‡	SEVERE HEMORRHAGE§
Cardiovascular	Normal or mildly increased heart rate	Tachycardia	Significant tachycardia	Severe tachycardia
	Normal pulse rate	Peripheral pulses may be diminished	Thready peripheral pulses	Thready central pulses
	Normal blood pressure	Normal blood pressure	Hypotension	Significant hypotension
	Normal pH	Normal pH	Metabolic acidosis	Significant acidosis
Respiratory	Normal rate	Tachypnea	Moderate tachypnea	Severe tachypnea
Central nervous system	Slight anxiousness	Irritability, confusion Combative affect	Irritability or lethargy Diminished pain response	Lethargy Coma
Skin	Warm, pink color	Cool extremities, mottling	Cool extremities, mottling or pallor	Cold extremities, pallor or cyanosis
	Brisk capillary refill	Delayed capillary refill	Prolonged capillary refill	Prolonged capillary refill
Kidneys	Normal urine output	Oliguria, increased specific gravity	Oliguria, increased blood urea nitrogen level	Anuria

*<15% blood volume loss.
†15% to 25% blood volume loss.
‡25% blood volume loss.
§40% blood volume loss.

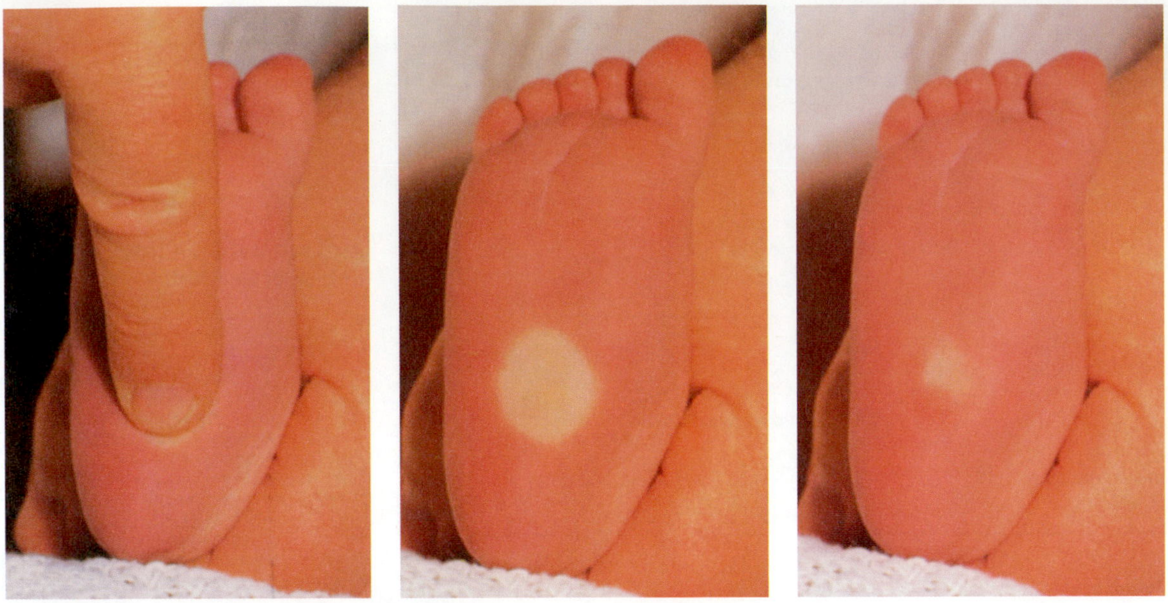

FIGURE 44-7 ■ Capillary refill in a child in shock.

20% range, vital signs should improve after this infusion. If improvement occurs, IV therapy should be continued at a maintenance rate during patient transport. The child may show little response to the first bolus. (For example, a slight improvement in color and capillary refill and a decreased heart rate may be evident (Fig. 44-7). If this is the case or if the patient does not respond to the initial infusion, the paramedic should give a second bolus of 20 mL/kg.

▶**NOTE** Establishing an intravenous line in a child through a peripheral vein (described in Chapter 18) can be difficult even in the most controlled settings. As a result, medical direction may advise that the paramedic establish an intraosseous infusion for the child in shock. They also may advise that the child be stabilized without establishing venous access and rapidly transported to a proper facility.

DISTRIBUTIVE SHOCK

As described in Chapter 21, distributive shock is used to refer to septic shock, neurogenic shock, and anaphylactic shock. This type of shock results in peripheral pooling because of loss of vasomotor tone. The vasodilation that occurs causes the blood pressure to fall. Vasodilation also allows plasma to leak from the vascular space. This type of shock is fairly uncommon in children.

Septic shock usually is caused by a systemic bacterial infection. Septic shock sometimes is associated with illnesses such as meningitis and pneumonia. Toxins released by the pathogen affect arterioles, capillaries, and venules, altering microcirculatory pressure and capillary permeability. These children usually appear very ill. They may have signs and symptoms that include those of decompensated shock. Characteristic findings in septic shock include skin that is warm in the early stages, and skin that is cool in the late stages of the illness.

Neurogenic shock results from sudden peripheral vasodilation caused by a traumatic injury. Most often this injury is to the spinal cord. The loss of sympathetic impulses and resultant vasodilation increase the size of the vascular compartment. The normal intravascular volume is not enough to fill the vascular compartment and to perfuse tissues. Characteristic findings in neurogenic shock include warm skin, bradycardia, and impaired neurological function.

Anaphylactic shock occurs when a person is exposed to a substance that produces a severe allergic reaction (see Chapter 33). Common causes of allergic reactions include antibiotic agents, venoms, and insect stings. The bodily response to the antigen causes a release of histamine. This release results in peripheral vasodilation and the leak of intravascular fluid into the interstitial space; this results in a decrease in intravascular volume. Characteristic findings in anaphylactic shock include vomiting and diarrhea, hives, allergic rash, erythema, airway swelling and wheezing (from bronchoconstriction) and hypotension.

Emergency care for patients with distributive shock is directed at ensuring the patient's vital functions through airway, ventilatory, and circulatory support, and rapid transport to an appropriate medical facility. Medical direction may advise IV fluid therapy and drugs to manage specific forms of distributive shock. (For example, ***dopamine*** may be given for neurogenic shock; ***epinephrine*** may be given for anaphylaxis.) Aids that often are used to calculate drug and fluid doses for pediatric patients were described in Chapter 18. These aids include the Pedi-Wheel and the Broselow tape (Fig. 44-8).

Cardiomyopathy. *Cardiomyopathy* refers to any disease of the heart muscle that causes a reduction in the force of

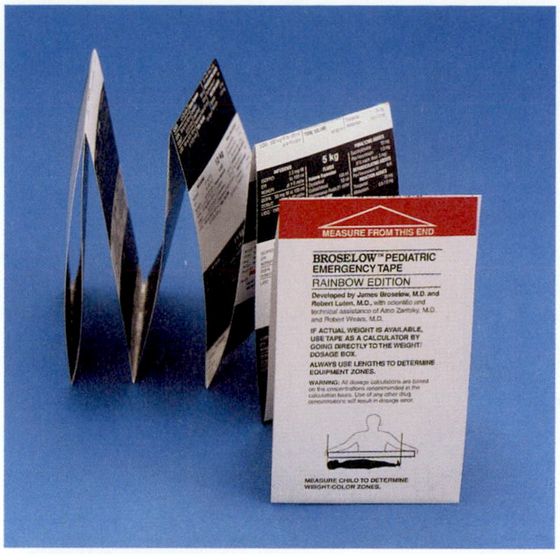

FIGURE 44-8 ■ Pediatric Broselow tape.

heart contractions. Decrease in the force of contractions decreases the amount of blood circulated to the lungs and to the rest of the body. In children, the condition usually results from viral infection or congenital abnormalities that affect both ventricles of the heart. Symptoms include fatigue, chest pain, and dysrhythmias. In severe cases, they include signs of heart failure and cardiogenic shock, such as the following:

- Crackles
- Hypotension
- Jugular vein distention (difficult to determine in young children)
- Peripheral edema
- Tachycardia
- Tachypnea

Patients in stable condition are managed with supportive care, administration of oxygen, and transport for evaluation by a physician. Children who are hypotensive and show other signs and symptoms of decompensation may require vascular access for the administration of drugs (e.g., antidysrhythmics, diuretics, and vasopressors). Intravenous fluid therapy should be restricted in these patients. This will help to avoid volume overload.

Rhythm Disturbances

As discussed in Chapter 43, most children have healthy hearts. When rhythm disturbances occur, they usually are the result of hypoxia, acidosis, hypotension, or structural heart disease.[5] The most common dysrhythmias in pediatric patients are sinus tachycardia, supraventricular tachycardia, bradycardia, and asystole. Ventricular tachycardia and ventricular fibrillation are not common but do occur.[2] The recommended management for these dysrhythmias is outlined in Figures 44-9 to 44-12. Drug treatments and specific guidelines for use of airway equipment during pediatric life support are listed in Tables 44-8 and 44-9.

Dysrhythmias and basic and advanced life support procedures (including cardiopulmonary resuscitation) are addressed in Chapter 29. The reader should refer to that chapter for review. The following discussions outline the unique aspects of abnormal rhythms in children.[5]

BRADYDYSRHYTHMIAS

Clinically significant bradycardia is defined as a heart rate less than 60 beats/min (or a rapidly dropping heart rate) associated with poor systemic perfusion. This bradycardia occurs despite adequate oxygenation and ventilation. Bradydysrhythmias may be caused by hypoxemia, acidosis, hypotension, hypoglycemia, central nervous system injury, or excessive vagal stimulation (e.g., from endotracheal intubation or pharyngeal suctioning). In infants and children, sinus bradycardia, sinus node arrest with slow junctional or idioventricular rhythm, and atrioventricular block are the most common preterminal rhythms. The paramedic should consider drug-induced causes (e.g., digitalis toxicity) and myocarditis with bradycardia caused by heart block. Infants and children with a history of heart surgery may have injury at the atrioventricular node or conduction system. This injury would produce sick sinus syndrome or heart block. All symptomatic bradycardias require treatment. Important electrocardiogram findings include the following:

- Heart rate is less than 60 beats/min.
- P waves may or may not be visible.
- QRS complex duration may be normal or prolonged.
- The P wave and QRS complex often are unrelated.

Treatment. The initial management of bradycardia should ensure that breathing is adequate and the patient is receiving supplemental oxygen (Fig. 44-9). If drug therapy is required, ***epinephrine*** is the drug of choice. Bradycardia caused by heart block or increased vagal tone (both of which are rare in pediatric patients) should be managed with ***atropine.*** In cases where bradycardia is caused by problems with the sinus node, external cardiac pacing may be lifesaving. External cardiac pacing is uncomfortable. Its use in children is reserved for profound symptomatic bradycardia that does not respond to advanced life support and basic life support treatments.

PULSELESS ELECTRICAL ACTIVITY

Pulseless electrical activity often precedes asystole. It usually is caused by prolonged periods of hypoxia, ischemia, or hypercarbia. Reversible causes of pulseless electrical activity include the four *H*'s (hypovolemia, hypoxemia, hypothermia, and hyperkalemia) and the four *T*'s (tension pneumothorax, pericardial tamponade, toxins, and thromboembolus) described in Chapter 29. Important electrocardiogram findings include the following:

- A slow, wide-complex rhythm
- The presence of some electrical activity (other than ventricular tachycardia/ventricular fibrillation) and the absence of a detectable pulse

Treatment. Pulseless electrical activity is managed in the same way as asystole (Fig. 44-10) with drug therapy ***(epinephrine)*** and cardiopulmonary resuscitation. Defibrillation is not effective in the treatment of asystolic arrest.[5] Reversible causes of the condition (the four *H*'s and four *T*'s) should be considered and corrected if possible.

Text continued on p. 1140

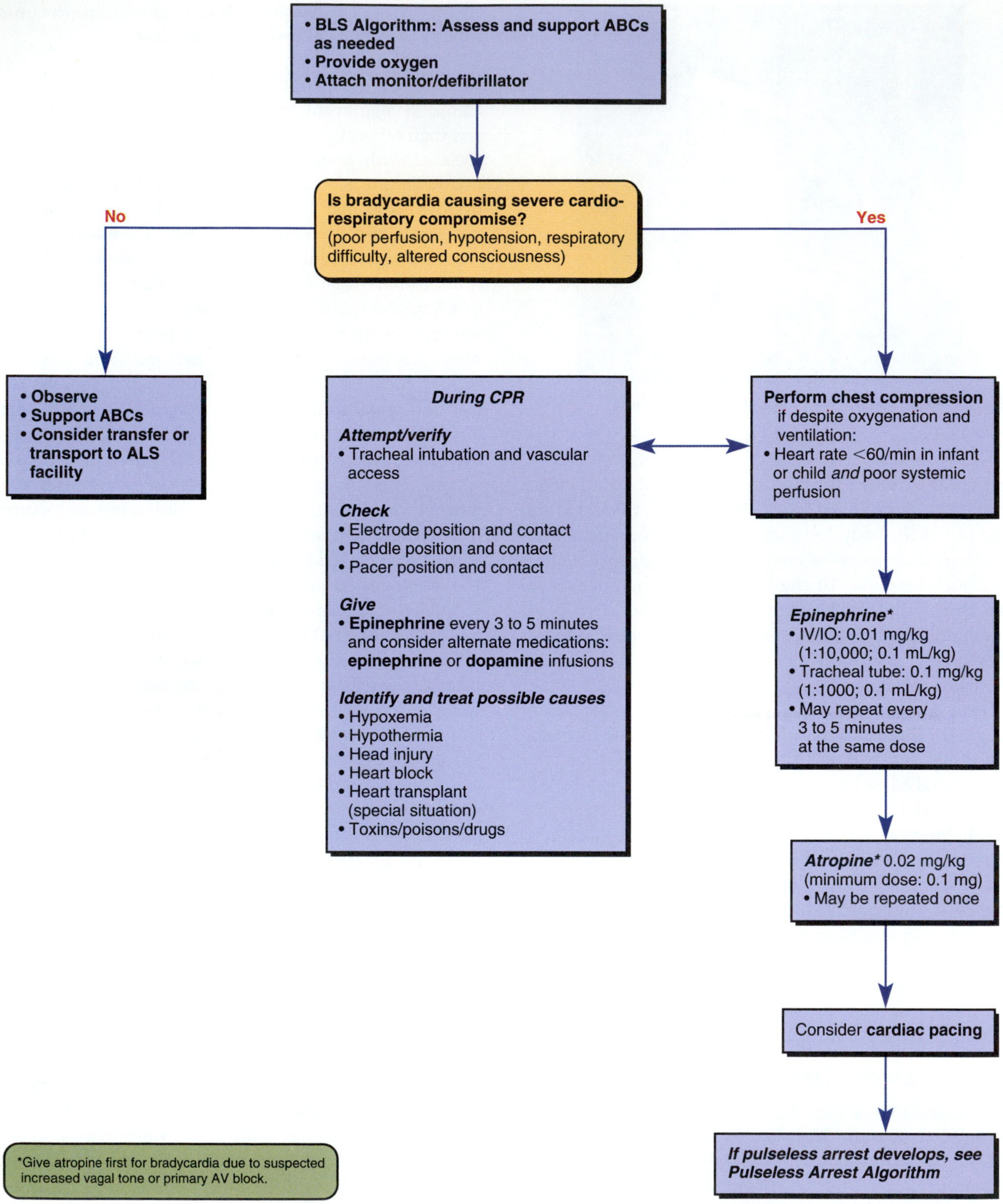
• BLS Algorithm: Assess and support ABCs as needed
• Provide oxygen
• Attach monitor/defibrillator
Is bradycardia causing severe cardio-respiratory compromise?
(poor perfusion, hypotension, respiratory difficulty, altered consciousness)
No
Yes
• Observe
• Support ABCs
• Consider transfer or transport to ALS facility
During CPR
Attempt/verify
• Tracheal intubation and vascular access
Check
• Electrode position and contact
• Paddle position and contact
• Pacer position and contact
Give
• Epinephrine every 3 to 5 minutes and consider alternate medications: epinephrine or dopamine infusions
Identify and treat possible causes
• Hypoxemia
• Hypothermia
• Head injury
• Heart block
• Heart transplant (special situation)
• Toxins/poisons/drugs
Perform chest compression if despite oxygenation and ventilation:
• Heart rate <60/min in infant or child and poor systemic perfusion
Epinephrine*
• IV/IO: 0.01 mg/kg (1:10,000; 0.1 mL/kg)
• Tracheal tube: 0.1 mg/kg (1:1000; 0.1 mL/kg)
• May repeat every 3 to 5 minutes at the same dose
Atropine* 0.02 mg/kg (minimum dose: 0.1 mg)
• May be repeated once
Consider cardiac pacing
If pulseless arrest develops, see Pulseless Arrest Algorithm
*Give atropine first for bradycardia due to suspected increased vagal tone or primary AV block.

FIGURE 44-9 ■ Algorithm for bradycardia in a pediatric patient.

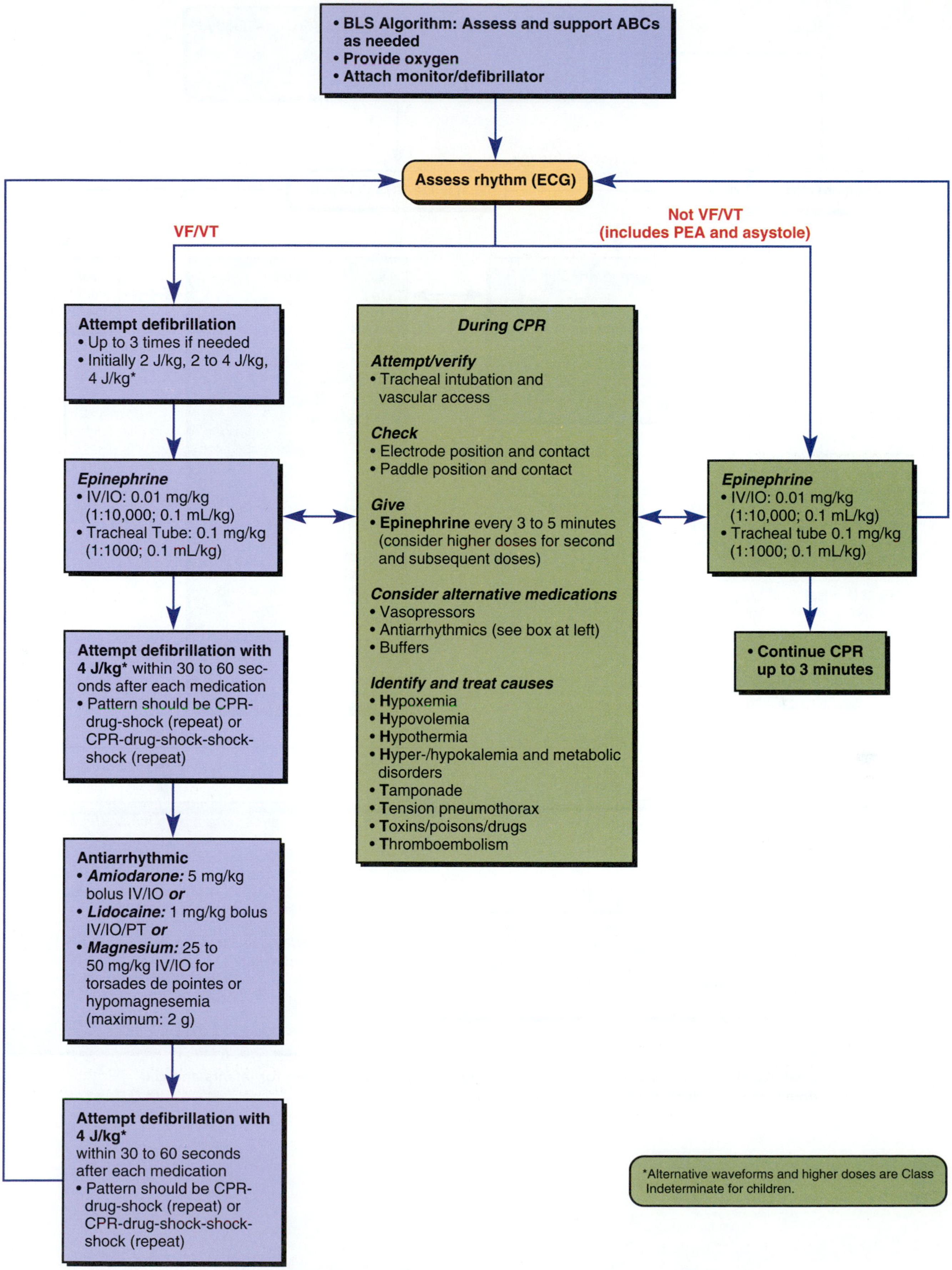

FIGURE 44-10 ■ Pediatric advanced life support pulseless arrest algorithm.

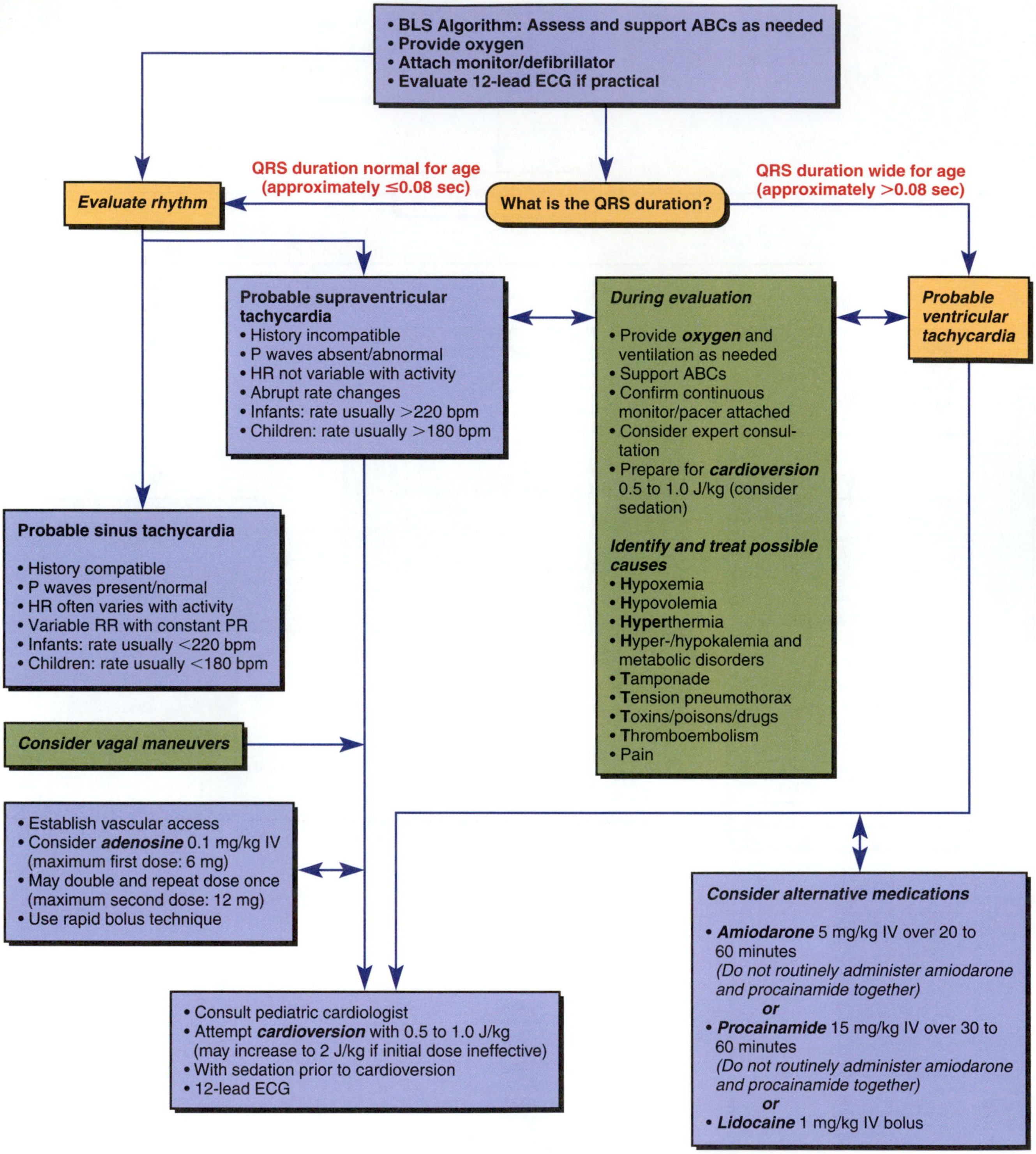
• BLS Algorithm: Assess and support ABCs as needed
• Provide oxygen
• Attach monitor/defibrillator
• Evaluate 12-lead ECG if practical
Evaluate rhythm
QRS duration normal for age (approximately ≤0.08 sec)
What is the QRS duration?
QRS duration wide for age (approximately >0.08 sec)
Probable supraventricular tachycardia
• History incompatible
• P waves absent/abnormal
• HR not variable with activity
• Abrupt rate changes
• Infants: rate usually >220 bpm
• Children: rate usually >180 bpm
During evaluation
• Provide oxygen and ventilation as needed
• Support ABCs
• Confirm continuous monitor/pacer attached
• Consider expert consultation
• Prepare for cardioversion 0.5 to 1.0 J/kg (consider sedation)
Identify and treat possible causes
• Hypoxemia
• Hypovolemia
• Hyperthermia
• Hyper-/hypokalemia and metabolic disorders
• Tamponade
• Tension pneumothorax
• Toxins/poisons/drugs
• Thromboembolism
• Pain
Probable ventricular tachycardia
Probable sinus tachycardia
• History compatible
• P waves present/normal
• HR often varies with activity
• Variable RR with constant PR
• Infants: rate usually <220 bpm
• Children: rate usually <180 bpm
Consider vagal maneuvers
• Establish vascular access
• Consider adenosine 0.1 mg/kg IV (maximum first dose: 6 mg)
• May double and repeat dose once (maximum second dose: 12 mg)
• Use rapid bolus technique
Consider alternative medications
• Amiodarone 5 mg/kg IV over 20 to 60 minutes
(Do not routinely administer amiodarone and procainamide together)
or
• Procainamide 15 mg/kg IV over 30 to 60 minutes
(Do not routinely administer amiodarone and procainamide together)
or
• Lidocaine 1 mg/kg IV bolus
• Consult pediatric cardiologist
• Attempt cardioversion with 0.5 to 1.0 J/kg (may increase to 2 J/kg if initial dose ineffective)
• With sedation prior to cardioversion
• 12-lead ECG

FIGURE 44-11 ■ Pediatric advanced life support tachycardia algorithm for infants and children with rapid rhythm and adequate perfusion.

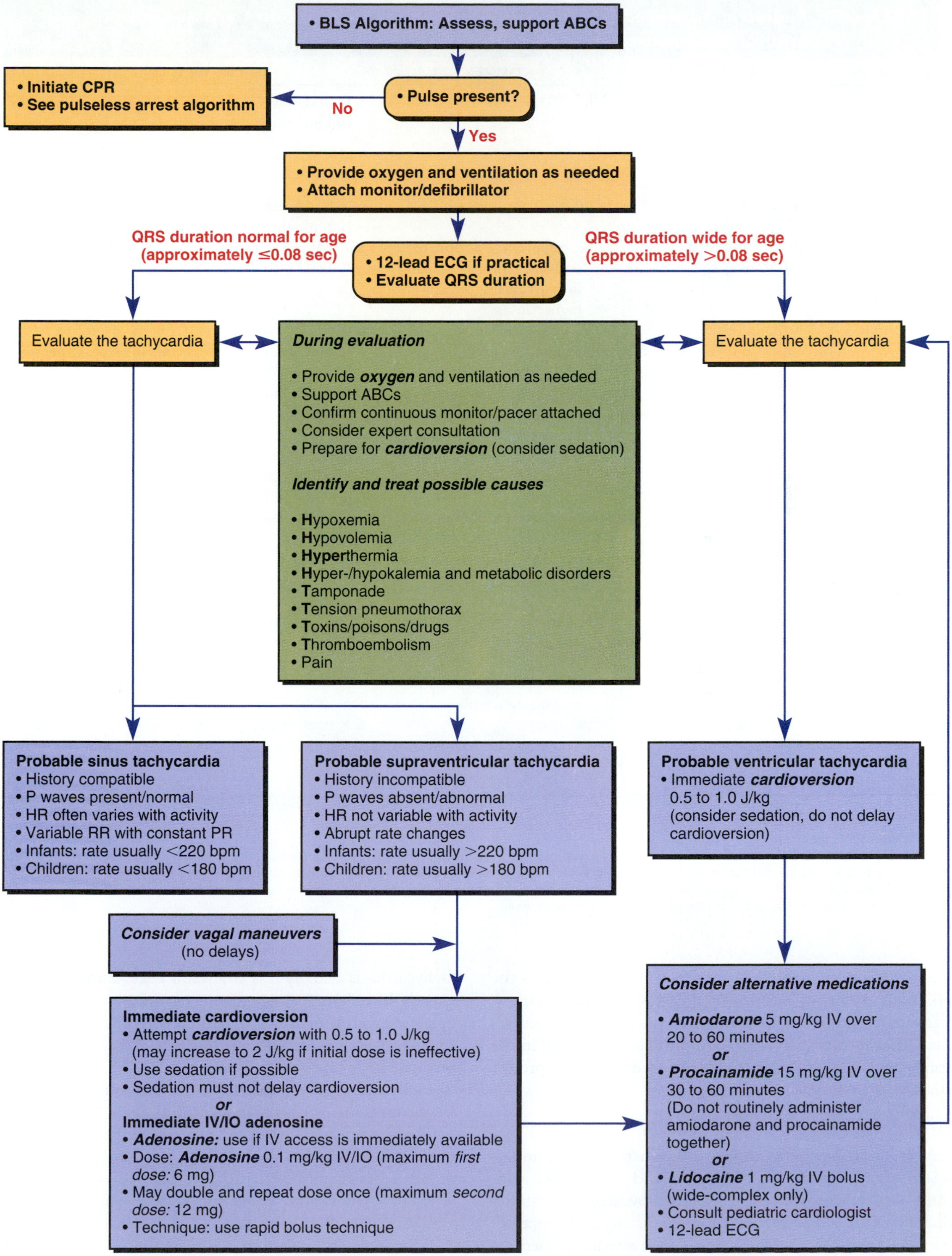
• BLS Algorithm: Assess, support ABCs
• Initiate CPR
• See pulseless arrest algorithm
No
• Pulse present?
Yes
• Provide oxygen and ventilation as needed
• Attach monitor/defibrillator
QRS duration normal for age
(approximately ≤0.08 sec)
• 12-lead ECG if practical
• Evaluate QRS duration
QRS duration wide for age
(approximately >0.08 sec)
Evaluate the tachycardia
During evaluation
• Provide oxygen and ventilation as needed
• Support ABCs
• Confirm continuous monitor/pacer attached
• Consider expert consultation
• Prepare for cardioversion (consider sedation)
Identify and treat possible causes
• Hypoxemia
• Hypovolemia
• Hyperthermia
• Hyper-/hypokalemia and metabolic disorders
• Tamponade
• Tension pneumothorax
• Toxins/poisons/drugs
• Thromboembolism
• Pain
Evaluate the tachycardia
Probable sinus tachycardia
• History compatible
• P waves present/normal
• HR often varies with activity
• Variable RR with constant PR
• Infants: rate usually <220 bpm
• Children: rate usually <180 bpm
Probable supraventricular tachycardia
• History incompatible
• P waves absent/abnormal
• HR not variable with activity
• Abrupt rate changes
• Infants: rate usually >220 bpm
• Children: rate usually >180 bpm
Probable ventricular tachycardia
• Immediate cardioversion
0.5 to 1.0 J/kg
(consider sedation, do not delay
cardioversion)
Consider vagal maneuvers
(no delays)
Immediate cardioversion
• Attempt cardioversion with 0.5 to 1.0 J/kg
(may increase to 2 J/kg if initial dose is ineffective)
• Use sedation if possible
• Sedation must not delay cardioversion
or
Immediate IV/IO adenosine
• Adenosine: use if IV access is immediately available
• Dose: Adenosine 0.1 mg/kg IV/IO (maximum first
dose: 6 mg)
• May double and repeat dose once (maximum second
dose: 12 mg)
• Technique: use rapid bolus technique
Consider alternative medications
• Amiodarone 5 mg/kg IV over
20 to 60 minutes
or
• Procainamide 15 mg/kg IV over
30 to 60 minutes
(Do not routinely administer
amiodarone and procainamide
together)
or
• Lidocaine 1 mg/kg IV bolus
(wide-complex only)
• Consult pediatric cardiologist
• 12-lead ECG

FIGURE 44-12 ■ Pediatric advanced life support tachycardia algorithm for infants and children with rapid rhythm and evidence of poor perfusion.

TABLE 44-8 Pediatric Advanced Life Support Medications to Maintain Cardiac Output and for Postresuscitation Stabilization

MEDICATION	DOSE RANGE	COMMENT	PREPARATION*
Amrinone	IV/IO loading dose: 0.75-1 mg/kg IV over 5 min; may repeat 2 times IV/IO infusion: 5-10 mcg/kg per min	Inodilator	6 × body mass (kg) = No. of mg diluted to total 100 mL; then 1 mL/hr delivers 1 mcg/kg per min
Dobutamine	IV/IO infusion: 2-20 mcg/kg per min	Inotrope; vasodilator	6 × body mass (kg) = No. of mg diluted to total 100 mL; then 1 mL/hr delivers 1 mcg/kg per min
Dopamine	IV/IO infusion: 2-20 mcg/kg per min	Inotrope; chronotrope; renal and splanchnic vasodilator in lower doses; pressor in higher doses	6 × body mass (kg) = No. of mg diluted to total 100 mL; then 1 mL/hr delivers 0.1 mcg/kg per min
Epinephrine	IV/IO infusion: 0.1-1 mcg/kg per min	Inotrope; chronotrope; vasodilator in lower doses and pressor in higher doses	0.6 × body mass (kg) = No. of mg diluted to total 100 mL; then 1 mL/hr delivers 0.1 mcg/kg per min
Lidocaine	IV/IO loading dose: 1 mg/kg IV/IO infusion: 20-50 mcg/kg per min	Antidysrhythmic, mild negative inotrope; use lower infusion rate if poor cardiac output or poor hepatic function	60 × body mass (kg) = No. of mg diluted to total 100 mL; then 1 mL/hr delivers 10 mcg/kg per min *or* **alternative premix:** 120 mg/100 mL at 1 to 2.5 mL/kg per hour
Milrinone	IV/IO loading dose: 50-75 mcg/kg IV/IO infusion: 0.5-0.75 mcg/kg per min	Inodilator	0.6 × body mass (kg) = No. of mg diluted to total 100 mL; then 1 mL/hr delivers 0.1 mcg/kg per min
Norepinephrine	IV/IO infusion: 0.1-2 mcg/kg per min	Vasopressor	0.6 × body mass (kg) = No. of mg diluted to total 100 mL; then 1 mL/hr delivers 0.1 mcg/kg per min
Prostaglandin E_1	IV/IO infusion: 0.05-0.1 mcg/kg per min	Maintains patency of ductus arteriosus in cyanotic congenital heart disease; monitor for apnea, hypotension, and hypoglycemia	0.3 × body mass (kg) = No. of mg diluted to total 50 mL; then 1 mL/hr delivers 0.1 mcg/kg per min
Sodium nitroprusside	IV/IO infusion: 1-8 mcg/kg per min	Vasodilator Prepare only in dextrose in water	6 × body mass (kg) = No. of mg diluted to total 100 mL; then 1 mL/hr delivers 1 mcg/kg per min

From American Heart Association: Guidelines 2000 for cardiopulmonary resuscitation and emergency cardiovascular care, International Consensus on Science, *Circulation* 102(8):328, 2000.
IV, Intravenous; *IO,* intraosseous.
*Most infusions may be calculated based on the rule of 6 as illustrated in the table. Alternatively, a standard concentration may be used to provide more dilute or more concentrated drug solution, but then an individual dose must be calculated for each patient and each infusion rate as follows: Infusion rate (mL/hr) = (mass [kg] × dose [mcg/kg per minute] × 60 min/hr)/concentration (mcg/mL). Diluent may be 5% dextrose in water, 5% dextrose in half-normal saline, normal saline, or lactate Ringer's unless noted otherwise.

Identification and treatment of the underlying cause is the only true means of reversal of pulseless electrical activity. Early recognition and treatment of pulseless electrical activity that results in a return of a pulse before arrival in the emergency department is associated with improved chances for survival.

SUPRAVENTRICULAR TACHYCARDIA

Supraventricular tachycardia is the most common nonarrest dysrhythmia during childhood and is the most common dysrhythmia that produces cardiovascular instability during infancy.[5] Two factors can help distinguish supraventricular tachycardia from sinus tachycardia caused by shock. They include patient history (e.g., dehydration or hemorrhage associated with shock) and heart rate. (Sinus tachycardia is usually less than 220 beats/min in infants, usually less than 180 beats/min in children, and usually greater than those rates with supraventricular tachycardia.) Important electrocardiogram findings in supraventricular tachycardia include the following:

- Heart rate is greater than 220 beats/min in infants and greater than 180 beats/min in children.
- The rhythm usually is regular because associated atrioventricular block is rare.
- P waves may not be identifiable, especially when the ventricular rate is high. If present, P waves usually are negative in leads II, III, and aV_F.
- QRS complex duration is normal in most children (<0.10 second). Supraventricular tachycardia with aberrant conduction (wide-complex supraventricular tachy-

TABLE 44-9 Pediatric Tracheal Tube and Suction Catheter Sizes*

APPROXIMATE AGE/SIZE (KG)	INTERNAL DIAMETER OF TRACHEAL TUBE (MM)	SUCTION CATHETER SIZE (FRENCH)
Premature infant (<1 kg)	2.5	5
Premature infant (1-2 kg)	3.0	5 or 6
Premature infant (2-3 kg)	3.0-3.5	6 or 8
Birth to 1 year/infant (3-10 kg)	3.5-4.0	8
1 year/small child (10-13 kg)	4.0	8
3 years/child (14-16 kg)	4.5	8 or 10
5 years/child (16-20 kg)	5.0	10
6 years/child (18-25 kg)	5.5	10
8 years/child to small adult (24-32 kg)	6.0 cuffed	10 or 12
12 years/adolescent (32-54 kg)	6.5 cuffed	12
16 years/adult (50+ kg)	7.0 cuffed	12
Adult female	7.0 cuffed	12 or 14
Adult male	7.0-8.0 cuffed	14

From American Heart Association: Guidelines 2000 for cardiopulmonary resuscitation and emergency cardiovascular care, International Consensus on Science, *Circulation* 102(8):328, 2000.

*These are approximations and should be adjusted based on clinical experience. Tracheal tube selection for a child should be based on the child's size or age. One size larger and one size smaller should be allowed for individual variation. Color-coding based on length or size of the child may facilitate approximation of correct tracheal tube size.

cardia) may be difficult to distinguish from ventricular tachycardia (but this form of ventricular tachycardia is rare in infants and children).

Treatment. Signs and symptoms during supraventricular tachycardia are affected by the child's age, duration of supraventricular tachycardia, prior ventricular function, and ventricular rate (Figs. 44-11 and 44-12). If the child is hemodynamically stable and cooperative, vagal maneuvers such as ice water being applied to the child's face, blowing through a straw, and carotid sinus massage may be successful in terminating the rhythm. Unstable supraventricular tachycardia is best managed with synchronized cardioversion or drug therapy. (***Adenosine*** is the drug of choice.)

Wide-complex tachycardias with signs of compromised tissue perfusion and impaired level of consciousness require immediate care. The paramedic should treat these tachycardias as if they are ventricular tachycardia. Urgent treatment includes synchronized cardioversion if pulses are present, and defibrillation if pulses are absent.

VENTRICULAR TACHYCARDIA AND VENTRICULAR FIBRILLATION

As stated before, ventricular tachycardia and ventricular fibrillation are uncommon in children. If present, the paramedic should consider causes of these dysrhythmias that include congenital heart disease, cardiomyopathies, myocarditis, reversible causes (e.g., drug toxicity), metabolic causes (e.g., hypoglycemia), or hypothermia. Important electrocardiogram findings include the following:

1. *Ventricular tachycardia*
   Ventricular rate at least 120 beats/min and regular
   Wide QRS complex
   P waves that often are not identifiable
2. *Ventricular fibrillation*
   No identifiable P wave, QRS complex, or T wave
   Ventricular fibrillation waves that may be coarse or fine

NOTE Automated external defibrillators with pediatric cable-pad systems have been approved by the Food and Drug Administration. They may be used for children under 8 years of age. These children must have no signs of circulation (Class IIb) and shockable rhythms (ventricular fibrillation and pulseless ventricular tachycardia). Ideally, the device should deliver a pediatric dose. The device also should be able specifically to identify pediatric dysrhythmias that require a shock. Currently, not enough evidence exists to support recommendation for or against the use of automated external defibrillators in children less than 1 year of age. For a lone rescuer responding to a child with no signs of circulation, 1 minute of cardiopulmonary resuscitation is still advised before any other action, such as activating emergency medical services or using an automated external defibrillator. (Information from Samson RA et al: Use of automated external defibrillators for children: an update—an advisory statement from the pediatric advanced life support task force, International Liaison Committee on Resuscitation, *Circulation* 107[25]:3250-3255, 2003.)

Treatment

Ventricular Tachycardia with a Pulse. Hemodynamically stable ventricular tachycardia should be managed under the advice of medical direction and with caution (Figs. 44-10 to 44-12). The initial efforts are aimed at determining the origin of the tachycardia. They also are focused on obtaining a full history. Drug therapy usually is delayed in the stable patient. Drug therapy is delayed until arrival in the emergency department. In the hospital, adminstration of ***amiodarone, procainamide,*** or ***lidocaine*** may be considered. Ventricular tachycardia that produces a palpable pulse and signs of shock (low cardiac output, poor perfusion) requires immediate synchronized cardioversion.

Pulseless Ventricular Tachycardia and Ventricular Fibrillation. Pulseless ventricular tachycardia and ventricular fibrillation are managed with immediate defibrillation, cardiopulmonary resuscitation, intubation with ventilatory support, and drug therapy (e.g., ***epinephrine*** and ***vasopressin, amiodarone, lidocaine,*** and ***procainamide***). Infant paddles (4.5 cm) generally should be used during defibrillation for infants up to about 1 year of age or 10 kg. Adult

CRITICAL THINKING

Are you comfortable using the pediatric paddles on the defibrillators you will be using in clinicals and on the ambulance?

BOX 44-3 Terminating Resuscitative Efforts

Most children who have a cardiac arrest will not survive—even with a transient return of spontaneous circulation. In the absence of recurring or refractory ventricular fibrillation or ventricular tachycardia, history of toxic drug exposure, or a primary hypothermic insult, medical direction may advise that resuscitative efforts be discontinued if there is no return of spontaneous circulation despite 30 minutes of advanced life support interventions.[5] Family members are sometimes present during the resuscitation efforts. If this is the case, one person should be assigned to the family. This person can answer questions and provide comfort measures.

TABLE 44-10 Summary of Postresuscitation Care

VITAL FUNCTION	INTERVENTION
Airway	Tracheal intubation with confirmation of tube position and repeat confirmation on movement/transport
	Secure tube before transport
	Gastric decompression
Breathing	100% inspired oxygen
	Provide mechanical ventilation targeting normal ventilation goals (P_{CO_2} 35 to 40 mm Hg)
	Monitor continuous pulse oximetry and exhaled CO_2 (or capnography) if available
Circulation	Ensure adequate intravascular volume (volume titration)
	Optimize myocardial function and systemic perfusion (inotropes, vasopressors, vasodilators)
	Monitor capillary refill, blood pressure, continuous electrocardiogram, urine output; measure arterial blood gas and lactate to assess degree of acidosis, if available
	Ideally maintain two routes of functional vascular access
Disability	Perform secondary assessment including brief neurological assessment
	Avoid hyperglycemia, treat hypoglycemia (monitor glucose)
	If seizures are observed, medicate with anticonvulsant agents
	Obtain laboratory studies (if available): arterial blood gases, glucose, electrolytes, hematocrit, chest radiograph
Exposure	Avoid and correct hyperthermia (monitor temperature)
	Avoid profound hypothermia ($<33°$ C)

From American Heart Association: Guidelines 2000 for cardiopulmonary resuscitation and emergency cardiovascular care, International Consensus on Science, *Circulation* 102(8):328, 2000.

paddles[6] (8 to 13 cm) generally should be used for patients older than 1 year of age or more than 10 kg (Box 44-3).

Postresuscitation Stabilization

The postresuscitation phase begins after initial stabilization of the patient with shock or respiratory failure. It also includes the time after return of spontaneous circulation in a patient who was in cardiac arrest. The goals of postresuscitation stabilization are as follows[5]:

- Preserve brain function.
- Avoid secondary organ injury.
- Seek and correct causes of illness.
- Enable the patient to arrive at an appropriate care facility in the best possible physiological state.

Postresuscitation stabilization continues assessment and support of the airway, breathing, and circulation. It also focuses on preserving neurological function and avoiding multisystem organ failure (Table 44-10). Postresuscitation stabilization requires knowledge and experience in the evaluation of all organ systems. It includes stabilizing the airway and supporting oxygenation, ventilation, and perfusion; performing a thorough secondary assessment; and obtaining a medical history.

The paramedic should be sure to communicate to the family what has been done and how the patient is responding to care. The paramedic also should make frequent reports to the receiving hospital.

Seizure

A seizure (described in Chapters 31 and 43) is an episode of sudden abnormal electrical activity in the brain. It results in abnormalities in motor, sensory, or autonomic function usually associated with abnormal behavior, changes in level of consciousness, or both. Common causes of seizure in adults and children include noncompliance with a drug regimen for the treatment of epilepsy, head trauma, intracranial infection, brain tumor, metabolic disturbance, or poisoning. The most common cause of new onset of seizure in children is fever.

FEBRILE SEIZURES

A febrile seizure is a seizure associated with fever but without evidence of intracranial infection or other definable cause; such seizures usually occur between the ages of 6 months and 5 years. About 2% to 5% of children under 7 years of age experience a febrile seizure. About 30% of those who have a seizure experience a recurrence. More than half of febrile seizures occur in children age 9 to 20 months. In 60% of cases, a family history of febrile seizures is a factor.[4]

Febrile seizures usually are associated with an underlying viral infection (most often of the upper respiratory tract), gastroenteritis, roseola, otitis media, or another febrile illness. The seizures usually occur in vulnerable patients during a rapid rise in body temperature. However, the intensity of the seizure is not related to the severity of the fever.

Febrile seizures may manifest with generalized tonic-clonic activity. Or they may have a more subtle presentation. As a rule, classic febrile seizures are of short duration. (They usually last less than 5 minutes.) They also have an uncomplicated and short postictal period. Seizures that last longer than 20 minutes call for extensive investigation. These should never be considered benign. Regardless of the suspected cause, all children who have suffered a seizure should be transported for evaluation by a physician per protocol.

Assessment and Management. In most cases the seizure has stopped before emergency medical services arrives. In many instances, the child is in a postictal state. As in any emergency, the first priorities are airway management and ventilatory and circulatory support. This includes airway positioning, suctioning of the airway, and administration of oxygen. Repeated assessment of the adequacy of ventilation is necessary. Special emphasis should be placed on respiratory rate and depth. If the airway cannot be maintained with manual maneuvers, airway adjuncts should be used.

After initial stabilization of the patient's condition, the paramedic should assess vital signs and obtain a history. Important elements of the history include the following:

- Previous seizures
- Number of seizures in this episode
- Description of seizure activity
- Presence of vomiting during the seizure (aspiration risk)
- Condition of the child when first found
- Recent illness
- Potential for toxic ingestion
- Potential head injury (as primary cause or secondary complication)
- Significant medical problems
- Recent headache or stiff neck (which may suggest meningitis)
- Medication use and compliance with anticonvulsant medication

During transport to the emergency department, the paramedic should monitor the child continuously. The paramedic should be alert for recurrent seizures. Medical direction may advise that a febrile patient be given an antipyretic if the patient is alert. The antipyretic will reduce the fever en route to the receiving hospital. The paramedic should not apply ice or submerge the patient in cool bath in an effort to reduce fever.

STATUS EPILEPTICUS

Status epilepticus is continuous seizure activity that lasts 30 minutes or longer. *Status epilepticus* also may be defined as a recurrent seizure without an intervening period of consciousness. Such a seizure is a true emergency. It can lead to hypotension and cardiovascular, respiratory, and renal failure, in addition to permanent brain damage. Children in status epilepticus should be managed with the following initial interventions:

1. Provide adequate airway, ventilatory, and circulatory support. Intubation for airway protection or mechanical ventilation seldom is needed. Intubation should be withheld unless the child fails to respond to the initial management.
2. Per protocol, obtain vascular access through an IV or intraosseous route. Measure the blood glucose level to screen for hypoglycemia. If the value is less than 60 mg/dL (40 mg/dL in an infant[4]), administer ***dextrose*** 10%, 25%, or 50% (per medical direction). (Hypoglycemia also can be treated with an intramuscular injection of ***glucagon*** if IV or intraosseous access cannot be established.) If seizures do not stop, consult medical direction regarding IV, intraosseous, or rectal administration of the anticonvulsants ***diazepam*** or ***lorazepam.***
3. Attach a cardiac monitor. Observe for rhythm or conduction abnormalities that may suggest hypoxia.

Diazepam. ***Diazepam*** breaks active seizures in 75% to 90% of cases.[7] The drug has a short duration of action (15 minutes). It may require repeat administration to a maximum of three doses. In addition, the paramedic should be ready for sudden respiratory depression or hypotension when using this drug. If IV or intraosseous access cannot be obtained, ***diazepam*** may be administered rectally (Box 44-4). Transport of the patient should not be delayed so as to attempt vascular access.

Lorazepam. An alternative to the IV or intraosseous administration of ***diazepam*** is ***lorazepam.*** Some physicians prefer it. ***Lorazepam*** may be injected intramuscularly. It also may be given intravenously, intraosseously, or rectally. The

BOX 44-4 Procedure for Rectal Administration of Diazepam

1. Carefully restrain the child. If possible, place the child in a knee-chest or decubitus position with the legs flexed at the hip and knee.
2. Draw the calculated diazepam dose into a syringe. A higher dose of 0.5 mg/kg is required because absorption is incomplete.
3. Introduce a lubricated 1-mL syringe just beyond the external sphincter (aimed just above the junction of the skin and mucous membranes and directed toward the rectal wall).
4. Inject the solution into the rectum and clear the syringe with 1 mL of normal saline.
5. Facilitate drug retention by squeezing the buttocks together with manual pressure.
6. Transport the patient for evaluation by a physician. Remove excessive clothing. En route, continually monitor the patient for recurrent seizures and the need for airway, ventilatory, and circulatory support.

side effects are similar to those of ***diazepam*** in terms of cardiorespiratory and central nervous system depression. The paramedic should be alert for these complications.

> **NOTE** Midazolam is being used by some emergency medical services systems to treat status epilepticus and refractory seizures in pediatric patients. Midazolam also is used when seizures do not respond to diazepam or lorazepam. The drug may be administered intramuscularly, intravenously, buccally or intranasally. The use of midazolam to control pediatric seizures is controversial; it may cause respiratory depression. (Information from Center for Pediatric Emergency Medicine: Scenario: seizures. http://www.cpem.org/trippals/SCEN13.PDF. Accessed October 18, 2004.)

Hypoglycemia

As described in Chapter 32, hypoglycemia is an abnormally low concentration of glucose in the blood. In children, hypoglycemia is usually the result of excessive response to glucose absorption, illness, physical exertion, or decreased dietary intake. In diabetic children, hypoglycemia usually is caused by too large of an insulin dose, a delayed or missed meal, or unusual or vigorous physical activity. The condition most commonly occurs in the prehospital setting in infants and children with type 1 diabetes, a disease that affects about 10 in 100,000 children.[8]

The signs and symptoms of hypoglycemia can be classified as *mild, moderate,* and *severe.* Mild symptoms include hunger, weakness, tachypnea, and tachycardia. Moderate symptoms include sweating, tremors, irritability, vomiting, mood disorders, blurred vision, stomachache, headache, and dizziness. Severe symptoms include decreased level of consciousness and seizure activity. This is an emergency that calls for prompt treatment with ***dextrose*** to prevent brain damage.

The prehospital care is directed first at ensuring adequate airway, ventilatory, and circulatory support. A blood glucose measurement should be obtained in any child with an altered level of consciousness that has no explainable cause. Conscious children who are mildly hypoglycemic should receive an oral glucose solution or paste. Unconscious children or those with moderate or severe hypoglycemia require IV/intraosseous ***dextrose*** or intramuscular ***glucagon*** administration. This should be followed by a repeat blood glucose measurement in 10 to 15 minutes. All children with signs and symptoms of hypoglycemia should be transported for physician evaluation.

Hyperglycemia

Hyperglycemia is an abnormally high concentration of glucose in the blood. It results from an absence or resistance to insulin. The low insulin level prevents glucose from entering the cells. This causes glucose to build up in the blood. If not treated, hyperglycemia can lead to dehydration, diabetic ketoacidosis, and coma. In children with type 1 diabetes, the condition often is the result of too small an insulin dose in relation to food intake, failure to take ***insulin***, illness, or a malfunctioning insulin-delivery system (e.g., insulin pump).

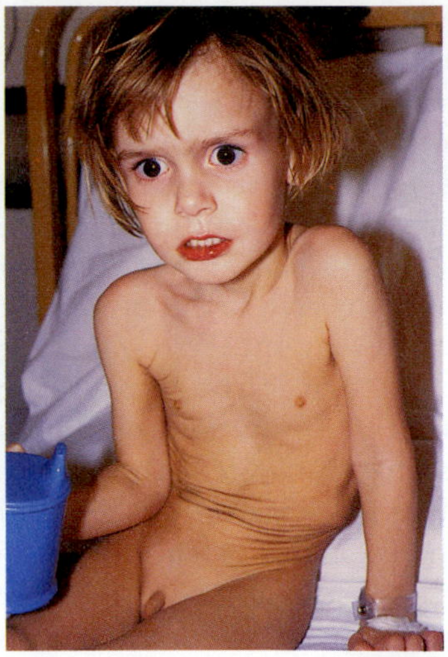

FIGURE 44-13 ■ Severe dyhydration and weight loss from diabetic ketoacidosis.

The signs and symptoms of hyperglycemia are classified as *early* or *late.* Early signs and symptoms include increased thirst (polydipsia), increased hunger (polyphagia), and increased urination (polyuria). (Weight loss also is considered an early sign of the illness.) Late signs and symptoms associated with dehydration and early ketoacidosis include weakness, abdominal pain, generalized aches, loss of appetite, nausea, vomiting, signs of dehydration (with the exception of urinary output), fruity breath odor, tachypnea, hyperventilation, and tachycardia. If untreated, Kussmaul's respirations and coma may occur.

Children suspected of being hyperglycemic should receive adequate airway, ventilatory, and circulatory support. This should be followed by glucose testing. These patients also may require IV fluid therapy if signs of dehydration are present (Fig. 44-13). The administration of ***insulin*** usually is reserved as an in-hospital procedure. If hyperglycemia cannot be confirmed through glucose testing, the diabetic patient should be given glucose or ***dextrose*** orally as described previously in case hypoglycemia is the true cause of the illness.

> **CRITICAL THINKING**
> Why do you think type I diabetes may go undetected until a child is seriously ill?

Infection

Children with infection may have a variety of signs and symptoms. The symptoms depend on the source and extent of infection and the length of time since the patient was exposed (Box 44-5). Often the parent or caregiver provides a history of recent illness. (This may include, for example, fever, upper respiratory tract infection, or otitis media [Fig.

BOX 44-5 Signs and Symptoms of Infection in Pediatric Patients

Bulging fontanelle (infants)	Nasal congestion
Chills	Poor feeding
Cool or clammy skin	Respiratory distress
Cough	Seizure
Dehydration	Severe headache
Fever	Sore throat
Hypoperfusion	Stiff neck
Hypothermia (neonates)	Tachycardia
Irritability	Tachypnea
Lethargy	Vomiting or diarrhea (or both)
Malaise	

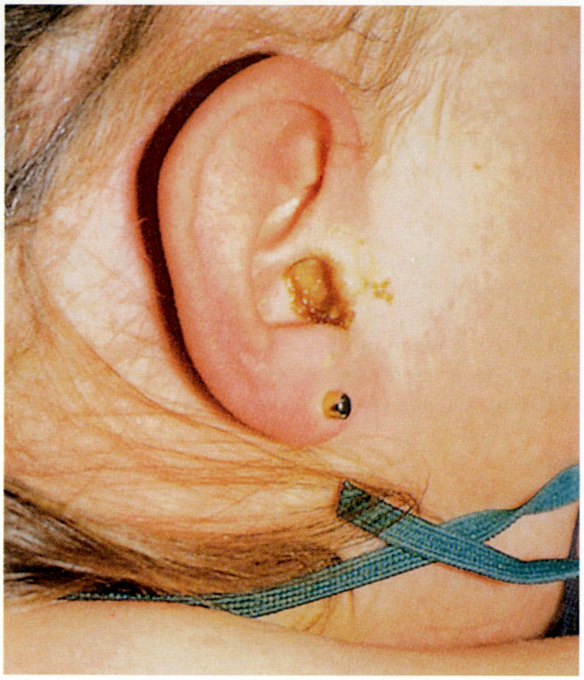

FIGURE 44-14 ■ Otitis media.

44-14].) When caring for any patient who may have an infectious disease, the paramedic must strictly adhere to body substance isolation because of the unknown cause of the infection.

Most children with infection need only supportive care while being transported for evaluation by a physician. However, in very sick children, support of the airway, ventilation, and circulation may be needed. If signs of decompensated shock are present, IV therapy may be needed (per medical direction). Active seizure activity may require the use of anticonvulsant agents. When possible, a child in stable condition should be transported in the child's position of comfort. The child also should be transported in the company of the parent or caregiver.

Poisoning and Toxic Exposure

As discussed in Chapter 36, most poisoning in the United States involves children and is a major cause of preventable death in children under 5 years of age.[9]

Common sources of poisoning (unintentional and intentional) include the following[2]:

- Acetaminophen
- Alcohol
- Anticholinergics
- ***Aspirin***
- Barbiturates
- Cold medicines
- Corrosives
- Digitalis, beta-blocker agents
- Hydrocarbons
- Narcotics
- Organic solvents (inhaled)
- Organophosphates
- Sedatives
- Vitamins (especially iron)

The signs and symptoms of poisoning vary. They depend on the toxic substance and the length of time since the child was exposed. These signs and symptoms may include cardiac and respiratory depression, central nervous system stimulation or depression, gastrointestinal irritation, and behavioral changes. Emergency care should be directed first at ensuring adequate airway, ventilatory, and circulatory support (Box 44-6). The paramedic should contact medical direction and the poison control center for specific treatments. All pills, substances, and containers associated with the poisoning should be transported with the child to the receiving hospital.

CRITICAL THINKING

For what critical signs or symptoms of poisoning should you be alert?

Pediatric Trauma

Blunt and penetrating trauma are major causes of injury and death in children.[9] These and other significant injuries in children often result from falls, motor vehicle crashes, pedestrian-vehicle collisions, drowning/submersion, penetrating injuries, burns, and abuse. The following common injuries highlight the value of injury prevention programs (see Chapter 3):

Falls: Falls are the single most common cause of injuries in children. Fortunately, serious injury or death from truly unintentional falls is uncommon; that is, unless the fall is from a significant height.

CRITICAL THINKING

Why are children at risk for injuries related to falls?

BOX 44-6 Toxicological Emergencies in Pediatric Patients

The most important agents associated with cardiac arrest or requiring advanced life support in children are cocaine, narcotics, tricyclic antidepressants, calcium channel blockers, beta-adrenergic blockers, and opioids.[5] Regardless of the drug, the initial approach in toxicological emergencies is to ensure adequate oxygenation, ventilation, and circulation. Subsequent priorities include reversing the adverse effects of the toxin (if possible) and preventing further absorption of the agent (see Chapter 36). This is an overview of these drugs, their effects, and specific treatment that may be required in the prehospital setting. (*Note:* All drug therapy referenced in this box is based on patient presentation and should be guided by medical direction.)

Cocaine

Effects are complex and are related to route of administration and form of cocaine used.

Signs and Symptoms

May include tachycardia, tremor, diaphoresis, mydriasis, mood elevation, movement disorders, hypertension, and acute coronary syndrome (chest pain and dysrhythmias)

Specific Treatment

Oxygen administration and ventilatory support
Continuous electrocardiogram monitoring
Benzodiazepines (diazepam or lorazepam) for anticonvulsant and central nervous system depressant effect
Aspirin and heparin to reverse platelet-activating effects of cocaine
Nitroglycerin to reduce coronary vasoconstriction
Sodium bicarbonate and lidocaine for ventricular dysrhythmias and cocaine-induced myocardial infarction
Epinephrine to increase coronary perfusion pressure during cardiopulmonary resuscitation

Tricyclic Antidepressants (and Other Sodium Channel Blocking Agents)

Effects result from inhibition of fast sodium channels in the brain and myocardium.

Signs and Symptoms

May include cardiac rhythm disturbances, including preterminal sinus bradycardia and heart block with junctional or ventricular wide-complex escape beats

Specific Treatment

Oxygen administration and ventilatory support
Continuous electrocardiogram monitoring
Sodium bicarbonate and lidocaine to increase myocardial contractility and to manage ventricular dysrhythmias
Normal saline boluses (10 mL/kg) to manage hypotension
Vasopressors (norepinephrine or dopamine) to maintain vascular tone and blood pressure

Calcium Channel Blockers

Effects result from inhibiting the influx of calcium into cells leading to bradydysrhythmias and hypotension.

Signs and Symptoms

May include bradycardia, hypotension, and altered mental status (including syncope, seizure, coma) from cerebral hypoperfusion

Specific Treatment

Oxygen administration and ventilatory support
Continuous electrocardiogram monitoring
Normal saline boluses (5 to 10 mL/kg) to manage hypotension (avoid pulmonary edema)
Calcium chloride 10% (controversial) to overcome channel blockade
High-dose vasopressor therapy with norepinephrine or epinephrine to treat bradycardia and hypotension
Insulin-glucose therapy to maintain serum glucose concentration (avoid hypoglycemia)

Beta-Adrenergic Blockers

Effects result from competition at beta-adrenergic receptors resulting in bradycardia and decreased cardiac contractility.

Signs and Symptoms

May include hypotension with bradycardia, varying degrees of heart block, and altered mental status (including seizures and coma)

Specific Treatment

Oxygen administration and ventilatory support
Continuous electrocardiogram monitoring
Treat for shock
Epinephrine infusions and glucagon may be effective in managing beta-adrenergic blockade and overdose
Insulin-glucose therapy to maintain serum glucose concentration (avoid hypoglycemia)
Sodium bicarbonate to manage intraventricular conduction delay
Calcium chloride to improve heart rate if glucagon and catecholamine are not effective (controversial)

Opioids

Effects produce central nervous system depression.

Signs and Symptoms

May include altered level of consciousness, hypoventilation, apnea, and respiratory failure

Specific Treatment

Oxygen administration and ventilatory support
Continuous electrocardiogram monitoring
Naloxone to reverse narcotic toxicity (normalize partial pressure of P_{CO_2} with ventilations before administration)

Motor vehicle crashes: Motor vehicle crashes are the leading cause of permanent brain injury, serious injury, and death in children.

Pedestrian-vehicle collisions: Pedestrian-vehicle collisions are an often lethal form of trauma in children. The initial injury is caused by impact with the vehicle. (The impact usually occurs to the extremity or trunk.) The child often is thrown from the force of the first impact. This causes additional injury (e.g., head and spine) upon a second impact with other objects. These objects may include the ground, another vehicle, or nearby objects. (See Chapter 20.)

Drowning/submersion: Drowning/submersion incidents are the third leading cause of death in children from birth to 4 years of age. Each year, about 2000 children die from drowning; 5% to 20% of children who are hospitalized for submersion suffer severe, permanent brain damage.

Penetrating injuries: Penetrating injuries are a major cause of trauma in children. They occur especially during adolescence. Penetrating injuries that are intentional (e.g., from violent crime) are more common in inner cities; however, unintentional penetrating injuries in rural areas also occur often. Stab wounds and firearm injuries make up about 10% to 15% of all pediatric trauma admissions. The risk of death from these injuries increases with the age of the patient. As with penetrating injuries to adults, the appearance of the external wounds cannot be used to determine the extent of internal injury in children.

Burns: Burns are the leading cause of unintentional death in the home for children under 14 years of age. Survival from burn trauma is determined by the size and depth of the burn, the presence of inhalation injury, and the nature of other injuries that may have occurred during the event. (See Chapter 23.)

CRITICAL THINKING

What types of situations cause burn injuries to children in the home?

Child abuse: Injuries to children may result from physical abuse, sexual abuse, emotional abuse, and child neglect. Physical abuse often is associated with lower socioeconomic status, domestic disturbances, younger-aged parents, substance abuse, and community violence. Physical abuse of children occurs in all levels of society, however. When caring for a child who may have been abused, thorough documentation of pertinent findings, treatment, and interventions are critical for legal purposes. (Physical abuse is described later in this chapter.)

SPECIAL CONSIDERATIONS FOR SPECIFIC INJURIES

Special considerations for managing pediatric injury are addressed in the chapters of Part 6. The following is a review of some of the more important elements in assessment and management for children with head and neck injury, traumatic brain injury, chest injury, abdominal injury, extremity injury, and burns.

Head and Neck Injury

1. Larger relative mass of the head and lack of neck muscle strength provide increased momentum in acceleration-deceleration injuries.
2. Fulcrum of cervical mobility in the younger child is at the C2 to C3 level (60% to 70% of fractures in children occur in C1 or C2).
3. Head injury is the most common cause of death in pediatric trauma victims.
4. Diffuse head injuries are common in children; focal injuries are rare.
5. Soft tissues, skull, and brain are more compliant in children than in adults.
6. Because of open fontanelles and sutures, infants up to 12 months of age may be more tolerant to increased ICP and can have delayed signs.
7. Subdural bleeding in an infant can produce hypotension (rare).
8. Significant blood loss can occur through scalp lacerations, and such bleeding should be controlled immediately.
9. The modified Glasgow Coma Scale (GCS) should be used for assessing infants and young children.

Traumatic Brain Injury

1. Early recognition and aggressive management can reduce mortality and morbidity.
2. Traumatic brain injury may be classified as *mild* (GCS score of 13 to 15), *moderate* (GCS of 9 to 12), or *severe* (GCS of 8 or lower).
3. Signs of increased ICP include elevated blood pressure, bradycardia, irregular respirations progressing to Cheyne-Stokes respirations, and bulging fontanelle in infants.
4. Signs of herniation include asymmetrical pupils and abnormal posturing.
5. Management
   a. Administer high-concentration oxygen for mild to moderate head injury (GCS score of 9 to 15).
   b. Intubate and ventilate at normal breathing rate with 100% oxygen for severe head injury (GCS score of 3 to 8).
   c. Hyperventilate only with signs of increased ICP.
   d. Some authorities recommend the use of ***lidocaine*** before intubation to blunt the rise in ICP. This, however, is controversial. Use of ***lidocaine*** should be guided by medical direction.

CRITICAL THINKING

What are some early signs of increasing intracranial pressure in a child?

Chest Injury

1. Chest injuries in children under 14 years of age usually are the result of blunt trauma.
2. Because of flexibility of the chest wall, severe intrathoracic injury can be present without signs of external injury such as rib fractures.
3. Tension pneumothorax is poorly tolerated and is an immediate threat to life.

BOX 44-7 Pain Management

Pain management is important when caring for children. It should be considered when indicated to relieve pain associated with traumatic injury such as fractures and burns. Children do not always express their pain as clearly as adults. As a result, they are less likely to receive appropriate pain therapy in an emergency situation. Thus the paramedic should perform a systematic pain assessment. A memory aid for one type of pain assessment is QUESTT*:

Q: Question the child about his or her pain, using age-appropriate language (e.g., "owie" or "boo-boo" for young children).

U: Use pain rating scales (e.g., the Faces Pain Rating Scale for young children; a numeric pain scale from 0 to 10 for older children).

E: Evaluate the child's behavior (e.g., facial grimace, rigidity, crying, and anxious behavior).

S: Secure the parent or caregiver's involvement in assessing the child's pain. (The parent will have seen the child in pain or discomfort before and will be aware of subtle changes.)

T: Take cause of the pain into account (e.g., type of injury and expected intensity of pain).

T: Take action to provide comfort and to relieve pain (e.g., narcotic and nonnarcotic drugs, comfort measures such as application of cold, elevation, and distraction techniques).

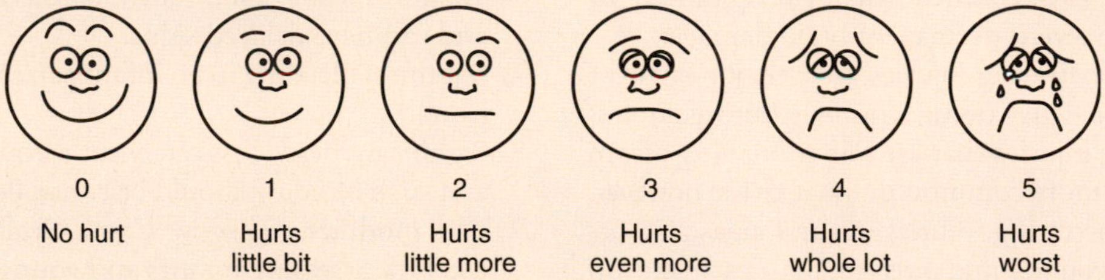

FIGURE 44-15 ■ Wong-Baker Pain Scale. Explain to the child that each face is for a person who feels happy because there is no pain (hurt) or sad because there is some or a lot of pain. Face 0 is very happy because there is no hurt. Face 1 hurts just a little bit. Face 2 hurts a little more. Face 3 hurts even more. Face 4 hurts a whole lot, but Face 5 hurts as much as you can imagine, although you do not have to be crying to feel this bad. Ask child to choose the face that best describes the child's own pain. Record the number under chosen face on patient care report.

*Wong D and Hess C: *Clinical manual of pediatric nursing,* ed 5, St Louis, 2000, Mosby.

4. Flail segment is an uncommon injury in children; when noted without a significant mechanism of injury, child abuse should be suspected.
5. Many children with cardiac tamponade have no physical signs other than hypotension.

Abdominal Injury

1. Musculature is minimal and poorly protects the viscera.
2. Organs most commonly injured are the liver, kidneys, and spleen.
3. Onset of symptoms may be rapid or gradual.
4. Because of the small size of the abdomen, palpation should be performed in one quadrant at a time.
5. Any child who is hemodynamically unstable without an obvious source of blood loss should be considered to have an abdominal injury until it is proved otherwise.

Extremity Injury

1. Extremity injury is relatively more common in children than adults.
2. Growth plate injuries are common.
3. Compartment syndrome is an emergency in children.
4. Management includes the following:
   a. Control any sites of active bleeding.
   b. Perform splinting to prevent further injury and blood loss.
   c. Pneumatic antishock garment may be useful for an unstable pelvic fracture with hypotension (per protocol).

Burns

1. Burns may be thermal, chemical, or electrical.
2. Management priorities include the following:
   a. Prompt management of the airway is required because swelling can develop rapidly.
   b. If intubation is indicated, an endotracheal tube one half size smaller than expected may be required.
   c. Suspect musculoskeletal injuries in electrical burn patients, and perform spine immobilization.

TRAUMA MANAGEMENT CONSIDERATIONS FOR PEDIATRIC PATIENTS

In addition to the general patient care guidelines appropriate for all injured persons, injured children require special consideration for airway control, immobilization techniques, fluid management, and pain relief. The following discussion reviews the highlights of management guidelines presented in the chapters of Part 6.

Airway Control. The airway of an injured child should be maintained in an in-line or neutral position. (The sniffing position is appropriate for older children and adults.) (Padding may need to be placed under the shoulders in some children. This will help to maintain a neutral airway position.) High-concentration oxygen should be given to all patients. Jaw-thrust positioning and suctioning can be used to keep the airway open. Endotracheal intubation (followed by insertion of a gastric tube) should be done when airway and ventilation remain inadequate. Cricothyroidotomy rarely is indicated for traumatic upper airway obstruction.

All paramedics who provide care for infants and children must be able to provide effective oxygenation and ventilation using the bag-mask technique. Endotracheal intubation sometimes may be needed when caring for injured children. When tracheal intubation is required, endotracheal tube placement should be confirmed by monitoring exhaled carbon dioxide, especially in children who have a pulse.

Immobilization. Spinal immobilization devices must be the right size for infants and children. Equipment that may be used includes the following:

- Child safety seat
- Long spine board
- Padding
- Pediatric immobilization device
- Rigid cervical collar
- Straps, cravats
- Tape
- Towel/blanket roll
- Vest-type/short spine board

The patient should be placed supine and immobilized in a neutral in-line position. This is achieved most effectively by using a backboard with a recess for the head or by using padding under the back from the shoulders to the buttocks.[5]

Fluid Management. Management of the child's airway and breathing takes priority over management of circulation. Circulatory compromise is less common in children than adults. When vascular access is indicated, the paramedic should consider the following:

- Large-bore IV catheters should be inserted into large peripheral veins.
- Transport should not be delayed to obtain vascular access.
- Intraosseous access in children can be used if IV access fails.
- An initial fluid bolus of 20 mL/kg of lactated Ringer's solution or normal saline should be given. This will help to manage volume depletion.
- Vital signs should be reassessed and the bolus (20 mL/kg) repeated if needed; vital signs that do not improve after a second bolus indicate the need for rapid surgical intervention.

Pain Relief. Injuries are often painful. Relief from pain should be a priority when providing care to an injured child (Box 44-7). Drugs that may be used to manage some forms of pain and to alter the emotional response in pediatric patients include ***meperidine, morphine,*** and ***ketorolac*** (in the absence of hemorrhage).[4] Pain medicines can mask signs and symptoms of illness or injury. Thus pain medication should be given to children only under medical direction. Other indications for pain relief or sedation in pediatric patients include some airway management procedures (e.g., rapid sequence intubation), entrapment requiring extended extrication time, and cardioversion or other uncomfortable procedures.

BOX 44-8 Sleep Positions and Other Factors That May Reduce the Risk of Sudden Infant Death Syndrome

In 1994 the Association of SIDS and Infant Mortality Programs joined with the U.S. Public Health Service, the American Academy of Pediatrics, the SIDS Alliance, and others to launch a national public health campaign titled Back to Sleep to reduce the risk of sudden infant death syndrome (SIDS). This initiative was based on research reports from Australia, New Zealand, England, Norway, and the United States. The data indicated that placing healthy newborns to sleep on the back or side was a means of reducing the risk of SIDS. In 1996 this recommendation was revised to endorse "back sleeping" as the best position for infants. Since the inception of this campaign, the SIDS rate has declined 30% to 40% in the United States, the greatest decline in the SIDS rate since statistics began to be compiled. Although such a dramatic decline suggests that a change in the sleeping position to back sleeping may reduce the risk of SIDS, it also has demonstrated that sleeping position, in and of itself, is not a cause of SIDS. Other recommendations for reducing the risk include the following:

- Starting medically recommended prenatal care early
- Avoiding drugs, alcohol, and smoking during pregnancy
- Forbidding smoking around the infant
- Breast-feeding when possible
- Avoiding overdressing or overheating the baby
- Maintaining regular well-baby health visits
- Obtaining immunizations on schedule
- Maintaining immunizations
- Placing the baby to sleep on a firm mattress and avoiding the use of beanbag cushions; waterbeds; soft, fluffy blankets; comforters; sheepskins; pillows; stuffed toys; or other soft materials

Note: Paramedics can play an important role in prevention by conveying this information to parents, other caregivers, and family members.

From Association of SIDS and Infant Mortality Programs: Infant sleep positioning and SIDS: counseling implications. http://www.asip1.org/isp.html. Accessed October 25, 2004.

Sudden Infant Death Syndrome

Sudden infant death syndrome is the leading cause of death in American infants under 1 year of age.[7] The syndrome is defined as the sudden death of a seemingly healthy infant that remains unexplained by history and an autopsy. Sudden infant death syndrome occurs an average of 1.1 times for every 1000 live births and is responsible for more than 7000 deaths in the United States each year.[4] The syndrome cannot be predicted or prevented. However, positioning during sleep may be a factor (Box 44-8).

Sudden infant death syndrome occurs during periods of sleep. It usually occurs between midnight and 6 AM. The typical age for SIDS is the first year of life, but most SIDS deaths (85%) occur within the first 6 months.[4]

The seasonal distribution for SIDS is October through March (in the northern hemisphere). The infant often has a history of minor illness, such as a cold, within 2 weeks before death. Classic signs that usually are present include lividity; frothy, blood-tinged drainage from the nose and mouth; and rigor mortis. With most SIDS cases, no external signs of injury are found. Often evidence indicates that the baby was active just before the death (e.g., rumpled bed clothes, unusual position or location in the bed).

PATHOPHYSIOLOGY

The cause of SIDS is unknown. Studies have failed to confirm a number of physiological, environmental, genetic, and social factors as causes. The studies have confirmed, however, that SIDS is not caused by external suffocation, regurgitation or aspiration of vomitus, hereditary factors, or allergies. (A small percentage of SIDS deaths are thought to be abuse related.[2]) Various physiological aspects that have been suggested to explain SIDS include immaturity of the central nervous system following a prenatal event, idiopathic apnea, brainstem abnormalities, upper airway obstruction, hyperactive upper airway reflexes, cardiac conduction disorders, abnormal responses to hypoxia and hypercarbia, abnormal responses to hyperthermia, and alterations in fat metabolism. Although no specific cause has been identified, a number of risk factors have been associated with the syndrome. These factors including the following:

- Maternal smoking
- Young maternal age (under age 20)
- Infants of mothers who received poor or no prenatal care
- Social deprivation
- Premature births and low-birth-weight infants
- Infants of mothers who used cocaine, methadone, or heroin during pregnancy

Sudden infant death syndrome is confirmed by excluding other causes of death. Autopsy findings that occur in most SIDS deaths include smooth muscle thickening in small pulmonary arteries and right ventricular hypertrophy. Both of these are thought to occur following hypoxia and constriction of the pulmonary vasculature. Other findings include brainstem tumors, which may be associated with respiratory center dysfunction, and neuroepithelial bodies in the tracheobronchial tree, along with distal atelectasis. About 80% of SIDS victims also have intrathoracic petechiae, especially on the thymus, pleura, and pericardium.[4]

MANAGEMENT

Emergency medical services providers can do little to help the SIDS infant. The main role of the paramedic is to offer emotional support for parents or other caregivers and loved ones. If the infant possibly could be viable, resuscitation should proceed as for any other infant in cardiac arrest. Resuscitation most likely will be unsuccessful. Still, for the parents or other caregivers to see that everything possible is being done for their child is crucial. The paramedic should follow pediatric resuscitation protocols and should consult with medical direction on decisions to initiate or continue efforts.

A variety of grief reactions should be expected from those who witness the event (parents, family members, neighbors, babysitters). These reactions may vary from shock and disbelief to anger, rage, and self-blame. Arrangements should be made for a relative or neighbor to stay with the family or accompany them to the hospital so that they are not left alone. Many areas have SIDS resource services. These services provide immediate counseling and support for the family of an infant who dies of SIDS.

Sudden infant death syndrome victims may appear to have been abused or neglected. The mysterious nature of SIDS deaths and classic signs such as postmortem lividity and frothy fluid in the infant's nose and mouth give such appearance. Regardless of the circumstances, the paramedic should avoid comments or questions that may imply a suspicion of improper child care. Determining the cause of death is not the duty of the emergency medical services crew. (However, careful scene observation is crucial.) The paramedic should document all findings objectively, accurately, and completely. Medical direction and other authorities (per protocol) should be advised if inappropriate child care is suspected.

The death of an infant has a powerful effect on all who are involved. Rescuers commonly have a range of emotional reactions after a SIDS death. Some emergency medical services, working with medical direction and SIDS resource agencies, provide counseling and formal debriefing programs. If these services are not available, the emergency medical services crew should discuss the event openly with others involved in the response (e.g., co-workers and law enforcement officers). This may help relieve normal feelings of anxiety and stress.

CRITICAL THINKING

What factors do you think influence the reactions of each crew member to a sudden infant death syndrome death?

Child Abuse and Neglect

More than 2.4 million cases of suspected child abuse and neglect are reported each year in the United States.[7] Child abuse and neglect results in about 4000 deaths each year. Paramedics should follow local protocol in reporting suspected abuse. They should discuss any suspicions of child abuse or neglect with medical direction as well. Agencies that may be involved in cases of child abuse or neglect include state, regional, and local child protection services. Also included are hospital social service departments.

Child abuse and neglect is a crime that must be reported by law in all 50 states. In some states persons have a legal duty to report child abuse or neglect (mandate reporter). Failure to report these cases may result in criminal prosecution. In fact, the failure may be punishable by fine or imprisonment or both. As a rule, reporting in good faith provides immunity from legal liability as a consequence of reporting, which may be raised as a defense if one is sued for negligent reporting.

ELEMENTS OF CHILD ABUSE

Child abuse and neglect is the maltreatment of children by their parents, guardians, or other caregivers. Forms of maltreatment include infliction of physical injury (battered child syndrome, shaken baby syndrome), sexual exploitation, and infliction of emotional pain and neglect (medical neglect, safety neglect, and nutritional deprivation). A number of factors come into play in the potential for child abuse. These include a caregiver with the potential to abuse, a child with particular characteristics that place him or her at risk for abuse, and an element of crisis.

Characteristics of Abusers. Child abuse usually reflects a pattern of unstable behavior. Child abuse is typically not a single act of violence. In many cases the abuser is the child's parent. However, other caregivers may be responsible. (For example, others may include family members, a boyfriend of the child's mother, an unrelated babysitter, or a sibling of the abused child.) In the case of physical abuse, most abusers tend to be unhappy, angry adults. They often are under extreme stress. They usually are isolated. Often they are incapable of using support agencies or an extended family in times of crisis. Often the abusers were the victim of physical or emotional abuse as children. Abusers come from all ethnic, geographical, religious, educational, occupational, and socioeconomic groups. Other factors that are characteristic of abusers include poverty and alcohol or other drug dependence.

> **CRITICAL THINKING**
>
> Can you make a determination that someone is not an abuser if they do not fit this profile based on your prehospital assessment?

Characteristics of an Abused Child. Abused children often have certain characteristics that increase their risk for abuse. Common traits include demanding and difficult behavior, decreased level of functioning (e.g., a handicapped child or preterm infant requiring extra parenting), hyperactivity, and precociousness with intellectual ability equal to or superior to the parent. Often the parent sees the abused child as "special" or "different" from other siblings. Other factors that tend to increase the potential for child abuse are age (the child is usually under 5 years old), gender (boys are involved more often than girls), and illegitimacy.

Crises That May Precipitate Abuse. Physical abuse or neglect can occur constantly during a child's life. More often, though, abuse and neglect are intermittent and unpredictable. The abuse often is brought on by stressors in the adult caregiver's life, especially when the caregiver expects the child to fill emotional needs created by the stress. Failure of the child to respond in an ideal way to the caregiver's needs may lead to abuse. Common crises associated with an episode of child abuse include the following:

- Financial stress
- Loss of employment
- Eviction from housing
- Marital or relationship stress
- Physical illness in a child that leads to intractable crying
- Death of a family member
- Diagnosis of an unwanted pregnancy
- Birth of a sibling

HISTORY OF INJURIES SUSPICIOUS FOR ABUSE

Physical abuse or neglect often is hard to determine. The ultimate diagnosis usually begins with suspicions based on unexplained injuries, discrepant history, delays in seeking medical care, and repeated episodes of suspicious injuries. If at any time an injured child indicates that an adult caused him or her physical harm, the paramedic should take this report seriously and advise medical direction. The paramedic should contact the proper authorities as well. In many cases these accusations are true. The following are 15 indicators of possible abuse[10]:

1. Any obvious or suspected fractures in a child under 2 years of age
2. Injuries in various stages of healing, especially burns and bruises
3. More injuries than are usually seen in other children of the same age
4. Injuries scattered on many areas of the body
5. Bruises or burns in patterns that suggest intentional infliction
6. Suspected increased intracranial pressure in an infant
7. Suspected intraabdominal trauma in a young child
8. Any injury that does not fit the description of the cause
9. An accusation that the child injured himself or herself intentionally
10. Long-standing skin infections
11. Extreme malnutrition
12. Extreme lack of cleanliness
13. Inappropriate clothing for the situation
14. Child who withdraws from parent
15. Child who responds inappropriately to the situation (e.g., quiet, distant, and withdrawn)

PHYSICAL FINDINGS SUGGESTIVE OF ABUSE

Some physical findings, such as multiple, widely dispersed bruises; welts; and burns, are suggestive of abuse. Such physical findings, along with a vague history or delays in seeking medical care for the child, should alert the paramedic to the possibility of abuse or neglect (Fig. 44-16).

Bruises (Table 44-11)

- Bruises that predominate on the buttocks or lower back are almost always related to punishment.
- Genital area or inner thigh bruises usually are inflicted for toileting mishaps.

A B C D E F

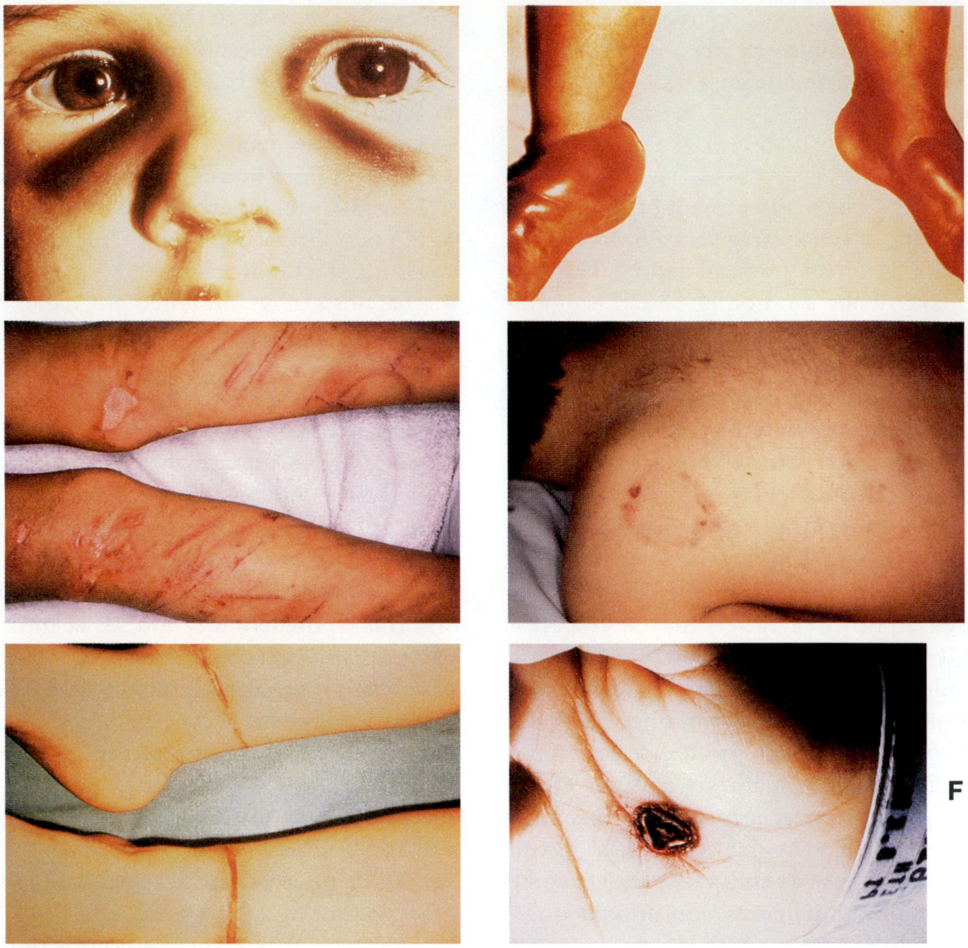

FIGURE 44-16 ■ Cutaneous manifestations of child abuse. **A,** "Raccoon eyes," or periorbital bruising, possible indication of anterior fossa skull fracture. **B,** "Dunking" burns of the feet. **C,** Welts and abrasions to legs as a result of an electrical cord. **D,** Human bites. **E,** Fresh abrasions of restraint injury. **F,** Fresh cigarette burn to palm.

TABLE 44-11 General Guidelines for Dating of Bruises by Color

COLOR OF BRUISE	AGE OF BRUISE
Reddish blue or purple	Less than 24 hours
Dark blue to purple	1 to 5 days
Green	5 to 7 days
Yellow	7 to 10 days
Brown	10 to 14 days or longer
Resolution	2 to 4 weeks

- Facial bruises or a number of petechiae on the ear lobe usually are caused by slapping.
- Bruises of the upper lip and labial frenulum usually are caused by forced feedings or from forcing a pacifier into the mouth of a screaming infant.
- Human hand marks resulting from squeezing are pressure bruises in shapes resembling fingertips, fingers, or the entire hand of the abuser.
- Human bite marks result in paired, crescent-shaped bruises. These bruises often contain individual teeth marks. The size of the arc distinguishes adult bites from child bites.

CRITICAL THINKING

Consider an infant under 3 months of age. Based on the physical capabilities of this age group, where would you expect to see "normal bruises"?

Welts

- Strap marks 1 to 2 inches wide are almost always caused by a belt.
- Bizarre-shaped welts or bruises usually are inflicted by a blunt object that resembles its shape (e.g., a toy or shoe).
- Choke marks may be seen on the neck.
- Circumferential bruising or abrasions on the ankles or wrists may be caused by rope, cord, or a dog leash.

Burns

- Cigarette burns often are found on the palms, soles, or abdomen.
- A lighted cigarette, a hot match, or burning incense sometimes is applied to the hand to stop the child from sucking the thumb or to the genital area to discourage masturbation.
- Burns may be inflicted with lighters or other sources of open flame (e.g., a gas stove) to teach a child not to play with fire.
- Dry contact burns may result from forcibly holding a child against a heating device (e.g., a radiator, hot iron, or electric hot plate).
- The most common hot-water burns or scalds occur from forcible immersion of the hands, feet, or buttocks in scalding water. These injuries often involve both arms or both legs, or they may be circular burns restricted to the buttocks; such burns are incompatible with falling or stepping into a tub of hot water.

Other less visible injuries may indicate child abuse. These include brain injury, abdominal visceral injury, and bone fractures.

Subdural Hematoma. Brain injury is the leading cause of death in battered children. The various pathological lesions include cerebral contusions, intraparenchymal hemorrhage, and subdural or even epidural hematomata. Subdural hematomata are among the most common injuries associated with intentionally inflicted head injury in children. They should be suspected in any young child who is in a coma or having convulsions. They should be suspected particularly if the child has no history of seizure disorder. In many cases, bleeding into the brain tissue occurs as a result of skull fractures or scalp bruises. These commonly result from a direct blow from a hand or by being thrown against a wall or door.

Subdural hematomata also can result from vigorous shaking of the child (shaken baby syndrome). The acceleration and deceleration forces on the brain associated with shaking cause tearing of the bridging cerebral veins. This leads to bleeding into the subdural space. Signs and symptoms of the shaken baby syndrome include retinal hemorrhages, irritability, altered level of consciousness, vomiting, and a full fontanelle.

CRITICAL THINKING

Why is it critical that your documentation be clear, objective, and complete in cases of suspected abuse?

Abdominal Visceral Injury. Intraabdominal injuries are the second most common cause of death in battered children. These injuries usually are produced by a blunt force such as a punch or blow to the abdomen. Children with an abdominal injury often have recurrent vomiting, abdominal distention, absent bowel sounds, and localized tenderness with or without abdominal bruising. Caregivers routinely deny a history of trauma to the child's abdomen in these cases.

Bone Injury. More than 20% of physically abused children have a positive result on radiological bone survey from previous abusive episodes.[7] Injuries that may be obvious only through radiography include fractures of the ribs, lateral portion of the clavicle, scapula, sternum, and extremities. Multiple fractures in various stages of healing are highly suspicious for physical abuse.

INJURIES FROM SEXUAL ABUSE

Sexual abuse of a child is a symptom of a seriously disturbed family relationship. Sexual abuse usually is associated with physical or emotional neglect or abuse. Often the sexually abusive adult received similar abuse as a child. The adult may justify this behavior in his or her mind. Family relationships are complex, and silent complicity by at least one parent often is involved.

Injuries from sexual abuse may be physical and psychological. Sexual abuse may include vaginal intercourse, sodomy (anal intercourse), oral-genital contact, or molestation (fondling, masturbation, or exposure). In many cases the victimized child is a girl. More than half of the victims are under 12 years of age at the time of the first offense. Many of these incidents are chronic and occur without force. Thus an emergency medical services response seldom is initiated. If, however, a physical injury results from the abuse, emergency care may be summoned. Physical findings suggestive of sexual abuse include the following:

- Pregnancy or venereal disease in a child 12 years of age or younger
- Painful urination or defecation
- Tenderness or lacerations to the perineal area
- Bleeding from the rectum or vagina
- Presence of dried blood, semen, or pubic hair in the genital area of a child

Emergency care for child victims of sexual abuse should be limited to managing injuries that pose a threat to life and giving emotional support during transport. These children undergo extensive interviews and examination by the emergency department physician and others. The paramedic should carefully document any statements made by the patient, family member, or caregiver. Any findings should be reported to medical direction. These children require compassionate support. A sexually abused child should never be made to feel that he or she is responsible for any of the abuse. The child also should not be given the impression that discussion of the event is inappropriate. If possible, a paramedic of the same sex should interview and care for the child.

INFANTS AND CHILDREN WITH SPECIAL NEEDS

Some infants and children are born with or develop conditions that pose special needs. These children may require special medical equipment to sustain life. Examples of these conditions include infants born prematurely, those who have altered functions from birth, and those who have chronic or acute disease of the lung, heart, or central nervous system. Often these children are cared for at home by family and home health services. Many are dependent on special medical equipment such as tracheostomy tubes, home artificial ventilators, central venous lines, gastrostomy tubes, and shunts (see Chapter 48). The parents and other family members of a child with special medical needs often are "experts" in caring for the child and maintaining the required medical equipment. Their knowledge, skills, and experience are valuable. The paramedic should use the skills and expertise of these parents when managing these emergencies.

CRITICAL THINKING

How can an emergency medical services agency prepare crews to care for these special needs children before a call is even received?

Tracheostomy Tubes

A patient with a complete tracheostomy has had the airway surgically interrupted. The larynx is no longer connected to the trachea. Modern tracheostomy tubes are flexible. They are relatively comfortable for the patient as well. They have few associated risks (Fig. 44-17). Complications that can occur with the tracheostomy tube include obstruction, air leak, bleeding, dislodgment, and infection. All of these may lead to inadequate ventilation. (Bleeding around a tracheostomy usually occurs within 24 hours of the surgery and is not commonly seen in the prehospital setting.) Aseptic technique and respiratory support are always high priorities in caring for these patients.

MANAGEMENT

The tracheostomy tube may become blocked or dislodged. In these cases, the paramedic must clear the tube with sterile water or saline or remove and reinsert it as described in Chapter 19. (Medical direction may advise that a tracheostomy tube be replaced with an endotracheal tube as a temporary measure.) Tracheal suctioning (using sterile technique) may be required to remove secretions and mucus. If tracheal intubation becomes necessary in these patients, it must be performed via the stoma.

NOTE Tracheal suctioning is a difficult procedure and often is traumatic for the patient. It can easily lead to hypoxia. Tracheal suctioning should be performed only when absolutely necessary. It should be performed for only a period of 10 to 15 seconds. After that, high-concentration supplemental oxygen should be administered by mask to stoma or via a bag-valve mask.

Home Artificial Ventilators

When a patient needs help breathing, the child may be put on a mechanical ventilator. This can simulate the normal movement of the diaphragm and thoracic cage. The type of home ventilator used depends on the patient's specific needs. Ventilators are classified by function. This is based on the amount of air and pressure they are set to deliver during certain phases of the respiratory cycle (Fig. 44-18). Complications can occur from malfunction of the machine and alarms, airway obstruction, and respiratory distress (Table 44-12).

MANAGEMENT

The many types of artificial ventilators work differently. Thus the paramedic should never try to troubleshoot a ventilator problem. The paramedic also should not try to adjust the settings of the ventilator. Rather, the emergency medical services crew should always treat the patient and not try to correct the malfunction of the machine. Steps in managing a patient with a home artificial ventilator problem are presented in Chapter 48.

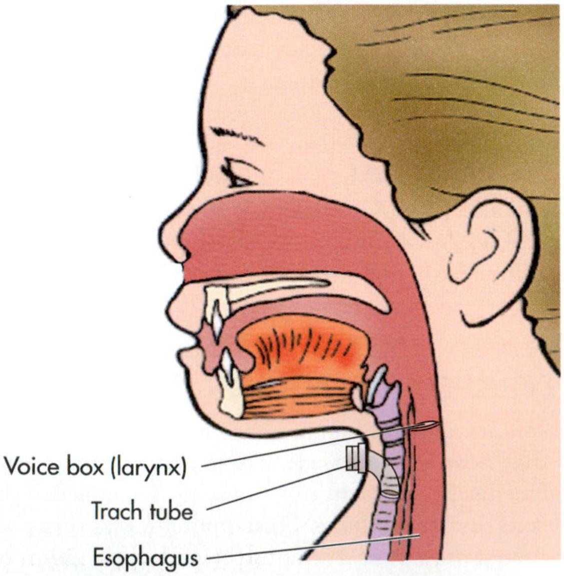

FIGURE 44-17 ■ Pediatric tracheostomy tube.

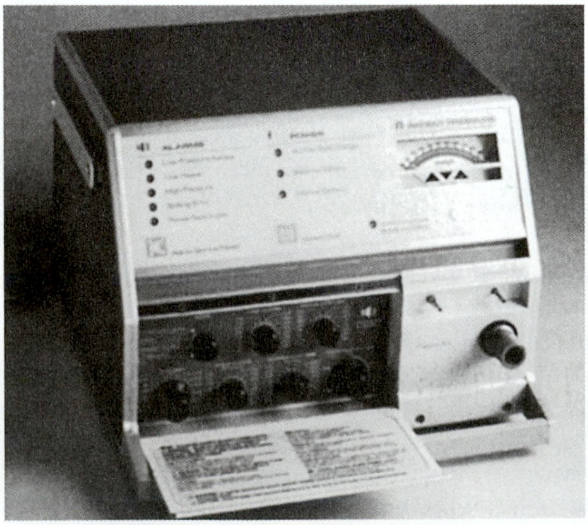
FIGURE 44-18 ■ Home ventilator.

Central Venous Lines

Some patients with chronic illnesses need prolonged and frequent access to venous circulation for drug or fluid therapy. This is made possible through vascular access devices. These devices are seen often in the prehospital setting in child and adult patients who are cared for in the home (Fig. 44-19).

TABLE 44-12 Complications Seen with Home Artificial Ventilators

COMPLICATION	POSSIBLE CAUSE
Airway obstruction	Bronchospasm, mucus or secretions, tracheostomy or endotracheal tube malfunction, patient cough, fear, anxiety
Barotrauma	
Pneumothorax	High-pressure volumes
Atelectasis	Improper deep breathing, pneumothorax
Cardiovascular impairment	Reduction in venous return to the heart caused by positive intrathoracic pressure, which compresses pulmonary circulation
Gastrointestinal complications	Swallowing air, gastrointestinal bleeding, gastric distention
Tracheal trauma	Cuff pressure on trachea
Respiratory infection	Bypass of natural defenses of upper airway, poor aseptic technique
Oxygen toxicity	High concentration of oxygen over prolonged periods

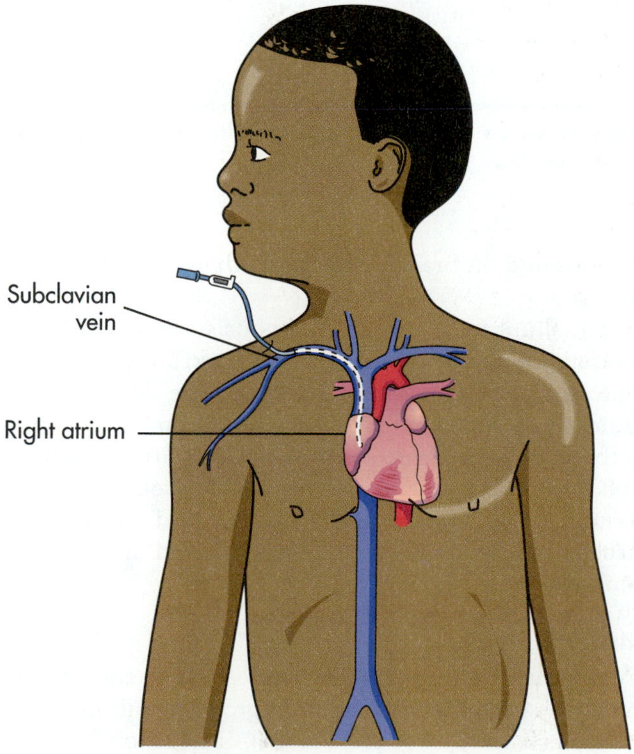

FIGURE 44-19 ■ Central venous line.

These devices include surgically implanted medication delivery devices (e.g., Mediports), peripheral vascular access devices (e.g., peripherally inserted central catheters, Intracath), and central venous access devices (e.g., Hickman and Groshong) (see Chapters 18 and 48). Complications that may occur with vascular access devices include a cracked line, air embolism, bleeding, obstruction, and local infection. Patients with vascular access devices often have a serious illness such as cancer or acquired immunodeficiency syndrome. The effects of these illnesses may complicate the assessment and management of emergencies associated with central venous lines.

MANAGEMENT

A torn or leaking catheter (cracked line) may allow fluids or drugs to infiltrate into the surrounding tissues. This can lead to an air embolism. A torn catheter is evidenced by leaking fluid, a complaint of a burning sensation, or swollen and tender skin near the insertion site. If a torn catheter is suspected, the paramedic should stop the infusion immediately. The paramedic should clamp the catheter between the tear and the patient. The patient who develops an altered level of consciousness (indicating a possible air embolism) should be positioned on the left side. The patient's head should be slightly lowered to help prevent the embolism from traveling to the brain. High-concentration oxygen, IV access, and rapid transport for evaluation by a physician are indicated. Any bleeding at the site should be controlled with direct pressure.

Occasionally, the lumen port becomes obstructed by a blood clot that disrupts the flow of fluids or drugs. (Signs and symptoms of obstruction include a sluggish flow and swelling and tenderness at the site.) When this occurs, the patient should be transported to the hospital so that the catheter can be cleared with thrombolytics or replaced. Attempts to clear a vascular access device require special training and authorization from medical direction. The technique is described in Chapter 48.

Gastric Tubes and Gastrostomy Tubes

A gastric tube (Fig. 44-20) is used as a temporary measure to provide liquid feeding to a patient who cannot swallow or absorb nutrients (often used for feeding premature infants). The tubes are inserted through the nose or mouth into the stomach and can cause irritation to the nasal and mucous membranes. They are designed for short-term use.

A gastrostomy tube (Fig. 44-21) provides a permanent route for gastric feeding in patients who usually cannot be fed by mouth (e.g., a patient with facial burns or paralysis). The tube is surgically placed into the stomach. The tube can be visualized in the upper left quadrant of the abdomen. The opening (stoma) has a flexible, silicone "button." (This is covered with a protective cap.) The stoma allows for regular feedings.

MANAGEMENT

Serious complications with gastric or gastrostomy tubes are rare. They seldom require emergency care. Potential complications include obstruction, pulmonary aspiration,

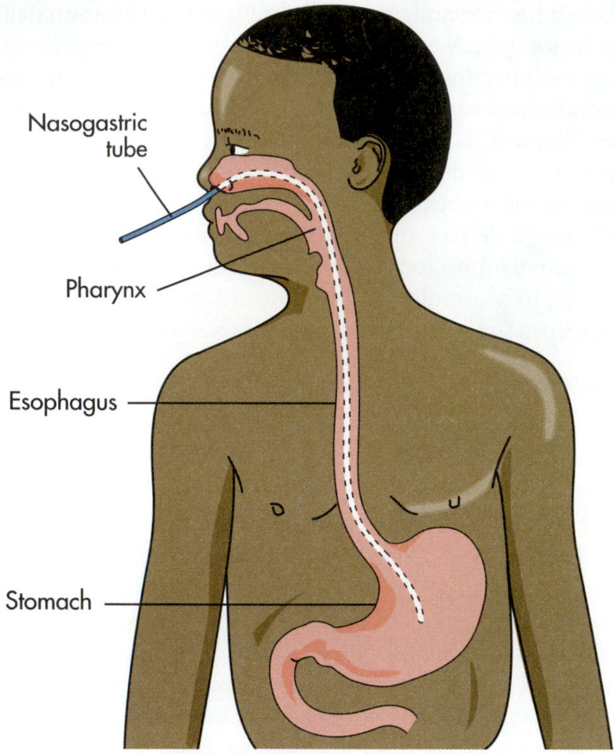

FIGURE 44-20 ■ Nasogastric tube.

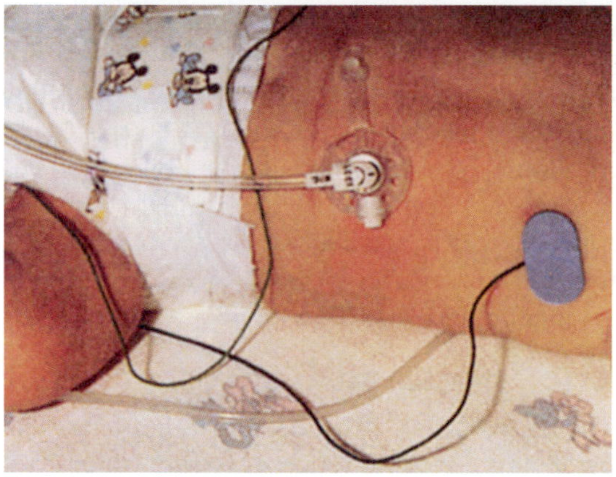

FIGURE 44-21 ■ Gastrostomy tube.

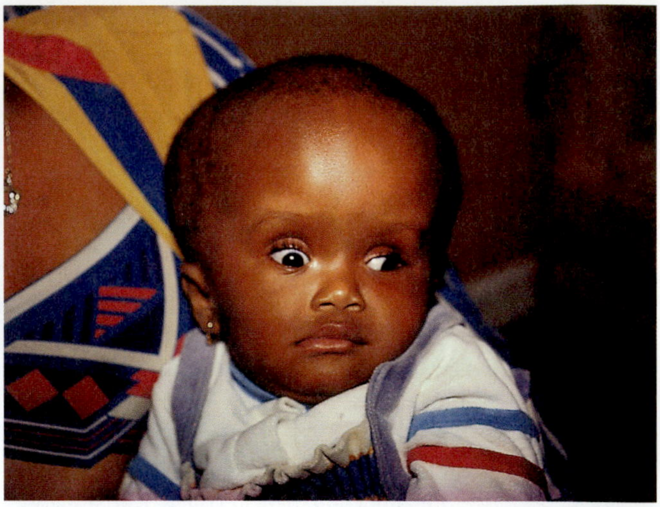

FIGURE 44-22 ■ Untreated hydrocephalus.

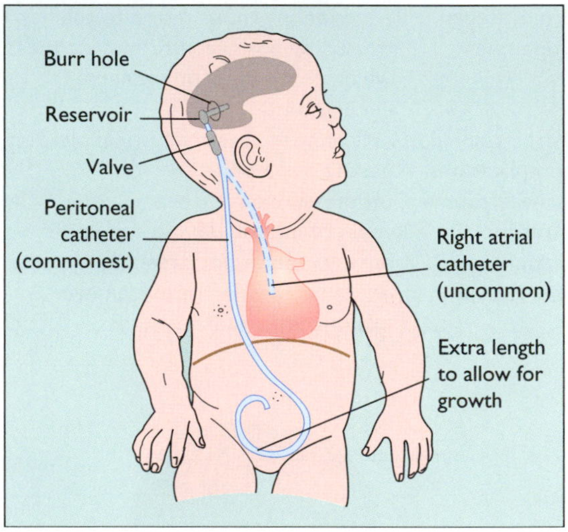

FIGURE 44-23 ■ Ventricular shunt for drainage of symptomatic hydrocephalus.

gastrointestinal disturbances (vomiting and diarrhea), irritation to the mucous membrane, and electrolyte imbalances. All of these can result in inadequate nutrition and fluid needs. Emergency care mainly is supportive. Care may include transport for evaluation by a physician. If not contraindicated, the patient will be most comfortable lying on the right side with the head elevated.

Shunts

A **shunt** is a tube or device that is implanted surgically in the body. The shunt redirects body fluid from one cavity or vessel to another. An example of a shunt is one used to relieve abnormal fluid pressures from excess cerebrospinal fluid around the brain in children with hydrocephalus (Fig. 44-22).

The shunt for hydrocephalus consists of two catheters, a reservoir, and a valve to prevent backflow (Fig. 44-23). The first catheter is inserted through the skull. It drains fluid from the ventricles of the brain. The second catheter is passed into another body cavity (usually the abdomen or right atrium of the heart through the jugular vein), where the excess fluid is absorbed. The reservoir usually can be palpated over the mastoid area, just behind the ear.

MANAGEMENT

Complications from this procedure include the need for catheter replacement as the child grows (requiring several surgeries in the first 10 years of life), obstruction from clotted blood or fluid, and catheter displacement. Infection may occur within several weeks of surgical placement. The signs and symptoms of obstruction or displacement are those of increased ICP. They include the following:

- Headache
- Nausea and vomiting
- Visual disturbances
- Cushing's triad (elevated systolic pressure, irregular respirations, bradycardia)

Children who have complications from a ventricular shunt need emergency surgery to prevent brainstem herniation. The paramedic first should ensure adequate airway, ventilatory, and circulatory support for these patients. Medical direction may recommend endotracheal intubation and hyperventilation to lower ICP, and IV access. These patients are prone to respiratory arrest. They need immediate transport to a proper facility for evaluation by a physician. If possible, the patient's head should be elevated during transport.

SUMMARY

- The Emergency Medical Services for Children program was designed to enhance and expand emergency medical services for acutely ill and injured children. The program has defined 12 basic components of an effective Emergency Medical Services for Children system.
- Children have unique anatomical, physiological, and psychological characteristics, which change during their development.
- Some childhood diseases and disabilities can be predicted by age group.
- Many elements of the initial evaluation can be done by observing the child. The child's parent or guardian also should be involved in the initial evaluation. The three components of the pediatric assessment triangle are appearance, work of breathing, and circulation.
- Obstruction of the upper or lower airway by a foreign body usually occurs in toddlers or preschoolers. Obstruction may be partial or complete.
- Croup is a common inflammatory respiratory illness. It usually is seen in children between the ages of 6 months and 4 years. Symptoms are caused by inflammation in the subglottic region.
- Bacterial tracheitis is an infection of the upper airway and subglottic trachea often seen in infants and toddlers; it often occurs with or after croup.
- Epiglottitis is a rapidly progressive, life-threatening bacterial infection. It causes edema and swelling of the epiglottis and supraglottic structures. It often affects children between 3 and 7 years of age.
- Asthma is common in children over 2 years of age. Asthma is characterized by bronchoconstriction that results from autonomic dysfunction or sensitizing agents.
- Bronchiolitis is a viral disease frequently caused by respiratory syncytial virus infection of the lower airway; it usually affects children age 6 to 18 months of age.
- Pneumonia is an acute infection of the lower airways and lungs involving the alveolar walls and the alveoli.
- Several special differences must be remembered when caring for a child in shock. These include circulating blood volume, body surface area and hypothermia, cardiac reserve, and vital signs and assessment. A child in shock may appear normal and stable until all compensatory mechanisms fail. At that point, pediatric shock progresses rapidly, with serious deterioration.
- When dysrhythmias occur in children, they usually result from hypoxia or structural heart disease.
- The most common causes of seizure in adult and pediatric patients is noncompliance with a drug regimen for the treatment of epilepsy, in addition to head trauma, intracranial infection, metabolic disturbance, or poisoning. The most common cause of new onset of seizure in children is fever.
- Hypoglycemia and hyperglycemia should be suspected whenever a child has an altered level of consciousness with no explainable cause.
- Children with infection may have a variety of signs and symptoms. These depend on the source and extent of infection and the length of time since the patient was exposed.
- Most poisoning events in the United States involve children. Signs and symptoms of accidental poisoning vary, depending on the toxic substance and the length of time since the child was exposed.
- Blunt and penetrating trauma is a chief cause of injury and death in children. Head injury is the most common cause of death in pediatric trauma patients. Early recognition and aggressive management can reduce morbidity and mortality caused by traumatic brain injury in children.
- Because of the pliability of the chest wall, severe intrathoracic injury can be present without signs of external injury. The liver, kidneys, and spleen are the most frequently injured abdominal organs. Extremity injuries are more common in children than adults.

Continued

- Sudden infant death syndrome is the leading cause of death in American infants under 1 year of age. The syndrome is defined as the sudden death of a seemingly healthy infant. The death cannot be explained by history and an autopsy.
- Child abuse and neglect is the maltreatment of children by their parents, guardians, or other caregivers. Forms of maltreatment include infliction of physical injury, sexual exploitation, and infliction of emotional pain and neglect.
- Some infants and children are born with or develop conditions that pose special needs. These children may require special medical equipment to sustain life. Often these children are cared for at home. Many are dependent on specialized medical equipment such as tracheostomy tubes, home artificial ventilators, central venous lines, gastrostomy tubes, and shunts.

REFERENCES

1. Tsai A, Kallsen G: Epidemiology of pediatric prehospital care, *Ann Emerg Med* 16:284, 1987.
2. US Department of Transportation, National Highway Traffic Safety Administration: *EMT-Paramedic national standard curriculum,* Washington, DC, 1998, The Department.
3. National Center for Education in Maternal and Child Health: *Emergency medical services for children: a report to the nation,* Washington, DC, 1991, The Center.
4. Hoekelman R et al: *Primary pediatric care,* ed 3, St Louis, 1997, Mosby.
5. American Heart Association: *Guidelines 2000 for cardiopulmonary resuscitation and emergency cardiovascular care,* International Consensus on Science, Dallas, 2000, The Association.
6. American Heart Association: *Pediatric advanced life support,* Dallas, 1997, The Association.
7. Rosen P, Barkin R: *Emergency medicine: concepts and clinical practice,* ed 4, St Louis, 1998, Mosby.
8. Volugaropoulos C: Type I diabetes in childhood: before and after diagnosis. In *Pediatric endocrinology and diabetes care,* St Louis, 1998, Unity Health Systems.
9. National Safety Council: *Injury facts,* Itasca, Ill, 1999, The Council.
10. Touloukian R: *Pediatric trauma,* ed 2, St Louis, 1990, Mosby.

APPENDIX 44-1

RECOMMENDED CHILDHOOD IMMUNIZATION SCHEDULE

Recommended Childhood and Adolescent Immunization Schedule — United States, 2003

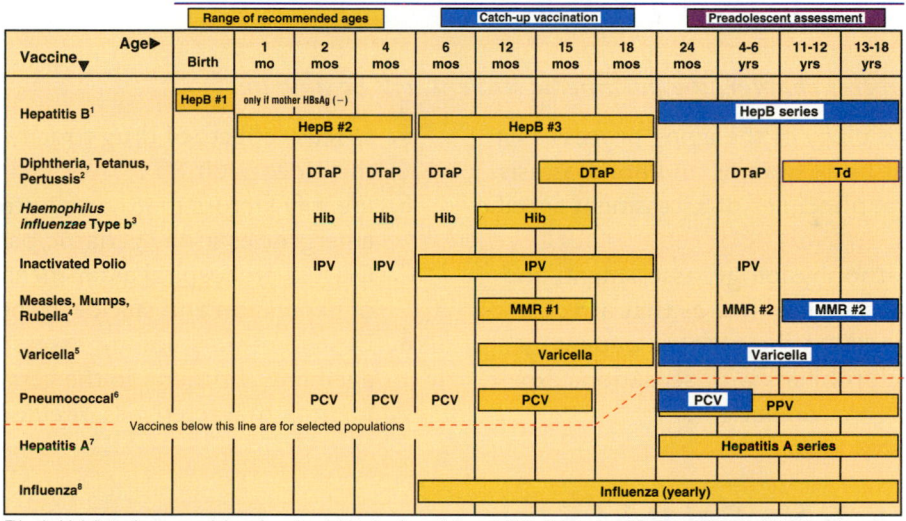

Range of recommended ages | Catch-up vaccination | Preadolescent assessment

Vaccine ▼ / Age ▶	Birth	1 mo	2 mos	4 mos	6 mos	12 mos	15 mos	18 mos	24 mos	4-6 yrs	11-12 yrs	13-18 yrs
Hepatitis B[1]	HepB #1	only if mother HBsAg (−) HepB #2			HepB #3				HepB series			
Diphtheria, Tetanus, Pertussis[2]			DTaP	DTaP	DTaP		DTaP			DTaP	Td	
Haemophilus influenzae Type b[3]			Hib	Hib	Hib	Hib						
Inactivated Polio			IPV	IPV	IPV					IPV		
Measles, Mumps, Rubella[4]						MMR #1				MMR #2	MMR #2	
Varicella[5]						Varicella			Varicella			
Pneumococcal[6]			PCV	PCV	PCV	PCV			PCV PPV			
Vaccines below this line are for selected populations												
Hepatitis A[7]									Hepatitis A series			
Influenza[8]					Influenza (yearly)							

This schedule indicates the recommended ages for routine administration of currently licensed childhood vaccines, as of December 1, 2002, for children through age 18 years. Any dose not given at the recommended age should be givenat any subsequent visit when indicated and feasible. ■ Indicates age groups that warrant special effort to administer those vaccines not previously given. Additional vaccines may be licensed and recommended during the year. Licensed combination vaccines may be used whenever any components of the combination are indicated and the vaccine's other components are not contraindicated. Providers should consult the manufacturers' package inserts for detailed recommendations.

1. Hepatitis B vaccine (HepB). All infants should receive the first dose of hepatitis B vaccine soon after birth and before hospital discharge; the first dose may also be given by age 2 months if the infant's mother is HBsAg-negative. Only monovalent HepB can be used for the birth dose. Monovalent or combination vaccine containing HepB may be used to complete the series. Four doses of vaccine may be administered when a birth dose is given. The second dose should be given at least 4 weeks after the first dose, except for combination vaccines which cannot be administeredbefore age 6 weeks. The third dose should be given at least 16 weeks after the first dose and at least 8 weeks after the second dose. The last dose in the vaccination series (third or fourth dose) should not be administered before age 6 months.

Infants born to HBsAg-positive mothers should receive HepB and 0.5 mL Hepatitis B Immune Globulin (HBIG) within 12 hours of birth at separate sites. The second dose is recommended at age 1-2 months. The last dose in the vaccination series should not be administered before age 6 months. These infants should be tested for HBsAg and anti-HBs at 9-15 months of age.

Infants born to mothers whose HBsAg status is unknown should receive the first dose of the HepB series within 12 hours of birth. Maternal blood should be drawn as soon as possible to determine the mother's HBsAg status; if the HBsAg test is positive, the infant should receive HBIG as soon as possible (no later than age 1 week). The second dose is recommended at age 1-2 months. The last dose in the vaccination series should not be administered before age 6 months.

2. Diphtheria and tetanus toxoids and acellular pertussis vaccine (DTaP). The fourth dose of DTaP may be administered as early as age 12 months, provided 6 months have elapsed since the third dose and the child is unlikely to return at age 15-18 months. **Tetanus and diphtheria toxoids (Td)** is recommended at age 11-12 years if at least 5 years have elapsed since the last dose of tetanus and diphtheria toxoid-containing vaccine. Subsequent routine Td boosters are recommended every 10 years.

3. *Haemophilus influenzae* type b (Hib) conjugate vaccine. Three Hib conjugate vaccines are licensed for infant use. If PRP-OMP (PedvaxHIB® or ComVax®[Merck]) is administered at ages 2 and 4 months, a dose at age 6 months is not required. DTaP/Hib combination products should notbe used for primary immunization in infants at ages 2, 4 or 6 months, but can be used as boosters following any Hib vaccine.

4. Measles, mumps, and rubella vaccine (MMR). The second dose of MMR is recommended routinely at age 4-6 years but may be administered during any visit, provided at least 4 weeks have elapsed since the first dose and that both doses are administered beginning at or after age 12 months. Those who have not previously received the second dose should complete the schedule by the 11-12 year old visit.

5. Varicella vaccine. Varicella vaccine is recommended at any visit at or after age 12 months for susceptible children, i.e. those who lack a reliable history of chickenpox. Susceptible persons aged ≥13 years should receive two doses, given at least 4 weeks apart.

6. Pneumococcal vaccine. The heptavalent **pneumococcal conjugate vaccine (PCV)** is recommended for all children age 2-23 months. It is also recommended for certain children age 24-59 months. **Pneumococcal polysaccharide vaccine (PPV)**is recommended in addition to PCV for certain high-risk groups. See *MMWR* 2000;49(RR-9);1-38.

7. Hepatitis A vaccine. Hepatitis A vaccine is recommended for children and adolescents in selected states and regions, and for certain high-risk groups; consult your local public health authority. Children and adolescents in these states, regions, and high risk groups who have not been immunized against hepatitis A can begin the hepatitis A vaccination series during any visit. The two doses in the series should be administered at least 6 months apart. See *MMWR* 1999;48(RR-12);1-37.

8. Influenza vaccine. Influenza vaccine is recommended annually for children age 6 months with certain risk factors (including but not limited to asthma, cardiac disease, sickle cell disease, HIV, diabetes, and household members of persons in groups at high risk; see *MMWR* 2002;51(RR-3);1-31), and can be administered to all others wishing to obtain immunity. In addition, healthy children age 6-23 months are encouraged to receive influenza vaccine if feasible because children in this age group are at substantially increased risk for influenza-related hospitalizations. Children aged ≤12 years should receive vaccine in a dosage appropriate for their age (0.25 mL if age 6-35 months or 0.5 mL if aged 3 years). Children aged 8 years who are receiving influenza vaccine for the first time should receive two doses separated byat least 4 weeks.

For additional information about vaccines, including precautions and contraindications for immunization andvaccine shortages,pleasevisit the National Immunization Program Website at www.cdc.gov/nip or call the National Immunization Information Hotlineat 800-232-2522 (English) or 800-232-0233 (Spanish).

Approved by the Advisory Committee on Immunization Practices (www.cdc.gov/nip/acip), the American Academy of Pediatrics (www.aap.org), and the American Academy of Family Physicians (www.aafp.org).

CHAPTER

45

Geriatrics

OBJECTIVES

Upon completion of this chapter, the paramedic student will be able to:

1. Explain the physiology of the aging process as it relates to major body systems and homeostasis.
2. Describe general principles of assessment specific to older adults.
3. Describe the pathophysiology, assessment, and management of specific illnesses that affect selected body systems in the geriatric patient.
4. Identify specific problems with sensations experienced by some geriatric patients.
5. Discuss effects of drug toxicity and alcoholism in the older adult.
6. Identify factors that contribute to environmental emergencies in the geriatric patient.
7. Discuss prehospital assessment and management of depression and suicide in the older adult.
8. Describe epidemiology, assessment, and management of trauma in the geriatric patient.
9. Identify characteristics of elder abuse.

KEY TERMS

cataract: A loss of transparency of the lens of the eye that results from changes in the delicate protein fibers within the lens.

continence: The ability to control bladder or bowel function.

elder abuse: The infliction of physical pain, injury, debilitating mental anguish, unreasonable confinement, or willful deprivation by a caregiver of services that are necessary to maintain mental and physical health of a geriatric person.

fecal impaction: An accumulation of hardened feces in the rectum or sigmoid colon that the person is unable to move.

gerontology: The study of the problems of all aspects of aging.

glaucoma: A condition in which intraocular pressure increases and causes damage to the optic nerve.

incontinence: The inability to control bladder or bowel function.

pressure ulcers: Sores or ulcers in the skin over a bony prominence that occurs most frequently on the sacrum, elbows, heels, outer ankles, inner knees, hips, and shoulder blades of high-risk patients especially those who are obese, elderly, or suffering from chronic diseases, infections, injuries, or a poor nutritional state.

retinopathy: A group of inflammatory eye disorders often caused by diabetes, hypertension, and atherosclerotic vascular disease.

The "graying" of American society includes the prospect that the health care needs of older adults will continue to increase in all areas. This includes prehospital care. About 25% of Americans will be 65 years of age or older by the year 2030 and will represent 70% of all ambulance transports.[1] This chapter addresses anatomical and physiological changes that accompany the aging process, special considerations in assessing and managing geriatric patients, and common emergencies that may result from normal aging and chronic illness.

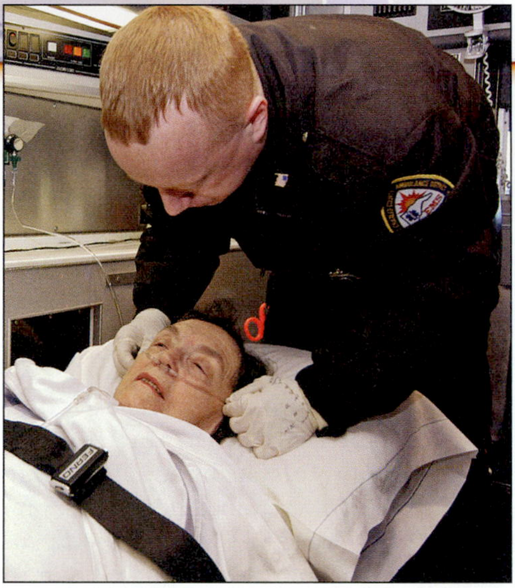

DEMOGRAPHICS, EPIDEMIOLOGY, AND SOCIETAL ISSUES

More than 34 million Americans (12% of the U.S. population) are 65 years of age or older. The size of this group has soared during the last 100 years. At the same time, fertility rates in the United States have dropped. Thus there will be fewer persons under 65 years of age to support the cost of heath care and living expenses of those over 65 years of age.

By the year 2050, nearly 25% of Americans will be eligible for Medicare. Also, the population over 85 years of age will have grown from 4 million to 19 million. This creates many challenges. Society will have to try to provide quality, cost-effective health care and support the increasing health and living expenses for the elderly. To meet the needs of this aging population properly, society must achieve the following[2]:

- The public must become better educated about the needs of the elderly because caregiving often falls to families and friends.
- Current and new health care professionals must be educated on the special needs of the aging population. Older adults have unique qualities. These qualities distinguish them from younger populations. Two examples are a higher level of adverse drug reactions and urinary incontinence. Thus health care professionals need special training to treat this population.
- The aging of the U.S. population demands continued and expanded research efforts into chronic diseases that affect the aged and their families.
- Health care professionals need to reform heath care financing, delivery, and administrative structures to accommodate the predominance of chronic illness among the aging population.
- Health care professionals must develop solutions for the long-term care needs of the growing aging population. These solutions must address the emotional and financial needs of older adults and their families. They also must address the financial influence of long-term care in the United States.

Other key issues to consider in caring for the aging population include legal ones such as advance directives, durable power of attorney, and do-not-resuscitate orders. These were discussed in Chapter 4.

LIVING ENVIRONMENTS AND REFERRAL SOURCES

Many older Americans enjoy independent living. They enjoy this lifestyle with the help of spousal or family support and home health care programs. Others live dependently in nursing care facilities, assisted-living environments, and nursing homes. The elderly often receive assistance in independent and dependent living environments. They receive this help through local, state, and national programs and other resource agencies (Box 45-1). The paramedic should be familiar with the programs in the community that offer assistance to the elderly.

BOX 45-1 Sampling of Support and Assistance Programs for the Geriatric Patient

- Community-based services
- Home health care services
- Hospice programs
- In-home services
- Institutional services
- Multipurpose senior centers
- Nutrition services
- Religious and pastoral services
- State advisory councils
- State and national aging organizations
- Volunteer organizations

PHYSIOLOGICAL CHANGES OF AGING

Gerontology is the study of the problems of all aspects of aging. The aging process proceeds at different rates in different persons. In addition, organ systems age at differing rates within the individual. However, in certain areas, predictable functional declines occur in all persons with increasing age. As a rough guideline, these changes begin to occur at a rate of 5% to 10% for each decade of life after 30 years of age. The aging process affects all body systems. However, the effects on specific organ systems particularly relevant to the older adult occur in the respiratory, cardiovascular, renal, nervous, and musculoskeletal systems (Table 45-1).

CRITICAL THINKING

Consider your family members and friends who are in their 40s, 60s, or 80s. What age-related changes have you noticed?

Respiratory System Changes

Respiratory function in the older adult generally declines as the lung tissue ages. Reduced pulmonary capacity results from changes in lung and chest wall compliance. With aging, the chest wall becomes stiffer as the bony thorax becomes more rigid. Lung elastic recoil also decreases. Despite the loss of elasticity, which would tend to increase total lung capacity, total lung capacity remains the same. This is due to the opposing loss of chest wall compliance and weakened respiratory muscles. The diameter of the alveoli increases. The distal airways tend to collapse on expiration. These changes lead to an increase in residual volume and a decrease in vital capacity. Consequently, by 75 years of age, vital capacity may decrease by as much as 50%, maximum breathing capacity by as much as 60%, and maximum work rate and maximum oxygen uptake by as much as 70%.[3]

Arterial oxygen pressure (Pa_{O_2}) also slowly decreases with age. But arterial carbon dioxide pressure stays the same. (This is most likely related to the much greater reserve in carbon dioxide elimination than in oxygen absorption.) At 30 years of age the Pa_{O_2} of a healthy person breathing ambient air at sea level is about 90 torr. At 70 years of age the expected Pa_{O_2} is 70 torr. These findings, along with the normal decline in chemoreceptor function, produce a diminished ventilatory response to hypoxia and hypercapnia.

Other factors that affect the respiratory system are the loss of cilia in the airways and a diminished cough reflex and impaired gag reflex. These can impair the bodily defense against inhaled bacteria and particulate matter. The decline in these defense mechanisms makes infectious pulmonary diseases of the older adult more common. It also makes these infections harder to resolve.

Cardiovascular System Changes

Cardiac function declines with age as a result of nonischemic physiological changes and the high incidence of atherosclerotic coronary artery disease.[4] Sorting out changes that are solely due to aging from those associated with ischemia is difficult because coronary artery disease is so prevalent in the older adult. However, even with aging alone, changes occur in the cardiovascular system that cause a decrease in cardiac function. These changes include a diminished ability to raise the heart rate even in response to exercise or stress, a decrease in compliance of the ventricle, a prolonged duration of contraction, and a decreased responsiveness to catecholamine stimulation. Between 30 and 80 years of age, resting cardiac output decreases about 30%. Combined with the progressive increase in peripheral vascular resistance that occurs after 40 years of age, this decrease in cardiac output yields a significant drop in organ perfusion.[3] Myocardial hypertrophy, coronary artery disease, and hemodynamic changes predispose the geriatric patient to dysrhythmias, heart failure, and sudden cardiac arrest when the cardiovascular system is placed under unexpected stress.

Changes also occur in the electrical conduction pathways of the heart. These changes occur as cells in the sinoatrial and atrioventricular nodes and the rest of the conduction system lose the ability to function. These physiological changes often lead to dysrhythmias. These include chronic atrial fibrillation, sick sinus syndrome, and various types of bradycardias and heart blocks. All of these can contribute to the decline in cardiac output.

CRITICAL THINKING

What lifestyle choices can slow down these physiological changes of aging?

Renal System Changes

Structural and functional changes in the kidneys occur during the aging process. For example, renal blood flow falls an average of 50% between 30 and 80 years of age.[3] This reduction in renal blood flow is associated with a proportional decrease in the glomerular filtration rate of about 8 mL/min per decade. Renal mass decreases by about 20% between 40 and 80 years of age. The steady decline in kid-

TABLE 45-1 Physiological Changes of Aging

CHANGE	RESULT
Overall Appearance	
Skin	Wrinkling
Loss of elasticity	Wrinkling, thinning of skin
Loss of collagen	Increased susceptibility to injury
Shrinking of sweat glands	Dryness
Pigment deposition	Age spots
Sun damage	Senile keratosis
Eyes	
Clouding of lens	Cataracts (decreased visual acuity)
	Poor peripheral vision
Pigment deposition	Arcus senilis (bluish circle that forms around the outer edge of the iris of the eye)
Cardiovascular System	
Increased internal thickening of arteries	Hypertension
	Increased risk of stroke or heart attack
	Varicosities and clots
	Dysrhythmias
Increased cholesterol deposits (atherosclerotic heart disease)	Coronary artery disease and peripheral vascular disease
Decreased rate of cardiac hypertrophy	Decreased cardiac output
Decreased cardiac output	Loss of exercise tolerance
	Diminished activity
	Increased work to heart
	Increased risk of myocardial infarction
Pulmonary System	
Decreased elasticity	Diminished breathing capacity
Decreased compliance and surface area	Decreased maximal oxygen uptake
Decreased ciliary activity	Increased risk of infection/toxicity
Gastrointestinal Tract	
Decreased hydrochloric acid production	Difficulty with digestion
	Food absorption problems and constipation
Delay in intestinal motility	Feeling full early, causing weight loss
Decreased saliva flow	Dry mouth, difficulty chewing
Fewer taste buds	Loss of food enjoyment, decreased appetite
Gum atrophy (shrinkage)	Tooth loss
Decreased liver function	Risk of toxicity from drugs
	Alcohol damage
	Loss of blood clotting
Central Nervous System	
Decreased cortical cell count	Memory impairment (dementia)
Increased synapse time	Decreased complex learning
Decreased nerve conduction velocity	Slower psychomotor skills
	Increased reflex time leading to risk of falling
Brain atrophy (shrinkage)	Prone to subdural hematomata
Vision	
Growth of lens	Decreased focusing ability
Cataract deposition	Hyperopia (farsightedness)
	Opacification of vision
Decreased pupil size	Decreased acuity and color perception
Loss of accommodation (focusing ability)	Decreased depth perception
	All cause increased risks of accidents and falls

From MedicAlert: *Geriatric emergencies: an EMT teaching manual,* Turlock, Calif, 1994, MedicAlert Foundation.

Continued

TABLE 45-1 Physiological Changes of Aging, cont'd

CHANGE	RESULT
Hearing	
Ossicle degeneration	Loss of high-frequency range of hearing
Atrophy (shrinkage) of auditory meatus	Loss of high-frequency range of hearing
Atrophy (shrinkage) of cochlear hair cells and auditory neurons	Decreased keenness and pitch discrimination Decreased sense of balance All cause increased risks of accidents and falls
Renal Function	
Decreased glomerular function	Decreased renal clearance
Decreased renal blood flow	Increased risk of toxicity from all drugs and toxins processed in the kidneys
Genitourinary System	
Loss of bladder control	Urinary infections
Prostate enlargement	Tumors and urinary retention
Endocrine Function	
Decrease in thyroid, ovarian, and testicular function	Decreased energy, decreased metabolic rate Decreased heat/cold tolerance Decreased reproductive function
Increased insulin	Predisposition for hypoglycemia
Musculoskeletal System	
Decreased muscle mass	Loss of strength
Increased joint/tendon breakdown	Arthritis, stiffness, loss of flexibility Increased risk of falls Loss of bone strength and size
Bone demineralization	Increased risk of fracture
Psychological/Social	
Loss of physical function	Decreased activity
Loss of friends/family	Depression
Loss of social support	Increased isolation and anxiety Increased risk of suicide attempts
Immune System	
Loss of T cell function	Increased infection

From MedicAlert: *Geriatric emergencies: an EMT teaching manual,* Turlock, Calif, 1994, MedicAlert Foundation.

ney function places the geriatric patient at greater risk for renal failure from trauma, obstruction, infection, and vascular occlusion.

As the patient ages, significant impairment develops in renal concentrating ability, sodium conservation, free water clearance (diuresis), glomerular filtration, and renal plasma flow. Hepatic blood flow decreases as well. This limits the effectiveness of liver metabolism. Decreases in kidney and liver function and loss of muscle and body water make the geriatric patient more susceptible to electrolyte disturbances. They also make the geriatric patient more likely to experience problems with medications or drugs.

Nervous System Changes

Although it was long thought that mental dysfunction in the geriatric patient was caused solely by senility, it is now well known that intellectual functioning deteriorates selectively and may result from many organic causes.[5] For example, beginning at about 30 years of age, the total number of neurons in certain cortical areas decreases gradually, so by 70 years of age, a 10% reduction in brain weight has occurred.[3] These factors, decreased cerebral blood flow, and changes in the location and amounts of specific neurotransmitters probably contribute to changes in the central nervous system (CNS). The velocity of nerve conduction in the peripheral nervous system decreases with aging as well. This may lead to changes in motor or position sense and delays in reaction time and motor responses. Other gradual changes in the patient's nervous system can result in decreased visual acuity and auditory keenness. They also can result in changes in sleep.

Toxic or metabolic factors that can affect mental functioning include the use of medications (e.g., anticholinergics, antihypertensives, antidysrhythmics, and analgesics); electrolyte imbalances; hypoglycemia; acidosis; alkalosis;

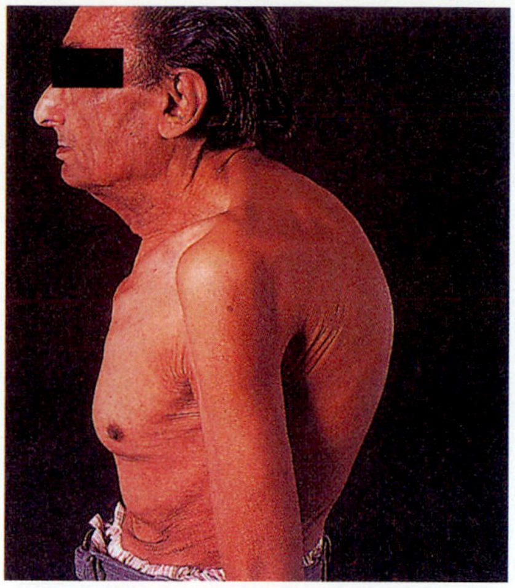

FIGURE 45-1 ■ Kyphosis.

hypoxia; liver, kidney, and lung failure; pneumonia; congestive heart failure (CHF); cardiac dysrhythmias; infection; and the development of benign or malignant tumors.

Musculoskeletal System Changes

As the body ages, muscles shrink, muscles and ligaments calcify, and intervertebral disks become thin. Osteoporosis is common in geriatric patients (especially in women). An estimated 68% of geriatric patients show some degree of kyphosis (Fig. 45-1). (This is a humpback posture.) These musculoskeletal changes result in a decrease in total muscle mass, a decrease in height of 2 to 3 inches, widening and weakening of certain bones, and a posture that impairs mobility and alters the balance of the body. As a result, falls are common. Moreover, the falls often are associated with significant morbidity and mortality.

Prevention strategies (described in Chapter 3) that can decrease injuries associated with falls include the following:

- Using assistive devices (e.g., walker or cane)
- Removing scatter rugs and securing loose carpeting
- Removing items that may cause tripping
- Providing and using handrails
- Ensuring adequate lighting
- Removing clutter from the environment
- Arranging furniture for walking ease
- Using nonslip decals in the bathtub or shower
- Providing handrails on bathtubs, showers, and commodes

CRITICAL THINKING

Consider a patient who has significant kyphosis. What aspects of care will you need to alter to immobilize the spine of this patient?

Other Physiological Changes

Other physiological changes that occur with aging include changes in body mass and total body water, a decreased ability to maintain internal homeostasis, a decrease in the function of immunological mechanisms, nutritional disorders, and decreases in hearing and visual acuity.

As an individual approaches 65 years of age, lean body mass may decrease as much as 25%, and fat tissue may increase as much as 35%.[3] These changes in body makeup can affect the dosage and frequency of administration of fat-soluble drugs. This is because there is more drug per weight of metabolically active tissue and a larger reservoir for buildup of the drug. In the same way, the decrease in total body water is likely to increase the concentration of water-soluble drugs.

The ability of the body to maintain normal temperature declines over time. The decline begins at about 30 years of age. Because of this, the geriatric patient is at greater risk for cold- and heat-related conditions. These include hypothermia, heat exhaustion, and hyperthermia. Several factors contribute to the increased risk of thermoregulatory disorders, including impaired sympathetic nervous system function, causing decreased capacity for peripheral vasoconstriction, lowered metabolic rate, poor peripheral circulation, and chronic illness. Because of the decline in many body functions, including blood pressure, cardiac output, and temperature regulation, a specific illness or injury often puts the geriatric patient "over the edge."

Aging causes a decrease in primary antibody response and cellular immunity and elevations in the amount of abnormal immunoglobulins and immune complexes.[3] These physiological changes increase the risk of infection, autoimmune disorders, and perhaps cancer. In addition, infections may not produce the usual signs and symptoms.

About one in eight deaths in geriatric patients results from cancer.[6] In younger patients, cancer often is the main or only disease from which they suffer. However, geriatric patients often have more than one disease and disability. Thus signs and symptoms such as a change in bowel habits, rectal bleeding, malaise, fatigue, weight loss, and anorexia may result from other maladies. Treatment with chemotherapy often results in immunosuppression. This increases the risk of infection and often masks the typical signs and symptoms associated with infection.

Many geriatric patients consume less than the minimum daily requirement of most vitamins,[7] which may be a result of loneliness and depression, decreased sensitivity to taste, decreased appetite, financial difficulties, physical infirmity, decreased vision, or a combination of these elements. All of these elements may act to reduce the motivation to shop for and prepare fresh food. Other factors associated with poor nutrition are poor dentition and reduced mastication, decreased esophageal motility, frequent hypochlorhydria, and decreased intestinal secretions that reduce absorption. Geriatric patients easily can become victims of malnutrition. Malnutrition in turn can cause dehydration and hypoglycemia.

CRITICAL THINKING

What effects can poor nutrition have on body function?

GENERAL PRINCIPLES IN ASSESSMENT OF THE GERIATRIC PATIENT

Normal physiological changes and underlying acute or chronic illness may make evaluation of an ill or injured geriatric patient a challenge. In addition to the components of a normal physical assessment (described in Chapter 12), the paramedic should consider special characteristics of geriatric patients that can complicate the clinical evaluation[8]:

- Geriatric patients are likely to suffer from more than one illness at a time.
- Chronic problems can make assessment for acute problems difficult.
- Signs or symptoms of chronic illness can be confused with signs or symptoms of an acute problem.
- Aging can affect an individual's response to illness or injury.
- Pain may be diminished or absent.
- The patient or paramedic can underestimate the severity of a condition.
- Social and emotional factors may have a greater influence on health in geriatric patients than in any other age group.
- The patient fears losing autonomy.
- The patient fears the hospital environment.
- The patient has financial concerns about health care.

Patient History

Gathering a history from a geriatric patient usually requires more time than with younger patients (see Chapter 10). In addition to a longer medical history because of the patient's age, chronic illness, and medication use, the geriatric patient may have physical impediments such as hearing loss and visual impairment. Questioning a patient who is fatigued or easily distracted also may lengthen the interview process. The paramedic should use the following techniques when communicating with geriatric patients:

- Always identify yourself.
- Speak at eye level to ensure that the patient can see you as you communicate.
- Locate a hearing aid, eyeglasses, and dentures (if needed).
- Turn on lights.
- Speak slowly, distinctly, and respectfully.
- Use the patient's surname, unless the patient requests otherwise.
- Listen closely.
- Be patient.
- Preserve dignity.
- Use gentleness.

> **CRITICAL THINKING**
> Why should you ask geriatric patients to bring all of their medications to the hospital?

Physical Examination

When conducting the physical examination of a geriatric patient, the paramedic should consider the following six points:

1. The patient may tire easily.
2. Geriatric patients often wear many layers of clothing for warmth. This may hamper the examination.
3. Respect the patient's modesty and need for privacy unless it interferes with the care.
4. Explain actions clearly before examining all geriatric patients. This is important with patients with diminished sight.
5. Be aware that the patient may minimize or deny his or her symptoms. Denial may be due to a fear of being bedridden or institutionalized or losing self-sufficiency.
6. Try to distinguish symptoms of chronic disease from acute problems.

If time allows, the paramedic should assess the geriatric patient's immediate surroundings for evidence of alcohol or medication use (e.g., insulin syringes, "vial of life," or MedicAlert information), presence of food, general condition of housing, and signs of adequate personal hygiene. These and other observations help provide information to the physician about the patient's general health and ability for self-care after release from the hospital.

The paramedic should question friends or family members who are present about the patient's appearance and responsiveness *now* versus the patient's normal appearance, responsiveness, and other characteristics. The paramedic also should discreetly ask about advance directives and initiation of care for the patient (described in Chapter 4). If these documents are available, the paramedic should obtain them and convey the information to medical direction. Finally, the paramedic should ensure gentle handling and padding for patient comfort if transport is needed.

SYSTEM PATHOPHYSIOLOGY, ASSESSMENT, AND MANAGEMENT

The pathophysiology, assessment, and management of specific illnesses described in this section include those of the pulmonary system, cardiovascular system, CNS, endocrine system, gastrointestinal system, integumentary system, musculoskeletal system, and problems associated with special senses. Toxicology, environmental considerations, behavioral and psychiatric disorders, trauma, and **elder abuse** also are discussed in this section.

Pulmonary System

Specific illnesses of the pulmonary system that are common in elderly patients include bacterial pneumonia, chronic obstructive pulmonary disease, and pulmonary embolism. These conditions were described in Chapter 30. They are presented here as a review.

BACTERIAL PNEUMONIA

Pneumonia is a leading cause of death in the geriatric age group and often is fatal in frail adults.[8] In addition, geriatric patients are more likely to develop bacteremia. They also are more susceptible to several respiratory germs (e.g., gram-negative bacilli). This susceptibility, associated with the presence of chronic disease, impairs the ability of older adults to keep the respiratory tract clean. It also allows germs to grow in the throat that then may travel to or be aspirated into the lungs. Because of the decreased lung function, pneumonia often may be associated with respiratory failure. Risk factors for bacterial pneumonia include institutional environments, chronic diseases, and compromise of the immune system.

Unlike in younger patients with bacterial pneumonia, the usual clinical picture of fever, productive cough, pleurisy, and signs of pulmonary congestion often is absent in the geriatric patient. This atypical presentation is responsible for the common delay in diagnosis. The following are possible signs and symptoms:

- Alterations in mental status
- Cough
- Fever (variable)
- Shortness of breath
- Tachycardia
- Tachypnea

Geriatric patients with pneumonia may be too weak to cough or produce sputum. They also may not be able to breathe deeply. Therefore breath sounds may be misleading because of preexisting emphysema or chronic CHF. Tachycardia and tachypnea often are the most reliable indicators of bacterial pneumonia in the prehospital setting.

Emergency care for geriatric patients with bacterial pneumonia focuses on managing life threats, maintaining oxygenation, and providing transport for physician evaluation. Bacterial pneumonia is linked to a high rate of hospital admission. Pneumonia generally is managed with antibiotics.

> **CRITICAL THINKING**
> Why is flu season linked to an increase in pneumonia in the elderly?

CHRONIC OBSTRUCTIVE PULMONARY DISEASE

Chronic obstructive pulmonary disease (COPD) in the geriatric patient is a major health problem in the United States. Chronic obstructive pulmonary disease is a common finding in the geriatric patient with a history of smoking. It usually is associated with various diseases that result in reduced expiratory air flow. (Examples of such diseases are asthma, emphysema, and chronic bronchitis.) An exacerbation of COPD often follows an acute respiratory infection that causes airway edema, bronchial smooth muscle irritability, and increased mucus secretion. These airway abnormalities may lead to factors associated with acute decompensation, including the following:

- Limited air flow
- Increased work of breathing
- Dyspnea
- Ventilation-perfusion mismatching
- Hypoxemia
- Respiratory acidosis
- Hemodynamic compromise

Signs and symptoms of COPD in the geriatric patient include extreme anxiety, cyanosis, wheezing, and abnormal or diminished breath sounds associated with marked dyspnea and the use of accessory muscles. Other signs and symptoms include dysrhythmias, paradoxical breathing, jugular vein distention, and decreased oxygen saturation levels (per pulse oximetry). The paramedic should obtain a full history of the event. (This should include a past history of intubation or steroid therapy.) The paramedic also should be prepared for aggressive airway management. The care for a patient with COPD is aimed at correcting life-threatening hypoxemia and improving air flow. To achieve these goals, the use of airway and ventilatory support with supplemental oxygenation and the administration of bronchodilators by inhalation or injection (per medical direction) is indicated. Failure to begin aggressive treatments to correct the acidosis and hypoxia from COPD can lead to a fast decline in the patient's condition.

PULMONARY EMBOLISM

Pulmonary embolism is a life-threatening cause of dyspnea. The condition is associated with venous stasis, heart failure, COPD, malignancy, and immobilization. All of these are common in older adults. Most pulmonary emboli in geriatric patients form in the veins of the legs. From there they travel through the femoral veins to the inferior vena cava and the heart. The clinical presentation of pulmonary embolism often is misleading in geriatric patients and frequently is misdiagnosed.[3]

Signs and symptoms of pulmonary embolism may range from a presentation of left ventricular failure with sudden tachypnea, unexplained tachycardia (a hallmark sign), and atrial fibrillation to signs and symptoms solely of the underlying venous thrombosis (calf discomfort without tenderness, mild calf or ankle edema, increased warmth, and dilation of superficial veins in one foot or leg). Pulmonary embolism can cause CHF to develop. Pulmonary embolism also may be mistaken for bacterial pneumonia in geriatric patients.

> **CRITICAL THINKING**
> What other conditions have similar cardiovascular signs and symptoms?

Emergency care focuses on ensuring adequate airway, ventilatory, and circulatory support; immobilizing and elevating an affected extremity; and rapidly transporting the patient for physician evaluation. In-hospital care may include analgesics, bed rest, hemodynamic stabilization with intravenously administered fluids and vasopressors to support blood pressure, and efforts to prevent further embolization. The physician may give some patients thrombolytics to dissolve the clot. The physician also may treat them with anticoagulants to prevent further emboli.

Cardiovascular System

Cardiovascular disorders were described in Chapter 29. Specific disorders reviewed in this section include myocardial infarction, heart failure, dysrhythmias, abdominal and thoracic aneurysm, and hypertension.

MYOCARDIAL INFARCTION

Chest pain as a symptom of myocardial infarction (MI) becomes less frequent by 70 years of age. Only 45% of patients over 85 years of age with MI have this complaint. Lack of typical chest pain can cause MI to go unrecognized in the geriatric patient.[4] The following are six major risk factors that the paramedic should evaluate when assessing a patient for MI:

1. Previous MI
2. Angina
3. Diabetes
4. Hypertension
5. High cholesterol level
6. Smoking

Some geriatric patients have chest pain or discomfort. However, many complain only of vague symptoms. Examples of such include dyspnea (the most common sign in patients over 85 years of age), abdominal or epigastric distress, and fatigue.

The mortality rate associated with acute MI doubles after 70 years of age.[8] For many geriatric patients the event is totally "silent." This may be a result of decreased visceral sensory function or a higher incidence of mental deterioration in this age group. Silent MIs are almost always marked by an atypical complaint. This may include fatigue, breathlessness, nausea, or abdominal pain. Thus the paramedic must maintain a high index of suspicion for MI in elderly patients with unusual warning signs or symptoms.

> **CRITICAL THINKING**
> What hormonal change in older women increases their risk for heart disease?

Emergency care includes airway, ventilatory, and circulatory support; oxygen administration and pain management therapy; management of serious dysrhythmias according to advanced life support protocol; and rapid and gentle transportation for physician evaluation.

HEART FAILURE

Heart failure is more frequent in geriatric patients. It also has a larger incidence of noncardiac causes. Heart failure occurs when the ventricular output cannot meet the metabolic demands of the body. Heart failure often is caused by ischemic heart disease, valvular heart disease, cardiomyopathy, dysrhythmias, hyperthyroidism, and anemia. The following are common signs and symptoms of heart failure:

- Dyspnea
- Fatigue (often the first symptom of left-sided heart failure)
- Orthopnea
- Dry, hacking cough progressing to productive cough with frothy sputum
- Dependent edema caused by right-sided heart failure
- Nocturia
- Anorexia, hepatomegaly, ascites

> **NOTE** Differentiating among the causes of dyspnea is difficult in the prehospital setting. However, such differentiation is important. If the patient has had acute episodes of heart failure in the past, the current emergency event also is likely to be heart failure.[9] A thorough patient history is important.

The emergency care is aimed at reversing the conditions associated with heart failure as soon as possible. This will help to prevent cardiac damage. In addition to oxygen administration and electrocardiograph monitoring, management may include intubation, intravenous (IV) therapy, and drug therapy ***(furosemide, nitroglycerin, morphine)***.

> **CRITICAL THINKING**
> How do furosemide, nitroglycerin, and morphine work to relieve the signs and symptoms of heart failure?

DYSRHYTHMIAS

The most common cause of dysrhythmias in the geriatric patient is hypertensive heart disease.[8] But any condition that decreases blood flow to the heart can cause rhythm irregularities. When assessing dysrhythmias in the geriatric patient, the paramedic should consider the following:

- Premature ventricular contractions are common in most adults over 80 years of age.
- Atrial fibrillation is the most common dysrhythmia.
- Dysrhythmias may result from electrolyte imbalances.

In addition to the serious implications of some dysrhythmias, associated complications may include traumatic injury from falls that result from cerebral hypoperfusion, transient ischemic attacks, and heart failure. The paramedic should focus emergency care on ensuring adequate airway, ventilatory, and circulatory support; administering oxygen; and transporting the patient for physician evaluation. The paramedic should manage serious dysrhythmias as described in Chapter 29.

ABDOMINAL AND THORACIC ANEURYSM

Atherosclerotic disease is a common cause of abdominal and thoracic aneurysm. Abdominal aortic aneurysm affects about 2% to 4% of the U.S. population over 50 years of age.[5]

BOX 45-2 Signs and Symptoms of Abdominal and Thoracic Aneurysm

Absent or reduced pulses	Pulsatile, tender mass
Acute myocardial infarction	Stroke
Chest pain	Sudden onset of abdominal or back pain
Diminished distal pulses	Syncope
Heart failure	Syncope
Hypotension	Unexplained hypotension
Low back pain or flank pain	
Pericardial tamponade	

Acute dissecting aortic aneurysm is more common than abdominal aneurysm and is associated with a high mortality rate. Signs and symptoms vary according to the site of rupture or extent of dissection (Box 45-2).

The goals of prehospital care are relief of pain and immediate transport to a hospital. Airway, ventilatory, and circulatory support may be required if the patient's condition deteriorates. Other prehospital care measures include the following:

- Gentle handling of the patient
- Allaying anxiety
- High-concentration oxygen administration
- Small-bore IV access to restrict fluids unless severe hypotension is present
- Pain medication per medical direction

HYPERTENSION

Geriatric patients who have atherosclerosis frequently have hypertension also. Associated risk factors for hypertension include advanced age, diabetes, and obesity. Hypertension[10] often is defined by a resting blood pressure consistently greater than 140/90 mm Hg. (Blood pressure greater than 160/95 mm Hg doubles the mortality rate in men.[8]) Chronic hypertension is associated with many medical conditions, including the following:

NOTE Systolic blood pressure gradually increases with age. However, diastolic pressure often stays normal or slightly decreases. Thus in persons over age 50, systolic pressure is a better indicator of risk for heart disease and stroke (American Heart Association: New high blood pressure guidelines say start early, treat aggressively, May 15, 2003. http://www.americanheart.org/presenter.jhtml?identifier=3011728. Accessed October 26, 2004). Current guidelines recommend that physicians treat older patients who have systolic hypertension with antihypertensive drugs. The goal of treatment is to achieve a blood pressure less than 140/90 mm Hg or less than 130/80 mm Hg in patients with diabetes or kidney disease. For patients with stage one hypertension (systolic pressure of 140 to159 mm Hg) and additional cardiovascular risk factors, a sustained reduction in systolic pressure for more than 10 years will decrease mortality rates.

BOX 45-3 Signs and Symptoms of Stroke and Transient Ischemic Attack

Ataxia	Numbness
Diplopia	Unilateral paralysis
Language disturbance	Vertigo
Monocular blindness	Visual disturbance

- Aneurysm formation
- Blindness
- Cardiac hypertrophy and left ventricular failure
- Kidney failure
- Myocardial ischemia and infarction
- Peripheral vascular disease
- Stroke

Hypertension in the geriatric patient may manifest only in nonspecific complaints such as headache, forgetfulness, and general malaise. Other signs and symptoms that may indicate chronic hypertension include epistaxis, tremors, and nausea and vomiting. Care is mainly supportive. In severe cases, medical direction may advise to use antihypertensives (e.g., ***labetalol***). After physician evaluation, the patient with chronic hypertension often is managed with oral medications, dietary sodium reduction, weight loss, and exercise.

Nervous System

Neurological disorders were described in Chapter 31. Specific disorders described in this section for review include cerebral vascular disease, delirium, dementia, Alzheimer's disease, and Parkinson's disease.

CEREBRAL VASCULAR DISEASE

Stroke is the third leading cause of death in most countries and the leading cause of brain injury in adults.[4] As described in Chapter 29, the neurological impairment is caused by an ischemic or hemorrhagic interruption in the blood supply to the brain. Associated risk factors for cerebral vascular disease in the older adult include smoking, hypertension, diabetes, atherosclerosis, hyperlipidemia, polycythemia, and heart disease. Box 45-3 provides a review of the signs and symptoms of stroke and transient ischemic attack.

Once the paramedic suspects stroke, the paramedic must *minimize time in the field*. The reason is the limited time to initiate therapy. (Less than 3 hours from onset is recommended for fibrinolytic therapy.) The paramedic should focus on managing the patient's airway, breathing, and circulation and on monitoring vital signs. Aside from supporting vital functions, the most important element of pre-

CRITICAL THINKING

What factors can cause a delay between the onset of signs and symptoms of stroke in the geriatric patient and when an emergency telephone call is made?

hospital care for a stroke victim is identification of the patient with stroke and rapid transportation of the patient to a stroke center that can provide treatment within 1 hour after arrival at the emergency department door.[11]

DELIRIUM

Delirium is an abrupt disorientation to time and place. It usually includes illusions and hallucinations. The patient's mind may "wander." The patient's speech may be incoherent. The patient may be in a state of mental confusion or excitement as well. Delirium commonly is a result of physical illness. Signs and symptoms vary according to personality, environment, and severity of illness. Causes of delirium are associated with organic brain dysfunction and include the following:

- Alcohol intoxication or withdrawal
- Drug reactions
- Fever
- Metabolic disorders
- Tumor

Delirium can be life threatening. It requires emergency care. The condition may be reversible if it is diagnosed early. Yet delirium can progress to chronic mental dysfunction. Prehospital care includes the following measures[9]:

1. Ensure adequate airway, breathing, and circulatory support.
   a. Manage hypoxia with oxygen.
   b. Manage hypotension with IV fluids if appropriate.
2. Reduce agitation and anxiety.
3. Avoid patient injury, and ensure personal safety.
   a. Restrain the patient if needed, per protocol.
   b. Sedate the patient as a last resort.
4. Consider hypoglycemia or a narcotic state.
   a. Measure blood glucose level.
   b. Administer ***dextrose 50%*** or ***naloxone*** per protocol.
5. Assess for CNS injury (e.g., trauma or stroke). Perform a careful neurological examination.
6. Look for signs of CNS infection (e.g., encephalitis).
7. Transport the patient for physician evaluation.

DEMENTIA

Dementia is a slow, progressive loss of awareness of time and place. It usually involves an inability to learn new things or recall recent events. Dementia often is a result of brain disease caused by strokes, genetic or viral factors, and Alzheimer's disease. Dementia generally is considered irreversible. Dementia eventually results in full dependence on others as a result of the progressive loss of cognitive functioning. During the course of the disease, patients often try to cover up their memory loss. They do this by *confabulation* (making up stories to fill gaps in memory). Sudden outbursts or embarrassing conduct may be the first clear signs of dementia. Some patients eventually regress to a "second childhood." At that point, they need full care for feedings, toileting, and physical activity. Dementia is present in about 50% of nursing home residents and affects, to some degree, about 20% of those over 80 years of age.[5]

TABLE 45-2 Differential Diagnosis for Delirium and Dementia

	DELIRIUM	DEMENTIA
Onset	Abrupt	Gradual
Characteristics	Reduced attention span Disorganized thinking Hallucinations	Impaired recent memory Regression Poor judgment

Dementia can be difficult to differentiate from delirium in the prehospital setting. The key difference between the two is that delirium is new with rapid onset, and dementia is progressive (Table 45-2). Thus a history of the event from a reliable witness (e.g., friend or family member) is the best source of information. A history provided by the patient may be unreliable. If a good witness is not available, the paramedic should manage the patient for delirium that may be a life-threatening emergency.

ALZHEIMER'S DISEASE

Alzheimer's disease is a condition in which nerve cells in the cerebral cortex die and the brain substance shrinks. The disease is the single most common cause of dementia and is responsible for the majority of cases in persons over 75 years of age.[3] Alzheimer's disease does not cause death directly; patients ultimately stop eating and become malnourished and immobilized. Then they are prone to intercurrent infections.

The cause of Alzheimer's disease is not known. Possible causes include abnormalities in glutamate metabolism, chronic infection, toxic poisoning by metals, reduction in brain chemicals (e.g., acetylcholine), and genetics. Atherosclerosis is *not* a cause of Alzheimer's disease. The primary disorder is in the nerve cells, not the blood vessels.

Early symptoms of Alzheimer's disease mainly are related to memory loss, especially the ability to make and recall new memories (Box 45-4).

As the disease progresses, agitation, violence, and impairment of abstract thinking occur. Judgment and cognitive abilities begin to interfere with work and social relations. In the advanced stages of Alzheimer's disease, patients often become bedridden. They often become totally unaware of their surroundings as well. Once the patient is bedridden, bed sores, feeding problems, and pneumonia shorten the patient's life.

No specific treatment exists for Alzheimer's disease. Treatment mainly consists of nursing and social care for the patient and relatives. The paramedic manages patients with this disease the same as for dementia.

PARKINSON'S DISEASE

As described in Chapter 31, Parkinson's disease is a brain disorder. (The disease is caused by degeneration of or damage to nerve cells in the basal ganglia.) The disorder causes

BOX 45-4 The Seven Warning Signs of Alzheimer's Disease

1. Asking the same question over and over again.
2. Repeating the same story, word for word, again and again.
3. Forgetting how to cook, or how to make repairs, or how to play cards—activities that were previously done with ease and regularity.
4. Losing one's ability to pay bills or balance one's checkbook.
5. Getting lost in familiar surroundings, or misplacing household objects.
6. Neglecting to bathe or wearing the same clothes over and over again even as patients insist that they have taken a bath or that their clothes are still clean.
7. Relying on someone else, such as a spouse, to make decisions or answer questions they previously would have handled themselves.

From Alzheimer's Disease Education & Referral Center: The Seven warning signs of Alzheimer's disease. http://www.alzheimers.org/pubs/sevensigns.htm. Accessed September 23, 2003. Reprinted with the permission of the Suncoast Gerontology Center, University of South Florida. Revised September 1, 1999.

muscle tremor, stiffness, and weakness. Characteristic signs of Parkinson's disease are trembling (usually beginning in one hand, arm, or leg), a rigid posture, slow movements, and a shuffling, unbalanced walk. If left untreated, the disease progresses over 10 to 15 years to severe weakness and incapacity. Parkinson's disease affects about 1 person in 200 (mostly older adults), with 50,000 new cases diagnosed in the United States each year.[8]

The emergency care for these patients mainly is supportive. It includes airway, ventilatory, and circulatory support and transport for physician evaluation. Parkinson's disease has no cure. However, counseling, exercise, special aids in the home, and drug therapy can improve the patient's morale, mobility, and quality of life.

Endocrine System

Two common endocrine disorders often are seen in geriatric patients. These disorders are diabetes and thyroid disease (described in Chapter 32). The following is a review of these conditions.

DIABETES

About 20% of older adults have diabetes, and almost 40% have some impaired glucose tolerance.[8] Type 2 (non–insulin-dependent) diabetes is most common in geriatric patients. Type 2 diabetes is especially common when the person is overweight. The following are associated risk factors in older adults for complications related to diabetes:

- Decreased ability to care for self
- Living alone
- Intercurrent illness
- Decline in renal function
- Polydrug use

A combination of dietary measures, weight reduction, and oral hypoglycemic agents can usually keep type 2 diabetes under control. In most cases, insulin injections are not required for type 2 diabetes. However, if not controlled, diabetes can lead to complications. These include **retinopathy,** peripheral neuropathy (ulcers on the feet are common), and kidney damage. Diabetic patients also have a higher-than-average risk for atherosclerosis, hypertension and other cardiovascular disorders and for cataracts. Emergency care for diabetic patients is outlined in Chapter 32 and includes airway, ventilatory, and circulatory support; blood glucose screening; IV ***dextrose*** (if indicated and in the absence of cerebral damage); and transport for physician evaluation.

Hyperglycemic hyperosmolar nonketotic coma, described in Chapter 32, is a serious complication of elderly type 2 diabetic patients with a mortality rate of 20% to 50%.[3] The paramedic often finds the type 2 diabetic patient comatose. If awake, the patient may complain of profound thirst and frequent urination. Frequent urination results from osmotic diuresis and leads to dehydration and electrolyte loss. Predisposing factors that make the geriatric patients susceptible to hyperglycemic hyperosmolar nonketotic coma include infection, noncompliance with medications, polydrug use, pancreatitis, stroke, hypothermia, heat stroke, and MI. If the paramedic suspects hyperglycemic hyperosmolar nonketotic coma, the paramedic should ensure adequate airway, ventilatory, and circulatory support; should search vigorously for an underlying cause; should initiate IV therapy; and should transport the patient rapidly for physician evaluation.

CRITICAL THINKING

What finding is present in the patient with diabetic ketoacidosis yet is absent in the patient with hyperglycemic hyperosmolar nonketotic coma?

THYROID DISEASE

Thyroid disease is more common in geriatric patients. It may be related to the aging process. The classic signs and symptoms of thyroid disorders (e.g., fullness in the neck, goiter, muscle or joint pain) often are not present in the geriatric patient. Thus the paramedic should suspect thyroid dysfunction in any geriatric patient who is ill.

The older patient often attributes the signs and symptoms of hypothyroidism to "growing old." Common complaints include weight loss, nonspecific musculoskeletal complaints, and confusion. More serious conditions associated with this disorder include CHF, anemia, hyponatremia, depression, dementia, seizures, and coma. Hyperthyroidism is less common than hypothyroidism in elderly patients. Hyperthyroidism may result from medication errors (e.g., too many doses of a thyroid hormone replacement). Signs and symptoms of hyperthyroidism include weight loss, constipation, mental status changes, CHF, tachydysrhythmias, and lethargy.

The emergency care mainly is supportive to ensure vital functions. The physician evaluates the patient with thyroid disease and treats the patient with various thyroid drugs, radioactive iodine treatments, and sometimes surgery. Severe complications from thyroid disease include thyroid storm and myxedema coma (described in Chapter 32). These complications can be made worse in a patient who has heart disease.

Gastrointestinal System

Gastrointestinal emergencies (described in Chapter 34) are common in the elderly. The paramedic should always consider abdominal pain a serious complaint in a geriatric patient. Life-threatening causes of abdominal pain in this age group include abdominal aortic aneurysm, gastrointestinal hemorrhage, ruptured viscus, dead or ischemic bowel, and acute bowel obstruction. Specific disorders discussed in this section are gastrointestinal hemorrhage, bowel obstruction, problems with **continence,** and problems with elimination.

GASTROINTESTINAL HEMORRHAGE

Gastrointestinal bleeding most commonly affects patients between 60 and 90 years of age. It has a mortality rate of about 10%. The older the patient, the higher the risk of death. This higher risk is because of the following[9]:

- Geriatric patients are less able to compensate for acute blood loss.
- They are less likely to feel symptoms and therefore seek treatment at later stages of disease.
- They are more likely to be taking ***aspirin*** or nonsteroidal antiinflammatory drugs, which places them at higher risk for ulcer disease and bleeding.
- They are at higher risk for colon cancer, intestinal vascular abnormalities, and diverticulitis.
- They are more likely to be on blood-thinning medications.

Signs and symptoms of gastrointestinal bleeding include vomiting of blood or coffee-ground emesis; blood-tinged stools or black, tarry stools; and weakness, syncope, or pain. If the paramedic suspects or confirms bleeding in a patient with signs and symptoms of shock, the paramedic should begin measures to ensure adequate airway, ventilatory, and circulatory support. The paramedic also should transport the patient rapidly for definitive care.

BOWEL OBSTRUCTION

Bowel obstruction generally occurs in patients with prior abdominal surgeries or hernias. Obstruction occurs in those with colonic cancer as well. Most complain of constipation, abdominal cramping, and an inability to pass gas. Other signs and symptoms include protracted vomiting of food or bile and vomiting of fecal material. The patient's heart rate and blood pressure often are in normal ranges. The abdomen also may be mildly distended and tender in all four quadrants. (Abdominal pain is variable.)

The prehospital care mainly is supportive to ensure vital functions. After physician evaluation, patient care may include bowel rest, nasogastric suction, and volume replacement. Some patients may need surgery to lyse the offending adhesions. Surgery may result in a cycle of new scarring and obstruction. They also may need surgery for hernia repair (most often in men).

PROBLEMS WITH CONTINENCE

Continence is the ability to control bladder or bowel function. It requires anatomically correct gastrointestinal and genitourinary tracts, competent sphincter mechanisms, cognitive and physical function, and motivation. Some factors associated with continence are affected by age. These factors include a decrease in bladder capacity, involuntary bladder contractions, decreased ability to postpone voiding, and medications that can affect bladder and bowel control. **Incontinence** of urine or bowel is abnormal at any age.

Urinary incontinence can vary in severity. It can be only mild incontinence (the escape of small amounts of urine). Or it can be total incontinence, with complete loss of bladder control. Causes of urinary incontinence include injury or disease of the urinary tract, prolapse of the uterus, a decline in sphincter muscle control surrounding the urethra (common in the elderly), CNS injury or disease, pelvic fracture, prostate cancer, and dementia.

Bowel incontinence in the geriatric patient usually is the result of **fecal impaction.** This occurs when feces lodged in the rectum irritate and inflame the lining. This allows fecal fluid and small feces to pass involuntarily. Other causes of bowel incontinence include severe diarrhea, injury to anal muscles (from childbirth or surgery), CNS injury or disease, and dementia.

All forms of incontinence usually are embarrassing for the patient. If incontinence is chronic, it can lead to skin irritation, tissue breakdown, and urinary tract infection. Some cases are managed with surgery to restore sphincter function. Patients with mild cases often wear absorptive undergarments to relieve discomfort and embarrassment.

> **CRITICAL THINKING**
> Consider the incontinent patient. How can you minimize the patient's embarrassment and discomfort?

PROBLEMS WITH ELIMINATION

Causes of difficulty in urination usually result from enlargement of the prostate (in men), urinary tract infection, urethral strictures, and acute or chronic renal failure. Difficulty in bowel elimination often is associated with diverticular disease, constipation, and colorectal cancer. Problems with elimination can cause great pain for geriatric patients. They can cause anxiety as well. The paramedic should take their complaints seriously. These conditions call for physician evaluation to identify the cause. The evaluation also will lead to the appropriate therapy.

Integumentary System

As persons age, the skin gradually becomes dry, transparent, and wrinkled. These integumentary changes are associated with a loss of elasticity, uneven pigmentation, and various benign and malignant lesions. In addition, aging results in a gradual decrease in epidermal cellular turnover. Aging results in a reduced rate of nail and hair growth as well. The associated loss of deep, dermal vessels and capillary circulation leads to common complaints such as dry, itchy skin; changes in thermal regulation; and skin-related complications. Some of these complications include the following:

- Slow healing
- Increased risk of secondary infection
- Increased risk of fungal or viral infections
- Increased susceptibility to abrasions and tears

The paramedic should always be gentle with the skin of a geriatric patient. Examples include use of aseptic technique during wound management, gentle placement and removal of electrocardiogram electrodes, and using careful taping procedures when securing IV catheters or tubing.

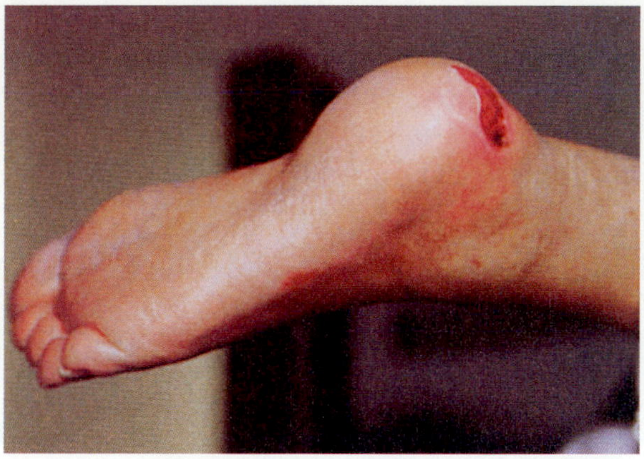

FIGURE 45-2 ■ Pressure ulcer.

CRITICAL THINKING

Consider a geriatric patient who has a burn injury. How do these changes influence the patient's recovery?

PRESSURE ULCERS

Pressure ulcers are common in geriatric patients (Fig. 45-2). They often develop on the skin of patients who are bedridden or immobile (e.g., *decubitus ulcers*). Most pressure ulcers occur in the lower legs, back, and buttocks, and over bony areas such as the greater trochanter or the sacrum. They often affect victims of stroke or other illnesses that result in a loss or change in the sensation of pain. Skin exposure to moisture (e.g., from incontinence), poor nutrition, and friction or shear also may be factors for developing pressure ulcers. Other causes of pressure ulcers in geriatric patients include vascular and metabolic disorders (e.g., venous stasis and diabetes), trauma, and cancer.

Pressure ulcers result from tissue hypoxia. They generally start as red, painful areas that become purple before the skin breaks down. Then they develop into open sores. Once integrity of the skin has been breached, the sores often become infected. Then they are slow to heal. Pressure ulcers should be covered with sterile dressing using aseptic technique. The paramedic then should transport the patient for physician evaluation and wound care to facilitate healing.

Musculoskeletal System

As described in Chapter 8 and earlier in this chapter, musculoskeletal changes occur as part of the aging process. Two musculoskeletal conditions that are common in elderly patients are osteoarthritis and osteoporosis.

OSTEOARTHRITIS

Osteoarthritis is a common form of arthritis in geriatric patients. Osteoarthritis is a degenerative condition. It results from cartilage loss and wear and tear on the joints (Fig. 45-3). The condition leads to pain, stiffness, and sometimes loss of function of the affected joint. Often the affected joint becomes large and distorted from outgrowths of new bone (*osteophytes*) that tend to develop at the margins of the joint surface. Osteoarthritis evolves in the middle years. It occurs to some extent in almost all persons over 60 years of age. However, some pesons have no symptoms. After physician evaluation, treatment may include medications (analgesics, nonsteroidal antiinflammatory drugs, corticosteroids), physical therapy, and sometimes joint replacement surgery. Newer drugs (cyclooxygenase-2 inhibitors) relieve the inflammation and pain associated with arthritis. These newer drugs have less risk of causing stomach irritation than traditional medications such as ***aspirin,*** nonsteroidal antiinflammatory drugs, and ibuprofen. An example of these newer drugs is celecoxib (Celebrex).

OSTEOPOROSIS

Osteoporosis is a natural part of aging. It especially is common in older women after menopause. This is because of a decrease in the estrogen hormone that helps maintain bone mass. Osteoporosis is present in most persons by 70 years of age, by which time the density of the skeleton has diminished by one third. Most persons with osteoporosis have some degree of kyphosis.

The loss of bone density causes bones to become brittle. Brittle bones can fracture easily, which often is the first sign of osteoporosis. Typical sites for fractures are just above the wrist, at the head of the femur, and at one of several vertebrae (often a spontaneous fracture). Osteoporosis is treated with preventive measures. These include a diet high in calcium, calcium supplements, exercise, and hormone replacement therapy after menopause (controversial).

Special Problems with Sensations

As persons age, they may experience problems with vision, hearing, and speech.

PROBLEMS WITH VISION

Vision changes begin to occur at around 40 years of age. They gradually increase over time. Vision impairments can severely limit daily activities. They can lead to a loss of in-

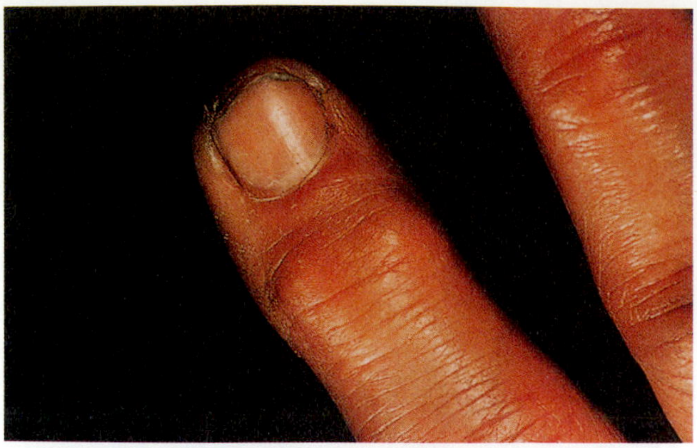

FIGURE 45-3 ■ Osteoarthritis.

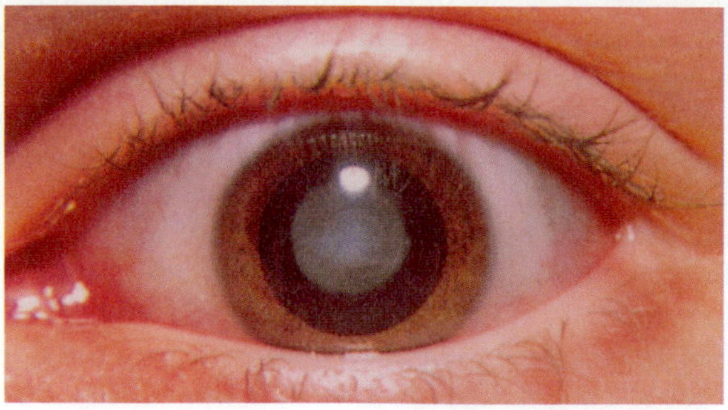

FIGURE 45-4 ■ Appearance of an eye with a cataract.

dependence in geriatric patients. The following are some effects of aging on vision:

- Reading difficulties
- Poor depth perception
- Poor adjustment of the eyes to variations in distance
- Altered color perception
- Sensitivity to light
- Decreased visual acuity

Two common eye conditions that develop with age are cataracts and **glaucoma.** A **cataract** is a loss of transparency of the lens of the eye. It results from changes in the delicate protein fibers within the lens (Fig. 45-4). A cataract never causes full blindness. Yet clarity and detail of an image progressively are lost. Cataracts usually occur in both eyes. In most cases, though, one eye is affected more severely than the other. Almost everyone over 65 years of age has some degree of cataract. Also, most persons over 75 years of age have minor visual deterioration from the disorder. Surgery to remove the cataract is a common procedure in the United States.

Glaucoma is a condition in which intraocular pressure increases. This pressure causes damage to the optic nerve. The result is nerve fiber destruction and partial or full loss of peripheral and central vision (Fig. 45-5). Glaucoma may result from aging (rarely seen before 40 years of age), a congenital abnormality, or trauma to the eye. Glaucoma is the most common major eye disorder in persons over 60 years of age and is the leading cause of preventable blindness in the United States.[12] Symptoms of acute glaucoma include dull, severe, aching pain in and above the eye; fogginess of vision; and the perception of "rainbow rings" (halos) around lights at night. Testing for glaucoma is part of most eye examinations in adults. If detected early, the condition can be treated with oral medications and eye drops to relieve pressure.

CRITICAL THINKING

Consider the patient who has glaucoma. What prehospital cardiac medication should not be given to this patient?

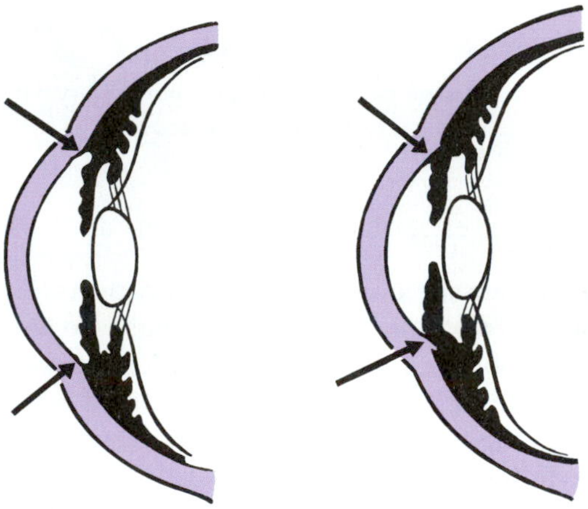

FIGURE 45-5 ■ Glaucoma. **A,** Open-angle glaucoma. The obstruction to aqueous flow lies in the trabecular meshwork. **B,** Closed-angle glaucoma. The trabecular meshwork is covered by the root of the iris. (From Stein HA, Slatt BJ, Stein RM: *The ophthalmic assistant: fundamentals in clinical practice,* St Louis, 1988, Mosby.)

PROBLEMS WITH HEARING

Not all geriatric patients have hearing loss. However, overall hearing tends to decrease with age. This results from degeneration of the hearing mechanism (*sensorineural* deafness). *Meniere's disease* (increased fluid pressure in the labyrinth), certain drugs, tumors, and some viral infections also can cause hearing problems. Hearing loss can interfere with the ability to perceive speech. Thus it can limit the ability to communicate. Hearing aid devices and surgical implants sometimes can restore or improve hearing.

Tinnitus can occur as a symptom of many ear disorders. The noise in the ear (e.g., ringing, buzzing, or whistling) sometimes may change in nature and intensity. However, in most cases it is present at all times with intermittent awareness by the person. Tinnitus is almost always associated with hearing loss, especially hearing loss that develops from aging.

CRITICAL THINKING

What common analgesic, when taken in excess, can cause tinnitus?

PROBLEMS WITH SPEECH

Speech is the most often used method of communication. Common problems with speech in geriatric patients often are associated with difficulty in word retrieval, decreased fluency of speech, slowed rate of speech, and changes in voice quality. These disorders may occur from damage to the language centers of the brain (usually as a result of stroke, head injury, or brain tumor), degenerative changes in the nervous system, hearing loss, disorders of the larynx, and poor-fitting dentures.

Toxicology

As described in Chapters 17 and 36, geriatric patients are at increased risk for adverse drug reactions. This is the result of age-related changes in body composition, drug absorption, distribution, metabolism, and excretion.

Age-related changes that affect absorption include increased gastric pH and decreased gastrointestinal motility. Both of these may increase or decrease absorption of various drugs. This depends on the chemical properties of the drug. Drug distribution may be affected by decreased cardiac output (e.g., as seen in CHF), total body water, changes in the ratio of lean mass to fat, and increased body fat. Metabolic changes may result from decreased liver blood flow; diseases such as thyroid disease, CHF, and cancer; smoking; and drug interactions. (Drug-induced metabolic changes are especially significant in the elderly. This is because they often take several different drugs for multiple diseases and conditions. This further increases their risk for adverse drug reactions.) Renal function decreases with age in the majority of adults. This can lead to a buildup of drugs that normally are cleared through the renal system. In addition, the action of drugs affecting the CNS (e.g., benzodiazepines, anesthetics, and narcotics) and the cardiovascular system (e.g., beta-blockers, calcium channel blockers, and diuretics) often is altered in older adults. Because of these changes, drugs may not produce the desired effect or may cause major drug toxicity in older adults. Drugs that commonly cause toxicity in the geriatric patient include the following:

- Analgesics
- Angiotensin-converting enzyme inhibitors
- Antidepressants
- Antihypertensives
- Beta-blockers
- Digitalis
- Diuretics
- Psychotropics

The adverse reactions associated with these and other drugs often result from "accidents" or "mishaps" in the prescribed drug regimen. Other common reasons for drug-induced illness in the geriatric patient include dispensing errors, noncompliance, confusion, forgetfulness, vision impairment, and the self-selection of drugs. In addition, older adults commonly have several prescriptions from more than one physician; improperly resume an old medication in addition to a newly prescribed one; or take prescribed medications along with over-the-counter drugs that may have synergistic or cumulative effects. Finally, changes in habits regarding alcohol, diet, and exercise also can affect drug metabolism. These changes can increase the risk for adverse drug reactions. The emergency care for geriatric patients with adverse drug reactions varies. Care may range from transport only to full advanced cardiac life support measures. Box 45-5 lists symptoms of drug toxicity and adverse reactions that can occur in the geriatric patient.

BOX 45-5 Symptoms of Drug Toxicity and Adverse Drug Reactions in the Geriatric Patient

Acute delirium	Glaucoma
Akathisia	Hypokalemia
Altered vision	Orthostatic hypotension
Bradycardia	Paresthesias
Cardiac dysrhythmias	Psychological disturbances
Chorea	Pulmonary edema
Confusion	Severe bleeding
Constipation	Tardive dyskinesia
Coma	Urinary hesitancy
Fatigue	

Substance Abuse

As described in Chapter 36, substance abuse involving alcohol and other drugs is common in the elderly population. Up to 17% of U.S. citizens aged 60 and older are estimated to be addicted to substances, and this number is expected to rise as the baby boomer population enters older age.[13]

Substance abuse in the geriatric patient often is attributed to severe stress as the primary risk factor.[8] This stress may result from life changes. These changes include age-related changes in health or appearance, loss of employment, loss of spouse or life partner, illness, malnutrition, loneliness, loss of independent living arrangements, and others. Box 45-6 lists signs of substance abuse.

BOX 45-6 Signs of Substance Abuse

Alcohol Abuse	Other Drug Abuse
Anorexia	Altered level of consciousness
Confusion	Falling
Denial	Hallucinations
Frequent falling	Memory changes
Hostility	Orthostatic hypotension
Insomnia	Poor coordination
Mood swings	Restlessness
Note: Ingestion of even small amounts of alcohol by the geriatric patient can cause intoxication.	Weight loss
	Note: Individuals often have a history of alcohol *and* other drug abuse.

If the paramedic suspects substance abuse, the paramedic should ask about this possibility with friends and family at the scene. The paramedic should ask them discreetly about the patient's alcohol or drug use. The cornerstones of therapy for these patients are identifying the problem and arranging referral to a physician for treatment. Treatment for the acutely intoxicated patient is described in Chapter 36 and may include resuscitative measures to manage the patient's airway, ventilation, and circulation. In addition, the paramedic should carefully assess the geriatric patient who has signs and symptoms of alcohol or other drug intoxication for hidden trauma injuries and any underlying medical conditions. These conditions may include hypoglycemia, cardiomyopathy and dysrhythmias, gastrointestinal bleeding, polydrug use (especially barbiturates and tranquilizers), and ethylene glycol or methanol ingestion.

Environmental Considerations

Elderly patients are at risk for developing illness from extremes in the environment. This is a result of the aging process and other factors. (See Chapter 38.) Two emergencies that relate to the environment are most common in geriatric patients. These are hypothermia and hyperthermia.

HYPOTHERMIA

Patients who are younger often develop hypothermia from extremes in the environment. In contrast, an older patient may develop hypothermia while indoors. This may occur as a result of cold surroundings and/or an illness that alters heat production or conservation. This is due in part to the following characteristics of older adults:

- They are less able to make up for environmental heat loss.
- They have a decreased ability to sense changes in temperature.
- They have less total body water to store heat.
- They are less likely to develop tachycardia to increase cardiac output in response to cold stress.
- They have a decreased ability to shiver to increase body heat.

In addition to these physical changes, geriatric patients are more prone to develop hypothermia as a result of socioeconomic factors. For instance, a fixed income may inhibit an older person from paying for the cost of properly heating and insulating his or her home. Poor nutrition that results in a decrease in fat stores may contribute to hypothermia in geriatric patients who live alone. The following are other medical causes of hypothermia in geriatric patients:

- Arthritis
- Drug overdose
- Hepatic failure
- Hypoglycemia
- Infection
- Parkinson's disease
- Stroke
- Thyroid disease
- Uremia

The signs and symptoms of hypothermia may be subtle. They may include an altered mental state, slurred speech, ataxia, and dysrhythmias. In severe cases, coma without signs of life may be present. Hypothermia in the geriatric patient carries a high mortality rate. The paramedic should manage these patients as described in Chapter 38. Rapid and gentle transport for in-hospital rewarming and life support measures is crucial for the patient's survival.

HYPERTHERMIA

Hyperthermia in the geriatric patient is less common than hypothermia. Yet hyperthermia carries a significant mortality rate. The condition most likely results from exposure to high temperatures. These temperatures most likely continue for several days (e.g., during a heat wave). As in hypothermia, geriatric patients are unable to control body temperature even in moderate heat. Hyperthermia also may result from medical conditions such as hypothalamic dysfunction and spinal cord injury. Certain medications (e.g., antidysrhythmics, beta-blockers, and cyclic antidepressants) can lead to hyperthermia. They do this by inhibiting heat dissipation, increasing motor activity, and impairing cardiovascular function.

As described in Chapter 38, hyperthermic illness may present as heat cramps, heat exhaustion, or heat stroke. Emergency care includes removing the patient from the warm environment, cooling the patient, and ensuring the patient's vital functions through airway, ventilatory, and circulatory support. Rapid transport for physician evaluation is indicated to manage the problems resulting from serious heat-related illness.

Behavioral and Psychiatric Disorders

Fifteen million elderly persons are expected to suffer from some kind of psychiatric illness by the year 2030.[14] In addition to the neurological disorders such as dementia and Alzheimer's disease, depression and suicide are common in geriatric patients.

DEPRESSION

Depression is a serious illness. It calls for physician evaluation. In the geriatric patient, depression can result from physiological and psychological causes. Examples include cognitive disorders with physical causes (e.g., dementia) and various personality disorders such as schizophrenia. (See Chapter 40.) Box 45-7 lists other physiological and psychological causes of depression in the geriatric patient. The signs and symptoms of depression vary by individual. They may include the following:

- Decreased libido
- Deep feelings of worthlessness and guilt
- Extreme isolation
- Feelings of hopelessness
- Irritability
- Loss of appetite
- Loss of energy (fatigue)
- Recurrent thoughts of death
- Significant weight loss
- Sleeplessness
- Suicide attempts

BOX 45-7 Common Causes of Depression in the Geriatric Patient

Physiological	Psychological
Dehydration	Fear of dying
Electrolyte imbalance	Financial insecurity
Fever	Loss of a spouse
Hyponatremia	Loss of independence
Hypoxia	Significant illness
Medications	
Metabolic disturbances	
Organic brain disease	
Reduced cardiac output	
Thyroid disease	

CRITICAL THINKING

What endocrine disorder can produce signs or symptoms that are similar to those of depression?

A major goal of care is to identify the patient who may be depressed. These patients need to be evaluated by a physician. The physician will rule out medical illness, especially thyroid disease, stroke, malignancy, and dementia; or medication use (e.g., beta-blockers) that may be responsible for the patient's depression. After determining that there are no physical threats to life, the paramedic should try to establish a rapport with the patient who is depressed. The paramedic should encourage the patient to talk openly about feelings, especially any thoughts of suicide. If possible, the paramedic should interview the family about the patient's mental state and question family members about any history of depression in the patient.

SUICIDE

The rate of completed suicides for geriatric patients is higher than that of the general population, and most of these persons visited their primary care physician in the month before the suicide.[15] Most were suffering from their first episode of major depression, which was only moderately severe, yet the depressive symptoms went unrecognized and untreated. Thus the paramedic should be aware of the increased risk for suicide when evaluating geriatric patients who are depressed. Clues and indicators for suicide in the geriatric patient that may be obtained through a patient history or observed by friends and family include[16]:

- Talking about or seemingly preoccupied with death and "getting affairs in order"
- Giving away prized possessions (e.g., family heirlooms, photographs, and keepsakes)
- Taking unnecessary risks (e.g., walking alone in unsafe areas or driving without personal restraints)
- Increased use of alcohol or other drugs
- Nonadherence to medical regimen (e.g., failure to take prescribed medications)
- Acquiring a weapon, especially firearms

As described in Chapter 40, there is no evidence that questions about suicidal thoughts and feelings increase the risk of suicide. Many depressed persons are willing to discuss their suicidal thoughts; therefore the paramedic should question the patient about suicidal thoughts if he or she suspects that the patient is at high risk. The following questions are appropriate for the paramedic to ask the patient:

1. Do you have thoughts about killing yourself?
2. Have you ever tried to kill yourself?
3. Have you thought about how you might kill yourself?

Most suicides committed by older adults involve firearms. Therefore safety of those at the scene and the emergency medical services crew is a priority when caring for a patient with suicidal tendencies. When indicated, law enforcement personnel should be available at the scene. After assessing the risk for suicidal tendencies, the paramedic should transport the patient for physician evaluation. While en route to the hospital, the paramedic should encourage the patient to discuss his or her feelings and reassure the patient that he or she can be helped through the crisis.

Trauma

Trauma (described in detail in Part 6) is the fifth leading cause of death for persons over 65 years of age. One third of traumatic deaths in persons 65 to 74 years of age are caused by vehicular trauma, and 25% result from falls. In those older than 80 years of age, falls account for 50% of injury-related deaths.[17] Burns also are a major cause of disability and death in geriatric patients. Contributing factors that increase the severity of traumatic injury in geriatric patients include the following[8]:

- Osteoporosis and muscle weakness that increase the likelihood of falls and fractures
- Reduced cardiac reserve that decreases the ability to compensate for blood loss
- Decreased respiratory function that increases the likelihood of adult respiratory distress syndrome
- Impaired renal function that decreases the ability to adapt to fluid shifts

VEHICULAR TRAUMA

More than 15 million licensed drivers are over 65 years of age. In 2001, more than 3000 deaths in this age group were attributed to motor vehicle crashes.[17] Most of these vehicle collisions are not related to high speed or alcohol. Rather, they are related to errors in perception or judgment or to delayed reaction time. A large number of older adults are injured as drivers or passengers in moving vehicles. In addition, more than 2000 pedestrian fatalities among older adults occur each year in the United States. This accounts for 20% of all pedestrian deaths from trauma.

The risk of death from multiple trauma is estimated to be 3 times greater at 70 years of age than at 20 years of age. This is mainly because the geriatric patient is more susceptible to serious injury from equivalent degrees of trauma. This patient also is less capable of an appropriate, protective physiological response. Prompt identification of injuries and sources of hemorrhage is critical in any trauma patient but is especially important in the geriatric patient. The geriatric patient has much less cardiac reserve. The patient will succumb more quickly to shock.

HEAD TRAUMA

A head injury with loss of consciousness in geriatric patients often has a poor outcome. The brain becomes smaller in size with age (cerebral atrophy). This atrophy produces an increase in distance between the surface of the brain and the skull. As veins are stretched across this space, they more easily are torn. This results in subdural hematomata. The extra space within the skull often allows a large amount of bleeding to occur before signs and symptoms of increased intracranial pressure are seen.

> **CRITICAL THINKING**
>
> Consider geriatric patients with head trauma. What home medications also can lead to an increased risk of intracerebral bleeding in these patients?

Geriatric patients also are at high risk for injuries of the cervical spine because of the arthritic and degenerative changes associated with aging. These structural changes lead to increased stiffening and decreased flexibility of the spine with narrowing of the spinal canal. This makes the spinal cord much more at risk for damage from fairly minor trauma.

CHEST INJURIES

Any mechanism of injury that produces thoracic trauma in a geriatric patient can be potentially lethal. The aged thorax is less elastic. Thus the thorax is more susceptible to injury. The pulmonary system also has marginal reserve because of a reduced alveolar surface area, decreased patency of small airways, and diminished chemoreceptor response.

Injuries to the heart, aorta, and major vessels are a greater risk to geriatric patients than they are to younger patients. Again, this is due to decreased functional reserve in older patients. It also is due to anatomical changes that make injury in these areas of greater significance. Myocardial contusion may be a complication of blunt injury to the chest. If severe, myocardial contusion may result in pump failure or life-threatening dysrhythmias. Rarely, cardiac tamponade occurs after blunt thoracic trauma. Cardiac rupture, valvular injury (e.g., flail valves), and aortic dissection also may occur with significant blunt chest injury. The first two entities are rare but rapidly fatal. When the mechanism of injury produces rapid deceleration, the paramedic should always consider the possibility of dissecting aortic aneurysm. Aortic dissections often are not immediately fatal. Proper evaluation and treatment can be lifesaving (see Chapter 29).

> **CRITICAL THINKING**
>
> Consider the patient who has a dissecting aortic aneurysm. What specific signs and symptoms may the paramedic see in this patient?

In the geriatric patient the heart cannot respond as effectively to increased demand for oxygen as in the younger person. This coupled with a slowed conduction system may cause ischemia and dysrhythmias when the geriatric patient has a significant trauma. These problems may occur even if the heart has not been damaged directly by the trauma. The paramedic should watch these patients' oxygenation and circulatory status closely.

ABDOMINAL INJURIES

Abdominal injuries in geriatric patients have more serious consequences than injuries to any other body area. Abdominal injuries often are less obvious. Thus they call for a high degree of suspicion. The geriatric patient is less likely to tolerate abdominal surgery well. This patient is more likely to develop lung problems and infection following surgery.

MUSCULOSKELETAL INJURIES

The osteoporotic bones of geriatric patients are more at risk for fractures. They can fracture with even mild trauma. Pelvic fractures are highly lethal in this age group. They can cause severe hemorrhage and soft tissue injury. When assessing for skeletal trauma, the paramedic should recall that the geriatric patient may have decreased pain perception. Often these patients have amazingly little tenderness with major fractures. Even with proper care, the mortality rate for geriatric patients with musculoskeletal injury is increased by delayed complications such as adult respiratory distress syndrome, sepsis, renal failure, and pulmonary embolism.

FALLS

Falls are a major cause of morbidity and mortality in older adults, accounting for more than 10,000 deaths each year.[17] About one third of older adults living at home fall each year. One in 40 of these persons is hospitalized. A major cause of falls in older adults results from the use of prescribed sedative-hypnotics. These drugs affect balance and postural control. Some examples are alprazolam, ***diazepam,*** chlordiazepoxide, and flurazepam.

> **CRITICAL THINKING**
>
> Consider geriatric patients who have fallen. What common problems may contribute to an increased death rate in these patients?

Fractures are the most common fall-related injuries. The hip fractures are the ones that most often result in hospitalization. In those who survive hip fracture, most will have significant problems with walking and moving about. They may become more dependent on others for help. Falls that do not result in physical injury may lead to self-imposed immobility from the fear of falling again. When immobility is strict and prolonged, joint contractures, pressure sores, urinary tract infection, muscle atrophy, depression, and functional dependency may result.

The paramedic should assume that any fall indicates an underlying problem until it is proved otherwise. The paramedic should try to uncover the medical, psychological, and environmental factors that may have been responsible for the fall. Thus the patient history should include a full review of all medical problems and medications. It also should include precise details of the fall. (This includes history of falling, time of fall, location, symptoms experienced, activity in which the victim was engaged, use of devices, and presence of witnesses.) The paramedic also should evaluate the patient's cardiovascular, neurological, and musculoskeletal systems.

BURNS

More than 1000 older adults die from fires and burns in the United States each year.[17] The increased risk of morbidity and mortality from burn trauma in older adults is due to preexisting disease, skin changes that result in increased burn depth, altered nutrition, and decreased ability to fight infection. The initial care and resuscitation of geriatric patients with thermal injury is described in Chapter 23. Geriatric burn patients need special approaches to fluid therapy to prevent damage to the kidneys. The patient's fluid status will need to be assessed in the initial hours after a burn injury by monitoring pulse and blood pressure, and striving to maintain a urine output of at least 50 to 60 mL per hour.

Trauma Management Considerations

The priorities of trauma care for geriatric patients are similar to those for all trauma patients described in Part Six. However, the paramedic should give special consideration to transport strategies and the geriatric patient's cardiovascular, respiratory, and renal systems.

CARDIOVASCULAR SYSTEM

Special considerations for cardiovascular problems include the following:

- Recent or past MI contributes to the risk of dysrhythmias and CHF.
- Adjustment of heart rate and stroke volume may be decreased in response to hypovolemia.
- Geriatric patients may need higher arterial pressures than younger patients for perfusion of vital organs. This is because of atherosclerotic peripheral vascular disease.
- Rapid IV fluid administration to geriatric patients may cause volume overload. The paramedic must take care not to overhydrate these patients. Older adults as a group are more susceptible to CHF. However, hypovolemia and hypotension are also poorly tolerated. The paramedic should consider hypovolemia in any geriatric patient whose systolic blood pressure is less than 120 mm Hg. Tachycardia may not occur if the patient takes beta-blockers. The paramedic should monitor lung sounds and vital signs carefully and frequently during fluid administration.

RESPIRATORY SYSTEM

Special considerations for respiratory problems include the following:

- Physical changes decrease chest wall compliance and movement. Thus they diminish vital capacity as well.
- PaO_2 decreases with age.
- Lower PO_2 at the same fractional inspired oxygen concentration occurs with each passing decade.
- All organ systems have less tolerance to hypoxia.
- Chronic obstructive pulmonary disease (common in geriatric patients) requires that the paramedic carefully adjust airway management and ventilation support for appropriate oxygenation and carbon dioxide removal. High-concentration oxygen may suppress hypoxic drive in some patients. However, oxygen should never be withheld from a patient with clinical signs of cyanosis. The paramedic may need to remove the patient's dentures for adequate airway and ventilation management

RENAL SYSTEM

Special considerations for renal problems include the following:

- The kidneys have decreased ability to maintain normal acid-base balance. They have decreased ability to compensate for fluid changes as well.
- Kidney disease may decrease further the ability of the kidneys to compensate.
- Decreased kidney function (along with decreased cardiac reserve) places the injured geriatric patient at risk for fluid overload and pulmonary edema following IV fluid therapy.

TRANSPORTATION STRATEGIES

Special considerations for transportation of geriatric patients include the following:

- Positioning, immobilization, and transport of a geriatric trauma patient may require modifications to accommodate physical deformities (e.g., arthritis or spinal abnormalities).
- Packaging should include bulk and extra padding to support and give comfort to the patient.
- The paramedic can prevent hypothermia by keeping the patient warm.

Elder Abuse

Elder abuse refers to the infliction of physical pain, injury, debilitating mental anguish, unreasonable confinement, or willful deprivation by a caregiver of services that are necessary to maintain mental and physical health of a geriatric person. Elder abuse has become more and more rec-

BOX 45-8 Signs and Symptoms of Elder Abuse and Neglect

Physical Abuse

Abandonment

Bruises, black eyes, welts, lacerations, and rope marks
Bone fractures, skull fractures
Open wounds, untreated injuries in various stages of healing
Sprains, dislocations, and internal injuries/bleeding
Broken eyeglasses/frames, physical signs of being subjected to punishment, and signs of being restrained
An elder's report of being hit, slapped, kicked, or mistreated
An elder's sudden change in behavior
The caregiver's refusal to allow examination of an elder without the caregiver being present
The desertion of an elder at a hospital, a nursing facility, or other similar institution
The desertion of an elder at a shopping center or other public location
An elder's own report of being abandoned

Financial or Material Exploitation

Sudden changes in bank account or banking practice, including an unexplained withdrawal of large sums of money by a person accompanying the elder
The inclusion of additional names on an elder's bank signature card
Unauthorized withdrawal of the elder's funds using the elder's automatic teller machine card

Sexual Abuse

Abrupt changes in a will or other financial documents
Bruises around the breasts or genital area
Unexplained venereal disease or genital infections
Unexplained vaginal or anal bleeding
Torn, stained, or bloody underclothing
An elder's report of being sexually assaulted or raped
Unexplained disappearance of funds or valuable possessions
Substandard care being provided or bills unpaid despite the availability of adequate financial resources
Discovery of an elder's signature being forged for financial transactions or for the titles of his or her possessions

Emotional or Psychological Abuse

Sudden appearance of previously uninvolved relatives
Being emotionally upset or agitated
Being extremely withdrawn and noncommunicative or nonresponsive
Unusual behavior usually attributed to dementia (e.g., sucking, biting, or rocking)
An elder's report of being verbally or emotionally mistreated claiming their rights to an elder's affairs and possessions
Unexplained sudden transfer of assets to a family member or someone outside the family
The provision of services that are not necessary
An elder's report of financial exploitation

Neglect

Self-neglect

Dehydration, malnutrition, untreated bed sores, and poor personal hygiene
Unattended or untreated health problems
Hazardous or unsafe living condition/arrangements (e.g., improper wiring and lack of heat or running water)
Unsanitary and unclean living conditions (e.g. dirt, fleas, body lice, soiled bedding, fecal/urine smell, and inadequate clothing)
An elder's report of being mistreated
Dehydration, malnutrition, untreated or improperly attended medical conditions, and poor personal hygiene
Hazardous or unsafe living conditions/arrangements (e.g., improper wiring, no indoor plumbing, and lack of heat or running water)
Unsanitary or unclean living quarters (e.g., animal/insect infestation, no functioning toilet, and fecal/urine smell)
Inappropriate and/or inadequate clothing, lack of the necessary medical aids (e.g., eyeglasses, hearing aids, and dentures)
Grossly inadequate housing or homelessness

Adapted from National Center on Elder Abuse: The basics: major types of elder abuse. http://www.elderabusecenter.org/default.cfm?p=basics.cfm. Accessed October 1, 2003.

ognized as a growing problem in the United States. Elder abuse is estimated to affect more than 500,000 older adults each year.[18]

Elder abuse takes many forms. These include physical abuse, sexual abuse, emotional or psychological abuse, neglect, abandonment, financial or material exploitation, and self-neglect. Box 45-8 lists the signs and symptoms of each type of elder abuse as defined by the National Center on Elder Abuse.

All 50 states have elder abuse statutes. Also, reporting of suspected elder abuse is mandatory under law in most states. If the paramedic suspects abuse or neglect of an older adult, the paramedic should advise medical direction. Moreover, the paramedic should follow the procedures that are established by local protocol. Emergency care is aimed at managing injuries that pose a threat to life and transporting the patient for physician evaluation. Abuse and neglect are discussed further in Chapter 46.

SUMMARY

- The aging process proceeds at different rates in different persons. Respiratory function in the older adult generally is compromised. This is a result of changes in pulmonary physiology that go along with the aging process. Cardiac function also declines with age. This is a result of normal physiological changes and the high incidence of coronary artery disease. Renal blood flow falls an average of 50% between 30 and 80 years of age. A gradual decrease in neurons, decreased cerebral blood flow, and changes in the location and amounts of specific neurotransmitters probably contribute to changes in the CNS. As the body ages, muscles shrink, muscles and ligaments calcify, and the intervertebral disks become thin. Other physiological changes that occur with aging include changes in body mass and total body water, a decreased ability to maintain internal homeostasis, a decrease in the function of immunological mechanisms, nutritional disorders, and decreases in hearing and visual acuity.
- Normal changes with aging and existing illnesses may make evaluation of an ill or injured geriatric patient a challenge.
- Pneumonia is a leading cause of death in the geriatric age group. It often is fatal in frail adults. Chronic obstructive pulmonary disease is a common finding in the geriatric patient who has a history of smoking. The disease usually is associated with various other diseases that result in reduced expiratory airflow. Pulmonary embolism is a life-threatening cause of dyspnea. Pulmonary embolism is associated with venous stasis, heart failure, COPD, malignancy, and immobilization. All of these are common in older adults.
- A lack of the typical chest pain can cause MI to go unrecognized in the geriatric patient. Heart failure is more frequent in geriatric patients and has a larger incidence of noncardiac causes. The most common cause of dysrhythmias in the geriatric patient is hypertensive heart disease. Abdominal aortic aneurysm affects 2% to 4% of the U.S. population over 50 years of age. This aneurysm is most prevalent between 60 and 70 years of age. The incidence of hypertension in the geriatric patient increases when atherosclerosis is present.
- Risk factors for cerebral vascular disease in the older adult include smoking, hypertension, diabetes, atherosclerosis, hyperlipidemia, polycythemia, and heart disease.
- Delirium is an abrupt disorientation of time and place. Delirium is commonly a result of physical illness.
- Dementia is a slow, progressive loss of awareness of time and place. It usually involves an inability to learn new things or remember recent events. This condition often is a result of brain disease. Alzheimer's disease is the most common cause of dementia. Alzheimer's disease is a condition in which nerve cells in the cerebral cortex die and the brain substance shrinks.
- Parkinson's disease is a brain disorder. It causes muscle tremor, stiffness, and weakness.
- About 20% of older adults have diabetes. Almost 40% have some impaired glucose tolerance. Hyperglycemic hyperosmolar nonketotic coma is a serious complication of elderly type 2 diabetic patients. It has a mortality rate of 20% to 50%. Thyroid disease is more common in geriatric patients. It may not present in the classic manner.
- Gastrointestinal bleeding most often affects patients between 60 and 90 years of age. It has a mortality rate of about 10%. Bowel obstruction generally occurs in patients with prior abdominal surgeries or hernias. It also occurs in those with colonic cancer. Some geriatric patients may have problems with continence or with elimination as well.
- Aging results in a gradual decrease in epidermal cellular turnover. It also results in loss of deep, and dermal vessels. Capillary circulation leads to changes in thermal regulation and skin-related complications.
- Osteoarthritis is a common form of arthritis in geriatric patients. It results from cartilage loss and wear and tear on the joints. The loss in bone density from osteoporosis causes bones to become brittle. These bones may fracture easily.
- As persons age, they may experience problems with vision, hearing, and speech.
- Geriatric patients are at an increased risk for adverse drug reactions. This is due to age-related changes in body makeup and drug distribution. It also is the result of metabolism and excretion. Moreover, the risk for adverse drug reactions often stems from multiple prescribed drugs. Alcohol abuse is a common problem in geriatric patients.
- The geriatric patient may develop hypothermia while indoors. This may be the result of cold surroundings and/or an illness that alters heat production or conservation. Hyperthermia most likely results from exposure to high temperatures that continue for several days.
- Depression is common in geriatric patients. It can result from physiological and psychological causes. The rate of completed suicides for geriatric patients is higher than that of the general population.
- One third of traumatic deaths in persons 65 to 74 years of age result from vehicular trauma. Twenty-five percent result from falls. In those older than 80 years of age, falls account for 50% of injury-related deaths. The risk of fatality from multiple trauma is estimated to be 3 times greater at 70 years of age than at 20 years of age.
- Elder abuse is classified as physical abuse, psychological abuse, financial or material abuse, and neglect.

REFERENCES

1. US Senate Special Committee on Aging: *Aging America: trends and projections,* Washington, DC, 1988, US Department of Health and Human Services.
2. Modified from American Geriatrics Society Foundation for Health in Aging: 2000-2010 decade of health in aging: the challenge–the aging of the U.S. population. http://www.healthinaging.org/the challenge.html. Accessed November 3, 2004.
3. Bosker G et al: *Geriatric emergency medicine,* St Louis, 1990, Mosby.
4. American Heart Association: *Advanced cardiac life support,* Dallas, 1997, The Association.
5. Rosen P, Barkin R: *Emergency medicine: concepts and clinical practice,* ed 4, St Louis, 1998, Mosby.
6. National Centers for Health Statistics, Centers for Disease Control and Prevention: Health, United States, 1999 with health and aging chartbook. http://www.cdc.gov/nchs/data/hus99.pdf. Accessed September 9, 2004.
7. Family health almanac: fitness, food, and medicine, *US News and World Report* 1998.
8. US Department of Transportation, National Highway Traffic Safety Administration: *EMT-Paramedic national standard curriculum,* Washington, DC, 1998, The Department.
9. Hogan T: *Geriatric emergencies,* Turlock, Calif, 1994, Medic Alert Foundation.
10. Joint National Committee on Hypertension: *The sixth report of the Joint National Committee on prevention, detection, evaluation, and treatment of high blood pressure,* Washington, DC, 1998, National Institutes of Health, National Heart Lung and Blood Institute.

11. American Heart Association: Guidelines 2000 for cardiopulmonary resuscitation and emergency cardiovascular care, International Consensus on Science, *Circulation* 102(8):204, 2000.
12. The Glaucoma Foundation: What is glaucoma? http://www.glaucomafoundation.org/education_content.php?i=7. Accessed December 10, 2004.
13. Results from the 2002 National Survey on Drug Use and Health. http://www.samhsa.gov/oas/nhsda/2k2nsduh/Results/2k2Results.htm#toc. Accessed January 4, 2005.
14. Waters M: Mental illness among elderly Americans expected to become a greater concern, *APA Monitor Online* 30:11, Dec 1999. http://www.apa.org/monitor/dec99/nl4.html.
15. National Institute of Mental Health: Frequently asked questions about suicide. http://www.nimh.nih.gov/suicideprevention/suicidefaq.cfm. Accessed January 25, 2004.
16. Snyder D, Christmas C, editors: *Geriatric education for emergency medical services,* American Geriatric Society, National Council of EMS Training Coordinators, Sudbury, Mass, 2003, Jones and Bartlett.
17. National Safety Council: *Injury facts,* Chicago, 2002, The Council.
18. Tatara T et al: *Domestic elder abuse information series,* Washington, DC, 1997, National Center on Elder Abuse.

CHAPTER

46

Abuse and Neglect

OBJECTIVES

Upon completion of this chapter, the paramedic student will be able to:

1. Define battering.
2. Describe the characteristics of abusive relationships.
3. Outline findings that indicate a battered patient.
4. Describe prehospital considerations when responding to and caring for battered patients.
5. Identify types of elder abuse.
6. Discuss legal considerations related to elder abuse.
7. Describe characteristics of abused children and their abusers.
8. Outline the physical examination of the abused child.
9. Describe the characteristics of sexual assault.
10. Outline prehospital patient care considerations for the patient who has been sexually assaulted.

KEY TERMS

battering: A form of domestic violence that establishes control and fear in a relationship through violence and other forms of abuse.

emotional abuse: The infliction of anguish, pain, or distress through verbal or nonverbal acts.

financial/material exploitation: The illegal or improper use of funds, properties, or assets.

neglect: The refusal or failure of the caregiver to fulfill obligations or duties to a person.

patterned injuries: Injuries that result from an identifiable object.

physical abuse: The use of physical force that may result in bodily injury, physical pain, or impairment.

self-neglect: A type of elder abuse; behaviors of an older adult that intentionally threaten personal health or safety.

sexual abuse: Nonconsensual sexual contact of any kind.

shaken baby syndrome: A serious form of child abuse that describes injuries to infants that occur after being shaken violently.

Partner, elder, and child abuse are growing problems in the United States. Paramedics will encounter victims of domestic violence in their careers. Abuse and neglect can result in mental and physical illness. They also can result in injury and even death. Education programs for emergency medical services personnel must include information about these violent crimes. This information includes identification of victims, special aspects of care, scene safety, and documentation requirements. This chapter addresses the types of abuse and neglect, the personality traits of those who abuse, and legal considerations in providing emergency care.

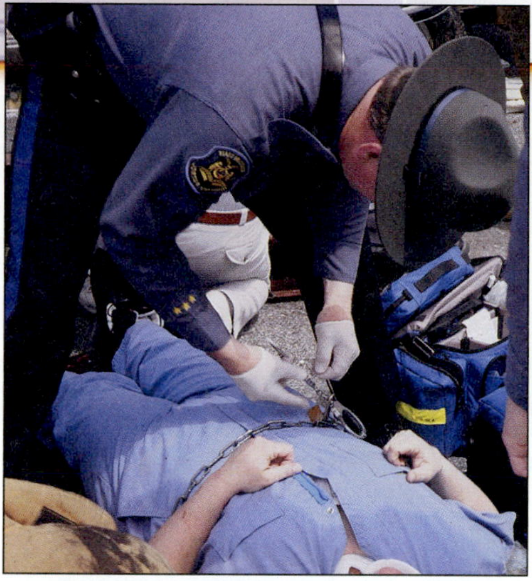

BATTERING

Battering is a form of domestic violence. Battering is the establishment of control and fear in a relationship through violence and other forms of abuse. The batterer uses acts of violence and series of behaviors to coerce and control the other person. These behaviors include intimidation, threats, psychological abuse, and isolation. Types of abuse and neglect include the following:

Emotional abuse: Infliction of anguish, pain, or distress through verbal or nonverbal acts
Financial/material exploitation: Illegal or improper use of funds, properties, or assets
Neglect: Refusal or failure of the caregiver to fulfill obligations or duties to a person
Physical abuse: Use of physical force that may result in bodily injury, physical pain, or impairment
Sexual abuse: Nonconsensual sexual contact of any kind

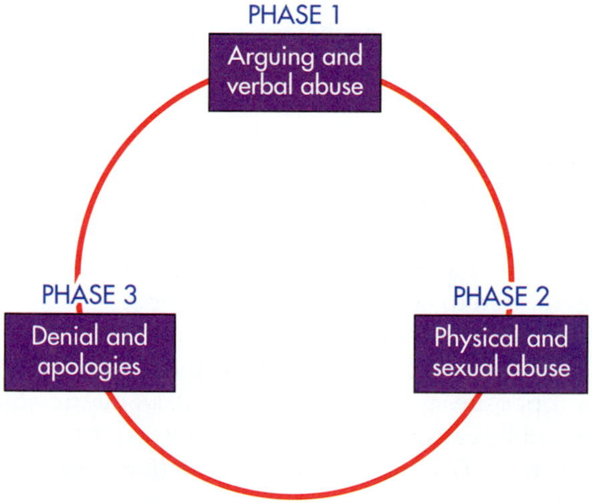

FIGURE 46-1 ■ Cycle of violence.

The violence associated with battering may not happen often. Yet battering is a hidden and constant terrorizing factor in some relationships. Over time the beatings usually become more severe and more frequent. They often occur without provocation. If children are present in a marriage or relationship, often the violence eventually turns toward them.[1] Persons involved in abusive relationships often fail to see other options. They often feel powerless to change.

Domestic violence follows a cycle of three phases[2] (Fig. 46-1). Phase one involves arguing and verbal abuse; phase two progresses to physical and sexual abuse; and phase three consists of denial and apologies (the "honeymoon phase"). The paramedic best achieves intervention in

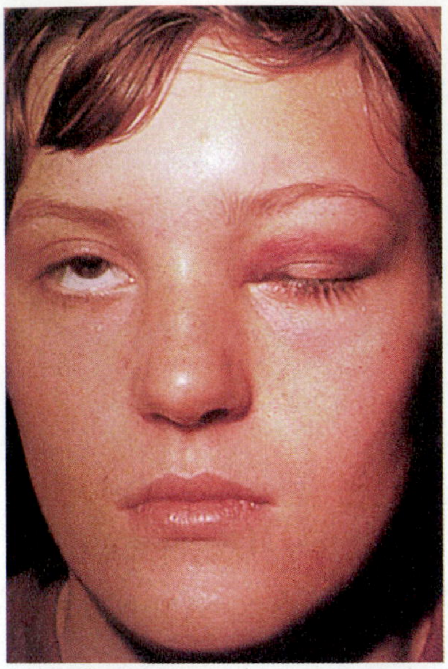

FIGURE 46-2 ■ A woman struck in the face.

phase two or three. The cycle repeats itself without intervention. The cycle also usually increases in frequency and severity. Understanding this cycle of violence will help the paramedic assess the situation and care for the victim.

Battered Women

A woman is battered by her husband, boyfriend, or live-in partner approximately every 15 seconds in the United States[3] (Box 46-1). Less than 10% of women report battering incidents for reasons that include the following[1]:

1. Personal fear or fear for her children
2. Belief that the offender's behavior will change (abusers often appear charming and loving after the battering incident)
3. Lack of financial and/or emotional support
4. Belief that she is the cause of the violent behavior
5. Belief that battering is "part of the marriage" and must be endured to keep the family together

Women of all cultures, races, occupations, income levels, and ages are battered by their husbands, boyfriends, and lovers (opposite- and same-sex partners). Domestic violence is the leading cause of injury to women who are between 15 and 44 years of age in the United States (Fig. 46-2).

Battered Men

In about 95% of domestic assaults the batterer is a man.[2] However, women are not the only battering victims. More than 150,000 men in the United States each year are victims of physical violence by a spouse or partner (from opposite- and same-sex relationships; Fig. 46-3).[4] Men report physical violence by a spouse or partner less often than women. This is probably as a result of humiliation, guilt, and/or fear to admit loss of control. In addition, society seems to be less empathetic toward battered men than battered women and has allocated fewer resources for support.

BOX 46-1 Domestic Violence: Facts and Statistics

- Battered women often are severely injured. At least one third of all emergency department visits by women are due to battering.
- Every year an estimated 4 million to 6 million women are beaten by a spouse or partner. This is more than are hurt in auto crashes, rapes, and muggings combined.
- One half of all homeless women and children are homeless as a result of domestic violence.
- About 15% to 25% of pregnant women are battered.
- Battered women are more likely to suffer miscarriages. They also are more likely to give birth to infants with low birth weights.
- Living in suburban and rural areas does not decrease a woman's risk of experiencing an act of violence by a spouse or partner.
- Up to 75% of domestic assaults reported to law enforcement agencies were inflicted after the couples had separated.
- Between 50% and 70% of the men who batter their spouse or partner also abuse their children.
- About 63% of young men between 11 and 20 years of age who are serving time for homicide have killed their mother's abuser.
- Domestic violence is the sixth most dangerous call for law enforcement officers killed in the line of duty.
- The United States has nearly 3 times as many animal shelters as it does shelters for battered women and their children.
- Compared with males, females experience more than 10 times as many incidents of violence by a spouse or partner each year.
- Children are present in 40% to 55% of homes when police intervene in domestic violence calls.
- In 85% to 90% of domestic homicides, the police had been called to the home at least once during the 2 years before the incident. In more than half of these cases the police had been called 5 times or more.
- Almost 6 times as many women victimized by spouses or partners, compared with those victimized by strangers, did not report their violent victimization to police because they feared reprisal from the offender.

From Federal Bureau of Investigation; National Coalition Against Domestic Violence; National Woman Abuse Prevention Project; US Senate, Committee on the Judiciary; US Department of Justice; Bureau of Justice Statistics, May 1999.

Characteristics of Persons in Abusive Relationships

Certain personality traits may draw persons into abusive relationships. The following are characteristics of one or both persons in an abusive relationship[1]:

1. Intense need for love and affection
2. Low self-esteem
3. Alcohol or other drug dependence
4. Difficulty in finances, job security, and possible legal issues

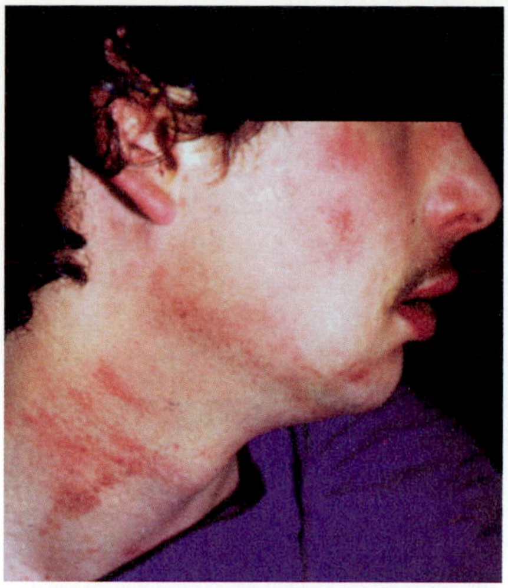

FIGURE 46-3 ■ Soft tissue injury to the face from blows and to the neck from a firm grip.

5. Background of physical, emotional, or sexual abuse; abusers are often survivors of abuse
6. Belief that abuse is demonstrating discipline
7. Fear of being "out of control"
8. Uncontrolled temper, extreme jealousy, and insecurity
9. Inability to set and enforce personal boundaries
10. Unrealistic expectations of a relationship
11. Difficulty in expressing anger
12. Loyalty to the abuser that takes precedence over emotional or physical safety
13. Repeated attempts to leave the relationship
14. Clinical depression
15. Suicidal ideation or attempts

Identification of the Battered Patient

The paramedic may have difficulty identifying the battered patient. Often the description of the injuries may be incorrect, inaccurate, and protective of the attacker. Injuries that are unintentional often involve the extremities and the periphery of the body. However, injuries from domestic violence often involve contusions and lacerations of the face, head, neck, breast, and abdomen. Bruises and lacerations may appear to be "old." This is because many victims of abuse do not seek medical help for their injuries. Other clues of domestic violence are the following:

- Excessive delays between injury and seeking treatment
- Repeated requests for emergency medical services assistance
- Injuries during pregnancy
- Substance abuse
- Frequent suicide gestures

Scene Safety

The paramedic must ensure scene and personal safety in domestic violence events. If dispatch reveals that the scene involves domestic violence, the paramedic should call on law enforcement personnel. The EMS crew also should not enter the scene until it has been secured. If the paramedic does not suspect domestic violence until after arriving at the scene, the paramedic should remove the victim from the scene. This should occur as soon as possible. Violence often is aimed at EMS personnel. This is especially the case if the abuser feels that the paramedic is giving too much empathy to the victim. Thus the paramedic should not question the victim regarding possible violence. The paramedic also should make no display of sympathy until the victim is in the ambulance or has been separated from the suspected batterer.

Care of the Victim

All injuries should be managed according to standard protocols. The paramedic should direct special attention to the emotional needs of the victim. The abuser often is unwilling to allow the victim to give a history. The abuser also may not want to allow the victim to be alone with EMS personnel. Thus the paramedic should question the patient privately about the incident when possible.

CRITICAL THINKING

If you suspect abuse, what can you say to invite the victim to talk about it?

The paramedic should obtain information about events that led to physical injury by using direct questions. Often the patient will avoid eye contact and be hesitant or evasive about details of an injury. Some may offer clues by saying, "Things haven't been going well lately," or "There have been problems at home." The paramedic should convey to the patient his or her awareness that the injuries may have resulted from battering. The patient may be relieved to know that someone else is aware of the abuse.

During the patient interview, the paramedic should be nonjudgmental and avoid comments such as "How awful" or "Why don't you leave?" The paramedic should listen carefully to the victim and offer emotional support. The patient should be encouraged to gain control of his or her life and to consider the best interests and needs of any children who may be involved in the abusive relationship. The paramedic also should provide access to community resources such as battered spouse programs, victim-witness assistance programs, and other support agencies for abused victims and their families. Finally, the paramedic should discuss safety measures with the victim who elects not to be transported for evaluation. This may include helping the patient identify a quick way out of a dangerous situation (e.g., where to go and whom to call). It also may include providing an approved written list or a small card (that can be hidden easily from the abuser) of community resources. These may include shelters and hotline numbers (Box 46-2).

CRITICAL THINKING

How would you feel if you respond to a call in which a woman has been injured by a batterer but chooses not to leave?

BOX 46-2 National Domestic Violence Hotline

In 1996 the U.S. government established a nationwide 24-hour toll-free domestic violence hotline through the Violence Against Women Act of 1994. The voice number for the hotline is 1-800-799-SAFE. The TDD number for the hearing impaired is 1-800-787-3224. The hotline is available 365 days a year. It operates throughout the United States, Puerto Rico, and the Virgin Islands. The hotline is staffed by trained advocates. These advocates offer crisis intervention, support, and referrals to local services in the caller's community.

Other components of the act include the allocation of funds for training prosecutors and police, maintaining shelters, and providing educational programs in schools and communities. These programs work with the hotline to treat domestic violence as a serious crime. They also help to prevent domestic violence before it starts.

Some patients who have suffered abuse eventually leave the abusive relationship. This often is made possible by health care providers and support agency personnel who do the following:

- Treat the victim in a sensitive and sympathetic manner.
- Confirm that the victim is not at fault and does not deserve to be abused.
- Ensure the victim's safety.
- Become "agents of change" in helping provide the support needed for the victim to leave the abusive environment.

Legal Considerations

Physical assault is a crime that may be a misdemeanor or a felony. This depends on state law, the amount of injury inflicted, and devices that the attacker uses during the assault. Often the attacker is arrested but is released from custody within hours on his or her own recognizance. If early release from custody is likely, the patient must be made aware of this. The patient also should be encouraged to take personal safety precautions.

Most states do not have mandatory reporting requirements for acts of domestic violence. Paramedics should be aware of the requirements in their state. Emergency medical services personnel are bound professionally to advise medical direction of their suspicions and observations about acts of violence.

Any act of physical abuse against a spouse, partner, elder, or child is a crime. So the paramedic must treat the scene as a crime scene. Paramedics should be careful not to disturb the scene or destroy possible evidence. Documentation is key. It should include a precise account of injuries, reported mechanisms of injuries, and a description of the behavior of the victim and alleged abuser. Using body diagrams in the patient care report may be helpful. The paramedic should record the victim's own words in the narrative when possible and record the names of police officers and witnesses at the scene. These details are important in cases of litigation. (See Chapter 16.)

ELDER ABUSE

Elder abuse (described in Chapter 45) is a prevalent medical and social problem in the United States. Although it is difficult to say how many older Americans are abused, neglected, or exploited, studies suggest that there may be as many as 5 million victims every year.[5] Factors that contribute to elder abuse include the following:

- Increased life expectancy
- Physical and mental impairment
- Decreased productivity
- Increased dependence
- Limited resources for care of the elderly
- Economic factors
- Stress of the middle-age caregiver responsible for two generations

CRITICAL THINKING

Do you think that the problem of elder abuse will increase or decrease during your career in emergency medical services? Why?

Types of Elder Abuse

As described in Chapter 45, elder abuse is classified into four categories: physical abuse (Fig. 46-4), psychological abuse, financial or material abuse, and neglect (active and passive) (Box 46-3). **Self-neglect** is another type of elder abuse. In this type the behaviors of an older adult intentionally threaten personal health or safety. (Examples include poor nutrition and not taking prescribed drugs.) Elder abuse also is classified by where it occurs. It occurs in domestic settings or in institutions.

DOMESTIC SETTINGS

The average victim of elder abuse in domestic settings is about 78 years of age. This person usually has multiple, chronic health conditions that make him or her dependent on others for care. Widows over 75 years of age carry the greatest risk of elder abuse. Neglect is the most common form of elder abuse in domestic settings; unexplained trauma is the most common finding. Evidence suggests that elder abuse is associated more with the personality of the abuser than with the burden of caring for a sick, dependent person. The National Aging Resource Center on Elder Abuse provides percentages of who the perpetrators are most likely to be in domestic settings[1] (Box 46-4).

Four major theories of causes of domestic elder abuse are as follows[1]:

1. Elder abuse occurs in settings where the caregiver is under a great amount of stress. This stress is a result of personal problems and/or a lack of knowledge about how to provide care to an older adult.

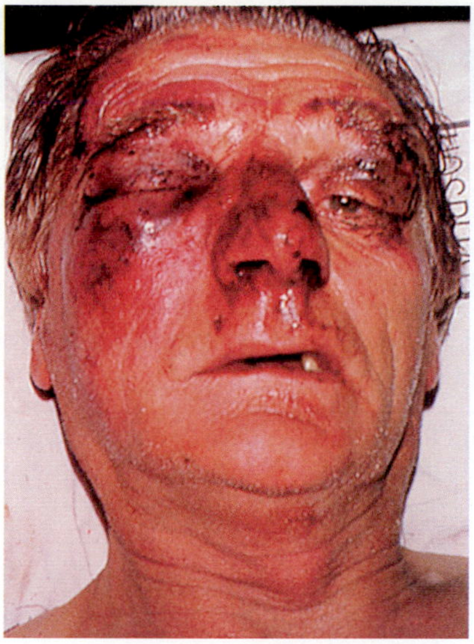

FIGURE 46-4 ■ Injuries from facial blows to an older adult.

2. Mental and/or physical impairments common in many older adults make them more likely to be abused than older adults who are in good health.
3. A "cycle of violence" often occurs in elder abuse. The cycle begins with ongoing tension. This tension escalates in a crisis in which abuse occurs. The abuse generally is followed by a period of calm, reconciliation, and denial, after which the cycle repeats.
4. Abusers of older adults often have more personal problems than nonabusers. (For example, they may have job insecurity and/or financial troubles.)

Older adults often are repeatedly abused by family members. The abusers most often are the children of the abused. Because of this familial relationship, many older adults do not report the abuse. Many also do not seek medical care for their injuries.

INSTITUTIONAL ABUSE

More than 1.6 million persons are currently residents in nursing homes and other heath care facilities. These individuals are at risk for intentional harm, physical violence, verbal aggression, or neglect from other residents and paid caregivers, staff, and professionals. Clues that may indicate institutional abuse include the following:

- Burns caused by cigarettes, caustics, or acids
- Caregiver who cannot explain the victim's condition adequately
- Dehydration, malnutrition, or pressure sores
- Emotional abuse
- Loss of weight
- Neglect
- Open wounds, cuts, bruises, welts, or discoloration
- Physical abuse
- Unsanitary and unclean conditions (dirt, soiled bed, or fecal or urine odor)
- Unusual behavior by the victim (sucking, biting, or rocking)
- Victim who is begging for food
- Victim who is emotionally upset or agitated
- Victim who is extremely withdrawn and noncommunicative
- Victim with poor personal hygiene
- Victim's sudden change in behavior

BOX 46-3 Types of Elder Abuse

Physical Abuse
Biting
Hitting
Physically restraining
Sexually molesting

Psychological Abuse
Causing fear
Humiliating
Insulting
Intimidating
Isolating
Name calling
Threatening verbally

Financial or Material Abuse
Forcing relocation from one dwelling to another
Stealing or misusing money
Stealing or misusing property

Neglect (Active and Passive)
Ignoring the person
Withholding medication, food, exercise, companionship, or bathroom assistance

BOX 46-4 Percentage of Those Who Abuse Elders

Adult children: 32.5%	Other relative: 12.5%
Grandchildren: 4.2%	Friend or neighbor: 7.5%
Spouse: 14.4%	All others: 18.2%
Sibling: 2.5%	Unknown: 2.0%

From US Department of Transportation, National Highway Traffic Safety Administration: *EMT-Paramedic national standard curriculum,* Washington, DC, 1997, The Department.

Legal Considerations

All 50 states have elder abuse statutes. Reporting of suspected elder abuse is mandatory under law in most states as well. If the paramedic suspects abuse or neglect, the paramedic should document all findings carefully, advise medical direction, and follow the procedures established by local protocol.

CHILD ABUSE

In 2001, child protective service agencies investigated more than 3 million reports alleging maltreatment of children, and these agencies determined that an estimated 903,000 children were victims of substantiated or indicated abuse or neglect.[6] As described in Chapter 44, various forms of child abuse—including physical injury, sexual exploitation, infliction of emotional pain, and neglect—can result in physical or emotional impairment.

BOX 46-5 Characteristics of Child Abusers

- Demonstrate immature behavior
- Show personal preoccupation (self-centeredness)
- Have little perception of how a child feels (physically or emotionally)
- Are critical of the child
- Seldom touch or look at the child
- Are unconcerned about the child's injury, treatment, or prognosis
- Show no feeling of guilt or remorse
- Blame the child for the injury or illness

BOX 46-6 Who Are the Child Victims of Abuse?

- More than 50% are 7 years of age or younger.
- Twenty-five percent are younger than 4 years of age.
- Twenty-five percent are 8 to 12 years of age.
- Twenty-one percent are 13 to 18 years of age.
- Fifty-two percent are female.
- Twenty-three percent of sexual abuse victims are boys.
- Children younger than 4 years of age account for 76% of fatalities from abuse.

From National Clearinghouse on Child Abuse and Neglect Information, Washington, DC, 1998.

Neglect is the most common form of child abuse. However, many children suffer more than one type of abuse. Neglect is the failure to provide physical care (e.g., medical care, nutrition, shelter, and clothing) or the failure to provide emotional care (i.e., indifference and disregard). Most substantiated reports of child abuse or neglect come from professional sources (educators, social services, law enforcement, and medical personnel). Persons in the family of the victim report only 18% of child abuse cases.

Characteristics of Abusers

The characteristics of abusers are not related to social class, income, or level of education. Most child abusers are the child's parents (77%). Eleven percent are other relatives of the victim. Most abusers are under 40 years of age. Two thirds are female (usually the child's mother). Persons who are in other caregiving relationships to the victim (e.g., childcare providers, foster parents, and facility staff) account for only 2% of perpetrators. About 10% of all abusers are noncaregivers or unknown. Neglect often is attributed to female perpetrators, whereas sexual abuse most often is attributed to males.[6] Box 46-5 provides other characteristics of child abusers.

CRITICAL THINKING

How does it make you feel when you hear a story about child abuse on the news? Think about how you will manage those feelings when you are at a scene with such a child.

A family history of rigorous discipline accounts for the cyclical nature of child abuse.[1] Many abusers were severely punished and beaten as children by their parents. Thus they often prefer to use other forms of discipline for their children. But the stresses of child rearing eventually culminate in some parents regressing to the earliest patterns of discipline that they experienced as a child. The abusive adult sometimes is aware of this cyclical nature. The adult may even try to seek help to prevent abusive behavior toward his or her children. This is known as the preabuse state, during which the following pattern often occurs[1]:

1. The adult makes several calls for help within a 24-hour period to 911 or support agencies.
2. The adult frequently calls EMS for trivial symptoms.
3. The adult begins to exhibit behavior of being unable to handle an impending crisis.

The preabuse state is important in identifying the potential for abuse. The pattern is often repetitive. It often results in frequent calls for EMS to the patient's home. The paramedic should remember that this behavior indicates the adult's awareness that child abuse is likely to occur. It also means that the adult is actively seeking help to prevent the abuse.

Characteristics of the Abused Child

Abused children often display behavior that provides important clues about abuse and neglect (Box 46-6). Although this behavior may be age-related, the paramedic should observe carefully the child under 6 years of age who is excessively passive, the child over 6 years of age who is excessively aggressive, and the child with the following characteristics:

- Does not mind (at any age) if his or her parents leave the room
- Cries hopelessly during treatment or cries very little
- Does not look at parents for reassurance
- Is wary of physical contact
- Is extremely apprehensive
- Appears constantly on the alert for danger
- Constantly seeks favors, food, or comfort items (e.g., blankets and toys)

Physical Examination

Injuries during childhood are common. Most are unintentional and not the result of abuse. Distinguishing between an intentional and accidental injury can be challenging for the paramedic. The paramedic obtains the most important clues by observing the child and his or her relationship with the parent or caregiver. The paramedic also obtains key clues by matching the history of the event to the injury. If the child volunteers the history of the event without hesitation and matches the history that the parent provides (and the history is suitable for the injury), child abuse is unlikely.[1]

LEGAL CONSIDERATIONS

When possible, the paramedic should perform the examination of a child who is a suspected victim of abuse with another colleague. This will help verify that the taking of notes is objective. The exam also will help ensure that assumptions and personal perceptions do not taint findings. The report must be succinct and legible. The paramedic should document all relevant findings and observations. Child abuse is a crime that is reportable under law in all 50 states. Paramedics should follow local protocol in reporting suspected child abuse. In addition, they should discuss any suspicions of child abuse or neglect with medical direction.

COMMON TYPES OF INJURIES

Common types of injuries associated with child abuse were described in Chapter 44. These injuries include the following:

Soft tissue injuries: Soft tissue injuries are the most common injury seen in cases of child abuse. They are often found in early abuse. They may present in various forms such as multiple bruises and ecchymosis, especially if bruises are extensive and are a mixture of old and new bruises. Defense wounds may be found on multiple body planes. They often are **patterned injuries** that result from an identifiable object. (For example, they might be bites, loop marks from a cord or belt [Fig. 46-5], cigarette burns, or bristle marks from a hairbrush.) In addition, scalds are a common form of abuse in the young and old (Fig. 46-6).

Fractures: Fractures are the second most common injury in cases of child abuse. They often are caused by twisting and jerking forces and may be of different ages (fresh and healed), indicating repeated injury. Rib fractures and multiple fractures are common findings.

Head injuries: Head injury is the most common cause of death in cases of child abuse; and children who survive head injury often have permanent disability (Fig. 46-7). Often there is a visible progression of injury that begins at the child's trunk and extremities and moves toward the head. Associated injuries include scalp wounds, skull fractures, subdural or subgaleal hematomata, and repeated concussions.

Abdominal injuries: Abdominal injures in cases of child abuse are less common than those injuries just described. However, they often are serious. Blunt trauma to the abdomen may lead to rupture of the liver. Trauma also may result in injuries to the intestines and mesentery.

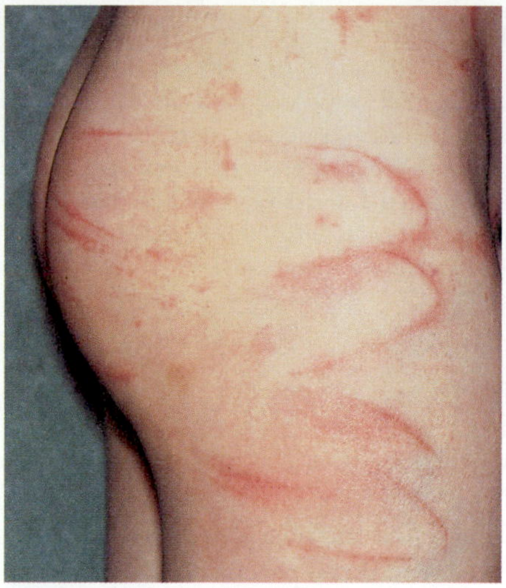

FIGURE 46-5 ■ Patterned injury from being struck with a belt.

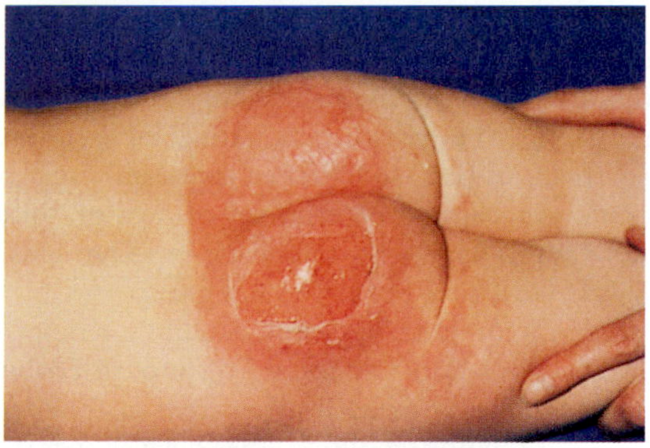

FIGURE 46-6 ■ "Bath dipping" typically produces scalds on the buttocks and feet.

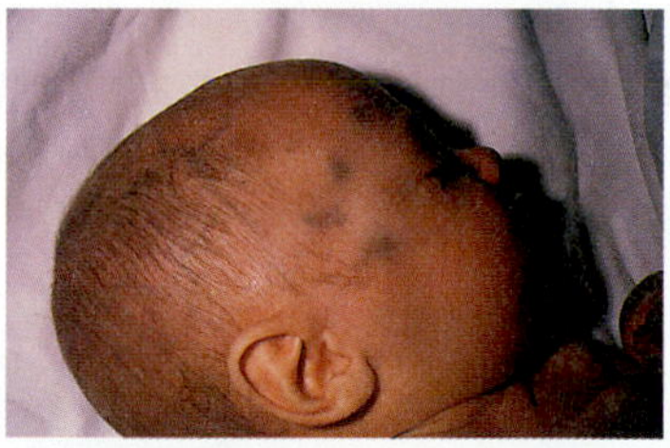

FIGURE 46-7 ■ Multiple bruises on an infant's head from finger pressure.

Children Who Die from Abuse and Neglect

More than 1000 children die from child abuse and neglect in the United States each year.[6] Fatal injuries from maltreatment result from many different acts, including the following:

- Severe head trauma
- **Shaken baby syndrome**
- Trauma to the abdomen and thorax
- Scalding

> **NOTE** Shaken baby syndrome is a serious form of child abuse. It refers to injuries to infants that occur after being violently shaken. These rapid shakes can cause cerebral hemorrhage, brain damage, blindness, paralysis, and death. Shaken baby syndrome most often occurs before 1 year of age and less often between 1 and 2 years of age. The shaking episode usually results from inconsolable crying.

- Drowning
- Suffocation
- Poisoning

Types of neglect that can result in death include the following:

1. *Supervision neglect* includes death that involves a critical moment in which the parent or caregiver is absent and the child is killed by a suddenly arising danger (e.g., leaving a child unattended in a bathtub).
2. *Chronic neglect* includes death that is caused by slowly building problems (e.g., malnutrition).
3. Deaths that result from *child physical abuse* involve fatal parental assaults on infants and children. These assaults are triggered by events such as inconsolable crying, feeding difficulties (Fig. 46-8), failed toilet training, and the parent's exaggerated perceptions of acts of "disobedience." Parents may have unrealistic expectations for the child's behavior for the child's age group.

Another factor that increases a child's risk of being killed is living in a home where spouse or partner abuse occurs. Acts of domestic violence often are transferred to children living in the household. Studies have shown that frequently the following characteristics identify an abusive parent who kills a child[7]:

- Is a young male in his mid-20s
- Lives near or below poverty level
- Has not finished high school
- Is depressed and unable to cope with stress
- Has experienced violence firsthand

> **CRITICAL THINKING**
> How can you calm yourself after caring for a child killed by abuse before writing a patient care report that likely will be called to court?

SEXUAL ASSAULT

Sexual assault is one of the fastest growing and most serious crimes in the United States. More than 400,000 persons age 12 and older report sexual assault each year.[8] Sexual assault is more often committed than other forms of abuse. It can result in mental or physical injury and death.

Legal Aspects of Sexual Assault

Each state has different interpretations of sexual assault. The term generally refers to any genital, anal, oral, or manual penetration of the victim's body by way of force and without the victim's consent. Lack of consent includes the

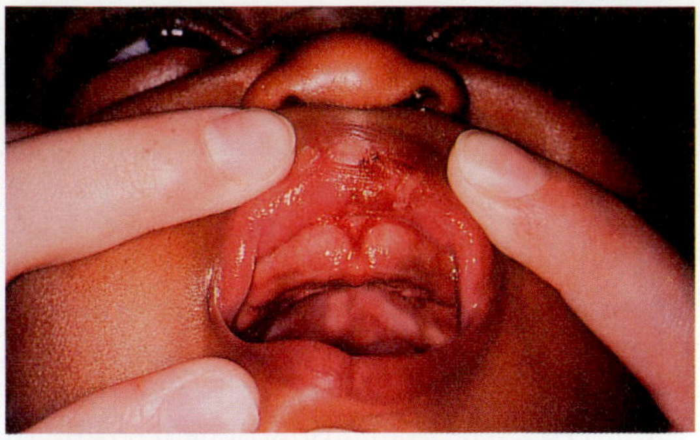

FIGURE 46-8 ■ A torn frenulum that may have been caused by forced bottle-feeding

inability to give consent. This inability may be as a result of impaired mental function caused by alcohol and other drugs, sleep, or unconsciousness.

In many cases, sexual assault is a felony crime that must be proved by evidence. Legal considerations for providing care to a patient who has been sexually assaulted include the following:

1. Take steps to preserve evidence.
2. Discourage the patient from urinating or defecating, douching, or bathing.
3. Do not remove evidence from any part of the body that was subjected to sexual contact unless necessary to provide urgent medical care.
4. Notify law enforcement personnel as soon as possible.
5. Be aware that there will be a "chain of evidence" with specific requirements of proof.
6. Follow local and state requirements in reporting these cases. Consult with medical direction and follow established protocols.

Characteristics of Sexual Assault

Anyone can be a victim of sexual assault at any age. The highest incidence of sexual assault occurs in women who live alone in isolated areas. The victim often knows the assailant. Sometimes the victim feels shame and personal responsibility for the attack. The methods that the assailant uses to gain control over male and female victims include entrapment, intimidation, and physical force. The assailant commonly uses threats of harm and a weapon to gain submission. Male victims are more likely to suffer significant physical trauma from sexual assault by other men than are female victims (Box 46-7). The following are common injuries that result from sexual assault:

- Abrasions and bruises on the upper limb, head, and neck
- Forcible signs of restraint (e.g., rope burns and mouth injuries)
- Petechiae of the face and conjunctiva caused by choking
- Broken teeth, swollen jaw or cheekbone, and eye injuries from being punched or slapped in the face
- Muscle soreness or stiffness in the shoulder, neck, knee, hip, or back from restraint in postures that allow sexual penetration

BOX 46-7 Five Myths and Misconceptions about Sexual Assault

Myth. All victims of sexual assault are women, and all perpetrators are men.
Fact. Most sexual assaults are perpetrated by men. However, men can be assaulted by other men. Sometimes women perpetrate sexual assaults against men and other women.
Myth. Rape is an impulsive act.
Fact. Fifty-eight percent to 71% of rapes clearly are planned.
Myth. Rape is motivated by sexual desire.
Fact. Rape is a crime of violence, motivated by anger and the desire for power and control.
Myth. Most women are raped by strangers.
Fact. Most women are victims of "acquaintance rape" by a known, trusted assailant.
Myth. According to the law, a husband cannot be charged with rape against his wife.
Fact. The law stipulates circumstances in which the husband can be charged with rape against his wife.

CRITICAL THINKING

How do you feel when you hear others say, "That rape victim brought it on herself?"

Psychosocial Aspects of Care

The trauma of sexual assault creates physical and psychological distress. Victims may behave in various ways. Some may be surprisingly calm and seem in control of their emotions. In contrast, others may be agitated, apprehensive, distraught, or tearful. After managing all threats to life, the paramedic should proceed with care by providing emotional support to the victim. As described in Chapter 41, the paramedic should not question victims of sexual assault in detail about the incident in the prehospital setting. The paramedic should limit the patient history to only what is required to provide care. The initial contact with the victim should include the following:

- Nonjudgmental and supportive attitude
- Empathetic and sensitive comments
- Quiet speech
- Slow movements
- Considerate gestures (ensure privacy and respect modesty)

The paramedic should move the patient to a safe and quiet environment. This will help to avoid further exposure and embarrassment. When possible, a paramedic of the same sex should provide care. If this is not possible, a chaperone should be present. The paramedic should not leave the patient alone. The paramedic should ask for permission to call a friend, family member, or sexual assault crisis advocate. Concerns of the victim about pregnancy and contracting human immunodeficiency virus and other sexually transmitted diseases should be relayed to medical direction. After the patient recovers from physical injury, the goal of treatment is for the patient to regain control of his or her life. Often this takes long-term counseling and support.

Child Victims

Children are particularly vulnerable to sexual assault. They also usually have frequent contact with the assailant. Often the assault occurs in a trusted person's home. Most sexual assaults involve a male assailant and female victim.[1] About 30% of acquaintance sexual assaults occur when the victim is between 11 and 17 years of age. Many young victims do not think of their experience as a sexual assault since they often are fondled or physically explored without intercourse. As a result, they rarely report the attack. In fact, they often assume that they are to blame. (Children often conceal sexual assault out of fear of punishment.) Victims involved in a same-sex assault also are unlikely to report the incident because of confusion or embarrassment. For these reasons, most victimized children do not receive proper treatment, including prophylaxis and counseling.

ASSESSMENT AND PATIENT CARE CONSIDERATIONS

Assessment for children of sexual assault should proceed as described before for other victims. The assessment should include age-related considerations that are appropriate for all children. The paramedic should be aware of the following symptoms. These symptoms may indicate behavior or physical manifestations as a result of sexual assault:

- Abrupt behavior changes
- Sleep difficulties, sleep disorders, and nightmares
- Withdrawal from and avoidance of friends and family
- Low self-esteem or desire to be invisible
- Phobias related to the offender
- Hostility
- Self-destructive behaviors
- Mood swings, depression, and anxiety
- Regression (e.g., bed-wetting)
- Truancy
- Eating disorders
- Alcohol or other drug use

The attitude and behavior of adults, including health care providers, greatly influence a child's impression of the assault. The paramedic should try to lessen the emotional influence of the assault by reassuring the child that he or she is not responsible for the attack. The child should also be assured that he or she did nothing wrong. The paramedic also should encourage the child to talk openly about the assault and any concerns that he or she may have.

LEGAL CONSIDERATIONS

If the paramedic suspects or confirms sexual assault, the paramedic must follow the laws that apply to the crime. Local and state laws affect the confidentiality of children. Paramedics should be aware of the regulations in their community. In addition, they should consult with medical direction.

SUMMARY

- Battering is the establishment of control and fear in a relationship through violence and other forms of abuse.
- Domestic violence follows a cycle of three phases. Phase one involves arguing and verbal abuse. Phase two progresses to physical and sexual abuse. Phase three consists of denial and apologies. Certain personality traits may predispose a person to abusive relationships.
- The paramedic may have a hard time identifying a battered patient. Injuries from domestic violence often involve contusions and lacerations of the face, neck, head, breast, and abdomen.
- The paramedic must ensure scene and personal safety in domestic violence events. The paramedic should manage physical injuries according to standard protocols. The paramedic should direct special attention toward the emotional needs of the victim as well.
- Elder abuse is classified into four categories: physical abuse, psychological abuse, financial or material abuse, and neglect.
- All 50 states have elder abuse statutes. Reporting of suspected elder abuse also is mandatory under law in most states.
- Most child abusers are the child's parents (77%). Eleven percent are other relatives of the victim. Abused children often exhibit behavior that provides key clues about abuse and neglect. The paramedic should observe carefully the child under 6 years of age who is passive or the child over 6 years of age who is aggressive.
- If the child volunteers the history of the event without hesitation and matches the history that the parent provides (and the history is suitable for the injury), child abuse is unlikely.
- Injuries may include soft tissue injuries, fractures, head injuries, and abdominal injuries.
- *Sexual assault* generally refers to any genital, anal, oral, or manual penetration of the victim's body by way of force and without the victim's consent. The highest incidence of sexual assault occurs in women who live alone in isolated areas.
- After managing all threats to life, the paramedic should provide emotional support to the victim. The paramedic should deliver care in a way that preserves evidence.

REFERENCES

1. US Department of Transportation, National Highway Traffic Safety Administration: *EMT-Paramedic national standard curriculum,* Washington, DC, 1998, The Department.
2. American College of Emergency Physicians: Guidelines for the role of EMS personnel in domestic violence (policy resource and education paper, March 2000). http://www.acep.org/1,443,0.html. Accessed March 11, 2005.
3. US Department of Justice, Bureau of Justice Statistics: *Violence against women: a national crime victimization report,* Washington, DC, 1994, The Department.
4. Department of Justice, Centers for Disease Control and Prevention: *Third annual report on the national violence against women survey,* Washington, DC, 1998, The Department.
5. National Center on Elder Abuse. http://www.elderabusecenter.org/default.cfm?p=nas.cfm. Accessed September 2, 2004.
6. US Department of Health and Human Services: *Child maltreatment 2001: summary of key findings,* Washington, DC, 2003, US Government Printing Office.
7. National Clearinghouse on Child Abuse and Neglect Information: Child fatalities fact sheet. http://www.calib.com/nccanch/pubs/factsheets/fatality.htm. Accessed October 16, 2004.
8. US Department of Justice, Office of Justice Programs, Bureau of Justice Statistics: *Selected findings: rape and sexual assault—reporting to police and medical attention, 1992-2000,* Washington, DC, August 2002, NCJ 194530.

CHAPTER

47

Patients with Special Challenges

OBJECTIVES

Upon completion of this chapter, the paramedic student will be able to:

1. Identify considerations in prehospital management related to physical challenges such as hearing, visual, and speech impairments; obesity; and patients with paraplegia or quadriplegia.
2. Identify considerations in prehospital management of patients who have mental illness, are developmentally disabled, or are emotionally or mentally impaired.
3. Describe special considerations for prehospital management of patients with selected pathological challenges.
4. Outline considerations in management of culturally diverse patients.
5. Describe special considerations in the prehospital management of terminally ill patients.
6. Identify special considerations in management of patients with communicable diseases.
7. Describe special considerations in the prehospital management of patients with financial challenges.

KEY TERMS

bariatrics: The field of medicine that focuses on the treatment and control of obesity and diseases associated with obesity.

cerebral palsy: A general term for nonprogressive disorders of movement and posture.

deafness: A complete or partial inability to hear.

diversity: Differences of any kind: race, class, religion, gender, sexual preference, personal habitat, and physical ability.

Down syndrome: A congenital condition characterized by varying degrees of mental retardation and multiple defects.

emotional/mental impairment: Impaired intellectual functioning that results in an inability to cope with normal responsibilities of life.

mental illness: Any form of psychiatric disorder.

mental retardation: A disorder characterized by below-average intellectual function with deficits or impairments in the ability to learn and adapt socially.

myasthenia gravis: An autoimmune disorder in which muscles become weak and tire easily.

obesity: A condition in which a person is 30% above ideal body weight.

paraplegia: A weakness or paralysis of both legs and sometimes, part of the trunk.

quadriplegia: A weakness or paralysis of all four extremities and the trunk.

terminally ill patients: Patients with advanced stage of disease with an unfavorable prognosis and no known cure.

Paramedics often provide care to patients with special challenges. The patient groups to be discussed in this chapter include those who have physical, emotional, or pathological challenges; patients who are culturally diverse, have terminal illness, and communicable diseases; and those with financial challenges that may hinder access to health care.

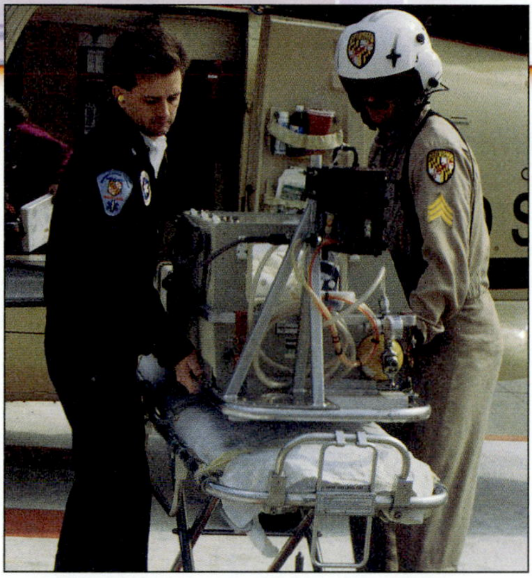

PHYSICAL CHALLENGES

Patients who are physically challenged may require special considerations in patient assessment and management. The physical challenges presented in this chapter include hearing, visual, and speech impairments; **obesity;** and patients with **paraplegia** or **quadriplegia.**

Hearing Impairments

Deafness is a complete or partial inability to hear. Total deafness is rare and usually congenital. Partial deafness may range from mild to severe. It most commonly results from an ear disease, injury, or degeneration of the hearing mechanism that occurs with age. All deafness is conductive or sensorineural.

Conductive deafness refers to the faulty transportation of sound from the outer to the inner ear. This type of deafness often is curable. In adults, conductive deafness commonly results from the buildup of earwax that blocks the outer ear canal. Conductive deafness also may result from infection (e.g., otitis media) and from injury to the eardrum or middle ear (e.g., from barotrauma).

Sensorineural deafness often is incurable. In this type of deafness, sounds that reach the inner ear fail to be transmitted to the brain. This is because of damage to the structures within the ear or to the acoustic nerve, which connects the inner ear to the brain. Sensorineural deafness that is present in early life may be congenital. It also can result from a birth injury or from damage to the developing fetus (e.g., from a mother who has rubella during pregnancy). Sensorineural deafness that occurs in later life may be caused by prolonged exposure to loud noise, disease (e.g., Meniere's disease), tumors, medications, viral infections, or natural degeneration of the cochlea or labyrinth in old age.

SPECIAL CONSIDERATIONS

The paramedic can use several helpful techniques for recognizing a patient who has a hearing impairment. One of these is noting the presence of hearing aids. Another is observing the patient for poor diction or the inability to respond to verbal communication in the absence of direct eye contact. Some accommodations may be needed. One includes retrieving the patient's hearing aid or other amplified listening device. Another is providing paper and pen to aid in communication.

When providing care to these patients, the paramedic should not shout or exaggerate lip movement. The emergency medical services (EMS) provider should speak softly and directly into the patient's ear canal. The provider should use a low-pitched voice. (About 80% of hearing loss is related to the inability to hear high-pitched sounds.) Another method to aid in communication includes asking family members to assist. The paramedic also can use pictures to illustrate basic needs and routine medical procedures.

Finally, the paramedic must notify the hospital as soon as possible if the patient has severe deafness. Some patients with severe hearing impairments will speak with unusual syntax. Some may use American Sign Language. Personnel with special training (e.g., an interpreter) may need to be summoned to assist with patient care.

Visual Impairments

Estimates indicate that more than 1 million Americans are blind and that 3 million are visually impaired, even with the best correction.[1] Normal vision depends on the uninterrupted passage of light from the front of the eye to the light-sensitive retina at the back. Any condition that obstructs the passage of light from the retina can cause vision loss. Vision impairment may be present at birth from a congenital disorder. It also may result from a number of other causes. These causes include the following:

- Cataracts
- Degeneration of the eyeball, optic nerve, or nerve pathways
- Diseases such as diabetes and hypertension
- Eye or brain injury (e.g., trauma, chemical burns, and stroke)
- Infections such as those that are caused by cytomegalovirus, herpes simplex virus, and bacterial ulcers
- Vitamin A deficiency in children living in developing countries

Patients with visual impairments may be totally blind or have a partial loss of vision that affects central vision, peripheral vision, or both. A patient who has central loss of vision is usually aware of the condition. Those who have a loss of peripheral vision may be more difficult to identify. This is because the loss often goes unnoticed by the person until it is well advanced.

SPECIAL CONSIDERATIONS

Techniques in assessing and managing patients with vision loss are described in Chapter 9. To review, accommodations for these patients that may be necessary include retrieving visual aids, describing all procedures before performing them, and providing sensory information (e.g., location of obstacles) as needed. The paramedic should guide ambulatory patients by "leading," not by "pushing." The paramedic should allow a guide dog used by the patient to accompany the patient to the hospital. The paramedic also should advise medical direction of the patient's special needs. That way, the appropriate personnel can be made available.

Speech Impairments

Speech impairments include disorders of language, articulation, voice production, or fluency (blockage of speech). All of these can lead to an inability to communicate well (Box 47-1).

Language disorders result from damage to the language centers of the brain. (They usually result from stroke, head injury, or brain tumor.) These patients often exhibit aphasia (loss of power of speech) with a slowness to understand speech and problems with vocabulary and sentence structure. Aphasia can affect children and adults. It may affect their ability to speak and to comprehend written or spoken words. Delayed development of language in a child may result from hearing loss, lack of stimulation, or emotional disturbance.

An articulation disorder is an inability to produce speech sounds. (The disorder sometimes is referred to as *dysarthria.*) These disorders result from damage to nerve pathways passing from the brain to the muscles of the larynx, mouth, or lips. Often the patient's speech will be slurred, indistinct, slow, or nasal. Disorders of articulation may result from brain injury. They also may result from diseases such as multiple sclerosis and Parkinson's disease. In children, articulation disorders commonly result from delayed development from hearing problems.

BOX 47-1 Types of Speech Impairments

Language Disorders
Brain tumor
Delayed development
Emotional disturbance
Head injury
Hearing loss
Lack of stimulation
Stroke

Articulation Disorders
Damage to nerve pathways passing from the brain to muscles in the larynx, mouth, or lips
Delayed development from hearing problems
Slow maturation of nervous system

Voice Production Disorders
Disorders affecting closure of vocal cords
Hormonal or psychiatric disturbance
Severe hearing loss

Fluency Disorders
Stuttering (for example)
Patient is not fully understood.

CRITICAL THINKING

What may cause a paramedic to become impatient when caring for a patient with this type of disorder?

Voice production disorders are characterized by hoarseness, harshness, inappropriate pitch, and abnormal nasal resonance. They often result from disorders that affect closure of the vocal cords. Some disorders are caused by hormonal or psychiatric disturbances and by severe hearing loss.

Fluency disorders are not well understood. They are marked by repetitions of single sounds or whole words and by the blocking of speech. An example of a fluency disorder is stuttering.

SPECIAL CONSIDERATIONS

Once a speech impairment has been identified, history taking and assessment need to be modified. Methods include allowing extra time for the patient to respond to questions, clarifying what the patient says or asking the patient to repeat an answer if it was not clearly understood, and offering appropriate aids (e.g., pen and paper) to assist in communications. Moreover, the paramedic should advise the hospital if a patient has a severe speech impairment. That way, the proper personnel (e.g., audiologist or speech specialist) can be made available.

Obesity

Obesity is defined as being 30% above ideal body weight. The disease affects nearly one third of the adult American population and is responsible for at least 300,000 deaths in the United States each year.[2]

Obesity is an abnormal increase in the proportion of fat and cells. The increase is mainly in the viscera and the subcutaneous tissues of the body. Although reasons for obesity in some persons are unclear, known causes for the condition include the following[3]:

- Caloric intake that exceeds calories burned
- Low basal metabolic rate
- Genetic disposition for obesity

The complications of obesity are many. Obesity increases a person's chance of becoming seriously ill. For example, obesity is associated with an increased risk for hypertension, stroke, heart disease, diabetes, and some cancers.[4] Osteoarthritis also is aggravated by increased body weight. The condition is treated with weight loss programs, exercise, counseling, medications, and sometimes surgery. The goal of treatment is lasting weight loss. The field of medicine that focuses on the treatment and control of obesity and diseases associated with it is known as **bariatrics.**

> **CRITICAL THINKING**
>
> Consider this situation. A crew member makes an insensitive remark about a patient's obesity within hearing range of the patient or the patient's family. How will you respond?

SPECIAL CONSIDERATIONS

The paramedic needs to give special considerations to caring for an obese patient. These include the need to obtain a thorough history. The history often will be extensive because of associated health problems. The paramedic should be aware that symptoms the patient may credit to obesity (e.g., fatigue, shortness of breath at rest or on exertion) may be a sign of an acute illness. (For example, the illness may be congestive heart failure or myocardial infarction.)

The examination of an obese person also may call for some modifications. These may include using large blood pressure cuffs, positioning the patient to better allow for hearing lung sounds, and placing electrocardiogram leads on areas of the body with less fat (e.g., the arms and thighs versus the chest wall). In addition, more personnel and special equipment may be needed to assist with moving the patient for transport. (For example, stretchers that can accommodate excessive weight and wide girth may be needed.)

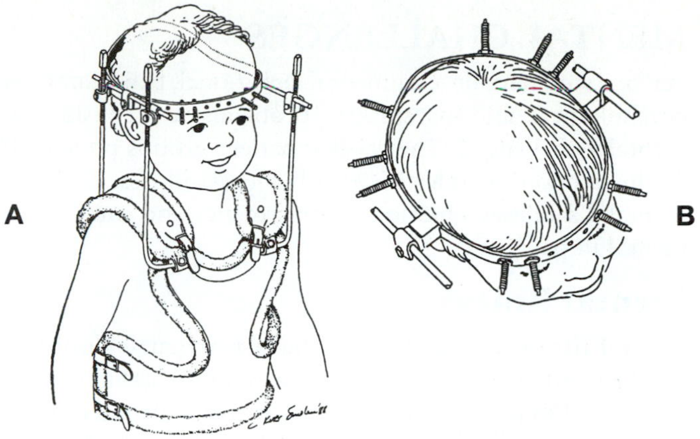

FIGURE 47-1 ■ **A,** Custom halo vest and light superstructure. **B,** Ten pin placement sites for infant halo ring attachment using multiple-pin, low-torque technique. Usually, four pins are placed anteriorly, avoiding temporal area, and the remaining six pins are placed in the occipital area.

Obese patients often are self-conscious about their weight. They may worry about the hardships they place on the EMS crew and other rescuers. Paramedics must maintain professionalism during these patient care encounters.

> **NOTE** One should note that weight limits vary widely for helicopters. When requesting an emergency rotary aircraft flight, the paramedic should inform the dispatcher if the patient is obese. This will help to determine whether the patient can be transported safely by air.

Patients with Paraplegia/Quadriplegia

Paraplegia is weakness or paralysis of both legs and sometimes part of the trunk; quadriplegia is weakness or paralysis of all four extremities and the trunk. The conditions result from nerve damage in the brain and spinal cord. These conditions usually are caused by a crash, sports injury, fall, or gunshot wound. (Medical illnesses such as lupus, multiple sclerosis, and stroke also can result in weakness and paralysis.) Paraplegia and quadriplegia are accompanied by a loss of sensation and loss of urinary control.

SPECIAL CONSIDERATIONS

Patients with extremity and trunk paralysis may require accommodations in patient care. For example, the patient may have a halo traction device to stabilize the spine (Fig. 47-1). Or the patient may rely on a home ventilator to assist with breathing. Both of these situations can complicate airway management. They also can make patient transport more difficult. Some patients who are paralyzed will have special equipment (e.g., walkers or wheelchairs); ostomies for the trachea, bladder, or colon; and medical devices that rely on electricity or a battery supply. (See Chapter 48.) Additional personnel may be required to assist with moving special equipment and to prepare the patient for ambulance transport.

MENTAL CHALLENGES

Persons who have developmental, emotional, behavioral, or psychological and psychiatric problems are considered mentally challenged. The specific patient groups presented in this section include those with mental illness, developmental disabilities, emotional impairments, and emotional/mental impairments.

Mental Illness

Mental illness refers to any form of psychiatric disorder. As described in Chapter 40, most forms of mental illness result from biological, psychosocial, or sociocultural causes. A person's mental illness may result from more than one of these factors. To review, examples of biological causes of mental illness are schizophrenia and depression that result from biochemical imbalance; and organic causes such as trauma, illness, and dementia. Psychosocial causes of mental illness can result from childhood trauma, child abuse or neglect, a dysfunctional family structure or other issues that cause an inability to resolve situational conflicts in a person's life. Sociocultural causes of mental illness may be related to personal relationships, family stability, economic status and other factors, that result in situational stress.

SPECIAL CONSIDERATIONS

Recognizing a patient with mental illness may be difficult, especially if the patient has only mild symptoms of the disease. Other patients with more serious disorders may have signs and symptoms that are consistent with mental illness. (An example is paranoid behavior in patients with schizophrenia.) When obtaining the patient history, the paramedic should not hesitate to ask about the following:

- History of mental illness
- Prescribed medications
- Compliance with prescribed medications
- Use of over-the-counter herbal products (e.g., St. John's wort)
- Concomitant use of alcohol or other drugs

If the patient acts anxiously, the paramedic should ask the patient's permission before performing any assessment or any procedure. This will help to establish rapport and trust during the care. Unless the call is related specifically to the mental illness, care should proceed in the same manner as for any other patient. Patients with mental illness experience medical illness and injury like all other patient groups. If the patient acts aggressively or combatively, the paramedic should retreat from the scene and call on law enforcement to secure the scene.

Developmentally Disabled

A person who is developmentally disabled has impaired or insufficient development of the brain. This causes an inability to learn at the usual rate *(developmental delay)*. Developmental delay has many causes, including the following:

- Lack of stimulation (as seen with child abuse or neglect)
- Severe vision or hearing impairment
- **Mental retardation**
- Brain damage before, during, or after birth
- Severe diseases of body organs and systems

Persons who are developmentally disabled often function well with daily activities, hold jobs, and live on their own (or with their family or in residential group homes). However, some delays may be severe and may affect any or all of the major areas of human achievement: walking upright; fine eye-hand coordination; listening, language, and speech; and social interaction.

The accommodations that may be needed when caring for these patients will vary depending on the severity of disability. The paramedic should allow extra time for obtaining a history and performing an examination. The paramedic also should allow extra time for preparing the patient for transport. When possible, a member of the patient's family or a caregiver should remain with the patient during the care.

> **CRITICAL THINKING**
> Do you think a patient with developmental delays should have any input into their care? Why?

Down Syndrome

Down syndrome results from an abnormal chromosome. This abnormality causes mild to severe mental retardation and a characteristic physical appearance (Fig. 47-2). The child with Down syndrome has features that typically include the following:

- Eyes that slope upward at the outer corners
- Folds of skin on either side of the nose that cover the inner corners of the eyes
- A small face and small facial features
- A large and protruding tongue
- Flattening on back of the head
- Hands that are short and broad

In most cases, Down syndrome occurs from the failure of the two chromosomes numbered 21 in a parent cell to go into separate daughter cells during the first stage of sperm or egg cell formation. This results in a triplet of chromosomes 21 (trisomy 21) rather than the usual pair. The extra number 21 chromosome is passed on to the child. This leads to Down syndrome. The incidence of affected fetuses increases with increased maternal age (mothers over age 35). It also increases in those with a family history of Down syndrome.

> **NOTE** In the general population, trisomy 21 occurs in only 1 of about 600 live births. After age 35, a mother's chances of having a Down syndrome child increases dramatically to as high as 1 in 80 by age 40.[5] Because of this increased risk, pregnant mothers over age 35 usually are tested to assess for the abnormality.

Persons with Down syndrome usually do not survive past their middle age. Many are cared for at home, and oth-

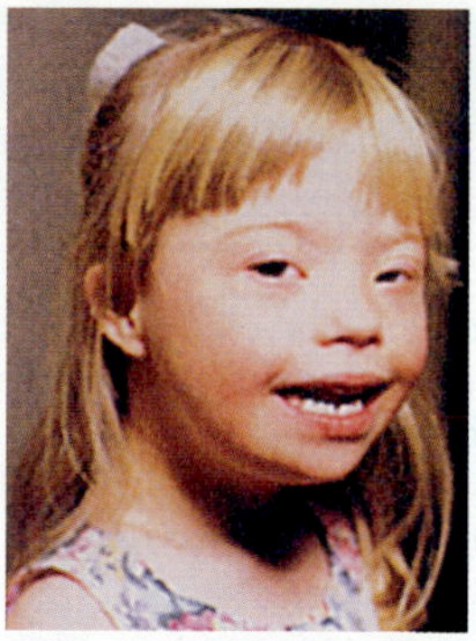

FIGURE 47-2 ■ Child with Down syndrome.

ers live in long-term nursing care facilities. About 25% of children born with Down syndrome have a heart defect at birth. Many have congenital intestinal disorders, hearing defects, and other illnesses. The degree of mental disability varies with an intelligence quotient (IQ) that ranges from 30 to 80. (An IQ of 80 to 120 is considered average.) Persons with Down syndrome are capable of limited learning and often are affectionate and friendly. Extra time must be allowed for obtaining a history and for performing assessment and patient care procedures.

Emotionally Impaired

Persons with emotional problems often suffer from anxiety disorders. These disorders were described in Chapter 40. They can result in a wide range of physical or mental symptoms attributed to mental stress.

SPECIAL CONSIDERATIONS

Distinguishing between symptoms produced by stress and those that indicate serious medical illness may be difficult. Thus management should always focus on the presenting complaint. The paramedic also should assume the most serious cause. As described in Chapter 40, signs and symptoms that may result from emotional impairment include somatic complaints such as chest discomfort, tachycardia, dyspnea, choking, and syncope. Hence the paramedic must gather a full history from the patient. A thorough examination also is essential to rule out serious illness. The prehospital care for these patients (in the absence of serious illness) mainly is supportive. It includes calming measures and transport for physician evaluation.

Emotionally/Mentally Impaired

Emotional/mental impairment refers to persons who have impaired intellectual functioning (mental retardation). This impairment results in an inability to cope with the normal responsibilities of life. Mental retardation can be classified further with IQ assessment as mild (IQ 50 to 70), moderate (IQ 35 to 59), and profound (IQ less than 20).[6] The more severe grades of emotional/mental impairment usually have a specific physical cause (e.g., brain damage or Down syndrome). In contrast, mild emotional/mental impairment often has no specific cause. However, poverty, malnutrition, and heredity may play a role (Box 47-2). Mild mental retardation is the most common form of emotional/mental impairment. It accounts for about 85% of the retarded population.

BOX 47-2 Causes of Mental Retardation

Genetic Conditions

Phenylketonuria: a single-gene disorder causing an enzyme deficiency

Chromosomal disorder (e.g., Down syndrome)

Fragile X syndrome (a single gene disorder on the Y chromosome; the leading inherited cause of mental retardation)

Problems during Pregnancy

Use of alcohol or other drugs by the mother

Use of tobacco

Illness and infection (toxoplasmosis, cytomegalovirus, rubella, syphilis, human immunodeficiency virus)

Problems at Birth

Brain injury

Prematurity

Low birth weight

Problems after Birth

Childhood diseases (whooping cough, chickenpox, measles, Hib disease)

Injury (e.g., head injury or near drowning)

Exposure to lead, mercury, and other environmental toxins

Poverty and Cultural Deprivation

Malnutrition

Disease-producing conditions

Inadequate medical care

Environmental health hazards

Lack of stimulation

From Arc National Headquarters: *Introduction to mental retardation,* Arlington, Texas, 2000, The Association.

SPECIAL CONSIDERATIONS

Changes to normal patient care vary based on the patient's level of retardation. Many with mild retardation show no symptoms other than slowness in carrying out mental tasks. Others with moderate to severe retardation may have limited to absent speech. Neurological problems are common. These patients may require extra time and care in patient assessment, management, and transportation.

PATHOLOGICAL CHALLENGES

Certain pathological conditions may require special assessment and management skills. Specific pathological conditions presented in this section include arthritis, cancer, **cerebral palsy,** cystic fibrosis, multiple sclerosis, muscular dystrophy, poliomyelitis, previous head injury, spina bifida, and **myasthenia gravis.**

Arthritis

As described in Chapters 32 and 45, arthritis is the inflammation of a joint. Arthritis is characterized by pain, stiffness, swelling, and redness. The disease has many forms and varies widely in its effects. Two forms of arthritis are common. One is osteoarthritis that results from cartilage loss and wear and tear of the joints (common in elderly patients). The other is rheumatoid arthritis (an au-

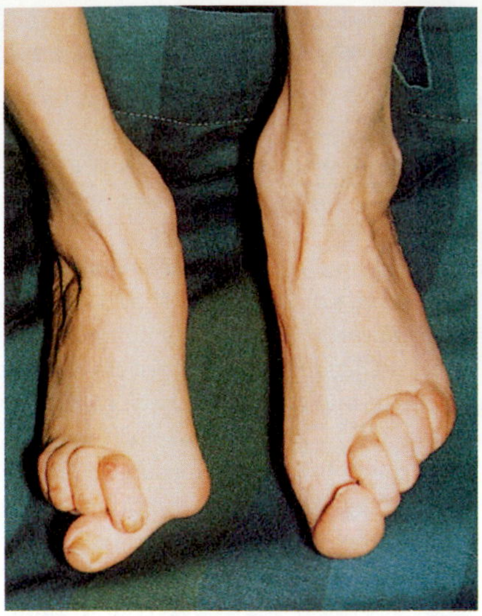

FIGURE 47-3 ■ Rheumatoid arthritis of the feet.

toimmune disorder that damages joints and surrounding tissues; Fig. 47-3).

SPECIAL CONSIDERATIONS

Patients with arthritis often have decreased range of motion and mobility. This may limit the physical exam. (It is important to ensure patient comfort whenever possible.) The paramedic also should determine current medication use (e.g., analgesics) before giving drugs to these patients. Transport strategies must take into account the patient's limited mobility. The paramedic also must adjust the equipment (e.g., backboards and splints) to fit the patient (not vice versa). This can be achieved by supplying adequate padding to fill all voids.

Cancer

Cancer is a group of diseases that allows for an unrestrained growth of cells in one or more of the body organs or tissues (see Chapter 37). The malignant tumors most often develop in major organs. These include the lungs, breasts, intestine, skin, stomach, and pancreas. However, they also may occur in cell-forming tissues of the bone marrow and in the lymphatic system, muscle, or bone.

SPECIAL CONSIDERATIONS

Patients with cancer often are very ill. The signs and symptoms of their disease depend on the site of origin of the cancer (Box 47-3). Often no signs of the disease are visible. However, medical treatment (e.g., chemotherapy or radiation) for many of the cancers can produce obvious signs and symptoms and various illnesses that may initiate an EMS response. These signs and symptoms include the following:

- Anorexia
- Depression
- Fatigue
- Gastrointestinal upset
- General malaise
- Loss of appetite
- Loss of hair (alopecia)
- Pain

BOX 47-3 Common Examples of Site of Origin Classifications for Cancer

Adenocarcinoma: originates in glandular tissue
Blastoma: originates in embryonic tissue of organs
Carcinoma: originates in epithelial tissue (i.e., tissue that lines organs and tubes)
Leukemia: originates in tissues that form blood cells
Lymphoma: originates in lymphatic tissue
Myeloma: originates in bone marrow
Sarcoma: originates in connective or supportive tissue (e.g., bone, cartilage, muscle)

Requests for emergency services for patients with advanced cancer often are related to the patient's pain medication. An example is patients whose pain is no longer relieved by the medicine. Another example is patients who have taken an accidental overdose of pain medicine. This may result in an altered level of consciousness or respiratory depression. If the patient's pain is not being relieved, the paramedic should consult with medical direction. (Larger than normal doses may need to be given to provide pain relief.) If an overdose is suspected, the paramedic should initiate the standard care for narcotic overdose.

The paramedic should try to obtain a full history from the patient. This should include a list of all medications. Many cancer patients take anticancer drugs and pain medications. They take these through transdermal skin patches that contain analgesic agents and through surgically implanted ports (e.g., mediports). If intravenous therapy is necessary, the paramedic should allot extra time to access the patient's peripheral veins. The veins often are scarred from chemotherapy and may be difficult to cannulate. (Aseptic technique is especially important in these patients. They often are immunocompromised as a result of the treatment for their disease.) As described in Chapter 18, paramedics should consult with medical direction and follow protocols before using a surgically implanted port for fluid or drug therapy.

The course of the disease and the medical regimen of care for cancer patients can be devastating for the patient, family, and loved ones. The paramedic must provide emotional support for all involved. Also essential is to ensure the patient's comfort. Finally, patients should be transported to the hospital where they are being treated for their cancer, when possible.

Cerebral Palsy

Cerebral palsy is a general term for nonprogressive disorders of movement and posture. The disease results from damage to the fetal brain during later months of pregnancy, during birth, during the newborn period, or in early childhood. The most common cause of cerebral palsy is cerebral dysgenesis (abnormal cerebral development) or cerebral malformations.[7] Other less common causes include fetal hypoxia, birth trauma, maternal infection, kernicterus (excessive fetal bilirubin, associated with hemolytic disease), and postpartum encephalitis, meningitis, or head injury. Cerebral palsy often is diagnosed during the child's first year of life when parents notice unusual muscle tone during holding. Sometimes they notice feeding difficulties. No cure exists for the disease. But those persons with moderate disability may live with relative independence and have a near-normal life expectancy.

TYPES OF CEREBRAL PALSY

Three distinct types of cerebral palsy exist. They are spastic paralysis, athetosis, and ataxia. Spastic paralysis produces abnormal stiffness and contraction of groups of muscles. With this type of cerebral palsy, the child may be categorized as diplegic, hemiplegic, or quadriplegic. With diplegic, all four limbs are affected. The legs are affected more severely than the arms. With hemiplegic, the limbs on only one side of the body are affected. The arm is usually more severe than the leg. With quadriplegic, all four limbs are severely affected, not necessarily symmetrically. Athetosis produces involuntary writhing movements. Ataxia produces a loss of coordination and balance. Hearing defects, epilepsy, and other central nervous system disorders are often present with the disease. Although some with athetosis and diplegia are highly intelligent, about 60% of all persons with cerebral palsy have mental retardation.[7] Most persons with quadriplegia are severely retarded.

CRITICAL THINKING

How can you determine the patient's normal level of functioning?

SPECIAL CONSIDERATIONS

Weakness, paralysis, and developmental delay vary by the type and severity of disease. For example, some children with mild cerebral palsy attend regular schools. Others with more severe forms of the disease never learn to walk or communicate well. They may require lifelong skilled nursing care. Accommodations that may be needed during a call include allowing extra scene time for the examination and extra resources and personnel to aid transport.

Cystic Fibrosis

Cystic fibrosis (mucoviscidosis) is an inherited metabolic disease of the lungs and digestive system that manifests in childhood. The disease is caused by a defective, recessive gene. The gene is inherited from each parent. The defective gene causes the glands in the lining of the bronchi to produce excessive amounts of thick mucus. This predisposes the person to chronic lung infections. In addition, the pancreas of a patient with cystic fibrosis fails to produce the enzymes required for the breakdown of fats and their absorption from the intestine. These alterations in metabolism cause classic symptoms of cystic fibrosis that include pale, greasy-looking, foul-smelling stools (often noticeable soon after birth); persistent cough and breathlessness; and lung infections that often develop into pneumonia, bronchiectasis, and bronchitis. Other features of the disease include stunted growth and sweat glands that produce abnormally salty sweat. In some cases the child with cystic fibrosis may fail to thrive; many patients survive into adulthood, although poor health is common.

NOTE If only one defective gene is inherited, that person will be a carrier of the disease. However, the person will have no symptoms. Often, these persons are unaware that they carry the defective gene. Genetic counseling and testing are appropriate for persons who have a family history of cystic fibrosis.

SPECIAL CONSIDERATIONS

Older patients (and parents of children) with cystic fibrosis generally are aware of their disease. Some may be oxygen-dependent. They may need respiratory support and suctioning to clear the airway of mucus and secretions. Many will use inhalants. The paramedic should expect a lengthy history and physical exam because of the nature of the disease and associated medical problems. Some patients will have received heart and lung transplants. They may require transfer to specialized medical facilities for treatment. If parents are unaware of the possibility of cystic fibrosis in the presence of signs and symptoms described previously, the paramedic should advise the physician at the hospital of his or her suspicions.

Multiple Sclerosis

Multiple sclerosis is a progressive and incurable autoimmune disease of the central nervous system that destroys patches of myelin in the brain and spinal cord. Scarring and destruction of the tissues cause symptoms that range from numbness and tingling to paralysis and incontinence. The cause of multiple sclerosis is unknown; however, it may have a heritable or viral component. (Many persons with multiple sclerosis lead active, normal lives between exacerbations of their illness.) The disease usually begins early in adult life. It becomes active for a brief time. Then it resumes years later. As described in Chapter 31, the symptoms of multiple sclerosis vary with the affected areas of the central nervous system. The symptoms may include the following:

Brain Involvement

- Ataxia
- Blurred or double vision
- Clumsiness
- Fatigue
- Muscle weakness

- Numbness, weakness, or pain in the face
- Slurred speech
- Vertigo

Spinal Cord Involvement

- Extremities that feel heavy and become weak
- Spasticity
- Tingling, numbness, or feeling of constriction in any part of the body

The symptoms of multiple sclerosis may occur singly or in combination. They may last from several weeks to several months. Attacks vary in intensity. They may be brought on by injury, infection, or physical or emotional stress. Some patients become disabled, bedridden, and incontinent early in middle life. Disabled patients also often suffer from painful muscle spasms, constipation, urinary tract infection, skin ulcerations, and mood swings. The disease is managed with medications, physical therapy, and counseling.

SPECIAL CONSIDERATIONS

Some patients with multiple sclerosis may be difficult to examine. They may be unable to provide a complete medical history because of the nature of their illness. The paramedic should allow extra time for patient assessment and to prepare the patient for transport. (The patient should not be expected to ambulate.) In severe cases, respiratory support may be indicated.

Muscular Dystrophy

Muscular dystrophy (see Chapter 31) is an inherited muscle disorder that results in a slow but progressive degeneration of muscle fibers. The disease is classified according to the age that symptoms first appear, the rate at which the disease progresses, and the way in which it is inherited. Muscular dystrophy is incurable. Genetic counseling and testing is appropriate for persons with a family history of muscular dystrophy.

The most common form of the disease is Duchenne's muscular dystrophy, caused by a sex-linked recessive gene that affects only males. Duchenne's muscular dystrophy rarely is diagnosed before age 3. Signs and symptoms of the disease include a child who is slow in learning to sit up and walk; an unusual gait; curvature of the spine; and muscles that become bulky as they are replaced by fat. Eventually, most children will be unable to walk. Many do not live past their teenage years as a result of chronic lung infections and congestive heart failure. With other less common forms of muscular dystrophy, patients may live well into their middle years with varying degrees of muscle weakness.

SPECIAL CONSIDERATIONS

Accommodations that may be required during emergency care depend on the person's age, weight, and severity of disease. For example, young children will be fairly easy to examine and prepare for transport. When caring for older patients, extra personnel may be needed to move the patient to the ambulance. In severe cases the patient may need respiratory support.

Poliomyelitis

Poliomyelitis (polio) is an infectious disease caused by *Poliovirus hominis*. The virus is spread through direct and indirect contact with infected feces and by airborne transmission. Poliovirus attacks with variable severity. The severity can range from asymptomatic infection to a febrile illness without neurological complications to aseptic meningitis and finally to paralytic disease (including respiratory paralysis) and possible death.

As described in Chapter 31, the incidence of polio cases has declined since the Salk and Sabin vaccines were made available in the 1950s. The disease, however, may affect nonimmune adults and indigent children. Signs and symptoms of polio in the nonparalytic and paralytic forms include fever, malaise, headache, and intestinal upset. In the majority of cases, persons with the nonparalytic form of polio recover fully. In the paralytic form, extensive paralysis of muscles of the legs and lower trunk can occur.

SPECIAL CONSIDERATIONS

Caring for a patient with paralytic polio who has respiratory paralysis may call for advanced airway support to ensure adequate ventilation. (Patients on home ventilators typically have a tracheostomy.) If the lower body is paralyzed, catheterization of the bladder may be needed (see Chapter 48). Extra resources and personnel may be needed to prepare the patient for transport.

Previously Head-Injured Patients

Traumatic brain injury can result from many types of trauma (see Chapter 24). These injuries can affect many cognitive, physical, and psychological skills. Physical deficit can include ambulation, balance and coordination, fine motor skills, strength, and endurance. Cognitive deficits of language and communication, information processing, memory, and perceptual skills are common. Psychological status also often is altered (Table 47-1).

SPECIAL CONSIDERATIONS

Depending on the patient's area of brain injury, obtaining a history and performing assessment and care may be difficult. Some patients may need restraint. Family and other caregivers should be involved in managing the patient (when appropriate). The paramedic also should interview them to determine whether the patient's actions and responses are "normal" for the patient. The paramedic should expect to spend extra time at the scene to provide care to these patients.

CRITICAL THINKING

Why is this group of patients at high risk for injury?

TABLE 47-1 Brain Injury Deficits

INJURY	INJURY DEFICITS
Cerebral Cortex	
Frontal lobe	Paralysis of various body parts
	Inability to plan a sequence of complex movements
	Inability to focus on tasks
	Mood changes
	Personality changes
	Inability to express language
Parietal lobe	Inability to name an object
	Problems with reading and writing
	Difficulty in distinguishing right from left
	Difficulty with math skills
	Difficulty with eye and hand coordination
Occipital lobe	Defects in vision
	Production of hallucinations
	Visual illusions
	Inability to recognize words
	Difficulties in reading and writing
Temporal lobe	Difficulty in recognizing faces
	Difficulty in understanding spoken words
	Short-term memory loss
	Interference with long-term memory
	Persistent talking
	Aggressive behavior
Brainstem	Decreased vital capacity in breathing
	Difficulty in swallowing food and water
	Difficulty with organization
	Problems with balance and movement
	Dizziness and nausea
	Sleeping difficulties
Cerebellum	Loss of ability to coordinate fine movements
	Loss of ability to walk
	Tremors
	Dizziness
	Slurred speech

Spina Bifida

Spina bifida (see Chapter 31) is a congenital defect. With this condition, part of one or more vertebrae fail to develop. This leaves a portion of the spinal cord exposed. The condition ranges in severity from that of minimal evidence of a defect to a child who is severely disabled. In severe cases the legs of some children may be deformed with partial or full paralysis and loss of sensation in all areas below the level of the defect. Associated abnormalities may include hydrocephalus with brain damage (Fig. 47-4), cerebral palsy, epilepsy, and mental retardation.

SPECIAL CONSIDERATIONS

Because of the varying degrees of spina bifida, care must be tailored to the patient's specific needs. Some patients require no special accommodations. Others need extra on-scene time for assessment and management. Additional resources and personnel to prepare the patient for transport may be needed as well.

> **NOTE** Between 18% and 73% of children and adolescents with spina bifida are estimated to be sensitive to latex.[8] Thus all patients with spina bifida should be considered at high risk for having an allergic reaction to rubber. These persons should avoid contact with rubber products. They should avoid contact especially during medical procedures. The paramedic should use only nonlatex gloves. Alternative products can be substituted safely. These other products usually are made of silicone, plastic, or vinyl.

Myasthenia Gravis

Myasthenia gravis is an autoimmune disorder. In this disorder, muscles become weak and tire easily. The damage occurs to muscle receptors that are responsible for transmitting nerve impulses. The disease commonly affects muscles of the eyes, face, throat, and extremities (Fig. 47-5). Myasthenia gravis is a rare disease that can begin suddenly or gradually. Myasthenia gravis can occur at any age but usually appears in women between age 20 and 30 and in men between 70 and 80 years of age.[9] Classic signs and symptoms include the following:

- Drooping eyelids, double vision
- Difficulty speaking
- Difficulty in chewing and swallowing
- Difficult extremity movement
- Weakened respiratory muscles

The affected muscles become worse with use. However, they may recover completely with rest. The condition may be worsened by infection, stress, medications, and menstruation. Myasthenia gravis often can be controlled with drug therapy to enhance the transmission of nerve impulses in the muscles. (Removal of the thymus gland may improve the condition.) In a small number of patients the disease will progress to paralysis of the throat and respiratory muscles and may lead to death.

SPECIAL CONSIDERATIONS

Accommodations required for care will vary based on the patient's presentation. In most cases, supportive care and transport will be all that is required. In the presence of respiratory distress, the paramedic should take measures to ensure adequate airway and ventilatory support.

CULTURALLY DIVERSE PATIENTS

Individuals vary in many ways, and huge diversity exists in populations of all cultures. **Diversity** is a term that once was used mainly to describe "racial awareness." Now it refers to differences of any kind. These differences include race, class, religion, gender, sexual preference, personal habitat, and physical ability. Good health care depends on sensitivity toward these differences.

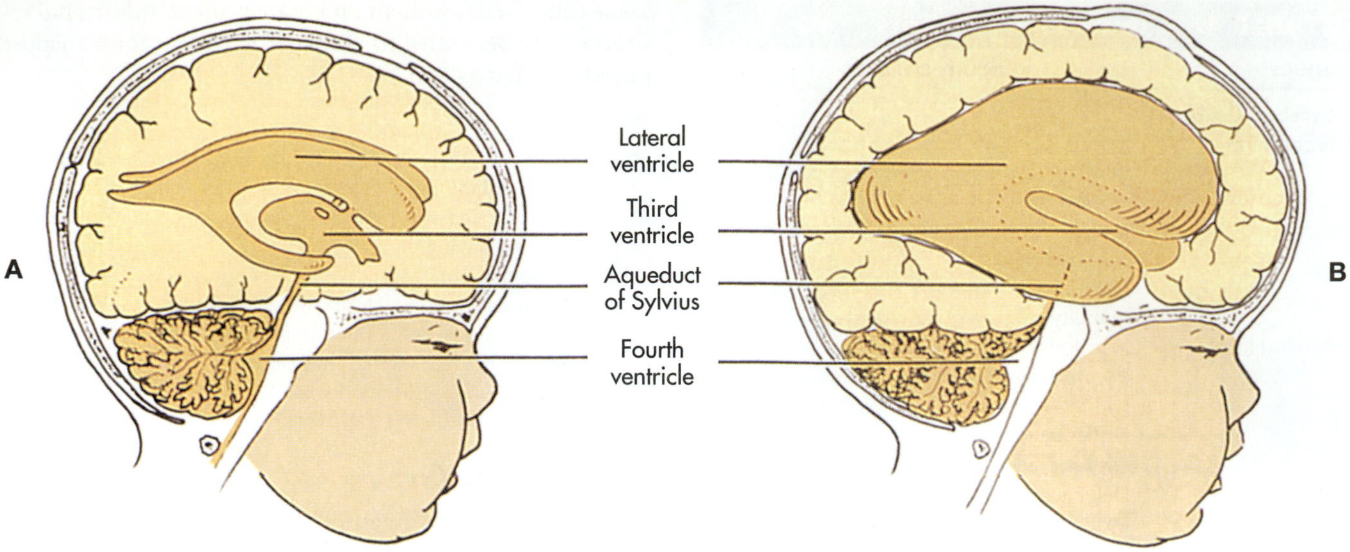

FIGURE 47-4 ■ Hydrocephalus: a block in flow of cerebrospinal fluid. **A,** Patent cerebrospinal fluid circulation. **B,** Enlarged lateral and third ventricles caused by obstruction of circulation—stenosis of aqueduct of Sylvius.

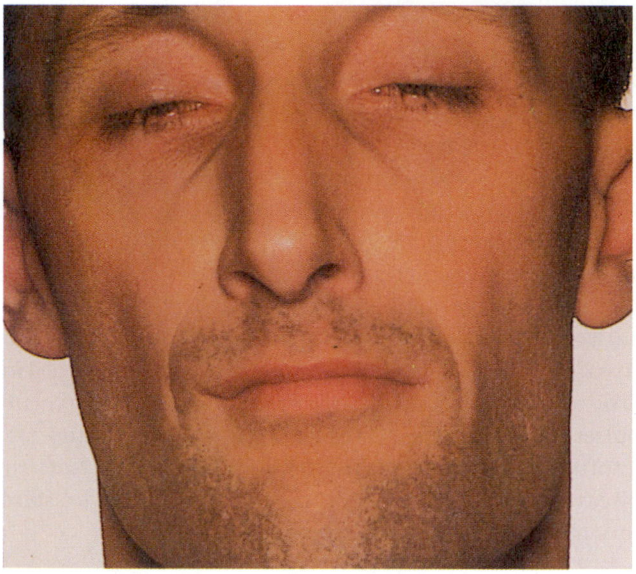

FIGURE 47-5 ■ A patient with myasthenia gravis.

CRITICAL THINKING

What kinds of diversity are there in your classroom? How do you feel about that diversity?

Experiences of health and illness vary widely as a result of different beliefs, behaviors, and past experiences. These experiences may conflict with learned medical practice of the paramedic. By revealing awareness of cultural issues, the paramedic conveys interest, concern, and respect. When dealing with patients from different cultures, the paramedic should recall the following eight key points:

1. The individual is the "foreground," the culture is the "background."
2. Different generations and individuals within the same family may have different sets of beliefs.
3. Not all persons identify with their ethnic cultural background.
4. All persons share common problems or situations.
5. Respect the integrity of cultural beliefs.
6. Realize that persons may not share your explanations of the causes of their ill health but may accept conventional treatments. (You do not have to "convert" a patient to your way of thinking to get the desired result.)
7. You do not have to agree with every aspect of another's culture, nor does the person have to accept everything about yours for effective and culturally sensitive health care to occur.
8. Recognize your personal cultural assumptions, prejudices, and belief systems. Do not let them interfere with patient care.

Special Considerations

Regardless of the patient's cultural background, education, occupation, or ability to speak English, most patients will be anxious during an emergency event. If the paramedic does not speak the patient's language, the paramedic should try to communicate in English first. The patient may understand or speak some English words or phrases. (Bystanders, co-workers, or family members may be available to assist.) In some areas, special translator devices (e.g., a telephone language line) for non–English-speaking patients are available. If the patient does not speak or understand English, the paramedic should try to communicate with signs or gestures. The hospital should be notified as soon as possible. That way, arrangements for an interpreter can be made.

If time allows, the paramedic should perform all assessment procedures slowly and with the patient's permission. The paramedic should be aware that "private space" is culturally defined. (See Chapter 9.) Therefore the best approach is to point to the area of the body to be examined before touching the patient. The paramedic must respect the patient's need for modesty and privacy at the scene and during transport.

TERMINALLY ILL PATIENTS

As health care professionals, paramedics will care for **terminally ill patients.** (These are patients with advanced stage of disease with an unfavorable prognosis and no known cure.) Often, these calls will be emotionally charged events. They will require a great deal of empathy and compassion for the patient and his or her loved ones. If emotions at the scene are out of control, the paramedic must take control. The paramedic should try to calm the persons involved.

If EMS has been called during the late stages of a patient's terminal illness or for a change in the patient's condition, a full history should be obtained. The patient or family should be asked about advance directives and the appropriateness of resuscitation procedures (see Chapter 4). The paramedic should review carefully any documentation made available concerning advance directives (e.g., a do-not-resuscitate order). The paramedic also should discuss advance directives with medical direction so that care decisions can be made.

Special Considerations

Care of a terminally ill patient often is mainly supportive and limited to calming and comfort measures. Care may include transport for physician evaluation. (Many terminally ill patients and their families will be involved in hospice care to help them deal with death and dying.) Pain assessment and the management of pain are important aspects of caring for these patients. The paramedic should try to gather a full pain medication history and examine the patient for the presence of transdermal drug patches or other pain-relief devices. Following an assessment of the patient's vital signs, level of consciousness, and medication history, medical direction may advise the use of analgesics or sedatives (e.g., ***morphine*** and ***midazolam***) to ensure the patient's comfort.

PATIENTS WITH COMMUNICABLE DISEASES

As described in Chapter 39, exposure to some infectious diseases can be a significant health risk to EMS providers. Thus it is crucial to ensure personal protection on *every* response. The required precautions depend on the mode of transmission. They also depend on the ability of the pathogen to cause disease. For example, in some cases gloves provide the required protection. In other cases, respiratory barriers also are needed. Paramedics cannot have an environment that is totally free of risk. But simple measures of protection greatly reduce exposure to pathogens.

Special Considerations

Some infectious diseases (e.g., acquired immunodeficiency syndrome) take a toll on the emotional well-being of affected patients, their families, and loved ones. The psychological aspects of providing care to these patients include an emphasis on recognizing each patient as an individual with unique health care needs, respecting each person's personal dignity, and providing considerate, respectful care focused upon the person's individual needs.

> **CRITICAL THINKING**
> How do you think you'll feel when called to care for a patient who is positive for human immunodeficiency virus or has acquired immunodeficiency syndrome?

FINANCIAL CHALLENGES

More than 41 million Americans and one third of persons living in poverty are estimated to have no health insurance,[10,11] and insurance coverage held by many others would not carry them through a catastrophic illness. Financial challenges for health care can quickly result from loss of a job and depletion of savings. Financial challenges that are combined with medical conditions that require uninterrupted treatment (e.g., tuberculosis, human immunodeficiency virus/acquired immunodeficiency syndrome, diabetes, hypertension, and mental disorders) or that occur in the presence of unexpected illness or injury, can deprive the patient of basic health care. Most medical providers recognize their ethical duty to provide services immediately, without regard to payment, in emergencies.

Poor health also is associated closely with homelessness. Many homeless persons have multiple health problems. In addition to chronic illness, frostbite, leg ulcers, and respiratory infections are common. These often are the direct result of homelessness. Homeless persons also are at greater risk for trauma from muggings, beatings, and rape. Homelessness precludes good nutrition, good personal hygiene, and basic first aid. In addition, some homeless persons with mental disorders may use alcohol or other drugs to self-medicate. Those with addictive disorders often are at risk of human immunodeficiency virus and other communicable diseases. Paramedics should be familiar with services in their community for the homeless. They should know where to refer the homeless for food and shelter.

> **CRITICAL THINKING**
> Consider patients with chronic illness and no insurance. How do you think that financial pressures influence medication compliance in these patients?

Special Considerations

Persons with financial challenges often are anxious about seeking medical care. Fortunately, the ability to pay for emergency care generally is not a concern for EMS providers (see Chapter 5). According to *Emergency Medical Services: Agenda for the Future,* "the focus of public access is the ability to secure prompt and appropriate EMS care regardless of socioeconomic status, age, or special need. For all those who contact EMS with a perceived requirement for care, the subsequent response and level of care provided must be commensurate with the situation."[12] When caring for a patient with financial challenges who is concerned about the cost of receiving needed health care, the paramedic should explain the following:

1. The patient's ability to pay should never be a factor in obtaining emergency care.
2. Federal law requires that care be provided, regardless of the patient's ability to pay.
3. Payment programs for health care services are available in most hospitals.
4. Government services are available to help patients in paying for health care.
5. Free (or near-free) health care services are available through local, state, and federally funded organizations.

In cases in which no life-threatening condition exists, the paramedic should ask the patient which hospital is covered through the patient's health plan or insurance policy. When the patient does not have insurance coverage, the paramedic should tell the patient about alternative facilities for health care for the patient's present condition. The paramedic also should counsel the patient about future situations that do not require transport for emergency department evaluation. As an example, the paramedic should provide an approved list of alternative heath care sites (e.g., a minor-emergency center or health clinic) that can provide medical care at costs that are much less than those charged by emergency departments.

SUMMARY

- Certain accommodations may be needed for a hearing-impaired patient. These include helping with a patient's hearing aid, providing paper and pen to aid in communication, speaking softly into the patient's ear, and speaking in clear view of the patient.
- When caring for the visually impaired patient, the paramedic should help the patient use his or her glasses or other visual aids. The paramedic also should describe all procedures before performing them.
- Allow extra time for the history of a patient with a speech impairment. If appropriate, provide aids such as a pen and paper to assist in communication.
- When caring for an obese patient, use the proper sized diagnostic devices. Also, secure extra personnel if needed to move the patient for transport.
- When transporting patients with paraplegia or quadriplegia, extra personnel may be needed to move special equipment.
- Once rapport and trust have been established with a patient who has mental illness, the paramedic should proceed with care in the standard manner.
- When caring for a patient with developmental delays, the paramedic should allow enough time to obtain a history, perform an assessment, deliver care, and prepare for transport.
- The challenge in assessing patients with emotional impairments is distinguishing between symptoms produced by stress and those caused by serious medical illness.
- Pathological conditions may call for special assessment and management skills. The paramedic should ask about current medications and the patient's normal level of functioning.
- Diversity refers to differences of any kind. These include race, class, religion, gender, sexual preference, personal habitat, and physical ability. Good health care depends on sensitivity toward these differences.
- Often, calls involving the care of a terminally ill patient will be emotionally charged. They require a great deal of empathy and compassion for the patient and his or her loved ones.
- Some infectious diseases will take a toll on the emotional well-being of affected patients, their families, and loved ones. Paramedics should be sensitive to the psychological needs of the patient and his or her family.
- Financial challenges can deprive a patient of basic health care services. These patients may be reluctant to seek care for illness or injury.

REFERENCES

1. American Academy of Ophthalmology: Statistics on blindness. http://upshawinst.org/mehrc/statistics.htm. Accessed March 29, 2005.
2. American Obesity Association: AOA fact sheets. http://www.obesity.org/subs/fastfacts/obesity_what2.shtml. Accessed November 3, 2004.
3. US Department of Transportation, National Highway Traffic Safety Administration: *EMT-Paramedic national standard curriculum,* Washington, DC, 1998, The Department.
4. American Heart Association: *Basic life support for healthcare providers,* Dallas, 1997, The Association.
5. Thibodeau G, Patton K: *Anatomy and physiology,* ed 2, St Louis, 1993, Mosby.
6. PsyWeb.com: Mental retardation (developmental disability). http://www.psyweb.com/Mdisord/menret.html. Accessed August 6, 2004.
7. Lissauer T, Clayden C: *Illustrated textbook of pediatrics,* St Louis, 1997, Mosby.
8. Spina Bifida Association of America. http://www.sbaa.org/html/sbaa_latex.html.
9. Howard JF Jr: *Myasthenia gravis: a summary,* St Paul, Minn, 1997, Myasthenia Gravis Foundation of America. http://www.myasthenia.org/information/summary.htm.
10. Department of Health and Human Services: *Statement by Dr. Claude Earl Fox,* Health Resources and Services Administration, on Fiscal Year 1999 President's Budget Request for the Health Resources and Services Administration. http://commdocs.house.gov/committees/approps/hapLABPAR3.000/hapLABPAR3_0.HTM. Accessed March 10, 2004.
11. National Coalition for the Homeless: *Healthcare and homelessness,* Washington, DC, 1999, The Coalition.
12. US Department of Transportation, National Highway Traffic Safety Administration, US Department of Health and Human Services: *Emergency medical services: agenda for the future,* Washington, DC, 1996, The Department.

CHAPTER

48

Acute Interventions for the Home Health Care Patient

OBJECTIVES

Upon completion of this chapter, the paramedic student will be able to:

1. Discuss general issues related to the home health care patient.
2. Outline general principles of assessment and management of the home health care patient.
3. Describe medical equipment, assessment, and management of the home health care patient with inadequate respiratory support.
4. Identify assessment findings and acute interventions for problems related to vascular access devices in the home health care setting.
5. Describe medical equipment, assessment, and management of the patient with a gastrointestinal or genitourinary crisis in the home health care setting.
6. Identify key assessments and principles of wound care management in the home health care patient.
7. Outline maternal/child problems that may be encountered early in the postpartum period in the home health care setting.
8. Describe medical therapy associated with hospice and comfort care in the home health care setting.

KEY TERMS

bronchopulmonary dysplasia: A chronic respiratory disorder characterized by scarring of lung tissue, thickened pulmonary arterial walls, and ventilation-perfusion mismatch; often occurs in infants who have long-term dependence on artificial ventilation.

colostomy: A surgical opening into the large intestine.

failure to thrive: The abnormal retardation of the growth and development of an infant resulting from conditions that interfere with normal metabolism, appetite, and activity.

ileostomy: A surgical opening into the small intestine.

obstructive apnea: A form of sleep apnea involving a physical obstruction of the upper airways that can lead to pulmonary failure, chronic fatigue, and cardiac abnormalities.

ostomy: An artificial opening into the urinary tract, gastrointestinal tract, or trachea; any surgical procedure in which an opening is created between two hollow organs or between a hollow viscus and the abdominal wall.

palliative care: A unique form of health care primarily directed at providing relief to terminally ill persons through symptom management and pain management; also known as comfort care.

urosepsis: Septic poisoning caused by retention and absorption of urinary products in the tissues.

The cost-driven allocation of health care resources and advances in technology have led to shortened hospital stays. This also has allowed many patients to be treated in the home setting. An estimated 7.6 million persons in the United States require home health care services because of acute illness, long-term health conditions, personal preference, permanent disability, or terminal illness.[1] Paramedics likely will play a key role in providing acute interventions to these patients.

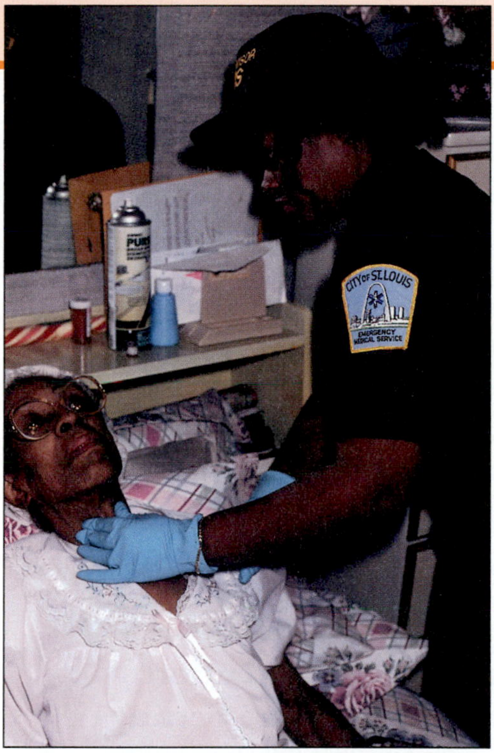

OVERVIEW OF HOME HEALTH CARE

Home health care started in the United States in the late 1800s as a direct result of rapid city growth and an increase in the number of immigrants moving into large cities.[2] The emphasis of home health care at that time was on personal hygiene and preventive care. The health services were provided by visiting nurses. These nurses worked in tenements to assist the poor. They also cared for wealthy and middle-class families after births or discharges from hospitals. At first, few physicians were associated with most of these home health care groups.

Until the mid-1960s, home health care continued to focus on the poor. The rest of the population received care in hospitals and doctors' offices. With the passage of the Social Security Act Amendments (commonly known as Medicare) in 1965, home health care became a benefit to older adult patients receiving Medicare. This greatly accelerated growth of the industry. (In 1973, these services were extended to certain disabled younger Americans; hospice benefits were added in 1983.) By 1997, an estimated 38.5 million older adult and disabled Americans were enrolled in Medicare programs, and 3.4 million Medicare recipients received home health services.[3] Medicare is the single largest payer of home care services in the United States. Other funding sources include Medicaid, the Older Americans Act, Title XX Social Services Block Grants, the Veterans Administration, TRICARE/CHAMPUS for military personnel, private insurance, and managed care organizations.

In recent years, federal health care reform has led to the development of managed care services that are provided to members by managed care organizations (see Chapter 1).

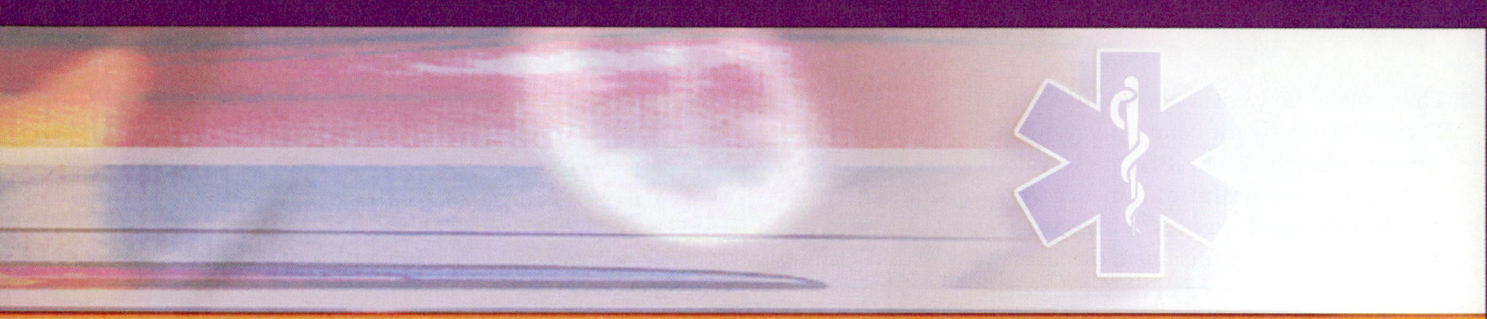

These plans now cover about 40% of the U.S. population. They have greatly influenced methods of health care delivery (including home health care services).

Today, home health care incorporates a wide variety of health and social services. These services are provided at home to recovering, disabled, or chronically ill and terminally ill persons in need of medical, nursing, social, or therapeutic treatment and help with the essential activities of daily living. The following is a sampling of services provided to home health care patients:

- Skilled nursing services
- Physical, speech, and occupational therapy
- Medical social services
- Home health aides
- Nutritional counseling

Advanced Life Support Response to Home Health Care Patients

About 25% of home health care patients have conditions related to diseases of the circulatory system as their primary diagnosis.[4] (Persons with heart disease, including congestive heart failure, make up about half of this group.) Other common diagnoses of home health care patients include cancer, diabetes, chronic lung disease, renal failure/dialysis, and hypertension. Thus emergency responses for home health care patients likely will be more common for emergency medical services (EMS) agencies. Typical emergencies may include respiratory failure, cardiac decompensation, septic complications, equipment malfunction, and other conditions that worsen in the home health care setting (Box 48-1).

Injury Control and Prevention in the Home Health Care Setting

The scientific approach to illness and injury prevention as a means to minimize morbidity and mortality is discussed in Chapter 3. Readers should refer to these areas to review primary prevention, acute care, and rehabilitation (tertiary prevention); their concepts; and their strategies.

INFECTION CONTROL

As with all other patient encounters, the paramedic should practice infection control in the home health care setting. Infection control includes using standard precautions and body substance isolation (or transmission-based precautions) when indicated. This practice, along with treating all patients as though they have an infectious disease, forms the basis for infection control guidelines recommended by the Centers for Disease Control and Prevention. The Occupational Safety and Health Administration, Centers for Disease Control and Prevention, and Environmental Protection Agency recommend the same infection control standards for the treatment of home health care patients as for acute care patients. Equipment set forth by these agencies for infection control in the home setting includes the following:

- Mask
- Gown
- Goggles, glasses, or face shield
- Resuscitation mask
- Specimen bags
- Environmental Protection Agency–approved disinfectant effective against hepatitis B virus, human immunodeficiency virus, and tuberculosis
- Soap and water
- Disposable paper towels
- Impervious trash bags and labels

This text assumes that the proper personal protection will be used by paramedics. The nature of the emergency and the patient's condition will dictate what protection to use.

BOX 48-1 Examples of Home Health Care Problems

Home Care Services Requiring Intervention by a Home Health Care Practitioner or Physician

Acquired immunodeficiency syndrome
Cardiopulmonary care
Catheter management/intravenous therapy infusion
Chemotherapy
Dermatological and wound care
Gastroenterological and ostomy care
Hospice care
Organ transplantation
Orthopedic care
Pain management
Rehabilitative care
Specimen collection
Urological and renal care

Home Health Care Problems Requiring Acute Intervention

Acute cardiac events
Acute infections
Acute respiratory events
Gastrointestinal/genitourinary crisis
Hospice/comfort care
Inadequate respiratory support
Maternal/child conditions
Vascular access complications

CRITICAL THINKING

What factors decrease the risks of spreading infection within a home health care setting versus a hospital?

Types of Home Care Patients

The need to reduce the costs of health care and technological advances in medicine have allowed many types of patients to receive home care. Many EMS agencies ask their communities to notify them when someone is on a complex home health care program. That way, a visit can be made to the home. This allows EMS providers to become familiar with the patient's condition and special equipment before an emergency. Classifications of home health care patients include those with the following conditions[5]:

- Pathological conditions of the airway causing inadequate pulmonary toilet or inadequate alveolar ventilation and/or oxygenation
- Circulatory pathological conditions causing alterations in peripheral circulation (e.g., pressure ulcers, delayed healing, or infection)
- Gastrointestinal/genitourinary conditions requiring special devices such as ostomies, feeding catheters, and special equipment needed for home dialysis
- Infection from cellulitis or systemic illness (e.g., sepsis)
- Wounds that require care (e.g., surgical wound closure, decubitus wounds, and surgical drains)

Other patient groups the paramedic may encounter in the home health care setting include patients receiving hospice care, expectant or new mothers, patients with dementia or other conditions that require psychological support for the patient or family, patients receiving chemotherapy or home care for chronic pain, and patients with organ transplants or those who are waiting for organ transplantation (transport candidate).

GENERAL PRINCIPLES AND MANAGEMENT

Scene Size-up

When paramedics arrive at the scene of a home health care patient, the scene size-up should include standard precautions, elements of scene safety, and an assessment of the patient's environment (environmental setting).

STANDARD PRECAUTIONS

As with all patient care, paramedics should use standard precautions to guard against communicable disease. Equipment that may be found in the home health care setting includes containers of medical waste, ostomy collection bags, tracheostomy tubes, sharps, soiled dressings, and other equipment (e.g., emesis basins, walkers, and wheelchairs) that may be contaminated with the patient's body fluids. In addition to personal precautions, the EMS crew should ensure that any infectious waste found in the home is contained properly. The waste should be disposed of per protocol.

SCENE SAFETY

Whenever an EMS response is made to a person's home, the paramedic should evaluate the scene for the presence of dangerous pets, firearms and other home protection devices, and for any home hazards (e.g., inadequate lighting, icy sidewalks, or steep stair wells). For the safety of the EMS crew, the patient, and others at the scene, all potential hazards found in a home must be contained or remedied. For example, it may be necessary to request law enforcement to help with unruly or hostile bystanders; and extra personnel and special equipment may be needed to help move a patient down a flight of steps for transport.

ENVIRONMENTAL SETTING

The paramedic should assess the setting for the patient's ability to maintain a healthy environment. Examples include cleanliness of the home; evidence of basic nutritional support; and needs of heat, water, shelter, and electricity. The EMS crew also should note any signs of abuse or neglect. Other factors to note are the cleanliness and condition of any medical devices. (For example, this includes clean oxygen and ventilation equipment and wheelchairs and hospital beds that are in good repair.)

Patient Assessment

The initial patient assessment should focus on illness or injury that poses a threat to life and take the appropriate measures as indicated (see Chapter 12). After the initial assessment, the paramedic should obtain a focused history and perform a physical examination. The paramedic should make use of any medical documents found in the home (e.g., patient records kept by home health care providers and do-not-resuscitate orders). The paramedic also should gather information from family and health care professionals (e.g., a home care nurse or physical or respiratory therapist) who may be present at the scene. Critical findings should alert the paramedic to forgo a detailed assessment and proceed with resuscitation measures and rapid transport for physician evaluation. If there are no critical findings, the paramedic should perform a physical examination that considers the possibility of medication interactions, compliance with the treatment regimen, and the possibility of dementia or a metabolic disturbance in a patient with an altered mental status.

A comprehensive assessment may include a physical examination using inspection, palpation, auscultation, and percussion (as indicated by the patient's condition and chief complaint). The ongoing assessment should evaluate any changes in the patient's status while at the scene or en route to the hospital. These assessment strategies can aid in differential diagnosis, treatment, and direction of patient management.

Management and Treatment Plan

Depending on the patient's condition, the home health care treatment may need to be replaced with advanced life support measures. These measures may include airway, ventilatory, and circulatory support and pharmacological and nonpharmacological therapy (e.g., electrical therapy).

Some patients with acute illness or injury need to be transported to the hospital for evaluation. When transport is needed, the paramedic must give special consideration for patient packaging and for moving the patient's equipment. Examples include properly securing intravenous (IV) catheters, urinary catheters, and feeding tubes; and ensuring available personnel to assist with moving patient care devices such as ventilation equipment. Family members at the scene often are well versed on the patient's medical devices. They usually will be eager to help when asked by the

EMS crew. If there is no family at the scene, the EMS crew should attempt to contact a family member or caregiver and advise this person of the patient's condition and hospital destination.

Other patients need only home care follow-up by home health care practitioners, or they may need a referral to other public service agencies. The paramedic should follow protocol and consult with medical direction about referrals and the need for notifying private physicians or home health care agencies. Regardless of the need for EMS transport, the paramedic should document completely all findings and any care provided on the care report.

CRITICAL THINKING

What feelings may a patient's family member (or caregiver) in the home setting have if there is a problem and the patient's condition worsens?

SPECIFIC ACUTE HOME HEALTH CARE INTERVENTIONS

Acute home health care emergencies may occur from equipment failure or malfunction, drug reactions, complications related to home treatment, and worsening medical conditions. This section discusses acute interventions for respiratory support, vascular access devices, gastrointestinal/genitourinary crisis, acute infections, maternal/child conditions, and hospice/**palliative care.**

Respiratory Support

More than 630,000 patients are discharged to home health care with diseases of the respiratory system each year.[1] These patients are at increased risk for airway infections. The progression of some respiratory diseases also may lead to an increased respiratory demand, making current support inadequate. Examples of chronic pathological conditions that require home respiratory support include the following:

- Asthma
- Awaiting lung transplant
- **Bronchopulmonary dysplasia**
- Chronic lung disease
- Cystic fibrosis
- Infection causing exacerbation of condition
- Sleep apnea

Acute interventions may be required for these patients. Any patient with respiratory distress should receive high-concentration oxygen and ventilatory support as priorities in care. Problems that may lead to a request for EMS assistance include increased respiratory demand, increased bronchospasm, increased secretions, obstructed or malfunctioning respiratory devices, or improper application of medical devices to support respirations.

OXYGEN THERAPY IN THE HOME SETTING

Three common ways to provide oxygen therapy in the home are compressed gas, liquid oxygen, and oxygen concentrators. Compressed gas is oxygen stored under pressure in oxygen cylinders equipped with a regulator that controls flow rate. Liquid oxygen is cold and is stored in a container similar to a thermos. When released, the liquid converts to gas and is used like compressed gas. An oxygen concentrator is an electrically powered device that separates oxygen from air, concentrates it, and stores it (Fig. 48-1). This system does not have to be resupplied and is not as costly as liquid oxygen. A cylinder of oxygen must be available as a backup, however, in case of power failure.

CRITICAL THINKING

What safety precautions for administering oxygen should be in place in the home setting?

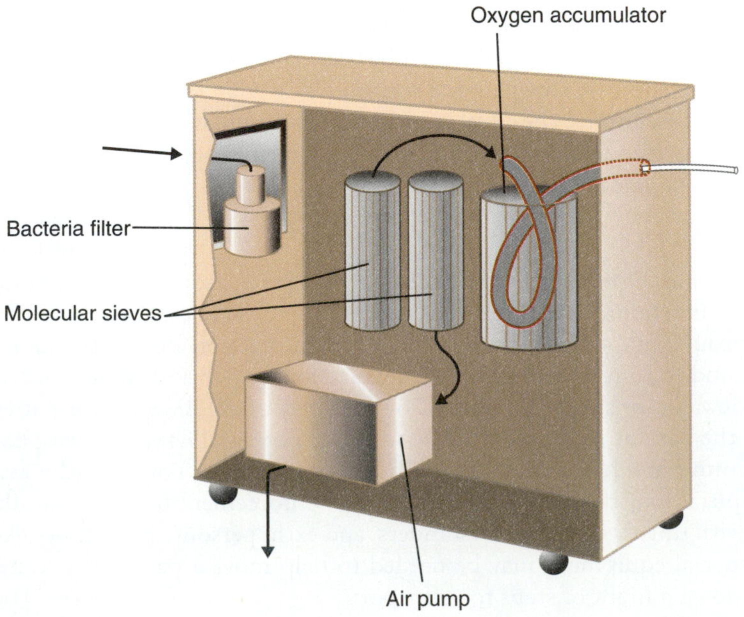

FIGURE 48-1 ■ Oxygen concentrator.

Oxygen is delivered to patients via nasal cannulae, oxygen masks, tracheostomy collars (devices that deliver high humidity and oxygen to patients with surgical airways), and ventilators. Some patients may require continuous positive airway pressure (CPAP) delivered by ventilatory support systems through mask CPAP, nasal CPAP, or biphasic positive airway pressure (BIPAP). As described in Chapter 30, the BIPAP ventilatory support system (designed for mask-applied ventilation in the home) delivers two different levels of positive airway pressure. The system cycles spontaneously between a preset level of inspiratory positive airway pressure and expiratory positive airway pressure. The BIPAP ventilatory support system is intended only to augment the patient's breathing; it does not provide for total ventilatory requirements. The BIPAP system is used by some patients with sleep apnea or chronic obstructive pulmonary disease.

Supportive ventilator management may be indicated to achieve the following:

- Prevent nocturnal hypoxemia caused by sleep hypoventilation in patients with neuromuscular disorders (e.g., muscular dystrophy or myasthenia gravis).
- Prevent respiratory fatigue in patients with chronic obstructive pulmonary disease.
- Improve ventilation and oxygen saturation in patients with **obstructive apnea,** a form of sleep apnea involving a physical obstruction of the upper airways that can lead to pulmonary failure, chronic fatigue, and cardiac abnormalities.

Home Ventilators. Home ventilators can be classified as *volume ventilators, pressure ventilators,* and *negative-pressure ventilators.* Most ventilators have a number of controls and ventilator settings. Box 48-2 describes some of these settings.

Volume ventilators (volume-preset) deliver a predetermined volume of gas with each cycle, after which inspiration is terminated. These types of ventilators deliver a constant tidal volume regardless of changes in airway resistance or compliance of the lungs and thorax. The volume remains the same unless very high peak airway pressures are reached. In that case, safety release valves stop the flow (Box 48-3; Table 48-1).

Pressure ventilators (pressure-preset) are pressure-cycled devices that terminate inspiration when a preset pressure is achieved. When the preset pressure is reached, the gas flow stops, and the patient passively exhales. These ventilators most often are used for patients whose ventilatory resistance is not likely to change.

Negative-pressure ventilators have settings for the respiratory rate and pressure of the negative force exerted. These devices use negative pressure to raise the rib cage and lower the diaphragm. This creates negative pressure within the lungs so that air flows into the lungs. Negative-pressure ventilators often are used for patients with healthy lungs who have a muscular inability to inhale. (For example, this may include patients with spinal cord injury or neuromuscular disease.) Examples of this type of ventilator are the "iron lung" and plastic wrap, or poncho, ventilators.

ASSESSMENT FINDINGS

When caring for a patient who requires oxygen therapy, the paramedic should evaluate the patient's work of breathing, tidal volume, peak flow, oxygen saturation, and quality of breath sounds. This assessment can be performed with visual inspection (chest rise and fall), peak flow meters, pulse oximetry, and auscultation (described in Chapters 19 and 30). The paramedic should be alert for signs and symptoms of hypoxia, including the following:

- Confusion and mental status changes
- Cyanosis
- Dyspnea
- Headache
- Hypertension
- Hyperventilation
- Restlessness
- Tachycardia

MANAGEMENT

Management goals for a patient receiving oxygen therapy who requires acute intervention are to improve airway patency, ventilation, and oxygenation.

BOX 48-2 Standard Initial Ventilator Settings

FiO_2 (fraction of inspired oxygen)	100%
Tidal volume	10 to 15 mL/kg body mass
Respiratory rate	10 to 15 breaths/min
Inspiratory flow	40 to 60 L/sec
Sensitivity	12 cm H_2O
Sigh rate (optional)	1 to 2/min

BOX 48-3 Ventilator Alarms

Ventilators are equipped with alarms. These alarms signal that there are problems with ventilator function. There are alarms for loss of power, frequency alarms (indicating changes in respiratory rate), volume alarms (indicating low-exhaled volume or low/high minute-ventilation), and high-pressure alarms. If alarms are sounding, the paramedic should check for the following possible causes:

- Kinks in endotracheal tube
- Disconnected ventilator tubing or poor connections
- Water in ventilator tubing
- Excessive secretions
- Pneumothorax
- Patient anxiety

After consulting with medical direction, acute interventions may include providing temporary ventilation assistance with a bag-valve-mask device, repositioning the endotracheal tube, correcting poor ventilator tube connections, emptying water from tube or water traps, suctioning the airway, thoracic decompression, and possible sedation.

TABLE 48-1 Ventilator Alarms

ALARM TYPE	CAUSES	INTERVENTIONS
High pressure	Increased secretions	Suction secretions from patient.
High pressure	Kinked tubing	Unkink tubing.
High pressure	Water in tubing	Disconnect tubing and allow it to drain.
High pressure	Anxiety	Decrease anxiety by providing a calm environment.
Low pressure	Disconnected tubing	Reconnect tubing.
Low pressure	Cuff leak	Add 1 mL of air at a time to pilot balloon of tracheostomy tube.
Low pressure	Tracheostomy tube out	Reinsert new tracheostomy tube.
Oxygen	Insufficient oxygen supply	Manually ventilate patient and prepare for transport.
Ventilator not operating	Power failure	Manually ventilate patient and prepare for transport.

Note: A memory aid useful for identifying possible causes of ventilator malfunction is DOPE. This stands for *d*isplacement of the tube, *o*bstruction of the tube, *p*neumothorax, and *e*quipment failure.

Improving Airway Patency. To improve airway patency, the paramedic first should reposition airway devices (e.g., face masks and nasal cannulae) to ensure they are applied properly and are well fitted. The paramedic should clear secretions that obstruct airflow from the airway with suction. The paramedic should clear secretions from any airway device using sterile water. If needed, the home airway device should be replaced with a new device. A tracheostomy tube that has become blocked and cannot be cleared may need to be replaced with another tracheostomy tube to ensure adequate ventilation. (Or the tube can be replaced temporarily with an endotracheal tube.) (See Chapter 19.)

Improving Ventilation and Oxygenation. If ventilation does not improve after providing a patent airway, the paramedic should remove the home ventilator care device. The paramedic then should assist the patient's ventilations with positive-pressure ventilation via a bag-valve-mask device and supplemental oxygen. Oxygen saturation should be monitored with pulse oximetry. The paramedic also should administer supplemental oxygen as needed to maintain oxygen saturation at 90% or higher. Medical direction may advise adjusting the settings of a home care device or changing the flow rate of an oxygen delivery device to improve ventilation and oxygenation. Extra personnel may be needed to assist in moving the patient who has a ventilator device to the ambulance for transport for evaluation.

On some ventilators the inspiratory flow rate is determined by tidal volume, respiratory rate, and the inspiratory/expiratory ratio. (This ratio is generally 1:2. This allows for complete exhalation and prevents air trapping.) On other ventilators the flow rate is set independently. This allows for adjustment of air flow to the flow wave pattern that is most comfortable for the patient. If the patient is having difficulty with spontaneous breathing, an increase in the flow rate may be indicated. However, a higher flow rate means a shorter inspiratory time and usually a higher respiratory pressure because of increased resistance. A lower flow rate requires a longer inspiratory time with a decreased inspiratory pressure. The paramedic should always consult with medical direction before changing the flow rate on any ventilator.

PSYCHOLOGICAL SUPPORT AND COMMUNICATION STRATEGIES

Difficulty breathing can be a horrifying experience for the patient, especially for a patient who depends on a ventilator. The paramedic crew should try to calm the patient and family. The crew should assure them that respirations will be supported adequately by other means while at the scene and during transport.

Some patients with tracheostomies have special valves attached to the tracheostomy tube ("talking trachs") that redirect exhaled air around the tracheostomy tube, through the vocal cords, and out of the mouth and nose. This allows for normal speech. Loss of verbal communication is a major source of anxiety in patients who have tracheostomies. The ability to communicate with these patients will be based on the patient's cognition, level of consciousness, language, and fine and gross motor skills. Methods of communication may include signing and writing on notepads. The paramedic should enlist the help of family and other caregivers in communicating with the patient.

Vascular Access Devices

Many patients in the home care setting have indwelling vascular access devices (VADs). Vascular access devices are used to provide nutritional support. They also are used to administer medications. In addition, VADs are used for patients who need long-term vascular access. (For example, this includes patients receiving dialysis or chemotherapy.). Those with indwelling vascular devices may experience problems, including the following:

- Anticoagulation associated with percutaneous or implanted devices
- Embolus formation associated with indwelling devices, stasis, and inactivity

NOTE Congestive heart failure is a common reason for hospitalization. Attempts often are made to manage these patients at home when possible. Thus paramedics may find patients with congestive heart failure receiving medications (e.g., ***dobutamine*** or ***furosemide***) intravenously in the home setting.

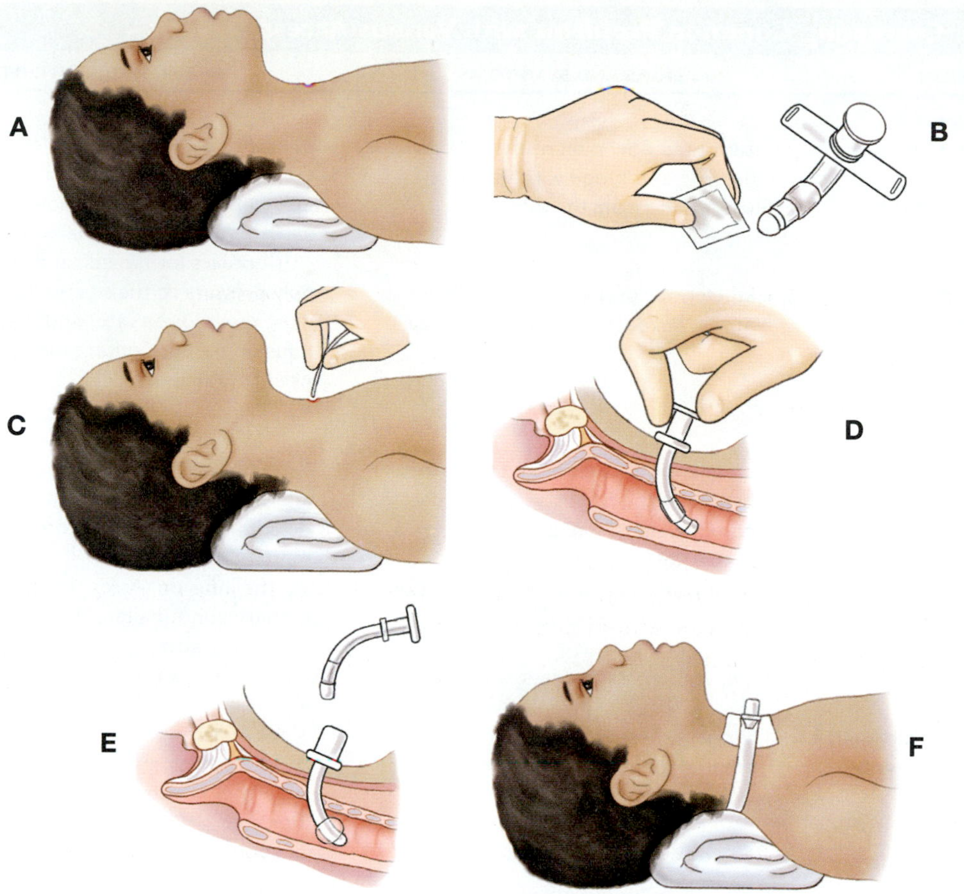

FIGURE 48-2 ■ Replacement of a tracheostomy tube. **A,** Position the child with padding under the shoulders. **B,** Select a tube the same size or one size smaller than the one removed and moisten with sterile, water-soluble lubricant. **C,** Suction the stoma and trachea before insertion of the new tube. **D,** Insert the tube gently into the trachea with the curve pointing downward. **E,** If the tube has an obturator, remove it; if it is a cuffed tube, inflate the cuff. **F,** Assess for correct tube placement and secure the tube.

- Air embolus associated with central venous access devices
- Obstructed or malfunctioning VADs
- Infection at the access site
- Infiltration and extravasation
- Obstructed dialysis shunts

TYPES

A variety of VADs are encountered in home health care patients. These include surgically implanted subcutaneous VADs, medication delivery devices (e.g., Mediports, as described in Chapter 18), peripheral VADs (e.g., peripherally inserted central catheters and midline catheters), central venous tunneled catheters (e.g., Hickman, Groshong, or Broviac), and dialysis shunts (Fig. 48-2).

ASSESSMENT FINDINGS AND ACUTE INTERVENTIONS

Certain assessment findings may require acute interventions in patients with VADs. These findings include infection, hemorrhage, hemodynamic compromise from circulatory overload or embolus, obstruction of the vascular device, catheter breakage, and leakage of medication (e.g., chemotherapeutic agents) (Table 48-2).

Infection. Home health care patients who have VADs generally are instructed to examine the area for infection. They also are instructed to change the dressings around their device often. Often this is done by family members and home health care practitioners. All types of dressings must be changed immediately if they become wet, soiled, contaminated, or unocclusive. A common problem of VADs is infection near the exit site, tunnel, or port. Signs and symptoms of site infection include pain, redness, warmth, and purulence. Signs and symptoms of systemic infection (which may result from a site infection) include fever, tachycardia, general weakness, malaise, mental status changes, body aches, and possibly septicemia. General principles in managing the site infection are as follows:

CRITICAL THINKING

Will it always be possible to identify the catheter as the source of sepsis while on the scene?

TABLE 48-2 Correcting Common Problems with Venous Access Devices

COMPLICATION	SIGNS AND SYMPTOMS	PREHOSPITAL INTERVENTIONS
Mechanical Problems		
Clotted intravenous catheter	Interrupted flow rate, resistance to flushing and blood withdrawal	Attempt to aspirate the clot. If unsuccessful, contact medical direction.
Cracked or broken tubing	Fluid leaking from the tubing	Apply padded hemostat above the break to prevent air from entering the line and change the tubing (with orders from medical direction).
Dislodged catheter	Catheter out of the vein	Apply pressure to the site with a sterile gauze pad.
Too-rapid infusion	Nausea, headache, lethargy, dyspnea	Adjust the infusion rate, and if applicable, check the infusion pump. Contact medical direction about need to transport.
Other Problems		
Air embolism	Apprehension, chest pain, tachycardia, hypotension, cyanosis, seizures, loss of consciousness, and cardiac arrest	Clamp the catheter. Place the patient in a steep, left lateral Trendelenburg position. Give oxygen as ordered. If cardiac arrest occurs, begin cardiopulmonary resuscitation.
Extravasation	Swelling and pain around the insertion site	Stop the infusion. Assess the patient for cardiopulmonary abnormalities. Notify medical direction for further advice.
Phlebitis	Pain, tenderness, redness, and warmth	Apply gentle heat to the area; elevate insertion site if possible.
Pneumothorax and hydrothorax	Dyspnea, chest pain, cyanosis, and decreased breath sounds	If signs and symptoms of tension pneumothorax are present, consider needle decompression after consulting with medical direction. Rapid transport is indicated.
Septicemia	Red and swollen catheter site, chills, fever	Transport for physician evaluation.
Thrombosis	Erythema and edema at the insertion site; ipsilateral swelling of the arm, neck, face, and upper chest; pain at the insertion site and along the vein; malaise; fever; tachycardia	Apply warm compresses to insertion site; elevate affected extremity. Transport patient.
Hemorrhage	Bleeding at site of venous access device or from broken device	Apply pressure to site. Clamp venous access device and treat for shock.

1. Use aseptic technique when examining the line.
2. Clean the site with alcohol (per protocol).
3. Apply antimicrobial ointment (per protocol). (This is controversial.)
4. Cover the site with a transparent, sterile dressing (per protocol).
5. Document the procedure. Label the dressing with the date, time, and paramedic's initials.
6. Consult with medical direction.

Hemorrhage. Bleeding at the site of a VAD should be controlled by applying gentle, direct pressure with aseptic technique. These patients need to be transported for physician evaluation. Blood loss from a broken or dislodged VAD can be significant. If blood loss is severe, the patient should be treated for hemorrhagic shock.

Hemodynamic Compromise. Hemodynamic compromise may result from circulatory overload or embolus. Circulatory overload can develop from too much IV fluid delivered too fast. Signs and symptoms of circulatory overload include a rise in blood pressure, distended neck veins, pulmonary congestion (crackles and wheezes), and dyspnea. If circulatory overload is suspected, the paramedic should do the following:

1. Slow the infusion to a keep-open rate.
2. Provide high-concentration oxygen.
3. Elevate the patient's head.
4. Maintain body warmth. This will promote peripheral circulation. It also will ease the stress on the central veins.
5. Monitor vital signs.
6. Consult with medical direction for patient management and disposition.

CRITICAL THINKING

What drug(s) may the physician order if this happens?

Displacement of a surgically implanted catheter or port is rare. However, an embolus that occurs from air, throm-

BOX 48-4 Causes of Embolus Formation

Air Embolism
Intravenous fluid containers that run dry
Air in intravenous tubing
Loose connections in catheter tubing
Catheter tears and breakage

Thrombus
Clot formation from inactivity or stasis

Plastic or Catheter Tip Migration
Plastic or catheter fragment from tugging or shearing forces
Wire from central line placement

bus, or plastic or catheter tip entering the circulation can develop (Box 48-4). Signs and symptoms of an embolus include hypotension; cyanosis; weak, rapid pulse; and loss of consciousness. A patient suspected of having an embolism should be managed as follows (described in Chapter 18):

1. Stop the IV infusion.
2. Position the patient on the left side with the head down (in an attempt to keep the embolus in the right side of the heart).
3. Administer high-concentration oxygen.
4. Notify medical direction.

If a plastic or catheter tip embolism is suspected, medical direction may advise that a constricting band be applied above the VAD site. This should stop the embolus from further movement.

Obstruction of the Vascular Device. An indwelling vascular device may become obstructed. This would disrupt the flow of fluids and medications. When this occurs, immediate intervention is needed. The device must be cleared by irrigation or the administration of fibrinolytic agents. The paramedic should always consult with medical direction before trying to clear an obstruction from a VAD. The most experienced paramedic should perform this procedure.

Flushing and Irrigation. Vascular access devices and medication ports need regular irrigation with normal saline and/or ***heparin.*** The solution used depends on the type of VAD (Table 48-3). The frequency of irrigation depends on the specific device and on the frequency of medication administration. If a VAD is obstructed, the paramedic should consult with medical direction. The paramedic also should follow these steps:

1. Explain the procedure to the patient.
2. Prepare prescribed irrigation solutions (normal saline or normal saline and ***heparin***).
3. Clean the injection cap(s) with an antiseptic and alcohol wipe (per protocol) and allow to air dry.
4. Release the clamp from the catheter (if present).
5. Irrigate the lumen with an appropriate volume of solution using a 10-mL syringe (no faster than 0.5 mL/sec). If resistance is persistent, stop the irrigation, or the catheter may rupture. *Note:* The paramedic must never try to force or dislodge a clot or other obstruction. Fibrinolytic agents may be required. The application of force could dislodge the obstruction and cause it to enter the circulatory system.
6. Aspirate blood back into the syringe; this removes clots or fibrin sheaths.
7. Flush with normal saline (10 to 20 mL) to clear system.
8. Use a heparin lock if necessary (e.g., Broviac, Hickman, or peripherally inserted central catheter).
9. Clamp catheter if needed.
10. Loop the catheter with the cap pointing upward on the dressing. Secure with tape.
11. Properly dispose of all equipment.

TABLE 48-3 Irrigation for Vascular Access Devices

DEVICE	SYRINGE SIZE	SOLUTION	AMOUNT
Peripheral Access Devices			
	3 mL	Heparin flush solution 10 units/mL	2.5-3.0 mL
Central Venous Access Devices			
Groshong	10 mL	0.9% sodium chloride (normal saline)	5 mL; 10-20 mL following blood draws
Mediports	10 mL	Sodium chloride 0.9% (normal saline)	10 mL
		Heparin 100 units/mL	5 mL

From Terry J: *Intravenous therapy: clinical principles and practice,* Philadelphia, 1995, Saunders.

Anticoagulant Therapy. At times, a medication port or other vascular device may require declotting with fibrinolytic agents. The paramedic should always consult with medical direction before using anticoagulant therapy. The following are the steps to follow in declotting a Port-A-Cath device:

1. Explain the procedure to the patient.
2. Prepare the necessary solutions and 1 mL of normal saline solution in a 3-mL syringe with a noncoring (Huber) needle.
3. Using sterile technique, clean the injection cap or area of skin over the Port-A-Cath septum with alcohol (per protocol). Allow it to air dry.
4. Connect the syringe to the integrated extension tubing. Unclamp the tubing.
5. Slowly inject the solution into the occluded lumen and port of the Port-A-Cath. Wait 30 minutes (if the patient is not being transported).
6. Try to aspirate the residual clot.
7. Repeat the procedure with a 15-minute dwell time if patency is not achieved.

8. Notify medical direction if the catheter cannot be aspirated. If patency is achieved, follow the previously described procedure for flushing and irrigation.
9. Properly dispose of all equipment.

Catheter Damage. A damaged (e.g., cracked or torn) catheter can allow fluids or medications to infiltrate into the surrounding tissues. This can lead to an air embolism. Signs and symptoms of a damaged catheter include leaking fluid, complaint of a burning sensation, or swollen and tender skin near the insertion site. If catheter damage is suspected, the infusion should be stopped immediately. The catheter should be clamped between the crack or tear in the catheter and the patient. These patients are managed with high-concentration oxygen, IV access through a peripheral vein, and transport for physician evaluation. A patient who develops an altered level of consciousness (indicating a possible air embolism) should be positioned on the left side. The head should be slightly lowered. This positioning will help to prevent the embolism from traveling to the brain.

BOX 48-5 Medical Therapy Found in the Home Setting for Patients with Gastrointestinal/Genitourinary Disease

Devices for Gastric/Intestinal Emptying or Feeding

Colostomy
Feeding tube
Nasogastric tube
Percutaneous endoscopic gastrostomy tubes, jejunostomy tubes, gastrostomy tubes

Devices for the Urinary Tract

External urinary catheters (e.g., condom catheter or Texas catheter)
Indwelling urinary catheter (e.g., Foley catheter or Coudé catheter)
Surgical urinary catheters (e.g., suprapubic catheters)
Urostomy

Gastrointestinal/Genitourinary Crisis

More than 500,000 patients with diseases of the digestive or genitourinary system are discharged to home health care each year.[1] Some of these patients have medical devices such as urinary catheters or urostomies, indwelling nutritional support devices (e.g., percutaneous endoscopic gastrostomy tube or gastrostomy tube), colostomies, and nasogastric tubes (Box 48-5). Acute interventions that may be required for these patients can result from urinary tract infection (UTI), **urosepsis,** urinary retention, and problems with gastric emptying or feeding.

URINARY TRACT INFECTION, UROSEPSIS, AND URINARY RETENTION

Urinary tract infection is common. It occurs in all age groups and both sexes (see Chapter 35). The organisms most often associated with UTI are gram-negative organisms normally found in the gastrointestinal tract. These include *Escherichia coli, Klebsiella, Proteus, Enterobacter,* and *Pseudomonas.* These frequently are introduced from the hands of health care personnel at the time of bladder catheterization.[6] (About 75% of UTIs are the result of urological instrumentation. Sterile technique during these procedures is crucial.) Other factors that increase the risk of UTI include the following:

- Obstructions (e.g., urethral strictures, calculi, tumors, or blood clots)
- Trauma (e.g., abdominal injury, ruptured bladder, or local trauma related to sexual activity)
- Congenital anomalies (e.g., polycystic kidneys, horseshoe kidney, or spina bifida)
- Abdominal or gynecological surgery
- Acute or chronic renal failure
- Immunocompromised state (e.g., patients with human immunodeficiency virus or older adults)
- Postpartum state
- Aging changes, particularly in women

If UTI is allowed to progress, it may lead to septic complications (urosepsis). This disease is managed with antibiotics.

Urinary Retention. Urinary retention may result from urethral stricture, inflammation, enlarged prostate, central nervous system dysfunction, foreign body obstruction, and use of certain drugs, such as parasympatholytic or anticholinergic agents. These patients need to be evaluated by a physician to determine the cause of the retention. If the cause is not easily correctable, the patient may need to be hospitalized.

Some patients may require bladder catheterization with an indwelling Foley catheter device. This procedure may be indicated to empty the bladder of a patient with urinary retention or replace an indwelling urinary catheter that is not functioning. Bladder catheterization is an invasive procedure. It carries some associated risks. These include the introduction of bacteria, which may lead to UTI; hematuria; and the creation of a false urethral passage, which may result in significant blood loss and the need for surgical repair. Special training and authorization from medical direction is required to perform bladder catheterization.

Indwelling Foley Catheter Insertion. To insert a Foley catheter, the paramedic should prepare the required equipment (e.g., Foley catheter insertion set). The paramedic also should follow closely the recommendations of the manufacturer (Box 48-6). Steps in bladder catheterization for male and female patients are described in this section. Most patients will be anxious and frightened of the procedure. The paramedic should provide a full explanation of the procedure, reassure the patient, and make every effort to ensure privacy.

CRITICAL THINKING

What measure should you take to protect yourself legally when inserting a Foley catheter into a patient in a home?

BOX 48-6 Necessary Equipment for Bladder Catheterization

Personal protective equipment
Urinary catheterization set containing the following:
- Sterile gloves
- Antiseptic solution
- Sterile cleansing sponges
- Sterile drapes or towels
- Syringe containing 5 mL sterile water
- Connecting tubing and collection bag
- Water-soluble sterile lubricant

Urinary catheter with 5-mL Foley balloon:
- Catheter usually is a number 16 Foley for males or a 14 Foley for females.
- Standard length is 18 inches.

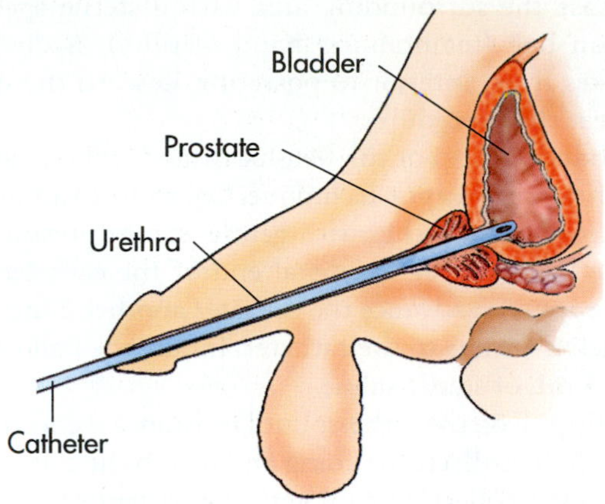

FIGURE 48-3 ■ Male catheterization.

Male Catheterization (Fig. 48-3)

1. Explain the procedure to the patient.
2. Wash hands.
3. Place the patient in supine position and remove the patient's pants and undergarments.
4. Wash hands.
5. Open the catheterization set using sterile technique.
6. Wash hands and don sterile gloves.
7. Place one sterile drape under the patient's penis and another above the penis to cover the abdomen.
8. Open a package of antiseptic solution and saturate sterile sponges (or cotton balls).
9. Attach the syringe to the catheter and test the balloon to make sure it inflates.
10. Open a package of water-soluble lubricant and lubricate the first several inches of the catheter.
11. Grasp the patient's penis with one hand and retract the foreskin (if present).
12. With the other hand, cleanse the glans with a sterile sponge (maintaining hand sterility) and then discard the sponge. Repeat the procedure.
13. Raise the shaft of the penis upright to straighten the penile urethra and pass the tip of the catheter through the meatus.
14. Continue passing the catheter with gentle, steady pressure, advancing the catheter 7 to 9 inches or until urine flows out the distal end of the catheter. Once urine appears, advance the catheter another 2 inches. If mild resistance is felt at the external sphincter, slightly increase traction on the penis and continue with steady, gentle pressure on the catheter. *If significant resistance is met, withdraw the catheter and consult with medical direction.*
15. Attach the syringe to the catheter and inflate the balloon with 3 to 5 mL of sterile saline.
16. Gently pull back on the catheter until the balloon rests against the prostatic urethra. (Resistance will be encountered.) Reposition the retracted foreskin of an uncircumcised patient. Attach the drainage bag to the catheter.

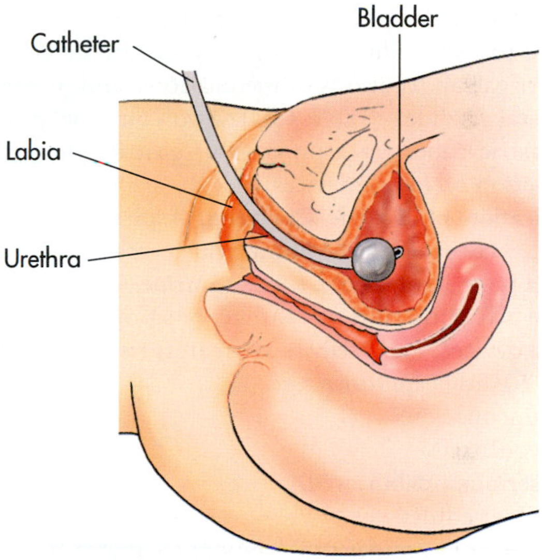

FIGURE 48-4 ■ Female catheterization.

17. Run the catheter tubing along the patient's leg and tape the connecting tubing to the patient's thigh. Do not place any tension on the catheter.
18. Attach the collection bag to the bed or stretcher at a level below that of the patient to facilitate drainage by gravity.

Female Catheterization (Fig. 48-4)

1. Prepare the patient and equipment as described in steps 1 to 4 and 6 to 8 of the previous procedure. Female patients should be positioned with knees bent, hips flexed, and feet resting about 24 inches apart. The patient should be draped appropriately by placing one sterile drape just under the patient's buttocks; position the fenestrated drape over the perineum, exposing the labia.
2. With one hand, separate the patient's labia to expose the urethral meatus.

3. Cleanse the surrounding area with a sterile sponge or cotton ball (maintaining hand sterility) in downward strokes from anterior to posterior. Discard the sponge. Repeat the procedure.
4. Introduce the tip of the well-lubricated catheter into the urethra using aseptic technique. Continue to advance the catheter 2 to 3 inches with gentle, steady pressure until urine flows out of the distal end of the catheter. Once urine appears, advance the catheter another 2 inches.
5. Attach a syringe to the catheter. Inflate the balloon with 3 to 5 mL of sterile saline.
6. Gently pull on the catheter until resistance is encountered.
7. Attach the collection tubing and bag to the catheter and secure the collection tubing to the patient's thigh as described above in steps 14 and 16 of the previous procedure. Position the collection bag to facilitate drainage.

TABLE 48-4 Feeding Tubes: Types and Placement

TYPE OF TUBE	PLACEMENT
Nasogastric	Passed via nose into stomach
Nasointestinal	Passed via nose into intestine
Esophagostomy	Passed into the esophagus tube though a surgically created opening in the anterior neck
Gastrostomy	Passed directly into the stomach through an opening created in the abdominal wall
Jejunostomy, percutaneous endoscopic gastrostomy	Passed into the jejunum through an opening created in the abdominal wall

PROBLEMS WITH GASTRIC EMPTYING OR FEEDING

Gastric tubes used in the home health care setting are devices that are inserted into the stomach or intestines. They are used to remove fluids and gas by suction or gravity, to instill irrigation solutions or medications, and to administer enteral feedings (Table 48-4). Two common problems with gastric tubes are aspiration of gastric contents and malfunction of gastric devices.

Aspiration of Gastric Contents. Aspiration of gastric contents may occur in the home health care patient as a result of a nonpatent gastric tube, improper nutritional support via a feeding tube, or patient positioning with these medical devices. The patients at greatest risk for aspiration of tube feedings are those who

- Are unconscious.
- Are confused.
- Are seriously debilitated.
- Are older adults.
- Have tracheostomies or large-bore feeding tubes.
- Have impaired gag reflexes.
- Cannot sit upright.

The paramedic should monitor patients with feeding tubes closely for signs of increased respiratory effort. Lung sounds should be clear on auscultation. Respiratory difficulty or tachypnea may indicate developing aspiration pneumonitis. Other problems that can occur in patients with feeding tubes include diarrhea, choking, irritable bowel syndrome, and bowel obstruction.

Obstruction or Malfunction of Gastric Devices. A gastric device may become obstructed or malfunction for different reasons. For example, there may be a kinked or clogged tube, or a surgically implanted feeding tube may become displaced. Acute interventions that may be required include unkinking a tube, irrigating a clogged tube, and reinserting a displaced tube (per medical direction; Table 48-5). When transporting a patient with a gastric device, the paramedic must ensure patient comfort. The paramedic should position the device to allow for proper drainage and to prevent reflux.

Ostomies. An **ostomy** is an artificial opening into the urinary tract, gastrointestinal tract, or trachea. An ostomy may be temporary or permanent. (An **ileostomy** is an opening into the small intestine. A **colostomy** is an opening into the large intestine.) The bowel usually discharges liquid or solid feces into the bag (pouch) once or twice a day; the bag then is changed. Potential complications associated with ostomies include infection, hemorrhage, obstruction, and stomal problems (e.g., necrosis, retraction, stenosis, and prolapse).

Colostomy irrigation, ostomy care, and pouch changes usually are performed for home health care patients by the patients themselves, family members, and home health care practitioners. These procedures require special training. They usually are not considered an acute intervention for paramedic practice. Bowel perforation and significant fluid/electrolyte imbalances may accidentally occur from colostomy irrigation performed by the patient or caregiver.

ASSESSMENT AND MANAGEMENT OF PATIENTS WITH GASTROINTESTINAL/GENITOURINARY CRISIS

The paramedic should evaluate a patient with gastrointestinal/genitourinary complaints by obtaining a focused history and performing a physical examination to determine the need for immediate transport for physician evaluation. Depending on the patient's chief complaint, the physical examination may include assessment for the following:

- Abdominal distention
- Abdominal pain
- Aspiration
- Fever
- Intestinal obstruction
- Peritonitis
- Urinary tract infection
- Urinary retention

Acute Infections

More than 160,000 patients with infectious and parasitic diseases are discharged to home health care in the United States each year.[1] Home health care patients with acute infections have an increased death rate from sepsis and severe peripheral infections. They also may have a decreased ability to perceive pain or perform self-care. Patients with chronic diseases, poor nutrition, or an inability to perform self-care are at increased

TABLE 48-5 Managing Tube-Feeding Problems*

COMPLICATION	INTERVENTIONS
Aspiration of gastric secretions	Discontinue feeding immediately. Perform tracheal suction of aspirated contents if possible. Notify the doctor. Check tube placement before feeding to prevent complications.
Tube obstruction	Flush the tube with warm water. If necessary, replace the tube. Flush the tube with 50 mL of water after each feeding to remove excess sticky formula, which could occlude the tube.
Nasal or pharyngeal irritation or necrosis	Provide frequent oral hygiene using mouthwash or lemon-glycerin swabs. Use petroleum jelly on cracked lips. Change the position of the tube. If necessary, replace the tube.
Vomiting, bloating, diarrhea, or cramps	Reduce the flow rate. Warm the formula. For 30 minutes after feeding, position the patient on the right side with the head elevated to facilitate gastric emptying. Notify the doctor. The doctor may want to reduce the amount of formula being given during each feeding.
Constipation	Provide additional fluids if the patient can tolerate them. Administer a bulk-forming laxative. Increase fruit, vegetable, or sugar content of the feeding.

*This table lists some interventions that the nurse, paramedic, patient, or caregiver may use to solve home tube-feeding problems.

risk for infection and impaired healing. Conditions that may result in the need for acute interventions in the home health care population include the following[5]:

- Airway infections in the immunocompromised patient
- Delayed healing and increased peripheral infection from poor peripheral perfusion
- Skin breakdown and peripheral infections from immobility or sedentary lifestyle
- Infection and sepsis from implanted medical devices
- Wounds and incisions
- Abscesses
- Cellulitis

OPEN WOUNDS

Patients with open wounds who are discharged to home health care may have a variety of dressings, wound packings, and drains that permit drainage of fluid or air. They also may have a variety of wound closure devices (Box 48-7). (Dressings, packings, and wound closure devices can become contaminated; drains can become occluded or displaced.) Wound healing greatly depends on wound management. The patient must be made aware of the importance of taking all prescribed medications (especially antibiotics). The patient also should be informed of the importance of completing all wound care procedures. Wound repair generally is believed to be enhanced by the following:

- Moist environment
- Wound bed free of necrotic tissue, eschar, and environmental contamination or infection
- Adequate blood supply to meet metabolic demands for tissue generation
- Sufficient oxygen and nutrition for cellular metabolism and tissue generation

BOX 48-7 Sampling of Wound Care Devices Found in Home Health Care Patients

Dressings and Wound Packing Material
Combination dressings
Cotton dressings (gauze)
Exudate absorptive dressings
Foam dressings
Hydrocolloid dressings
Hydrogel dressings
Hydrophilic powder dressings
Impregnated cotton dressings
Paste bandages
Transparent film (adhesive or nonadhesive)

Drains
Jackson-Pratt drains
Penrose drains

Wound Closure Techniques
Skin adhesive
Staples
Sutures
Tape
Wires

GENERAL PRINCIPLES IN WOUND CARE MANAGEMENT

Wound care requires assessment of the wound and the surrounding tissues. It also requires evaluation for infection or sepsis. General principles in wound care management include an assessment for the following[7]:

1. Location and size.
2. Color of the wound bed. A red or pink granular wound bed indicates healing. A green, yellow, or black wound bed suggests infection or necrosis (tissue death).
3. Drainage. Clear or blood-tinged drainage is common in a healing wound. Green or yellow drainage suggests infection.
4. Wound odor. A sweet smell may indicate decay. A foul smell may indicate infection.
5. Surrounding skin. The paramedic should assess the skin for redness, inflammation, or signs of tissue breakdown.

If the dressing is wet or contaminated, the paramedic should change it after wound evaluation. Medical direction may advise cleaning the wound with normal saline and/or antiseptic solution before redressing it. The débridement of necrotic tissue may be required. Mechanical débridement is achieved by gently rubbing the tissue with a gauze pad moistened with sterile, normal saline. Some patients may need transport for physician evaluation if severe infection or sepsis is suspected.

Maternal/Child Conditions

In the early 1990s, many insurance companies began paying only for 24-hour hospital stays for uncomplicated vaginal childbirth. (These sometimes were called "drive-by deliveries.") In the wake of complaints about inadequate care, states began passing laws in 1995 and 1996. These laws required insurance to pay for 48-hour stays. A similar federal law was passed in 1996. This law took effect in January 1998. Under this law, health plans must cover hospital stays of at least 48 hours for women who give birth naturally. They must cover up to 4 days for those who deliver by cesarean section. Problems that may be encountered when these patient groups return to the home health care setting include the following:

- Postpartum pathophysiologies (e.g., hemorrhage, infection, and pulmonary embolism)
- Postpartum depression
- Septicemia in the newborn
- Infantile apnea
- **Failure to thrive**
- Sudden infant death syndrome

POSTPARTUM PATHOPHYSIOLOGIES

Postpartum pathophysiologies include hemorrhage, infection, and pulmonary embolism. (Acute interventions for these patients are presented in Chapter 42.) Postpartum hemorrhage occurs in about 5% of all deliveries. It frequently takes place within the first few hours after delivery, but it can be delayed up to 6 weeks.[6] Causes of postpartum hemorrhage include incomplete contraction of uterine muscle fibers, retained pieces of placenta or membranes in the uterus, and vaginal or cervical tears during delivery (which are rare).

Postpartum infection affects 2% to 8% of all pregnancies. (The most common infection is endometritis.) The condition occurs when bacteria grow and invade the uterus or other tissues along the birth canal. The symptoms usually develop on the second or third day after delivery. Fever and abdominal pain are the most common signs of infection.

Pulmonary embolism during pregnancy, labor, or the postpartum period is one of the most common causes of maternal death. The embolus often results from a blood clot in the pelvic circulation; it more commonly is associated with cesarean section than with vaginal delivery.

> **CRITICAL THINKING**
> A mother is having a postpartum complication that requires urgent transport. What will you do with the baby if they are home alone?

POSTPARTUM DEPRESSION

Postpartum depression affects 10% to 15% of mothers. The depression most likely is caused by a combination of sudden hormonal changes and psychological and environmental factors. The disease can be a short-lived attack of mild depression ("baby blues"). Or, in contrast, it can manifest as a depressive illness that requires in-hospital supervision. Risk factors for postpartum depression include the following:

- Adverse socioeconomic conditions
- Anxiety
- Complicated pregnancy or delivery
- Fetal complications
- Low self-esteem
- Poor marital adjustment
- Previous episodes of depression
- Recent life stressors

Recognizing and treating postpartum depression is important. The depression can interfere with the bonding between the mother and infant. It also can seriously affect the mother's ability to care for her newborn (Box 48-8). Many women with postpartum depression fear they will harm their babies. They often feel ashamed and guilty for these feelings. Sensitivity to the possibility of depression is crucial. Such sensitivity also is necessary for successful diagnosis and treatment. (Interventions for depression are presented in Chapter 40.)

SEPTICEMIA IN THE NEWBORN

Healthy newborns are vulnerable to several conditions that can require hospital treatment (see Chapters 43 and 44). Examples include jaundice that results from physiological immaturity of bilirubin metabolism, dehydration that can lead to serious electrolyte abnormalities, and sepsis. In addition, neonates are highly susceptible to infection because of diminished nonspecific (inflammatory) and specific (humoral) immunity.

Septicemia in the newborn usually is caused by group B streptococci, *Listeria monocytogenes,* or gram-negative enteric organisms (especially *Escherichia coli*).[8] Signs and symptoms of sepsis may be minimal and nonspecific. ("In the newborn, anything can be a sign of anything.")[5] Examples of

BOX 48-8 Signs and Symptoms of Postpartum Depression

Anxiety
Change of appetite (loss of appetite or overindulgence)
Desire to leave or feelings of being trapped
Difficulty making decisions
Excessive concern or lack of concern for baby
Fantasies of disaster or bizarre fears
Fatigue or exhaustion
Fear of harming self or baby
Forgetfulness or memory loss
Hatred of spouse, self, or baby
Hopelessness
Hostility
Inability to care for baby
Increased alcohol consumption or other drug use
Irritability
Lack of interest in previously enjoyed activities
Lack of sexual interest
Loss of hope
Panic attacks
Rapid mood swings
Severe sleep disturbance
Unexplainable crying (in joy or sadness)

signs and symptoms of sepsis in the newborn include the following:

- Temperature instability
- Respiratory distress
- Apnea
- Cyanosis
- Gastrointestinal changes (e.g., vomiting, distention, diarrhea, and anorexia)
- Central nervous system features (e.g., irritability, lethargy, and weak suck)

Risk factors for sepsis include prematurity, prolonged rupture of membranes, and chorioamnionitis (an inflammatory reaction in the amniotic membranes caused by bacterial viruses in the amniotic fluid). The diagnosis generally is confirmed after physician evaluation by a positive blood, urine, or cerebrospinal fluid culture.

INFANTILE APNEA

Apnea involves periods of cessation of respirations for more than 10 to 15 seconds with or without cyanosis, pallor, hypotonia (diminished tone), and/or bradycardia or for less than 10 seconds accompanied by bradycardia.[9] The condition often reflects the immature respiratory control centers in some infants. Other causes of infantile apnea include the following[10]:

- Metabolic derangements (e.g., hypoglycemia, hypocalcemia, or hypothermia)
- Infection (e.g., sepsis, pneumonia, or meningitis)
- Central nervous system damage (e.g., hemorrhage, hypoxic injury, or seizures)
- Pulmonary disorders (e.g., respiratory distress, hyaline membrane disease, pneumonia, obstruction, or upper respiratory abnormalities)
- Intentional poisoning

The paramedic must assess the presence of apnea carefully and document it. Most infants with the diagnosis of apnea will be hospitalized and observed closely. They are observed using electronic apnea monitoring devices. These devices detect changes in thoracic or abdominal movement and heart rate. Managing apnea in these patients may include the home health care use of apnea monitors, oscillating waterbeds, and CPAP with supplemental oxygen. Some patients also may be prescribed respiratory stimulants (e.g., doxapram or methylxanthines).

FAILURE TO THRIVE

Failure to thrive is an abnormally slow rate of growth and development of an infant. It results from conditions that interfere with normal metabolism, appetite, and activity. Causative factors include the following:

- Chromosomal abnormalities
- Major organ system defects that lead to deficiency or malfunction
- Systemic disease or acute illness
- Physical deprivation (primarily malnutrition related to insufficient breast milk, poverty, or poor knowledge of nutrition)
- Various psychosocial factors (e.g., maternal deprivation)

Failure to thrive can result in permanent and irreversible retardation of physical, mental, or social development. Any suspicions of failure to thrive should be documented carefully. The paramedic should report these suspicions to medical direction as well.

WELL-BABY CARE

Some infants and children have periodic health assessments through well-baby care programs. These programs specialize in medical supervision and services for healthy infants. Well-baby care promotes optimal physical, emotional, and intellectual growth and development. Such health care measures include the following:

- Routine immunizations to prevent disease
- Screening procedures for early detection and treatment of illness
- Parental guidance and instruction in proper nutrition, injury prevention, and specific care and rearing of the child at various stages of development

The recommended preventative health care schedule for children who are developing normally is monthly for the first 6 months of life; every 2 months until 1 year of age; every 3 months during the second year; and every 6 months during the third year; followed by annual visits. Well-baby care may be provided in a clinic ("well-baby clinics"), a doctor's office, the office of a community health nursing center, or a school. Nurses or nurse practitioners often provide the care in these programs.

Hospice/Palliative Care

In 2002, hospices served more than 579,000 patients throughout the United States.[11] Hospice services include supportive social, emotional, and spiritual services for the terminally ill. They also provide support for the patient's family. Hospice care relies on the combined knowledge and skill of a team of professionals. This team includes physicians, nurses, medical social workers, therapists, counselors, chaplains, and volunteers. These persons work together to provide a personal plan of care for each patient and family. The need for hospices likely will continue to rise because of an aging population, the increasing number of persons with acquired immunodeficiency syndrome, and rising health care costs. Medical professionals and the general public more and more are choosing hospice care over other forms of health care for terminally ill patients. The holistic, patient-family, in-home-centered philosophy is one reason for this.

PALLIATIVE CARE

Palliative care is a unique form of health care. It mainly is directed at providing relief to terminally ill persons through symptom management and pain management. (Palliative care also is called *comfort care.*) This specialty focuses on the needs of the patient and family when a life-threatening illness such as cancer or acquired immunodeficiency syndrome has reached the terminal stage. A chief goal of palliative care is to improve the quality of a person's life as death approaches and to help patients and their families move toward this reality with comfort, reassurance, and strength. Palliative care is not focused on death; it is about specialized care for the living. Well-rounded palliative care programs also address mental health and spiritual needs. Palliative care may be delivered in hospice, home care settings, and hospitals. Medical needs vary depending on the disease that is leading toward death. Thus specialized palliative care programs exist for common conditions such as cancer and acquired immunodeficiency syndrome (Box 48-9).

Emergency medical services and medical direction should work closely with the families and physicians of terminally ill patients in private homes and hospice programs so that they will make the best use of the EMS system. (For instance, they will know when to call 911.) Even though resuscitation may not be indicated, EMS may be needed to manage pain, treat acute medical illness or traumatic injury, and provide transport to a hospital. If the patient is not to receive medical intervention to prolong life, the paramedic should provide measures of comfort to the patient. In addition, the paramedic should provide emotional support to family members and loved ones. (See Chapter 2.)

BOX 48-9 Essential Elements of a Palliative Care Program

Palliative care is an accepted specialty of medicine and nursing that concentrates on the total care of patients suffering from any form of terminal illness. Its development, as part of the health care services, is a recognition that dying is a normal consequence of living. The support of health professionals and use of modern medical technology can relieve much of the distress normally associated with dying. Essential elements of a palliative care program are the following:

1. The coordination of care for patients with a terminal illness, at home or in hospital, by a distinct service.
2. The unit of care is the patient and the patient's family, who have the right to make choices and decisions based on an understanding of the illness and to have those decisions respected.
3. The care is provided by an interdisciplinary team.
4. The care is coordinated and delivered by specifically selected and trained nurses.
5. The service is directed by a physician.
6. The emphasis is on control of symptoms, be they physical, social, or emotional.
7. The services are available on a 24 hours a day, 7 days a week, on-call basis.
8. The program must be sensitive to differences in faith and culture and must incorporate the patients' beliefs into decisions on their care.
9. Following the death of a patient, the program should ensure that grief support is available for the family. This may be provided by the program itself or by other community services.
10. There is a system of structured staff support and communication.
11. The program is integrated and coordinated with other services, and continuity of care for the patient is provided.
12. Evaluation of the program and its services must be regular. This evaluation may extend into the area of research.
13. The program will provide education for its own staff, other health care providers, and the public.

From *Essential elements of a palliative care program,* Health Canada, Minister of Public Works and Government Services, 2000, Ottawa, Canada.

HOSPICE CARE IN THE HOME SETTING

A patient receiving hospice care may be receiving medication delivery for the relief of pain (e.g., narcotic infusion devices). The patient also will have medical and legal documents such as do-not-resuscitate orders and advance directives (see Chapter 4). The paramedic should discuss any concerns about effective pain management, overmedication, or interpreting medical or legal documents with medical direction (Box 48-10).

BOX 48-10 Bill of Rights and Responsibilities for Terminally Ill Patients

A. Personal Dignity and Privacy

1. You have the right to considerate, respectful service and care, with full recognition of your personal dignity and individuality, without regard to gender, age, ethnicity, income level, lifestyle, educational background, or spiritual philosophy.
2. You have the right to be dressed as you wish and not to be disrobed or uncovered any longer than necessary for your care.
3. You have the right to privacy and the assurance of confidentiality when receiving care, to refuse visitors or persons not directly involved in your care, and to choose who will receive information about your condition.
4. You have the right to request the presence of a person of your choice during interactions with health care professionals.
5. You have the right to experience all emotions, including anger, sadness, confusion, guilt, depression, impatience, fear, and loss.
6. You have the right to have your end-of-life choices respected by health care professionals, including continuing or discontinuing treatment or requesting medications to self-administer for a hastened death.
7. You have the right to die with your loved ones present and to request the presence of a health care professional, if desired.
8. You have the responsibility to treat your caregiver with respect and to follow their directions when consistent with your wishes.
9. You have the responsibility to make certain that your right to privacy and confidentiality is clearly understood by all parties involved in your care and to communicate to your health care providers when you feel that your rights to privacy and confidentiality are in jeopardy.

B. Informed Participation

1. You have the right to honest, accurate, and understandable information about your current diagnosis and prognosis; the recommended treatment and what it is expected to do; the possibility of success; and the possible risks of complications and side effects, including the probability of their occurrence.
2. You have the right to be informed about alternative forms of treatment, including hospice and home care, and to participate in all decisions affecting your care.
3. You have the right to request and receive a second opinion. When curative care is no longer indicated or desired, you have the right to access palliative care, including pain medication in whatever dosage or schedule you deem necessary to alleviate pain and suffering, even at the risk of hastening death.
4. You have the right to make your own decisions regarding what constitutes your human dignity, as long as you are mentally competent and continue to have basic decision-making capacity. You will be considered mentally competent if you can understand the nature of your condition, the treatment alternatives available, the likely outcomes of treatment versus nontreatment, and can accept responsibility for your decisions.
5. You have the right to access information in your medical record and to know if your health care providers believe that your condition or course of disease will result in death. This information may be needed to make informed decisions about your future.
6. You have the right to forgo eating and drinking naturally in order to permit the process of dying to proceed unencumbered.
7. You have the right and responsibility to complete a directive to physicians (living will).
8. You have the right and responsibility to execute a durable power of attorney for health care so that someone you choose can make health care decisions for you, if needed.

C. Competent Care

1. You have the right to competent medical, nursing, and social services care.
2. You have the right to choose your personal physician and to change your physician at any time.
3. You have the right to know who is responsible for coordinating and supervising your care and to know how to contact that person.
4. You have the right to be informed about who owns and controls the agency or facility involved with your care and the right to referral to institutions, facilities, and practitioners who can provide the care you need.
5. You have the responsibility to choose a primary care physician who is able and willing to carry out your wishes.
6. You have the responsibility to communicate your end-of-life wishes to family, friends, and health care providers.

From Compassion In Dying Federation, Portland, Oregon.

SUMMARY

- About 25% of home health care patients have heart and circulatory diseases as their primary diagnosis. Other common diagnoses of home health care patients include cancer, diabetes, and hypertension. Typical EMS calls to a home health care setting may include respiratory failure, cardiac decompensation, septic complications, equipment malfunction, and other medical problems.
- After arrival at the scene of a home health care patient, the scene size-up should include standard precautions, elements of scene safety, and environmental setting. The initial assessment should focus on illness or injury that pose a threat to life. The paramedic should take appropriate measures as indicated.
- Patients with diseases of the respiratory system being cared for at home are at increased risk for airway infections. In addition, the progression of their illnesses may lead to difficulty breathing, making current support equipment inadequate.
- Assessment findings that may require acute interventions in patients with VADs include infection, hemorrhage, hemodynamic compromise from circulatory overload or embolus, obstruction of the vascular device, and catheter damage with leakage of medication.
- Patients with diseases of the digestive or genitourinary system may have medical devices such as urinary catheters or urostomies, indwelling nutritional support devices (e.g., percutaneous endoscopic gastrostomy tube, or gastrostomy tube), colostomies, and nasogastric tubes. Acute interventions required for these patients can result from UTI, urosepsis, urinary retention, and problems with gastric emptying or feeding.
- Home health care patients with acute infections have an increased death rate from sepsis and severe peripheral infections. Many also have a decreased ability to perceive pain or perform self-care.
- Maternal/child conditions that one may encounter in the home health care setting during the postpartum period include postpartum hemorrhage, infection, pulmonary embolism, postpartum depression, septicemia in the newborn, infantile apnea, and failure to thrive.
- Hospice services include supportive social, emotional, and spiritual services for the terminally ill. They also provide support for a patient's family. Palliative care is directed mainly at providing relief to a terminally ill person. They do this through symptom and pain management.

REFERENCES

1. National Association of Home Care: *Basic statistics about home care: 1999 home care stats,* Washington, DC, 2001, The Association.
2. *Home health care: history and philosophy*, Kansas City, Kan, 1997, Spectrum Home Health Agency.
3. Health Care Financing Administration: *Managed care in Medicare and Medicaid,* Washington, DC, 1998, Department of Health and Human Services.
4. National Center for Health Statistics: *An overview of home health and hospice care patients: 1996 national home and hospice care survey,* Hyattsville, Md, 1996, The Center.
5. US Department of Transportation, National Highway Traffic Safety Administration: *EMT-Paramedic national standard curriculum,* Washington, DC, 1998, The Department.
6. Rosen P, Barkin R: *Emergency medicine: concepts and clinical practice,* ed 4, St Louis, 1998, Mosby.
7. Rice R: *Handbook of home health nursing procedures,* St Louis, 1995, Mosby.
8. Hoekelman R: *Primary pediatric care,* ed 3, St Louis, 1997, Mosby.
9. Polin R, Ditmar M: *Pediatric secrets,* ed 2, Philadelphia, 1997, Hanley & Belfus.
10. Barkin R et al: *Pediatric emergency medicine: concepts and clinical practice,* St Louis, 1992, Mosby.
11. National Association of Home Care: *Basic statistics about hospice, 2002,* Washington, DC, 2002. The Association.

PART TEN

IN THIS PART

CHAPTER 49 Ambulance Operations

CHAPTER 50 Medical Incident Command

CHAPTER 51 Rescue Awareness and Operations

CHAPTER 52 Crime Scene Awareness

CHAPTER 53 Hazardous Materials Incidents

CHAPTER 54 Bioterrorism and Weapons of Mass Destruction

CHAPTER 49

Ambulance Operations

OBJECTIVES

Upon completion of this chapter, the paramedic student will be able to:

1. List standards that govern ambulance performance and specifications.
2. Discuss the tracking of equipment, supplies, and maintenance on an ambulance.
3. Outline the considerations for appropriate stationing of ambulances.
4. Describe measures that can influence safe operation of an ambulance.
5. Identify aeromedical crew members and training.
6. Describe the appropriate use of aeromedical services in the prehospital setting.

KEY TERMS

ambulance: A generic term that describes the various land-based emergency vehicles used by emergency medical services (EMS) personnel, including basic and advanced life support units, paramedic units, mobile intensive care units, and others.

KKK A-1822D standards: The national standards that provide the foundation of uniformity for the design of ambulance vehicles.

landing zone: An area prepared for the landing of an aircraft; generally 100 by 100 feet.

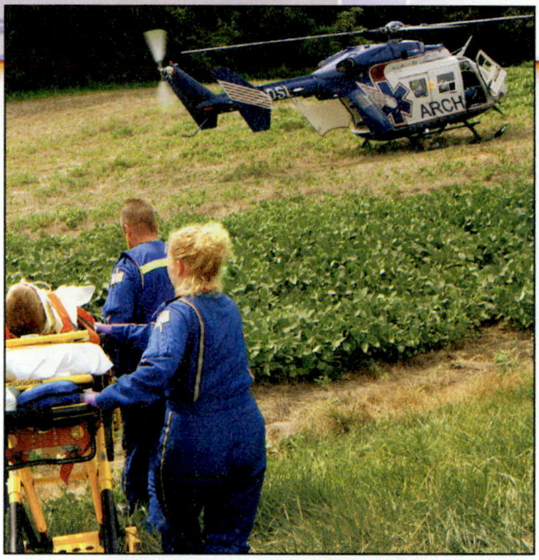

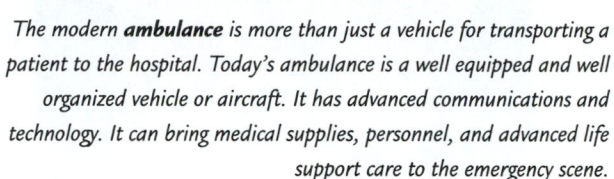

*The modern **ambulance** is more than just a vehicle for transporting a patient to the hospital. Today's ambulance is a well equipped and well organized vehicle or aircraft. It has advanced communications and technology. It can bring medical supplies, personnel, and advanced life support care to the emergency scene.*

AMBULANCE STANDARDS

In 1968 the National Academy of Sciences–National Research Council (NAS-NRC) recommended ambulance design standards. These standards included the size, shape, color, electrical systems, and emergency equipment. They led to the development of the federal specifications that many states now use as ambulance standards. The national standards developed by NAS-NRC and the National Highway Traffic Safety Administration (NHTSA) are known as the **KKK A-1822D standards.** These standards and their revisions provide the basis for uniformity in the design of ambulance vehicles. They cover the three basic ambulance designs: type I, type II, and type III (Fig. 49-1). Also, because of the extra weight of equipment used in rescue and emergency care and the space needed for this equipment, medium-duty truck chassis are used for some ambulances. Many fire service vehicles (e.g., pumpers, rescue units, and fire trucks) also carry EMS equipment.

The federal standards of design and performance for ambulance vehicles are augmented by other federal standards, state statutes, administrative rules, and city, county, and district ordinances. These influence ambulance design, equipment, and staffing. These additional requirements include the following:

- Air ambulance standards
- Operational staffing standards
- Operational driver standards
- Operational driving standards
- Operational equipment standards

CRITICAL THINKING

Consider your state or regional standards. What do they require for ambulance design, performance, and equipment?

CHECKING AMBULANCES

Completing an equipment and supply checklist at the start of every work shift is important. It is essential for safety, patient care, and risk management. It also helps to ensure proper handling and safekeeping of scheduled medications (Fig. 49-2). Either paper checklists or special computer software can be used for this purpose. Some equipment (e.g., glucometers and defibrillators) require routine maintenance, testing, and cleaning (Box 49-1). This ensures safe, effective operation.

The procedures for vehicle maintenance vary by EMS agency. These procedures are in place to improve the vehicles' reliability and extend their life. The paramedic should follow all agency guidelines and procedures for checking vehicles, equipment, and supplies.

AMBULANCE STATIONING

In the 1970s the methods for estimating the need for ambulance service and where they should be located in a community were based on the availability of ambulances. They also were based on the average response time to the emergency scene. Methods for estimating needs have changed. They have shifted toward determining the percentage of

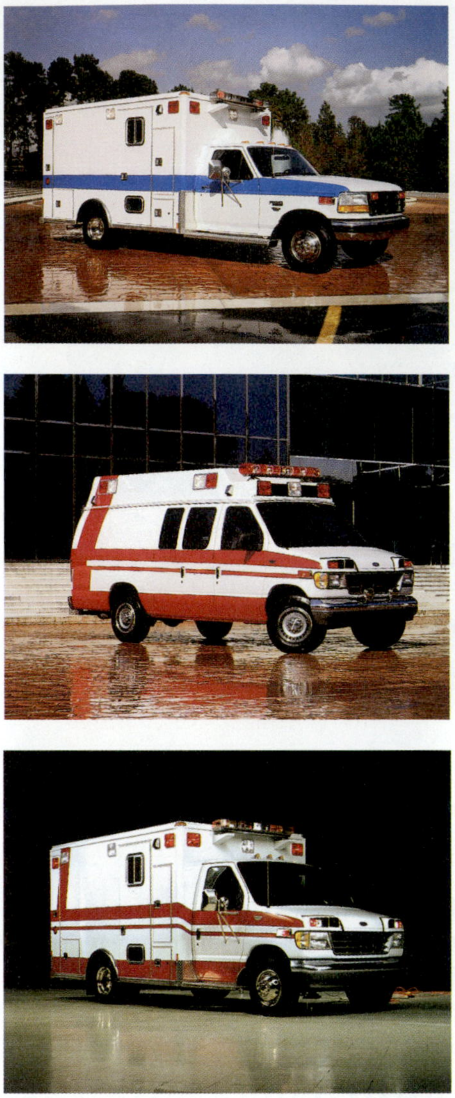

FIGURE 49-1 ■ Basic ambulance designs. **A,** Type I. **B,** Type II. **C,** Type III.

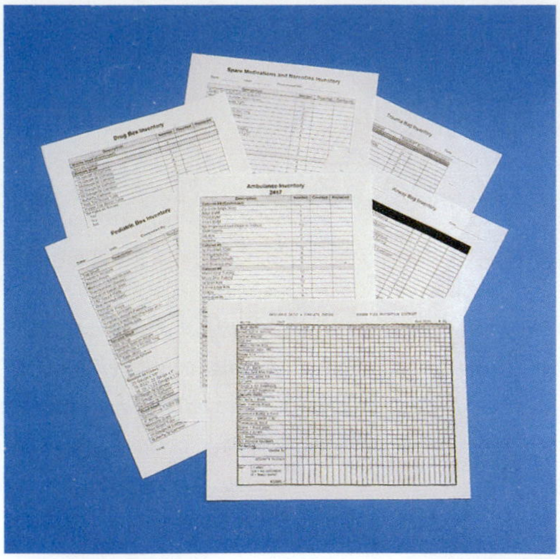

FIGURE 49-2 ■ Ambulance checklists.

> **BOX 49-1 Examples of Equipment Checks on an Emergency Medical Services (EMS) Vehicle**
>
> **General Operations**
> Airway equipment (basic and advanced)
> Burn supplies
> Drug inventory
> Extrication/rescue supplies
> Infection control supplies
> Immobilization equipment
> Obstetrical/childbirth supplies
> Patient assessment equipment
> Stretchers and related equipment
> Vehicle safety and operations
> Wound care supplies
>
> **Specific Medical Equipment**
> Automated transport ventilator (ATV)
> Cardiac monitor/defibrillator
> Glucometer
> Pulse oximetry equipment
> Telemetry equipment

compliance *(standard of reliability)* in providing EMS services within time frames that meet national guidelines. (For example, the American Heart Association recommends that advanced life support [ALS] be available at the scene within 8 minutes of a cardiac arrest.[1]) Factors that may affect an EMS system's standard of reliability include the geographical area, population and patient demand, traffic conditions, time of day, and appropriate placement of emergency vehicles.

Strategies for ambulance stationing often are based on areas with the highest volume of calls *(peak load)*. These strategies take into consideration the day of the week and the time of day. Computers and other technological devices may be used to formalize strategic unit deployment and reduce response times. Deployment strategies vary by EMS agency. They range from simple deployment of one vehicle stationed in the middle of a response area to full automated deployment plans for each hour of the day and each day of the week. The comprehensive plans include "minideployment" plans within each hour, depending on the number of ambulances left in the system. The best deployment system usually is a compromise between these two extremes.[2]

SAFE AMBULANCE OPERATION

Between 1991 and 2000, there were 300 fatal crashes involving occupied ambulances. These resulted in the deaths of 82 ambulance occupants and 275 occupants of other vehicles and pedestrians.[3]

Safe operation of ambulances is crucial. It is essential for the safety of patients, the EMS crew, and others in the vicin-

BOX 49-2 Guidelines for Safe Ambulance Driving

1. Be tolerant and observant of other motorists and pedestrians.
2. Always use occupant safety restraints (both driver and passenger).
3. Be familiar with the characteristics of the emergency vehicle.
4. Be alert to changes in weather and road conditions.
5. Exercise caution in the use of audible and visual warning devices.
6. Drive within the speed limit except in circumstances allowed by law.
7. Select the fastest and most appropriate route to and from the incident scene.
8. Maintain a safe following distance.
9. Drive with due regard for the safety of all others.
10. Always drive in a manner consistent with managing acceptable levels of risk.

ity of a response. Many EMS agencies require their personnel to take an emergency driving course. Many also are required to undergo periodic evaluations of their emergency driving skills (Box 49-2). In addition to the size and weight of the emergency vehicle and the driver's experience, a number of factors influence safe operation of an ambulance. These include the following:

- Appropriate use of escorts
- Environmental conditions
- Appropriate use of warning devices
- Proceeding safely through intersections
- Parking at the emergency scene
- Operating with due regard for the safety of others
- Safely moving a patient into and out of the ambulance

CRITICAL THINKING

How do you think you would feel if you struck another vehicle while driving an ambulance?

Appropriate Use of Escorts

Police escorts during an emergency response can be dangerous. They should be used sparingly. Collisions can occur as a result of confusion. Motorists in the area may wrongly assume that only one emergency vehicle is on the road. As a rule, paramedics should use escorts only when the EMS crew is responding to a scene in an unfamiliar area. Even then the EMS driver should keep a safe distance between the ambulance and the escort. The use of audible and visual warning devices during escorts should be guided by local protocol. If the paramedic uses audible and visual warning devices, the ambulance and police escort should use different siren tones (per protocol). This alerts other motorists to the fact that a second emergency vehicle is in the area.

Some communities use a *tiered response system.* In such a system, several units and sometimes several agencies respond to emergency calls. The tiered response system allows for a safer emergency response. It also helps to ensure that the proper resources and personnel are available during an emergency. For example, a fire service unit staffed with basic-level emergency medical technicians (EMT-Bs) responds to a car crash with full use of audible and visual warning devices. The EMT-Bs determine that the patient's injury is minor. They request a basic life support (BLS) ambulance (either public or private) to respond to the scene in a nonemergency mode (at normal speed and without warning devices). The BLS ambulance assumes care and provides transport to the hospital.

Environmental Conditions

Poor weather conditions can create significant dangers when paramedics respond to a call. Factors that can affect safe ambulance operation include road and weather conditions, such as fog and heavy rain that reduce visibility, and slippery pavement caused by ice, snow, mud, oil, or water that can cause the ambulance to hydroplane.

When poor environmental conditions are present, the driver of the emergency vehicle should proceed at safe speeds. These speeds should be appropriate for the road and weather conditions. The driver should use low-beam headlights during all responses. This increases visibility for the EMS crew. It also makes it easier for other motorists to recognize the ambulance.

Dry roads and clear weather do not guarantee a safe response. About 69% of all emergency vehicle crashes occur on dry roads, and about 77% occur during clear weather.[4]

Appropriate Use of Warning Devices

As noted before, during an emergency response and patient transport, lights and sirens should be used according to protocol and state motor vehicle laws. Most EMS agencies authorize the use of these devices during all responses when the cause or severity of the emergency is unknown. In these cases, audible and visual warning devices should be used at the same time. (If one is indicated, so is the other.) The use of warning devices during patient transport usually is reserved for patients with limb- or life-threatening illness or injury.

When using lights and sirens, paramedics should keep in mind that motorists who drive with the car windows rolled up or who are using an audio device, air conditioning, or the heating system may not be able to hear the sirens or air horns. Therefore the EMS crew should always proceed with caution. They should never assume that the vehicle's lights, sirens, and air horns provide an absolute right-of-way or privileged immunity to proceed. It should be noted that some state and motor vehicle laws grant privileged immunity only to drivers of emergency vehicles that respond using *all* available lights and sirens. Paramedics should be familiar with the motor vehicle laws in their state that cover an emergency response.

CRITICAL THINKING

In what situations do you think the crew member driving an ambulance may be tempted to drive too fast?

Proceeding Safely through Intersections

Approximately 53% of ambulance crashes in the United States occur in intersections where an ambulance proceeds against a red light.[5] It is important that the driver of an emergency vehicle stop at all controlled intersections. The driver should try to make eye contact with all motorists before going through the intersection. Another safety measure for going through an intersection is making a secondary stop to assess the intersection before crossing. A final measure is using the siren's "yelp" mode or air horn to alert nearby traffic. Some emergency vehicles now have traffic signal preempting devices. These devices can change the traffic light at an intersection to green (in the ambulance's direction of travel).

Parking at the Emergency Scene

When parking the ambulance at a scene, the paramedic should make sure that the vehicle's location allows for traffic flow around the area. If law enforcement and fire service personnel have secured the scene, the paramedic should position the ambulance about 100 feet past the scene. (This should be on the same side of the road.) The ambulance should be positioned uphill (about 200 feet). It also should be positioned upwind if the presence of hazardous materials is suspected. If law enforcement and fire service personnel have not secured the scene, the paramedic should position the ambulance about 50 feet in front of the scene. This is the "fend-off" position. (Fig. 49-3). In this position, the emergency vehicle deflects and averts from the scene other vehicles that may strike the ambulance or providers.

Other safety precautions a paramedic can take when parking an ambulance at an emergency scene include the following:

- Emergency lighting should be used when the vehicle blocks traffic.
- The parking brake should be set. (Setting the parking brake before putting the transmission in "Park" allows the entire weight of the vehicle to be shared between the emergency brake and the transmission.)
- Another person should be asked to help guide the vehicle when it is backing up. (This person should be visible in the vehicle mirrors at all times while the ambulance is slowly backing up.)
- Reflective gear should be worn when paramedics work near the roadway.

When choosing a parking area for the ambulance, the paramedic also should consider the possibility of collapsing structures, fires, explosive hazards, and downed electrical wires.

Operating with Due Regard for the Safety of All Others

Most states allow privileges for drivers of emergency vehicles. For instance, they are allowed to drive slightly above the speed limit. They also are allowed to proceed through a controlled intersection (after a stop) during an emergency response (Box 49-3). However, these privileges must take into consideration the safety of all people using the roads. This "due regard for the safety of all others" carries legal responsibility. The paramedic and the EMS agency can incur liability if damage, injury, or death results from failure to observe this principle (see Chapter 4). The paramedic should be aware of local and state laws and regulations that cover the operation of an emergency vehicle.

Safely Moving a Patient Into and Out of an Ambulance

After initial stabilization at the scene, the patient must be packaged and safely placed in the emergency vehicle for transport. The paramedic crew should use safe lifting practices (see Chapter 2). These techniques help to prevent personal injury. They also ensure that the patient is positioned securely on the ambulance stretcher. The patient compartment of the ambulance is equipped with locking devices. These prevent the stretcher from moving while the ambulance is in motion. Unnecessary equipment should be stowed before transport. Also, objects such as monitors should be secured in a locking device. This minimizes the risk of injuries in a collision. All those traveling in the ambulance (except for the paramedic providing patient care) should have their personal restraints securely fastened. Before the vehicle leaves the scene, the driver of the ambulance should be signaled that it is safe to put the vehicle in motion.

▶NOTE Whenever possible, children should be transported secured in a proper child safety seat. Except in the most critical cases, care can be delivered effectively when the child is restrained in this way.

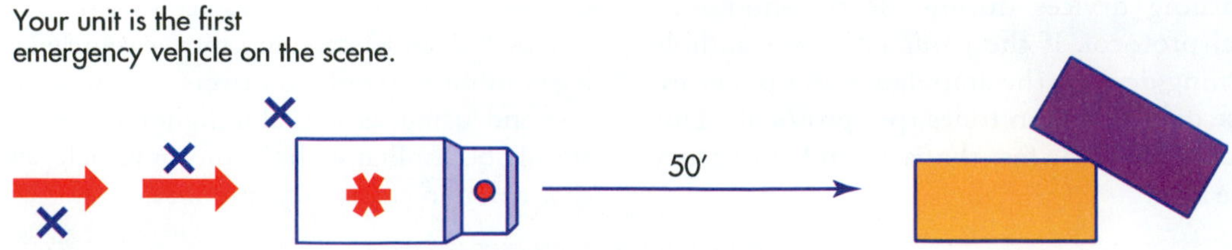
Your unit is the first
emergency vehicle on the scene.
50′

FIGURE 49-3 ■ The "fend-off" position.

During transport, the patient should be closely monitored for any changes in status. If emergency care is required while the ambulance is in motion (e.g., intubation, defibrillation), the driver of the vehicle should be advised to slow the vehicle. When possible, the driver should safely park the vehicle and stay parked until the procedure has been successfully performed.

Upon arrival at the hospital, the ambulance should come to a full stop. At that point, personal restraints can be removed and the vehicle can be exited. All patient care equipment must be secured before the stretcher is released from the locking device. (This includes, for example, immobilization devices, intravenous [IV] lines, and airway adjuncts.) Using safe lifting techniques, the patient's stretcher should be removed from the ambulance. The patient should be appropriately transferred to health care personnel at the facility.

BOX 49-3 The Two-Second Rule and Braking Distance Chart

Most rear-end collisions are caused by drivers who follow too closely behind the vehicle in front of them. Therefore it is important that the paramedic keep enough space (following distance) between the emergency vehicle and the vehicle in front to avoid a crash if the car in front brakes suddenly.

A quick method for gauging the recommended distance is the 2-second rule. It works like this:

1. You (the driver of the emergency vehicle) note an object by the side of the road (e.g., a tree or sign) that the vehicle in front of you will soon pass.
2. Count "one thousand and one, one thousand and two." If you reach the object before the phrase is complete, you are too close to the vehicle in front of you.
3. This rule applies with good road and weather conditions. If the road and weather conditions are not good, the following distance should be increased to a 4- or 5-second count.

Braking distance is based on average reaction time, average vehicle weight, average road conditions, and average brakes. Wet roadways, poor brakes, poor tires, heavy vehicle weight, and poor reaction times lengthen the braking distance. The following chart shows braking distance at various speeds.

Note: Larger emergency vehicles (e.g., those mounted on a freightliner-type chassis) have different handling characteristics and longer braking and stopping distances than conventional type I, II, or III emergency vehicles.

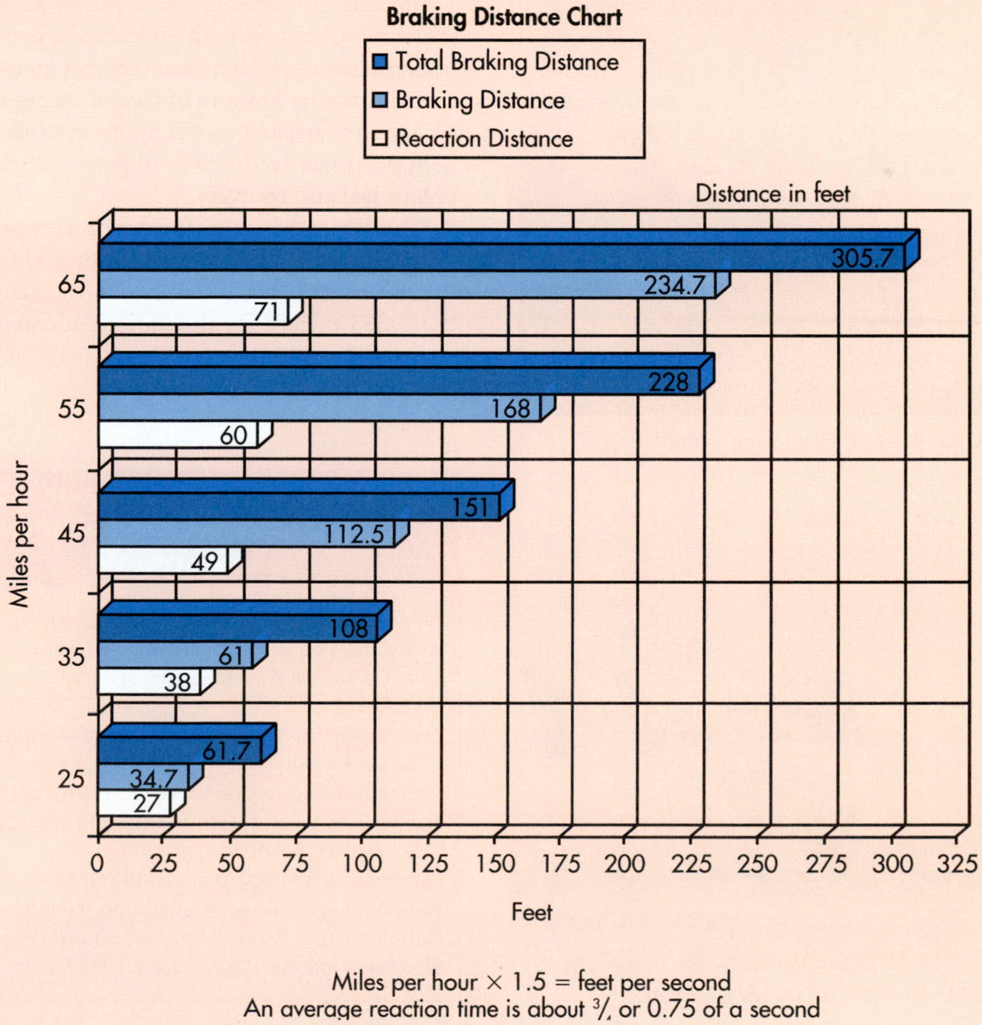

From Los Angeles Unified School District Police Department, Braking Distance Chart, Los Angeles, Calif., 1999.

AEROMEDICAL TRANSPORTATION

Like many other aspects of prehospital emergency care, air evacuation is rooted in military history. During the Prussian siege of Paris in 1870, soldiers and civilians were evacuated by a hot-air balloon. In 1928 a Marine pilot used an engine-powered aircraft to evacuate the wounded in Nicaragua.[6] However, the first full-scale use of aircraft for medical evacuation did not occur until 1950, during the Korean conflict. The experience gained in Korea formed the basis for helicopter rescue in Vietnam. In Vietnam, nearly 1 million casualties were transported by air. In the more recent military confrontations involving the United States in Panama, Grenada, and the Middle East, massive advanced aeromedical support capabilities and plans were on site before the conflicts began. Response times of 25 minutes were achieved for air evacuation of wounded solders in the Persian Gulf. Field surgical units were set up to handle the 1500 to 3000 casualties estimated to occur within the first 24 hours of the war; most of the injured soldiers arrived by air transportation.[7]

Currently, more than 406 air medical service programs using fixed wing aircraft (Fig. 49-4) and/or rotary wing (helicopter) aircraft (Fig. 49-5) have been established throughout the United States.[8] Fixed wing aircraft services are not usually as high profile as helicopters. Often they are used for interhospital transfer of patients and to deliver organs for transplantation when the distance is greater than 100 miles.

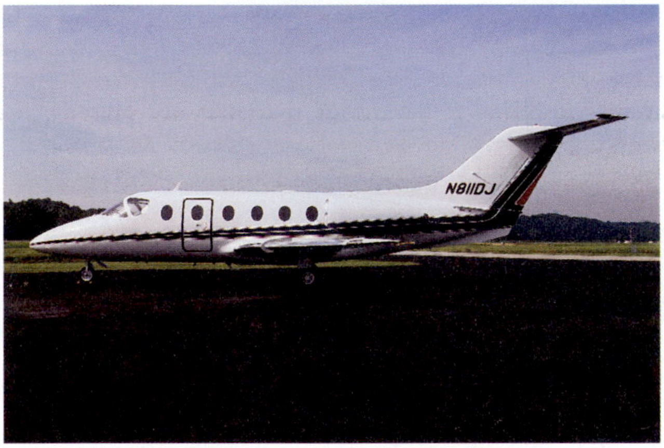

FIGURE 49-4 ■ Fixed wing aircraft.

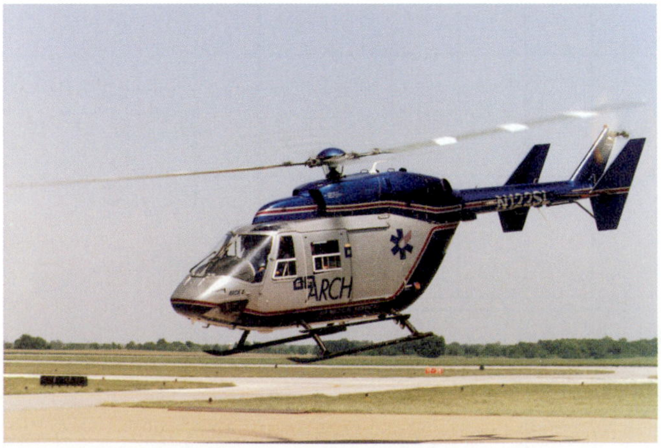

FIGURE 49-5 ■ Rotary wing aircraft.

Aeromedical Crew Members and Training

The staffing of air ambulances includes a pilot and various health care professionals. (These may include EMTs, paramedics, respiratory therapists, nurses, and physicians.) Air ambulance crews undergo specialized training in flight physiology and advanced medical equipment and procedures. The American College of Surgeons (ACS) Committee on Trauma and the Association of Air Medical Services have established guidelines for personnel qualifications. The Department of Transportation (DOT) and the NHTSA funded the development of the *Air Medical Crew National Standard Curriculum* in 1988. Many flight programs have used this curriculum to teach flight physiology, aircraft components and construction, safety regulations, aviation and navigation terminology, and operational safety (Box 49-4).

Use of Aeromedical Services

The local EMS system develops the criteria for requesting aeromedical services to the scene of an emergency. As described in Chapter 20, the paramedic generally should consider air transport when emergency personnel have determined that one or more of the following is a factor:

- The time needed to transport a patient by ground to an appropriate facility would pose a threat to the patient's survival and recovery.
- Weather, road, or traffic conditions would seriously delay the patient's access to advanced life support.
- Critical care personnel and specialized equipment are needed to care for the patient adequately during transport (Box 49-5).

BOX 49-4 Selected Organizations Associated with the Air Medical Industry

Air Medical Physicians Association (AMPA)
Association of Air Medical Services (AAMS)
Commission on Accreditation of Air Medical Services (CAAMS)
Commission on the Accreditation of Medical Transport Services (CAMTS)
International Society of Air Medical Services (Australasia) (ISAS)
National Association of Air Medical Communications Specialists (NAACS)
National EMS Pilots Association (NEMSPA)
National Flight Nurses Association (NFNA)
National Flight Paramedics Association (NFPA)
Shock Trauma Air Rescue Society (STARS)

NOTIFICATION OF AEROMEDICAL SERVICES

Most aeromedical transportation providers accept requests for medical services from physicians, EMS and fire service personnel, or other on-scene public service agency personnel. Local and state guidelines cover aeromedical activation. The paramedic should consult with medical direction and follow all state laws, administrative rules, and city, county, and district ordinances and standards when using aeromedical services. When notified that an aeromedical response may be needed, the flight crews of some services move to the aircraft so that they are ready for the flight. (They are placed on *stand-by*.) If paramedics determine that the situation does not require an aeromedical response, the appropriate agency should be notified as soon as possible. This makes the crew available for other flights.

If paramedics request air service for medical, trauma, or search and rescue events, they should advise the flight crew of the type of emergency response, the number of patients, the location of a **landing zone** (LZ), and any prominent landmarks and hazards (e.g., vertical structures or power lines). Direct ground to air communication must be available between a designated LZ officer and the aeromedical staff on the responding aircraft. If possible, the fire department should be dispatched to the LZ to provide fire-suppression support. Law enforcement personnel also should be available for securing the scene.

BOX 49-5 Advantages and Disadvantages of Air Medical Services

Advantages
- Transports are rapid and usually smooth.
- Access to accident sites is quick.
- Traffic, trains, mountains, ship canals, and other barriers can be avoided.
- Travel is still possible when road conditions are poor.
- Sophisticated communication equipment is available.
- Ground ambulances are not detained for long periods.
- Quality of care is improved in rural areas where only basic life support is available.
- Fewer air ambulance crashes occur than ground ambulance crashes.

Disadvantages
- In urban settings, ground ambulances are usually faster within a 30-mile range.
- If the helicopter is on another flight, no other aircraft may be available.
- Inclement weather may prevent the aircraft from traveling.
- The high noise level may limit or prevent communication with the patient or crew.
- Space and weight restrictions may limit access to the patient and restrict the crew, patients, and equipment that can be carried.
- Helicopter transports are more expensive than transports by ground ambulance.
- Helicopter crashes have fewer survivors.

LANDING SITE PREPARATION

The space requirement for a helicopter LZ generally is 100 by 100 feet. The ideal LZ should have no vertical structures that can hamper takeoff or landing. It should be relatively flat. It should be free of high grass, crops, or other factors that can conceal uneven terrain or hinder access. The LZ also should be free of debris that can injure people or damage structures or the helicopter. If patients are close to the LZ, the paramedic should provide protection by covering wounds and eyes. Rescue personnel close to the landing site should wear protective equipment such as helmets with lowered face shields and safety glasses.

If a nighttime LZ is used, emergency vehicles with lighted bar lights should be situated at the perimeters of the LZ. If white lights are used, they should be directed *down* to the center of the LZ as spotlights because white lights (spotlights or headlights) directed toward the aircraft can temporarily blind the pilot. Traffic cones with reflectors can help identify the LZ. Flares should not be used because the helicopter rotor wash can blow the flares from the site and create a fire hazard. A fire crew should wet down dusty LZs, especially if vehicle traffic is moving in the area. This prevents the pilot and vehicle drivers from being temporarily blinded by the dust.

Helpful radio communications with the pilot include notification of wind direction and any possible obstructions or hazards. Wind direction can be determined by throwing grass or dirt, wetting a finger, or by smoke patterns from smoke canisters. If hazardous materials are present, the paramedic should advise the flight crew of the substance, the location of the hazardous materials site, and the possibility of patient contamination. The pilot generally does not land the aircraft until all danger of fire or explosion has been eliminated. When the aircraft is coming in to land, one emergency responder should stand facing the LZ. That way, the pilot will see the landing area. LZ hand signals that may be useful to the pilot are shown in Fig. 49-6.

SAFETY PRECAUTIONS

Everyone should be clear of the landing area during takeoffs and landings. A distance of 100 to 200 feet is best (Fig. 49-7). In addition, paramedics should take the following precautions:

- Never allow ground personnel to approach the helicopter unless the pilot or flight crew asks them to do so.
- Allow only necessary personnel to help load or unload patients.
- Secure any loose objects or clothing that could be blown by rotor downwash (e.g., stretcher, sheets, or blankets).
- Do not allow smoking.
- After the aircraft is parked, move to the front beyond the perimeter of the rotor blades and *wait for a signal from the pilot* to approach.
- Approach the helicopter in a crouched position, staying in view of the pilot or other crew members.
- *Never approach the rear of the aircraft from any direction.* The tail rotors on most aircraft are near the ground and spin

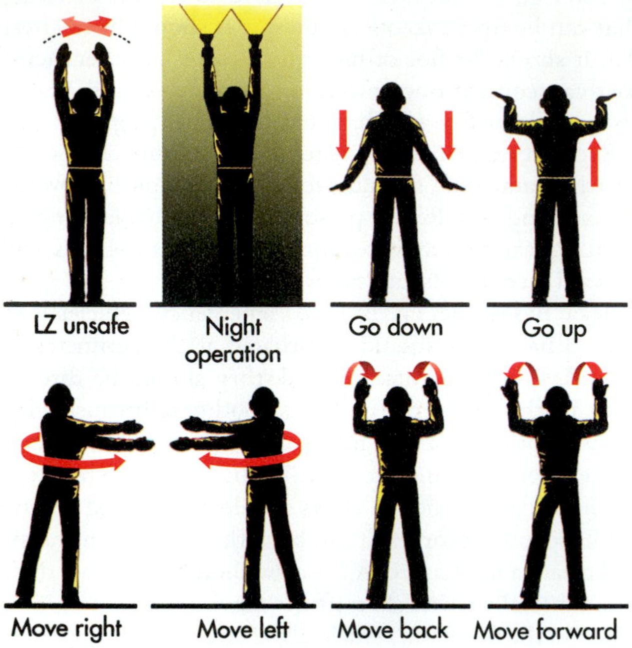

FIGURE 49-6 ■ Landing zone hand signals.

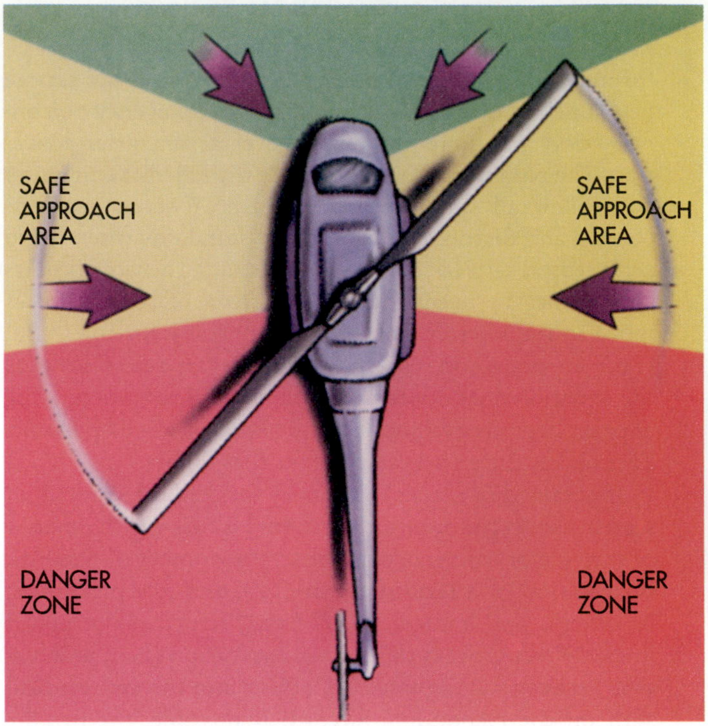

FIGURE 49-7 ■ Safe-approach zones.

at 3400 revolutions per minute. This makes them virtually invisible. Tail rotor injuries are often fatal.

- Carry long objects horizontally and no higher than waist high.
- Depart the helicopter from the front and within view of the pilot.

PATIENT PREPARATION

Preparing a patient for air transport requires special measures. Some medical procedures must be done *before* the patient is loaded into the aircraft. For example, the patient's airway must be established and secured before loading. Also, application of a traction splint must be done before loading. Special equipment (e.g., automated chest compression devices) must be positioned according to the aircraft's configuration. Most aeromedical crews perform a brief patient assessment before liftoff. They do so to verify the patient's condition. Patients who are combative may require physical or chemical restraint during flight.

CRITICAL THINKING

How do you think an alert patient would feel while waiting for helicopter transportation?

SUMMARY

- The federal KKK A-1822D standards provide the foundation of uniformity for the design of ambulance vehicles.
- Completing an equipment and supply checklist at the start of every work shift is important. It is essential for safety, patient care, and risk management. It also helps to ensure proper handling and safekeeping of scheduled medications.
- The methods for estimating ambulance service needs and placement in a community have changed. Compliance in providing EMS services within time frames that meet national standards is the method that now is commonly used.
- Factors that influence safe ambulance operation include proper use of escorts, environmental conditions, proper use of warning devices, proceeding safely through intersections, parking at the emergency scene, and operating with due regard for the safety of all others.
- The staffing of air ambulances includes a pilot and various health care professionals. These individuals undergo specialized training in flight physiology and the use of special medical equipment and procedures.
- When paramedics request aeromedical service, the flight crew should be advised of the type of emergency response, the number of patients, and the location of the landing zone and any prominent landmarks and hazards. Paramedics should always follow strict safety measures during helicopter landings. This helps to prevent injury to air medical crews, ground crews, the patient, and bystanders.

REFERENCES

1. American Heart Association: *Textbook of advanced cardiac life support,* Dallas, 1997, The Association.
2. Ambulance crash-related injuries among emergency medical services workers: United States, 1991-2002. www.cdc.gov/mmwr/preview/mmrhtml/mm5208a3.htm. Accessed October 28, 2003.
3. Fitch J: *Prehospital care administration: issues, readings, cases,* St Louis, 1995, Mosby.
4. National Safety Council: *Injury facts*, Itasca, Ill, 2002, The Council.
5. Kahn C et al: Characteristics of fatal ambulance crashes in the United States: an 11-year retrospective, *Prehospital Emergency Care,* July-Sep, 5(3):261-269, 2001.
6. US Department of Transportation, National Highway Traffic Safety Administration: *Air medical crew national standard curriculum,* Washington, DC, 1988, The Department.
7. Burkle FM: Emergency medicine in the Persian Gulf. I. Preparations for triage and combat casualty care, *Ann Emerg Med* 23(4):742, 1994.
8. Air Medical Transport Registry. http://www.flightweb.com/AMT-Registry. Accessed March 17, 2005.

CHAPTER

50

Medical Incident Command

OBJECTIVES

Upon completion of this chapter, the paramedic student will be able to:

1. Identify the components of an effective incident command system.
2. Outline the activities of the preplanning, scene management, and postdisaster follow-up phases of an incident.
3. Identify the five major functions of the incident command system.
4. List command responsibilities during a major incident response.
5. Describe the section responsibilities in the incident command system.
6. Identify situations that may be classified as major incidents.
7. Describe the steps necessary to establish and operate the incident command system.
8. Given a major incident, describe the groups and/or divisions that would need to be established and the responsibilities of each.
9. List common problems related to the incident command system and to mass casualty incidents.
10. Outline the principles and technology of triage.
11. Identify resources for the management of critical incident stress.

KEY TERMS

divisions: Subdivisions of the incident command system that encompass specific geographical areas of responsibility as deemed necessary by the incident commander.

groups: Subdivisions of the incident command system that encompass specific functional areas of responsibility as deemed necessary by the incident commander.

incident command system: A management program designed to control, direct, and coordinate emergency response operations and resources.

major incident: An event for which available resources are insufficient to manage the nature of the emergency.

mass casualty incident: An event for which available resources are insufficient to manage the number of casualties.

mutual aid: An agreement with neighboring emergency agencies to exchange equipment and personnel when necessary.

*A **major incident** is an event for which the available resources are insufficient to manage the number of casualties or the type of emergency. Major incidents include highway crashes, air crashes, major fires, train derailments, building collapses, acts of violence or terrorism, search and rescue operations, hazardous materials releases, and natural disasters. These incidents stress and may overwhelm local, regional, state, and even national and international resources.*

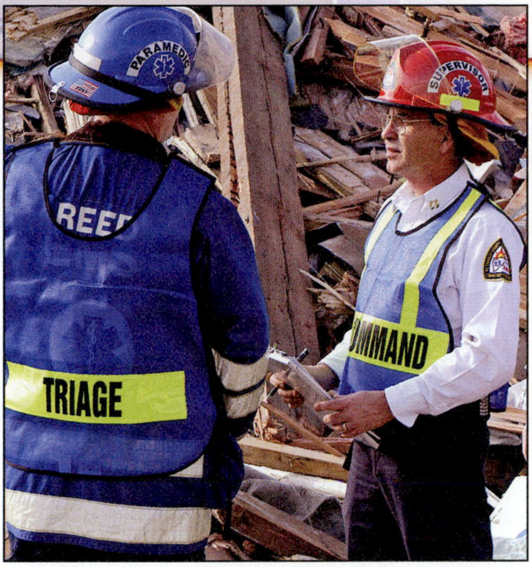

NOTE The term *disaster* usually is associated with a man-made or natural event. The event involves damage across a large area or to a community's infrastructure. (For example, this may include roads, power, communications, or housing.) A subcategory of a disaster is a **mass casualty incident** (MCI), which involves many injuries and/or fatalities. The mobilization of resources and the methods used to meet the needs of a disaster response constitute *disaster management*.

CRITICAL THINKING

What effect do you think lack of organization could have on rescue operations, scene safety, patient care, and transportation in a major incident?

INCIDENT COMMAND SYSTEM

In the past, the management of a **major incident** often involved a number of different agencies. For example, emergency medical services (EMS) agencies, the fire service, rescue organizations, law enforcement, and others may have responded. Each of these agencies operated independently. Interagency organization and personnel accountability were minimal to nonexistent. This made it difficult to determine who was in charge of the scene. It also made it difficult to determine what emergency services were needed or were being provided.

The **incident command system** (ICS) was developed to address these concerns. This system organizes interagency functions and responsibilities. In 2004 the ICS was included as part of the National Incident Management System (NIMS) of the Department of Homeland Security. All emergency response agencies at every level of government are required to use the incident command system at *all* incidents[1] regardless of the type, size, or complexity.

The ICS provides for a number of arrangements: (1) single jurisdiction and single agency involvement; (2) single jurisdiction and multiagency involvement; and (3) multijurisdiction and multiagency involvement. This allows the ICS to be adapted to the needs of any agency or to the particular incident requiring emergency management. The ICS also must be capable of being expanded from dealing with a nonmajor incident to a major one in a logical way. Use of the ICS as standard operating procedure for small incidents allows a smooth transition when a major incident occurs.[2] Other components of the ICS include common elements of organization, terminology (Box 50-1), and procedures. The system should be put into place with the least possible disruption to existing systems (EMS, fire, and law enforcement agencies). It should be simple enough to keep operating and upkeep costs to a minimum.

The ICS system can easily be used at a minor incident in which the units dispatched to the scene are sufficient to handle the event. It can be expanded if more units are needed for a minor incident that becomes a major one. Use of the ICS is critical whenever it becomes apparent that the need for extended operations will quickly overwhelm the

BOX 50-1 Important Terminology for Medical Incident Command Systems

apparatus: A vehicle used for fire suppression or rescue; this category does not include staff vehicles.
command: The act of directing, ordering, or controlling by virtue of explicit, statutory, regulatory, or delegated authority.
command post: The area from which command directs operations for an incident.
communications center: A facility used to dispatch emergency equipment and coordinate communications between field units and personnel.
division: A subdivision of the incident command system (ICS) that encompasses a specific geographic area of responsibility as deemed necessary by the incident commander.
group: A subdivision of the ICS that encompasses a specific functional area of responsibility as deemed necessary by the incident commander.
medical direction: A process of ensuring that actions taken on behalf of ill or injured people are medically appropriate, including prospective, concurrent, and retrospective aspects of emergency medical services (EMS) quality improvement, hiring, and education.
mutual aid: An agreement with neighboring emergency agencies to exchange equipment and personnel when necessary.
staging area: A designated area where incident-assigned vehicles are directed and held until needed.

responding units. (An example is an event that involves many patients or one that may last several hours to days.)

Federal law now requires use of the ICS in response to all types of incidents. The ICS is a flexible system. It is used in both the public and private sectors in some routine and most large-scale emergencies. Much of the success of the ICS is due to its application of a common organizational structure and key principles in a standardized way. ICS organization is built around the following five major components (Fig. 50-1)[3]:

1. Command
2. Finance/Administration
3. Logistics
4. Operations
5. Planning

The five major components of ICS are also known as *C-FLOP* (command, finance/administration, logistics, operations, planning). They are the foundation on which organization develops. They apply during a major event, in preparation for a major event, or in management of the response to a major event.

Command Function

At most incidents the responsibility of command should belong to *one* person. This should be an individual with the ability to coordinate a variety of emergency activities. This is the cornerstone of the ICS structure.

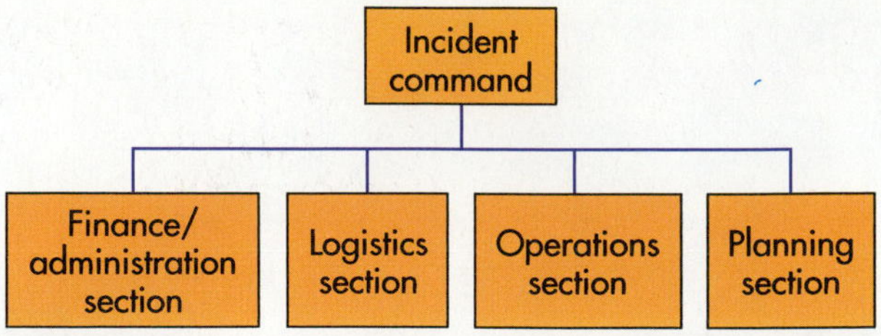

FIGURE 50-1 ■ Incident command system organization (C-FLOP).

The initial command should be determined by a preplanned system of arriving emergency units and personnel (e.g., the first or second arriving EMS, fire, or law enforcement unit). The person assuming command is the *incident commander (IC)*. This person must be familiar with the ICS structure. The IC also must be familiar with the operating procedures of other responding agencies. The IC need not be the person with the highest rank or the most medical training (although this is commonly the case). Rather, the IC should be the person best able to manage the emergency scene effectively.

Command must be established immediately. The commander must be clearly identified. Also, all others at the scene must be informed as to who is in command. As a more qualified person arrives, command may be transferred per standard operating procedures (SOPs). Once established, command should take the following steps:

- Assume an effective command mode and position
- Transmit brief initial radio reports to the communications center, identifying the location of the command post
- Evaluate the situation quickly
- Develop a management strategy
- Request more resources and provide assignments as needed
- Implement a personal accountability system
- Control and assign **divisions** and/or **groups** as required (these should be consistent with the needs of the incident, SOPs, or disaster plans); also, provide these units with operating objectives
- Provide ongoing effective command and progress reports until relieved by a higher ranking person
- Develop the command organization by delegating authority to subordinates (this helps to accomplish incident needs and objectives)
- Review and evaluate the effectiveness of site operations and revise these operations as needed
- Return units to service and end command when appropriate

TYPES OF COMMAND

Command may take a single or unified form (Box 50-2). With single command, one person is responsible for the entire operation. This type of command often works well for incidents with limited jurisdictions or responsibilities. It also works best in small events of short duration.

BOX 50-2 Single and Unified Command Structures

- In a *single command structure,* a single incident commander (IC) is solely responsible (within the confines of authority) for establishing objectives and for devising the overall management strategy for the incident. The incident commander is directly responsible for follow-through. The IC must ensure that all functional area actions are directed toward accomplishment of the strategy. Implementation of the overall strategy is the responsibility of a single individual (section chief). This person reports directly to the incident commander.
- In a *unified command structure,* the individuals designated by their jurisdictions (or by departments within a jurisdiction) must jointly determine objectives, strategies, and priorities. As in the single command structure, the section chief is responsible for carrying out the plan.

Unified command may be needed in large events or as a small incident evolves. In unified command, specialized organizations are identified (e.g., EMS, fire, police, health department, American Red Cross), and personnel unify to complement command. This type of command stimulates cooperation (the "right" agency leads command at the "right" time) and provides for balanced decision making. It also facilitates *interoperability* (the ability of multiple organizations to communicate effectively) when many different radio frequencies and types of communications equipment are used by responding agencies. The concept of unified command means that all involved agencies contribute to the command process by (1) determining the overall objectives; (2) planning jointly for operational activities while conducting integrated operations; and (3) maximizing the use of all assigned resources (Fig. 50-2). Unified command may be indicated in incidents such as those involving the following factors:

- More than one political jurisdiction is affected.
- A number of agencies within a jurisdiction are involved.
- The incident affects several geographical and functional agencies.

CRITICAL THINKING

Where do you think command should be located in a major incident that is confined to one area?

In either single or unified command, the IC may delegate authority for certain activities by activating additional sections (operations, planning, logistics, or finance/administration). These sections help to meet the needs of the situation. The incident commander bases the decision to expand (or contract) the ICS organization on three major incident priorities[3]:

1. *Life safety.* The IC's first priority is *always* the safety of the responders and the public.

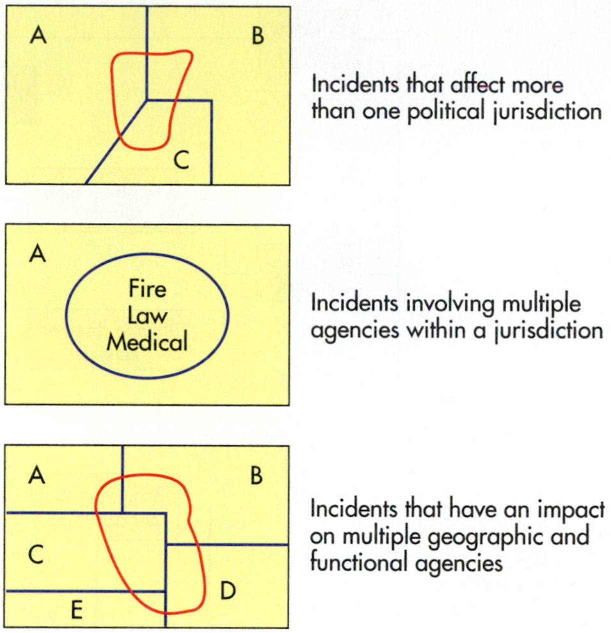

FIGURE 50-2 ■ Application of unified command.

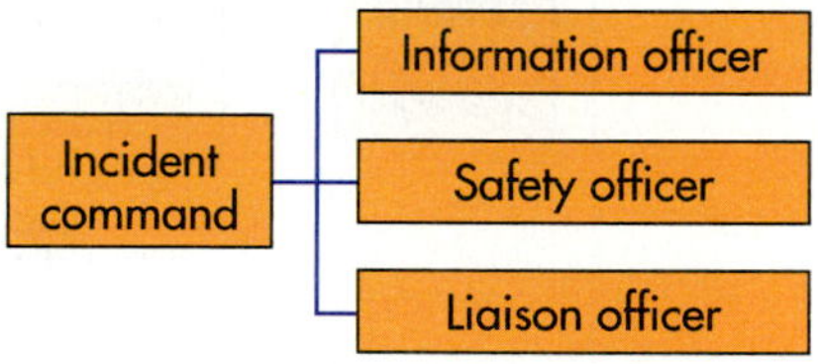

FIGURE 50-3 ■ Command staff positions. The information officer handles all media inquiries and coordinates the release of information to the media with the public affairs officer at the emergency operations center (EOC). The safety officer monitors safety conditions and develops measures for ensuring the safety of all assigned personnel. The liaison officer is the on-scene contact for other agencies assigned to the incident.

2. *Incident stability.* The IC is responsible for deciding on strategies to minimize the effect of the incident on the area. These strategies also should maximize the response effort while using resources effectively.
3. *Property conservation.* The IC is responsible for minimizing damage to property while achieving the incident objectives.

When expansion of command is required, the IC establishes the other general staff positions (Fig. 50-3).

Section Responsibilities

In the ICS, a manageable *span of control* (the number of people one section chief can manage effectively) falls within the range of three to seven, with five being the optimum.[2]

In some cases the span of control indicates that the incident organization must be expanded to allow effective management of the situation. In such cases the IC assigns one or more of the general staff sections (planning, operations,

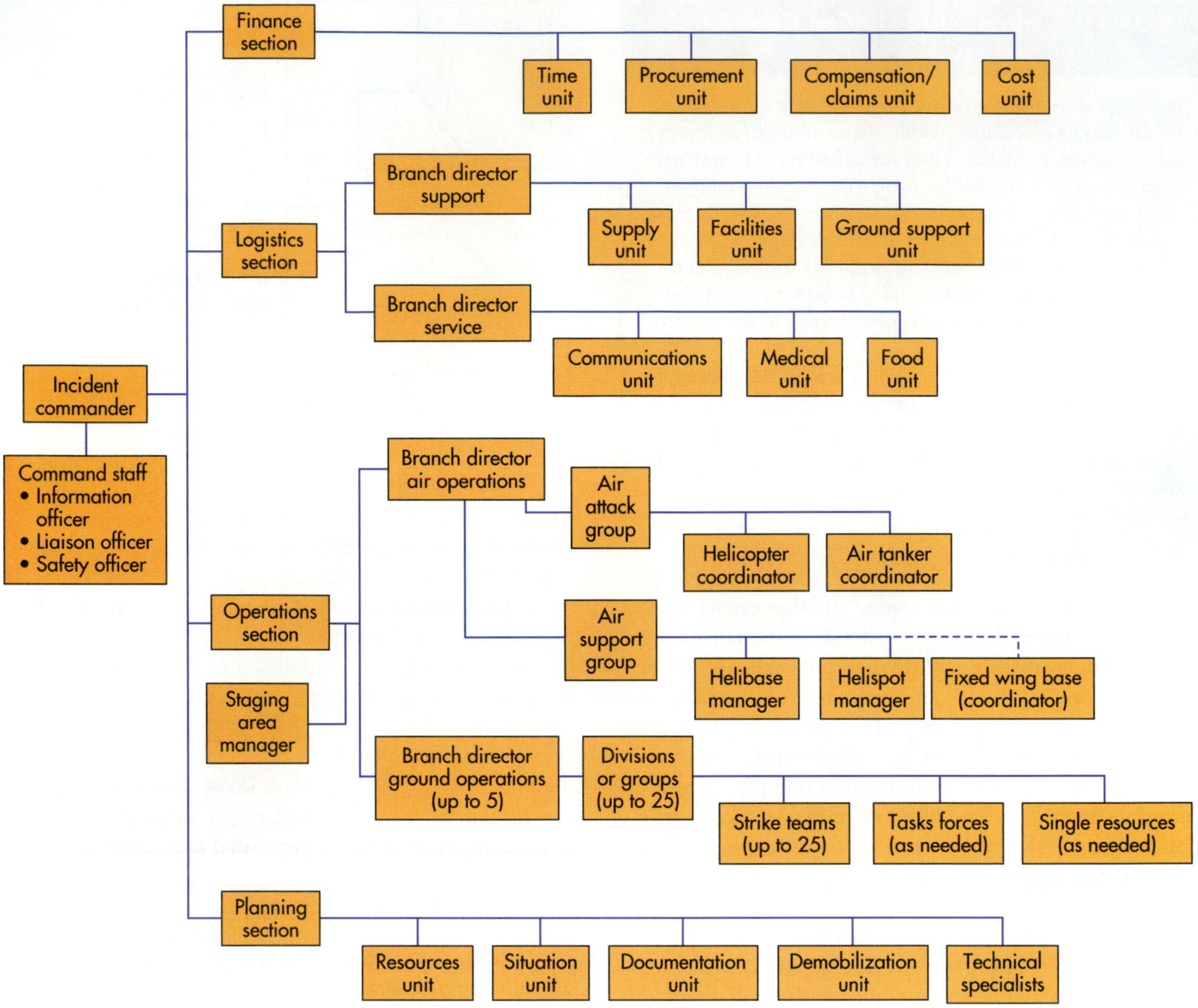

FIGURE 50-4 ■ Command section organizational plan.

logistics, and/or finance/administration) to sections chiefs. Section chiefs must be strong supervisors and managers. Their chief role in the ICS is to "make things happen." They enact the plans and strategies of the incident commander. They also ensure that all rescuers in their sections are working toward a common goal. Which of the four sections may be needed varies, depending on the scope of the incident. The IC makes this determination (Fig. 50-4).

Section chiefs should not become involved in physical tasks. (Examples of such tasks are carrying litters or operating rescue equipment.) This allows them to maintain control and supervise the section. General responsibilities of section chiefs include the following:

- Accomplishing the objectives set by command
- Monitoring work progress
- Redirecting activities as necessary
- Coordinating related activities with other sections
- Requesting additional resources as needed for the section
- Monitoring the welfare of personnel from each section
- Providing command with frequent reports
- Reallocating resources within the section

The section chief should report to command when a job is assigned, when a job is accomplished, or if a job cannot be accomplished.

FINANCE/ADMINISTRATION SECTION

The finance/administration section (Fig. 50-5) is important for tracking costs and the way reimbursement is handled. This section is seldom used in small-scale incidents. However, it is considered essential if the incident grows in magnitude and costs (e.g., a presidential declaration of a disaster). Functions of the finance/administration section during a major incident may include time accounting, procurement, payment of claims, and estimation of costs.

LOGISTICS SECTION

The logistics section (Fig. 50-6) is responsible for providing supplies and equipment (including personnel to operate the equipment), facilities, services, food, and communications

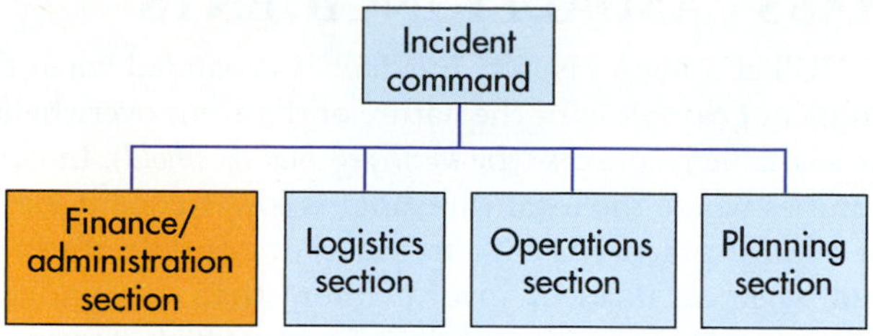

FIGURE 50-5 ■ Finance/administration section.

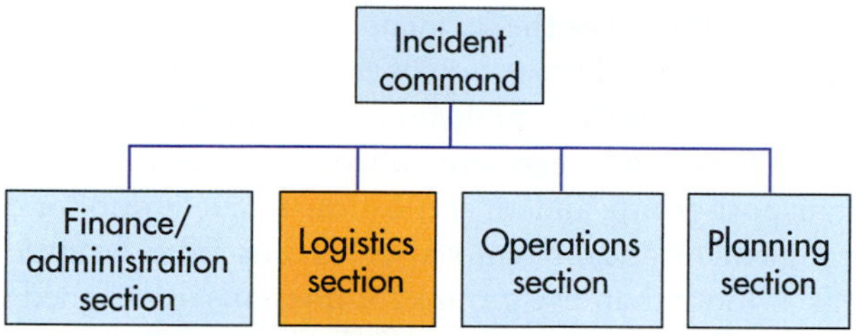

FIGURE 50-6 ■ Logistics section.

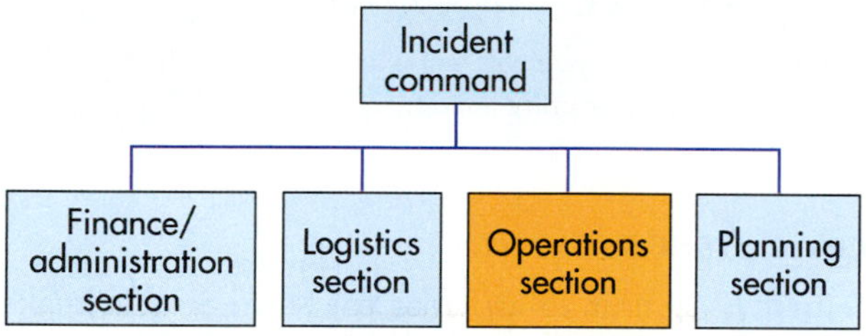

FIGURE 50-7 ■ Operations section.

support. The main function of this section is to provide gear and support to the responders. The essential equipment for supporting a medical incident includes supplies for airway, respiratory, and hemorrhage control, burn management, and patient packaging and immobilization. Resources for moving and transporting patients (people, ambulances, buses) also may be needed. The medical unit of the logistics section cares for the incident responders; it does not care for the civilian victims. Often part of the logistics section is used for routine daily incidents. For example, responder rehabilitation and the support branch are parts of the logistics section.

OPERATIONS SECTION

The operations section (Fig. 50-7) directs and coordinates all emergency scene operations. It also ensures the safety of all personnel. (EMS operation areas generally fall under this section.) The operations section chief is in charge of the tactical operations at an incident. This person is responsible for the following activities:

- Accomplishing tactical objectives
- Directing front-end activities
- Participating in planning
- Modifying action plans as needed
- Maintaining discipline

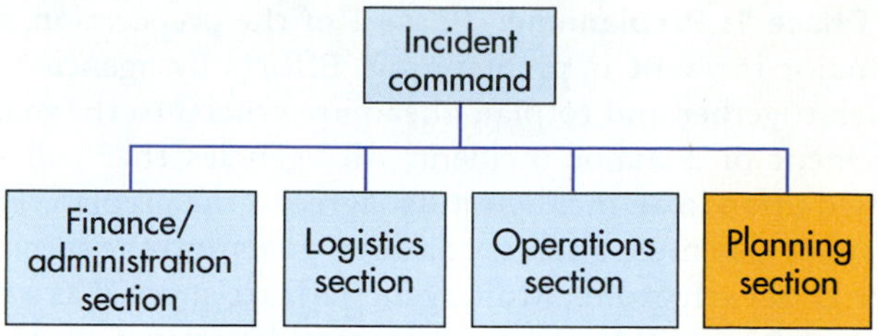

FIGURE 50-8 ■ Planning section.

- Accounting for personnel
- Updating command on the progress or lack of progress of an operation

PLANNING SECTION

The staff function of the planning section (Fig. 50-8) is to provide past, present, and future information about the incident and the status of resources. This section's duties also may include the creation of a written or verbal incident action plan (IAP). (The incident commander determines the need for an IAP.) The IAP defines the response activities and use of resources for a specified period. These operational periods can vary in length; however, they should be no longer than 24 hours (12-hour operational periods are common for large-scale incidents). IAPs may be indicated when (1) resources from several agencies are used; (2) several jurisdictions are involved; or (3) the incident is complex (e.g., changes in shifts or personnel are required).

Declaring a Major Incident

Declaring a major incident is a critical phase of the response. If an EMS unit is dispatched to a scene that has this potential, the crew should be advised or should declare (per established protocol) that they are responding to a possible major incident or **mass casualty incident** (MCI) and will confirm on arrival. This information allows other agencies to be contacted, and those agencies can be placed on standby. It also allows time for determination of the availability of other resources. Medical direction and area hospitals should also be alerted. The receiving hospitals need information on the number of patients and the severity of injuries as soon as possible. That way, they can begin to prepare for the patients' arrival. A possible major incident should be declared when

- More than two ambulance units are required for adequate treatment, particularly in rural areas where communities may have only one ambulance
- Hazardous or radioactive materials or chemicals in significant quantity are involved
- An MCI results in a large number of patients and requires special EMS resources, such as helicopters, rescue teams, or several rescue or extrication units

PREPARING FOR A MAJOR INCIDENT

Preparation for a major incident involves three phases: preplanning, scene management, and postdisaster follow-up (or after-action review).[3]

Phase 1: Preplanning. Phase 1 of the preparation for a major incident is preplanning. Efforts by agencies to work together and to plan ahead are crucial to the management of a major incident. All agencies that will be called upon in an incident must agree to the preplan. The preplan also must address common goals and the specific duties of each group. Multiagency efforts succeed as a result of frequent meetings and practice sessions or exercises (drills or "tabletop" exercises). The preplan should include a system of sorting or prioritizing care, treatment, and transportation.

▶NOTE The details of the preplan can be found through the community's local emergency planning committee (LEPC).

Another component of the preplan is the identification of hazards in a community (a risk assessment). Such hazards may include the manufacture, storage, and transport of hazardous materials; fire threats; the population base at various times of the day; and violence and other potential social problems. An inventory of resources that may be needed during a major incident includes the following:

- Shelter and mass feeding
- Air evacuation
- Medical equipment and supplies
- Heavy equipment, power generators, and lighting
- Communications equipment
- Law enforcement personnel
- Specialized rescue services

Phase 2: Scene Management. Phase 2 of preparation involves the development of a strategy to manage the incident scene. Some major incidents can be managed with local resources and personnel (closed or contained incidents). However, other incidents may affect large geographical areas and many jurisdictions (open or uncontained incidents). In these incidents, many federal, state, and local agencies become involved. Regardless of the size of the incident or the number of agencies involved, scene management calls for a coordinated effort. This effort must ensure an effective response and the efficient and safe use of resources.

▶NOTE The procedure for managing a major multiagency, multijurisdictional incident is outlined in the federal National Incident Management System (NIMS). This procedure should be adopted for local use.

Phase 3: Postdisaster Follow-up. Phase 3 involves a postdisaster (or after-action) review. This includes the "lessons learned" from the incident. It also includes methods of improvement. These may include improvement of emergency response, planning, and community protection. This phase also should assess stress-related anxiety and illness among emergency workers that may have resulted from the incident.

MASS CASUALTY INCIDENTS

The ICS at a mass casualty incident is expanded when the number of casualties or the nature of the event overwhelms the available resources (the *local/regional threshold*). In communities where the local threshold is low, frequent use of the ICS for practice is encouraged. (For example, it can be used when an incident involves more than one patient.) When a mass casualty incident is identified, command must quickly determine how best to expand the ICS to meet the needs of the event. In other words, sections, groups, and divisions must be put into place according to the size and scope of the incident.

Typically, initial expansion of the ICS for a mass casualty incident requires the establishment of a medical group (including triage and treatment subcomponents, called *units*); a transport group; and an extrication/rescue group for disentanglement and/or removal of victims from hazardous areas. If more than five groups (or divisions, if assigned geographically) are activated, an operations section typically is established (Fig. 50-9).

CRITICAL THINKING

How do you think you will feel when you arrive first on the scene of a mass casualty incident?

Scene Assessment

The first EMS unit to arrive at the scene should make a quick and rapid assessment (size-up) of the situation. A more precise and full assessment should be performed as soon as safety and time allow. This fuller assessment should include the following:

- The type of incident and the potential duration
- Whether entrapment or special rescue resources may be needed
- The number of patients in each triage category (described later in this chapter)
- Initial assignments for incoming units
- The need for any additional resources to manage the incident

▶NOTE The scene assessment must be updated continually. This helps in the identification of specific or changing needs.

Communications

Command must immediately establish radio contact with the main communications center or the emergency operations center (EOC). Most jurisdictions maintain an EOC as part of their community's preparedness program. An EOC is where department heads, government officers and officials, and volunteer agencies gather to coordinate their response to an emergency event. Command and the EOC

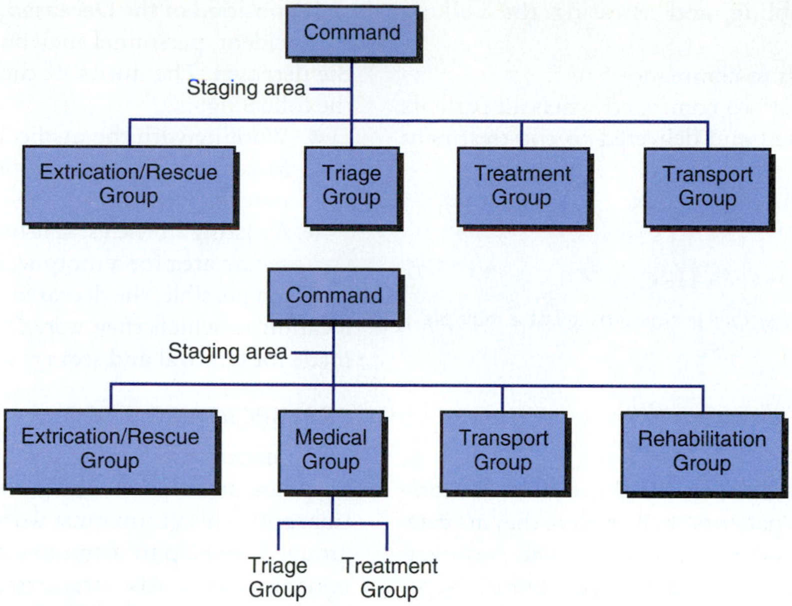

FIGURE 50-9 ■ Two examples of ICS for mass casualty incidents.

share similar goals. However, they function at different levels of responsibility. The incident commander is responsible for on-scene activities. The EOC is responsible for the entire community-wide response to the event. Radio traffic can be very distracting; therefore incident personnel must observe strict radio and/or phone procedures. Moreover, they should use clear, plain English. All transmissions should be short and to the point.

Obtaining Resources

More units should be requested as soon as the need has been identified or anticipated. (The communications center should have a written SOP for requesting **mutual aid.**) Support may include obtaining food, shelter, and clothing for victims. The IC is responsible for providing instructions for the deployment of the resources. (Personnel should stay with their vehicle until instructions are received.) Staging techniques that may be used to deploy resources effectively include the following:

- Lining vehicles up at the scene to facilitate egress
- Staging away from a limited access highway
- Identifying a formal staging area with an assigned staging officer

The "tool box" theory of strategic deployment of resources can be used. It involves identifying the resources ("tools") specific to the incident, using only the needed resources, and issuing instructions for the deployment of resources.

Group or Division Functions

As stated before, the number of groups or divisions needed at a major medical incident varies. Common groups and their responsibilities include extrication/rescue, treatment, and transportation. The staging area, rehabilitation area, and support branch are also important parts of an incident organization.

EXTRICATION/RESCUE GROUP

The extrication/rescue group is responsible for managing patients who are trapped at the scene. This involves rescue, initial triage, tagging, and treatment before transfer of the patients to the treatment group. Patient care for this group includes only assessment and treatment of life-threatening injuries. Examples include the need to secure airways, control severe bleeding, and cover open chest wounds. In addition, the rescue/extrication group is responsible for site safety and personnel safety (e.g., supplying self-contained breathing apparatus; atmospheric monitoring if indicated for explosive or oxygen-deficient atmospheres; protective clothing) and for evaluating and directing the resources needed for extrication and rescue. Rescue/extrication group responsibilities include the following:

- Determining whether triage and the primary treatment will be conducted on site or in the treatment group area
- Attaching tagging assignments to injured patients
- Evaluating the resources needed for extrication of trapped patients and for their delivery to the treatment group
- Ensuring site safety
- Evaluating resources needed for triage and the primary treatment of patients
- Communicating resource requirements to command
- Allocating assigned resources
- Supervising assigned personnel and resources

- Collecting, assembling, and assessing the walking wounded
- Reporting progress to command
- Reporting "all clear" to command when all patients have been extricated and delivered to the treatment group
- Coordinating with other groups

CRITICAL THINKING

What dilemmas might you face in doing triage at a multiple casualty incident?

TREATMENT GROUP

The treatment group works closely with the rescue/extrication group in patient care. As patients are delivered, they are categorized according to their medical needs. The treatment group provides advanced care and stabilization until the patients are transported to a medical facility. Most paramedics and hospital personnel are assigned to this group.

With a large number of patients, the area usually is further divided into immediate and delayed treatment zones. This helps in the determination of priorities for patient transport. Immediate treatment patients include those with life-threatening injuries; delayed treatment patients include the walking wounded and those whose care and transport can be delayed if necessary. It should be noted that triage monitoring is a function of all groups involving ill or injured patients. It is a continuing component of the ICS. Treatment group responsibilities include the following:

- Locating a suitable treatment area that satisfies hazardous material (hazmat) concerns, if applicable (e.g., uphill/upwind/upstream) and reporting that location to the rescue/extrication group and command
- Evaluating resources required for patient treatment and reporting these needs to command
- Providing continued triage of patients arriving in the treatment area
- Providing suitable immediate and delayed treatment areas
- Allocating resources
- Assigning, supervising, and coordinating personnel in the group
- Reporting progress to command
- Coordinating with other divisions and groups

On-Scene Physicians. Physicians who are on scene can provide valuable help during an MCI. The roles of the physicians may include providing on-scene medical direction, making difficult triage decisions and secondary triage decisions in a treatment area, and performing emergency surgery to facilitate extrication. Physicians also can perform specialized invasive procedures at the scene, as well as a more detailed patient assessment. In addition, they may provide direction for specific treatments that may be beyond the scope of normal paramedic practice.

Disposition of the Deceased. Depending on the scale of the incident, personnel may be assigned to disposition of the deceased. The duties of these individuals may include the following:

- Working with the medical examiner, coroner, law enforcement, and other appropriate agencies to coordinate disposition
- Assisting in the establishment of an appropriate and secure area for a morgue, if needed

When possible, the deceased victims should be left in the location in which they were found until a plan has been made for removal and storage of the bodies.

TRANSPORTATION GROUP

The transportation group communicates with the receiving hospitals, ambulances, and aeromedical services for patient transport. This group must work closely with the treatment group. They help to determine appropriate destinations for injured patients. Also, the arrival and departure of transfer vehicles must be coordinated with the staging area. Transportation group responsibilities include the following:

- Determining patient transportation needs and obtaining appropriate transportation
- Evaluating resources required to manage patient transportation
- Establishing an ambulance staging area (if command has not already done so) and patient loading areas
- Establishing and operating a helicopter landing zone
- Communicating with hospitals to determine capabilities
- Coordinating patient transportation allocations with the treatment group and hospitals
- Tracking patients leaving the site with a written log (including patient identification, the transporting unit, and the destination facility)
- Reporting resource requirements to command
- Coordinating with other divisions and groups
- Advising command when the last patient has been transported

Staging Area

Staging areas are needed for large incidents. They help to prevent vehicle congestion and delays in response. All emergency vehicles (fire, law enforcement, EMS) should report to this area for direction. Other agencies, such as disaster relief services and news media, also may be supervised by the staging area manager. The responsibilities of the staging area manager include the following:

- Coordinating with law enforcement personnel to block streets, intersections, and other areas to allow the set-up of a staging area
- Ensuring that all equipment and vehicles are parked in an appropriate manner
- Maintaining a log of all equipment in the staging area and an inventory of all specialized equipment and medical equipment that may be needed

- Reviewing with command the resources that must be maintained in staging, as well as coordinating this request with the dispatching center
- Assuming a visible position for incoming equipment and vehicles (e.g., leaving emergency lights operating on one vehicle and wearing an identification vest)
- Coordinating with other divisions and groups

Rehabilitation Area

A rehabilitation (rehab) area is part of the major incident response plans of many fire and EMS agencies. This area usually is set up outside the operational area. It allows rescue personnel to get physical and psychological rest. With smaller incidents, the rehab unit leader usually reports directly to command. In large-scale incidents or whenever a logistics group is established, the rehab unit leader reports to the logistics chief. (In large-scale incidents, more than one rehab area may be needed.)

One duty of the rehab unit leader is to ensure that personnel get medical care and treatment as needed. Another duty is to keep accurate logs of those who enter and leave the area. Records of medical care and treatments are kept for each person who enters the rehab area. (Medical care of rescue personnel is further addressed in Chapter 53.)

CRITICAL THINKING

Why do you think a rehabilitation area is important?

Support Branch

The support branch is in charge of gathering and distributing equipment and supplies. This branch may be responsible for obtaining medical supplies from area hospitals, rescue supplies, and other equipment needed at the incident. Support branch responsibilities include the following:

- Determining the medical supply needs of other divisions and groups
- Establishing a suitable location for supply operations
- Coordinating procurement of medical supplies from hospitals with the transportation group
- Coordinating procurement of medical supplies that are not available from hospitals
- Reporting additional resource requirements to command
- Allocating supplies and equipment as needed
- Reporting progress to command
- Coordinating with other divisions and groups

NOTE Often only specific parts of the logistics group are needed at an incident. One of these is the rehabilitation unit; the other is the support branch. Depending on the span of control, these two units can be implemented without the establishment of a logistics group section chief; they report directly to command.

Identification and Communication

When an ICS is in place, all responders must know its organizational structure and the lines of radio communication. Although clothing and identification vary by system, the following guidelines usually apply:

- Color-coded vests identify personnel. For example, the commander may wear a white vest; EMS group managers, blue vests; fire group managers, red; law enforcement group managers, green; and so on.
- With the exceptions of command and division/group communications, most communications are face to face. Radio use is intended for command operations.
- Radio communications use operation titles instead of personal or unit names: "Treatment group to command" or "Rescue/extrication group to treatment group." This system ensures that all participants can reach the appropriate person by one radio designation.

RADIO COMMUNICATIONS

Communications is a key function during a major incident. Preplanning includes identifying the radio frequencies to be used in major incident responses. It also includes planning for the ways these frequencies are to be used. For example, all responding units should have multichannel radios that use a common frequency. Within this common frequency, separate frequencies should be used for EMS, fire, and other support operations. Division and group officers should have portable radios set on a channel that permits direct communication with command. These channels may be assigned in advance or by the dispatching agency at the time of the incident. In addition, state, regional, and local communications systems should undergo a periodic review. This review should include the controls for activating communications, system frequencies, and portable and mobile radio equipment. Other communications considerations include the following:

- Radio traffic must be clear, concise, and in plain English.
- Messages should be given thought and prepared before transmission.
- The speaker should clearly identify the unit number or division or group.
- All radio traffic should be minimized.
- Face to face communication is preferable and encouraged.

Common Problems at Mass Casualty Incidents

In addition to common failures of incident command systems (Box 50-3), there are common problems specific to mass casualty incidents. These include the following[1]:

- Failure to adequately provide widespread notification of the event

BOX 50-3 Common Failures Seen in the Incident Command System

Incident Command Failures
- To establish a single, unified command
- To establish staging
- To request additional resources early
- To delegate authority
- To wear identification vests

Dispatch Failure
- To coordinate the response of on-duty and off-duty emergency personnel to the scene

Communications Failures
- To designate a single radio channel for disaster operations
- To adopt standard operating procedures that limit radio traffic during incident operations

Staging Operation Failures
- To establish a central staging area (command)
- To select a large or easily accessible staging area (staging manager)
- To frequently inventory specialized equipment and personnel (staging manager)

General Division/Group Failures
- To provide adequate progress reports to command
- To become involved in physical tasks, such as carrying litters or operating rescue equipment (division/group supervisor)
- To control the perimeter (law enforcement)
- To advise command of available personnel

Extrication/Rescue Group Failures
- To triage and tag patients
- To treat patients where they are found (as opposed to stabilizing them and moving them to a treatment area) (rescuers)
- To provide adequate safety precautions

Treatment Group Failures
- To collect patients into an organized treatment area
- To establish a sufficiently large treatment area
- To organize the treatment area and monitor patients
- To effectively coordinate transportation arrangements with the transportation group

Transportation Group Failures
- To establish adequate access and egress routes for vehicles
- To have adequate personnel to assist in transportation
- To alert or update hospitals
- To advise hospitals when the last patient has been transported

Support Branch Failures
- To plan for the medical supply needs of mass casualty events
- To provide rapid transport of supplies to the scene

- Failure to provide rapid initial stabilization of all patients
- Failure to move, collect, and organize patients quickly in a treatment area
- Failure to provide proper triage
- Provision of overly time-consuming care
- Transport of patients prematurely
- Improper use of personnel in the field
- Failure to distribute patients to medical facilities properly
- Failure to communicate with local hospitals regarding patient flow and hospital capacity
- Lack of proper preplanning and of adequate training for all personnel

PRINCIPLES AND TECHNOLOGY OF TRIAGE

Triage is a method of categorizing patients according to priorities of treatment. Assessment of the severity of injury is based on abnormal physiological signs, obvious anatomical injury (including the mechanism of injury), and concurrent disease factors that might affect the patient's prognosis. It should be stressed that triage is an ongoing process during a major incident. Constant monitoring of the patient's condition may reveal a need to change the initial grouping and priority of treatment. The criteria for triage classifications are determined by the size of the incident, the number of injured patients, and the available personnel. No national standards have been established yet for field triage. However, the most widely recognized model is the simple triage and rapid treatment (START) technique. The paramedic must be familiar with local methods of triage categorization.

Primary versus Secondary Triage

Triage may be classified as primary or secondary. *Primary triage* is used at the site to rapidly categorize patient conditions for treatment. During primary triage, the paramedic records the location of the patient and the transport needs. A triage label, tag, ribbon, or tape is then attached to the patient. No care is given during primary triage except for immediate life-saving measures to ensure an airway or control hemorrhage. The goal is to sort patients quickly.

Secondary triage is used at the treatment area, where patients are triaged again. They are labeled (usually with pa-

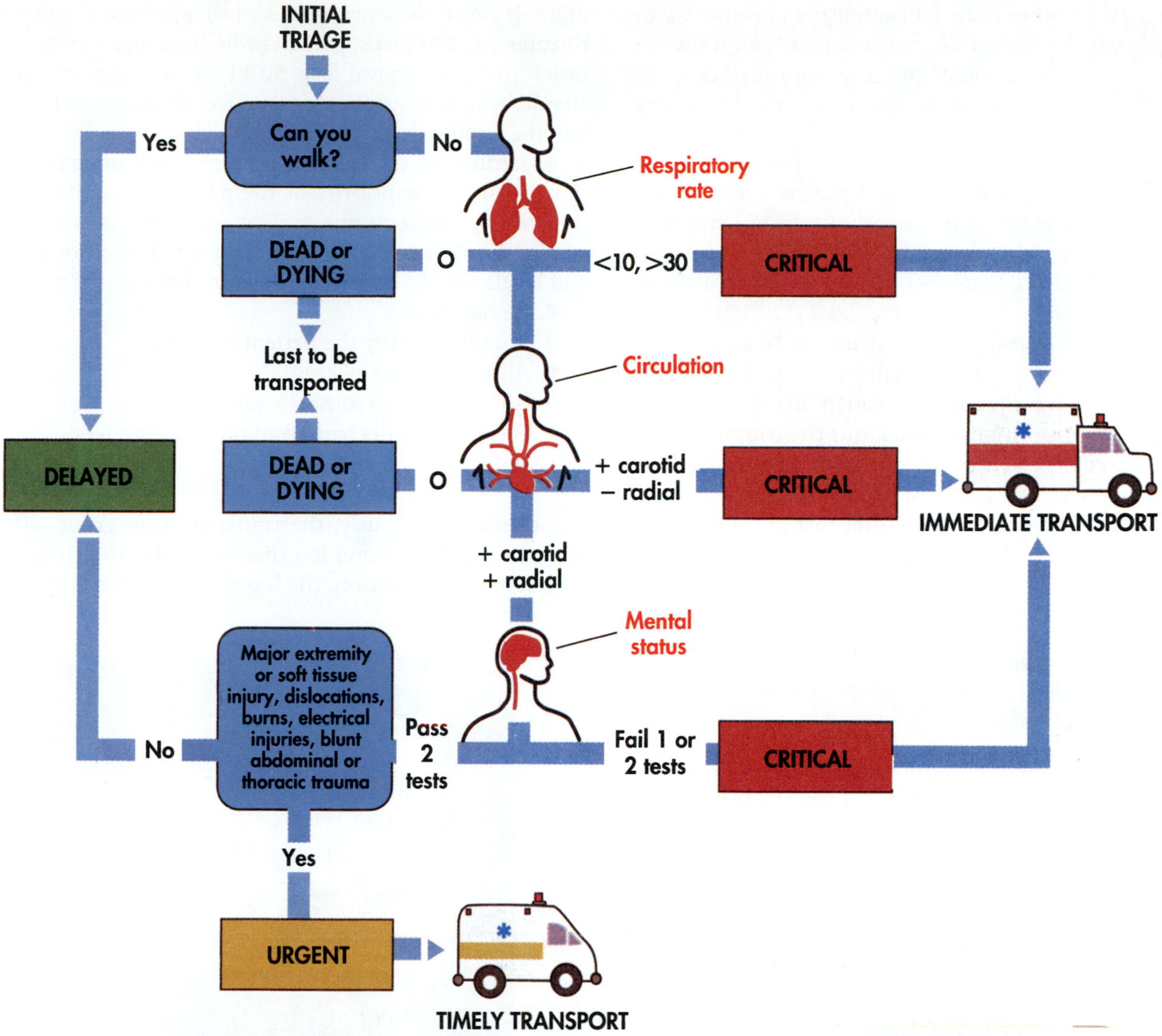

FIGURE 50-10 ■ The simple triage and rapid treatment (START) system sorts patients into critical or delayed categories. Patients are quickly removed from the scene according to their triage group.

per tags) to assign priorities of care. Secondary triage often is not needed at small-scale incidents.

START Technique of Primary Triage

The *START Field Guide* was developed by Hoag Memorial Hospital Presbyterian in Newport Beach, California. It describes a 60-second assessment. This assessment focuses on the patient's ability to walk, respiratory effort, pulses/perfusion, and neurological status (Fig. 50-10). This assessment is used to classify a victim's status as delayed, urgent, critical, or dead/dying. The *START Field Guide* allows rescuers to quickly identify victims at greatest risk of early death. Rescuers can then advise other rescuers of the patient's need for stabilization by tagging the patient with color-coded triage tags (described below).

Procedure. START triage has four basic assessment steps. Paramedics and other rescue personnel should do the following:

1. *Assess the patient's ability to walk.* Patients who can walk and understand basic commands are classified as *delayed* (walking wounded). Direct delayed patients to remain in their location for further assistance or to walk to a treatment or transportation site. If the patient cannot walk, assess the respiratory rate (step 2). (*Note:* The initial triage is directed toward patients who cannot walk.)
2. *Evaluate breathing and rate.* If breathing is absent, the patient is classified as *dead/dying.* A rate of fewer

than 10 or more than 30 breaths per minute in an adult patient indicates *critical* status. Based on the respiratory assessment and the paramedic's intuition, these patients also can be classified as *urgent* or *delayed.*

3. *Assess pulses/perfusion.* If no pulse is present, the patient is classified as *dead/dying.* A present carotid pulse and an absent radial pulse indicate *critical* status. If both the carotid and radial pulses are present, assess the mental status (step 4) before assigning a triage classification.
4. *Assess mental status.* Mental status can be assessed by asking the patient to perform two simple tasks. For example, have the patient touch his or her nose with the index finger or stick out the tongue; in addition, assess orientation with name, date, and year. Patients who can perform both tasks are classified as *delayed.* Those who fail either test are considered *critical.*

CRITICAL THINKING

What conditions might a patient have if the respiratory rate is fewer than 10 or more than 30 breaths per minute?

As mentioned before, repositioning the airway and controlling severe hemorrhage are the only treatments given in primary triage. However, in a mass casualty event, these measures should not delay the triage of other patients. Depending on the circumstances and the number of casualties, the walking wounded may be able to help provide airway support and control severe hemorrhage for more seriously wounded victims.

Triage Tagging/Labeling

Many types of tags, tapes, ribbons, and labels are used to indicate a victim's triage category. One labeling method is the METTAG system. This system uses the international agreement on color coding and priorities to alert emergency care personnel and staff members of the receiving hospital to the patient's category (Table 50-1). Red identifies the victims who are most critically injured; yellow, those less critically injured; green, those with injuries that are not life or limb threatening; and black, patients who have died or whose injuries preclude survival (Fig. 50-11). Triage tags and labels should be used routinely, for practice. That way, EMS crews become familiar with their use.

Regardless of the labeling system used, categorization must identify the priority of the patient's condition, prevent retriage of the same patient, and serve as a tracking system during treatment and transport. Therefore all tags and labels should have the following characteristics:

- Be easy to use
- Rapidly identify the patient's priority
- Allow for easy tracking
- Allow room for some documentation
- Prevent patients from retriaging themselves

TABLE 50-1 International Color Coding and Priorities

PATIENT STATUS	COLOR CODE	PRIORITY
Immediate	Red	Priority no. 1 (P-1)
Delayed	Yellow	Priority no. 2 (P-2)
Hold	Green	Priority no. 3 (P-3)
Deceased	Black	Priority no. 0 (P-0)

From US Department of Transportation, National Highway Traffic Safety Administration: *EMT-paramedic national standard curriculum,* Washington, DC, 1998, The Department.

Tracking Systems for Patients

As described previously, the transportation group officer must keep a destination log that integrates the triage tagging system. In addition, the log should have the patient's

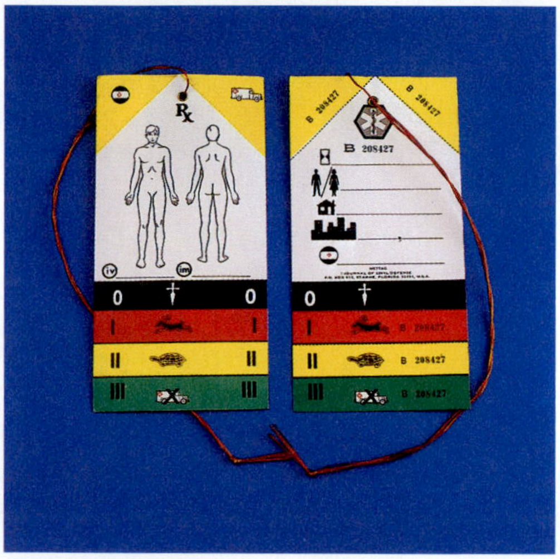

FIGURE 50-11 ■ METTAG card.

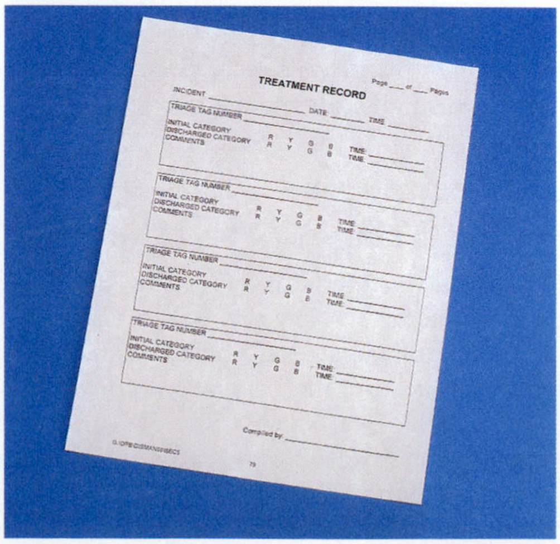

FIGURE 50-12 ■ Incident command system (ICS) patient log.

name or triage label identification number. A tracking log (Fig. 50-12) is similar to a shipping manifest. It must have the following information:

- Patient identification
- Transporting unit
- Patient priority
- Hospital destination

Transportation of Patients

The way patients are transported depends on their triage priority and situation. Ambulances typically are used. However, buses may be used to transport a large number of stable patients. Air ambulances are usually reserved for the transport of patients in critical condition.

CRITICAL INCIDENT STRESS MANAGEMENT

As described in Chapter 2, critical incident stress is a potential hazard for rescue personnel. For this reason, critical incident stress debriefings often are conducted after a disaster. To review, the basic types of services that should be made available include the following[4]:

- Preincident stress training for all personnel
- On-scene support for obviously distressed personnel
- Individual consults when only one or two rescuers are affected by an incident
- Defusing services immediately after a large-scale incident
- Mobilization services after a large-scale incident
- Critical incident stress debriefing 24 to 72 hours after an event for any emergency personnel involved in a stressful incident
- Follow-up services to ensure that personnel are recovering
- Specialty debriefings to nonemergency groups when no other timely resources are available in the community
- Support during routine discussions of an incident by emergency personnel
- Advice to command staff during large-scale events

Other approaches that can aid stress management include employee assistance programs, counseling, spouse support programs, family life programs, pastoral services, and periodic stress evaluations.

SUMMARY

- The ICS organizational structure should be adaptable to any agency or to any incident requiring emergency management. The ICS also must be expandable. It must be able to expand from dealing with a nonmajor incident to a major one in a logical way.
- All participating response agencies must agree to the preplan (phase 1 of the ICS). The preplan must address common goals and the specific duties of each group. Phase 2 requires the development of a strategy to manage the emergency scene. Phase 3 includes a postdisaster review of lessons learned from the incident and the determination of ways to improve.
- The five major functions of the ICS organization are command, planning, operations, logistics, and finance/administration.
- The responsibility of command should belong to one person. This should be a person who can effectively manage the emergency scene. In multiagency and/or multijurisdictional incidents, unified command may be used.
- The planning section should provide past, present, and future information about the incident and the status of resources. The operations section directs and coordinates all operations. It also ensures the safety of all personnel. The logistics section is responsible for providing supplies and equipment (including personnel to operate the equipment), facilities, services, food, and communications support. The finance/administration section tracks incident and reimbursement costs.
- The need to expand the ICS at a medical incident is based on the number of casualties and the nature of the event.
- The first EMS unit to arrive at the scene should make a quick and rapid assessment of the situation. Command must immediately establish radio contact with the communications center or emergency operations center. Additional units should be requested as soon as the need has been identified.
- Common divisions or groups that may need to be established include extrication/rescue, treatment, and transportation. A staging area and support branch may also be needed. The rescue/extrication group is responsible for managing trapped patients at the scene. The treatment group provides advanced care and stabilization until the patients are transported to a medical facility. The transportation group communicates with the receiving hospital, ambulances, and aeromedical services for patient transport. The staging area is used in large incidents to prevent vehicle congestion and delays in response. The rehabilitation area allows rescue personnel to receive physical and psychological rest. The support branch coordinates the gathering and distribution of equipment and supplies for all divisions and groups.

- Problems of mass casualty incidents and incident command systems stem from numerous issues related to communication, resource allocation, and delegation.
- Triage is a method used to categorize patients for priorities of treatment. START triage uses a 60-second assessment. It focuses on the patient's ability to walk, respiratory effort, pulses/perfusion, and neurological status. The METTAG system is one of a number of tape, tag, and label systems used to categorize patients during triage.
- Critical incident stress debriefing is part of a critical incident stress management program. Such debriefing should be part of postdisaster standard operating procedures.

REFERENCES

1. US Department of Homeland Security, National Incident Management System, Washington, DC, 2004.
2. US Department of Transportation, National Highway Traffic Safety Administration: *EMT-paramedic national standard curriculum,* Washington, DC, 1998, The Department.
3. Federal Emergency Management Agency: *Incident command system for emergency medical services,* Emmitsburg, MD, 1996, US Fire Administration.
4. Mitchell J, Bray G: *Emergency services stress,* Englewood Cliffs, NJ, 1990, Brady Publishing.

SUGGESTED READING

FIRESCOPE: field operations guide (420-1) Incident Command System Publication, Mather, Calif., 2004, California Office of Emergency Services.

US Department of Homeland Security: *Protecting emergency responders:* vol 3, *safety management in disaster and terrorism response,* vol 3, Washington, DC, 2004, National Institute for Occupational Safety and Health.

CHAPTER

51

Rescue Awareness and Operations

OBJECTIVES

Upon completion of this chapter, the paramedic student will be able to:

1. Describe factors that must be considered to ensure appropriate timing of medical and mechanical skills during a rescue.
2. Outline each phase of a rescue operation.
3. Identify the appropriate personal protective equipment (PPE) for rescue operations.
4. Describe important considerations for emergency medical services (EMS) crews in a surface water rescue.
5. Discuss important considerations for EMS crews in rescues associated with hazardous atmospheres, including confined spaces and trench or cave-in situations.
6. Describe hazards that may be present during an EMS rescue operation on a highway.
7. Describe important considerations for EMS crews in a rescue involving hazardous terrain.
8. Outline special considerations for prehospital assessment and management during a rescue operation.

KEY TERMS

disentanglement: The process of making a pathway through the wreckage of an accident and removing wreckage from patients.

hazard control: The phase of rescue that involves managing, reducing, and minimizing risks from uncontrollable hazards; ensuring scene safety; and providing personal protective equipment appropriate for the incident.

patient packaging: Completion of emergency care procedures needed to transfer a patient from the scene to the emergency vehicle.

rescue: The act of delivery from danger or imprisonment.

__Rescue__ is defined as "the act of delivery from danger or imprisonment."[1] Many of the day-to-day activities of EMS crews and other public service agencies meet this definition. For example, paramedics are called to care for people who have been traumatized or stranded. Rescue requires specialized medical and mechanical skills. It also requires a knowledge of the appropriate time to use these skills.

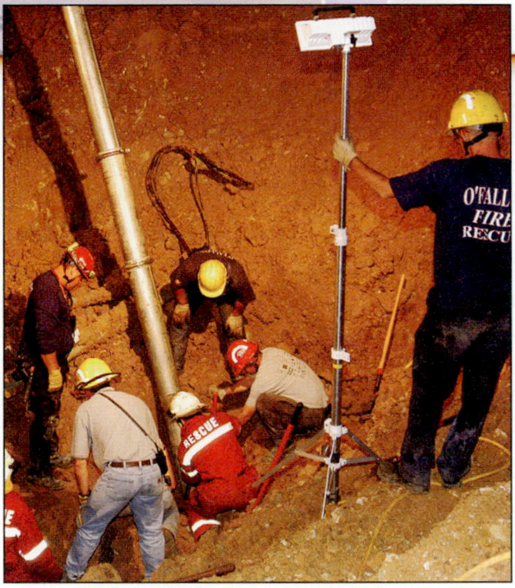

NOTE Rescue skills have become highly specialized. Techniques have been devised and refined for farm rescue, high-angle rescue, rescue in confined spaces, search and recovery, and others. In addition, many rescue agencies require training and certification by an authority or jurisdiction. A number of rescue skills may be needed in a specific area. Also, many different techniques may be involved in a rescue. This chapter focuses on concepts that are basic to all rescue operations.

APPROPRIATE TRAINING FOR RESCUE OPERATIONS

Rescue work requires training and expertise. The medical and mechanical skills are carefully balanced. This helps to ensure that patients get effective treatment and timely extrication.

The rescue effort must be driven by the patient's needs, both medical and physical. The success of any rescue depends on a coordinated effort between medical care and specialized rescue efforts. A coordinated effort allows the following:

- Patient access and assessment for treatment needs
- Initiation of treatment at the site
- Release of the patient from entrapment or imprisonment
- Continuous medical care throughout the incident

Role of the Paramedic in Rescue Operations

Most rescues in the United States are accomplished through a systems operations approach. In this form of management, extrication is performed by fire service personnel, specialized units, or both. Patient care is the duty of the emergency medical services (EMS) provider. In another type of rescue system, rescue services are provided by fire, EMS, or law enforcement agencies that have cross-trained personnel. In this system, the roles and responsibilities for rescue and patient care are shared.

The main role of the paramedic in a rescue is to have proper training and appropriate personal protective equipment (PPE). These allow for safe access to the patient and treatment at the site and throughout the rescue. Paramedics often are the first responders to many scenes that require rescue. Therefore they should

- Understand the hazards associated with various environments
- Know when it is safe to gain access or attempt rescue
- Have the skills to perform a rescue when it is safe and necessary
- Understand the rescue process and know when certain techniques are indicated or contraindicated
- Be skilled in patient packaging techniques to allow safe extrication and medical care

CRITICAL THINKING

What kind of emotions do you think you would see in a critical life-threatening rescue?

Safety

Safety during any rescue is paramount because of the potential for associated risks. For example, rescues may involve hazardous materials, inclement weather, temperature extremes, fire, electrical hazards, toxic gases, unstable structures, heavy equipment, road hazards, and sharp edges and fragments. Initial scene assessment for hazards, personal protective measures, and constant monitoring throughout the operation are essential for every rescue response.

The priorities for safety in any rescue are (1) personal safety, (2) the safety of the crew, (3) the safety of bystanders, and (4) rescue of the trapped and injured. The reasons for this order of priority are as follows:

- When well-trained and properly equipped rescuers act safely, remaining vigilant for hazards, they minimize the risk of personal injury and of complicating the scene by becoming another patient who requires care and possibly extrication.
- The crew is the support team for the rescuer. Therefore crew safety is essential to ensure an effective rescue and to provide mutual support for each team member. Operating with disregard for the safety of fellow team members increases the risk of injuries. It also complicates the operation.
- Uninvolved people must be evacuated and kept clear of hazards. Bystanders or untrained "helpers" only increase the risk of additional injuries. They also complicate the rescue operation.
- Rescue of the trapped or injured is the last priority. These people are already trapped or injured. Carrying out the first three priorities safely maximizes the chance for a successful rescue.

PHASES OF A RESCUE OPERATION

A rescue operation has seven phases[1]: (1) arrival and scene size-up, (2) hazard control, (3) gaining access to the patient, (4) medical treatment, (5) disentanglement, (6) patient packaging, and (7) transportation. As is stressed throughout this text, paramedics should not enter a scene until it has been secured and made safe by trained personnel. Personal safety is always a priority.

Arrival and Scene Size-Up

The first phase of a rescue is the arrival and scene size-up. That is, paramedics must decide what is needed at a specific emergency. This involves quickly gathering facts about the situation, analyzing the problems, and determining the appropriate response. During this phase, the EMS crew must

- Understand the environment and risks
- Establish command and conduct a scene assessment
- Determine the number of patients and triage as necessary
- Determine whether the situation is a search, rescue, or body recovery
- Perform a risk versus benefit analysis that considers personal safety before rescue is attempted
- Request additional information
- Make a realistic time estimate in accessing and evaluating patients or other people at the scene

Scene size-up is an ongoing evaluation of the emergency scene. It begins when the call is received and when information is obtained from the dispatch center. The paramedic must constantly be alert to situations that may change the needs of a particular incident. If power lines are downed during an extrication, for example, electrical utility services may be needed that were not initially required.

Three elements of the assessment phase are response, other factors, and resources.

RESPONSE

During the initial response to a scene, information often is limited. En route, the EMS crew and the dispatcher should gather as much detail about the situation as possible. Essential information includes exact location, type of occupancy (manufacturing, mercantile, residence), number of victims, type of situation, and hazards involved. Weather conditions (e.g., extreme heat or cold, rising water, rain, high winds) also can affect rescue attempts, the patient's condition, and the need to expedite the operation.

Standardized dispatch protocols guide the initial emergency response. This system is based on the details of the reported emergency. For example, if the event is a single-car crash, a first-responder fire company and EMS unit may be dispatched. If the event involves a bus wreck with many patients, several fire companies and EMS units may respond. As the dispatch center receives information about the actual severity of the event, the dispatch protocol upgrades or downgrades the response as needed. The center advises the responding units of the updated reports.

CRITICAL THINKING

Is there any disadvantage to routinely sending too much emergency equipment to a scene?

OTHER FACTORS

Other factors to be considered in determining the type of response needed are the description of the scene and the time of day. An emergency in a highly populated area may call for special vehicles and equipment for extrication and fire suppression. Examples of such a scene would be a high-rise apartment, a school, or a shopping mall. An emergency in a rural or wilderness setting may require helicopter rescue or other resources. If hazardous materials are present, special response and decontamination equipment may be needed for bystanders, patients, and rescue personnel.

The time of day may affect on-scene needs. For example, rush-hour traffic and crowd control may be a concern; extra lighting may be needed for early morning, evening, or night rescue. These and other factors determine the personnel requirements and the scene management operations.

RESOURCES

The ability to assess an emergency quickly and correctly requires preplanning. It also requires the development of a systems approach to the response. The available resources are a critical part of any response. The responding crew may not have the personnel, training, or expertise to handle the event. Resources that may be required include the following:

- Additional emergency vehicles for a large number of patients
- Area hospital availability and personnel
- Aeromedical services
- Law enforcement
- Fire service for automobile extrication, fire suppression, or lighting
- Water rescue, teams with self-contained underwater breathing apparatus (SCUBA), and other specialized rescue units
- Hazardous materials teams
- Urban search and rescue teams

Hazard Control

Hazard control is the phase of rescue in which on-scene dangers are quickly identified and managed by the first-arriving crew. This involves minimizing risks from uncontrollable hazards, making sure the scene is as safe as possible, and ensuring that all personnel are equipped with PPE appropriate for the incident. Examples of possible hazards at a scene include fire, unstable structures, confined spaces, poisonous substances, and unruly crowds. Hazard control for specific types of incidents is discussed throughout this chapter.

Gaining Access to the Patient

Rapid access to an ill or injured patient who requires extrication or rescue can be critical to the patient's eventual outcome. For patients who have multisystem trauma, assessment, stabilization, and extrication should be rapid. However, these procedures must be accomplished with the safety of both the patient and the rescue team as a top priority. To safely gain access, the paramedic must determine the best method of reaching the patient, deploy appropriate personnel to the patient, and stabilize the patient's physical location.

Extrication tools and equipment (Fig. 51-1) can cause injuries. To reduce the risk, paramedics should use the least amount of force needed. They should clear the area of unnecessary people. In addition, extraneous noise should be kept to a minimum. Also, a safety officer should remain alert to the stress of the operation on the rescuers. This officer should rotate personnel to prevent heat exposure disorders and injuries resulting from fatigue. Rescuers should wear approved protective clothing. Also, protective covering for the patient should be supplied.

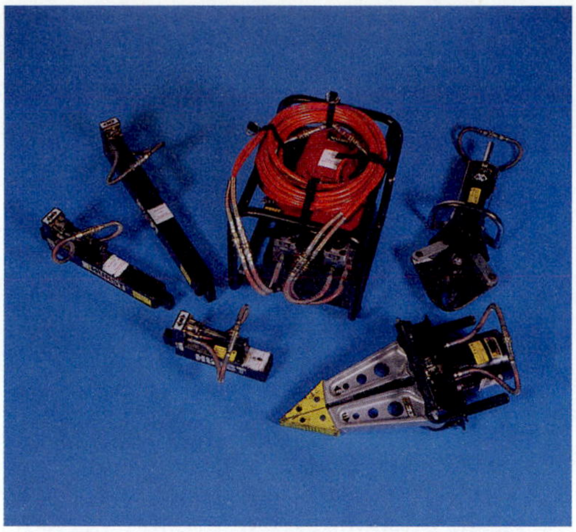

FIGURE 51-1 ■ Extrication tools and equipment.

Paramedics may not directly take part in freeing the patient. However, they have chief responsibility for patient care. In addition, they serve a key role as observers for potentially hazardous procedures. The team concept is the most important element in any rescue or operation. Teamwork maximizes safety, efficiency, and effectiveness. It is a basic element of prehospital care. In addition, it has powerful implications for the safety of responders.

Medical Treatment

After the team has gained access to the patient, medical treatment can begin. The paramedic should perform a rapid initial assessment; this helps to identify and manage any life-threatening situations. Care may be limited by circumstances and the working area. However, the paramedic may be able to start some stabilization procedures, such as spinal immobilization, airway management, oxygen administration, and intravenous (IV) fluid therapy. If the paramedic recognizes rapidly fatal or potentially fatal conditions, a "load and go" approach must be taken. In these cases, rapid extrication and transport are indicated.

A physical examination should be performed after the initial assessment has been completed and life-threatening conditions have been stabilized. Another crew member may perform the examination at the same time if it does not interrupt the initial assessment and emergency care.

Disentanglement

Disentanglement involves making a pathway through the wreckage of an incident and removing wreckage from patients. The main responsibilities of the paramedic during disentanglement are to release the patient from entrapment and to perform a *risk versus benefit* analysis. This analysis should take personal safety into account. This phase of rescue is driven by the needs of the patient. It may call for specialized rescue personnel and equipment. Paramedics should be aware of the available resources in their area. They also should know how to mobilize these resources. Disentanglement often is time-consuming; the EMS crew should be prepared for extended scene time.

CRITICAL THINKING

What rescue teams are accessible to your community?

Patient Packaging

Stabilizing a patient physically and preparing the person for transport is known as **patient packaging.** This may call for special rescue capabilities. For instance, the patient may need to be moved over hazardous terrain or lifted by hoist to a helicopter. As with all other aspects of rescue, the coordination of activities and patient care among the various agencies offers the greatest chance of a successful outcome.

It is the paramedic's duty to make sure the patient is ready to be removed from the scene. It also is the paramedic's duty to protect the patient from additional injury during disentanglement and egress. The patient should be covered with blankets or tarpaulins and provided with ear and eye protection. In addition, a face mask with supplemental oxygen or air should be applied. This protects the patient from toxic fumes, if present.

For minimum packaging for transport, the patient's airway and cervical spine must be stabilized, IV lines and oxygen tubing must be secured, and the patient must be immobilized on a long spine board. When time allows, extremity fractures should be immobilized and open wounds covered with sterile dressings and secured with bandages. A scene delay for patients who require rapid stabilization and transport may lessen the patient's chances of survival.

Use of other patient care equipment should be considered as the patient is removed from the area of entrapment. Communication and coordination with other rescuers must continue during this process. The exit pathway must be clear and secure. No additional danger for the patient or the rescuers should exist during the removal phase.

During disentanglement and patient packaging, the paramedic should consider the patient's emotional needs. Patients often are anxious and frightened by the rescue operations. When possible, paramedics should maintain a rapport with the patient. They should (1) provide reassurance that the patient is well cared for; (2) prepare the patient for unexpected movements or procedures that may cause discomfort; and (3) explain all rescue situations.

Transportation

If the patient is to be transported immediately to the ambulance, a wheeled stretcher, basket stretcher, or long spine board should be available. While the patient is transported to the emergency vehicle, the terrain, equipment, and personnel requirements for moving the patient should be considered (e.g., the need for air evacuation, specialized resources and extra personnel). The ambulance should be appropriately warmed or cooled, based on the patient's needs and the rescue setting. The rescue is considered complete once the patient is en route to the hospital. As in any other patient transport, the EMS crew continues emergency care, and medical direction is advised of the patient's status.

RESCUER PERSONAL PROTECTIVE EQUIPMENT

Personal protective equipment for EMS personnel historically has been adapted from other fields (e.g., the fire service). The standards for protective clothing and PPE established by the National Fire Protection Association[2] and the federal Occupational Safety and Health Administration (OSHA)[3] have been adopted by many fire and EMS agencies, including a number of municipal and industrial fire services throughout the United States. It generally is agreed that, at minimum, EMS providers involved in rescue and other rescue personnel should have access to the following PPE:

- Impact-resistant protective helmet with ear protection and chin strap
- Safety goggles with elastic strap and vents to prevent fogging
- Lightweight, puncture-resistant turnout coat
- Slip-resistant, waterproof gloves
- Boots with steel insoles and steel toe protection
- Self-contained breathing apparatus (SCBA)

Different situations require different PPE. Adequate protection depends on the level of rescuer involvement and the nature of the incident. Other PPE may be appropriate in some rescue events (Box 51-1).

Personal Protection from Blood-Borne Pathogens

OSHA has established criteria for workplace protection from blood-borne and airborne diseases.[4,5] These measures for personal protection (see Chapter 39) should be observed whenever the potential exists for exposure to a patient's body fluids or to communicable diseases.

SURFACE WATER RESCUE

People are drawn to moving water for recreation. Many, including rescuers, underestimate the power and hazards of water. The hydraulics of moving water are affected by several variables. These include the depth and velocity of water and any obstructions to flow. Water rescue is very dangerous and requires special training and skills. Water rescue should never be attempted by a single rescuer or by an untrained one.

Obstructions to Flow

Water that moves over a uniform obstruction can create recirculating currents ("drowning machines") (Fig. 51-2). These can trap victims and make escape difficult.

BOX 51-1 Supplemental Personal Protective Equipment

Head Protection that Meets Safety Standards for the Appropriate Use
- Compact firefighters' helmet that meets National Fire Protection Association (NFPA) standards for most vehicle/structural applications
- Climbing helmet for confined space and technical rescue uses
- Padded rafting/kayaking helmet for water rescue

Eye Protection
- Adequate face shield (face shields on most fire helmets are inadequate)
- American National Standards Institute (ANSI)-approved safety glasses or goggles with solid shields (preferred)

Hearing Protection
- Required for high-noise areas
- Ear plugs or ear muffs should be available.

Hand Protection
- Gloves that allow adequate dexterity and protect against cuts and punctures

Foot Protection
- Gear that provides ankle support to limit range of motion
- Tread that provides traction and prevents slips
- Insulation from environmental extremes
- Steel toe/shank that meets safety requirements

Flame/Flash Protection (when Fire Is Possible)
- Nomex/PBI/flame-retardant cotton to provide limited flash protection, turnout clothing, jumpsuits/flyers/coveralls (*Note:* This clothing does not provide complete protection from punctures or cuts. The thermal protection offered by turnout clothing may increase heat stress.)

Personal Flotation Device (when Operating on or Around Water)
- Meets Coast Guard standards for flotation
- Type II or type III (preferred for most water rescue work)
- Attached whistle and strobe light
- Attached knife for cutting

Visibility
- Reflective trim on all outerwear
- Orange clothing or safety vests for use during highway operations

Extended, Remote, or Wilderness Protection
- Additional or different personal protective equipment, if needed, for bad weather conditions not normally encountered (e.g., cold, rain, snow, wind)
- Personal drinking water and snacks
- Possible shelter needs

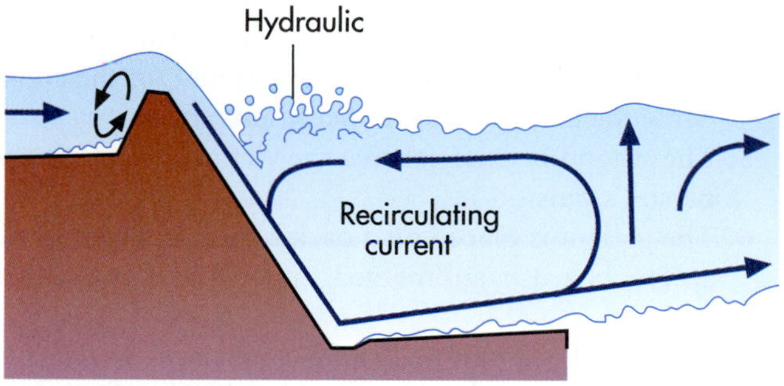

FIGURE 51-2 ■ Low-head dams range in height from 6 inches to 10 feet. They can create dangerous hydraulics.

Recirculating currents commonly are found in rivers and on low-head dams and often appear harmless. (The height of the dam is no indication of the degree of hazard.) The force of the moving water is very deceptive and makes for a hazardous rescue. Trapped victims often succumb to fatigue, hypothermia, and drowning.

Strainers are obstructions (e.g., trees, grating wire, or mesh) that allow current to flow through but that can trap objects such as boats or people. The force of the water against the victim makes escape difficult. Rescue teams must approach strainers cautiously to avoid becoming entrapped themselves.

Foot or Extremity Pin

It generally is considered unsafe to walk in fast-moving water that is over knee-high depth. Doing so may lead to entrapment of an extremity in a strainer, and the victim can be dragged under the water's surface. With a foot or extremity pin, it is crucial to remember that *the body part must be extricated in the same way it went in.*

Flat Water

About 3900 deaths occur each year in flat (static) water (lakes, ponds, and marsh) as a result of drowning.[6] Factors that contribute to these deaths include alcohol or other drug use. Another factor is a cool water temperature, which leads to hypothermia. These factors can quickly incapacitate a victim and result in drowning. Most people who drown never planned on being in the water, and personal flotation devices (PFDs) that are worn routinely and fastened properly when a person is on or around the water can save lives by reducing the likelihood of drowning.[1] PFDs are required during water rescue operations. Type I or type II PFDs are preferred for water rescue work. Specialty type III PFDs are suitable for some rescue situations.[7]

Water Temperature

As described in Chapter 38, immersion in water with a temperature below 98° F (37° C) can cause hypothermia. A person cannot maintain body heat when the water tempera-

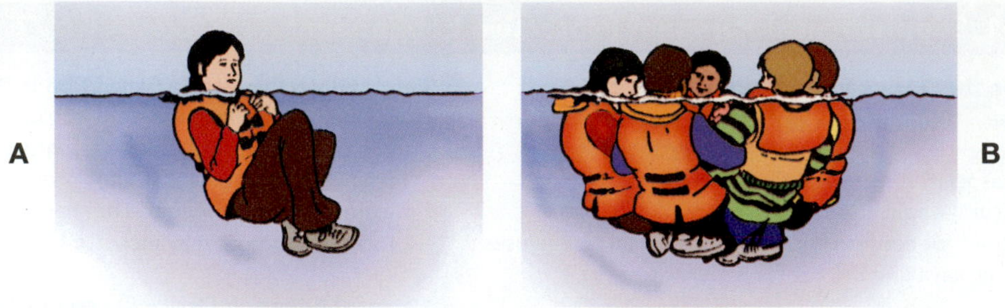

FIGURE 51-3 ■ HELP and HUDDLE. When a person is floating in cold water, body heat can be conserved by using a body position that reduces the escape of heat. **A,** If the person is alone, the HELP position should be used. **B,** If several people are present, they should *huddle* together.

ture is below 92° F (33° C). Water causes heat loss 25 times faster than exposure to air at the same temperature. (The colder the water, the faster the rate of heat loss.) At a water temperature of 35° F (1.7° C), a person immersed for 15 to 20 minutes likely will die of hypothermia and drowning.[1]

Sudden immersion in cold water may trigger laryngospasm. This can lead to aspiration, severe hypoxia, and unconsciousness. If hypothermia develops, the victim often is unable to follow directions (e.g., grab a safety device). Also, the victim often is unable to help himself or herself to safety. PFDs lessen heat loss and the energy required for flotation. In cases of sudden immersion, a single victim should assume a fetal position (the heat escape–lessening posture [HELP]). Multiple victims should *huddle* together to reduce heat loss (Fig. 51-3).

COLD PROTECTIVE RESPONSE

The cold protective response is the *mammalian diving reflex* (see Chapter 38). This response increases the chance of a victim's survival in cold water. To review, this protective response includes parasympathetic stimulation from immersion of the face in cold water. It leads to bradycardia, peripheral vasoconstriction that shunts blood to the core, and hypotension. The effectiveness of this protective response depends on the victim's age, posture in the water, and lung volume, as well as the water temperature.

The rapid development of hypothermia sometimes can improve brain viability in patients who suffer prolonged submersion. Therefore hypothermic patients should be presumed salvageable. ("A victim is never cold and dead—only warm and dead.") The patient must be rewarmed in a hospital before an accurate assessment can be made.

Rescue versus Body Recovery

In addition to temperature, other factors affect the outcome of a patient who has been submerged in water. These include the length of time the victim has been submerged, known or possible trauma, environmental conditions, the victim's age and physical condition, and the time until rescue or removal is achieved. Because successful resuscitation with full neurological recovery has occurred in victims of prolonged submersion in extremely cold water, resuscitation should be initiated by rescuers at the scene unless physical evidence of death is obvious (e.g., putrefaction, dependent lividity, or rigor mortis).[8]

In-Water Spinal Immobilization

In-water spinal immobilization (see Chapter 25) requires special training. Only rescuers trained in water rescue should enter the water. To review, the steps required for in-water spinal immobilization are as follows:

1. The primary rescuer maintains spinal immobilization and the patient's airway.
2. The second rescuer determines the cervical collar size and holds the collar open under the victim's neck.
3. The second rescuer brings the collar up to the back of the victim's neck. The primary rescuer maintains the airway while allowing the second rescuer to bring the collar around the victim's neck and throat.
4. The second rescuer secures the fastener on the collar while the primary rescuer maintains the airway.
5. The second rescuer secures the victim's hands at the person's waist.
6. The patient is placed on a back board and extricated.
   a. The board is submerged under the victim at the waist.
   b. The board is allowed to float up to the victim; the victim is *never* lifted to the board.
   c. The victim is secured with straps, cravats, or other devices.
   d. The victim is moved to an extrication point on shore or a boat.
   e. The victim is extricated head first so that body weight does not compress the spinal cord and aggravate any spinal trauma.
   f. The victim should not be extricated through surf because the board could collapse.
   g. The patient's airway is maintained during extrication.

Overview of Rescue Techniques

As stated before, rescuers should never underestimate the power of moving water. Also, they should never attempt water rescue without highly specialized training. The recommended water rescue model is *reach-throw-row-go*.

- *Reach.* If the victim is close to shore, the paramedic should try to reach out to the person. An oar, a large branch, a pole, or some other rescue device should be used for this purpose. Before a rescue attempt, paramedics should put on a PFD. They also should make sure their footing is secure so that they are not pulled into the water by the victim.
- *Throw.* While the paramedic remains on the shore, a flotation device (e.g., a water throw bag attached to polypropylene rope) should be thrown to the victim. That way, the victim can be pulled to shore.
- *Row.* If reach and throw methods are unsuccessful or if the victim is unconscious, trained rescuers should row out to the victim in a boat if one is available.
- *Go.* If a boat is unavailable and reach and throw methods are not viable options, trained rescuers should go to the patient by wading or swimming.

A shore-based rescue attempt by a first responder, either by coaching the victim in self-rescue or by reaching or throwing, is the method of choice. Boat-based or "go" techniques require specialized training.

SELF-RESCUE TECHNIQUES

If paramedics inadvertently enter dangerous water, they should use self-rescue techniques as follows:

1. Cover your mouth and nose during entry.
2. Protect your head and keep your face out of the water.
3. If in flat water, assume the HELP position.
4. If in moving water, do not attempt to stand up.
5. Float on your back with your feet downstream and your head pointed toward the nearest shore at a 45-degree angle.

HAZARDOUS ATMOSPHERES

Hazardous atmospheres are oxygen-deficient environments that may occur in confined spaces. (Such spaces have limited access or egress and are not designed for human occupancy or habitation.) According to the National Institute of Occupational Safety and Health (NIOSH), nearly 60% of the deaths associated with confined spaces are people attempting rescue of a victim.[1] Examples of confined spaces include the following:

- Grain bins and silos
- Wells and cisterns
- Storage tanks
- Manholes and pumping stations
- Drainage culverts
- Underground vaults
- Trenches and cave-ins

Hazards Associated with Confined Spaces

Six major hazards are associated with confined spaces.[1] These include low oxygen in the space, chemical/toxic exposure or explosion, engulfment, machinery entrapment, electricity, and structural concerns.

BOX 51-2 Toxic Gases that May Be Found in Confined Spaces

Hydrogen sulfide (H_2S)	Methane (CH_4)
Carbon dioxide (CO_2)	Ammonia (NH_3)
Carbon monoxide (CO)	Nitrogen dioxide (NO_2)
Chlorine (Cl)	
Low- or high-oxygen (O_2) concentrations	

LOW-OXYGEN ATMOSPHERES

Low-oxygen atmospheres are not a visible problem. Therefore rescuers often presume that an atmosphere is safe. The available oxygen in confined spaces must be tested by trained personnel. They use an atmospheric monitoring meter at the top, middle, and bottom of a confined space before entry. Any confined space that has an oxygen concentration less than 19.5% must be considered an atmospheric hazard.[9] An oxygen level that is too high (above 22%) in a confined space may produce rapid combustion. This also is a serious safety hazard.

Chemical/Toxic Exposure or Explosion

Oxygen can be removed from the atmosphere by certain chemical reactions. Examples include reactions that occur during the formation of rust on steel structures and while pouring concrete, and natural decaying processes that displace oxygen by producing dangerous gases (e.g., methane). In addition, the presence of some chemicals and gases can lead to toxic exposure (see Chapter 53) (Box 51-2). They also may pose a high risk of explosion. Some dusts and particulate materials found in grain bins, silos, and storage tanks can be highly explosive when mixed with air. Many gases are heavier than air. Therefore these gases are found in higher concentrations at the bottom of storage vessels. As with oxygen content, trained personnel should monitor for toxic or explosive gases in confined spaces using an appropriate testing device.

CRITICAL THINKING

Why can workers easily become disabled in situations that may involve exposure to toxic gases?

NOTE Some silos are designed to produce a low-oxygen condition. This aids the fermentation process. These silos usually can be identified by their blue exteriors.

ENGULFMENT

Entrapment can occur when earth, grain, coal, or any other dry material engulfs a person in a confined space. Engulfment can produce an atmosphere that is low in oxygen. As a result, a person can suffocate. In addition, those trapped by engulfment may be victims of physical injury (crushing). They also are at an increased risk from explosive hazards.

MACHINERY ENTRAPMENT

Some structures, such as grain bins and silos, often have augers, screws, conveyors, and other machinery to move material stored in them. These and other mechanical devices can entrap a person. Before rescue is attempted, trained and experienced personnel should identify and secure all such devices.

ELECTRICITY

Electrical hazards from the power supply of motors and materials-management equipment may be present in some situations. Like machinery, all electrical devices must be identified and secured by experienced personnel. (These devices include electrical boxes and switches.) This helps to ensure the safety of the rescuer. This *lock-out process* must prevent any unauthorized person from entering the area or gaining access to the controls that have been shut off. Motors and other electrical devices can "store" power that can lead to entrapment or injury. Chemical, steam, and water lines also must be secured or blocked by trained personnel during all rescues.

STRUCTURAL CONCERNS

The supporting structures of a confined space must be identified before entry to aid in safe rescue and extrication. For example, most cylindrical structures are supported by central I beams. These beams make for relatively easy maneuvering. However, noncylindrical structures may have L-, T-, and X-shaped spaces. These can affect entry and rescue procedures. They also can complicate the extrication pathway.

CRUSH COMPARTMENT SYNDROMES SECONDARY TO ENTRAPMENT

As described in Chapter 22, compartment syndrome can be caused by crushing mechanisms, which lead to ischemic muscle damage, tissue necrosis, and crush syndrome. These injuries can be severe. They are associated with rupture of internal organs, major fractures, and hemorrhagic shock. The degree of injury produced by the crushing force depends on three elements: (1) the amount of pressure applied to the body; (2) the length of time the pressure is exerted on the body; and (3) the specific body region where the injury occurs. A massive crush injury to vital organs may cause immediate death.

Patients with crush syndrome are victims of compressive forces that crush tissue. This causes prolonged hypoxia. The patient may appear stable for hours or days, as long as the compressive forces remain in place. When the patient is released from the entrapment, the reperfusion of the trapped body part may lead to detrimental processes. These include volume loss into the tissue and the release of myoglobin, lactic acid, and other toxins into the circulation. As described in Chapter 22, these events occur at the same time and ultimately may lead to death. If the patient's condition or the mechanism of injury is suspicious for compartment syndrome or crush injury, the paramedic should consult with medical direction. Management of crush syndrome is controversial. Prehospital care must be supervised through a medical direction physician familiar with this pathological process.

Emergencies in Confined Spaces

OSHA requires a permit before workers may enter a confined space.[9] This standard has forced industrial, municipal, and government response teams to be better prepared to manage confined-space incidents. Requirements for obtaining a permit include the following:

1. The area must be made safe or workers must wear PPE.
2. Fall-arresting and retrieval devices must be in place.
3. Environmental monitoring must be available at the site before entry.

Sites without permits at which no atmospheric monitoring is performed are likely locations for emergencies. At these sites, rescuers often may encounter atmospheres that are low in oxygen. Other types of emergencies that can occur in confined spaces (in both permitted and nonpermitted locations) include the following:

- Falls
- Medical emergencies
- Explosion
- Entrapment
- Exposure to toxic gases and chemicals

SAFE ENTRY FOR RESCUERS

As stated before, safe entry for rescuers in a confined-space operation requires specialized training. No rescuer should enter the space until a rescue team has made the area safe. Safe entry cannot be made without the following[1]:

- Proper and thorough training in confined-space rescue
- Atmospheric monitoring to determine the oxygen concentration, hydrogen sulfide level, carbon monoxide level, explosive limits, flammable atmosphere, and toxic air contaminants
- Proper ventilation
- Secured electrical systems (lock-out/tag-out of all power)
- Dissipation of stored energy
- Disconnection of all pipes (blinding/blanking) to prevent flow into the site
- Appropriate respiratory protection

Supplied-Air Breathing Apparatus. Close quarters make access and extrication difficult in confined-space rescue. Because of this, use of the typical "bottle on back" SCBA is usually dangerous. The device provides a limited air supply, can cause entrapment, and may have to be removed in order to reach the victim. The supplied-air (airline) breathing apparatus (SABA) is preferred in confined-space operations (Fig. 51-4). These lightweight devices

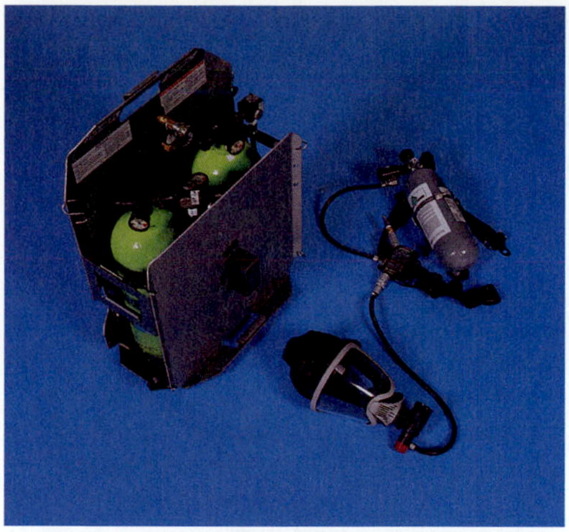

FIGURE 51-4 ■ Supplied-air (air-line) breathing apparatus (SABA).

provide a nearly unlimited supply of air from a device located outside the confined space.

Potential complications of the SABA include equipment malfunction, damaged or entangled air lines, and limitations imposed by the length of the air hose. Trained rescuers carry a small, personal reserve air supply (escape bottle) that can be used for a short time if needed.

ARRIVING AT THE SCENE

An EMS crew that arrives at the scene of a confined-space emergency should proceed as follows:

1. Perform a scene size-up and determine the nature of the emergency by obtaining a copy of the OSHA permit (Fig. 51-5) for the site from the permit/entry supervisor. Determine the number of workers (victims) in the confined space.
2. Request specialized rescue teams.
3. Establish a safe perimeter away from the incident. Allow only rescue team members to enter the space.
4. Assist workers at the site with any remote retrieval devices they may be using.

Note: Scene safety is of prime importance for all involved in the rescue. Only specialized rescue personnel should directly perform rescue activities. EMS personnel who are not trained in specialized rescue should assist the rescue team only if they can do so safely without entering the space.

Rescue from Trenches and Cave-Ins

Most trench collapses occur in trenches less than 12 feet deep and 6 feet wide.[1] Federal law requires either shoring or a trench box for evacuations that are 5 feet or deeper. Often these collapses occur when contractors forsake safety measures because of the increased cost of providing them. Factors that contribute to collapse include the following:

- Cave-in of lips on one or both sides of the trench
- Walls that shear away and cave in
- Piling of excavated dirt too close to the edge, causing collapse
- The presence of intersecting trenches
- Ground vibrations
- Water seepage

> **NOTE** One cubic foot of soil weighs 100 pounds; 2 feet of soil on a person's chest or back is equal to 700 to 1000 pounds of pressure, which can cause burial and can rapidly lead to suffocation.[1]

ARRIVAL AT THE SCENE

On arrival at the scene of a collapse that has resulted in burial, paramedics should keep in mind that a second collapse is likely and should not approach the lip. EMS personnel should not attempt a rescue unless the trench is less than waist deep. Instead, they should take the following steps in scene management:

1. Secure the scene, establish command, and secure a safe perimeter.
2. Shut down nonessential equipment that can cause vibrations.
3. Request specialized rescue teams.
4. Prevent entry into the trench or cave-in area.

Access to the patient should be attempted by trained personnel only after proper shoring is in place. The process of shoring and excavating can be labor and time intensive. However, scene safety is necessary for a successful recovery.

> **CRITICAL THINKING**
> Consider an EMS and rescue team that, for safety reasons, will be unable to go in after a person who is buried in a trench collapse. How do you think they will feel?

HIGHWAY OPERATIONS

Traffic flow is the largest hazard in EMS highway operations.[1] Factors associated with highway hazards include emergency responses to limited and unlimited access highways, emergency vehicle crashes, and the backup of traffic that impedes flow to and from the scene. Because of the potential problems in traffic flow, EMS personnel must work closely with law enforcement to help ensure a safe response. Paramedics can take the following steps to reduce traffic hazards:

- Position an apparatus (pumper, rescue, or other emergency vehicle) across the traffic way in the fend-off position. This protects the scene from traffic hazards.
- Stage unnecessary apparatus off the highway (this is essential on limited access highways); establish a staging area away from scene.
- Position an apparatus to reduce traffic flow and provide for a safe ambulance loading area.
- Use only essential warning lights so that drivers are not distracted or confused. (Consider the use of amber scene lighting.) Turn off headlights that might blind nearby motorists.

APPENDIX IV - MOBIL OIL CONFINED SPACE RESCUE FORM

CONFINED SPACE ENTRY PERMIT

SCOPE

Effective date ________ 19 ____ Time ______ [AM PM] Expiration date ______ Time ______ [AM PM]

Permit Issued to ______________________

Description of Work ______________________

Lease or Area ____________ Specific Location ______________________

PREP

- ☐ Equipment/piping depressurized & vented
- ☐ Powered(forced air) ventilation
- ☐ Other ______________________
- ☐ Equipment/piping blinded, blanked, or misaligned
- ☐ Electric, hydraulic,pneumatic & mechanical energy sources shut-off & locked out
- ☐ Vessel/space steamed,cleaned,or washed

ATMOSPHERE TESTING

Type	☐ Flammable			☐ Oxygen			☐ Hydrogen sulfide			☐ Other ______			☐ Continuous Monitoring
Time													Instrument
%, LEL or PPM													Most Recent Calibration date
Tested by			CO. VERIFY			CO. VERIFY			CO. VERIFY			CO. VERIFY	Field Calibration O.K. ☐
Action Levels	10% L.E.L. <10% evaluate for toxicity			LESS THAN 19.5% MORE THAN 23%			10 PPM			Carbon Monoxide(35ppm),Aromatic Hydrocarbon(10ppm) Ammonia(25ppm),Mineral Spirits(100ppm),Methanol(200ppm)			

PROTECTIVE EQUIPMENT

OPERATIONAL AND PROTECTIVE EQUIPMENT

- ☐ Warning signs, barricades
- ☐ Barricade tape/cones
- ☐ Ventilation Fan or blower
- ☐ Fire extinguisher
- ☐ Ground fault circuit interupter
- ☐ Lighting(hazardous location rated)
- ☐ Static protection
- ☐ Ladder
- ☐ Other ______________

PERSONAL PROTECTIVE EQUIPMENT

- ☐ Self Contained Breathing Apparatus
- ☐ Airline supplied respirator
- ☐ Chemical splash goggles
- ☐ Impervious gloves
- ☐ Impervious clothing
- ☐ Boots
- ☐ Hearing protection
- ☐ Safety glasses
- ☐ Fall protection/arresting equipment
- ☐ Other ______________

EMERGENCY ACTION

RESCUE PROCEDURES AND EQUIPMENT

Emergency Phone Number [ ] Base Station ______________

Location of Phone/Radio ______________________

RESCUE EQUIPMENT NEEDED

- ☐ Full body harness/lifeline
- ☐ Rescue winch
- ☐ Wristlets
- ☐ Personal motion alarm
- ☐ Davit/Tripod
- ☐ Other ______________

CSE COMMUNICATION

- ☐ Radio communication
- ☐ Rope signals
- ☐ Visual hand signals
- ☐ Other ______________

POTENTIAL EMERGENCY SITUATION(S) ______________________

ACTIONS TO BE TAKEN ______________________

SIGNATURE

CONFINED SPACE ENTRANT(S) We(I) have reviewed the potential emergency situations and actions to be taken. We(I) are familiar with all rescue equipment, and communication methods.

X ____________ X ____________ X ____________

CONFINED SPACE OBSERVER/STANDBY I have checked all rescue and communication equipment and reviewed all emergency actions to be taken with entrant personnel. X ____________

CONTRACT SUPERVISOR I have evaluated and completed all portions of this permit. All personnel have reviewed the conditions of the permit and are adequately trained to perform this job. I have reviewed the site to ensure compliance with the requirements of this permit. X ____________

MOBIL REPRESENTATIVE I have evaluated and completed all portions of this permit. All personnel have reviewed the conditions of the permit and are adequately trained to perform this job. I have reviewed the site to ensure compliance with the requirements of this permit. X ____________

DEBRIEF

Were any Hazards or Potential Hazards Encountered During the CSE? NO ☐ YES ☐ If yes, Explain ______________________

White - Local Safety Dept. Manila Tag - Post at Job Site

BAKCSE 93

iv - xii

CMC Confined Space Rescue Manual

FIGURE 51-5 ■ Example of a confined-space entry permit.

- Use traffic cones and flares to redirect traffic away from workers and to create a safe zone. (Use flares safely in proximity to the scene. Do not extinguish them once they have been ignited.)
- Make sure that all rescuers wear high-visibility clothing (e.g., orange highway vests, reflective trim).

Other scene hazards associated with highway operations include fuel and fire hazards, electrical power, unstable vehicles, airbags and supplemental restraint systems (SRS), and hazardous cargoes.

Fuel and Fire Hazards

Gasoline spills from crashes are a common fire hazard encountered by EMS providers. The chances that flammable liquids will ignite can be reduced by turning off the vehicle ignition switch, forbidding smoking, and avoiding use of flares near the spill. Alternate fuel systems (e.g., natural gas and electrical power) also are capable of producing fire hazards and injury from explosion of high-pressure cylinders and storage cells. EMS personnel should approach the scene with fire extinguishers and should keep the extinguishers ready throughout extrication (Box 51-3). Ideally, a fire apparatus with a charged hose line should be at the scene.

The battery of a crashed car generally should be left connected so that power electric door locks, windows, seat mechanisms, and trunks can be operated. However, if the battery is to be disabled, the ground cable should be disconnected first to reduce the chance of sparking. Sparking may ignite spilled fuel or leaking battery gases. Most newer American cars have positive ground cables that can be identified by battery markings or by locating the ground wires attached to the frame, engine, or body of the vehicle. The battery cable can be cut with wire cutters or disconnected with battery pliers. The disconnected cable should be folded back onto itself. Then it should be securely taped to insulate it from any bare metal contact that might reestablish the electrical ground to the system. Both cables should be disconnected and secured.

Vehicle fires associated with crashes usually are caused by ruptured fuel tanks and fuel lines ignited during the crash. (Catalytic converters are capable of igniting spilled fuel.) Paramedics should not try to fight fully involved vehicle fires unless they have been trained to do so. If the fire service has not arrived and victims are in a burning vehicle, the EMS crew should quickly determine whether the victims can be safely removed. If the victims are trapped and the vehicle is not fully engulfed by flames, an attempt should be made to stop the fire from spreading. This should be done using fire extinguishers.

Burning vehicles present very serious potential hazards. They may explode with deadly force at any time. All actions must be directed toward rescuer safety and protection. When paramedics must approach a burning vehicle, they should crouch low and approach from the side, staying clear of bumpers that may fly off during explosions. PPE also should be worn to guard against dangerous and caustic smoke.

BOX 51-3 Fire Extinguishers

Portable fire extinguishers are classified by their anticipated effectiveness in suppressing four classes of fires:

- Class A—Ordinary combustibles
- Class B—Flammable liquids
- Class C—Energized electrical equipment
- Class D—Combustible metals

ABC-all purpose extinguishers are suitable for more than one class of fire. They should be carried by EMS crews. These dry chemical extinguishers can be used to suppress fires of ordinary combustible materials, flammable liquids, and electrical equipment.

Class A and class B fire extinguishers are given a numerical rating in addition to the letter classification. This rating designates the size of fire the extinguisher can be expected to suppress. A 20-B extinguisher generally extinguishes 20 times as much fuel as a 1-B extinguisher.

Fire suppression agents work by reducing heat and eliminating the oxygen needed to maintain combustion. Eliminating oxygen may present a danger to the rescuer and patient; therefore paramedics must work carefully in confined spaces. In addition, crew members and patients should avoid undue exposure to the fumes of any fire suppression agent. All rescuers should use an appropriate breathing apparatus.

Electrical Power

Downed electrical wires are dangerous. Modern transformers are programmed to retest broken circuits at certain time intervals. The dead lines can suddenly surge with lethal current. Rescuers must be familiar with the power system in their area. They should check with the local power company for information and the availability of training sessions for the response team. Only utility workers and trained rescuers using proper equipment should secure downed electrical wires.

Rescuers should never approach the patient until the scene is safe. Rescuers who experience tingling sensations in the soles of the feet, legs, or thorax as they enter an area should not proceed. Rather, they should retreat from the area. Victims inside a vehicle that is in contact with downed wires should be advised to remain inside unless they are at additional risk of injury (e.g., explosion, fire). Leaving the vehicle is dangerous and poses a significant risk of electrical injury.

When it is absolutely necessary to touch a patient who is in contact with a source of electricity, trained personnel may use nonconductive equipment such as leather gauntlets, wooden poles, polypropylene rope, and other specially designed equipment. However, none of these measures provides absolute safety from electrical injury.

Unstable Vehicles

Unstable vehicles are a common hazard in rescue events. All unstable vehicles must be stabilized before access is gained. The mechanism of the crash, the position and number of

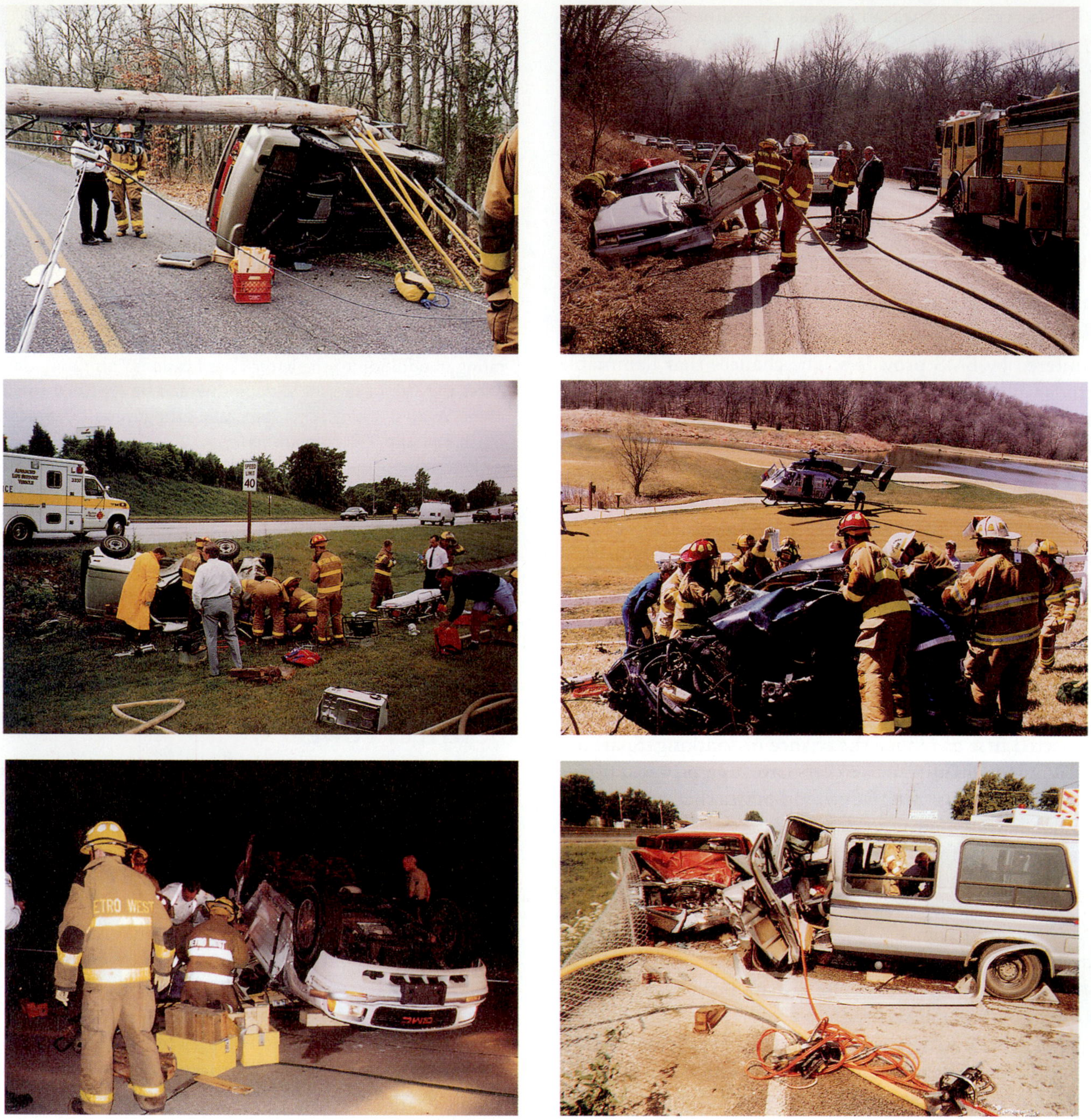

FIGURE 51-6 ■ Vehicle stabilization.

vehicles, and the environment of the scene must all be considered when assessing the stability of vehicles.

Some vehicles are obviously unstable. (For example, a vehicle may be on its side or on its roof.) However, even a car on its wheels that appears to be stable may be unstable from possible movement of the tires and swaying of the vehicle's suspension system. All wrecked vehicles should be approached cautiously. Standard methods of stabilizing vehicles include supporting the vehicle with wooden cribbing, wheel chocks, and airbags and securing the vehicle with ropes, cables, and chains to poles, trees, and other vehicles and structures (Fig. 51-6). Fig. 51-7 shows equipment used to stabilize vehicles. Specialized training is required for paramedics involved in this aspect of rescue management.

Airbags and Supplemental Restraint Systems

Airbags as a supplemental restraint system (SRS) are required safety features in all cars manufactured in the United States. The three types of airbags are frontal impact, side impact, and head protection bags. Airbags generally

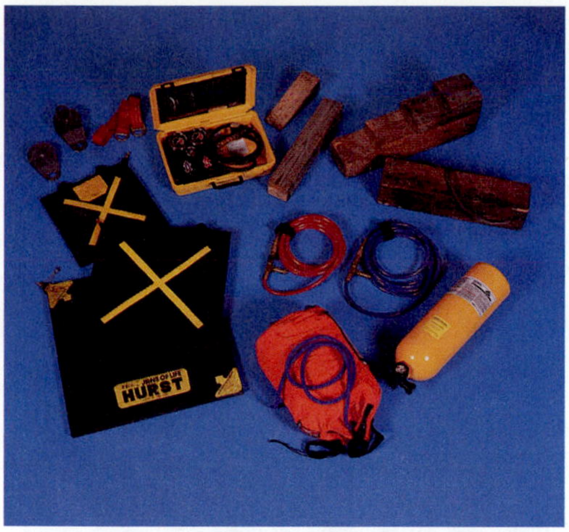

FIGURE 51-7 ■ Equipment used to stabilize vehicles.

are considered an effective safety device in crashes. However, children and small adults in the passenger seat have been fatally injured after airbag deployment.[10]

Once deployed, airbags are not dangerous. However, they do produce a residue that can cause minor skin or eye irritation. Irritation from this residue is temporary. It can be avoided by wearing gloves and eye protection; by keeping the residue away from the patient's eyes and wounds; and by thoroughly washing after exposure. Emergency personnel should be trained in detection and scene management of SRS equipment. Rescue guidelines for airbag-equipped cars have been provided by the National Highway Traffic Safety Administration and automobile and airbag manufacturers and have been coordinated with the U.S. Fire Administration (Box 51-4).[11]

Hazardous Cargoes

Most hazardous substances transported in the United States travel by road.[1] Therefore paramedics should be suspicious of crashes that involve commercial vehicles. Methods that can be used to identify carriers of hazardous cargoes (e.g., United Nations class identification number and North American number [UN/NA number] and placards) and the management of hazardous materials incidents are discussed in Chapter 53.

BOX 51-4 Rescue Guidelines for Airbag-Equipped Cars

Incident with a Deployed Airbag

Deployed airbags are not dangerous. However, not all airbags deploy during a crash. Also, side impact airbags operate independent of the frontal airbags. Rescuers should practice the *5-10-20 rule* for safe distancing to reduce the severity and risk of injury should unintentional deployment occur. The rule is as follows:

- Side impact curtain and airbags—Maintain a safe distance of 5 inches or more.
- Driver side frontal airbags—Maintain a safe distance of 10 inches or more.
- Passenger side frontal airbags—Maintain a safe distance of 20 inches or more.

In addition, rescuers should not place any hard board or device between an airbag and a patient or rescuer.

Once the airbag is deployed, it will not deploy again.

Incident with an Undeployed Airbag

Undeployed airbags can suddenly deploy during a rescue. This releases a tremendous amount of energy. The energy can be dangerous to both the patient and rescuer. If a patient is pinned behind an undeployed airbag, the car battery should be deactivated as soon as possible. Before they disconnect the battery, paramedics should determine whether they will need to move a power seat, unlock electric doors, or power down electric windows. The procedure for deactivating the battery is as follows:

1. Turn off all electrical units and the ignition switch. Carefully disconnect both battery cables (disconnect the negative cable first).
2. Cables that need to be cut should be cut twice to ensure that the cut ends will not touch and arc. Make sure the battery terminals cannot make contact with metal body parts that could reactivate an electrical circuit. Do not attempt to turn on the ignition switch to test a battery disconnect; verify it by attempting to turn on the lights.
3. For additional safety, maintain the 5-10-20 rule near airbags that have not deployed.

Note: If the incident involves fire, normal fire extinguishing procedures should be used. Heat may trigger an undeployed airbag. However, it will not cause the activating canister to explode.

Automobile Anatomy

Vehicle rescue operations require a basic understanding of the anatomy of automobiles (Fig. 51-8). The following are several important features:

- *Construction, roof,* and *support posts.* Most vehicles are of unibody rather than frame construction. The support posts (A, B, C, and D posts), floor fire wall, and trunk are integral to the integrity of unibody construction. Cutting the support posts can threaten the stability of these vehicles.
- *Fire wall* and *engine compartment.* A fire wall separates the engine and occupant compartments. The fire wall often collapses onto the occupant's legs during high-speed, head-on collisions. The car battery is usually located in the engine compartment.
- *Glass.* Safety glass is composed of glass-plastic and laminate glass and is usually found in the windshield. It is designed to stay intact when the glass is broken or shattered (it fractures into long strands). Tempered glass has high tensile strength and may not stay intact when it is shattered or broken (it fractures into small pieces).
- *Doors.* Most car doors contain a reinforcing bar. They are designed to provide structural integrity to the vehicle and protection to the occupants during front- and side-impact collisions. Doors also have a case-hardened steel "Nader" pin or latch that is designed to prevent the car door from opening during impact.

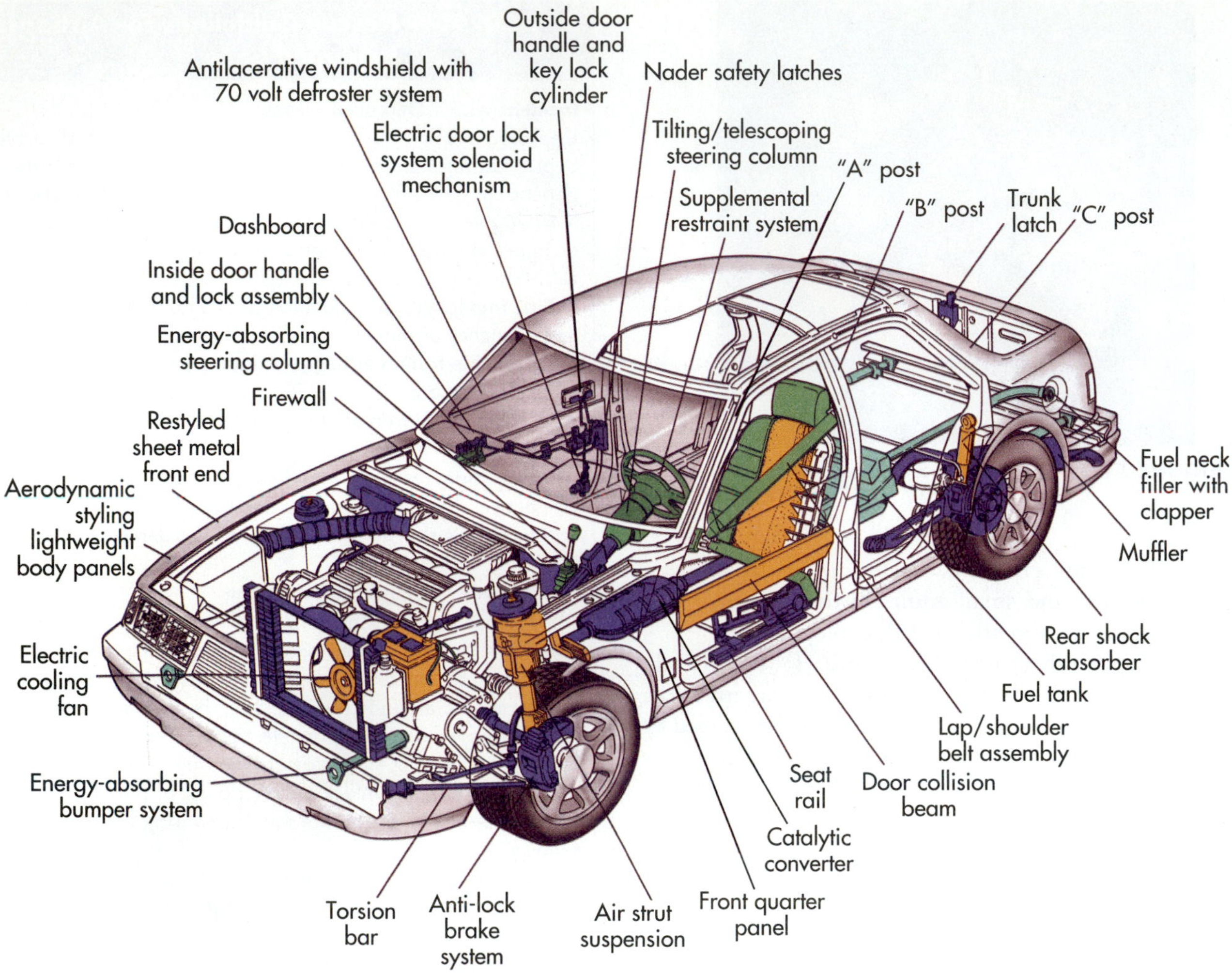

FIGURE 51-8 ■ Anatomy of a car.

If the pin is engaged, it may be difficult to pry open the door; it must be disengaged first.

RESCUE STRATEGIES

Rescue strategies for vehicle crashes should begin during the initial scene size-up. They sometimes can be based on the details provided by the dispatching center before arrival. On arriving at the scene, the EMS crew should begin hazard control, establish command, and call for appropriate backup. Important elements of the scene size-up include the following:

- Scene safety (including protecting the scene from traffic hazards)
- Location of the crash
- Vehicle stability
- Electrical hazards
- Fire hazards
- Hazardous materials
- Special rescue needs
- Number and location of patients

After the initial scene size-up and ensuring scene safety, the responding crew should assess the degree of entrapment. They also should assess the fastest means of extrication. The paramedic should try to gain access to trapped victims by first trying to open all car doors. When a door cannot be readily opened by the patient or rescuer, another option is the side windows. (Glass windows can be shattered by striking the glass in a lower corner or by using a spring-loaded center punch.) Initial patient care can then be provided. This is done until trained rescue personnel with extrication tools can safely remove the patient from the vehicle by door removal, roof removal, front or rear windshield openings, or a dash roll-up maneuver (Fig. 51-9). Paramedics involved in the rescue or who are near the site should wear PPE. The PPE should provide adequate hand, eye, and body protection. Clothing with reflective striping improves safety during day and night operations.

HAZARDOUS TERRAIN

Hazardous terrain can pose major difficulties during rescue operations. An example is a car crash that occurs on an embankment. Other examples are rescues for sport enthusiasts such as rock climbers, snow skiers, and moun-

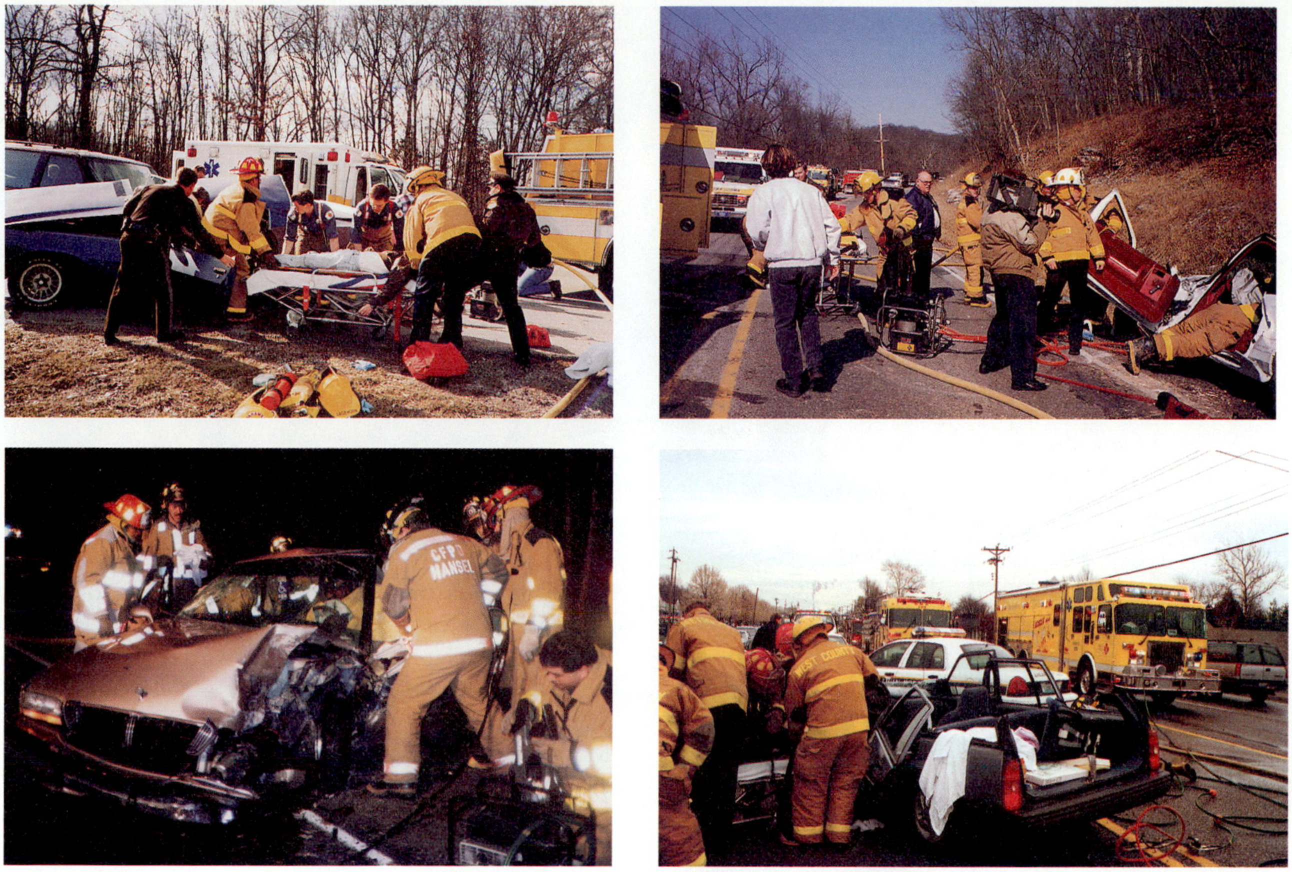

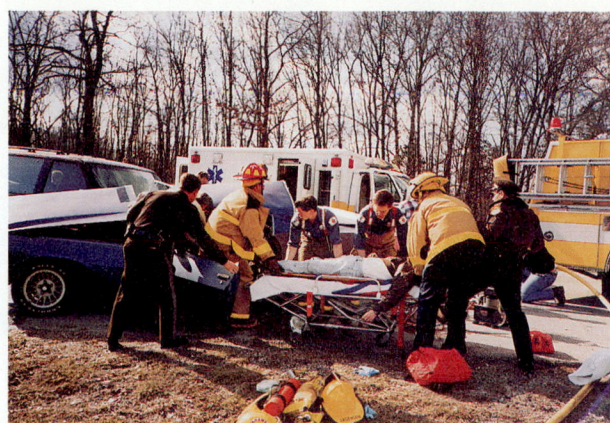

FIGURE 51-9 ■ Extrication scenes.

tain bikers. Three common classifications of hazardous terrain are *low-angle, high-angle,* and *flat terrain with obstructions* (Box 51-5). Highly specialized training and equipment are required for rescues in both low-angle (weight supported by ground) and high-angle (weight supported by rope) environments.

The term *low angle* (steep slope) refers to terrain that can be walked on without the use of the hands. However, secure footing may be difficult on steep slopes. This makes it hazardous to carry a litter even with several rescuers. In these situations, low-angle rescue is used to prevent falls and tumbles through the use of ropes to counteract gravity during litter carrying (Fig. 51-10).

CRITICAL THINKING

What factors in the environment can increase the danger of steep-slope rescue?

The term *high angle* (vertical) refers to terrain (cliffs, sides of buildings) that is so steep the hands must be used to maintain balance (slopes of more than 40 degrees). In these situations, rescuers are completely dependent on rope or aerial apparatus for litter movement. High-angle rescue requires rappelling by trained personnel to retrieve victims. Falls are likely to result in serious injury or death (Fig. 51-11).

BOX 51-5 Terms and Definitions Related to Rescue over Hazardous Terrain

anchoring: Attaching a high-angle rope to a secure point.

belay: A method of attaching a safety rope and controlling the rope so that if the person or load starts to fall, the belay rope prevents the fall.

high angle: An environment in which rescuers need to be secured with rope for safety. Most of the rescue load is supported by the rope system.

low angle: An environment in which the weight of the stretcher is supported primarily by the tender's legs, but rope systems are required to facilitate movement and for protection against falls.

rappelling: A method of descent that involves lowering oneself with a rope.

scrambling: Movement over rough terrain that is not steep enough to require the use of a rope.

Flat terrain may have various obstructions that can make rescue difficult. Examples include level land with large rocks, loose soil (scree), and waterbeds or creeks. In these situations, extra personnel and resources may be needed to extricate a victim safely and to ensure safe litter movement.

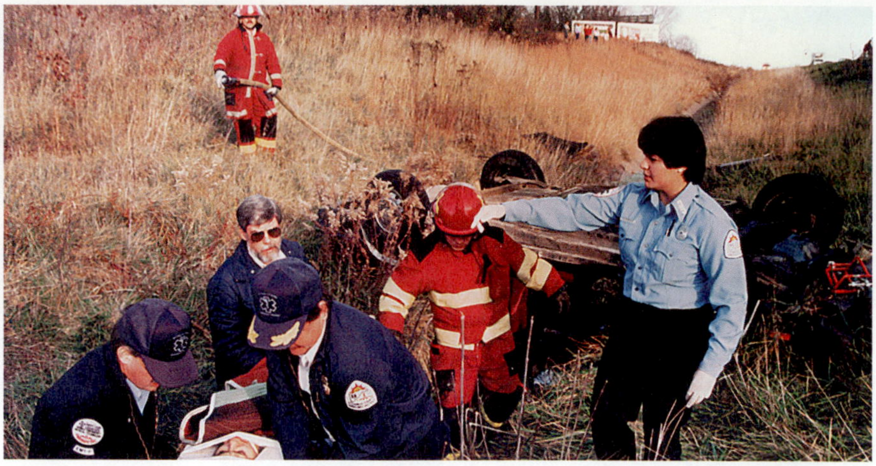

FIGURE 51-10 ■ Low-angle rescue.

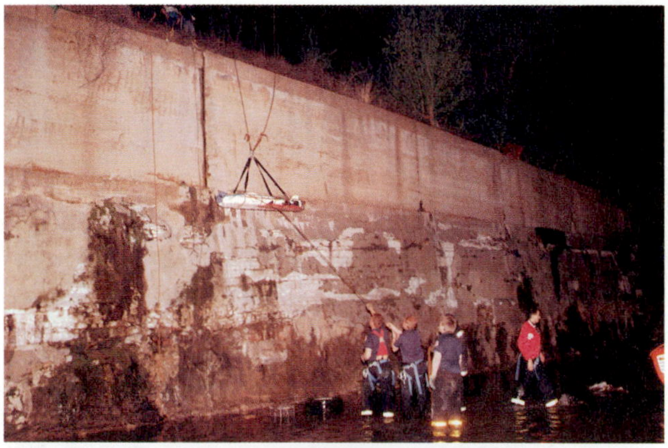

FIGURE 51-11 ■ High-angle rescue.

Patient Packaging with Litters

The basket stretcher is the standard for rough terrain evacuation. The rigid frame of this device offers protection for the victim. It also is relatively easy to carry with enough personnel. Patients generally are immobilized on a long back board and secured in the basket. Alternative spinal immobilization devices (e.g., vest-type devices) also can be used in conjunction with the basket stretcher. Using the basket stretcher itself as a spinal immobilization device should be considered a last resort. The older "military style" devices do not provide adequate spinal immobilization.

Basket stretchers have two basic designs: wire mesh (Stokes) and plastic. Wire mesh generally is the stronger of the baskets. It also is relatively inexpensive. The design allows for air and water to flow through the device. This makes it ideal in water rescue when used with supplemental flotation. Plastic basket stretchers generally are weaker than steel mesh. However, they provide better protection for the patient. (Plastic bottoms with steel frames are considered superior designs.) Most basket stretchers are equipped with adequate restraints. However, all require additional strapping or lacing (e.g., harness, leg stirrups) to prevent movement, as well as padding for rough-terrain evacuation or extraction. A plastic helmet or litter shield should be available to protect the patient.

PATIENT MOVEMENT

Methods of moving a patient over rough terrain may include evacuation and litter-carrying over flat terrain. However, special rescue equipment may be required for low-angle and high-angle evacuation. Such equipment may include load-lifting straps, anchors, and rope-lowering and rope-hauling systems. In addition, the use of aerial apparatus (e.g., tower-ladder or bucket trucks, aerial ladders) also may be required in some high-angle rescue operations. Moving a patient during low-angle and high-angle evacuations requires specialized knowledge and skills.

LITTER-CARRYING PROCEDURES

Carrying a litter across rough, flat terrain requires a minimum of six rescuers: four to carry the litter and two to observe or "scout" for potential hazards (e.g., loose rocks, holes, tree branches). Team members should be matched in height. This ensures that equal weight is shared and that the litter remains level. Load-lifting straps sometimes are used to spread the weight of the load over other parts of the rescuer's body (e.g., around the rescuer's shoulders and back). Proper lifting techniques should be used to protect and support the rescuer's back. Figure 51-12 shows a basic litter-carrying sequence.

Helicopter Use in Hazardous Terrain Rescue

As described in Chapter 49, helicopters can be used for transport and for rescues. When they are used for rescue, the helicopter team (civilian and military) is geared toward performing the rescue rather than providing medical care and transport. The rescue helicopter team has specialized knowledge and skills. They are required to hover or land in tight places and to transport people and equipment. Special rescue

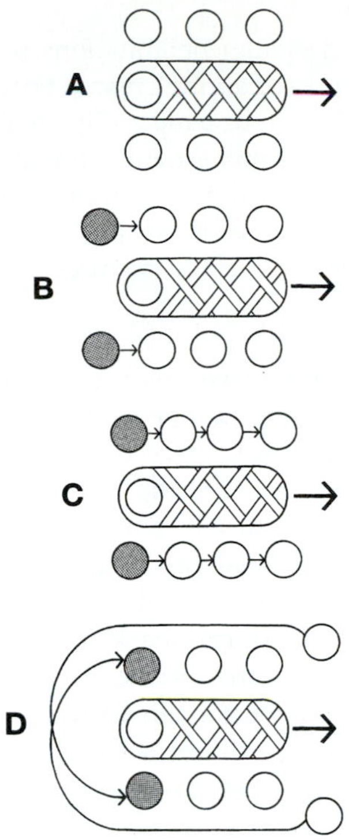

FIGURE 51-12 ■ Litter-carrying sequence. **A,** Six rescuers are usually required to carry a litter; they may need relief over long distances (more than ¼ mile). **B,** Relief rescuers can rotate into position while the litter is in motion by approaching from the rear. As relief rescuers move forward, others progressively move forward **(C)** until the forwardmost rescuers can release the litter (peel out) and move to the rear **(D).** Rescuers in the rear can rotate sides so that they can alternate carrying arms. Carrying straps (webbing) can also be used to distribute the load over the rescuers' shoulders. In most cases the litter is carried feet first with a medical attendant at the head monitoring airway, breathing, level of consciousness, and so on.

BOX 51-6 Paramedic Equipment

Airway
- Oral and nasal airways
- Manual suction device
- Intubation equipment

Breathing
- Thoracic decompression device
- Small oxygen tank and regulator
- Masks and cannulas
- Pocket mask and bag-valve-mask device

Circulation
- Bandages and dressings
- Triangular bandages
- Occlusive dressings
- Intravenous fluid administration set
- Blood pressure cuff and stethoscope

Disability
- Extrication collars

Exposure of Body Surface
- Scissors

Miscellaneous
- Headlamp and flashlight
- Space blanket
- Pneumatic splints

Personal Protective Equipment
- Leather gloves
- Latex gloves
- Eye shields
- Other equipment as indicated

techniques that these helicopters use may include cable hoisting to extract people from the ground, and short-haul (sling load) operations that allow personnel and equipment to be carried beneath the helicopter as an external load. Rescue helicopters have the same safety concerns and limitations as those used for medical transport (see Chapter 49). All personnel at the scene should be familiar with the elements of scene safety, hazards, and restrictions for helicopter use.

ASSESSMENT PROCEDURES DURING RESCUE

Patient assessment during rescue operations often is complicated by factors such as weather and temperature extremes, available access, equipment limitations, patient entrapment, and cumbersome PPE that affects rescuer mobility. Other factors that can affect the paramedic's ability to perform a thorough assessment and that can result in a compromised physical examination include the following:

- Difficulty completing exposing a patient
- Restrictive clothing and PPE required for personal safety
- Working in a cramped space
- Limited lighting
- Difficulty transporting medical equipment to the patient

Specific Assessment and Management Considerations

During rescues, paramedics may need to downsize medical equipment. They may not be able to carry the normal bags and "street packaging." Ideally, paramedics should be able to carry the equipment hands free. In addition to ensuring adequate lighting to perform assessment and treatment, paramedics should have access to the equipment listed in Box 51-6.[1]

EXPOSURE OF PATIENTS

Patients who need to be rescued may be at high risk for developing hypothermia. They should be covered to ensure thermal protection. Also, the patient should be protected with shields (e.g., back boards or blankets) to prevent injury from equipment and debris during the extrication.

ADVANCED LIFE SUPPORT MEASURES

Advanced life support (ALS) measures should be provided only if necessary. However, good basic life support (BLS) techniques are mandatory. As a rule, ALS equipment such as IV lines, endotracheal (ET) tubes, and electrocardiographic (ECG) leads complicate the extrication process. However, advanced airway support and volume replacement may be needed. Airway control with administration of supplemental oxygen must always be a priority during the rescue.

PATIENT MONITORING

Monitoring of the patient's vital signs and level of consciousness is necessary throughout the rescue. In high-noise and tight spaces, blood pressure may need to be measured by palpation. It also may be necessary to use compact devices such as a pulse oximeter. Paramedics should create and continue a rapport with the patient when possible. They should explain the procedures performed and why they are necessary. Providing emotional support during the rescue is crucial.

IMPROVISATION

Because of space and equipment limitations, some patient care may have to be improvised during a rescue. For example, an upper extremity fracture can be temporarily stabilized by tying it to the patient's torso; a lower extremity fracture can be tied to the patient's uninjured leg (buddy splinting). Formable splints (e.g., structural aluminum malleable [SAM] splint) also can be very useful for securing extremity fractures or dislocations.

PAIN CONTROL

Pain control for patients who require rescue may include drugs and other methods. For example, splinting, distraction (talking to the patient and asking questions), and methods such as creating sensory stimuli (e.g., mildly scratching the patient) when a painful procedure or maneuver is performed can help control pain. Drug therapy may be used to control pain that results from trauma. Pain medication can mask serious injury and alter a patient's level of consciousness. Therefore the paramedic should consult with medical direction or follow established protocol regarding the use of drug therapy in these situations.

SUMMARY

- Rescue is a patient-driven event. It calls for specialized medical and mechanical skills. The right amount of each must be applied at the right time. The main role of the paramedic in rescues is to have the proper training and the appropriate PPE. These allow safe access to the patient and the provision of treatment at the site and throughout the incident.
- The seven phases of a rescue operation are arrival and scene size-up, hazard control, gaining access to the patient, medical treatment, disentanglement, patient packaging, and transportation.
- The standards for protective clothing and personal protection equipment established by the National Fire Protection Association and OSHA have been adopted by many fire and EMS agencies. The appropriate PPE depends on the level of rescuer involvement and the nature of the incident.
- Water rescue should never be attempted by a single rescuer or by one who is untrained.
- Water hazards include obstructions to flow and foot or extremity pins that can trap victims and drag them under water. Some factors that contribute to flat water drowning are alcohol or other drug use. Also, cool water temperatures contribute to such drownings.
- Hazardous atmospheres are environments with low oxygen. These environments can occur in confined spaces. The six major hazards associated with confined spaces are oxygen-deficient atmospheres, chemical/toxic exposure and explosion, engulfment, machinery entrapment, electricity, and structural concerns.
- Traffic flow is the biggest hazard in EMS highway operations. Other scene hazards associated with highway operations include fuel or fire hazards, electrical power, unstable vehicles, airbags and supplemental restraint systems, and hazardous cargoes.
- Hazardous terrain can create major difficulties during rescue events. Three common classifications of hazardous terrain are low-angle, high-angle, and flat terrain with obstructions.

REFERENCES

1. US Department of Transportation, National Highway Traffic Safety Administration: *EMT-paramedic national standard curriculum,* 1998, Washington, DC, The Department.
2. National Fire Protection Association: *Standard on protective clothing for medical operations (NFPA 1999),* Quincy, MA, 2003.
3. Occupational Safety and Health Administration: *Hazardous waste operations and emergency response (HAZWOPER).* Standard 1910.120, Washington, DC, 2003, The Administration.
4. Occupational Safety and Health Administration: *Occupational exposure to bloodborne pathogens* (29 CFR 1910.1030), Washington, DC, 2001, The Administration.
5. Occupational Safety and Health Administration: *Enforcement policy and procedures for occupational exposure to tuberculosis,* Washington, DC, 1995, The Administration.
6. National Safety Council: *Accident facts,* Itasca, Ill., 2002, The Council.
7. American Academy of Orthopaedic Surgeons: *Basic rescue and emergency care,* Park Ridge, Ill., 1990, The Academy.
8. American Heart Association: *Advanced cardiac life support,* Dallas, Tex., 1997, The Association.
9. Occupational Safety and Health Administration: *Permit required confined spaces for general industry,* (29 CFR 1910.146), Washington, DC, 1997, The Administration.
10. National Highway Traffic Safety Administration: *Special crash investigation study,* Washington, DC, 1999, The Administration.
11. *Emergency response guidelines for air-bagged equipped cars,* Washington, DC, 1990, US Government Printing Office.

CHAPTER 52

Crime Scene Awareness

OBJECTIVES

Upon completion of this chapter, the paramedic student will be able to:

1. Describe general techniques for determining whether a scene is violent and choosing the appropriate response.
2. Outline techniques for recognizing and responding to potentially dangerous residential calls.
3. Outline techniques for recognizing and responding to potentially dangerous calls on the highway.
4. Describe signs of danger and emergency medical services (EMS) response to violent street incidents.
5. Identify characteristics of and EMS response to situations involving gangs, clandestine drug labs, and domestic violence situations.
6. Outline general safety tactics EMS personnel can use if they find themselves in a dangerous situation.
7. Describe special EMS considerations in the provision of tactical patient care.
8. Discuss EMS documentation and preservation of evidence at a crime scene.

KEY TERMS

avoidance: The act of keeping away from someone, something, or a situation, or of preventing the occurrence of something; it requires the paramedic to continually be aware of the scene by remaining observant and being knowledgeable about warning signs that may indicate a dangerous situation.

concealment: A means of keeping out of sight; it provides no ballistic protection.

cover: A type of concealment that hides the body and offers ballistic protection.

crime scene: A location where any part of a criminal act has occurred, or a location where evidence relating to a crime may be found.

distraction: A self-defense measure in which a diversion is created to draw a person's attention.

evasive tactics: A self-defense measure in which an aggressor's moves and actions are anticipated, and unconventional pathways are used during retreat for personal safety.

tactical EMS: Emergency medical services provided by EMS personnel who are specially trained and equipped to provide prehospital emergency care in tactical environments.

tactical patient care: Patient care activities that occur inside the scene perimeter, or hot zone, of a dangerous scene.

tactical retreat: Leaving the scene when danger is observed or when violence or indicators of violence are displayed; requires immediate and decisive action.

Many violent crimes require an EMS response. In fact, EMS crews often arrive at the scene before law enforcement personnel. Consequently, awareness and avoidance of dangerous situations are issues of concern for responders. National studies have reported a decline in violent crimes in recent years. However, violence against EMS personnel from street gangs, threat groups, domestic disputes, and drug users is on the rise.[1,2] Personal safety and crime scene awareness must be the top priorities on every call of this nature.

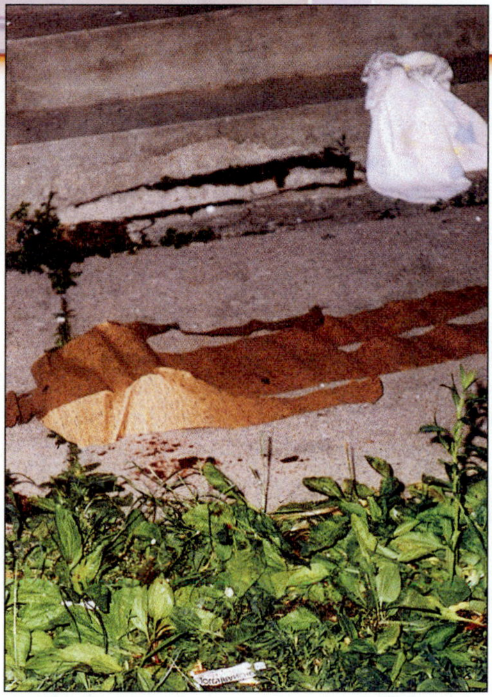

CRITICAL THINKING

Why isn't it always possible to identify a dangerous scene before arriving at the scene?

APPROACHING THE SCENE

For paramedics and other responders, determining personal safety is a basic part of analyzing a scene. It begins before paramedics arrive at the scene with information provided by a dispatching center. *A key point in ensuring personal safety is identifying and responding to potential dangers before they develop.* Certain types of information may be available from a dispatching center. This information should alert the EMS crew to possible dangers. Such information includes known locations of unsafe scenes (e.g., through computer-aided dispatch systems) and/or the presence of the following:

- Large crowds
- People under the influence of alcohol or other drugs
- On-scene violence
- Weapons

Other information can sometimes be gathered en route to the scene from crew members and other responders monitoring the call. Some of these people may have had previous experience with a particular area or address. The paramedic also should be aware of additional inherent hazards that may exist at the scene. Examples include downed power lines, busy roadways, toxic substances, the potential for fire, dangerous pets, and vehicle hazards and dangers. If the scene is not safe, the EMS crew should retreat. The crew should stage at a safe location to await the arrival of law enforcement and/or other rescuers.

When responding to a scene with a potential for danger, the EMS crew should begin observation several blocks from the scene. They also should use audible and visual warning (AVW) devices that are appropriate for the call. For example, responding with AVW devices to an urban scene may draw a crowd of bystanders; lights generally are required for safety at highway scenes. When possible, joint fire-EMS-law enforcement responses should be defined through preplanning (e.g., fire-EMS response with full use of AVW devices; law enforcement responding without AVW devices and at normal speed) (see Chapter 49).

Scene safety considerations for all types of danger must continue throughout the EMS response. A scene that has been made safe can become unsafe, even when the police are present. This can happen if violence resumes, crowds gather or turn violent, or other people enter the scene. Violence against EMS providers also may occur if they are mistaken for police officers (because of uniform colors or badges) or when they exit an emergency vehicle that has AVW devices. The paramedic crew must be familiar with local protocols when intervening in violent situations. They also must have a strategic escape plan ready.

Scenes Known to Be Violent

If the scene is known to be violent, the EMS crew should remain at a safe, out-of-sight distance from the area ("out of sight—out of scene"). They should remain at this distance until the area has been secured by law enforcement personnel. Remaining at a safe staging area away from a violent scene is important for several reasons:

- If paramedics can be seen, people will come to them.
- Entering an unsafe scene adds one or more potential victims.
- Paramedics may be injured or killed.
- Paramedics may be taken hostage.
- Paramedics may become additional patients in a scene that is already a multiple casualty incident.

It must be stressed that if the scene is unsafe, the EMS crew should retreat to a staging area and wait for resource personnel who can provide scene safety.

DANGEROUS RESIDENCE

A response to a residence is an everyday occurrence for most EMS providers. However, even calls that appear routine require a size-up. This should begin before the EMS crew leaves the emergency vehicle. Warning signs of danger in residential calls include the following:

- A history of problems or violence
- A known drug or gang area
- Loud noises (e.g., screams, items breaking, possible gunshots)
- Seeing or hearing acts of violence
- The presence of alcohol or other drug use
- The smell of chemicals or the presence of empty chemical containers
- Evidence of dangerous pets (e.g., exotic snakes and reptiles, breeds of dogs that are often trained to be vicious)
- Unusual silence or darkened residence

If any of these or other warning signs are present, the EMS crew should retreat from the scene and call for law enforcement assistance.

When approaching a suspicious residence, the EMS crew should choose tactics that match the threat or situation. For example, they should not use AVW devices; they should take unconventional pathways (rather than using the sidewalk, for example); and they should not stand in front of the ambulance lights (backlighting). In addition, paramedics should listen for sounds indicating danger before announcing their presence or entering the home. They should stand on the side of the entry door opposite the hinges (doorknob side) (Fig. 52-1). If danger becomes evident, paramedics should immediately retreat from the scene.

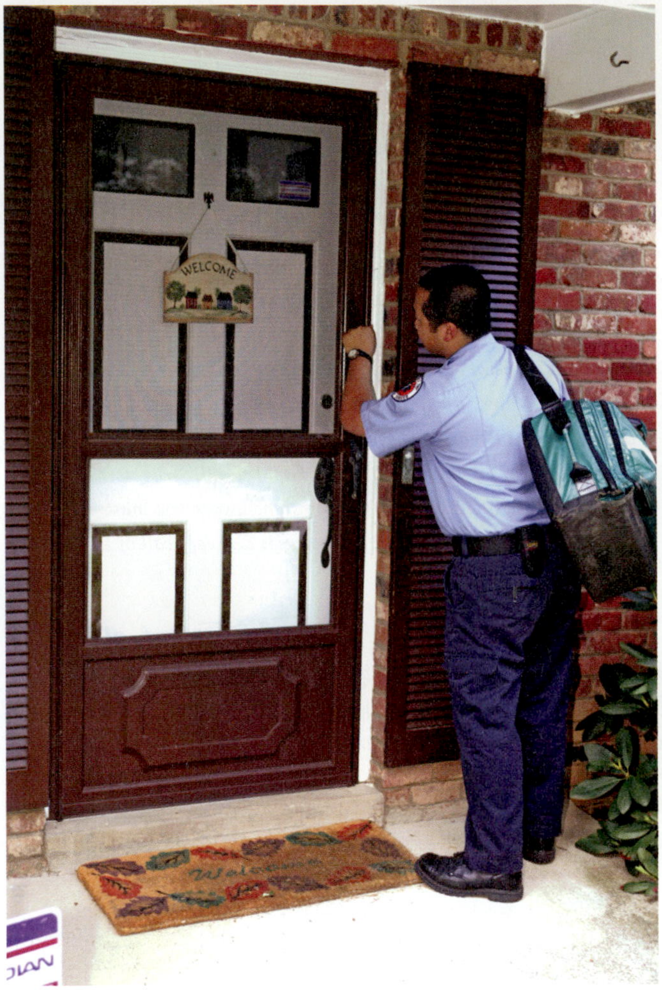

FIGURE 52-1 ■ If danger from inside a residence is suspected, paramedics should stand on the side of an entry door opposite the hinges (i.e., the doorknob side).

DANGEROUS HIGHWAY ENCOUNTERS

As with calls to residences, a response to a traffic incident should never be considered routine. Such calls involve inherent dangers associated with traffic flow, emergency vehicle positioning, and extrication. Also, the danger of violence may exist. For example, a vehicle's occupants may be armed, wanted, or fleeing felons; intoxicated or drugged; or violent and abusive because of an altered mental state (Box 52-1).

For approaching a vehicle, a one-person approach is recommended.[2] This allows the partner who remains in the ambulance to notify dispatch of the situation, location, license plate number, and state registration of suspicious vehicles. (Because the ambulance is elevated, it provides greater visibility.) At night, the ambulance's lights should be used to illuminate the interior of the vehicle. They also can be used to illuminate the surrounding area.

BOX 52-1 Street-Smart Safety Tips

- When working in a trafficway, always wear reflective clothing and make sure you can leave the scene quickly and safely if required.
- At nighttime, use the ambulance lights to illuminate a vehicle's interior.
- Before approaching a vehicle, consider using the public address (PA) system to get a response from passengers in the car.
- If a passenger in the car is adjusting the side or rear view mirror as you approach, retreat to safety. (This is a sign of danger.)
- Open or unlatched trunks may indicate that people are hiding or have been restrained in the compartment. If the trunk is slightly open, slam it shut without opening it further.
- Retreat to the ambulance (or another place of safety) at the first sign of danger.

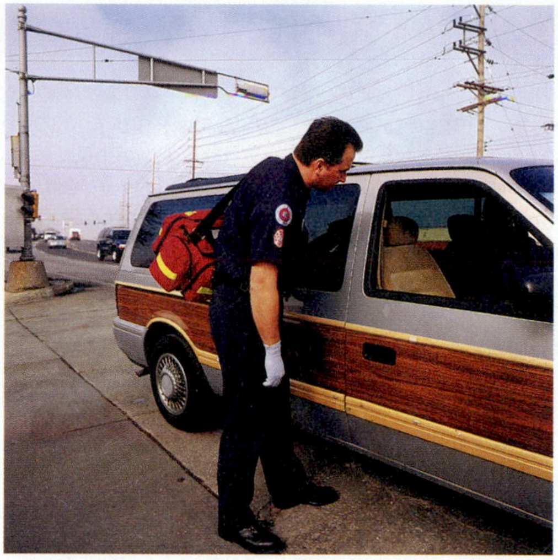

FIGURE 52-2 ■ In approaching a car with potentially dangerous occupants, paramedics should observe the front seat from behind post B. They should move forward only after ensuring their safety.

The paramedic who approaches the car should do so from the passenger side of the vehicle. This provides protection from vehicular traffic. Furthermore, it usually is the opposite approach a driver would expect from law enforcement personnel. As another safety precaution, the paramedic should not walk between the ambulance and the other vehicle, to avoid being trapped and injured if the vehicle backs up. Also, the paramedic should walk around the rear of the ambulance and then to the passenger side of the vehicle.

Car posts A, B, and C (see Chapter 51) may provide the best ballistic protection. The paramedic should observe for unusual activity in the rear seat. He or she should not move forward of the post nearest the threat unless no threats exist in these areas. The paramedic should observe the front seat from behind post B. He or she should move forward only after making sure it is safe to do so (Fig. 52-2). If signs of danger are present (e.g., weapons, suspicious behavior or movements in the vehicle, arguing or fighting among passengers), paramedics should immediately retreat to a safe staging area. From that area, they should request the help of law enforcement.

CRITICAL THINKING

In your community, what type of EMS calls routinely merit a law enforcement response?

VIOLENT STREET INCIDENTS

Murder, assault, and robbery are common occurrences in the United States. Many of these crimes involve dangerous weapons. Violence may be directed toward EMS personnel from perpetrators at the scene or who return to the scene. The violence may even come from injured and distraught patients. In addition, dangerous crowds and bystanders quickly can become large in number and volatile. They may direct violence toward everyone and everything in the surrounding area. Warning signs of potential danger in violent street incidents include the following:

- Voices that become louder, escalating in tone
- Pushing and shoving
- Hostility toward people at the scene (e.g., perpetrator, police, victim)
- A rapid increase in the size of the crowd
- The use of alcohol or other drugs by people at the scene
- Inability of law enforcement personnel to control the crowd

Paramedic crews should constantly monitor crowds and retreat from the scene if necessary. The location and careful parking of the emergency vehicle is important for personal safety. The EMS crew should position the ambulance so that it cannot be blocked by other vehicles (allowing for easy retreat from the scene). When possible and when it is safe to do so, the patient should be removed from the scene as the crew retreats. (This may eliminate the need to return to the scene.)

VIOLENT GROUPS AND SITUATIONS

According to a study completed by the Department of Justice's Office of Juvenile Justice and Delinquency Prevention (OJJDP), more than 750,000 gang members currently belong to more than 24,500 gangs throughout the United States[3] (Box 52-2). Most gangs and other threat groups operate through intimidation and extortion (Box 52-3).

Gang Characteristics

A *gang* can be defined as any group of people who engage in socially disruptive or criminal behavior. They usually are territorial. Often, but not always, a gang is all male or all fe-

BOX 52-2 Short History of Gangs

Modern-era gangs first emerged in the United States in the late 1960s. Two of the best-known gangs, the Crips and the Bloods, started in Compton, California, when two rival high schools began to sport their school colors. The Bloods wore red to denote their gang affiliation; the Crips wore blue. Other gangs sprouted from roots in the prison system. The Black Gangster Disciples (now known as the Gangster Disciple Nation) was the most noteworthy of these. This gang started in the Chicago prison system and competed for the drug market in that city. In recent years, gangs have evolved to include all ethnic origins and backgrounds (e.g., Asian, Hispanic, Latin, and white threat groups). Most operate in secrecy with codes of honor and pledges that frequently involve acts of violence. Gang membership often is a lifetime commitment.

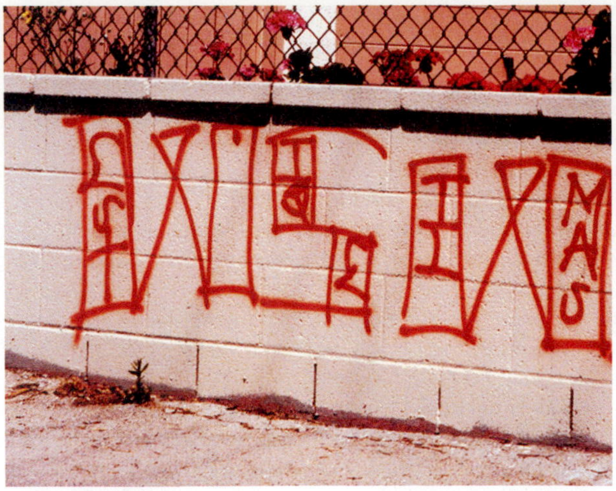

FIGURE 52-3 ■ Blood graffiti on a wall in Los Angeles.

BOX 52-3 Some Gangs and Other Threat Groups in the United States

Bad Boy Club	Latin Kings (Almighty Latin King & Queen Nation)
Banditos	Mexican Posse (MP)
Bloods	Pagans
Crips	Skin Heads
Gangs for Disciples	Outlaws
Hell's Angels	

male. Gangs also operate by creating an atmosphere of fear in a community. The gang may choose a name, logo, specific color, or method of dress to identify its own members and counterparts.

CRITICAL THINKING

In addition to consulting police sources and familiarizing yourself with gang markings, dress, and colors, how can you obtain information about gang activity in your community?

GRAFFITI AND CLOTHING

Graffiti ("tagging") is probably the most visible sign of gang criminal activity. It can be seen in neighborhood parks, the backs and side walls of stores, fences, retaining walls, and any other prominent structure that is paintable (Fig. 52-3). Gang graffiti usually marks territorial boundaries. (This is known as *turf.*) Gang-related clothing often is unique and specific to a group. It is worn to identify affiliation and rank. Common gang-related clothing and styles are listed in Box 52-4.

SAFETY ISSUES IN GANG AREAS

Common gang activities include fighting, vandalism, armed robbery, weapon offenses, automobile theft, battery, and drug dealing. (Not all gang members are engaged in illegal activities.) The criminal activity usually is committed for monetary benefit, either for the gang in general or for a single member. Violent acts from gangs are highly likely. Because the uniforms of EMS personnel often look like those of law enforcement officials, paramedics must be very cautious about personal safety when working in gang areas.

Clandestine Drug Labs

As described in Chapter 36, the illegal manufacture of drugs can pose major hazards for emergency providers. In some clandestine labs, drugs are created from chemical precursors (e.g., lysergic acid diethylamide [LSD], methamphetamine). (This is known as *synthesis.*) Also, a drug's form can be changed. (This is known as *conversion.*) For example, cocaine hydrochloride may be changed to a base form. The processes of drug synthesis and conversion can produce low-oxygen atmospheres. They also can create highly explosive and toxic gases (e.g., phosgene). These gases can readily be absorbed through the skin in amounts that can be fatal. Toxic solvents involved in drug-making processes also can lead to lab explosions and exposure to dangerous chemicals.

Booby traps are another safety hazard associated with clandestine drug labs. These can maim or kill an intruder. Also, those who operate these labs are sometimes armed or otherwise violent. Clandestine labs usually are located in an area that ensures privacy. They generally are well ventilated. They also usually have access to water, electric, and gas utilities, which are required for the drug-making process. Suspicious individuals, activities, and deliveries often are at the site.

CRITICAL THINKING

What type of calls might EMS crews respond to at a drug lab?

When responding to a scene that may be a site of illegal drug manufacture, EMS crews should be alert for signs. These may include chemical odors and the presence of chemical

BOX 52-4 Gang Clothing and Styles

Male
- Shaved, bald head or extremely short hair
- Tattoos (variable) and jewelry
- Bandanas
- White, oversized T-shirt that is creased in the middle
- White, athletic-type undershirt
- Polo-type knit shirts (oversized), usually worn buttoned to the top and not tucked in; other types of oversized shirts
- Oversized Dickie, Ben Davis, or Solos pants
- Pants worn low, or "sagging," and cuffed inside at the bottom or dragging on the ground
- Baseball caps worn backward (usually black and sometimes having the gang's initials)
- Cutoff, below-the-knee short pants worn with knee-high socks
- A predominance of dark or dull clothing or clothing of one particular color
- Black stretch belt with chrome or silver gang initial belt buckle
- Clothing a mixture of gang colors, black and silver, or white

Female
- Exaggerated use of mousse, gel, or baby oil in the hair
- Tattoos (variable) and jewelry
- Black or dark clothing and shoes
- Black oversized jackets, sweatshirts, or athletic football jerseys
- Oversized shirts worn outside of pants
- Oversized T-shirts
- Dark jackets with lettering (cursive or Old English style)
- Baggy, long pants that drag on the ground
- Heavy makeup, dark and excessive eye shadow, shaved eyebrows, dark lipstick, dark fingernail polish
- Tank tops or revealing blouses
- Stretch belt with initial on belt buckle

equipment (e.g., glassware, chemical containers, heating mantles, burners). If a drug lab is identified, the EMS crew should[2]

1. Leave the area at once
2. Notify law enforcement and request appropriate agencies and personnel (e.g., hazardous materials [HAZMAT] teams, fire service personnel, Drug Enforcement Administration [DEA] personnel, chemistry specialists)
3. Initiate an incident management system and HAZMAT procedures per protocol
4. Help law enforcement personnel to evacuate the surrounding area in an orderly fashion (to ensure public safety)

NOTE EMS crews should never touch anything found in or around a drug lab. Only specially trained personnel should try to alter drug-making equipment or stop chemical reactions in a drug lab.

Domestic Violence

As described in Chapter 46, *domestic violence* is violence that occurs between people in a relationship. The perpetrator may be male or female. The individuals may be in an opposite-sex or same-sex relationship. Domestic violence results in physical, emotional, sexual, verbal, or economic abuse. It may occur in several combinations. To review, many signs indicate domestic violence and abuse. Some of these include the following:

- Apparent fear of a household member
- Different or conflicting accounts by parties at the scene
- One party preventing another from speaking
- A patient who is reluctant to speak
- Injuries that do not match the reported mechanism of injury
- Unusual or unsanitary living conditions or personal hygiene

EMS personnel who respond to a scene of domestic violence should be aware that acts of violence may be directed toward them by the perpetrator. They should take all safety precautions. If the scene is considered safe for the EMS crew, paramedics should treat the patient's injuries. They also should notify medical direction and other authorities consistent per standard procedures and protocol. (Mandatory reporting may be required.) To help ensure scene safety for the crew and the abused person, paramedics should not be judgmental about the relationship. They should not direct accusations toward the abuser. When appropriate, paramedics should supply the victim with phone numbers for domestic violence hotlines, community support programs, and available shelters.

SAFETY TACTICS

Tactics that help ensure personal safety include avoidance, tactical retreat, cover and concealment, and distraction and evasive maneuvers. Many programs in the United States teach tactics for safety and patient care. Some EMS providers are specially trained and equipped to work in tactical law enforcement settings (Box 52-5).

Avoidance

Avoidance is always preferable to confrontation. To practice avoidance, paramedics must continually be aware of the scene. They can stay aware by being observant and by being knowledgeable about warning signs that may indicate a dangerous situation. In addition, they must be knowledgeable about tactical responses for avoiding danger or for dealing with danger that cannot be avoided. An example of avoidance is *staging*. With staging, the dispatching center learns of danger and advises the EMS crew not to approach the scene. They do not approach until the scene has been secured by the appropriate authorities.

Tactical Retreat

Tactical retreat means leaving the scene when danger is observed or when violence or indicators of violence are displayed. Tactical retreat requires immediate and decisive ac-

BOX 52-5 Tactical EMS

The term *tactical EMS (TEMS)* refers to EMS personnel who are specially trained and equipped to provide prehospital emergency care in tactical law enforcement settings. Such settings may include hostage-barricaded situations, high-risk search warrants, and other adverse situations involving law enforcement and/or rescue operations in which standard EMS units may be inappropriate.

The concept of training emergency medical technicians (EMTs) and paramedics in TEMS started in the late 1980s. It has since expanded nationwide. Forward-thinking law enforcement departments have adopted TEMS programs as a way to increase the safety of their special weapons and tactics (SWAT) officers and the innocent hostage or bystander. They also are a means of addressing liability exposure. Tactical training for EMS personnel also is recognized as a valuable tool for personal safety when EMS personnel find themselves in an unsafe situation.

Many tactical medical teams use the Counter Narcotics Tactical Operations Medical Support (CONTOMS) program for initial training of their personnel. CONTOMS is a joint federal program supported by the Department of Defense and the Department of the Interior, with assistance from the Department of Justice and the Department of the Treasury, as well as many state and local law enforcement agencies. The CONTOMS program leads to certification as an EMT-Tactic (EMT-T) or SWAT medic. The focus of the training is to integrate specific skills to complement an agency's standard operating procedures. These skills include the ability to

- Assess and plan for preventive medicine needs in sustained operations
- Provide preventive medical care in sustained operations
- Recognize and treat unique wound patterns resulting from deliberate interpersonal aggression
- Use medical care skills appropriate to hostile and austere environments
- Explain medical and physiological parameters that lead to performance decrement and implement plans that minimize those effects
- Develop and apply injury control strategies
- Access and analyze medical information and make a medical threat assessment
- Apply special law enforcement principles to the delivery of medical care

tion. Retreat on foot or by vehicle (in a calm, safe manner) involves choosing the mode and route of retreat that provides the least exposure to danger. During tactical retreat, the EMS crew should be aware that the risks they faced are now located behind them. They must stay alert for associated dangers. Of course, the required distance from danger for a safe tactical retreat must be guided by the nature of the incident. In general, a safe distance must

- Protect the crew from any potential danger
- Keep the crew out of the immediate line of sight
- Protect the crew from gunfire (i.e., provide cover)
- Keep the crew far enough away to give them time to react if danger reappears

CRITICAL THINKING

Could the EMS crew be charged with abandonment if they make a tactical retreat and leave the patient?

Once tactical retreat has been achieved, the EMS crew must notify other responding units and agencies of the danger. They notify other units using interagency EMS and law enforcement standard operating procedures and agreements. (Interagency procedures that deal with violent situations should be established in the preplanning stages. That way, each agency is aware of its specific duties.)

Documentation also is essential to reducing liability if injuries or deaths occur. Thorough documentation should include observations of danger at the scene; who was notified of the danger; actions at the scene; and accurate times that retreat or return to the scene occurred. Tactical retreat for appropriate circumstances is not considered patient abandonment.[2]

Cover and Concealment

Cover and **concealment** provide protection from injury. *Cover* involves large, heavy structures and thus provides ballistic protection. Examples of such structures include large trees, telephone poles, and a vehicle's engine block. *Concealment* hides the body. However, it offers little or no ballistic protection. Examples of concealment include bushes, wallboards, and the doors of vehicles.

Cover and concealment should be integrated into tactical retreat or used when the EMS crew is pinned down (e.g., by gunfire) or in other dangerous settings. When the need for cover or concealment arises, paramedics should

- Constantly be aware of their surroundings
- Place as much of the body as possible behind adequate cover
- Constantly look for ways to improve protection and location
- Be aware of reflective clothing (e.g., trim, badges) that may draw attention or serve as a target

CRITICAL THINKING

What parts of your ambulance provide cover?

Distraction and Evasive Maneuvers

Distraction and **evasive tactics** can be used as self-defense measures during retreat. They also can be used when retreat and cover and concealment are impossible (Box 52-6). For example, equipment may be used to provide distraction; a stretcher may be wedged in a doorway to block an aggressor, or equipment may be thrown to trip or slow a pursuer. These actions may allow the EMS crew to make a safe retreat or gain adequate cover and concealment. Evasive tactics involve anticipating the moves of the aggressor (Box 52-7) and using unconventional pathways during retreat.

BOX 52-6 Self-Defense Measures

Training in self-defense is probably appropriate for all emergency responders. Avoidance is always superior to confrontation. However, some violent situations may call for self-defense. Examples include physical attacks that cannot be avoided, armed confrontation or robbery, hostage situations, and dangerous animals. A person can be controlled with physical or chemical restraints (see Chapter 40). Equipment (e.g., metal clipboards, jump kits, stretchers) or other items (e.g., furniture) can be used to block an aggressor. In addition to these techniques, self-defense measures may include training in the use of pepper sprays or other chemical deterrents and defensive physical maneuvers that can allow escape.

Sometimes escape is impossible, and paramedics may be caught in a dangerous situation. (For example, they may be held as a hostage.) In such cases paramedics should

- Remain as calm as possible
- Avoid any confrontation
- Play an active role with the captor in resolving the incident
- Focus on a peaceful resolution and escape

BOX 52-7 Warning Signs of Possible Violent Aggression

People who are about to escalate to violence often give subtle warning signs of this development. Such a person may

- Conspicuously ignore emergency responders
- Be verbally abusive
- Invade the responder's personal space
- Have a violent history or background
- Shift the body weight from side to side or foot to foot (boxer stance)
- Clench the fists
- Tighten the muscles (e.g., have stiff arms and/or shoulders)
- Maintain eye contact by staring

Paramedic crews trained in **tactical EMS** often use preassigned roles for distraction and evasive maneuvers. One paramedic usually is the *contact provider.* This person initiates and provides direct patient care. This includes patient assessment and most elements of interpersonal scene contact. Another crew member serves as the *cover provider.* In a tactical context, the cover provider's role is to ensure safe cover for the contact providers while they perform patient care. This role includes monitoring the scene for danger. The cover provider generally does not perform patient care duties. These would prevent this individual from observing the scene. The cover provider also may be responsible for ensuring the safekeeping of equipment, drugs, and supplies while at the scene.

Methods of communication between the contact and cover providers should be developed in advance. That way, they can alert team members of potential dangers without alerting the aggressor. This often can be done with subtle verbal and nonverbal signals, such as using coded terms, scratching the neck, or rubbing the nose. It is crucial in these situations to maintain radio contact with the dispatching center. The crew also should involve the dispatcher in the danger signal process. For example, if the dispatcher hears a coded term that means danger, a priority response of the proper personnel can be initiated.

TACTICAL PATIENT CARE

The term **tactical patient care** describes patient care activities that occur inside the scene perimeter. This is also known as the *hot zone.* The provision of emergency medical services in the hot zone requires special training and authorization, body armor and a tactical uniform, compact and functional equipment and, in some operations, personal defensive weapons. Tactical EMS in the hot zone often requires risks not taken in standard EMS situations. *Tactical medics* provide immediate medical care to the injured during a special weapons and tactics (SWAT) operation. These medics treat the injured on site or stabilize them and extract them from the scene. Tactical medics generally work alongside law enforcement officers. Some agencies use individuals who are cross-trained in law enforcement and tactical EMS.

Body Armor

As described in Chapter 20, soft body armor (also known as *bulletproof vests*) offers protection from some blunt and penetrating trauma. It absorbs and distributes the impact of a ballistic missile or penetrating object. This equipment is effective against most handgun bullets and knives. However, they do not provide protection from high-velocity rifle bullets or thin or dual-edged weapons (e.g., ice picks). Like all other protective clothing, body armor is effective only when it is properly worn. It also must be in good condition. Some body armor (e.g., Kevlar) degrades with age. This armor may carry a ballistic expiration date that should be observed. Wet or worn vests do not provide optimum protection. A type III or higher level of protection generally is recommended for tactical EMS providers.

When wearing body armor, paramedics should take care not to develop a false sense of security. *A general rule is, never try a maneuver that wouldn't normally be done without body armor.* Also, paramedics should keep in mind that body armor does not cover the entire body. Severe injury can still result from the forces of blunt trauma (in the absence of penetration) even when the vest is properly worn.

EMS CARE IN THE HOT ZONE

As stated before, the provision of EMS care in tactical situations calls for special training and authorization. Most tactical medics (EMT-Ts and SWAT medics) are trained in the following[4]:

- Team health and management
- Care under fire
- Officer rescue
- Medical operations planning and medical intelligence
- Responding to the active shooter
- Special medical gear for tactical operations
- Personal protective gear
- Special needs for extended operations
- Preventive medicine

- Management of weapons of mass destruction and toxic hazards

Most programs involve training exercises. Some of these include the following:

- Physical assessment under sensory deprivation/overload conditions
- Medical threat assessment
- Advanced medical-tactical techniques
- Field expedient decontamination
- New technologies for safe searches
- Management of dental injuries
- "Officer down" rescue and extraction
- Aeromedical evacuation
- Medical management of clandestine drug lab raids
- Safe search techniques
- Remote physical assessment

Patient care in dangerous settings involves a number of special concerns. These include the frequent need to remove a patient from the area safely; the frequent care of trauma patients; the need to modify patient care; and medical and transport actions that must be coordinated with the incident commander. Often tactical EMS providers work under protocols and standing orders that are different from those of "standard" EMS practice. These medical direction issues regarding patient care are dictated by the nature of the event. They also are determined by the uncontrolled and hazardous scene in which emergency medical services are provided. Awareness programs are available for those who supervise or manage personnel assigned to a tactical team. Programs are also available for physicians (and others) who provide medical direction for rescuers who work with tactical law enforcement teams. Quality assurance programs and direct physician involvement at the local level are recommended.

EMS AT CRIME SCENES

A **crime scene** is a location where any part of a criminal act has occurred. It also can be a location where evidence relating to a crime may be found. Important physical evidence that may be found at a crime scene includes fingerprints, footprints, and blood and other body fluids. Fingerprints and footprints are unique to an individual. No two people have identical prints. These ridge characteristics often are left behind on a surface, along with oil and moisture from the skin. Blood and other body fluids can be tested for deoxyribonucleic acid (DNA) and ABO blood typing. They also have characteristics that may be unique to the individual. In addition, particulate evidence (e.g., hair, carpet, and clothing fibers) can provide useful information and is considered valuable at a crime scene.

The paramedic's observations at a crime scene are important. They should be documented carefully on the patient care report or other appropriate form. For example, victims' positions, their injuries, and conditions at the scene may be helpful to law enforcement personnel in solving the crime. Documentation also should include any statements made by the patient or other people at the scene and any dying declarations. Paramedics should be careful to (1) record their observations objectively; (2) record patients' or bystanders' words in quotes; and (3) avoid personal opinions that are not relevant to patient care. Paramedics must keep in mind that patient care reports are legal documents; they may be used in court.

BOX 52-8 Considerations for Crime Scene Preservation

Paramedics should observe the following rules when called to a known or a possible crime scene:

1. Approach no crime scene until it has been secured for your safety.
2. Park your vehicle as far away as conveniently possible to preserve skid marks, tire prints, or other evidence.
3. Survey and assess the scene before proceeding to the victim.
4. Try to approach the victim from a route different from the assailant's probable route.
5. Follow the same path to and from the victim.
6. Avoid stepping on blood stains or spatter if possible.
7. Disturb the victim and the victim's clothing as little as possible while performing your assessment and during treatment.
8. When cutting clothing from a victim, try to do it in a way that preserves the points of wounding.
9. Report your actions and any disturbances you make to the crime scene investigator.
10. Keep all unnecessary people away from the victim.
11. Do not smoke or eat at the crime scene.
12. Do not touch any evidence if at all possible.
13. Make no comments to bystanders about the situation.
14. Save the victim's clothes and personal items in a paper bag. The bag should be labeled, sealed, and turned over to law enforcement personnel.
15. Be alert to any dying declarations the patient makes.
16. Keep accurate, detailed records.
17. Keep in mind that law enforcement personnel are in charge of the crime scene; you are in charge of the patient.

Modified from Vollrath R: Crime scene preservation: it's everybody's concern, *Journal of Emergency Medical Services* 20(1):53, 1995.

NOTE A *dying declaration* is a statement(s) made by a person who believes he or she is about to die. The statement concerns the cause or circumstance surrounding his or her impending death. An example is an assault victim who makes a dying declaration implicating a certain person as being her attacker.

Preserving Evidence

Patient care is the paramedic's top priority, even at crime scenes. However, evidence can be protected during patient care. Paramedics can do this by being careful not to disturb the scene unnecessarily and not destroying evidence. For example, paramedics should be observant of the scene and surroundings; they should touch only what is required for patient care; and they should wear latex gloves for infection control and to avoid leaving additional fingerprints at the scene. Other measures that aid crime scene preservation are listed in Box 52-8.

CRITICAL THINKING

If the main goal is caring for the patient, why should a paramedic be concerned about preserving evidence?

SUMMARY

- A key point in ensuring scene safety is to identify and respond to dangers before they threaten. If the scene is known to be violent, the EMS crew should remain at a safe distance and out of sight of the area. They should remain at this distance until the scene has been secured.
- Paramedics should look for warning signs of violence during a response to a residence. They should retreat from the scene if danger becomes evident.
- A response to a highway incident may involve the dangers associated with traffic and extrication. It also may present the danger of violence. The occupants of a vehicle may be armed, may be wanted or fleeing felons, may be intoxicated or drugged, or may be violent or abusive because of an altered mental state.
- Paramedics should monitor for warning signs of danger in violent street incidents. They should retreat from the scene if necessary.
- A gang is any group of people who take part in socially disruptive or criminal behavior. Some gangs are involved in violent criminal activities. EMS personnel often look like law enforcement officers. Therefore they should be very cautious about personal safety when working in gang areas.
- Clandestine labs can produce explosive and toxic gases. Other risks include armed or violent occupants and booby traps that can maim or kill an intruder.
- EMS personnel who respond to a scene of domestic violence should keep alert for any acts of violence toward them by the perpetrator and should take all safety precautions.
- Tactics for safety include avoidance, tactical retreat, cover and concealment, and distraction and evasive maneuvers.
- The term *tactical patient care* refers to care activities that occur inside the scene perimeter (the *hot zone*). To provide care in this area, a paramedic must have special training and authorization, body armor and a tactical uniform, compact and functional equipment, and, in some operations, personal defensive weapons.
- The paramedic's observations at a crime scene are important and should be carefully documented. Paramedics should try to protect evidence while caring for the patient. This can be done by not destroying evidence and by taking care not to disturb the scene unnecessarily.

REFERENCES

1. Maggiore WA, Palmer RB: Medical and legal issues you must understand to protect the patient and yourself, *Journal of Emergency Medical Services,* 2(3), 2002.
2. US Department of Transportation, National Highway Traffic Safety Administration: *EMT-paramedic national standard curriculum,* Washington, DC, 1998, The Department.
3. Egley A, Jr: *National Youth Gang Survey Trends from 1996 to 2000.* Fact Sheet (2002-2003), Washington, DC: U.S. Department of Justice, Office of Juvenile Justice and Delinquency Prevention, http://www.ncjrs.org/pdffiles1/ojjdp/fs200203.pdf. Accessed March 22, 2005.
4. EMT-T Tactical Course, U.S. Immigration and Customs Enforcement, Federal Protective Service Office of Protective Medicine, U.S. Department of Homeland Security, http://www.casualtycareresearchcenter.org/emt-t_provider_program.htm. Accessed March 20, 2005.

CHAPTER 53

Hazardous Materials Incidents

OBJECTIVES

Upon completion of this chapter, the paramedic student will be able to:

1. Define hazardous materials terminology.
2. Identify legislation about hazardous materials that influences emergency health care workers.
3. Describe resources to assist in identification and management of hazardous materials incidents.
4. Identify the protective clothing and equipment needed to respond to selected hazardous materials incidents.
5. Describe the pathophysiology, signs, and symptoms of internal damage caused by exposure to selected hazardous materials.
6. Identify the pathophysiology, signs and symptoms, and prehospital management of selected hazardous materials that produce external damage.
7. Outline the prehospital response to a hazardous materials emergency.
8. Describe medical monitoring and rehabilitation of rescue workers who respond to a hazardous materials emergency.
9. Describe emergency decontamination and management of patients who have been contaminated by hazardous materials.
10. Outline the eight steps to decontaminate rescue personnel and equipment at a hazardous materials incident.

KEY TERMS

decontamination: The process of making patients, rescuers, equipment, and supplies safe by eliminating harmful substances.

placards: Four-sided, diamond-shaped signs displayed on hazardous materials containers that usually are yellow, orange, white, or green. They have a four-digit United Nations identification number and a legend to indicate the contents of the container.

primary contamination: Exposure to a hazardous substance that is harmful only to the person exposed and that poses little risk of exposure to others.

secondary contamination: Exposure to a hazardous substance whereby liquid and particulate substances are transferred easily to others by touching.

shipping papers: Descriptions of the hazardous materials that include the substance name, classification, and United Nations identification number.

Hazardous materials incidents create added responsibilities for emergency service providers. Large incidents may involve a number of political jurisdictions. In addition, cooperation in mass evacuations and mass decontamination may be required. Specialized roles and responsibilities include, among others, recognition and identification of hazardous material, scene safety, responsibilities to stage at major scenes, containment and cleanup of the material, extrication and decontamination of exposed individuals, provision of emergency care, and continual medical assessment of team members involved in the incident.

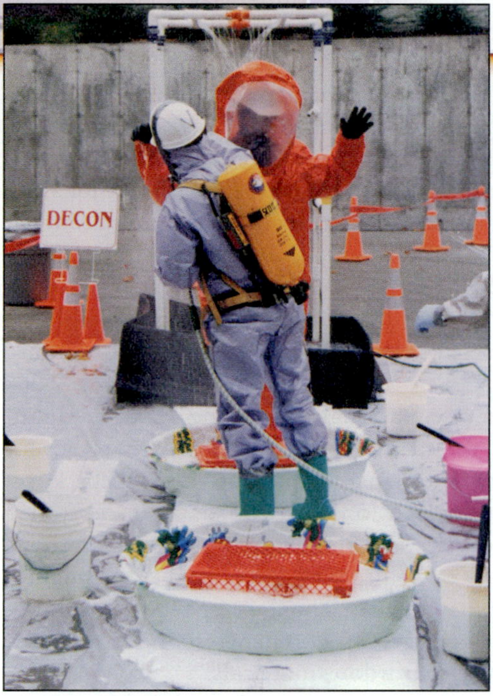

SCOPE OF HAZARDOUS MATERIALS

A *hazardous material* is defined as "any substance or material capable of posing an unreasonable risk to health, safety, and property."[1] More than 50 billion tons of hazardous materials are made in the United States each year. About 4 billion tons are shipped within the United States.[2] An estimated 5% to 15% of all trucks on the road at any time carry hazardous materials. Emergency responses to vehicular crashes are common; thus the potential for exposure to hazardous materials is great. Other possible causes of hazardous materials incidents include mishaps in the storage of materials and manufacturing operations, illicit drug manufacturing (e.g., "meth labs"), and acts of terrorism (see Chapter 54.)

CRITICAL THINKING

Consider the industries in your area. Do any of these have the potential for a hazardous materials exposure?

Injury or illness also may result from exposure to household chemicals, pesticides, and industrial toxins. The following statistics emphasize the importance of emergency medical service (EMS) personnel knowing how to manage hazardous materials exposure[3]:

- About 9000 deaths occur each year from exposure to poisonous solids, liquids, and gases.
- An estimated 100,000 industrial workers are exposed to respiratory irritants each year.
- Pesticide poisoning accounts for more than 3000 hospitalizations each year.
- Most fire-related deaths result from inhalation of toxic products of combustion.

LAWS AND REGULATIONS

In recent years much focus has been placed on the handling of hazardous materials. Major incidents have attracted the attention of employee and citizen groups. These incidents also have drawn the attention of local, state, and federal officials. Some of these incidents include the Union Carbide disaster in Bhopal, India (1984); the Chernobyl nuclear accident in the Soviet Union (1986); the Three Mile Island incident in the United States (1979); and the Criticality accident in Tokaimura, Japan (1999); threats and acts of bioterrorism (e.g., the sarin gas attack on Tokyo subways in 1995); and the need for proper disposal of hazardous wastes.

This attention has resulted in more laws and regulations. These laws and regulations have helped to ensure strict control of hazardous materials.

The Superfund Amendments and Reauthorization Act (the Superfund Act) of 1986 established requirements for federal, state, and local governments and industry regarding emergency planning and the reporting of hazardous materials–related incidents. This act was intended to help communities better manage a chemical emergency. The Superfund Act helped increase public knowledge about hazardous materials in communities and helped to improve public access to this information. The act required owners and operators of facilities using or storing any of the extremely hazardous substances identified by the Environmental Protection Agency (EPA) to notify the local fire department, the local emergency planning committee, and the state emergency response commission.

In 1989 the Occupational Safety and Health Administration (OSHA) and the EPA published rules to govern training requirements, emergency plans, medical checkups, and other safety precautions for workers at uncontrolled hazardous waste sites and those responding to hazardous chemical releases or spills.[4] The Superfund Act mandates that states adopt these rules. The training requirements apply to five groups of persons who may respond to an emergency that involves hazardous materials.

In addition to these training levels outlined by OSHA, the National Fire Protection Association (NFPA) has published standards that address competencies for EMS personnel at hazardous materials (hazmat) scenes.[5] According to these standards, paramedics who transport patients who pose no risk of **secondary contamination** must be trained to NFPA standard 473 Level I. Paramedics who may have to decontaminate rapidly or assist in the **decontamination** area must be trained to NFPA standard 473 Level II[6] (see chapter appendix).

IDENTIFICATION OF HAZARDOUS MATERIALS

At the center of dealing with hazardous materials is identifying the substance. Two methods can be used to identify such materials. The first one is informal product identification. The second one is formal product identification. (The second method involves **placards, shipping papers,** and other hazmat information resources.)

Informal Product Identification

Arriving emergency personnel may be able to determine the presence and type of hazardous materials at the scene. Informal methods of identification include the following:

- Visual inspection of the scene with binoculars before entering the site
- Verbal reports by bystanders or other responsible individuals
- Occupancy type (intended use of a particular structure such as fuel storage or pesticide plant)
- Incident location (probable location for presence of hazardous materials)
- Location within a building (what is stored in that area)
- Visual indicators (vapor clouds, smoke, leakage)
- Vehicle types (named carriers or company)
- Container characteristics (size, shape, color, deformed containers)
- Senses (peculiar smell)
- Signs and symptoms of victims of exposure

These informal ways to identify a product should be used as a quick means to determine the presence of any hazardous materials. The paramedic should always identify a product formally before taking any action that may pose a threat to the safety of all responders.

NOTE Personal safety is the primary priority when responding to a hazardous materials incident. If the scene is not safe, the emergency medical services crew should retreat. They should not enter the scene until it has been made safe by trained personnel.

Formal Product Identification

Traditionally, hazardous materials have been labeled by one or more of the following six systems:

1. The American National Standards Institute uses a label to identify a specific hazard (e.g., explosives, flammable liquids, radioactive materials) rather than a specific chemical.
2. The U.S. Department of Transportation (DOT) uses labels and placards with pictographs and printed hazard categories. In addition, DOT requires specific information on shipping manifests.
3. The United Nations Labeling System uses pictographs, symbols, or both, similar to those used by DOT, to identify a specific hazard rather than a specific chemical.
4. The International Air Transport Association uses the United Nations pictographs and indicates written emergency precaution measures in case of an incident.
5. The National Fire Protection Association uses color and a numerical rating scale (NFPA 704 System) to identify the degree of hazard for health, fire, and reactivity. Many state and local fire codes require the diamond-shaped identification symbols on fixed facilities (Fig. 53-1). The numbering system rates each category from 1 (least harmful) to 4 (most harmful).
6. The U.S. Department of Labor requires material safety data sheets (also known as MSDSs) for hazardous chemicals that are stored, handled, or used in the workplace.

CRITICAL THINKING

The next time you are on the highway, see if you can easily spot the placards on large trucks.

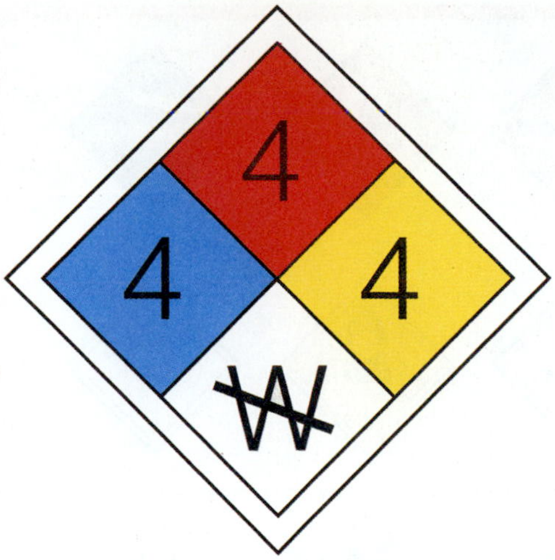

FIGURE 53-1 ■ A National Fire Protection Association placard. The numbers correspond to health, flammability, and reactivity hazards.

PLACARDS AND SHIPPING PAPERS

A number of identification systems may be used. However, hazardous materials usually are identified by placards (Fig. 53-2) and shipping papers.

The United Nations class (or division) identification number and North American number (UN/NA number) may be displayed on the bottom of a placard. Or the number may be displayed on the shipping paper after the listed shipping name or names. In certain cases this class or division number may replace the written name of the hazard class in the shipping paper description. Box 53-1 shows the meanings of the class and division numbers.

The location and type of paperwork that identifies hazardous materials varies according to the mode of transport. Most shipping papers are kept near the operator (e.g., driver, pilot, or captain) of the vehicle, aircraft, train, or ship. Several chemical agents may have the same UN/NA number. Thus it is important to refer to specific guidelines for hazardous material by chemical name in addition to this number.

> **NOTE** Shippers are responsible to track hazardous loads in transit. If shipping papers are not easy to obtain or too dangerous to recover, law enforcement personnel can contact the shipper by phone with a description of the vehicle (e.g., truck or car number and license plate number). This will help identify the type of hazardous material.

MATERIAL SAFETY DATA SHEETS

Material safety data sheets are required by OSHA for each chemical produced, stored, or used in the United States. Material safety data sheets are supplied by the manufacturer. They contain information for the safe and proper handling and storage of the material. They also have information on emergency actions to take. Material safety data sheets also classify the potential of significant health hazards from exposure to a material.

The potential health hazard of a material may be defined in a number of different ways. This may depend on the degree of inherent toxicity and type of exposure. Material safety data sheets provide useful information. However, they should not be used as the sole source of chemical information, information on health risks, or treatment recommendations. Paramedics should consult with medical direction, a poison control center, or another appropriate authority.

OTHER SOURCES OF INFORMATION ON HAZARDOUS MATERIALS

A number of resources are available for reference on hazardous materials. Product information should be referenced through more than one source. (Preferably three sources should be used, if time and availability permit.) One such reference is the *North American Emergency Response Guidebook* published by the DOT, Transport Canada, and the Secretariat of Communications and Transportation of Mexico. This guidebook lists more than 1000 hazardous materials. It also lists the proper emergency procedures. It includes names and identification numbers of substances. The book is cross-referenced in alphabetical and numerical order. This free reference is carried in emergency vehicles by many EMS, fire, and other public service agencies. One should note that the *Emergency Response Guidebook* is designed to assist first responders with initial actions for evacuation only. The book also includes the distance and area from the incident that should be evacuated. The book is not a stand-alone guide for dealing with hazmat emergencies.

Regional poison control centers have been established throughout most of the United States. They are a valuable asset in any EMS system. Many of these centers are available 24 hours a day. They are staffed with specialists. These individuals provide information, consultation, treatment recommendations, patient follow-up, and data collection. Poison control centers are linked to many agencies that deal with toxic substances. In addition, they are tied closely to all area hospitals. These centers maintain a listing of more than 450,000 drugs, toxic substances, and other products. The Universal Poison Control number is 1-800-222-1222.

The Chemical Transportation Emergency Center (CHEMTREC) is a public service of the Chemical Manufacturers Association. The center provides immediate advice to on-scene personnel about the management of known or unknown hazardous materials. The agency also contacts the shipper of the material for more information or assistance when needed. The Chemical Transportation Emergency Center operates 24 hours a day, 7 days a week. The center can be reached in the United States and Canada through the emergency toll-free number: 1-800-424-9300 (in Alaska 0-202-483-7616). The paramedic should contact the CHEMTREC as soon as possible during a hazmat incident. The paramedic should supply the name of the substance, its identification number, and the nature of the problem. Involving CHEMTREC in the management of a hazmat

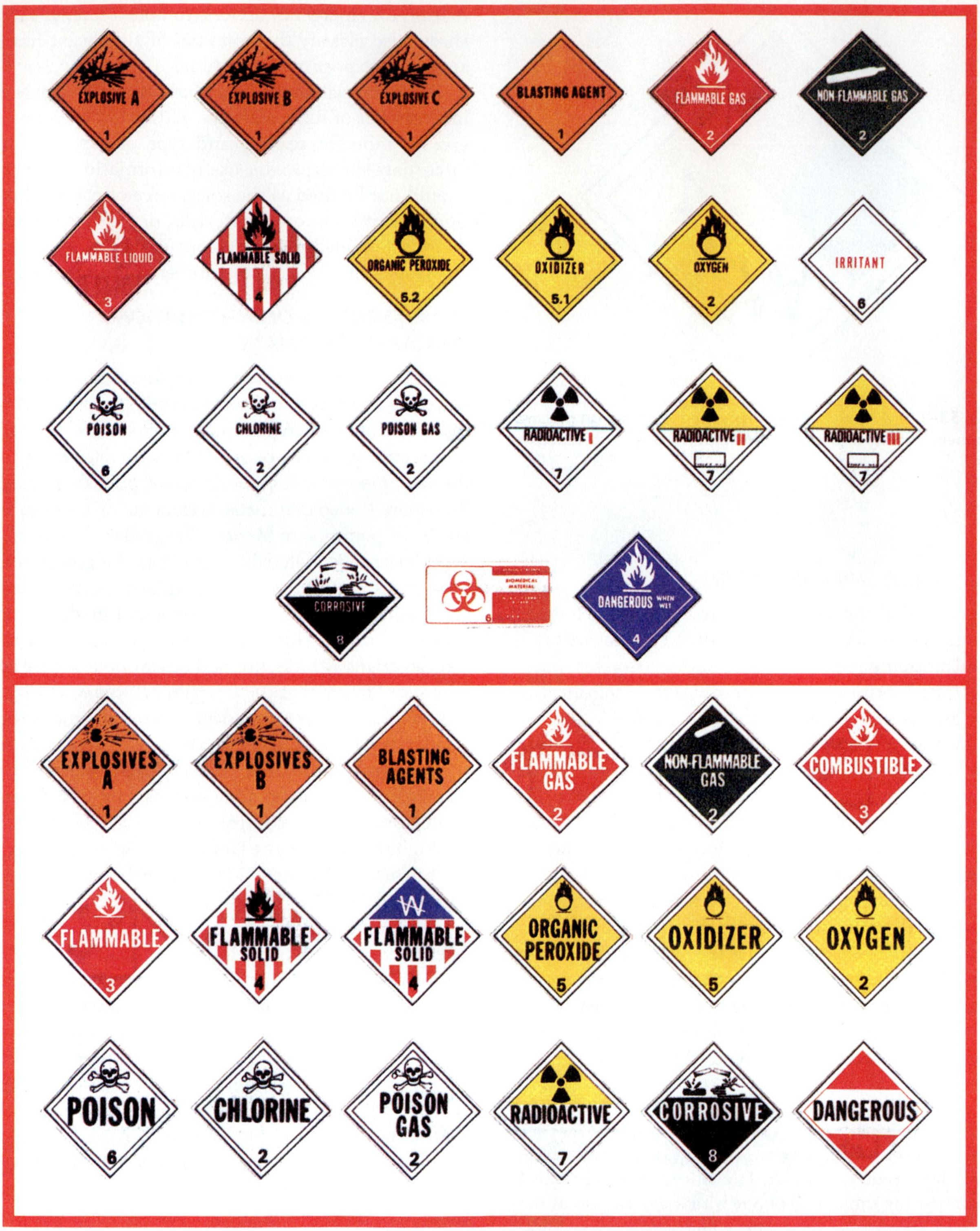

FIGURE 53-2 ■ Hazardous materials warning placards and labels.

BOX 53-1 International Classification System for Hazardous Materials

Class or division numbers may be displayed in the bottom of placards, or they may be displayed in the hazardous materials description on shipping papers. In certain cases a class or division number may replace the written name of the hazard class description on the shipping paper. The class and division numbers have the following meanings:

Class 1	Explosives
Division 1.1	Explosives with a mass explosion hazard
Division 1.2	Explosives with a projection hazard
Division 1.3	Explosives with predominantly a fire hazard
Division 1.4	Explosives with no significant blast hazard
Division 1.5	Very insensitive explosives
Division 1.6	Extremely insensitive explosive articles
Class 2	Gases
Division 2.1	Flammable gases
Division 2.2	Nonflammable gases
Division 2.3	Poison gases
Division 2.4	Corrosive gases (Canadian)
Class 3	Flammable Liquids
Division 3.1	Flashpoint below −18° C (0° F)
Division 3.2	Flashpoint −18° C and above but less than 23° C (73° F)
Division 3.3	Flashpoint of 23° C and up to 61° C (141° F)
Class 4	Flammable Solids, Spontaneously Combustible Materials, Materials That Are Dangerous When Wet
Division 4.1	Flammable solids
Division 4.2	Spontaneously combustible materials
Division 4.3	Materials that are dangerous when wet
Class 5	Oxidizers and Organic Peroxides
Division 5.1	Oxidizers
Division 5.2	Organic peroxides
Class 6	Poisonous and Etiological (Infectious) Materials
Division 6.1	Poisonous materials
Division 6.2	Etiological (infectious) materials
Class 7	Radioactive Materials
Class 8	Corrosives
Class 9	Miscellaneous Hazardous Materials

From US Department of Transportation, National Highway Traffic Safety Administration: *EMT-Paramedic national standard curriculum,* Washington, DC, 1997, The Department.

BOX 53-2 Agencies that Assist in Hazardous Materials Incidents Federal Agencies*

Federal Agencies
Centers for Disease Control and Prevention
Department of Transportation
Environmental Protection Agency
Federal Aviation Administration
National Response Center
U.S. Armed Forces (Army, Navy, Air Force, Marines)
U.S. Coast Guard
U.S. Department of Energy

Regional and State Agencies
National Guard
State emergency management agencies
State Environmental Protection Agency
State health departments
State police

Local Agencies
Emergency management
Fire service (hazardous materials units)
Law enforcement agencies
Poison control center
Public utilities
Sewage and treatment facilities

Commercial Agencies
American Petroleum Institute
Association of American Railroads and Hazardous Materials Systems
Chemical Manufacturers Association
Chevron (provides assistance with Chevron products)
HELP (the Union Carbide Emergency Response System for company shipments)
Local industry
Local contractors
Local: carriers and transporters
Railway industry

*This box lists only a sampling of the agencies; the list is not all-inclusive.

incident is usually part of the standard operating procedure of any emergency response team.

CHEMTEL, Inc., is an emergency response communications center. It serves the United States and Canada. The office can provide specific product information. It also can provide referral to the proper state and federal authorities for incidents that involve radioactive material. CHEMTEL can be reached 24 hours a day, 7 days a week, through the toll-free number 1-800-255-3924.

Computer-aided management of emergency operations (CAMEO) systems are designed to assist emergency responders quickly in the management of hazmat incidents. The program is available to municipalities. It uses computers to predict the effects of chemical spills and toxins released in plumes of smoke. The system helps communities prepare emergency response plans. The system currently provides information on more than 83,000 chemicals. Box 53-2 lists other government and private sector agencies that may assist in a hazmat incident.

PERSONAL PROTECTIVE CLOTHING AND EQUIPMENT

The potential for injury from exposure to hazardous materials is related to the toxicity, flammability, and reactivity of a particular substance. Use of the right protection is crucial for anyone dealing with hazardous materials. This includes the use of the proper respiratory protection and personal protective equipment (PPE).

Protective Respiratory Devices

The emergency responder must remember the potential for damage to the respiratory system from an unknown hazardous material. However, the paramedic can protect the respiratory system by air purification devices and respiratory equipment that supplies clean air (atmosphere supplying device).

Air purification relies on respirators or filtration devices. These devices remove particulate matter, gases, or vapors from the atmosphere. These devices do not use a separate source of air. They also require constant monitoring for contaminants and oxygen levels. As a rule, they are not recommended for use in a hazardous materials release and must be fitted to the wearer. Filtration devices are material specific ("must match the gas"). They are not used in the presence of multiple types of chemicals.

Atmosphere supplying devices rely on a separate source of positive pressure to supply air. They provide the highest level of respiratory protection. Two basic types are available. One is the self-contained breathing apparatus (SCBA). The other is the supplied air breathing apparatus (SABA), or air lines. The use of either requires training, recertification, and proper fit-testing as governed by regulations from OSHA.

Self-contained breathing apparatus provides respiratory protection in oxygen-deficient and toxic atmospheres. Only SCBAs that maintain positive pressure in the face piece during inhalation and exhalation should be used when working with hazardous materials. The SCBA usually is considered excellent protection in hazardous environments. However, the rescuer should be aware of potential face piece penetration and contamination by certain toxic substances, such as methyl bromide, Telone (1,3-dichloropropene and chloropicrin; DowElanco, Indianapolis, Indiana), and ethyleneimine.

Supplied air breathing apparatus supplies air to the rescuer via an air line hose away from the scene. These devices often are used at hazardous material sites when extended working times are required. Supplied air breathing apparatus must have an escape capability for operations in atmospheres classified as immediately dangerous to life and health. Respiratory protection devices that combine SCBAs and air line hose units are available. However, because of their dependence on air supply via a line, they limit the distance entry personnel can enter into a hot zone.

Classifications of Protective Clothing

Protective clothing is categorized in two ways: disposable or reusable. The clothing is made from a variety of materials that are designed specifically for certain chemical exposures. (Training in the use of this clothing should take place in a safe environment before it is used at emergency scenes.) Examples of this material include Tyvek/Saranex, nitrile rubber, Teflon, and Viton. No single material is compatible with all chemicals. Thus the manufacturer's guidelines and recommendations must be followed (Box 53-3). Protective clothing is classified in several ways. The classifications defined by OSHA and the EPA areas follows[7]:

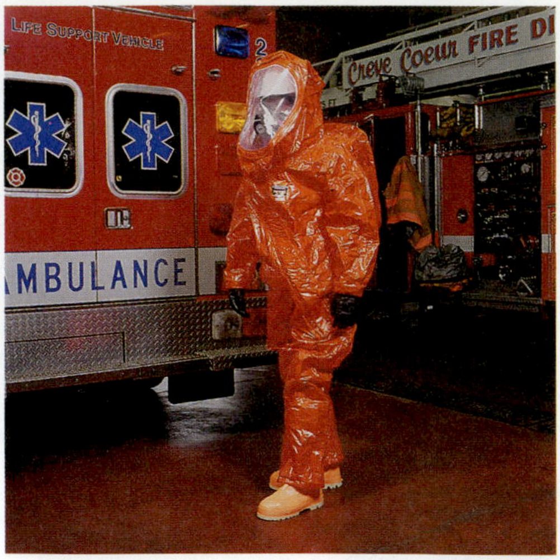

FIGURE 53-3 ■ Level A protective clothing.

BOX 53-3 Forms of Chemical Intrusion

Degradation: The physical destruction or decomposition of a clothing material caused by exposure to chemicals, use, or ambient conditions.

Penetration: The flow of a hazardous liquid chemical through zippers, stitched seams, pinholes, or other imperfections in a material.

Permeation: The process by which a hazardous liquid chemical moves through a material on a molecular level.

Level A: Level A provides the highest level of skin, respiratory, and eye protection (Fig. 53-3). Level A equipment typically is used by hazmat teams for entry into the incident site. Level A equipment includes a positive-pressure, full-face piece SCBA or positive-pressure supplied air respirator with escape SCBA, approved by the National Institute of Occupational Safety and Health (NIOSH). This level of protection also includes a totally encapsulating (gastight) chemical protective suit, coveralls and long underwear (optional), outer and inner gloves that are chemical resistant, an undersuit hard hat (optional), and a disposable protective suit (including gloves and boots) that may be worn over a totally encapsulating suit. (Unless specified by the manufacturer, these disposable suits are not to be worn in flammable atmospheres.)

Level B: Level B provides the highest level of respiratory protection. However, it provides a lower level of skin protection (Fig. 53-4). Level B protection typically is worn by the decontamination team. Level B equipment includes positive-pressure, full-face piece SCBA or positive-pressure sup-

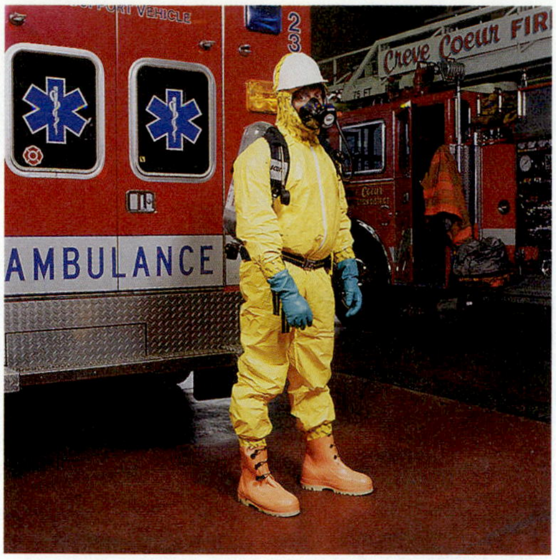

FIGURE 53-4 ■ Level B protective clothing. It offers the highest level of respiratory protection and a higher level of skin protection than Level C protective clothing.

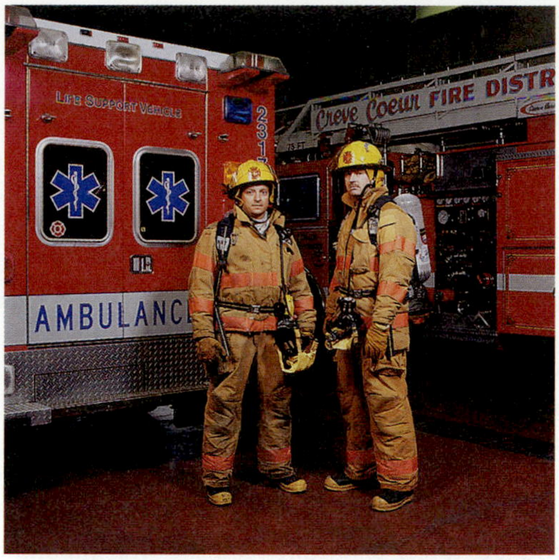

FIGURE 53-5 ■ Level D protective clothing.

plied air respirator with escape SCBA (NIOSH approved); hooded, chemical-resistant clothing (overalls, long-sleeved jacket, coveralls, one- or two-piece chemical splash suit, disposable chemical overalls); coveralls (optional); inner and outer chemical-resistant gloves; chemical-resistant boots with steel toe and shank; outer chemical-resistant boot covers (optional); an optional hard hat and face shield.

Level C: Level C protection is used during the transport of contaminated patients. Level C protection is used when the concentration and type of airborne substance (or substances) is known and the criteria for using air-purifying respirators are met. Level C equipment includes full face or half mask air-purifying respirators (NIOSH approved); hooded, chemical-resistant clothing (overalls, two-piece chemical splash suit, disposable chemical-resistant overalls); coveralls (optional); outer and inner chemical-resistant gloves; outer chemical-resistant boots with steel toe and shank (optional); disposable outer chemical-resistant boot covers (optional); and optional escape mask and face shield.

Level D: Level D is a work uniform that affords minimal protection (used for nuisance contamination only; Fig. 53-5). Level D protection commonly is known as firefighter "turnout" gear. (Turnout gear with SCBA may be considered level B protection for some chemicals that do not pose danger for skin contact or absorption.) Level D equipment includes coverall; optional gloves, chemical-resistant boots or shoes with steel toe and shank; disposable outer chemical-resistant boots (optional); safety glasses or chemical splash goggles; and optional hard hat, escape mask, and face shield.

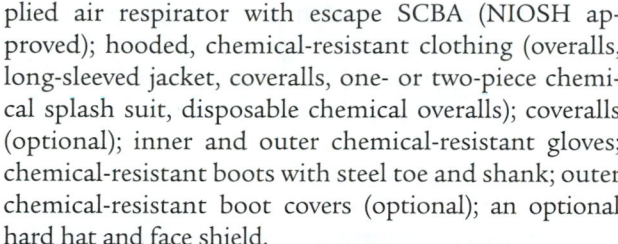

> **CRITICAL THINKING**
>
> What types of patient care do you think you will be able to provide when wearing each of the levels of hazardous materials protective gear?

Regardless of the type of PPE used during a hazmat incident, all avenues through which hazardous materials can enter the body must be protected. The following points should be of particular concern to any rescuer involved in hazmat response:

- Protective clothing should not be affected adversely by the hazardous materials involved.
- Protective clothing should seal all exposed skin.
- Contact with the hazardous materials should be of the absolute minimal duration required.
- Protective clothing and equipment should be decontaminated properly. Or it should be discarded properly.
- The safety standards and methods for cleaning and disposing of clothing and equipment should be followed strictly.
- Contaminated patient clothing should be left at the scene. It should not be transported with the patient. This will limit the contamination of the ambulance.

HEALTH HAZARDS

Hazardous materials may enter the human body by inhalation, ingestion, injection, and absorption (see Chapter 36). Entry by means of any of these routes may result in internal and external damage to the rescuer. Exposure to dangerous substances may affect the body in several different ways. It may produce numerous injuries or illnesses.

Exposure to poisons can produce acute toxicity, delayed toxicity, and local and systemic effects. How the body responds depends on the concentration of the chemical to which the body is exposed (also called the *dose response*). The paramedic also should be aware that drug treatment can result in synergistic effects. Thus all treatment methods must be guided by medical direction, a poison control center, or other appropriate authority.

Internal Damage

Internal damage to the human body from exposure to hazardous materials may involve the respiratory tract, the central nervous system, or other internal organs. Some substances injure all cells on contact. Others have a more direct effect on specific organs (target organs), such as the kidneys and liver.

Depending on the hazardous materials, the physical injury may vary. It may range from minor irritation to more serious complications. The more serious ones may include cardiac and respiratory compromise and death. Chronic illness (e.g., chronic obstructive pulmonary disease) and various forms of cancer also may result. Some substances can cause abnormal fetal development and changes in gene structure. For example, penetrating radiation (described in Chapter 23) can lead to cell and chromosomal changes and can cause genetic changes, cell death, and sterility.

IRRITANTS

Respiratory problems are a common complaint of rescuers and patients who have been exposed to hazardous materials. Chemical irritants emit vapors that affect the mucous membranes of the body. These include the surfaces of the eyes, nose, mouth, and throat. As these irritants combine with moisture, acidic or alkaline reactions may occur. Exposure to these irritants may result in damage to the upper, lower, and deep respiratory tract. Examples of chemical irritants are hydrochloric acid, halogens, and ozone. Self-defense chemical sprays used by some civilians and law enforcement officers are common. They present a hazard to responders. These sprays are irritants and produce excessive tearing of the eyes. They include chloroacetophenone, orthochlorobenzalmalononitrile, and capsicum oleoresin.

ASPHYXIANTS

Asphyxiants are gases. They displace the oxygen in the air and also dilute the oxygen concentration of the air. Examples of simple asphyxiants are carbon dioxide, methane, and propane. Other gases not only displace oxygen in the air but also interfere with tissue oxygenation; these are referred to as *blood poisons* or *chemical asphyxiants.* They tend to interrupt the transport or use of oxygen by tissue cells. Through various mechanisms, these toxic gases deprive body tissue of needed oxygen. Examples include hydrogen cyanide, carbon monoxide, and hydrogen sulfide.

NERVE POISONS, ANESTHETICS, AND NARCOTICS

Nerve poisons, anesthetics, and narcotics act on the nervous system. They change the ability of the brain to regulate the heart and the respiratory system. They also can interfere with the ability to transmit nerve impulses to the heart and lungs.

Nerve poisons were developed by the military. They often are referred to as *war gases, nerve gases,* or *nerve agents* (see Chapter 54). Similar substances are used in solid pesticides. Exposure to these chemicals may result in fatal complications. Examples of these poisons include carbamates, organophosphates, parathion, and malathion. Anesthetics and narcotics are less hazardous than nerve poisons. However, continuous exposure or exposure to large amounts may result in unconsciousness or death. Examples include ethylene, nitrous oxide, and ethyl alcohol.

HEPATOTOXINS

Hepatotoxins are substances that damage the liver. The poisons build up in the body and destroy the ability of the liver to function. Examples include chlorinated and halogenated hydrocarbons.

CARDIOTOXINS

Cardiotoxins are hazardous materials that can cause myocardial ischemia and dysrhythmias. Examples include some nitrates and ethylene glycol. Acute myocardial infarction and sudden death have been reported in healthy young persons who were exposed to these substances. Short-term exposure to fluorocarbons and other halogenated hydrocarbons also has been known to cause cardiac abnormalities.

NEPHROTOXINS

Nephrotoxins are hazardous materials that are especially destructive to the kidneys. Examples include carbon disulfide, lead, high concentrations of organic solvents, and inorganic mercury. Exposure to carbon tetrachloride used as a solvent for dry cleaning or fire-extinguishing agent can damage the kidneys.

NEUROTOXINS

Neurological and behavioral toxicity may result from exposure to hazardous substances such as arsenic, lead, mercury, and organic solvents. In some cases, cerebral hypoxia may occur as a result of decreased oxygen in the blood.

HEMOTOXINS

Hemotoxins are hazardous substances that may cause the destruction of red blood cells. This destruction can result in hemolytic anemia (see Chapter 37). Substances that can produce hemolytic anemia include aniline, naphthol, quinones, lead, mercury, arsenic, and copper. Pulmonary edema and cardiac and liver injury also may be caused by hemotoxin exposure.

CARCINOGENS

Carcinogens are cancer-causing agents. Many hazardous materials are carcinogenic or are suspected carcinogens. The exact amount of hazardous materials exposure required for cancer to develop is unknown. However, short-term exposure to specific agents is known to produce long-term effects. Disease and complications have been reported 20 years after exposure to hazardous materials.[6]

Of particular interest to rescuers involved in firefighting is that all fossil and organic fuels when burned produce dioxins. Many of the dioxins are carcinogens. (For example, burning wood produces carcinogenic formaldehyde.) A positive-pressure SCBA is the most important piece of protective equipment to protect against these carcinogenic vapors and respiratory poisons. All rescuers should avoid exposure to smoke or clouds of fumes as a standard practice in scene safety.

> **NOTE** An important sign of a critical exposure is several persons having the same symptoms at the same time. Any time two or more members of the team report that they "feel" similar symptoms, the team should suspect a toxic gas or agent. Emergency medical services responders should always immediately report the onset of symptoms. They should report the onset to their crew members and other emergency responders at the scene.

GENERAL SYMPTOMS OF EXPOSURE

Health effects from exposure to hazardous materials vary by individual. They also depend on the chemical involved, the concentration of the chemical, the duration of exposure, the number of exposures, and the route of entry (inhalation, ingestion, injection, absorption). In addition, a person's age, gender, general health, allergies, smoking habits, alcohol consumption, and medication use influence how that person is affected

Various symptoms may result from exposure to hazardous materials. Some symptoms may be delayed or masked by common illnesses such as influenza or by smoke inhalation. If any of the following symptoms is present after exposure to hazardous materials, the rescuer or patient should seek immediate medical attention:

- Changes in skin color or blushing
- Chest tightness
- Confusion, light-headedness, anxiety, dizziness
- Coughing or painful respiration
- Diarrhea and involuntary urination or defecation (or both)
- Dim, blurred, or double vision; photophobia
- Loss of coordination
- Nausea, vomiting, abdominal cramping
- Salivation, drooling, rhinorrhea
- Seizure
- Shortness of breath, burning of the upper airway
- Tingling or numbness of extremities
- Unconsciousness

> **CRITICAL THINKING**
> Two rescuers complain of similar symptoms on the scene of a rescue that may involve hazardous materials. What actions should be taken immediately?

External Damage

Body surface tissue may be injured by hazardous materials. Many substances have corrosive properties. Many substances also become corrosive when mixed with water. Exposure to these substances may produce chemical burns and severe tissue damage. Examples include hydrochloric acid, hydrofluoric acid, and caustic soda.

SOFT TISSUE DAMAGE

Corrosives are acids or bases (alkaline). Exposure to either may cause pain on contact. However, alkalis generally burn more extensively than acids. Exposing human tissue to a base corrosive such as lye may result in a breakdown of fatty tissue (liquefaction) that produces a greasy or slick feeling to the skin. These signs should alert the rescuer to decontaminate immediately and seek medical attention. Unless the substance is identified, decontamination should begin by brushing off the dry powder and flushing the skin with copious amounts of water. (Different areas of the skin absorb chemicals at different rates.) Paramedics should never try to neutralize an acid or base; doing so could produce great heat and cause further burns. The area should be flushed copiously with water, and the patient should be transported for care. Rescuers should be aware of possible "off-gassing" or fumes resulting from the decontamination of a wound site.

Cryogenics are refrigerant liquid gases that can freeze human tissue on contact. These liquids vaporize as soon as they are released from their containers. They may cause tissue damage. Extreme caution should be used when near any refrigerated liquids. They can produce freeze burns, frostbite, and other cold-related injuries. Examples include freon, liquid oxygen, and liquid nitrogen.

CHEMICAL EXPOSURE TO THE EYES

Chemical exposure to the eyes (described in Chapter 23) may cause damage. The damage may range from superficial inflammation to severe burns. Patients with these conditions have local pain, visual disturbance, tearing, edema, and redness of surrounding tissues. Basic management guidelines include flushing the eyes with water. This should be done using a mild flow from a hose, intravenous tubing, water from a container, or irrigation lens (per protocol). A rapid assessment of visual acuity is important. However, assessment should not delay flushing or irrigation of the eyes.

RESPONSE TO HAZARDOUS MATERIALS EMERGENCIES

When an EMS crew is dispatched to a scene involving the potential for hazardous materials, decisions must be made about rescuer safety, the type and degree of the potential hazard, the involvement of other agencies, and protection for the general public. As discussed in Chapter 50, preplanning and early coordination of activities in these major inci-

BOX 53-4 Hazardous Materials Terminology and Definitions

Toxicological Terms Used to Determine Toxicity of a Compound

IDLH (immediately dangerous to life and health): Any atmosphere that poses an immediate hazard to life or that produces immediate, irreversible debilitating effects on health.

LD_{50} (lethal dose, 50% kill): The amount of a dose that, when administered to laboratory animals, kills 50% of them.

PEL (permissible exposure limit): The maximum time-weighted concentration at which 95% of exposed, healthy adults suffer no adverse effects over a 40-hour workweek.

ppm/ppb: Parts per million/parts per billion.

TLV-C (threshold limit value—ceiling level): The maximum concentration that should not be exceeded even instantaneously.

TLV-STEL (threshold limit value–short-term exposure limit): A 15-minute, time-weighted average exposure that should not be exceeded at any time nor repeatedly more than 4 times a day, with 60-minute rest periods required between each STEL exposure.

Specific Terminology for Medical Hazardous Materials Operations

Alpha radiation: Large radioactive particles that have minimal penetrating ability.

Beta radiation: Small radioactive particles that can penetrate subcutaneous tissue and usually enter the body through damaged skin, ingestion, or inhalation.

Boiling point: The temperature at which a liquid changes to a vapor or a gas; the temperature at which the pressure of the liquid equals atmospheric pressure.

Flammable/exposure limits: The range of gas or vapor concentration that will burn or explode if an ignition source is present.

Flash point: The minimum temperature at which a liquid gives off enough vapors to ignite and flash-over but not to continue to burn without additional heat.

Gamma radiation: The most dangerous form of penetrating radiation, which can produce internal and external hazards.

Ignition temperature: The minimum temperature required to ignite gas or vapor without a spark or flame being present.

Specific gravity: The weight of a material as compared with the weight of an equal volume of water.

Vapor density: The weight of a pure vapor or gas compared with the weight of an equal volume of dry air at the same temperature and pressure.

Vapor pressure: The pressure exerted by the vapor within the container against the sides of a container.

Vapor solubility: The ability of a vapor to mix with water.

From Noll G et al: *Hazardous materials: managing the incident,* Stillwater, Okla, 1988, Fire Protection Publications.

dents is important. In addition, medical direction should be advised of the incident as soon as possible. That way, they can prepare personnel and facilities. Not all hazmat incidents are large-scale events. Sometimes, a single event involving only one patient may require a full hazmat response.

The first rescue personnel to arrive at the scene of a hazmat incident may not be the most qualified or best equipped. However, most communities look to the first responders to provide immediate safety and direction. Thus the EMS crew must be capable of the initial management of hazmat incidents.

Hazard and Risk Assessment

While en route to the scene, EMS personnel should begin to research hazmat references. They also should begin a *hazard and risk assessment.* In hazmat incidents, hazards are the chemical properties of a material that may cause danger or peril (Box 53-4). *Risk* refers to the possibility of suffering harm or loss. Risk levels vary and are influenced by several factors, including the following[8] (Fig. 53-6):

- Hazardous nature of the material involved
- Worst-case scenario situations
- Quantity of the material involved
- Weather conditions that might affect the scene adversely
- Containment system and type of stress applied to the container
- Proximity of exposures (e.g., schools, nursing homes, and shopping centers)
- Level of available resources
- Lead time for mutual aid

A hazard and risk assessment also includes consideration of the potential hazards to the public and environment, the potential risk of **primary contamination** to patients, and the potential risk for secondary contamination to rescuers (Box 53-5).

If the product can be identified through hazmat references, the EMS crew should familiarize themselves with potential health hazards, recommended PPE, initial first aid, and the "safe distance" factor as outlined in the reference guides. Most emergency response guides offer only general management actions. After formal product identification, the appropriate hazmat agencies (e.g., CHEMTREC and poison control) can give more exact information.

Approaching the Scene

The paramedics should approach the scene cautiously from uphill and upwind. The EMS crew should be alert to environmental clues. These include wind direction, unusual odors, leakage, and vapor clouds. Other environmental clues that are good indicators for the presence of hazardous materials include affected or afflicted wildlife and plant life (e.g., dead birds and wilted or discolored plants). Paramedics can use binoculars initially to observe the scene from a safe distance. Emergency vehicles should never be driven through leakage or vapor clouds or smoke. In addition, personnel should not enter the incident area until it has

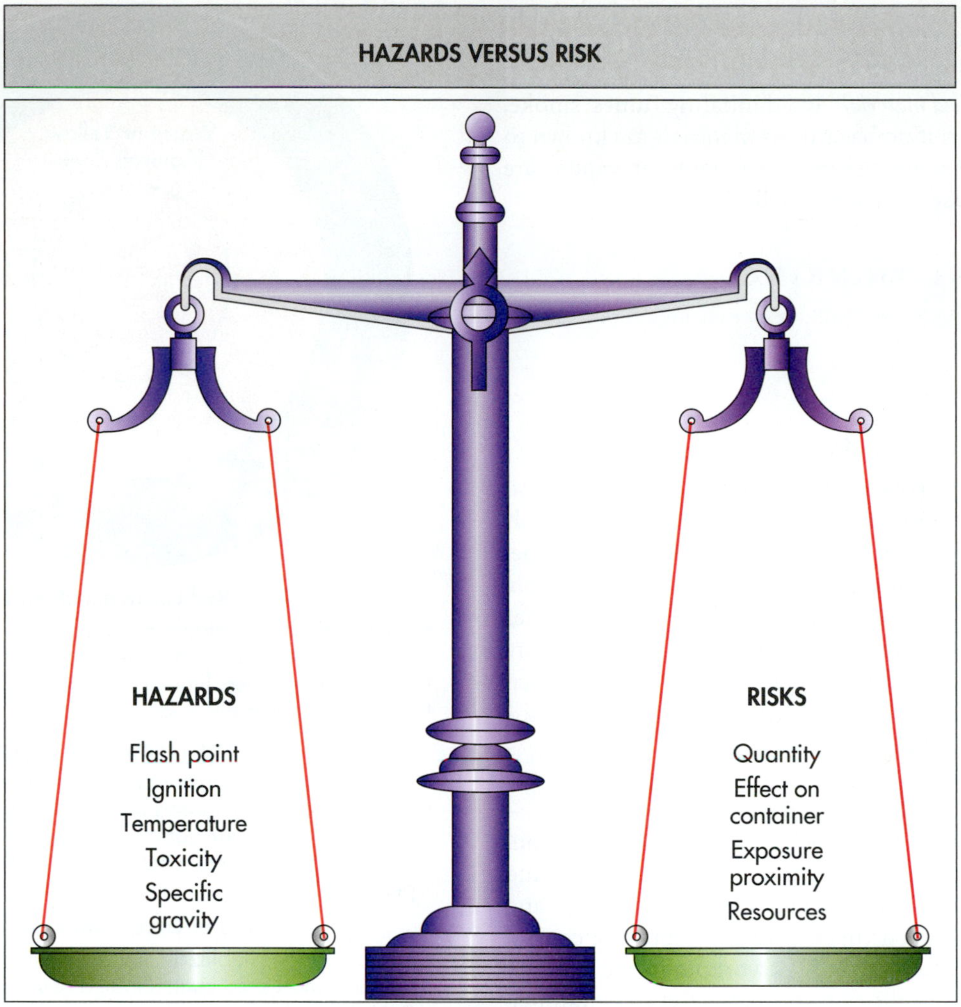

FIGURE 53-6 ■ Hazards versus risk.

> **BOX 53-5 Types of Contamination**
>
> **Primary Contamination**
> Exposure to substance
> Substance only harmful to exposed person
> Little chance of exposure to others
>
> **Secondary Contamination**
> Exposure to substance
> Liquid and particulate substances easily transferred by touching

been determined to be safe. In addition to these guidelines, rescuers should do the following as recommended in the *Emergency Response Guidebook*[9]:

- *Approach cautiously.* Resist the urge to rush in; you cannot help others until you know what you are facing.
- *Identify the hazards.* Placards, container labels, shipping papers, and knowledgeable persons on the scene are valuable sources of information. Evaluate all of them and then consult the recommended guide page before you place yourself or others at risk. Do not be alarmed if new information from a CHEMTREC expert changes some of the emphasis or details of the guide page warnings. You must remember that the guide page provides only the most important information for your initial response with a family or class of hazardous materials. As more accurate, material-specific information becomes available, your response becomes more appropriate for the situation.
- *Secure the scene.* Without entering the immediate hazard zone, do what you can to isolate the area and ensure the safety of persons and the environment. Move and keep persons away from the scene and the perimeter. Allow enough room to move and remove your own equipment.
- *Obtain help.* Advise your headquarters to notify responsible agencies and call for assistance from trained experts through CHEMTREC and the National Response Center, which can be reached through CHEMTREC or dialed directly.
- *Decide on site entry.* Any efforts you make to rescue persons or protect property or the environment must be

weighed against the possibility that you could become part of the problem. Enter the area with the appropriate protective gear (if trained to do so). Above all, *do not walk into or touch spilled material.* Avoid inhaling fumes, smoke, and vapors, even if no hazardous materials are known to be involved. Do not assume that gases or vapors are harmless because of lack of smell.

CRITICAL THINKING

Which of these guidelines would it be easy for the first arriving crew to miss?

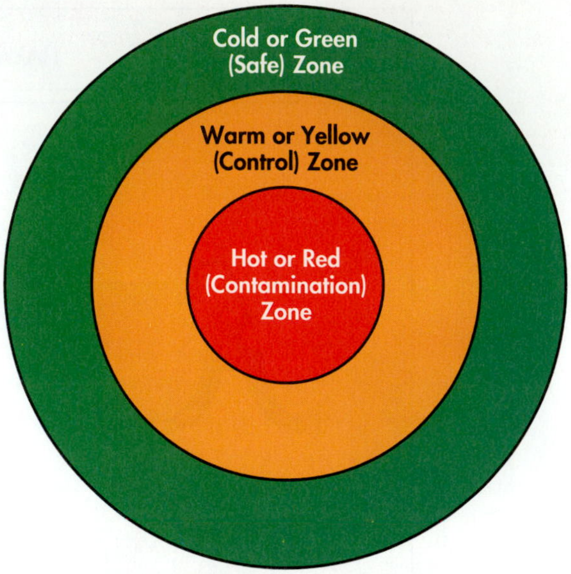

Hot or Red (Contamination) Zone

- Contamination is actually present.
- Personnel must wear appropriate protective gear.
- Number of rescuers limited to those absolutely necessary.
- Bystanders never allowed.

Warm or Yellow (Control) Zone

- Area surrounding the contamination zone.
- Vital to preventing spread of contamination.
- Personnel must wear appropriate protective gear.
- Life-saving emergency care and decontamination are performed.

Cold or Green (Safe) Zone

- Normal triage, stabilization, and treatment are performed.
- Rescuers must shed contaminated gear before entering the cold zone.

FIGURE 53-7 ■ Zones at a hazmat incident.

Control of the Scene

The first agency to arrive at the scene has several responsibilities. Its members must detect and identify the materials involved, assess the risk of exposure to rescue personnel and others, consider the potential risk of fire or explosion, gather information from on-site personnel or other sources, and confine and control the incident. In addition, a command post should be established per the preplanned incident command structure. Members also must define the safety distances and zones.

Safety Zones

After the presence of hazardous materials has been confirmed, the scene should be separated into hot, warm, and cold zones (Fig. 53-7). These zones should have access and egress corridors between them. (Corridors provide control points. They also allow responders working in the zones to know where they should exit and enter for decontamination, accountability, and debriefing.) Safety zones should be established and enforced early in the incident (Box 53-6). The dispatch center and responding units should be advised of the location of the hot zone and safe approach directions.

The *hot zone* is the area of the incident that includes the hazardous material. It also includes any surrounding area that may be exposed to gases, vapors, mist, dust, or runoff. All rescue personnel and vehicles should be stationed outside this zone. Anyone entering this zone must wear high-level PPE. Only specially trained EMS personnel should attempt patient care activities in this area. Some EMS agencies and incident command system structures refer to the hot zone as the *exclusion zone,* a *restricted area,* or the *red zone.*

The *warm zone* is a larger, buffer area that surrounds the hot zone with "cold" and "hot" end corridors. Although protective clothing is required, it usually is considered a safer environment for workers. However, if the hot zone becomes unstable, the warm zone may be exposed to the hazardous materials. This zone is where most EMS activities, such as decontamination and patient care activities, are performed. Some agencies refer to this zone as the *limited-access zone,* the *containment reduction corridor,* or the *yellow zone.*

The *cold zone* is the area that encompasses the warm zone. The cold zone also is restricted to emergency personnel. This area usually is considered safe, requiring only minimal protective clothing. The cold zone contains the command post and other support agencies necessary to control the incident. This area is referred to by some agencies as a *support zone* or the *green zone.*

MEDICAL MONITORING AND REHABILITATION

The safety of rescue personnel is of top importance in any emergency. Situations that involve hazardous materials are among the most dangerous. Thus a medical monitoring program should be part of any EMS/hazmat system and all hazmat incidents.

The Occupational Safety and Health Administration requires medical examinations for members of hazmat response teams and employees who may have been exposed to hazardous substances during an emergency. Other parts of a hazmat medical monitoring program may include any needed medical care, medical monitoring during a hazmat incident, record keeping, and periodic evaluation of the surveillance program.

BOX 53-6 Hazardous Materials Zones

Hot Zone
Contamination present
Site of incident
Entry with high-level personal protective equipment
Entry limited

Warm Zone
Buffer zone outside hot zone
Contains decontamination corridor with "hot" and "cold" end

Cold Zone
Safe area
Staging area for personnel and equipment
Site of medical monitoring
One end of corridor

Medical monitoring should include a medical examination just before entering a hazardous area. This examination is done to establish health history for any rescuer who will be exposed to a hazardous substance. It also is done to establish the person's normal vital sign readings. Individuals should be told of the expected symptoms of illness or exposure before entering the hazardous area.

In addition to injury from exposure, responders working in protective clothing and equipment can become dehydrated and develop heat illnesses. Rescue protective suits protect, but they also prevent cooling through evaporation, conduction, convection, or radiation. Heat-stress factors are affected by the prehydration of the rescuer, degree of physical fitness, ambient air temperature, and the degree and duration of physical activity. The parameters of the presuit evaluation should include the following:

- Temperature, pulse, respiration, and blood pressure measurements
- Cardiac rhythm
- Body weight
- Cognitive and motor skills
- Hydration
- Significant recent medical history (e.g., medications or illnesses)

After entry into the hazardous area, medical monitoring should note the amount of time a rescuer has been in protective clothing. Rescuers should be observed for any signs of heat-related illness or exposure. If illness or injury occurs to any team member, all entry team members should be removed from the hot zone for treatment. A backup team should be ready to assist the entry team members in the hot zone at all times.

After the incident, rescue personnel should be reevaluated in the "rehab sector." They should be reevaluated using the same parameters as in the presuit examination. This exam determines the rescuer's ability to reenter the operation if needed. As a rule, rescuers are not allowed to reenter the site until vital signs and hydration are normal. Body weight generally is used to estimate fluid loss and the need for oral or intravenous fluid replacement (per protocol).

CRITICAL THINKING

What might prevent personnel from seeking out emergency medical services for medical monitoring unless there is a strict procedure to guarantee they are monitored?

Documentation

Detailed records are a necessary part of hazmat medical monitoring and rehabilitation. At a minimum, records should include the following[6]:

- The hazardous substance
- The toxicity and danger of secondary contamination
- Use of appropriate PPE and any permeation ("breakthrough") that occurred
- The level of decontamination performed or required
- Use of antidotes and other medical treatment
- The method of transportation and destination

Baseline statistics from preentry and postentry screenings also should be included in the records. (Many agencies use preprinted forms for these.)

EMERGENCY MANAGEMENT OF CONTAMINATED PATIENTS

Patient care activities, triage, and evacuation should be part of a preplanned incident command system structure. Identification of a specific hazardous substance may take some time. Thus rescue efforts, decontamination, possible evacuation, and timely treatment of toxic exposures are important. The primary goals of decontamination are to reduce the patient's dosage of material, decrease the threat of secondary contamination, and reduce the risk of rescuer injury.[6] The specific substance and route of contamination affect triage and decontamination methods. The following guidelines for rapid decontamination are general. They should not supersede any organizational approach in scene management of hazmat incidents or treatment recommendations for chemical exposures:

1. The paramedic should not enter a contaminated area or initiate care without adequate PPE. The paramedic also must possess training that is specific to the incident. Victims who can walk should be encouraged to extricate themselves from the scene. They should be advised to stay together for treatment or until they are escorted individually to decontamination.
2. Patients who cannot walk should be removed from the hot zone by trained personnel. Removal usually is performed by fire department personnel, specialized hazmat teams, or both. Patient care activities in the hot zone should be limited to gross airway management, spinal immobilization, and hemorrhage control. Decontamination and further patient care should be done in the warm zone by a properly equipped decontamination team.

3. All patients exposed to the hot zone should be considered contaminated. They should be treated as such until they have been properly assessed, triaged, and decontaminated.
4. Patient care provisions of airway, breathing, and circulatory support should begin as soon as the patient is contacted and conditions allow. The rescuer safety information received from hazmat agencies should be used when performing basic life support procedures.
5. Intravenous therapy should be administered only under a physician's direction. This and other invasive procedures may allow the hazardous materials to enter the patient.
6. Decontamination procedures should avoid any unnecessary exposure to the rescuer. Emergency medical services providers assisting in decontamination should be well protected with two or three layers of gloves, head coverings, positive-pressure SCBA, and proper protective clothing. (As a rule of thumb for personal safety, decontamination teams or anyone working in the warm zone, should be wearing equal PPE. Or they should be wearing no less than one protection level down from the level of protection worn by those working in the hot zone.)
7. When the hazardous material is a dry agent, lightly brush the material off the patient. Make sure the dry agent does not get into the patient's airway. Cutting off or removing clothing often removes most of the contaminating material. After the dry agent has been removed, the decontamination should continue as follows:
   a. Wash the patient with copious amounts of water and mild detergent soap. Make sure that all water and runoff is contained in the warm zone. Depending on the exposure, other patient decontamination procedures may be warranted. Pay special attention to irrigation of the eyes, hair, ears, underarms, and pubic areas and thorough cleaning of the body creases of the neck, groin, elbows, and knees. Be careful not to abrade the skin, which may promote absorption of the material involved.
   b. Leave all patient clothing, rescuer clothing, and decontamination equipment in the decontamination area. Safely move the patient to the support zone for further triage, treatment, and transport.

NOTE Water is considered the universal decontamination solution. Water is used to dilute the concentration of a substance. Water generally does not alter the chemical structure of a compound. Degradation solutions may be recommended for some exposures. These include water and mild soap, isopropyl alcohol, and vegetable oil (among others). These solutions should be used only when advised by medical direction or other appropriate authority. They should not be applied directly to the skin.

One should note that the field decontamination procedures described represent only a gross decontamination. The resources needed for full decontamination usually are not available at the scene. Thus the patient should be isolated from the environment. This will help to contain any contamination that has been missed during these steps. This is accomplished by placing the patient in a body bag to the neck and covering the patient's hair. In the absence of body bags, the victim may be packaged for transport by folding one side of a sheet or blanket over the patient. Use the other side to overlap and package the patient. If necessary, the patient's arm may be exposed through an opening in the sheet for vital sign assessment and fluid and drug administration.

NOTE Rapid decontamination is a two-step process. In the first step, remove the patient from danger. In the second step, provide gross decontamination.

Decontamination Decision Making

Hazardous materials incidents often are fast breaking. Therefore they may require rapid decision making. For example, a group of walking, contaminated persons at the scene may be trying to reach rescuers; others self-rescue by walking out of the hot zone; and some may become impatient and leave the hot zone while waiting for rescue teams to arrive. In these situations the paramedic crew must be prepared for quick gross decontamination and treatment, rapid application of PPE, and quick transport and isolation procedures.

If the patient's condition is critical (and whether the exposure involved a life-threatening material is unknown), the paramedic should perform decontamination and treatment at the same time. This is done by removing the patient's clothing, treating life-threatening problems, lavaging the patient with copious amounts of water, and providing for isolation and transportation. Patients who are not in critical condition can be managed in the same manner with a more contemplative approach, particularly if the hazardous substance is known.

A hazmat incident that is well controlled (not a fast-breaking event) can be managed over longer duration. In these cases, rescue should not be attempted for patients in the hot zone. Rather the paramedic crew should wait for a hazmat team and for a decontamination corridor to be established (Fig. 53-8). (This may take an hour or more.) Longer-duration events allow for more thorough decontamination, better PPE, less chance of secondary contamination, and better environmental protection.

CRITICAL THINKING
What type of hazardous materials response resources does your community have?

Preparing the Ambulance for Patient Transfer

Contamination of ambulances and equipment can be minimized by preparing the vehicle before transporting a partly decontaminated patient. These measures include using as much disposable equipment as necessary. They also include removing all items from cabinets that will not be needed

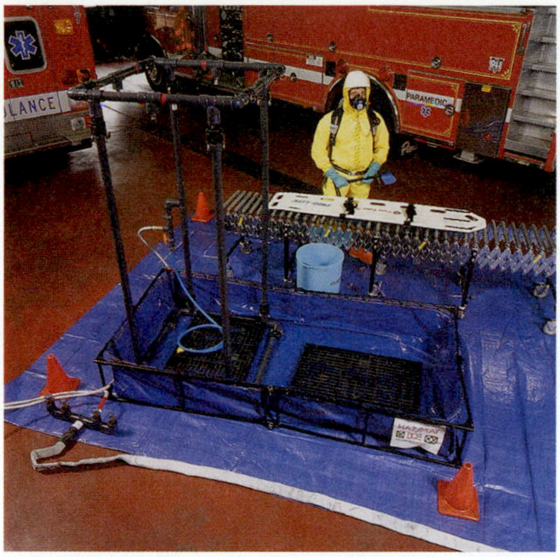

FIGURE 53-8 ■ Patient decontamination area.

for patient use. Ideally, the patient should be isolated completely in a stretcher decontamination pool. This should be covered in plastic and secured to the stretcher. Immediate notification of the hospital staff that they will be receiving contaminated patients is crucial. The emergency department will need time to prepare and do research to manage the patients adequately and efficiently.

On arrival at the hospital, the EMS crew should follow the decontamination protocols of the hospital. The EMS crew should not return to regular service until rescue personnel, vehicle, and equipment have been monitored for contamination. Equipment decontamination should follow the recommendations of local, state, and federal authorities or standard operating procedures of medical direction. Specific solutions may be required for a particular hazmat exposure. However, most equipment can be cleaned adequately and made ready for use with soap and water.

DECONTAMINATION OF RESCUE PERSONNEL AND EQUIPMENT

Decontamination of rescue personnel involves eight steps and begins in the decontamination corridor[6] (Fig. 53-9). These steps include the following:

1. An entry point is established at the "hot" end of the corridor where "dirty" personnel and equipment are set up to start the decontamination process.
2. A tool drop is designated. Outer gloves and boots are removed and placed in a receptacle.
3. Gross surface contamination is removed. Generally this is done by washing with copious amounts of water.
4. Contaminated SCBA bottles are removed (doffed) for personnel who must reenter the dirty area; at this step they receive clean SCBA bottles.
5. Protective clothing is removed and handled (stored, decontaminated) as required.
6. Other clothing is removed. This step depends on the seriousness of the hazardous materials involved.
7. Personnel wash their bodies using overhead showers. Usually two washings are required. Personnel dry off and receive new or clean, uncontaminated clothing.
8. Personnel going through the decontamination system receive medical evaluation. (Medical evaluation continues at a medical facility.)

In addition, the following safety precautions should be followed by any rescuer exposed to hazardous materials:

- Do not touch your face, mouth, nose, or genital area before full body decontamination.
- Shower first with a cold rinse (no scrubbing) to wash off potential contaminants without opening up pores of the skin and then thoroughly wash with warm water, surgical soap, sponge, and brush; pay particular attention to hair, body orifices (especially the ears), and any body parts that come in contact with each other (arms and chest, thighs, fingers, toes, and buttocks). Repeat shower and rinse.
- Shampoo hair several times and rinse thoroughly.

CRITICAL THINKING

Why do you think that extensive preplanning and drills are needed to make this system work well?

Care and Maintenance of Clothing and Equipment

After the hazmat incident, the rescuer should take the following precautions:

- Properly dispose of any protective clothing that has been torn or worn through.
- Properly and thoroughly clean all clothing and equipment. This will help to avoid the risk of chemical reactions at future incidents. It also will lessen the potential for chronic exposure to absorbed chemicals. Some hazardous materials can destroy or penetrate protective clothing and equipment. For this reason, product compatibility tables should be evaluated during the decontamination procedure. Decontamination provides no assurance that protective clothing is clean or that the process of chemical penetration has stopped.
- Do not wash or dispose of clothing or equipment at home. This helps to avoid exposing family members and contaminating home articles.
- Follow all local codes and laws regarding disposal or decontamination of equipment and clothing.
- Carefully maintain personal SCBA.

When the incident is over, all personnel operating at the scene (in any capacity) should be debriefed. The debriefing session should include what the substances were. It also should include what possible acute and chronic health issues may arise. Finally, it should include any associated signs and symptoms. Information on how to follow up regarding long-term effects also should be provided. The documentation for possible work-related exposures should follow standard department/company policies.

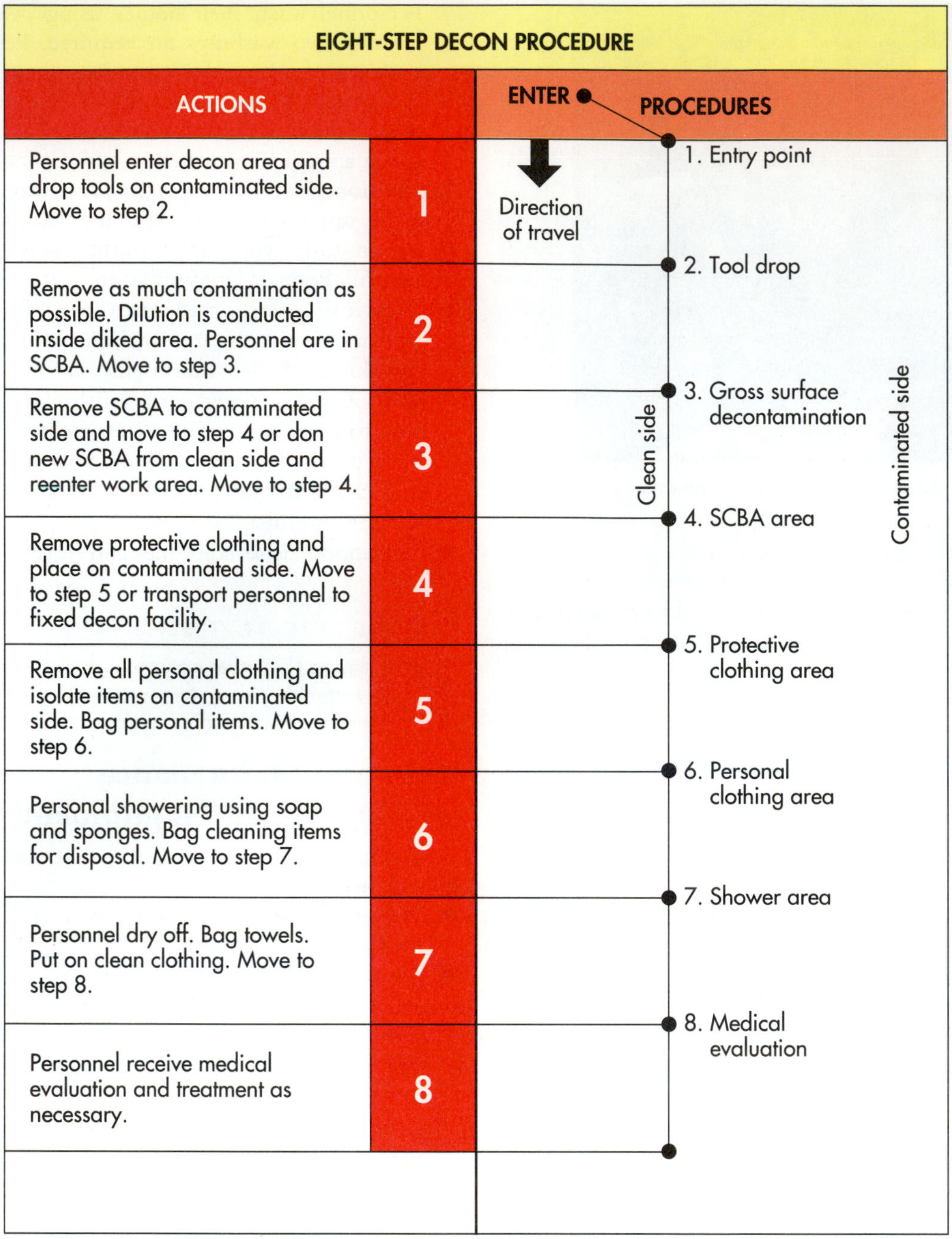

FIGURE 53-9 ■ Eight-step decontamination process.

SUMMARY

- A hazardous material is any substance or material that is capable of posing an unreasonable risk to health, safety, and property.
- The Superfund Amendments and Reauthorization Act of 1986 established requirements for federal, state, and local governments and industry regarding emergency planning and the reporting of hazardous materials–related incidents. In 1989 OSHA and the EPA published rules to govern training requirements, emergency plans, medical checkups, and other safety precautions for workers at uncontrolled hazardous waste sites and those responding to hazardous chemical spills. In addition, the NFPA has published standards that address competencies for EMS workers at hazmat scenes.
- Two methods are used to identify hazardous materials. One is informal product identification. (This includes vi-

sual, olfactory, and verbal clues.) The other is formal product identification. (This includes, for example, placards and shipping papers.) Resources for hazmat reference include the *North American Emergency Response Guidebook,* regional poison control centers, CHEMTREC, CHEMTEL, and CAMEO.

- Use of proper protection is crucial for anyone dealing with hazardous materials. This includes using the proper respiratory devices and wearing protective clothing. This clothing is made of a variety of materials. The clothing is designed for certain chemical exposures. Thus the paramedic must follow the manufacturer's guidelines.
- Hazardous materials may enter the body through inhalation, ingestion, injection, and absorption. Internal damage to the human body from hazmat exposure may involve the respiratory tract, central nervous system, or other internal organs. Chemicals producing internal damage include irritants, asphyxiants, nerve poisons, anesthetics, narcotics, hepatotoxins, cardiotoxins, nephrotoxins, neurotoxins, and carcinogens.
- Exposure to hazardous materials may result in burns and in severe tissue damage.
- The first agency to arrive at the scene of a hazmat incident must detect and identify the materials involved, assess the risk of exposure to rescue personnel and others, consider the potential risk of fire or explosion, gather information from on-site personnel or other sources, and confine and control the incident.
- A hazmat medical monitoring program may include medical examination for members of hazmat response teams, providing medical care, record keeping, and periodic evaluation of the surveillance program.
- The primary goals of decontamination are to reduce the patient's dosage of material, decrease the threat of secondary contamination, and reduce the risk of rescuer injury.
- Rescuers should follow strict protocols for proper decontamination of themselves, their clothing, and any contaminated equipment.

REFERENCES

1. General Services Administration, National Archives and Records Service, Office of the Federal Register: *Code of federal regulations,* 49 CFR, 173.500, parts 100-177, Washington, DC, 1981, The Administration.
2. Dickinson E (validated by International Fire Service Training Association): *Fire service emergency care,* Upper Saddle River, NJ, 1999, Brady/Prentice Hall.
3. National Safety Council: *Injury facts,* Itasca, Ill, 2002, The Council.
4. General Services Administration: *Hazardous waste operations and emergency response standards,* 29 CFR, 1910.120, Washington, DC, 2003, The Administration.
5. National Fire Protection Association: *Standard for competencies for EMS personnel responding to hazardous materials incidents,* NFPA 473 (rev 2002), Quincy, Mass, 2002, The Association.
6. US Department of Transportation, National Highway Traffic Safety Administration: *EMT-Paramedic national standard curriculum,* Washington, DC, 1998, The Department.
7. US Department of Health and Human Services, Occupational Safety and Health Administration: *General description and discussion of the levels of protection and protective gear,* 20 CFR, 1926.65, Appendix B, Washington, DC, 1994, The Administration.
8. Noll G et al: *Hazardous materials: managing the incident,* Stillwater, Okla, 1988, Fire Protection Publications.
9. US Department of Transportation: *North American emergency response guidebook,* Washington, DC, 2000, The Department.

APPENDIX

Overview of Training Requirements for EMS Personnel Responding to a Hazardous Materials Incident as Established by OSHA/EPA and the NFPA*

OSHA/EPA TRAINING REQUIREMENTS

1. *First responder awareness.* This category pertains to individuals who are likely to witness or discover a hazardous substance release but who do not have emergency response duties pertaining to hazardous materials as part of their job functions. This applies to most law enforcement officers. Individuals in this category must have sufficient training to demonstrate the following:
   a. An understanding of what hazardous materials are and the risks associated with them in an accident
   b. An understanding of the possible outcomes of an emergency in which hazardous materials are present
   c. The ability to recognize the presence of hazardous materials in an emergency
   d. The ability to identify the hazardous materials (if possible)
   e. An understanding of the role of the first responder in the emergency response plan
   f. The ability to recognize the need for additional resources
2. *First responder operations.* Individuals are included in this category if they respond to hazardous materials incidents to protect nearby persons, property, or the environment without trying to stop the hazardous release. Firefighters and emergency medical services (EMS) personnel are in this category. In addition to the knowledge base of first responder awareness, these individuals must have training in the following:
   a. Basic hazard and risk assessment techniques
   b. Personal protective clothing and equipment
   c. Basic control, containment, and confinement operations
   d. Basic decontamination procedures
3. *Hazardous material technicians.* Individuals in this category respond to hazardous materials emergencies for the purpose of stopping the release. Hazardous materials technicians usually are considered members of a hazardous materials response team. These individuals have additional training in the following:
   a. Emergency response plans
   b. The use of survey instruments and equipment to identify hazardous materials
   c. Incident command systems
   d. Specialized protective clothing and equipment
   e. Specialized containment and confinement operations
4. *Hazardous materials specialists.* The duties of these individuals require specific knowledge of the various hazardous substances. Hazardous materials specialists respond with and provide support to hazardous materials technicians and act as site liaisons with federal, state, and local government authorities. In addition to the knowledge base of the hazardous materials technician, hazardous materials specialists have training in the following:
   a. The use of advanced survey instruments and equipment
   b. In-depth hazard and risk assessment
   c. Implementation of decontamination procedures
   d. Site safety and control
   e. Chemical, radiological, and toxicological terminology relevant to hazardous substance behaviors
5. *On-scene incident commander.* The on-scene incident commander is trained to assume control of a hazardous materials event. In addition to the first responder awareness level of training, the on-scene incident commander's responsibilities include the following:
   a. Implementation of an incident command system
   b. Implementation of emergency response plans
   c. Knowledge of state and federal regional response teams
   d. Knowledge of medical hazards and risks for individuals working in protective clothing and equipment

NPFA 473: COMPETENCIES FOR EMS PERSONNEL RESPONDING TO HAZARDOUS MATERIALS INCIDENTS†

Level I Responders

The goal of the competencies at EMS/HM Level I shall be to provide the individual with knowledge and skills necessary to safely deliver emergency medical care in the cold zone [and meet the following requirements]:

1. Analyze a hazardous materials emergency to determine what risks are present to the provider and the patient by completing the following tasks:

**OSHA,* Occupational Safety and Health Administration; *EPA,* Environmental Protection Agency; *NFPA,* National Fire Protection Association.

†From National Fire Protection Association: *NPFA 473: Competencies for EMS personnel responding to hazardous materials incidents,* Quincy, Mass, 1997, The Association.

a. Determine the hazards present to the Level I responder and the patient in a hazardous materials incident
b. Assess the patient to determine the risk of secondary contamination
2. Plan a response to provide emergency medical care to persons involved in hazardous materials incidents by completing the following tasks:
a. Describe the role of the Level I responder in a hazardous materials incident
b. Plan a response to provide the appropriate level of emergency medical care in a hazardous materials incident
c. Determine if the personal protective equipment provided is appropriate
d. Determine if the equipment and supplies provided are adequate [that is, will meet the patient care needs]
3. Implement the planned response by completing the following tasks:
a. Perform the necessary preparations for receiving the hazardous materials patient and preventing secondary contamination
b. Treat the hazardous materials patient
c. Transport the patient as appropriate
d. Terminate the incident

Level II Responders

The goal of the competencies at EMS/HM Level II shall be to provide the Level II responder with the knowledge and skills necessary to perform and/or coordinate patient care activities and medical support of hazardous materials response personnel in the warm zone. The Level II responder should be able to [perform the following]:

1. Analyze a hazardous materials incident to determine the magnitude of the problem in terms of outcomes by completing the following tasks:
a. Determine the hazards present to the Level II responder and the patient in a hazardous material incident
b. Assess the patient to determine the patient care needs and the risk of secondary contamination
2. Plan a response to provide the appropriate level of emergency medical care to persons involved in hazardous materials incidents and to provide medical support to hazardous materials response personnel by completing the following tasks:
a. Describe the role of the Level II responder in a hazardous materials incident
b. Plan a response to provide the appropriate level of emergency medical care in a hazardous materials incident
c. Determine if the personal protective equipment provided to EMS personnel is appropriate
3. Implement the planned response by completing the following tasks:
a. Perform the preparations for receiving the patient
b. Provide treatment to the hazardous materials patient
c. Coordinate and manage the EMS component of the hazardous materials incident
d. Perform medical support of hazardous materials incident response personnel
4. Terminate the incident

CHAPTER 54

Bioterrorism and Weapons of Mass Destruction

OBJECTIVES

Upon completion of this chapter, the paramedic student will be able to:

1. List five types of weapons of mass destruction.
2. Identify actions, signs and symptoms, methods of distribution and management of biological weapons of mass destruction.
3. Identify actions, signs and symptoms, methods of distribution and management of chemical weapons of mass destruction.
4. Identify actions, signs and symptoms, methods of distribution and management of nuclear weapons of mass destruction.
5. Describe security threat levels as defined by the Department of Homeland Security.
6. Identify measures to be taken by paramedics who respond to incidents with suspected weapons of mass destruction involvement.

KEY TERMS

anthrax: An acute infectious disease caused by the spore-forming bacterium *Bacillus anthracis.*

bioterrorism: The use of biological agents, such as pathogenic organisms or agricultural pests, for the express purpose of causing death or disease, to instill a sense of fear and panic in the victims, and to intimidate governments or societies for political, financial, or ideological gain.

B-NICE: An acronym used for identifying five categories of weapons of mass destruction: *B*iological, *N*uclear, *I*ncendiary, *C*hemical, and *E*xplosives.

chlorine: A poisonous, yellow-green gas with an odor that has been described as a mixture of pineapple and pepper.

phosgene: A poisonous gas that appears as a grayish white cloud and smells of newly mowed hay.

plague: A disease caused by the bacteria *Yersinia pestis,* found in rodents (e.g., chipmunks, prairie dogs, ground squirrels, and mice) and their fleas in many areas around the world.

ricin: A potent protein cytotoxin derived from the beans of the castor plant *(Ricinus communis).*

riot control agents: Chemicals that can produce sensory irritation or disabling physical effects that disappear within a short time after termination of exposure.

sarin: A clear, colorless, and tasteless liquid that has no odor in its pure form; may be used as a nerve agent.

soman: A clear, colorless, tasteless liquid with a slight camphor odor; may be used as a nerve agent.

tabun: A clear, colorless, tasteless liquid with a faint fruity odor; may be used as a nerve agent.

tularemia: A serious illness that is caused by the bacterium *Francisella tularensis* found in animals (especially rodents, rabbits, and hares).

vesicants: Chemicals with severely irritating properties that produce fluid-filled pockets on the skin and damage to the eyes, lungs, and other mucous membranes.

viral hemorrhagic fevers: A group of illnesses caused by several distinct families of viruses that include arenaviruses, filoviruses, bunyaviruses, and flaviviruses.

VX: A thick, amber-colored, odorless liquid that resembles motor oil; may be used as a nerve agent.

weapons of mass destruction: Large conventional biological, nuclear, incendiary, chemical, or explosive weapons (B-NICE).

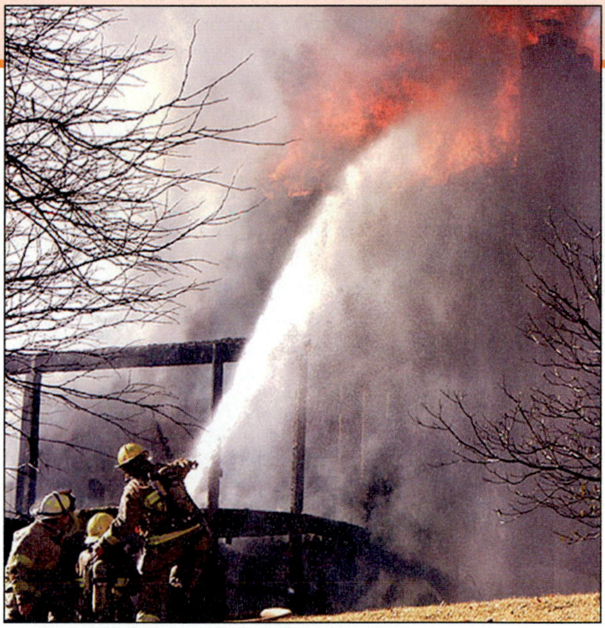

International conventions have long prohibited the use of chemicals and biological agents during war and bar any country from making or acquiring biological weapons.[1] A number of countries and terrorist groups, however, maintain them. This chapter serves as an overview of ***bioterrorism*** *and* ***weapons of mass destruction*** *(WMD). It also provides general guidelines for emergency response.*

NOTE B-NICE is an acronym that can be used for identifying the five categories of weapons of mass destruction. It stands for *B*iological, *N*uclear, *I*ncendiary, *C*hemical, and *E*xplosives.

HISTORY OF BIOLOGICAL WEAPONS

The use of biological agents as weapons has occurred throughout history, dating back to 184 BC when Hannibal ordered that pots filled with venomous snakes be thrown onto the decks of enemy ships (Box 54-1).[2] However, many countries agreed to stop biological weapons research and development in 1972. Some of these countries included the United States, the previous Soviet Union, Canada, and the United Kingdom. But some countries continue to have biological warfare programs. In addition, the use of biological agents against civilians through acts of bioterrorism recently has appeared. The serious reality of bioterrorism

NOTE Acts of terrorism can pose significant risk to civilian populations. If airplanes sprayed chemical and biological agents on a city on a clear, breezy night, thousands and perhaps millions of persons would be killed. For example, 200 lb of anthrax sprayed over a city the size of Omaha would kill as many as 2.5 million persons; 200 lb of botulinum toxin would kill as many as 40,000 persons in an area the size of the Mall of America; and 200 lb of VX sprayed over an area the size of Disneyland would kill about 12,500 persons.[3]

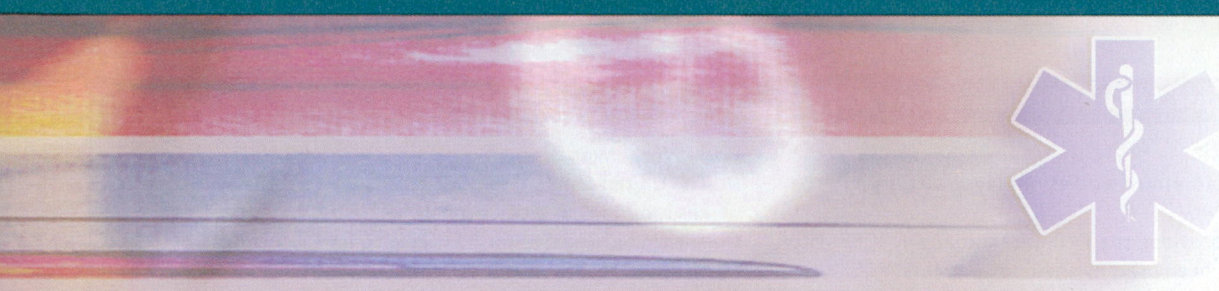

BOX 54-1 Time Line of Suspected or Reported Use of Biological Weapons

Early Examples
- The Tartar army catapulted bodies of plague victims into the city of Caffa in 1346.
- The British army provided the Delaware Indians in 1763 with blankets that had been used by smallpox patients.

Pre-World War II
- The Germans used various human and animal pathogens as agents of germ warfare in Europe during World War I. They are reported to have shipped horses, sheep, and cattle inoculated with *Bacillus anthracis* and *Pseudomonas pseudomallei* to the United States and other countries.
- Germany was accused of spreading cholera in Italy and plague in Russia in 1915.

World War II
- The Japanese used germ warfare against the Chinese and the Soviets by scattering *Yersinia pestis*–contaminated rice and fleas by airplane. This was followed by an outbreak of bubonic plague in those areas.
- The Japanese experimented with biological agents by exposing prisoners of war to anthrax, botulism, brucellosis, cholera, dysentery, gas gangrene, meningococcal infection, and plague. More than 1000 prisoners died from the experiments.
- The British performed trials with *Bacillus anthracis* off the coast of Scotland.
- The United States prepared about 5000 anthrax bombs at Camp Detrick, Maryland, in 1942 (although none were used during the war).

Post–World War II
- The United States dispersed stimulant aerosols over large areas around U.S. cities from 1949 to 1968.
- The United States exposed willing volunteer members of the Seventh Day Adventist Church (who were religious objectors to taking up arms) to aerosols of *Francisella tularensis* and *Coxiella burnetii* in 1953. (No deaths occurred and all recovered.)
- An unintentional release of anthrax spores from a biological warfare facility in the Soviet Union resulted in 66 deaths from inhalational anthrax in 1979.

The Gulf War
- The Iraqi government admitted that it had conducted research into the offensive use of *B. anthracis, Clostridium botulinum* toxin, and *C. perfringens* and had filled warheads with biological agents.

The Aum Shinrikyo
- The religious cult intentionally contaminated the Tokyo subway system with sarin in 1995, resulting in 5500 health care visits and 12 deaths.
- Several unsuccessful attempts were made to release anthrax or botulinum toxin to other areas around Tokyo.

Recent Terrorist Group Activities
- A religious commune deliberately contaminated several community salad bars in the United States with *Salmonella typhimurium,* resulting in more than 750 illnesses in 1984.
- Anthrax-laden envelopes were sent via U.S. mail in 2001, resulting to date in 11 cases of inhalational anthrax (including 5 deaths) and 12 cases of cutaneous anthrax.

From Darling R et al: *Bioterrorism: the May 2002 issue of the Emergency Medicine Clinics of North America,* Philadelphia, 2002, Saunders.

became clear in the United States in 2001 when **anthrax** cases occurred following exposure to contaminated mail in New York, New Jersey, and Washington, D.C.

CRITICAL BIOLOGICAL AGENTS

The Centers for Disease Control and Prevention[4] published a list of critical biological agents in 2000. The list is divided into categories A, B, and C (Box 54-2).

Category A agents are the highest priority. They pose a risk to national security. They can be spread easily by person-to-person contact. They cause a high death rate and have the potential to cause a major public health problem. They might cause public panic and disruption. Category A agents require special action for public health preparedness. An example of a category A agent is *Bacillus anthracis* (anthrax).

Category B agents are the second highest priority. They are fairly easy to disseminate. They cause moderate illnesses and have a lower death rate than Category A agents. These agents call for specific enhancements of diagnostic capacity and disease surveillance. An example of a category B agent is *Coxiella burnetii* (Q fever).

Category C agents are the third highest priority. They include new pathogens that could be engineered for mass dissemination in the future. These agents are widely available. They also are easy to produce and dispense. They have the potential to cause a high rate of death and sickness. An example of a category C agent is Nipah virus.

METHODS OF DISSEMINATION

Most biological agents used in bioterrorism are designed to enter the body through one of three ways. One of these is the inhalation of small particles into the lungs. Another is through the ingestion of contaminated food or water. The third way is by contamination of the skin that allows for absorption of the toxins. Because all Category A agents can be disseminated through aerosolization, the inhalation route is of greatest concern.

Aerosols can be delivered in wet or dry form in closed or open spaces. Equipment that may be used to disseminate aerosols includes crop-dusting planes for open spaces, aerosol-generating devices for enclosed areas (e.g., subways and enclosed malls), ventilation systems in buildings, and

BOX 54-2 Critical Biological Agents

Category A
Anthrax *(Bacillus anthracis)*
Botulism (*Clostridium botulinum* toxin)
Plague *(Yersinia pestis)*
Smallpox (variola major)
Tularemia *(Francisella tularensis)*
Viral hemorrhagic fevers (filoviruses [e.g., Ebola and Marburg] and arenaviruses [e.g., Lassa and Machupo])

Category B
Brucellosis (*Brucella* species)
Epsilon toxin of *Clostridium perfringens*
Food safety threats (e.g., *Salmonella* species, *Escherichia coli* O157:H7, and *Shigella*)
Glanders *(Burkholderia mallei)*
Melioidosis *(Burkholderia pseudomallei)*
Psittacosis *(Chlamydia psittaci)*
Q fever *(Coxiella burnetii)*
Ricin toxin from *Ricinus communis* (castor beans)
Staphylococcal enterotoxin B
Typhus fever *(Rickettsia prowazekii)*
Viral encephalitis (alphaviruses [e.g., Venezuelan equine encephalitis, eastern equine encephalitis, and western equine encephalitis])
Water safety threats (e.g., *Vibrio cholerae* and *Cryptosporidium parvum*)

Category C
Nipah virus
Hantaviruses
Tick-borne hemorrhagic fever viruses
Tick-borne encephalitis viruses
Yellow fever
Multidrug-resistant tuberculosis

From Centers for Disease Control and Prevention: Bioterrorism agents/diseases. http://www.bt.cdc.gov/agent/agentlist-category.asp#a. Accessed December 30, 2003.

contamination of items in the environment with fine powders that are aerosolized easily when disrupted. (The last example is what occurred with the recent anthrax cases in the United States. Those were caused by opening contaminated mail.)

CRITICAL THINKING
Why would aerosolized agents of mass destruction pose a great risk to first responders?

SPECIFIC BIOLOGICAL THREATS

Hundreds of biological and chemical agents can be used in a bioterrorism attack. This section provides a brief overview of certain agents. These agents are considered to be the ones most likely to be used as a threat to civilian populations. The most common biological threats are thought to be anthrax, botulism, **plague, ricin, tularemia,** smallpox, and **viral hemorrhagic fevers.**

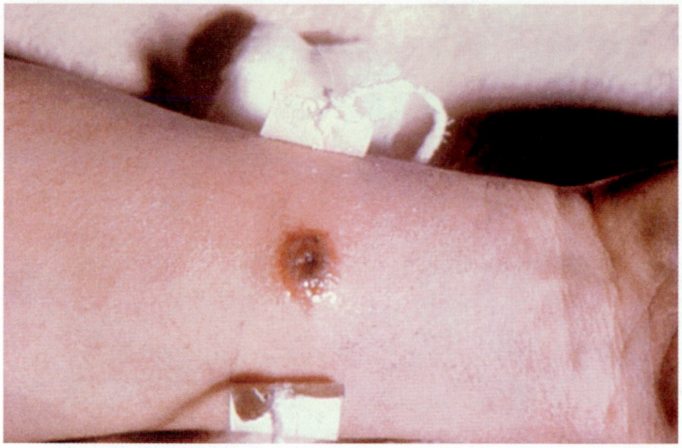

FIGURE 54-1 ■ Cutaneous anthrax.

NOTE Like all other hazardous materials incidents, it is assumed that all responders will wear the proper personal protective equipment. It also is assumed that they will use standard precautions at the scene and during patient care. (See chapter appendix.) No emergency service providers should enter a scene with known or suspected biological/chemical threats. They should not enter the scene until it has been made safe by the proper personnel.

Anthrax

Anthrax is an acute infectious disease caused by the spore-forming bacterium *B. anthracis.* Anthrax most often occurs in warm-blooded animals. However, it also can infect human beings. Symptoms of disease vary. Usually, though, symptoms appear within 7 days after exposure. The most common form of anthrax is cutaneous anthrax. It results from direct contact with spores or bacilli. Cutaneous anthrax causes localized itching. This is followed by a papular lesion that turns vesicular and subsequent development of black eschar within 7 to 10 days of the initial lesion (Fig. 54-1). Symptoms of inhalational anthrax often resemble a common cold in the initial stages. This is followed by severe respiratory distress and sepsis (Fig. 54-2). (Inhalational anthrax usually results in death within 36 hours after onset of the acute symptoms.) Other, less common forms of anthrax include intestinal anthrax from consuming contaminated meat and oropharyngeal anthrax (rare).

TREATMENT

Direct person-to-person spread of anthrax most likely does not occur. Thus immunization or treatment of persons who have come in contact with a patient (e.g., household members, friends, and co-workers) is unnecessary. These persons do not need to be treated unless they also were exposed to the aerosol at the time of the attack. The disease is

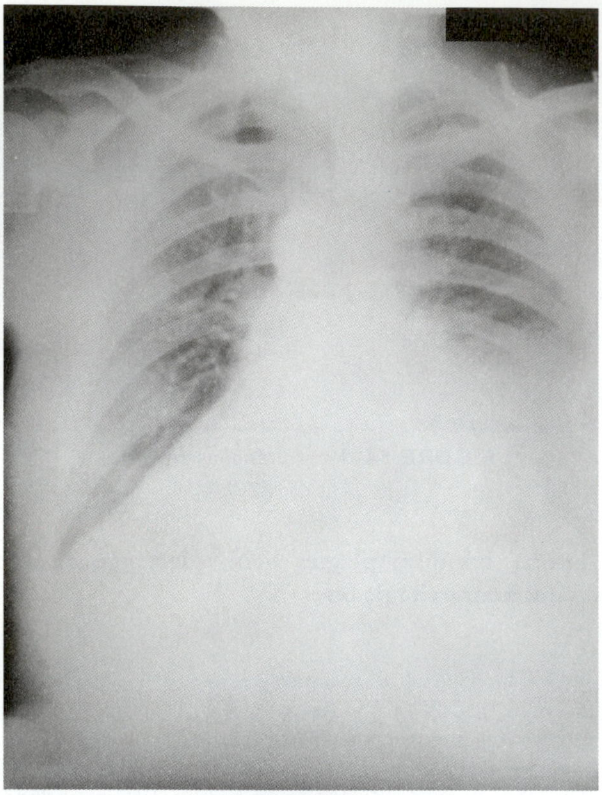

FIGURE 54-2 ■ Respiratory distress and sepsis in anthrax.

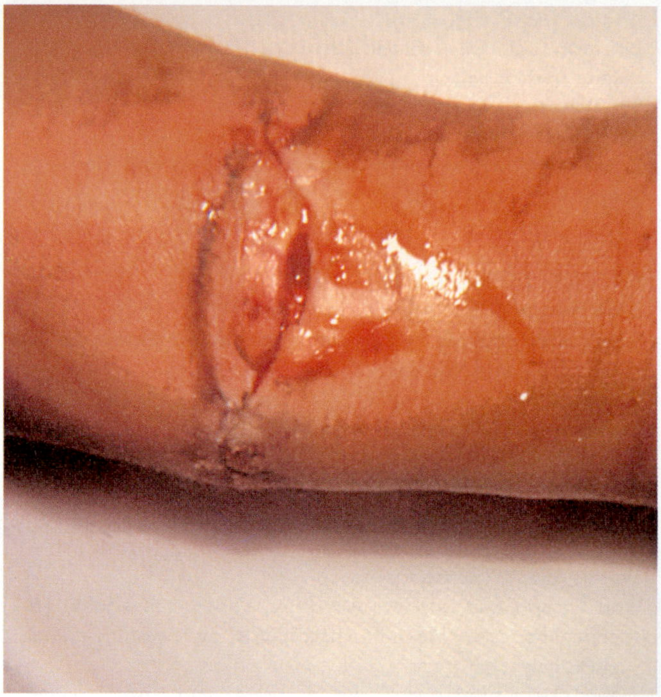

FIGURE 54-3 ■ Wound botulism.

diagnosed by isolating *B. anthracis* from the blood, skin lesions, or respiratory secretions or by measuring specific antibodies in the blood of suspected cases. Treatment with antibiotics should be early; if left untreated, the disease can be fatal. Human anthrax vaccines (controversial) are available and are reported to be 93% effective against cutaneous anthrax.[5] Vaccination to protect against inhalational anthrax is recommended only for those at high risk. This includes, for example, military personnel and workers in research laboratories that handle anthrax bacteria routinely.

Botulism

As described in Chapter 36, botulism is a rare but serious paralytic illness. The bacterium *Clostridium botulinum* produces a nerve toxin that causes paralysis. Botulinum toxin is the most potent, lethal substance known to man. There are three main types of botulism. One type is food-borne botulism. Eating foods that contain the botulism toxin causes it. The second type is wound botulism (Fig. 54-3). This type is caused by toxin produced from a wound infected with *C. botulinum*. The third type is infant botulism. This type is caused by consumption of the spores of the botulinum bacteria, which then grow in the intestines and release toxin. All forms of botulism can be fatal and are considered medical emergencies.

In a bioterrorism attack, breathing in the toxin as an aerosol weapon or ingesting the toxin via contaminated food or water are the most likely routes of exposure for serious illness. Food-borne botulism can be especially dangerous because small amounts of the bacterium in contaminated food can poison many persons. Signs and symptoms of the illness include nausea, dry mouth, blurred vision, dysphagia, fatigue, and dyspnea that may begin several hours to several days after the exposure.

TREATMENT

Botulism is not spread from person to person. If diagnosed early, food-borne and wound botulism can be treated with an antitoxin. The antitoxin blocks the action of toxin circulating in the blood. Recovery may take several weeks. As a result of the paralysis and respiratory failure that occur with botulism, the patient may be placed on a ventilator.

CRITICAL THINKING

What kind of resources would your community need to support hundreds of patients who need care on a ventilator?

Plague

Plague is caused by the bacteria *Yersinia pestis.* The bacteria are found in rodents (e.g., chipmunks, prairie dogs, ground squirrels, and mice) and their fleas in many areas of the world. The bacteria also can be grown in large amounts and disseminated by aerosol in a bioterrorism attack. This would result in an epidemic of the pneumonic form of the disease with the potential for secondary contamination. Signs and symptoms include fever, extreme weakness, shortness of breath, chest pain, cough, and bloody sputum. Gastrointestinal symptoms often accompany the others, including nausea, vomiting, abdominal pain, and diarrhea. The illness can lead to septic shock within 2 to 4 days. Without treatment, plague has a high mortality rate. A bioterrorism attack with the bacteria would be characterized by pneumonic plague occurring at the same time in persons following a common exposure. A secondary outbreak of illness would occur in others who had close contact with an infected person's respiratory droplets.

TREATMENT

The disease is diagnosed through testing for the bacteria. Plague must be treated early (within 24 hours). Plague is treated with antibiotic or antimicrobial agents to help ensure a successful outcome. Persons who have been in close contact with the patient should be identified. These persons must be evaluated for postexposure drug therapy. Pneumonic plague is spread through the respiratory droplets of an infected person. Thus patients with the disease should be isolated. Standard precautions and personal respiratory protection for all caregivers are critical.

> **CRITICAL THINKING**
>
> Your service notices a sudden increase in patients with severe respiratory distress. These patients also have pneumonia-like signs and symptoms. Would you initially consider bioterrorism as a cause of the outbreak?

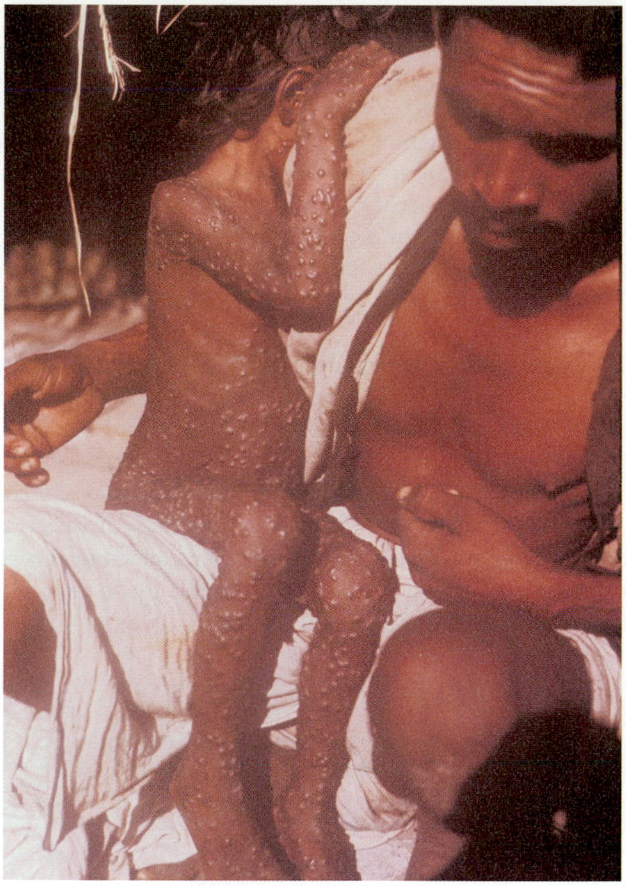

FIGURE 54-4 ■ Smallpox lesions.

Ricin

Ricin is a potent protein cytotoxin. Ricin is derived from the beans of the castor plant *(Ricinus communis)*. Castor beans are widely available throughout the world. The toxin also is relatively easy to extract. Ricin can be made into a mist, powder, or pellet. When ricin is inhaled as an aerosol, it results in pulmonary toxicity with severe respiratory symptoms within 8 hours. This is followed by acute hypoxic respiratory failure in 36 to 72 hours. (Nonspecific findings of weakness, fever, vomiting, cough, hypoxemia, hypothermia, and hypotension in large numbers of patients might suggest exposure to several respiratory pathogens.) If ricin is ingested, severe gastrointestinal symptoms occur with rapid onset of nausea, vomiting, abdominal cramps, and severe diarrhea. This is followed by vascular collapse and death.

TREATMENT

No antidote exists for ricin poisoning. Treatment is aimed at avoiding exposure and eliminating the toxin from the body as quickly as possible. Patients who have inhaled ricin should be moved to an area with fresh air; clothing contaminated with the toxin should be removed, and the patient should be decontaminated (see Chapter 53). The prehospital care may include airway, ventilatory, and circulatory support. Seizures, hypotension, and respiratory failure should be anticipated.

Smallpox

Smallpox was declared extinct by the World Health Organization in 1980 because of near-universal vaccination. However, the virus could be used as a biological weapon. The variola virus that causes smallpox is fairly stable. The infectious dose also is small. Moreover, an aerosol release of the virus would be widely spread. The incubation period for smallpox is about 12 days following exposure. The virus usually is spread by an infected person releasing infected saliva from the mouth into the air. Persons in close or prolonged contact to the infected person inhale the virus. Smallpox also can be spread through direct contact with infected body fluids or contaminated objects such as bedding or clothing. Signs and symptoms of the disease include high fever, fatigue, and head and back aches. These are followed within 2 to 3 days with the smallpox rash and skin lesions. These lesions finally form crusts. Upon healing, the lesions leave depressed, depigmented scars (Fig. 54-4). Permanent joint deformities and blindness may follow recovery. The death rate from smallpox is about 35% in unvaccinated persons.

Vaccine immunity may prevent or modify the illness. At this time, however, the federal government does not recommend prophylactic vaccination for health care workers or the general public because of the possibility of toxic or allergic reactions.[6] If an attack is known or imminent, smallpox response teams whose members have received the vaccine will administer the vaccine to others. They also will care for victims who have been exposed. Currently, the United States has enough smallpox vaccine in storage to vaccinate everyone in the country who might need it in the event of an emergency.[7] Production of a new vaccine is also under way.

TREATMENT

There is no proven treatment for smallpox. However, several antiviral drugs are being studied. Patients with smallpox should receive supportive care provided by vaccinated personnel. The personnel must use universal precautions. (This includes appropriate respiratory protection.) Objects that come in contact with the patient require disinfection. (Examples of such objects are bed linens, clothing, ambulances, and equipment.) This disinfection must be by fire, steam, or sodium hypochlorite solution.

> **CRITICAL THINKING**
> Your employer asks you to get the smallpox vaccination. Where can you look to find information about the side effects and risks of immunization with this vaccine?

Tularemia

Tularemia is a serious illness caused by the bacterium *Francisella tularensis.* This bacterium is found in animals (especially rodents, rabbits, and hares). The disease is highly infectious. Some strains are resistant to antibiotics. The bacterium responsible for tularemia can be delivered in a bioterrorism attack by aerosol. Infection may result from inhalation of the aerosol. It also may result from the skin, mucous membranes, respiratory tract, or gastrointestinal tract (via contaminated soil, water, food, or animals) being exposed to the virus. Transmission of the disease from person to person does not occur. The development of signs and symptoms varies widely (from 1 day to 2 weeks). This is based on the strength of the strain and the route of exposure. Following a bioterrorism attack with the agent, patients may complain of an abrupt onset of an acute febrile illness (headache, chills, general malaise). They also may complain of gastrointestinal illness that includes nausea, vomiting, and diarrhea. If left untreated, septic tularemia may lead to disseminated intravascular coagulation with bleeding, acute respiratory failure, and death.

TREATMENT

The disease is managed with antibiotics. The patient may require airway, ventilatory, and circulatory support. A vaccine for tularemia is under review by the Food and Drug Administration. However, the vaccine is not currently available in the United States.

Viral Hemorrhagic Fevers

Viral hemorrhagic fevers (VHFs) refer to a group of illnesses caused by several distinct families of viruses that include arenaviruses, filoviruses, bunyaviruses, and flaviviruses. The viruses all have lipid envelopes and limited geographic ranges. Most are highly infectious if spread as an aerosol. These viruses naturally reside in animals (e.g., cotton rat and deer mouse) or arthropods (e.g., ticks and mosquitoes). The viruses are fully dependent on these living hosts for reproduction and survival. Viruses that cause hemorrhagic fever usually are transmitted to human beings during contact with urine, fecal matter, saliva, or other body excretions from an infected rodent or from a bite from an infected mosquito or tick. Some VHFs (e.g., Ebola and Marburg) also can be spread from person to person following an initial infection. This type of infection most often results from close contact with infected persons through their body tissues and fluids.

Viral hemorrhagic fevers cause a multisystem syndrome. The syndrome is characterized by hemorrhage and life-threatening disease. Signs and symptoms vary by the type of VHF. However, they often include fever, fatigue, dizziness, muscle aches, loss of strength, and exhaustion. Patients with severe cases of VHF may bleed from mucous membranes, internal organs, or from the mouth, eyes, or ears. (Death rarely results from this blood loss.) Shock, renal failure, central nervous system dysfunction, coma, and seizures may develop with severe infection. These may lead to a fatal outcome.

TREATMENT

Therapy for patients with VHFs is supportive. With the exception of yellow fever and Argentine hemorrhagic fever, for which vaccines have been developed, no vaccines exist that can protect against these diseases. The goals of therapy are to maintain vital functions. This may allow for recovery in some patients.

NUCLEAR AND RADIOLOGICAL THREATS

Nuclear explosions can cause deadly effects from blinding light, intense heat (thermal radiation), initial nuclear radiation, blast, fires started by the heat pulse, and secondary fires caused by destruction. A radiological dispersion device (RDD) is also called a "dirty nuke" or "dirty bomb." The use of such a device as a terrorist weapon is considered far more

> **NOTE** Radiological attacks are a credible threat. However, they would not result in the hundreds of thousands of deaths that could be caused by a crude nuclear weapon that requires a fission reaction. A radiological attack, however, could cause serious illness in persons in the immediate area, contaminate several city blocks, and require costly cleanup (if even possible).

likely than use of a true nuclear device. (A true nuclear device uses weapons-grade uranium or plutonium.)[8] These dirty bombs appeal to terrorists. They require little technical knowledge to build and deploy compared with that of a true nuclear device. These radioactive materials also are used widely in medicine, agriculture, industry, and research. They are readily available and easy to obtain.

The main type of RDD combines an explosive, such as dynamite, with a radioactive material. The extent of contamination would depend on a number of factors. These include the size of the explosive, the amount and type of radioactive material used, and weather conditions (e.g., wind). The detonation of an RDD releases radioactive fallout. This could cause radiation sickness, severe burns, and long-term cancer fatalities. In most cases the conventional explosive itself would result in more deaths than from exposure to the radioactive material.[9] A second type of RDD might involve a powerful radioactive source hidden in a public place. It may be hidden, for example, in a trash can in a busy train or subway station. In such a place, persons passing close to the source might receive a significant dose of radiation.

CRITICAL THINKING

What emergency medical services groups or divisions should you consider setting up if there is a report of a dirty bomb explosion?

Emergency Care

As described in Chapter 23, the principles of *time, distance,* and *shielding* should be used for personal protection and for the protection of others:

1. Limit the amount of time at a radiological scene. Fallout radiation loses its intensity fairly rapidly.
2. Increase the distance between you and the scene.
3. Shield yourself with appropriate personal protective equipment, geography, or structural materials whenever possible. The more heavy, dense materials between you and the fallout particles, the better.

After dealing with the initial blast, the top priorities are the treatment of radiation sickness, the containment and monitoring of radioactive fallout, evacuation, and decontamination.

INCENDIARY THREATS

Incendiary devices are firebombs. These devices range from a simple Molotov cocktail (a bottle containing a rag soaked in gasoline that is ignited) to much larger and sophisticated devices. Their main use in terrorism is to generate panic (a *weapon of mass disruption*). However, they are also capable of causing loss of life and property damage from fire. Depending on the severity of the attack, primary concerns may include the following:

- The possibility for large numbers of injured victims and fatalities
- Significant damage to buildings and the infrastructure of a community
- Overwhelming of local resources (emergency response agencies, hospitals, mental health agencies)
- The involvement of law enforcement at local, state, and federal levels because of the criminal nature of the event
- The closing of workplaces and schools
- Possible restrictions on domestic and international travel
- The need for evacuation and extended cleanup
- Public fear that can continue for a prolonged period

Emergency Care

Emergency care depends on the nature of the attack. Care may include providing initial wound care for injured victims at a small-scale event. However, care also may include managing a scene with multiple patients at a large-scale event. (See Chapter 50.)

As with any emergency response, EMS crews should not approach the scene until it has been made safe by the proper personnel. Following the initial explosion, detonation of a second device is possible. The second device is designed to injure or kill emergency response personnel or bystanders. In addition, biological, chemical, or nuclear materials may have been used in the explosion. Thus it is critical to personal safety not to enter the scene until the area is determined to be safe.

SPECIFIC CHEMICAL THREATS

Specific chemicals that may be used in war and acts of terrorism include nerve agents, poisonous gases, and blister agents. The deliberate release of these chemicals in the form of toxic gas, liquid, or solid can poison persons or the environment (Box 54-3).

Nerve Agents

Nerve agents were used in military conflicts in the Persian Gulf in the 1980s. They also were used in terrorist attacks in Japan in 1995. They are the most toxic and rapidly acting of the known chemical warfare agents.[10] Nerve agents are similar to organophosphates in terms of how they work and what kinds of harmful effects they cause. (However, they are more potent.) (See Chapter 36.) Nerve agents inhibit the effects of acetylcholinesterase, which causes a cholinergic "overdrive" *(cholinergic crisis).* This disrupts the nerve transmissions in the central and peripheral nervous systems. The extent of poisoning caused by nerve agents depends on the amount, route, and length of exposure. Mildly or moderately exposed persons usually recover fully. Severely exposed persons are not likely to survive. The nerve agents discussed in this chapter are **sarin, soman, tabun,** and **VX.**

CRITICAL THINKING

Would you expect a fast or slow heart rate if the patient has been exposed to a nerve agent?

BOX 54-3 Riot Control Agents

Riot control agents are solid chemicals with low vapor pressure that are dispersed in the air as fine particles. They produce sensory irritation or disabling physical effects that disappear within a short time after termination of exposure. Riot control agents often are referred to as "tear gas" and sometimes are used in military exercises, by law enforcement personnel for crowd control, and by individuals and the general public for personal protection (e.g., mace and pepper spray). Paramedics and other emergency responders likely will encounter exposure to these agents during their careers. Personal protective equipment is needed to guard against the effects of these agents.

The most common riot control agent compounds are chloroacetophenone and chlorobenzylidenemalononitrile. Other examples include chloropicrin, bromobenzylcyanide, dibenzoxazepine, and combinations of various agents. Riot control agents cause irritation to the area of contact (e.g., eyes, skin, and nose) within seconds of exposure. Signs and symptoms vary, depending on the location of exposure (open versus enclosed spaces) and the duration of contact with the agent and may include some or all of the following:

- Eyes: excessive tearing, burning, blurred vision, redness
- Nose: runny nose, burning, swelling
- Mouth: burning, irritation, difficulty swallowing, drooling
- Lungs: chest tightness, coughing, choking sensation, wheezing, shortness of breath
- Skin: burns, rash
- Gastrointestinal: nausea and vomiting

Although most effects from exposure to riot control agents are minor and last only 15 to 30 minutes, exposure to large doses or exposure in an enclosed area rarely may result in blindness, glaucoma, severe burns to airway structures, and life-threatening respiratory failure. Emergency care consists of moving persons away from the source to fresh air. In severe cases, oxygen administration, ventilatory support, burn care, and decontamination may be required.

Source: Centers for Disease Control and Prevention: Facts about riot control agents. http://www.bt.cdc.gov/agent/riotcontrol/factsheet.asp. Accessed February 4, 2004.

Sarin (also known as "BG") is a clear, colorless, and tasteless liquid that has no odor in its pure form. However, sarin can evaporate into a vapor (gas) and spread into the environment. The agent also mixes easily with water. This allows for contamination by persons touching or drinking water. Symptoms may begin within minutes to hours after exposure. They may include headache, salivation, chest pain, abdominal cramps, wheezing, fasciculations, seizure, and respiratory failure that possibly can lead to death.

Soman (also known as "GD") is a clear, colorless, tasteless liquid with a slight camphor odor. The odor is similar to the smell of Vicks Vapo-Rub or a rotting fruit odor. The agent can vaporize if heated. Compared with other nerve agents, soman is more volatile than VX but less volatile than sarin. (The higher the volatility of a chemical, the more likely it will evaporate and disperse into the environment.) Persons can be exposed to the vapor even if they do not come in contact with the liquid form. Symptoms may begin within seconds to hours after exposure. They include headache, salivation, chest pain, abdominal cramps, wheezing, fasciculations, seizure, and respiratory failure that possibly can lead to death.

Tabun (also known as "GA") is a clear, colorless, tasteless liquid with a faint fruity odor. The chemical can vaporize if heated. Thus persons can be exposed to the nerve agent by skin or eye contact or by inhalation. The agent also mixes easily with water. This allows for possible cutaneous exposure and exposure to the gastrointestinal tract if contaminated food or water is ingested. Moreover, secondary contamination is possible. This would occur from clothing or personal articles that have been contaminated by tabun vapor. Symptoms generally appear within a few seconds after exposure to tabun vapor. They generally appear within 18 hours after exposure to liquid tabun. Signs and symptoms of mild to moderate exposure to tabun include watery eyes, blurred vision, headache, weakness, cough, drooling, polyuria, excessive sweating, fasciculations, hypotension or hypertension, and cardiac abnormalities. With severe exposure, patients may experience loss of consciousness, seizures, and cardiorespiratory arrest. Severely poisoned patients are not likely to survive.

VX

VX is a thick, amber-colored, odorless liquid. It resembles motor oil and is the most potent of all nerve agents. VX is considered to be much more toxic when absorbed through the skin and somewhat more toxic by inhalation than are other nerve agents. VX is primarily a liquid exposure hazard. However, if heated to very high temperatures, it can turn into small amounts of vapor. Following release of VX into the air, persons can be exposed through skin contact, eye contact, or inhalation. VX also can be released into the water. This allows for exposure by ingestion or absorption. Symptoms will appear within a few seconds after exposure to the vapor form of VX. They will appear within a few minutes to up to 18 hours after exposure to the liquid form. Signs and symptoms of exposure are the same as for other nerve agents.

TREATMENT

Treatment for exposure to nerve agents consists of quickly removing the agent from the body. Treatment also consists of supporting the patient's vital functions. If vapor exposure has occurred, the patient should be moved quickly to an area of fresh air. If the exposure occurred in an open-air environment, the patient should be moved uphill and upwind from the contamination site. Many nerve agents are heavier than air and will settle in low-lying areas. The patient's clothing should be removed. Then the patient should be decontaminated by trained personnel. A person's clothing and other contaminated surfaces can release nerve agents for about 30 minutes after exposure. Thus secondary contamination is possible. ***Atropine*** and ***pralidoxime chloride*** are antidotes (available in autoinjector kits, e.g., MARK I kits) for nerve agent toxicity (Table 54-1). They

TABLE 54-1 Recommendations for Prehospital Nerve Agent Therapy

PATIENT'S AGE	ANTIDOTES* MILD/MODERATE SYMPTOMS†	SEVERE SYMPTOMS‡	OTHER TREATMENT
Infant (0-2 yr)	Atropine: 0.05 mg/kg IM; 2-PAM Cl: 15 mg/kg IM	Atropine: 0.1 mg/kg IM; 2-PAM Cl: 25 mg/kg IM	For severe exposures, assisted ventilation should be started after administration of antidotes.
Child (2-10 yr)	Atropine: 1 mg IM; 2-PAM Cl: 15 mg/kg IM	Atropine: 2 mg IM; 2-PAM Cl: 25 mg/kg IM	
Adolescent (>10 yr)	Atropine: 2 mg IM; 2-PAM Cl: 15 mg/kg IM	Atropine: 4 mg IM; 2-PAM Cl: 25 mg/kg IM	**Repeat atropine (2 mg IM)** at 5- to 10-min intervals until secretions have diminished and breathing is comfortable or airway resistance has returned to near normal.
Adult	Atropine: 2-4 mg IM; 2-PAM Cl: 600 mg/kg IM *or* 1 MARK I kit IM	Atropine: 6 mg IM; 2-PAM Cl: 1800 mg/kg IM *or* 3 MARK I kits IM	
Elderly, frail	Atropine: 1 mg IM; 2-PAM Cl: 10 mg/kg IM	Atropine: 2-4 mg IM; 2-PAM Cl: 25 mg/kg IM	

Modified from Agency For Toxic Substances and Disease Registry: Medical management *guidelines (MMGs) for nerve agents.* www.atsdr.cdc.gov.
*2-PAM Cl solution must be prepared from the ampule containing 1 g of desiccated 2-PAM Cl: inject 3 mL of saline, 5% distilled or sterile water into ampule and shake well. The resulting solution is 3.3 mL of 300 mg/mL.
†Mild to moderate symptoms include localized sweating, muscle fasciculations, nausea, vomiting, weakness, and dyspnea.
‡Severe symptoms include unconsciousness, convulsions, apnea, and flaccid paralysis

work by blocking the effects of acetylcholine. (See Chapter 36 and the EDI.) Large doses of these drugs and repeated administration may be required. ***Diazepam*** or ***lorazepam*** may be indicated if seizures are present. (The paramedic should consult with medical direction before administering these drugs if muscle twitching is present.) Once seizures begin, they can be almost impossible to stop. Caring for patients who have ingested a nerve agent should be guided by medical direction, a poison control center, or other authority.

Poisonous Gases

Poisonous gases were popular weapons in World War I. Although they have not been used as toxic pulmonary inhalants by the military since 1918,[10] they are produced in large quantities worldwide for use in the industrial sector. They are widely available. Thus use of these gases for acts of terrorism is a possibility. The gases described in this section are **chlorine** and **phosgene.**

Chlorine is a yellow-green gas with an odor that has been described as a mixture of pineapple and pepper. Chlorine gas can be pressurized and condensed to change it into a liquid. In liquid form, chlorine can be shipped and stored. When liquid chlorine is released, it quickly vaporizes into a gas that stays close to the ground and spreads rapidly. If chlorine is released into the air, persons may be exposed to chlorine gas through skin or eye contact or by inhalation. If chlorine liquid is released into water, exposure can occur by touching or drinking contaminated water or by ingesting food that was prepared with the contaminated water. Like other chemical agents, the extent of poisoning depends on the amount, route, and duration of exposure to the agent. Signs and symptoms may include cough; chest pain; burning sensation in the nose, eyes, or throat; watery eyes; blurred vision; gastrointestinal disturbances; dermal burns from skin contact; and shortness of breath and dyspnea. Pulmonary edema can develop within 2 to 4 hours following inhalation of the gas.

Phosgene (also know as "CG") is a poisonous gas that appears as a grayish white cloud and smells of newly mowed hay. With cooling and pressure, the gas can be condensed into a liquid so that it can be shipped and stored. When liquid phosgene is released, it quickly vaporizes into a gas that stays close to the ground and spreads rapidly. Inhaled phosgene damages the lungs, producing a burning sensation, cough, and labored breathing. Pulmonary edema with frothy sputum production may develop. Cutaneous exposure to the gas can result in skin or eye injury. Exposure also can occur by touching or drinking water contaminated with the gas or by ingesting food that was prepared with the contaminated water. In addition to the signs and symptoms noted previously for chlorine exposure, phosgene poisoning may cause hypotension and heart failure. In lethal doses, death can occur within 48 hours.

TREATMENT

No antidotes exist for chlorine or phosgene poisoning. Treatment for exposure to these gases consists of removing them from the body as soon as possible and providing supportive medical care. All patients should be moved to an area of fresh air and to the highest ground possible (if exposure occurred in an open air space). The patient's clothing should be removed. Then the patient should be decontaminated by trained personnel.

Blister Agents

Blister agents or **vesicants** are chemicals with highly irritating properties that produce fluid-filled pockets on the skin and damage to the eyes, lungs, and other mucous membranes. In addition to cutaneous effects from exposure to these agents, blister agents also can cause loss of vision, convulsions, and respiratory failure. The gastrointestinal system, central nervous system, and bone marrow also can be affected through systemic absorption. Symptoms of exposure may be delayed until hours after exposure. The major chemicals in this category are sulfur mustard (H, HD, HT), nitrogen mustard (HN-1, HN-2, HN-3), and lewisite (L, L-1, L-2, L-3). Phosgene oxime is more of an urticant, producing irritation without blisters. However, the gas still is classified as a vesicant.

Mustard is an oily liquid that comes in a variety of colors ranging from brown to yellow. It may smell like garlic, onion, horseradish, or mustard itself. Lewisite is an oily, odorless liquid. Lewisite is more volatile than mustard and smells like geraniums in its gaseous state. (Unlike mustard, in which symptoms may be delayed, lewisite causes immediate pain and irritation on contact.) Phosgene oxime is a colorless solid or yellowish brown liquid. It may have a peppery or pungent odor. Like lewisite, this agent causes immediate pain and irritation on contact with the skin or mucous membranes.

TREATMENT

After ensuring personal safety (including the use of appropriate personal protective equipment), the initial assessment and treatment of the patient should begin with airway, ventilatory, and circulatory support as needed. Immediate decontamination may reduce damage to tissue. All skin exposures should be treated with standard burn care. Advanced cardiac life support protocols should be followed for any patient with cardiac or breathing problems. Advanced trauma life support protocols should be followed for any trauma patient. The signs and symptoms may not develop for several hours following exposure to some blister agents. Thus a patient with a significant exposure should be evaluated by a physician. Patients who have only mild symptoms should be advised to seek physician evaluation if signs and symptoms worsen.

EXPLOSIVE THREATS

An explosive is a bomb. Bombs can be made from a variety of dangerous materials and can be made in a variety of sizes weighing several ounces to several thousand pounds. Explosives used by terrorists are often classified by the following categories[11]:

- Unconventional use: a conventional object used in an unconventional way to create mass destruction. In the September 11, 2001, attack on the World Trade Center and Pentagon, hijackers flew passenger planes into their intended targets, relying on the impact of the planes and their full fuel tanks to create havoc.
- Vehicle bomb: usually large powerful devices that consist of a large quantity of explosives fitted with a timed or remotely triggered detonator packed onto a car or truck.
- Pipe bomb: a quantity of explosives sealed into a length of metal or plastic pipe. A timing fuse usually controls detonation, but other methods can be used, including electronic timers, remote triggers, and motion sensors. These are the most common explosive devices and are at the opposite end of the scale from vehicle bombs in terms of size and power.
- Satchel charge: an old military term for an explosive device in a canvas-carrying bag. In recent history, "daypacks" or knapsacks have been used for the carrying device, and the explosives have contained antipersonnel materials such as nails and glass to inflict more casualties.
- Package or letter bomb: explosive material contained in a package or letter that usually is triggered by opening of the package.

Emergency Care

Like the incendiary devices described before, the care for victims of an explosion may vary. Treatment may require only minor wound care to several persons. Or treatment could be a large-scale event. The larger events may have many patients and casualties. The incident may involve secondary explosions and chemical and biological threats. Thus it is critical to personal safety not to enter the scene until the area is determined to be safe by the proper personnel.

DEPARTMENT OF HOMELAND SECURITY

Following the terrorist attacks on the World Trade Center in New York City on September 11, 2001, the Department of Homeland Security was established through the Homeland Security Act of 2002 (H.R. 5005).[12] The three primary missions of the Department of Homeland Security are to (1) prevent terrorist attacks within the United States, (2) reduce America's vulnerability to terrorism, and (3) minimize the damage from potential attacks and natural disasters. To help meet these goals, a uniform national threat advisory system (Homeland Security Advisory System) was developed to inform federal agencies, state and local officials, and the private sector of terrorist threats and appropriate protective actions. The Homeland Security Advisory System establishes five threat conditions with associated suggested protective measures[13]:

1. Low Condition (Green). This condition is declared when there is a low risk of terrorist attacks. Federal departments and agencies should consider the following general measures in addition to the agency-specific protective measures they develop and implement:
    - Refining and exercising preplanned protective measures
    - Proper training on the Homeland Security Advisory System and specific preplanned department or agency protective measures
    - Developing a process to ensure that all facilities and regulated sectors are assessed regularly for vulnerabilities to terrorist attacks and that all reasonable measures are taken to prevent these vulnerabilities.
2. Guarded Condition (Blue). This condition is declared when there is a general risk of terrorist attacks. In addi-

tion to the protective measures taken in the previous threat condition, federal departments and agencies should consider the following general measures:

- Checking communications with designated emergency response or command locations
- Reviewing and updating emergency response procedures
- Providing the public with any information that would strengthen its ability to act appropriately

3. Elevated Condition (Yellow). This condition is declared when there is a significant risk of terrorist attacks. In addition to the protective measures taken in the previous threat conditions, federal departments and agencies should consider the following measures:
   - Increasing surveillance of critical locations
   - Coordinating emergency plans as appropriate with nearby jurisdictions
   - Assessing whether the characteristics of the threat require the further refinement of preplanned protective measures
   - Implementing, as appropriate, contingency and emergency response plans
4. High Condition (Orange). This condition is declared when there is a high risk of terrorist attacks. In addition to the protective measures taken in the previous threat conditions, federal departments and agencies should consider the following general measures:
   - Coordinating security efforts with federal, state, and local law enforcement agencies or other appropriate armed forces organizations
   - Taking additional precautions at public events and possibly considering alternative venues or even cancellation
   - Preparing to execute contingency procedures, such as moving to an alternate site or dispersing their workforce
   - Restricting threatened facility access to essential personnel only
5. Severe Condition (Red). This condition reflects a severe risk of terrorist attacks. Under most circumstances, the protective measures for a severe condition are not intended to be sustained for long periods of time. In addition to the protective measures in the previous threat conditions, federal departments and agencies also should consider the following general measures:
   - Increasing or redirecting personnel to address critical emergency needs
   - Assigning emergency response personnel and prepositioning and mobilizing specially trained teams or resources
   - Monitoring, redirecting, or constraining transportation systems
   - Closing public and government facilities

GENERAL GUIDELINES FOR EMERGENCY RESPONSE

General guidelines for responding to a scene that may involve hazardous materials were described in Chapter 53. Many aspects of a WMD incident are comparable to other medical, trauma, and hazardous materials incidents. However, there are some significant differences. For example, terrorists have been known to time secondary events (e.g., booby traps, additional bombs, and armed resistance) to injure emergency responders. Secondly, a terrorist act is a criminal event. This means that the site becomes a crime scene. Thus everything is considered evidence of the crime. Fear and panic can be expected from the public, patients, and emergency responders. This makes scene safety, security, and crowd control major issues with which to contend. Finally, contingency plans for emergency responders at the scene and at destination facilities will need to be in place. These plans will help emergency responders to deal with the large numbers of upset, agitated, frightened, and injured patients.

> **CRITICAL THINKING**
>
> Why will correct, prompt information to the media be critical during a weapons of mass destruction event?

Emergency Responder Guidelines

Emergency responder guidelines have been established by the Office of Justice Program, Office for Domestic Preparedness, to prepare for and respond to incidents of domestic terrorism. These incidents may involve chemical and biological agents and nuclear, radioactive, and explosive devices. Recommended guidelines for EMS providers are as follows[14]:

- Recognize hazardous materials incidents.
- Know the protocols used to detect the potential presence of WMD agents or materials.
- Know and follow self-protection measures for WMD events and hazardous materials events.
- Know procedures for protecting a potential crime scene.
- Know and follow agency/organization scene security and control procedures for WMD and hazardous material events.
- Possess and know how to use equipment properly to contact dispatchers or higher authorities to report information collected at the scene and to request additional assistance or emergency response personnel. Know how to characterize a WMD event and be able to identify available response assets within the affected jurisdiction(s).

Finally, EMS agencies must be prepared to implement incident operations, provide personal and public safety measures, perform appropriate decontamination, and provide emergency medical care specific to the incident.

SUMMARY

- The five categories of weapons of mass destruction are biological, nuclear, incendiary, chemical, and explosives.
- Biological agents include anthrax, botulism, plague, ricin, tularemia, and smallpox.
- Person-to-person spread is possible in patients who are infected with plague or smallpox.
- Nerve agents include sarin, soman, tabun, and VX. Exposure causes a cholinergic overdrive. The antidote for nerve agent exposure is atropine and pralidoxime chloride.
- Poisonous gases such as chlorine and phosgene cause severe respiratory problems. They also can cause skin and eye injury. Move exposed patients to safety, remove their clothing, and treat their symptoms.
- Dirty bombs could cause heat damage and radiation sickness, severe burns, and cancer.
- The Department of Homeland Security has identified five terrorist threat levels. Each level has specific community-wide emergency preparedness activities to be taken.
- Emergency responders at a WMD incident should recognize hazardous materials incidents, know protocols to detect WMD, use personal protective equipment, know crime scene procedures, know how to activate more resources, and implement incident operations.

REFERENCES

1. Geissler E, editor: *Biological and toxin weapons today,* Oxford, England, 1986, Oxford University Press.
2. Osterholm MT, Schwartz J: *Living terrors: what America needs to know to survive the coming bioterrorist catastrophe,* New York, 2000, Delacorte Press.
3. Cowley G, Rogers A: The terrors of toxins, *Newsweek,* Nov 1997.
4. Centers for Disease Control and Prevention: Biological and chemical terrorism: strategic plan for preparedness and response–recommendations of the CDC strategic planning workgroup, *MMWR* 49(RR04):1-14, 2000.
5. Centers for Disease Control and Prevention: Fact sheet: anthrax information for health care providers. http://www.bt.cdc.gov/agent/anthrax/anthrax-hcp-factsheet.asp#Cutaneous. Accessed December 30, 2003.
6. Centers for Disease Control and Prevention: Protecting Americans: smallpox vaccination program. http://www.bt.cdc.gov/agent/smallpox/vaccination/vaccination-program-statement.asp. Accessed January 7, 2004.
7. Darling R et al: *Bioterrorism: the May 2002 issue of the Emergency Medicine Clinics of North America,* Philadelphia, 2002, Saunders.
8. Federal Emergency Management Agency: Nuclear and radiological attack: are you ready? a guide to citizen preparedness. http://www.fema.gov/areyouready/nuclear_blast.shtm. Accessed March 23, 2005.
9. US Nuclear Regulatory Commission: Fact sheet on dirty bombs. http://www.nrc.gov/reading-rm/doc-collections/fact-sheets/dirty-bombs.html. Accessed January 13, 2004.
10. Centers for Disease Control and Prevention: Facts about tabun. http://www.bt.cdc.gov/agent/tabun/basics/facts.asp. Accessed January 8, 2004.
11. Virginia Department of Emergency Management: Terrorist information: the facts–how to prepare, how to respond. http://www.vaemergency.com/prepare/terrorismtoolkit/terrguide/weapons/incendiary.htm. Accessed November 9, 2004.
12. Homeland Security Act of 2002 (HR 5005), Nov 25, 2002.
13. US Department of Homeland Security: Homeland Security Advisory System. http://www.dhs.gov/dhspublic/display?theme=29. Accessed January 20, 2004.
14. US Department of Homeland Security, Office of Domestic Preparedness: *Emergency responder guidelines,* Washington, DC, Aug 2002, The Office.

APPENDIX

Personal Protective Equipment for Chemical, Biological, Radiological, and Nuclear Agents

Recent terrorist events in the United States underscore the importance of emergency response procedures for dealing with terrorist-related events involving chemical, biological, radiological, or nuclear (CBRN) agents. OSHA [Occupational Safety and Health Administration] and NIOSH [National Institute of Occupational Safety and Health] continue to work with other Federal response agencies to provide accurate, current information to help prepare these on-scene responders.

PERSONAL PROTECTIVE EQUIPMENT FOR CBRN RESPONSE

Emergency response to hazardous substance releases including CBRN are guided under OSHA's *Hazardous Waste Operations and Emergency Response (HAZWOPER) Standard (29 CFR 1910.120[q])*. Personal protective equipment is selected to meet the requirements of this standard and Subpart I. NIOSH has developed a *respiratory protection approval specifically for CBRN exposures,* and the Department of Homeland Security also provides *guidelines* of appropriate personal protective equipment.

SITE CONTROL

The OSHA zones of Red, Yellow, and Green described next are available to be used by incident commanders as complementary guidance for personal protective equipment selection based on the level of knowledge about the [weapons of mass destruction] WMD events. The use of the Red, Yellow, and Green zones is not mandatory nor exclusionary of other site control concepts. It is intended to offer flexibility to an incident commander managing a large WMD event within the limitations of current first responder monitoring capabilities.

RED ZONE: Areas where significant contamination with chemical, biological, radiological, or nuclear agents has been confirmed or is strongly suspected, but the area has not been characterized. The area is presumed to be life threatening from both skin contact and inhalation.

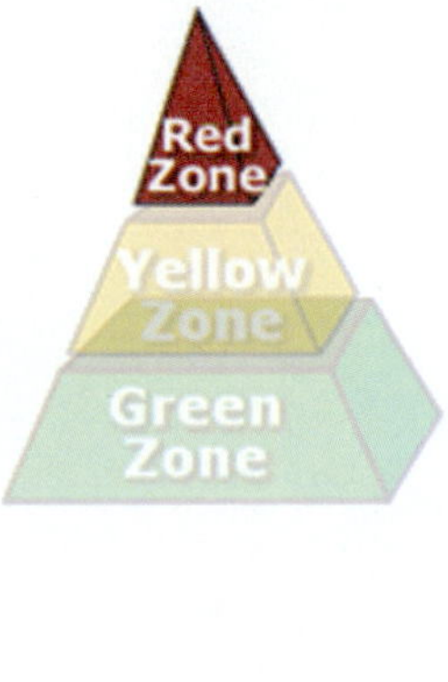

Level A protection is generally needed when the active release is still occurring or the release has stopped but there is no information about the duration of the release or the airborne concentrations of CBRN agents. Respirators chosen initially for responders going into a known release area where CBRN are suspected should be a positive-pressure self-contained breathing apparatus (SCBA) with a fully encapsulating protective suit until monitoring results allow for other decisions. Level A protection should be consistent with the description in *HAZWOPER Appendix B,* and suits should be appropriate for CBRN agents; for example, meets the requirements of *NFPA 1994-2001*, has been tested by a third party such as the U.S. Army and Soldier and Biological Chemical Command (SBCCOM), or has undergone other manufacturer testing. A *NIOSH-certified CBRN SCBA respirator* should be used, if available. Other prudent work practices should include minimizing exposure time to that essential for lifesaving or initial monitoring, avoiding any unnecessary contact with surfaces or potentially contaminated material, use of natural ventilation flows to reduce exposure, mandatory decontamination, and postexit evaluation for signs and symptoms of exposure.

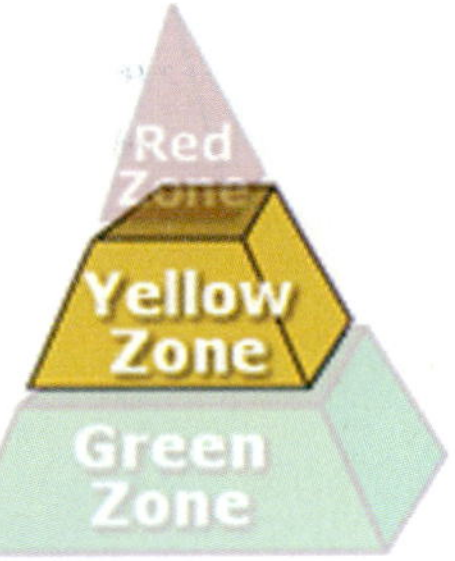

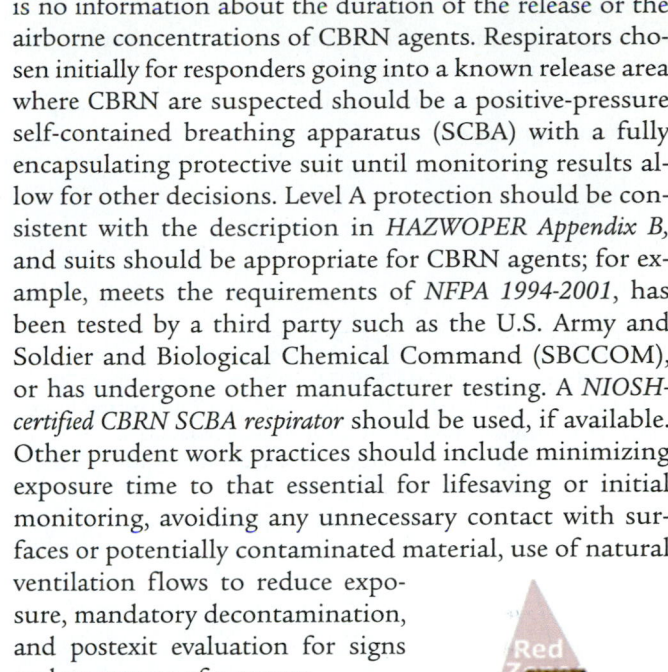

YELLOW ZONE: Areas where contamination with chemical, biological, radiological, or nuclear agents is possible, but active release has ended and initial monitoring exists.

Areas in proximity to the release area or that are known to be contaminated and certain job activities on the periphery of the event area should be considered for this zone. Risk factors that should be considered include determining the relative risk for job activities from inhalation based on available air monitoring results, skin contact and absorption potential, proximity to the event, and wind directions. Refer to the specific hazard information [see Web page] to select personal protective equipment and limited work durations to reduce exposure to safe levels. Use prudent work practices listed for red zone exposures.

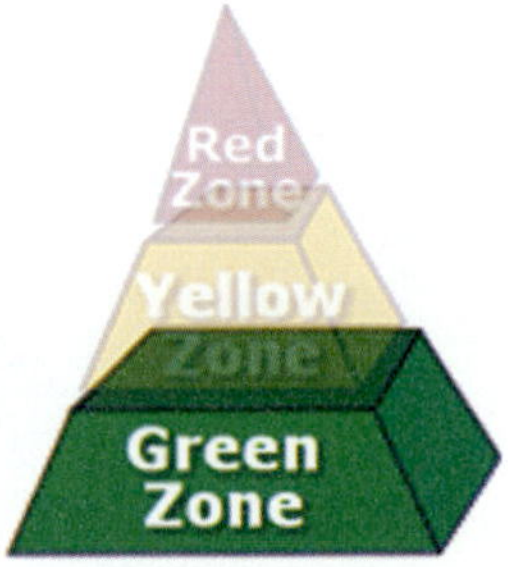

GREEN ZONE: Areas where contamination with chemical, biological, radiological, or nuclear agents is unlikely. This zone covers the area beyond the expected significant dispersal range of the initial event and secondary contamination range caused by traffic and emergency responders.

Even in areas which are not thought to pose a hazard, there may be a concern or potential for a minimal level of transient or unknown exposures in the aftermath of an event. The following suggestions for prudent work practices may reduce the amount of concern regarding this potential:

- Inform people of location of event and control zones.
- Provide information regarding signs and symptoms of exposure.
- Suggest a means for reporting suspected exposures.
- Suggest attention to general hygiene practices.
- Provide information on voluntary use of personal protective equipment.

Modified from US Department of Labor, Occupational Safety and Health Administration: OSHA/NIOSH interim guidance–August 30, 2004: chemical–biological–radiological–nuclear (CBRN) personal protective equipment selection matrix for emergency responders. http://www.osha.gov/SLTC/emergencypreparedness/cbrnmatrix/index.html. Accessed November 9, 2004.

EMERGENCY DRUG INDEX

Activated charcoal
Adenosine
Albuterol
Amiodarone
Amrinone
Amyl nitrite
Aspirin
Atenolol
Atropine sulfate
Calcium chloride
Dexamethasone
Dextrose 50%
Diazepam
Digoxin
Diltiazem
Diphenhydramine
Dobutamine
Dopamine
Epinephrine
Epinephrine racemic
Etomidate
Fentanyl
Flumazenil
Furosemide
Glucagon
Haloperidol lactate
Heparin sodium
Hydralazine
Hydroxyzine
Ibutilide
Insulin
Ipratropium
Isoproterenol
Ketamine
Ketorolac tromethamine
Labetalol
Lidocaine
Lorazepam
Magnesium sulfate
Mannitol
Meperidine
Metaproterenol
Methylprednisolone
Metoprolol
Midazolam hydrochloride
Morphine sulfate
Nalmefene
Naloxone
Nitroglycerin
Nitropaste
Nitrous oxide:oxygen
Norepinephrine
Oxygen
Oxytocin
Pancuronium
Phenytoin
Pralidoxime
Procainamide
Promethazine
Propranolol
Reteplase
Sodium bicarbonate
Streptokinase
Succinylcholine
Syrup of ipecac
Tetracaine
Thiamine
Tissue plasminogen activator
Vasopressin
Verapamil

DRUG IDENTIFICATION GUIDE

The *Emergency Drug Index* is a list of commonly prescribed medications that are used in prehospital care; it is not intended to be a complete guide to all emergency medications. For additional drug information, consult other standard references or pharmacology textbooks. Drugs included in this index are listed alphabetically by generic name. The trade name(s) are shown in parentheses following the generic listing.

PREGNANCY CATEGORY RATINGS FOR DRUGS

Drugs have been categorized by the Food and Drug Administration according to the level of risk to the fetus. These categories are listed for each drug herein under Pregnancy Safety and are interpreted as follows:

Category A: Controlled studies in women fail to demonstrate a risk to the fetus in the first trimester, and there is no evidence of risk in later trimesters; the possibility of fetal harm appears to be remote.

Category B: Either (1) animal reproductive studies have not demonstrated a fetal risk but there are no controlled studies in pregnant women or (2) animal reproductive studies have shown an adverse effect (other than decreased fertility) that was not confirmed in controlled studies on women in the first trimester and there is no evidence of risk in later trimesters.

Category C: Either (1) studies in animals have revealed adverse effects on the fetus and there are no controlled studies in women or (2) studies in women and animals are not available. Drugs in this category should be given only if the potential benefit justifies the risk to the fetus.

Category D: Positive evidence of human fetal risk exists, but the benefits for pregnant women may be acceptable despite the risk, as in life-threatening diseases for which safer drugs cannot be used or are ineffective. An appropriate statement must appear in the "Warnings" section of the labeling of drugs in this category.

Category X: Studies in animals or human beings have demonstrated fetal abnormalities, there is evidence of fetal risk based on human experience, or both; the risk of using the drug in pregnant women clearly outweighs any possible benefit. The drug is contraindicated in women who are or may become pregnant. An appropriate statement must appear in the "Contraindications" section of the labeling of drugs in this category.

ACTIVATED CHARCOAL (AQUA, ACTIDOSE, LIQUI-CHAR)

CLASS

Adsorbent, antidote

DESCRIPTION

Activated charcoal is a fine black powder that binds and adsorbs ingested toxins. Once the drug binds to the activated charcoal, the combined complex is excreted in the feces.

ONSET AND DURATION

Onset: Immediate
Duration: Continual while in gastrointestinal tract; reaches equilibrium once saturated.

INDICATIONS

Many oral poisonings and medication overdoses

CONTRAINDICATIONS

Corrosives, caustics, petroleum distillates (relatively ineffective and may induce vomiting)

ADVERSE REACTIONS

May indirectly induce nausea and vomiting
May cause constipation or mild, transient diarrhea

DRUG INTERACTIONS

Syrup of ipecac (adsorbed by activated charcoal and will result in vomiting of the charcoal)

HOW SUPPLIED

25 g (black powder)/125-mL bottle (200 mg/mL)
50 g (black powder)/250-mL bottle (200 mg/mL)

Other sizes include 15 g and 30 g, bottles and squeeze tubes. Most products come premixed (not powder) with water (aqueous preparations) or with sorbitol, a cathartic.

DOSAGE AND ADMINISTRATION

From 1 to 2 g/kg body mass (larger amounts if food is also present), prepared in a slurry and administered PO or slowly via nasogastric or orogastric tube
Adult: 30-100 g
Pediatric (1-12 yr): 15-30 g
Infant (less than 1 yr): 1 g/kg

SPECIAL CONSIDERATIONS

Pregnancy safety: Category C
Charcoal frequently is administered to pregnant patients, and the potential benefit versus risk is very high. Because charcoal remains within the gastrointestinal tract, its risk to the fetus virtually is eliminated, unless the charcoal and other stomach contents are aspirated.
Activated charcoal also may be known as "AC."
Activated charcoal is relatively insoluble in water.
Activated charcoal may blacken feces.
Activated charcoal must be stored in a closed container.
Different charcoal preparations may have varying adsorptive capacity.
Activated charcoal does not adsorb all drugs and toxic substances (e.g., phenobarbital, aspirin, cyanide, lithium, iron, lead, and arsenic).

ADENOSINE (ADENOCARD)

CLASS

Endogenous nucleoside, miscellaneous antidysrhythmic

DESCRIPTION

Adenosine primarily is formed from the breakdown of adenosine triphosphate. Adenosine triphosphate and adenosine are found in every cell of the human body and have a wide range of metabolic roles. Adenosine slows supraventricular tachycardias by decreasing electrical conduction through the atrioventricular node without causing negative inotropic effects. It also acts directly on sinus pacemaker cells and vagal nerve terminals to decrease chronotropic (heart rate) activity. Adenosine is recommended as the drug of choice for paroxysmal supraventricular tachycardia and can be used diagnostically for stable, wide-complex tachycardias of unknown type, following two doses of lidocaine.

ONSET AND DURATION

Onset: Immediate
Duration: 10 sec

INDICATIONS

First drug for most forms of narrow-complex paroxysmal supraventricular tachycardia and dysrhythmias associated with bypass tracts such as Wolff-Parkinson-White syndrome in adults and pediatric patients.

CONTRAINDICATIONS

Second- or third-degree atrioventricular block, or sick sinus syndrome

Hypersensitivity to adenosine
Atrial flutter, atrial fibrillation, ventricular tachycardia (Adenosine is not effective in converting these rhythms to sinus rhythm.)

ADVERSE REACTIONS

Light-headedness
Paresthesias
Headache
Diaphoresis
Palpitations
Chest pain
Hypotension
Shortness of breath
Transient periods of sinus bradycardia, sinus pause, or bradyasystole
Ventricular ectopy (fibrillation, flutter, tachycardia, torsades de pointes)
Nausea
Metallic taste

DRUG INTERACTIONS

Methylxanthines (e.g., caffeine and theophylline) antagonize the action of adenosine.
Dipyridamole potentiates the effect of adenosine; reduction of adenosine dose may be required.
Carbamazepine may potentiate the atrioventricular-nodal blocking effect of adenosine.

HOW SUPPLIED

Parenteral for IV injection
3 mg/mL in 2-mL and 5-mL flip-top vials

DOSAGE AND ADMINISTRATION

Adult:
Initial dose: 6-mg rapid IV bolus over 1-3 sec, followed by a 20-mL saline flush; elevate extremity
Repeat dose: If no response is observed after 1-2 min, administer a 12-mg repeat dose in the same manner; may repeat once in 1-2 min (max single dose: 12 mg)
Pediatric: Initial dose 0.1 mg/kg; may be doubled once (max first dose: 6 mg); rapid IV bolus, followed by a 5-mL saline flush

SPECIAL CONSIDERATIONS

Pregnancy safety: Category C
Place patient in mild reverse Trendelenburg position before drug administration.
A brief period of asystole (up to 15 sec) following conversion, followed by resumption of normal sinus rhythm, is common after rapid administration.
Patients taking theophylline may require larger doses of adenosine; cardiac transplant recipients may require only a small dose.
Adenosine may produce bronchoconstriction in patients with asthma and in patients with bronchopulmonary disease.
Monitor electrocardiogram during administration.

ALBUTEROL (PROVENTIL AND OTHERS)

CLASS

Sympathomimetic, bronchodilator, $beta_2$-agonist

DESCRIPTION

Albuterol is a sympathomimetic that is selective for $beta_2$-adrenergic receptors. It relaxes smooth muscles of the bronchial tree and peripheral vasculature by stimulating adrenergic receptors of the sympathetic nervous system.

ONSET AND DURATION

Onset: 5-15 min after inhalation
Duration: 3-4 hr after inhalation

INDICATIONS

Relief of bronchospasm in patients with reversible obstructive airway disease
Prevention of exercise-induced bronchospasm

CONTRAINDICATIONS

Prior hypersensitivity reaction to albuterol
Cardiac dysrhythmias associated with tachycardia

ADVERSE REACTIONS

Usually dose related
Restlessness, apprehension
Dizziness
Palpitations, tachycardia
Dysrhythmias

DRUG INTERACTIONS

Other sympathomimetics may exacerbate adverse cardiovascular effects.
Antidepressants may potentiate effects on the vasculature (vasodilation).
Beta-blockers may antagonize albuterol.
Albuterol may potentiate diuretic-induced hypokalemia.

HOW SUPPLIED

Metered dose inhaler: 90 mcg/metered spray (17-g canister with 200 inhalations)
Solution for aerosolization: 0.5% (5 mg/mL); 0.083% (2.5 mg) in 3-mL unit dose/nebulizer

DOSAGE AND ADMINISTRATION

Bronchial asthma
Adult:
Metered dose inhaler: 1-2 inhalations (90-180 mcg) q 4-6 hr (wait 5 min between inhalations); max 12 inhalations/day
Solution: 2.5 mg (0.5 mL of 0.5% solution) diluted to 3 mL with 0.9% NS (0.083% solution); administer over 5-15 min; 3-4 times/day by nebulizer
Note: In settings of severe asthma exacerbation, 4 inhalations or 5 mg in 2.5-3 mL is indicated.

Pediatric:
Metered dose inhaler: Same as for adult
Solution: 0.01-0.03 mL (0.05-0.15 mg)/kg/dose to max of 0.50 mL/dose diluted in 2 mL of 0.9% NS; may be repeated q 20 min 3 times

SPECIAL CONSIDERATIONS

Pregnancy safety: Category C
Albuterol may precipitate angina pectoris and dysrhythmias.
Albuterol should be used with caution in patients with diabetes mellitus, hyperthyroidism, prostatic hypertrophy, seizure disorder, or cardiovascular disorder.
In prehospital emergency care, albuterol should be administered only via inhalation.

AMIODARONE (CORDARONE)

CLASS

Class III antidysrhythmic

DESCRIPTION

Amiodarone is a unique antidysrhythmic agent with multiple mechanisms of action. The drug prolongs duration of the action potential and effective refractory period, and when given short-term IV, probably includes noncompetitive beta-adrenoreceptor and calcium channel blocker activity.

ONSET AND DURATION

Onset: Within minutes
Duration: Variable

INDICATIONS (IV USE)

Initial treatment and prophylaxis of frequently recurring ventricular fibrillation and hemodynamically unstable ventricular tachycardia in patients refractory to other therapy.
Refractory paroxysmal supraventricular tachycardia in conjunction with electrical cardioversion

CONTRAINDICATIONS

Pulmonary congestion
Cardiogenic shock
Hypotension
Sensitivity to amiodarone
Bradycardia

ADVERSE REACTIONS

Hypotension
Headache
Dizziness
Bradycardia
Atrioventricular conduction abnormalities
Flushing
Abnormal salivation

DRUG INTERACTIONS

May potentiate bradycardia and hypotension with beta-blocker and calcium channel blockers
May increase risk of atrioventricular block and hypotension with calcium channel blockers
May increase anticoagulant effects of warfarin
May decrease metabolism and increase serum levels of phenytoin, procainamide, quinidine, and theophyllines
Routine use in combination with drugs that prolong the Q-T interval is not recommended
Y-site incompatibilities with furosemide, heparin, and sodium bicarbonate

HOW SUPPLIED

50-mg/mL vials

DOSAGE AND ADMINISTRATION

Adult:
Pulseless arrest: 300 mg IV push (diluted in 20-30 mL of NS or D_5W. Consider repeating 150 mg IV push in 3-5 min (max cumulative dose: 2.2 g IV/24 hr)
Wide-complex tachycardia: May be given as rapid infusion 150 mg IV over first 10 min (15 mg/min) repeated every 10 min as needed; or by slow infusion 360 mg IV over 6 hr (1 mg/min). Maintenance infusion: 540 mg IV over 18 hr (0.5 mg/min)
Pediatric:
Pulseless arrest: 5 mg/kg rapid IV bolus
Perfusing tachycardias: Loading dose 5 mg/kg IV/IO over 20-60 min (max dose: 15 mg/kg/day IV)

SPECIAL CONSIDERATIONS

Pregnancy safety: Category D
Continuous electrocardiogram monitoring is required.
Slow infusion or discontinue if bradycardia or atrioventricular block occurs.
Maintain at room temperature and protect from excessive heat.

AMRINONE (INOCOR)

CLASS

Inotropic, vasodilator

DESCRIPTION

Amrinone is a rapid-acting inotropic agent that increases cardiac output after IV administration. Amrinone is a phosphodiesterase (class III) inhibitor that increases myocardial contractility and produces systemic vasodilation without stimulating alpha- or beta-adrenergic receptors.

ONSET AND DURATION

Onset: Less than 15 min IV
Duration: $4\frac{1}{2}$ hr

INDICATIONS

Severe congestive heart failure refractory to diuretics, vasodilators, and conventional inotropic agents

CONTRAINDICATIONS

Hypotension
Idiopathic hypertrophic subaortic stenosis
Hypersensitivity to amrinone or bisulfite
Valvular obstructive disease

ADVERSE REACTIONS

Tachydysrhythmias
Increase in myocardial ischemia
Hypotension
Thrombocytopenia (dose related)
Fever, flulike symptoms
Increase in liver enzyme levels

DRUG INTERACTIONS

Hypotension may develop when amrinone is used with agents with negative inotropic or vasodilatory effects.
Amrinone potentiates inotropic, chronotropic, and arrhythmogenic response to catecholamine and theophylline.
Amrinone is incompatible with furosemide.

HOW SUPPLIED

5 mg/mL (20-mL ampules)

DOSAGE AND ADMINISTRATION

Adult: 0.75 mg/kg IV given over 2-3 min; follow with infusion of 5-15 mcg/kg/min titrated to clinical response.
Pediatric: 0.75-1 mg/kg IV/IO over 5 min; may repeat twice (max 3 mg/kg); follow with infusion 5-10 mcg/kg/min

SPECIAL CONSIDERATIONS

Pregnancy safety: Category D
Do not mix with dextrose solutions or other drugs.
Optimal use requires hemodynamic monitoring.

AMYL NITRITE

CLASS

Coronary vasodilator

DESCRIPTION

Amyl nitrite is related chemically to nitroglycerin and has been used for many years to treat angina pectoris. Amyl nitrite is also effective in the emergency management of cyanide poisoning by causing the oxidation of hemoglobin to the compound methemoglobin. Cyanide preferentially binds methemoglobin, thus freeing hemoglobin to react with oxygen.

ONSET AND DURATION

Onset: 30 sec inhaled
Duration: 3-20 min

INDICATIONS

Cyanide poisoning (only until sodium nitrate can be given IV)

CONTRAINDICATIONS

None when used for cyanide poisoning
Severe anemia
Hypersensitivity to nitrates

ADVERSE REACTIONS

Hypotension
Tachycardia
Palpitations
Syncope
Headache
Nausea

DRUG INTERACTIONS

None significant
Alcohol can increase toxicity.

HOW SUPPLIED

0.3 mL/glass ampule (capsule covered with woven gauze)

DOSAGE AND ADMINISTRATION

Adult: Glass ampule should be broken (crush ampule and hold under patient's nostrils) and inhaled for 30-60 sec; may be repeated as necessary; one to six inhalations from one ampule usually is sufficient
Pediatric: Same as adult

SPECIAL CONSIDERATIONS

Pregnancy safety: Category X
Amyl nitrite frequently is abused (claimed to be an aphrodisiac).
The drug also is known as "amy."
Cyanide poisoning often produces a bitter almond breath odor (not all persons can detect the odor).
Patient should be supine during administration, and blood pressure should be monitored.

ASPIRIN (A.S.A., BAYER, ECOTRIN, ST. JOSEPH, OTHERS)

CLASS

Analgesic, antiinflammatory, antipyretic, antiplatelet

DESCRIPTION

Aspirin decreases inflammation, blocks pain impulses in the central nervous system, dilates peripheral vessels, and decreases platelet aggregation. The use of aspirin is strongly recommended for all patients with acute myocardial infarction.

ONSET AND DURATION

Onset: 15-30 min
Duration: 4-6 hr

INDICATIONS

Mild to moderate pain or fever
Prevention of platelet aggregation in ischemia and thromboembolism
Unstable angina
Prevention of myocardial infarction or reinfarction

CONTRAINDICATIONS

Hypersensitivity to salicylates
Gastrointestinal bleeding
Active ulcer disease
Hemorrhagic stroke
Bleeding disorders
Children with flulike symptoms

ADVERSE REACTIONS

Stomach irritation
Heartburn or indigestion
Nausea or vomiting
Allergic reaction

DRUG INTERACTIONS

Decreased effects with antacids and steroids
Increased effects with anticoagulants, insulin, oral hypoglycemics, fibrinolytic agents

HOW SUPPLIED

Tablets (65, 81, 325, 500, 650, 975 mg)
Capsules (325, 500 mg)
Controlled-release tablets (800 mg)
Suppositories (varies from 60 mg to 1.2 g)

DOSAGE AND ADMINISTRATION

Adult:
Mild pain and fever: 325-650 mg PO q 4 hr
Myocardial infarction: 160-325 mg PO (chewing is preferable to swallowing)
Pediatric (over 12 years of age): Mild pain and fever—40-100 mg/kg/day in divided doses

SPECIAL CONSIDERATIONS

Pregnancy safety: Category D
Should be given as soon as possible to the patient with acute myocardial infarction

ATENOLOL (TENORMIN)

CLASS

Beta-blocking agent

DESCRIPTION

Atenolol competes with beta-adrenergic agonists for available beta receptor sites on the membranes of cardiac muscle, bronchial smooth muscle, and the smooth muscle of blood vessels. The $beta_1$ blocking action on the heart decreases heart rate, conduction velocity, myocardial contractility, and cardiac output. Atenolol is used to control ventricular response in supraventricular tachydysrhythmias (paroxysmal supraventricular tachycardia, atrial fibrillation, atrial flutter). Atenolol is considered a second-line agent after adenosine, diltiazem, or digitalis derivative.

ONSET AND DURATION

Onset: Within 10 min
Duration: 2-4 hr

INDICATIONS

Paroxysmal supraventricular tachycardia
Atrial flutter
Atrial fibrillation
To reduce myocardial ischemia and damage in acute myocardial infarction patients

CONTRAINDICATIONS

Heart failure
Cardiogenic shock
Bradycardia
Lung disease associated with bronchospasm
Hypersensitivity to atenolol
Hypotension
Second- or third-degree heart block

ADVERSE REACTIONS

Bradycardia
Atrioventricular conduction delays
Hypotension

DRUG INTERACTIONS

Atenolol may potentiate antihypertensive effects when given to patients taking calcium channel blockers or MAO inhibitors; catecholamine-depleting drugs may potentiate hypotension; sympathomimetic effects may be antagonized; signs of hypoglycemia may be masked.

HOW SUPPLIED

5 mg in 10-mL ampules

DOSAGE AND ADMINISTRATION

Adult: 5 mg slow IV (over 5 min); wait 10 min and then give second dose of 5 mg over 5 min
Pediatric: Not recommended

SPECIAL CONSIDERATIONS

Pregnancy safety: Category C
Atenolol must be given slowly IV over 5 min.
Concurrent IV administration with IV calcium channel blockers such as verapamil or diltiazem can cause severe hypotension.
Atenolol should be used with caution in persons with liver or renal dysfunction.

ATROPINE SULFATE (ATROPINE AND OTHERS)

CLASS

Anticholinergic agent

DESCRIPTION

Atropine sulfate (a potent parasympatholytic) inhibits actions of acetylcholine at postganglionic parasympathetic (primarily muscarinic) receptor sites. Small doses inhibit salivary and bronchial secretions; moderate doses dilate pupils and increase heart rate. Large doses decrease gastrointestinal motility, inhibit gastric acid secretion, and may block nicotinic receptor sites at the autonomic ganglia and at the neuromuscular junction. Blocked vagal effects result in increased heart rate and enhanced atrioventricular conduction with limited or no inotropic effect. In emergency care, atropine primarily is used to increase the heart rate in life-threatening or symptomatic bradycardia and to antagonize excess muscarinic receptor stimulation caused by organophosphate insecticides or chemical nerve agents (e.g., sarin and soman).

ONSET AND DURATION

Onset: Rapid
Duration: 2-6 hr

INDICATIONS

Hemodynamically significant bradycardia
Asystole
Pulseless electrical activity with absolute bradycardia
Organophosphate or nerve gas poisoning

CONTRAINDICATIONS

Tachycardia
Hypersensitivity to atropine
Obstructive disease of gastrointestinal tract
Obstructive uropathy
Unstable cardiovascular status in acute hemorrhage with myocardial ischemia
Narrow-angle glaucoma
Thyrotoxicosis

ADVERSE REACTIONS

Tachycardia
Paradoxical bradycardia when pushed too slowly or when used at doses less than 0.5 mg
Palpitations
Dysrhythmias
Headache
Dizziness
Anticholinergic effects (dry mouth/nose/skin, photophobia, blurred vision, urinary retention, constipation)
Nausea and vomiting
Flushed, hot, dry skin
Allergic reactions

DRUG INTERACTIONS

Use with other anticholinergic agents may increase vagal blockade.
Potential adverse effects may occur when administered with digitalis, cholinergics, neostigmine.
The effects of atropine may be enhanced by antihistamines, procainamide, quinidine, antipsychotics and antidepressants, and thiazides.
Increased toxicity: Amantadine

HOW SUPPLIED

Parenteral: There are various injection preparations.
In emergency care, atropine usually is supplied in prefilled syringes containing 1 mg in 10 mL of solution.

DOSAGE AND ADMINISTRATION

Bradydysrhythmias
Adult: 0.5-1 mg IV; every 3-5 min for desired response (max total dose: 0.04 mg/kg)
Pediatric: 0.02 mg/kg IV/IO/endotracheal tube (diluted to 3-5 mL); min dose: 0.1 mg; max single dose of 0.5 mg for a child and 1 mg for an adolescent; may be repeated in 5 min for a max total dose of 1 mg for a child and 2 mg for an adolescent
Asystole or Pulseless Electrical Activity
Adult: 1 mg IV, endotracheal tube (2-3 mg diluted to a total of 10 mL of NS); may be repeated every 3-5 min (max: 0.03-0.04 mg/kg)
Pediatric: Efficacy has not been established.
Anticholinesterase Poisoning
Adult: 1-2 mg IV push every 5-15 min until atropine effects are observed; then every 1-4 hr for at least 24 hr
Pediatric: 0.02-0.05 mg/kg/dose (usual dose 1-5 mg) IV; may be repeated every 10-20 min until atropine effect is observed; then 1-4 hr for at least 24 hr

SPECIAL CONSIDERATIONS

Pregnancy safety: Category C
Follow endotracheal tube administration with several positive-pressure ventilations.
Atropine causes pupillary dilation, rendering the pupils nonreactive; pupil response may not be useful in monitoring central nervous system status.

CALCIUM CHLORIDE

CLASS

Electrolyte

DESCRIPTION

Calcium is an essential component for functional integrity of the nervous and muscular systems, for normal cardiac contractility, and the coagulation of blood. Calcium chloride contains 27.2% elemental calcium. Calcium chloride is a hypertonic solution and should be administered only IV (slowly, not exceeding 1 mL/min).

ONSET AND DURATION

Onset: 5-15 min
Duration: Dose dependent (effects may persist for 4 hr after IV administration)

INDICATIONS

Hyperkalemia (except when associated with digitalis toxicity)
Hypocalcemia (e.g., after multiple blood transfusions)
Calcium channel blocker toxicity
Hypermagnesemia
To prevent hypotensive effects of calcium channel blocking agents (IV verapamil and diltiazem)

CONTRAINDICATIONS

Ventricular fibrillation during cardiac resuscitation
In patients with digitalis toxicity
Hypercalcemia
Renal or cardiac disease

ADVERSE REACTIONS

Bradycardia (may cause asystole)
Hypotension
Metallic taste
Severe local necrosis and sloughing following intramuscular use or IV infiltration

DRUG INTERACTIONS

Calcium may worsen dysrhythmias caused by digitalis
Calcium may antagonize the peripheral vasodilatory effects of calcium channel blockers.

HOW SUPPLIED

10% solution in 10 mL (100 mg/mL) ampules, vials, and prefilled syringes

DOSAGE AND ADMINISTRATION

Hyperkalemia, Hypocalcemia, Hypermagnesemia, and Calcium Channel Blocker Overdose
Adult: 8-16 mg/kg (usually 5-10 mL) of 10% solution slow IV; may be repeated in 10 minutes if needed
Pediatric: 20 mg/kg (0.2 mL/kg) of 10% solution IV/IO push; may repeat in 10 minutes for documented conditions

SPECIAL CONSIDERATIONS

Pregnancy safety: Category C
Calcium may produce vasospasm in coronary and cerebral arteries.
Do not use routinely in cardiac arrest.
Hypertension and bradycardia may occur with rapid administration.
Monitor heart rate during administration.

NOTE It is important to flush IV line between administration of calcium chloride and sodium bicarbonate to avoid precipitation.

DEXAMETHASONE (DECADRON, HEXADROL, AND OTHERS)

CLASS

Glucocorticoid

DESCRIPTION

Dexamethasone is a synthetic steroid that is related chemically to the natural hormones secreted by the adrenal cortex. The drug suppresses acute and chronic inflammation, potentiates the relaxation of vascular and bronchial smooth muscle by beta-adrenergic agonists, and possibly alters airway hyperreactivity. In emergency care, dexamethasone generally is used in the treatment of allergic reactions and asthma and to reduce swelling in the central nervous system.

ONSET AND DURATION

Onset: 4-8 hr after parenteral administration
Duration: 24-72 hr

INDICATIONS

Endocrine, rheumatic, hematological disorders
Allergic states
Septic shock
Chronic inflammation

CONTRAINDICATIONS

Hypersensitivity to the product
Active untreated infections (relative)

ADVERSE REACTIONS

Decreased wound healing
Hypertension
Gastrointestinal bleeding
Hyperglycemia

DRUG INTERACTIONS

Barbiturates and phenytoin can decrease dexamethasone effects.

HOW SUPPLIED

Common preparations used in emergency care are for IV administration and are as follows:
4 mg/mL in 1-, 5-, 10-, 25-, 30-mL vials
10 mg/mL in 10-mL vials, 1-mL syringe, 1-mL ampule
20 mg/mL in 5-mL vials (IV or IM), 5-mL syringe (IV)
24 mg/mL (IV only) in 5- and 10-mL vials

DOSAGE AND ADMINISTRATION

Adult: There is considerable variance in recommended dexamethasone doses. The usual range in emergency care is 4-24 mg IV. Some physicians may prefer significantly higher doses (up to 100 mg) for unusual indications.
Pediatric: 0.25-0.5 mg/kg/dose IV/IO

SPECIAL CONSIDERATIONS

Pregnancy safety: Category C. Dexamethasone crosses the placenta and may cause fetal damage.
Medication should be protected from heat.
Because of onset of action (4-8 hr), dexamethasone should not be considered a first-line medication for allergic reactions.

DEXTROSE 50%

CLASS

Carbohydrate, hypertonic solution

DESCRIPTION

The term *dextrose* is used to describe the six-carbon sugar *d-glucose,* the principal form of carbohydrate used by the body. 50% dextrose solution is used in emergency care to treat hypoglycemia and in the management of coma of unknown origin.

ONSET AND DURATION

Onset: 1 min
Duration: Depends on the degree of hypoglycemia

INDICATIONS

Hypoglycemia
Altered level of consciousness
Coma of unknown origin
Seizure of unknown origin

CONTRAINDICATIONS

Intracranial hemorrhage
Increased intracranial pressure
Known or suspected cerebral vascular accident in the absence of hypoglycemia

ADVERSE REACTIONS

Warmth, pain, burning from medication infusion, hyperglycemia, thrombophlebitis

DRUG INTERACTIONS

None significant

HOW SUPPLIED

25 g/50 mL prefilled syringe (500 mg/mL)

DOSAGE AND ADMINISTRATION

Adult: 12.5-25 g slow IV; may be repeated once
Pediatric: 0.5-1 g/kg IV/IO
1-2 mL/kg 50%
2-4 mL/kg 25%
5-10 mL/kg 10%

SPECIAL CONSIDERATIONS

Pregnancy safety: Category C
Draw blood sample before administration if possible.
Perform blood glucose analysis before administration if possible.
Extravasation may cause tissue necrosis; use large vein and aspirate occasionally to ensure route patency.
50% dextrose solution sometimes may precipitate severe neurological symptoms (Wernicke's encephalopathy) in thiamine-deficient patients—for example, alcoholics. (This can be prevented by administering 100 mg of thiamine IV.)

DIAZEPAM (VALIUM AND OTHERS)

CLASS

Benzodiazepine

DESCRIPTION

Diazepam is a frequently prescribed medication to treat anxiety and stress. In emergency care, diazepam is used to treat alcohol withdrawal and grand mal seizure activity. Diazepam acts on the limbic, thalamic, and hypothalamic regions of the central nervous system to potentiate the effects of inhibitory neurotransmitters, raising the seizure threshold in the motor cortex. It also may be used in conscious patients during cardioversion and transcutaneous pacing to induce amnesia and sedation. Its use as an anticonvulsant may be short-lived because of rapid redistribution from the central nervous system. Rapid IV administration may be followed by respiratory depression and excessive sedation, particularly in elderly patients.

ONSET AND DURATION

Onset: (IV) 1-5 min
(IM) 15-30 min
Duration: (IV) 15 min-1 hr
(IM) 15 min-1 hr

INDICATIONS

Acute anxiety states
Acute alcohol withdrawal
Skeletal muscle relaxation
Seizure activity
Premedication before countershock or transcutaneous pacing

CONTRAINDICATIONS

Hypersensitivity to the drug
Substance abuse (use with caution)
Coma (unless the patient has seizures or severe muscle rigidity or myoclonus)
Shock
Central nervous system depression as a result of head injury
Respiratory depression

ADVERSE REACTIONS

Hypotension
Reflex tachycardia (rare)
Respiratory depression
Ataxia
Psychomotor impairment
Confusion
Nausea

DRUG INTERACTIONS

Diazepam may precipitate central nervous system depression and psychomotor impairment when the patient is taking other central nervous system depressant medications.

Diazepam should not be administered with other drugs because of possible precipitation (incompatible with most fluids; should be administered into an IV of NS solution).

HOW SUPPLIED

Parenteral: 5 mg/mL vials, ampules, Tubex

DOSAGE AND ADMINISTRATION

Seizure Activity

Adult: 5 mg over 2 min (up to 10 mg for most adults) IV q 10-15 min prn (max dose: 30 mg)

Pediatric: Dose for infants 30 days to 5 yr is 0.2 mg to 0.5 mg slow IV q 2-5 min to max 5 mg; children 5 yr or older is 1 mg q 2-5 min to max 10 mg slow IV

Premedication for Cardioversion or Transcutaneous Pacing

Adult: 5-15 mg IV, 5-10 min before procedure

SPECIAL CONSIDERATIONS

Pregnancy safety: Category D

Diazepam may cause local venous irritation.

Diazepam has short duration of anticonvulsant effect.

Reduce dose by 50% in elderly patients.

Resuscitation equipment should be readily available.

DIGOXIN (LANOXIN)

CLASS

Cardiac glycoside, miscellaneous antidysrhythmic

DESCRIPTION

Digoxin (digitalis) is a cardiac glycoside derived primarily from the foxglove plant. Its primary action involves alteration of ion transport across cardiac cell membranes. Increased intracellular calcium improves myocardial contractility. Digoxin increases vagal tone and therefore indirectly decreases sinus node rate, reduces sympathetic tone and decreases atrioventricular node conduction velocity (with an increase in atrioventricular node refractory period). Sodium pumped out of cells may cause increased automaticity.

ONSET AND DURATION

Onset: (IV) 5-30 min

Duration: 3-4 days

INDICATIONS

Supraventricular tachycardias, especially atrial flutter and atrial fibrillation

Congestive heart failure

Cardiogenic shock

CONTRAINDICATIONS

Ventricular fibrillation

Ventricular tachycardia

Atrioventricular block

Digitalis toxicity

Hypersensitivity to digoxin

Second- or third-degree heart block in the absence of artificial pacing

ADVERSE REACTIONS (MOSTLY RELATED TO DIGITALIS TOXICITY)

Headache

Weakness

Visual disturbances (blurred, yellow or green vision)

Confusion

Seizures

Dysrhythmias (virtually any disturbance, but junctional tachycardias are most common)

Nausea and vomiting

Skin rash

DRUG INTERACTIONS

Amiodarone, verapamil, and quinidine may increase serum digoxin concentrations by 50%-70%.

Concurrent administration of IV digoxin and IV verapamil may lead to severe heart block.

Erythromycin and tetracycline may increase serum digoxin concentrations by reducing hepatic breakdown.

Diuretics may potentiate digoxin cardiotoxicity via loss of potassium.

Sympathomimetics may augment the inotropic and cardiotoxic effects of digoxin.

Concomitant administration of kaolin, pectin, and antacids may reduce digoxin absorption from the gastrointestinal tract.

HOW SUPPLIED

In emergency care, the common form of digoxin is supplied in 2-mL ampules, containing 0.5 mg of the drug (0.25 mg/mL)

DOSAGE AND ADMINISTRATION

Adult: Loading dose 10-15 mcg/kg; maintenance dose affected by body size and renal function

Pediatric: Not recommended in prehospital setting

SPECIAL CONSIDERATIONS

Pregnancy safety: Category C

Patient should be monitored constantly for signs of digitalis toxicity.

Patients with myocardial infarction and/or renal failure are prone to developing digitalis toxicity.

Digitalis toxicity is potentiated in patients with hypokalemia, hypomagnesemia, and hypercalcemia.

Avoid use in patients with Wolff-Parkinson-White syndrome because of possible ventricular dysrhythmias.

DILTIAZEM (CARDIZEM) INJECTABLE

CLASS

Slow calcium channel blocker or calcium channel antagonist

DESCRIPTION

Diltiazem is a calcium channel blocking agent that slows conduction, increases refractoriness in the atrioventricular node, and causes coronary and peripheral vasodilation. The drug is used to control ventricular response rates in patients with atrial fibrillation or flutter, multifocal atrial tachycardias, and paroxysmal supraventricular tachycardia.

ONSET AND DURATION

Onset: 2-5 min
Duration: 1-3 hr

INDICATIONS

Atrial fibrillation
Atrial flutter
Multifocal atrial tachycardias
Paroxysmal supraventricular tachycardia

CONTRAINDICATIONS

Sick sinus syndrome
Second- or third-degree atrioventricular block (except with a functioning pacemaker)
Hypotension (less than 90 mm Hg)
Cardiogenic shock
Hypersensitivity to diltiazem
Atrial fibrillation or atrial flutter associated with Wolff-Parkinson-White syndrome or a short P-R interval syndrome
Concomitant use of IV beta-blockers
Ventricular tachycardia
Wide-complex tachycardia of unknown origin
Acute myocardial infarction

ADVERSE REACTIONS

Atrial flutter
First- and second-degree atrioventricular block
Bradycardia
Hypotension
Chest pain
Congestive heart failure
Peripheral edema
Syncope
Ventricular dysrhythmias
Sweating
Nausea and vomiting
Dizziness
Dry mouth
Dyspnea
Headache

DRUG INTERACTIONS

Caution is warranted in patients receiving medications that affect cardiac contractility and/or sinoatrial or atrioventricular node conduction.
Diltiazem is incompatible with simultaneous furosemide injection.

HOW SUPPLIED

25 mg (5-mL vial); 50 mg (10-mL vial)

DOSAGE AND ADMINISTRATION

Bolus injection: 0.25 mg/kg (15-20 mg for the average patient) IV over 2 min; may be repeated in 15 min (0.35 mg/kg; 20-25 mg for the average patient) IV over 2 min
Maintenance infusion: Dilute 125 mg (25 mL) in 100 mL of solution; infuse 5-15 mg/hr, titrated to heart rate
Pediatric: Safety not established

SPECIAL CONSIDERATIONS

Pregnancy safety: Category C
Use with caution in patients with impaired renal or hepatic function.
Hypotension occasionally may result (carefully monitor vital signs).
Premature ventricular contractions may be present on conversion of paroxysmal supraventricular tachycardia to sinus rhythm.
Shelf-life at room temperature is 1 month.

DIPHENHYDRAMINE (BENADRYL)

CLASS

Antihistamine

DESCRIPTION

Antihistamines prevent the physiological actions of histamine by blocking H_1 (e.g., diphenhydramine and cimetidine) and H_2 (e.g., cimetidine, ranitidine, and famotipine) receptor sites. Antihistamines are indicated for conditions in which histamine excess is present (e.g., acute urticaria) and are used as adjunctive therapy (with epinephrine, for example) in the treatment of anaphylactic shock. Antihistamines also are effective in the treatment of certain extrapyramidal (dystonic) reactions and for relief of upper respiratory and sinus symptoms associated with allergic reactions.

ONSET AND DURATION

Onset: Max effects 1-3 hr
Duration: 6-12 hr

INDICATIONS

Moderate to severe allergic reactions (after epinephrine)
Anaphylaxis
Acute extrapyramidal (dystonic) reactions

CONTRAINDICATIONS

Patients taking MAO inhibitors
Hypersensitivity
Narrow-angle glaucoma (relative)
Newborns and nursing mothers

ADVERSE REACTIONS

Dose-related drowsiness
Disturbed coordination
Hypotension
Palpitations
Tachycardia, bradycardia
Thickening of bronchial secretions
Dry mouth and throat
Paradoxical excitement in children

DRUG INTERACTIONS

Central nervous system depressants may increase depressant effects.
MAO inhibitors may prolong and intensify anticholinergic effects of antihistamines.

HOW SUPPLIED

Parenteral: 10 and 50 mg/mL vials, prefilled syringe

DOSAGE AND ADMINISTRATION

Adult: The standard dose of diphenhydramine is 10-50 mg IM, IV every 6-8 hr (max: 400 mg/day)
Pediatric (greater than 10 kg): 1.25 mg/kg/dose q 6 hr (max: 300 mg/day)

SPECIAL CONSIDERATIONS

Pregnancy safety: Category C
Use cautiously in patients with central nervous system depression or lower respiratory diseases such as asthma.

DOBUTAMINE (DOBUTREX)

CLASS

Sympathomimetic

DESCRIPTION

Dobutamine is a synthetic catecholamine that primarily stimulates $beta_1$-adrenergic receptors, and has much less significant effects on $beta_2$- and alpha-adrenergic receptors. The clinical effects of this drug include positive inotropic effects with minimal changes in chronotropic activity or systemic vascular resistance. For these reasons, dobutamine is useful in the management of congestive heart failure when an increase in heart rate is not desired.

ONSET AND DURATION

Onset: 1-2 min; peak after 10 min
Duration: 10-15 min

INDICATIONS

Inotropic support for patients with left ventricular dysfunction

CONTRAINDICATIONS

Tachydysrhythmias (atrial fibrillation, atrial flutter)
Severe hypotension with signs of shock
Idiopathic hypertrophic subaortic stenosis
Suspected or known drug-induced shock

ADVERSE REACTIONS

Headache
Dose-related tachydysrhythmias
Hypertension
Ventricular ectopy

DRUG INTERACTIONS

Beta-adrenergic antagonists may blunt inotropic responses.
Sympathomimetics and phosphodiesterase inhibitors may exacerbate dysrhythmia responses.
Dobutamine is incompatible with sodium bicarbonate and furosemide in same IV line; it may be given in separate IV lines.

HOW SUPPLIED

12.5 mg/mL injectable

DOSAGE AND ADMINISTRATION

Adult: Usual dose is 2-20 mcg/kg/min IV, based on inotropic effect
Pediatric: 2-20 mcg/kg/min IV/IO, titrated to desired effect

SPECIAL CONSIDERATIONS

Pregnancy safety: Category C
Administer via an infusion pump to ensure precise flow rates.
Dobutamine may be administered through a Y-site with concurrent dopamine, lidocaine, nitroprusside, and potassium chloride infusions.
Blood pressure should be monitored closely.
Increases in heart rate of more than 10% may induce or exacerbate myocardial ischemia.
Lidocaine should be readily available.
Correct hypovolemia before using dobutamine in hypotensive patients.

DOPAMINE (INTROPIN)

CLASS

Sympathomimetic

DESCRIPTION

Dopamine is related chemically to epinephrine and norepinephrine. It acts primarily on $alpha_1$- and $beta_1$-adrenergic receptors in dose-dependent fashion. At low doses, dopamine acts on dopaminergic receptors, causing renal, mesenteric, and cerebral vascular dilation. At moderate doses ("cardiac doses"), dopamine stimulates beta-adrenergic receptors, causing enhanced myocardial contractility, increased cardiac output, and a rise in blood pressure. At high doses ("vasopressor doses"), dopamine has an alpha-adrenergic effect, producing peripheral arterial and venous constriction. Dopamine commonly is used in the treatment of hypotension associated with cardiogenic shock.

ONSET AND DURATION

Onset: 2-4 min
Duration: 10-15 min

INDICATIONS

Hemodynamically significant hypotension in the absence of hypovolemia

CONTRAINDICATIONS

Tachydysrhythmias
Ventricular fibrillation
Patients with pheochromocytoma

ADVERSE REACTIONS

Dose-related tachydysrhythmias
Hypertension
Increased myocardial oxygen demand (e.g., ischemia)

DRUG INTERACTIONS

Dopamine may be deactivated by alkaline solutions (sodium bicarbonate and furosemide).
MAO inhibitors may potentiate the effect of dopamine.
Sympathomimetics and phosphodiesterase inhibitors exacerbate dysrhythmia response.
Beta-adrenergic antagonists may blunt inotropic response.
When administered with phenytoin, hypotension, bradycardia, and seizures may develop.

HOW SUPPLIED

200 mg, 400 mg, 800 mg in 5-mL prefilled syringe and ampule for IV infusion (IV piggyback)

DOSAGE AND ADMINISTRATION

Adult:
Low dose: 1-5 mcg/kg/min
Moderate dose: 5-10 mcg/kg/min (cardiac doses)
High dose: 10-20 mcg/kg/min (vasopressor doses)
Pediatric: 2-20 mcg/kg/min IV/IO, titrated to patient response (not to exceed 20 mcg/kg/min)

SPECIAL CONSIDERATIONS

Pregnancy safety: Category C
Infuse through large, stable vein to avoid the possibility of extravasation injury.
Use infusion pump to ensure precise flow rates.
Monitor patient for signs of compromised circulation.
Correct hypovolemia before using dopamine in hypotensive patients.

EPINEPHRINE (ADRENALIN)

CLASS

Sympathomimetic

DESCRIPTION

Epinephrine is an endogenous catecholamine that directly stimulates alpha-, $beta_1$-, and $beta_2$-adrenergic receptors in dose-related fashion. Epinephrine is the initial drug of choice for treating bronchoconstriction and hypotension resulting from anaphylaxis and all forms of cardiac arrest. Epinephrine is useful in the management of reactive airway disease, but beta-adrenergic agents usually are considered the drugs of choice because they are inhaled and have fewer side effects. Rapid injection produces a rapid increase in blood pressure, ventricular contractility, and heart rate. In addition, epinephrine causes vasoconstriction in the arterioles of the skin, mucosa, and splanchnic areas, and antagonizes the effects of histamine.

ONSET AND DURATION

Onset: (SQ) 5-10 min
(IV/endotracheal tube) 1-2 min
Duration: 5-10 min

INDICATIONS

Acute allergic reaction (anaphylaxis)
Cardiac arrest
Asystole
Pulseless electrical activity
Ventricular fibrillation and pulseless ventricular tachycardia unresponsive to initial defibrillation
Profound symptomatic bradycardia
Bronchial asthma

CONTRAINDICATIONS

Hypersensitivity (not an issue especially in emergencies—the dose should be lowered or given slowly in non-cardiac arrest patients with heart disease)
Hypovolemic shock (as with other catecholamines, correct hypovolemia before use)
Coronary insufficiency (use with caution)

ADVERSE REACTIONS

Headache
Nausea
Restlessness
Weakness
Dysrhythmias, including ventricular tachycardia and ventricular fibrillation
Hypertension
Precipitation of angina pectoris
Tachycardia

DRUG INTERACTIONS

MAO inhibitors may potentiate the effect of epinephrine.
Beta-adrenergic antagonists may blunt inotropic response.
Sympathomimetics and phosphodiesterase inhibitors may exacerbate dysrhythmia response.
May be deactivated by alkaline solutions (sodium bicarbonate, furosemide).

HOW SUPPLIED

Parenteral: 1 mg/mL (1:1000), 0.1 mg/mL (1:10,000) ampule and prefilled syringe
Autoinjector (EpiPen): 0.5 mg/mL (1:2000)

DOSAGE AND ADMINISTRATION

Profound Bradycardia or Hypotension
Adult: See IV infusion dose
Pediatric: 0.01 mg/kg (1:10,000, 0.1 mL/kg) IV/IO
Pulseless Arrest
Adult:
Initial: 1 mg (10 mL, 1:10,000) IV push or endotracheal tube (2-2.5 mg diluted in 10 mL of NS), repeated every 3-5 min during resuscitation (follow each IV dose with a 20-mL saline flush); higher doses (up to 0.2 mg/kg) may be used if 1-mg doses fail
Pediatric:
First dose: 0.01 mg/kg (1:10,000, 0.1 mL/kg) IV/IO or endotracheal tube (0.1-0.2 mg/kg of 1:1000 [0.1-0.2 mL/kg]).
Subsequent doses: Repeat initial dose or may increase up to 10 times (0.1 mg/kg, 1:1000, 0.1 mL/kg); administer every 3-5 min; IV/IO/endotracheal tube doses as high as 0.2 mg/kg of 1:1000 may be effective
Epinephrine infusions for pulseless arrest and symptomatic bradycardia with profound hypotension refractory to other interventions
Adult: Add 30 mg epinephrine (30 mL of 1:1000 solution) to 250 mL of NS or D_5W; run at 100 mL/hr and titrate to response
Pediatric: 0.1-1 mcg/kg/min IV/IO; calculate dose by 0.6 × body mass (kilograms) equals number of milligrams diluted to total 100 mL; then 1 mL/hr delivers 0.1 mcg/kgs/min
Anaphylactic Reaction or Bronchoconstriction
Adult: (Mild)—0.3-0.5 mL (1:1000) SQ
(Moderate to severe)—1-2 mL (1:10,000) slow IV over 5 minutes
Pediatric: (Mild)—0.01 mL/kg SQ (1:1000), max 0.3 mL
(Moderate to severe)—0.05-0.15 mcg/kg/min IV infusion

SPECIAL CONSIDERATIONS

Pregnancy safety: Category C
Do not use prefilled syringes for epinephrine infusions.
Syncope has occurred following epinephrine administration to asthmatic children.
Epinephrine may increase myocardial oxygen demand.

NOTE Complications of IV administration of epinephrine are significant and include the development of uncontrolled systolic hypertension, vomiting, seizures, dysrhythmias, and myocardial ischemia. This route should be used only in patients with a critical life-threatening condition. Intravenous administration of epinephrine rarely is performed in conscious patients. Intravenous administration is performed with extreme caution in rare circumstances and only with authorization from medical direction.

EPINEPHRINE RACEMIC (MicroNefrin)

CLASS

Sympathomimetic

DESCRIPTION

As with other forms of epinephrine, racemic epinephrine acts as a bronchodilator that stimulates $beta_2$ receptors in the lungs, resulting in relaxation of bronchial smooth muscle. This alleviates bronchospasm, increases vital capacity, and reduces airway resistance. Racemic epinephrine is also useful in treating laryngeal edema. Racemic epinephrine also inhibits the release of histamine.

ONSET AND DURATION

Onset: Within 5 min
Duration: 1-3 hr

INDICATIONS

Bronchial asthma
Treatment of bronchospasm
Croup (laryngotracheobronchitis)
Laryngeal edema

CONTRAINDICATIONS

Hypertension
Underlying cardiovascular disease
Epiglottitis

ADVERSE REACTIONS

Tachycardia
Dysrhythmias

DRUG INTERACTIONS

MAO inhibitors may potentiate the effect of epinephrine.
Beta-adrenergic antagonists may blunt the bronchodilating response.
Sympathomimetics and phosphodiesterase inhibitors may exacerbate dysrhythmia response.

HOW SUPPLIED

Metered dose inhaler: 0.16-0.25 mg/spray
Solution: 7.5, 15, 30 mL in 1%, 2.25% solution

DOSAGE AND ADMINISTRATION

Metered dose inhaler
Adult: 2-3 inhalations, repeat once in 5 min prn
Solution
Adult: Dilute 5 mL (1%) in 5 mL saline, administer over 15 min
Pediatric: Dilute 0.25 mL (0.1%) in 2.5 mL saline (if less than 20 kg); 0.5 mL in 2.5 mL saline (if 20-40 kg); 0.75 mL in 2.5 mL saline (if greater than 40 kg); administer by aerosolization

SPECIAL CONSIDERATIONS

Pregnancy safety: Category C
Racemic epinephrine may produce tachycardia and other dysrhythmias.
Monitor vital signs closely.
Excessive use may cause bronchospasm.
Rebound exacerbation of severe croup may occur following drug administration.

ETOMIDATE (AMIDATE)

CLASS

Nonbarbiturate hypnotic, anesthetic

DESCRIPTION

Etomidate is a short-acting drug that acts at the level of the reticular activating system to produce anesthesia. Etomidate may be administered for conscious sedation to relieve apprehension or impair memory before tracheal intubation or cardioversion.

ONSET AND DURATION

Onset: Within 30 sec
Duration: 3-5 min

INDICATIONS

Premedication for tracheal intubation or cardioversion

CONTRAINDICATIONS

Hypersensitivity to etomidate
Labor/delivery

ADVERSE REACTIONS

Nausea and vomiting
Dysrhythmias
Breathing difficulties
Hypotension
Hypertension
Involuntary muscle movement
Pain at injection site

DRUG INTERACTIONS

Effects may be enhanced when given with other central nervous system depressants.

HOW SUPPLIED

2 mg/mL vials

DOSAGE AND ADMINISTRATION

Adult: 0.2-0.6 mg/kg IV over 30-60 sec
Pediatric (over 10 years of age): 0.2-0.6 mg/kg over 30-60 sec

SPECIAL CONSIDERATIONS

Pregnancy safety: Category C
Carefully monitor vital signs.
Etomidate can suppress adrenal gland production of steroid hormones, which can cause temporary gland failure.

FENTANYL (SUBLIMAZE)

CLASS

Opioid analgesic

DESCRIPTION

Fentanyl (like other opioids) combines with receptor sites in the brain to produce potent analgesic effects. The drug often is given in combination with benzodiazepines for conscious sedation.

ONSET AND DURATION

Onset: 7-8 min
Duration: ½-1 hr

INDICATIONS

Pain control
Sedation for invasive airway procedures (e.g., rapid-sequence induction)

CONTRAINDICATIONS

Respiratory depression
Hypotension
Head injury
Cardiac dysrhythmias
Myasthenia gravis
Hypersensitivity to opiates

ADVERSE REACTIONS

Respiratory depression
Bradycardia
Hypotension or hypertension
Nausea and vomiting

DRUG INTERACTIONS

Effects may be increased when given with other central nervous system depressants or skeletal muscle relaxants.

HOW SUPPLIED

0.05-mg/mL ampules

DOSAGE AND ADMINISTRATION

Adult: 0.05-0.1 mg IM every 1-2 hr as needed to control pain
Child (over 2 years of age): 0.02-0.03 mg/9 kg IM one time; rarely used in the prehospital setting

SPECIAL CONSIDERATIONS

Pregnancy safety: Category C
Fentanyl is a schedule II drug with the potential for abuse.
Fentanyl should be used (if at all) with caution in elderly patients and in those with severe respiratory disorders, seizure disorders, cardiac disorders, or pregnancy.
Naloxone or nalmefene should be available to reverse respiratory depression.

FLUMAZENIL (ROMAZICON)

CLASS

Benzodiazepine receptor antagonist, antidote

DESCRIPTION

Flumazenil antagonizes the actions of benzodiazepines in the central nervous system. It has been shown to reverse sedation, impairment of recall, and psychomotor impairment produced by benzodiazepines. Flumazenil is not, however, as effective in reversing hypoventilation. Flumazenil does not antagonize central nervous system effects of ethanol, barbiturates, or opioids.

ONSET AND DURATION

Onset: 1-2 min
Duration: Related to plasma concentration of benzodiazepine

INDICATIONS

Reversal of excessive or prolonged benzodiazepine sedation or overdose

CONTRAINDICATIONS

Hypersensitivity to flumazenil or to benzodiazepines
Cyclic antidepressant overdose
Cocaine or other stimulant intoxication
Known seizure disorder (relative)

ADVERSE REACTIONS

Nausea and vomiting
Dizziness
Headache
Agitation
Injection-site pain
Cutaneous vasodilation
Abnormal vision
Seizures

DRUG INTERACTIONS

Toxic effects of mixed drug overdose (especially cyclic antidepressants) may emerge with the reversal of the benzodiazepine effects.

HOW SUPPLIED

5- and 10-mL vials (0.1 mg/mL)

DOSAGE AND ADMINISTRATION

For suspected benzodiazepine overdose:
Adult: 0.2 mg (2 mL) IV over 15 sec; an additional dose of 0.3 mg (3 mL) may be given in 30 sec, followed by 0.5 mg (5 mL) over 30 sec at 1-min intervals (max dose: 3 mg)
Pediatric: Not recommended

SPECIAL CONSIDERATIONS

Pregnancy safety: Category C
To minimize the likelihood of injection-site pain, administer through an IV infusion established in a large vein.
Be prepared to manage seizures in patients who are physically dependent on benzodiazepines to control seizures or who have ingested large doses of other drugs.
Flumazenil may precipitate withdrawal syndromes in patients who are dependent on benzodiazepines.
Patients should be monitored for possible resedation, respiratory depression, or other residual benzodiazepine effects.
Be prepared to establish and assist ventilation.

FUROSEMIDE (LASIX)

CLASS

Loop diuretic

DESCRIPTION

Furosemide is a potent diuretic that inhibits the reabsorption of sodium and chloride in the proximal tubule and loop of Henle. Intravenous doses also can reduce cardiac preload by increasing venous capacitance.

ONSET AND DURATION

Onset: (IV) diuretic effects within 15-20 min; vascular effects within 5 min
Duration: 2 hr

INDICATIONS

Pulmonary edema associated with congestive heart failure, hepatic or renal disease

CONTRAINDICATIONS

Anuria (though loop diuretics can be used in patients with reduced creatinine clearance)
Hypersensitivity
Hypovolemia/dehydration
Known hypersensitivity to sulfonamides
Severe electrolyte depletion (hypokalemia)

ADVERSE REACTIONS

Hypotension
Electrocardiogram changes associated with electrolyte disturbances
Dry mouth
Hypochloremia
Hypokalemia
Hyponatremia

Hypercalcemia
Hyperglycemia
Hearing loss can occur rarely after too rapid infusion of large doses especially in patients with renal impairment.

DRUG INTERACTIONS

Digitalis toxicity may be potentiated because of potassium depletion, which can result from furosemide administration.
Furosemide increases ototoxic potential of aminoglycoside antibiotics.
Lithium toxicity may be potentiated because of sodium depletion.
Furosemide may potentiate therapeutic effect of other antihypertensive drugs.

HOW SUPPLIED

Parenteral: 10 mg/mL in 2-, 4-, 8-mL ampule, 10 mg/mL in 10-mL vial

DOSAGE AND ADMINISTRATION

Adult: 20-40 mg (0.5-1 mg/kg) slow IV over 1-2 min (not to exceed 20 mg/min); may repeat in 1-2 hr
Pediatric: 1 mg/kg/dose (max total dose: 6 mg/kg)

SPECIAL CONSIDERATIONS

Pregnancy safety: Category C
Furosemide has been known to cause fetal abnormalities.
Furosemide should be protected from light and stored at room temperature; do not use if solution is discolored or yellow.

GLUCAGON

CLASS

Pancreatic hormone, insulin antagonist

DESCRIPTION

Glucagon is a protein secreted by the alpha cells of the pancreas. When released, glucagon results in blood glucose elevation by increasing the breakdown of glycogen to glucose (glycogenolysis) and stimulating glucose synthesis (gluconeogenesis). The drug is only effective in treating hypoglycemia if liver glycogen is available and therefore may be ineffective in chronic states of hypoglycemia, starvation, and adrenal insufficiency. In addition, glucagon exerts positive inotropic action on the heart and decreases renal vascular resistance. For this reason, glucagon also is used in managing patients with beta-blocker and calcium channel blocker cardiotoxicity who do not respond to saline infusions or other conventional therapy.

ONSET AND DURATION

Onset: Within 1 min
Duration: 60-90 min

INDICATIONS

Persistent hypoglycemia despite glucose supplementation
Calcium channel blocker or beta-blocker toxicity

CONTRAINDICATIONS

Hypersensitivity (allergy to proteins)

ADVERSE REACTIONS

Tachycardia
Hypotension
Nausea and vomiting
Urticaria

DRUG INTERACTIONS

Effect of anticoagulants may be increased if given with glucagon.
Do not mix with saline.

HOW SUPPLIED

Glucagon must be reconstituted (with provided diluent) before administration. Dilute 1 unit (1 mg) white powder in 1 mL of diluting solution (1 mg/mL).

DOSAGE AND ADMINISTRATION

Hypoglycemia
Adult: 0.5-1 mg IM; may repeat in 7-10 min
Pediatric: 0.025-1 mg IM; may repeat in 7-10 min
Calcium Channel Blocker or Beta-Blocker Toxicity
Adult: 1-5 mg over 2-5 min (IV)
Pediatric: Safety and efficacy have not been established

SPECIAL CONSIDERATIONS

Pregnancy safety: Category B
Glucagon should not be considered a first-line choice for hypoglycemia.
Intravenous glucose will need to be administered if the patient does not respond to a second dose of glucagon.
Do not use the provided diluent to mix continuous infusions.

HALOPERIDOL LACTATE (HALDOL)

CLASS

Antipsychotic/neuroleptic

DESCRIPTION

Haloperidol has pharmacological properties similar to those of the phenothiazines. The drug is thought to block dopamine (type 2) receptors in the brain, altering mood and behavior. In emergency care, haloperidol usually is administered IM but also may be given IV.

ONSET AND DURATION

Onset: (IM) 30-60 min
Duration: 12-24 hr

INDICATIONS

Acute psychotic episodes
Emergency sedation of severely agitated or delirious patients

CONTRAINDICATIONS

Central nervous system depression
Coma
Hypersensitivity
Pregnancy
Severe liver or cardiac disease

ADVERSE REACTIONS

Dose-related extrapyramidal reactions:
Pseudoparkinsonism
Akathisia
Dystonias
Hypotension
Orthostatic hypotension
Nausea, vomiting
Allergic reactions
Blurred vision

DRUG INTERACTIONS

Other central nervous system depressants may potentiate effects.
Haloperidol may inhibit vasoconstrictor effects of epinephrine.

HOW SUPPLIED

5-, 50-, 100-mg/mL ampule

DOSAGE AND ADMINISTRATION

Adult: 2-5 mg IM every 4-8 hr as needed
Pediatric: Safety not established

SPECIAL CONSIDERATIONS

Pregnancy safety: Category C

HEPARIN SODIUM

CLASS

Anticoagulant

DESCRIPTION

Heparin inhibits the clotting cascade by activating specific plasma proteins. The drug is used in the prevention and treatment of all types of thromboses and emboli, disseminated intravascular coagulation, arterial occlusion, and thrombophlebitis and is used prophylactically to prevent clotting before surgery. Heparin also is considered part of the antithrombotic package (along with aspirin and fibrinolytic agents) administered to patients with acute myocardial infarction and acute coronary syndromes including unstable angina and non–Q wave myocardial infarction.

ONSET AND DURATION

Onset: (IV) Immediate
(SQ) 20-60 min
Duration: 4-8 hr

INDICATIONS

Acute myocardial infarction
Prophylaxis and treatment of thromboembolic disorders (e.g., pulmonary emboli and deep venous thrombosis)

CONTRAINDICATIONS

Hypersensitivity
Active bleeding
Recent intracranial, intraspinal, or eye surgery
Severe hypertension
Bleeding tendencies
Severe thrombocytopenia

ADVERSE REACTIONS

Allergic reaction (chills, fever, back pain)
Thrombocytopenia
Hemorrhage
Bruising

DRUG INTERACTIONS

Salicylates, ibuprofen, dipyridamole, and hydroxychloroquine may increase risk of bleeding.

HOW SUPPLIED

10, 100, and 1000-40,000 U/mL

DOSAGE AND ADMINISTRATION

If used with fibrinolytic therapy, always obtain a blood sample for control of partial thromboplastin time before heparin administration. (Heparin along with aspirin is part of the antithrombotic package.) Heparin is given as an IV bolus of 60 IU/kg max 4000 IU (weight adjusted). A continuous infusion is given following the bolus at a rate of 12 IU/kg/hr (max: 4000 IU or 1000 units/hr). (Follow medical direction and local protocol.)

SPECIAL CONSIDERATIONS

Pregnancy safety: Category C
Heparin does not lyse existing clots.

HYDRALAZINE (APRESOLINE)

CLASS

Antihypertensive, vasodilator

DESCRIPTION

Hydralazine is an older antihypertensive medication that is a direct vasodilator. Hydralazine is used today almost exclusively for treatment of preeclampsia and eclampsia. The effects of the drug include a decrease in arterial pressure, a decrease in peripheral resistance, and an increase in cardiac output (as a result of reflex tachycardia).

ONSET AND DURATION

Onset: (IV) 5-30 min
(IM) 10-40 min
Duration: 2-6 hr

INDICATIONS

Hypertensive crisis (other agents preferred)
Hypertension associated with renal failure, preeclampsia, and eclampsia
Primary pulmonary hypertension

CONTRAINDICATIONS

Compensatory hypertension
Coronary artery disease
Dissecting aneurysm
Hypersensitivity
Mitral valve/rheumatic heart disease

ADVERSE REACTIONS

Reflex tachycardia
Palpitations
Hypotension
Facial flushing
Headache
Diaphoresis
Anxiety
Nausea and vomiting
Diarrhea

DRUG INTERACTIONS

Concurrent use of diazoxide may result in severe hypotension.
Color changes may occur when given with glucose solutions.
MAO inhibitors may result in significant hypotension.

HOW SUPPLIED

20 mg in 1-mL ampule (20 mg/mL)

DOSAGE AND ADMINISTRATION

Adult: 10-40 mg IM or IV; may be repeated in 10 min prn
Infusion: 20 mg in 250 mL NS or lactated Ringer's at 5-20 mg/hr
Pediatric: 0.1-0.2 mg/kg/dose q 4-6 hr IM, IV; may be repeated prn
Infusion: 0.75-3 mg/kg q 6-12 hr

SPECIAL CONSIDERATIONS

Pregnancy safety: Category C
Blood pressure and electrocardiogram should be monitored continuously.

HYDROXYZINE (ATARAX, VISTARIL)

CLASS

Antihistamine

DESCRIPTION

Hydroxyzine is a H_1 receptor antagonist that is used to treat allergy-induced pruritus and is used perioperatively for its antiemetic and sedative properties. It can be used for treatment of anxiety. Concomitant use with analgesics may potentiate their effects.

ONSET AND DURATION

Onset: (IM) 15-30 min
Duration: 4-6 hr

INDICATIONS

To potentiate the effects of analgesics
Nausea and vomiting
Anxiety reactions
Motion sickness
Pruritus

CONTRAINDICATIONS

Hypersensitivity to hydroxyzine

ADVERSE REACTIONS

Dry mouth
Drowsiness

DRUG INTERACTIONS

The potentiating action of hydroxyzine must be considered when the drug is used along with central nervous system depressants such as narcotics, barbiturates, and alcohol and with anticholinergics.

HOW SUPPLIED

25, 50 mg/mL in 1-mL vials

DOSAGE AND ADMINISTRATION

Adult: 25-100 mg deep IM
Pediatric: 1 mg/kg/dose, deep IM

SPECIAL CONSIDERATIONS

Pregnancy safety: Category C
Hydroxyzine should be administered by deep IM injection only (not for SQ or IV use).
Localized burning at the injection site is a common complaint.

IBUTILIDE (CORVERT)

CLASS

Short-acting antidysrhythmic

DESCRIPTION

Ibutilide prolongs the action potential duration and increases the refractory period of cardiac tissue. Ibutilide is recommended for acute pharmacological conversion of atrial flutter or atrial fibrillation or as an adjunct to electrical cardioversion.

ONSET AND DURATION

Onset: ½-1½ hr
Duration: 10-12 hr

INDICATIONS

Supraventricular dysrhythmias
Conversion of atrial fibrillation and atrial flutter of brief duration

CONTRAINDICATIONS

History of heart failure or ventricular tachycardia
Sensitivity to ibutilide

ADVERSE REACTIONS

Ventricular dysrhythmias
Hypotension and hypertension

DRUG INTERACTIONS

Avoid concurrent administration of ibutilide with other antidysrhythmics that prolong the refractory period (e.g., amiodarone) or drugs that induce Q-T interval prolongation (e.g., procainamide).

HOW SUPPLIED

1 mg in 10-mL ampules

DOSAGE AND ADMINISTRATION

Adult (60 kg or more): 1 mg (10 mL) IV over 10 min. A second dose may be administered at the same rate 10 min later. The initial dose for adults who weigh less than 60 kg is 0.01 mg/kg IV.
Pediatric: Not recommended

SPECIAL CONSIDERATIONS

Pregnancy safety: Category C
Ibutilide must be given slowly IV over 10 min. This may make it impractical for use in emergent situations.
Ventricular dysrhythmias develop in 2% to 5% of patients who are given ibutilide; continuous electrocardiogram monitoring is essential.
Use with caution in patients with impaired left ventricular function.

INSULIN (REGULAR, NPH, ULTRALENTE, AND OTHERS)

CLASS

Antidiabetic agent

DESCRIPTION

Insulin is secreted by the beta cells (islets of Langerhans) of the pancreas and is required for proper glucose utilization by the body. If insulin secretion is diminished (as in diabetes mellitus), supplemental insulin must be obtained by injection. Insulin preparations are classified as *rapid-acting* (regular), *intermediate-acting* (NPH), and *long-acting* (Ultralente). Insulin seldom is administered in the prehospital setting, even when ketoacidosis is present. (Large amounts of normal saline solution is considered the first-line treatment.) Insulin may be required for long transport times.

ONSET AND DURATION

Onset: ½-1 hr (rapid-acting)
1-1½ hr (intermediate-acting)
4-6 hr (long-acting)
Duration: 6-8 hr (rapid-acting)
18-24 hr (intermediate-acting)
More than 36 hr (long-acting)

INDICATIONS

Type I diabetes mellitus
Type II diabetes mellitus if oral hypoglycemic agents do not control blood glucose adequately
Diabetic ketoacidosis
Nonketotic hyperosmolar coma
Insulin and 50% dextrose solution are given together to lower potassium levels in hyperkalemia.

CONTRAINDICATIONS

Hypoglycemia

ADVERSE REACTIONS

Hypoglycemia
Fatigue
Weakness
Confusion
Headache
Tachycardia
Rapid, shallow breathing
Nausea
Diaphoresis
Allergic reaction

DRUG INTERACTIONS

Corticosteroids, dobutamine, epinephrine, and thiazide diuretics may antagonize (decrease) the hypoglycemic effects of insulin.
Alcohol, beta-adrenergic blockers, MAO inhibitors, and salicylates may potentiate (increase) the hypoglycemic effects of insulin.

HOW SUPPLIED

100 units/mL in 10-mL vials

DOSAGE AND ADMINISTRATION

Insulin may be administered SQ, IM, or IV, and dosage is governed by the clinical presentation of the patient. A standard dose of insulin administration in diabetic coma is as follows:

Adult: 10-25 units regular insulin IV, followed by an infusion of 0.1 units/kg/hr

Pediatric: 0.1-0.2 units/kg/hr IM

Infusion: 50 units of regular insulin mixed in 250 mL of NS (0.2 units/mL), infused at a rate of 0.1-0.2 units/kg/hr (use infusion pump)

SPECIAL CONSIDERATIONS

Pregnancy safety: Category B

Insulin is the drug of choice for control of diabetes in pregnancy.

Regular insulins are clear, whereas modified insulins are cloudy.

Insulin injected into the abdominal wall is absorbed most rapidly, insulin in the arm is absorbed more slowly, and insulin is absorbed slowest when injected into the thigh.

IPRATROPIUM (ATROVENT)

CLASS

Anticholinergic, bronchodilator

DESCRIPTION

Ipratropium inhibits interaction of acetylcholine at receptor sites on bronchial smooth muscle, resulting in decreased cyclic guanosine monophosphate and bronchodilation.

ONSET AND DURATION

Onset: 5-15 min
Duration: 4-6 hr

INDICATIONS

Persistent bronchospasm
Chronic obstructive pulmonary disease exacerbation

CONTRAINDICATIONS

Hypersensitivity to ipratopium, atropine, alkaloid, soybean protein, peanuts

ADVERSE REACTIONS

Nausea and vomiting
Coughing
Headache
Tachycardia
Dry mouth
Blurred vision

DRUG INTERACTIONS

None reported

HOW SUPPLIED

Aerosol 18 mcg/actuation

DOSAGE AND ADMINISTRATION

Note: When used in combination with beta-agonists (e.g., metaproterenol and albuterol), the beta-agonist is always administered first with a 5-min wait before administering ipratropium.

Adult: 1-2 inhalations

Pediatric (over 12 years of age): Same as adult

SPECIAL CONSIDERATIONS

Pregnancy safety: Category B
Shake well before use.
Use with caution in patients with urinary retention.

ISOPROTERENOL (ISUPREL)

CLASS

Sympathomimetic

DESCRIPTION

Isoproterenol is a synthetic catecholamine that stimulates both $beta_1$- and $beta_2$-adrenergic receptors (no alpha receptor stimulation). The drug affects the heart by increasing inotropic and chronotropic activity. In addition, isoproterenol causes arterial and bronchial dilation and sometimes is administered via aerosolization as a bronchodilator to treat bronchial asthma and bronchospasm. (Because of the undesirable $beta_1$ cardiac effects, the use of this drug as a bronchodilator is uncommon in the prehospital setting.)

ONSET AND DURATION

Onset: 1-5 min
Duration: 15-30 min

INDICATIONS

Hemodynamically significant bradycardias unresponsive to atropine, transcutaneous pacing, dopamine, and epinephrine.

Management of torsades de pointes

CONTRAINDICATIONS

Ventricular tachycardia
Ventricular fibrillation
Hypotension (relative)
Pulseless idioventricular rhythm
Ischemic heart disease/angina (relative)
Cardiac arrest

ADVERSE REACTIONS

Dysrhythmias
Hypotension
Precipitation of angina pectoris
Facial flushing
Restlessness
Dry throat
Discoloration of saliva (pinkish red)

DRUG INTERACTIONS

MAO inhibitors potentiate the effects of catecholamines.
Beta-adrenergic antagonists may blunt inotropic response.
Sympathomimetics and phosphodiesterase inhibitors may exacerbate dysrhythmia response.

HOW SUPPLIED

5-mL (0.2 mg/mL) vial; 0.02 mg/mL in 1- and 10-mL vials

DOSAGE AND ADMINISTRATION

Adult: Dilute 1 mg in 250 mL of D_5W (4 mcg/mL); infuse at 2-10 mcg/min or until the desired heart rate is obtained; in torsades de pointes, titrate to increase heart rate until ventricular tachycardia is suppressed
Pediatric: Not recommended

SPECIAL CONSIDERATIONS

Pregnancy safety: Category C
Isoproterenol increases myocardial oxygen demand and can induce serious dysrhythmias (including ventricular tachycardia and ventricular fibrillation).
Administer via infusion pump to ensure precise flow rates.
Isoproterenol may exacerbate tachydysrhythmias caused by digitalis toxicity or hypokalemia.
Newer inotropic agents have replaced isoproterenol in most clinical settings.
If electronic pacing is available, it should be used instead of isoproterenol or as soon as possible after drug administration has been initiated.

KETAMINE (KETALAR)

CLASS

Nonbarbiturate anesthetic

DESCRIPTION

Ketamine acts on the limbic system and cortex to block afferent transmission of impulses associated with pain perception. It produces short-acting amnesia without muscular relaxation. Ketamine is a derivative of the drug of abuse, phencyclidine.

ONSET AND DURATION

Onset: Within 30 sec
Duration: 5-10 minutes

INDICATIONS

Pain control
As an adjunct to nitrous oxide

CONTRAINDICATIONS

Stroke
Increased intracranial pressure
Severe hypertension
Cardiac decompensation
Hypersensitivity to ketamine

ADVERSE REACTIONS

Hypertension
Increased heart rate
Hallucinations, delusions, explicit dreams
Less common side effects include hypotension, bradycardia, and respiratory depression

DRUG INTERACTIONS

No significant drug interactions have been reported.

HOW SUPPLIED

10-, 50-, and 100-mg/mL ampules

DOSAGE AND ADMINISTRATION

Adult: 1-2 mg/kg IV over 1 min or 5-10 mg IM
Child (over 2 years of age): Same as adult

SPECIAL CONSIDERATIONS

Pregnancy safety: Category C
Ketamine may increase blood pressure, muscle tone, and heart rate.
Ketamine should not be given to patients with kidney or renal failure.
As with any anesthetic, the dosage needs to be assessed carefully and individualized.
Keep patient in a quiet environment (if possible).

KETOROLAC TROMETHAMINE (TORADOL)

CLASS

Nonsteroidal antiinflammatory

DESCRIPTION

Ketorolac tromethamine is an antiinflammatory drug that also exhibits peripherally acting nonnarcotic analgesic activity by inhibiting prostaglandin synthesis.

ONSET AND DURATION

Onset: Within 10 min
Duration: 6-8 hr

INDICATIONS

Short-term management (less than 5 days) of moderate to severe pain

CONTRAINDICATIONS

Hypersensitivity to the drug
Patients with allergies to aspirin or other nonsteroidal antiinflammatory drugs
Bleeding disorders
Renal failure
Active peptic ulcer disease

ADVERSE REACTIONS

Anaphylaxis from hypersensitivity
Edema
Sedation
Bleeding disorders
Rash
Nausea
Headache

DRUG INTERACTIONS

Ketorolac may increase bleeding time when administered to patients taking anticoagulants.
Effects of lithium and methotrexate may be increased.

HOW SUPPLIED

15 mg or 30 mg in 1 mL
60 mg in 2 mL

DOSAGE AND ADMINISTRATION

Adult: IM: 30-60 mg; then 15-30 mg every 6 hr as needed up to 5 days (max dose: 150 mg in first 24 hr)
IV: 30 mg over 1 min (for patients less than 65 years of age); one-half dose (15 mg) for patients over 65 years and in those with renal impairment
Pediatric: Not recommended

SPECIAL CONSIDERATIONS

Pregnancy safety: Category C
Solution is clear and slightly yellow.
Use with caution and reduce dose when administering to elderly patients.

LABETALOL (NORMODYNE, TRANDATE)

CLASS

Alpha- and beta-adrenergic blocker

DESCRIPTION

Labetalol is a competitive $alpha_1$ receptor blocker and a nonselective beta receptor blocker that is used for lowering blood pressure in hypertensive crisis. Labetalol is a more potent beta-blocker than alpha-blocker. Blood pressure is reduced without reflex tachycardia, and total peripheral resistance is decreased, helping maintain cardiac output. In emergency care, labetalol is administered IV.

ONSET AND DURATION

Onset: Within 5 min
Duration: 3-6 hr

INDICATIONS

Hypertensive emergencies

CONTRAINDICATIONS

Bronchial asthma (relative)
Uncompensated congestive heart failure
Second- and third-degree heart block
Bradycardia
Cardiogenic shock
Pulmonary edema

ADVERSE REACTIONS

Headache
Dizziness
Edema
Fatigue
Vertigo
Ventricular dysrhythmias
Dyspnea
Allergic reaction
Facial flushing
Diaphoresis
Dose-related orthostatic hypotension (most common)

DRUG INTERACTIONS

Bronchodilator effects of beta-adrenergic agonists may be blunted by labetalol.
Nitroglycerin may augment hypotensive effects.

HOW SUPPLIED

5 mg/mL in 4-, 8-, 20-, and 40-mL vials

DOSAGE AND ADMINISTRATION

Adult: 10 mg IV over 1-2 min. May repeat or double labetalol every 10 minutes to a max dose of 150 mg.
Infusion: Mix 200 mg in 250 mL of D_5W (0.8 mg/mL); infuse at a rate of 2-8 mg/min, titrated to supine blood pressure (max: 300 mg)
Pediatric: Safety has not been established; initiate cautiously with careful dosage adjustments and blood pressure monitoring.

SPECIAL CONSIDERATIONS

Pregnancy safety: Category C
Blood pressure, pulse rate, and electrocardiogram should be monitored continuously.
Observe for signs of congestive heart failure, bradycardia, and bronchospasm.
Labetalol should be administered only with the patient in a supine position.

LIDOCAINE (XYLOCAINE)

CLASS

Antidysrhythmic (Class I-B), local anesthetic

DESCRIPTION

Lidocaine decreases phase 4 diastolic depolarization (which decreases automaticity) and has been shown to be effective in suppressing premature ventricular complexes. In addition, lidocaine is used to treat ventricular tachycardia and some cases of ventricular fibrillation. Lidocaine also raises the ventricular fibrillation threshold.

ONSET AND DURATION

Onset: 30-90 sec
Duration: 10-20 min

INDICATIONS

Ventricular tachycardia
Ventricular fibrillation
Wide-complex tachycardia of uncertain origin
Significant ventricular ectopy in the setting of myocardial ischemia/infarction

CONTRAINDICATIONS

Hypersensitivity
Adams-Stokes syndrome
Second- or third-degree heart block in the absence of an artificial pacemaker

ADVERSE EFFECTS

Light-headedness
Confusion
Blurred vision
Hypotension
Cardiovascular collapse
Bradycardia
Altered level of consciousness, irritability, muscle twitching, seizures with high doses

DRUG INTERACTIONS

Metabolic clearance of lidocaine may be decreased in patients taking beta-adrenergic blockers or in patients with decreased cardiac output or liver dysfunction.
Apnea induced with succinylcholine may be prolonged with large doses of lidocaine.
Cardiac depression may occur if lidocaine is given concomitantly with IV phenytoin.
Additive neurological effects may occur with procainamide and tocainide.

HOW SUPPLIED

Prefilled syringes: 100 mg in 5 mL of solution
1- and 2-g additive syringes
Ampules: 100 mg in 5 mL of solution
1- and 2-g vials in 30 mL of solution
5 mL containing 100 mg/mL

DOSAGE AND ADMINISTRATION

Ventricular Tachycardia/Ventricular Fibrillation/Cardiac Arrest
Adult: 1-1.5 mg/kg IV bolus or endotracheal tube (at 2-2.5 times the IV dose); consider repeat in 3-5 min (max total dose: 3 mg/kg); a single dose of 1.5 mg/kg is acceptable; for refractory ventricular tachycardia/ventricular fibrillation, an additional bolus of 0.5-0.7 mg/kg can be given; repeat in 5-10 min if necessary
Pediatric: 1 mg/kg IV/IO or endotracheal tube (diluted to 3-5 mL)
Maintenance Infusion after Resuscitation from Ventricular Tachycardia/Ventricular Fibrillation/Cardiac Arrest
Adult: 1-4 mg/min
Pediatric: 20-50 mcg/kg/min (1-2.5 mL/kg/hr)
Wide-Complex Paroxysmal Supraventricular Tachycardia/Wide-Complex Tachycardia of Uncertain Type/Stable Ventricular Tachycardia
Adult: Initial loading dose of 1-1.5 mg/kg IV; if needed, give 0.5-0.75 mg/kg in 5-10 min (max total dose: 3 mg/kg); after conversion, start a lidocaine drip (1-4 mg/min)
Pediatric: Initial loading dose of 1 mg/kg IV/IO, followed by an infusion of 20-50 mcg/kg/min

SPECIAL CONSIDERATIONS

Pregnancy safety: Category B
A 75-100 mg bolus will maintain adequate blood levels for only 20 min (in absence of shock).
If bradycardia occurs along with premature ventricular contractions, always treat the bradycardia first with atropine.
Exceedingly high doses of lidocaine can result in coma or death.
Decrease dose in the elderly.
Avoid lidocaine for reperfusion dysrhythmias following fibrinolytic therapy.
Use extreme caution in patients with hepatic disease, heart failure, marked hypoxia, severe respiratory depression, hypovolemia or shock, incomplete heart block, or bradycardia and atrial fibrillation.

LORAZEPAM (ATIVAN)

CLASS

Benzodiazepine

DESCRIPTION

Lorazepam is a benzodiazepine with antianxiety and anticonvulsant effects. When given by injection, it appears to suppress the propagation of seizure activity produced by foci in the cortex, thalamus, and limbic areas.

ONSET AND DURATION

Onset: 20-30 min
Duration: 6-8 hr

INDICATIONS

Agitation requiring sedation
Initial control of status epilepticus or severe recurrent seizures (investigational)

CONTRAINDICATIONS

Hypersensitivity to the drug
Substance abuse (relative)
Coma (unless seizing)
Severe hypotension
Shock
Preexisting central nervous system depression

ADVERSE REACTIONS

Respiratory depression
Tachycardia/bradycardia
Hypotension
Sedation
Ataxia
Psychomotor impairment
Confusion

DRUG INTERACTIONS

Lorazepam may precipitate central nervous system depression and psychomotor impairment when the patient is taking central nervous system depressant medications

HOW SUPPLIED

2 and 4 mg/mL concentrations in 1-mL vials

DOSAGE AND ADMINISTRATION

Before IV administration, lorazepam must be diluted with an equal volume of sterile water or sterile saline. When given IM, lorazepam is not to be diluted.
Adult: 1-4 mg slow IM/IV over 2-10 min; may be repeated in 15-20 min to a max dose of 8 mg
Pediatric (not FDA-approved): 0.05-0.15 mg/kg slow IV/IO/IM over 2 min; may be repeated once in 5-10 min to a max dose of 4 mg; 0.1-0.2 mg/kg (rectal dose)

SPECIAL CONSIDERATIONS

Pregnancy safety: Category D
Monitor respiratory rate and blood pressure during administration.
Have suction and intubation equipment available.
Inadvertent intraarterial injection may produce arteriospasm, resulting in gangrene that may require amputation.
Lorazepam expires in 6 weeks when not refrigerated; do not use if discolored or if solution contains precipitate.

MAGNESIUM SULFATE

CLASS

Electrolyte, anticonvulsant

DESCRIPTION

Magnesium sulfate reduces striated muscle contractions and blocks peripheral neuromuscular transmission by reducing acetylcholine release at the myoneural junction. In emergency care, magnesium sulfate is used in the management of seizures associated with toxemia of pregnancy. Other uses of magnesium sulfate include uterine relaxation (to inhibit contractions of premature labor), as a bronchodilator after beta-agonist and anticholinergic agents have been used, and replacement therapy for magnesium deficiency. Magnesium sulfate is gaining popularity as an initial treatment in the management of various dysrhythmias, particularly torsades de pointes, and dysrhythmias caused by tricyclic antidepressant overdose or digitalis toxicity. The drug also is considered as a Class IIA agent (American Heart Association guidelines; probably helpful) for ventricular fibrillation/ventricular tachycardia refractory to lidocaine.

ONSET AND DURATION

Onset: (IV) Immediate
(IM) 3-4 hr
Duration: 30 min (IV)
3-4 hr (IM)

INDICATIONS

Seizures of eclampsia (toxemia of pregnancy)
Torsades de pointes
Suspected hypomagnesemia
Refractory ventricular fibrillation
Status asthmaticus not responsive to beta-adrenergic drugs

CONTRAINDICATIONS

Heart block or myocardial damage

ADVERSE REACTIONS

Diaphoresis
Facial flushing
Hypotension
Depressed reflexes
Hypothermia
Reduced heart rate
Circulatory collapse
Respiratory depression
Diarrhea

DRUG INTERACTIONS

Central nervous system depressant effects may be enhanced if the patient is taking other central nervous system depressants.
Serious changes in cardiac function may occur with cardiac glycosides (avoid excess magnesium administration).

HOW SUPPLIED

10%, 12.5%, 50% solution in 40, 80, 100, and 125 mg/mL

DOSAGE AND ADMINISTRATION

Seizure Activity Associated with Pregnancy

Adult: 1-4 g (8-32 mEq) IV; max dose of 30-40 g/day

Pulseless Arrest (for Hypomagnesemia or Torsades de Pointes)

Adult: 1-2 g (2-4 mL of a 50% solution) diluted in 10 mL of D_5W IV push

Pediatric: 25-50 mg/kg (max 2 g) over 10-20 min

Torsades de Pointes (Not in Cardiac Arrest) and Acute Myocardial Infarction (If Indicated)

Adult: Loading dose of 1-2 g in 50-100 mL of D_5W over 5-60 min IV; follow with 0.5-1 g/hr/IV (titrate dose to control the torsades)

Pediatric: Same as pulseless arrest

SPECIAL CONSIDERATIONS

Pregnancy safety: Category B.

Magnesium sulfate is administered for the treatment of toxemia of pregnancy. It is recommended that the drug not be administered in the 2 hr before delivery, if possible. IV calcium gluconate or calcium chloride should be available as an antagonist to magnesium if needed

Convulsions may occur up to 48 hr after delivery, necessitating continued therapy.

The "cure" for toxemia is delivery of the baby.

Magnesium must be used with caution in patients with renal failure because it is cleared by the kidneys and can reach toxic levels easily in those patients.

MANNITOL (OSMITROL)

CLASS

Osmotic diuretic

DESCRIPTION

Because of the osmotic properties of mannitol, the drug promotes the movement of fluid from the intracellular into the extracellular space. In emergency care, mannitol most often is used to decrease cerebral edema and intracranial pressure caused by head injury or mass lesions.

ONSET AND DURATION

Onset: 1-3 hr (for diuretic effect)

Within 15 min (for reduction of intracranial pressure)

Duration: 4-6 hr (for diuretic effect)

3-8 hr (for reduction of intracranial pressure)

INDICATIONS

Cerebral edema

Other causes of increased intracranial pressure (space-occupying lesions)

Rhabdomyolysis (myoglobinuria)

Blood transfusion reactions

Promoting urinary excretion of toxic substances

Contraindications

Severe hypotension

Active intracranial bleeding

Dehydration

Hyponatremia

Severe pulmonary edema or congestion

Profound hypovolemia

Severe renal disease (anuria)

ADVERSE REACTIONS

Transient volume overload

Pulmonary edema

Renal failure

Congestive heart failure

Hypotension (from excessive diuresis)

Sodium depletion

DRUG INTERACTIONS

When given concurrently with digitalis glycosides, an increase in digitalis toxicity may develop.

HOW SUPPLIED

250 and 500 mL of a 20% solution for IV infusion (200 mg/mL) 25% solution in 50 mL for slow IV push

DOSAGE AND ADMINISTRATION

Adult: 0.5-1 g/kg in a 20% solution over 5-10 min; usual adult dose is 20-200 g/24 hr

Pediatric: 0.2-0.5 g/kg/dose IV infusion over 30-60 min (max dose: 1 g/kg) every 4-6 hr

SPECIAL CONSIDERATIONS

Pregnancy safety: Category C

Mannitol may crystallize at low temperatures and may need to be warmed in boiling water until clear (cool to body temperature before use).

In-line filter should always be used.

Effectiveness depends on large doses and an intact blood-brain barrier.

The use of mannitol and its dosages in emergency care are controversial.

MEPERIDINE (DEMEROL)

CLASS

Opioid analgesic

DESCRIPTION

Meperidine is a synthetic opioid agonist that works at opioid receptors to produce analgesia and euphoria. Excessive doses can cause respiratory and central nervous system depression and seizures. It has high potential for physical dependence and abuse and is classified as a Schedule II drug.

ONSET AND DURATION

Onset: (IM) 10-15 min

(IV) Within 5 min

Duration: 2-4 hr

INDICATIONS

Moderate to severe pain
Preoperative medication
Obstetrical analgesia

CONTRAINDICATIONS

Hypersensitivity to narcotics
Patients taking MAO inhibitors or selective serotonin reuptake inhibitors
During labor or delivery of a premature infant
Head injury

ADVERSE REACTIONS

Respiratory depression
Nausea and vomiting
Euphoria
Delirium
Agitation
Hallucination
Seizures
Headache
Hypotension
Visual disturbances
Coma
Facial flushing
Circulatory collapse
Dysrhythmias
Allergic reaction

DRUG INTERACTIONS

Respiratory depression, hypotension or sedation may be potentiated by central nervous system depressants.
Therapeutic doses of meperidine have caused fatal reactions in patients taking MAO inhibitors within the previous 14 days.
Phenytoin may decrease analgesic effects.

HOW SUPPLIED

Parenteral: 25, 50, 100 mg/mL in 1- and 5-mL prefilled syringe and Tubex

DOSAGE AND ADMINISTRATION

Adult: 50-100 mg IM every 3-4 hr as needed; 15-35 mg IV per hour (dose should be individualized)
Elderly: 25 mg IM every 4 hr as needed
Pediatric: 1-2 mg/kg/dose IM every 3-4 hr as needed

SPECIAL CONSIDERATIONS

Pregnancy safety: Category B (if not used for prolonged periods or in high doses at term)
Use with caution in patients with asthma and chronic obstructive pulmonary disease.
Meperidine may aggravate seizures in those with convulsive disorders (especially in patients with renal insufficiency).
Use with caution in those susceptible to central nervous system depression.
Naloxone should be readily available.
Protect from light and freezing.

METAPROTERENOL (ALUPENT)

CLASS

Sympathomimetic, bronchodilator

DESCRIPTION

Metaproterenol relaxes the smooth muscles of the bronchial tree and peripheral vasculature by stimulating $beta_2$-adrenergic receptors of the sympathetic nervous system.

ONSET AND DURATION

Onset: 1 minute after inhalation
Duration: 3-6 hr

INDICATIONS

Bronchial asthma
Reversible bronchospasm (bronchitis, emphysema)

CONTRAINDICATIONS

Hypersensitivity
Cardiac dysrhythmias
Tachycardia caused by digitalis toxicity

ADVERSE REACTIONS

Restlessness, apprehension
Palpitations
Tachycardia
Dysrhythmias
Decreased blood pressure
Coughing
Tremor
Facial flushing
Diaphoresis

DRUG INTERACTIONS

Other sympathomimetics may exacerbate adverse cardiovascular effects.
Tricyclic antidepressants and MAO inhibitors may potentiate hypotensive effects.
Beta-blockers may antagonize the effects of metaproterenol.

HOW SUPPLIED

Metered dose inhaler: 0.65/mg/spray (15-mL inhaler)
Solution: 0.4%, 0.6%, and 5%
Syrup: (10 mg/5 mL)

DOSAGE AND ADMINISTRATION

Metered dose inhaler
Adult: 2-3 inhalations q 3-4 hr (2 min between inhalations); max dose of 12 inhalations/day
Pediatric (over 12 years of age): Same as adult
Solution
Adult: 5-15 inhalations of 5% solution
Pediatric (over 6 yr of age): Same as adult

SPECIAL CONSIDERATIONS

Pregnancy safety: Category C
Monitor vital signs for hypotension and tachycardia.
Use with caution in patients with coronary artery disease and diabetes mellitus.
Shake well.
Do not use if solutions are brown or contain precipitate.

METHYLPREDNISOLONE (SOLU-MEDROL)

CLASS

Glucocorticoid

DESCRIPTION

Methylprednisolone is a synthetic steroid that suppresses acute and chronic inflammation. In addition, it potentiates vascular smooth muscle relaxation by beta-adrenergic agonists and may alter airway hyperactivity. It currently is used for reduction of posttraumatic spinal cord edema, but this indication is controversial.

ONSET AND DURATION

Onset: 1-2 hr
Duration: 8-24 hr

INDICATIONS

Anaphylaxis
Bronchodilator: unresponsive asthma
Shock (controversial)
Acute spinal cord injury (controversial)
Adrenal insufficiency (hydrocortisone [Solu-Cortef] also may be used)

CONTRAINDICATIONS

Use with caution in patients with gastrointestinal bleeding, diabetes mellitus, or severe infection.

ADVERSE REACTIONS

Headache
Hypertension
Sodium and water retention
Hypokalemia
Alkalosis

DRUG INTERACTIONS

Hypoglycemic responses to insulin and oral hypoglycemic agents may be blunted.
Potassium-depleting agents may potentiate hypokalemia induced by corticosteroids.

HOW SUPPLIED

20, 40, 80 mg/mL

DOSAGE AND ADMINISTRATION

Adult: Variable; usually within the range of 40-125 mg IV, except for spinal cord injury where the initial dose is 30 mg/kg IV bolus followed by an IV infusion of 5.4 mg/kg/hr
Pediatric: 1-2 mg/kg/dose IV

SPECIAL CONSIDERATIONS

Pregnancy safety: Category C

METOPROLOL (LOPRESSOR)

CLASS

Beta-blocking agent

DESCRIPTION

Beta-adrenergic blocking agents compete with beta-adrenergic agonists for available beta receptor sites on the membrane of cardiac muscle, bronchial smooth muscle, and the smooth muscle of blood vessels. The $beta_1$ blocking action on the heart decreases heart rate, conduction velocity, myocardial contractility, and cardiac output. Metoprolol is used to control ventricular response in supraventricular tachydysrhythmias (paroxysmal supraventricular tachycardia, atrial fibrillation, atrial flutter). Metoprolol is considered a second-line agent after adenosine, diltiazem, or a digitalis derivative.

ONSET AND DURATION

Onset: 1-2 min
Duration: 3-4 hr

INDICATIONS

Paroxysmal supraventricular tachycardia
Atrial flutter
Atrial fibrillation
To reduce myocardial ischemia and damage in patients with acute myocardial infarction

CONTRAINDICATIONS

Heart failure
Second- or third-degree heart block
Cardiogenic shock
Hypotension
Bradycardia
Lung disease associated with bronchospasm
Hypersensitivity to metoprolol

ADVERSE REACTIONS

Bradycardia
Atrioventricular conduction delays
Hypotension

DRUG INTERACTIONS

Metoprolol may potentiate antihypertensive effects when given to patients taking calcium channel blockers or MAO inhibitors.
Catecholamine-depleting drugs may potentiate hypotension.
Sympathomimetic effects may be antagonized; signs of hypoglycemia may be masked.

HOW SUPPLIED

1-mg/mL ampules

DOSE AND ADMINISTRATION

Adult: 5 mg slow IV at 5-min intervals to a total of 15 mg
Pediatric: Safety not established

SPECIAL CONSIDERATIONS

Pregnancy safety: Category C
Metoprolol must be given slowly IV over 5 min.
Concurrent IV administration with IV calcium channel blockers such as verapamil or diltiazem can cause severe hypotension
Metoprolol should be used with caution in persons with liver or renal dysfunction.

MIDAZOLAM HYDROCHLORIDE (VERSED)

CLASS

Short-acting benzodiazepine

DESCRIPTION

Midazolam hydrochloride is a water-soluble benzodiazepine that may be administered for conscious sedation to relieve apprehension or impair memory before tracheal intubation or cardioversion.

ONSET AND DURATION

Onset: 1-3 min (IV); dose dependent
Duration: 2-6 hr; dose dependent

INDICATIONS

Premedication for tracheal intubation, cardioversion, or other painful procedures

CONTRAINDICATIONS

Hypersensitivity to midazolam
Glaucoma (relative)
Shock
Coma
Alcohol intoxication (relative; may be used for alcohol withdrawal)
Depressed vital signs
Concomitant use of barbiturates, alcohol, narcotics, or other central nervous system depressants

ADVERSE REACTIONS

Respiratory depression
Hiccup
Cough
Oversedation
Pain at the injection site
Nausea and vomiting
Headache
Blurred vision
Fluctuations in vital signs
Hypotension
Respiratory arrest

DRUG INTERACTIONS

Sedative effect of midazolam may be accentuated by concomitant use of barbiturates, alcohol, or narcotics (and therefore should not be used in patients who have taken central nervous system depressants).

HOW SUPPLIED

2-, 5-, 10-mL vials (1 mg/mL)
1-, 2-, 5-, 10-mL vials (5 mg/mL)

DOSAGE AND ADMINISTRATION

Adult: 1-2.5 mg slow IV (over 2-3 min); may be repeated if necessary in small increments (total max dose not to exceed 0.1 mg/kg)
Elderly: 0.5 mg slow IV (max: 1.5 mg in a 2-min period)
Pediatric: Loading dose 0.05-0.2 mg/kg; then continue infusion 1-2 mcg/kg/min

SPECIAL CONSIDERATIONS

Pregnancy safety: Category D
Provide continuous monitoring of respiratory and cardiac function.
Have resuscitation equipment and medication readily at hand.
Never administer medication as IV bolus.

MORPHINE SULFATE (ASTRAMORPH/PF AND OTHERS)

CLASS

Opioid analgesic

DESCRIPTION

Morphine sulfate is a natural opium alkaloid that has a primary effect of analgesia. It also increases peripheral venous capacitance and decreases venous return (chemical phlebotomy). Morphine sulfate causes euphoria and respiratory and central nervous system depression. Secondary pharmacological effects of morphine include depressed responsiveness of alpha-adrenergic receptors (producing peripheral vasodilation) and baroreceptor inhibition. In addition, because morphine decreases preload and afterload, it may decrease myocardial oxygen demand. The properties of this medication make it extremely useful in emergency care. Morphine sulfate is a Schedule II drug.

ONSET AND DURATION

Onset: 1-2 min after administration
Duration: 2-7 hr

INDICATIONS

Chest pain associated with myocardial infarction
Pulmonary edema, with or without associated pain
Moderate to severe acute and chronic pain

CONTRAINDICATIONS

Hypersensitivity to narcotics
Hypovolemia
Hypotension
Head injury or undiagnosed abdominal pain
Increased intracranial pressure
Severe respiratory depression
Patients who have taken MAO inhibitors within 14 days

ADVERSE REACTIONS

Hypotension
Tachycardia
Bradycardia
Palpitations
Syncope
Facial flushing, diaphoresis, itching
Respiratory depression
Euphoria
Bronchospasm
Dry mouth
Allergic reaction

DRUG INTERACTIONS

Central nervous system depressants may potentiate effects of morphine (respiratory depression, hypotension, sedation).
Phenothiazines may potentiate analgesia.
MAO inhibitors may cause paradoxical excitation.

HOW SUPPLIED

Morphine is supplied in tablets, suppositories, and solution. In emergency care, morphine sulfate usually is administered IV.
Parenteral preparations are available in many strengths. A common preparation is 10 mg in 1 mL of solution, ampules and Tubex syringes.

DOSAGE AND ADMINISTRATION

Adult: 2-4 mg slow IV over 1-5 min every 5-30 min; titrated to effect
Pediatric: 0.1-0.2 mg/kg/dose IV (max total dose: 15 mg)

SPECIAL CONSIDERATIONS

Pregnancy safety: Category B (if not used for prolonged periods or in high doses at term); narcotics rapidly cross the placenta
Safety in neonates has not been established.
Use with caution in the elderly, those with asthma, and in those susceptible to central nervous system depression.
Morphine should be used with caution in chronic pain syndromes.
Morphine may worsen bradycardia or heart block in inferior myocardial infarction (vagotonic effect).
Naloxone should be readily available.

NALMEFENE (REVEX)

CLASS

Opioid antagonist

DESCRIPTION

Nalmefene is a competitive opioid antagonist used in the management of known or suspected opioid overdose, including respiratory depression induced by natural or synthetic opioids.

ONSET AND DURATION

Onset: Within 2 min
Duration: Up to 8 hr

INDICATIONS

For the complete or partial reversal of central nervous system and respiratory depression induced by opioids including propoxyphene, nalbuphine, pentazocine, and butorphanol

CONTRAINDICATIONS

Hypersensitivity to nalmefene
Use with caution in narcotic-dependent patients who may experience withdrawal syndrome (including neonates of narcotic-dependent mothers).

ADVERSE REACTIONS

Tachycardia
Hypertension
Dysrhythmias
Nausea and vomiting
Diaphoresis
Blurred vision
Withdrawal (opiate)

DRUG INTERACTIONS

May be an increased risk for seizure with flumazenil

HOW SUPPLIED

Available in two concentrations: Blue label (100 mcg/mL) used postoperatively, and Green label (1 mg/mL) in 2-mL ampule to manage or reverse narcotic overdose

DOSAGE AND ADMINISTRATION (GREEN LABEL)

Adult: 0.5-1 mg/70 kg; may be repeated once in 2-5 min
Pediatric: Safety not established

SPECIAL CONSIDERATIONS

Pregnancy safety: Category B
Exercise caution when administering nalmefene to narcotic addicts (may precipitate withdrawal with hypertension, tachycardia, and violent behavior).

NALOXONE (NARCAN)

CLASS

Opioid antagonist

DESCRIPTION

Naloxone is a competitive narcotic antagonist used in the management of known or suspected overdose caused by narcotics. Naloxone antagonizes all actions of morphine. Naloxone is the preferred first-line agent in suspected opioid overdose.

ONSET AND DURATION

Onset: Within 2 min
Duration: 30-60 min

INDICATIONS

For the complete or partial reversal of central nervous system and respiratory depression induced by opioids including the following:

Narcotic Agonist
Morphine sulfate
Heroin
Hydromorphone
Methadone
Meperidine
Paregoric
Fentanyl citrate
Oxycodone
Codeine
Propoxyphene
Narcotic Agonist/Antagonist
Butorphanol tartrate
Pentazocine
Nalbuphine
Decreased Level of Consciousness
Coma of Unknown Origin

CONTRAINDICATIONS

Hypersensitivity
Use with caution in narcotic-dependent patients who may experience withdrawal syndrome (including neonates of narcotic-dependent mothers).

ADVERSE REACTIONS

Tachycardia
Hypertension
Dysrhythmias
Nausea and vomiting
Diaphoresis
Blurred vision
Withdrawal (opiate)

DRUG INTERACTIONS

Incompatible with bisulfite and alkaline solutions

HOW SUPPLIED

0.4 mg/mL (1-mL, 10-mL), 1 mg/mL (2-mL) vials

DOSAGE AND ADMINISTRATION

Adult: 0.4-2 mg IM/IV/SQ (or endotracheal tube diluted); may be repeated in 5-min intervals to a max of 10 mg over a short period (less than 10 min)
Infusion: Mix 8 mg in 1000 mL of D_5W; infuse at two thirds of the initial reversal dose titrated to desired effect
Pediatric: 0.04-0.16 mg/kg/hr (IV/IO/SQ, or endotracheal tube diluted)
Infusion: If 5 years old or younger or 20 kg or less: 0.1 mg/kg; if more than 5 years old or greater than 20 kg: 2 mg; titrate to desired effect

SPECIAL CONSIDERATIONS

Pregnancy safety: Category B
Seizures have been reported (no causal relationship has been established).
Naloxone may not reverse hypotension.
Exercise caution when administering naloxone to narcotic addicts (may precipitate withdrawal with hypertension, tachycardia, and violent behavior).

NITROGLYCERIN (NITROSTAT AND OTHERS)

CLASS

Vasodilator

DESCRIPTION

Nitrates and nitrites dilate arterioles and veins in the periphery (and coronary arteries in high doses). The resultant reduction in preload, and to a lesser extent in afterload, decreases the workload of the heart and lowers myocardial oxygen demand. Nitroglycerin is lipid soluble and is thought to enter the body from the gastrointestinal tract through the lymphatics rather than the portal blood.

ONSET AND DURATION

Onset: 1-3 min
Duration: 30-60 min

INDICATIONS

Ischemic chest pain
Congestive heart failure
Hypertensive emergencies
Pulmonary hypertension

CONTRAINDICATIONS

Volume depletion
Hypersensitivity
Hypotension
Head injury

Cerebral hemorrhage
Recent use of tadalafil (Cialis), vardenafil (Levitra), or sildenafil (Viagra)
Aortic stenosis

ADVERSE REACTIONS

Transient headache
Reflex tachycardia
Hypotension
Nausea and vomiting
Postural syncope
Diaphoresis

DRUG INTERACTIONS

Other vasodilators may have additive hypotensive effects.

HOW SUPPLIED

Tablets: 0.15 mg ($^1/_{400}$gr), 0.3 mg ($^1/_{200}$ gr), 0.4 mg ($^1/_{150}$ gr), 0.6 ($^1/_{100}$ gr), and extended-release capsules and transdermal preparations
Metered spray: 0.4 mg per spray
Parenteral: 5 mg/mL, 10, 20, 40 mg/100 mL

DOSAGE AND ADMINISTRATION

Adult: Tablet: 0.3-0.4 mg sublingually; may repeat twice q 5 min
Metered spray: Spray onto oral mucosa using a lingual aerosol canister for ½-1 sec q 5 min for max of 3 doses delivers 0.4 mg/spray
Infusion: 200-400 mcg/mL at a rate of 10-20 mcg/min; increase by 5-10 mcg/min q 5-10 min until desired effect is achieved
Pediatric: Not recommended

SPECIAL CONSIDERATIONS

Pregnancy safety: Category C
Nitroglycerin is associated with increased susceptibility to hypotension in the elderly.
Nitroglycerin decomposes when exposed to light or heat.
Nitroglycerin must be kept in airtight containers.
Active ingredient of nitroglycerin will "sting" when administered sublingually.
Use with caution in patients with inferior acute myocardial infarction.
Administer IV nitroglycerin by infusion pump to ensure precise flow rate.
PVC tubing may absorb up to 80% of available drug; non-PVC tubing should be used.

NITROPASTE (NITRO-BID OINTMENT)

CLASS

Vasodilator

DESCRIPTION

Nitropaste contains a 2% solution of nitroglycerin in an absorbent paste.

ONSET AND DURATION

Onset: 15-60 min
Duration: 2-12 hr

INDICATIONS

Angina pectoris
Chest pain associated with acute myocardial infarction (less easily titratable than IV nitroglycerin).

CONTRAINDICATIONS

Same as nitroglycerin
Hypersensitivity
Hypotension
Head injury
Cerebral hemorrhage

ADVERSE REACTIONS

Transient headache
Postural syncope
Reflex tachycardia
Hypotension
Nausea and vomiting
Allergic reaction

DRUG INTERACTIONS

Other vasodilators may have additive hypotensive effects.

HOW SUPPLIED

20-, 60-g tubes of 2% nitroglycerin paste (measuring applicators are supplied)

DOSAGE AND ADMINISTRATION

Adult: Apply 1-2 inches over 2- to 4-inch area of skin that is free of hair (usually the chest wall); cover with transparent wrap and secure with tape
Pediatric: Not recommended

SPECIAL CONSIDERATIONS

Pregnancy safety: Category C
Wear gloves when applying paste.
Do not massage or rub paste (rapid absorption will interfere with the sustained action of the drug).
Store paste in a cool place with the tube tightly capped.
Although the adverse effects for nitropaste are the same as for sublingually administered nitroglycerin, their frequency and severity usually are considerably less with the sustained-release preparations because of the slower absorption and less erratic serum levels.

NITROUS OXIDE:OXYGEN (50:50) (NITRONOX)

CLASS

Gaseous analgesic/anesthetic

DESCRIPTION

Nitrous oxide:oxygen is a blended mixture of 50% nitrous oxide and 50% oxygen. When inhaled, nitrous oxide/oxygen depresses the central nervous system, causing anesthesia. In addition, the high concentration of oxygen delivered along with the nitrous oxide increases oxygen tension in the blood, thereby reducing hypoxia. Nitrous oxide:oxygen is self-administered.

ONSET AND DURATION

Onset: 2-5 min
Duration: 2-5 min

INDICATIONS

Moderate to severe pain
Anxiety
Apprehension

CONTRAINDICATIONS

Impaired level of consciousness
Head injury
Chest trauma (pneumothorax)
Inability to comply with instructions
Decompression sickness (nitrogen narcosis, air embolus, air transport)
Undiagnosed abdominal pain or marked distention
Bowel obstruction
Hypotension
Shock
Chronic obstructive pulmonary disease (with history or suspicion of CO_2 retention)

ADVERSE REACTIONS

Dizziness
Apnea
Cyanosis
Nausea and vomiting
Malignant hyperthermia (rare but dangerous)

DRUG INTERACTIONS

None significant

HOW SUPPLIED

D and E cylinders (blue and white in Canada, blue and green in United States) of 50% nitrous oxide and 50% oxygen compressed gas

DOSAGE AND ADMINISTRATION

Adult: Invert cylinder several times before use; instruct the patient to inhale deeply through a patient-held mask or mouthpiece
Pediatric: Same as adult

SPECIAL CONSIDERATIONS

Pregnancy safety: Nitrous oxide has been shown to increase the incidence of spontaneous abortion.
Nitrous oxide is 34 times more soluble than nitrogen and will diffuse into pockets of trapped gas in the patient (intestinal obstruction, pneumothorax, blocked middle ear). As the nitrogen leaves and is replaced by larger amounts of nitrous oxide, increased pressures or volumes may cause serious damage, for example, intestinal rupture.
Nitrous oxide is a nonexplosive gas.
Patient must hold mask and self-administer.

> **NOTE** When delivering nitrous oxide and oxygen from a single tank, the paramedic must ensure that enough oxygen remains in the tank to provide adequate oxygenation. Inverting the cylinder several times to mix the gases is important for this reason. Monitoring of oximetry during administration of nitrous oxide also is reasonable.

NOREPINEPHRINE (LEVOPHED)

CLASS

Sympathomimetic

DESCRIPTION

Norepinephrine is an alpha- and beta$_1$-adrenergic agonist. Norepinephrine is a potent vasoconstrictor that also increases myocardial contractility. Because norepinephrine tends to constrict the renal and mesenteric blood vessels, it rarely is used in the prehospital setting.

ONSET AND DURATION

Onset: 1-3 min
Duration: 5-10 min

INDICATIONS

Cardiogenic shock
Neurogenic shock
Inotropic support
Hemodynamically significant hypotension refractory to other sympathomimetic amines

CONTRAINDICATIONS

Hypotensive patients with hypovolemia

ADVERSE REACTIONS

Headache
Dysrhythmias
Tachycardia
Reflex bradycardia
Angina pectoris
Hypertension

DRUG INTERACTIONS

Norepinephrine can be deactivated by alkaline solutions.
MAO inhibitors and bretylium may potentiate the effects of catecholamines.
Beta-adrenergic antagonists may blunt inotropic response.
Sympathomimetics and phosphodiesterase inhibitors may exacerbate dysrhythmia response.

HOW SUPPLIED

1 mg/mL, 4-mL ampule

DOSAGE AND ADMINISTRATION

Adult: Dilute 4 mg in 250 mL of D_5W or D_5NS (16 mcg/mL); begin infusion at 0.5-1 mcg/min (up to 30 mcg/min) titrated to desired effect (average adult dose is 8-12 mcg/min)
Pediatric: 0.1-2 mcg/kg/min IV/IO

SPECIAL CONSIDERATIONS

Pregnancy safety: Category D
Norepinephrine may cause fetal anoxia when used in pregnancy.
Infuse norepinephrine through a large, stable vein to avoid extravasation and tissue necrosis.
Use infusion pump to ensure precise flow rate.
Do not administer in same IV line as alkaline solutions.

OXYGEN

CLASS

Naturally occurring atmospheric gas

DESCRIPTION

Oxygen is an odorless, tasteless, colorless gas that is present in room air at a concentration of approximately 21%. Oxygen is an important emergency drug used to reverse hypoxemia; in doing so, it helps oxidize glucose to produce adenosine triphosphate (aerobic metabolism). Oxygen may help reduce the size of infarcted tissue during an acute myocardial infarction (in patients who are hypoxemic on room air).

ONSET AND DURATION

Onset: Immediate
Duration: Less than 2 min

INDICATIONS

Confirmed or suspected hypoxia
Ischemic chest pain
Respiratory insufficiency
Prophylactically during air transport
Confirmed or suspected carbon monoxide poisoning and other causes of decreased tissue oxygenation (cardiac arrest)

CONTRAINDICATIONS

Oxygen should never be withheld in any critically ill patient.

ADVERSE REACTIONS

High-concentration oxygen may cause decreased level of consciousness and respiratory depression in patients with chronic carbon dioxide retention.

DRUG INTERACTIONS

None significant

HOW SUPPLIED

Oxygen cylinders (usually green and white) of 100% compressed oxygen gas

DOSAGE AND ADMINISTRATION

Adult:
High-concentration: 10-15 L/min via non-rebreather mask or high-flow oxygen delivery device
Low concentration: 1-4 L/min via nasal cannula
Venturi mask concentrations (e.g., 24%, 28%, 32%, 36%) for intermediate rates of oxygen administration in patients with chronic obstructive pulmonary disease
Pediatric: Same as for adult

SPECIAL CONSIDERATIONS

Pregnancy safety: NA
Oxygen vigorously supports combustion.

OXYTOCIN (PITOCIN)

CLASS

Pituitary hormone

DESCRIPTION

Oxytocin means "rapid birth" and is a synthetic hormone named for the natural posterior pituitary hormone. It stimulates uterine smooth muscle contractions and helps expedite the normal contractions of a spontaneous labor. As with all significant uterine contractions, a transient reduction in uterine blood flow occurs. Oxytocin also stimulates the mammary glands to increase lactation, without increasing the production of milk. The drug is administered in the prehospital setting to control postpartum bleeding.

ONSET AND DURATION

Onset: (IV) Immediate
(IM) Within 3-5 min
Duration: (IV) 20 min after the infusion is stopped
(IM) 30-60 min

INDICATIONS

Postpartum hemorrhage after infant and placental delivery

CONTRAINDICATIONS

Hypertonic or hyperactive uterus
Presence of a second fetus
Fetal distress

ADVERSE REACTIONS

Hypotension
Tachycardia
Hypertension
Dysrhythmias
Angina pectoris
Anxiety
Seizure
Nausea and vomiting
Allergic reaction
Uterine rupture (from excessive administration)

DRUG INTERACTIONS

Vasopressors may potentiate hypertension

HOW SUPPLIED

10 USP units/1-mL ampule (10 U/mL) and prefilled syringe
5 USP units/1-mL ampule (5 U/mL) and prefilled syringe

DOSAGE AND ADMINISTRATION

Control of Postpartum Hemorrhage
IM: 3-10 units IM following delivery of placenta
Bleeding Following Incomplete or Elective Abortion
IV: Mix 10-40 units (1-4 mL) in 1000 mL NS or lactated Ringer's; infuse at 10-40 mU/min via microdrip tubing, titrated to severity of bleeding and uterine response

SPECIAL CONSIDERATIONS

Pregnancy safety: Category X
Vital signs and uterine tone should be monitored closely.
Oxytocin should be administered only in the prehospital setting after delivery of all fetuses.

PANCURONIUM (PAVULON)

CLASS

Neuromuscular blocker (nondepolarizing)

DESCRIPTION

Pancuronium produces complete muscular relaxation by binding to the receptor for acetylcholine at the neuromuscular junction, without initiating depolarization of the muscle membrane. As the concentration of acetylcholine rises in the neuromuscular junction, pancuronium is displaced and muscle tone is regained. Neuromuscular blocking agents are used to provide muscle relaxation during surgery (particularly relaxation of the abdominal muscles) usually with general anesthesia and to prevent convulsive muscle spasms during electroconvulsive therapy. In emergency care, pancuronium is used to optimize conditions for endotracheal intubation and assisted ventilations.

ONSET AND DURATION

Onset: Paralysis in 3-5 min
Duration: 45-60 min

INDICATIONS

Induction or maintenance of paralysis after intubation to assist ventilations

CONTRAINDICATIONS

Known hypersensitivity to the drug
Inability to control airway and/or support ventilations with oxygen and positive pressure
Neuromuscular disease (e.g., myasthenia gravis)

ADVERSE REACTIONS

Transient hypotension
Tachycardia
Dysrhythmias
Hypertension
Excessive salivation
Pain, burning at IV injection site

DRUG INTERACTIONS

Positive chronotropic drugs may potentiate tachycardia.

HOW SUPPLIED

1, 2 mg/mL, 4 mg/2 mL

DOSAGE AND ADMINISTRATION

Adult: 0.04-0.1 mg/kg slow IV; repeat q 30-60 min prn
Pediatric: 0.04-0.1 mg/kg slow IV
(Newborn 0.02 mg/kg/dose)

> **NOTE** If the patient is conscious, explain the effects of the medication before administration, and always sedate the patient before using a neuromuscular blocking agent.

SPECIAL CONSIDERATIONS

Pregnancy safety: Category C
Patients must be sedated completely and have an artificial airway during paralysis.
Carefully monitor the patient and be prepared to resuscitate.
The effects of pancuronium are antagonized by neostigmine (Prostigmin) 0.05 mg/kg and should be accompanied by atropine (0.6-1.2 mg IV).
Pancuronium has no effect on consciousness or pain.
Pancuronium will not stop neuronal seizure activity or decrease central nervous system damage caused by seizures.
Heart rate and cardiac output will be increased.
Pancuronium is excreted in the urine; doses should be decreased for patients with renal disease.

> **NOTE** Neuromuscular blocking agents produce respiratory paralysis. Therefore intubation and ventilatory support must be readily available.

PHENYTOIN (DILANTIN)

CLASS

Anticonvulsant

DESCRIPTION

Phenytoin (a hydantoin) is a drug of choice in controlling grand mal and focal motor seizure activity. It was developed as an alternative anticonvulsant that would cause less sedation than barbiturates. Phenytoin appears to inhibit the spread of seizure activity by promoting sodium efflux from neurons, thereby stabilizing the threshold of the neuron against excitability caused by excess stimulation. Phenytoin also has been used to treat digitalis-induced atrial and ventricular dysrhythmias by stabilizing the sodium influx in Purkinje fibers of the heart, decreasing abnormal ventricular automaticity, and increasing atrioventricular node conduction.

ONSET AND DURATION

Onset: 20-30 min for seizure disorder
Duration: Several days

INDICATIONS

Major motor seizures (generalized grand mal, simple partial and complex partial seizures)
Status epilepticus

CONTRAINDICATIONS

Hypersensitivity
Sinus bradycardia
Second- and third-degree heart block
Sinoatrial block

ADVERSE REACTIONS

Hypotension with rapid IV push (greater than 50 mg/min)
Cardiovascular collapse (with rapid IV use)
Dysrhythmias
Bradycardia
Respiratory depression
Central nervous system depression
Ataxia
Nystagmus
Thrombophlebitis
Nausea and vomiting
Pain from injection site

DRUG INTERACTIONS

Anticoagulants, cimetidine, sulfonamides, and salicylates may increase serum phenytoin levels.
Chronic alcohol consumption or use induces metabolism of the drug.
Lidocaine, propranolol, and other beta-blocking agents may increase cardiac depressant effects.
Xanthines may result in decreased phenytoin absorption.
Precipitation may occur when mixed with D_5W.
Phenytoin is incompatible with many solutions and medications.
Anticoagulation is enhanced with warfarin administration.

HOW SUPPLIED

50 mg/mL in 2- and 5-mL ampules, 2-mL prefilled syringe
May be diluted in NS (1-10 mg/mL, per protocol); use in-line filter
IV line should be flushed with 0.9% NS before and after the drug is administered

DOSAGE AND ADMINISTRATION

Seizures

Adult: 1000 mg or 15-20 mg/kg (usual loading dose) slow IV; not to exceed 1 g or rate of 50 mg/min; followed by 100-150 mg/dose at 30-min intervals (max of 1500 mg/24 hrs)
Pediatric: 10-20 mg/kg slow IV (<0.5 mg/kg/min) loading dose

SPECIAL CONSIDERATIONS

Pregnancy safety: Category D
Phenytoin normally may have slight yellow color.
Carefully monitor vital signs.
Venous irritation can occur because of the alkalinity of the solution.
Use with caution in patients with pulmonary, cardiovascular, hepatic, or renal insufficiency.
Use large, stable vein for injection (extravasation may cause tissue necrosis).

PRALIDOXIME (2-PAM, PROTOPAM)

CLASS

Cholinesterase reactivator and antidote

DESCRIPTION

Pralidoxime reactivates the enzyme acetylcholinesterase, which allows acetylcholine to be degraded, thus relieving the parasympathetic overstimulation caused by excess acetylcholine.

ONSET AND DURATION

Onset: Within minutes
Duration: Variable

INDICATIONS

Organophosphate poisoning (after atropine)

CONTRAINDICATIONS

Hypersensitivity to pralidoxime

ADVERSE REACTIONS

Tachycardia
Hypertension
Laryngospasm

Hyperventilation
Muscle weakness
Nausea

DRUG INTERACTIONS

Pralidoxime should not be mixed in the same syringe or solution with any other drug.

HOW SUPPLIED

Emergency single-dose kit containing one 20-mL vial of 1 g of the sterile drug, one 20-mL ampule of sterile diluent, and a 20-mL syringe with needle

DOSAGE AND ADMINISTRATION

Adult: 600 mg IM (usually by autoinjector) or 1-2 g IV over 15-30 min
Pediatric: 20-50 mg/kg IV over 15-30 min

SPECIAL CONSIDERATIONS

Pregnancy safety: Category C
Each 1 g of sterile powder is diluted with 20 mL of sterile water for injection.
Pralidoxime should be diluted further in 100 mL of NS and given as an IV infusion. Use promptly after reconstitution.
Medical direction may recommend the almost simultaneous administration of atropine.
Pralidoxime is not recommended in carbamate poisoning.
Reduce dosage in cases of known renal insufficiency.

PROCAINAMIDE (PRONESTYL)

CLASS

Antidysrhythmic (Class IA)

DESCRIPTION

Procainamide suppresses phase 4 depolarization in normal ventricular muscle and Purkinje fibers, reducing the automaticity of ectopic pacemakers. It also suppresses reentry dysrhythmias by slowing intraventricular conduction. Procainamide may be effective in treating premature ventricular contractions and recurrent ventricular tachycardia that cannot be controlled with lidocaine.

ONSET AND DURATION

Onset: 10-30 min
Duration: 3-6 hr

INDICATIONS

Suppressing premature ventricular contractions refractory to lidocaine
Suppressing ventricular tachycardia (with a pulse) refractory to lidocaine
Suppressing ventricular fibrillation refractory to lidocaine
Paroxysmal supraventricular tachycardias with wide-complex tachycardia of unknown origin

CONTRAINDICATIONS

Second- and third-degree atrioventricular block (without functioning artificial pacemaker)
Digitalis toxicity
Torsades de pointes
Complete heart block
Tricyclic antidepressant toxicity

ADVERSE REACTIONS

Hypotension
Bradycardia
Reflex tachycardia
Atrioventricular block
Widened QRS complex
Prolonged P-R or Q-T interval
Premature ventricular contractions
Ventricular tachycardia, ventricular fibrillation, asystole
Central nervous system depression
Confusion
Seizure

DRUG INTERACTIONS

Increases effects of skeletal muscle relaxants
Increases plasma/NAPA (active metabolites) concentrations with cimetidine, ranitidine, beta-blockers, amiodarone, trimethoprim, and quinidine

HOW SUPPLIED

1 g in 10-mL vial (100 mg/mL)
1 g in 2-mL vials (500 mg/mL) for infusion

DOSAGE AND ADMINISTRATION

Adult: 20 mg/min slow IV infusion in recurrent
Ventricular fibrillation/pulseless ventricular tachycardia (max total: 17 mg/kg; max dose usually 1 g); 100 mg IV push doses given every 5 min in refractory ventricular fibrillation/ventricular tachycardia are acceptable
Maintenance: Infusion (after resuscitation from cardiac arrest): mix 1 g in 250 mL solution (4 mg/mL), infuse at 1-4 mg/min
Pediatric: Loading dose 15 mg/kg IV/IO; infuse over 30-60 min

SPECIAL CONSIDERATIONS

Pregnancy safety: Category C
Procainamide has potent vasodilating and negative inotropic effects.
Rapid injection may cause procainamide-induced hypotension.
Carefully monitor vital signs and electrocardiogram (a small amount of QRS complex widening is expected).
Routine use in combination with other drugs that prolong the Q-T interval is not recommended.
Administer cautiously to patients with asthma, digitalis-induced dysrhythmias, acute myocardial infarction, or cardiac, hepatic, or renal insufficiency.

NOTE Discontinue if the dysrhythmia is suppressed, hypotension develops, the QRS complex is widened by 50% of its original width, or a total of 1 g has been administered.

PROMETHAZINE (PHENERGAN)

CLASS

Phenothiazine, antihistamine

DESCRIPTION

Promethazine is an H_1 receptor antagonist that blocks the actions of histamine by competitive antagonism at the H_1 receptor. In addition to antihistaminic effects, promethazine also possesses sedative, antimotion, antiemetic, and considerable anticholinergic activity. Promethazine often is administered with analgesics, particularly narcotics, to potentiate their effects, though the occurrence of potentiation is controversial.

ONSET AND DURATION

Onset: IV (rapid)
Duration: 4-6 hr

INDICATIONS

Nausea and vomiting
Motion sickness
Preoperative and postoperative, obstetric (during labor) sedation
To potentiate the effects of analgesics
Allergic reactions

CONTRAINDICATIONS

Hypersensitivity
Comatose states
Central nervous system depression from alcohol, barbiturates, or narcotics
Signs associated with Reye's syndrome

ADVERSE REACTIONS

Sedation
Dizziness
May impair mental and physical ability
Allergic reactions
Dysrhythmias
Nausea and vomiting
Hyperexcitability
Dystonias
Use in children may cause hallucinations, convulsions, and sudden death

DRUG INTERACTIONS

Concomitant use of central nervous system depressants may have an additive sedative effect.
Increased incidence of extrapyramidal effects occurs when given with some MAO inhibitors.
Concomitant use of epinephrine may decrease blood pressure further.

HOW SUPPLIED

25, 50 mg/mL in 1-mL ampules and Tubex syringes

DOSAGE AND ADMINISTRATION

Adult: 12.5-25 mg IV, deep IM
Pediatric: Not indicated in the prehospital setting

SPECIAL CONSIDERATIONS

Pregnancy safety: Category C (generally considered safe for use during labor)
Use caution in patients with asthma, peptic ulcer, and bone marrow depression.
Take care to avoid accidental intraarterial injection.
IM injections are the preferred route of administration.
Give slow IV administration over 1 min.

PROPRANOLOL (INDERAL)

CLASS

Beta-adrenergic blocker, antidysrhythmic (Class II)

DESCRIPTION

Propranolol is a nonselective beta-adrenergic blocker that inhibits chronotropic, inotropic, and vasodilator response to beta-adrenergic stimulation. It slows the sinus rate, depresses atrioventricular conduction, decreases cardiac output, and reduces blood pressure. In addition, propranolol decreases myocardial oxygen demand and reduces the risk of sudden death in patients with acute myocardial infarction.

ONSET AND DURATION

Onset: Within 1-2 hr
Duration: 6-12 hr

INDICATIONS

Hypertension
Angina pectoris
Ventricular tachycardia, ventricular fibrillation, and rapid supraventricular dysrhythmias refractory to other therapies

CONTRAINDICATIONS

Sinus bradycardia
Second- or third-degree atrioventricular block
Asthma
Cardiogenic shock
Pulmonary edema
Uncompensated congestive heart failure
Chronic obstructive pulmonary disease (relative)

ADVERSE REACTIONS

Bradycardia
Heart blocks
Bronchospasm (in susceptible persons)
Dyspnea
Dizziness
Weakness, dizziness
Nausea and vomiting
Visual disturbances

DRUG INTERACTIONS

Catecholamine-depleting drugs may potentiate hypotension.
Sympathomimetic effects may be antagonized.
Verapamil may worsen atrioventricular conduction abnormalities.
Succinylcholine effects may be enhanced.
Isoproterenol, norepinephrine, dopamine, and dobutamine may reverse effects of propranolol.
Epinephrine may cause a rise in blood pressure, a decrease in heart rate, and severe vasoconstriction.
Signs of hypoglycemia may be masked.

HOW SUPPLIED

1-mg/mL vials

DOSAGE AND ADMINISTRATION

Adult: 1-3 mg IV over 2-5 min (not to exceed 1 mg/min); can be repeated after 2 min (total dose of 0.1 mg/kg)
Pediatric: Not recommended.

SPECIAL CONSIDERATIONS

Pregnancy safety: Category C
Propranolol may produce life-threatening side effects; closely monitor patient during administration.
Use with caution in elderly patients.
Use with caution in patients with impaired hepatic or renal function.
Atropine should be readily available.

> **NOTE** Beta$_1$-selective drugs now available are used more commonly for cardiac emergencies.

RETEPLASE (RETAVASE)

CLASS

Fibrinolytic

DESCRIPTION

Reteplase is a recombinant plasminogen activator. Fibrinolytic action occurs by generating plasmin from plasminogen. Plasmin degrades the fibrin matrix of a thrombus. The drug is used in the management of acute myocardial infarction in adults, for the improvement of ventricular function following acute myocardial infarction, and for a reduction in the incidence of congestive heart failure. Treatment with reteplase should be initiated as soon as possible after the onset of acute myocardial infarction symptoms.

ONSET AND DURATION

Onset: Causes reperfusion within 90 min for most patients
Duration: Variable

INDICATIONS

Management of acute myocardial infarction in adults (must be confirmed with 12-lead electrocardiogram)

CONTRAINDICATIONS

Active internal bleeding
History of stroke
Recent intracranial or intraspinal surgery or trauma
Intracranial neoplasm, atrioventricular malformation, or aneurysm
Bleeding disorders
Severe uncontrolled hypertension

ADVERSE REACTIONS

Bleeding (internal and at superficial sites)
Reperfusion dysrhythmias
Allergic reaction (rare)
Nausea and vomiting
Hypotension

DRUG INTERACTIONS

Risk of bleeding will be increased if used concurrently with drugs that alter platelet function.
Risk of bleeding with concomitant use of heparin, vitamin K antagonist (e.g., warfarin) is greatly increased.
Reteplase is incompatible with heparin; do not administer in the same IV line.

HOW SUPPLIED

Supplied in kit with components for reconstitution: single-use reteplase vials (10.8 units each), single-use diluent vials of sterile water (10 mL each), sterile 10-mL syringes with 20-gauge needles, sterile dispensing pins, sterile 20-gauge needles for administration, and alcohol swabs. Reconstitute by withdrawing 10 mL of diluent; open the package containing the dispensing pin; remove the needle from the syringe and discard the needle; remove the connective cap from the dispensing pin and connect the syringe to the pin; remove the flip cap from one vial of reteplase; remove the protective cap from the spike end of the dispensing pin and insert the spike into the vial of reteplase; transfer the diluent through the dispensing pin into the vial of reteplase; with the dispensing pin and syringe still attached, swirl (not shake) the vial gently to dissolve the reteplase; withdraw 10 mL of the reconstituted solution back into the syringe; detach the syringe from the dispensing pin, and attach a sterile 20-gauge needle; the 10-mL bolus dose is now ready to administer.

DOSAGE AND ADMINISTRATION

Adult: Administered as 10 + 10 U double-bolus injection. Each bolus is administered IV over 2 min. (The second bolus is given 30 min after the first bolus.) Heparin and aspirin should be administered concomitantly.
Pediatric: Safety not established.

SPECIAL CONSIDERATIONS

Pregnancy safety: Category C
Reteplase should be given in an IV line in which no other medication is being injected or infused simultaneously.
Protect contents of package from light.

SODIUM BICARBONATE

CLASS

Buffer, alkalinizing agent, electrolyte supplement

DESCRIPTION

Sodium bicarbonate reacts with hydrogen ions to form water and carbon dioxide and thereby can act to buffer metabolic acidosis. As the plasma hydrogen ion concentration decreases, blood pH rises.

ONSET AND DURATION

Onset: 2-10 min
Duration: 30-60 min

INDICATIONS

Tricyclic antidepressant overdose
Known preexisting bicarbonate responsive acidosis
Intubated patient with continued long arrest interval, pulseless electrical activity
Upon return of spontaneous circulation after long arrest interval
Alkalinization for treatment of specific intoxications/rhabdomyolysis
Management of metabolic acidosis
Diabetic ketoacidosis

CONTRAINDICATIONS

In patients with chloride loss from vomiting and gastrointestinal suction
Metabolic and respiratory alkalosis
Severe pulmonary edema
Abdominal pain of unknown origin
Hypocalcemia
Hypokalemia
Hypernatremia
When administration of sodium could be detrimental

ADVERSE REACTIONS

Metabolic alkalosis
Hypoxia
Rise in intracellular P_{CO_2} and increased tissue acidosis
Electrolyte imbalance (hypernatremia)
Seizures
Tissue sloughing at injection site

DRUG INTERACTIONS

Sodium bicarbonate may precipitate in calcium solutions.
Alkalinization of urine may shorten elimination half-lives of certain drugs.
Vasopressors may be deactivated.

HOW SUPPLIED

50 mEq in 50 mL, and 0.5, 0.6 mEq/mL

DOSAGE AND ADMINISTRATION

Urgent Forms of Metabolic Acidosis
Adult: 1 mEq/kg IV; repeat with 0.5 mEq/kg q 10 min
Pediatric: Same as adult; infuse slowly and only if ventilations are adequate

SPECIAL CONSIDERATIONS

Pregnancy safety: Category C
When possible, blood gas analysis should guide bicarbonate administration.
Bicarbonate administration produces carbon dioxide, which crosses cell membranes more rapidly than bicarbonate (potentially worsening intracellular acidosis).
Sodium bicarbonate may increase edematous or sodium-retaining states.
Sodium bicarbonate may worsen congestive heart failure.
Maintain adequate ventilation (gas exchange).

STREPTOKINASE (STREPTASE)

CLASS

Fibrinolytic agent

DESCRIPTION

Streptokinase combines with plasminogen to produce an activator complex that converts free plasminogen to the proteolytic enzyme plasmin. The plasmin in turn functions as an enzyme that degrades fibrin threads and fibrinogen, causing lysis of the blood clot. Streptokinase is administered to selected patients with acute myocardial infarction.

ONSET AND DURATION

Onset: 10-20 min (fibrinolysis, 10-20 min; clot lysis, 60-90 min)
Duration: 3-4 hr (prolonged bleeding times up to 24 hr)

INDICATIONS

Acute myocardial infarction
Massive pulmonary emboli
Arterial thrombosis and embolism
To clear arteriovenous cannulas
Deep venous thrombosis (rare)

CONTRAINDICATIONS

Hypersensitivity
Active bleeding
Recent surgery (within 2-3 weeks)
Recent cerebral vascular accident
Prolonged cardiopulmonary resuscitation
Intracranial or intraspinal surgery
Recent significant trauma (particularly head trauma)
Uncontrolled hypertension (systolic pressure equal to or greater than 180 mm Hg; diastolic pressure equal to or greater than 110 mm Hg)

ADVERSE REACTIONS

Bleeding (gastrointestinal, genitourinary, intracranial, other sites)
Allergic reactions
Hypotension
Chest pain
Reperfusion dysrhythmias
Abdominal pain

DRUG INTERACTIONS

Acetylsalicylic acid may increase risk of bleeding (and may be beneficial in improving overall effectiveness).
Heparin and other anticoagulants may increase risk of bleeding and improve overall outcome.

HOW SUPPLIED

250,000-, 750,000-, 1.5 million-IU vials
Reconstitute by slowly adding 5 mL of sodium chloride or D_5W, directing the stream toward the side of the vial, rather than into the powder. Gently roll—do not shake—the vial for reconstitution. Slowly dilute the entire contents of the vial to a total of 45 mL.

DOSAGE AND ADMINISTRATION

Acute Myocardial Infarction
Adult: 1.5 million U diluted to 45 mL (IV) over 1 hr (use infusion pump)
Pediatric: Safety not established

SPECIAL CONSIDERATIONS

Pregnancy safety: Category C
Do not administer IM injections to patients receiving fibrinolytic drugs.
Obtain blood sample for coagulation studies before administration.
Carefully monitor vital signs.
Observe the patient for bleeding.
Use caution when moving patient to avoid bruising or bleeding.
Do not draw arterial blood gas specimens in fibrinolytic therapy candidates.
Use one IV line exclusively for fibrinolytic administration.

SUCCINYLCHOLINE (ANECTINE)

CLASS

Neuromuscular blocker (depolarizing)

DESCRIPTION

Succinylcholine has the quickest onset and briefest duration of action of all neuromuscular blocking drugs, making it a drug of choice for procedures such as endotracheal intubation, electroconvulsive shock therapy, and terminating laryngospasm. Like nondepolarizing blockers, depolarizing drugs also bind to the receptors for acetylcholine. However, because they cause depolarization of the muscle membrane, they often lead to fasciculations and some muscular contractions.

ONSET AND DURATION

Onset: Less than 1 min
Duration: 5-10 min after single IV dose

INDICATIONS

To facilitate intubation
Terminating laryngospasm
Muscle relaxation

CONTRAINDICATIONS

Burns or injuries in the first 12 hours
Hypersensitivity
Skeletal muscle myopathies
Inability to control airway and/or support ventilations with oxygen and positive pressure
Personal or family history of malignant hyperthermia
Acute rhabdomyolysis
Intraocular (globe rupture) injuries

ADVERSE REACTIONS

Hypotension
Respiratory depression
Bradycardias
Dysrhythmias
Initial muscle fasciculation
Excessive salivation
Malignant hyperthermia
Allergic reaction
Succinylcholine may exacerbate hyperkalemia in trauma patients (hours after trauma)

DRUG INTERACTIONS

Oxytocin, beta-blockers, chronic contraceptive use, and organophosphates may potentiate effects.
Diazepam may reduce duration of action.
Cardiac glycosides may induce dysrhythmias.

HOW SUPPLIED

20, 50, 100 mg/mL, 1-g multidose vial

DOSAGE AND ADMINISTRATION

NOTE If the patient is conscious, explain the effects of the medication before administration. Premedication with atropine should be strongly considered, particularly in the pediatric age group. Premedicating with lidocaine may blunt any increase in intracranial pressure associated with intubation. Finally, diazepam or another sedative should be used in any conscious patient undergoing neuromuscular blockade.

Adult: 0.3-1.1 mg/kg (25-75 mg) over 10-30 sec IV; 0.04-0.07 mg/kg to maintain relaxation
Pediatric: 1-2 mg/kg dose rapid IV

SPECIAL CONSIDERATIONS

Pregnancy safety: Category C

> **NOTE** Neuromuscular blocking agents will produce respiratory paralysis. Therefore intubation and ventilatory support must be readily available.

Carefully monitor the patient and be prepared to resuscitate.
Administer with caution to patients with severe trauma, burns, and electrolyte imbalances (high potassium levels).
Brain or spinal cord injury may prolong effects.
Patients must have a patent or artificial airway and adequate sedation during paralysis. Children are not as sensitive to succinylcholine on a weight basis as adults and may require higher doses.
Succinylcholine has no effect on consciousness or pain.
Succinylcholine will not stop neuronal seizure activity.
Succinylcholine rarely may cause ventricular dysrhythmias/cardiac arrest in infants and children.

SYRUP OF IPECAC

CLASS

Emetic, antidote

DESCRIPTION

Syrup of ipecac acts as a local irritant on the gastric mucosa and on emetic centers of the brain. Vomiting induced by syrup of ipecac occurs in 80%-90% of patients. The drug is available over-the-counter; however, medical direction and/or a poison control center should be consulted before administration.

ONSET AND DURATION

Onset: Generally 15-20 min
Duration: Up to 1-2 hr

INDICATIONS

Acute oral drug or toxin overdose in alert patients

CONTRAINDICATIONS

Caustics, corrosives, petroleum distillates
Tricyclic antidepressant overdose
Camphor ingestion
Unprotected airway/absent gag reflex
Unconscious patient greater than 1 hr time elapsed since exposure
Unknown ingestion
Children less than 1 year of age
Rapidly acting central nervous system depressants (causing decreased level of consciousness faster than ipecac can work) or stimulants (causing seizures)
Upper gastrointestinal bleeding

ADVERSE REACTIONS

Prolonged vomiting
Muscle aching, weakness
Drowsiness

DRUG INTERACTIONS

Activated charcoal adsorbs ipecac.

HOW SUPPLIED

15-, 30-mL vials

DOSAGE AND ADMINISTRATION

Adult: 15-30 mL PO followed by 3-4 glasses of water; may repeat with 15 mL once in 20 min if ineffective
Pediatric (1-12 years): 5-15 mL PO followed by $1^1/_2$-2 glasses of water; may repeat with 15 mL once in 20 min if ineffective

SPECIAL CONSIDERATIONS

Pregnancy safety: Category C
Carefully monitor patient's airway.
90% of patients vomit within one-half hour of administration (average time is 20 min).
Activated charcoal should be administered only after vomiting has ceased for 1-2 hr.
A disadvantage of syrup of ipecac is that persistent vomiting may preclude use of activated charcoal.
Save emesis sample for evaluation.
Patients usually vomit 2-3 times per dose over one to two periods. Keep patient awake NPO for 2 hr.
Ipecac should not be given unless overdose was witnessed (e.g., acetaminophen ingestion witnessed by parent) and is recommended by medical direction or a poison control center.

> **NOTE** Syrup of ipecac is less effective than activated charcoal in decreasing toxin absorption. Syrup of ipecac is seldom indicated for use in the prehospital setting.

TETRACAINE (PONTOCAINE)

CLASS

Topical ophthalmic anesthetic

DESCRIPTION

Tetracaine is used for rapid, brief, superficial anesthesia. The agent inhibits conduction of nerve impulses from sensory nerves.

ONSET AND DURATION

Onset: Within 30 sec
Duration: 10-15 min

INDICATIONS

Short-term relief from eye pain or irritation
Patient comfort before eye irrigation

CONTRAINDICATIONS

Hypersensitivity to tetracaine
Open injury to the eye

ADVERSE REACTIONS

Burning or stinging sensation
Irritation

DRUG INTERACTIONS

Incompatible with mercury or silver salts often found in ophthalmic products

HOW SUPPLIED

0.5% solution

DOSAGE AND ADMINISTRATION

Adult: 1-2 drops
Pediatric: Same as adult

SPECIAL CONSIDERATIONS

Pregnancy safety: Category C
Tetracaine can cause epithelial damage and systemic toxicity.
Tetracaine is not recommended for prolonged use.

THIAMINE (BETAXIN)

CLASS

Vitamin (B_1)

DESCRIPTION

Thiamine combines with adenosine triphosphate to form thiamine pyrophosphate, a coenzyme necessary for carbohydrate metabolism. Most vitamins required by the body are obtained through diet; however, certain states such as alcoholism and malnourishment may affect the intake, absorption, and utilization of thiamine. The brain is extremely sensitive to thiamine deficiency.

ONSET AND DURATION

Onset: Rapid
Duration: Depends on the degree of deficiency

INDICATIONS

Coma of unknown origin (with administration of dextrose 50% or naloxone)
Delirium tremens
Beriberi (rare)
Wernicke's encephalopathy

CONTRAINDICATIONS

None significant

ADVERSE REACTIONS

Hypotension (from rapid injection or large dose)
Anxiety
Diaphoresis
Nausea and vomiting
Allergic reaction (usually from IV injection; rare); angioedema

DRUG INTERACTIONS

None significant

HOW SUPPLIED

1-, 2-mL vials (100 mg/mL)

DOSAGE AND ADMINISTRATION

Adult: 100 mg slow IV or IM
Pediatric: Not recommended in the prehospital setting

SPECIAL CONSIDERATIONS

Pregnancy safety: Category A (Category C if dose exceeds recommended daily allowance)
Large IV doses may cause respiratory difficulties.
Anaphylactic reactions have been reported.

TISSUE PLASMINOGEN ACTIVATOR (t-PA, ACTIVASE, RECOMBINANT ALTEPLASE)

CLASS

Fibrinolytic

DESCRIPTION

Tissue plasminogen activator is a naturally occurring enzyme that has been mass produced using recombinant DNA technology. The enzyme binds to fibrin-bound plasminogen at the site of an arterial clot, thus converting plasminogen to plasmin. Plasmin digests the fibrin strands of the clot, causing clot lysis and restoration of perfusion to the occluded artery. In emergency care, fibrinolytic agents are used in treating selected patients with acute evolving myocardial infarction.

ONSET AND DURATION

Onset: Clot lysis often occurs within 60-90 min
Duration: 30 min (80% cleared in 10 min)

INDICATIONS

Same as other fibrinolytic agents
Acute evolving myocardial infarction
Massive pulmonary emboli
Deep venous thrombosis
Arterial thrombosis and embolism
To clear arteriovenous cannulas
Acute stroke

CONTRAINDICATIONS

Active bleeding
Recent surgery (within 2-3 weeks)
Recent cerebral vascular accident
Prolonged cardiopulmonary resuscitation
Intracranial or intraspinal surgery
Recent significant trauma (particularly head trauma)
Uncontrolled hypertension
Recent gastrointestinal bleeding

ADVERSE REACTIONS

Bleeding (gastrointestinal, genitourinary, intracranial, other sites)
Allergic reactions
Hypotension
Chest pain
Reperfusion dysrhythmias
Abdominal pain

DRUG INTERACTIONS

Acetylsalicylic acid may increase risk of bleeding (and may be beneficial in improving overall effectiveness).
Heparin and other anticoagulants also may increase risk of bleeding and improve overall effectiveness

HOW SUPPLIED

50, 100 mg/vial with 50, 100 mL of diluent, respectively
May dilute further with equal amounts of 0.9% sodium chloride or D_5W

DOSAGE AND ADMINISTRATION

Adult (for acute myocardial infarction): Give 15 mg IV bolus, then 0.75 mg/kg over next 30 min (not to exceed 50 mg), and then 0.5 mg/kg over next 60 min (not to exceed 35 mg) (Other doses may be prescribed by medical direction.)
Pediatric: Safety not established

SPECIAL CONSIDERATIONS

Pregnancy safety: Category C
Gently roll—do not shake—the vial to mix powder with liquid.
Closely monitor vital signs.
Observe for bleeding.
Obtain blood sample for coagulation studies before administration.
Do not administer IM injections to patients receiving fibrinolytic drugs.
No arterial blood gas specimens should be drawn on potential fibrinolytic therapy candidates due to bleeding tendency.
Use caution when moving patient to avoid bleeding or bruising.
Use one IV line exclusively for fibrinolytic administration.

VASOPRESSIN (PITRESSIN)

CLASS

Naturally occurring antidiuretic hormone

DESCRIPTION

Vasopressin acts by direct stimulation of smooth muscle V_1 receptors. When given in extremely high doses, it acts as a nonadrenergic peripheral vasoconstrictor.

ONSET AND DURATION

Onset: Immediate
Duration: Variable

INDICATIONS

As an alternative pressor to epinephrine in adult shock-refractory ventricular fibrillation
Vasodilatory shock

CONTRAINDICATIONS

Responsive patients with coronary artery disease

ADVERSE REACTIONS

Ischemic chest pain
Abdominal distress
Sweating
Nausea and vomiting
Tremors
Bronchial constriction
Uterine contraction

DRUG INTERACTIONS

No significant drug reactions have been reported

HOW SUPPLIED

5 U/mL

DOSAGE AND ADMINISTRATION

Adult: Ventricular fibrillation/cardiac arrest: 40 U IV push one time
Child and infant: Not recommended

SPECIAL CONSIDERATIONS

Pregnancy safety: Category C
Vasopressin may increase peripheral vascular resistance and provoke cardiac ischemia and angina.
Vasopressin may be given IO.

VERAPAMIL (ISOPTIN)

CLASS

Calcium channel blocker (Class IV antidysrhythmic)

DESCRIPTION

Verapamil is used as an antidysrhythmic, antianginal, and antihypertensive agent. It works by inhibiting the movement of calcium ions across cell membranes. The slow calcium ion current blocked by verapamil is more important for the activity of the sinoatrial node and atrioventricular node than for many other tissues in the heart. By interfering with this current, calcium channel blockers achieve some selectivity of action. Verapamil decreases atrial automaticity, reduces atrioventricular conduction velocity, and prolongs the atrioventricular nodal refractory period. In addition, verapamil depresses myocardial contractility, reduces vascular smooth muscle tone, and dilates coronary arteries and arterioles in normal and ischemic tissues.

ONSET AND DURATION

Onset: 2-5 min
Duration: 30-60 min (up to 4 hr is possible)

INDICATIONS

Paroxysmal supraventricular tachycardias
Atrial flutter with a rapid ventricular response
Atrial fibrillation with a rapid ventricular response
Vasospastic and unstable angina
Chronic stable angina

CONTRAINDICATIONS

Hypersensitivity
Sick sinus syndrome (unless the patient has a functioning pacemaker)
Second- or third-degree heart block
Sinus bradycardia
Hypotension
Cardiogenic shock
Severe congestive heart failure
Wolff-Parkinson-White with atrial fibrillation or flutter
Patients receiving IV beta blockers
Wide-complex tachycardias (Ventricular tachycardia can deteriorate into ventricular fibrillation when calcium channel blockers are given.)

ADVERSE REACTIONS

Dizziness
Headache
Nausea and vomiting
Hypotension
Bradycardia
Complete atrioventricular block
Peripheral edema

DRUG INTERACTIONS

Verapamil increases serum concentration of digoxin.
Beta-adrenergic blockers may have additive negative inotropic and chronotropic effects.
Antihypertensives may potentiate hypotensive effects.

HOW SUPPLIED

Parenteral: 5 mg/2 mL in 2-, 4-, 5-mL vials, or 2-, 4-mL ampules

DOSAGE AND ADMINISTRATION

Adult:
Initial dose: 2.5-5 mg IV bolus over 2 min
Repeat dose: 5-10 mg in 15-30 min after initial dose; or 5 mg q 15 min until a desired response is achieved (max dose: 30 mg)
Pediatric: Not recommended in the prehospital setting

SPECIAL CONSIDERATIONS

Pregnancy safety: Category C
Closely monitor patient's vital signs.
Give smaller amounts (2-4 mg) over longer periods of time (3-4 min) when treating the elderly or when the blood pressure is in the lower range of normal.
Be prepared to resuscitate.
Atrioventricular block or asystole may occur because of slowed atrioventricular conduction.

> **NOTE** Some physicians recommend slow IV administration of 500 mg calcium chloride before dose of verapamil to minimize the untoward results of hypotension and bradycardia.

REFERENCES

American Health Association: *2000 Handbook of emergency cardiovascular care for healthcare providers,* Dallas, 2000, The Association.

American Heart Association: *Advanced cardiac life support,* Dallas, 1997, The Association.

American Heart Association: *Pediatric advanced life support,* Dallas, 1997, The Association.

Clark J et al: *Pharmacologic basis of nursing practice,* ed 4, St Louis, 1993, Mosby.

Gonzalez E et al: Intravenous amiodarone for ventricular arrhythmias: overview and clinical use, *Resuscitation* 39:31, 1998.

Guidelines for cardiopulmonary resuscitation and emergency cardiac care, *JAMA* 16:2171, 1992.

Hoekelman R: *Primary pediatric care,* ed 3, St Louis, 1997, Mosby.

McKenry L, Salerno E: *Mosby's pharmacology in nursing,* ed 18, St Louis, 1992, Mosby.

Physician's desk reference, ed 53, Oradell, NJ, 1999, Medical Economics.

Ryan T et al: *Guidelines for the management of patients with acute myocardial infarction: report of the American College of Cardiology/American Heart Association Task Force on Practice Guidelines (Committee on Management of Acute Myocardial Infarction),* Dallas, 1998, The Association.

Salerno E: *Pharmacology for health professionals,* St Louis, 1999, Mosby.

Skidmore-Roth L: *Mosby's 1999 nursing drug reference,* St Louis, 1999, Mosby.

GLOSSARY

abandonment Terminating medical care without legal excuse or turning care over to personnel who do not have training and expertise appropriate for the medical needs of the patient.

abdominal Pertaining to the abdomen.

abdominal aorta The portion of the descending aorta that passes from the aortic hiatus of the diaphragm into the abdomen, where it divides into the two common iliac arteries.

abdominal cavity The space within the abdominal walls between the diaphragm and the pelvic area; it contains the liver, stomach, intestines, spleen, kidneys, and associated tissues and vessels.

abdominopelvic cavity The space between the diaphragm and the groin.

abduction Movement away from the midline.

abnormal Deviating from the normal.

abnormal presentation A type of vaginal delivery in which the newborn's head does not deliver first.

abortion The spontaneous or induced termination of a pregnancy before the fetus has developed into a stage of viability.

abrasion A partial-thickness injury caused by scraping or rubbing away of a layer or layers of skin.

abruptio placentae Separation of the placenta implanted in a normal position in a pregnancy of 20 weeks or more; it occurs during labor or delivery of the fetus.

absolute refractory period The portion of the action potential during which the membrane is insensitive to all stimuli regardless of strength.

absorption The process by which drug molecules are moved from the site of entry into the body into the general circulation.

accelerated atrioventricular conduction See *anomalous conduction*.

acclimatization Physical adjustment to a different climate or to changes in altitude or temperature.

acetabulum The large, cup-shaped articular cavity at the juncture of the ilium, the ischium, and the pubis that contains the ball-shaped head of the femur.

acetoacetic acid A colorless, oily ketone body produced by the metabolism of lipids and pyruvates; it is excreted in trace amounts in normal urine and in elevated amounts with diabetes mellitus, especially in ketoacidosis.

acetonemia The presence of acetone in the blood, characterized by the fruity breath odor of ketoacidosis.

acetylcholine A neurotransmitter, widely distributed in body tissues, with the primary function of mediating the synaptic activity of the nervous system.

acetylcholinesterase An enzyme found in the synaptic cleft that causes the breakdown of acetylcholine into acetic acid and choline, thereby limiting the stimulatory effect of acetylcholine.

acid A compound that yields hydrogen ions when dissociated in solution.

acidosis A condition marked by a high concentration of hydrogen ions (i.e., a pH below 7.35).

acinus A small lobule of a compound gland; the exocrine portion of the pancreas that produces pancreatic juice.

acquired immunodeficiency syndrome A disease that results from infection with the human immunodeficiency virus; the syndrome impairs the immune system, giving rise to opportunistic infections and malignancies.

acromegaly A chronic metabolic condition characterized by a gradual, marked enlargement and elongation of the bones of the face, jaw, and extremities.

acromion process The lateral extension of the spine of the scapula; it gives attachment to the deltoideus and trapezius muscles.

actin A protein found in muscle fibers that acts with myosin to bring about contraction and relaxation.

actinomycosis A chronic systemic disease characterized by deep, lumpy abscesses that extrude a granular pus through multiple sinuses.

action plan A plan of action based on the patient's condition and the environment.

action potential A change in membrane potential in an excitable tissue that acts as an electrical signal and is propagated in an all-or-none fashion.

active transport A carrier-mediated process that can move substances against a concentration gradient.

active tubular secretion Secretion that involves the transport of free drug from the blood across the proximal tubular cell and into the tubular urine by an active process against a concentration gradient.

acute dystonia A sudden impairment of muscle tone; it commonly involves the head, neck, or tongue and often occurs as an adverse effect of medication.

acute gastroenteritis Inflammation of the stomach and intestines with an associated sudden onset of vomiting, diarrhea, or both.

acute hepatitis An inflammatory condition of the liver associated with the sudden onset of malaise, weakness, anorexia, intermittent nausea and vomiting, and dull right upper quadrant pain, usually followed within 1 week by the onset of jaundice, dark urine, or both, characterized by jaundice.

acute mountain sickness A common high-altitude illness that results when an unacclimatized person rapidly ascends to high altitudes.

acute pain Severe pain such as may follow trauma or may accompany myocardial infarction or other conditions and diseases.

acute renal failure A clinical syndrome that results from a sudden and significant decrease in filtration through the glomeruli, leading to the accumulation of salt, water, and nitrogenous wastes within the body.

adaptation A cellular response to stress of any kind to escape and protect from injury; a central part of the response to changes in the physiological condition.

addiction A compulsive, uncontrollable dependence on a substance, habit, or practice to such a degree that cessation causes severe emotional, mental, or physiological reactions.

Addison disease A rare and potentially life-threatening disorder caused by a deficiency of the corticosteroid hormones normally produced by the adrenal cortex.

adduction Movement toward the midline.

adenohypophysis The anterior lobe of the pituitary gland.

adenoma A tumor of glandular epithelium in which the cells of the tumor are arranged in a recognizable glandular structure.

adenosine A compound derived from nucleic acid and composed of adenine and a sugar.

adenosine diphosphate A product of the hydrolysis of adenosine triphosphate.

adenosine monophosphate A compound that affects energy release in work done by muscles.

adenosine triphosphate Adenosine, an organic base, with three phosphate groups attached to it; it stores energy in muscles.

adhesion The quality of remaining in close contact with or stuck to another entity; also, a structure that joins several parts, sometimes abnormally.

adipose tissue A specialized connective tissue that stores lipids; also known as fat tissue.

adrenal gland Either of two secretory glands perched atop the kidneys; each gland consists of two parts, the cortex and medulla, which have independent functions.

adrenal medullary mechanism The mechanism by which epinephrine and norepinephrine are released from the adrenal medulla as a result of the same stimuli that increase sympathetic stimulation of the heart and blood vessels.

adrenaline An endogenous adrenal hormone that helps prepare the body for energetic action.

adrenergic Of or pertaining to the sympathetic nerve fibers of the autonomic nervous system, which use epinephrine or epinephrine-like substances as neurotransmitters.

adrenocorticotropic hormone A hormone of the anterior pituitary gland that stimulates growth of the adrenal gland cortex and secretion of corticosteroids.

adsorption The capacity of a substance to attract and hold other materials or particles on its surface.

adult respiratory distress syndrome A group of symptoms that accompany fulminant pulmonary edema, resulting in acute respiratory failure; also known as *noncardiogenic pulmonary edema.*

advanced cardiac life support Clinical care or guidelines for care of life-threatening cardiovascular and respiratory disorders.

advanced life support The provision of care that paramedics or allied health professionals render, including advanced airway management, defibrillation, intravenous therapy, and medication administration.

aerobic Of or pertaining to the presence of air or oxygen.

aerobic oxidation A biochemical reaction that increases the positive charges on an atom or the loss of negative charges in the presence of oxygen.

aerosol Pressurized gas that contains a finely nebulized medication for inhalation therapy.

affect An outward manifestation of a person's feelings or emotions.

affective disorder Any of a group of psychotic disorders characterized by severe and inappropriate emotional responses, prolonged and persistent disturbances of mood and related thought distortions, and other symptoms associated with depressed or manic states.

afferent division Nerve fibers that send impulses from the periphery to the central nervous system.

affinity The propensity of a drug to bind or attach itself to a given receptor site.

afterdrop phenomenon A sudden return of cold blood and waste products to the core of the body as a result of rewarming methods used to treat hypothermia.

afterload The total resistance against which blood must be pumped. Also known as *peripheral vascular resistance.*

agglutinated Reference to cells that have clumped together. See *agglutination.*

agglutination A clumping together of cells as a result of their interaction with specific antibodies called agglutinins.

agglutinin A kind of antibody; its interaction with antigens is manifested as agglutination.

agonal rhythm A ventricular escape complex or rhythm that occurs when the electrical impulses from the sinoatrial node, atria, or atrioventricular junction fail to reach the ventricles because of sinus arrest or high-degree atrioventricular block; frequently seen as the last rhythm in an unsuccessful resuscitation.

agonists Drugs that combine with receptors and initiate the expected response.

air trapping The result of a prolonged but inefficient expiratory effort, usually caused by chronic obstruction of the pulmonary tree, as is seen commonly in chronic obstructive pulmonary disease or asthma.

akathisia An abnormal condition characterized by restlessness and agitation.

albumin A water-soluble protein containing carbon, hydrogen, oxygen, nitrogen, and sulfur.

aldosterone A steroid hormone produced by the adrenal cortex to regulate the sodium and potassium balance in the blood.

aliquot A sample that is representative of the whole.

alkaline Having the reactions of an alkali.

alkalosis A condition marked by a low concentration of hydrogen ions (i.e., a pH above 7.45).

allergens Substances that can produce hypersensitivity reactions in the body.

allergic reaction A hypersensitivity response to an allergen to which a person previously was exposed and to which the person has developed antibodies.

allergy A hypersensitivity reaction to intrinsically harmless antigens, most of which are environmental.

all-or-none principle The principle that when a stimulus is applied to a cell, an action potential is produced or is not produced.

alpha cell A constituent of the islets of Langerhans that produces glucagon.

alpha-adrenergic receptor Any one of the postulated adrenergic components of receptor tissues that responds to norepinephrine and to various blocking agents.

alveolar duct Part of the respiratory passages beyond a respiratory bronchiole; alveolar sacs and alveoli arise from it.

alveoli Small outpouchings of walls of alveolar space through which gas exchange takes place between alveolar air and pulmonary capillary blood.

alveolus A small cavity; the terminal ending of a secretory gland. Alveoli of the lungs are microscopic, saclike dilations of terminal bronchioles.

Alzheimer's disease A disease characterized by confusion, memory failure, disorientation, speech disturbances, and inability to carry out purposeful movements.

amaurosis fugax Unilateral vision loss as a result of internal carotid artery plaque emboli.

ambulance A generic term that describes the various land-based emergency vehicles used by emergency medical services personnel, including basic and advanced life support units, paramedic units, mobile intensive care units, and others.

amenorrhea The absence of menstruation.

amino acid An organic chemical compound composed of one or more basic amino groups and one or more acidic carboxyl groups.

ammonia A colorless, aromatic gas consisting of nitrogen and hydrogen.

amnestic Causing amnesia.

amniocentesis An obstetrical procedure in which a small amount of amniotic fluid is removed for laboratory analysis; it aids in diagnosis of fetal abnormalities.

amniotic fluid embolism An embolism that occurs when particulate matter in amniotic fluid forms an embolus and gains access to maternal circulation during labor or delivery or immediately after delivery.

amniotic sac A thin-walled bag that contains the fetus and amniotic fluid during pregnancy.

amplitude modulation A transmitted radio frequency carrier fixed in frequency but increasing or decreasing in amplitude in accordance with the strength of the applied audio.

ampulla A round, saclike dilation of the uterine tube.

amputation A complete or partial loss of a limb caused by mechanical force.

amylase A starch-splitting enzyme.

amyotrophic lateral sclerosis One of a group of rare disorders in which the nerves that control muscular activity degenerate in the brain and spinal cord; also called Lou Gehrig's disease.

anabolic steroid Any of several compounds derived from testosterone or prepared synthetically to promote general body growth, to oppose the effects of endogenous estrogen, or to promote masculinizing effects.

anaerobic Of or pertaining to the absence of oxygen.

anaerobic metabolism Metabolism that occurs in the absence of oxygen.

anal canal The final portion of the alimentary tract between the rectal ampulla and the anus.

anal fissure A linear ulceration or laceration of the skin of the anus.

anal fistula An abnormal opening of the cutaneous surface near the anus.

anal triangle The posterior portion of the perianal region through which the anal canal opens.

anaphylactic shock Shock that occurs when the body is exposed to a substance that produces a severe allergic reaction.

anaphylaxis An exaggerated, life-threatening hypersensitivity reaction to a previously encountered antigen.

anasarca Generalized, massive edema.

anastomosis The joining of two parts.

anatomical dead space The volume of the conducting airways from the external environment down to the terminal bronchioles.

anatomical position A position standing erect with the feet and palms facing the examiner.

anchoring Attaching a high-angle rope to a secure point.

androgen Any steroid hormone that increases male characteristics.

anemia A decrease in blood hemoglobin.

anesthesia Without sensation.

aneurysm A localized dilation of a wall of a blood vessel.

angina pectoris Ischemic chest pain most often caused by myocardial anoxia as a result of atherosclerosis of the coronary arteries.

angioedema A localized edematous reaction of the deep dermal or subcutaneous or submucosal tissues that appears as giant wheals.

angiogram A study of vessels.

angioplasty Repair of damaged vessels.

angiotensin I The inactive form of angiotensin, formulated by the stimulation of renin, which is converted to angiotensin II.

angiotensin II A potent vasoconstrictor that also acts to stimulate the secretion of antidiuretic hormone.

angle of Louis See *sternal angle.*

anhedonia The inability to enjoy what is usually pleasurable.

anion An ion with a negative charge.

anisocoria Normal or congenital unequal pupil size.

anomalous conduction A preexcitation syndrome; a clinical condition associated with abnormal conduction pathways between the atria and ventricles that bypass the atrioventricular node and bundle of His and allow the electrical impulses to initiate depolarization of the ventricles earlier than usual. Also known as *accelerated atrioventricular conduction*.

anorexia Lack or loss of appetite, resulting in an inability to eat.

anorexia nervosa A disorder characterized by a prolonged refusal to eat, resulting in emaciation, amenorrhea, emotional disturbance concerning body image, and an abnormal fear of becoming obese.

anovulation Failure of the ovaries to produce, mature, or release eggs.

antagonism The opposition between two or more medications; it occurs when the combined (conjoint) effect of two drugs is less than the sum of the drugs acting separately.

antagonist muscle A muscle that works in opposition to another muscle.

antagonists Agents designed to inhibit or counteract the effects of other drugs or undesired effects caused by normal or hyperactive physiological mechanisms.

antecubital fossa See *antecubital space*.

antecubital space The depressed area in front of the elbow or at the bend of the elbow; also known as the *antecubital fossa*.

antegrade amnesia The loss of memory for events that occurred immediately after recovery of consciousness.

antenatal Occurring or formed before birth.

antepartum The period before labor and delivery.

anterior The front, or ventral, surface.

anterior chamber of the eye The chamber of the eye between the cornea and the iris.

anterior communicating artery The artery that connects with the anterior cerebral arteries and completes the circle of Willis.

anterior cord syndrome A spinal cord injury usually seen in flexion injuries; caused by pressure on the anterior aspect of the spinal cord by a ruptured intervertebral disk or fragments of the vertebral body extruded posteriorly into the spinal canal.

anterior superior iliac spine One of two bony segments that form the iliac crest.

anthrax An acute infectious disease caused by the spore-forming bacterium *Bacillus anthracis*.

antibody A substance produced by the body that destroys or inactivates a specific substance (antigen) that has entered the body.

anticholinergic Of or pertaining to the blocking of acetylcholine receptors, resulting in inhibition of transmission of parasympathetic nerve impulses.

anticoagulant A substance that prevents or delays coagulation of the blood.

antidiuretic hormone A hormone produced in the posterior pituitary gland to regulate the balance of water in the body by accelerating the resorption of water.

antidote A drug or other substance that opposes the action of a poison.

antigenic site A site capable of binding to and reacting with an antibody.

antigens Substances (usually proteins) that cause the formation of an antibody and react specifically with that antibody.

antiplatelet drug A drug that interferes with platelet aggregation.

antipyretic Something that works against fever.

antivenin A suspension of venom-neutralizing antibodies prepared from the serum of immunized horses.

anuria The inability to urinate; the cessation of urine production; a diminished urinary output of less than 100 to 250 mL per day.

anus The distal end or outlet of the rectum.

anxiety A state or feeling of apprehension, uneasiness, agitation, uncertainty, and fear resulting from the anticipation of some threat or danger.

aorta The main and largest artery in the body.

aortic aneurysm A localized dilation of the wall of the aorta.

aortic body Any of the specialized nerve cells located in the arch of the aorta, where they monitor levels of oxygen and hydrogen ions in the cardiovascular system.

aortic semilunar valve A valve that guards the orifice between the left ventricle and the aorta.

apex of the heart The top or tip of the heart opposite the base.

Apgar score The evaluation of a newborn's physical condition, usually performed at 1 minute and 5 minutes after birth, including heart rate, respiratory effort, muscle tone, reflex irritability, and color.

aphasia Loss of the power of speech.

apical impulse A pulsation of the left ventricle of the heart, palpable and sometimes visible at the fifth intercostal space to the left of the midline.

apnea An absence of spontaneous respirations.

apneustic center A group of neurons in the pons that has a stimulatory effect on the inspiratory center.

apocrine gland A gland that has cells that contribute cytoplasm to its secretion, such as a mammary gland.

apothecary A system of graduated liquid volumes arranged in order of heaviness; it is based on the grain.

apparatus A vehicle used for fire suppression or rescue that does not include staff vehicles.

appendicitis An acute inflammation of the appendix.

appendicular region The limbs or extremities.

appendicular skeleton The bones of the upper and lower extremities.

appendix A wormlike, blunt process extending from the cecum; also known as the *vermiform appendix*.

application of principle A component of critical thinking in which the examiner makes patient care decisions based on conceptual understanding of the situation and the interpretation of data gathered from the patient.

aqueous humor The clear, watery fluid circulating in the anterior and posterior chambers of the eye.

Arachnida A large class of arthropods that includes spiders, scorpions, mites, and ticks.

arachnoid layer A delicate, weblike middle membrane that covers the brain.

areflexia A neurological condition characterized by absence of the reflexes.

areola The circular, pigmented area surrounding the nipple.

areolar connective tissue A loose tissue that consists of delicate webs of fibers and a variety of cells embedded in a matrix of soft, sticky gel.

areolar gland A gland that forms small, rounded projections from the surface of the areola of the mamma.

arrector pili Smooth muscles of the skin attached to hair follicles; when contraction occurs, the hair rises, resulting in gooseflesh.

arterial capillary The ends of capillaries closest to arterioles.

arteriogram A study of arteries.

arteriole A small branch of an artery.

arteriovenous anastomosis A vessel that allows blood to flow from arteries to veins without passing through capillaries; also known as an *arteriovenous shunt*.

arteriovenous shunt See *arteriovenous anastomosis*.

artery A vessel that carries blood away from the heart.

arthritis An inflammatory condition of the joints, characterized by pain and swelling.

arthroscopy Inspection of a joint.

artifact A deflection on the electrocardiogram display or tracing produced by factors other than the electrical activity of the heart.

arytenoid cartilages Small, pyramidal laryngeal cartilages that articulate with the cricoid cartilage.

asbestosis A chronic lung disease caused by the inhalation of asbestos fibers; it results in the development of alveolar, interstitial, and pleural fibrosis.

ascending colon The segment of the colon that extends from the cecum in the right lower quadrant of the abdomen to the transverse colon at the hepatic flexure on the right side; usually at the level of the umbilicus.

ascites An abnormal intraperitoneal accumulation of fluid containing large amounts of protein and electrolytes.

aseptic Sterile, without germs.

asphyxiation A state of suffocation, caused by severe hypoxia, that leads to hypoxemia and hypercapnia, loss of consciousness, and if not corrected, death.

aspiration Inhalation of foreign substances into the pulmonary system.

assault Creating apprehension, or unauthorized handling and treatment of a patient.

asthma A respiratory disorder characterized by recurring episodes of paroxysmal dyspnea, wheezing on expiration caused by constriction of the bronchi, coughing, and viscous mucoid bronchial secretions.

asthma exacerbation An aggravation of asthma, usually associated with severe symptoms.

astigmatism An abnormal condition of the eye in which the light rays cannot be focused clearly on a point on the retina because the spherical curve of the cornea is not equal in all meridians.

astrocyte gliosis A tumor composed of glial cells within the nervous system; it may be associated with respiratory center dysfunction and neuroepithelial bodies in the tracheobronchial tree, along with distal atelectasis.

asystole A life-threatening cardiac condition characterized by the absence of electrical and mechanical activity of the heart.

ataxia Failure of muscle coordination.

ataxic breathing A type of cluster or irregular breathing pattern characterized by a series of inspirations and expirations.

atelectasis An abnormal condition characterized by the collapse of lung tissue, which prevents the respiratory exchange of oxygen and carbon dioxide.

atelectatic breathing A modified respiratory effort thought to be a protective reflex to hyperinflate the lungs and reexpand alveoli that might have been collapsed.

atheroma An abnormal accumulation of fat or lipids as a cyst or a deposit in an arterial wall; a hard, atherosclerotic plaque.

atherosclerosis A common arterial disorder characterized by yellowish plaques of cholesterol, lipids, and cellular debris in the inner layers of the walls of large and medium-sized arteries.

athetosis A neuromuscular condition characterized by slow, continuous, and involuntary movement of the extremities.

atlantooccipital joint One of a pair of condyloid joints formed by the articulation of the atlas of the vertebral column with the occipital bone of the skull.

atlas The first cervical vertebra, which articulates with the occipital bone and the axis.

atmospheric pressure The pressure exerted by the weight of the atmosphere; at sea level this pressure is 760 mm Hg.

atom The smallest division of an element that exhibits all the properties and characteristics of the element; atoms comprise neutrons, electrons, and protons.

atony Weak muscle tone.

atria Chambers or cavities, such as the atria of the heart.

atrial natriuretic factor A peptide released from the atria when atrial blood pressure is increased; it lowers blood pressure by increasing urine production, thus reducing blood volume.

atrial natriuretic hormone A hormone secreted by specialized muscle fibers in the atrial wall of the heart that influences water reabsorption in the kidney; it acts as an antagonist of aldosterone.

atrial synchronous ventricular pacemaker An artificial pacemaker synchronized with the patient's atrial rhythm; it paces the ventricles only when an atrioventricular block occurs.

atrial-ventricular demand pacemaker An artificial pacemaker that paces the atria or ventricles when the intrinsic rate of the paced chamber drops dangerously low.

atrioventricular canal The path through which the atria open into the ventricles.

atrioventricular dissociation A conduction disturbance in which atrial and ventricular contractions occur rhythmically but are unrelated to each other.

atrioventricular node An area of specialized cardiac muscle that receives the cardiac impulse from the sinoatrial node and conducts it to the bundle of His.

atrioventricular sequential pacemaker An artificial pacemaker that paces the atria first and then the ventricles when spontaneous activity is absent or slowed in the atria and ventricles.

atrioventricular valve A valve in the heart through which blood flows from the atria to the ventricles.

atrophy Decrease in size (shrinkage) of a cell, which adversely affects cell function.

attention deficit disorder A syndrome that affects children, adolescents, and, in rare cases, adults and is characterized by learning and behavioral disabilities.

auditory Of or pertaining to hearing or the organs of hearing.

auditory meatus A tubelike channel of the external ear extending from the auricle to the tympanum of the middle ear.

auditory ossicles The incus, malleus, and stapes; small bones in the middle ear that articulate with each other and the tympanic membrane.

auditory tube The auditory canal; it extends from the middle ear to the nasopharynx; also known as the *eustachian tube.*

aura A sensation that may precede a migraine or seizure activity.

auricle The part of the external ear that protrudes from the head; also known as the *pinna.*

auscultation A technique that requires the use of a stethoscope and is used to assess body sounds produced by the movement of various fluids or gases in organs or tissues.

autoimmune pericarditis Inflammation of the pericardium associated with the production of antibodies directed against one's own tissues.

autoimmunity An abnormal characteristic or condition in which the body reacts against constituents of its own tissues.

autolysis The spontaneous disintegration of tissues or cells by the action of their own autogenous enzymes.

automatic external defibrillator A device used in cardiac arrest to perform a computer analysis of the patient's cardiac rhythm and deliver defibrillatory shocks when indicated.

automatic implantable cardioverter-defibrillator A surgically implanted device that monitors a person's heart rate; it is designed to deliver defibrillatory shocks as needed.

automatic vehicle location A radio communications subsystem that uses one or more electronic methods periodically to determine the position of a land, marine, or air vehicle and relay that information via radio to a communications center.

automaticity A property of specialized excitable tissue that allows self-activation through spontaneous development of an action potential.

automatism Abnormal repetitive motor behavior such as lip smacking, chewing, or swallowing during which the patient is amnestic.

autonomic hyperreflexia syndrome A neurological disorder characterized by a discharge of sympathetic nervous system impulses as a result of stimulation of the bladder, large intestine, or other visceral organs.

autonomic nervous system The part of the nervous system that regulates involuntary vital functions, including the activity of cardiac muscle, smooth muscle, and glands.

autophagia Nutrition of the body by consumption of its own tissues.

avascular Having blood vessels.

Avogadro's number The number of molecules in a gram mole of any chemical substance.

avoidance The act of keeping away from someone, something, or a situation, or of preventing the occurrence of something; it requires the paramedic to continually be aware of the scene by being observant and knowledgeable about warning signs that may indicate a dangerous situation.

avulsion A full-thickness skin loss in which the wound edges cannot be approximated.

axial loading Vertical compression of the spine that results when direct forces are transmitted along the length of the spinal column.

axial region The head, neck, thorax, abdomen, and pelvis.

axial skeleton The bones of the head, neck, and torso.

axillae Armpits.

axillary node One of the lymph glands of the axillae that help fight infections in the chest, armpit, neck, and arm and drain lymph nodes from those areas.

axis The second cervical vertebra about which the atlas rotates, allowing the head to be turned, extended, or flexed.

axon The main central process of a neuron that normally conducts action potentials away from the neuron cell body.

azotemia The retention of excessive amounts of nitrogenous compounds in the blood.

B lymphocytes The lymphocytes responsible for antibody-mediated immunity.

Babinski reflex A reflex movement in which the great toe bends upward when the outer edge of the sole is scratched.

bacteremia The presence of bacteria in the blood.

bacteria Single-celled microorganisms that cause an infection characteristic of that species.

bacterial tracheitis A bacterial infection of the upper airway and subglottic trachea.

bacteriocidal Destructive to bacteria.

bacteriophage Any virus that causes lysis of host bacteria.

bacteriostatic Tending to restrain the development or the reproduction of bacteria.

ball-and-socket joint A joint that consists of a ball (head) at the end of one bone and a socket in an adjacent bone into which a portion of the ball fits.

bariatrics The field of medicine that focuses on the treatment and control of obesity and diseases associated with obesity.

baroreceptor A sensory nerve ending in the walls of the atria of the heart, venae cavae, aortic arch, and carotid sinuses; it is sensitive to stretching of the walls caused by an increase in blood pressure.

barotitis An inflammation of the ear caused by changes in atmospheric pressure.

barotrauma A physical injury sustained as a result of exposure to increased environmental pressure.

Bartholin's gland One of two small, mucus-secreting glands located on the posterior and lateral aspect of the vestibule of the vagina.

Barton's bandage A circumferential head dressing applied to restrict jaw movement and minimize pain.

base A chemical compound that combines with an acid to form a salt; also known as an alkali.

base of the heart The portion of the heart opposite the apex, directed to the right side of the body.

base station A grouping of radio equipment consisting of at least a transmitter, a receiver, a transmission line, and an antenna located at a specific, fixed location.

basic life support Care provided by persons trained in first aid, cardiopulmonary resuscitation, and other noninvasive care.

basilar artery The single arterial trunk formed by the junction of the two vertebral arteries at the base of the skull.

basilar fracture A fracture that may occur when the mandibular condyles perforate the base of the skull but that more commonly results from extension of a linear fracture into the floor of the anterior and middle fossae.

basophil A white blood cell that promotes inflammation; it readily stains with specific dyes.

battering A form of domestic violence that establishes control and fear in a relationship through violence and other forms of abuse.

battery Physical contact with a person without consent and without legal justification.

Battle's sign Ecchymosis over the mastoid process caused by a fracture of the temporal bone.

Beck triad A combination of three symptoms that characterize cardiac tamponade: elevated central venous pressure, muffled heart sounds, and hypotension.

behavior indicator Nonspecific behavioral changes that may suggest that a child is being maltreated. Behavior indicators for sexual abuse are called nonspecific because children may display such behavior changes because of other traumatic conditions. Prompt evaluation is warranted when these nonspecific behavior indicators occur to rule out maltreatment; appropriate assistance for the child must be obtained.

behavioral emergency A change in mood or behavior that cannot be tolerated by the involved person or others and requires immediate attention.

belay Method of attaching a safety rope and controlling the rope so that if the person or load starts to fall, the belay rope will prevent the fall.

Bell palsy A condition in which paralysis of the facial muscles is caused by inflammation of the seventh cranial nerve; usually is one sided and temporary and often develops suddenly.

beta cell A constituent of the islets of Langerhans that produces insulin.

beta-adrenergic receptor Any of the postulated adrenergic components of receptor tissues that respond to epinephrine and various blocking agents.

beta-hydroxybutyric acid One of the ketone bodies that occur in abnormal amounts in diabetic ketoacidosis as a result of fatty acid oxidation.

bicarbonate buffer system The principal mechanism for stabilizing acid-base balance.

biceps brachii The biceps muscle of the arm that flexes and supinates the forearm.

bicuspid valve One of the two atrioventricular valves located between the left atrium and ventricle; also known as the *mitral valve.*

bifurcate To divide into two branches.

bilateral Having or occurring on two sides.

bile A bitter, yellow-green secretion of the liver that is stored in the gallbladder.

bilirubin The orange-yellow pigment of bile, formed principally from the breakdown of hemoglobin in red blood cells after termination of their normal life span.

bioethics The systematic study of moral dimensions including moral vision, decisions, conduct, and policies of the life sciences and health care.

biological half-life The time required to metabolize or eliminate half the total amount of a drug in the body.

biology The study of life.

biosynthesis A chemical reaction that continually occurs throughout the body in which molecules form more complex molecules.

Biot's respiration A respiratory pattern consisting of irregular respirations that vary in depth and that are interrupted by intervals of apnea.

bioterrorism The use of biological agents, such as pathogenic organisms or agricultural pests, for the express purpose of causing death or disease, to instill a sense of fear and panic in the victims, and to intimidate governments or societies for political, financial, or ideological gain.

biotransformation The process by which a drug is converted chemically to a metabolite.

biphasic complex A QRS complex that is partly positive and partly negative.

bipolar disorder A disorder marked by alternating periods of mania and depression; also known as *manic-depressive disorder.*

bipolar lead A lead composed of two electrodes of opposite polarity.

blast injury A general term used to describe damage to a person exposed to a pressure field.

blastocyst The stage of mammalian embryos in which the embryo consists of the inner cell mass and a thin trophoblast layer.

bleb An accumulation of fluid under the skin.

blood The fluid and its suspended, formed elements that circulate through the heart, arteries, capillaries, and veins.

blood clot The end result of the clotting process in blood; a blood clot normally consists of red cells, white cells, and platelets enmeshed in an insoluble fibrin network.

blood colloid osmotic pressure Osmotic pressure caused by the presence of plasma proteins (mostly albumin) that are too large to pass through the wall of the capillary; also known as *oncotic pressure.*

blood-brain barrier An anatomical-physiological feature of the brain thought to consist of walls of capillaries in the central nervous system and surrounding glial membranes; its function is to prevent or slow the passage of chemical compounds from the blood into the central nervous system.

blowout fracture A fracture of the floor of the orbit caused by a blow that suddenly increases the intraocular pressure.

blunt trauma An injury produced by the wounding forces of compression and change of speed, both of which can disrupt tissue.

B-NICE An acronym used for identifying five categories of weapons of mass destruction: *B*iological, *N*uclear, *I*ncendiary, *C*hemical, and *E*xplosives.

body The largest or main part of any organ or structure.

bone A highly specialized form of hard, connective tissue; it consists of living cells and mineralized matrix.

bone marrow Specialized soft tissue that fills the spaces in the cancellous bone of the epiphyses.

bony labyrinth Part of the inner ear; it contains the membranous labyrinth.

borderline personality disorder A pervasive pattern of instability of interpersonal relationships, self-image, and affect, in addition to considerable impulsivity that begins by early adulthood.

botulism An often fatal form of food poisoning caused by the bacillus *Clostridium botulinum.*

bowel obstruction An occlusion of the intestinal lumen that results in blockage of normal flow of intestinal contents.

Bowman's capsule The expanded beginning of a renal tubule.

boxer's fracture Fracture of the fifth metacarpal bone from direct trauma to a closed fist.

Boyle's law See *general gas law.*

brachial plexus A network of nerves in the neck that passes under the clavicle and into the axilla, originating in the fifth, sixth, seventh, and eighth cervical nerves and the first two thoracic spinal nerves; the brachial plexus innervates the muscles and the skin of the chest, shoulders, and arms.

bradycardia A heart rate of less than 60 beats per minute.

bradykinin A peptide of nonprotein origin that contains nine amino acid residues; a potent vasodilator.

bradypnea A persistent respiratory rate slower than 12 breaths per minute.

brainstem The midbrain, pons, and medulla.

brand name See *trade name.*

Braxton-Hicks contraction Irregular tightening of the pregnant uterus that begins in the first trimester and increases in frequency, duration, and intensity as pregnancy progresses.

breech presentation The intrauterine position of the fetus in which the buttocks or feet present.

broad ligament A folded sheet of peritoneum draped over the uterine tubes, uterus, and ovaries.

bronchial tree An anatomical complex of the bronchi and bronchial tubes.

bronchiectasis An abnormal dilation of the bronchi caused by a pus-producing infection of the bronchial wall.

bronchiole A small branch of a bronchus.

bronchiolitis An acute viral infection of the lower respiratory tract that occurs primarily in infants under 18 months of age; it is characterized by expiratory wheezes, respiratory distress, inflammation, and obstruction at the level of the bronchioles.

bronchopulmonary dysplasia A chronic respiratory disorder characterized by scarring of lung tissue, thickened pulmonary arterial walls, and ventilation-perfusion mismatch; often occurs in infants who have dependence on long-term artificial ventilation.

brow presentation See *face presentation.*

Brown-Séquard syndrome A hemitransection of the spinal cord. In the classic presentation, pressure on half of the spinal cord results in weakness of the upper and lower extremities on the ipsilateral (same) side and loss of pain and temperature sensation on the contralateral (opposite) side.

bruit An abnormal sound or murmur heard while auscultating an artery, organ, or gland.

buccal Of or pertaining to the inside of the cheek.

buccal route A route for administering medication in which the agent is placed between the teeth and mucous membrane of the cheek.

bulbourethral glands Small glands located just below the prostate gland that lubricate the terminal portion of the urethra and contribute to seminal fluid; also known as *Cowper's glands.*

bulimia nervosa A disorder characterized by an insatiable craving for food, often resulting in episodes of binge eating followed by purging (through self-induced vomiting or use of laxatives), depression, and self-deprivation.

bullae Thin-walled blisters of the skin or mucous membranes that contain clear, serous fluid.

bullet tumble See *bullet yaw.*

bullet yaw The forward rotation of a bullet around its center of mass, which causes an end-over-end motion, producing a greater energy exchange and greater tissue damage; also known as *bullet tumble.*

bundle of His A band of fibers in the myocardium through which the cardiac impulse is transmitted from the atrioventricular node to the ventricles.

bundle of Kent Fibers that connect atrial muscle to ventricular muscle, bypassing the AV node; also known as *Kent fibers.*

burette An intravenous device used to deliver a wide range of accurate, specific volumes.

bursitis An inflammation of the bursa, the connective tissue structure surrounding a joint.

calcaneus The heel bone, the largest of the tarsal bones.

calcium The fifth most abundant element in the human body; it occurs mainly in bone.

calipers An instrument with two hinged, adjustable legs used to measure components of the electrocardiogram.

canaliculus A very small tube or channel.

cancellous bone Latticelike tissue normally present in the interior of many bones where spaces usually are filled with marrow; also known as spongy bone.

cancer A neoplasm characterized by the uncontrolled growth of anaplastic cells that tend to invade surrounding tissue and to metastasize to distant body sites.

Candida A genus of yeastlike fungi.

candidiasis An infection caused by a species of *Candida* organisms that is characterized by pruritus, exudate, and easy bleeding.

cannulation The insertion of a cannula into a body duct or cavity.

capillaries Tiny vessels that connect arterioles to venules.

capillary refill test A test used to evaluate the rate of blood flow through peripheral capillary beds.

capitation A method of payment to cover all health care expenses for each member of a managed care organization.

capitulum The lateral aspect of the humerus; it articulates with the head of the radius.

capnography Measuring of the proportion of carbon dioxide in expired air.

capsid A protein coat that encloses a virus.

carbaminohemoglobin A chemical complex formed by carbon dioxide and hemoglobin after the release of oxygen by the hemoglobin to a tissue cell.

carbohydrate Any group of organic compounds composed of carbon, hydrogen, and oxygen; it is primarily obtained from plant foods.

carbonic acid An aqueous solution of carbon dioxide.

carbonic anhydrase The enzyme that converts carbon dioxide into carbonic acid.

carboxyhemoglobin A compound produced by the exposure of hemoglobin to carbon monoxide.

carcinogenic Cancer causing.

cardiac cycle The complete round of cardiac systole and diastole.

cardiac ejection fraction The percentage of ventricular blood volume released during a contraction.

cardiac muscle A special striated muscle of the myocardium that contains dark, intercalated disks at the junctions of the abutting fibers; cardiac muscle is characterized by special contractile abilities.

cardiac myopathy An abnormal condition of the heart characterized by weakness of the myocardium.

cardiac output The volume of blood pumped each minute by the ventricle.

cardiac plexus One of several nerve complexes situated close to the arch of the aorta.

cardiac sphincter A ring of muscle fibers at the juncture of the esophagus and stomach.

cardiogenic shock Shock that results when cardiac action is unable to deliver sufficient circulating blood volume for tissue perfusion.

cardiography Recording the movements of the heart.

cardiomyopathy Any disease that affects the myocardium.

cardiopulmonary Of or pertaining to the heart and lungs.

cardiopulmonary resuscitation An emergency procedure for life support consisting of artificial respiration and manual external cardiac massage.

carina of the trachea A downward and backward projection of the lowest tracheal cartilage, forming a ridge between the openings of the right and left primary bronchi.

carotid body A small structure containing neural tissue at the bifurcation of the carotid arteries; it monitors the oxygen content of the blood and helps regulate respiration.

carotid sinus massage See *carotid sinus pressure.*

carotid sinus pressure A technique used to increase vagal tone to convert paroxysmal supraventricular tachycardia to sinus rhythm; also known as *carotid sinus massage.*

carpal Pertaining to the carpus, or wrist.

carpometacarpal joint The joint of the thumb.

carrier A radio signal of specific frequency generated by a transmitter without audio information imposed on it.

carrier molecule A protein that combines with solutes on one side of a membrane, transporting the solute to the other side; it is used in mediated transport mechanisms.

cartilage Firm, smooth, nonvascular connective tissue.

cartilaginous joint See *joint.*

catabolic Pertaining to the destruction of complex substances by living cells to form simple compounds.

cataract A loss of transparency of the lens of the eye that results from changes in the delicate protein fibers within the lens.

catecholamine Any of a group of sympathomimetic amines, including dopamine, epinephrine, and norepinephrine.

cathartic Causing evacuation of the bowel.

cation An ion with a positive charge.

cavitation A temporary or permanent opening produced by a force that pushes body tissues laterally away from the track of a projectile.

cecum A cul-de-sac constituting the first part of the large intestine.

cell body The part of the cell that contains the nucleus and surrounding cytoplasm, exclusive of any projections or processes; it is concerned more with metabolism of the cell than with a specific function.

cell-mediated immunity Immunity characterized by the formation of a population of lymphocytes that attack and destroy foreign material.

cellular phone An 800- to 900-MHz radio communications system used to gain access to dial-up telephone circuits and vice versa. The system usually is divided into small coverage areas called cells, which are interconnected via microwave or dedicated telephone circuits.

cellulitis An inflammation of the skin characterized most commonly by local heat, redness, pain, swelling, and occasionally fever, malaise, chills, and headache.

cementum The bonelike connective tissue that covers the roots of the teeth and helps to support them.

centigram A metric unit of mass equal to $\frac{1}{100}$ of a gram.

centimeter A metric unit of length equal to $\frac{1}{100}$ of a meter, or 0.3937 inches.

central cord syndrome A spinal cord injury commonly seen with hyperextension or flexion cervical injuries; characterized by greater motor impairment of the upper than lower extremities.

central nervous system The brain and spinal cord.

central nervous system ischemic response An increase in blood pressure caused by vasoconstriction that occurs when oxygen levels are too low, carbon dioxide levels are too high, or pH is too low in the medulla.

central pain syndrome Infection or disease of the trigeminal nerve (cranial nerve V).

central thermoreceptors Nerve endings located in or near the anterior hypothalamus that are sensitive to heat.

centrifugation The process of separating components of different densities contained in a liquid by spinning them at high speeds.

centriole Usually paired organelles lying in the centrosome.

centrosome A specialized zone of cytoplasm close to the nucleus that contains two centrioles.

cephalic presentation A classification of fetal position in which the head of the fetus is at the uterine cervix; also known as *vertex presentation.*

cephalopelvic disproportion An obstetrical condition in which a newborn's head is too large or a mother's birth canal too small to permit normal labor or birth.

cephalothorax The united head and thorax of a spider.

cerebellar cortex The outer portion of the cerebellum.

cerebellum The second largest part of the brain, which plays an essential role in producing normal movements.

cerebral Pertaining to the brain.

cerebral aqueduct The narrow conduit between the third and fourth ventricles in the midbrain that conveys cerebrospinal fluid.

cerebral cortex A thin layer of gray matter, made up of neuron dendrites and cell bodies, that composes the surface of the cerebrum.

cerebral edema An accumulation of fluid in the brain tissue.

cerebral palsy A general term for nonprogressive disorders of movement and posture.

cerebral perfusion pressure A measure of the amount of blood flow to the brain calculated by subtracting the intracranial pressure from the mean systemic arterial blood pressure.

cerebrospinal fluid Fluid that fills the subarachnoid space in the brain and spinal cord and in the cerebral ventricles.

cerebrospinal fluid rhinorrhea Leakage of cerebrospinal fluid caused by fracture of the ethmoid cribriform plate.

cerebrovascular accident An abnormal condition of the blood vessels of the brain characterized by occlusion by an embolus, thrombus, or cerebral hemorrhage; also known as *stroke* and brain attack.

cerebrum The largest and uppermost part of the brain; it controls consciousness, memory, sensations, emotions, and voluntary movements.

certification (or registration) The process by which an agency or association grants recognition to an individual for meeting specific requirements to participate in an activity.

cerumen A yellowish or brownish waxy secretion produced in the external ear canal; also known as earwax.

ceruminous gland The gland that produces a waxy substance, cerumen (earwax).

cervical Pertaining to the neck.

cervical node One of the lymph glands in the neck.

cervical plexus The network of nerves formed by the ventral primary divisions of the first four cervical nerves.

cervical spondylosis A form of degenerative joint and disk disease that affects the cervical vertebrae and results in compression of the associated nerve roots.

cervical vertebrae The first seven segments of the vertebral column, designated C1 to C7.

cervicitis Acute or chronic inflammation of the uterine cervix.

cervix The lower part of the uterus.

cesarean delivery A surgical procedure in which the abdomen and uterus are incised and the baby is delivered transabdominally.

Chadwick's sign The bluish coloration of the vulva and vagina that develops after the sixth week of pregnancy as a normal result of local venous congestion; an early sign of pregnancy.

chancre A skin lesion, usually of primary syphilis, that begins at the site of infection as a papule and develops into a red, bloodless, painless ulcer with a craterlike appearance.

channel An assigned frequency or pair of frequencies used to carry voice or data communications or both. In emergency medical services, an advanced life support "MED" channel is a pair of radio frequencies, one used for transmitting, the other for receiving.

chemical name The exact designation of a chemical structure as determined by the rules of chemical nomenclature.

chemoreceptor A sensory cell stimulated by a change in the concentration of chemicals to produce action potentials.

chemotactic factors Biochemical mediators that are important in activating the inflammatory response.

chemotaxis The response of leukocytes to products formed in immunological reactions; a part of the inflammatory response.

CHEMTREC (Chemical Transportation Emergency Center) A public service of the Chemical Manufacturers Association, the center provides immediate advice to on-scene personnel regarding management of hazardous materials.

Cheyne-Stokes respiration A regular, periodic pattern of breathing with equal intervals of apnea followed by a crescendo-decrescendo sequence of respirations.

chickenpox See *varicella.*

chief complaint A patient's primary complaint.

child abuse The physical, sexual, or emotional maltreatment of a child.

Chlamydia A genus of microorganisms that live as intracellular parasites; a common cause of sexually transmitted diseases and a frequent cause of sterility.

chlorine A poisonous, yellow-green gas with an odor that has been described as a mixture of pineapple and pepper.

choanal atresia A bony or membranous occlusion that blocks the passageway between the nose and pharynx; it can result in serious ventilation problems in the neonate.

cholecystitis Inflammation of the gallbladder, most often associated with the presence of gallstones.

cholecystokinin A hormone that stimulates the contraction of the gallbladder and the secretion of pancreatic juice.

cholesterol A fat-soluble compound found in animal fats and oils that is distributed widely in the body.

cholinergic Of or pertaining to the effects produced by the parasympathetic nervous system or drugs that stimulate or antagonize the parasympathetic nervous system.

chondrocytes Cartilage cells.

chorioamnionitis An inflammatory reaction in the amniotic membranes caused by organisms in the amniotic fluid.

chorionic gonadotropin A chemical component of the urine of pregnant women.

choroid The portion of the vascular tunic associated with the sclera of the eye.

choroid plexus A network of brain capillaries that are involved in producing cerebrospinal fluid.

chromatin granules The material within the cell nucleus from which chromosomes are formed.

chronic bronchitis Obstructive airway disease of the trachea and bronchi.

chronic gastroenteritis Inflammation of the stomach and intestines that accompanies numerous gastrointestinal disorders.

chronic obstructive pulmonary disease A progressive, irreversible condition characterized by diminished inspiratory and expiratory capacity of the lungs.

chronic pain Pain that continues or recurs over a prolonged period; it is caused by various disease or abnormal conditions.

chronic pulmonary hypertension A condition of abnormally high pressure within the pulmonary circulation.

chronic renal failure A progressive, irreversible systemic disease caused by kidney dysfunction that leads to abnormalities in blood counts and blood chemistry levels.

chronotropic Pertaining to agents that affect the heart rate; a drug that increases the heart rate is said to have a positive chronotropic effect.

chyme The semifluid mass of partly digested food passed from the stomach into the duodenum.

cilia Small, hairlike processes on the outer surfaces of some cells.

ciliary body A structure continuous with the choroid layer that contains smooth muscle cells and that functions in accommodation.

ciliated tissue Any tissue that projects cilia from its surface, such as portions of the epithelium in the respiratory tract.

circadian rhythm A pattern based on a 24-hour cycle, especially repetition of certain physiological phenomena, such as sleeping and eating.

circle of Willis The circle of interconnected blood vessels at the base of the brain.

circulatory shock Failure of the cardiovascular system to supply the cells with enough oxygenated blood to meet metabolic demands.

circumduction Movement in a circular motion.

circumflex artery The subdivision of the left coronary artery that feeds the lateral and posterior portions of the left ventricle and part of the right ventricle.

cirrhosis A chronic degenerative disease of the liver.

citrate Any salt or ester of citric acid.

classic heat stroke A severe, sometimes fatal condition resulting from the failure of the temperature-regulating capacity of the body; it is caused by prolonged exposure to the sun or to high temperatures.

claudication Cramplike pains in the calves caused by poor circulation of blood to the leg muscles.

clavicle A long, curved, horizontal bone just above the first rib that forms the ventral portion of the shoulder girdle.

clinical perineum The portion of the perineum between the vaginal and anal openings.

clinical reasoning Use of the results of questions to think about associated problems and body system changes related to the patient's complaint.

clitoris Erectile tissue located in the vestibule of the vagina.

closed pneumothorax A collection of air or gas in the pleural space that causes the lung to collapse without exposing the pleural space to atmospheric pressure.

cluster headache A type of headache that occurs in bursts (clusters); also known as histamine headache.

coagulation Formation of a clot.

coarse ventricular fibrillation Fibrillatory waves greater than 3 mm in amplitude.

coccygeal bone The four segments of the sacral vertebral column that fuse to form the adult coccyx.

coccygeal plexus A network of coccygeal nerves.

cochlea Part of the bony labyrinth of the inner ear.

coitus See *copulation.*

colitis An inflammatory condition of the large intestine characterized by severe diarrhea, bleeding, and ulceration of the mucosa of the intestine.

collagen The ropelike protein of the extracellular matrix.

collecting duct A straight tubule that extends from the cortex of the kidney to the tip of the renal pyramid.

Colles' fracture A fracture of the radius at the epiphysis within 1 inch of the joint of the wrist; it is easily recognized by the resultant dorsal and lateral position of the hand.

colloid A state of matter in which large molecules or aggregates of molecules that do not precipitate are dispersed in another medium.

colon The portion of the large intestine that extends from the cecum to the rectum.

colorectal cancer A malignant disease of the large intestine characterized by a change in bowel habits and the passing of blood.

colostomy A surgical opening into the large intestine.

command The act of directing, ordering, or controlling by virtue of explicit, statutory, regulatory, or delegated authority.

command post The area from which command directs operations for an incident.

communicability period A stage of infection that begins when the latent period ends and continues as long as the agent is present and can spread to other hosts.

communicable disease An infectious disease that can be transmitted from one person to another.

communications The transmission and reception of information, resulting in common understanding.

communications center A facility used to dispatch emergency equipment and coordinate communications between field units and personnel.

community health assessment An assessment of a target community to identify needs and resources required to provide prevention and wellness promotion activities.

compact bone Hard, dense bone that usually is found at the surface of skeletal structures, as distinguished from cancellous bone.

compartment syndrome The result of a crush injury, usually caused by compressive forces or blunt trauma to muscle groups confined in tight fibrous sheaths with minimal ability to stretch.

competitive antagonist An agent with an affinity for the same receptor site as an agonist. The competition with the agonist for the site inhibits the action of the agonist; increasing the concentration of the agonist tends to overcome the inhibition.

complement One of 11 complex, enzymatic serum proteins; complement causes lysis in an antigen-antibody reaction.

complement system A group of proteins that coats bacteria; the proteins then either help kill the bacteria directly, or they assist neutrophils (in the blood) and macrophages (in the tissues) to engulf and destroy the bacteria.

complete abortion An abortion in which the patient has passed all the products of conception.

complete breech A delivery presentation that occurs when the fetus has both knees and hips flexed; the buttocks are the presenting part.

compliance The ease with which the lungs and thorax expand during pressure changes. The greater the compliance, the easier the expansion.

components of skeletal survey An x-ray study comprising a two-view chest with bone technique, two-view skull technique, views of the lateral lumbar spine and anteroposterior pelvis, and anteroposterior views of the upper and lower extremities, including anteroposterior views of the feet and posteroanterior views of the hands.

computer-aided dispatching An enhanced dispatch system in which computerized data are used to assist the dispatcher in selecting and routing emergency equipment and resources.

concealment A means of keeping out of site; it provides no ballistic protection.

concentration gradient The concentration difference between two points in a solution divided by the distance between the points.

concept formation A component of critical thinking that refers to all elements that are gathered to form a general impression of the patient.

concha The three bony ridges on the lateral wall of the nasal cavity.

concussion A head injury that results from violent jarring or shaking, such as that caused by a blow or explosion.

condyle A rounded projection on a bone, usually for articulation with another bone.

cone A photoreceptor in the retina of the eye; it is responsible for color vision.

confabulation The invention of stories to make up for gaps in memory.

congenital Present at birth.

congenital anomalies Defects that occur during fetal development.

congenital rubella syndrome A serious disease that affects about 25% of infants born to women infected with rubella during the first trimester of pregnancy; it is associated with multiple congenital anomalies, mental retardation, and an increased risk of death from congenital heart disease and sepsis during the first 6 months of life.

congestive heart failure An abnormal condition that reflects impaired cardiac pumping, usually a result of myocardial infarction, ischemic heart disease, or cardiomyopathy.

conjugate gaze Deviation of both eyes to either side at rest; the condition implies a structural lesion.

conjunctiva A mucous membrane that covers the anterior surface of the eyeball and the lining of the eyelids.

conjunctivitis Inflammation of the conjunctiva, caused by bacterial or viral infection, allergy, or environmental factors.

connective tissue Tissue that supports and binds other body tissues and parts.

conservation of energy law The principle that energy can be neither created nor destroyed; it can only change from one form (mechanical, thermal, electrical, or chemical) to another.

constipation Difficulty passing stools, or incomplete or infrequent passage of hard stools.

contact dermatitis Skin rash that results from exposure to an irritant or sensitizing antigen.

continence The ability to control bladder or bowel function.

continuous quality improvement A management approach to customer service and organizational performance that includes constant monitoring, evaluation, decisions, and actions.

contracture deformity An abnormal, usually permanent condition of a joint characterized by flexion and fixation and caused by atrophy and shortening of muscle fibers or by loss of elasticity of the skin.

contraindications Medical or physiological factors that make it harmful to administer a medication that would otherwise have a therapeutic effect.

contralateral Affecting or originating in the opposite side of the body.

contrastimulant A factor that works against stimulation.

contrecoup An injury that occurs at a site opposite the side of impact.

control console Typically, a desk-mounted, enclosed piece of equipment that contains the mechanical and electronic controls used to operate a radio base station.

controlled substance Any drug defined in the categories of the Comprehensive Drug Abuse Prevention and Control Act (also known as the Controlled Substances Act) of 1970.

contusion A closed, soft tissue injury characterized by swelling, discoloration, and pain.

copulation The sexual union of two persons of the opposite sex in which the penis is introduced into the vagina; also known as *coitus.*

cor pulmonale An abnormal cardiac condition characterized by hypertrophy of the right ventricle of the heart as a result of hypertension of the pulmonary circulation.

cord presentation A presentation that occurs when the cord slips down into the vagina or appears externally after the amniotic membranes have ruptured.

core body temperature The temperature of deep structures of the body as compared with temperatures of peripheral tissues.

cornea The convex, transparent, anterior part of the eye.

corneal abrasion The rubbing off of the outer layers of the cornea.

corniculate cartilage A conical nodule of elastic cartilage that surrounds the apex of each arytenoid cartilage.

coronal plane See *frontal plane.*

coronary artery One of two arteries that arise from the base of the aorta and carry blood to the muscle of the heart.

coronary artery disease One of several abnormal conditions that affect the arteries of the heart and reduce the flow of oxygen and nutrients to the myocardium.

coronary sinus A short trunk that receives most of the veins of the heart and empties into the right atrium.

corpus callosum An arched mass of white matter in the depths of the longitudinal fissure; it is made up of the transverse fibers that connect the cerebral hemispheres.

corpus luteum A yellow endocrine body formed in the ovary at the site of a ruptured vesicular follicle immediately after ovulation.

corpus luteum cyst A type of cyst prone to rupture that forms as a result of hemorrhage in a mature corpus luteum.

cortisol A steroid hormone that occurs naturally in the body.

costal margin The margin of the lower limit of the ribs.

costochondral Pertaining to the junction of the ribs and cartilage.

countershock A high-intensity, short-duration electrical shock applied to the area of the heart, resulting in total cardiac depolarization.

coup Local damage that occurs at the site of impact.

couplet Two premature ventricular contractions in a row.

cover A type of concealment that hides the body and offers ballistic protection.

coverage The area covered by radio communication. The generally accepted national emergency system standard is the "90/90" standard. This means that 90% of the coverage area will have communication 90% of the time. Coverage usually is expressed as dead (no coverage), marginal (spotty), good (few problems), or excellent (no problems).

Cowper's glands See *bulbourethral glands.*

coxae The hip joints; the head of the femur and the acetabulum of the innominate bone.

crackle A fine, bubbling sound heard on auscultation of the lung; it is produced by air entering distal airways and alveoli that contain serous secretions.

cranial nerve One of 12 pairs of nerves that originate from a nucleus within the brain.

cranial vault The eight skull bones that surround and protect the brain; the brain case.

craniectomy Surgical removal of bone fragments from the cranium.

cremaster muscle A thin muscle layer spreading out over the spermatic cord in a series of loops; it functions to draw the testis up toward the superficial inguinal ring in response to cold or stimulation of the nerve.

crenate The shrinking of red blood cells caused by exposure to a hypertonic solution.

crepitus A grating sound associated with rubbing of bone fragments.

cricoid cartilage The most inferior laryngeal cartilage.

cricothyroid membrane The membrane joining the thyroid and cricoid cartilages.

cricothyrotomy An emergency incision into the larynx.

crime scene A location where any part of a criminal act has occurred, or a location where evidence relating to a crime may be found.

Crohn's disease A chronic, inflammatory bowel disease of unknown origin, usually affecting the ileum, the colon, or both structures.

croup An acute viral infection of the upper and lower respiratory tract that occurs primarily in infants and young children 3 months to 3 years of age; it is characterized by hoarseness, fever, a harsh, brassy cough, inspiratory stridor, and varying degrees of respiratory distress; also known as *laryngotracheobronchitis.*

crown The portion of the human tooth covered by enamel.

crowning The phase at the end of labor in which the fetal head is seen at the opening of the vagina.

crush injury Injury from exposure of tissue to a compressive force sufficient to interfere with the normal structure and metabolic function of the involved cells and tissues.

crush syndrome A life-threatening and sometimes preventable complication of prolonged immobilization; a pathologic process that causes destruction, alteration, or both of muscle tissue.

crystalloid A substance in a solution that can be diffused through a semipermeable membrane.

crystalluria The presence of crystals in the urine.

cubic centimeter A metric unit of length equal to $^{1}/_{100}$ of a meter.

Cullen's sign The appearance of irregularly formed hemorrhagic patches on the skin around the umbilicus.

cumulative action The effect that occurs when several doses of a drug are administered or when absorption occurs more quickly than removal by excretion or metabolism or both.

cuneiform cartilage A small rod of elastic cartilage above the corniculate cartilages in the larynx.

CUPS system A method of patient status coding that assigns patients to one of four categories: *c*ardiopulmonary resuscitation, *u*nstable, *p*otentially unstable, and *s*table.

current health status A focus on the patient's current state of health, environmental conditions, and personal habits.

Cushing's reflex An attempt by the body to compensate for a decline in cerebral perfusion pressure by a rise in mean arterial pressure.

Cushing's disease A metabolic disorder resulting from the chronic and excessive production of cortisol by the adrenal cortex or by the administration of glucocorticoids in large doses for several weeks or longer; also known as *Cushing's syndrome.*

Cushing's syndrome A condition caused by an abnormally high circulating level of corticosteroid hormones, produced naturally by the adrenal glands.

Cushing's triad Increased systolic pressure, widened pulse pressure, and decrease in the pulse and respiratory rate, which result from increased intracranial pressure.

cutaneous Of or pertaining to the skin.

cuticle The skinfold covering the root of the nail.

cyanotic Having bluish discoloration.

cystic medial necrosis Degenerative changes in the connective tissue of the aortic media.

cystitis Inflammation of the urinary bladder and ureters.

cytochrome oxidase A respiratory enzyme that functions in the transfer of electrons from cytochromes to oxygen, thus activating oxygen, which unites with hydrogen to form water.

cytology The study of cells.

cytomegalovirus A member of a group of large, species-specific, herpes-type viruses with a wide variety of disease effects.

cytoplasm All of the substance of a cell other than the nucleus.

cytoplasmic membrane The plasma membrane.

cytotoxic Pertaining to a pharmacological compound or other agent that destroys or damages tissue cells.

dartos muscle A layer of smooth muscle in the skin of the scrotum; it raises and lowers the testes in the scrotum in response to changes in ambient temperature.

data interpretation A component of critical thinking in which the examiner gathers the necessary data to form a field impression and working diagnosis.

DCAP-BTLS An acronym for wound assessment: deformity, contusions, abrasions, penetrations or punctures, burns, tenderness, lacerations, and swelling.

deafness A complete or partial inability to hear.

debriefing An activity in which rescuers and others involved in an emergency event discuss their feelings to relieve emotions and anxiety; it usually takes place 24 to 72 hours after the event.

decerebrate posturing A position in which a comatose patient's arms are extended and internally rotated and the legs are extended with the feet in forced plantar flexion; usually observed in patients who have compression of the brainstem.

deciduous tooth Any of the 20 teeth that appear normally during infancy.

decoding The act of interpreting symbols and format.

decompression sickness A multisystem disorder that results when nitrogen in compressed air converts back from solution to gas, forming bubbles in the tissues and blood.

decontamination The process of making patients, rescuers, equipment, and supplies safe by eliminating harmful substances.

decorticate posturing A position in which the comatose patient's upper extremities are rigidly flexed at the elbows and at the wrists; usually observed in patients who have a lesion in the mesencephalic region of the brain.

dedicated line A special telephone circuit designated for specific point-to-point communication purposes, such as alerting emergency medical services quarters.

deep frostbite A cold injury that results in significant tissue loss even with appropriate therapy; it is associated with subdermal layers and deep tissues.

deep vein thrombosis A disorder involving a thrombus in one of the deep veins of the body, most commonly the iliac and femoral veins.

defecation The elimination of feces from the digestive tract through the rectum.

defense mechanism An unconscious, intrapsychic reaction to protect the self from a stressful situation.

defibrillation The delivery of direct electrical current in an attempt to terminate ventricular fibrillation or pulseless ventricular tachycardia.

defibrillator A device used to depolarize fibrillating myocardial cells, thus allowing them to repolarize uniformly.

defusing An informal gathering of the persons involved in an emergency event to allow an initial release of feelings and an opportunity for persons to share their experiences.

degloving injury An injury usually involving the hand or finger in which the soft tissue is removed down to the bone.

degradation The physical destruction or decomposition of clothing material caused by use, ambient conditions, or exposure to chemicals.

degranulation The release of internal substances.

dehydration An excessive loss of water from the body tissues; it may follow prolonged fever, diarrhea, vomiting, acidosis, and other conditions.

delirium An abrupt disorientation for time and place, usually with illusions and hallucinations.

delirium tremens An acute and sometimes fatal psychotic reaction caused by cessation of excessive intake of alcohol over a long period of time; also known as DTs.

delta cell A constituent of the islets of Langerhans; it secretes somatostatin.

delta wave Widened, abnormal slurring or notching of the onset of the QRS complex; it indicates anomalous spread of the impulse and is a diagnostic finding for Wolff-Parkinson-White syndrome.

deltoid muscle A large, thick, triangular muscle that covers the shoulder joint.

delusions Persistent beliefs or perceptions held by a person despite evidence that refutes them (i.e., false beliefs).

dendrite The branching processes of a neuron that receive stimuli and conduct potentials toward the cell body.

dentin The chief material of teeth, surrounding the pulp and situated inside the enamel and cementum.

deoxyribonucleic acid A type of nucleic acid that comprises the genetic material of cells.

dependent lividity A red or bluish-purple tissue condition in dependent areas of the body caused by venous congestion.

depersonalization Forced emotional estrangement.

depolarization A change in electrical charge difference across the cell membrane that causes the difference to be smaller or closer to 0 mV; a phase of the action potential in which the membrane potential moves toward zero or becomes positive.

depressant A substance that decreases or lessens a body function or activity.

depressed skull fracture Any fracture of the skull in which fragments are depressed below the normal surface of the skull.

depression A mood disturbance characterized by feelings of sadness, despair, and discouragement.

dermatitis Inflammation of the skin.

dermatome The skin surface area supplied by a single spinal nerve.

dermis Dense, irregular connective tissue that forms the deep layer of the skin.

descending colon The segment of the colon that extends from the end of the transverse colon at the splenic flexure on the left side of the abdomen down to the beginning of the sigmoid colon in the pelvis.

desensitization Emotional insensitivity.

designated officer A person who serves as a liaison between the public safety agency and community health agencies involved in monitoring and responding to communicable diseases.

diabetes insipidus A metabolic disorder characterized by extreme polyuria and polydipsia, caused by deficient production or secretion of antidiuretic hormone or inability of the kidney tubules to respond to antidiuretic hormone.

diabetes mellitus A complex disorder of carbohydrate, fat, and protein metabolism that primarily results from partial or complete lack of insulin secretion by the beta cells of the pancreas or of defects of the insulin receptors.

diabetic ketoacidosis An acute, life-threatening complication of uncontrolled diabetes characterized by hyperglycemia, hypovolemia, electrolyte imbalance, and a breakdown of free fatty acids, causing acidosis; also known as diabetic coma.

diad The combination of sarcoplasmic reticulum and T tubules.

diagnosis Identification of a disease or condition by an evaluation of physical signs, symptoms, history, laboratory tests, and procedures.

dialysate A solution used in dialysis.

dialysis A technique used to normalize blood chemistry in patients with acute or chronic renal failure and to remove blood toxins in some patients who have taken a drug overdose.

dialysis fistula An artificial passage, as in an arteriovenous fistula, used to gain access to the patient's bloodstream for hemodialysis.

diaphoresis Profuse secretion of sweat.

diaphragm The dome-shaped, musculofibrous partition that separates the thoracic and abdominal cavities.

diaphragmatic hernia A herniation in the diaphragm caused by the improper fusion of structures during fetal development.

diaphysis The shaft of a long bone, consisting of a tube of compact bone that encloses the medullary cavity.

diarrhea The frequent passage of loose, watery stools; it is generally the result of increased motility in the colon.

diastolic blood pressure The minimum level of blood pressure measured between contractions of the heart.

diencephalon The parts of the brain between the cerebral hemispheres and the mesencephalon.

differentiation A process in which cells become specialized in one type of function or act in concert with other cells to perform a more complex task.

diffusion The process in which solid, particulate matter in a fluid moves from an area of higher concentration to an area of lower concentration, resulting in an even distribution of the particles in the fluid.

dilation and curettage A gynecological procedure that refers to widening of the uterine cervix and scraping away of the endometrium of the uterus.

diphtheria An acute contagious disease characterized by the production of a systemic toxin and a false membrane lining of the mucous membranes of the throat.

diplopia Double vision.

direct laryngoscopy Visual examination of the larynx with a laryngoscope.

disease period A stage of infection that follows the incubation period; the duration of which varies with the disease.

disentanglement The process of making a pathway through the wreckage of an accident and removing wreckage from patients.

disequilibrium Unstable equilibrium; motion sickness.

disequilibrium syndrome A group of neurological findings that sometimes occur during or immediately after dialysis; thought to result from a disproportionate decrease in osmolality of the extracellular fluid compared with that of the intracellular compartment in the brain or cerebrospinal fluid.

disoriented Unaware of surroundings.

dispositional hearing The phase of the family court process in which appropriate placement for a child and appropriate treatment, if any, for the parent of a child are determined and ordered.

dissecting aortic aneurysm Localized dilation of the aorta characterized by a longitudinal dissection between the outer and middle layers of the vascular wall.

disseminated intravascular coagulation A grave coagulopathy that results from the overstimulation of the clotting and anticlotting processes in response to disease or injury.

dissolution The rate at which a solid drug goes into solution after ingestion; the faster the rate of dissolution, the more quickly the drug is absorbed.

distraction 1. A self-defense measure in which a diversion is created to draw a person's attention. 2. A spinal injury that occurs if the cervical spine is suddenly stopped while the weight and momentum of the body pull away from it.

distress Negative, debilitating, or harmful stress.

distribution The transport of a drug through the bloodstream to various tissues of the body and ultimately to its site of action.

disulfiram-ethanol reaction A potentially life-threatening physiological response caused by disulfiram and ethanol that produces ill effects on the gastrointestinal, cardiovascular, and autonomic nervous systems; disulfiram is prescribed to some alcoholic patients to help them maintain abstinence.

diuresis The increased formation and secretion of urine.

diversity Differences of any kind: race, class, religion, gender, sexual preference, personal habitat, and physical ability.

diverticulitis Inflammation of one or more diverticula.

diverticulosis The presence of pouchlike herniations through the muscular layer of the colon.

diverticulum A pouchlike herniation through the muscular wall of a tubular organ; it may be present in the stomach, small intestine, or most commonly, the colon.

divisions Subdivisions of the incident command system that encompass specific geographical areas of responsibility as deemed necessary by the incident commander.

do not resuscitate A physician order instructing emergency care providers not to attempt resuscitation of a patient in the event of cardiac or respiratory failure; also known as a "no code" order.

dorsal root A sensory component that conveys afferent nerve processes to the spinal cord.

dorsal root ganglia See *spinal ganglia.*

dorsogluteal site An area made up of several gluteal muscles; it is used as an injection site.

Down syndrome A congenital condition characterized by varying degrees of mental retardation and multiple defects.

dram A unit of mass equal to an apothecaries' measure of 60 gr or ⅛ oz.

dromotropic Pertaining to agents that affect conduction velocity through the conducting tissues of the heart; a drug that speeds conduction is said to have a positive dromotropic effect.

drowning A mortal event in which a submersion victim is pronounced dead at the scene of the attempted resuscitation, or within 24 hours after arrival in the emergency department or hospital.

drug Any substance taken by mouth; injected into a muscle, blood vessel, or cavity of the body; or applied topically to treat or prevent a disease or condition.

drug absorption A process in which drug molecules move from the site of entry into the body to the general circulation.

drug abuse Self-medication or self-administration of a drug in chronically excessive amounts, resulting in psychological or physical dependence (or both), functional impairment, and deviation from approved social norms.

drug allergy A systemic reaction to a drug resulting from previous sensitizing exposure and the development of an immunological mechanism.

drug dependence A state in which intense physical or emotional disturbance is produced if a drug is withdrawn; previously called *habituation.*

drug interaction Modification of the effects of one drug by the previous or concurrent administration of another drug, thereby increasing or diminishing the pharmacological or physiological action of one or both drugs.

drug receptors Parts of a cell (usually an enzyme or large protein molecule) with which a drug molecule interacts to trigger its desired response or effect.

drug-protein complex A complex formed by the attachment of a drug to proteins, mainly albumin.

ductus arteriosus A vascular channel in the fetus that joins the pulmonary artery directly to the descending aorta.

ductus deferens A thick, smooth muscular tube that allows sperm to exit from the epididymis through the ejaculatory duct; also known as the *vas deferens.*

ductus venosus The continuation of the umbilical vein through the liver to the inferior vena cava.

duodenum The first subdivision of the small intestine.

duplex mode A communications mode with the ability to transmit and receive traffic simultaneously through two different frequencies, one to transmit and one to receive.

duplex/multiplex system A communications system with the ability to transmit and receive simultaneously with concurrent transmission of voice and telemetry.

dura mater The outermost layer of the meninges.

duration of action The period from the onset of drug action to the time when a drug effect is no longer seen.

dysarthria Difficult and poorly articulated speech resulting from poor control over the muscles of speech.

dysconjugate gaze Deviation of the eyes to opposite sides at rest; it implies a structural brainstem dysfunction in the pathways that traverse the brainstem from the upper midbrain to at least the level of the lower pons.

dyshemoglobinemia Hemoglobin saturated with compounds other than oxygen, such as carbon monoxide or methemoglobin.

dyskinesia An impairment of the ability to execute voluntary movements; often an adverse effect of prolonged use of antipsychotic medications.

dysmenorrhea Pain associated with menstruation.

dyspareunia Pain with intercourse.

dysphagia Inability or difficulty in swallowing because of medical or traumatic causes.

dysphonia An abnormality in the speaking voice, such as hoarseness.

dysplasia Abnormal cellular growth.

dyspnea Difficulty breathing.

dysrhythmia Variation from a normal rhythm.

dystonia A condition characterized by local or diffuse changes in muscle tone, resulting in painful muscle spasms, unusually fixed postures, and strange movement patterns.

EACOM/HEAR The Emergency Administrative Communications (by General Electric) or Hospital Emergency Administrative Radio (by Motorola). These radio systems use 1500-Hz rotary-pulse dialing, which transmits specific groups of rotary tone pulses for the purpose of selectively addressing hospital-based receivers in particular regions throughout the United States. Most ambulance services have access to this system.

eardrum The cellular membrane that separates the external ear from the middle ear; also known as the *tympanic membrane.*

eating disorders A term referring to anorexia nervosa and bulimia nervosa, conditions in which dissatisfaction with weight and body shape cause an individual to develop disordered eating behaviors.

eclampsia A grave form of pregnancy-induced hypertension, characterized by convulsions, coma, proteinuria, and edema.

ectoparasite An organism that lives on the outside of the body of the host, such as a louse.

ectopic Out of place.

ectopic foci Cardiac dysrhythmias caused by irritation of an excitation impulse at a site other than the sinus node.

ectopic pregnancy An abnormal pregnancy in which the conceptus implants outside the uterine cavity.

eczema Superficial dermatitis of unknown cause.

edema The accumulation of fluid within the interstitial spaces.

effacement The shortening of the vaginal portion of the cervix and the thinning of its walls as it is stretched and dilated by the fetus during labor.

efferent division Nerve fibers that send impulses from the central nervous system to the periphery.

efficacy An intrinsic activity that refers to the ability of a drug to initiate biological activity as a result of such binding.

Einthoven's triangle An equilateral triangle formed by the patient's right arm, left arm, and left leg; it is used in electrode sensor placement for electrocardiogram monitoring.

ejaculatory duct A duct formed by the joining of the ductus deferens and the duct from the seminal vesicle that allows sperm to enter the urethra.

ejection The forceful expulsion of blood from the ventricle of the heart.

elastin The major connective tissue protein of elastic tissue; it has a structure like a coiled spring.

elder abuse The infliction of physical pain, injury, debilitating mental anguish, unreasonable confinement, or willful deprivation by a caregiver of services that are necessary to maintain mental and physical health of a geriatric person.

electroconvulsive therapy Induction of a brief convulsion by passing an electrical current through the brain to treat affective disorders.

electrolyte A cation or anion in solution that conducts an electrical current.

elevation Movement of a structure in a superior direction.

ellipsoid joint A modified ball-and-socket joint in which the articular surfaces are ellipsoid rather than spherical.

emaciated To be abnormally lean from disease or lack of nutrition.

embolectomy A surgical incision into an artery for the removal of an embolus or clot.

embryo In human beings the stage of prenatal development between the time of implantation of the fertilized ovum until the end of the seventh or eighth week.

emergency medical services A national network of services coordinated to provide aid and medical assistance from primary response to definitive care; the network involves personnel trained in rescue, stabilization, transportation, and advanced management of traumatic and medical emergencies.

emergency medical technician—paramedic A person who has completed training based on the EMT-Paramedic National Standard Curriculum. A paramedic has advanced training in patient assessment, cardiac rhythm interpretation, defibrillation, drug therapy, and airway management.

emissary veins The small vessels in the skull that connect the sinuses of the dura with the veins on the exterior of the skull through a series of anastomoses.

emotional abuse The infliction of anguish, pain, or distress through verbal or nonverbal acts.

emotional/mental impairment Impaired intellectual functioning that results in an inability to cope with normal responsibilities of life.

emphysema An abnormal condition of the pulmonary system characterized by overinflation and destructive changes in the alveolar walls, resulting in a loss of lung elasticity and a decrease in gases.

EMS communications The delivery of patient and scene information (either in person, in writing, or through communications technology) to other members of the emergency response team.

EMT-Paramedic See *emergency medical technician—paramedic.*

enamel A hard white substance that covers the dentin of the crown of the tooth.

encephalitis An inflammatory condition of the brain, usually caused by an infection transmitted by the bite of an infected mosquito; it also may result from lead or other poisoning or from hemorrhage.

encoding The act of placing a message in an understandable format (either written or verbal).

endolymph Fluid found within the membranous labyrinth.

endometriosis An abnormal gynecological condition characterized by ectopic growth and function of endometrial tissue; it is thought to result when, during menstruation, fragments of endometrium from the lining of the uterus are regurgitated backward through the fallopian tubes into the peritoneal cavity, where they attach and grow as small cystic structures.

endometritis An inflammatory condition of the endometrium, usually caused by bacterial infection.

endometrium The mucous membrane lining of the uterus, which changes in thickness and structure with the menstrual cycle.

endoplasmic reticulum A network of connecting sacs or canals that wind through the cytoplasm of a cell serving as a miniature circulatory system for the cell.

endorphin Any of several peptides secreted in the brain that have a pain-relieving effect like morphine.

endotoxin A toxin contained in the cell walls of some microorganisms, especially gram-negative bacteria.

endotracheal intubation An airway management procedure in which an endotracheal tube is inserted through the mouth or nose into the trachea. Intubation is used to maintain a patent airway, to prevent aspiration of material from the digestive tract, to permit suctioning of tracheobronchial secretions, to administer positive-pressure ventilation, and to administer certain medications when other means of vascular access are unavailable.

endotracheal route Refers to drugs administered through an endotracheal tube.

enhanced automaticity The cause of dysrhythmias in Purkinje fibers and other myocardial cells with a high resting membrane potential; it results from an acceleration of phase 4 depolarization commonly caused by abnormally high leakage of sodium ions into the cells, which causes the cells to reach threshold prematurely.

enophthalmos Recessed globe.

enteral route A route of drug administration along any portion of the gastrointestinal tract.

envenomation The injection of snake, arachnid, or insect venom into the body.

enzyme A protein produced by living cells that catalyzes chemical reactions in organic matter.

eosinophil A white blood cell that inhibits inflammation; it readily stains with acidic dyes.

eosinophil chemotactic factor of anaphylaxis A group of active substances, including histamine and leukotrienes, that are released during an anaphylactic reaction.

epicardium See *visceral pericardium.*

epicondyle A projection on the surface of a bone above its condyle.

epidermis The outer portion of skin; it is formed of epithelial tissue that rests on or covers the dermis.

epididymis A tightly coiled tube that lies along the top of and behind the testes, where sperm mature.

epididymitis An inflammation of the epididymis, a tubular section of the male reproductive system that carries sperm from the testicles to the seminal vesicles.

epidural hematoma Accumulation of blood between the dura mater and the cranium.

epidural space The space above or on the dura.

epiglottis A lidlike cartilage that overhangs the entrance to the larynx.

epiglottitis Inflammation of the epiglottis; a severe form of the condition that affects primarily children is characterized by fever, sore throat, stridor, croupy cough, and an erythematous epiglottis.

epilepsy A condition characterized by a tendency of the individual to have recurrent seizures (excluding those that arise from correctable or avoidable circumstances).

epinephrine Adrenaline; the secretion of the adrenal medulla.

epiphyseal line A dense plate in a bone that is no longer growing, indicating the former site of the epiphyseal plate.

epiphyseal plate See *growth plate.*

epiphysis The head of a long bone that is separated from the shaft of the bone by the epiphyseal plate until the bone stops growing, the plate is obliterated, and the shaft and the head are united.

epistaxis Bleeding from the nose.

epithelial tissue The cellular covering of internal and external surfaces of the body, including the lining of vessels and other small cavities.

Epstein-Barr virus The herpes virus that causes infectious mononucleosis.

erection The condition of hardness, swelling, and elevation observed in the penis and to a lesser degree in the clitoris, usually caused by sexual arousal.

erythrocyte A red blood cell.

escape beat An automatic beat of the heart that occurs after an interval longer than the duration of the dominant heartbeat cycle.

eschar A scab or dry crust resulting from a thermal or chemical burn.

escharotomy Surgical incision into necrotic tissue caused by a severe burn; escharotomy sometimes is necessary to prevent edema from building up sufficient interstitial pressure to impair capillary filling and cause ischemia.

esophageal reflux A chronic disease manifested by various sequelae associated with reflux of the stomach and duodenal contents into the esophagus.

esophageal stricture An abnormal temporary or permanent narrowing of the esophagus caused by inflammation, external pressure, or scarring.

esophagitis Inflammation of the esophagus.

esophagogastric varices A complex of longitudinal, tortuous veins at the lower end of the esophagus that become large and swollen as a result of portal hypertension; also known as esophageal varices.

esophagus The muscular canal extending from the pharynx to the stomach.

estimated date of confinement Delivery date for the fetus.

estrogen One of a group of hormonal steroid compounds that promote the development of female secondary sex characteristics.

ethics The discipline relating to right and wrong, moral duty and obligation, moral principles and values, and moral character; a standard for honorable behavior designed by a group with expected conformity.

ethmoid bone The very light, spongy bone at the base of the cranium that forms most of the walls of the superior part of the nasal cavity.

ethmoid sinus One of the numerous small, thin-walled cavities in the ethmoid bone of the skull, rimmed by the frontal maxilla and the lacrimal, sphenoidal, and palatine bones.

ethylene glycol A chemical used in automobile antifreeze preparations.

eukaryote A cell with a true nucleus, found in all higher organisms and in some microorganisms.

eustachian tube See *auditory tube.*

eustress Positive, performance-enhancing stress.

evaluation A component of critical thinking in which the examiner assesses the patient's response to care.

evasive tactics A self-defense measure in which an aggressor's moves and actions are anticipated, and unconventional pathways are used during retreat for personal safety.

eversion Turning outward.

evisceration The protrusion of an internal organ through a wound or surgical incision, especially in the abdominal wall.

excitability The property of a cell that enables it to react to irritation or stimulation.

excretion The elimination of toxic or inactive metabolites, primarily by the kidneys; the intestines, lungs, and mammary, sweat, and salivary glands also may be involved.

excursion Movement from side to side.

exertional heat stroke An abnormal condition characterized by weakness, vertigo, nausea, muscle cramps, and loss of consciousness; caused by depletion of body fluid and electrolytes resulting from exposure to intense heat or inability to acclimatize to heat.

exocrine Secreting into a duct.

exophthalmos An abnormal condition characterized by marked protrusion of the eyeballs.

exothermic Marked or accompanied by the evolution of heat.

exotoxin A toxin secreted or excreted by a living organism.

expiration Breathing out (exhalation), normally a passive process.

expiratory center The region of the medulla that is electrically active during nonquiet expiration.

expiratory reserve volume The maximum volume of air that can be exhaled after a normal expiration.

exposure incident Any specific contact of the eyes, the mouth, other mucous membranes, nonintact skin, or parenteral contact with blood, blood products, bloody body fluids, or other potentially infectious materials.

expressed consent Verbal or written consent to the treatment.

extended scope of practice The expansion of health care services provided by emergency medical technicians and paramedics in the prehospital setting.

extension Stretching out.

external anal sphincter A sphincter muscle located at the tip of the coccyx and surrounding fascia; it prevents the movement of feces out of the rectum until it is relaxed.

external auditory canal The passage for sound impulses passing through the ear.

external auditory meatus The canal of the external ear; also known as the *external auditory canal.*

external cardiac pacing The delivery of repetitive electrical currents to the heart, substituting for a natural pacemaker that has become blocked or dysfunctional; also known as *transcutaneous cardiac pacing.*

external ear The portion of the ear that includes the auricle and external auditory meatus; it terminates at the eardrum.

external jugular vein One of a pair of large vessels in the neck that receive most of the blood from the exterior of the cranium and deep tissues of the face.

external urinary sphincter The smooth muscle that surrounds the urethra as the urethra extends through the pelvic floor; it controls the flow of urine through the urethra.

extracellular Occurring outside of a cell or cell tissues or in cavities or spaces between cell layers or groups of cells.

extracellular fluid The water found outside the cells, including that in the intravascular and interstitial compartments.

extracellular matrix Nonliving chemical substances located between connective tissue cells.

extrapyramidal reaction A response to a treatment or drug characterized by involuntary movement, changes in muscle tone, and abnormal posture.

extravasate The passage or escape of blood, serum, or lymph into the tissues.

extubation Removal of an endotracheal tube.

exudate Fluid, cells, or other substances that have been discharged slowly from cells or blood vessels through small pores or breaks in cell membranes.

face presentation An abnormal presentation in which the brow or forehead of the fetus is the first part of the body to enter the birth canal; also known as *brow presentation.*

facial bones The 14 bones that form the structure of the face in the anterior skull; they do not contribute to the cranial vault.

facial nerve palsy Partial or total loss of the functions of the facial muscles or loss of sensation in the face.

facies A facial expression or appearance.

facilitated diffusion A carrier-mediated process that moves substances into or out of cells from a high to a low concentration.

failure to thrive The abnormal retardation of the growth and development of an infant resulting from conditions that interfere with normal metabolism, appetite, and activity.

fallopian tube See *uterine tube.*

false imprisonment Intentional and unjustifiable detention of a person.

false movement An unnatural movement of an extremity, usually associated with fracture.

false rib See *rib.*

false vocal cord See *vestibular fold.*

family court Sometimes referred to as juvenile court; the court is authorized to handle proceedings involving claims of abuse and neglect, dependency, delinquency, and requests for the termination of parental rights.

family history Illness or disease in a patient's family or a family's background that may be relevant to the patient's complaint.

fascia The loose areolar connective tissue found beneath the skin or dense connective tissue that encloses and separates muscle.

fascicle A small bundle or cluster of nerve or muscle fibers that provides pathways for impulse conduction.

fasciculation A localized, uncoordinated, uncontrollable twitching of a single muscle group that can be palpated and seen under the skin.

fasciotomy Incision of a fascia to relieve elevated intracompartmental pressure.

fat A substance composed of lipids or fatty acids.

febrile seizure A seizure that results from fever.

fecal impaction An accumulation of hardened feces in the rectum or sigmoid colon that the person is unable to move.

fecalith A hard, impacted mass of feces in the colon.

feces Waste material discharged from the intestines.

Federal Communications Commission A federal agency with jurisdiction over interstate and international telephone and telegraph services and satellite communications.

femoral vein A large vein in the thigh that originates in the popliteal vein and accompanies the femoral artery in the proximal two thirds of the thigh.

femur The thigh bone, which extends from the pelvis to the knee; the largest and strongest bone in the body.

fetal membrane disorder One of several disorders that pertain to the fetus or to the period during its development, including premature rupture of membranes, amniotic fluid embolism, and meconium staining.

fetus Unborn young, from the third month of the intrauterine period until birth.

fibrinogen A soluble blood protein converted into insoluble fibrin during clotting.

fibrocartilage Cartilage that consists of a dense matrix of white collagenous fibers.

fibrosis An abnormal condition in which fibrous connective tissue spreads over or replaces normal smooth muscle or other normal organ tissue.

fibrous connective tissue A connective tissue that consists mainly of bundles of strong, white collagenous fibers arranged in parallel rows.

fibrous joint See *joint.*

fibrous pericardium Fibrous outer layer of the heart.

fibrous tunic The sclera and cornea.

fibula The bone of the leg, lateral to and smaller than the tibia.

Fick principle The principle used to determine cardiac output. It assumes that the quantity of oxygen delivered to an organ is equal to the amount of oxygen consumed by that organ plus the amount of oxygen carried away from that organ.

field impression An impression of the patient's condition that the paramedic makes from pattern recognition and gut instinct that results from experience.

filtrate A filtered liquid.

filtration Movement caused by a pressure gradient of a liquid through a filter that prevents some or all of the substances in the liquid from passing through.

fimbria A fringelike structure located at the border of the uterine tube.

financial/material exploitation The illegal or improper use of funds, properties, or assets.

fine ventricular fibrillation Fibrillatory waves less than 3 mm in amplitude.
first stage of labor The stage of labor that begins with the onset of regular contractions and ends with complete dilation of the cervix.
first-degree burn A burn injury in which only a superficial layer of epidermal cells is destroyed.
first-pass metabolism The initial biotransformation of a drug during passage through the liver from the portal vein that occurs before the drug reaches the general circulation.
fistula An abnormal passage from an internal organ to the body surface.
flail chest A chest wall injury in which three or more adjacent ribs are fractured in two or more places.
flat bones Bones that have a thin, flattened shape, such as certain skull bones, the ribs, the sternum, and scapulae.
flatulence Excessive air or gas in the stomach or intestinal tract, causing distention of the organs and in some cases mild to moderate pain.
flexion Bending.
floating rib See *rib.*
flora Microorganisms that live on or in the body to compete with disease-producing microorganisms and provide a natural immunity against certain infections.
flutter waves Abnormal P waves in a sawtooth or picket fence pattern; they represent atrial depolarization in an abnormal direction followed by atrial repolarization.
focal seizure See *Jacksonian seizure.*
focused history A component of patient assessment to ascertain the patient's chief complaint, history of present illness, medical history, and current health status.
fontanelle A space covered by a tough membrane between the bones of an infant's cranium.
food poisoning Poisoning that results from food contaminated by toxic substances or by bacteria containing toxins.
foramen ovale An opening in the septum between the right and left atria in the fetal heart; it provides a bypass for blood that would otherwise flow to the fetal lungs.
foreign body airway obstruction A disturbance in normal function or a pathological condition caused by an object lodged in the airway.
formed elements Cells and cell fragments of blood.
formic acid A colorless, pungent liquid found in nature in ants and other insects.
fourth ventricle The ventricle located in the superior region of the medulla; continuous with the central canal of the spinal cord.
fourth-degree burn A full-thickness burn injury that penetrates the subcutaneous tissue, muscle, fascia, periosteum, or bone.
fracture A break in the continuity of bone or cartilage.
frank breech See *front breech.*
fraternal twins Two offspring born of the same pregnancy from two ova released simultaneously from the ovary and fertilized at the same time.
French scale system A scale used to denote the size of catheters and other tubular instruments; each unit is roughly equivalent to 0.33 mm in diameter.
frequency The number of repetitive cycles per second completed by a radio wave.
frequency modulation A deviation of carrier frequency in accordance with the strength of applied audio. Frequency modulation is less susceptible to some types of interference than amplitude modulation and typically is used in emergency medical services communications.
front breech A presentation that occurs when the fetal hips are flexed and the legs extend in front of the fetus, making the buttocks the presenting part; also known as a *frank breech.*
frontal bone The single cranial bone that forms the front of the skull.
frontal lobe The largest of the five lobes that comprise each of the two cerebral hemispheres; it significantly influences personality and is associated with higher mental activities such as planning, judgment, and conceptualization.
frontal plane An imaginary plane that divides the body into front and back or anterior and posterior positions; also known as the *coronal plane.*
frontal sinus One of a pair of small cavities in the frontal bone of the skull that communicates with the nasal cavity.
frostbite A localized injury that results from environmentally induced freezing of body tissues.
frostnip The mildest form of cold injury; it may be treated without loss of tissue.
full-thickness burn A burn injury in which the entire thickness of the epidermis and dermis is destroyed; also known as a *third-degree burn.*
functional residual capacity The expiratory reserve volume plus the residual volume; it reflects the amount of gas remaining in the lungs at the end of a normal expiration.
fundus The bottom or rounded end of a hollow organ, such as the fundus of the uterus.
fusion beat A premature ventricular contraction that occurs at approximately the same time that an electrical impulse of the underlying rhythm is activating the ventricles, thereby causing ventricular depolarization to occur simultaneously in two directions; it results in a QRS complex that has the characteristics of the premature ventricular contraction and the QRS complex of the underlying rhythm.
gag reflex A normal neural response triggered by touching the soft palate or posterior pharynx.
gallbladder A pear-shaped excretory sac on the visceral surface of the right lobe of the liver; it serves as a reservoir for bile.
gallows humor Morbid or cynical humor.
ganglia A group of nerve cell bodies in the peripheral nervous system.
gap junction A small channel between cells that allows the passage of ions and small molecules between cells.
gastric gland A gland located in the stomach mucosa.
gastric lavage Irrigation of the stomach with sterile water or normal saline.
gastrin A polypeptide hormone that stimulates the flow of gastric juice and contributes to the stimulus that causes bile and pancreatic enzyme secretion.
gastritis Inflammation of the lining of the stomach; it may be acute or chronic.

gastroenteritis The inflammation of the stomach and intestines that accompanies numerous gastrointestinal disorders.
gastrointestinal Of or pertaining to the organs of the gastrointestinal tract from mouth to anus.
gastrostomy An artificial opening into the stomach.
gating protein A protein that controls the rate at which ions move through an ion channel.
general gas law The characteristic of gas that it flows from an area of higher pressure or concentration to an area of lower pressure or concentration; also known as *Boyle's law.*
general impression An immediate assessment of the environment and the patient's chief complaint used to determine if the patient is ill or injured and the nature of the illness or the mechanism of injury.
generic name The official, established name assigned to a drug.
genitalia Reproductive organs.
genitourinary Of or pertaining to the genital and urinary systems of the body, the organ structures, the organ functions, or both.
German measles See *rubella.*
gerontology The study of the problems of all aspects of aging.
gestation The period from fertilization of the ovum until birth.
gestational diabetes mellitus A disorder characterized by impaired ability to metabolize carbohydrates, usually caused by a deficiency of insulin; it occurs in pregnancy and disappears after delivery but in some cases returns years later.
gingiva The portion of the oral mucosa surrounding the tooth.
gingival hypertrophy Swelling of the gums; it often is associated with chronic phenytoin therapy.
gingivostomatitis Multiple, painful ulcers on the gums and mucous membranes of the mouth; the result of a herpes virus infection.
Glasgow Coma Scale A standardized system for assessing the degree of conscious impairment in the critically ill and for predicting the duration and ultimate outcome of coma.
glaucoma A condition in which intraocular pressure increases and causes damage to the optic nerve.
glia limitans A supporting structure of nervous tissue consisting of large, star-shaped cells.
gliding joint See *plane joint.*
globule A small, spherical mass.
globulin One of a broad category of simple proteins classified by solubility, mobility, and size.
glomerular filtration rate The amount of plasma that filters into Bowman's capsules per minute.
glomerulus The mass of capillary loops at the beginning of each nephron.
glossopharyngeal nerve Either of a pair of cranial nerves essential to the sense of taste, to sensation in some viscera, and to secretion from certain glands.
glottic opening The vocal cords and the space between them.
glottis The space between the vocal cords.
glucagon A hormone produced by the alpha cells in the islets of Langerhans that stimulates the conversion of glycogen to glucose in the liver.
glucocorticoid An adrenocortical steroid hormone that increases glyconeogenesis, exerts an antiinflammatory effect, and influences many body functions.
gluconeogenesis The formation of glycogen from fatty acids and proteins rather than carbohydrates.
glucosuria The abnormal presence of glucose in the urine resulting from large amounts of carbohydrates, from kidney disease, or from a metabolic disease such as diabetes mellitus.
gluteus medius muscle The muscle that originates between the anterior and posterior gluteal lines of the ilium and inserts into the greater trochanter of the femur.
glycogenolysis The breakdown of glycogen to glucose.
glycolysis An anaerobic process during which glucose is converted to pyruvic acid.
glycoprotein Any of a large group of conjugated proteins in which the nonprotein substance is a carbohydrate.
goblet cell One of the many specialized cells that secrete mucus and form glands of the epithelium of the stomach, intestine, and parts of the respiratory tract.
goiter A hypertrophic thyroid gland, usually evident as a pronounced swelling in the neck.
golden hour The critical period during which surgical intervention for a trauma patient can enhance survival and reduce complications.
Golgi apparatus Specialized endoplasmic reticulum that concentrates and packages materials for secretion from the cell.
gomphosis An articulation by the insertion of a conic process into a socket, such as the insertion of the root of a tooth into an alveolus of the mandible or maxilla.
gonad A gamete-producing gland, such as an ovary or testis.
gonorrhea A sexually transmitted disease that results from contact with the causative organism *Neisseria gonorrhoeae.*
gout A disease associated with an inborn error of uric acid metabolism that increases production of or interferes with excretion of uric acid; also known as *hyperuricemia.*
gouty arthritis A type of arthritis caused by excess uric acid, which is converted to sodium urate crystals that are deposited in the joints.
graafian follicle See *vesicular follicle.*
grain The smallest unit of mass in apothecaries' weights equal to 64.8 mg.
gram A metric unit of mass equal to $^1/_{1000}$ of a kilogram.
gram-negative sepsis Sepsis caused by gram-negative bacteria when the bacterium dies and is broken down in the body.
grand mal seizure A seizure characterized by a generalized involuntary muscular contraction and cessation of respiration followed by tonic and clonic spasms of the muscles.
grand multipara A woman who has had seven deliveries or more.
granulosa cell A cell in the layer surrounding the primary follicle.
gravida The number of all current and past pregnancies.
gray matter The gray tissue that makes up the inner core of the spinal column.
great vessels The large arteries and veins entering and leaving the heart; they include the aorta, the pulmonary arteries and veins, and the superior and inferior venae cavae.

groups Subdivisions of the incident command system that encompass specific functional areas of responsibility as deemed necessary by the incident commander.

growth plate The site of bone elongation; also known as the *epiphyseal plate.*

Guillain-Barré syndrome A rare disease that affects the peripheral nervous system, especially the spinal nerves, but also the cranial nerves; it is associated with a viral infection or immunization.

habituation See *drug dependence.*

hair follicle An invagination of the epidermis into the dermis that contains the root of the hair and receives the ducts of sebaceous and apocrine glands.

hair papilla A small, cup-shaped cluster of cells located at the base of the follicle where hair growth begins.

hair root The part of the hair that lies hidden in the follicle.

hair shaft The visible part of the hair.

half duplex The use of two different frequencies, one to transmit and one to receive, that cannot be used simultaneously.

half-life The amount of time required to reduce a drug level to one half its initial value.

hallucinations The apparent perception of sights, sounds, and other sensory phenomena that are not actually present.

Hantavirus A cause of several different forms of hemorrhagic fever with renal syndrome.

hard palate The floor of the nasal cavity that separates the nasal cavity from the oral cavity.

hazard control The phase of rescue that includes managing, reducing, and minimizing risks from uncontrollable hazards; ensuring scene safety; and providing personal protective equipment that is appropriate for the incident.

head of bone An eminence on a bone by which it articulates with another bone.

heart The muscular, cone-shaped organ that pumps blood throughout the body by coordinated nerve impulses and muscular contractions.

heart murmur An abnormal heart sound caused by altered blood flow into a chamber or through a valve.

heat cramps Brief, intermittent, and often severe muscular cramps that frequently occur in muscles fatigued by heavy work or exercise.

heat exhaustion A form of heat illness characterized by minor aberrations in mental status, dizziness, nausea, headache, and mild to moderate increase in core body temperature.

heat stroke A syndrome that occurs when the thermoregulatory mechanisms normally in place to meet the demands of heat stress break down entirely. As a result, the body temperature increases to extreme levels. Multisystem tissue damage and physiological collapse also occur.

hemasite A small, button-shaped indwelling vascular device usually placed in the upper arm or proximal, anterior thigh; it is similar to an arteriovenous graft but has an external rubber septum sutured to the skin through which a dialysis catheter is inserted for treatment.

hematemesis Vomiting of bright red blood, indicating upper gastrointestinal bleeding.

hematochezia The passage of red blood through the rectum.

hematology The scientific study of blood and blood-forming tissues.

hematoma A closed injury characterized by blood vessel disruption and swelling beneath the epidermis.

hematuria The abnormal presence of blood in the urine.

hemiblock Failure in conduction of cardiac impulse in either of two main divisions of the left branch of the bundle of His; interruption may occur in the anterior (superior) or posterior (inferior) division.

hemiparesis One-sided weakness.

hemiplegia Paralysis of one side of the body.

hemitransection A cut across the long axis of tissue, such as the spinal cord.

hemoagglutinin An agglutinin that clumps red blood corpuscles.

hemochromatosis A rare disease of iron metabolism characterized by excess deposition of iron throughout the body.

hemodialysis A procedure in which impurities or wastes are removed from the blood; it is used in treating renal insufficiency and various toxic conditions.

hemoglobin A complex protein-iron compound in the blood that carries oxygen to the cells from the lungs and carbon dioxide away from the cells to the lungs.

hemolysis The breakdown of red blood cells and the release of hemoglobin.

hemolytic anemia A condition in which delivery of oxygen to tissues is reduced because of an increase in hemolysis of erythrocytes.

hemopericardium An accumulation of blood within the pericardial sac surrounding the heart.

hemoperitoneum The presence of extravasated blood in the peritoneal cavity.

hemophilia A group of hereditary bleeding disorders in which one of the factors necessary for blood coagulation is deficient.

hemophilia A A condition caused by a deficiency of coagulation factor VIII; it is considered the classic type of hemophilia.

hemophilia B A condition caused by a deficiency of coagulation factor IX.

hemopneumothorax See *pneumohemothorax.*

hemopoietic tissue Tissue related to the process of formation and development of various types of blood cells.

hemoptysis Coughing up of blood from the respiratory tract.

hemorrhage Flowing of blood.

hemorrhagic shock Hypoperfusion associated with the sudden and rapid loss of significant amounts of blood.

hemorrhoids Swollen, distended veins (internal, external, or both) in the rectoanal area.

hemostasis The cessation of bleeding by mechanical or chemical means or by substances that arrest the blood flow.

hemostatic An agent that reduces bleeding by speeding clot formation.

hemothorax The accumulation of blood in the pleural space caused by bleeding from the lung parenchyma or damaged vessels.

hemotympanum Blood behind the tympanic membrane from fractures of the temporal bone.

heparin A substance that inhibits blood clotting; it is obtained from the liver.

heparin lock A peripheral vascular access device that has no attached intravenous tubing; it is used to ensure ready access to peripheral veins for brief administration of medications or when frequent intravenous therapy is indicated on an outpatient basis (e.g., chemotherapy).

hepatic artery The branch of the aorta that delivers blood to the liver.

hepatic encephalopathy A type of brain damage caused by liver disease and consequent ammonia intoxication.

hepatic portal system The system that transports blood from the digestive tract to the liver.

hepatitis An inflammatory condition of the liver characterized by jaundice, hepatomegaly, anorexia, abdominal and gastric discomfort, abnormal liver function, clay-colored stools, and dark urine. Viruses responsible for hepatitis are *hepatitis A virus, hepatitis B virus, hepatitis C virus,* hepatitis D virus, and hepatitis E virus.

hepatitis A virus See *hepatitis.*

hepatitis B virus See *hepatitis.*

hepatitis C virus See *hepatitis.*

hepatomegaly Enlargement of the liver.

Hering-Breuer reflex A reflex in which afferent impulses from stretch receptors in the lungs arrest inspiration; expiration then occurs.

hernia Protrusion of any organ through an abdominal opening in the muscle wall of the cavity that surrounds it.

herniation A protrusion of a body organ or portion of an organ through an abnormal opening in a membrane, muscle, or other tissue.

herpes Any of several acute inflammatory viral diseases characterized by the eruption of small blisters on the skin and mucous membranes.

herpes simplex virus type 1 An infection caused by the herpes simplex virus; it tends to occur in the facial area, particularly around the mouth and nose.

herpes simplex virus type 2 An infection caused by the herpes simplex virus; it usually is limited to the genital region.

hertz A unit of frequency equal to 1 cycle per second.

hexaxial reference system The system of intersecting lines of the standard limb leads and three other intersecting lines of reference: aV_R, aV_L, and aV_F leads.

hiatal hernia Protrusion of a portion of the stomach upward through the diaphragm.

Hickman catheter A long indwelling catheter sometimes used by patients with cancer, gastrointestinal dysfunction, or debilitating disease and by those who need intermittent intravenous administration of antibiotics, nutritional supplements, or other intravenous medications.

high angle An environment in which rescuers need to be secured with rope for safety. The majority of the rescue load is supported by the rope system.

high-altitude cerebral edema The most severe form of acute high-altitude illness. It is characterized by a progression of global cerebral signs in the presence of acute mountain sickness.

high-altitude pulmonary edema A high-altitude illness thought to be caused at least partly by an increase in pulmonary artery pressure that develops in response to hypoxia.

high-grade atrioventricular block Occurs when at least two consecutive atrioventricular impulses (atrial P waves) fail to be conducted to the ventricles.

hilum A depression or pit at the part of an organ where the vessels and nerves enter.

hinge joint A joint that consists of a convex cylinder in one bone applied to a corresponding concavity in another bone; this type of joint allows movement in one plane only.

histamine An amine released by mast cells and basophils that promotes inflammation.

history taking Information gathered during the patient interview.

Hodgkin's disease A malignant disorder characterized by pain and progressive enlargement of lymphoid tissue.

homeopathic Pertaining to homeopathy, a system of therapeutics in which diseases are treated with small doses of drugs that, in larger doses, are capable of producing in healthy persons symptoms like those of the disease to be treated.

homeostasis A state of equilibrium in the body with respect to functions and composition of fluids and tissues.

horizontal plane Any place of the erect body parallel to the horizon; dividing the body into upper and lower parts.

human immunodeficiency virus The viral agent responsible for acquired immunodeficiency syndrome.

humerus The largest bone of the upper arm, comprising a body, head, and condyle.

humoral immunity One of the two forms of immunity that respond to antigens such as bacteria and foreign tissue.

Huntington's disease A rare, hereditary disease characterized by quick, involuntary movements, speech disturbances, and mental deterioration; it is caused by degenerative changes in the cerebral cortex and basal ganglia; also known as Huntington's chorea.

hyaline cartilage Gelatinous, glossy cartilage tissue; it thinly covers the articulating ends of bones, connects the ribs to the sternum, and supports the nose, trachea, and part of the larynx.

hydrocephalus A pathological condition characterized by an abnormal accumulation of cerebrospinal fluid, usually under increased pressure, within the cranial vault, resulting in dilation of the ventricles.

hydrochloric acid The acid in gastric juice.

hydrogen ion The acidic element in a solution.

hymen A mucous membrane that may partly or entirely occlude the vaginal outlet.

Hymenoptera A large, highly specialized order of insects that includes wasps, bees, and ants.

hyoid bone The U-shaped bone between the mandible and the larynx.

hyperbilirubinemia Larger than normal amounts of the bile pigment bilirubin in the blood, often characterized by jaundice, anorexia, and malaise.

hypercalcemia A higher than normal concentration of calcium in the blood.

hypercholesterolemia Increased serum cholesterol.

hypercoagulability A tendency of the blood to coagulate more rapidly than normal.

hyperglycemia A greater than normal amount of glucose in the blood.

hyperkalemia A higher than normal concentration of potassium in the blood.

hyperkaluria A high potassium concentration in the urine.

hyperlipidemia An excess of lipids in the plasma.

hypermagnesemia A higher than normal concentration of magnesium in the blood.

hypernatremia A greater than normal concentration of sodium in the blood.

hyperosmolar hyperglycemic nonketotic coma A diabetic coma in which the level of ketone bodies is normal. It is caused by hyperosmolarity of extracellular fluid and results in dehydration of intracellular fluid.

hyperparathyroidism A condition of increased parathyroid function.

hyperphosphatemia High levels of alkaline phosphate in the blood.

hyperplasia An excessive increase in the number of cells.

hyperpolarization An increase in the charge difference across the cell membrane; it causes the charge difference to move away from 0 mV.

hypersensitivity reaction An altered immunological response to an antigen that results in a pathological immune response upon reexposure.

hypersomina Excessive drowsiness; a sleep disorder of excessive depth or duration.

hypertension A disorder characterized by elevated blood pressure, which persistently exceeds 140/90 mm Hg.

hypertensive crisis A sudden, severe increase in blood pressure greater than 200/120 mm Hg.

hypertensive encephalopathy A set of symptoms—including headache, convulsions, and coma—that result solely from elevated blood pressure.

hyperthermia Abnormal elevation of body temperature.

hyperthyroidism A condition characterized by increased activity of the thyroid gland.

hypertonic A term used to describe a solution that causes cells to shrink.

hypertrophy An increase in the size of a cell.

hyperuricemia See *gout.*

hyperventilation syndrome Abnormally deep or rapid breathing that results in excessive loss of carbon dioxide (producing respiratory alkalosis).

hyphema A hemorrhage into the anterior chamber of the eye; it usually is a result of blunt trauma.

hypocalcemia A lower than normal concentration of calcium in the blood.

hypocarbia A state of diminished carbon dioxide in the blood; also known as hypocapnia.

hypochlorhydria A deficiency of hydrochloric acid in the gastric juice of the stomach.

hypoglycemia A lower than normal amount of glucose in the blood.

hypokalemia A lower than normal concentration of potassium in the blood.

hypomagnesemia A lower than normal concentration of magnesium in the blood plasma.

hyponatremia A lower than normal concentration of sodium in the blood.

hyponatremic A term describing a lower than normal concentration of sodium in the blood.

hypoparathyroidism A condition of diminished parathyroid function.

hypoperfusion Severely inadequate circulation that results in insufficient delivery of oxygen and nutrients necessary for normal tissue and cellular function. Also known as *shock.*

hypopituitarism An abnormal condition caused by diminished activity of the pituitary gland; it is marked by excessive deposits of fat or acquisition of adolescent characteristics.

hypopyon An accumulation of pus in the anterior chamber of the eye.

hypotension An abnormal condition in which the blood pressure is not adequate for normal perfusion and oxygenation of the tissues.

hypothalamus A portion of the diencephalon of the brain that activates, controls, and integrates the peripheral autonomic nervous system, endocrine processes, and many somatic functions such as body temperature, sleep, and appetite.

hypothermia An abnormal body temperature below 95° F (35° C).

hypothyroidism A condition characterized by decreased activity of the thyroid gland.

hypotonia A condition of diminished tone or tension that may involve any body structure.

hypotonic A term used to describe a solution that causes cells to swell.

hypotonicity of the muscles Decreased muscle tone or tension.

hypovolemia An abnormally low circulating blood volume.

hypovolemic shock A form of shock most frequently caused by hemorrhage but also caused by dehydration.

hypoxemia A state of decreased oxygen content of arterial blood.

hypoxia A state of decreased oxygen content at the tissue level.

hypoxic drive The low arterial oxygen pressure stimulus to respiration that is mediated through the carotid bodies.

hysterectomy The surgical removal of the uterus.

iatrogenic Caused by treatment or diagnostic procedures.

identical twins Two offspring born of the same pregnancy and developed from a single fertilized ovum that splits into equal halves during the early phase of embryonic development, giving rise to separate fetuses.

idiopathic epilepsy See *primary epilepsy.*

idiosyncrasy An abnormal or peculiar response to a drug.

idioventricular rhythm A ventricular escape rhythm that results when impulses from higher pacemakers fail to reach the ventricles or when the rate of discharge of higher pacemakers become less than that of the ventricles.

ileocecal sphincter The valve between the ilium of the small intestine and the cecum of the large intestine.

ileostomy A surgical opening into the small intestine.

ileum The distal portion of the small intestine.

ileus An obstruction of the intestines.

iliac crest The upper free margin of the ilium.

iliac spine A portion of the iliac crest; the flaring portion of the hipbone.
ilium One of the three bones that make up the innominate bone.
immersion hypothermia Hypothermia from immersion in cold water.
immune response A defense function of the body that produces antibodies to destroy invading antigens and malignancies.
immunity Insusceptibility to a particular disease or condition.
immunization The process of rendering a person immune or of becoming immune.
immunogen Any agent or substance capable of an immune response or of producing immunity.
immunoglobulin Any of five structurally and antigenically distinct antibodies present in the serum and external secretions of the body; they are IgA, IgD, IgE, IgG, and IgM.
implied consent The presumption that an unconscious or incompetent person would consent to lifesaving care.
incident command system A management program designed to control, direct, and coordinate emergency response operations and resources.
incomplete abortion An abortion in which the patient has passed some but not all of the products of conception.
incomplete breech The presentation that occurs when the fetus has one or both hips incompletely flexed, resulting in the presentation of one or both lower extremities, often a foot.
incontinence The inability to control bladder or bowel function.
incubation period The stage of infection during which an organism reproduces; it begins with invasion of an agent and ends when the disease process begins.
incus The middle of the three ossicles in the middle ear.
induced abortion The intentional termination of a pregnancy.
infectious disease Any illness that is caused by a specific microorganism.
infectious pericarditis Inflammation of the pericardium associated with infection.
inferior Toward the feet; below a point of reference in the anatomical position.
inferior nasal concha One of three bony ridges on the lateral wall of the nasal cavity.
inferior vena cava The vein that returns blood from the lower limbs and the greater part of the pelvic and abdominal organs to the right atrium.
infertility The inability to produce offspring.
infiltration The process whereby a fluid passes into tissues.
inflammatory response A tissue reaction to injury or an antigen; it may include pain, swelling, itching, redness, heat, and loss of function.
influenza A highly contagious infection of the respiratory tract transmitted by airborne droplet infection. Researchers have identified three main types of the virus (types A, B, and C).
informed consent Consent obtained from a patient after explaining all facts necessary for the patient to make a reasonable decision.
inguinal canal The passage through the lower abdominal wall that transmits the spermatic cord in the male and the round ligament in the female.
inguinal node One of approximately 18 nodes in the group of lymph glands in the upper femoral triangle of the thigh.
inhalation injury An upper and/or lower airway injury that results from thermal and/or chemical exposure.
initial assessment A component of the patient assessment to recognize and manage all immediate life-threatening conditions.
injury risk Real or potentially hazardous situations that put individuals at increased risk for sustaining an injury.
injury surveillance The ongoing systematic collection, analysis, and interpretation of injury data essential to the planning, implementation, and evaluation of public health practice.
inner ear The part of the ear that contains the sensory organs for hearing and balance.
inotropic Pertaining to the force or energy of muscle contraction, particularly contractions of the heart.
insertion The more movable attachment point of a muscle.
insomnia A chronic inability to sleep or to remain asleep throughout the night.
inspection A visual assessment of the patient and surroundings.
inspiration The act of drawing air into the lungs.
inspiratory capacity The sum of the tidal volume and the inspiratory reserve volume.
inspiratory center The region of the medulla that stimulates inspiration.
inspiratory reserve volume The maximum volume of air that can be inspired after a normal inspiration.
insulin A hormone secreted by the pancreatic islets.
integumentary system The largest organ system in the body, consisting of the skin and accessory structures.
interatrial septum Tissue that separates the right and left atria of the heart.
intercalated disk Cell-to-cell attachment with gap junctions between cardiac muscle cells.
intercellular Occurring between or among cells.
interference Any undesired radio signal on a radio frequency. It may arise from other radio transmitters or other sources of electromagnetic radiation. "Nuisance interference" is interference that can be heard but does not override system signals. "Destructive interference" overrides system signals.
internal anal sphincter A sphincter muscle located at the caudal end of the rectum.
internal carotid artery Each of two arteries that enter the cranial vault through the carotid canals.
internal jugular vein One of a pair of veins in the neck; each collects blood from one side of the brain, the face, and the neck, and both unite with the subclavian vein to form the brachiocephalic vein.
internal mammary artery One of the pair of arteries that arise from the first portions of the subclavian arteries; it supplies the pectoral muscles, breasts, pericardium, and abdominal muscles; also known as the *internal thoracic artery.*
internal thoracic artery See *internal mammary artery.*
internal urinary sphincter The smooth muscle of the bladder located at the junction of the urethra with the urinary bladder; it controls the flow of urine through the urethra.
interneuron See *motor neuron.*
internodal tract Pathways between the segments of a nerve fiber.
interpolated premature ventricular contraction A premature ventricular contraction that falls between two sinus beats without interrupting the rhythm.

interstitial fluid Fluid that occupies the space outside the blood vessels and/or outside of cells of an organ or tissue.

interventricular foramen One of two passageways between the two lateral ventricles and the third ventricle.

interventricular septum The tissue that separates the right and left ventricles of the heart.

intervertebral disk One of the fibrous disks between all adjacent spinal vertebrae except the atlas and axis; it serves as a shock absorber for the vertebral column and provides additional support for the body; it also prevents the vertebral bodies from rubbing against each other.

intracellular Occurring within cell membranes.

intracellular fluid The fluid found in all body cells.

intracerebral hematoma An accumulation of blood or fluid within the tissue of the brain.

intradermal injection The introduction of a substance (e.g., serum or vaccine) with a hypodermic needle into the dermis.

intramuscular injection The introduction of medication with a hypodermic needle into muscle.

intraocular pressure Pressure within the eye that keeps the eye inflated.

intraosseous infusion Placement of a rigid needle into a bone and the infusion of fluid and medication directly into the bone marrow.

intraosseous injection The introduction of medication or fluid into the bone marrow.

intrapartum The period during labor and delivery.

intrapleural Within the pleura.

intrapleural pressure See *intrathoracic pressure.*

intrapulmonic pressure The pressure of the gas within the alveoli.

intrathecal injection The introduction of medication with a hypodermic needle into the subarachnoid space.

intrathoracic pressure The pressure in the pleural space; also known as *intrapleural pressure.*

intravenous injection The introduction of medication with a hypodermic needle into a vein.

intrinsic factor The factor secreted by the parietal cells of the gastric glands; it is required for adequate absorption of vitamin B_{12}.

invagination Infolding or in-pocketing.

invasion of privacy Making public, without legal justification, details about a person's private life that might reasonably expose that person to ridicule, notoriety, or embarrassment.

inversion Turning inward.

involuntary Occurring without conscious control or direction.

involuntary consent Treatment that is granted by authority of law.

involuntary guarding An unconscious rigid contraction of the abdominal muscles; a sign of peritoneal inflammation.

involuntary muscle A muscle that is not normally consciously controlled; see *smooth muscle.*

ion An atom or group of atoms carrying a charge of electricity by virtue of having gained or lost one or more electrons.

ipsilateral Pertaining to the same side of the body.

iris The colored contractile membrane of the eye that can be seen through the cornea.

iron deficiency anemia Anemia caused by inadequate supplies of iron needed to synthesize hemoglobin.

irregular bones Bones that are not representative of the other three categories (long, short, or flat bones); examples include vertebrae and facial bones.

ischemia A state of insufficient perfusion of oxygenated blood to a body organ or part.

ischium One of the three parts of the hipbone, which joins the ilium and the pubis to form the acetabulum.

islets of Langerhans Clusters of cells within the pancreas that produce insulin, glucagon, and pancreatic polypeptide.

isoimmunity An immune response directed against beneficial foreign tissues.

isolette A self-contained incubator unit that provides controlled heat, humidity, and oxygen for the isolation and care of premature and low-birth-weight neonates.

isometric contraction A muscle contraction in which the length of the muscle does not change, but the tension produced increases.

isotonic A term used to describe a solution that causes cells neither to shrink nor to swell.

isotonic contraction A muscle contraction in which the tension produced by the muscle stays the same, but the muscle length becomes shorter.

J point The point at which the T wave takes off from the QRS complex.

Jacksonian seizure A transitory disturbance in motor, sensory, or autonomic function resulting from abnormal neuronal discharges in a localized part of the brain; also known as a *focal seizure.*

jaundice A yellow discoloration of the skin, mucous membranes, and sclerae of the eyes caused by a greater than normal amount of bilirubin in the blood.

jejunum One of the three portions of the small intestine.

joint Any one of the connections between bones that are classified according to structure and movability as fibrous, cartilaginous, or synovial. *Fibrous joints* are immovable, *cartilaginous joints* are slightly movable, and *synovial joints* are freely movable.

joint capsule A well-defined structure that encloses a joint.

joint dislocation An injury that occurs when the normal articulating ends of two or more bones are displaced.

Joule's law The principle that the amount of heat produced is directly proportional to the square of the current strength times the resistance of the tissue times the duration of the current flow.

jugular notch The superior margin of the manubrium; it is palpated easily at the anterior base of the neck; also known as the *suprasternal notch.*

jugular vein distention Engorgement of jugular veins caused by an increase in central venous pressure; it is estimated by positioning the head of a supine patient at a 45-degree angle and observing the neck veins.

kallikrein/kinin system A proposed hormonal system that functions within the kidneys, mediating production of bradykinin, which acts as a vasodilator peptide.

Kaposi's sarcoma A malignant, multifocal neoplasm of reticuloendothelial cells that begins as soft, brownish or purple papules on the feet and slowly spreads in the skin, metastasizing to the lymph nodes and viscera; it is associated with diabetes, malignant lymphoma, acquired immunodeficiency syndrome, and other disorders.

Kehr sign Pain in the left shoulder thought to be caused by referred pain secondary to irritation of the adjacent diaphragm.

Kent fibers See *bundle of Kent.*

keratitis Any inflammation of the cornea.

ketoacidosis Acidosis accompanied by the accumulation of ketones in the body, resulting from faulty carbohydrate metabolism.

ketoacids Compounds containing the carbonyl and carboxyl groups.

ketogenesis The formation or production of ketone bodies.

ketone bodies The normal metabolic products of lipid and pyruvate within the liver; excessive production leads to their excretion in urine.

ketonuria Presence in the urine of excessive amounts of ketone bodies.

kidney The organ that cleanses the body of the waste products continually produced by metabolism.

kilogram A metric unit of mass equal to 1000 grams or 2.2046 pounds.

kilohertz A unit of frequency equal to 1000 cycles per second.

kinematics The process of predicting injury patterns that can result from the forces and motions of energy.

kinin Serum protein that causes vasodilation and increases vascular permeability.

KKK standards The national standards that provide the foundation of uniformity among ambulance vehicles.

Koplik's spots Small red spots with bluish white centers on the lingual and buccal mucosa, characteristic of measles.

Korsakoff's psychosis A form of amnesia often seen in alcoholics, characterized by a loss of short-term memory and an inability to learn new skills.

Krebs cycle A sequence of enzymatic reactions involving the metabolism of carbon chains of sugar, fatty acids, and amino acids to yield carbon dioxide, water, and high-energy phosphate bonds.

Kussmaul's respiration An abnormally deep, rapid sighing respiratory pattern characteristic of diabetic ketoacidosis or other metabolic acidosis.

kyphosis An abnormal condition of the vertebral column characterized by increased convexity in the curvature of the thoracic spine as viewed from the side.

labia majora Two rounded folds of skin surrounding the labia minora and the vestibule.

labia minora Two longitudinal folds of mucous membrane enclosed by the labia majora and bounding the vestibule.

labial frenulum A medial fold of mucous membrane connecting the inside of each lip to the corresponding gum.

laceration A torn or jagged wound.

lacrimal bone One of the smallest and most fragile bones of the face; it is located in the anterior part of the medial wall of the orbit.

lacrimal canal The canal that carries excess tears away from the eye.

lacrimal gland The tear gland located in the superolateral corner of the orbit.

lacrimal sac An enlargement of the lacrimal canal that leads into the nasolacrimal duct.

lacrimation Excessive tear production.

lactate A salt of lactic acid.

lactation The secretion of milk from the breasts to nourish an infant or child.

lactic acid A three-carbon molecule derived from pyruvic acid as a product of anaerobic respiration.

lactic acidosis A disorder characterized by an accumulation of lactic acid in the blood, resulting in a lowered pH in muscle and serum.

lactiferous duct The duct that drains the grapelike cluster of milk-secreting glands in the breast.

lactose intolerance A sensitivity disorder resulting in the ability to digest lactose because of a deficiency of or defect in the enzyme lactase.

landing zone An area prepared for the landing of an aircraft; generally 100 by 100 feet.

lanugo hair Soft, downy hair covering a normal fetus.

laparoscopy Examination of the abdominal cavity with a laparoscope.

large intestine The portion of the digestive tract comprising the cecum, the appendix, the ascending, transverse, and descending colons, and the rectum.

laryngectomy Surgical removal of the larynx, performed to treat cancer of the larynx.

laryngopharynx The lowest part of the pharynx.

laryngoscope An endoscope for visualization of the larynx.

laryngoscopy Examination of the larynx via a laryngoscope.

laryngotracheobronchitis See *croup.*

larynx The voice box, located just below the pharynx.

latent period A stage of infection that begins when a pathogenic agent invades the body and ends when the agent can be shed or communicated.

latent period of drug action See *onset of action.*

lateral malleolus The rounded process on the lateral side of the ankle joint.

lateral recumbent position The position in which the patient is lying on his or her right or left side.

lateral ventricle A large, fluid-filled space in each cerebral hemisphere.

laxative A substance that causes evacuation of the bowel by increasing the bulk of the feces, by softening the stool, or by lubricating the intestinal wall.

lead An electrode sensor attached to the body to record electrical activity, especially of the heart and brain.

Le Fort fracture A fracture pattern that can be produced in the midface region.

left anterior descending artery The subdivision of the left coronary artery that supplies the left auricle and its appendix and supplies branches to both ventricles and numerous small branches to the pulmonary artery and commencement of the aorta.

left coronary artery One of a pair of branches from the ascending aorta that supplies both ventricles and the left atrium.

legend A prescription drug.

legionellosis An acute bacterial pneumonia caused by infection with *Legionella pneumophila;* it is characterized by an influenza-like illness followed within a week by high fever, chills, muscle aches, and headache.

legionnaires' disease See *legionellosis.*

Lenègre's disease See *Lev's disease.*

lens The crystalline portion of the eye.

lethargy A state of indifference, apathy, or sluggishness.

leukemia A malignant neoplasm of blood-forming organs.

leukocyte White blood cell.

leukocytosis An abnormal increase in the number of circulating white blood cells.

leukotrienes A class of biologically active compounds that occur naturally in leukocytes and that produce allergic and inflammatory reactions.

Lev's disease Third-degree block in the elderly from chronic degenerative changes in the conduction system; it usually is not associated with increased parasympathetic tone or drug toxicity; also known as *Lenègre's disease.*

libel Publishing in writing false statements about someone, knowing them to be false, with malicious intent or with reckless disregard for their falsity.

libido The drive associated with sexual desire, pleasure, or creativity.

licensure The process by which a government agency grants permission to an individual to engage in an occupation or profession.

life threat An illness or injury that threatens survival.

ligament A band of white, fibrous tissue that connects bones.

ligamentum arteriosum A fibrous cord from the pulmonary artery to the branch of the aorta; the remains of the ductus arteriosus of the fetus.

limbic system The part of the brain involved with emotions and olfaction.

linear fracture A fracture that extends parallel to the long axis of a bone but does not displace the bone tissue.

lingual tonsil A collection of lymphoid tissue on the posterior portion of the dorsum of the tongue.

lipid Any of the free fatty acid fractions in the blood.

lipid bilayer The central layer of the cytoplasmic membrane; it is composed of a double layer of lipid molecules.

lipodystrophy Any abnormality in the metabolism or distribution of fats.

lipoprotein A conjugated protein in which lipids form an integral part of the molecule; it is synthesized primarily in the liver.

liquefaction Conversion of solid tissues to a fluid or semifluid state.

liter A metric unit of capacity equal to 1 cubic decimeter, 61.025 cubic inches, or 1.0567 liquid quarts.

Littre's gland The inner surface of the membrane lining the urethra.

loading dose A large quantity of drug that temporarily exceeds the capacity of the body to excrete the drug.

lobule A small lobe or subdivision of a lobe.

long bones Bones that are longer than they are wide, such as the humerus, ulna, radius, femur, tibia, fibula, and phalanges.

long saphenous vein See *saphenous vein.*

loop diuretic A group of powerful, short-acting agents that inhibit sodium and chloride reabsorption in the loop of Henle, resulting in an excessive loss of potassium and water and an increase in the excretion of sodium.

loop of Henle The U-shaped portion of the renal tubule.

lordosis An inward curvature in the lumbar spine that is normally present to some degree.

low angle An environment in which the weight of the stretcher is supported primarily by the tender's legs, but rope systems are required to facilitate movement and for fall protection.

lower esophageal sphincter The ring of muscle located at the inferior end of the esophagus that regulates the passage of materials out of the esophagus.

lucid interval A period of relative mental clarity between periods of decreased consciousness or irrationality.

lumbar vertebrae The five largest segments of the movable part of the vertebral column; they are designated L1 to L5.

lumbosacral plexus The combination of all the ventral primary divisions of the lumbar, sacral, and coccygeal nerves.

lumen A cavity or channel within any organ or structure of the body.

Lund and Browder chart A method to estimate burn injury that assigns specific numbers to each body part and that accounts for developmental changes in percentages of body surface area.

lung One of a pair of light, spongy organs in the thorax; the main component of the respiratory system.

lunula The crescent-shaped white area of the nail; it is most visible on the thumbnail.

luxation A complete dislocation.

Lyme disease An acute, recurrent inflammatory infection transmitted by a tick.

lymph node An encapsulated mass of lymph tissue found among lymph vessels.

lymphangitis An inflammation of one or more lymphatic vessels.

lymphatic system The network of vessels, ducts, nodes, valves, and organs involved in protecting and maintaining the internal fluid environment of the body.

lymphocyte A type of white blood cell formed in lymphoid tissue.

lymphokine One of the chemical factors produced and released by T lymphocytes that attract macrophages to the site of infection or inflammation.

lymphoma A group of diseases that range from slowly growing chronic disorders to rapidly evolving acute conditions.

lyse To cause decomposition.

lysis The process by which a cell swells and ruptures.

lysosome A membranous-walled organelle that contains enzymes, which enable it to function as an intracellular digestive system.

macrodrip tubing An apparatus used to deliver measured amounts of intravenous solutions at specific flow rates based on the size of drops of the solution. The drops delivered by a macrodrip are larger than those delivered by a microdrip.

macromolecule A molecule of colloidal size, such as a protein, nucleic acid, or polysaccharide.

macrophage A phagocytic cell in the immune system.

macula A small pigmented area that appears separate or different than the surrounding tissue.

maintenance dose The amount of a drug required to keep a desired steady state of drug concentration in tissues.

major incident An event for which available resources are insufficient to manage the nature of the emergency.

malaise A vague feeling of weakness or discomfort.

malar eminence The zygomatic bone or cheekbone.

malaria A serious infectious illness caused by one or more of at least four species of the protozoan genus *Plasmodium;* it is characterized by chills, fever, anemia, and an enlarged spleen.

malignant Very dangerous or virulent; likely to cause death.

malleolus A rounded, bony process, such as the protuberance on each side of the ankle.

malleus The largest of the three ossicles in the middle ear.

Mallory-Weiss syndrome A condition characterized by massive bleeding after a tear in the mucous membrane at the junction of the esophagus and the stomach.

mamma The breast; the organ of milk secretion.

mammalian diving reflex A reflex triggered by immersing the face in cold water; it diverts blood from the arms and legs to the central circulation and lowers the heart rate as a result of vagal stimulation.

mammary gland An external accessory sex organ in females; breasts.

managed care Patient care services that are provided to members by managed care organizations.

managed care organizations Networks that provide patient care services to their members, including health maintenance organizations and preferred provider organizations.

mandible A large bone that constitutes the lower jaw.

mania A mood disorder characterized by extreme excitement, hyperactivity, agitation, and sometimes violent and self-destructive behavior.

manic Pertaining to a specific psychosis.

manic-depressive disorder See *bipolar disorder.*

manubriosternal junction The point at which the manubrium joins the body of the sternum; the location of the second rib; also known as the *sternal angle.*

manubrium One of the three bones of the sternum; it has a broad, quadrangular shape that narrows caudally at its articulation with the superior end of the body of the sternum.

Marfan syndrome An abnormal condition characterized by elongation of the bones, often with associated abnormalities of the eyes and cardiovascular system.

mass casualty incident An event for which available resources are insufficient to manage the number of casualties.

mastectomy Surgical removal of one or both breasts, performed to remove a malignant tumor.

mastication Chewing, tearing, or grinding food with the teeth while it is mixed with saliva.

mastoid air cell One of several spaces within the mastoid process of the temporal bone; it is connected to the middle ear by ducts.

maxilla One of a pair of large bones that form the upper jaw.

maxillary sinus One of the pair of large air cells that form a pyramidal cavity in the body of the maxilla.

McBurney point A site of extreme sensitivity in acute appendicitis situated in the normal area of the appendix, approximately 2 inches from the right anterior-superior spine of the ilium, on a line between that spine and the umbilicus.

mean arterial pressure The arithmetic mean of the blood pressure in the arterial portion of the circulation.

measles An acute, highly contagious viral disease involving the respiratory tract that is characterized by a spreading, maculopapular, cutaneous rash.

meconium aspiration syndrome Inhalation of meconium by the fetus or newborn; the meconium can block the air passages and result in failure of the lungs to expand or cause other pulmonary dysfunction.

meconium staining The presence of fetal stool in amniotic fluid.

medial malleolus The rounded process on the medial side of the ankle joint.

mediastinitis Inflammation of the mediastinum.

mediastinum A portion of the thoracic cavity in the middle of the thorax between the pleural sacs containing the two lungs; it extends from the sternum to the vertebral column and contains all the thoracic viscera except the lungs.

mediated transport mechanisms Mechanisms that use carrier molecules to move large, water-soluble molecules or electrically charged molecules across cell membranes.

medical asepsis The removal or destruction of disease-causing organisms or infected material.

medical direction A process of ensuring that actions taken on behalf of ill or injured persons are medically appropriate, including prospective, concurrent, and retrospective aspects of emergency medical services quality improvement, hiring, and education.

medulla The lowest part of the brainstem, which controls vital functions; an enlarged extension of the spinal cord; also known as the *medulla oblongata.*

medulla oblongata See *medulla.*

medullary cavity A large, marrow-filled cavity in the diaphysis of a long bone.

megahertz A unit of frequency equal to 1 million cycles per second; emergency medical services radios transmit and receive on frequencies measured in megahertz.

melanocyte A body cell capable of producing melanin.

melatonin The only hormone secreted in the bloodstream by the pineal gland; it lightens skin pigmentation and may inhibit numerous endocrine functions.

melena Abnormal black, tarry stools containing digested blood.

membrane channel A tunnel through which specific molecules may pass.

membranous labyrinth A membranous structure within the inner ear; it forms the cochlea, vestibule, and semicircular canals.

menarche The first menstruation and commencement of the cyclic menstrual function.
meninges Fluid-containing membranes surrounding the brain and spinal cord.
meningitis Inflammation of the meninges.
menopause The cessation of menses.
menstruation The periodic discharge through the vagina of a blood secretion containing tissue debris from the shedding of the endometrium from the nonpregnant uterus.
mental illness Any form of psychiatric disorder.
mental retardation A disorder characterized by below-average intellectual function with deficits or impairments in the ability to learn and adapt socially.
mental status examination An evaluation tool that includes an assessment of appearance and behavior, speech and language, emotional stability, and cognitive abilities.
merocrine gland A gland that secretes products with no loss of cellular material, such as a water-producing sweat gland.
mesencephalon See *midbrain.*
mesentery The double layer of peritoneum extending from the abdominal wall to the abdominal viscera; it conveys vessels and nerves.
mesovarium A short peritoneal fold connecting the ovary with the broad ligament of the uterus.
metabolic acidosis A disorder that results when excess acid is added to the body fluids or bicarbonate is lost from them.
metabolic alkalosis A disorder that results from a significant loss of acid in the body or increased levels of base bicarbonate.
metabolism The culmination of all chemical processes that take place in living organisms.
metabolite A substance that is produced by metabolic action or that is necessary for the metabolic process.
metacarpal One of five bones extending from the carpus to the phalanges.
metaplasia A change from one cell type to another that is better able to tolerate adverse conditions; a conversion into a form that is not normal for that cell.
metarteriole One of the small peripheral blood vessels that contain scattered groups of smooth muscle fibers in their walls; they are located between the arterioles and the true capillaries.
metatarsal Any one of the five bones comprising the metatarsus.
meter A metric unit of length equal to 1000 millimeters.
methanol A chemical widely used as a solvent and in the production of formaldehyde.
methemoglobin A form of hemoglobin in which the iron component has been oxidized from the ferrous to the ferric state.
methemoglobinemia The presence of methemoglobin in the blood, causing cyanosis as a result of the inability of the red blood cells to release oxygen.
microdrip tubing An apparatus for delivering relatively small amounts of intravenous solutions at specific flow rates; the drops delivered by a microdrip are smaller than those delivered by a macrodrip.
microgram A metric unit of mass equal to $^{1}/_{1,000,000}$ of a gram.
microinfarct A small infarct caused by obstruction of circulation in capillaries, arterioles, or small arteries.
microorganism Any tiny, usually microscopical entity capable of carrying on living processes, such as bacteria, fungi, protozoa, and viruses.
microthrombus A minute thrombus.
microtubule A hollow tube that helps to support the cytoplasm of the cell; a component of certain cell organelles such as centrioles, spindle fibers, cilia, and flagella.
microwave Radio waves with frequencies of 890 MHz and upward. The signals are generated by special equipment that depends on line of sight placement to operate properly. Microwave channels may have a wide band to carry a large number of simultaneous transmissions.
midbrain One of the three parts of the brainstem; also known as the *mesencephalon.*
middle cerebral artery The artery that supplies a large portion of the lateral cerebral cortex.
middle ear An air-filled space within the temporal bone that contains the auditory ossicles.
migraine A severe, incapacitating headache that often is preceded by visual and/or gastrointestinal disturbances.
milliequivalent $^{1}/_{1000}$ of a gram equivalent.
milligram A metric unit of mass equal to $^{1}/_{1000}$ of a gram.
milliliter A metric unit of capacity equal to $^{1}/_{1000}$ of a liter.
millimeter A metric unit of length equal to $^{1}/_{1000}$ of a meter.
mineral An inorganic substance usually referred to by the name of the compound of which it is a part; minerals are important in regulating many body functions.
mineralocorticoid A hormone secreted by the adrenal cortex that maintains normal blood volume, promotes sodium and water retention, and increases urine secretion of potassium and hydrogen ions.
minim A measure of volume in the apothecaries' system, originally 1 drop of water; 60 minims equal 1 fl dr, and 1 minim equals 0.06 mL.
minimal effective concentration The lowest plasma concentration that produces the desired drug effect.
minute alveolar ventilation The amount of inspired gas available for gas exchange during 1 minute.
minute volume The amount of gas inhaled or exhaled in 1 minute. It is found by multiplying the tidal volume by the respiratory rate.
miscarriage See *spontaneous abortion.*
missed abortion The retention of the fetus in utero for 4 or more weeks after fetal death.
mitochondria Small, spherical, rod-shaped, or thin filamentous structures in the cytoplasm of cells; a site of adenosine triphosphate production.
mitosis Cell division resulting in two daughter cells with exactly the same number and type of chromosomes as the mother cell.
mitral valve See *bicuspid valve.*
mitral valve prolapse Protrusion of one or both cusps of the mitral valve back into the left atrium during ventricular systole, resulting in incomplete closure of the valve and mitral insufficiency.

mittelschmerz Abdominal pain in the region of the ovary during ovulation; it usually occurs midway through the menstrual cycle.

MMR vaccine The abbreviation for live measles, mumps, and rubella virus vaccine.

mobile data terminal A computer connected through a modem ("black box") with a radio that sends and receives pretyped messages to printers, computer screens, or both. Some mobile data terminals have graphics (floor plans) and database (hazardous materials) capabilities. Mobile data terminals rely on a host computer interfaced to a base station.

mobile relay station A fixed base station that automatically retransmits mobile or portable radio communications back to the receiving frequency of other portables, mobiles, and base stations operating in the same system; also known as a repeater.

mobile repeater A mobile radio unit capable of automatically retransmitting any radio traffic originated by a handheld portable, by other mobiles, or by base stations. This repeater may be one-way or two-way and may be known as a PAC-RAT (Motorola) or an extender. Also known as a vehicle repeater.

mole A standard unit used to measure the amount of a substance.

monocyte A type of white blood cell found in lymph nodes, spleen, bone marrow, and loose connective tissue.

monomorphic Existing only in one form.

mons pubis The prominence caused by a pad of fatty tissue over the symphysis pubis in the female.

morals Social standards or customs; dealing with what is right or wrong in a practical sense.

Moro reflex A normal infant response elicited by a sudden loud noise. The infant flexes the legs, makes an embracing gesture with the arms, and usually gives a brief cry.

morphology The study of the physical shape and size of a specimen, plant, or animal.

motor neuron A neuron that innervates skeletal, smooth, or cardiac muscle fibers; also known as an *interneuron.*

mucin The chief ingredient in mucus.

mucosa Mucous membrane.

mucus The viscous, slippery secretion of mucous membranes and glands.

multifocal premature ventricular contraction A premature ventricular complex that originates from multiple sites in the ventricles.

multigravida A woman who has had two or more pregnancies.

multipara A woman who has had two or more deliveries.

multiple gestation A pregnancy with more than one fetus.

multiple myeloma A malignant neoplasm of the bone marrow.

multiple organ dysfunction syndrome The progressive failure of two or more organ systems after a severe illness or injury.

multiple sclerosis A progressive disease of the central nervous system in which scattered patches of myelin in the brain and spinal cord are destroyed.

multiplex mode A communications mode with the ability to transmit two or more different types of information simultaneously, in either or both directions, over the same frequency.

mumps An acute viral disease characterized by swelling of the parotid glands.

muscarinic receptor A class of cholinergic receptor molecule specifically activated by muscarine in addition to acetylcholine.

muscular dystrophy An inherited muscle disorder of unknown cause marked by a slow but progressive degeneration of muscle fibers.

muscular tissue A primary tissue type characterized by its contractile abilities.

mutagenic Any chemical or physical environmental agent that induces a genetic mutation or increases the mutation rate.

mutual aid An agreement with neighboring emergency agencies to exchange equipment and personnel when necessary.

myalgia Diffuse muscle pain, usually accompanied by malaise; it occurs in many infectious diseases.

myasthenia Muscle weakness.

myasthenia gravis An autoimmune disorder in which muscles become weak and tire easily.

Mycobacterium leprae A genus of gram-positive bacteria that causes leprosy.

Mycobacterium tuberculosis A genus of gram-positive bacteria that causes tuberculosis.

Mycoplasma A genus of microscopic organisms lacking rigid cell walls; they are considered to be the smallest free-living organisms.

myelinated axon A nerve fiber having a myelin sheath.

myeloblast Bone marrow cell.

myocardial hypertrophy An abnormal increase in the size of cardiac muscle.

myocardial infarction Necrosis of a portion of cardiac muscle caused by obstruction in a coronary artery from atherosclerosis or an embolus.

myoclonus A condition characterized by rapid, uncontrollable muscular contractions or spasms of muscles that occur at rest or during movement.

myoepithelium Tissue made up of contractile epithelial cells.

myofibril A slender, striated strand of smooth muscle.

myofilament An extremely fine, molecular, threadlike structure that helps to form the myofibril of muscle; thick myofibrils are formed of myosin, and thin myofilaments are formed of actin.

myoglobinuria The presence of myoglobin in the urine.

myometrium The muscular wall of the uterus.

myosin A cardiac and skeletal muscle protein; it makes up about half of the proteins that occur in muscle tissue.

myxedema A condition that results from a deficiency in thyroid hormone.

nail bed The end of a finger or toe covered by the nail; it is abundant in blood vessels.

nail body The visible part of the nail.

narcolepsy A syndrome characterized by sudden sleep attacks and visual or auditory hallucinations at the onset of sleep.

nares Nostrils.

narrative The portion of the patient care report that allows for a chronological description of the call.

nasal bone The bony partition that separates the nasal cavity into left and right parts; also known as the *nasal septum.*

nasal septum A partition that separates the right and left nasal cavities.

nasogastric decompression The management of gastric distention or emesis control by means of a nasogastric tube.

nasogastric tube Any tube passed into the stomach through the nose.

nasolacrimal duct A duct that leads from the lacrimal sac to the nasal cavity.

nasopharynx The uppermost portion of the pharynx just behind the nasal cavities.

nasotracheal Accessing the trachea through the nasal cavity.

near-drowning Submersion with at least temporary survival.

nebulizer A device for producing a fine spray of medication for inhalation therapy.

necrosis Death of a cell or group of cells as the result of disease or injury.

negative feedback mechanisms Any mechanism that tends to produce a response that balances a change in a system.

neglect The refusal or failure of the caregiver to fulfill obligations or duties to a person.

negligence Failure to use such care as a reasonably prudent emergency medical services provider would use in similar circumstances.

nematocyst A capsule containing threadlike, venomous stinging cells found in some coelenterates.

neonate An infant in the first 28 days of life.

neoplasia The new and abnormal development of cells, which may be benign or malignant.

neoplasm Abnormal growth; a malignant or benign tumor.

nephron The functional unit of the kidney.

nerve A bundle of nerve fibers and accompanying connective tissue located outside the central nervous system.

nerve tract Bundles of parallel axons with associated sheaths in the central nervous system.

nervous tissue A major tissue type characterized by its conductile abilities.

nervous tunic The retina.

neuralgia Pain along a nerve.

neurogenic hypotension Hypotension following spinal shock; caused by a loss of sympathetic tone to the vessels.

neurogenic shock Shock resulting from vasomotor paralysis below the level of injury; also known as *spinal cord shock.*

neuroglia Cells in the nervous system other than neurons.

neurohormone A junction hormone secreted by a neuron.

neuromuscular A specialized synapse between a motor neuron and a muscle fiber.

neuromuscular junction The area of contact between the ends of a large myelinated nerve fiber and a fiber of skeletal muscle.

neuron The functional unit of the nervous system, consisting of the nerve cell body, the dendrites, and the axon.

neuropathy A disease of the peripheral nerves.

neurosis Any faulty or inefficient way of coping with anxiety or inner conflict; it may ultimately lead to a neurotic disorder.

neutrophil A small, phagocytic white blood cell with a lobed nucleus and small granules in the cytoplasm; it stains readily with neutral dyes.

newborn An infant in the first few hours of life.

Newton's first law of motion The principle that an object, whether at rest or in linear motion, remains in that state unless force is applied.

Newton's second law of motion The principle that force is equal to mass times acceleration or deceleration.

nicad batteries Nickel cadmium rechargeable batteries, which are used in portable radios.

nicotinic receptor A class of cholinergic receptor molecules that are activated specifically by nicotine and acetylcholine.

nit The egg of a parasitic insect, particularly a louse.

nitrogen narcosis An illness associated with scuba diving in which nitrogen becomes dissolved in solution as a result of greater than normal atmospheric pressure; also known as rapture of the deep.

nocturia Particularly excessive urination at night.

node of Ranvier The short interval in the myelin sheath of a nerve fiber between adjacent Schwann cells.

noncardiogenic pulmonary edema See *adult respiratory distress syndrome.*

noncompensatory pause The pause that occurs when the next expected P wave of the underlying cardiac rhythm appears earlier than it would have if the sinoatrial node had not been disturbed by a conduction abnormality.

noncompetitive antagonist An agent that combines with different parts of the receptor mechanism and inactivates the receptor so that the agonist cannot be effective regardless of its concentration.

nonconducted premature atrial complex A premature atrial complex blocked at the atrioventricular node.

nonelectrolyte A substance with no electrical charge.

nonproprietary name See *generic name.*

nonstriated muscle See *smooth muscle.*

noradrenalin An adrenergic hormone produced by the adrenal medulla, similar in chemical and pharmacological properties to epinephrine. It acts to increase blood pressure by vasoconstriction but does not affect cardiac output; also known as norepinephrine.

nuclear membrane A double membrane structure surrounding and enclosing the nucleus; also known as the nuclear envelope.

nucleic acids Extremely complex, long-chain compounds of high molecular weight that occur naturally in the cells of all living organisms; they form the genetic material of the cell and direct the synthesis of protein within the cell.

nucleolus Any one of the somewhat rounded, dense, well-defined nuclear bodies with no surrounding membrane; the nucleolus contains ribosomal RNA and protein.

nucleoplasm The protoplasm of the nucleus, as contrasted with that of the cell.

nucleus The central controlling body within a living cell.

nullipara A woman who has never borne a child.

nutrient Any substance that nourishes and aids the growth and development of the body.

nystagmus Involuntary rhythmic movements of the eyes.

obesity A condition in which a person is 30% above ideal body weight.

obligate Necessary; compulsory.

obsessive compulsive disorder A psychiatric disorder in which the person feels stress or anxiety about thoughts or rituals over which he or she has little control.

obstructive apnea A form of sleep apnea involving a physical obstruction of the upper airways that can lead to pulmonary failure, chronic fatigue, and cardiac abnormalities.

obtundation A state of being insensitive to unpleasant or painful stimulation associated with a reduced level of consciousness, such as by anesthesia or a strong narcotic analgesic.

obturator foramen A large opening on each side of the lower portion of the hipbone, formed posteriorly by the ischium, superiorly by the ilium, and anteriorly by the pubis.

occipital bone The cuplike bone at the back of the skull, marked by a large opening (the foramen magnum), that communicates with the vertebral canal.

occipital foramen A passage in the occipital bone through which the spinal cord enters the spinal column.

occipital lobe One of the five lobes of each cerebral hemisphere.

occiput posterior presentation An abnormal presentation in which the infant's head is delivered face up instead of face down.

oculomotor nerve The third cranial nerve, which contains sensory and motor fibers; it provides for movement in most of the muscles of the eye, for constriction of the pupil, and for accommodation of the eye to light.

odontoid process The toothlike projection that rises perpendicularly from the upper surface of the body of the second cervical vertebra or axis, which serves as a pivot point for the rotation of the atlas.

official name The name of a drug that is followed by the initials USP *(United States Pharmacopeia)* or NF *(National Formulary)*, denoting its listing in one of the official publications; usually the same as the generic name.

off-line (indirect) medical direction The establishment and monitoring of all medical components of an emergency medical services system, including protocols, standing orders, educational programs, and the quality and delivery of online (direct) medical direction.

olecranon fossa The depression in the posterior surface of the humerus that receives the olecranon of the ulna when the forearm is extended.

olecranon process The large bony process of the ulna; also known as the olecranon.

olfactory Of or pertaining to the sense of smell.

olfactory bulb The tissue that receives the olfactory nerves from the nasal cavity.

olfactory membranes Membranes that contain the receptors for the sense of smell; they are located in the roof of the nasal cavity.

olfactory recess The extreme superior region of the nasal cavity.

olfactory tract The nerve tract that projects from the olfactory bulb to the olfactory cortex.

oliguria A diminished capacity to form or pass urine.

omphalocele Congenital herniation of intraabdominal viscera through a defect in the abdominal wall around the umbilicus.

oncotic pressure See *blood colloid osmotic pressure.*

ongoing assessment A repeat of the initial assessment that is performed throughout the paramedic-patient encounter.

online (direct) medical direction The medical direction physician or designee who directly supervises prehospital care activities via radio or phone. Online (direct) medical direction may also be responsible for the activities of the emergency department staff and others at the medical direction hospital.

onset of action The interval between the time a drug is administered and the first sign of its effects; also known as the *latent period of drug action.*

oocyte An incompletely developed ovum.

open pneumothorax A chest wall injury that exposes the pleural space to atmospheric pressure.

open vault fracture A fracture that results in direct communication between a scalp laceration and cerebral substance.

opiate A narcotic drug that contains opium, derivatives of opium, or any of several semisynthetic or synthetic drugs with opium-like activity.

opioid Any synthetic narcotic that has opiate-like activities but is not derived from opium.

opposition Movement of the thumb and little finger toward each other for the purpose of grasping objects.

optic nerve The nerve that carries visual signals from the eye to the crossing of the optic tracts.

orchitis Painful inflammation of the testicle.

organ A structure made up of two or more kinds of tissues organized to perform a more complex function than any one tissue alone.

organ of Corti The organ of hearing; it is located in the cochlea and filled with endolymph.

organelle Any one of various particles of living substance bound within most cells, such as the mitochondria, the Golgi apparatus, the endoplasmic reticulum, the lysosomes, and the centrioles.

oriented Aware of one's surroundings.

origin The less movable attachment point of a muscle.

orogastric decompression The management of gastric distention or emesis control by means of an orogastric tube.

oropharyngeolaryngeal axis The three axes of the mouth, pharynx, and trachea; a patient position used for direct visualization of the larynx.

oropharynx The portion of the pharynx located behind the mouth.

orotracheal Gaining access to the trachea through the oral cavity.

orthostatic hypotension Abnormally low blood pressure that occurs when an individual assumes the standing posture; also called postural hypotension.

osmolality The osmotic concentration of a solution.

osmosis Diffusion of solvent (water) through a membrane from a less concentrated solution to a more concentrated solution.

osmotic pressure The force required to prevent the movement of water across a selectively permeable membrane.

ossified To be changed or developed into bone.

osteoarthritis A form of arthritis in which one or many joints undergo degenerative changes.

osteomyelitis Local or generalized infection of bone and bone marrow, usually caused by bacteria introduced by trauma or surgery.

osteoporosis A disorder characterized by a reduction in bone density; it occurs most often in postmenopausal women.

ostomy An artificial opening into the urinary tract, gastrointestinal tract, or trachea; any surgical procedure in which an opening is created between two hollow organs or between a hollow viscus and the abdominal wall.

otorrhea Any discharge from the external ear.

ounce A unit of weight equal to $^{1}/_{16}$ lb, or 28.349 g.

ovarian follicle The spherical cell aggregation in the ovary that contains an oocyte.

ovarian ligament The bundle of fibers that passes to the uterus from the ovary.

ovarian torsion Twisting of an ovary around its vascular pedicle.

ovary One of the pair of female gonads found on each side of the lower abdomen beside the uterus.

ovulation The release of an ovum or secondary oocyte from the vesicular follicle.

oxyhemoglobin Oxygenated hemoglobin.

P wave The first complex of the electrocardiogram, representing depolarization of the atria.

pacemaker cell Certain myocardial cells capable of initiating an electrical impulse.

packaging See *patient packaging.*

Paget's disease A common, nonmetabolic disease of bone of unknown cause characterized by excessive bone destruction and unorganized bone repair.

paging equipment Equipment typically using tone activation with one-way transmission to receive-only units.

palate A structure that forms the roof of the mouth; it is divided into the hard and soft palates.

palatine bone One of a pair of bones of the skull forming the posterior part of the hard palate, part of the nasal cavity, and the floor of the orbit of the eye.

palatine tonsil One of two large oval masses of lymphoid tissue embedded in the lateral wall of the oropharynx.

palliative care A unique form of health care primarily directed at providing relief to terminally ill persons through symptom management and pain management; also known as comfort care.

palmar grasp A normal infant response. The infant curls the fingers in response to a touch on the palm of the hand.

palpation A technique in which an examiner uses the hands and fingers to gather information from a patient by touch.

pancreas A fish-shaped nodular gland located across the posterior abdominal wall in the epigastric region of the body; it secretes various substances, including digestive enzymes, insulin, and glucagon.

pancreatic juice The fluid secretion of the pancreas produced by the stimulation of food in the duodenum.

pancreatitis Inflammation of the pancreas, which causes severe epigastric pain.

para The number of past pregnancies that have remained viable to delivery.

parainfluenza virus One of a group of viruses isolated from patients with upper respiratory tract disease of varying severity in infants and young children; it may cause croup, tracheobronchitis, bronchiolitis, bronchopneumonia, pharyngitis, and the common cold.

paralytic ileus The decrease in or absence of intestinal peristalsis that may occur after abdominal surgery, illness, or injury; the most common cause of intestinal obstruction.

parametritis An inflammatory condition of tissue of the structures around the uterus.

paranoia A condition characterized by an elaborate, overly suspicious system of thinking.

paraplegia A weakness or paralysis of both legs and sometimes part of the trunk.

parasagittal plane An imaginary vertical plane passing through the body parallel to the medial plane; it divides the body into left and right portions.

parasympathetic Of or pertaining to the craniosacral division of the autonomic nervous system.

parasympathetic nervous system The subdivision of the autonomic nervous system usually involved in activating vegetative functions such as digestion, defecation, and urination.

parasympatholytic agent Anticholinergic; producing effects resembling those of interruption or blockade of the parasympathetic nerve supply to effector organs or tissues.

parasympathomimetic agent An agent with effects that mimic those resulting from stimulation of parasympathetic nerves, especially the effects produced by acetylcholine.

parasystole An independent ectopic rhythm the pacemaker of which cannot be discharged by impulses of the dominant rhythm because of an area of depressed conduction surrounding the parasystolic focus.

parenchyma The essential or functional elements of an organ.

parens patriae A term that refers to the authority of the state to intervene over the objections of parents to protect children.

parenteral Of or pertaining to any medication route other than the alimentary canal.

paresthesia A sensation of numbness, tingling, or "pins and needles."

parietal bone One of a pair of bones that form the side of the cranium.

parietal lobe The portion of each cerebral hemisphere that occupies the parts of the lateral and medial surfaces covered by the parietal bone.

parietal Of or pertaining to the outer wall of a cavity or organ.

parietal pericardium The portion of serous pericardium lining the fibrous pericardium.

parietal peritoneum The layer of peritoneum lining the abdominal walls.

parkinsonism A neurological disorder characterized by tremor, muscle rigidity, hypokinesia, a slow shuffling gait, and difficulty in chewing, swallowing, and speaking; it frequently occurs in patients treated with antipsychotic drugs.

Parkinson disease A disease caused by degeneration or damage (of unknown origin) to nerve cells within the basal ganglia in the brain.

parotitis Inflammation or infection of one or both parotid salivary glands.

paroxysm A sudden attack or recurrence of symptoms of a disease.

paroxysmal nocturnal dyspnea An abnormal condition of the respiratory system characterized by sudden attacks of shortness of breath, profuse sweating, tachycardia, and wheezing that awaken a person from sleep; often associated with left ventricular failure and pulmonary edema.

paroxysmal supraventricular tachycardia An ectopic rhythm in excess of 100 beats per minute and usually faster than 170 beats per minute that begins abruptly with a premature atrial or junctional beat and is supported by an atrioventricular nodal reentry mechanism or by an atrioventricular reentry involving an accessory pathway.

partial antagonist An agent that has affinity and some efficacy but that may antagonize the action of other drugs that have greater efficacy.

partial pressure The pressure exerted by a single gas.

partial reabsorption The amount of drug reabsorbed from the renal tubule by passive diffusion.

partial-thickness burn A burn injury that extends through the epidermis to the dermis; considered a deep partial-thickness injury if it extends to the basal layers of the skin; also known as a *second-degree burn.*

parturition The process of giving birth.

passive glomerular filtration The renal process whereby fluid in the blood is filtered across the capillaries of the glomerulus and into the urinary space of Bowman's capsule.

patella A flat, triangular bone at the front of the knee joint; the kneecap.

patient care report A document used in the prehospital setting to record all patient care activities and circumstances related to an emergency response.

patient packaging Completion of emergency care procedures needed to transfer a patient from the scene to the emergency vehicle.

pattern recognition The process of comparing gathered information with the paramedic's knowledge base of medical illness and disease.

patterned injuries Injuries that result from an identifiable object.

peak plasma level The highest plasma concentration attained from a dose.

pectoral girdle See *shoulder girdle.*

pectus deformity Malformation of the chest wall.

pediatric trauma score An injury severity index that grades six components commonly seen in pediatric trauma patients: size (weight), airway, central nervous system, systolic blood pressure, open wound, and skeletal injury.

pelvic cavity The area of the body enclosed by the bones of the pelvis.

pelvic girdle The encircling bony structure supporting the lower limbs.

pelvic inflammatory disease Any inflammatory condition of the female pelvic organs, especially one caused by bacterial infection.

penetrating trauma An injury produced by crushing and stretching forces of a penetrating object that results in some form of tissue disruption.

penetration The flow of a hazardous liquid chemical through zippers, stitched seams, pinholes, or other imperfections in a material.

penis The external reproductive organ of the male.

pepsin The principal digestive enzyme of gastric juice.

pepsinogen A proenzyme formed and secreted by certain cells of the gastric mucosa.

peptic ulcer A sharply circumscribed loss of the mucous membrane of the stomach, duodenum, or any other part of the gastrointestinal system.

peptic ulcer disease Illness that results from a complex pathological interaction among the acidic gastric juice and proteolytic enzymes and the mucosal barrier.

peptide bond A chemical bond between amino acids.

percussion A technique used to evaluate the presence of air or fluid in body tissues.

perfusion The circulation of blood to the tissues.

periappendiceal abscess A cavity containing pus and inflamed tissue around the vermiform appendix.

pericardial cavity The area of the body that surrounds the heart.

pericardial fluid A viscous fluid contained within the pericardial cavity between the visceral and parietal pericardium; it serves as a lubricant.

pericardial friction rub A dry, grating sound heard with a stethoscope during auscultation; suggestive of pericarditis.

pericardial sac The sac that surrounds the heart.

pericardial tamponade Compression of the heart produced by the accumulation of fluid or blood in the pericardial sac.

pericardiocentesis A procedure for withdrawing fluid from the pericardial sac.

pericarditis Inflammation of the pericardium.

pericardium The membrane that surrounds the heart.

perilymph The fluid contained within the bony labyrinth.

perinatal Occurring at or near the time of birth.

perineum The pelvic floor and associated structures occupying the pelvic outlet, bounded anteriorly by the pubic symphysis, laterally by the ischial tuberosities, and posteriorly by the coccyx.

periodontal membrane The membrane that surrounds the root of the tooth.

periosteum Tough connective tissue that covers the bone.

periostitis Inflammation of the periosteum characterized by tenderness and swelling of the affected bone, pain, fever, and chills.

peripheral nervous system A subdivision of the nervous system consisting of nerves and ganglia.

peripheral neuropathy Diseases and disorders that affect the peripheral nervous system, including spinal nerve roots, cranial nerves, and peripheral nerves.

peripheral thermoreceptors Nerve endings sensitive to heat, located in the skin and some mucous membranes; they usually are categorized as cold or warm receptors.

peripheral vascular disease Any abnormal condition that affects the blood vessels outside the heart and lymphatic vessels.
peripheral vascular resistance The total resistance against which blood must be pumped; also known as *afterload.*
peristalsis The coordinated, rhythmic, and serial contraction of smooth muscle that forces food through the digestive tract, bile through the bile duct, and urine through the ureters.
peristaltic Pertaining to peristalsis.
peritoneal cavity The potential space between the parietal and visceral layers of the peritoneum; the two layers normally are in contact.
peritoneal dialysis A dialysis procedure that uses the peritoneum as a diffusible membrane; performed to correct an imbalance of fluid or electrolytes in the blood or to remove toxins, drugs, or other wastes normally excreted by the kidney.
peritoneal Pertaining to the peritoneum.
peritoneum The serous membrane that covers the abdominal wall of the body and is reflected over the contained viscera.
peritonitis Inflammation of the serous membrane that covers the abdominal wall.
peritubular capillary The capillary network located in the cortex of the kidney.
permeable A condition of being pervious so that fluids and other substances can pass through, as occurs in a semipermeable membrane.
permeation The process by which a hazardous liquid chemical moves through a material on a molecular level.
persistent generalized lymphadenopathy Enlarged lymph nodes involving two noncontiguous sites other than inguinal nodes; a common feature in early human immunodeficiency virus infection.
pertinent negative findings Findings that warrant no medical care or intervention but that, by seeking them, show evidence of the thoroughness of the examination and history of the event.
pertussis An acute, highly contagious respiratory disease characterized by paroxysmal coughing that ends in a loud, whooping inspiration; also known as whooping cough.
petit mal seizure An epileptic seizure characterized by a sudden, momentary loss of consciousness occasionally accompanied by minor muscle spasms of the neck or upper extremities.
pH An inverse logarithm of the hydrogen ion concentration.
phagocytic Pertaining to phagocytosis.
phagocytosis The process of ingestion by cells of solid substances such as other cells, bacteria, bits of necrosed tissue, and foreign particles.
phalanges Any bone of a finger or toe.
pharmaceutics The science of dispensing drugs.
pharmacodynamics The study of how a drug acts on a living organism.
pharmacokinetics The study of how the body handles a drug over a period of time, including the processes of absorption, distribution, biotransformation, and excretion.
pharmacology The science of drugs used to prevent, diagnose, and treat disease.
pharyngeal tonsil One of two collections of aggregated lymphoid nodules on the posterior wall of the nasopharynx.
pharyngitis Inflammation or infection of the pharynx.
phase 0 The rapid depolarization phase; it represents the rapid upstroke of the action potential that occurs when the cell membrane reaches the threshold potential (approximately −70 mV).
phase 1 The early rapid repolarization phase; the phase in which the fast sodium channels close, the flow of sodium ions into the cell terminates, and loss of potassium from the cell continues.
phase 2 The plateau phase; the prolonged phase of slow repolarization of the action potential.
phase 3 The terminal phase of rapid repolarization; it results in the inside of the cell becoming considerably negative and the membrane potential returning to approximately −90 mV, or its resting level.
phase 4 The period between action potentials when the membrane has returned to its resting membrane potential.
phencyclidine psychosis A true psychiatric emergency with clinical syndromes ranging from a catatonic and unresponsive state to bizarre and violent behavior; it may occur after a single low-dose exposure to phencyclidine and may last several days to weeks.
phlebitis Inflammation of a vein, often accompanied by formation of a clot; also known as *thrombophlebitis.*
phlebotomy The incision of a vein for the letting of blood.
phobia An anxiety disorder characterized by an obsessive, irrational, and intense fear of a specific object or activity.
phonation The production of speech sounds.
phosgene A poisonous gas that appears as a grayish white cloud and smells of newly mowed hay.
phospholipid One of a class of compounds, widely distributed in living cells, that contains phosphoric acid, fatty acids, and a nitrogenous base.
photophobia Abnormal sensitivity to light.
physical abuse The use of physical force that may result in bodily injury, physical pain, or impairment.
physical dependence An adaptive physiological state that occurs after prolonged use of many drugs; discontinuation causes withdrawal syndromes that are relieved by readministering the same drug or a pharmacologically related drug.
physical examination An assessment of a patient that includes examination techniques, measurement of vital signs, an assessment of height and weight, and the skillful use of examination equipment.
physiological dead space The sum of the anatomical dead space plus the volume of any nonfunctional alveoli.
pia mater The innermost layer of the meninges that directly covers the brain.
Pickwickian syndrome An abnormal condition characterized by obesity, decreased pulmonary function, somnolence, and polycythemia.
pigmented retina The pigmented portion of the retina.
piloerection Erection of the hairs of the skin in response to cold environment, emotional stimulus, or irritation of the skin.
pineal gland A cone-shaped structure in the brain that secretes the hormone melatonin.
pinna See *auricle.*

pituitary gland A small gland attached to the hypothalamus; it supplies numerous hormones that govern many vital processes.

pivot joint A joint that consists of a relatively cylindrical bony process that rotates within a ring composed partly of bone and partly of ligament.

placards Four-sided, diamond-shaped signs displayed on hazardous materials containers that usually are yellow, orange, white, or green. They have a four-digit United Nations identification number and a legend to indicate the contents of the container.

placebo An inactive substance or a less than effective dose of a harmless substance; it is used in experimental drug studies to compare the effects of the inactive substance with those of the experimental drug.

placenta A highly vascular fetal-maternal organ through which the fetus absorbs oxygen, nutrients, and other substances and excretes carbon dioxide and other wastes.

placenta previa A condition of pregnancy in which the placenta is implanted abnormally in the uterus so that it impinges on or covers the internal os of the uterine cervix.

placental barrier A protective biological membrane that separates the blood vessels of the mother and the fetus.

plague A disease caused by the bacteria *Yersinia pestis,* found in rodents (e.g., chipmunks, prairie dogs, ground squirrels, and mice) and their fleas in many areas around the world.

plane joint A joint that consists of two opposed flat surfaces that are approximately equal in size; also known as a *gliding joint.*

plasma The fluid portion of blood.

plasma membrane The outer covering of a cell that contains the cellular cytoplasm; also known as the cell membrane.

plasma-protein binding A type of drug reservoir in which drugs attach to proteins, mainly albumin, and form a drug-protein complex.

plateau phase Prolongation of the depolarization phase of cardiac muscle cell membrane; it results in a prolonged refractory period.

platelet A fragment of a cell; it contains granules in the central part and clear protoplasm peripherally but has no definite nucleus.

pleural cavity The area of the body that surrounds the lungs.

pleural fluid Serous fluid found in the pleural cavity; it helps to reduce friction when the pleural membranes rub together.

pleural friction rub A rubbing or grating sound that occurs as one layer of the pleural membrane slides over the other during breathing.

pleural lavage A rewarming technique that uses warm saline to irrigate the thorax; it is used to treat some patients with severe hypothermia.

pleural space The potential space between the visceral and parietal layers of the pleura.

pleurisy Inflammation of the parietal pleura of the lungs, characterized by dyspnea and stabbing chest pain.

plexus A network of intersecting nerves and blood vessels or lymphatic vessels.

pneumatic antishock garment A garment used to manage some forms of hypovolemia and to stabilize some fractures.

pneumococcus A gram-positive diplococcal bacterium of the species *Diplococcus pneumoniae;* the most common cause of bacterial pneumonia.

***Pneumocystis carinii* pneumonia** A bacterial pneumonia caused by infection with the parasite *Pneumocystis carinii;* it usually is seen in infants or debilitated or immunosuppressed persons and is characterized by fever, cough, tachypnea, and, frequently, cyanosis.

pneumohemothorax A collection of air and blood in the pleural space; also known as a *hemopneumothorax.*

pneumomediastinum The presence of air or gas in the mediastinal tissues.

pneumonia An acute inflammation of the lungs, usually caused by inhaled pneumococci of the species *Streptococcus pneumoniae.*

pneumopericardium The presence of air or gas in the pericardial cavity.

pneumoperitoneum The presence of air or gas within the peritoneal cavity of the abdomen.

pneumotaxic center A group of neurons in the pons that have an inhibitory effect on the inspiratory center.

pneumothorax A collection of air or gas in the pleural space that causes the lung to collapse.

poikilothermy Variation in body temperature according to the ambient temperature.

point of maximum impulse The location or area where the apical pulse is palpated the strongest, often in the fifth intercostal space of the thorax just medial to the left midclavicular line.

poison Any substance that produces harmful physiological or psychological effects.

polio See *poliomyelitis.*

poliomyelitis An infectious disease caused by one of three polio viruses; asymptomatic, mild, and paralytic forms of the disease occur.

poliovirus hominis The causative organism of poliomyelitis.

polyarthritis Inflammation of several joints.

polycythemia A condition characterized by an unusually large number of red cells in the blood as a result of their increased production by the bone marrow.

polydipsia Excessive thirst.

polymorphic Occurring in many forms.

polyp A small, tumorlike growth that projects from a mucous membrane surface.

polyphagia Excessive eating.

polysaccharide A carbohydrate that contains three or more molecules of simple carbohydrates.

polyuria Excessive secretion of urine.

pons The part of the brainstem between the medulla and the midbrain.

portal hypertension An increased venous pressure in the portal circulation caused by compression or by occlusion in the portal or hepatic vascular system.

portal vein A vein that ramifies like an artery in the liver and ends in capillary-like sinusoids that convey the blood to the inferior vena cava through the hepatic veins.

positive end-expiratory pressure Ventilation controlled by a flow of air delivered in cycles of constant pressure through the respiratory cycle.

posterior The back, or dorsal, surface.

posterior cerebral artery The artery that supplies the posterior portion of the cerebrum.

posterior chamber of the eye The chamber of the eye between the iris and the lens.

posterior communicating artery The artery that branches off each internal carotid artery and connects with the ipsilateral posterior cerebral artery.

posterior superior iliac spine One of two bony segments that form the iliac crest.

postictal phase The phase that usually follows a seizure in which the person is drowsy and lethargic.

postpartum The maternal period after delivery.

postpartum hemorrhage Blood loss of more than 500 mL after delivery of the newborn.

postsynaptic neuron The membrane of a nerve that is in close association with a presynaptic terminal.

posttraumatic syndrome An anxiety reaction to a severe psychosocial event; also known as posttraumatic stress disorder.

potassium ion The predominate intracellular cation; it helps to regulate neuromuscular excitability and muscle contraction.

potassium-sparing agent A group of medications that promote sodium and water loss without an accompanying loss of potassium.

potential difference The difference in electrical potential, measured as the charge difference across the cell membrane.

potentiation Enhancement of the effect of a drug, caused by concurrent administration of two drugs in which one drug increases the effect of the other.

pound A unit of measure equal to 16 oz, or 0.45359 kg.

P-R interval The time elapsing between the beginning of the P wave and the beginning of the QRS complex in the electrocardiogram.

precapillary sphincter The smooth muscle sphincter that regulates blood flow through a capillary.

precipitous delivery A rapid, spontaneous delivery of less than 3 hours from onset of labor to birth; it results from overactive uterine contractions and little maternal soft tissue or bony resistance. Childbirth that occurs with such speed that usual preparations cannot be made.

precordial thump A cardiopulmonary resuscitation technique used to restore circulation in monitored ventricular fibrillation or unstable ventricular tachycardia.

preeclampsia An abnormal disease of pregnancy characterized by the onset of acute hypertension after the twenty-fourth week of gestation.

pregravid Before pregnancy.

preload The amount of blood returning to the ventricle.

premature atrial complex A cardiac dysrhythmia characterized by an atrial beat occurring before the expected excitation and indicated on the electrocardiogram as an early P wave.

premature birth Refers to an infant who is born before 37 weeks of gestation.

premature junctional contraction A cardiac dysrhythmia that occurs during sinus rhythm earlier than the next expected sinus beat and is caused by premature discharge of an ectopic focus in the atrioventricular junctional tissue.

premature rupture of membranes Rupture of the amniotic sac before the onset of labor, regardless of gestational age.

premature ventricular contraction A cardiac dysrhythmia characterized by a ventricular beat preceding the expected electrical impulse and indicated on the electrocardiogram as an early, wide QRS complex without a preceding related P wave.

prenatal Existing or occurring before birth.

prepuce In males, the free fold of skin that covers the glans penis; the foreskin. In females, the external fold of the labia minora that covers the clitoris.

present illness Identification of the chief complaint and a full, clear, chronological account of the symptoms.

presenting part The part of the fetus that lies closest to the internal os of the cervix.

presenting the patient The effective communication and transfer of patient information in the course of out-of-hospital and hospital care.

pressure ulcers Sores or ulcers in the skin over a bony prominence that occurs most frequently on the sacrum, elbows, heels, outer ankles, inner knees, hips, and shoulder blades of high-risk patients, especially those who are obese, elderly, or suffering from chronic diseases, infections, injuries, or a poor nutritional state.

presynaptic neuron The nerve terminal that contains neurotransmitter vesicles.

presynaptic terminal The enlarged axon terminal.

preterm infant An infant born before 37 weeks of gestation.

priapism Painful, persistent erection of the penis.

primary bronchus One of the two tubes arising at the inferior end of the trachea; each primary bronchus extends into one of the lungs.

primary contamination Exposure to a hazardous substance that is harmful only to the person exposed and that poses little risk of exposure to others.

primary epilepsy Epilepsy for which the cause is unknown; also known as *idiopathic epilepsy*.

primary follicle The ovarian follicle that contains the primary oocyte.

primary injury prevention The practice of preventing an injury from occurring.

primary oocyte The oocyte before the first meiotic division.

primary pulmonary hypertension Abnormally high pressure within the pulmonary circulation.

prime mover A muscle that plays a major role in accomplishing movement.

primigravida A woman who is pregnant for the first time.

primipara A woman who has given birth only one time.

Prinzmetal's angina An atypical form of angina that occurs at rest rather than with effort; it is associated with gross ST segment elevation in the electrocardiogram that disappears when the pain subsides.

priority patients Patients who need immediate care and transport.

proarrhythmia A new or worsened rhythm disturbance seemingly generated by antidysrhythmic therapy.

prodromal stage The early period of labor before uterine contractions become forceful and frequent enough to result in progressive dilation of the uterine cervix.

progesterone A steroid sex hormone prescribed to treat various menstrual disorders, functional uterine bleeding, and repeated spontaneous abortions.

progestin Any group of hormones secreted by the corpus luteum, placenta, or adrenal cortex that have a progesterone-like effect on the uterus.

prokaryote A cell without a true nucleus and with nuclear material scattered throughout the cytoplasm.

prolapsed umbilical cord An umbilical cord that protrudes beside or ahead of the presenting part of the fetus.

proliferative phase The time between the end of menses and ovulation characterized by rapid division of endometrial cells and the development of follicles in the ovary.

pronation Rotation of the forearm so that the anterior surface is down.

prone The position in which the patient is lying on the stomach (face down).

proprietary name See *trade name.*

proprioception Information about the position of the body and its various parts.

prostaglandin A class of naturally occurring fatty acids that affect body functions such as vasodilation, stimulation and contraction of uterine smooth muscle, and promotion of inflammation and pain.

prostate gland The gland that lies just below the male bladder; its secretion is one of the components of semen.

prostatic hypertrophy Hypertrophy or enlargement of the prostate gland.

prostatitis Acute or chronic inflammation of the prostate gland.

prosthesis An artificial replacement for a missing part of the body, such as an artificial limb.

protein Any of a large group of naturally occurring, complex, organic nitrogen compounds.

prothrombin A chemical that is part of the clotting cascade; the precursor of thrombin.

protoplasm The living substance of a cell.

protraction Movement in the anterior direction

pseudoaneurysm A condition resembling an aneurysm, caused by enlargement and tortuosity of a vessel.

pseudomembranous colitis A life-threatening form of diarrhea caused by *Clostridium difficile.*

psoas muscle A long muscle originating from the transverse processes of the lumbar vertebrae and the fibrocartilage and sides of the vertebral bodies of the lower thoracic vertebrae and the lumbar vertebrae.

psoriasis A common, chronic, inheritable skin disorder characterized by circumscribed red patches covered by thick, dry, adherent scales that result from excessive development of epithelial cells.

psychological dependence Emotional reliance on a drug; manifestations range from a mild desire for a drug to craving and drug-seeking behavior to repeated compulsive use of a drug for its subjectively satisfying or pleasurable effects.

psychology The science or study of behavior.

psychomotor seizure A seizure manifested by impaired consciousness of variable degree; the patient carries out a series of coordinated acts that are inappropriate, bizarre, and serve no useful purpose, about which the patient is amnesic.

psychosis Maladaptive behavior involving major distortions of reality.

puberty The period of life when the ability to reproduce begins.

pubis One of a pair of pubic bones that, with the ischium and the ilium, form the hipbone and join the pubic bone from the opposite side at the pubic symphysis.

public duty doctrine or rule The provision that a public official is generally not liable to individuals for his or her negligence in discharging public duties.

public service answering point A communications center that coordinates the deployment of emergency personnel and other resources required for an emergence response.

pulmonary artery The artery that carries deoxygenated blood from the right ventricle into the lung.

pulmonary capacity The sum of two or more pulmonary volumes.

pulmonary contusion Bruising of the lung tissue that results in rupture of the alveoli and interstitial edema.

pulmonary edema The accumulation of extravascular fluid in lung tissues and alveoli.

pulmonary embolism The blockage of a pulmonary artery by foreign matter such as fat, air, tumor tissue, or a thrombus that usually arises from a peripheral vein.

pulmonary hypertension A condition of abnormally high pressure within the pulmonary circulation.

pulmonary overpressurization syndrome A condition that results from expansion of trapped air in the lungs; it may lead to alveolar rupture and extravasation of air into extraalveolar locations.

pulmonary semilunar valve A valve that guards the orifice between the right ventricle and the pulmonary artery.

pulmonary surfactant Certain lipoproteins that reduce the surface tension of pulmonary fluids, allowing the exchange of gases in the alveoli of the lungs and contributing to the elasticity of pulmonary tissue.

pulmonary trunk The large elastic artery that carries blood from the right ventricle of the heart to the right and left pulmonary arteries.

pulmonary vein Any vein that carries oxygenated blood from the lung to the left atrium.

pulmonary ventilation The movement of air in and out of the lungs. This process brings oxygen into the lungs and removes carbon dioxide.

pulmonic pressure Pressure generated by the right side of the heart.

pulp The soft, spongy chamber of the tooth.

pulse deficit A condition that exists when the radial pulse is less than the ventricular rate; it indicates a lack of peripheral perfusion.

pulse pressure The difference between systemic and pulmonic pressure.

pulsus paradoxus An abnormal decrease in systolic blood pressure that drops more than 10 to 15 mm Hg during inspiration compared with expiration.

punctate Spotted; marked with points of puncture.

punctum The opening of each lacrimal canal.

puncture wound An open injury that results from contact with a penetrating object.

pupil The opening in the center of the iris that regulates the amount of light entering the eye.

purified protein derivative A dried form of tuberculin used in testing for past or present infection with tubercle bacilli.

Purkinje fibers Myocardial fibers that are a continuation of the bundle of His and that extend into the muscle walls of the ventricles.

pustule A small, circumscribed elevation of skin containing fluid, which is usually purulent.

pyelolithotomy Removal of a stone from a kidney by surgical incision.

pyelonephritis An inflammation of the kidney parenchyma associated with microbial infection.

pyloric sphincter A thickened, muscular ring in the stomach that separates the pylorus from the duodenum.

pyorrhea Discharge of pus.

pyrogen Any substance or agent that tends to cause a rise in body temperature.

pyrogenic A substance or agent that produces fever.

pyruvate The end product of glycolysis; it may be metabolized to lactate or acetyl coenzyme A.

QRS complex The principal deflection in the electrocardiogram, representing ventricular depolarization.

Q-T interval The time elapsing from the beginning of the QRS complex to the end of the T wave, representing the total duration of electrical activity of the ventricles.

quadriplegia A weakness or paralysis of all four extremities and the trunk.

R prime A subsequent positive deflection in the QRS complex that extends above the baseline and that is taller than the first R wave.

rabies An acute, usually fatal viral disease of the central nervous system of animals; it is transmitted from animals to human beings by infected blood, tissue, or most commonly, saliva.

raccoon's eyes Ecchymosis of one or both orbits caused by fracture of the base of the sphenoid sinus.

radial tuberosity A large, oblong elevation at the distal end of the radius.

radioulnar syndesmosis The articulation of the radius and ulna, consisting of a proximal articulation, a distal articulation, and three sets of ligaments.

radius One of the bones of the forearm, lying parallel to the ulna.

range The general perimeter of communications coverage, beyond which coverage is nonexistent or severely degraded to an unusable level; it is measured in miles.

rapid sequence induction An airway management technique that involves the virtually simultaneous administration of a potent sedative agent and a neuromuscular blocking agent for the purpose of endotracheal intubation; it provides optimal intubation conditions while minimizing the risk of aspiration of gastric contents.

rappelling A method of descent that involves lowering oneself with a rope.

reabsorption The process of absorbing again that occurs in the kidneys.

reactive airway disease An inflammatory airway condition that develops as a reaction to an antigen.

reactive hyperemia Increased blood flow associated with increased metabolic activity.

rebound tenderness A sign of peritoneal inflammation in which pain is caused by the sudden release of fingertip pressure on the abdomen.

receptor molecule A reactive site on the cell surface or within the cell that combines with a drug molecule to produce a biological effect.

reciprocal socialization A term that refers to a child's temperament and the responses it obtains from adults and family members. This interaction forms the basis for early social interactions with others and with the child's environment.

reciprocity The practice of granting an individual licensure or certification/registration based on licensure or certification/registration by another state, agency, or association.

rectum The segment of the large intestine continuous with the descending sigmoid colon just proximal to the anal canal.

rectus femoris muscle A muscle of the anterior thigh; one of the four parts of the quadriceps femoris.

red marrow Specialized soft tissue found in many bones of infants and children, in the spongy bone of the proximal epiphyses of the humerus and femur, and in the sternum, ribs, and vertebral bodies of adults. It is essential in the manufacture of red blood cells.

red measles See *rubeola.*

reentry The reactivation of tissue by a returning impulse; the sustaining mechanism in some cases of ventricular bigeminy or trigeminy, ventricular tachycardia, and paroxysmal supraventricular tachycardia.

referred pain Visceral pain felt at a site distant from its origin.

reflection on action A component of critical thinking (usually performed after the event) in which the examiner evaluates a patient care episode for possible improvement in similar future responses.

reflex An automatic response to a stimulus that occurs without conscious thought; produced by a reflex arc.

reflex arc The smallest portion of the nervous system capable of receiving a stimulus and producing a response.

refractory period The period after effective stimulation during which excitable tissue fails to respond to a stimulus of threshold intensity.

refractory shock Shock that is resistant to treatment but is still reversible.

relative hypovolemia Inadequate preload as a result of vasodilation.

relative refractory period The portion of the action potential after the absolute refractory period during which another action potential can be produced with a greater than threshold stimulus strength.

renal calculus Kidney stone.

renal calyx The first unit in the system of the ducts of the kidney carrying urine from the renal pyramid of the cortex to the renal pelvis for excretion through the ureters.

renal capsule The cortical substance that separates the renal pyramids.

renal corpuscle The glomerulus and its enclosing Bowman's capsule.

renal cortex The outer layer of the kidney, which contains approximately 1.25 million renal tubules, which remove body waste in the form of urine.

renal failure Inability of the kidneys to secrete wastes, concentrate urine, and conserve electrolytes; it may be chronic or acute.

renal medulla The inner layer of the kidney.

renal papilla The apex of the renal pyramid.

renal pelvis The funnel-shaped expansion of the upper end of the ureter that receives the calyces.

renal pyramid One of a number of pyramidal masses seen on longitudinal section of the kidney; it contains part of the loop of Henle and the collecting tubules.

renal tubule One of the collecting tubules in the kidney.

renin A proteolytic enzyme that surrounds each arteriole as it enters a glomerulus; it affects blood pressure by catalyzing the change of angiotensin I to angiotensin II.

renin-angiotensin-aldosterone mechanism Renin, released from the kidneys in response to low blood pressure, converts angiotensinogen to angiotensin I. Angiotensin I is converted by angiotensin-converting enzyme to angiotensin II, which causes vasoconstriction, resulting in increased blood pressure. Angiotensin II also increases aldosterone secretion, which increases blood pressure by increasing blood volume.

repolarization The phase of the action potential in which the membrane potential moves from its maximum degree of depolarization toward the value of the resting membrane potential.

reposition To move a structure to its original position.

rescue The act of delivery from danger or imprisonment.

residual volume The volume of air remaining in the lungs after a maximum expiratory effort.

respiration The process of the molecular change of oxygen and carbon dioxide within the body's tissues.

respiratory acidosis An abnormal condition characterized by an increased arterial P_{CO_2}, excess carbonic acid, and an increased plasma hydrogen ion concentration.

respiratory alkalosis An abnormal condition characterized by decreased P_{CO_2}, decreased hydrogen ion concentration, and increased blood pH.

respiratory bronchiole The smallest bronchiole that connects the terminal bronchiole to the alveolar duct.

respiratory membrane The membrane in the lungs across which gas exchange occurs with the blood.

respiratory syncytial virus A single-strand virus that is a common cause of epidemics of acute bronchiolitis, bronchopneumonia, and the common cold in young children and sporadic acute bronchitis and mild upper respiratory tract infections in adults.

resting membrane potential The electrical charge difference inside a cell membrane measured relative to just outside the cell membrane.

reticular activating system A functional system in the brain essential for wakefulness, attention, concentration, and introspection.

reticular formation A small, thick cluster of neurons nestled within the brainstem that controls breathing, the heartbeat, blood pressure, level of consciousness, and other vital functions.

reticular Relating to a fine network of cells or collagen fibers.

retina The nervous tunic of the eye; it is continuous with the optic nerve.

retinopathy A group of inflammatory eye disorders often caused by diabetes, hypertension, and atherosclerotic vascular disease.

retraction Movement in the posterior direction

retrograde amnesia The loss of memory for events that occurred before the event that precipitated the amnesia.

retroperitoneal Of or pertaining to the organs closely attached to the abdominal wall and partly covered by peritoneum.

retroperitoneum Behind the peritoneum.

retrovirus Any of a family of viruses that converts genetic RNA to DNA after entering the host cell.

Revised Trauma Score An injury severity index that uses the Glasgow Coma Scale and measurements for systolic blood pressure and respiratory rate.

Reye's syndrome A combination of acute encephalopathy and fatty infiltration of the internal organs that may follow acute viral infections.

Rh factor An antigenic substance present in the erythrocytes of most persons; a person lacking the Rh factor is Rh negative.

rhabdomyolysis An acute, sometimes fatal, disease characterized by destruction of skeletal muscle.

rheumatic fever An inflammatory disease that may develop as a delayed reaction to streptococcal infection of the upper respiratory tract.

rheumatoid arthritis A chronic, sometimes deforming destructive collagen disease that has an autoimmune component.

rheumatoid lungs Rheumatoid arthritis with emphasis on nonarticular changes; for example, pulmonary interstitial fibrosis, pleural effusion, and lung nodules.

rhinitis Inflammation of the mucous membranes of the nose.

rhinorrhea The free discharge of watery nasal fluid.

rhonchi Abnormal sounds heard on auscultation of a respiratory airway obstructed by thick secretions, muscular spasm, neoplasm, or external pressure.

rib One of the 12 pairs of elastic arches of bone forming a large part of the thoracic skeleton. The first seven ribs on each side are called *true ribs* because they articulate directly with the sternum. The remaining five ribs are called *false ribs*; the first three attach ventrally to the ribs, and the last two ribs are free at their ventral extremities and are called *floating ribs*.

ribonucleic acid A nucleic acid found in the nucleus and the cytoplasm of cells that transmits genetic instructions from the nucleus to the cytoplasm. In the cytoplasm, RNA functions in the assembly of proteins.

ribosome The "factory" of a cell where protein is synthesized.

ricin A potent protein cytotoxin derived from the beans of the castor plant *(Ricinus communis)*.

right lymphatic duct A vessel that conveys lymph from the right upper quadrant of the body into the bloodstream in the neck at the junction of the right internal jugular and the right subclavian veins.

rigor mortis The rigid stiffening of skeletal and cardiac muscle shortly after death.

riot control agents Chemicals that can produce sensory irritation or disabling physical effects which disappear within a short time after termination of exposure.

Rocky Mountain spotted fever A serious tick-borne infectious disease, characterized by chills, fever, severe headache, mental confusion, and rash.

rod A photoreceptor in the retina of the eye; it is responsible for noncolor vision in low-intensity light.

R-on-T phenomenon The occurrence of a ventricular depolarization during a vulnerable period of relative refractoriness.

root The lowest part of the tooth; it is covered by cementum.

rooting reflex A normal infant response elicited by touching or stroking the side of the cheek or mouth; this causes the infant to turn the head toward the stimulated side and to begin to suck.

rotation Movement of a structure about its axis.

rouleau formation An aggregation of red cells in what looks like a stack of coins or checkers.

round ligament The remains of the umbilical vein.

rubella A contagious viral disease characterized by fever, symptoms of mild upper respiratory tract infection, lymph node enlargement, and a diffuse, fine, red maculopapular rash; it is spread by droplet infection; also known as *German measles*.

rubeola An acute, highly contagious viral disease involving the respiratory tract; it is characterized by a spreading, maculopapular, cutaneous rash and occurs primarily in young children who have not been immunized; also known as *red measles*.

rule of nines A method to estimate burn injury that divides the total body surface area into segments that are multiples of 9%.

rupture of membranes Rupture of the amniotic sac; it usually occurs toward the end of the first stage of labor.

ruptured diaphragm A tear or break in the diaphragm, usually as a result of injury.

ruptured ovarian cyst A ruptured globular sac filled with fluid or semisolid material that develops in or on the ovary.

S prime A subsequent negative deflection in the QRS complex that extends below the baseline.

sacral bone A bone composed of the five segments of the vertebral column that are fused in the adult to form the sacrum; the segments are designated S1 to S5.

sacral promontory The projecting portion of the pelvis at the base of the sacrum.

sacral sparing The preservation of sensory or voluntary motor function of the perineum, buttocks, scrotum, or anus.

sacrum The large, triangular bone at the dorsal part of the pelvis; it is inserted like a wedge between the two hipbones.

saddle joint A joint that consists of two saddle-shaped articulating surfaces oriented at right angles to each other.

sagittal plane An imaginary plane that runs vertically through the middle of the body, producing right and left sections.

salicylate Any one of several widely prescribed drugs derived from salicylic acid (e.g., aspirin).

salivary amylase A digestive enzyme found in saliva that begins the chemical digestion of carbohydrates.

salivary gland One of the three pairs of glands that pour their secretions into the mouth, thus aiding the digestive process.

salpingitis An inflammation or infection of the fallopian tube.

saltatory conduction Conduction in which action potentials jump from one node of Ranvier to the next node of Ranvier.

saphenous vein One of a pair of the longest veins in the body; it begins in the medial marginal vein in the dorsum of the foot and ends in the femoral vein.

sarcoidosis A chronic disorder of unknown origin characterized by the formation of lesions in the lung, spleen, liver, skin, and mucous membranes and in the lacrimal and salivary glands.

sarcolemma Part of a myofibril between adjacent Z lines.

sarcomere The contractile unit of skeletal muscle, which contains thick and thin myofilaments.

sarcoplasmic reticulum Endoplasmic reticulum of the muscle.

sarin A clear, colorless, and tasteless liquid that has no odor in its pure form; may be used as a nerve agent.

scanning A component of attention that refers to one's ability to review a large amount of sensory input rapidly. Different individuals have different capacities for scanning and may use various approaches and styles in their scanning.

scapula One of the pair of large, flat, triangular bones that form the dorsal part of the shoulder girdle.

scene size-up An assessment of the scene to ensure scene safety for the paramedic crew, patient(s), and bystanders; a quick assessment to determine the resources needed to manage the scene adequately.

schizophrenia A group of disorders characterized by recurrent episodes of psychotic behavior.

Schwann cell A cell that forms a myelin sheath around each nerve fiber of the peripheral nervous system.

sciatic nerve A long nerve that originates in the sacral plexus and extends through the muscles of the thigh, leg, and foot with numerous branches.

sciatica Inflammation of the sciatic nerve.

sclera The opaque membrane covering the eyeball.

scoliosis A lateral curvature of the spine.

scrambling Movement over rough terrain that is not steep enough to require the use of a rope.

scrotum The sac of skin that contains the testes.

sebaceous gland A gland of the skin, usually associated with a hair follicle that produces sebum.

sebum The secretion of sebaceous glands; it prevents drying and protects against some bacteria.

second stage of labor The stage of labor measured from full dilation of the cervix to delivery of the newborn.

secondary bronchus A branch from a primary bronchus that conducts air to each lobe of the lungs.

secondary contamination Exposure to a hazardous substance whereby liquid and particulate substances are transferred easily to others by touching.

secondary epilepsy Epilepsy that can be traced to trauma, infection, a cerebrovascular disorder, or another illness that contributes to or causes the seizure disorder.

secondary follicle The follicle in which the secondary oocyte is surrounded by granulosa cells.

second-degree burn A burn injury that extends through the epidermis to the dermis (superficial partial thickness); it is considered a deep partial-thickness injury if it extends to the basal layers of the skin.

secretin The hormone that stimulates secretion of pancreatic juice.

secretion A general term for a substance produced inside a cell and released from the cell.

secretory phase The portion of the menstrual cycle extending from the time of formation of the corpus luteum after ovulation to the time when menstrual flow begins.

sedative-hypnotic A drug that reversibly depresses the activity of the central nervous system; these drugs are used chiefly to induce sleep and relieve anxiety.

seizure A temporary alteration in behavior or consciousness caused by abnormal electrical activity of one or more groups of neurons in the brain.

selectivity A component of attention that refers to a person's ability to pick or choose specific components of the sensory input that the person is reviewing and then focus on that input.

self-contained breathing apparatus A respiratory protection device that provides an enclosed system of air.

self-neglect A type of elder abuse; behaviors of an older adult that intentionally threaten personal health or safety.

Sellick maneuver Cricoid cartilage pressure directed posteriorly to compress the trachea against the cervical vertebra, thereby occluding the esophagus; this maneuver is useful for limiting the risk of aspiration during an intubation procedure.

semen Male reproductive fluid.

semicircular canal A structure located in the inner ear that generates a nerve impulse when the head moves.

semi-Fowler position An inclined position with the upper half of the body raised by elevating the head or a stretcher about 30 degrees to prevent reflux of gastric contents.

semilunar valve A valve with a half-moon shape, such as the aortic valve and the pulmonary valve.

seminal vesicle One of two glandular structures that empty into the ejaculatory ducts; its secretion is one of the components of semen.

semipermeable membranes A membrane that allows some fluids and substances to pass through it but not others, usually depending on size, shape, electrical charge, or other chemical properties.

senile dementia An organic mental disorder of the aged resulting from generalized atrophy of the brain with no evidence of cerebrovascular disease.

sensitization An acquired reaction in which specific antibodies develop in response to an antigen.

sensory layer The portion of the retina that contains rods and cones; also known as the *sensory retina.*

sensory Pertaining to a part or all of the sensory nerve network of the body.

sensory retina See *sensory layer.*

sepsis Infection.

septic shock A form of shock that most often results from a serious systemic bacterial infection.

septicemia Systemic infection in which the pathogens are present in the bloodstream, having spread from an infection in any part of the body.

septum A thin wall dividing two cavities or masses of soft tissue.

serotonin A hormone and neurotransmitter released from platelets when blood vessel walls are damaged.

serous membrane One of the many thin sheets of tissue that line closed cavities of the body, such as the pleura lining the thoracic cavity, the peritoneum lining the abdominal cavity, and the pericardium lining the sac that encloses the heart.

serous pericardium The thin inner layer of the pericardium that surrounds the heart.

serum Blood plasma without its clotting factors.

sexual abuse Nonconsensual sexual contact of any kind.

sexual assault The forcible perpetration of an act of sexual contact on the body of another person, male or female, without his or her consent.

shaken baby syndrome A serious form of child abuse that describes injuries to infants that occur after being violently shaken.

shingles An acute infection caused by reactivation of the latent varicella zoster virus; it is characterized by painful vesicular eruptions that follow the underlying route of cranial or spinal nerves inflamed by the virus; also known as herpes zoster.

shipping papers Descriptions of the hazardous materials that include the substance name, classification, and United Nations identification number.

shock An abnormal condition of inadequate blood flow to the body's peripheral tissues that is associated with life-threatening cellular dysfunction; also known as *hypoperfusion.*

short bones Bones that are approximately as broad as they are long, such as the carpal bones of the wrist and the tarsal bones of the ankle.

shoulder dystocia An obstacle to delivery that occurs when the fetal shoulders press against the maternal symphysis pubis, blocking shoulder delivery.

shoulder girdle The encircling bony structure that supports the upper limbs; also known as the *pectoral girdle.*

shoulder presentation The presentation that results when the long axis of the fetus lies perpendicular to that of the mother; also known as *transverse presentation.*

shunt A tube or device surgically implanted in the body to redirect body fluid from one cavity or vessel to another.

shunting The redirection of a flow of body fluid from one cavity or vessel to another.

sickle cell anemia See *sickle cell disease.*

sickle cell crisis An acute episodic condition that occurs in individuals with sickle cell anemia.

sickle cell disease A debilitating and unpredictable recessive genetic illness that produces an abnormal type of hemoglobin with an inferior oxygen-carrying capacity.

side effect An often unavoidable and undesirable effect of using therapeutic doses of a drug; actions or effects other than those for which the drug was originally given.

sighing An occasional deep, audible inspiration that usually is insignificant.

sigmoid colon The segment of the colon that extends from the end of the descending colon in the pelvis to the juncture with the rectum.

significant medical history A patient's medical background that may offer insight into the patient's current problem.

silicosis A lung disorder caused by continued long-term inhalation of the dust of an inorganic compound, silicon dioxide; the disorder is characterized by dyspnea and the development of nodular fibrosis in the lungs.

simplex mode A communications mode with the ability to transmit or receive in one direction at a time. Simultaneous transmission cannot occur.

sinoatrial node An area of specialized heart tissue that generates the cardiac electrical impulse.

sinus headache A headache characterized by pain in the forehead, nasal area, and eyes.

sinus One of several cavities in the bones of the skull that connect to the nasal cavities by small channels.

sinusitis Inflammation of one or more paranasal sinuses.

sinusoid A form of terminating blood channel, somewhat larger than a capillary, lined with reticuloendothelial cells.

size-up See *scene size-up.*

skeletal muscle Muscle tissue that appears microscopically to consist of striped myofibrils; also known as *striated muscle* and *voluntary muscle.*

Skene's glands The largest of the glands that open into the urethra of women.

skin graft A portion of skin implanted to cover areas where skin has been lost through burns or injury or by surgical removal of diseased tissue.

slander Verbally making false statements to others about a person, knowing that the statements are false, and with malicious intent or reckless disregard for their falsity.

sleep apnea A sleep disorder characterized by periods in which attempts to breathe are absent.

slough To shed or cast off; tissue that has been shed.

slow reactive substance of anaphylaxis A bronchoconstrictor mediator released from mast cells; it increases the production of prostaglandins.

small intestine The longest portion of the digestive tract; it is divided into the duodenum, jejunum, and ileum.

smallpox A highly contagious viral disease characterized by fever, prostration, and a vesicular, pustular rash.

smooth muscle One of two kinds of muscle; it is composed of elongated, spindle-shaped cells in muscles not under voluntary control, such as smooth muscle of the intestines, stomach, and other visceral organs; also known as *visceral muscle, involuntary muscle,* and *nonstriated muscle.*

sniffing position The patient position used during orotracheal intubation in which the patient's neck is flexed at C5 and C6 and the head is extended at C1 and C2.

SOAP format A memory aid used to organize written and verbal patient reports; it includes subjective data, objective data, assessment data, and plan of patient management.

sodium bicarbonate An antacid, electrolyte, and urinary alkalinizing agent.

sodium ions Ions involved in acid-base balance, water balance, nerve impulse transmission, and muscle contraction.

sodium-potassium exchange pump The biochemical mechanism that uses energy derived from adenosine triphosphate to achieve the active transport of potassium ions opposite to that of sodium ions.

soft palate The posterior muscular portion of the palate, which forms an incomplete septum between the mouth and the oropharynx and between the oropharynx and the nasopharynx.

solutes Substances dissolved in solution.

soman A clear, colorless, tasteless liquid with a slight camphor odor; may be used as a nerve agent.

somatic nervous system The part of the nervous system composed of nerve fibers that send impulses from the central nervous system to skeletal muscle.

somatic pain Pain that arises from skeletal muscles, ligaments, vessels, or joints.

somatoform disorder Any of a group of neurotic disorders characterized by symptoms suggesting physical illness or disease, for which there are no organic or physiological causes.

somatomotor nerves Motor nerves to the skeletal muscles.

somatomotor Refering to cranial nerves that control the skeletal muscles through motor neurons.

spasm An involuntary muscle contraction of sudden onset.

spastic colon Abnormally increased motility of the small and large intestines, generally associated with stress; also known as irritable bowel syndrome.

special emergency radio service A specific group of radio frequencies designated by the Federal Communications Commission for use by emergency agencies.

sperm See *spermatozoon.*

spermatic cord A structure that extends from the deep inguinal ring in the abdomen to the testes; each cord comprises arteries, veins, lymphatics, nerves, and the excretory duct of the testis.

spermatogenesis The process of development of spermatozoa.

spermatozoa See *spermatozoon.*

spermatozoon The male sex cell, composed of a head and tail; it contains genetic information transmitted by the male.

sphenoid bone The bone at the base of the skull anterior to the temporal bones and the basilar part of the occipital bone.

sphenoid sinus One of a pair of cavities in the sphenoid bone that are lined with mucous membrane continuous with that of the nasal cavity.

sphincter Ring-shaped muscle.

sphygmomanometer The device used to measure blood pressure.

spina bifida A congenital defect in which part of one or more vertebrae fail to develop completely, leaving a portion of the spinal cord exposed.

spinal cord shock See *neurogenic shock.*

spinal ganglia The structures that contain the cell bodies of sensory neurons; also known as *dorsal root ganglia.*

spinal nerve One of 31 pairs of nerves formed by the joining of the dorsal and ventral routes that arise from the spinal cord.

spinal shock A temporary loss of all types of spinal cord function distal to a cord injury.

spinous process A part of the vertebrae that projects backward from the vertebral arch, giving attachment to muscles of the back.

spleen A large, highly vascular lymphatic organ situated in the upper part of the abdominal cavity between the stomach and the diaphragm; it responds to foreign substances in the blood, destroys worn-out erythrocytes, and is a storage site for red blood cells.

splenomegaly An abnormal enlargement of the spleen.

spondylosis A condition of the spine characterized by fixation or stiffness of the vertebral joint.

spontaneous abortion An abortion that usually occurs before the twelfth week of gestation; the lay term is *miscarriage.*

spontaneous pneumothorax A condition that results when a subpleural bleb ruptures, allowing air to enter the pleural space from within the lung.

sprain A partial tearing of a ligament caused by a sudden twisting or stretching of a joint beyond its normal range of motion.

sputum Material coughed up from the lungs and expectorated from the mouth.

squelch A radio receiver circuit used to suppress the audio portion of unwanted radio signals or radio noises below a predetermined carrier strength level.

ST segment The early part of repolarization in the electrocardiogram of the right and left ventricles.

staging area A designated area where incident-assigned vehicles are directed and held until needed.

standing orders Specific treatment protocols used by prehospital emergency care providers in the absence of online (direct) medical direction when delay in treatment would harm the patient.

stapes The smallest of the three ossicles in the middle ear.

staphylococcal infection An infection caused by any one of several pathogenic species of *Staphylococcus,* commonly characterized by the formation of abscesses of the skin or other organs.

starch The principal molecule used for the storage of food in plants.

Starling hypothesis The concept that describes the movement of fluid back and forth across the capillary wall (net filtration).

Starling's law of the heart A rule that the force of the heartbeat is determined by the length of the fibers making up the myocardial walls.

stasis A disorder in which the normal flow of fluid through a vessel of the body is slowed or halted.

status asthmaticus A severe, prolonged asthma exacerbation that has not been broken with repeated doses of bronchodilators.

status epilepticus Continuous seizure activity lasting 30 minutes or longer, or a recurrent seizure without an intervening period of consciousness.

stellate wound A star-shaped wound.

stenosis Abnormal constriction or narrowing of an opening or passageway in a body structure.

sternal angle The point at which the manubrium joins the body of the sternum; also known as the *angle of Louis.*

sternoclavicular joint The double gliding joint between the sternum and the clavicle.

sternomanubrial joint See *sternal angle.*

sternum The elongated, flattened bone forming the middle portion of the thorax.

steroid A member of a large family of lipids, including some reproductive hormones, vitamins, and cholesterol.

stimulant A drug that enhances or increases body function or activity.

Stokes-Adams syndrome A condition characterized by sudden episodes of loss of consciousness caused by incomplete heart block; seizures may accompany the episodes.

stoma A surgically created artificial opening of an internal organ on the surface of the body.

stomach The major organ of digestion, located in the right upper quadrant of the abdomen.

strain An injury to the muscle or its tendon from overexertion or overextension.

stratum basale The innermost layer of the epidermis.

stratum corneum The most superficial layer of the epidermis.

stratum granulosum The layer of the epidermis that lies just beneath the stratum corneum except in the palms of the hands and soles of the feet, where it lies just beneath the stratum lucidum.

stratum lucidum The layer of the epidermis that lies just beneath the stratum corneum; it is present only in the thick skin of the palms of the hands and soles of the feet.

stratum spinosum The layer of the epidermis that lies on top of the stratum basale and beneath the stratum granulosum.

streptococcal infection An infection caused by pathogenic bacteria of one of several species of the genus *Streptococcus* or their toxins.

stress A nonspecific mental or physical strain caused by any emotional, physical, social, economic, or other factor that initiates a physiological response.

stressor Any factor that causes wear and tear on the physical or mental resources of the body.

stretch mark See *stria.*

stria A streak or linear scar that often results from rapidly developing tension in the skin; also known as a *stretch mark.*

striated Having striped or parallel lines, as in skeletal muscle.

striated muscle See *skeletal muscle.*

stridor An abnormal, high-pitched musical sound caused by obstruction in the trachea or larynx.

stroke See *cerebrovascular accident.*

stroke volume The volume of blood ejected from one ventricle in a single heartbeat.

stupor A state of lethargy and unresponsiveness in which a person seems unaware of his or her surroundings.

stylet A thin metal probe for inserting into or passing through a needle, tube, or catheter; it sometimes is used to change the configuration of an endotracheal tube.

styloid process A bony projection.

subarachnoid hematoma A collection of blood or fluid in the subarachnoid space.

subarachnoid space The area below the arachnoid membrane but above the pia matter that contains cerebrospinal fluid.

subclavian vein The continuation of the axillary vein in the upper body; it extends from the lateral border of the first rib to the sternal end of the clavicle, where it joins the internal jugular to form the brachiocephalic vein.

subcutaneous injection The introduction of medicine through a hypodermic needle into the subcutaneous tissue beneath the skin.

subcutaneous tissue The adherent layer of adipose tissue just below the dermal layer; also known as the hypodermis.

subdural hematoma A collection of blood in the subdural space.

subdural space The space between the dura mater and arachnoid.

subendocardial infarction See *transmural infarction.*

subgaleal hematoma A collection of blood beneath the strong sheet of fibrous connective tissue that joins the frontal and occipitofrontal muscles.

sublingual route The route of medication administration in which the medication is placed under the tongue so that the tablet dissolves in salivary secretions.

subluxation A partial dislocation.

submersion An incident in which a person experiences some swimming-related distress that is sufficient to require support in the prehospital setting and transportation to a medical facility for further observation and treatment.

substrate A substance acted upon and changed by an enzyme in any chemical reaction.

sucking reflex A normal infant response in which touching the infant's lips with the nipple of a breast or bottle causes involuntary sucking movements.

sudden death A death that occurs within the first 2 hours after the onset of illness or injury.

sudden infant death syndrome The unexpected and sudden death of an apparently normal and healthy infant that occurs during sleep.

sudoriferous gland See *sweat gland.*

summation The combined effects of two drugs that equal the sum of the individual effects of each agent.

superficial burn A burn injury where only a superficial layer of epidermal cells is destroyed; also known as a *first-degree burn.*

superficial frostbite A cold injury with at least some minimal tissue loss; it usually involves the dermis and shallow subcutaneous layers.

superficial pain Pain that arises from the skin or mucous membrane.

superior Situated above or higher than a point of reference in the anatomical position.

superior vena cava The vein that returns blood from the head and neck, upper limbs, and thorax to the right atrium.

supination Rotation of the forearm so that the anterior surface is up.

supine The position in which the patient is lying on the back (face up).

supine hypotension syndrome Hypotension that occurs in pregnant women who are in a supine position; it results when the uterus compresses the inferior vena cava, decreasing cardiac filling and cardiac output.

suprasternal notch The superior margin of the manubrium, which can be felt easily at the anterior base of the neck; also known as the *jugular notch.*

surface tension The tendency of the surface of a liquid to minimize the area of its surface by contracting.

surfactant Lipoproteins that reduce the surface tension of pulmonary fluids.

suspensory ligament The band of peritoneum that extends from the ovary to the body wall; it contains the ovarian vessels and nerves.

suture A border or joint between two bones of the cranium.

sweat gland A structure that produces sweat or viscus organic secretions; also known as a *sudoriferous gland.*

sympathetic nervous system A subdivision of the autonomic nervous system that usually is involved in preparing the body for physical activity.

sympatholytic Antiadrenergic; blocking transmission of impulses from the adrenergic postganglionic fibers to effector organs or tissues.

sympathomimetic A pharmacological agent that mimics the effects of sympathetic nervous system stimulation of organs and structures by acting as an agonist or by increasing the release of the neurotransmitter norepinephrine at postganglionic nerve endings.

symphysis A cartilaginous joint.

symphysis pubis The slightly movable, interpubic joint of the pelvis; it consists of two bones separated by a disk of fibrocartilage and connected by two ligaments; also known as the pubic symphysis.

synapse Functional membrane-to-membrane contact of a nerve cell with another nerve cell, muscle cell, gland cell, or sensory receptor; it functions in transmitting action potentials from one cell to another.

synaptic cleft The space between the presynaptic and postsynaptic membranes.

synaptic vesicle A secretory vesicle in the presynaptic terminal that contains neurotransmitter substances.

synchondrosis A cartilaginous joint between two immovable bones, such as the symphysis pubis, the sternum, and the manubrium.

syncope A brief lapse in consciousness caused by transient cerebral hypoxia.

syncytium Cardiac muscle cells that are bound together so tightly and their membranes are so permeable to electrical impulse that they act as a mass of merged cells or a single cell.

syndesmosis A fibrous articulation in which two bones are connected by interosseous ligaments.

synergism The combined action of two drugs that is greater than the sum of each agent acting independently.

synergist A muscle that works with other muscles to cause movement.

synovial fluid A thin, lubricating film that allows considerable movement between articulating bones.

synovial joint See *joint.*

synovial membrane The inner layer of an articular capsule that surrounds a freely movable joint.

syphilis A sexually transmitted disease characterized by distinct stages of effects over a period of years; any organ system may be involved.

system Interconnected functions or organs in which a stimulus or an action in one area affects all other areas.

systemic circulation Blood flow from the left ventricle to all parts of the body and back to the right atrium.

systemic lupus erythematosus A chronic inflammatory disease that affects many systems of the body; it is characterized by severe vasculitis, renal involvement, and lesions of the skin and nervous system.

systemic pressure Pressure generated by the left side of the heart.

systolic blood pressure The blood pressure measured during the period of ventricular contraction.

T lymphocytes The lymphocytes responsible for cell-mediated immunity.

T tubule Tubelike invagination of the sarcolemma that conducts action potentials toward the center of the cylindrical muscle fibers.

T wave A deflection in the electrocardiogram after the QRS complex, representing ventricular repolarization.

tabes dorsalis An abnormal condition characterized by the slow degeneration of all or part of the body and the progressive loss of peripheral reflexes.

tabun A clear, colorless, tasteless liquid with a faint fruity odor; may be used as a nerve agent.

tachycardia A heart rate that exceeds 99 beats per minute.

tachyphylaxis A phenomenon in which the repeated administration of some drugs results in a significant decrease in their effectiveness.

tachypnea A persistent respiratory rate that exceeds 20 breaths per minute.

tactical EMS Emergency medical services provided by EMS personnel who are specially trained and equipped to provide prehospital emergency care in tactical environments.

tactical patient care Patient-care activities that occur inside the scene perimeter, or hot zone, of a dangerous scene.

tactical retreat Leaving the scene when danger is observed or when violence or indicators of violence are displayed; requires immediate and decisive action.

talus The second largest tarsal bone; the ankle bone.

tardive dyskinesia An abnormal condition characterized by involuntary, repetitious movements of the muscles of the face, limbs, and trunk.

tarsal Pertaining to the area of articulation between the foot and the leg.

taste bud Any one of many peripheral taste organs distributed over the tongue and roof of the mouth.

teachable moment The time after an injury has occurred when the patient and observers remain acutely aware of what has happened and may be more receptive to being taught ways that the event or illness could have been prevented.

telecommunicator A person trained in public safety telecommunications; the term applies to call takers, dispatchers, radio operators, data terminal operators, or any combination of such functions in a public service answering point.

telemedicine Refers to technological communications that allow for the transmission of photographs, video, and other information to be sent directly from the scene to a hospital for physician evaluation and consultation.

telemetry The transmission and reception of physiological data by radio or telephone; for example, electrocardiograms.

temperament A person's style of behavior; the way the person interacts with the environment. It is the basis on which children develop relationships.

temporal bone One of a pair of large bones that form part of the lower cranium and that contain various cavities and recesses associated with the ear.

temporal lobe The lateral region of the cerebrum; it contains the center for smell and some association areas for memory and learning.

ten code (10 code) A code sometimes used in radio communications that uses the number 10 plus another number to relay a particular message.

tendon A band or cord of dense connective tissue that connects muscle to bone or other structures; it is characterized by strength and nonstretchability.

tendonitis An inflammatory condition of a tendon, usually caused by a sprain.

tenosynovitis Inflammation of a tendon sheath.

tension headache A headache caused by muscle contractions of the face, neck, and scalp.

tension pneumothorax An accumulation of air or gas in the pleural cavity that can lead to collapse of the lung.

teratogenic Any substance, agent, or process that interferes with normal prenatal development.

term A pregnancy that has reached 40 weeks of gestation.

terminal bronchiole The end of the conducting airway.

terminal drop A theory that a decline in intelligence in older adulthood may be caused by a person's conscious or unconscious perception of coming death.

terminally ill patients Patients with advanced stage of disease with an unfavorable prognosis and no known cure.

termination of action The point at which a drug effect is no longer seen.

tertiary segmental bronchus The bronchus that extends from the secondary bronchus and conducts air to each lobule of the lung.

testes The male gonads, which produce the male sex cells, or sperm.

testicular torsion A condition in which a testicle twists on its spermatic cord, disrupting its own blood supply.

testosterone The male sex hormone.

tetanus An acute, potentially fatal infection of the central nervous system caused by the tetanus bacillus *Clostridium tetani;* it is characterized by muscle spasms and convulsions.

tetralogy of Fallot A congenital cardiac anomaly that consists of four defects: pulmonic stenosis, ventricular septal defect, malposition of the aorta so that it rises from the septal defect or the right ventricle, and right ventricular hypertrophy.

thalamus Tissue located just above the hypothalamus; it helps to produce sensations, associates sensations with emotions, and plays a part in arousal.

therapeutic abortion The legal termination of a pregnancy for reasons of maternal well-being.

therapeutic action The desired, intended action of a drug.

therapeutic communications A planned, deliberate, professional act that involves the use of communications techniques to achieve two purposes: (1) a positive relationship with a patient and (2) a shared understanding of information for desired patient care goals.

therapeutic index A measurement of the relative safety of a drug.

therapeutic range The range of plasma concentrations that is most likely to produce the desired drug effect with the least likelihood of toxicity; the range between minimal effective concentration and toxic level.

thermogenesis Production of heat, especially by the cells of the body.

thermolysis The dissipation of heat by means of radiation, evaporation, conduction, or convection.

thiazide A group of diuretics that are moderately effective in lowering blood pressure.

third stage of labor The stage of labor that begins with delivery of the infant and ends when the placenta has been expelled and the uterus has contracted.

third ventricle The ventricle located in the center of the diencephalon between the two halves of the thalamus.

third-degree burn A burn injury in which the entire thickness of the epidermis and dermis is destroyed.

thoracentesis Puncturing of pleural space.

thoracic aorta The large upper portion of the descending aorta; it supplies many parts of the body such as the heart, ribs, chest muscles, and stomach.

thoracic cavity The area of the body enclosed by the ribs.

thoracic duct The common trunk of all the lymphatic vessels of the body except those on the right side of the head and neck, the thorax, right upper limb, right lung, right side of the heart, and the diaphragmatic surface of the liver.

thoracic vertebrae The 12 bony segments of the spinal column of the upper back, designated T1 to T12.

thoroughfare channel The channel for blood through a capillary bed from an arteriole to a venule.

threatened abortion An abortion diagnosed when a patient has some uterine bleeding with an intrauterine pregnancy in which the internal cervical os is closed; it may stabilize and end in normal delivery or progress to an incomplete or complete abortion.

threshold potential The value of the membrane potential at which an action potential is produced as a result of depolarization in response to a stimulus.

thrill A fine vibration felt by an examiner's hands over the site of an aneurysm or on the pericardium.

thrombectomy The removal of a thrombus from a blood vessel.

thrombin An enzyme formed in plasma as part of the clotting process; it causes fibrinogen to change to fibrin, which is essential in the formation of a clot.

thrombocytes Cell fragments.

thrombocytopenia An abnormal hematological condition in which the number of platelets is reduced; the most common cause is a bleeding disorder.

thromboembolism A condition in which a blood vessel is blocked by an embolus carried in the bloodstream from the site of formation of the clot.

thrombogenesis Clot formation.

thrombolytic agent A drug that dissolves clots after their formation by promoting the digestion of fibrin.

thrombophlebitis See *phlebitis.*

thrombosis An abnormal formation of a thrombus within a blood vessel of the body.

thromboxanes Antagonistic prostaglandin derivatives that are synthesized and released by degranulating platelets, causing vasoconstriction and promoting the degranulation of other platelets.

thrombus An aggregation of platelets, fibrin, clotting factors, and the cellular elements of the blood attached to the interior wall of a vein or artery, which sometimes occludes the lumen of the vessel.

thymectomy Excision of the thymus.

thymus A single, unpaired gland located in the mediastinum; the primary central gland of the lymphatic system.

thyroid cartilage The largest laryngeal cartilage; it forms the laryngeal prominence, or Adam's apple.

thyroid membrane The fibrous membrane that joins the hyoid and the thyroid cartilages.

thyrotoxicosis A term that refers to any toxic condition that results from thyroid hyperfunction.

tibia The second longest bone of the skeleton; it is located at the medial side of the leg.

tibial tuberosity A large, oblong elevation at the proximal end of the tibia that attaches to the ligament of the patella.

tick paralysis A rare, progressive, reversible disorder caused by several species of ticks that release a neurotoxin that causes weakness, incoordination, and paralysis.

tidal volume The volume of gas inhaled or exhaled in a single, resting breath.

tinea A group of fungal skin diseases characterized by itching and scaling and sometimes by painful lesions.

tissue binding A type of drug reservoir in which drug pooling occurs in fat tissue and bone.

tolerance A physiological response that requires that a drug dosage be increased to produce the same effect formerly produced by a smaller dose.

tone The audio signal or carrier wave of controlled amplitude and frequency used for equipment control purposes or to selectively signal a receiver, such as activating a pager; tones are measured in hertz.

tonsil A large collection of lymphatic tissue beneath the mucous membrane of the oral cavity and pharynx.

tonsillectomy Surgical removal of the tonsils.

tonsillitis Inflammation of the tonsils.

torr A measurement in millimeters of mercury.

torsades de pointes An unusual bidirectional ventricular tachycardia.

total body water All the water within the body, including intracellular and extracellular water and the water in the gastrointestinal and urinary tracts.

total lung capacity The sum of the inspiratory and expiratory reserve volumes plus the tidal volume and residual volume.

total pressure The combination of pressures exerted by all the gases in any mixture of gas.

Tourette's syndrome An abnormal condition characterized by facial grimaces, tics, and involuntary arm and shoulder movements.

toxic level The plasma concentration at which a drug is likely to produce serious adverse effects.

toxic shock A severe, acute disease caused by infection with strains of *Staphylococcus aureus.*

toxin A poison usually produced by or occurring in a plant or microorganism.

toxoid A toxin that has been treated with chemicals or with heat to reduce its toxic effects but that retains its antigenic power.

trachea A cylindrical tube in the neck composed of cartilage and membrane; it conveys air to the lungs.

tracheal stenosis Constriction of the trachea.

tracheostomy An opening through the neck into the trachea through which an indwelling tube may be inserted.

trade name The trademark name of a drug, designated by the drug company that sells the medication.

tragus A projection of the cartilage of the auricle at the opening of the external auditory meatus.

transceiver A combination transmitter and receiver with a switching circuit or duplexer to use a single antenna.

transcutaneous cardiac pacing The use of an artificial pacemaker to substitute for a natural pacemaker of the heart that is blocked or dysfunctional. In the prehospital setting a transcutaneous pacemaker is used to treat symptomatic bradycardia, heart block associated with reduced cardiac output that is unresponsive to atropine, pacemaker failure, and asystole.

transection A complete or incomplete lesion to the spinal cord.

transfusion hepatitis Hepatitis that results from a transfusion with infected blood.

transient dysphagia A temporary impairment of speech.

translaryngeal cannula ventilation An advanced airway procedure that provides high-volume, high-pressure oxygenation of the lungs through cannulation of the trachea below the glottis; also known as needle percutaneous transtracheal ventilation and needle cricothyrotomy.

transmembrane potential The difference in electrical charge between inside and outside the plasma membrane.

transmural infarction A myocardial infarction that extends through the full thickness of the myocardium, including the endocardium and epicardium.

transudate A fluid passed through a membrane as a result of a difference in hydrostatic pressure.

transverse At right angles to the long axis of any common part.

transverse colon The segment of the colon that extends from the end of the ascending colon at the hepatic flexure on the right side across the midabdomen to the beginning of the descending colon at the splenic flexure on the left side.

transverse plane An imaginary plane that divides the body into top and bottom or superior and inferior sections; also known as the *horizontal plane.*

transverse presentation See *shoulder presentation.*

transverse process The bony segment that extends laterally from each side of the vertebral arch.

trauma An injury caused by a transfer of energy from some external source to the human body.

trauma index An early measurement that used a numerical injury rating system based on a patient's injured body region, type of injury, and cardiovascular, central nervous system, and respiratory status.

trauma score An injury severity index used to predict the outcome for patients with blunt or penetrating injuries.

traumatic asphyxia A severe crushing injury to the chest and abdomen that causes an increase in intrathoracic pressure. The increased pressure forces blood from the right side of the heart into the veins of the upper thorax, neck, and face.

traumatic hyphema See *hyphema.*

traumatic iridoplegia Traumatic dilation or, less commonly, constriction of the pupil.

treatment protocols Guidelines that define the scope of prehospital intervention practiced by emergency care providers.

Trendelenburg's position A position in which the head is low and the body and legs are on an inclined plane.

triage A method used to sort or categorize patients according to severity of injury.

triaxial reference system Three intersecting lines of reference used in standard limb leads.

trichomoniasis A vaginal infection caused by the protozoan *Trichomonas vaginalis;* it is characterized by itching, burning, and a frothy, pale yellow to green vaginal discharge.

tricuspid valve The valve located between the right atrium and ventricle.

trigeminal nerve Either of the largest pair of cranial nerves, which are essential for chewing and the general sensibility of the face.

triglyceride A compound consisting of a fatty acid and glycerol.

trigone The triangular smooth area at the base of the bladder between the openings of two ureters and that of the urethra.

trimester One of three periods of approximately 3 months into which pregnancy is divided.

triphosphate bond Energy sources for the muscles, nerves, and overall function of the body; an example is adenosine triphosphate.

triplets Three premature ventricular contractions in a row.

trochanter One of the two bony projections at the proximal end of the femur that serve as the attachment point for various muscles.

trochlea The medial aspect of the humerus; it articulates with the ulna.

trophoblast A cell layer that forms the outer layer of the blastocyst, which erodes the uterine mucosa during implantation; it contributes to the formation of the placenta.

true rib See *rib.*

true vocal cord See *vocal cord.*

truncal obesity Obesity that preferentially affects or is isolated in the trunk of the body rather than the extremities.

trunking system A radio system consisting of base stations on different channels connected to each other with small computers that work with special mobile and portable signaling to allow multiple simultaneous conversations.

tubal ligation One of several sterilization procedures in which both fallopian tubes are blocked to prevent conception from occurring.

tubercle A nodule or small eminence, such as that on a bone or that produced by infection from tubercle bacilli.

tuberculosis A chronic granulomatous infection caused by *Mycobacterium tuberculosis;* it usually affects the lungs and generally is transmitted by inhalation or ingestion of infected droplets.

tuberosities Elevations or protuberances, especially of bones.

tuboovarian abscess An abscess involving the ovary and fallopian tube.

tularemia A serious illness that is caused by the bacterium *Francisella tularensis* found in animals (especially rodents, rabbits, and hares).

tunic One of the enveloping layers of a part; one of the coats of a blood vessel; one of the coats of the eye; one of the coats of the digestive tract.

tunica adventitia The outermost fibrous coat of a vessel or an organ that is derived from the surrounding connective tissue.

tunica intima The innermost coat of a blood vessel.

tunica media The middle coat, usually muscular, of an artery or other tubular structure.

turbinate The concha nasalis.

turgor The normal resiliency of the skin caused by the outward pressure of the cells and interstitial fluid.

Turner's sign Bruising of the skin of the flanks or loin in acute hemorrhagic pancreatitis; also known as Grey Turner's sign.

Turner's syndrome A chromosomal anomaly characterized by the absence of one X chromosome and characterized by short stature, undifferentiated gonads, and various other abnormalities.

tympanic membrane See *eardrum.*

type and crossmatch A test used to determine the patient's ABO group and Rh type.

U wave The gradual deviation from the T wave in the electrocardiogram, thought to represent the final stage of repolarization of the ventricles.

ulceration The formation of a craterlike lesion on the skin or mucous membranes.

ulcerative colitis An inflammatory condition of the large intestine characterized by severe diarrhea and ulceration of the mucosa of the intestine.

ulna One of the bones of the forearm.

ultrahigh frequency Radio frequency between 300 and 3000 MHz; the 460 MHz range commonly is used for emergency medical services communications.

umbilical cord A flexible structure connecting the umbilicus with the placenta and giving passage to the umbilical arteries and vein.

umbilicus The point on the abdomen at which the umbilical cord joined the fetal abdomen.

unethical Conduct that fails to conform to moral principles, values, or standards.

unifocal premature ventricular contraction A premature ventricular complex that originates from a single ectopic pacemaker site.

unipolar lead A lead composed of a single positive electrode and a reference point.

universal donor A person with blood of type O, Rh factor negative.

universal precautions Infection control practices in health care that are observed with every patient and procedure and that prevent exposure to blood-borne pathogens.

universal recipient A person with blood type AB who can receive any of the four types of blood.

unmyelinated axon A nerve fiber lacking a myelin sheath.

untoward effects Side effects that prove harmful to the patient.

upper esophageal sphincter The ring of muscle located at the superior opening of the esophagus that regulates the passage of materials into the esophagus.

urea A nitrogen-containing waste product.

uremia The presence of excessive amounts of urea and other nitrogenous wastes produced in the blood.

uremic frost A pale, frostlike deposit of white crystals on the skin caused by kidney failure and uremia.

ureter One of a pair of tubes that carry the urine from the kidney into the bladder.

urethra A small tubular structure that drains urine from the bladder; in men, it also serves as a passageway for semen during ejaculation.

urethritis An inflammatory condition of the urethra.

uric acid A product of the metabolism of protein present in the blood and excreted in the urine.

urinary bladder The muscular, membranous sac in the pelvis that stores urine for discharge through the urethra.

urinary retention The inability to urinate.

urinary tract infection An infection of one or more structures of the urinary tract.

urogenital triangle The anterior portion of the perianal region; it contains the openings of the urethra and vagina in the female and the root structures of the penis in the male.

urosepsis Septic poisoning caused by retention and absorption of urinary products in the tissues.

urticaria A pruritic skin eruption characterized by transient wheals of various shapes and sizes with well-defined margins and pale centers.

uterine Pertaining to the uterus.

uterine inversion A rare event in which the uterus turns inside out after birth.

uterine rupture A rare event in which the wall of the uterus ruptures when it is unable to withstand the strain placed on it.

uterine tube One of a pair of ducts opening at one end into the uterus and the other end into the peritoneal cavity, over the ovary; also known as a *fallopian tube.*

uterosacral ligament A primary ligament that holds the uterus in place.

uterus The hollow, pear-shaped internal female organ of reproduction.

uvula The cone-shaped process hanging down from the soft palate that helps prevent food and liquid from entering the nasal cavities.

vagina The part of the female genitalia that forms a canal from the orifice through the vestibule to the uterine cervix.

vaginitis An inflammation of the vaginal tissues.

vagus nerve Either of the longest pair of cranial nerves essential for speech, swallowing, and the sensibilities and functions of many parts of the body.

vallecula A furrow between the glossoepiglottic folds on each side of the posterior oropharynx.

Valsalva maneuver A vagal maneuver used to slow the heart and decrease the force of atrial contraction by stimulating postganglionic parasympathetic nerve fibers in the wall of the atria and specialized tissues of the sinoatrial and atrioventricular nodes via the vagus nerve.

varicella An acute, highly contagious viral disease caused by a herpes virus, varicella-zoster virus; it occurs primarily in young children and is characterized by crops of pruritic vesicular eruptions on the skin; also known as *chickenpox.*

varicella-zoster virus A member of the herpes virus family that causes the disease varicella (chickenpox) and herpes zoster (shingles).

varicocele A collection of varicose veins in the scrotum.

vas deferens See *ductus deferens.*

vascular tunic The choroid, ciliary body, and iris.

vasoconstriction A narrowing of the lumen of any blood vessel.

vasodilation An increase in the diameter of a blood vessel caused by inhibition of its constrictor nerves or stimulation of dilator nerves.

vasomotor Of or pertaining to the nerves and muscles that control the diameter of the lumen of blood vessels.

vasopressin mechanism The mechanism by which antidiuretic hormone secretion increases when blood pressure drops or plasma osmolarity increases; it reduces urine production and stimulates vasoconstriction.

vastus lateralis muscle The largest of the four muscles of the quadriceps femoris; it is situated on the lateral side of the thigh.

vein A vessel that carries blood toward the heart.

venereal disease A contagious disease usually acquired by sexual intercourse or genital contact.

venostasis Retardation of venous flow in a part.

venous capillary The ends of capillaries closest to venules.

venous sinus One of many sinuses that collect blood from the dura mater and drain it into the internal jugular vein.

ventral root The nerve that conveys efferent nerve processes away from the spinal cord.

ventricle A small cavity; it usually refers to the right or left ventricle of the heart.

ventricular bigeminy A cardiac rhythm disturbance characterized by two ventricular beats in rapid succession followed by a longer interval.

ventricular fibrillation A cardiac dysrhythmia marked by rapid, disorganized depolarization of the ventricular myocardium.

ventricular quadrigeminy A cardiac dysrhythmia that occurs when every fourth complex is a premature ventricular complex.

ventricular tachycardia A tachycardia that usually originates in the Purkinje fibers.

ventricular trigeminy A cardiac dysrhythmia characterized by three ventricular beats in rapid succession followed by a longer interval.

ventrogluteal muscle The muscle that overlies the iliac crest and the anterior-superior iliac spine.

venule Small blood vessels that collect blood from the capillaries and join to form veins.

vermiform appendix See *appendix.*

vertebra Any one of 33 bones of the spinal column.

vertebral arch The dorsal, bony arch of a vertebra composed of the laminae and pedicles; it protects the spinal cord.

vertebral artery Each of the two arteries branching from the subclavian arteries.

vertebral body A bony disk that serves as the weight-bearing portion of the vertebra.

vertex presentation See *cephalic presentation.*

vertigo A sensation of faintness or an inability to maintain normal balance in a standing or seated position.

very high frequency Radio frequencies between 30 and 300 MHz (usually in the 150 MHz range). The very high frequency spectrum is divided further into high and low bands.

vesicants Chemicals with severely irritating properties that produce fluid-filled pockets on the skin and damage to the eyes, lungs and other mucous membranes.

vesicular Pertaining to a blisterlike condition.

vesicular follicle The secondary follicle in which the oocyte attains its full size; also known as the *graafian follicle.*

vesiculation The formation of vesicles.

vestibular fold One of two folds of mucous membrane that stretch across the laryngeal cavity; it helps close the glottis; also known as the *false vocal cord.*

vestibule The portion of the inner ear adjacent to the oval window between the semicircular canals and the cochlea.

vestibule of the ear The middle region of the middle ear.

vestibule of the vagina The space behind the labia minora that contains the opening of the vagina, the urethra, and the vestibular glands.

vestibulocochlear nerve The eighth cranial nerve, formed by the cochlear and vestibular nerves; it extends to the brain.

viral hemorrhagic fevers A group of illnesses caused by several distinct families of viruses that include arenaviruses, filoviruses, bunyaviruses, and flaviviruses.

virulence The relative strength of a pathogen.

virus A minute, parasitic microorganism without independent metabolic activity that can replicate only within a cell of a living plant or animal host.

visceral Pertaining to internal organs enclosed within a body cavity, primarily the abdominal organs.

visceral pain Deep pain that arises from smooth vasculature or organ systems.

visceral pericardium The portion of the serous pericardium that covers the heart surface; also known as the *epicardium.*

visceral peritoneum The layer of peritoneum that covers the abdominal organs.

vital capacity The volume of gas moved on deepest inspiration and expiration, or the sum of the inspiratory reserve volume, the tidal volume, and the expiratory reserve volume.

vitamin An organic compound essential in small quantities for normal physiological and metabolic functioning of the body.

vitamin D A fat-soluble vitamin essential for the normal formation of bones and teeth and for absorption of calcium and phosphorus from the gastrointestinal tract.

vitamin K A fat-soluble compound essential for the synthesis of several related proteins involved in the clotting of blood.

vitreous humor The transparent, jellylike material that fills the space between the lens and the retina.

vocal cord One of two folds of elastic ligaments covered by mucous membrane that stretch from the thyroid cartilage to the arytenoid cartilage; vibration of the vocal cords is responsible for voice production; also known as a *true vocal cord.*

Volkmann's contracture A serious, persistent flexion contraction of the forearm and hand caused by ischemia.

voluntary Action originated or accomplished by a person's free will or choice.

voluntary muscle A muscle that is controlled consciously; see *skeletal muscle.*

vomer bone The bone forming the posterior and inferior part of the nasal septum.

vulva The external genitals of the female.

VX A thick, amber-colored, odorless liquid that resembles motor oil; may be used as a nerve agent.

wandering atrial pacemaker The passive transfer of pacemaker sites from the sinus node to other latent pacemaker sites in the atria and atrioventricular junction.

water vapor pressure The partial pressure exerted by water molecules after they have been converted into a gas.

watt The unit of measurement of a transmitter's power output.

weapons of mass destruction Large conventional biological, nuclear, incendiary, chemical, or explosive weapons (B-NICE).

Wenckebach heart block Type I second-degree atrioventricular block; a progressive, beat-to-beat prolongation of the P-R interval that finally results in a nonconducted P wave; at this point, the sequence recurs.

Wernicke-Korsakoff syndrome A disease that results from chronic thiamine deficiency combined with an inability to use thiamine because of a heritable disorder or because of a reduction in intestinal absorption and metabolism of thiamine by alcohol.

Wernicke's encephalopathy A stage of Wernicke-Korsakoff syndrome that usually develops suddenly with the clinical manifestations of ataxia, nystagmus, disturbances of speech and gait, signs of neuropathy, stupor, or coma.

West Nile virus A potentially serious mosquito-borne illness that affects the central nervous system.

wheeze A form of rhonchus characterized by a high-pitched, musical quality; it is caused by high-velocity airflow through narrowed airways.

windchill chart An index developed to calculate the cooling effects of the ambient temperature based on thermometer readings and the wind speed.

withdrawal syndrome A predictable set of signs and symptoms that occurs after a decrease in the usual dose of a drug or its sudden cessation.

xiphoid process The smallest of three parts of the sternum; it articulates caudally with the body of the sternum and laterally with the seventh rib.

years of productive life The calculation obtained by subtracting the victim's age at death from 65 (the average age of retirement).

yellow fever An acute infection transmitted by mosquitoes; it is characterized by headache, fever, jaundice, vomiting, and bleeding.

yellow marrow Specialized soft tissue (mainly adipose) found in the compact bone of most adult epiphyses.

Z line The delicate, membrane-like structure found at either end of a sarcomere.

zone of coagulation In a burn wound, the central area that has sustained the most intense contact with the thermal source; in this area coagulation necrosis of the cells has occurred and the tissue is nonviable.

zone of hyperemia An area in which blood flow is increased as a result of the normal inflammatory response to injury; it lies at the periphery of the zone of stasis.

zone of stasis The area of burn tissue that surrounds the critically injured area; it consists of tissue that is potentially viable despite the serious thermal injury.

zygomatic bone One of a pair of bones that forms the prominence of the cheek, the lower part of the orbit of the eye, and parts of the temporal bone; also known as the *zygomatic process.*

zygomatic process See *zygomatic bone.*

zygote The developing ovum from the time it is fertilized until it is implanted in the uterus as a blastocyst.

APPENDIX

ADVANCED PRACTICE PROCEDURES FOR THE CRITICAL CARE PARAMEDIC

Some critically ill or injured patients require a level of interhospital service and care that is beyond the scope of the paramedic as defined in the *National EMS Education and Practice Blueprint*. For example, a patient may have special needs that require continuous medical supervision by one or more health professionals in a specialty area such as nursing, emergency medicine, respiratory care, cardiovascular care, or care provided by paramedics with advanced levels of training.

Critical care transport (CCT) (also known as *specialty care transport [SCT]*) is the term used for the delivery of medical services for a critically ill or injured patient during transport. This type of care normally could be provided only in intensive care units and other specialty care areas in the hospital setting. Most paramedics who are members of a CCT team have completed a training program, such as Critical Care EMT–Paramedic (CCEMT-P), and have additional clinical experience working with critical care patients. Through this education, they are trained and become skilled in advanced practice procedures that may be performed infrequently by most prehospital providers. Such procedures include invasive hemodynamic monitoring and arterial line placement, insertion of an intraaortic balloon pump (IABP), blood administration, use of IV infusion devices, tube thoracostomy, pericardiocentesis, and other advanced life support (ALS) skills described elsewhere in this text. The following descriptions of these advanced practice procedures are intended as an overview. All procedures carry significant complications and risks and require special training and authorization from medical direction.

INVASIVE HEMODYNAMIC MONITORING

Invasive hemodynamic monitoring requires placement of a catheter (central venous line, arterial line) in a vein, artery, or heart chamber. Knowledgeable health care providers can obtain and interpret many different pieces of information from this tool, depending on the type of catheter used. Box A-1 lists potential risks and complications associated with hemodynamic monitoring.

BOX A-1 Possible Complications and Risks Associated with Hemodynamic Monitoring

- Air embolism
- Arterial spasm
- Bleeding
- Dysrhythmias (with heart chamber catheterization)
- Hematoma
- Pneumothorax (with some insertion sites)
- Systemic infection
- Thrombosis
- Tissue and blood vessel injury

Hemodynamic monitoring is most useful for assessing and managing patients with hypertensive emergencies, shock, pulmonary edema, sepsis, and multiple organ failure. In particular, a pulmonary artery (PA) catheter can help distinguish among the various types of shock (cardiogenic, hypovolemic, obstructive, and distributive). Hemodynamic monitoring requires special equipment to produce visible waveforms on an oscilloscope and pressure monitor (Fig. A-1). These waveforms reflect the phases of the cardiac cycle and can be used to monitor systemic arterial pressure, right atrial pressure (central venous pressure), left atrial pressure, and pulmonary artery pressure.

Systemic Arterial Pressure Monitoring

The placement of an arterial line in a peripheral artery allows for continuous and accurate measurement of arterial pressure. It may be indicated for monitoring drug therapy (e.g., titration of vasopressors, inotropics), blood pressure, or for frequent arterial blood gas sampling. Indwelling arterial catheters may be inserted into the radial, femoral, brachial, or dorsalis pedis artery. The radial or brachial artery is most commonly used for continuous pressure monitoring.

Right Atrial Pressure (RAP) Monitoring

RAP monitoring (also known as *central venous pressure [CVP] monitoring*) allows direct measurement of pressure in the right atrium and *reflects* right ventricular pressure. It is used to monitor blood volume, right ventricular function, and

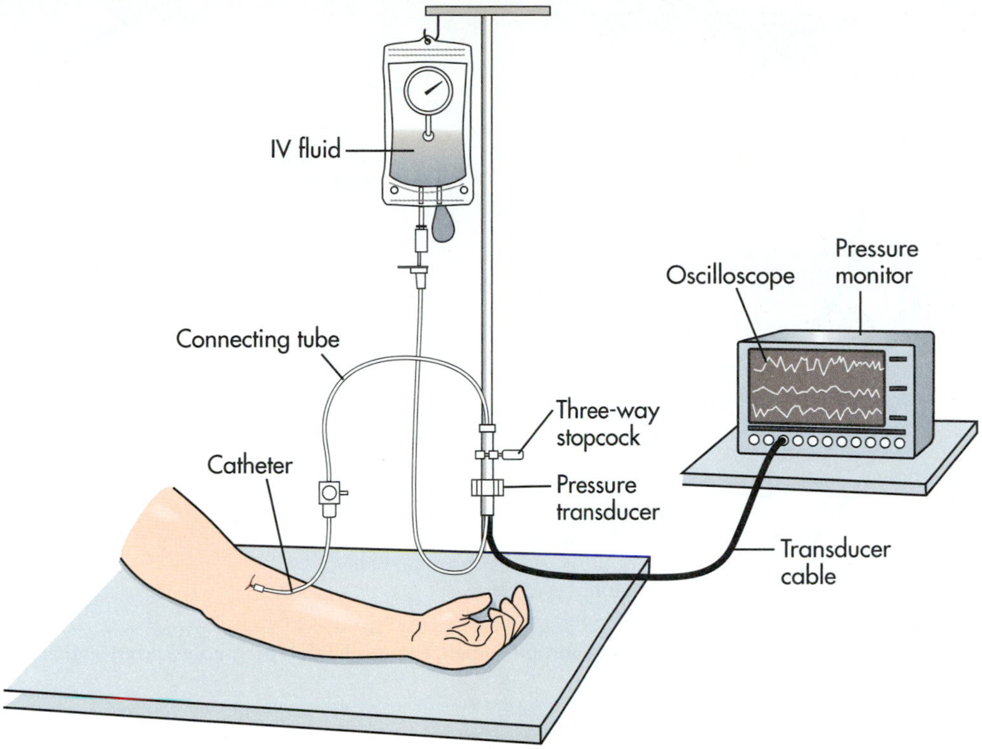

FIGURE A-1 ■ Hemodynamic monitoring equipment.

central venous return. The vascular access device also can be used to administer IV fluids, medications, blood, and to obtain blood samples. Although monitoring RAP measures the pressure in the right atrium, this is used to indirectly determine the volume of blood in the right atrium and thus the right ventricular preload. Common insertion sites for RAP monitoring are the internal jugular vein and the subclavian vein.

Left Atrial Pressure (LAP) Monitoring

LAP monitoring measures the pressure of the blood as it returns to the left side of the heart. It is a reliable indicator of left ventricular end-diastolic pressure, and therefore, of left ventricular function. Short-term LAP monitoring is usually performed in the operating room during cardiac surgery, when a catheter is placed directly into the left atrium. In other settings, LAP more often is indirectly monitored through a pulmonary artery catheter.

Pulmonary Artery Pressure (PAP) Monitoring

PAP monitoring provides an indirect measure of left ventricular function. The catheter used for PAP monitoring has four lumens (and sometimes a fifth proximal infusion port) that contain a balloon inflation port, proximal and distal injection ports, and a thermistor lumen for obtaining cardiac output measurements (Fig. A-2). Some PAP devices also are designed for transvenous pacing.

The catheter is usually inserted in the subclavian or internal jugular vein and is passed through the right atrium and right ventricle into the pulmonary artery. PAP monitoring is useful in treating shock, congestive heart failure (CHF), pulmonary edema, pulmonary embolism, and for monitoring patients who are undergoing cardiac surgery. The PAP reflects venous pressure in the lungs, the mean filling pressure for the left side of the heart, and indicates left ventricular end-diastolic pressure (in the absence of mitral valve disease). In addition to measuring pulmonary artery pressure, PAP monitoring provides a measurement of RAP, pulmonary capillary wedge pressure (PCWP), cardiac output, and mixed venous oxygen saturation.

PULMONARY CAPILLARY WEDGE PRESSURE (PCWP)

PCWP (also known as *pulmonary artery wedge pressure [PAWP]*) helps to determine left ventricular function. It is measured when the pulmonary balloon of the PA catheter is inflated and occludes a pulmonary artery branch, allowing the distal lumen in front of the balloon to register left heart pressure. Once the measurement is obtained, the balloon is deflated and the catheter will float back into the pulmonary artery. (The balloon is only inflated for PCWP readings; it remains deflated for continuous PAP monitoring.) PCWP usually is measured every 4 hours.

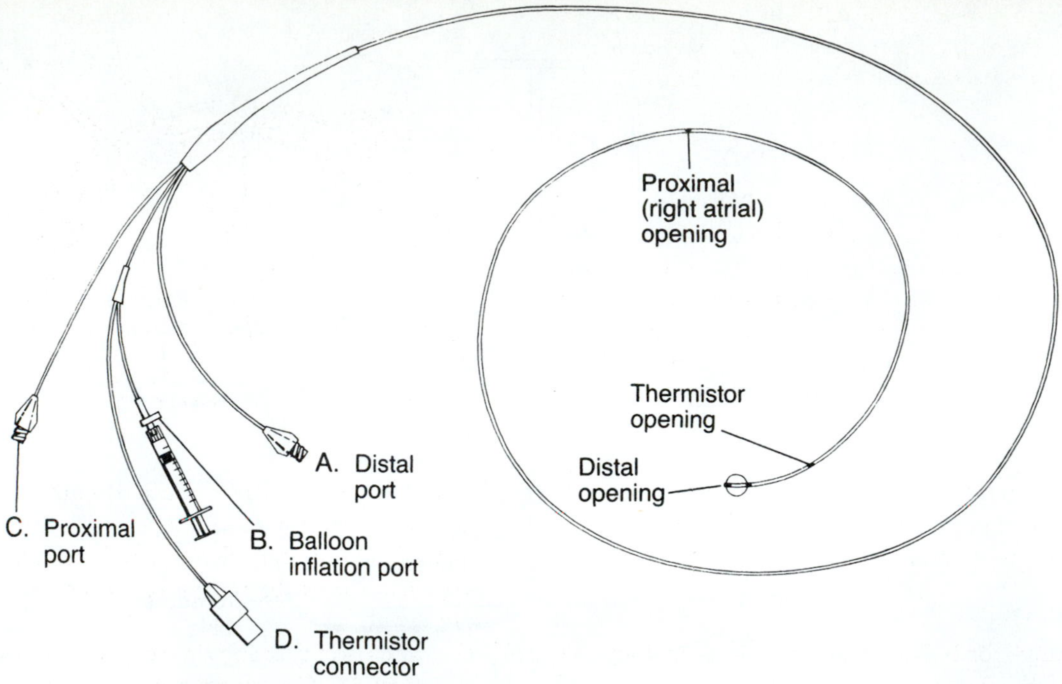

FIGURE A-2 ■ Number 7 French quadruple-lumen, thermodilution pulmonary artery catheter.

CARDIAC OUTPUT

The thermistor lumen measures cardiac output (CO) through a special computer. It also aids in assessing left ventricular function and the function of heart valves. This measure is taken (as needed) by injecting a solution called *injectate* at a known temperature (iced or room temperature) into the proximal lumen port of the PA catheter or through a closed injectate delivery system. The solution then mixes with blood from the superior vena cava or the right atrium (depending on the location of the catheter), and lowers the temperature of the heart's blood. The thermistor detects the drop in temperature, which is analyzed by the computer, calculating cardiac output of the right and left ventricle. Continuous CO measurements also can be obtained by special catheters and equipment that change the temperature of the heart's blood at specific intervals without injectate, calculating CO over several minutes.

MIXED VENOUS OXYGEN SATURATION

Mixed venous oxygen saturation (SVO2) can be measured from a PA catheter to determine if the oxygen supply adequately meets the oxygen demands of the tissues. Mixed venous blood from organs and tissues flows back to the lungs and can be sampled through the PA catheter where oxygen saturation can be measured. This measurement can be taken intermittently by withdrawing blood from the port of a PA catheter, or continuously by using fiberoptic catheters and an oximetry system that assesses cardiac and pulmonary function.

Intraaortic Balloon Pump (IABP)

An intraaortic balloon pump is a mechanical cardiac assist device that benefits patients with actual or potentially life-threatening circulatory problems. Indications for its use include patients:

- With cardiogenic shock as a bridge to reperfusion therapy
- With ventricular septal defect and acute mitral regurgitation
- Who are candidates for cardiac transplant
- Who are high-risk surgical patients
- Who are high risk and undergoing angiography or angioplasty
- Who have refractory ventricular dysrhythmias complicating AMI
- Who have recurrent post-infarction angina

The catheter with balloon usually is inserted in the patient's femoral artery and is advanced until the catheter lies just distal to the left subclavian artery. The balloon is at the distal end of the catheter, and when inflated by a computerized pump, it fills the patient's descending thoracic aorta. The balloon inflates during diastole causing blood in the balloon to be forced back toward the extremities and proximally into the coronary arteries and main branches of the aortic arch. This allows increased perfusion of the myocardium, helping alienate myocardial ischemia. Just before systole, the balloon deflates, causing a decrease of the pressure in the aorta, making it easier for the left ventricle to expel blood during contraction. This results in decreased workload for the left ventricle, and increases cardiac output and perfusion of vital organs.

As a rule, the IABP is initially set to an inflation/deflation cycle for each cardiac cycle (1:1 ratio) and then is gradually reduced, based on the patient's condition.

INTRACRANIAL PRESSURE MONITORING

As described in Chapter 24, a rise in intracranial pressure (ICP) can decrease cerebral perfusion. ICP monitoring is often used in patients with brain lesions, head trauma with bleeding or edema, hydrocephalus, encephalitis, and those who have an overproduction and/or insufficient absorption of cerebrospinal fluid. ICP can be monitored using an intraventricular cannula (the most common method), an epidural catheter, a subdural or subarachnoid monitoring device, or by a fiberoptic transducer tipped probe (Fig. A-3). All devices must be placed by a physician, and all monitoring systems require calibration.

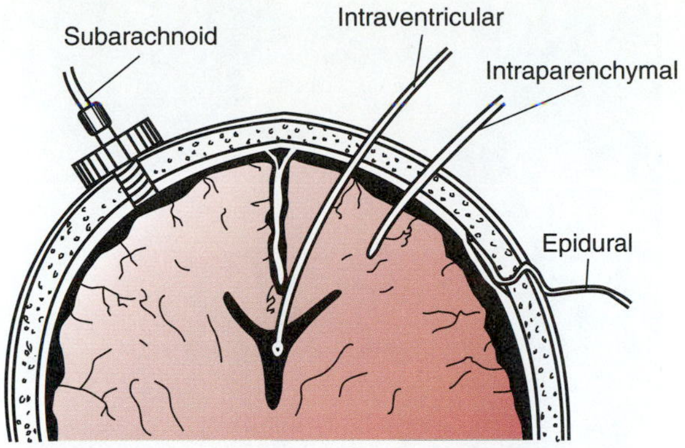

FIGURE A-3 ■ Intracranial pressure monitoring sites.

ICP Waveforms

The normal range for ICP in an adult is between 4 and 15 mm Hg, but this can vary by individual with position changes and activity level. Therapies that may be needed to control increasing ICP include:

- Maintaining oxygenation to improve gas exchange
- Hyperventilating the patient to decrease C_{O2} and to stimulate cerebral vasoconstriction (controversial)
- Avoiding hypoxia and/or hypercapnia
- Positioning the patient by elevating the patient's head or the head of the stretcher to optimize cerebral perfusion pressure (CPP) and to lower ICP
- Avoiding maneuvers that might increase intrathoracic or intraabdominal pressure (e.g., coughing, Valsalva maneuver, patient movement, hip flexion)
- Preventing sudden variation in systemic blood pressure
- Administering osmotic diuretics and/or steroids to reduce cerebral edema and inflammation
- Restricting IV fluid therapy
- Providing sedation to prevent agitation
- Maintaining normal body temperature

BLOOD ADMINISTRATION

As described in Chapter 7 and Chapter 17, blood replacement therapy may be indicated when caring for patients who have suffered acute blood loss and in some patients who have symptomatic anemia or other disorders. Blood products that commonly are administered to critical patients include packed red blood cells, fresh frozen plasma, and platelets. (Whole blood is not commonly available, but it is still used occasionally.) Because of the risk of transfusion reactions and the possible transmission of infectious disease, blood products should be given only when specifically indicated. Before administering a blood transfusion:

1. The patient and blood product must be identified by two health care professionals.
2. Blood containing RBCs must be compared to the patient's ABO group and Rh type.
3. The name and identification number on the patient's wrist band must be compared to the slip on the blood bag.
4. The expiration date and time on the blood product must be identified. The blood bag should be turned upside down to gently mix it and inspect its contents for color and consistency.
5. The label must remain attached to the blood product until the transfusion is complete.

Blood and blood products can be safely administered through a peripheral IV line, Portacath, and most central lines. Optimally, the tubing of the administration set should be connected directly to the access line and should not be piggy-backed into an existing IV line (which can increase the risk of contamination). Peripheral IV access must be sufficient to maintain an adequate flow rate for the transfusion. Straight-type blood administration sets contain a standard filter in the tubing and are adequate for the administration of most blood products (Fig. A-4). Y type blood/solution administration sets contain a standard filter in the tubing with a Y-tubing above the filter to permit a dual connection for a blood component (e.g., red blood cells) and saline.

IV INFUSION DEVICES

IV infusion devices maintain a more accurate flow rate when providing fluid and medication therapy than the more common gravity systems. Many IV infusion devices are available, and all require familiarity with the operating instructions for the specific device (Fig. A-5). Most models can be operated by battery as well as electric current. They incorporate warnings and alarms of low or high occlusion pressure, air in tubing, infusion complete, and low battery. All infusion devices require frequent monitoring to ensure that they are accurately calibrated. During the infusion, a periodic assessment should include ensuring the flow rate corresponds to the rate displayed on the IV infusion device, and that the infusion site is patent. If any problems occur during IV therapy, the paramedic should check all alarms

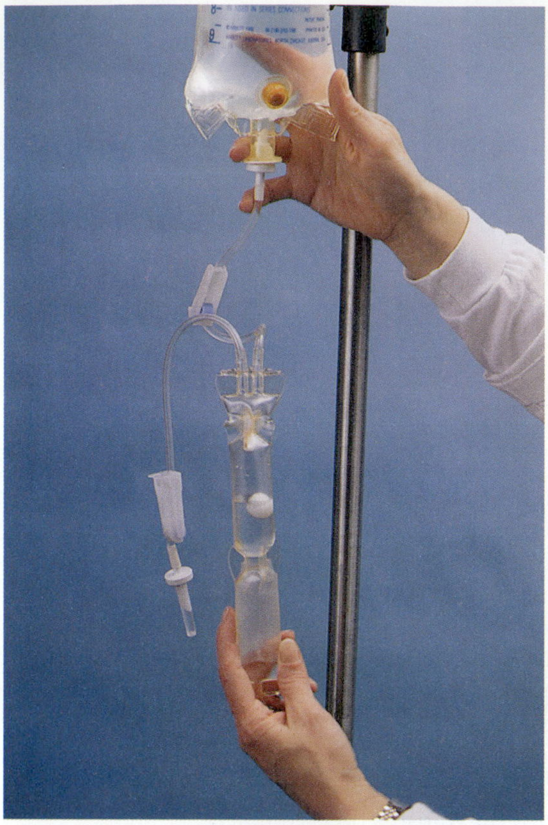

FIGURE A-4 ■ Blood administration set primed with normal saline.

(per the manufacturer's instructions), stop the IV infusion if necessary, and contact medical direction.

TUBE THORACOSTOMY

As described in Chapter 26, chest wall injury can result in pneumothorax, hemothorax, or hemopneumothorax. These conditions can be life threatening and may need to be managed with pleural decompression. Pleural decompression can be achieved though needle thoracostomy (described in Chapter 26) or through tube thoracostomy.

Tube thoracostomy involves the insertion of a catheter ("chest tube") through the chest wall. The tube is usually secured to the chest wall with sutures, and is attached to suction to help with drainage. It remains in place until all or most of the air or fluid has been drained from the pleural space (usually a few days). Tube thoracostomy also is helpful in collecting infected fluid (e.g., pus) that has accumulated in the pleural space from bacterial infection or tuberculosis.

PERICARDIOCENTESIS

Pericardiocentesis is an invasive procedure in which a needle is inserted in the pericardial sac to aspirate blood or fluid. The primary indication for pericardiocentesis is pericardial tamponade. Pericardiocentesis carries significant risk, including penetration of the inferior surface of the heart. Other complications include laceration of a coronary artery, laceration of the lung or liver, cardiac dysrhythmias, and increased tamponade.

A

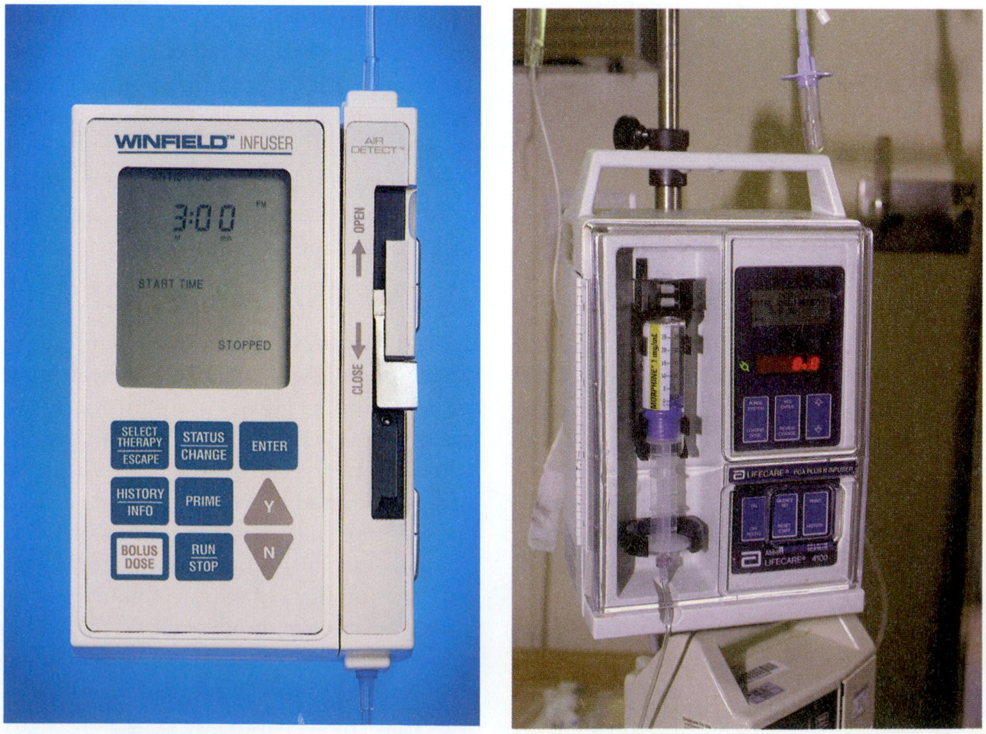

B

FIGURE A-5 ■ A, Electronic infusion device. B, Ambulatory infusion pump.

SUGGESTED READINGS

Dalton A et al: *Advanced medical life support: a practical approach to adult medical emergencies,* 1999, Brady/Prentice Hall.

Daly E, Schroeder J: *Techniques in bedside hemodynamic monitoring,* ed 5, St Louis, 1994, Mosby.

Darovic G: *Hemodynamic monitoring: invasive and noninvasive clinical application,* ed 3, Philadelphia, 2002, WB Saunders.

Holleran R, editor: *Air and surface care transport: principles and practice,* ed 3, St Louis, 2003, Mosby.

Marx J, editor: *Rosen's emergency medicine: concepts and clinical practice,* ed 5, St Louis, 2002, Mosby.

Sole M et al: *Introduction to critical care nursing,* ed 3, Philadelphia, 2001, WB Saunders.

ILLUSTRATION CREDITS

Chapter 1

Chapter opener photo. Courtesy Ray Kemp.

Fig. 1-1, 1-2. National Highway Traffic Safety Administration, US Department of Transportation: Emergency medical services: *NHTSA leading the way*, Washington, DC, 1995, The Administration; accessed at www.nhtsa.dot.gov/people/injury/ems/ agenda/ emsman.html#SERVICES.

Fig. 1-3. US Department of Health and Human Services, Health Resources and Services Administration, Maternal and Child Health Bureau: *Emergency medical services agenda for the future*, Washington, DC, 1999, The Administration.

Chapter 3

Chapter opener photo. Courtesy Kim McKenna.

Fig. 3-1 From National Safety Council: *Injury facts*, Itasca, Ill, 2002, The Council.

Chapter 4

Fig. 4-2 Courtesy Missouri Department of Health, Bureau of Emergency Medical Services, Jefferson City, Mo.

Chapter 5

Fig. 5-1 Modified from Iserson KV: *An approach to ethical problems in emergency medicine*, Baltimore, 1986, Williams and Wilkins.

Chapter 6

Fig. 6-2, 6-5, 6-7, 6-13, 6-33, 6-35, 6-38, 6-40, 6-50, 6-52, 6-53, 6-56, 6-66. Thibodeau, GA: *Anatomy and physiology*, ed 5, St Louis, 2003, Mosby.

Fig. 6-61. Seidel HM et al: *Mosby's guide to physical examination,* ed 5, St Louis, 2003, Mosby.

Fig. 6-6, 6-28, 6-30, 6-31, 6-32, 6-34, 6-37, 6-42, 6-49, 6-59, 6-60, 6-62,6-63, 6-64. Thibodeau GA: *Structure and function of the body,* ed 9, St Louis, 1992, Mosby.

Fig. 6-36, 6-45, 6-46, 6-54, 6-55, 6-65. McCance, KL, Huether, SE: *Pathophysiology: the biologic basis for disease in adults and children,* ed 4, St. Louis, 2003, Mosby.

Chapter 7

Chapter opener photo. Courtesy Kim McKenna.

Fig. 7-11-7-15, 7-25. McCance, KL, Huether, SE: *Pathophysiology: the biologic basis for disease in adults and children,* ed 4, St. Louis, 2003, Mosby.

Fig. 7-15 Lewis SM et al: *Medical-surgical nursing: assessment and management of clinical problems,* ed 5, St Louis, 2000, Mosby.

Fig. 7-16 Baron EJ, Peterson, LR, Finegold SM: *Bailey and Scott's diagnostic microbiology*, ed 9, St Louis, 1994, Mosby.

Fig. 7-17 US Department of Health Education and Welfare; Public Health Service, Centers for Disease Control, Atlanta, Georgia.

Fig. 7-21 Carr JH, Rodak BF: *Clinical hematology atlas*, ed 2, Philadelphia, 2005, WB Saunders.

Fig. 7-22 Redrawn from Crowley L: *Introduction to human disease*, ed 3, Boston, 1992, Jones and Bartlett.

Chapter 9

Chapter opener photo. Courtesy Ray Kemp.

Chapter 10

Chapter opener photo. Courtesy Ray Kemp.

Chapter 11

Fig. 11-8, 11-12 to 11-14, 11-19, 11-20, 11-23 to 11-26, 11-28, 11-31. Seidel HM et al: *Mosby's guide to physical examination,* ed 5, St Louis, 2003, Mosby.

Fig. 11-9. Developed by the National Center for Health Statistics in collaboration with the National Center for Chronic Disease Prevention and Health Promotion (2000).

Fig. 11-16. Potter PA, Perry AG: *Fundamentals of nursing: concepts, process, and practice,* ed 3, St Louis, 1993, Mosby.

Fig. 11-38. Snell RS, Smith MS: *Clinical anatomy for emergency medicine,* St Louis, 1993, Mosby.

Chapter 12

Chapter opener photo. Courtesy Ray Kemp.

Chapter 14

Chapter opener photo. Courtesy Ray Kemp.

Chapter 15

Chapter opener photo. Courtesy Ray Kemp.

Chapter 16

Fig. 16-3 Courtesy of Grande Prairie Regional EMS.

Chapter 17

Chapter opener photo. Courtesy Ray Kemp.

Chapter 18

Chapter opener photo. Courtesy Ray Kemp.

Chapter 19

Chapter opener photo. Courtesy Ray Kemp.

Fig. 19-1, 19-3, 19-4, 19-8, 19-12 to 19-18. Thibodeau GA, Patton KT: *Anatomy and physiology*, ed 5, St. Louis, 2003, Mosby.

Fig. 19-5. Seidel H: *Mosby's guide to physical examination*, ed 2, St Louis, 1991, Mosby.

Fig. 19-6. Seely R: *Anatomy and physiology*, ed 2, St Louis, 1992, Mosby.

Fig. 19-9. Wilson S: *Respiratory disorders*, St Louis, 1990, Mosby.

Fig. 19-19, 19-21. McCance, KL, Huether, SE: *Pathophysiology: the biologic basis for disease in adults and children*, ed 4, St. Louis, 2003, Mosby.

Fig. 19-20. Hockenberry MJ, Wilson D, Winkelstein M, et al. *Wong's nursing care of infants and children*, St Louis, 1999, Mosby.

Fig. 19-74, 19-78. Shade B: *Mosby's EMT-intermediate textbook*, St Louis, 1997, Mosby.

Chapter 20

Chapter opener photo. Courtesy Ray Kemp.

Fig. 20-1. *National Safety Council Accident Facts*, 1997 edition, p. v, National Safety Council, United States, 1996.

Fig. 20-2 to 20-4, 20-6, 20-8 to 20-11. NAEMT: *PHTLS basic and advanced prehospital trauma life support*, St Louis, 2003, Mosby.

Fig. 20-14. Moylan J: *Principles of trauma surgery*, ed 2, New York, 1992, Gower Medical Publishing.

Fig. 20-15. London PS: *A colour atlas of diagnosis after recent injury*, Ipswich, England, 1990, Wolfe Medical Publications.

Chapter 21

Chapter opener photo. Courtesy Ray Kemp.

Fig. 21-2. Adapted from Hardaway R, editor: *Shock: the reversible stage of dying*, Littleton, Mass, 1988, PSG Publishing.

Fig. 21-6. Courtesy Jobst Institute, Inc., Toledo, Ohio

Chapter 22

Fig. 22-2, 22-3. Thibodeau GA, Patton KT: *Structure and function of the body*, ed 9, St Louis, 1992, Mosby.

Figs. 22-4 to 22-14. London PS: *A colour atlas of diagnosis after recent injury*, Ipswich, England, 1990, Wolfe Medical Publications, Ltd.

Fig. 22-16 Beattie T et al: *Pediatric emergencies*, London, 1997, Mosby-Wolfe.

Fig. 22-20 doCarmo P: *Basic EMT skills and equipment*, St Louis, 1988, Mosby.

Chapter 23

Fig. 23-3, 23-4, 23-5. St John's Mercy Medical Center, St Louis, Mo.

Fig. 23-6. Rosen P, Barkin R: *Emergency medicine: concepts and clinical practice,* ed 4, St Louis, 1998, Mosby.

Fig. 23-7. Lee G: *Flight nursing: principles and practice,* St Louis, 1991, Mosby.

Fig. 23-11. Beattie TF, Hendry GM, Duguid KP: *Pediatric emergencies,* London, 1997, Mosby-Wolfe.

Fig. 23-14. Michael Graham, MD.

Chapter 24

Fig. 24-1, 24-2, 24-4, 24-6, 24-10, 24-12, 24-14, 24-16. London PS: A *colour atlas of diagnosis after recent injury,* Ipswich, England, 1990, Wolfe Medical Publications, Ltd.

Figs. 24-3, 24-19. Sheehy S: *Emergency nursing,* ed 3, St. Louis, 1992, Mosby.

Figs. 24-5, 24-7, 24-8. Ragge N: *Immediate eye care,* London, 1990, Wolfe Medical Publications, Ltd.

Fig. 24-9 Thibodeau GA, Patton KT: *Structure and function of the body,* ed 9, St. Louis, 1992, Mosby.

Fig. 24-11. Moore EE: *Early care of the injured patient,* ed 4, Philadelphia, 1990, Decker.

Fig. 24-15, 24-17, 24-21 to 24-23. Ferrera, Colucciella, Marx, et al: *Trauma management: an emergency medicine approach*, St. Louis, 2001, Mosby.

Chapter 25

Chapter opener photo. Courtesy Ray Kemp.

Fig. 25-1, 25-15 From National Association of Emergency Medical Technicians: *PHTLS: basic and advanced prehospital life support,* ed 5, St Louis, 2003, Mosby.

Fig. 25-2, 25-4, 25-5. Rosen P, Barkin R: *Emergency medicine: concepts and clinical practice*, ed 4, St Louis, 1998, Mosby.

Fig. 25-3. From Moore EE, editor: *Early care of the injured patient,* ed 4, Philadelphia, 1990, BC Decker.

Fig. 25-6. Courtesy Gary Quick, M.D.

Chapter 26

Fig. 26-1, 26-2, 26-4, 26-11. London PS: *A colour atlas of diagnosis after recent injury,* Ipswich, England, 1990, Wolfe Medical Publications, Ltd.

Fig. 26-13. NAEMT: *PHTLS: Basic and advanced prehospital life support*, ed 5, St. Louis, 2003, Mosby.

Chapter 27

Chapter opener photo. Courtesy Ray Kemp.

Fig. 27-3 to 27-6 London PS: *A colour atlas of diagnosis after recent injury,* Ipswich, England, 1990, Wolfe Medical Publications, Ltd.

Chapter 28

Fig. 28-1 McKinney, ES et al: *Maternal-child nursing,* Philadelphia, 2000, WB Saunders.

Fig. 28-2, 28-4, 28-20 C, E, Fig. 28-21, Fig. 28-22, Fig. 28-24, Fig. 28-26, Fig. 28-28, Fig. 28-30. Ferrera PC, Colucciello SA, Marx JA, et al: *Trauma management—an emergency medicine approach*, St. Louis, 2001, Mosby.

Fig. 28-3, 28-5, 28-6, 28-12. Ferguson DG and Fodden DI: *Accident and emergency medicine*, 1998, Churchill Livingstone.

Fig. 28-7 Lewis SM, Collier IC, Heitkemper MM: *Medical-surgical nursing: assessment and management of clinical problems*, ed 4, St. Louis, 1996, Mosby.

Fig. 28-8 NAEMT: *PHTLS basic and advanced prehospital trauma life support*, ed 5, St. Louis, 2003, Mosby.

Fig. 28-12 C-H, Fig. 28-20 A-B, D, F. London PS: *A colour atlas of diagnosis after recent injury*, Ipswich, England, 1990, Wolfe Medical Publications, Ltd.

Chapter 29

Fig. 29-2. Thibideau GA: *Structure and function of the human body*, ed 9, St. Louis, 1992, Mosby.

Fig. 29-3, 29-9 Thibodeau GA, Patton KT: *Anatomy and physiology*, ed 2, St Louis, 1993, Mosby.

Fig. 29-15, 29-16, 29-23—29-26, 29-90, 29-98, 29-102 Grauer K: *Practical guide to ECG interpretation*, St. Louis, 1992, Mosby.

Fig. 29-17 Goldberger A: *Treatment of cardiac emergencies*, ed 5, St Louis, 1990, Mosby.

Fig. 29-18 American College of Emergency Physicians: *Paramedic field care: a complaint-based approach*, St Louis, 1997, Mosby.

Fig. 29-19, 29-20 Phalen T: *The 12-lead ECG in acute myocardial infarction*, St Louis, 1996, Mosby.

Fig. 29-22, 29-27—29-38, 29-60, 29-62—29-64, 29-78, 29-85, 29-86, 29-89. Huszar R: *Basic dysrhythmias*, ed 3, St Louis, 2002, Mosby.

Fig. 29-52, 29-67, 29-69, 29-99, 29-104, 29-105. Aehlert B: *ACLS quick review study guide*, ed 2, St Louis, 2002, Mosby.

Fig. 29-41, 29-47, 29-49, 29-58, 29-68, 29-70, 29-7, 29-80. Reproduced with permission. Guidelines 2000 for Cardiopulmonary Resuscitation and Emergency Cardiovascular Care. Copyright 2003, Copyright American Heart Association

Fig. 29-61. Atwood S: *Introduction to basic cardiac dysrhythmias*, St. Louis, 1990, Mosby.

Fig. 29-73, 29-76. Multi-lead medics, courtesy Bob Page, Springfield, Mo, 1997.

Chapter 30

Fig. 30-1, 30-3, 30-5, 30-10. Modified from Desjardins T, Burton GG: *Clinical manifestations and assessment of respiratory disease*, ed 3, St. Louis.

Figs. 30-2, 30-4, 30-7, 30-9. Wilson SF: *Respiratory disorders*, St Louis, 1990, Mosby.

Chapter 31

Chapter opener photo. Courtesy Ray Kemp.

Fig. 31-2, 31-3, 31-4, 31-5. Thibodeau GA: *Structure and function of the body*, ed 9, St Louis, 1992, Mosby.

Fig. 31-6. Modified from Thibodeau GA, Patton KI: *Anatomy and physiology*, ed 4, St. Louis, 1999, Mosby.

Fig. 31-1, 31-11. McSwain N: *The basic EMT: comprehensive prehospital patient care*, St Louis, 1996, Mosby.

Fig. 31-9. Patton KT, Thibodeau GA. *Mosby's handbook of anatomy & physiology*, St. Louis, 2000, Mosby.

Fig. 31-12. A London: *A colour atlas of diagnosis after recent injury*, Ipswich, England, 1990, Wolfe Medical Publications, Ltd. B courtesy Gary Quick, M.D.

Fig. 31-13.Guidelines 2000 for Cardiopulmonary Resuscitation and Emergency Cardiovascular Care. *Circulation, Volume 102, No 8*, Aug. 22, 2000. Copyright © American Heart Association.

Figs. 31-11, 31-14, 31-16. McCance KL, Huether SE: *Pathophysiology: the biologic basis for disease in adults and children*, ed 3, St Louis, 1998, Mosby.

Chapter 32

Chapter opener photo. Courtesy Ray Kemp.

Fig. 32-4. Thibodeau GA Patton KT: *Anatomy and physiology*, ed 5, St Louis, 2003, Mosby.

Fig. 32-9, 32-11, 32-14, 32-15. Epstein O, Perkin GD, Cookson J, et al: *Clinical examination*, ed 3, St Louis, 2003, Mosby.

Fig. 32-13 Lewis SM, Collier IC, Heitkemper MM: *Medical-surgical nursing: assessment and management of clinical problems*, ed 4, St Louis, 1996, Mosby.

Chapter 33

Fig. 33-1. Thibodeau GA, Patton KT: *Anatomy and physiology* ed 5, St Louis, 2003, Mosby.

Fig. 33-2. McCance KL, Huether SE: *Pathophysiology: the biologic basis for disease in adults and children*, ed 3, St Louis, 1998, Mosby.

Fig. 33-6. Courtesy Gary Quick.

Chapter 34

Fig. 34-1. Thibodeau G: *Structure and function of the body*, ed. 9, St Louis, 1992, Mosby.

Fig. 34-3. Epstein O, Perkin GD, Cookson J, et al: *Clinical examination*, ed 3, St Louis, 2003, Mosby.

Fig. 34-4. Modified from Stevens A, Lowe J: *Pathology*, London, 1995, Mosby.

Fig. 34-5. From Gitlin N, Strauss RM. *Atlas of clinical hepatology*, Philadelphia, 1995, WB Saunders.

Chapter 35

Fig. 35-3 Ferguson DG and Fodden DI: *Accident and emergency medicine*, 1998, Churchill Livingstone.

Chapter 36

Figs. 36-1, 36-5, 36-6. Courtesy Saint Louis Zoo, St Louis, Mo.

Figs. 36-2, 36-3, 36-4. Auerbach PS: *Management of wilderness and environmental emergencies*, ed 2, St Louis, 1989, Mosby.

Figs. 36-7, 36-8, 36-9. From Auerbach PS: *A medical guide to hazardous marine life*, ed 2, St Louis, 1991, Mosby.

Chapter 37

Fig. 37-2. McCance, KL, Huether, SE: *Pathophysiology: the biologic basis for disease in adults and children,* ed 4, St. Louis, 2003, Mosby.

Fig. 37-4-37-6. McKinney ES et al: *Maternal-child nursing,* Philadelphia, 2003, Saunders.

Fig. 37-8. Ferguson DG, Fodden DI: *Accident and emergency medicine: colour guide,* ed 2, Philadelphia, 1998, Churchill Livingstone.

Chapter 38

Fig. 38-1. McSwain N, Paturas J: *The basic EMT: comprehensive prehospital patient care*, ed 2, St. Louis, 2001, Mosby.

Fig. 38-2. Huszar R: *Basic dysrhythmias*, ed 3, St Louis, 2002, Mosby.

Fig. 38-3. Reproduced with permission, Guidelines 2000 for Cardiopulmonary Resuscitation and Emergency Cardiovascular Care, © 2003, Copyright American Medical Association.

Figs. 38-4-38-7. Auerbach PS: *Management of wilderness and environmental emergencies*, ed 4, St Louis, 2001, Mosby.

Chapter 39

Fig. 39-2—39-4. Grimes D: *Infectious diseases,* St Louis, 1991, Mosby.

Fig. 39-6, 39-10, 39-11, 39-12. Courtesy The Centers for Disease Control, 1990. In Grimes D: *Infectious diseases,* St Louis, 1991, Mosby.

Fig. 39-8, 39-16. Lissauer T, Clayden G. *Illustrated textbook of pediatrics,* ed 2, St. Louis, 2001, Mosby.

Fig. 39-9. London PS: *A colour atlas of diagnosis after recent injury,* Ipswich, England, 1990, Wolfe Medical Publications, Ltd.

Fig. 39-13. Courtesy Gary Quick, M.D.

Fig. 39-14, 39-17. Epstein, Perkin, Cookson & de Bono: *Clinical examination,* ed 3, St. Louis, 2003, Mosby.

Chapter 41

Fig. 41-2, 41-3. Thibodeau G: *Structure and function of the body*, ed 11, St Louis, 2000, Mosby.

Chapter 42

Fig. 42-1, Thibodeau, G, Patton, K *Anatomy and physiology,* ed 5, 2003, Mosby.

Fig. 42-2. McKinney ES Ashwill JW, et al: *Maternal-child nursing*, 2000, WB. Saunders.

Fig. 42-3. Thibodeau G: *Structure and function of the body,* ed 9, St Louis, 1992, Mosby.

Fig. 42-4, 42-5. Seidel HM et al: *Mosby's guide to physical examination,* ed 2, St Louis, 1991, Mosby.

Fig. 42-10, 42-11. Al-Azzawi F: *Color atlas of childbirth and* obstetric techniques, London, 1990, Wolfe.

Chapter 43

Fig. 43-1, 43-2. Lissauer T, Clayden G. *Illustrated textbook of pediatrics,* ed 2, St. Louis, 2001, Mosby.

Fig. 43-5. Reproduced with permission. CPR issue of JAMA, Oct 28, 1992. Copyright American Medical Association.

Fig. 43-8. Courtesy Nellcor Puritan Bennett, Minneapolis, Minnesota.

Chapter 44

Chapter opener photo. Courtesy Ray Kemp.

Fig. 44-2. Modified with permission from Silverman, W., Andersen, D. [1956]. A cold clinical trial of effects of water mist on obstructive respiratory signs, death rate, and necropsy findings among premature infants. *Pediatrics*, 17(4), 1-9.

Fig. 44-3. McKinney ES: *Maternal-child nursing,* ed 2, St. Louis, 2005, Mosby.

Fig. 44-4, 44-6, 44-13, 44-22, 44-23. Lissauer T, Clayden G: *Illustrated textbook of pediatrics*, ed 2, St. Louis, 2001, Mosby.

Fig. 44-5. Zitelli BJ, Davis HW: *Atlas of pediatric physical diagnosis,* ed 3, St Louis, 1997, Mosby-Wolfe.

Fig. 44-7, 44-14. Beattie T: *Pediatric emergencies,* London, 1997, Mosby-Wolfe.

Fig. 44-9, 44-10, 44-11, 44-12. Reproduced with permission. Guidelines 2000 for Cardiopulmonary Resuscitation and Emergency Cardiovascular Care. C, 2003. Copyright American Heart Association.

Fig. 44-15. Wong D, Baker C: *Pain in children: comparison of assessment scales, Pediatr Nurs* 14(1): 9-17, 1988.

Fig. 44-16. Courtesy Gary Quick, MD.

Fig. 44-18. Courtesy Puritan-Bennett LP6 from Mallinckrodt, St Louis, Mo.

Chapter 45

Chapter opener photo. Courtesy Ray Kemp.

Fig. 45-1, 45-3. Epstein O, Perkin DG, Cookson J, et al: *Clinical examination*, ed 3, St. Louis, 2003, Mosby.

Fig. 45-2. Potter PA, Perry AG: *Fundamentals of nursing,* ed 4, St Louis, 1997, Mosby.

Fig. 45-4. Black, Hawks, and Keene/Courtesy Ophthalmic Photography, University of Michigan W.K. Kellogg Eye Center, Ann Arbor, Mich.

Fig. 45-5 From Stein HA, Slatt BJ, Stein RM: *The ophthalmic assistant: fundamentals in clinical practice*, St. Louis, 1988, Mosby.

Chapter 46

Fig. 46-2, 46-3, 46-4. London PS: *A colour atlas of diagnosis after recent injury,* Ipswich, England, 1990, Wolfe Medical Publications, Ltd.

Fig. 46-5 Beattie T: *Color atlas of pediatric emergencies,* St. Louis, 1997, Mosby.

Fig. 46-6 Ferguson DG, Fodden, DI: *Accident and emergency medicine*, 1998, Churchill Livingstone.

Fig. 46-7, 46-8 Lissauer T, Clayden G: *Illustrated textbook of pediatrics*, ed 2, St. Louis, 2001, Mosby.

Chapter 47

Fig. 47-1. From Mubarak SJ, et al: *J Pediatr Orthop* 9:612, 1989.

Fig. 47-2. McCance KL, Huether SE: *Pathophysiology: the biologic basis for disease in adults and children,* ed 3, 1998, Mosby. Courtesy Drs. A. Olney and M. MacDonald, University of Nebraska Medical Center, Omaha, Neb.

Fig. 47-3, 47-5. Epstein O, Perkin GD, Cookson J, et al: *Clinical examination,* ed 3. St.Louis, 2003, Mosby.

Fig. 47-4. From Wong DL: *Nursing care of infants and children*, ed 5, St Louis, 1994, Mosby.

Chapter 48

Fig. 48-1. Wilkins, RL, Stoller JK, Scanlan CL: *Egan's fundamentals of respiratory care*, ed 8, St. Louis, 2003, Mosby.

Chapter 49

Chapter opener photo. Courtesy Ray Kemp.

Fig. 49-4, 49-5 Courtesy Air Rescue Consortium of Hospitals, St Louis, Mo.

Fig. 49-7 American College of Emergency Physicians: *Paramedic field care: a complaint-based approach,* St Louis, 1997, Mosby.

Chapter 50

Chapter opener photo. Courtesy Ray Kemp.

Fig. 50-10 From American College of Emergency Physicians: *Paramedic field care: a complaint-based approach,* St Louis, 1997, Mosby.

Fig. 50-12 Courtesy METTAG Products, Starke, Fla.

Chapter 51

Chapter opener photo. Courtesy Ray Kemp.

Fig. 51-1, 51-4, 51-7. Courtesy Eureka Fire Protection District, Eureka, Mo.

Fig. 51-5. Courtesy Mobil Oil Co.

51-8 From Moore RE: *Vehicle rescue and extrication*, St Louis, 1991, Mosby.

Chapter 52

Fig. 52-3 Courtesy Lisa Taylor-Austin.

Chapter 53

Fig. 53-1. From National Fire Protection Association, Quincy, Mass, 1996.

Fig. 53-2. From Bronstein A: *Mosby's emergency care for hazardous material exposure,* St Louis, 1988, Mosby.

Fig. 53-3, 53-4, 53-8. Courtesy Creve Coeur Fire Protection District, Creve Coeur, Mo.

Fig. 53-6 Redrawn from Noll G et al: *Hazardous materials: managing the incident,* Stillwater, Okla., 1998, Fire Protection Publications.

Chapter 54

Fig. 54-1 to 54-4. Centers for Disease Control and Prevention. http://phil.cdc.gov.

CCT Appendix

Fig. A-2. Darovic GO: *Hemodynamic monitoring, invasive and noninvasive clinical application*, ed 3, Philadelphia, 2003, WB Saunders.

Fig. A-3. Kee JT: *Youman's neurological surgery*, ed 4, Philadelphia, 1996, WB Saunders.

Fig. A-4. Elkin MK, Perry AG, Potter PA: *Nursing interventions and clinical skills*, ed 3, St Louis, 2004, Mosby.

INDEX

A

Abandonment
  definition of, 54
  legal complications with, 64
Abbreviations in documentation, 323b–325b
Abdomen. *See also* Acute abdominal pain
  physical examination of, 262–265, 263f, 264b, 264f, 265f, 279
Abdominal trauma, 644–650, 645b, 645n, 649b, 649f, 656f, 657f, 658b, 658f
  assessment of, 649, 649b, 650
  blunt trauma as, 645, 645b, 650
  hollow organ injury with, 646, 647f, 648b
    colon, 646
    small intestine, 646
    stomach, 646
  management of, 649–650
  mechanisms of, 645–646, 645b
  pelvic organ injury with, 648–649, 649f, 650
    urethra, 649
    urinary bladder, 648
  penetrating trauma as, 645–646, 650
  retroperitoneal organ injury with, 646–648, 648f, 648n, 650
    duodenum, 648
    kidneys, 648
    pancreas, 648
    ureters, 648
  solid organ injury with, 646, 646f, 647f, 650
    hemoperitoneum in, 646
    Kehr sign in, 646
    liver, 646, 647f, 650
    spleen, 646, 646f, 650
  vascular structure injury with, 649, 650
Abrasion
  assessment of, 543, 543f
  definition of, 538
Abruptio placentae
  complications of pregnancy with, 1085, 1085t
Absorption
  drug, 332, 338–341, 339b, 340b, 341b, 343f, 350, 382
Abuse/neglect, 1184–1194
  battering with, 1185–1186, 1185f–1187f, 1186b, 1194
    men in, 1186
    women in, 1186, 1186f, 1187f
  characteristics of persons in, 1186–1188, 1187f
  child, 1116, 1150–1153, 1152f, 1152t, 1158, 1189–1192, 1190b, 1191f, 1192f, 1192n, 1194
  elder, 1160, 1166, 1179–1180, 1180t, 1181, 1188–1189, 1189b, 1189f, 1194
  legal considerations in, 1188, 1191, 1192, 1193
  sexual assault as, 1192–1193, 1193b, 1194
Accelerated junctional rhythm
  cardiology dysrhythmias with, 738, 739f
Acid-base balance in cells, 164–172, 165b, 166f–168f, 170f, 171b, 171f, 172t
  acidosis with, 166–169, 167f, 168f, 170f, 194
  alkalosis with, 169–170, 171f
  buffering systems with, 165, 166f
  imbalance with, 165–166
  mixed disturbances of, 170–172, 171b, 172t
  ph with, 165, 165b, 166f
Acidosis, 150, 166–169, 167f, 168f, 170f
  definition of, 150
  diabetes mellitus with, 872–873
  diabetic ketoacidosis, 169
  lactic, 168–169
  metabolic, 167–168, 168f, 194
  renal failure causing, 169
  respiratory, 167, 167f, 194
  toxins failure causing, 169
Acquired immunodeficiency syndrome (AIDS), 186, 186n, 187b
  public health principles related to, 1006b
Action plan
  assessment-based patient management with, 298, 299–300, 300f
Active transport, 150, 154
Acute abdominal pain
  management of, 897, 897b
  patient assessment for, 893–897, 905
    appendicitis in, 895
    auscultation in, 896
    cholecystitis in, 895
    history in, 893–894
    involuntary guarding in, 895
    pain location/type in, 894–895, 895b
    palpation in, 897
    pancreatitis in, 895
    percussion in, 897
    physical examination for, 896–897, 896f
    rebound tenderness in, 895
    referred pain in, 895, 896f
    signs/symptoms in, 895
    somatic pain in, 895
    visceral pain in, 894–895
    vital signs in, 895
Acute arterial occlusion, 795–797, 796f, 797f, 797n, 811
  management of, 796–797, 797n
  signs/symptoms of, 796
Acute coronary syndromes
  emergency cardiac for drug-induced, 966
Acute deep vein thrombosis, 797–798, 811
Acute gastroenteritis, 898
  definition of, 892
Acute hepatitis, 903, 904b, 905
  definition of, 892
Acute mountain sickness, 1000–1001, 1000b
  definition of, 984
Acute renal failure, 912–913, 913t, 918
  definition of, 908
Addison disease, 880, 880f, 880t, 881
  definition of, 864
Adolescence
  development characteristics of, 204–206, 205b, 205f, 206b, 210
  psychosocial development of, 205–206, 206b
Adrenal medullary mechanism, 179
Adrenergic drugs, 332, 351, 356
Adult respiratory distress syndrome (ARDS)
  management of, 829–830, 829f, 829n
    biphasic positive airway pressure in, 830
    continuous positive airway pressure in, 829–830
    positive end-expiratory pressure in, 829, 829f
  pulmonary emergencies from, 828–830, 829b, 829f, 829n, 834
Advance directives
  legal issues with, 66–68, 67f
Advanced life support (ALS)
  definition of, 2
  funding for, 5
Aeromedical transportation, 1236–1238, 1236b, 1236f, 1237b, 1238f, 1239
  advantages/disadvantages with, 1237b
  crew members/training with, 1236, 1236b
  hazardous terrain rescue helicopter use in, 1272–1273
  landing site preparation with, 1237, 1238f
  patient preparation for, 1238
  safety precautions with, 1237–1238
Affect, 1045
  definition of, 1042
Afferent division
  definition of, 82
Age-related disorders, 191, 192t
Agonist, 332, 337
AIDS. *See* Acquired immunodeficiency syndrome
Airway management
  advanced procedures for, 472–490, 498
    complications from intubation in, 480
    digital intubation as, 480, 480f
    endotracheal intubation as, 473–476, 473f, 474f, 474t, 475f, 476n, 483
    intubation with spinal precautions in, 481, 481n, 483
    laryngeal mask airway as, 486, 488–489, 488n, 489f
    multilumen airway as, 489–490, 490f
    nasotracheal intubation as, 480–481, 481n, 482f
    orotracheal intubation as, 476–480, 476b, 476f, 477f, 478f, 478n, 479f, 479n, 483, 484f
    pediatric considerations in, 483, 485, 485n
  cricothyrotomy in, 494–497, 495f, 496f
    complications possible for, 497
    contraindications for, 497
    description of, 494
    equipment for, 494–496, 495f
    removal of, 497
    technique for, 496, 496f, 496n
  evaluation parameters in, 453–455, 497
    auscultation/palpation techniques with, 453–454, 453n, 454f
    inadequate ventilation with, 454
    observation techniques with, 453
    patient history with, 454
    problem recognition with, 453–454, 453n, 454f
    rate/regularity/effort, 453
    respiratory pattern changes with, 454, 455f, 456b
  manual techniques for, 464–466, 466f, 497
  mechanical adjuncts in, 469–472
    nasopharyngeal airway, 469–471, 470f, 471f
    oropharyngeal airway, 471–472, 472f
  pathophysiology of, 449–453, 449n, 450t, 451n
    airway obstruction as, 449–451, 450t, 451n

Airway management *(Continued)*
aspiration by inhalation in, 452–453, 497
fractured larynx as, 451
laryngeal spasm as, 451
tracheal trauma as, 452
pharmacological adjuncts to, 490–492, 490n, 491f, 492b
paralytic agents in emergency intubation with, 490–491
rapid sequence intubation with, 491–492, 492b
rescue breathing in, 459–461, 460f–463f, 461b, 462b
automatic transport ventilators with, 454, 454f, 454n
bag-valve devices with, 462–463, 462f
infants/children with, 460
mouth-to-mask devices with, 461–462, 461f, 462b, 462f
mouth-to-mouth method of, 459–460
mouth-to-nose method of, 460
mouth-to-stoma method of, 460–461, 460f, 461b
suction in, 466–469
catheters for, 466–467, 467f
devices for, 466, 467f
gastric distention with, 468
gastric tubes with, 468–469, 469f, 470f
tracheobronchial, 467–468, 468f, 468n
supplemental oxygen therapy in, 455–459
oxygen delivery devices with, 457–459, 457f, 457t, 458f, 458t, 459f
oxygen sources with, 455–457, 456b, 456f, 457f
translaryngeal cannula ventilation in, 492–494, 493f, 494f, 494n
advantages/disadvantages to, 494
complications with, 494
description of, 492
equipment for, 492
removal of, 494
technique of, 492–494, 493f, 494f, 494n
ventilation in, 459–464, 461b, 461f, 462b, 462f, 463f
Alcohol, 359–361
Alcoholism, 955–961, 964
acute alcohol intoxication with, 959
alcohol withdrawal syndromes with, 959–960
blood alcohol content with, 956, 956n
cardiac/skeletal muscle myopathy with, 959
cirrhosis with, 958
delirium tremens with, 960
dependence in, 955–956
disulfiram-ethanol reaction with, 960–961
emergencies with, 959–961
ethanol with, 956, 956b
fluid/electrolyte imbalances with, 958
gastrointestinal disorders with, 958–959
gastrointestinal hemorrhage with, 958
immune suppression with, 959
medical consequences with, 956–959, 957t
metabolism with, 956
neurological disorders with, 957, 957t
nutritional deficiencies with, 957–958
pancreatitis with, 958–959
trauma with, 959
Wernicke-Korsakoff syndrome with, 958
withdrawal hallucinations with, 960
withdrawal seizures with, 960
Alkalosis, 169–170, 171f
Allergens, 150, 185
Allergies/anaphylaxis, 882–891
antigen-antibody reaction of, 883, 884f, 885b, 891
Allergies/anaphylaxis *(Continued)*
assessment findings for, 887–888, 887b, 887t, 888f, 888n
cardiovascular effects in, 887
cutaneous effects in, 888, 888f, 888n
gastrointestinal effects in, 887–888
nervous system effects in, 888
respiratory effects in, 887, 887b
causative agents of, 884–885, 885b
drug therapy for, 889, 889b, 889n
eosinophil chemotactic factor of, 886
history of, 888–889
initial assessment for, 888
interventions during, 890
interventions preventing, 889, 889b, 889n
latex caused, 885b
leukotrienes with, 886
pathophysiology of, 885–887, 886b, 886f, 887f
physical examination for, 889
reaction with, 883–884, 883n, 885b, 885f, 886f
localized, 884, 885f
sensitization with, 883
thromboxanes with, 886
All-terrain vehicles
blunt trauma from, 510–511, 518
ALS. *See* Advanced life support
Ambulance
definition of, 1230
Ambulance operations, 1230–1239
aeromedical transportation in, 1236–1238, 1236b, 1236f, 1237b, 1238f, 1239
advantages/disadvantages with, 1237b
crew members/training with, 1236, 1236b
landing site preparation with, 1237, 1238f
patient preparation for, 1238
safety precautions with, 1237–1238
checking in, 1231, 1232b, 1232f, 1239
safe, 1232–1235, 1233b, 1234f, 1235b1239
driving guidelines for, 1233, 1233b
emergency scene parking in, 1234, 1234f
environmental conditions with, 1233
escorts for, 1233
moving patient in, 1234–1235, 1235n
proceeding through intersections in, 1234
warning device use with, 1233–1234
standards for, 1231, 1232f
stationing in, 1231–1232, 1239
American Burn Association
burns classifications with, 563–564, 564b
American Red Cross
EMS history with, 4
Amino acids, 24
Amniotic fluid embolism, 1095, 1096
Amniotic sac
specialized pregnancy structures of, 1074
Amphetamines, 362
Amputation
assessment of, 545, 545f
definition of, 538
special considerations for, 556
Amyotrophic lateral sclerosis, 860, 863
definition of, 836
Analgesics, 358–359, 359b
Anaphylactic shock, 526
management of, 536
Anaphylaxis. *See* Allergies/anaphylaxis
Anatomical dead space, 435
definition of, 430
Anatomical position
definition of, 82
Anatomy, 82–149
anatomical planes in, 84, 86f
body cavities in, 84, 87f
Anatomy *(Continued)*
body regions in, 84, 87f
cell structure, 84–85, 88–90, 88f, 88t
cell classes with, 90
cell functions with, 90
cell reproduction with, 90
cytoplasm in, 85, 88t, 89–90, 89f
cytoplasmic membrane in, 84–85, 88f, 88t
nucleus in, 88t, 90
organ system, 92–144, 93f, 149
cardiovascular system in, 123–128, 124f–127f, 149
circulatory system in, 119–128, 122t, 123t, 124f–127f, 129f, 130f, 149
digestive system in, 135–138, 137f, 149
endocrine system in, 119, 121f, 149
integumentary system in, 92–95, 94f, 149
muscular system in, 104–108, 105f–110f, 108t, 149
nervous system in, 108–119, 111f–118f, 118t, 119t, 120f, 149
reproductive system in, 140–144, 141f, 142f, 143f, 144f, 149
respiratory system in, 128, 131–135, 131f–135f, 149
skeletal system in, 95–104, 96f, 97f, 98f, 99f, 100f, 101f, 102f, 103f, 104b, 104f, 149
urinary system in, 138–140, 139f, 140f, 149
sense organ, 144–149
hearing, 146–148, 148f
olfactory, 144–145, 145f
taste, 145, 146f
visual, 145–146, 147f
terminology for, 83, 84f, 85t
tissue, 90–92
connective, 91–92, 91f
epithelial, 90–91
muscle, 92
Anemia, 972–975, 982
definition of, 970
diagnosis/treatment of, 975, 975n
hemolytic, 974
iron deficiency, 974, 974f
signs/symptoms of, 974–975, 975t
Anesthetics, 359, 359b
Angina pectoris, 778–779, 779b, 779n, 811
conditions mimicking, 779b
management of, 779
stable, 779
unstable, 779
Angiotensin II receptor antagonists, 368
Ankles
injury, 668, 669f
physical examination of, 267–268, 269f
Anorexia nervosa, 1056
Anorexiants, 361, 361n
Ant bites/stings. *See* Arthropod bites/stings
Antacids, 372
Antagonists, 332, 337, 358–359, 359b
Antegrade amnesia, 580, 596
Antepartum, 1100, 1101
Anterior cord syndrome
definition of, 606
spinal trauma with, 612
Anterior neck trauma, 509–593, 590f, 591f, 592n
esophageal injury, 592–593
evaluation of, 590–591, 591f
Anterior neck trauma *(Continued)*
hematomata, 591, 591n
laryngeal/tracheal injury, 592, 592n
soft tissue, 591–593, 591n, 592n
vascular injury, 591–592, 592n
Anthrax, 1306, 1309, 1309b, 1309f, 1310f
Antianxiety drugs, 359–361, 360b

Antibiotics, 378, 384
Anticholinergic agents, 332, 355
Anticoagulants, 368–369
Anticonvulsants, 361, 361b, 383
Antidepressants, 363, 363n
Antidiarrheal drugs, 374
Antiflatulent drugs, 372
Antifungal drugs, 378–379, 379b
Antiglaucoma drugs, 374–375, 384
Antihemophilic agents, 369
Antihemorrheologic agents, 368
Antihistamines, 372
Antihyperlipidemic drugs, 369, 369b
Antihypertensives, 366–368, 383
Antiinflammatory drugs, 380, 384
Antineoplastic disease agents, 377, 377b, 384
Antioxidants, 24b
Antipsychotic agents, 362–363
Antiserotonins, 372
Antiviral drugs, 378–379, 379b, 384
Anxiety
  definition of, 1042, 1043
  mental/emotional health with, 31
Anxiety disorders, 1050–1051, 1051b, 1060
  obsessive-compulsive, 1051, 1051b
  phobia, 1050–1051
  posttraumatic syndrome, 1051, 1051b
Aortic aneurysms, 792–795, 793f, 794b, 794f, 795n, 811
  abdominal, 793–794, 794b, 811
  acute dissecting, 794–795, 794f, 795n, 811
  management of, 793–794, 795
  signs/symptoms of, 795, 795n
Apgar score, 1072, 1089, 1091t, 1096
  definition of, 1072
  neonates assessment with, 1106
Apnea, 1100, 1103
  definition of, 1100
  neonatal life support needed for, 1109, 1114
Apothecary system, 389b, 391
Appendicitis, 895, 900, 905
  definition of, 892
Aquatic life
  poison from, 941–944, 941f, 943f, 963
Arachnida bites/stings, 937–939, 937f, 938f, 939b, 963
ARDS. *See* Adult respiratory distress syndrome
Arthritis
  musculoskeletal trauma with, 657–658, 657f, 671
  special considerations for, 1201–1202, 1202f
Arthropod bites/stings, 935–939, 936b, 937f, 938f, 939b
Aspiration pneumonia, 828
Assault
  definition of, 54
  legal complications with, 64
  paramedic protection from, 57
Assessment-based patient management, 293–294, 298–305
  action plan with, 298, 299–300, 300f
  clinical decision making with, 293–294
  effective assessment with, 299–302
  factors affecting, 300–301
  field impression with, 298, 299–300, 300f
  general approach to patient with, 303
  optional take-in equipment for, 302
  pattern recognition with, 298, 299, 300b, 300f
  presenting the patient in, 298, 303–304, 305
  right stuff for, 302, 302b
Asthma, 822–825, 822n, 823b, 823f–825f, 824n, 825n, 826t, 833
  assessment of, 822–824, 824n
  differential considerations for, 825, 827t
  management of, 824–825, 824b, 824n, 825f, 825n, 826t
Asthma *(Continued)*
  pathophysiology of, 822, 822n, 823f, 824f
  pulmonary function tests for, 824–825, 825f, 825n, 826t
Atelectasis, 441
  definition of, 430
Atherosclerosis, 778, 811
  effects of, 778
  risk factors with, 778
Atrial fibrillation
  cardiology dysrhythmias with, 730–735, 730n, 732f–734f, 734b, 810
  clinical significance of, 731
  description of, 731, 732f
  etiology of, 731
  interpretation rules for, 731, 731n
  management of, 731–735, 733f–734f, 734b
Atrial flutter
  cardiology dysrhythmias with, 729–730, 730f, 730n, 810
  clinical significance of, 731, 731n
  description of, 729, 730f
  etiology of, 729–730
  interpretation rules for, 730–731, 730n
  management of, 731–735, 733f–734f, 734b
Atrioventricular blocks
  cardiac conduction disorder dysrhythmias of, 763–770, 764f–770f, 764n
  first degree, 763, 764f, 768f
  second degree type I (Wenckebach), 763–764, 764n, 765f, 768f
  second degree type II, 765–767, 766f, 767f, 768f
  third degree, 767–770, 767n, 768f, 769f, 770f, 770n
Atrioventricular dissociation
  definition of, 674
Atrioventricular junction dysrhythmias, 735–738, 736f, 737f, 739f
Atrophy, 151, 172
ATV. *See* Automatic transport ventilators
Auscultation
  abdomen, 264
  acute abdominal pain assessment with, 896
  airway evaluation with, 453–454, 453n, 454f
  breath sounds in, 258–261, 259f, 260f, 261f
  chest, 256–261, 259f, 260f, 261f
  heart, 261–262, 262f
  technique of, 234, 235b, 236, 278
Automatic transport ventilators (ATV), 454, 454f, 454n
Automaticity, 674, 685
Autonomic hyperreflexia syndrome, 627, 629
Autonomic nervous system, 117–119, 118f, 118t, 119t, 120f
  pharmacology for, 351–369, 353f, 354f, 355t, 356t, 357b, 358t, 359b
Avoidance, 1276, 1281
Avulsion
  assessment of, 544–545, 545f
  definition of, 538
  special considerations for, 556
Axial loading, 610
  definition of, 606
Azotemia, 908

B

Babinski reflex, 196, 199t
Bacterial pneumonia, 827, 833
Bacterial tracheitis, 1116
Bag-valve devices, 462–463, 462f
Balance, 146–148, 148f
Ballistics
  considerations for specific injuries in, 516–517
    abdominal injuries in, 517
    extremity injuries in, 517
Ballistics *(Continued)*
    head in, 517
    thoracic injuries in, 517
  entrance/exit wounds in, 516, 516f, 517b
  medium/high-energy projectile wounding in, 515–516, 515f, 516n
  penetrating trauma in, 514–517, 514f, 515f, 516f, 517b
  projectile damage/energy levels in, 514, 514f
  shotgun wounds in, 516
  soft body armor and, 514–515
Barbiturates, 360–361
Bariatrics, 1196
Baroreceptor reflexes, 177, 177b, 178f
Barotrauma, 997–1000, 998b, 998n, 999b, 999f, 1000n, 1002
Basic life support, 2
Basilar skull fractures, 593–594, 594f, 594n, 595f
Battering, 1185–1186, 1185f–1187f, 1186b, 1194
  definition of, 1184
  men in, 1186
  women in, 1186, 1186f, 1187f
Battery
  definition of, 54
  legal complications with, 64
  paramedic protection from, 57
Battle's sign
  definition of, 580
  skull fractures with, 594, 595f
Beck triad
  definition of, 630
Bee bites/stings. *See* Arthropod bites/stings
Behavioral emergency, 1042, 1043
  definition of, 1042
Behavioral/psychiatric disorders, 1043–1061
  anxiety disorders as, 1050–1051, 1051b, 1060
    obsessive-compulsive, 1051, 1051b
    phobia, 1050–1051
    posttraumatic syndrome, 1051, 1051b
  assessment/management of, 1045–1048
    assessment in, 1045–1046, 1047t
    interview techniques with, 1046–1047, 1048b, 1060
    mental status examination with, 1046
    other patient care measures with, 1047
  classes of, 1048n
  cognitive disorders as, 1048–1049, 1049b, 1060
    delirium, 1048–1049
    dementia, 1049, 1049b
  dissociative disorders as, 1055–1056, 1060
  eating disorders as, 1056, 1056b, 1060
    anorexia nervosa, 1056
    bulimia nervosa, 1056
  emergencies with, 1042–1045, 1044b, 1045f, 1060
    biological causes for, 1042–1043, 1046b
    psychosocial causes for, 1043
    sociocultural causes for, 1043
  factitious disorders as, 1055, 1060
  impulse control disorders as, 1056, 1060
  mood disorders as, 1051–1054
    bipolar, 1052–1053, 1052f, 1053b, 1060
    depression, 1052, 1052b, 1060
    suicide/suicide threats with, 1053–1054, 1053b, 1060–1061
  personality disorders as, 1056–1057, 1060
  schizophrenia as, 1049–1050, 1049b, 1050b, 1060
    delusions with, 1049, 1050b

Behavioral/psychiatric disorders *(Continued)*
dyskinesia with, 1049
paranoia with, 1049, 1050b
somatoform disorders as, 1054–1055, 1055b, 1060
conversion, 1055, 1055b
somatization, 1055, 1055b
special patient consideration with, 1057–1060, 1059f
chemical restraint in, 1059–1060
elderly patients in, 1057
personal safety in, 1059, 1061
problem children in, 1057, 1061
restraints for, 1058–1060, 1059f, 1061
violent patients in, 1057–1060, 1057n, 1061
substance-related disorders as, 1054
dual diagnosis with, 1045b, 1054
Bell palsy, 860, 860f, 863
definition of, 836
Benzodiazepines, 360
Bioethics, 72, 73
Bioterrorism, 1306–1320
biological weapons as, 1307–1312
anthrax, 1309–1310, 1309b, 1310f
botulism, 1309b, 1310, 1310f
critical agents of, 1308, 1308b
dissemination methods in, 1308–1309
history of, 1307–1308, 1307n
plague, 1309b, 1310–1311
ricin, 1309b, 1311
smallpox, 1309b, 1311–1312, 1311f
tularemia, 1309b, 1312
definition of, 1306
Department of Homeland Security for, 1316–1317
emergency response guidelines for, 1317
explosive threats as, 1315–1316
incendiary threats as, 1313
nuclear/radiological threats as, 1312–1313, 1312n
personal protective equipment for, 1319–1320
specific chemical threats as, 1313–1315, 1314b
nerve agents, 1313–1314
VX, 1314–1315
Biotransformation
drug, 332, 342, 343f, 344f, 345b, 350
BiPAP. *See* Biphasic positive airway pressure
Biphasic positive airway pressure (BiPAP), 830
Bipolar mood disorders, 1052–1053, 1052f, 1053b, 1060
Bites
assessment of, 545–546, 545f, 546n
Blast injuries
blunt trauma from, 512–513, 512f, 518
soft tissue trauma from, 547, 547f
Blind intubation, 480, 480f
Blood group antigens, 184–185, 185f
Blood pressure cuff, 238, 238f
Blood sample
obtaining, 423–424, 424t, 426
Blunt trauma, 500, 504–513, 518
abdominal trauma as, 645, 645b, 650
all-terrain vehicles with, 510–511, 518
blast injuries, 512–513, 512f, 518
compression injuries as, 509–510, 509f
abdominal, 510
head, 509
thoracic, 509–510, 509f
deceleration injuries as, 508–510, 508f, 518
abdominal, 508–509, 509f
head, 508, 508f
thoracic, 508, 509f
definition of, 500
motor vehicle collision, 505–506, 505f
Blunt trauma *(Continued)*
head-on impact, 505–506, 505f
lateral impact, 506
rear-end impact, 506
rollover accidents in, 506
rotational impact, 506
motorcycle collision, 510, 510f, 511f, 518
organ collision injuries as, 508–510, 508f, 509f, 518
pedestrian injuries, 511, 518
restraints preventing, 506–508, 507f, 508b, 518
air bags as, 507
child safety seats as, 507–508, 508b
diagonal shoulder straps as, 507
lap belts as, 507, 507f
sports injuries, 511–512, 518
vertical falls with, 513
BMI. *See* Body mass index
B-NICE
definition of, 1306
Body mass index (BMI), 27, 27b
Bone marrow transplant
leukemia treated with, 976, 977b
Borrowed servants, 60
Botulism, 930
biological weapons of, 1309b, 1310, 1310f
definition of, 920
Bowel obstruction, 901, 901b, 901n, 905
definition of, 892
Bradycardia. *See also* Sinus bradycardia
emergency cardiac for drug-induced, 966
neonatal life support needed for, 1109–1110, 1114
Bradydysrhythmias
pediatric, 1135, 1136f
Brain abscess, 857–858, 857n, 858f, 862
Brain death criteria, 69b
Brain neoplasm, 857–858, 857n, 858f, 862
Brain trauma. *See* Head/facial trauma
Breach of duty, 59
Breech presentation
delivery complications with, 1092–1093, 1092f
Bronchiectasis, 820
definition of, 816
Bronchiolitis
pediatric, 1130, 1130t, 1157
Bronchitis
chronic, 820, 820f, 821t, 833
Bronchodilators, 370–371, 370b, 383
Bronchopulmonary dysplasia
definition of, 1210
Brown-Séquard syndrome
definition of, 606
Spinal trauma with, 612–613
Buccal drugs, 420
Buffering systems, 165, 166f
Bulb/syringe esophageal detector, 486, 488f
Bulimia nervosa, 1056
Bundle of Kent
definition of, 674
Wolff-Parkinson-White syndromes with, 775
Burns, 558–578
chemical injury with, 570–573, 571f, 572f, 578
alkali metals, 572
ammonia, 572
antidotes/neutralizing agents for, 571
assessment of, 571
eyes in, 571, 572f
hydrofluoric acid, 572
management of, 571
petroleum, 572
phenol, 572
classifications of, 561–565, 562f, 563f, 564b, 564f, 578
Burns, 558–578 *(Continued)*
American Burn Association in, 563–564, 564b
burn center referral criteria in, 565
depth in, 561–562, 562f, 563f
full-thickness burns in, 562, 563f
Lund and Browder chart in, 563, 564f
partial-thickness burns in, 562, 562f
rule of nines in, 563, 563f, 563n
severity in, 563–564, 563f, 564b, 564f
superficial burns in, 561–562, 562f
electrical injury with, 573–576, 573b, 574f, 575n, 576f, 578
assessment of, 574–575
effects of, 573–574
lightning injury as, 575–576, 576f, 576n
management of, 574–575
physical examination for, 575
types of, 573, 574f
general management principles for, 567–569, 568n, 578
airway/oxygen/ventilation in, 568
circulation in, 568–569
special considerations in, 569
stopping burning process in, 568, 568n
incidence/patterns of, 559–561, 559b, 561b, 561f
inhalation injury with, 569–570, 569b, 570f
above glottis, 570, 570f
below glottis, 570
carbon monoxide poisoning, 569–570, 569b, 569n
local response to, 560, 561f
pathophysiology of, 565–566, 565n, 566f
consensus formula in, 566
fluid replacement in, 565–566, 565n
patient assessment for, 566–567, 567f
initial, 567, 567f
physical examination in, 567
radiation exposure, 576–578, 577b
decontamination procedures for, 578
emergency care for, 577–578
emergency response for, 577
harmful effects from, 576–577, 577n
personal protection from, 577
types of, 577b
sources of, 559–560
chemical, 560
electrical, 560
radiation, 560
thermal, 559–560
systemic response to, 560–561, 561b
Bursitis
musculoskeletal trauma with, 656, 657f, 671

C

Calcium imbalance, 163–164
Call prioritization
communications with, 315
Cancer
prevention of, 28–29, 29b, 41
special considerations for, 1202, 1202b
Capillaries
definition of, 82
Capillary network anatomy
cell water movement with, 155–157, 157f, 158f
Capitation
definition of, 2
federal health care reform influencing, 6
Carbon monoxide poisoning, 569–570, 569b, 569n
Cardiac arrest
emergency cardiac for drug-induced, 969
EMS research on, 17b
Cardiac cycle, 677–679, 677n, 678f
ventricular systole/diastole in, 677–679

Cardiac ejection fraction, 729
definition of, 674
Cardiac glycosides, 365–366, 383
Cardiac tamponade, 792, 811
Cardiogenic shock, 526, 791–792, 811
management of, 536
Cardiology, 674–812
acute arterial occlusion in, 795–797, 796f, 797f, 797n, 811
management of, 796–797, 797n
signs/symptoms of, 796
acute deep vein thrombosis in, 797–798, 811
anatomy in, 676–677, 677f
angina pectoris in, 778–779, 779b, 779n, 811
conditions mimicking, 779b
management of, 779
stable, 779
unstable, 779
aortic aneurysms in, 792–795, 793f, 794b, 794f, 795n, 811
abdominal, 793–794, 794b, 811
acute dissecting, 794–795, 794f, 795n, 811
management of, 793–794, 795
signs/symptoms of, 795, 795n
atherosclerosis in, 778, 811
effects of, 778
risk factors with, 778
basic life support in, 799–802, 800t–801t, 801f, 802f, 802n, 812
cardiopulmonary resuscitation devices with, 801, 801f
cardiopulmonary resuscitation with, 799, 800t–801t, 801
chest compression circulation physiology with, 799, 800t–801t
monitor-defibrillators with, 801–802, 802n, 812
cardiac tamponade in, 792, 811
cardiogenic shock in, 791–792, 811
conduction disorder dysrhythmias in, 763–777, 764f–777f, 772b, 774t
anterior hemiblock with, 773, 773f
atrioventricular blocks as, 763–770, 764f–770f, 764n
bifascicular hemiblock with, 773
bundle branch anatomy with, 770–771, 771f
bundle branch block management with, 773–774
classifications of, 763
common electrocardiogram findings with, 771–773, 771n, 772b, 772f, 773f
left bundle branch block with, 772–773, 772b, 772f
multilead determination of hemiblock with, 773, 774t
posterior hemiblock with, 773, 774f
preexcitation syndromes with, 775–778, 776f, 777f
pulseless electrical activity with, 774–775, 775f
right bundle branch block with, 771, 772b, 772f
ventricular conduction disturbances as, 770–774, 771f, 772b, 772f, 773f, 774b, 774f
Wolff-Parkinson-White syndromes with, 775–778, 776f, 777f
congestive heart failure in, 787–791, 787b, 788f–790f, 791b
left ventricular failure in, 787–789, 787b, 787n, 788f–790f, 811
right ventricular failure in, 789–791, 791b, 791n, 811
Cardiology *(Continued)*
dysrhythmias, 713–778, 810
accelerated junctional rhythm with, 738, 739f
artificial pacemaker rhythms with, 759–763, 761f, 762b
atria originating, 722–735, 722f, 723f, 725f, 726f, 728f, 729b, 730f, 732f–734f, 734b, 810
atrial fibrillation with, 730–735, 730n, 732f–734f, 734b, 810
atrial flutter with, 729–730, 730f, 730n, 810
atrioventricular junction sustained/originating, 735–738, 736f, 737f, 739f
classifications algorithms for, 713–714
classifications of, 713–714, 713n, 714b
conduction disorder, 763–777, 764f–777f, 772b, 774t
junctional escape complexes/rhythms with, 735, 737f, 738
pacemaker site classifications of, 713
premature atrial complex with, 723–724, 723f, 724n
premature junctional contraction with, 735, 736f
premature ventricle complex with, 742–746, 744f–746f
rate classifications of, 713
R-on-T phenomenon with, 746, 746f
sinoatrial node, 714–722, 715f, 716f, 717b, 718f, 720f, 721f, 810
sinus arrest, 719–722, 721f, 810
sinus bradycardia, 714–717, 715f, 716f, 717b, 810
sinus dysrhythmia, 719–722, 720f, 721f, 810
sinus tachycardia, 718–719, 718f, 810
supraventricular tachycardia with, 724–729, 724n, 725f, 726f, 727n, 728f, 729b, 729n, 810
ventricle escape complexes/rhythms with, 740–742, 740f, 741f
ventricle originating, 738–763, 740f, 741f, 743f–754f, 755b, 756f–761f, 759b, 762b, 810
ventricular asystole with, 757–759, 759f, 760f, 761b
ventricular bigeminy with, 742, 745f
ventricular fibrillation with, 756–757, 757f, 757n, 758f, 759b
ventricular tachycardia with, 745f, 746–756
ventricular trigeminy with, 742, 745f
wandering pacemaker with, 722, 722f, 810
electrocardiogram interpretation for, 702–712, 703f–712f, 810
five step rhythm analysis in, 702–708, 703f–712f
heart rate calculator rulers with, 706, 706f
R-R method with, 706, 707f
6-second count method with, 708, 708f
step 1: QRS complex analysis in, 703, 704f, 810
step 2: P wave analysis in, 703, 705f, 810
step 3: rate analysis in, 703, 706–708, 706f–708f, 810
step 4: rhythm analysis in, 708, 709f, 710f, 810
step 5: P-R interval analysis in, 708, 711f
triplicate method with, 706, 706f
electrocardiogram monitoring for, 691–702, 810
artifacts with, 701–702
augmented limb leads with, 692, 693f
Cardiology *(Continued)*
basic concepts of, 691–699, 692t, 693f–699f, 694b
graph paper in, 698–699, 699f
leads with, 692, 692t, 693f
modified lead recording with, 692, 694f
monitoring electrode application in, 697–698
9-lead monitoring in, 697, 698f
P wave with, 700, 810
P-R interval with, 700
precordial leads in, 694–697, 694f–697f
QRS complex with, 700–701, 700f, 810
Q-T interval with, 701, 701n, 702f, 810
relation to electrical activity of, 699–702, 700f, 701f, 701n
routine monitoring in, 693, 694b
ST segment with, 701, 702f
standard limb leads with, 692, 693f
T wave with, 701, 810
torsades de pointes with, 701
12-lead monitoring in, 693, 694f
electrophysiology in, 680–688, 681f–687f
autonomic nervous system effects with, 687
cardiac cells electrical activity with, 681, 681f
cardiac muscle excitation sequence with, 686–687, 686f
cell excitability with, 682–685, 684f, 685f, 810
ectopic electrical impulse formation with, 687–688, 687f
electrical conduction system with, 685–688, 686f, 687f, 810
ion channel diffusion with, 681–682, 683f
membrane potential of, 681, 681f, 682f
pacemaker activity with, 685–686, 687
paroxysmal supraventricular tachycardia with, 688
pharmacological actions of, 682
premature atrial complex with, 687
premature junctional contraction with, 687
premature ventricular complex with, 687
refractory period with, 685, 685f
sodium-potassium exchange pump with, 682, 684f, 810
ventricular tachycardia with, 688
emergencies managed in, 799–809
basic cardiac life support with, 799–802, 800t–801t, 801f, 802f, 802n
cardiac arrest/sudden death with, 807–808, 808b
defibrillation with, 801, 802–805, 803f, 804b, 812
resuscitation termination with, 808–809, 812
synchronized cardioversion with, 805–806, 812
transcutaneous cardiac pacing with, 806–807, 806f, 808f, 812
hypertension in, 798–799, 798b, 798t, 812
blood pressure levels with, 798b, 812
chronic, 798
emergencies from, 798–799, 798b, 812
signs/symptoms of, 798b
myocardial infarction in, 779–787, 780f, 781f–786f, 783t, 811
death of myocardium with, 780, 781f
deaths following, 780–781, 781n
electrocardiogram findings with, 782, 782f, 782n
fibrinolytic therapy for, 784f–786f, 785–787
management of, 783–787, 784f–786f
precipitating events for, 779

Cardiology *(Continued)*
signs/symptoms of, 781–782
12-lead electrocardiogram used for, 782–783, 783f, 783n, 783t
types/locations of, 780, 780f
noncritical peripheral vascular condition in, 797–798, 811
patient assessment for, 688–691, 690f, 691b
abnormal heartbeat in, 689
chest pain/discomfort in, 688–689, 689n
chief complaint in, 688–689, 810
dyspnea in, 689
heart sounds in, 689–690, 690b
palpitations in, 689
physical examination in, 689–690, 689f, 690b
significant medical history in, 689
syncope in, 689
physiology in, 677–681, 677n, 678f, 679f, 680n
cardiac cycle within, 677–679, 677n, 678f
cardiac output within, 680
electrolytes within, 681, 810
hormonal regulation of heart within, 680–681
myocardial contractility within, 680
nervous system control of heart within, 680, 680n, 809
Starling's law of the heart within, 679, 679f
stroke volume within, 679–680, 679f, 679n
ventricular systole/diastole within, 677–679
prevention strategies with, 676
risk factors in, 676, 676b
Cardiopulmonary resuscitation (CPR)
legal issues with, 65–66, 66b
Cardiovascular disease
prevention of, 28, 29b
Cardiovascular endurance
paramedic well-being with, 27
Cardiovascular system, 123–128, 124f–127f, 149
coronary vessels of, 123–124
drugs for, 364–368, 365b, 383
heart anatomy of, 123, 124f
heart blood flow in, 125, 126f
heart chambers/valves of, 124–125
heart conduction system in, 125, 126f
pericardium of, 123
peripheral circulation in, 125–127
Cataract, 1174
definition of, 1160
Cavitation
definition of, 500
penetrating trauma with, 513, 514f
Cell
acid-base balance in, 164–172, 165b, 166f–168f, 170f, 171b, 171f, 172t
acidosis with, 166–169, 167f, 168f, 170f, 194
alkalosis with, 169–170, 171f
buffering systems with, 165, 166f
imbalance with, 165–166
mixed disturbances of, 170–172, 171b, 172t
ph with, 165, 165b, 166f
adaptation of, 172–173, 172f
injury in, 173–176
genetic factor with, 175
hypoperfusion, 176–179, 177b, 178f, 195
hypoxic, 173
infectious, 173–175, 174f, 175b, 175f
inflammatory, 175
manifestations of, 176

Cell *(Continued)*
multiple organ dysfunction syndrome with, 152, 180, 180b, 181f
nutritional imbalance with, 175
shock with, 179–180, 180b
metabolism impairment in, 180–181, 182f
physiology, 152–172, 194
intracellular/extracellular fluid in, 152
TBW distribution in, 152–153, 152n, 153t
self-defense mechanisms of, 181–185, 183f, 184f, 185f
immune response in, 151, 183–185, 185–187, 185f, 195
inflammatory response in, 151, 181–183, 183f, 184f, 185–187, 195
sodium/chloride balance in, 159–162, 160f–161f, 162t
water balance in, 159, 162
water movement in, 153–159
alterations in, 158–159
capillary network anatomy with, 155–157, 157f, 158f
capillary/membrane permeability with, 157
diffusion with, 154
edema with, 158–159, 159b
fluid replacement therapy with, 155f
intracellular/extracellular, 153–155, 153n, 154f, 154n, 155b, 155f
mediated transport mechanisms with, 154–155, 156f
osmosis with, 153, 154f
plasma/interstitial fluid, 155–157, 157f, 158f
Starling hypothesis with, 157
Cell excitability
action potential propagation with, 682–685, 684f, 685f
cardiology electrophysiology with, 682–685, 684f, 685f, 810
phase 0 of, 683
phase 1 of, 683
phase 2 of, 685
phase 3 of, 685
phase 4 of, 685
refractory period with, 685, 685f
threshold potential with, 682
Cell structure anatomy, 84–85, 88–90, 88f, 88t, 152
cell classes with, 90
cell functions with, 90
cell reproduction with, 90
cytoplasm in, 85, 88t, 89–90, 89f
cytoplasmic membrane in, 84–85, 88f, 88t
nucleus in, 88t, 90
Central cord syndrome
definition of, 606
spinal trauma with, 612
Central nervous system, 111–116, 111f, 112f, 113t, 114f, 115f
definition of, 82
Central pain syndrome, 859–860, 863
definition of, 836
Central venous cannulation, 410–413, 411f, 412f, 414, 425
complications of, 414
Central venous lines
special needs children with, 1155, 1155f
Cephalopelvic disproportion, 1091, 1096
Cerebral hematoma, 601
Cerebral palsy
definition of, 1196
special considerations for, 1202–1203
Cerebral perfusion pressure (CPP), 598
definition of, 580
neurology pathophysiology with, 842, 844

Certification
EMS, 11, 11n
paramedic, 56
Cervical spine
physical examination of, 255
Cesarean delivery, 1069
definition of, 1062
CHART format, 326–327
Chemical burn injury, 560, 570–573, 571f, 572f, 578
alkali metals, 572
ammonia, 572
antidotes/neutralizing agents for, 571
assessment of, 571
eyes in, 571, 572f
hydrofluoric acid, 572
management of, 571
petroleum, 572
phenol, 572
Chest
physical examination of, 255–261, 255f–261f
Chickenpox, 1030–1031, 1031f, 1040
Child abuse, 1150–1153, 1152f, 1152t, 1158, 1189–1192, 1190b, 1191f, 1192f, 1192n, 1194
definition of, 1116
elements of, 1151
physical findings suggestive of, 1151–1153, 1152f, 1152t
abdominal visceral injury, 1153
bone injury, 1153
bruises, 1152, 1152t
burns, 1153
subdural hematoma, 1153
welts, 1152
sexual, 1153
suspicious injuries for, 1151
Childhood infectious diseases, 1029–1031
chickenpox, 1030–1031, 1031f, 1040
mumps, 1030, 1030f, 1040
pertussis, 1031, 1040
rubella, 1029, 1029f, 1040
rubeola, 1029–1030, 1030f, 1040
Chlamydia, 1035, 1036f, 1040
Chlorine, 1306, 1314, 1315
Cholecystitis, 895, 903, 905
definition of, 892
Cholesterol, 23, 23n, 24b, 26, 28, 29b
Cholinergic drugs, 332, 351, 355
Chronic bronchitis, 820, 820f, 821t, 833
Chronic gastroenteritis, 898–899, 899n
Chronic obstructive pulmonary disease (COPD), 820–825, 820f, 821f, 821t, 823b, 823f–825f, 826t, 833
assessment of, 821–822
asthma in, 822–825, 822n, 823b, 823f–825f, 824n, 825n, 826t, 833
assessment of, 822–824, 824n
differential considerations for, 825, 827t
management of, 824–825, 824b, 824n, 825f, 825n, 826t
pathophysiology of, 822, 822n, 823f, 824f
pulmonary function tests for, 824–825, 825f, 825n, 826t
chronic bronchitis in, 820, 820f, 821t, 833
emphysema in, 820–822, 820f, 821f, 821t
Chronic renal failure, 913–915, 914t, 918
definition of, 908
Circulatory system, 119–128, 123t, 124f–127f, 129f, 130f, 149. *See also* Cardiovascular system
blood components, 120–121, 123t
peripheral circulation in, 125–127
pulmonary circulation in, 127
systemic circulation in, 127
CISM. *See* Critical incident stress management

Civil rights
negligence with, 60–61
Clavicular fractures, 630, 630f
Clinical decision making, 290–296
application of principle in, 290, 292, 292f
assessment-based patient management with, 293–294
concept formation in, 290, 291–292, 292f
critical thinking process with, 291–293, 292f
data interpretation in, 290, 292, 292f
evaluation in, 290, 292–293, 292f
fundamental elements of, 293
prehospital care spectrum, 291, 291b
reflection on action in, 290, 292f, 293
six R's with, 294–295
Closed pneumothorax, 633–634, 634f, 641
definition of, 630
Cluster headache, 856
definition of, 836
COBRA. *See* Consolidated Omnibus Budget Reconciliation Act
Coccygeal fractures
spinal trauma with, 612
Code of Hammurabi, 3, 4b
Cognitive disorders, 1048–1049, 1049b, 1060
delirium, 1048–1049
dementia, 1049, 1049b
Colon
abdominal trauma with, 646
Colostomy
definition of, 1210
Coma, 847–849, 848b, 848n, 862
assessment of, 848–849, 848n
causes of, 847, 848b
management of, 848–849, 848n
structural v. toxic-metabolic, 847–848, 848n, 862
Communicability period
definition of, 1004
infectious disease stages of, 1016, 1016f, 1016t
Communicable disease. *See also* Infectious disease
definition of, 1004, 1005
Communications, 306–317. *See also* Therapeutic communication
call prioritization with, 315
components/functions of, 314–315, 314b
dispatcher training for, 314, 314b
EMS procedures in, 315–316
EMS role of, 308–310, 308f
model of, 308–309, 308f
operation modes in, 312–314, 313f, 317
duplex, 306, 313, 313f
multiplex, 306, 313, 313f
simplex, 306, 313, 313f
trunked system, 313–314
patient information in, 315–316, 316n, 317
regulation of, 315, 317
SOAP format in, 306, 316
systems, 310–314
technological advances in, 309–310, 309f
terminology, 306, 310b–311b, 317
typical EMS event, 307–308, 307f
verbal, 309
written, 309
Community health, 50–52, 51b, 51f, 52f, 53
assessment
definition of, 42
injury prevention programs with, 50–51, 51f
education, 52
intervention into, 52
Community leadership
essential activities of, 46–47, 46b
EMS provider education in, 47
EMS provider protection in, 46–47
injury data collection in, 47
Compartment syndrome
crush injury with, 546–547, 546f, 547b
definition of, 538
Compensated shock, 527, 527b, 528f
Complement system, 151, 174
Compliance
definition of, 430
Compression injuries
blunt trauma from, 509–510, 509f
Concealment, 1276, 1282
Concussion, 596
Confidentiality
defamation with, 62
definition of, 62
ethics of, 77–78, 79
HIPPA with, 61b
improper information release with, 62
invasion of privacy with, 62
paramedic-patient relationships with, 61–62, 61b
Congenital anomalies
definition of, 1100
Congestive heart failure, 787–791, 787b, 788f–790f, 791b
left ventricular failure in, 787–789, 787b, 787n, 788f–790f, 811
right ventricular failure in, 789–791, 791b, 791n, 811
Consent
EMS research requiring, 19–20, 19n
ethics of, 78, 79
expressed, 54, 63
implied, 54, 63
informed, 54, 63
involuntary, 54, 63
legal complications with, 64
mentally incompetent adult, 63
minors, 63
paramedic-patient relationships with, 62–64
prisoners, 63
refusal of care with, 63–64
special situations of, 63
types of, 63–64
Consolidated Omnibus Budget Reconciliation Act (COBRA), 61
Contemplation
mental/emotional health with, 31–32, 32n
Continence
definition of, 1160
Continuous positive airway pressure (CPAP), 829–830
Continuous quality improvement (CQI)
definition of, 2
EMS with, 13, 16, 16b, 20
medical professional attributes with, 13
Controlled Substances Act, 332, 335–336, 335n, 336t, 337b
Contusions, 542–543, 543f
Conversion disorders, 1055, 1055b
COPD. *See* Chronic obstructive pulmonary disease
Cord injuries
spinal trauma with, 612–613
Cord presentation
delivery complications with, 1093
Core body temperature, 985
definition of, 984
Cough suppressants, 371–372, 372b
Cover, 1276, 1282
CPAP. *See* Continuous positive airway pressure
CPP. *See* Cerebral perfusion pressure
CPR. *See* Cardiopulmonary resuscitation
CQI. *See* Continuous quality improvement
Cranial nerve injuries
skull fractures with, 596
Cricothyrotomy, 494–497, 495f, 496f
complications possible for, 497
contraindications for, 497
Cricothyrotomy *(Continued)*
description of, 494
equipment for, 494–496, 495f
removal of, 497
technique for, 496, 496f, 496n
Crime scene, 1283, 1283b, 1284
definition of, 1276
Crime scene awareness, 1276–1285
approaching, 1277–1278, 1285
clandestine drug labs in, 1280–1281, 1281n, 1285
dangerous highway encounters in, 1278–1279, 1279b, 1279f, 1285
dangerous residence in, 1278, 1278f, 1285
domestic violence in, 1281
EMS at crime scene with, 1283, 1283b, 1284
gang characteristics in, 1279–1280, 1280b, 1280f, 1281b, 1285
legal issues with, 69, 70b
safety tactics in, 1281–1283, 1282b, 1283b
avoidance, 1281
cover/concealment, 1282
distraction/evasive maneuvers, 1282–1283, 1283b
tactical retreat, 1281–1282
tactical patient care with, 1283–1284, 1285
body armor for, 1283–1284
violent groups/situations in, 1279–1281, 1280b, 1280f, 1285
violent street incidents in, 1279, 1285
Critical incident stress management (CISM), 36–37, 37b, 41, 1253, 1254
Crohn's disease, 897, 901–902, 901n, 905
definition of, 892
Crowning
definition of, 1072
Crush injury, 543, 543f, 546–547, 546f, 547b
compartment syndrome with, 546–547, 546f, 547b
crush syndrome with, 547
definition of, 538
rhabdomyolysis with, 547
Crush syndrome
crush injury with, 547
definition of, 538
special considerations for, 556–557
Current health status, 226, 230–231, 230b
Cushing syndrome, 879–880, 879f, 881
definition of, 864
Cushing's triad, 598
definition of, 580
neurology pathophysiology with, 845, 845f
Cyanosis
neonatal life support needed for, 1110, 1114
Cystic fibrosis
special considerations for, 1203, 1203n
Cystitis
nontraumatic gynecology emergencies of, 1066b, 1067, 1071

D

DAI. *See* Diffuse axonal injury
DCAP-BTLS
definition of, 652
Deafness
definition of, 1196
Death/dying
dealing with, 37–39
developmental considerations with, 39
legal issues in determination of, 69, 69b
paramedic's needs with, 38–39
patient/family needs with, 37
recommended communication strategies with, 38b
Deceleration injuries
blunt trauma from, 508–510, 508f
Decerebrate posturing, 598
definition of, 580

Decompression sickness, 999–1000
  definition of, 984
Decontamination
  decision making for, 1300, 1301f
  definition of, 1286
  8 step process for, 1302b
  patient emergency with, 1299–1301, 1300n, 1301f
  rescue personnel/equipment, 1301, 1302b, 1303
Decorticate posturing, 598
  definition of, 580
Defamation, 62
Defense mechanisms, 35b
Defibrillation
  cardiac emergencies managed with, 801, 802–805, 802f, 803f, 804b, 812
  implantable cardioverter, 804–805, 805f
  monitor-defibrillators with, 801–802, 802f
    automated external, 802, 802f
    biphasic technology for, 802
  operator/personnel safety with, 804, 804b
  paddle electrodes for, 803, 803f
  procedure for, 803–804
  in special environments, 804
  stored/delivered energy with, 803
Degenerative disk disease, 628
Degenerative neurological diseases, 858–862
Dehydration, 162–163, 194
Delirium, 1048–1049, 1170, 1170t
Delirium tremens
  alcoholism with, 960
  definition of, 920
Delusions
  definition of, 1042
  schizophrenia with, 1049, 1050b
Dementia, 1049, 1049b, 1170, 1170t
Dental trauma, 589, 590f, 605
Department of Homeland Security, 1316–1317
Depressed skull fractures, 594–595, 594f, 595f
Depression, 1052, 1052b, 1060
  definition of, 1042
  elderly with, 1176–1177, 1177b, 1181
Designated officer (DO)
  definition of, 1005
Diabetes mellitus, 867–876, 867t, 868b, 868f, 869f, 870t, 871f, 874b, 875b, 875f, 876t, 881, 1171
  acidosis with, 872–873
  assessment of, 874–875
  diabetic ketoacidosis with, 874, 874b
  differential diagnosis of, 876, 876t
  effects of, 872–873
  emergencies with, 873–876, 874b, 875b, 875f, 876t
  gestational, 1084
  glucose metabolism with, 867–872, 870t, 871f
    dietary intake and, 867–868
    digestion process and, 868–870
    glucagon and, 869f, 870–872, 870t, 871f
  hyperosmolar hyperglycemic nonketotic with, 867t, 874, 875f
  hypoglycemia with, 873–874
  insulin for, 867, 868b, 873
  management of, 873, 875–876, 875b, 875f, 875n
  oral hypoglycemic agents for, 873
  pancreas anatomy with, 867, 868b, 868f, 869f
    glucagon in, 867, 869f
    islets of Langerhans in, 867
  pathophysiology of, 872
  urine glucose missing with, 872
Diabetic ketoacidosis (DKA), 169
  diabetes mellitus with, 874, 874b, 881
Dialysis, 915–917, 916f, 916n, 917b, 917n, 918
  air embolism with, 917, 917n
  chest pain with, 917
  definition of, 908
  disequilibrium syndrome with, 916, 917
  emergencies with, 915–916
  hemodialysis, 915, 916f
  hemorrhage with, 916
  hypotension with, 916–917, 917b
  peritoneal, 915
  severe hyperkalemia with, 917, 917n
  vascular access problems with, 916, 916n
Diaphragmatic hernia
  definition of, 1100
  neonatal life support needed for, 1109, 1114
Diaphragmatic rupture, 641, 641f, 642
Diarrhea
  neonatal life support needed for, 1112, 1114
Dietary fats, 23–24, 24b, 26, 26b
Dietary recommendations, 26, 26b. *See also* Nutrition
Diffuse axonal injury (DAI), 597
Diffusion, 151, 154
  definition of, 151
  pulmonary pathophysiology of, 817–818, 818t, 833
Digestant drugs, 373
Digestive system, 135–138, 137f, 149
  functions of, 136
  gallbladder of, 138
  large intestine of, 138
  liver of, 136–138
  oral cavity of, 136
  pancreas of, 138
  small intestine of, 136
  stomach of, 136, 137f
Digital intubation, 480, 480f
Dilation and curettage, 1069, 1069n
  definition of, 1062
Direct medical direction
  definition of, 3
  EMS, 15, 20
Disease period
  definition of, 1005
  infectious disease stages of, 1016–1017, 1016f, 1016t
Disease prevention
  cancer, 28–29, 29b
  cardiovascular, 28, 29b
  infectious, 29
  paramedic well-being with, 28–29, 29b
Disease transmission
  prevention of, 39–40
    documentation with, 40
    exposure management with, 40
    exposure sources with, 39
    protection from airborne/blood-borne pathogen with, 40
  terminology, 39b
Disentanglement, 1256, 1259–1260
Disequilibrium syndrome, 916, 917
  definition of, 908
Dislocations
  spinal trauma with, 612, 613f
Dispatch systems, 314, 314b
Dispatcher
  EMS, 8–9
Disseminated intravascular coagulation, 525
  definition of, 520
Disseminated intravascular coagulopathy, 978, 983
Dissociative disorders, 1055–1056, 1060
Distraction, 609, 610–611, 611f, 1276, 1282–1283, 1283b
  definition of, 606
Distress, 32, 41
Distribution
  drug, 333, 341–342, 343f, 344f, 345b, 350, 382
Diversity
  definition of, 1196
Diverticulitis, 900, 905
  definition of, 892
Diverticulosis, 897, 899–900, 899f, 905
  definition of, 892
Diving emergencies, 997–1000
  air embolism in, 998–999, 999b, 999f
  barotrauma in, 997–1000, 998b, 998n, 999b, 999f, 1000n, 1002
  decompression sickness in, 999–1000
  gas properties influencing, 997, 997n, 1002
  nitrogen narcosis in, 1000, 1000n
Divisions, 1240, 1242, 1242b, 1247–1248
DKA. *See* Diabetic ketoacidosis
DO. *See* Designated officer
Documentation, 318–329
  abbreviations used in, 323b–325b
  consequences of inappropriate, 328, 328b
  general considerations for, 320, 320b, 321f–322f, 323b–325b
  importance of, 318, 318b
  narrative in, 318, 320, 325–326
  narrative writing systems with, 326–327, 327n
    CHART format, 326–327
    SOAP format, 326–327
  paramedic's responsibility for, 328b
  pertinent negative findings in, 318, 320
  properly written, 326, 326f
  revision/correction, 328
  special considerations of, 327–328
Domestic violence
  crime scene awareness with, 1281
Down syndrome
  definition of, 1196
  special considerations for, 1200–1201, 1200n, 1201f
Dressings
  injuries not requiring closure with, 552, 552f–554f
  materials used for, 551–552, 557
Drowning
  definition of, 984
  submersion with, 995–996, 995f, 1001
Drug abuse. *See* Toxicology
Drug labs
  clandestine, 1280–1281, 1281n, 1285
Drugs. *See* Pharmacology
Dual diagnosis
  substance-related disorders with, 1045b, 1054
Duodenum
  abdominal trauma with, 648
Duplex mode, 306, 313, 313f
Dyskinesia
  definition of, 1042
  schizophrenia with, 1049
Dysmenorrhea
  nontraumatic gynecology emergencies of, 1066b, 1067, 1071
Dystonia, 859, 862
  definition of, 836

E

Ear(s)
  drugs for, 374–375, 384, 422–423
  physical examination of, 253–254, 253f, 254
Ear trauma, 585–586, 585f, 605
  barotitis, 585–586
  chemical injuries, 585
  lacerations/contusions, 585, 585f
  thermal injuries, 585
  traumatic perforations, 585

Early adulthood
development characteristics of, 206, 207f, 210
Eating disorders, 1056, 1056b, 1060
anorexia nervosa, 1056
bulimia nervosa, 1056
Eclampsia
complications of pregnancy with, 1083–1084, 1083b, 1096
definition of, 1072
Ectopic pregnancy
complications of pregnancy with, 1085
nontraumatic gynecology emergencies of, 1066b, 1068, 1068n, 1071
Edema
cell water movement with, 158–159, 159b
clinical manifestations of, 159
definition of, 15
pathophysiology of, 158–159
Education
continuing, 11, 20
curriculum model for, 12f
EMS, 11, 12f, 20
initial, 11
Efferent division
definition of, 82
Elbows
injury, 662, 663f
physical examination of, 267, 267f
Elder abuse, 1160, 1166, 1179–1180, 1180t, 1181, 1188–1189, 1189b, 1189f, 1194
definition of, 1160
Electrical burn injury, 560, 573–576, 573b, 574f, 575n, 576f, 578
assessment of, 574–575
effects of, 573–574
lightning injury as, 575–576, 576f, 576n
management of, 574–575
physical examination for, 575
types of, 573, 574f
Electrocardiogram
conduction disorder dysrhythmias in, 771–773, 771n, 772b, 772f, 773f
interpretation of, 702–712, 703f-712f, 810
five step rhythm analysis in, 702–708, 703f-712f
heart rate calculator rulers with, 706, 706f
R-R method with, 706, 707f
6-second count method with, 708, 708f
step 1: QRS complex analysis in, 703, 704f, 810
step 2: P wave analysis in, 703, 705f, 810
step 3: rate analysis in, 703, 706–708, 706f–708f, 810
step 4: rhythm analysis in, 708, 709f, 710f, 810
step 5: P-R interval analysis in, 708, 711f
triplicate method with, 706, 706f
monitoring of, 691–702, 810
artifacts with, 701–702
augmented limb leads with, 692, 693f
basic concepts of, 691–699, 692t, 693f–699f, 694b
electrode application in, 697–698
graph paper in, 698–699, 699f
leads with, 692, 692t, 693f
modified lead recording with, 692, 694f
9-lead, 697, 698f
P wave with, 700, 810
P-R interval with, 700
precordial leads in, 694–697, 694f–697f
QRS complex with, 700–701, 700f, 810
Q-T interval with, 701, 701n, 702f, 810
relation to electrical activity of, 699–702, 700f, 701f, 701n
routine, 693, 694b
Electrocardiogram *(Continued)*
ST segment with, 701, 702f
standard limb leads with, 692, 693f
T wave with, 701, 810
torsades de pointes with, 701
12-lead, 693, 694f
myocardial infarction in, 782–783, 783f, 783n, 783t
Electrolytes
cardiac function influenced by, 681, 810
imbalances, 163–164
Emergency medical services (EMS)
certification for, 11, 11n
components of, 8f
continuous quality improvement for, 13, 16, 16b, 21
crime scene with, 1283, 1283b, 1284
current, 7–9, 8f, 10b
definition of, 2
education for, 11, 12f, 20
federal health care reform influencing, 6
group involvement, 10, 10b
Hammurabi code and, 3, 4b
hazardous materials personnel training, 1304–1305
competencies in, 1304–1305
OSHA/EPA requirements in, 1304
health care elements with, 6f
history of, 3–7, 4b, 5b, 6f, 6n, 7b, 20
injury prevention involvement of, 46–50
community leadership activities for, 46–47, 46b
dangerous situations recognition for, 48
provider education with, 47
provider protection in, 46–47
licensure for, 11, 11n
medical direction for, 15–16, 15b, 15n, 16b
direct, 15, 20
indirect, 15, 20
offline, 15, 20
online, 15, 20
on-scene physicians in, 15–16, 15n
types of, 15
NHTSA with, 4, 5, 5b, 7
organizations, 10, 10b, 20
paramedic education, 11, 12f
continuing, 11
initial, 11
paramedic's role within, 13–15, 14b, 14n
additional responsibilities of, 14–15, 14n, 20
primary responsibilities of, 13–14, 14b, 20
poison control center for, 921–922
pre-twentieth century, 3–4, 4b, 20
professionalism with, 11–13, 20
attributes of, 13
CQI of, 13
provider levels, 8–10, 9n, 10b, 20
dispatcher in, 8–9
EMT-basic in, 9, 20
EMT-intermediate in, 10, 20
EMT-paramedic in, 10, 10b, 20
first responder in, 9
quality assurance for, 16, 16b
recommendations for, 4, 4b
registration for, 11
required components of, 5, 5b
research for, 16–20, 17b, 17n, 18n, 19n, 21
basic principles of, 17–18, 17b, 17n, 18n
cardiac arrest, 17b
consent with, 19–20, 19n
ethics of, 19–20, 19n
evaluating, 20b
format of, 20, 20b
statistics in, 18–19, 18n, 19n
steps in conducting, 17b
Emergency medical services (EMS) *(Continued)*
types of, 17b
Utstein style in, 17b
response teams for, 14n
roles/responsibilities of, 2–20, 4b, 5b, 6f, 6n, 7b, 8f, 12f, 14b, 17b, 20b
standing orders for, 15, 15b
system operations of, 7–8
citizen activation with, 8
hospital care with, 8
prehospital care with, 8
rehabilitation with, 8
tactical, 1276, 1282b, 1283
treatment protocols for, 15, 15b
twentieth century, 4–7, 4b, 5b, 6f, 6n, 7b, 20
Emergency Medical Services Systems Act (EMSS), 5
Emergency medical technicians (EMT), 6
Emetic drugs, 373
Emotional abuse
definition of, 1184
Emotional health. *See* Mental/emotional health
Emotional impairment
definition of, 1196
special considerations for, 1201, 1208
Emphysema, 820–822, 820f, 821f, 821t
assessment of, 821–822
management of, 822
EMS. *See* Emergency medical services
EMSS. *See* Emergency Medical Services Systems Act
EMT. *See* Emergency medical technicians
EMT-basic
EMS, 9, 20
EMT-intermediate
EMS, 10, 20
EMT-paramedic
definition of, 3
description of, 10b
EMS, 10, 10b, 20
Endocrinology, 119, 121f, 122t, 123t, 149, 864–881
Addison disease in, 880, 880f, 880t, 881
adrenal gland disorders in, 878–880, 879f, 880f, 880t
anatomy/physiology of, 865–866, 865f, 866f
gland functions in, 865–866, 866f
hormone secretion regulation in, 866
Cushing syndrome in, 879–880, 879f, 881
diabetes mellitus in, 867–876, 867t, 868b, 868f, 869f, 870t, 871f, 874b, 875b, 875f, 876t, 881
acidosis with, 872–873
assessment of, 874–875
diabetic ketoacidosis with, 874, 874b, 881
differential diagnosis of, 876, 876t
effects of, 872–873
emergencies with, 873–876, 874b, 875b, 875f, 876t
glucose metabolism with, 867–872, 870t, 871f
hyperosmolar hyperglycemic nonketotic with, 874, 875f, 881
hypoglycemia with, 873–874, 881
insulin for, 873
management of, 873, 875–876, 875b, 875f, 875n
oral hypoglycemic agents for, 873
pancreas anatomy with, 867, 868b, 868f, 869f
pathophysiology of, 872
urine glucose missing with, 872
drugs for, 375–376, 375b, 376b, 384
specific disorders of, 866–867, 867t

Endocrinology *(Continued)*
  thyroid gland disorders in, 877–878, 877b, 877f, 878f, 878n, 878t
    anatomy/physiology of, 877–878, 877b, 877f, 878n
    causes of, 877, 877b
    management of, 878, 878t
    myxedema as, 878, 878f
    thyrotoxicosis as, 877, 877f, 881
Endometriosis
  nontraumatic gynecology emergencies of, 1066b, 1068
Endometritis
  nontraumatic gynecology emergencies of, 1066b, 1067–1068, 1071
Endometrium
  definition of, 1062
Endotracheal drugs, 422, 422f
Endotracheal intubation, 473–476, 473f, 474f, 474t, 475f, 476n
  advantages of, 483
  anatomical considerations for, 476, 476n
  description of, 473, 473f
  necessary equipment for, 474–475, 474f, 475f
  pediatric considerations in, 485, 485n
  preparation for, 475–476, 475f
  tub sizes for, 473, 474t
  tube placement confirmation adjuncts for, 485–486, 485n, 486f
    bulb/syringe esophageal detector, 486, 488f
    end-tidal carbon dioxide detector, 485–486, 485n, 486f, 487b
    pulse oximetry, 486, 488b, 488f
End-tidal carbon dioxide detector, 485–486, 485n, 486f, 487b
Envenomation, 937
  definition of, 920
Environmental conditions, 984–1002
  diving emergencies with, 997–1000
    air embolism in, 998–999, 999b, 999f
    barotrauma in, 997–1000, 998b, 998n, 999b, 999f, 1000n, 1002
    decompression sickness in, 999–1000
    gas properties influencing, 997, 997n, 1002
    nitrogen narcosis in, 1000, 1000n
  frostbite with, 993–995, 994f, 1001
    deep, 994, 994f
    management of, 994–995
    pathophysiology of, 993–994
    superficial, 994, 994f, 994n
  high-altitude illness with, 1000–1001, 1000b, 1002
    acute mountain sickness in, 1000–1001, 1000b
    high-altitude cerebral edema in, 1000b, 1001
    high-altitude pulmonary edema in, 1000b, 1001
  hyperthermia with, 988–990
    heat cramps, 988, 1001
    heat exhaustions, 988, 1001
    heat stroke, 988–990, 988n, 1001
  hypothermia with, 909f, 990–993, 991t, 992f, 1001
    management of, 991–993, 992f
    pathophysiology of, 909f, 990–991, 991t
  submersion with, 995–997, 995f, 1001
    clinical outcome factors in, 996
    drowning in, 995–996, 995f, 1001
    management of, 996–997
  thermoregulation with, 985–987, 986b, 987b, 987f, 1001
    external environmental factors in, 986
Environmental conditions *(Continued)*
    heat loss regulation in, 986, 987b, 987f
    heat production regulation in, 986, 986b
Eosinophil chemotactic factor of anaphylaxis, 886
  definition of, 882
Epididymitis, 911, 918
  definition of, 908
Epidural hematoma, 598–600, 600f
Epilepsy. *See also* Status epilepticus
  definition of, 836
Equipment
  safety, 30–31, 30t
Eschar, 562
  definition of, 558
Esophageal injuries, 640–641, 641n, 642
Esophageal-tracheal Combitube. *See* Multilumen airway
Esophagogastric varices, 897, 902, 902f, 905
  definition of, 892
Ethics, 72–79
  confidentiality in, 77–78, 79
  consent in, 78, 79
  definition of, 72
  emergency problems of, 76, 76f
  EMT code of, 73, 74b
  futile situations, 78
  health care tests of, 76
  Hippocratic Oath, 74b
  legal accountability with, 75
  moral accountability with, 75–76, 76n
  obligation to provide care in, 78
  overview of, 73
  paramedic practice issues of, 77–79
  patient advocacy in, 78
  physician extender role in, 79
  principles of medical, 75b
  professional accountability with, 73–75, 74b, 75b
  rapid approach to, 76, 76f
  resolving dilemmas of, 76–77
  resource allocation, 77
  resuscitation decisions, 77, 79
Eustress, 32, 41
Evasive tactics, 1276, 1282–1283, 1283b
Excretion
  drug, 333, 342–344, 343f, 344f, 350, 351
Exposure incident
  definition of, 1005
Expressed consent
  definition of, 54
  paramedic-patient relationships with, 63
Extended scope of practice
  definition of, 3
  federal health care reform influencing, 6
External medication administration, 397–399, 399b, 425
  gastric tube in, 398–399, 399b
  oral route of, 397–398, 399b
  rectal, 399, 399b
Extracellular fluid
  cell water movement of, 153–155, 153n, 154f, 154n, 155b, 155f
  definition of, 151
Eye(s)
  anatomy, 145–146, 147f
  drugs for, 374–375, 384, 422–423, 423f
  physical examination of, 251–253, 251b, 252f, 253f
Eye trauma, 586–589, 587f, 588b, 588f, 589b, 605
  contact lenses, 588, 588b
  evaluation of, 586, 586n, 587–589, 587f, 588b, 588f
  extraocular movements in, 586–587
  pupillary reaction in, 586
  signs/symptoms of, 587b

F

Facilitated diffusion, 151, 154
Factitious disorders, 1055, 1060
Failure to thrive
  definition of, 1210
False imprisonment
  definition of, 54
  legal complications with, 64
False movement
  definition of, 652
Familial diseases, 189–193, 189b, 190t, 191f, 191t, 192f, 192t, 193t
  factors causing, 189–190, 189b, 190t, 191t
    age, 190
    environmental, 189b, 190, 190t, 191t
    gender, 190
    genetic, 189
  risk analysis of, 189, 192, 193t
Family history, 226, 230
Family/peer/community connections
  mental/emotional health with, 32
FBAO. *See* Foreign body airway obstruction
Fecal impaction
  definition of, 1160
Feet. *See also* Lower extremity injuries
  injury, 668, 669f
  physical examination of, 267–268, 269f
Female genitalia
  physical examination of, 266, 279
Female reproductive system, 142–144, 142f, 143f, 144f, 149. *See also* Gynecology
Femoral fracture, 664, 666, 666n, 667f
Fever
  neonatal life support needed for, 1111, 1111n, 1114
Fibular injury, 668, 668f, 669f
Fick principle, 443
  definition of, 431
Field impression
  assessment-based patient management with, 298, 299–300, 300f
Financial challenges
  special considerations for, 1207, 1208
Financial exploitation
  definition of, 1184
Finger injury, 664, 664f
First responder
  curriculum for, 9
  EMS, 9
Fitness
  body mass index with, 27, 27b
  cardiovascular endurance, 27
  muscle flexibility, 27–28
  muscle strength, 27
  paramedic well-being with, 27–28, 27b, 27n, 41
Flail chest, 631–632, 631f, 631n
  definition of, 630
Flexion
  spinal trauma with, 610, 611f
Fluid replacement therapy, 155f
Focal injury. *See* Head/facial trauma
Focused history
  definition of, 280
  medical patients, 286
  trauma patients, 286–287
Foreign body airway obstruction (FBAO), 449–451, 450t, 451n
Fractures
  definition of, 652
  musculoskeletal trauma with, 652, 654f, 655b, 655f, 671
  spinal trauma with, 612, 613f

Free radicals, 24b
Frostbite, 993-995, 994f, 1001
deep, 994, 994f
definition of, 984
management of, 994-995
pathophysiology of, 993-994
superficial, 994, 994f, 994n
Full-thickness burns
burns classifications of, 562, 563f
definition of, 558

G

Gag reflex, 452
definition of, 431
Gallbladder, 138
Gang characteristics
crime scene awareness of, 1279-1280, 1280b, 1280f, 1281b, 1285
Gastric lavage
definition of, 920
Gastric tubes/gastrostomy tubes
special needs children with, 1155-1156, 1156f
Gastroenteritis, 905
acute, 898
chronic, 898-899, 899n
Gastroenterology, 892-907
acute abdominal pain patient assessment in, 893-897, 905
appendicitis with, 895
auscultation with, 896
cholecystitis with, 895
history with, 893-894
involuntary guarding with, 895
management of, 897, 897b
pain location/type with, 894-895, 895b
palpation with, 897
pancreatitis with, 895
percussion with, 897
physical examination for, 896-897, 896f
rebound tenderness with, 895
referred pain with, 895, 896f
signs/symptoms of, 895
somatic pain with, 895
visceral pain with, 894-895
vital signs with, 895
acute gastroenteritis in, 898
acute hepatitis in, 903, 904b, 905
anatomy of, 893, 894f
appendicitis in, 900, 905
bowel obstruction in, 901, 901b, 901n, 905
cholecystitis in, 903, 905
chronic gastroenteritis in, 898-899, 899n
Crohn's disease in, 897, 901-902, 901n, 905
diverticulitis in, 900, 905
diverticulosis in, 897, 899-900, 899f, 905
esophagogastric varices in, 897, 902, 902f, 905
gastrointestinal bleeding in, 897-898
hemorrhoids in, 897, 902-903, 903f, 905
hernia in, 901, 901b
nasogastric tube insertion with, 906-907, 906f, 907f
pancreatitis in, 902
peptic ulcer disease in, 897, 900, 905
ulcerative colitis in, 899, 899n, 905
Gastrointestinal bleeding, 897-898
Gastrointestinal system
drugs for, 372-374, 383-384
Gastrointestinal/genitourinary crisis
home health care patient with, 1220-1222, 1220b, 1221b, 1221f, 1222t, 1228
female catheterization in, 1221-1222, 1221f
gastric emptying/feeding in, 1222, 1222t
indwelling Foley catheter insertion in, 1220, 1221b
Gastrointestinal/genitourinary crisis *(Continued)*
male catheterization in, 1221, 1221f
urinary retention in, 1220
Genetic diseases. *See* Familial diseases
Geriatrics, 1160-1181
assistance programs for, 1161, 1162b
cardiovascular system of, 1168-1169
abdominal/thoracic aneurysm in, 1168-1169, 1169b
dysrhythmias in, 1168
heart failure in, 1168, 1168n
hypertension in, 1169, 1169b, 1169n
myocardial infarction in, 1168
demographics/societal issues with, 1161
elder abuse with, 1166, 1179-1180, 1180t, 1181
endocrine system of, 1171-1172
environmental considerations with, 1176
hyperthermia as, 1176, 1181
hypothermia as, 1176, 1181
gastrointestinal system of, 1172
integumentary system of, 1172-1173, 1173f
musculoskeletal system of, 1173
nervous system of, 1169-1171, 1170t, 1171b
patient history in, 1166
physical examination in, 1166
physiological changes with, 1162-1166, 1164t, 1165f
cardiovascular, 1162
musculoskeletal, 1165, 1165f
nervous system, 1164-1165
renal, 1162-1164
respiratory, 1162
psychiatric disorders with, 1176-1177
depression as, 1176-1177, 1177b, 1181
suicide as, 1177
pulmonary system of, 1166-1168
bacterial pneumonia in, 1167
chronic obstructive pulmonary disease in, 1167
pulmonary embolism in, 1167-1168
sensations in, 1173-1175
hearing, 1174, 1174f
speech, 1175
vision, 1173-1174, 1174f
substance abuse with, 1175-1176, 1175b, 1181
toxicology with, 1175, 1175b
trauma with, 1177-1179, 1181
Gerontology
definition of, 1160
Gestation, 1072, 1074
Glasgow Coma Scale, 603, 603t
Glaucoma, 1174
definition of, 1160
Gluconeogenesis, 867
definition of, 864
Glycogenolysis, 867
definition of, 864
Gonorrhea, 1035, 1040
Good Samaritan laws, 59
Gram, 388, 389b, 390, 390f
Gravida, 1072, 1077
Grieving process, 37-38
developmental considerations in dealing with, 39
paramedic needs dealing with, 38-39
patient/family needs with, 37
stages of, 37-38
acceptance, 38
anger, 38
bargaining, 38
denial, 37-38
depression, 38
Groups, 1240, 1242, 1242b, 1247-1248
Gynecology, 1062-1071
female reproductive organs in, 1063, 1063f
follicle/oocyte development in, 1063-1064, 1064f
menstruation in, 1063, 1064b, 1071
nontraumatic emergencies in, 1066-1068, 1066b
cystitis, 1066b, 1067, 1071
dysmenorrhea, 1066b, 1067, 1071
ectopic pregnancy, 1066b, 1068, 1068n, 1071
endometriosis, 1066b, 1068
endometritis, 1066b, 1067-1068, 1071
mittelschmerz, 1066b, 1067, 1071
pelvic inflammatory disease, 1066, 1066b, 1067f, 1071
ruptured ovarian cyst, 1066-1067, 1066b, 1067f, 1071
vaginal bleeding, 1066b, 1068, 1071
ovulation in, 1064-1066, 1065f
hormonal control of, 1065-1066, 1065f
sexual assault in, 1070-1071
traumatic emergencies in, 1066b, 1068-1070, 1069n, 1069t, 1071
vaginal bleeding, 1066b, 1068, 1071

H

Hallucinations
definition of, 1042
Hammurabi code, 3, 4b
Hand injury, 663-664, 663f
Hand-held nebulizer, 421-422, 422f
Hands
physical examination of, 267, 267f
Hantavirus, 1028-1029, 1040
Hazard control, 1256, 1259
Hazardous atmospheres rescue, 1263-1265, 1263b, 1265f, 1274
chemical/toxic exposure or explosion with, 1263-1264, 1263n
confined spaces emergencies with, 1264-1265, 1265f, 1266f
confined spaces with, 1263, 1263b
crush compartment syndromes with, 1264
trenches/cave-ins with, 1265, 1265n
Hazardous materials incidents, 1286-1305
chemical exposure to eyes with, 1295
contaminated patient emergency with, 1299-1301, 1300n, 1301f
EMS personnel training for, 1304-1305
competencies in, 1304-1305
OSHA/EPA requirements in, 1304
exposure symptoms with, 1295, 1295n
external damage with, 1295
identification in, 1288-1291, 1289f, 1290f, 1291b, 1302-1303
formal, 1288-1291, 1289f, 1289n, 1290f, 1291b
informal, 1288, 1288n
international, 1291b
placards for, 1289, 1289n, 1290f, 1291b
internal damage with, 1294-1295, 1295n, 1303
laws/regulations with, 1287-1288, 1302
medical monitoring/rehabilitation for, 1298-1299
personal protective clothing/equipment for, 1291-1293, 1292b, 1292f, 1293f, 1303
classification of, 1292-1293, 1292b, 1292f, 1293f
respiratory devices as, 1292, 1303
rescue personnel/equipment decontamination for, 1301, 1302b, 1303
response to, 1295-1298, 1296b, 1297b, 1297f, 1298f, 1299b
approaching scene for, 1296-1298
controlling scene for, 1298

Hazardous materials incidents *(Continued)*
risk assessment for, 1296, 1296b, 1297f
safety zones in, 1298, 1298f, 1299b
scope of, 1287
soft tissue damage with, 1295, 1304
terminology for, 1296b
Hazardous terrain rescue, 1270–1273, 1271b, 1272f, 1273f, 1274
helicopter use for, 1272–1273
patient packaging for, 1272
terminology of, 1271, 1271b
HDL. *See* High-density lipoproteins
Head
physical examination of, 251, 255
Headache, 856–857, 862
Head/facial trauma, 580–605
anterior neck trauma as, 509–593, 590–593, 590f, 591f, 592n
esophageal injury, 592–593
evaluation of, 590–591, 591f
hematomata, 591, 591n
laryngeal/tracheal injury, 592, 592n
soft tissue, 591–593, 591n, 592n
vascular injury, 591–592, 592n
brain trauma as, 596–603, 605
airway/ventilation with, 601
antegrade amnesia with, 596
assessment of, 601–603, 602b, 603n
cerebral blood flow in, 598
cerebral contusion with, 597, 597f
cerebral hematoma in, 601
circulation with, 601–602, 602b
concussion, 596
diffuse axonal injury, 597
drug therapy for, 603, 603n
edema with, 597
epidural hematoma in, 598–600, 600f
fluid therapy for, 602–603
focal injury, 597–603, 597f, 598n, 599b, 599f, 600f, 601f, 602b, 602n
hemorrhage with, 598–601, 598n, 599b, 599f, 600f
intracranial pressure in, 598, 599b, 599f
ischemia with, 597
mild diffuse injury, 596
moderate diffuse injury, 596
neurological evaluation of, 602, 602n
penetrating injury in, 601
respiratory patterns in, 598
retrograde amnesia with, 596
subarachnoid hematoma in, 600, 601f
subdural hematoma as, 598–600, 600f
ear trauma as, 585–586, 585f, 605
barotitis, 585–586
chemical injuries, 585
lacerations/contusions, 585, 585f
thermal injuries, 585
traumatic perforations, 585
eye trauma as, 586–589, 587f, 588b, 588f, 589b, 605
contact lenses, 588, 588b
evaluation of, 586, 586n, 587–589, 587f, 588b, 588f
extraocular movements in, 586–587
pupillary reaction in, 586
signs/symptoms of, 587b
injury rating systems for, 603–605, 603t, 604t
Glasgow Coma Scale as, 603, 603t
pediatric trauma score as, 604–605, 604t
trauma score/revised trauma score as, 603–604, 604t
maxillofacial injury as, 581–584, 582f, 583f, 584f, 605
facial fractures, 581–584, 582f, 583f, 584f
management of, 584
Head/facial trauma *(Continued)*
mandible fractures, 582
midface fractures, 582–583, 582f, 583f, 583n
nose fractures, 584
nose/ear foreign body insertion with, 584
orbit fractures, 583–584, 584f
soft tissue, 581, 582f
zygoma fractures, 583, 584f
skull fractures as, 593–596, 594f, 594n, 595f, 605
basilar, 593–594, 594f, 594n, 595f
Battle's sign with, 594, 595f
cranial nerve injuries with, 596
depressed, 594–595, 594f, 595f
linear, 593, 594f
open vault, 594f, 595, 595f
raccoon's eyes with, 594, 595f
soft tissue to scalp as, 593
Head-injured patients
special considerations for, 1204, 1205t
Health Insurance Portability and Accountability Act (HIPPA), 61b
Health maintenance organizations. *See* Managed care organizations
Hearing impairments
special considerations for, 1197–1198, 1208
Hearing sense organ, 146–148, 148f
Heart
physical examination of, 261–262, 261f, 262f
Heat cramps, 988, 1001
definition of, 984
Heat escape-lessening posture (HELP), 1262, 1262f
Heat exhaustion, 988, 1001
definition of, 984
Heat stroke, 988–990, 988n, 1001
definition of, 984
HELP. *See* Heat escape-lessening posture
Hematology, 970–983
anemia in, 972–975, 982
diagnosis/treatment of, 975, 975n
hemolytic, 974
iron deficiency, 974, 974f
signs/symptoms of, 974–975, 975t
assessment/management of disorders in, 981–982, 982t
prehospital care with, 981–982
blood/blood components in, 971–972, 972f, 973b, 973f, 974b, 982
plasma, 971
platelets, 972, 974b
red blood cells, 971–972, 973b, 973f
white blood cells, 972
definition of, 970
disseminated intravascular coagulopathy in, 978, 983
hemophilia in, 978–979, 978b, 979n, 979t, 983
Hodgkin's disease in, 976–977, 977f, 982
leukemia in, 975–976, 976f, 977b, 982
bone marrow transplant for, 976, 977b
lymphomas in, 976–977, 977f, 982
multiple myeloma in, 981, 983
non-Hodgkin's lymphomas in, 977, 982
polycythemia in, 977–978, 983
sickle cell disease in, 979–981, 979b, 980f, 981f, 983
Hematoma
definition of, 538
Hematomata, 542–543, 543f
anterior neck trauma with, 591, 591n
Hematuria
definition of, 644
Hemodialysis, 915, 916f
Hemoperitoneum, 646
definition of, 644
Hemophilia, 978–979, 978b, 979n, 979t, 983
definition of, 970
Hemorrhage, 520–522, 536, 537
assessment/treatment integration for, 536
brain trauma, 598–601, 598n, 599b, 599f, 600f
cerebral blood flow in, 598
cerebral hematoma as, 601
epidural hematoma as, 598–600, 600f
intracranial pressure in, 598, 599b, 599f
penetrating injury in, 601
respiratory patterns in, 598
subarachnoid hematoma as, 600, 601f
subdural hematoma as, 598–600, 600f
types of, 598–601, 599f, 600f, 601f
direct pressure for, 549, 549f
elevation for, 549, 549f
external, 521, 521n
immobilization by splinting for, 550, 550f
internal, 521
physiological response to, 521–522
pneumatic pressure devices for, 551, 551f
pressure point for, 549, 550f
soft tissue trauma, 549–551, 549f, 550f, 551f, 557
tourniquet for, 551, 551f
Hemorrhoids, 897, 902–903, 903f, 905
definition of, 892
Hemostasis, 521
definition of, 520
Hemostatic agents, 369, 383
Hemothorax, 637, 637f
definition of, 630
Hepatitis, 1020–1023, 1021t, 1022n, 1023b, 1040. *See also* Acute hepatitis
A, 1021t, 1023
B, 1021t, 1022–1023
C, 1021t, 1023
Hepatitis B
protective equipment for, 30t
Herbs, 385–386
Hernia, 901, 901b
Herniated intervertebral disk, 628
Herpes virus infections, 1035–1036, 1036f, 1041
HHNK. *See* Hyperosmolar hyperglycemic non-ketotic
High-altitude cerebral edema, 1000b, 1001
definition of, 984
High-altitude illness, 1000–1001, 1000b, 1002
acute mountain sickness in, 1000–1001, 1000b
high-altitude cerebral edema in, 1000b, 1001
high-altitude pulmonary edema in, 1000b, 1001
High-altitude pulmonary edema, 1000b, 1001
definition of, 985
High-density lipoproteins (HDL), 29b
Highway operations rescue, 1265–1270, 1267b, 1268f–1271f, 1269b, 1274
airbag/supplemental restraint systems in, 1268–1269, 1269b
automobile anatomy in, 1269–1270, 1270f
electrical power hazards in, 1267
fuel/fire hazards in, 1267, 1267b
hazardous cargoes in, 1269
unstable vehicles in, 1267–1268, 1268f, 1269f
Hip fracture, 664, 667f
HIPPA. *See* Health Insurance Portability and Accountability Act
Hips
physical examination of, 268, 269f

History taking, 226–233, 227b, 229b, 230b
  content in, 227–228, 227b
  definition of, 226
  special challenges of, 231–233
  techniques of, 228–231, 229b, 230b
    current health status in, 226, 230–231, 230b
    family history in, 226, 230
    present illness history, 226, 228–229, 229b
    significant past medical history in, 226, 229–230, 230b
HIV. *See* Human immunodeficiency virus
Hodgkin's disease, 976–977, 977f, 982
  definition of, 970
Home artificial ventilators
  special needs children with, 1154, 1154f, 1155t
Home health care patient, 1210–1228
  acute infections with, 1222–1224, 1223b, 1223t, 1228
  advanced life support response to, 1212, 1212b
  gastrointestinal/genitourinary crisis with, 1220–1222, 1220b, 1221b, 1221f, 1222t, 1228
  general management principles for, 1213–1214
  hospice/palliative care with, 1226, 1227b, 1228
  injury control with, 1212
  maternal/child conditions with, 1224–1225, 1225b, 1228
  overview of, 1211–1213, 1212b
  respiratory support for, 1214–1216, 1214f, 1215b, 1216t, 1228
  types of, 1212–1213
  vascular access devices for, 1216–1220, 1216n, 1217f, 1218t, 1219b, 1219t, 1228
Homeostasis
  definition of, 82
Hospice
  home health care patient with, 1226, 1227b, 1228
Hostile environments
  paramedic well-being and, 29–30
Household system, 389b, 391
Human immunodeficiency virus (HIV), 186, 186n, 187b, 1017–1020, 1017n, 1018t–1019t, 1020f, 1020n, 1040
  classification/categories of, 1017–1019, 1018t–1019t, 1020f
    category A, 1017–1019
    category B, 1019
    category C, 1019, 1020f
  pathophysiology of, 1017, 1017n
  personal protection from, 1019–1020
  postexposure prophylaxis with, 1020, 1020n
  precautions for, 427
  protective equipment for, 30t
  psychological reactions to, 1020
  transmission prevention principles related to, 1008b, 1009t
Humeral injury, 662, 663f
Huntington's disease, 364
Hymenoptera bites/stings, 935, 963
Hypercalcemia, 151, 164, 194
Hyperextension
  spinal trauma with, 610
Hyperglycemia
  pediatric, 1144, 1144f, 1157
Hyperkalemia, 151, 163, 194
Hypermagnesemia, 151, 164, 194
Hypernatremic dehydration, 151, 162
Hyperosmolar hyperglycemic nonketotic (HHNK)
  definition of, 864
  diabetes mellitus with, 874, 875f, 881
Hyperplasia, 151, 172
Hyperrotation
  spinal trauma with, 610
Hypersensitivity reaction, 151, 174
Hypertension, 798–799, 798b, 798t, 812
  blood pressure levels with, 798b, 812
  chronic, 798
  elderly with, 1169, 1169b, 1169n
  emergencies from, 798–799, 798b, 812
  signs/symptoms of, 798b
Hypertensive emergencies
  emergency cardiac for drug-induced, 966
Hypertensive encephalopathy
  definition of, 674
Hyperthermia, 988–990
  elderly with, 1176, 1181
  heat cramps, 988, 1001
  heat exhaustions, 988, 1001
  heat stroke, 988–990, 988n, 1001
Hypertonic solution, 151, 153, 155b, 155f
Hypertrophy, 151, 172
Hyperventilation syndrome
  definition of, 816
  management of, 832
  pulmonary emergency from, 832, 834
Hypocalcemia, 151, 164, 194
Hypocarbia, 444
  definition of, 431
Hypoglycemia
  diabetes mellitus with, 873–874, 881
  neonatal life support needed for, 1111–1112, 1112b, 1112n, 1114
  pediatric, 1144, 1157f
Hypokalemia, 151, 163, 194
Hypomagnesemia, 151, 164, 194
Hyponatremic dehydration, 151, 162–163
Hypoperfusion, 151, 176–179, 177b, 178f, 195
  cardiac output decreased in, 176–177, 177b, 178f
  compensatory mechanisms for, 177–179, 177b, 178f
    adrenal medullary, 179
    baroreceptor reflexes, 177, 177b, 178f
    chemoreceptor reflexes, 177
    hormonal, 179
    nervous system ischemic response, 177, 179
    vasopressin, 179
Hypothermia, 909f, 990–993, 991t, 992f, 1001
  elderly with, 1176, 1181
  management of, 991–993, 992f
  neonatal life support needed for, 1111, 1114
  pathophysiology of, 909f, 990–991, 991t
Hypotonic solution, 151, 154, 155b, 155f
Hypovolemia
  neonatal life support needed for, 1110, 1114
  pediatric shock with, 1132–1134, 1132f–1134f, 1133t
    blood loss in, 1132–1134, 1133t, 1134n
    dehydration in, 1132, 1132f, 1133t
Hypovolemic shock, 526, 526n
  management of, 536
Hypoxemia, 151, 170, 444
  definition of, 431
Hypoxia, 444
  definition of, 431
Hysterectomy, 1064b
  definition of, 1062
I
Ileostomy
  definition of, 1210
Immobilization, 615n, 616–626, 617f–626f, 629. *See also* Splinting
  diving incidents with, 625–626, 626f
  helmet issues with, 623–625, 624f, 625f, 625n
    helmet removal as, 624–625, 625f, 625n
  manual in-line, 615n, 616–618, 617f, 618f, 619f
    logroll with, 616–618, 618f, 619f
    sitting/standing patient in, 616, 617f
    supine patient in, 616, 617f
  mechanical devices for, 618–623, 619f–623f
    Kendrick extrication device, 619–620, 620f
    long spine boards, 620–623, 623f
    rigid cervical collars, 618, 619f
    short spine boards, 618–620, 620f, 620n
  pediatric patients with, 622f, 623, 624f
  splinting for, 550, 550f
Immune response, 151, 183–185, 185–187, 185f, 195
  blood group antigens with, 184–185, 185f
  deficiencies in, 186–187
  definition of, 151
  introduction to, 184
  Rh factor with, 185
  variances in, 185–187
Immune system
  drugs for, 381–382, 381f, 384
Immunoglobulins (Ig), 186, 186b
Impaired conduction
  emergency cardiac for drug-induced, 969
Implied consent
  definition of, 54
  paramedic-patient relationships with, 63
Impulse control disorders, 1056, 1060
Incident command system, 1241–1246, 1241n, 1242b, 1242f–1245f, 1243b. *See also* Medical incident command
  command function in, 1242–1243, 1242f, 1243b, 1243f
  declaring major incident in, 1245–1246, 1246n
  definition of, 1240
  section responsibilities with, 1243–1245, 1244f, 1245f
  terminology with, 1242b
Incontinence
  definition of, 1160
Incubation period
  definition of, 1005
  infectious disease stages of, 1016, 1016f, 1016t
Indirect medical direction
  definition of, 3
  EMS, 15, 20
Indwelling vascular devices, 417b–418b
Infant
  development characteristics of, 197–201, 198f, 199f–200f, 199t, 201b, 210
  drug dosage calculations for, 395–396, 396f
  growth/development review for, 1118, 1119b, 1120t
  physical examination of, 275–277, 276t, 277f
  premature, 1110, 1110n, 1114
  rescue breathing for, 460
  sudden infant death syndrome in, 1149–1150, 1149b, 1158
Infectious disease, 1004–1041
  childhood, 1029–1031
    chickenpox, 1030–1031, 1031f, 1040
    mumps, 1030, 1030f, 1040

Infectious disease *(Continued)*
pertussis, 1031, 1040
rubella, 1029, 1029f, 1040
rubeola, 1029–1030, 1030f, 1040
definition of, 1005
drugs for, 378–381, 378b, 379b, 380b, 384
hantavirus as, 1028–1029, 1040
hepatitis as, 1020–1023, 1021t, 1022n, 1023b, 1040
HIV as, 1017–1020, 1017n, 1018t–1019t, 1020f, 1020n, 1040
home health care patient with, 1222–1224, 1223b, 1223t, 1228
human physiology's response to, 1011–1015, 1012f, 1014f–1016f, 1015b, 1016t, 1040
influenza as, 1031–1032, 1032b, 1040
lice as, 1036–1037, 1037f, 1041
meningococcal meningitis as, 1025–1026, 1026f, 1026n, 1040
mononucleosis as, 1032, 1040
paramedic's role in preventing, 1039
pathophysiology of, 1009–1011, 1010b, 1010f, 1011b, 1039
host susceptibility in, 1011
transmission in, 1010f, 1011
pediatric, 1144–1145, 1145b, 1145f, 1157
pneumonia as, 1026–1027, 1040
prevention of, 29
public health principles related to, 1005–1009, 1006b–1009b, 1009t, 1039
agency responsibility in, 1006–1007, 1007b
AIDS in, 1006b
body substance isolation in, 1007, 1009b
decontamination methods in, 1007, 1009
HIV transmission prevention in, 1008b, 1009t
personal responsibility in, 1007–1009, 1008b, 1009b, 1009t
rabies as, 1028, 1040
reporting exposure to, 1038–1039, 1038n, 1041
medical evaluation/follow up with, 1038–1039
report for, 1038–1039
SARS as, 1032, 1033b–1034b, 1040
scabies as, 1036, 1037–1038, 1038b, 1038f, 1041
sexually transmitted, 1032, 1034–1036, 1040
chlamydia as, 1035, 1036f, 1040
gonorrhea as, 1035, 1040
herpes virus infections as, 1035–1036, 1036f, 1041
syphilis as, 1034–1035, 1034f, 1040
stages of, 1015–1017, 1015t, 1016f, 1040
communicability period in, 1016, 1016f, 1016t
disease period in, 1016–1017, 1016f, 1016t
incubation period in, 1016, 1016f, 1016t
latent period in, 1015–1016, 1016f, 1016t
tetanus as, 1027–1028, 1027t, 1040
tuberculosis as, 1023–1025, 1023n, 1024f, 1025b, 1040
Infectious disease exposure
paramedic legal issues with, 57
Inflammatory response, 151, 181–183, 183f, 184f, 185–187, 195
deficiencies in, 186–187
definition of, 151
drugs for, 378–381, 378b, 379b, 380b, 384
mast cells with, 183, 183f
stages of, 181–183
Inflammatory response *(Continued)*
stress with, 188, 195
systemic response to, 183, 184f
variances in, 185–187
Influenza, 825–827, 827b, 1031–1032, 1032b, 1040
Informed consent
definition of, 54
EMS research requiring, 19–20, 19n
paramedic-patient relationships with, 63
Inhalation injury, 569–570, 569b, 570f
definition of, 558
Inhaled drugs, 420–421
Initial assessment, 280, 281–286, 283f, 283t, 284f, 285b
definition of, 280
general impression in, 281, 282
life-threatening conditions in, 283–286
airway with, 285
breathing with, 285–286
circulation with, 286
level of consciousness with, 283
Injury
concepts, 43–45, 45t
Haddon's matrix, 43–45, 45t
injury triangle, 43–45, 45t
definition of, 43, 44b
epidemiology, 43, 44b, 44f, 44t
on-scene education with, 48–49
teachable moment in, 48
prevention, 42–53
community health for, 50–52, 51b, 51f, 52f, 53
community leadership activities for, 46–47, 46b
dangerous situations recognition for, 48
EMS involvement with, 46–50
EMS provider activities for, 47, 47b
EMS provider protection in, 46–47
EMS provider role in, 49
outside resources needed for, 48, 48b
overview of, 43–46
paramedic well-being with, 29–31, 30b, 30t, 41
patient care considerations for, 48
programs for, 50
strategies of, 47b, 48, 49b–50b
three E's of, 45–46
injury risk
definition of, 42, 44b
injury surveillance
definition of, 42, 44b
Inspection
abdomen, 263–264, 264f
chest, 255–256, 257f
technique of, 234, 235–236, 235b, 278
Insulin
diabetes mellitus with, 873
Integumentary system, 92–95, 94f, 149
definition of, 82
glands in, 94–95
hair in, 93–94
nails in, 94
skin in, 92–93, 94f
Interstitial fluid
cell water movement in, 155–157, 157f, 158f
definition of, 151
Intracellular fluid
cell water movement of, 153–155, 153n, 154f, 154n, 155b, 155f
definition of, 151
Intracerebral hematoma
definition of, 580
Intraosseous medications, 416–420, 417b–418b, 419f, 425
complications with, 420
contraindications for, 420
equipment for, 419
indwelling vascular devices with, 417b–418b
insertion technique for, 419–420, 419f
Intrapartum, 1101
definition of, 1100
Intrapulmonic pressure
definition of, 431
Intrathoracic pressure
definition of, 431
Intravenous fluid administration, 408–416, 408f, 409f, 410f, 411f, 412f, 413b, 415f, 416f, 425
catheter types for, 408, 408f
central venous cannulation for, 410–413, 411f, 412f, 414
complications of, 413–416, 413b, 415f, 416f
air embolism as, 413–414, 413b
infiltration as, 413, 413b
medications in, 414–416, 415f, 416f
peripheral insertion for, 408–410, 408f, 409f, 410f, 411f
Invasion of privacy, 62
Involuntary consent
definition of, 54
paramedic-patient relationships with, 63
Involuntary guarding, 895
definition of, 892
In-water spinal immobilization
rescue operations with, 1262
Irreversible shock, 527b, 528–529, 529n, 530f
Isotonic dehydration, 162, 194
Isotonic solution, 151, 154, 155b, 155f

J

Joint dislocations
definition of, 652
musculoskeletal trauma with, 656, 656f, 671
Junctional escape rhythms
cardiology dysrhythmias with, 735, 737f, 738

K

Kehr sign, 646
definition of, 644
Kendrick extrication device, 619–620, 620f
Ketogenesis
definition of, 864
Kidneys
abdominal trauma with, 648
Kilogram, 388, 389b, 390, 390f
Kinematics
definition of, 500
KKK standards, 1230, 1231, 1239
Knee injury, 666, 668f
Korsakoff's psychosis, 958
definition of, 920
Krebs cycle, 181, 182f

L

Laceration
assessment of, 543–544, 543f
Lactic acidosis, 152, 168–169
Landing zone, 1230, 1237
Large intestine, 138
Laryngeal mask airway, 486, 488–489, 488n, 489f
advantages/disadvantages of, 489
description of, 488
equipment for, 489
insertion of, 488–489, 489f

Late adulthood
development characteristics of, 207–210, 207f, 208f, 209b
Latent period
definition of, 1005
infectious disease stages of, 1015–1016, 1016f, 1016t
Lateral bending
spinal trauma with, 610
Laxative drugs, 373
LDL. *See* Low-density lipoproteins
Le Fort fracture
definition of, 580
Left ventricular failure, 787–789, 787b, 787n, 788f–790f, 811
Legal issues, 54–71
crime scene responsibilities, 69, 70b
death determination in field, 69, 69b
documentation in, 69–70, 71
ethical responsibilities, 55, 55f, 55n
legal system structure and, 55–56
negligence as, 58–61, 58n, 59n, 61b
borrowed servants with, 60
breach of duty in, 59
civil rights with, 60–61
COBRA/OBRA, 61
components of, 58–59, 58n, 59n
defenses to, 59–61
duty to act in, 58–59
Good Samaritan laws with, 59
liability insurance for, 60
protection against claims of, 61
proximate cause with, 59
punitive damages with, 59
organ donation, 68–69, 68b
paramedic, 56–58, 56n, 57b, 58f, 58n
assault/battery of, 57
infectious disease exposure with, 57
injury lawsuit with, 57–58, 58f, 58n
licensure/certification with, 56
mandatory reporting with, 56–57, 57b
medical direction with, 56
medical practice act with, 56
motor vehicle laws with, 56, 56n
protection for, 57
scope of practice with, 56
paramedic accountability, 58–61, 58n, 59n, 61b
paramedic-patient relationships, 61–65, 61b
confidentiality in, 61–62, 61b
consent in, 62–64
force used in, 64
transportation in, 64–65, 65b
paramedic's duties, 55, 55f, 55n
resuscitation, 65–68, 66b, 67f, 68n, 71
advance directive with, 66–68, 67f
CPR, 65–66, 66b
withholding/stopping, 65–66, 66b, 71
Leukemia, 975–976, 976f, 977b, 982
bone marrow transplant for, 976, 977b
Leukotrienes, 886
definition of, 882
Liability insurance
negligence, 60
Lice, 1036–1037, 1037f, 1041
Licensure
EMS, 11, 11n
paramedic, 56
Life span, 196–210
Lifting
injury prevention with, 29
Lightning injury, 575–576, 576f, 576n
Limbic system
definition of, 82
Linear skull fractures, 593, 594f
Liter, 388, 389b, 390, 390f
Liver, 136–138
abdominal trauma with, 646, 647f, 650
Loading dose, 333, 338
Lou Gehrig disease. *See* Amyotrophic lateral sclerosis
Low back pain, 627
prevention/rehabilitation of, 30b
Low-density lipoproteins (LDL), 29b
Lower extremity injuries, 664–668, 664n, 665f, 666f, 666n, 667f, 668f, 669f, 671
Lund and Browder chart
burns classifications with, 563, 564f
definition of, 558
Lung cancer
management of, 833
pathophysiology of, 832, 833f
pulmonary emergency from, 832–833, 833f, 834
signs/symptoms of, 832
Lyme disease, 939
definition of, 920
Lymphatic system
definition of, 83
Lymphomas, 976–977, 977f, 982
definition of, 970

M

Magnesium imbalance, 164
Major incident, 1240, 1241, 1245–1246, 1246n. *See also* Mass casualty incidents
definition of, 1240
preparing for, 1245–1246, 1246n
Male reproductive system, 140–142, 141f, 149
Managed care organizations
definition of, 3
federal health care reform influencing, 6
Mandatory reporting
paramedic legal issues with, 56–57, 57b
Mania
definition of, 1042
MAP. *See* Mean arterial pressure
Marine animals
poison from, 941–944, 941f, 943f, 963
Mass casualty incidents, 1246–1250, 1247f, 1250b, 1254
common problems at, 1249–1250, 1250b
communications with, 1246–1247
definition of, 1240
group/division functions with, 1247–1248
obtaining resources with, 1247
rehabilitation area for, 1249
scene assessment with, 1246, 1246n
staging area for, 1248–1249
support branch for, 1249, 1249n
Mast cells, 183, 183f
Material exploitation
definition of, 1184
Mathematical equivalents, 389–391, 389b, 390f, 390t, 391f
apothecary system, 389b, 391
household system, 389b, 391
metric system, 389–391, 389b, 390f, 390t, 391f
temperature conversions with, 391, 391f
Maxillofacial injury
head/facial trauma of, 581–584, 582f, 583f, 584f, 605
MDI. *See* Metered-dose inhaler
Mean arterial pressure (MAP), 598
definition of, 580
Meconium staining
definition of, 1100
neonatal life support needed for, 1103–1104, 1104f, 1104n, 1114
Mediated transport mechanisms, 152, 154–155, 156f
definition of, 152
Medical asepsis, 397, 397b, 425
Medical incident command, 1240–1254
critical incident stress management in, 1253, 1254
mass casualty incidents in, 1246–1250, 1247f, 1250b, 1254
common problems at, 1249–1250, 1250b
communications with, 1246–1247
group/division functions with, 1247–1248
obtaining resources with, 1247
rehabilitation area for, 1249
scene assessment with, 1246, 1246n
staging area for, 1248–1249
support branch for, 1249, 1249n
system for, 1241–1246, 1241n, 1242b, 1242f–1245f, 1243b
command function in, 1242–1243, 1242f, 1243b, 1243f
declaring major incident in, 1245–1246, 1246n
section responsibilities with, 1243–1245, 1244f, 1245f
terminology with, 1242b
triage principles/technology for, 1250–1253, 1251f, 1252f, 1252t, 1254
patient tracking systems in, 1252–1253, 1253f
patient transportation in, 1253
primary v. secondary, 1250–1251
START technique in, 1251–1252, 1251f
tagging/labeling in, 1252, 1252t, 1253f
Medical patients
focused history for, 286
trauma patients v., 288
Medical practice act, 56
Medication administration, 388–427. *See also* Pharmacology
blood sample obtained in, 423–424, 424t, 426
drug calculations in, 391–397, 392b, 393b, 395b, 396b, 396f, 425
basic formula for, 393–394
clock method for, 395b
conversion of units for, 393
dimensional analysis with, 394
doses assessment with, 393
infant/children dosage, 395–396, 396f
infusion rates with, 395
intravenous flow rates with, 395
methods for, 391–394, 392b, 393b
ratios/proportions with, 394
errors in, 397
external, 397–399, 399b, 425
gastric tube, 398–399, 399b
oral route, 397–398, 399b
rectal, 399, 399b
intraosseous, 416–420, 417b–418b, 419f, 425
complications with, 420
contraindications for, 420
equipment for, 419
indwelling vascular devices with, 417b–418b
insertion technique for, 419–420, 419f
intravenous fluid, 408–416, 408f–412f, 413b, 415f, 416f, 425
catheter types for, 408, 408f
central venous cannulation for, 410–413, 411f, 412f, 414
complications of, 413–416, 413b, 415f, 416f
medications in, 414–416, 415f, 416f
peripheral insertion for, 408–410, 408f, 409f, 410f, 411f
mathematical equivalents used in, 389–391, 389b, 390f, 390t, 391f

Medication administration *(Continued)*
apothecary system, 389b, 391
household system, 389b, 391
metric system, 389-391, 389b, 390f, 390t, 391f
temperature conversions with, 391, 391f
medical asepsis with, 397, 397b, 425
parenteral, 399-420, 425
containers for, 399-401, 401f, 402f, 403f
equipment used for, 399-403, 399b, 400b, 400f, 401f, 402f, 403f
injection site preparation for, 401
intradermal injection with, 403, 404f
intramuscular injection with, 405-408, 406f, 407f, 408f
subcutaneous injection with, 403-405, 404f, 405f
syringes/needles for, 399, 399b
pediatric patients with, 423
percutaneous, 420-423, 420f, 421f, 422f, 423f, 425
buccal drugs in, 420
ear drugs in, 422-423
endotracheal drugs in, 422, 422f
eye drugs in, 422-423, 423f
hand-held nebulizer in, 421-422, 422f
inhaled drugs in, 420-421
metered-dose inhaler in, 421, 421f
nose drugs in, 422-423, 423f
sublingual drugs in, 420
topical drugs in, 420, 420f
safety considerations/procedures for, 396-397, 425
universal precautions in, 397, 397n, 398t
Meditation
mental/emotional health with, 31-32, 32n
Menarche, 196, 204
definition of, 1062
Meningococcal meningitis, 1025-1026, 1026f, 1026n, 1040
Menopause, 196, 206, 1062, 1063
Menstruation
definition of, 1062
Mental illness
definition of, 1196
special considerations for, 1200, 1208
Mental impairment, 1196, 1201
definition of, 1196
Mental retardation
definition of, 1196
special considerations for, 1201, 1208
Mental status examination
behavioral disorders assessment with, 1046
definition of, 1042
Mental/emotional health, 31-32
anxiety with, 31
family/peer/community connections for, 32
meditation/contemplation for, 31-32, 32n
smoking cessation for, 31, 32b
spirituality for, 32n
substance misuse/abuse with, 31, 31b, 41
Metabolic acidosis, 167-168, 168f, 194
Metabolic alkalosis, 169-170, 171f
Metacarpal injury, 663-664, 663f
Meter, 390, 390f
Metered-dose inhaler (MDI), 421, 421f
Methamphetamine, 950b
Methicillin-resistant *Staphylococcus aureus* (MRSA), 1011b
Metric system, 389-391, 389b, 390f, 390t, 391f
Middle adulthood
development characteristics of, 206-207, 207f, 210
Migraine, 856
definition of, 836
Mild diffuse injury. *See* Head/facial trauma
Minerals, 24, 25t
Minute alveolar ventilation, 435-437
Minute volume, 435-437
definition of, 431
Mittelschmerz
nontraumatic gynecology emergencies of, 1066b, 1067, 1071
Moderate diffuse injury. *See* Head/facial trauma
Mononucleosis, 1032, 1040
Mood disorders, 1051-1054
bipolar, 1052-1053, 1052f, 1053b, 1060
depression, 1052, 1052b, 1060
suicide/suicide threats with, 1053-1054, 1053b, 1060-1061
Morals
definition of, 72, 73
Moro reflex, 196, 199t
Motor vehicle collision
blunt trauma from, 505-506, 505f
Motorcycle collision
blunt trauma from, 510, 510f, 511f
Mouth-to-mouth method
rescue breathing with, 459-460
Moving
injury prevention with, 29
MRSA. *See* Methicillin-resistant *Staphylococcus aureus*
MS. *See* Multiple sclerosis
Multilumen airway, 489-490, 490f
Multiple myeloma, 981, 983
definition of, 970
Multiple organ dysfunction syndrome, 152, 180, 180b, 181f
Multiple sclerosis (MS), 859, 862
definition of, 836
special considerations for, 1203-1204
Multiplex mode, 306, 313, 313f
Mumps, 1030, 1030f, 1040
Muscle flexibility
paramedic well-being with, 27-28
Muscle strength
paramedic well-being with, 27
Muscular dystrophy, 858-859, 862
definition of, 836
special considerations for, 1204
Muscular system, 104-108, 105f-110f, 108t, 149
muscle types comparison for, 108t
Musculoskeletal trauma, 652-671
assessment of, 658, 659b, 671
DCAP-BTLS in, 658, 671
six Ps of, 659b
classification of, 652-656, 654f, 655b, 655f, 656b, 656f, 671
fractures in, 652, 654f, 655b, 655f, 671
joint dislocations in, 656, 656f, 671
sprains in, 655, 656b, 656f, 671
strains in, 655-656, 671
inflammatory/degenerative conditions of, 656-658, 656b, 657f, 671
arthritis as, 657-658, 657f, 671
bursitis as, 656, 657f, 671
tendonitis as, 657, 657f, 671
lower extremity injuries as, 664-668, 664n, 665f, 666f, 666n, 667f, 668f, 669f, 671
femoral fracture in, 664, 666, 666n, 667f
foot/ankle injury in, 668, 669f
hip fracture in, 664, 667f
knee/patellar injury in, 666, 668f
pelvic fracture in, 664, 664n
phalangeal injury in, 668
tibial/fibular injury in, 668, 668f, 669f
open fractures as, 668-669
reducing dislocations with, 669-670, 669n
signs/symptoms of, 658, 658n, 671
splinting for, 658-660, 659f, 660b, 660f, 671
Musculoskeletal trauma *(Continued)*
general principles of, 658, 660b
types of, 658-660, 660f
straightening angular fractures for, 669-670, 669n
upper extremity injuries as, 660-664, 661f-663f, 664f, 671
elbow injury in, 662, 663f
finger (phalangeal) injury in, 664, 664f
hand (metacarpal) injury in, 663-664, 663f
humeral injury in, 662, 663f
radial injury in, 662, 663f
shoulder injury in, 660-662, 660n, 663f
ulnar injury in, 662, 663f
wrist injury in, 662, 663f
Mutual aid, 1240, 1247
Myasthenia gravis
definition of, 1196
special considerations for, 1205, 1206f
Mycoplasmal pneumonia, 827-828, 827n
Myocardial contractility, 680
Myocardial contusion
thoracic trauma with, 639, 642
Myocardial infarction, 779-787, 780f, 781f-786f, 783t, 811
death of myocardium with, 780, 781f
deaths following, 780-781, 781n
electrocardiogram findings with, 782, 782f, 782n
fibrinolytic therapy for, 784f-786f, 785-787
management of, 783-787, 784f-786f
precipitating events for, 779
signs/symptoms of, 781-782
12-lead electrocardiogram used for, 782-783, 783f, 783n, 783t
types/locations of, 780, 780f
Myoclonus, 861, 863
definition of, 836
Myxedema, 878, 878f, 881
definition of, 864

N

Narrative
documentation, 318, 320, 325-326
Nasal airway. *See* Nasopharyngeal airway
Nasal cannula, 457-458, 457f, 457t, 458t
Nasogastric tube insertion, 906-907, 906f, 907f
Nasopharyngeal airway (Nasal airway)
airway management with, 469-471, 470f, 471f
National Highway Traffic Safety Administration (NHTSA)
EMS with, 4, 5, 5b, 7
system elements of, 5, 5b
Neck
physical examination of, 254-255, 254f
Neglect. *See also* Abuse/neglect
definition of, 1184
Negligence, 58-61, 58n, 59n, 61b
borrowed servants with, 60
breach of duty in, 59
civil rights with, 60-61
COBRA/OBRA, 61
components of, 58-59, 58n, 59n
defenses to, 59-61
definition of, 54
duty to act in, 58-59
Good Samaritan laws with, 59
liability insurance for, 60
protection against claims of, 61
proximate cause with, 59
punitive damages with, 59
Nematocyst
definition of, 920

Neonates, 197, 1102
  Apgar score assessment of, 1106
  definition of, 1100
Neonatology, 1100–1114
  advanced life support situations of, 1109–1113, 1114
    apnea in, 1109, 1114
    bradycardia in, 1109–1110, 1114
    cyanosis in, 1110, 1114
    diaphragmatic hernia in, 1109, 1114
    diarrhea in, 1112, 1114
    fever in, 1111, 1111n, 1114
    hypoglycemia in, 1111–1112, 1112b, 1112n, 1114
    hypothermia in, 1111, 1114
    hypovolemia in, 1110, 1114
    premature infant in, 1110, 1110n, 1114
    respiratory distress in, 1110, 1114
    seizures in, 1110–1111, 1111b, 1114
    vomiting in, 1112, 1114
  birth physiological adaptations and, 1102–1103, 1113
  distressed newborn resuscitation in, 1106–1108, 1106f, 1106n, 1107f, 1108t
    drug administration routes with, 1106
    medications used with, 1108, 1108t
    umbilical vein access with, 1106–1107, 1106f
  initial resuscitation steps for, 1103–1105, 1103f, 1103n, 1104f, 1104n, 1113
    airway opening in, 1103
    Apgar score in, 1106
    infant evaluation in, 105n, 1104–1106, 1104f
    meconium staining in, 1103–1104, 1104f, 1104n, 1114
    preventing heat loss/hypothermia in, 1103
    tactile stimulation provided in, 1104
  neonatal transport in, 1108–1109, 1109f
  postresuscitation care in, 1108
  resuscitation need risk factors for, 1101–1102, 1102b, 1102f
    congenital anomalies as, 1101–1102, 1102f, 1113
Neoplasia, 152, 172
Nervous system, 108–119, 111f–118f, 118t, 119t, 120f, 149
  autonomic, 117–119, 118f, 118t, 119t, 120f
  central, 111–116, 111f, 112f, 113t, 114f, 115f
  divisions of, 111, 111f, 112f
  drugs for, 351–364, 351b, 352b, 352f
  parasympathetic, 119
  peripheral, 116–117, 116f, 117f
  physical examination of, 270–275, 271f–274f, 274t, 279
Neurogenic hypotension, 626, 627, 629
  definition of, 606
Neurogenic shock, 526, 526n
  management of, 536
Neurology, 836–863
  amyotrophic lateral sclerosis in, 860, 863
  anatomy/physiology of, 837–842
    blood supply in, 840–842, 841f, 842f
    brain divisions in, 842, 843f
    impulse transmission in, 838–840, 839f, 840f
    nervous system cells in, 837–838, 837f
    neuron types in, 838, 838f
    reflexes in, 840, 841f
    synapse in, 839–840, 840f
    ventricles in, 842, 843f
  Bell palsy in, 860, 860f, 863
  brain neoplasm/abscess in, 857–858, 857n, 858f, 862
Neurology *(Continued)*
  central pain syndrome in, 859–860, 863
  coma in, 847–849, 848b, 848n, 862
    assessment of, 848–849, 848n
    causes of, 847, 848b
    management of, 848–849, 848n
    structural v. toxic-metabolic, 847–848, 848n, 862
  degenerative neurological diseases in, 858–862
  dystonia in, 859, 862
  headache in, 856–857, 862
  multiple sclerosis in, 859, 862
  muscular dystrophy in, 858–859, 862
  myoclonus in, 861, 863
  Parkinson disease in, 859, 862
  pathophysiology for, 842–847
    assessment of, 844–847, 844b, 845f–847f, 847n
    cerebral perfusion pressure in, 842, 844
    Cushing triad with, 845, 845f
    extraocular movements with, 847, 847f
    history with, 844–845, 862
    muscle tone with, 846
    neurological evaluation of, 846–847, 846f, 847f, 847n
    physical examination for, 844–845, 844b, 845f, 862
    pupillary reflexes with, 846–847, 846f, 847n
    respiratory patterns with, 845
    vital signs with, 845, 845f, 862
  peripheral neuropathy in, 860–861, 863
  polio in, 861–862, 863
  seizure disorders in, 854–856, 855n, 856t, 862
    assessment of, 855
    history with, 855
    management of, 855–856
    physical examination for, 855
    status epilepticus, 856
    syncope v., 855, 856t
    types of, 854–855, 855n
  spina bifida in, 861, 861f, 863
  stroke in, 849–854, 849b, 850t, 851b, 852b, 853f, 862
    assessment of, 851, 851b, 852b
    cerebral embolus, 850
    Cincinnati Prehospital Stroke Scale for, 851, 851b
    hemorrhagic, 849b, 850, 850t, 862
    in-hospital treatment for, 854
    ischemic, 849–850, 849b, 850t, 862
    Los Angeles Prehospital Stroke Screen for, 851, 852b
    management of, 852–854, 852n, 853f
    paramedics' role caring for, 851–854, 851b, 851n, 852b, 853f
    pathophysiology of, 849
    transient ischemic attacks as, 850
    types of, 849–850, 849b
Newborn, 1101
  cardiovascular system of, 198
  definition of, 1100
  development characteristics of, 197–201, 198f, 199f–200f, 199t, 201b, 210
  growth/development review for, 1118, 1119b, 1120t
  immune system of, 199
  musculoskeletal system of, 198
  nervous system of, 198
  psychosocial development of, 199
  respiratory system of, 198
  resuscitation of distressed, 1106–1108, 1106f, 1106n, 1107f, 1108t
    drug administration routes with, 1106
Newborn *(Continued)*
    medications used with, 1108, 1108t
    umbilical vein access with, 1106–1107, 1106f
  vital signs, 197
  vital signs of, 197
  weight of, 197–198
NHTSA. *See* National Highway Traffic Safety Administration
Nitrogen narcosis, 1000, 1000n
  definition of, 985
Non-Hodgkin's lymphomas, 977, 982
Nose
  drugs for, 422–423, 423f
Nutrition, 23–27, 23n, 24b, 25t, 26b, 27b
  amino acids in, 24
  antioxidants in, 24b
  cholesterol in, 23, 23n, 24b, 26, 28, 29b
  dietary fats in, 23–24, 24b, 26, 26b
  dietary recommendations in, 26, 26b
  free radicals in, 24b
  minerals in, 24, 25t
  vitamins in, 24, 25t
Nystagmus
  definition of, 920

O

Obesity
  definition of, 1196
  special considerations for, 1199, 1208
OBRA. *See* Omnibus Budget Reconciliation Act
Obsessive-compulsive disorders, 1051, 1051b
Obstetrics, 1072–1096
  complications of pregnancy with
    abortion with, 1084, 1084b
    abruptio placentae with, 1085, 1085t
    ectopic pregnancy with, 1085
    gestational diabetes mellitus as, 1084
    labor/delivery with, 1086–1091, 1087f, 1088b, 1089f–1091f, 1091t, 1096
    maternal injury as, 1081
    medical conditions as, 1083–1091
    placenta previa with, 1085–1086, 1085t
    preeclampsia/eclampsia as, 1083–1084, 1083b, 1096
    trauma as, 1080–1083, 1082b, 1082f
    uterine rupture with, 1085t, 1086
    vaginal bleeding as, 1084–1086, 1084b, 1085t, 1096
  delivery complications with, 1091–1095, 1092b, 1092f, 1094b
    abnormal presentation in, 1092–1093, 1092f
    amniotic fluid embolism in, 1095, 1096
    breech presentation in, 1092–1093, 1092f
    cephalopelvic disproportion in, 1091, 1096
    cord presentation in, 1093
    fetal membrane disorders in, 1095
    multiple gestation in, 1094, 1094b, 1096
    precipitous delivery in, 1094, 1096
    premature birth in, 1093–1094, 1096
    premature membrane rupture in, 1095, 1096
    pulmonary embolism in, 1095, 1096
    shoulder dystocia in, 1093, 1096
    shoulder presentation in, 1093
    uterine inversion in, 1094–1095, 1096
  fetal growth/development in, 1074–1077, 1076f, 1077b
    adjustments of infant at birth with, 1075–1077
  normal pregnancy events of, 1073, 1074f
  patient assessment of, 1077–1080, 1079n, 1080f, 1081f

Obstetrics *(Continued)*
history in, 1079, 1079n, 1095
maternal changes in, 1077–1079, 1095
physical examination in, 1079–1080, 1080f, 1081f, 1095
specialized pregnancy structures of, 1073–1074, 1075f
amniotic sac/fluid as, 1074
placenta as, 1073–1074, 1095
umbilical cord as, 1074, 1075f
terminology of, 1077, 1077b
Obstructive apnea
definition of, 1210
Off-line medical direction
definition of, 3
EMS, 15, 20
Olfactory sense organ, 144–145, 145f
Omnibus Budget Reconciliation Act (OBRA), 61
Ongoing assessment, 280, 287–288
On-line medical direction
definition of, 3
EMS, 15, 20
Open fractures
musculoskeletal trauma with, 668–669
Open pneumothorax, 634–635, 634f, 634n, 635f, 641
definition of, 630
Open vault skull fractures, 594f, 595, 595f
Ophthalmoscope, 237, 237f
Oral airway. *See* Oropharyngeal airway
Oral cavity, 136
Oral hypoglycemic agents
diabetes mellitus with, 873
Organ collision injuries
blunt trauma from, 508–510, 508f, 509f
Organ donation
legal issues with, 68–69, 68b
Organ system anatomy, 92–144, 93f, 149
cardiovascular system in, 123–128, 124f–127f, 149
circulatory system in, 119–128, 122t, 123t, 124f–127f, 129f, 130f, 149
digestive system in, 135–138, 137f, 149
endocrine system in, 119, 121f, 149
integumentary system in, 92–95, 94f, 149
muscular system in, 104–108, 105f–110f, 108t, 149
nervous system in, 108–119, 111f–118f, 118t, 119t, 120f, 149
reproductive system in, 140–144, 141f, 142f, 143f, 144f, 149
respiratory system in, 128, 131–135, 131f–135f, 149
skeletal system in, 95–104, 96f–104f, 104b, 149
urinary system in, 138–140, 139f, 140f, 149
Oropharyngeal airway (Oral airway)
airway management with, 471–472, 472f
Orotracheal intubation, 476–480, 476b, 476f, 477f, 478f, 478n, 479f, 479n
confirmation methods for, 478–479, 479n
face-to-face, 483, 484f
sniffing position for, 476, 476f
transillumination technique for, 479–480, 479f
Osmolality, 152, 159
Osmosis, 152, 153, 154f
definition of, 152
Ostomy
definition of, 1210
Otoscope, 237–238, 238f
Overhydration, 163
Ovulation
definition of, 1062
Oxygen
airway management with, 455–459
delivery devices for, 457–459, 457f, 457t, 458f, 458t, 459f
nasal cannula as, 457–458, 457f, 457t, 458t
nonrebreather mask as, 458–459, 459f
partial rebreather mask as, 458, 458f
simple face mask as, 458, 458f
Venturi mask as, 459, 459f
flowmeters for, 457, 457f
regulators for, 457, 457f
sources for, 455–457, 456b, 456f, 457f
liquid oxygen, 455, 457

P

P wave
definition of, 674
electrocardiogram monitoring with, 700, 810
five step rhythm analysis with, 703, 705f, 810
Pacemakers
artificial rhythms with, 759–763, 761f, 762b
autonomic nervous system effects on, 687
cardiology electrophysiology of, 685–686, 686f
transcutaneous cardiac pacing with, 806–807, 806f
wandering, 722, 722f, 810
Palliative care
definition of, 1211
home health care patient with, 1226, 1227b, 1228
Palmar grasp reflex, 196, 199t
Palpation
abdomen, 264–265, 265f
acute abdominal pain assessment with, 897
airway evaluation with, 453–454, 453n, 454f
chest, 256, 257f
heart, 261, 261f
pelvis, 269f
spine, 271f
technique of, 234, 235b, 236, 236f, 278
Pancreas, 138
abdominal trauma with, 648
anatomy of, 867, 868b, 868f, 869f
Pancreatitis, 895, 902
definition of, 892
Para, 1072, 1077
Paramedic
education for, 11, 12f, 20
EMT
definition of, 3
description of, 10b
EMS with, 10, 10b, 20
rescue operations role of, 1257–1258
response teams of, 14n
role of, 13–15, 14b, 14n, 20
additional responsibilities in, 14–15, 14n, 20
primary responsibilities in, 13–14, 14b, 20
well-being of, 22–41
Paranoia
definition of, 1042
schizophrenia with, 1049, 1050b
Paraplegia
definition of, 1196
special considerations for, 1199, 1199f, 1208
Parasympathetic nervous system, 119
definition of, 83
Parenteral medication administration, 399–420
containers for, 399–401, 401f, 402f, 403f
equipment used for, 399–403, 399b, 400b, 400f, 401f, 402f, 403f
Parenteral medication administration *(Continued)*
injection site preparation for, 401
intradermal injection with, 403, 404f
intramuscular injection with, 405–408, 406f, 407f, 408f
subcutaneous injection with, 403–405, 404f, 405f
syringes/needles for, 399, 399b
Parkinson disease, 363, 859, 862, 1170–1171
definition of, 836
Paroxysmal nocturnal dyspnea
definition of, 674
Paroxysmal supraventricular tachycardia, 688
definition of, 675
Partial-thickness burns
burns classifications of, 562, 562f
definition of, 558
Patellar injury, 666, 668f
Patient advocacy
ethics with, 78
Patient assessment, 280–288
abnormal heartbeat in, 689
acute abdominal pain in, 893–897, 905
blood-borne pathogens in, 281, 283t
burns in, 566–567, 567f
chest pain/discomfort in, 688–689, 689n
chief complaint in, 688–689, 810
dyspnea in, 689
focused history with, 286–287
heart sounds in, 689–690, 690b
initial, 280, 281–286, 283f, 283t, 284f, 285b
maternal changes in, 1077–1079, 1095
medical v. trauma patients in, 288
ongoing, 280, 287–288
palpitations in, 689
priorities, 281
protective clothing in, 280, 281f
rapid trauma examination with, 287
scene size up in, 280–281
significant medical history in, 689
Patient care report (PCR). *See also* Documentation
general considerations with, 320
importance of, 319
photo image of, 321f–322f
Patient packaging, 1256, 1260
Pattern recognition
assessment-based patient management with, 298, 299, 300b, 300f
Patterned injuries
definition of, 1184
PCR. *See* Patient care report
Pedestrian injuries
blunt trauma from, 511, 518
Pediatric trauma score, 604–605, 604t
Pediatrics, 1116–1159
anatomy/physiology review for, 1120–1122
abdomen in, 1121
airway in, 1121
cardiovascular system in, 1122
chest/lungs in, 1121
extremities in, 1121
head in, 1120–1121
nervous system in, 1122
respiratory system in, 1122
skin in, 1121–1122
bronchiolitis in, 1130, 1130t, 1157
child abuse/neglect in, 1150–1153, 1152f, 1152t, 1158
EMS for children and, 1117–1118
general principles for, 1122–1125
focused history in, 1124
initial assessment in, 1123, 1123f
ongoing assessment in, 1124
patient management in, 1125

Pediatrics *(Continued)*
physical examination in, 1124
scene size-up in, 1122–1123
vital functions in, 1123–1124, 1123t
growth/development review for, 1118–1120, 1119b, 1120t
adolescent in, 1119b, 1120, 1120t
infant in, 1118, 1119b, 1120t
neonate in, 1118, 1119b, 1120t
newborn in, 1118, 1119b, 1120t
preschooler in, 1119b, 1120, 1120t
school age in, 1119b, 1120, 1120t
toddler in, 1118–1120, 1119b, 1120t
hyperglycemia in, 1144, 1144f, 1157
hypoglycemia in, 1144, 1157f
infection in, 1144–1145, 1145b, 1145f, 1157
medication administration for, 423
paramedic's role in, 1117
pneumonia in, 1130, 1157
poisoning/toxic exposure in, 1145, 1146b, 1157
postresuscitation stabilization in, 1142, 1142t
respiratory compromise with, 1125–1130, 1125n, 1127f–1130f
asthma in, 1130
bacterial tracheitis in, 1129–1130
croup in, 1126–1128, 1128f, 1129t, 1157
epiglottitis in, 1128–1129, 1128n, 1129t, 1157
foreign body airway obstruction in, 1125n, 1126–1130, 1127f–1130f
rhythm disturbances in, 1135–1142, 1136f–1139f, 1140t, 1141n, 1141t, 1142b, 1157
bradydysrhythmias as, 1135, 1136f
pulseless electrical activity as, 1135, 1137f, 1140
tachycardia as, 1138f, 1139f, 1140–1142, 1142n
seizure in, 1142–1144, 1143b, 1144n, 1157
shock in, 1130–1135, 1131b, 1132f–1135f, 1132n, 1133t, 1157
circulating blood volume with, 1131, 1131t
distributive, 1134–1135, 1135f
hypovolemia with, 1132–1134, 1132f–1134f, 1133t
special needs children in, 1153–1157, 1154f–1156f, 1155t
central venous lines for, 1155, 1155f
gastric tubes/gastrostomy tubes for, 1155–1156, 1156f
home artificial ventilators for, 1154, 1154f, 1155t
shunts for, 1156–1157, 1156f
tracheostomy tubes for, 1154, 1154f
status epilepticus in, 1143–1144, 1143b, 1144n
sudden infant death syndrome in, 1149–1150, 1149b, 1158
trauma in, 1145, 1147–1149, 1148b, 1157
PEEP. *See* Positive end-expiratory pressure
Pelvic inflammatory disease
nontraumatic gynecology emergencies of, 1066, 1066b, 1067f, 1071
Pelvis
fracture of, 664, 664n
physical examination of, 268, 269f
Penetrating trauma, 500, 513–518
abdominal trauma as, 645–646, 650
ballistics in, 514–517, 514f, 515f, 516f, 517b
cavitation in, 513, 514f
definition of, 500
thoracic trauma with, 638–639, 639n, 640, 642
Peptic ulcer disease, 897, 900, 905
definition of, 892
Percussion
abdomen, 264–265, 265f
acute abdominal pain assessment with, 897
chest, 256, 257f
technique of, 234, 235b, 236, 236b, 236f, 278
Percutaneous medication administration, 420–423, 420f, 421f, 422f, 423f, 425
buccal drugs in, 420
ear drugs in, 422–423
endotracheal drugs in, 422, 422f
eye drugs in, 422–423, 423f
hand-held nebulizer in, 421–422, 422f
inhaled drugs in, 420–421
metered-dose inhaler in, 421, 421f
nose drugs in, 422–423, 423f
sublingual drugs in, 420
topical drugs in, 420, 420f
Perfusion
pulmonary pathophysiology of, 818, 818t, 833
Peripheral nervous system, 116–117, 116f, 117f
definition of, 83
Peripheral neuropathy, 860–861, 863
definition of, 836
Peritoneal dialysis, 915
definition of, 908
Peritonitis
definition of, 644
Personality disorders, 1056–1057, 1060
Pertinent negative findings
documentation with, 318, 320
Pertussis, 1031, 1040
Ph, 152, 165, 165b, 166f
Phalangeal injury, 664, 664f, 668
Pharmacodynamics, 333, 345–347, 345b, 346b, 346f, 347f
Pharmacokinetics, 333, 338–345, 339b, 340b, 341b, 343f, 344f
Pharmacology, 332–386, 337–347, 337n, 338b, 339b, 340b, 341b, 343f, 344f, 345b, 346b, 346f, 347f. *See also* Medication administration
action mechanisms, 337–351
airway management with, 490–492, 490n, 491f, 492b
paralytic agents in emergency intubation with, 490–491
rapid sequence intubation with, 491–492, 492b, 498
antifungal/antiviral drugs within, 378–379, 379b, 384
autonomic nervous system in, 351–369, 353f, 354f, 355t, 356t, 357b, 358t, 359b
drugs affecting, 355–369, 356t, 357b, 358t, 359b
nerve impulse transmission with, 353–354, 354f, 355t
blood affecting drugs within, 368–369, 369b, 383
anticoagulant, 368–369
antihemophilic agents as, 369
antihyperlipidemic, 369, 369b
hemostatic agents as, 369, 383
cardiovascular system drugs within, 364–368, 365b, 383
angiotensin II receptor antagonist, 368
antihemorrheologic agents as, 368
antihypertensive, 366–368, 383
cardiac glycoside, 365–366, 383
emergency, 365b
terminology for, 365b
Pharmacology *(Continued)*
Controlled Substances Act for, 332, 335–336, 335n, 336t, 337b
drug absorption in, 332, 338–341, 339b, 340b, 341b, 343f, 350, 382
drug information sources within, 335, 335b
drug interactions in, 347
drug names in, 334–335, 334b, 382
chemical, 334–335, 334b
generic, 334–335
official, 334–335
trade, 334–335
drug preparations in, 348, 348b
drug profiles in, 348–349
ear drugs within, 374–375, 384
endocrine system drugs within, 375–376, 375b, 376b, 384
adrenal cortex, 375, 376b
pancreas, 376, 376b
parathyroid gland, 375, 375b
pituitary gland, 375, 375b
eye drugs within, 374–375, 384
antiglaucoma, 374–375, 384
gastrointestinal system drugs within, 372–374, 383–384
antacid, 372
antidiarrheal, 374
antiflatulent, 372
digestant, 373
emetic, 373
laxative, 373
general properties of, 337–347, 337n, 338b, 339b, 340b, 341b, 343f, 344f, 345b, 346b, 346f, 347f
herbs within, 385–386
historical trends in, 334–337, 334b, 335b, 336t, 337b
immune system drugs within, 381–382, 381f, 384
infectious disease/inflammation drugs within, 378–381, 378b, 379b, 380b, 384
neoplastic disease drugs within, 377, 377b, 384
nervous system drugs within, 351–364, 351b, 352b, 352f
alcohol as, 359–361
anesthetics, 359, 359b, 382
antianxiety, 359–361, 360b
anticonvulsants, 361, 361b, 383
central nervous system stimulants, 361–362
dopamine affecting, 364
narcotic analgesics/antagonists, 358–359, 359b, 382
neurochemical transmission with, 352–353
nonnarcotic analgesics, 359, 382
psychotherapeutic, 362–363, 362f, 383
sedative-hypnotic agents as, 359–361, 360b
specific dysfunction, 363–364
pharmaceutical phase of, 337–338, 338b
pharmacodynamic phase of, 345–347, 345b, 346b, 346f, 347f
biological half-life in, 346–347
drug-receptor interaction in, 345, 345b, 346f
drug-response assessment in, 345–346, 346b, 347f
therapeutic index in, 333, 347
pharmacokinetic phase of, 338–345, 339b, 340b, 341b, 343f, 344f
absorption in, 332, 338–341, 339b, 340b, 341b, 343f, 382
biotransformation in, 332, 342, 343f, 344f, 345b

Pharmacology *(Continued)*
distribution in, 333, 341–342, 343f, 344f, 345b, 382
excretion in, 333, 342–344, 343f, 344f
factors influencing drug action in, 344–345
routes of drug administration in, 339–341, 339b, 340b, 341b
regulatory agencies for, 336–337, 382
reproductive system drugs within, 376–377, 384
respiratory system drugs within, 370–372, 370b, 372b, 383
antihistamine, 372
antiserotonin, 372
bronchodilator, 370–371, 370b, 383
cough suppressant, 371–372, 372b
emergency, 370b
respiratory depressant, 371
respiratory stimulant, 371, 383
serotonin, 372
special considerations in, 348–351, 349b
older patients, 350–351
pediatric patients, 349–350
pregnant patients, 349, 349b
standards/legislation for, 335–336, 335n, 336t, 337b
terminology, 338b
Phobia
anxiety disorders with, 1050–1051
Phosgene, 1306, 1315
Physical abuse
definition of, 1184
Physical examination. *See also* Patient assessment
abdomen in, 262–265, 263f, 264b, 264f, 265f, 279
auscultation of, 264
inspection of, 263–264, 264f
percussion/palpation of, 264–265, 265f
acute abdominal pain in, 896–897, 896f
allergies/anaphylaxis in, 889
breath sounds in
auscultation of, 258–261, 259f, 260f, 261f
chest in, 255–261, 255f–261f
auscultation of, 256–261, 259f, 260f, 261f
inspection of, 255–256, 257f
palpation of, 256, 257f
percussion of, 256, 257f
pleural friction rub, 261
definition of, 234
detailed, 287
ears in, 253–254, 253f, 254
electrical burn injury in, 575
equipment, 237–238, 278
blood pressure cuff, 238, 238f
ophthalmoscope, 237, 237f
otoscope, 237–238, 238f
stethoscope, 237, 237f
extremities in, 266–270, 267f–270f, 279
ankles/feet, 267–268, 269f
elbows, 267, 267f
hands/wrists, 267, 267f
pelvis/hips/knees, 268, 269f
shoulders, 267, 268f
eyes in, 251–253, 251b, 252f, 253f
female genitalia in, 266, 279
general survey in, 240–250
geriatrics, 1166
head/cervical spine in, 255
head/face in, 251
heart in, 261–262, 261f, 262f
auscultation of, 261–262, 262f
palpation of, 261, 261f
height/build in, 240
infants/children in, 275–277, 276t, 277f
Physical examination *(Continued)*
male genitalia in, 266.279
mental status in, 238–240
mouth/pharynx in, 254
nails in, 251, 251b
neck in, 254–255, 254f
nervous system in, 270–275, 271f–274f, 274t, 279
cranial nerves with, 270–272, 271f
mental status/speech with, 270
motor system with, 272–273, 272f
reflexes with, 274–275, 274f, 275f
sensory system with, 273, 273f
neurology pathophysiology in, 844–845, 844b, 845f, 862
nose in, 254
obstetrics, 1079–1080, 1080f, 1081f, 1095
older adults in, 277–278
pediatrics, 1124
pulmonary emergencies in, 818–819
rapid trauma, 287
seizure disorders in, 855
shock in, 531–532
skin in, 250–251
color/lesions of, 240, 240b, 241f, 242t–244t, 245t–247t
color/temperature/moisture of, 248–250, 250f
soft tissue trauma in, 548
spine in, 255, 270, 279
technique, 235–236
auscultation, 234, 235b, 236, 278
inspection, 234, 235–236, 235b, 278
palpation, 234, 235b, 236, 236f, 278
percussion, 234, 235b, 236, 236b, 236f, 278
vital signs in, 240, 248–250, 249f, 249t, 250f
blood pressure, 248, 249f
pupils, 250
respirations, 248
skin color/temperature/moisture, 248–250, 250f
weight in, 240, 247f
Physical well-being, 23–31, 41
disease prevention in, 28–29, 29b
cancer, 28–29, 29b, 41
cardiovascular, 28, 29b
infectious, 29
fitness in, 27–28, 27b, 27n, 41
body mass index with, 27, 27b
cardiovascular endurance, 27
muscle flexibility, 27–28
muscle strength, 27
injury prevention in, 29–31, 30b, 30t, 41
nutrition in, 23–27, 23n, 24b, 25t, 26b, 27b
amino acids with, 24
antioxidants with, 24b
cholesterol with, 23, 23n, 24b, 26, 28, 29b
dietary fats with, 23–24, 24b, 26, 26b
dietary recommendations with, 26, 26b
free radicals with, 24b
minerals with, 24, 25t
vitamins with, 24, 25t
sleep's importance in, 28, 28b, 28n, 41
Physiological dead space, 435
definition of, 431
Placards
definition of, 1286
Placenta
definition of, 1072
specialized pregnancy structures of, 1073–1074, 1095
Placenta previa
complications of pregnancy with, 1085–1086, 1085t
Plague, 1306, 1309b, 1310–1311
Plasma
cell water movement with, 155–157, 157f, 158f
Plasma membrane
definition of, 83
Pneumatic pressure devices
hemorrhage controlled with, 551, 551f
Pneumonia, 1026–1027, 1040
aspiration, 828
bacterial, 827, 833
management of, 828
mycoplasmal, 827–828, 827n
pediatric, 1130, 1157
pulmonary emergency with, 825–828, 825n, 827b, 827f, 833–834
viral, 825–827, 827b, 833
Poison. *See also* Toxicology
definition of, 921, 962
emergency cardiac care in, 966–969, 967t–968t
Poison control center, 921–922
Polio, 861–862, 863
Poliomyelitis
special considerations for, 1204
Polycythemia, 977–978, 983
definition of, 970
Positive end-expiratory pressure (PEEP), 829, 829f
Posttraumatic syndrome, 1051, 1051b
Potassium imbalance, 163
P-R interval
definition of, 675
electrocardiogram monitoring with, 700
five step rhythm analysis with, 708, 711f, 810
Preeclampsia
complications of pregnancy with, 1083–1084, 1083b, 1096
definition of, 1072
Preexcitation syndromes
cardiac dysrhythmias, 775–778, 776f, 777f
Preferred provider organizations. *See* Managed care organizations
Premature atrial complex, 687
cardiology dysrhythmias with, 723–724, 723f, 724n
clinical significance of, 724
definition of, 675
description of, 723, 723f
etiology of, 724
interpretation rules for, 724, 724n
management of, 724
Premature birth
delivery complications with, 1093–1094, 1096
neonatal life support needed for, 1110, 1110n, 1114
Premature junctional contraction, 687
cardiology dysrhythmias with, 735, 736f
definition of, 675
Premature membrane rupture, 1095, 1096
Premature ventricle complex
cardiology dysrhythmias with, 742–746, 744f–746f
Premature ventricular complex, 687
definition of, 675
Preschool child. *See* Toddler
Present illness history, 226, 228–229, 229b
Presenting the patient
assessment-based patient management with, 298, 303–304, 305
Pressure ulcers
definition of, 1160
Preterm infant
apnea in, 1109
definition of, 1100

Primary contamination
  definition of, 1286
primary injury prevention
  definition of, 42, 44b
Proarrhythmia
  definition of, 675
Professionalism
  attributes of, 13
  EMS, 11–13, 20
Psychosis
  definition of, 1042
Psychotherapeutic drugs, 362–363, 362f, 383
Puberty, 196, 204
Pulmonary contusion, 637–638
  definition of, 630
Pulmonary emergencies, 816–834
  adult respiratory distress syndrome in, 828–830, 829b, 829f, 829n, 834
  asthma in, 822–825, 822n, 823b, 823f–825f, 824n, 825n, 826t, 833
    assessment of, 822–824, 824n
    differential considerations for, 825, 827t
    management of, 824–825, 824b, 824n, 825f, 825n, 826t
    pathophysiology of, 822, 822n, 823f, 824f
    pulmonary function tests for, 824–825, 825f, 825n, 826t
  chronic bronchitis in, 820, 820f, 821t, 833
  delivery complications with, 1095, 1096
  diagnostic testing in, 819–820
  emphysema in, 820–822, 820f, 821f, 821t
  focused history in, 818–819
  hyperventilation syndrome in, 832, 834
  initial assessment in, 818
  known pulmonary diagnosis in, 819–820, 819n
  lung cancer in, 832–833, 833f, 834
  obstructive airway disease in, 820–825, 820f, 821f, 821t, 823b, 823f–825f, 826t, 833
    assessment of, 821–822
  pathophysiology of, 817–818, 817n, 818b, 818t
    diffusion, 817–818, 818t, 833
    perfusion, 818, 818t, 833
    ventilation, 817, 818t, 833
  patient care in, 818–819
  physical examination in, 818–819
  pneumonia in, 825–828, 825n, 827b, 827f, 833
    aspiration, 828
    bacterial, 827
    management of, 828
    mycoplasmal, 827–828, 827n
    viral, 825–827, 827b
  pulmonary thromboembolism in, 830–831, 830b, 830f, 834
  scene size-up/rescuer safety with, 818–819
  spontaneous pneumothorax in, 831–832, 831n, 834
  upper respiratory infection in, 831, 834
Pulmonary injury, 633
Pulmonary thromboembolism
  contributing factors for, 830b
  management of, 831
  pulmonary emergencies with, 830–831, 830b, 830f, 834
  signs/symptoms of, 831
Pulmonary ventilation
  definition of, 431
Pulse oximetry, 486, 488b, 488f
Pulse pressure, 522
  definition of, 520
Puncture wound
  assessment of, 544, 544f
  definition of, 538
Punitive damages
  negligence, 59
Pyelonephritis, 910, 918
  definition of, 908

Q

QA. *See* Quality assurance
QRS complex
  definition of, 675
  electrocardiogram monitoring with, 700–701, 700f, 810
  five step rhythm analysis with, 703, 704f, 810
Q-T interval
  definition of, 675
  electrocardiogram monitoring with, 701, 701n, 702f, 810
Quadriplegia
  definition of, 1196
  special considerations for, 1199, 1199f, 1208
Quality assurance (QA)
  EMS, 16, 16b

R

Rabies, 1028, 1040
Raccoon's eyes
  definition of, 580
  skull fractures with, 594, 595f
Radial injury, 662, 663f
Radiation burn injury, 560
Radiation exposure, 576–578, 577b
  decontamination procedures for, 578
  emergency care for, 577–578
  emergency response for, 577
  harmful effects from, 576–577, 577n
  personal protection from, 577
  types of, 577b
Rapid sequence intubation (RSI), 491–492, 492b, 498
Rebound tenderness, 895
  definition of, 892
Reciprocity
  definition of, 3
Red Cross
  American, 4
Referred pain, 895, 896f
  definition of, 892
Refractory period, 685, 685f
  definition of, 675
Registration
  EMS, 11
Reproductive system, 140–144, 141f, 142f, 143f, 144f, 149
  drugs for, 376–377, 384
  female, 142–144, 142f, 143f, 144f, 149
  male, 140–142, 141f, 149
Reptile bites
  poison from, 939–941, 940b, 940f, 963
Rescue
  definition of, 1256
Rescue awareness/operations, 1256–1274
  assessment procedures during, 1273–1274, 1273b
  hazardous atmospheres, 1263–1265, 1263b, 1265f, 1274
    chemical/toxic exposure or explosion with, 1263–1264, 1263n
    confined spaces emergencies with, 1264–1265, 1265f, 1266f
    confined spaces with, 1263, 1263b
    crush compartment syndromes with, 1264
    trenches/cave-ins with, 1265, 1265n
  hazardous terrain, 1270–1273, 1271b, 1272f, 1273f, 1274
Rescue awareness/operations *(Continued)*
    helicopter use for, 1272–1273
    patient packaging for, 1272
    terminology of, 1271, 1271b
  highway operations, 1265–1270, 1267b, 1268f–1271f, 1269b, 1274
    airbag/supplemental restraint systems in, 1268–1269, 1269b
    automobile anatomy in, 1269–1270, 1270f
    electrical power hazards in, 1267
    fuel/fire hazards in, 1267, 1267b
    hazardous cargoes in, 1269
    unstable vehicles in, 1267–1268, 1268f, 1269f
  personal protective equipment for, 1260, 1261b, 1274
  phases of, 1258–1260, 1259f, 1274
    arrival/scene size-up in, 1258–1259
    disentanglement in, 1259–1260
    hazard control in, 1259
    medical treatment in, 1259
    patient access in, 1259, 1259f
    patient packaging in, 1260
    transportation in, 1260
  surface water, 1260–1263, 1261f, 1262f, 1274
    body recovery with, 1262
    flat, 1261
    flow obstructions in, 1260–1261, 1261f
    foot/extremity pin in, 1261, 1274
    in-water spinal immobilization with, 1262
    rescue techniques overview for, 1262–1263
    temperature of, 1261–1262, 1262f
  training for, 1257–1258, 1274
Rescue breathing, 459–461, 460f–463f, 461b, 462b
  automatic transport ventilators with, 454, 454f, 454n
  bag-valve devices with, 462–463, 462f
  infants/children with, 460
  mouth-to-mask devices with, 461–462, 461f, 462b, 462f
  mouth-to-mouth method of, 459–460
  mouth-to-nose method of, 460
  mouth-to-stoma method of, 460–461, 460f, 461b
Rescue situations
  paramedic well-being with, 30
Research
  basic principles of, 17–18, 17b, 17n, 18n
  cardiac arrest, 17b
  consent with, 19–20, 19n
  EMS, 16–20, 17b, 17n, 18n, 19n, 21
  ethics of, 19–20, 19n
  evaluating, 20b
  format of, 20, 20b
  statistics in, 18–19, 18n, 19n
    descriptive, 18, 18n
    inferential, 18–19, 18n, 19n
  steps in conducting, 17b
  types of, 17b
  Utstein style in, 17b
Respiratory acidosis, 167, 167f, 194
Respiratory alkalosis, 169
Respiratory depressants, 371
Respiratory distress
  neonatal life support needed for, 1110, 1114
Respiratory stimulants, 371, 383
Respiratory support
  home health care patient with, 1214–1216, 1214f, 1215b, 1216t, 1228

Respiratory system, 128, 131–135, 131f–135f, 149. *See also* Airway management
airway anatomy with, 128, 131f
definition of, 431
drugs for, 370–372, 370b, 372b, 383
lower airway structures with, 132–135, 134f, 135f
lungs in, 135, 135f
measurement of gases with, 437–438, 438f, 438t
mechanics of, 431–437, 432f, 433f, 434f, 4356
lung volumes/capacities in, 435, 437f
minute volume/minute alveolar ventilation in, 435–437
muscles used in, 432–433, 434f
pressure changes in, 431–432, 432f
ventilation in, 431–432, 432f
work of breathing in, 433–435, 434f, 436f
pathophysiology, 449–453, 449n, 450t, 451n
airway obstruction as, 449–451, 450t, 451n
aspiration in, 452–453, 497
fractured larynx as, 451
laryngeal spasm as, 451
tracheal trauma as, 452
physiology, 431–449
pulmonary circulation in, 438–449, 439f–444f, 445b, 446f, 448f, 449f
blood carbon dioxide content with, 442–443, 443n, 444f
blood oxygen content with, 442, 442f, 442n, 443f
blood oxygenation factors with, 443–444, 445b
chemical respiratory control with, 446–447, 448f
diffusion with, 439–442, 440f, 441f
gas exchange/transport with, 439
modified forms of respiration with, 447–449
nervous respiratory control with, 445–446, 445f
older patient considerations with, 449, 449f, 497
respiratory regulation with, 444
voluntary respiratory control with, 444–445
upper airway structures with, 128, 131–132, 132f, 133f
Response teams
EMS, 14n
Resting membrane potential, 681, 681f, 682f
definition of, 675
Resuscitation
advance directive on, 66–68, 67f
cardiopulmonary, 799, 800t–801t, 801
devices for, 801, 801f
CPR, 65–66, 66b
distressed newborn, 1106–1108, 1106f, 1106n, 1107f, 1108t
drug administration routes with, 1106
medications used with, 1108, 1108t
umbilical vein access with, 1106–1107, 1106f
ethics decisions with, 77, 79
ethics of, 77, 79
legal issues with, 65–68, 66b, 67f, 68n, 71
advance directive with, 66–68, 67f
neonatal
airway opening in, 1103
Apgar score in, 1106
infant evaluation in, 105n, 1104–1106, 1104f
initial steps for, 1103–1105, 1103f, 1103n, 1104f, 1104n, 1113
Resuscitation *(Continued)*
meconium staining in, 1103–1104, 1104f, 1104n, 1114
preventing heat loss/hypothermia in, 1103
tactile stimulation provided in, 1104
pediatrics postresuscitation stabilization for, 1142, 1142t
procedures, 285b
shock, 532–534, 532f, 533n, 534n
termination of, 808–809, 812
criteria for, 809
procedure for, 809
special considerations with, 809
withholding/stopping, 65–66, 66b, 71
Reticular activating system
definition of, 83
nervous system anatomy with, 113
Retinopathy
definition of, 1160
Retrograde amnesia, 596
definition of, 580
Rh factor, 185
Rhabdomyolysis
crush injury with, 547
definition of, 538
Rib fractures, 630–631, 631f
Ricin, 1306, 1309b, 1311
Right ventricular failure, 789–791, 791b, 791n, 811
Riot control agents, 1306, 1314b
Rocky Mountain spotted fever, 939
definition of, 921
R-on-T phenomenon
cardiology dysrhythmias with, 746, 746f
definition of, 675
Rooting reflex, 196, 199t
R-R method
five step rhythm analysis with, 706, 707f
RSI. *See* Rapid sequence intubation
Rubella, 1029, 1029f, 1040
Rubeola, 1029–1030, 1030f, 1040
Rule of nines
burns classifications with, 563, 563f, 563n
definition of, 558
Ruptured ovarian cyst
nontraumatic gynecology emergencies of, 1066–1067, 1066b, 1067f, 1071

S

Sacral fractures
spinal trauma with, 612
Safety
equipment, 30–31, 30t
Sarin, 1306, 1313
SARS. *See* Severe acute respiratory syndrome
Scabies, 1036, 1037–1038, 1038b, 1038f, 1041
Scene size up, 280–281, 288
Schizophrenia, 1049–1050, 1049b, 1050b, 1060
definition of, 1042
delusions with, 1049, 1050b
dyskinesia with, 1049
paranoia with, 1049, 1050b
School-age child
body systems of, 203–204
development characteristics of, 203–204, 210
Scope of practice
paramedic legal issues with, 56
Scorpion bites. *See* Arachnida bites/stings
Secondary contamination
definition of, 1286
Sedative-hypnotic agents, 359–361, 360b
Seizure(s)
definition of, 836
neonatal life support needed for, 1110–1111, 1111b, 1114
pediatric, 1142–1144, 1143b, 1144n, 1157
Seizure disorders, 854–856, 855n, 856t, 862
assessment of, 855
history with, 855
management of, 855–856
physical examination for, 855
status epilepticus, 856
syncope v., 855, 856t
types of, 854–855, 855n
Self-neglect
definition of, 1184
Sellick maneuver, 462, 462b
Sense organ anatomy, 144–149
hearing, 146–148, 148f
olfactory, 144–145, 145f
taste, 145, 146f
visual, 145–146, 147f
Sensitization
allergies/anaphylaxis with, 883
definition of, 882
Septic shock, 527
management of, 536
Serotonin, 372
Severe acute respiratory syndrome (SARS), 829b, 1032, 1033b–1034b, 1040
Sexual abuse
definition of, 1184
Sexual assault, 1070–1071, 1192–1193, 1193b, 1194
definition of, 1062
Sexually transmitted diseases, 1032, 1034–1036, 1040
chlamydia as, 1035, 1036f, 1040
gonorrhea as, 1035, 1040
herpes virus infections as, 1035–1036, 1036f, 1041
syphilis as, 1034–1035, 1034f, 1040
Shaken baby syndrome
definition of, 1184
Shipping papers
definition of, 1286
Shock, 520, 522–537
body as container with, 523–524, 523f
capillary-cellular relationship in, 524–526, 524f
disseminated intravascular coagulation with, 525
stage 1 (vasoconstriction) with, 524–525, 525n
stage 2 (capillary/venule opening) with, 525, 525n
stage 3 (disseminated intravascular coagulation) with, 525, 525n
stage 4 (multiple organ failure) with, 525–526, 526n
classifications of, 179–180, 180b, 526–527
anaphylactic, 526
cardiogenic, 526
hypovolemic, 526, 526n
neurogenic, 526, 526n
septic, 527
definition of, 152, 522
detailed physical examination with, 531–532
differential assessment findings with, 531
emergency cardiac for drug-induced, 969
initial assessment of, 529–531, 531n
airway in, 529
breathing in, 529–530
circulation in, 530
disability in, 530–531, 531n
exposure in, 531
management/treatment of, 529–536

Shock *(Continued)*
anaphylactic shock in, 536
assessment/treatment integration in, 536
cardiogenic shock in, 536
hypovolemic shock in, 536
key principles in, 534–536, 535f
neurogenic shock in, 536
septic shock in, 536
specific forms of shock in, 536
pediatric, 1130–1135, 1131b, 1132f–1135f, 1132n, 1133t, 1157
circulating blood volume with, 1131, 1131t
distributive, 1134–1135, 1135f
hypovolemia with, 1132–1134, 1132f–1134f, 1133t
resuscitation of, 532–534, 532f, 533n, 534n
colloids in, 533–534, 534n
crystalloids in, 533, 533n
fluid in, 533–534, 533n, 534n
pneumatic antishock garment in, 532–533, 532f
red blood cell oxygenation in, 532
volume/container size ratio in, 532
stages of, 527–529, 527b, 528f, 529f
compensated, 527, 527b, 528f
irreversible, 527b, 528–529, 529n, 530f
uncompensated, 527–528, 527b, 529f
tissue oxygenation with, 522–523, 537
heart in, 522
lungs in, 523
microcirculation in, 523
pulse pressure in, 522
vasculature in, 522–523
variations in physiological response to, 529
Shoulder dystocia
delivery complications with, 1093, 1096
Shoulder presentation
delivery complications with, 1093
Shoulders
injury of, 660–662, 660n, 663f
physical examination of, 267, 268f
Shunt
definition of, 1116
special needs children with, 1156–1157, 1156f
Sickle cell disease, 979–981, 979b, 980f, 981f, 983
definition of, 970
Significant past medical history, 226, 229–230, 230b
Simplex mode, 306, 313, 313f
Sinus arrest
cardiology dysrhythmias with, 719–722, 721f, 810
clinical significance of, 719
description of, 719, 721f
etiology of, 719
interpretation rules for, 719
management of, 722
Sinus bradycardia
algorithm, 716f
cardiology dysrhythmias with, 714–717, 715f, 716f, 717b, 810
care for, 717b
clinical significance of, 715
dopamine infusion for, 717, 717b
epinephrine infusion for, 717, 717b
etiology of, 714
interpretation rules for, 714–715
isoproterenol infusion for, 717, 717b
management of, 716f, 717, 717b
Sinus dysrhythmia
cardiology dysrhythmias with, 719, 720f, 810
clinical significance of, 719
Sinus dysrhythmia *(Continued)*
description of, 719, 720f
etiology of, 719
interpretation rules for, 719
management of, 719
Sinus headache, 856
definition of, 836
Sinus tachycardia
cardiology dysrhythmias with, 718–719, 718f, 810
clinical significance of, 719
description of, 718, 718f
etiology of, 718–719
interpretation rules for, 719
management of, 719
6-second count method
five step rhythm analysis with, 708, 708f
Skeletal muscle relaxants, 364, 383
Skeletal system, 95–104, 96f–104f, 104b, 149
appendicular, 95, 99, 100f, 101f, 102f, 103, 103f
arm bones with, 95, 99, 100f
axial, 95, 97f, 98f, 99f
body movement with, 103–104, 104t–107f
foot bones with, 99, 102f
leg bones with, 99, 101f
pelvic girdle with, 99, 100f
scull with, 95, 97f, 103f
thoracic cage with, 95, 99f
vertebral column with, 95, 98f
Skin
physical examination of, 250–251
Skull fractures, 593–596, 594f, 594n, 595f, 605
basilar, 593–594, 594f, 594n, 595f
Battle's sign with, 594, 595f
cranial nerve injuries with, 596
depressed, 594–595, 594f, 595f
linear, 593, 594f
open vault, 594f, 595, 595f
raccoon's eyes with, 594, 595f
Sleep
paramedic well-being with, 28, 28b, 28n, 41
Small intestine, 136
abdominal trauma with, 646
Smallpox
bioterrorism with, 1309b, 1311–1312, 1311f
Smoking cessation
mental/emotional health with, 31, 32b
Snakes
poison from, 939–941, 940b, 940f, 963
SOAP format, 306, 316, 326–327
Sodium/chloride balance
cellular, 159–162, 160f–161f, 162t
Sodium-potassium exchange pump, 682, 684f, 810
Soft tissue trauma, 538–557, 539n
anatomy/physiology of, 539–540, 540f
dermis in, 539–540, 540f, 557
epidermis in, 539, 540f, 557
anterior neck trauma as, 591–593, 591n, 592n
assessment of, 541–547
abrasion in, 543, 543f
amputation in, 545, 545f
avulsion in, 544–545, 545f
bites in, 545–546, 545f, 546n
blast injuries in, 547, 547f
closed wounds in, 542–543, 543f, 557
contusions in, 542–543, 543f
crush injury in, 543, 543f, 546–547, 546f, 547b
hematomata in, 542–543, 543f
laceration in, 543–544, 543f
open wounds in, 543–546, 543f, 544f, 545f, 546n, 557
puncture wound in, 544, 544f
Soft tissue trauma *(Continued)*
bandages improperly applied with, 552
dressing materials used with, 551–552, 557
hemorrhage/bleeding control for, 549–551, 549f, 550f, 551f, 557
direct pressure in, 549, 549f
elevation in, 549, 549f
immobilization by splinting in, 550, 550f
pneumatic pressure devices in, 551, 551f
pressure point in, 549, 550f
tourniquet in, 551, 551f
injuries not requiring closure as, 552–556
dressing/bandages for, 552, 552f–554f
evaluation of, 552
patient instructions for, 554, 555f
tetanus vaccine for, 554
wound healing assessment with, 556
wound infection with, 554–555
management principles for, 547–548, 548f
maxillofacial injury as, 581, 582f
open wound dressing with, 552
pathophysiology of, 540–547
inflammatory response with, 541–542, 557
wound healing alterations with, 542
wound healing hemostasis with, 540–541, 540f, 541f
physical examination for, 548
special considerations for, 556–557
amputations in, 556
avulsion in, 556
crush syndrome in, 556–557
penetrating chest/abdominal injury in, 556
treatment priorities for, 548, 548f
wound history for, 548
Soman, 1307, 1313
Somatic nervous system
definition of, 83
Somatic pain, 895
definition of, 892
Somatization disorders, 1055, 1055b
Somatoform disorders, 1054–1055, 1055b, 1060
conversion, 1055, 1055b
somatization, 1055, 1055b
Special needs patients, 1196–1208
arthritis with, 1201–1202, 1202f
cancer with, 1202, 1202b
cerebral palsy with, 1202–1203
cystic fibrosis with, 1203, 1203n
Down syndrome with, 1200–1201, 1200n, 1201f
emotionally impaired, 1201, 1208
financial challenges with, 1207, 1208
head-injured patients with, 1204, 1205t
hearing impairments with, 1197–1198, 1208
mental illness with, 1200, 1208
mental retardation in, 1201, 1208
multiple sclerosis with, 1203–1204
muscular dystrophy with, 1204
myasthenia gravis with, 1205, 1206f
obesity with, 1199, 1208
paraplegia/quadriplegia with, 1199, 1199f, 1208
poliomyelitis with, 1204
speech impairments with, 1198–1199, 1198b, 1208
spina bifida with, 1205, 1205n, 1206f
terminally ill patients with, 1207, 1208
visual impairments with, 1198, 1208
Speech impairments
special considerations for, 1198–1199, 1198b, 1208
Spiders bites. *See* Arachnida bites/stings

Spina bifida, 861, 861f, 863
definition of, 836
special considerations for, 1205, 1205n, 1206f
Spinal cord tumors, 628
Spinal shock, 627, 629
definition of, 606
Spinal stabilization. *See* Immobilization
Spinal trauma, 606–629
anatomy/physiology of, 609, 610f, 628
assessment criteria for, 606–609, 607f, 609b
indications for immobilization in, 608f
mechanism of injury as, 609, 609b
assessment of, 609–611, 611f, 614–615, 615f, 615t
axial loading in, 610
distraction in, 609, 610–611, 611f
flexion in, 610, 611f
hyperextension in, 610
hyperrotation in, 610
lateral bending in, 610
lower extremity neurological function in, 614
motor findings in, 614
reflex responses in, 615, 615f
sensory findings in, 614–615, 615t
upper extremity neurological function in, 614
autonomic hyperreflexia syndrome with, 627, 629
classifications of, 611–614, 613f, 628
anterior cord syndrome, 612
Brown-Séquard syndrome, 612–613
central cord syndrome, 612
coccygeal fractures, 612
cord injuries, 612–613
dislocations, 612, 613f
fractures, 612, 613f
sacral fractures, 612
sprains/strains, 612
incidence of, 606
management of, 615–623, 615n, 617f, 618f, 619f, 620f, 621f, 622f, 623f
morbidity/mortality of, 606
neurogenic hypotension with, 626, 627, 629
nontraumatic spinal conditions and
assessment/management of, 628
degenerative disk disease as, 628
herniated intervertebral disk as, 628
low back pain as, 627
spinal cord tumors as, 628
spondylosis as, 628
pharmacological therapy for, 613
presentation of, 626–627
spinal shock with, 627, 629
spinal stabilization/immobilization techniques for, 615n, 616–626, 617f–626f, 629
diving incidents with, 625–626, 626f
helmet issues with, 623–625, 624f, 625f, 625n
Kendrick extrication device, 619–620, 620f
long spine boards, 620–623, 623f
manual in-line, 615n, 616–618, 617f, 618f, 619f
mechanical devices for, 618–620, 619f, 620f
pediatric patients with, 622f, 623, 624f
rapid extrication, 620–623, 621f, 622f, 623f
rigid cervical collars for, 618, 619f
short spine boards, 618–620, 620f, 620n
Spirituality
mental/emotional health with, 32n
Spleen
abdominal trauma with, 646, 646f, 650
Splinting
general principles of, 658, 660b
immobilization with, 550, 550f
musculoskeletal trauma with, 658–660, 659f, 660b, 660f, 671
types of, 658–660, 660f
Spondylosis, 628
Spontaneous pneumothorax
definition of, 816
management of, 832
pulmonary emergency from, 831–832, 831n, 834
Sports injuries
blunt trauma in, 511–512, 518
Sprains/strains
definition of, 652
musculoskeletal trauma with, 655–656, 656b, 656f, 671
spinal trauma with, 612
ST segment
definition of, 675
electrocardiogram monitoring with, 701, 702f
Standing orders
definition of, 3
EMS, 15, 15b
Starling hypothesis
cell water movement in, 157
definition of, 152
Starling's law of the heart, 679, 679f
definition of, 675
START technique of triage, 1251–1252, 1251f
Statistics
descriptive, 18, 18n
EMS research, 18–19, 18n, 19n
inferential, 18–19, 18n, 19n
Status asthmaticus
definition of, 816
Status epilepticus
definition of, 836
pediatric, 1143–1144, 1143b, 1144n
Sternal fractures, 633, 633f
Stethoscope, 237, 237f
Stomach, 136, 137f
abdominal trauma with, 646
Stress
adaptation to, 34–36, 41
burnout with, 36n
critical incident management for, 36–37, 37b, 41
disease with, 188–189, 189t
immune system's role with, 188, 195
management techniques for, 36
neuroendocrine regulation of, 187–188, 187t, 188t
catecholamines in, 187, 187t
cortisol in, 187–188, 188t
pathophysiology of, 187–189, 187t, 188t, 189t
physiological/psychological effects of, 33f, 34, 34b
reactions to, 34
symptoms of, 34b
techniques for reducing, 37b
warning signs of, 34b
Stress response, 31, 32–38, 41
EMS causes of, 34
factors triggering, 34–37
phases of, 32
alarm reaction, 32–33, 32f
exhaustion, 33–34
resistance, 33, 33f
Stroke, 849–854, 849b, 850t, 851b, 852b, 853f, 862
assessment of, 851, 851b, 852b
cerebral embolus, 850
Cincinnati Prehospital Stroke Scale for, 851, 851b
hemorrhagic, 849b, 850, 850t, 862
in-hospital treatment for, 854
ischemic, 849–850, 849b, 850t, 862
Los Angeles Prehospital Stroke Screen for, 851, 852b
management of, 852–854, 852n, 853f
paramedics' role caring for, 851–854, 851b, 851n, 852b, 853f
pathophysiology of, 849
transient ischemic attacks as, 850
types of, 849–850, 849b
Stroke volume, 679–680, 679f, 679n
afterload in, 679, 679n
myocardial contractility in, 680
preload in, 679
Starling's law of the heart with, 679, 679f
Subarachnoid hematoma, 600, 601f
definition of, 580
Subdural hematoma, 598–600, 600f
Sublingual drugs, 420
Subluxation, 610
definition of, 606
Submersion, 995–997, 995f, 1001
clinical outcome factors in, 996
definition of, 985
drowning in, 995–996, 995f, 1001
management of, 996–997
Substance misuse/abuse
mental/emotional health with, 31, 31b, 41
Substance-related disorders, 1054
dual diagnosis with, 1045b, 1054
Sucking reflex, 196, 199t
Sudden infant death syndrome, 1149–1150, 1149b, 1158
definition of, 1116
Suicide, 1053–1054, 1053b, 1060–1061
elderly in, 1177
Superficial burns
burns classifications of, 561–562, 562f
definition of, 558
Supraventricular tachycardia. *See also* Paroxysmal supraventricular tachycardia
cardiac ejection fraction with, 729
cardiology dysrhythmias with, 724–729, 724n, 725f, 726f, 727n, 728f, 729b, 729n, 810
clinical significance of, 726–727, 727n
description of, 724, 724n, 725f, 726f
etiology of, 724
interpretation rules for, 724–726
management of, 727, 727n, 728f, 729, 729b, 729n
Sympathomimetics, 962, 962t
Synchronized cardioversion, 805–806, 812
Syphilis, 1034–1035, 1034f, 1040
Syringes. *See* Parenteral medication administration

T

T wave
definition of, 675
electrocardiogram monitoring with, 701, 810
Tabun, 1307, 1313
Tachycardia
emergency cardiac for drug-induced, 966
pediatric, 1138f, 1139f, 1140–1142, 1142n
Tactical EMS, 1276, 1282b, 1283
Tactical patient care, 1283–1284, 1285
body armor for, 1283–1284
definition of, 1276

Tactical retreat, 1276, 1281–1282
Taste sense organ, 145, 146f
Teachable moment
  definition of, 42, 44b
  injury on-scene education with, 48
Temperature conversions, 391, 391f
Tendonitis
  musculoskeletal trauma with, 657, 657f, 671
Tension headache, 856
  definition of, 836
Tension pneumothorax, 635–637, 635f, 635n, 636f
  closed trauma associated with, 636–637, 636f
  definition of, 630
  penetrating trauma associated with, 635–636
Terminal drop, 196, 210
Terminally ill patients
  definition of, 1196
  special considerations for, 1207, 1208
Testicular torsion, 911, 912f, 918
  definition of, 908
Tetanus, 1027–1028, 1027t, 1040
Therapeutic communication, 214–224, 215b, 215f, 217b, 218f, 219b, 220b, 222b, 223b
  definition of, 214
  effective, 216–218, 218f
    empathy for, 216
    eye contact for, 218
    listening ability for, 216–217
  elements of, 215–216
  good rapport with, 219
  information obtaining strategies in, 219–220
  mental status assessment in, 220–221
  patient interview in, 218
  personal space with, 223b
  special interview situations in, 221–223, 223b
    age difference with, 221–222
    blind patient as, 222
    hearing-impaired patient as, 222
    hostile patient as, 221
    non-talking patient as, 221
    sexually aggressive patient as, 222–223
  techniques for, 218–219, 219b
Therapeutic index, 333, 347
Thermal burn injury, 559–560
Thermogenesis, 986
  definition of, 985
Thermolysis, 986
  definition of, 985
Thermoregulation. *See* Environmental conditions
Thoracic trauma, 630–642
  clavicular fractures with, 630, 630f, 641
  closed pneumothorax with, 633–634, 634f, 641
  diaphragmatic rupture with, 641, 641f, 642
  esophageal injuries with, 640–641, 641n, 642
  flail chest with, 631–632, 631f, 631n
  heart/great vessel injury with, 638–640, 639n, 640f, 640n
  hemothorax with, 637, 637f
  myocardial contusion with, 639, 642
  open pneumothorax with, 634–635, 634f, 634n, 635f, 641
  penetrating trauma with, 638–639, 639n, 642
  penetrating wounds with, 640
  pulmonary contusion with, 637–638
  pulmonary injury with, 633
  rib fractures with, 630–631, 631f, 641
  skeletal injury with, 630–633, 631f, 632f, 633f
Thoracic trauma *(Continued)*
  sternal fractures with, 633, 633f, 641
  tension pneumothorax with, 635–637, 635f, 635n, 636f
  tracheobronchial injuries with, 640–641, 641n
  traumatic aortic rupture with, 639–640, 640f, 640n
  traumatic asphyxia with, 638
Threshold potential
  definition of, 675
Thromboxanes
  definition of, 882
Thyroid gland disorders, 877–878, 877b, 877f, 878f, 878n, 878t
  anatomy/physiology of, 877–878, 877b, 877f, 878n
  causes of, 877, 877b
  management of, 878, 878t
  myxedema as, 878, 878f, 881
  thyrotoxicosis as, 877, 877f, 881
Thyrotoxicosis, 877, 877f, 881
  definition of, 864
Tibial injury, 668, 668f, 669f
Ticks, 921, 939. *See also* Arachnida bites/stings
Tidal volume, 234, 256, 435
  definition of, 431
Tinnitus, 1174
Toddler
  body systems of, 201–202
  development characteristics of, 201–203, 202b, 202f, 210
  growth/development review for, 1118–1120, 1119b, 1120t
  parenting of, 202–203, 203t
  psychosocial development of, 202
  vital signs of, 201
Topical drugs, 420, 420f
Torsades de pointes
  definition of, 675
  electrocardiogram monitoring with, 701
  ventricular tachycardia with, 748f, 755n
Total body water (TBW), 152–153, 152n, 153t
Tourniquet
  hemorrhage controlled with, 551, 551f
Toxicology, 920–969. *See also* Hazardous materials incidents
  alcoholism, 955–961, 964
    acute alcohol intoxication with, 959
    alcohol withdrawal syndromes with, 959–960
    blood alcohol content with, 956, 956n
    cardiac/skeletal muscle myopathy with, 959
    cirrhosis with, 958
    delirium tremens with, 960
    dependence in, 955–956
    disulfiram-ethanol reaction with, 960–961
    emergencies with, 959–961
    ethanol with, 956, 956b
    fluid/electrolyte imbalances with, 958
    gastrointestinal disorders with, 958–959
    gastrointestinal hemorrhage with, 958
    immune suppression with, 959
    medical consequences with, 956–959, 957t
    metabolism with, 956
    neurological disorders with, 957, 957t
    nutritional deficiencies with, 957–958
    pancreatitis with, 958–959
    trauma with, 959
    Wernicke-Korsakoff syndrome with, 958
    withdrawal hallucinations with, 960
    withdrawal seizures with, 960
  drug abuse, 945–955, 964
    acetaminophen overdose, 954–955, 955b, 964
Toxicology *(Continued)*
    cardiac medications, 952–953, 952b, 964
    cocaine, 949–950, 950b
    common drug names of, 947t–948t
    general management principles for, 946–948
    hallucinogen overdose, 951, 964
    ibuprofen overdose, 953
    lithium, 952
    methamphetamine, 950b
    monoamine oxidase inhibitors, 953, 964
    nonsteroidal antiinflammatory drugs in, 953–955, 953n, 954b, 955b, 964
    opioid overdose, 948–949, 949b, 964
    phencyclidine overdose, 950–951, 964
    salicylate overdose, 953–954, 954b
    sedative-hypnotic overdose, 949, 964
    sexual gratification use with, 955, 955b, 964
    stimulant overdose, 949–951, 950b, 964
    terminology of, 946b
    tricyclic antidepressant overdose, 951–952, 951b, 964
    United States, 946b
  emergency cardiac care in, 966–969, 967t–968t
    drug-induced acute coronary syndromes with, 966
    drug-induced bradycardia with, 966
    drug-induced cardiac arrest with, 969
    drug-induced hypertensive emergencies with, 966
    drug-induced impaired conduction with, 969
    drug-induced shock with, 969
    drug-induced tachycardia with, 966
    drug-induced ventricular fibrillation with, 966
    severe poisoning guidelines for, 966–969, 967t–968t
  management principles for, 961–962, 961b, 961n
    anticholinergics in, 961
    cholinergics in, 961
    hallucinogens in, 961
    opiates in, 961–962
    sympathomimetics in, 962, 962t
  pediatric, 1145, 1146b, 1157
  poison absorption in, 944–945, 944b, 945n
  poison control center for, 921–922
  poison ingestion in, 922–931, 962
    activated charcoal for, 924, 924b
    antidotes for, 925t
    assessment/management of, 923, 923n
    cardiovascular complications with, 923
    ethylene glycol, 928, 963
    food, 930–931, 963
    gastric lavage for, 924–925, 924n, 925n
    hydrocarbons, 926–927, 926n, 963
    iron, 929, 963
    isopropanol, 928–929, 963
    lead, 929–930, 929b, 963
    mercury, 930, 963
    metals, 929–930, 929b
    methanol, 927–928, 963
    neurological complications with, 923
    plants, 931, 931b, 963
    respiratory complications with, 923
    strong acids/alkalis as, 925–926, 926b, 962–963
    syrup of ipecac for, 925, 925b
  poison inhalation in, 932–935, 963
    ammonia, 934–935, 963
    chemical properties with, 932, 963
    cyanide, 933–934, 934b, 934n, 963
    general management of, 932, 933t

Toxicology *(Continued)*
hydrocarbon, 935, 963
physical properties with, 932
poison injection in, 935–944
Arachnida (spiders, scorpions, ticks) with, 937–939, 937f, 938f, 939b, 963
arthropod bites/stings with, 935–939, 936b, 937f, 938f, 939b
hazardous aquatic life with, 941–944, 941f, 943f, 963
hymenoptera (wasps, bees, ants) with, 935, 963
reptile bites with, 939–941, 940b, 940f, 963
poison management guidelines in, 922, 922b
Tracheobronchial injuries, 640–641, 641n
Tracheostomy tubes
special needs children with, 1154, 1154f
Transcutaneous cardiac pacing, 806–807, 806f, 808f, 812
artificial pacemakers in, 806–807, 806f
electrode placement with, 807, 808f
indications/contraindications for, 807
procedure in, 807, 807n
Transection, 611
definition of, 606
Translaryngeal cannula ventilation, 492–494, 493f, 494f, 494n
advantages/disadvantages to, 494
complications with, 494
description of, 492
equipment for, 492
removal of, 494
technique of, 492–494, 493f, 494f, 494n
Transportation
destination choice with, 65
emergency vehicle operating privileges with, 64–65
paramedic-patient relationships with, 64–65, 65b
payer protocols with, 65
trauma considerations with, 503
Trauma, 500–518. *See also* Abdominal trauma; Head/facial trauma; Musculoskeletal trauma; Soft tissue trauma; Spinal trauma; Thoracic trauma
blunt, 500, 504–513, 518
all-terrain vehicles with, 510–511
blast injuries, 512–513, 512f, 518
compression injuries as, 509–510, 509f
deceleration injuries as, 508–510, 508f
motor vehicle collision, 505–506, 505f
motorcycle collision, 510, 510f, 511f, 518
organ collision injuries as, 508–510, 508f, 509f
pedestrian injuries, 511
restraints preventing, 506–508, 507f, 508b
sports injuries, 511–512, 518
vertical falls with, 513
centers, 502, 503b
complications of pregnancy with, 1080–1083, 1082b, 1082f
deaths from, 501, 501n, 502f, 503b, 518
elderly with, 1177–1179, 1181
epidemiology of, 500–503, 501n, 502b, 502f, 503b
kinematics with, 503–504
energy in, 503, 518
physical laws in, 504
pediatric, 1145, 1147–1149, 1148b, 1157
penetrating, 500, 513–518
ballistics in, 514–517, 514f, 515f, 516f, 517b
cavitation in, 513, 514f
phases of care for, 501–502, 502b, 503b
systems, 502
transportation considerations for, 503
trends in, 501, 501n, 502f
Trauma patients
focused history for, 286–287
medical patient v., 288
Trauma score, 603–604, 604t
Traumatic aortic rupture, 639–640, 640f, 640n
Traumatic asphyxia, 638
definition of, 630
Treatment protocols
definition of, 3
EMS, 15, 15b
Triage principles/technology, 1250–1253, 1251f, 1252f, 1252t, 1254
patient tracking systems in, 1252–1253, 1253f
patient transportation in, 1253
primary v. secondary, 1250–1251
START technique in, 1251–1252, 1251f
tagging/labeling in, 1252, 1252t, 1253f
Triplicate method
five step rhythm analysis with, 706, 706f
Trunked system communications, 313–314
Tuberculosis, 1023–1025, 1023n, 1024f, 1025b, 1040
pathophysiology of, 1023–1024
patient care/protective measures with, 1024, 1024f, 1025b
prophylactic isoniazid with, 1024–1025
testing for, 1024
treatment for, 1024, 1025b
Tularemia, 1307, 1309b, 1312

U

U wave
definition of, 675
Ulcerative colitis, 899, 899n, 905
definition of, 892
Ulnar injury, 662, 663f
Umbilical cord
specialized pregnancy structures of, 1074, 1075f
Uncompensated shock, 527–528, 527b, 529f
Upper extremity injuries, 660–664, 661f–663f, 664f, 671
Upper respiratory infection
management of, 831
pulmonary emergency from, 831, 834
Uremia
acute renal failure with, 912, 913
definition of, 908
Ureters
abdominal trauma with, 648
Urethra
abdominal trauma with, 649
Urinary bladder
abdominal trauma with, 648
Urinary calculus, 910–911, 911b, 918
Urinary retention, 909–910, 918
definition of, 908
Urinary system, 138–140, 139f, 140f, 149
kidneys in, 138, 139f
ureters in, 138–139
urethra in, 138–139
urinary bladder in, 138–139, 139f
urine production in, 139
urine regulation in, 139
Urinary tract infection, 910, 918
Urology, 908–918
acute renal failure in, 912–913, 913t, 918
intrarenal, 913
postrenal, 913
prerenal, 913
uremia with, 912, 913
anatomy/physiology of, 909–911, 909f, 911b, 912f
chronic renal failure in, 913–915, 914t, 918
epididymitis with, 911, 918
Urology *(Continued)*
genitourinary disorder examination in, 912, 918
pyelonephritis with, 910, 918
renal dialysis in, 915–917, 916f, 916n, 917b, 917n, 918
air embolism with, 917, 917n
chest pain with, 917
disequilibrium syndrome with, 916, 917
emergencies with, 915–916
hemodialysis, 915, 916f
hemorrhage with, 916
hypotension with, 916–917, 917b
peritoneal, 915
severe hyperkalemia with, 917, 917n
vascular access problems with, 916, 916n
renal failure in, 912, 918
testicular torsion with, 911, 912f, 918
urinary calculus with, 910–911, 911b, 918
urinary retention with, 909–910, 918
urinary tract infection with, 910, 918
Urosepsis
definition of, 1211
U.S. Department of Homeland Security, 1316–1317
Uterine rupture
complications of pregnancy with, 1085t, 1086
Utstein style
EMS cardiac research with, 17b

V

Vaginal bleeding, 1066b, 1068, 1071
complications of pregnancy with, 1084–1086, 1084b, 1085t, 1096
nontraumatic gynecology emergencies of, 1066b, 1068, 1071
Vascular access devices
correcting common problems with, 1218t
hemorrhage with, 1218
home health care patient with, 1216–1220, 1216n, 1217f, 1218t, 1219b, 1219t, 1228
infection with, 1217
types of, 1217, 1217f
Vasopressin mechanism, 179
Vehicle safety
paramedic well-being with, 30
Ventilation. *See also* Airway management
pulmonary pathophysiology of, 817, 818t, 833
Ventricle escape complexes/rhythms
cardiology dysrhythmias with, 740–742, 740f, 741f
Ventricular bigeminy
cardiology dysrhythmias with, 742, 745f
definition of, 675
Ventricular fibrillation
emergency cardiac for drug-induced, 966
Ventricular tachycardia, 688
cardiology dysrhythmias with, 746–756, 747f–754f, 755b, 756f
clinical significance of, 748, 748n
definition of, 675
description of, 746, 747f
electrical cardioversion algorithm with, 754f
etiology of, 747–748, 747n, 748n
interpretation rules of, 748, 748n
management of, 748–756, 748f–754f, 755b, 755n, 756f
monomorphic, 750f
polymorphic, 751f–752f
pulseless, 753f
torsades de pointes with, 748f, 755n
12-lead strategies for, 755–756, 755n, 756f, 756n
wide-complex, 749f

Ventricular trigeminy
cardiology dysrhythmias with, 742, 745f
definition of, 675
Venturi mask, 459, 459f
Vertical falls
blunt trauma from, 513
Vesicants
definition of, 1307
Viral pneumonia, 825–827, 827b, 833
Viruses, 174–175, 175b, 175f
Visceral pain, 894–895
definition of, 892
Visual impairments
special considerations for, 1198, 1208
Visual sense organ, 145–146, 147f
Vital signs
newborn, 197
physical examination of, 240, 248–250, 249f, 249t, 250f
blood pressure, 248, 249f
pupils, 250
respirations, 248
skin color/temperature/moisture, 248–250, 250f
physical examination with, 240, 248–250, 249f, 249t, 250f
toddler, 201
Vitamins, 24, 25t
Vomiting
neonatal life support needed for, 1112, 1114
VX, 1307, 1313, 1314–1315

W

Wandering pacemaker
cardiology dysrhythmias with, 722, 722f, 810
clinical significance of, 722
Wandering pacemaker *(Continued)*
description of, 722, 722f
etiology of, 722
interpretation rules for, 722
management of, 722
Wasp bites/stings. *See* Arthropod bites/stings
Water balance
cellular, 159, 162
Weapons of mass destruction. *See also* Bioterrorism
definition of, 1307
Wellness
disease transmission prevention in, 39–40
documentation with, 40
exposure sources with, 39
management of, 40
protection from airborne/blood-borne pathogen with, 40
terminology of, 39b
grieving process in, 37–38
developmental considerations in dealing with, 39
paramedic needs dealing with, 38–39
patient/family needs with, 37
stages of, 37–38
mental/emotional health, 31–32
anxiety with, 31
family/peer/community connections for, 32
meditation/contemplation for, 31–32, 32n
smoking cessation for, 31, 32b
spirituality for, 32n
substance misuse/abuse with, 31, 31b, 41
physical well-being, 23–31, 41
disease prevention in, 28–29, 29b
Wellness *(Continued)*
fitness in, 27–28, 27b, 27n, 41
injury prevention in, 29–31, 30b, 30t, 41
nutrition in, 23–27, 23n, 24b, 25t, 26b, 27b
sleep's importance in, 28, 28b, 28n, 41
stress response and, 31, 32–38, 41
adaptation with, 34–36, 41
alarm reaction with, 32–33, 32f
EMS causes of, 34
exhaustion with, 33–34
factors triggering, 34–37
phases of, 32
physiological/psychological effects of, 33f, 34, 34b
reactions to, 34
resistance with, 33, 33f
West Nile virus, 936b
definition of, 921
Wolff-Parkinson-White syndromes
bundle of Kent with, 775
cardiology conduction disorder dysrhythmias in, 775–778, 776f, 777f
clinical significance of, 776
description of, 775–776
etiology of, 776, 776f
management of, 776, 777f
Wound healing
alterations of, 542
anatomic factors in, 542
drug use with, 542
scar formation with, 542
hemostasis of, 540–541, 540f, 541f
high risk, 542
Wrist injury, 662, 663f